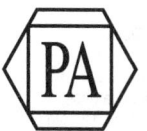

PHYSICIAN ASSISTANT'S
DRUG
HANDBOOK
SECOND EDITION

SPRINGHOUSE
Springhouse, Pennsylvania

Staff

Senior Publisher
Donna O. Carpenter

Editorial Director
William J. Kelly

Clinical Director
Marguerite Ambrose, RN, MSN, CS

Creative Director
Jake Smith

Art Director
Elaine Kasmer Ezrow

Drug Information Editor
Tracy A. Roux, PharmD

Senior Associate Editors
Karen C. Comerford, Jennifer P. Kowalak

Editors
Naina Chohan, Linda Jones

Clinical Editors
Theresa P. Fulginiti, RN, BSN, CEN (project editor); Eileen Cassin Gallen, RN, BSN; Carol Knauff, RN, MSN, CCRN; Nancy LaPlante, RN, BSN; Deanna H. McCarthy, RN, MSN, CCRN, CCTC; Pamela S. Messer, RN, MSN; Kimberly A. Zalewski, RN, MSN, CEN

Copy Editors
Caryl Knutsen, Louise Quinn

Designers
Arlene Putterman (associate design director), Joseph John Clark, Donald G. Knauss

Electronic Production Services
Diane Paluba (manager), Joy Rossi Biletz (technician)

Manufacturing
Patricia K. Dorshaw (manager), Otto Mezei (book production manager)

Editorial Assistants
Carol A. Caputo, Arlene Claffee

Indexer
Barbara Hodgson

Authorization to photocopy items for internal or personal use, or the internal or personal use of specific clients, is granted by Springhouse Corporation for users registered with Copyright Clearance Center (CCC) Transactional Reporting Services provided that the fee of $.75 per page is paid directly to CCC, 222 Rosewood Dr., Danvers, MA 01923. For those organizations that have been granted a photocopy license by CCC, a separate system of payment has been arranged. The fee code for users of the Transactional Reporting Service is 1582550786/00 $00.00 + $.75. Printed in the United States of America.

Visit our Web site at eDrugInfo.com

ISBN 1-58255-0786
ISSN 1522-4848
PADH—D N O S A J J M A M
04 03 02 01 10 9 8 7 6 5 4 3 2 1

Contents

Contributors and consultants

Gary J. Arnold, MD, FACS
Associate Professor, College
of Nursing
University of Louisiana at
Lafayette

John M. Bertoni, MD, PhD
Professor and Chair,
Department of Neurology
Creighton University
Omaha

Thomas A. Brabson, DO
EMS Fellowship Director,
Chief Division EMS
Albert Einstein Medical Center
Philadelphia

Terrill Bravender, MD, MPH
Assistant Professor of
Pediatrics, Director
of Adolescent Medicine
Duke University Medical
Center
Durham, N.C.

Lawrence Carey, BS,
PharmD
Clinical Pharmacy Supervisor
Jefferson Home Infusion
Service
Philadelphia

Laurie Chern, MD
Family Physician
Providence Medical Group—
Tarasbourne
Aloha, Ore.

Clayton T. Cowl, MD, MS
Chief, Section of Aviation
Medicine
Division of Preventive &
Occupational Medicine
and Internal Medicine
Mayo Clinic and Mayo Medical
School
Rochester, Minn.

Diane Dixon, PA-C, MA,
MMSC
Assistant Professor
University of Alabama
Mobile, Alabama

Susan Epp, PA-C, NCCPA,
MPAS
Broadlawns Medical Center
Des Moines, Iowa

Gary N. Fox, MD, FAAFP, CAQ
Geriatrics
Associate Director
Mercy Health Partners Family
Practice Residency
Toledo, Ohio

Edgar Gonzalez, PharmD
Associate Professor
Medical College of Virginia
Richmond

Fred Harchelroad, MD
Director, Medical Toxicology
Treatment Center
Allegheny General Hospital
Pittsburgh

Thomas E. Lafferty, MD
Rheumatologist
Ocala Orthopaedic Group,
P.A.
Ocala, Fla.

Henry R. Lemke, PA-C, MMS
Director, Physician Assistant
Studies
Health Science Center
Fort Worth, Tx.

Roger M. Morrell, MD, PhD,
FACP
Medical Consultant and
Clinical Investigator
Lathrup Village, Mich.

Joseph L. Neri, DO, FACC
Cardiologist
The Heart Care Group
Allentown, Pa.

Glenn H. Nordehn, DO
Assistant Professor
University of Minnesota,
Department of Family
Medicine
Duluth

William O'Hara, BS, PharmD
Clinical Team Leader
Thomas Jefferson Hospital
Philadelphia

Larry A. Pfeifer, RPh, MapST
Director, Pharmacy Services
National Hansen's Disease
Program
Baton Rouge, La.

Cathy Plooard-Colombo,
RPA-C, BS
Director, Infectious Diseases
(AIDS Program)
Bronx-Lebanon Hospital
Bronx

John Porter, MD
Private Practice
PHX Rehab, Inc.
Phoenix, Ariz.

Iris Reyes, MD, FACEP
Assistant Professor of
Emergency Medicine
Hospital of the University of
Pennsylvania
Philadelphia

Susan W. Sard, PharmD
Clinical Pharmacist
Anne Arundel Medical Center
Annapolis, Md.

Joel Shuster, PharmD
Associate Professor of Clinical
Pharmacy Practice; Clinical
Pharmacist
Temple University School of
Pharmacy; Medical College
of PA Hospital
Philadelphia

Rein Tideiksaar, PA-C, PhD
Director
Sierra Health Services, Inc.
Las Vegas, Nev.

Douglas N. Weismann, MD
Associate Professor,
Department of Pediatrics
University of Iowa College of
Medicine
Iowa City

George L. White, Jr., PhD,
MSPH, PA-C
Professor/Director Public
Health Programs
University of Utah, School of
Medicine
Salt Lake City

Foreword

When I wrote the Foreword for the first edition of this book, I told of my wish for a quick and user friendly drug reference after having been out of practice for two years. At that time I was amazed at how much drug therapy had changed, how many new drugs had become available, and how quickly my recall of even frequently used drugs had become shaky. Then, about the only reference available was a huge "tome" that was difficult to use for a quick reference. How I wished for a drug reference that was portable and gave me the information that I needed in a concise, direct format. When I reviewed the first edition of *The Physician Assistant's Drug Handbook*, I was convinced it was the answer to my prayers. Now, after using the handbook in my Family Medicine practice, I know it is a valuable adjunct to my prescriptive practice. Additionally, other providers (including physician assistants, faculty physicians, residents, nurse practitioners, and students of every type) in my clinic have "borrowed" my copy at times. I have heard many favorable comments about its format, style of information presentation, and how "handy" it is.

One of the things that makes the handbook even more valuable to the busy physician assistant (or any practitioner) is the presence of more than just drug information. The first edition had information on everything from abbreviations to contact numbers for pharmaceutical companies. The information on pediatric and geriatric drug therapy was particularly important to me because small children and infants make up a small portion of my practice. Even after 25 years as a physician assistant, I have some trepidation about prescribing for very small children. The immunization schedule was a great guide for those who deal with children.

The same is true for our older adult patients. Although I am very comfortable with prescribing for the geriatric patient, it was good to have a ready resource if questions arose. I often used the creatinine clearance calculations to help guide pharmacologic interventions. The picture guide was often used when patients would bring their medications all in one bottle or in unlabeled containers. As all of you know, this happens a lot and if you are like me, it is hard to say what that "red pill" is without some pictorial help.

Also included in the handbook, an overview of pharmacology, information on effective prescribing practices, pharmacologic classifications, topical drugs, and combination analgesics. All of these are useful to the practicing physician as-

sistant to confirm information. For a physician assistant student, the information in the handbook is key to understanding vital components of pharmacologic therapeutics and prescriptive practice.

A key piece of important information is the therapeutic drug monitoring guidelines. This is a very important concept to understand and to use with today's powerful and potentially harmful drugs. Along with the drug monitoring guidelines, the section on antidotes to poisoning or overdose will be invaluable, particularly for the physician assistant who does not deal with overdoses and poisonings on a regular basis.

I have used the handbook and found it to meet many of my practice needs, as well as using it as a reference for my teaching duties. That is why I am very pleased to have been given the opportunity to write the Foreword for this second edition. A quick perusal of the table of contents will reveal much of the first edition, but with some important additions. Two of the content items that I consider very important for the physician assistant are the antibiotic selection chart and information on the most commonly used herbals.

It is apparent that antibiotic prescribing is becoming more complicated as new antibiotics become available and bacterial resistance increases. Our armamentarium is large and complex, but so are the bacteria we must deal with in our infected patients. This guide helps you as you try to negotiate complicated and simple bacterial treatment programs. This chart and guide will help us in our judicious use of antibiotics.

The use of herbal and other alternative therapies are on the rise among our patients. Studies have shown a large percentage of the population use some type of non-medical therapy and often do not tell their medical providers about that use. While herbs may be "natural," they may not always be safe. Few physician assistants learn about herbs during their education, but there is no doubt that herbal compounds impact health care today. We need to have knowledge of what herbs do and how they interact with medications. This guide will be helpful.

Other additions to this new edition include a restructured drug interactions section that presents the interacting agent, the interaction, and a clinical tip to help avoid or minimize the effect. The Special Considerations section includes a subsection on Monitoring that covers important clinical signs and laboratory tests for monitoring and monitoring frequency. Patient education continues to be an important aspect of the book.

I have been more than pleased with the first edition of *The Physician Assistant's Drug Handbook*. This second edition will be even more useful. I think you will find many of the features helpful, particularly for problems you see infrequently or for medications and herbs that may be new to you. I also like the fact that the information on thousands of drugs is presented without bias. The information is succinct, regardless of the type of practice or specialty.

Pharmacology is a complex field with many confounding aspects. Safe and accurate prescribing is a public trust that each of us must hold sacred. When we prescribe we have to consider almost everything a patient may take, as well as the physical and psychological impacts on the patient. It is a challenge that is complicated by the rapid changes that occur in medicine every day. We need every tool to ensure that our prescribing is appropriate for the conditions treated and the patient taking the medications. This handbook is one of those tools. I think you will find it a valuable companion to your efforts.

More than any other reason, I think that the public trust and our duty to the social, mental, and physical health of our patients should drive us to be confident prescribers. Prescribing is more than writing a prescription. It is also over-the-counter recommendations, herbs, vitamins, mineral, diet, and exercise.

I invite you to review this edition of the handbook. I think you will find it to be a useful, ready to use, and versatile resource. As you review it, think about your own practice and the treatment demands it puts on you. You will find the contents of the handbook to be a vital part of your solutions to those demands. I have used the first edition extensively and found it to be everything it should be. The updates, additions, and changes in this edition will make the handbook another important component of your "peripheral brain." I strongly recommend it to you as a valuable resource component for physician assistant practice.

J. Dennis Blessing, Jr., PhD, PA-C
Associate Professor and Chair
Department of Physician Assistant Studies
University of Texas School of Allied Health
  Sciences
San Antonio

Guide to abbreviations

ACE	angiotensin converting enzyme		GI	gastrointestinal
AIDS	acquired immunodeficiency syndrome		GU	genitourinary
ALT	alanine aminotransferase		HIV	human immunodeficiency virus
ANC	absolute neutrophil count		hr	hour
APPT	activated partial thromboplastin time		h.s.	at bedtime
AST	aspartate aminotransferase		I.D.	intradermal
ATP	adenosine triphosphate		I.M.	intramuscular
AUC	adequate area under the curve		INR	International Normalized Ratio
AV	atrioventricular		IPPB	intermittent positive pressure breathing
b.i.d.	twice a day		IU	International Unit
BPH	benign prostatic hyperplasia		I.V.	intravenous
BUN	blood urea nitrogen		kg	kilogram
cAMP	cyclic 3', 5' adenosine monophosphate		L	liter
CBC	complete blood count		LD	lactate dehydrogenase
CDC	Centers for Disease Control and Prevention		m^2	square meter
CK	creatine kinase		mm^3	cubic millimeter
CNS	central nervous system		MOA	monoamine oxidase
COPD	chronic obstructive pulmonary disease		mcg	microgram
CPR	cardiopulmonary resuscitation		mcl	microliter
CSF	cerebrospinal fluid		mEq	milliequivalent
CV	cardiovascular		mg	milligram
CVA	cerebrovascular accident		MI	myocardial infarction
CVP	central venous pressure		min	minute
DIC	disseminated intravascular coagulation		ml	milliliter
dl	deciliter		N_2O	nitrous oxide
DNA	deoxyribonucleic acid		ng	nanogram (millimicrogram)
ECG	electrocardiogram		NSAID	nonsteroidal anti-inflammatory drug
EEG	electroencephalogram		O_2	oxygen
FDA	Food and Drug Administration		OTC	over-the-counter
g	gram		$Paco_2$	partial pressure of arterial carbon dioxide
G	gauge		Pao_2	partial pressure of arterial oxygen
GGT	gamma glutamyltransferase		pg	picogram
G6PD	glucose-6-phosphate dehydrogenase		P.O.	by mouth
			P.R.	per rectum

p.r.n.	as needed
PT	prothrombin time
PTT	partial thromboplastin time
PVC	premature ventricular contraction
q	every
q.d.	every day
q.i.d.	four times a day
RBC	red blood cell
RNA	ribonucleic acid
SA	sinoatrial
S.C.	subcutaneous
SIADH	syndrome of inappropriate antidiuretic hormone
S.L.	sublingual
T_3	triiodothyronine
T_4	thyroxine
t.i.d.	three times a day
tsp	teaspoon
WBC	white blood cell
wk	week

The *Physician Assistant's Drug Handbook,* 2nd Edition, provides exhaustively reviewed, completely updated drug information on virtually every drug in current clinical use. It covers all aspects of drug information from fundamental pharmacology to specific management of toxicity and overdose. It also includes several unique features: individual entries that describe major pharmacologic classes, a comprehensive listing of indications that includes clinically approved but unlabeled uses, and antidotes for poisoning and overdose.

Introductory chapters

Chapter 2 explains, in a general way, how drugs work. It also reviews adverse reactions and gives general guidelines about drug use during pregnancy and the presence of drugs in breast milk. Chapter 3 discusses the unique issues related to giving drugs to children and elderly patients. Chapter 4 describes how to take an effective drug history and write a proper prescription.

Generic drug entries

The individual drug entries provide detailed information on virtually all drugs in current clinical use, all arranged alphabetically by generic name for easy access. This new edition includes 32 new drug entries, most of which have been recently approved. A guide-word at the top of each page identifies the generic drug presented on that page. Each generic entry is complete where it falls alphabetically and doesn't need cross-referencing to other sections of the book.

In each drug entry, the generic name (with alternative generic names following in parentheses) precedes an alphabetically arranged list of current trade names. (An asterisk signals products available only in Canada.) Several drugs available solely as combinations—such as acetaminophen and oxycodone hydrochloride (Percocet)—are listed in an appendix.

Next, the pharmacologic and therapeutic classifications identify the drug's pharmacologic or chemical category and its major clinical uses. Listing both classifications helps the reader grasp the multiple, varying, and sometimes overlapping uses of drugs within a single pharmacologic class and among different classes. If appropriate, the next line identifies any drug that the Drug Enforcement Agency (DEA) lists as a controlled substance and specifies the schedule of control as II, III, IV, or V.

The pregnancy risk category identifies the potential risk to the fetus. Categories listed were determined by application of the FDA definitions to available clinical data in order to define a drug's potential to cause birth defects or fetal death. These categories, labeled A, B, C, D, and X, are listed below with an explanation of each. Drugs in category A usually are considered safe to use during pregnancy; drugs in category X usually are contraindicated.

● A: Adequate studies in pregnant women have failed to show a risk to the fetus in the first trimester of pregnancy, and there is no evidence of risk in later trimesters.

● B: Animal studies haven't shown an adverse effect on the fetus, but there are no adequate clinical studies in pregnant women.

● C: Animal studies have shown an adverse effect on the fetus, but there are no adequate studies in pregnant women. The drug may be useful in pregnant women despite its potential risks.

● D: There is evidence of risk to the fetus, but the potential benefits of use in pregnant women may be acceptable despite potential risks.

● X: Studies show fetal abnormalities, or adverse reaction reports indicate evidence of fetal risk. The risks involved clearly outweigh potential benefits.

● NR: Not rated.

Pregnancy risk classifications were assigned for all appropriate generic drugs according to the above criteria.

How supplied lists the preparations available for each drug (for example, tablets, capsules, solution, or injection), specifying available dosage forms and strengths.

Indications, route, and dosage presents all clinically accepted indications for use with general dosage recommendations for adults and children; dosage adjustments for specific patient groups, such as patients with renal or hepatic impairment, are included when appropriate. (Note that additional information may be found in the *Special considerations* section.) A preceding open diamond signals a clinically accepted but unlabeled use. Dosage instructions reflect current clinical trends in therapeutics and shouldn't be considered as absolute and universal recommendations. For individual application, dosage must be considered according to the patient's condition.

Pharmacodynamics explains the mechanism and effects of the drug's physiologic action.

Pharmacokinetics describes absorption, distribution, metabolism, and excretion of the drug; it specifies onset and duration of action, peak levels, and half-life, as appropriate.

Contraindications and precautions lists conditions that are associated with special risks in patients who receive the drug.

Interactions specifies the clinically significant additive, synergistic, or antagonistic effects that result when the drug is used with other drugs (drug-drug), herbs (drug-herb), foods (drug-food), or lifestyle activities (drug-lifestyle).

Adverse reactions lists the undesirable effects that may follow use of the drug; these effects are arranged by body systems (CNS, CV, EENT, GI, GU, Hematologic, Hepatic, Metabolic, Musculoskeletal, Respiratory, Skin, and Other). Local effects occur at the site of drug administration (by application, infusion, or injection); adverse reactions not specific to a single body system (for example, the effects of hypersensitivity) are listed under Other. Throughout, the most common adverse reactions (those experienced by at least 10% of people taking the drug in clinical trials) are in *italic* type; less common reactions are in roman type; life-threatening reactions are in ***bold italic*** type; and reactions that are both common and life-threatening are in BOLD CAPITAL letters. At the end of this section, severe and hazardous reactions that mandate discontinuation of the drug are listed, when appropriate.

Special considerations offers detailed recommendations specific to the drug for preparation and administration; for monitoring the patient; for care and teaching of the patient during therapy; and for use in elderly, pediatric, and breast-feeding patients. This section includes recommendations for preventing and treating adverse reactions, for treating overdose, for promoting patient comfort, and for storing the drug. Possible effects of the drug on diagnostic tests are also included. Recommendations that are common to all members of the drug's pharmacologic class are listed only in the relevant *pharmacologic class* entry. Thus, if specific considerations are unknown for geriatric, pediatric, or breast-feeding use of the generic drug, or if known information is listed in the pharmacologic class entry or elsewhere in the generic entry, these headings are omitted. For example, if the *Indications, route, and dosage* section lists detailed instructions for use in children and no additional considerations apply, the generic entry omits the heading *Pediatric patients*. However, relevant information that applies to all drugs in the drug's pharmacologic class may exist in the pharmacologic class entry.

Pharmacologic class entries

Listed alphabetically as a separate section, 49 entries describe the pharmacology, clinical indications and actions, adverse effects, and special implications of drugs that fall into a major phar-

macologic group. This allows the reader to compare the effects and uses of drugs within each class. Pharmacologic class entries list special considerations that are common to all generic members of the class, and include recommendations for geriatric, pediatric, and breast-feeding patients. If specific considerations are unknown, these headings are omitted.

Representative combinations at the end of each class entry list major combinations of generic drugs in the class with other generics of the same or of another class, followed by trade names of products that contain each combination of generics.

Photoguide

This extensive section provides full-color photographs of more than 320 of the most commonly prescribed tablets and capsules. Shown in actual size, the tablets and capsules are organized alphabetically for quick reference, along with their most common dosage strengths. A page reference to the text monograph appears with each drug shown.

Graphic enhancement

Selected charts and tables compare uses, effects, or dosages of drugs within a class.

Appendices

The appendices provide a charted summary of prescribing authority for physician assistants by state; a summary of combination analgesic drugs; creatinine clearance calculations; an antibiotic selection chart; an organized chart about topical drugs; an immunization schedule; guidelines for therapeutic drug monitoring; a list of antidotes to poisoning or overdose; a guide to common herbal medicines; and the contact numbers and Web site addresses of major pharmaceutical companies, agencies, and organizations.

Index

The index lists drugs by generic and trade names, plus diseases and pharmacologic classes.

2 Overview of pharmacology

Administration of a drug provokes a series of physicochemical events within the body. The first event, when a drug combines with cellular drug receptors, is known as the drug *action*. The result of this action is known as the drug *effect*.

Depending on the number of cellular drug receptors affected by a given drug, a drug effect can be local, systemic, or both. A local effect follows application to the skin; however, transdermal absorption can produce systemic effects. Moreover, local effects can follow systemic absorption. The antipeptic ulcer drug cimetidine acts solely by blocking histamine receptor cells in the parietal cells of the stomach. This is known as a local drug effect because the drug action is limited to one area and doesn't spread to other parts of the body. However, diphenhydramine produces a systemic effect in that it blocks histamine receptors in widespread areas of the body. Thus, local drug effects are specific to a limited number of organ systems, whereas systemic drug effects are generalized and affect different and diverse organ systems.

Drug properties
Drug absorption, distribution, metabolism, and excretion make up a drug's pharmacokinetic profile. This branch of pharmacology also describes a drug's onset of action, peak concentration level, duration of action, and bioavailablity.

Absorption
Before a drug can act within the body, it must be absorbed into the blood—usually after oral administration, the most commonly used route. For a drug that is contained in a tablet or capsule to be absorbed, the dosage form must disintegrate and dissolve in gastric juices. Absorption can occur only after a drug is dissolved. Most absorption of orally administered drugs occurs in the small intestine, where the mucosal villi provide extensive surface area. Once absorbed and circulated in the blood, the drug is bioavailable, or ready to produce an effect. Complete or partial absorption depends on the drug's physicochemical effects, dosage form, route of administration, and interactions with other substances in the GI tract, plus various patient characteristics. These factors also determine the speed of absorption. Thus, oral solutions and elixirs, which bypass the need for disintegration and dissolution, are usually absorbed more rapidly. Some tablets have enteric coatings that prevent disintegration in the acidic environment of the stomach; others may have coatings of varying thickness that delay disintegration.

Drugs administered I.M. must first be absorbed through the muscle into the blood. Rectal suppositories must dissolve to be absorbed through the rectal mucosa. I.V. drugs, which are injected directly into the blood, are completely and immediately bioavailable.

Distribution
After absorption, a drug moves from the bloodstream into various fluids and tissues within the body. Patient variations can greatly alter the amount of drug that is distributed throughout the body. For example, a given dose must be distributed to a larger volume in an edematous patient than in a nonedematous patient; the amount of drug may sometimes need to be increased. The dose should be decreased when the edema is corrected. Conversely, in an extremely dehydrated patient, the drug is distributed to a much smaller volume, so the dose must then be decreased. The total area to which a drug is distributed is known as volume of distribution.

Patients who are obese may present another problem in regard to drug distribution. Drugs such as digoxin, gentamicin, and tobramycin aren't well distributed to fatty tissue. Therefore, dosage based on actual body weight may lead to overdose and serious toxicity. Sometimes, dosage is based on lean body weight, which may be estimated from actuarial tables that give average weight range for height.

Metabolism
Most drugs are metabolized in the liver. Hepatic disease may affect one or more of the liver's metabolic functions. Therefore, the metabolism of a drug may be increased, decreased, or unchanged in patients with hepatic disease. These patients should be monitored closely for drug effect and toxicity.

The rate of drug metabolism varies with the individual. In some patients, drugs are metabolized so rapidly that their blood and tissue levels prove therapeutically inadequate, whereas the rate of metabolism is so slow in other patients that normal doses produce toxic results.

Excretion
The body eliminates drugs by metabolism (usually hepatic) and excretion (usually renal). Drug excretion refers to the movement of a drug or its metabolites from the tissues back into circulation

and from the circulation into the organs of excretion. Although most drugs are excreted by the kidneys, some can be removed via the lungs, exocrine glands (sweat, salivary, or mammary), liver, skin, and intestinal tract. Drugs may also be removed artificially by direct interventions such as hemodialysis.

Other modifying factors

An important factor that influences a drug's action and effect is its *binding to plasma proteins*, especially albumin, and other tissue components. Because only a free, unbound drug can act in the body, binding influences effectiveness and duration of effect. Protein-binding can be affected by malnutrition, renal failure, and other protein-bound drugs. When protein-binding occurs, drug dosage may need to be modified.

The *patient's age* also affects drug action and effect. Elderly patients often have decreased hepatic function, less muscle mass, and diminished renal function. They need lower doses and sometimes longer dosage intervals to avoid toxicity. With similar consequences, neonates have underdeveloped metabolic enzyme systems and inadequate renal function. These patients need highly individualized dosages and careful monitoring.

Another factor influencing drug action is *underlying disease*. For example, acidosis may cause insulin resistance. Genetic diseases, such as G6PD deficiency and hepatic porphyria, may turn drugs into toxins with serious consequences. Patients with G6PD deficiency may develop hemolytic anemia when given sulfonamides or other drugs. If given a barbiturate, a genetically susceptible patient can develop an acute porphyria attack. Also, patients who have highly active hepatic enzyme systems (for example, rapid acetylators), when treated with isoniazid, can develop hepatitis from the rapid intrahepatic buildup of a toxic metabolite.

Drug administration issues

Factors related to the administration of a drug can also influence a drug's action within the body. The dosage form of the drug is important. Some tablets and capsules are too large to be swallowed by ill patients. Although an oral solution may be substituted, it produces higher drug blood levels than a tablet because the liquid is more easily and completely absorbed. When a potentially toxic drug (such as digoxin) is given, the increased amount absorbed could cause toxicity. Sometimes a change in dosage form requires a change in dosage itself.

Routes of drug administration aren't therapeutically interchangeable. For example, diazepam is readily absorbed orally but is slowly and erratically absorbed I.M. However, gentamicin must be given parenterally because oral administration yields blood levels inadequate to treat systemic infections.

Improper storage can alter a drug's potency. Most drugs should be stored in tight containers and protected from direct sunlight and extremes in temperature and humidity to avoid deterioration. Some may need special storage conditions such as refrigeration.

The timing of drug administration is important. The administration of an oral drug during or shortly after meals may decrease the amount absorbed. This isn't clinically significant with most drugs and may sometimes be desirable with drugs such as aspirin. However, penicillins and tetracyclines shouldn't be given with meals because certain foods can inactivate their action. If the effect of food on a drug is uncertain, consult the pharmacist.

Consider the patient's age, height, and weight. This information may be needed when calculating the dosage for many drugs, and should be available in the patient's chart, along with current laboratory data (especially renal and liver function studies) for adjusting the dosage as needed.

Watch for metabolic changes. Monitor the patient for any physiologic change (depressed respiratory function, acidosis, or alkalosis) that might alter drug effect.

Know the patient's history. Obtain a comprehensive family history, when possible. Ask about past reactions to drugs, possible genetic traits that might alter drug response, and the current use of other drugs. Multiple drug therapy can cause drug interactions that can dramatically change the effects of many drugs.

Drug interactions

When one drug administered with or shortly after another drug alters the effect of either or both drugs, this is known as a *drug interaction*. Usually, the effect of one drug is increased or decreased. For instance, a drug may inhibit or stimulate the metabolism or excretion of the other, or it may release another from plasma protein–binding sites, freeing it for further action.

Combination therapy is based on drug interaction. A drug, for example, may be given to potentiate another drug's action. Probenecid, which blocks the excretion of penicillin, may be given with penicillin to maintain adequate blood levels of penicillin for a longer period. In most cases, two drugs with similar actions are given together precisely because of the additive effect that results. For instance, aspirin and codeine, both analgesics, are commonly given in combination because together they provide greater pain relief than either alone.

Drug interactions are sometimes used to prevent or antagonize specific adverse reactions. Hydrochlorothiazide and spironolactone, both diuretics, are commonly administered in combination because the former is potassium-depleting, whereas the latter is potassium-sparing.

However, not all drug interactions are beneficial. Multiple drugs can interact to produce effects that are undesirable and sometimes hazardous. Harmful drug interactions decrease efficacy or increase toxicity. For example, in a patient taking both diuretics and lithium, the diuretics may cause an increase in serum levels of lithium, resulting in lithium toxicity. Such a drug effect is known as antagonism. Drug combinations that produce these effects should be avoided. Another inhibiting effect occurs when a tetracycline is given with drugs or foods containing calcium or magnesium (such as antacids or milk). These combine with tetracycline in the GI tract and cause inadequate absorption of tetracycline.

Adverse reactions
Any drug effect other than what is therapeutically intended is called an adverse reaction. It may be expected and benign or unexpected and potentially harmful. Mild, but *predictable,* adverse reactions are sometimes called adverse effects; one such example is drowsiness caused by antihistamines. During hay fever season, a patient may have to contend with this drowsiness to obtain relief from symptoms of hay fever. In this case, the dosage may be adjusted up or down to balance therapeutic effects with adverse effects.

An adverse reaction may be tolerated for a necessary therapeutic effect, or it may be hazardous and unacceptable and require discontinuation of the drug. Some adverse reactions subside with continued use. For example, the drowsiness associated with paroxetine and the orthostatic hypotension associated with prazosin usually subside after several days, as the patient develops a tolerance to these effects. However, many adverse reactions are dose-related and lessen or disappear only if the dosage is reduced. Although most adverse reactions aren't therapeutically desirable, an occasional reaction can be put to clinical use. An example is the drowsiness associated with diphenhydramine, which makes it useful as a mild hypnotic.

Hypersensitivity, also known as drug allergy, is the result of an antigen-antibody immune reaction that occurs when a drug is given to a susceptible patient. The most dangerous hypersensitivity is penicillin allergy, which can be fatal.

Idiosyncratic reactions occur rarely. These are highly unpredictable, individual, and unusual reactions. The best known idiosyncratic drug reaction is aplastic anemia caused by chloramphenicol. This reaction only occurs in 1 out of 40,000 patients, but can be fatal. A common idiosyncratic reaction is extreme sensitivity to very low doses of a drug, or insensitivity to higher-than-normal doses.

To resolve adverse reactions, monitor minor changes in the patient's clinical status because these may be an early indication of pending toxicity. Listen to the patient's complaints about his reactions to a drug, and consider each complaint objectively. Adverse reactions may be reduced in many ways. Dosage reduction or a rescheduling of the same dose may be helpful. For example, pseudoephedrine may produce stimulation that won't be problematic if the drug is given early in the day; similarly, the drowsiness associated with antihistamines or tranquilizers can be harmless if the dose is taken at bedtime. It's important that the patient be informed of the expected adverse reactions so that he won't become worried or stop taking the drug. The patient should always report any unusual or unexpected adverse reactions promptly.

Recognizing drug allergies or serious idiosyncratic reactions can be lifesaving. Ask the patient about other drugs he has taken or is taking and if unusual reactions have occurred. If a patient claims to be allergic to a drug, ask him to relate exactly what happens after taking the drug. He may be referring to a harmless adverse effect such as upset stomach as an allergic reaction, or he may have a true tendency toward anaphylaxis. Record and report clinical changes during the patient's hospital stay. If a severe adverse reaction is suspected, withhold the drug and check with the pharmacist.

Toxic reactions
Chronic drug toxicities are usually caused by the cumulative effect and resulting accumulation of the drug in the body. These effects may be extensions of the desired therapeutic effect; for example, glyburide normalizes the blood glucose level when given in usual doses but in larger doses can produce undesired hypoglycemia.

Drug toxicities typically occur when drug blood levels rise because of impaired metabolism or excretion. For example, blood levels of theophylline rise when hepatic dysfunction impairs metabolism of the drug. Similarly, digoxin toxicity can follow impaired renal function because digoxin is eliminated from the body almost exclusively by the kidneys. Toxic blood levels also occur after excessive dosage. Tinnitus is usually a sign that the safe dose of aspirin has been exceeded.

Most drug toxicities are predictable and dose-related; fortunately, most are also readily reversible once the dosage is adjusted. Monitor patients carefully for physiologic changes that might alter drug effect. Watch especially for impaired hepatic and renal function. Warn the patient about signs of pending toxicity, and tell him what to do if a toxic reaction occurs. Also, be sure to emphasize the importance of taking a drug exactly as prescribed. Warn the patient about serious problems that could arise if he changes the dose or dosage schedule.

Drugs and pregnancy

Since the thalidomide tragedy of the late 1950s—when thousands of malformed infants were born after their mothers used the mild sedative-hypnotic during pregnancy—use of drugs during pregnancy has been a source of serious medical concern and controversy. To identify drugs that may cause such teratogenic effects, preclinical drug studies always include tests on pregnant laboratory animals. These tests point out gross teratogenicity but don't clearly establish safety. Because different species react to drugs differently, animal studies don't eliminate possible teratogenic effects in humans. For example, the preliminary studies on thalidomide gave no warning of teratogenic effects, and it was subsequently released for general use in Europe.

Although the placental barrier was believed to protect the fetus from drug effects, it really isn't much of a barrier. Except for drugs with exceptionally large molecular structures, such as heparin, virtually every drug administered to a pregnant woman crosses the placenta and enters the fetal circulation. Theoretically, heparin could be used in a pregnant woman without harming the fetus—but even heparin carries a warning for cautious use during pregnancy. Conversely, because a drug crosses the placenta doesn't necessarily mean it's harmful to the fetus.

Only one factor—the stage of fetal development—seems to be clearly related to exaggerated risk during pregnancy. During two stages of pregnancy—the first and third trimesters—the fetus is especially vulnerable to damage from maternal use of drugs. During these times, *all* drugs should be given with extreme caution.

The most sensitive period for drug-induced fetal malformation is the first trimester, when fetal organs are undergoing organogenesis. All drugs, except those labeled as pregnancy risk category A or B, should be withheld during this time unless the mother's health is in jeopardy. Theoretically, even aspirin may be harmful to the fetus. Stress that all self-prescribed drugs during early pregnancy should be avoided.

The last trimester is also a sensitive period with regard to the fetus. After birth, the neonate must rely on his own metabolism to eliminate any remaining drug. Because his detoxifying systems aren't fully developed, residual drug may take a long time to be metabolized and thus induce prolonged toxic reactions. Consequently, drugs should be used only when absolutely necessary during the last 3 months of pregnancy.

However, in some conditions pregnant women must continue to take certain drugs. A woman with a seizure disorder that is well controlled with an anticonvulsant should continue taking the drug even during pregnancy. The potential risk to the fetus is outweighed by the mother's need. The relative risk to the fetus is expressed by the drug's pregnancy risk category.

Follow these guidelines to avoid indiscriminate and potentially harmful use of drugs during pregnancy:
● Before a drug is prescribed for a woman of childbearing age, ask for the date of her last menstrual period and if she may be pregnant. If a drug is a known teratogen, some manufacturers may recommend special precautions to ensure that the drug not be given until pregnancy is ruled out.
● Tell pregnant patients, especially during the first and third trimesters, to avoid all drugs except those essential to maintain the pregnancy or maternal health.
● Topical drugs aren't exempt from the warning against indiscriminate use during pregnancy. Many topically applied drugs can be absorbed in large enough amounts to be harmful to the fetus.
● When a pregnant patient needs a drug, prescribe the safest possible drug in the lowest possible dose to minimize potential effects on the fetus.
● Tell pregnant patients to seek medical approval before taking any drug or herbal or "natural" agents.

Drugs and lactation

Most drugs taken by a breast-feeding woman appear in breast milk. Levels of drug in breast milk tend to be high when drug blood levels are high, usually after each dose has been taken. Therefore, advise the patient to breast-feed before taking her medication and not afterward.

Sometimes breast-feeding may continue with medical approval. However, it should be temporarily replaced with bottle-feeding when tetracyclines, chloramphenicol, sulfonamides (during first 2 weeks postpartum), oral anticoagulants, drugs containing iodine, or antineoplastics are being used.

To protect the infant, a breast-feeding woman should avoid taking drugs indiscriminately. She should first check with her health care provider or pharmacist to be sure of taking the safest drug at the lowest dosage.

Patient education

Use the following guidelines to educate the patient so that he obtains maximal therapeutic benefits and avoids adverse reactions, accidental overdose, or potentially harmful changes in drug effectiveness during therapy:
● Tell the patient to store the drug in its original container, at room temperature (unless directed otherwise), in a place that isn't accessible to children or exposed to sunlight. Avoid storage in the bathroom medicine cabinet, in the kitchen in close proximity to heat, or in the glove compartment or trunk of a car, where extremes of temperature and humidity will cause the drug to deteriorate.
● Instruct the patient to learn the trade and generic names of all drugs he is taking and to inform

his regular health care provider about their use. Before taking a drug, tell him also to report unusual reactions experienced in the past, any allergies to foods and other drugs, special medical problems, and drugs taken over the past few weeks, including OTC or herbal medicines. (This might be the appropriate time to tell the patient that herbal agents may cause toxic reactions; although some may have therapeutic use, these agents haven't been fully evaluated and aren't strictly regulated.)

• Inform the patient to always read the label before taking a drug, to take it exactly as prescribed, and to never share prescription drugs.

• Instruct the patient to check the expiration date before taking the drug.

• Warn the patient not to change brands of a drug without medical approval to avoid potentially harmful changes in effectiveness. Certain generic preparations aren't equivalent in effect to brand-name preparations of the same drug.

• Caution the patient never to mix different drugs in a single container, remove a drug from its original container, or remove the label. Relying on memory to identify a drug and specific directions for its use is hazardous.

• Instruct the patient to safely discard drugs that are outdated or no longer needed and to keep them out of reach of children and pets.

• Advise the patient to inform the health care professional about use of drugs before undergoing any surgery (including dental surgery).

• Stress the importance of informing the physician assistant, nurse, or pharmacist about any adverse reactions experienced during drug therapy.

• Instruct the patient to keep emergency numbers handy, including those for the health care professional, poison control center, and pharmacist and to call immediately if he or someone else has taken an overdose. Advise the patient to have syrup of ipecac available at home to induce vomiting, but only if advised to do so by these professionals.

• Tell the patient to have all prescriptions filled at the same pharmacy. The pharmacist can warn against possible harmful drug interactions.

• Tell the patient to have a sufficient supply of drugs when traveling and to carry them with him and not stow them in his luggage.

• Advise the patient to teach his children about safety and medicines. Tell him to show the children what a medicine container looks like and to never refer to medicine as candy. Instruct him to treat vitamins, especially those containing iron, as medicines.

Drug therapy in children and elderly patients

Drug action and its adverse effects may vary substantially among children and elderly patients, as opposed to those in the general adult population. Developmental differences or immature or declining body systems can exaggerate these variations and make a drug's effects less predictable and sometimes even risky. These variations must be kept in mind when administering a drug to a patient with particular developmental considerations.

This chapter outlines special considerations for drug therapy in children and elderly patients.

Drug therapy in children
Providing drug therapy to children and adolescents is challenging. Physiologic differences, including those in vital organ maturity and body composition, between children and adults can significantly influence a drug's effectiveness. It's therefore imperative to consider developmental physiology, physical assessment, and pharmacology in pediatric drug therapy.

Physiologic changes affecting drug action
A child's absorption, distribution, metabolism, and excretion processes undergo profound changes that affect drug dosage.

Absorption
Oral administration is the most common method of drug therapy in children. Drug absorption in children depends on the form and physical properties of the drug, other drugs or substances (such as food) taken simultaneously, physiologic changes, and the presence of disease.

The pH of neonatal gastric fluid affects drug absorption because it's neutral or slightly acidic and becomes more acidic as the infant matures. For example, nafcillin and penicillin G are better absorbed in an infant than an adult because of low gastric acidity.

Several infant formulas or milk products may increase gastric pH and impede absorption of acidic drugs. If possible, oral drugs should be given on an empty stomach.

Gastric emptying time and transit time through the small intestine—which is longer in children than in adults—can affect absorption. Also, intestinal hypermotility (as in diarrhea) can diminish absorption.

A child's comparatively thin epidermis allows increased absorption of topical drugs.

Rectal administration can also be used in neonates and children. Although absorption may sometimes be erratic, glycerin and acetaminophen are commonly administered in suppository form and generally are adequately absorbed.

Distribution
As with absorption, changes in body weight and physiology during childhood can significantly influence a drug's distribution and effects. In a premature infant, body fluid makes up about 85% of total body weight; in a full-term infant, 55% to 70%; and in an adult, 50% to 55%. Extracellular fluid (mostly blood) constitutes 40% of a neonate's body weight, compared with 20% in an adult. Intracellular fluid remains fairly constant throughout life and has little effect on drug dosage.

Extracellular fluid volume influences a water-soluble drug's level and effect because most drugs travel through extracellular fluid to reach their receptors. Children have a larger proportion of fluid to solid body weight, so their distribution area is proportionately greater.

Because the proportion of fat to lean body mass increases with age, the distribution of fat-soluble drugs is more limited in children than in adults. Consequently, a drug's lipid or water solubility affects the dosage for a child. For some drugs, such as anticancer chemotherapeutic drugs, drug dosing based on body surface area may be more accurate, as well as when using a drug with a narrow therapeutic index.

Binding to plasma proteins
Because of a decrease in albumin level or intermolecular attraction between drug and plasma protein, many drugs are less bound to plasma proteins in infants than in adults.

Moreover, preparations that bind plasma proteins may displace endogenous compounds, such as bilirubin or free fatty acids. Conversely, an endogenous compound may displace a weakly bound drug. For example, displacement of bound bilirubin can cause a rise in unbound bilirubin, which can lead to increased risk of kernicterus at normal bilirubin levels. Acidic drugs, such as phenytoin and sulfonamides, bind to serum albumin. Basic drugs, such as lidocaine and quinidine, bind to serum globulins.

Because only an unbound, or free, drug has a pharmacologic effect, alteration of the protein bound-to-unbound active drug ratio can significantly influence its effect.

Several diseases and disorders, such as nephrotic syndrome and malnutrition, can also decrease plasma protein and increase the level of an unbound drug, thus intensifying the drug's effect or producing a toxic effect.

Metabolism

The prevailing route for drug metabolism is the liver. A neonate's ability to metabolize a drug depends on the integrity of the hepatic enzyme system, the intrauterine exposure to the drug, and the nature of the drug itself.

Certain metabolic mechanisms are underdeveloped in neonates. Glucuronidation is a metabolic process that renders most drugs more water soluble, thereby facilitating renal excretion. This process is insufficiently developed to permit full pediatric doses until the infant is age 1 month. Thus, chloramphenicol may cause gray baby syndrome in a neonate, illustrating the infant's inability to metabolize the drug. Use of chloramphenicol in neonates, therefore, requires decreased dosage and monitoring of blood levels. Other metabolic mechanisms include sulfation (steroids and acetaminophen) and acetylation (sulfonamides and isoniazid).

Conversely, intrauterine exposure to drugs may induce precocious development of hepatic enzyme mechanisms, increasing the infant's capacity to metabolize potentially harmful substances.

Older children can metabolize drugs such as theophylline more rapidly than adults because of their increased hepatic metabolic activity. Larger doses than those recommended for adults may be needed.

Also, preparations given concurrently to a child may alter hepatic metabolism and induce production of hepatic enzymes. For example, phenobarbital can induce hepatic enzyme production and accelerate metabolism of drugs given concurrently.

Excretion

Renal excretion of a drug is the net effect of glomerular filtration, active tubular secretion, and passive tubular reabsorption. Because so many drugs are excreted in the urine, the degree of renal development or presence of renal disease can profoundly affect a child's dosage requirements.

If a child is unable to excrete a drug renally, drug accumulation and possible toxicity may result unless the dosage is reduced.

Physiologically, an infant's kidneys differ from an adult's in that they have a high resistance to blood flow and receive a smaller proportion of cardiac output; exhibit incomplete glomerular and tubular development and short, incomplete loops of Henle (glomerular filtration reaches adult values between 2 ¼ and 5 months; tubular secretion may reach adult values between 7 and 12 months); have low glomerular filtration rate (penicillins are eliminated by this route); demonstrate decreased ability to concentrate urine or reabsorb various filtered compounds; and have a reduced ability of the proximal tubules to secrete organic acids. If a child has decreased renal function, it's important to measure and calculate the creatinine clearance.

Drugs can also be eliminated by the biliary, GI, and respiratory tracts. However, the primary pathway of excretion is by means of the kidneys.

Special administration considerations

Biochemically, a drug displays the same mechanisms of action in all individuals. However, the response of a drug can be affected by a child's age and size as well as the maturity of the target organ. To ensure optimal drug effect and minimal toxicity, consider the following factors when prescribing drugs for children.

Adjusting pediatric dosages

When calculating pediatric dosages, avoid using formulas that modify adult dosages: A child isn't a scaled-down version of an adult. Pediatric dosages should be calculated on the basis of either body weight (mg/kg) or body surface area (mg/m^2).

Reevaluate dosages regularly to ensure necessary adjustments as the child develops. Although body surface area provides a useful standard for adults and older children, it shouldn't be used in premature or full-term infants. Use the body weight method instead. Don't exceed the maximum adult dosage when calculating amounts per kilogram of body weight (except with certain drugs such as theophylline).

Obtain an accurate maternal drug history—prescription and OTC drugs, vitamins, and herbal agents or other health foods taken during pregnancy. Drugs passed through breast milk can also have adverse effects on the breast-feeding infant. Before a drug is prescribed for a breast-feeding woman, the potential effects on the infant should be studied. For example, sulfonamides given to a breast-feeding mother for a urinary tract infection appear in breast milk and may cause kernicterus at lower-than-normal levels of unconjugated bilirubin.

Administering oral drugs

Consider the following when prescribing oral drug for a child.

If the patient is an infant, administer an oral drug in the liquid form if possible. For accuracy, the preparation should be measured and given by syringe; never in a vial or cup. The patient's head should be lifted to prevent aspiration of the drug, and his chin pressed down to prevent choking. The drug may also be placed in a nipple to allow the infant to suck the contents.

If the patient is a toddler, explain how he is to take the drug. If possible, have the parents enlist the child's cooperation. Drug shouldn't be mixed with food or called "candy," even if it has a pleasant taste. The child should drink liquids from a calibrated medication cup rather than from a spoon — it's easier and more accurate. If the preparation is available only in tablet form, it should be crushed and mixed with a compatible syrup. (Check with the pharmacist or a reference source to verify that the tablet can be crushed without compromising its effectiveness.)

If the patient is an older child who can swallow a tablet or capsule by himself, have him place the tablet or capsule on the back of his tongue and swallow it with water or fruit juice. Remember, milk or milk products may interfere with drug absorption.

Administering I.V. infusions
Drugs administered I.V. obtain the highest serum level because they are already in solution.

In infants, use a peripheral vein or a scalp vein in the temporal region for I.V. infusions. The scalp vein is safest in that the needle isn't likely to be dislodged; however, the head must be shaved around the site. Temporary disfigurement may result from the needle and infiltrated fluids. For these reasons, the scalp veins aren't used as commonly today as in the past.

The extremities are the most accessible insertion sites; however, because patients tend to move about, keep the following precautions in mind:
● Protect the insertion sites to prevent catheter or needle dislodgment.
● Place clamps out of the child's reach and secure any connections.
● Provide a simple explanation to a child who is to be restrained while asleep to allay anxiety and maintain trust.

During an I.V. infusion, check the child's condition. Flow rate may vary if a pump isn't used. Flow should be adequate because some drugs (calcium, for example) can be irritating at low flow rates. Infants, small children, and children with compromised cardiopulmonary status are particularly vulnerable to fluid overload with I.V. administration. Ensure that a limited amount of fluid is infused in a controlled manner; use a volume-control set and an infusion pump or syringe.

Administering I.M. injections
I.M. injections are the preferred route of administration when a drug can't be given by other parenteral routes and rapid absorption is necessary.

The vastus lateralis muscle is the preferred injection site in children under age 2; in older children, either the ventrogluteal area or the gluteus medius muscle can be used. To select the correct needle size, consider the patient's age, muscle mass, and nutritional status and the drug's viscosity; record and rotate injection sites. Explain to the patient that the injection will hurt or pinch, but that the drug will help him. Restrain him during the injection, if needed, and comfort him afterward.

Administering topical drugs and inhalants
Percutaneous absorption of drugs is inversely proportionate to skin thickness, but proportionate to skin hydration. Therefore, neonates absorb much more through their skin than do older children.

Consider the following when administering topical drugs or inhalants.

Use eardrops warmed to room temperature; cold drops can cause considerable pain and possibly vertigo. To administer drops, turn the child on his side, with the affected ear up. If the child is under age 3, pull the pinna down and back; if he is age 3 or over, pull the pinna up and back.

Avoid using inhalants in young children; obtaining their cooperation is difficult. Before attempting to administer drug through a metered-dose nebulizer to an older child, explain the inhaler to him. Then have him hold the nebulizer upside down and close his lips around the mouthpiece. Have him exhale, pinch his nostrils shut and, when he starts to inhale, release one dose of drug into his mouth. Tell the patient to continue inhaling until his lungs feel full. Most inhaled drugs aren't useful if taken orally; if you doubt the patient's ability to use the inhalant correctly, don't use it.

Use topical corticosteroids cautiously because delayed growth in children has been associated with chronic steroid use. When topical corticosteroids are used on the diaper area of infants, avoid covering this area with plastic or rubber pants, which will act as an occlusive dressing and enhance systemic absorption.

Administering parenteral nutrition
Administer I.V. nutrition to patients who are unable to take adequate food orally and to those with hypermetabolic conditions who need supplementation, including premature infants and children who have burns or other major trauma, intractable diarrhea, malabsorption syndromes, and emotional disorders (such as anorexia nervosa).

Before fat emulsions are given to infants and children, however, the potential benefits must be weighed against possible risks. Their use is limited by the child's ability to metabolize them; for example, a child with a diseased liver can't efficiently metabolize fats.

Some fats, however, must be supplied both to prevent essential fatty acid deficiency and to permit normal growth and development. A minimum of calories (2% to 4%) must be supplied as linoleic acid—an essential fatty acid found in lipids. In infants, fats are essential for normal neurologic development.

Fat solutions may decrease oxygen perfusion and may adversely affect children with pulmonary disease. Minimize this risk by providing only the minimum fat needed for essential fatty acid requirements and not the usual intake of 40% to 50% of the child's total calories.

Fatty acids can also displace bilirubin bound to serum albumin, causing an increase in free, unconjugated bilirubin and an increased risk of kernicterus. However, fat solutions may interfere with some bilirubin assays and cause falsely elevated levels. To prevent this, obtain a blood sample 4 hours after lipid infusion; if the emulsion is introduced over 24 hours, centrifuge the blood sample before the assay is performed.

Drug therapy in elderly patients
When prescribing drug therapy for elderly patients, consider the physiologic and pharmacokinetic changes that may alter appropriate drug dosage or cause common adverse reactions or compliance problems. It's also important to avoid complex drug regimens.

Physiologic changes affecting drug action
As a person ages, gradual physiologic changes occur. Some of these age-related changes may alter the therapeutic or toxic effects of drugs.

Body composition
Proportions of fat, lean tissue, and water in the body change with age. Total body mass and lean body mass tend to decrease; the proportion of body fat tends to increase.

Depending on the individual, these changes in body composition affect the relationship between a drug's level and distribution in the body. For example, a water-soluble drug such as gentamicin isn't distributed to fat. Because there is relatively less lean tissue in an elderly person, more drug remains in the blood.

GI function
In elderly patients, decreases in gastric acid secretion and GI motility slow the emptying of stomach contents and the movement of intestinal contents through the tract. Furthermore, research suggests that elderly patients may have more difficulty absorbing drugs. This is an especially significant problem with drugs that have a narrow therapeutic range, such as digoxin, in which any change in absorption can be crucial.

Hepatic function
The liver's ability to metabolize certain drugs decreases with age. This is caused by diminished blood flow to the liver, which results from the age-related decrease in cardiac output and from the diminished activity of certain liver enzymes. When an elderly patient takes certain sleep aids such as flurazepam, the liver's reduced ability to metabolize the drug may produce a hangover effect the next morning.

Decreased hepatic function may cause more intense drug effects due to higher blood levels, longer-lasting drug effects due to prolonged blood levels, and greater risk of drug toxicity.

Renal function
Although an elderly person's renal function is usually sufficient to eliminate excess body fluid and waste, the ability to eliminate some drugs may be reduced by 50% or more.

Many drugs commonly used by elderly patients, such as digoxin, are excreted primarily through the kidneys. If the kidneys' ability to excrete the drug is decreased, high drug blood levels may result. Digoxin toxicity, therefore, is relatively common in elderly patients who aren't receiving a reduced digoxin dosage that accommodates decreased renal function.

Drug dosages can be modified to compensate for age-related decreases in renal function. The drug dosage may be adjusted with the help of laboratory tests, such as for BUN and serum creatinine levels, so that the patient receives the expected therapeutic benefits without the risk of toxicity. Observe the patient for signs or symptoms of toxicity.

Special administration considerations
Aging is usually accompanied by a decline in organ function that can profoundly affect drug distribution and clearance. This physiologic decline is likely to be exacerbated by a disease or chronic disorder. Together, these factors can significantly increase the risk of adverse reactions, drug toxicity, and noncompliance. Be aware of these changes when prescribing a drug to an elderly patient.

Adverse reactions
Compared with younger people, elderly patients experience twice as many adverse drug reactions as a result of greater drug consumption, poor compliance with drug regimens, and numerous physiologic changes.

Signs and symptoms of adverse drug reactions—confusion, weakness, and lethargy—are often mistakenly attributed to senility or disease. If the adverse reaction isn't identified, the patient may continue to receive the drug. Furthermore, he may receive unnecessary additional drugs to treat complications caused by the original drug.

This can sometimes result in a pattern of inappropriate and excessive drug use. This problem may be exacerbated by visits to multiple health care professionals who may prescribe still more drugs.

Although any drug can cause adverse reactions, most of the serious reactions in elderly patients are caused by relatively few drugs. Be particularly alert for toxicities resulting from diuretics, antihypertensives, digoxin, corticosteroids, anticoagulants, sleeping aids, and OTC drugs.

Diuretic toxicity
Because total body water content decreases with age, normal dosages of potassium-wasting diuretics, such as hydrochlorothiazide and furosemide, may result in fluid loss and even dehydration in an elderly patient.

These diuretics may deplete serum potassium, causing weakness in the patient, and they may raise blood uric acid and glucose levels, complicating preexisting gout and diabetes mellitus.

Antihypertensive toxicity
Many elderly people experience light-headedness or fainting when using antihypertensives, partly in response to atherosclerosis and decreased elasticity of the blood vessels. Antihypertensives lower blood pressure too rapidly, resulting in insufficient blood flow to the brain. This may cause dizziness, fainting, or even stroke.

Consequently, dosages of antihypertensives must be carefully individualized. In elderly patients, too aggressive treatment of high blood pressure may do more harm, so treatment goals should be reasonable. Although bringing blood pressure down to 120/85 mm Hg may be appropriate in a young hypertensive patient, a more reasonable goal for an elderly hypertensive patient might be 150/95 mm Hg.

Digoxin toxicity
As the body's renal function and rate of excretion decline, digoxin levels in the blood may build to toxic levels, causing nausea, anorexia, vomiting, diarrhea, and—most serious—arrhythmias. Try to prevent severe toxicity by monitoring serum levels and by observing the patient for early signs or symptoms of digoxin toxicity, such as appetite loss, confusion, or depression.

Corticosteroid toxicity
Elderly patients on corticosteroids may experience short-term effects, including fluid retention and psychological manifestations ranging from mild euphoria to acute psychotic reactions. Long-term toxic effects such as osteoporosis can be especially severe in elderly patients who have been taking prednisone or related steroidal compounds for months or even years. To prevent serious toxicity, carefully monitor patients on long-term regimens. Observe them for subtle changes in appearance, mood, and mobility; signs of impaired healing; and fluid and electrolyte disturbances.

Anticoagulant effects
Elderly patients taking anticoagulants are at increased risk for bleeding, especially when they also take NSAIDs. Observe INRs carefully, and monitor these patients for bruising and other signs of bleeding.

Sleeping aid toxicity
Sedatives or sleeping aids may cause excessive sedation or residual drowsiness. Keep in mind that ingestion of alcohol may exaggerate such depressant effects, even if the sleeping aid was taken the previous evening. Delirium and gait disturbances may also occur.

OTC drug toxicity
When aspirin, analgesics containing aspirin, and other OTC NSAIDs are used in moderation, toxicity is minimal, but prolonged ingestion may cause GI irritation—even ulcers—and gradual blood loss resulting in severe anemia. Prescription NSAIDs may cause similar problems, especially in elderly patients. Although anemia from chronic aspirin consumption can affect all age-groups, elderly patients may be less able to compensate because of their already reduced iron stores. Acetaminophen, long marketed for its safety, may cause toxicity when taken with alcohol.

Laxatives may cause diarrhea in elderly patients who are extremely sensitive to such drugs as bisacodyl. Long-term oral use of mineral oil as a lubricating laxative may result in lipid pneumonia from aspiration of small residual oil droplets in the patient's mouth.

Noncompliance
Poor compliance can be a problem with patients of any age. A significant number of hospitalizations result from noncompliance to medical regimen. However, in elderly patients, specific factors linked to aging—such as diminished visual acuity, hearing loss, forgetfulness, the common need for multiple drug therapy, and socioeconomic factors—can combine to make compliance a special problem. About one-third of elderly patients fail to comply with their prescribed drug therapy. They may fail to take prescribed doses or to follow the correct schedule or they may take drugs prescribed for previous disorders, discontinue drugs prematurely, or indiscriminately use drugs that are to be given on an as needed basis. Elderly patients may also have multiple prescriptions for the same drug and, therefore, inadvertently take an overdose.

Review the patient's drug regimen with him. Make sure he understands the medication amount and the time and frequency of doses. Also, explain how he should take each medication—with food or water or by itself.

Provide the patient whatever help is needed to avoid drug therapy problems. Suggest that he use drug calendars, pill sorters, or other aids to help him comply with his prescribed drug regimen, and refer him to the pharmacist if he needs further information.

It's important to manage medical conditions without drugs as often as possible. When drugs are needed, always consider how the clinical status of each patient could influence the pharmacology of the drug. Start with smaller doses and gradually increase the dose only if necessary, making sure to monitor the elderly patient frequently.

Two components of drug therapy are essential for prescribers: taking a detailed medication history and writing prescriptions appropriately and accurately. A careful medication history can help identify the use, dosage, effectiveness, potential interactions, and adverse reactions for each drug used.

Proper prescription writing practices are essential in providing comprehensive patient care and ensuring patient safety. They also reduce the legal liability of the prescriber, making errors and misunderstandings less likely.

Taking a medication history
Before prescribing a drug for a patient, conduct a complete assessment of the patient's condition and medication history. Assess the patient's knowledge about drug therapy and its effectiveness. A beneficial outcome to current or past drug use improves the patient's health status and overall quality of life.

Interview the patient during the hospital admission or in an outpatient setting. Ask specific questions about the patient's background that can significantly influence drug therapy, including questions about allergies, medical history, habits, socioeconomic status, lifestyle and beliefs, sensory deficits, and specific prescription drugs, OTC preparations, and herbal agents being taken. During the assessment, observe the patient's cognitive status because the patient's ability to comply with a drug regimen influences the choice of drug and administration route.

Allergies
The patient may have had allergic or adverse reactions to drugs or foods. Obtain specific information about the drug name; a description of the reaction; its situation, time, and setting; and contributing factors, such as concurrent use of stimulants, tobacco, alcohol, or illegal drugs or a significant change in nutritional patterns. Tell the patient to describe the allergic reaction to help determine whether the reaction is an adverse effect or a dislike of taking the drug.

Allergies to foods can also affect drug therapy. Shellfish allergies, for instance, can contraindicate use of drugs that contain iodine or are byproducts of shellfish. Patients with allergies to eggs can't receive vaccines that are derived from chick embryos.

Medical history
When gathering the medical history, note the presence of chronic disorders and record the date of diagnosis, initial and current treatment, and the primary health care provider's name.

Careful attention to the patient's medical history can reveal important problems associated with drug therapy, such as conflicting and incompatible drug regimens. A patient who doesn't have a family health care provider to oversee and coordinate all care may seek the care of several specialists who may prescribe drug therapy without knowledge of other drugs being taken by the patient. You may find it helpful to contact the patient's pharmacist for a detailed list of drugs the patient is taking.

Habits
Consider the patient's dietary habits and nontherapeutic use of drugs. Certain foods can directly influence the effectiveness of a drug. A patient receiving the anticoagulant warfarin, for instance, shouldn't increase his intake of green leafy vegetables because they contain vitamin K, which can antagonize warfarin's anticoagulant effect.

Nontherapeutic uses of drugs can also affect a patient's health and impair the effectiveness of drug therapy. Consider the use of alcohol, tobacco, caffeine, and illegal drugs, such as marijuana, cocaine, or heroin. If the patient uses alcohol, note the frequency of use and the amount and type of alcohol consumed. Carefully document the intake of stimulants such as caffeine because these agents can adversely affect a patient's CV and CNS status. Record the type of stimulant used, frequency of intake, and amount consumed.

For the patient who uses tobacco, document the number of years the patient has smoked or chewed, type of tobacco used, and the quantity, frequency, and brand of tobacco product used each day.

Defining a patient's use of illicit drugs may be difficult. However, if such use is suspected, encourage the patient to discuss his use openly and honestly, emphasizing that these drugs have profound effects that may cause serious drug interactions. If the patient admits using illicit drugs, document the type of drug used, amount and frequency of use, and preferred route of administration.

Socioeconomic status
The patient's age, educational level, occupation, and insurance coverage may affect compliance. The patient's age determines the individuals (parents or family members) to be included in the plan of care and the level of information appropriate for patient teaching. For the elderly or impaired patient, also consider the availability and qualifications of caregivers and home health providers.

Knowing the patient's educational background and occupation is helpful when selecting appropriate interventions, planning a drug regimen that fits the patient's daily routine, and encouraging compliance. Knowledge of the patient's insurance status may help you anticipate the need for financial assistance and counseling. Remember that noncompliance commonly results from an inability to afford the drugs the patient has been prescribed.

Lifestyle and beliefs
Support systems, marital status, childbearing status, attitudes toward health and health care, whether the health care system is used, and daily activity patterns may affect the plan of care for a patient and the likelihood of compliance. For example, an 18-year-old single parent who has dropped out of high school, is on medical assistance, and has no family support will probably need more teaching and assistance to gain compliance than a 40-year-old affluent professional with a great deal of family support, who understands the reasons for using the drug, and can afford the cost of therapy.

Sensory deficits
Any sensory deficit can significantly shape an appropriate plan of care. Impaired vision, paralysis of one or more extremities, loss of a limb, or loss of sensation in an extremity can impair the patient's ability to administer a subcutaneous injection, break a scored tablet, or open a medication container. Color blindness may cause difficulty in distinguishing between two drugs. Hearing impairment can complicate effective patient instruction.

Always evaluate sensory deficits fully before planning drug therapy.

Special monitoring
Some drug regimens need special monitoring, such as monitoring the blood glucose level or checking the radial pulse. Make sure the patient knows how to accurately perform special monitoring procedures. Discuss the effects of drug therapy with the patient and determine if new symptoms or unforeseen adverse reactions have developed. Noting the patient's pattern of administration may provide insight into why a particular drug regimen succeeds or fails.

OTC drugs and herbal agents
A comprehensive drug history should also include determining what, if any, OTC products or herbal agents the patient is using. OTC preparations include a wide range of products, from nutritional supplements to herbal or natural products to homeopathic remedies. Many OTC drugs and herbal agents can inhibit or potentiate the effects of a prescribed drug. For example, aspirin potentiates the anticoagulant effects of warfarin, and goldenseal can interfere with the action of an antihypertensive. Include dosage and frequency information as well as the type of product used.

Cognitive status
A patient's intact cognitive abilities ensure that he can understand and implement the actions necessary for compliance. During the interview, note whether the patient is alert and oriented, able to interact appropriately with people, and exhibits appropriate conversation. Consider whether the patient can think clearly and express his thoughts coherently. Finally, check short- and long-term memory because the patient will need both to follow the prescribed drug regimen.

If such an evaluation identifies cognitive deficits, determine the probable cause, which can range from a transient drug-related effect to permanent neurologic impairments. Then determine whether the patient can comply with the prescribed drug regimen. If compliance isn't possible, find another way to ensure that the patient receives the prescribed therapy.

Effective prescription writing
The physician assistant can write prescriptions in accordance with state laws governing such practice. It's important that the prescription be correctly and safely written. (See *Components of a properly written prescription,* page 16.)

Prescription components
Write a prescription legibly, and include the following components: patient's full name and address, date of the prescription, prescribed drug name, dosage form (if more than one formulation exists), total amount of the drug to be dispensed, amount of each dose, administration route, administration schedule or time, number of times the prescription can be refilled, and your signature and credentials.

Prescription writing practices
Medication errors often stem from poorly written prescriptions. To prevent such errors from occurring, write clearly and precisely, and review all parts of the form before signing the prescription.

Effective prescription writing practices help ensure the accurate interpretation of your writ-

COMPONENTS OF A PROPERLY WRITTEN PRESCRIPTION

Prescriptions contain certain basic information and should be filled out properly to avoid misunderstandings. Here is an example of a correctly written prescription.

Lakeview Hospital
2000 N. Main Street
Lewistown, N.J. 00265

DATE 3/10/01

PATIENT'S
NAME *Kelly R. Weaver*
ADDRESS *1000 Limerick Lane*
Dresher, N.J. 00265

ADDRESSOPLATE OR COMPLETE ABOVE

This Rx NOT VALID For Schedule Drugs

Synthroid 0.2mg tab

Disp: #30

Sig: i tab P.O. daily

William Jackson PA-C

Refill _3_

IN ORDER FOR A BRAND NAME PRODUCT TO BE DISPENSED, THE PRESCRIBER MUST HAND-WRITE, "BRAND NECESSARY" OR "BRAND MEDICALLY NECESSARY" IN THE SPACE ABOVE.

Pharmacy will dispense a generic equivalent (under the formulary system) unless the particular drug is encircled.

PRESCRIBER'S PRINTED NAME _William Jackson, PA-C_

ten prescriptions. Remember the following considerations:
• Never abbreviate the names of drugs; abbreviations can be misinterpreted and the wrong drug given by mistake.
• Don't abbreviate the word "unit"; a sloppy, handwritten "U" or "u" could look like a zero and cause a tenfold drug overdose error.
• Don't use ambiguous abbreviations that could be misinterpreted, such as O.D., which could represent "once daily" or "right eye." When the accurate interpretation of an abbreviation is in question, write out the abbreviation completely.
• Avoid the unnecessary use of a decimal point and zero after a whole number. For instance, write "4 mg," not "4.0 mg." If the decimal point isn't seen, a tenfold drug overdose error could occur.

• Always place a zero before the decimal point when the quantity is less than 1. For instance, write "0.2 ml," not ".2 ml."
• Write instructions (including the reason the drug is being prescribed) on the prescription to prevent misinterpretation of the order and reduce the risk of error.

Besides enhancing patient safety and ensuring a beneficial outcome to treatment, a properly written prescription may also serve as an important legal protection.

abacavir sulfate
Ziagen

Pharmacologic classification: nucleoside analogue reverse transcriptase inhibitor (NRTI)
Therapeutic classification: antiviral
Pregnancy risk category C

How supplied
Available by prescription only
Tablets: 300 mg
Oral solution: 20 mg/ml

Indications, route, and dosage
HIV type 1 (HIV-1) infection
Adults: 300 mg P.O. b.i.d. with other antiretrovirals.
Children ages 3 months to 16 years: 8 mg/kg P.O. b.i.d. (maximum 300 mg P.O. b.i.d.) with other antiretrovirals.

Pharmacodynamics
Antiviral action: Converted intracellularly to an active metabolite, carbovir triphosphate, which inhibits the activity of HIV-1 reverse transcriptase by competing with the natural substrate deoxyguanosine-5′-triphosphate (dGTP) and by incorporation into viral DNA.

Pharmacokinetics
● *Absorption:* Rapidly and extensively absorbed after oral administration; mean absolute bioavailability of tablet is 83%.
● *Distribution:* Distributed in the extravascular space. About 50% of drug binds to plasma proteins.
● *Metabolism:* Primarily metabolized by alcohol dehydrogenase and glucuronyl transferase to form 2 metabolites that lack antiviral activity.
● *Excretion:* Primarily excreted in urine; about 16% of dose excreted in feces. Elimination half-life in single-dose studies was 1 to 2 hours.

Contraindications and precautions
Contraindicated in patients with hypersensitivity to the drug or its components. Use cautiously in patients with known risk factors for liver disease.

Interactions
Drug-lifestyle. *Alcohol:* Reduces elimination of abacavir, increasing overall exposure to drug. Monitor alcohol consumption. Use together cautiously.

Adverse reactions
CNS: insomnia and sleep disorders, headache.
GI: *nausea, vomiting,* diarrhea, loss of appetite (anorexia).
Skin: rash.
Other: *hypersensitivity reaction,* fever.

☑ Special considerations
● Always use drug with other antiretrovirals; don't add as a single drug when antiretroviral regimens are changed because of loss of virologic response.
● Drug can be given without regard to meals.
● Because drug is absorbed equally well from either solution or tablets, both forms can be used interchangeably.
● Drug has caused fatal hypersensitivity reactions. Patients developing signs or symptoms of hypersensitivity (fever, rash, fatigue, GI symptoms such as nausea, vomiting, diarrhea, or abdominal pain) should discontinue drug as soon as a reaction is first suspected and seek immediate medical attention.
● Don't restart drug after a hypersensitivity reaction because more severe symptoms will recur within hours and may include life-threatening hypotension and death. Symptoms usually appear within the first 6 weeks of treatment, but may occur at any time.
● To facilitate reporting of hypersensitivity reactions and collection of information on each case, an abacavir hypersensitivity registry has been established. Physicians should register patients by calling 1-800-270-0425.
● Lactic acidosis and severe (even fatal) hepatomegaly with steatosis have been reported with use of nucleoside analogues, such as abacavir and other antiretrovirals, alone or in combination. Stop treatment in patients who develop clinical or laboratory findings suggestive of lactic acidosis or pronounced hepatotoxicity (including hepatomegaly and steatosis even in the absence of marked transaminase elevations).
● No known antidote for toxicity exists. It's unknown if drug is removed by peritoneal dialysis or hemodialysis.

Monitoring the patient
● Monitor patient for signs or symptoms of hypersensitivity reaction.

● Monitor liver function studies in patients at risk for hepatic disease.

Information for the patient
● Advise patient of the risk of a life-threatening hypersensitivity reaction with this drug.
● Tell patient to stop taking drug and call physician immediately if signs or symptoms of hypersensitivity (fever, rash, severe tiredness, achiness, generally ill feeling, or GI symptoms such as nausea, vomiting, diarrhea, or stomach pain) develop.
● Instruct patient to always carry a medical alert card identifying symptoms of hypersensitivity reaction.
● Explain that drug isn't a cure for HIV infection nor does it reduce the risk of transmission of HIV to others. Advise patient to remain under a physician's care throughout therapy and to use safe sex practices.
● Urge patient to read medication guide that comes with each new prescription and refill.
● Inform patient that long-term effects of drug are unknown.
● Advise patient to take drug exactly as prescribed.
● Tell patient that drug may be taken without regard to meals.

Geriatric patients
● It's unknown if patients ages 65 and over respond to drug differently than younger patients. Determine dose selection for an elderly patient cautiously, taking into account greater risk of decreased hepatic, renal, or cardiac function and concomitant disease or other drug therapy.

Pediatric patients
● Safety and effectiveness have been established in children ages 3 months to 13 years.

Breast-feeding patients
● Because of the potential for HIV transmission and possible adverse effects, women shouldn't breast-feed while taking this drug.

abciximab
ReoPro

Pharmacologic classification: antiplatelet aggregator
Therapeutic classification: platelet aggregation inhibitor
Pregnancy risk category C

How supplied
Available by prescription only
Injection: 2 mg/ml

Indications, route, and dosage
Adjunct to percutaneous transluminal coronary angioplasty (PTCA) or atherectomy for prevention of acute cardiac ischemic complications in patients at high risk for abrupt closure of treated coronary vessel
Adults: 0.25 mg/kg as an I.V. bolus given 10 to 60 minutes before start of PTCA; then a continuous I.V. infusion of 10 mcg/minute for 12 hours.
Unstable angina not responding to conventional therapy with plans to undergo PTCA within 24 hours
Adults: 0.25 mg/kg I.V. bolus; then 18- or 24-hour I.V. infusion of 10 mcg/minute ending 1 hour after PTCA.

Pharmacodynamics
Platelet aggregation inhibiting action: As the Fab fragment of the chimeric human-murine monoclonal immunoglobulin antibody 7E3, abciximab binds selectively to platelet glycoprotein (GP IIb/IIIa) receptors and inhibits platelet aggregation.

Pharmacokinetics
● *Absorption:* Only given I.V.
● *Distribution:* No information available.
● *Metabolism:* No information available.
● *Excretion:* Initial half-life is less than 10 minutes, then a second phase of about 30 minutes.

Contraindications and precautions
Contraindicated in patients with hypersensitivity to any component of drug or to murine proteins and in those with active internal bleeding, significant GI or GU bleeding within 6 weeks, history of CVA within 2 years or CVA with significant residual neurologic deficit, bleeding diathesis, thrombocytopenia (less than 100,000/mm^3), major surgery or trauma within 6 weeks, intracranial neoplasm, intracranial arteriovenous malformation, intracranial aneurysm, severe uncontrolled hypertension, or history of vasculitis. Also contraindicated when oral anticoagulants have been administered within past 7 days unless PT is 1.2 times control or less, or when I.V. dextran is being used before or is intended to be used during PTCA.
   Use cautiously in patients who are at increased risk for bleeding, including those less than 165 lb (75 kg) or over age 65, those with history of GI disease, or those receiving thrombolytics. Conditions that also increase risk of bleeding include PTCA within 12 hours of onset of symptoms for acute MI, PTCA lasting over 70 minutes, or failed PTCA. Heparin anticoagulation used with abciximab may also increase risk of bleeding.

Interactions
Drug-drug. *Antiplatelet drugs, heparin, NSAIDs, thrombolytics, other anticoagulants:* Increased risk of bleeding. Monitor patient closely.

Adverse reactions
CNS: confusion, hypoesthesia.
CV: *bradycardia, hypotension,* peripheral edema.
EENT: abnormal vision.
GI: *nausea, vomiting.*
Hematologic: anemia, *bleeding,* leukocytosis, **thrombocytopenia.**
Respiratory: pleural effusion, pleurisy, pneumonia.
Other: pain.

☑ Special considerations
• Patients at risk for abrupt closure, and thus candidates for drug therapy, include those undergoing PTCA with at least 1 of the following conditions: unstable angina or a non-Q-wave MI, acute Q-wave MI within 12 hours of symptom onset, or the presence of 2 type B lesions in artery to be dilated, 1 type B lesion in artery to be dilated in women age 65 or older or diabetic patients, 1 type C lesion in artery to be dilated, or angioplasty of infarct-related lesion within 7 days of MI.
• Give drug with aspirin and heparin.
• Keep epinephrine, dopamine, theophylline, antihistamines, and corticosteroids readily available in case of anaphylaxis.
• Inspect solution for particulate matter before administration. If opaque particles are present, discard solution and obtain new vial. Withdraw necessary amount of drug for bolus injection through a sterile, nonpyrogenic, low-protein-binding, 0.2- or 0.22-millipore filter into a syringe. Administer bolus 10 to 60 minutes before procedure.
• Withdraw 4.5 ml of drug for continuous infusion through a sterile, nonpyrogenic, low-protein-binding, 0.2- or 0.22-micron filter into a syringe. Inject into 250 ml of sterile normal saline or 5% dextrose and infuse at 17 ml/hour for 12 hours through a continuous infusion pump equipped with an in-line filter. Discard unused portion at end of 12-hour infusion.
• Administer drug in a separate I.V. line; don't add other drugs to infusion solution.
• There have been no reports of overdose in humans. However, discontinue infusion after 12 hours to avoid effects of prolonged platelet receptor blockade.

Monitoring the patient
• Monitor patient closely for bleeding. Bleeding may be of 2 types: bleeding at the arterial access site for cardiac catheterization, and internal bleeding involving the GI or GU tracts or retroperitoneal sites.
• Institute bleeding precautions. Maintain patient on bed rest for 6 to 8 hours after sheath removal or drug discontinuation, whichever is later. Discontinue heparin at least 4 hours before sheath removal. Minimize or avoid, if possible, arterial and venous punctures, I.M. injections, nasotra-

cheal intubation, and use of urinary catheters, nasogastric tubes, and automatic blood pressure cuffs.
• Platelet function recovers in about 48 hours but drug remains in circulation for up to 10 days in a platelet-bound state.
• Platelet counts should be monitored before treatment, 2 to 4 hours after treatment, and at 24 hours after treatment or before discharge.
• Before infusion, platelet count, PT, activated clotting time, and APTT should be measured to identify preexisting hemostatic abnormalities.

Information for the patient
• Instruct patient to report bleeding promptly.

Geriatric patients
• Use drug cautiously in patients over age 65.

Pediatric patients
• Safety and effectiveness in pediatric patients haven't been established.

Breast-feeding patients
• It's unknown if drug appears in breast milk or is absorbed systemically after ingestion. Use cautiously.

acarbose
Precose

Pharmacologic classification: alpha-glucosidase inhibitor
Therapeutic classification: antidiabetic
Pregnancy risk category B

How supplied
Available by prescription only
Tablets: 50 mg, 100 mg

Indications, route, and dosage
Dietary adjunct to lower blood glucose levels in patients with type 2 diabetes mellitus whose hyperglycemia can't be managed by diet alone or by diet and a sulfonylurea
Adults: Initially, 25 mg P.O. t.i.d. with the first bite of each main meal. Adjust dosage at 4- to 8-week intervals based on 1-hour postprandial glucose levels and tolerance. Maintenance dose is 50 to 100 mg P.O. t.i.d. depending on patient's weight. Maximum dose for patients 60 kg (132 lb) or less is 50 mg P.O. t.i.d.; for patients over 60 kg, maximum is 100 mg P.O. t.i.d.
Adjunct to insulin or metformin therapy in patients with type 2 diabetes mellitus whose hyperglycemia can't be managed by diet, exercise, and insulin or metformin alone
Adults: Initially, 25 mg P.O. t.i.d. with first bite of each main meal. Adjust dosage at 4- to 8-week intervals based on 1-hour postprandial glucose levels and tolerance to determine minimum ef-

fective dosage of each drug. Maintenance dose is 50 to 100 mg P.O. t.i.d. based on patient's weight. Maximum dose for patients 60 kg (132 lb) or less is 50 mg P.O. t.i.d.; for patients over 60 kg, maximum is 100 mg P.O. t.i.d.

Pharmacodynamics
Antidiabetic action: Lowers blood glucose levels by a competitive, reversible inhibition of pancreatic alpha-amylase and membrane-bound intestinal alpha-glucoside hydrolase enzymes. In diabetic patients, this enzyme inhibition results in delayed glucose absorption and a lowering of postprandial hyperglycemia. Doesn't enhance insulin secretion.

Pharmacokinetics
- *Absorption:* Minimally absorbed.
- *Distribution:* Acts locally within the GI tract.
- *Metabolism:* Metabolized exclusively within the GI tract, principally by intestinal bacteria with some metabolized action caused by digestive enzymes.
- *Excretion:* Within 96 hours, 51% is excreted in feces as unabsorbed drug. The fraction of drug absorbed is almost completely excreted by the kidneys. Plasma elimination half-life is about 2 hours. Drug accumulation doesn't occur with t.i.d. oral dosing.

Contraindications and precautions
Contraindicated in patients with hypersensitivity to drug and in those with diabetic ketoacidosis, cirrhosis, inflammatory bowel disease, colonic ulceration, or partial intestinal obstruction. Also contraindicated in those predisposed to intestinal obstruction, in those with chronic intestinal diseases associated with marked disorders of digestion or absorption, and in those with conditions that may deteriorate because of increased gas formation in the intestine. Avoid drug in patients with serum creatinine levels exceeding 2 mg/dl and in breast-feeding or pregnant women. Use cautiously in patients with mild to moderate renal impairment.

Interactions
Drug-drug. *Calcium channel blockers, corticosteroids, estrogens, isoniazid, nicotinic acid, oral contraceptives, phenothiazines, phenytoin, sympathomimetics, thiazides, thyroid products, other diuretics:* May cause hyperglycemia or hypoglycemia when withdrawn. Monitor patient's blood glucose levels.
Insulin, sulfonylureas: Hypoglycemic potential of these drugs may be increased. Monitor patient's blood glucose level closely.
Intestinal adsorbents (activated charcoal), digestive enzyme preparations containing carbohydrate-splitting enzymes (amylase, pancreatin): May reduce effect of acarbose. Don't administer together.

Adverse reactions
GI: *abdominal pain, diarrhea, flatulence,* elevated serum transaminase levels.

☑ Special considerations
- If hypoglycemia occurs, treat with oral glucose (dextrose) rather than sucrose (cane sugar). Absorption of dextrose isn't inhibited by acarbose. Severe hypoglycemia may require I.V. glucose infusion or glucagon administration. Dosage adjustment of acarbose and sulfonylurea may be required to prevent further episodes of hypoglycemia.
- During periods of increased stress, such as infection, fever, surgery, or trauma, patient may require insulin therapy. Monitor patient closely for hyperglycemia in these situations.
- Unlike sulfonylureas or insulin, acarbose overdose doesn't result in hypoglycemia.
- An overdose may cause transient increases in flatulence, diarrhea, and abdominal discomfort, which quickly subside.

Monitoring the patient
- Monitor patient's 1-hour postprandial plasma glucose levels to determine therapeutic effectiveness of drug and to identify appropriate dose. Thereafter, measure glycosylated hemoglobin every 3 months. Treatment goals include decreasing both postprandial plasma glucose and glycosylated hemoglobin levels to normal or near normal by using the lowest effective dose of acarbose either as monotherapy or with sulfonylureas.
- Monitor serum transaminase levels every 3 months during first year of therapy, then periodically in patients receiving doses exceeding 50 mg t.i.d. Abnormalities may require dosage adjustment or withdrawal of drug.

Information for the patient
- Tell patient to take drug with first bite of each of 3 main meals daily.
- Make sure patient understands that therapy relieves symptoms but doesn't cure disease.
- Stress importance of adhering to specific diet, reducing weight, exercising, and following personal hygiene programs. Explain how and when to perform self-monitoring of blood glucose level, and teach recognition of and intervention for hyperglycemia.
- If a sulfonylurea is also taken, teach patient to recognize and intervene for hypoglycemia. Tell patient to treat symptoms of low blood glucose level with a form of dextrose instead of products containing table sugar.
- Advise patient to carry medical identification regarding diabetic status.

Pediatric patients
- Safety and effectiveness in pediatric patients haven't been established.

Reactions may be *common*, uncommon, **life-threatening**, or COMMON AND LIFE-THREATENING.

Breast-feeding patients
● It's unknown if drug appears in breast milk. Don't give drug to breast-feeding women.

acebutolol
Sectral

Pharmacologic classification: beta blocker
Therapeutic classification: antihypertensive, antiarrhythmic
Pregnancy risk category B

How supplied
Available by prescription only
Capsules: 200 mg, 400 mg

Indications, route, and dosage
Hypertension
Adults: 400 mg P.O. either as a single daily dose or 200 mg b.i.d. Patients may receive as much as 1,200 mg divided b.i.d.
Ventricular arrhythmias
Adults: 200 mg P.O. b.i.d. Increase dosage to provide adequate clinical response. Usual daily dose is 600 to 1,200 mg.
◇ *Angina*
Adults: Initially, 200 mg b.i.d. Increase up to 800 mg daily until angina is controlled. Patients with severe angina may require higher doses.
✦ *Dosage adjustment.* Reduce dose in elderly patients and in those with impaired renal function. If creatinine clearance is 25 to 49 ml/minute, decrease dose by 50%; if less than 25 ml/minute, decrease by 75%. Avoid doses over 800 mg/day in elderly patients.
Antihypertensive action: Exact mechanism unknown. Has cardioselective beta blocking properties and mild intrinsic sympathomimetic activity.
Antiarrhythmic action: Decreases heart rate and prevents exercise-induced increases in heart rate; also decreases myocardial contractility, cardiac output, and SA and AV nodal conduction velocity.

Pharmacokinetics
● *Absorption:* Well absorbed after oral administration. Plasma levels peak at about 2¼ hours.
● *Distribution:* About 26% protein-bound; minimal quantities are detected in CSF.
● *Metabolism:* Undergoes extensive first-pass metabolism in the liver; levels of its major active metabolite, diacetolol, peak at about 3¼ hours.
● *Excretion:* From 30% to 40% is excreted in urine; the remainder appears in feces and bile. Half-life of acebutolol is 3 to 4 hours; half-life of diacetolol is 8 to 13 hours.

Contraindications and precautions
Contraindicated in patients with persistent severe bradycardia, second- and third-degree heart block, overt cardiac failure, and cardiogenic shock. Use cautiously in patients at risk for heart failure and in patients with bronchospastic disease, diabetes, hyperthyroidism, and peripheral vascular disease.

Interactions
Drug-drug. *Alpha-adrenergic stimulants such as those in OTC cold remedies, indomethacin, NSAIDs:* Hypotensive effects of acebutolol may be antagonized. Use together cautiously.
Insulin, oral antidiabetics: Dosage changes may be needed. Monitor glucose levels.
Other antihypertensives: Increased hypotensive effects. Use together cautiously.

Adverse reactions
CNS: depression, dizziness, fatigue, headache, hyperesthesia, hypoesthesia, impotence, insomnia.
CV: *bradycardia,* chest pain, edema, *heart failure,* hypotension.
GI: abdominal pain, constipation, diarrhea, dyspepsia, flatulence, nausea, vomiting.
Musculoskeletal: arthralgia, myalgia.
Respiratory: *bronchospasm,* cough, dyspnea.
Skin: rash.

☑ Special considerations
Besides the recommendations for all beta blockers, consider the following.
● Don't discontinue drug abruptly.
● Drug may cause positive antinuclear antibody titers.
● Symptoms of overdose include severe hypotension, bradycardia, heart failure, and bronchospasm. After acute ingestion, empty stomach by emesis or gastric lavage; follow with activated charcoal to reduce absorption. Provide symptomatic and supportive treatment.

Monitoring the patient
● Monitor blood glucose levels in diabetic patients.
● Monitor thyroid functions in patients with thyroid dysfunction.

Information for the patient
● Advise patient to report wheezing promptly.

Geriatric patients
● Older patients have about a twofold increase in bioavailability and may require lower maintenance doses.

Pediatric patients
● Safety and efficacy in pediatric patients haven't been established.

Breast-feeding patients
• Acebutolol and its metabolite, diacetolol, appear in breast milk. Women receiving drug shouldn't breast-feed.

acetaminophen
Acephen, Anacin-3, Bromo-Seltzer, Feverall, Panadol, Tempra, Tylenol

Pharmacologic classification: para-aminophenol derivative
Therapeutic classification: nonnarcotic analgesic, antipyretic
Pregnancy risk category B

How supplied
Available without a prescription
Tablets: 160 mg, 325 mg, 500 mg, 650 mg
Tablets (chewable): 80 mg, 120 mg, 160 mg
Capsules: 325 mg, 500 mg
Suppositories: 80 mg, 120 mg, 125 mg, 300 mg, 325 mg, 650 mg
Solution: 48 mg/ml, 80 mg/ml*, 100 mg/ml, 80 mg/5 ml, 120 mg/5 ml, 160 mg/5 ml, 167 mg/5 ml, 500 mg/15 ml
Suspension: 48 mg/ml, 80 mg/ml*, 100 mg/ml, 80 mg/5 ml*, 160 mg/5 ml
Caplets: 160 mg, 500 mg, 650 mg
Syrup: 16 mg/ml
Sprinkle capsules: 80 mg, 160 mg

Indications, route, and dosage
Mild pain, fever
Adults and children over age 12: 325 to 650 mg P.O. or P.R. q 4 to 6 hours, p.r.n. Maximum dose shouldn't exceed 4 g daily. Maximum for long-term therapy is 2.6 g daily.
Children ages 11 to 12: 480 mg/dose q 4 to 6 hours.
Children ages 9 to 10: 400 mg/dose q 4 to 6 hours.
Children ages 6 to 8: 320 mg/dose q 4 to 6 hours.
Children ages 4 to 5: 240 mg/dose q 4 to 6 hours.
Children ages 2 to 3: 160 mg/dose q 4 to 6 hours.
Children ages 12 to 23 months: 120 mg/dose q 4 to 6 hours.
Children ages 4 to 11 months: 80 mg/dose q 4 to 6 hours.
Children age 3 months or less: 40 mg/dose q 4 to 6 hours.

Pharmacodynamics
Mechanism and site of action may be related to inhibition of prostaglandin synthesis in the CNS.
Analgesic action: Possibly related to an elevation of the pain threshold.
Antipyretic action: Possibly due to direct action on the hypothalamic heat-regulating center to block the effects of endogenous pyrogen, resulting in increased heat dissipation through sweating and vasodilation.

Pharmacokinetics
• *Absorption:* Absorbed rapidly and completely via the GI tract. Plasma levels peak in ¼ to 2 hours, slightly faster for liquid preparations.
• *Distribution:* 25% protein-bound. Plasma levels don't correlate well with analgesic effect, but do correlate with toxicity.
• *Metabolism:* About 90% to 95% is metabolized in the liver.
• *Excretion:* Excreted in urine. Average elimination half-life is from 1 to 4 hours. In acute overdose, prolongation of elimination half-life correlates with toxic effects. Half-life over 4 hours is associated with hepatic necrosis; over 12 hours, with coma.

Contraindications and precautions
No known contraindications. Use cautiously in patients with history of chronic alcohol abuse because hepatotoxicity has occurred after therapeutic doses. Also use cautiously in patients with hepatic or CV disease, renal function impairment, or viral infection.

Interactions
Drug-drug. *Antacids:* Delayed and decreased absorption of acetaminophen. Monitor patient for drug effect.
Anticoagulants, thrombolytics: May potentiate effects of these drugs. Monitor patient and coagulation laboratory test results.
Anticonvulsants, isoniazid: May increase risk of hepatotoxicity. Avoid concomitant use.
Phenothiazines: May result in hypothermia. Monitor patient's temperature.
Drug-food. *Any food:* Delayed and decreased absorption of acetaminophen. Don't administer with food.
Caffeine: May enhance therapeutic effect of acetaminophen. This is an advantageous use.
Drug-herb. *Watercress:* May inhibit oxidative metabolism of acetaminophen. Avoid concomitant use.
Drug-lifestyle. *Alcohol:* Increased risk of liver toxicity. Don't use together.

Adverse reactions
Hematologic: hemolytic anemia, neutropenia, leukopenia, ***pancytopenia.***
Hepatic: jaundice, ***severe liver damage with toxic doses.***
Metabolic: hypoglycemia.
Skin: rash, urticaria.

☑ Special considerations
• Although acetaminophen has no significant anti-inflammatory effect, it has proved beneficial for patients with osteoarthritis of the knee.
• When calculating total daily dose, remember that many OTC products contain acetaminophen.
• Patients unable to tolerate aspirin may be able to tolerate acetaminophen.

Reactions may be *common*, uncommon, ***life-threatening***, or COMMON AND LIFE-THREATENING.

- Assess patient's level of pain and response before and after drug administration.
- Store rectal acetaminophen suppositories in refrigerator.
- In acute overdose, plasma levels of 300 mcg/ml 4 hours postinjection or 50 mcg/ml 12 hours postinjection are associated with hepatotoxicity. Signs of overdose include cyanosis, anemia, jaundice, skin eruptions, fever, emesis, CNS stimulation, delirium, methemoglobinemia progressing to depression, coma, vascular collapse, seizures, and death.
- Acetaminophen poisoning develops in stages: Stage 1 (12 to 24 hours after ingestion)—nausea, vomiting, diaphoresis, anorexia. Stage 2 (24 to 48 hours after ingestion)—clinical improvement but elevated liver function test results. Stage 3 (72 to 96 hours after ingestion)—peak hepatotoxicity. Stage 4 (7 to 8 days after ingestion)—recovery.
- To treat toxicity, empty stomach immediately by inducing emesis with ipecac syrup if patient is conscious or by gastric lavage. Administer activated charcoal via nasogastric tube. Oral acetylcysteine (Mucomyst) is a specific antidote for acetaminophen poisoning and is most effective if started within 10 to 12 hours after ingestion, but it can help if started within 24 hours after ingestion. Administer a Mucomyst loading dose of 140 mg/kg P.O., then maintenance doses of 70 mg/kg P.O. every 4 hours for an additional 17 doses. Doses vomited within 1 hour of administration must be repeated. Remove charcoal before giving acetylcysteine because it may interfere with absorption of this antidote.
- Acetylcysteine minimizes hepatic injury by supplying sulfydryl groups that bind with acetaminophen metabolites. Hemodialysis may be helpful to remove acetaminophen from the body. Monitor laboratory parameters and vital signs closely. Provide symptomatic and supportive measures (respiratory support, correction of fluid and electrolyte imbalances). Determine plasma acetaminophen levels at least 4 hours after overdose. If plasma acetaminophen levels indicate hepatotoxicity, perform liver function tests every 24 hours for at least 96 hours.

Monitoring the patient
- Monitor vital signs, especially temperature, to evaluate drug's effectiveness.
- Monitor CBC and liver function studies if indicated.

Information for the patient
- Instruct patient in proper administration of prescribed form of drug.
- Advise patient on long-term, high-dose drug therapy to arrange for monitoring of laboratory parameters, especially BUN, serum creatinine, liver function tests, and CBC.

- Warn patient with current or past rectal bleeding to avoid using rectal acetaminophen suppositories. If they are used, they must be retained in the rectum for at least 1 hour.
- Warn patient that high doses or unsupervised long-term use of acetaminophen can cause liver damage. Use of alcoholic beverages increases the risk of liver toxicity.
- Tell patient to avoid using drug for a temperature above 102° F (39° C), a fever persisting longer than 3 days, or a recurrent fever. Acetaminophen may cause a false-positive test result for urinary 5-hydroxyindoleacetic acid.
- When prescribing buffered acetaminophen effervescent granules, consider sodium content for sodium-restricted patients.
- Tell patient not to take NSAIDs with acetaminophen on a regular basis.
- Warn patient to avoid taking tetracycline antibiotics within 1 hour after taking buffered acetaminophen effervescent granules.
- Tell patient not to use drug for arthritic or rheumatic conditions without medical approval. Drug may relieve pain but not other symptoms.
- Tell patient not to take drug for more than 10 days without medical approval.
- Tell patient on high-dose or long-term therapy that regular follow-up visits are essential.

Geriatric patients
- Elderly patients are more sensitive to drug. Use with caution.

Pediatric patients
- Children shouldn't take more than 5 doses per day or take drug for over 5 days unless prescribed.

Breast-feeding patients
- Low levels of drug appear in breast milk. No adverse effects have been reported.

acetazolamide
acetazolamide sodium
Dazamide, Diamox, Diamox Sequels

Pharmacologic classification: carbonic anhydrase inhibitor
Therapeutic classification: antiglaucoma drug, anticonvulsant, diuretic, altitude sickness drug (prevention and treatment)
Pregnancy risk category C

How supplied
Available by prescription only
Tablets: 125 mg, 250 mg
Capsules (extended-release): 500 mg
Injection: 500 mg

Indications, route, and dosage

Preoperative management of acute angle-closure glaucoma
Adults: 250 mg P.O. q 4 hours; 250 mg P.O. b.i.d.; or, for short-term rapid-relief therapy, 500 mg I.V., which may be repeated in 2 to 4 hours, if necessary; then 125 to 250 mg P.O. q 4 hours.

Edema in heart failure
Adults: 250 to 375 mg P.O. daily in morning.
Children: 5 mg/kg P.O. or I.V. daily in morning.

Drug-induced edema
Adults: 250 to 375 mg P.O. as single daily dose for 1 to 2 days alternating with 1 drug-free day.

Open-angle glaucoma, secondary glaucoma
Adults: 250 mg to 1 g P.O. or I.V. daily, divided q.i.d.

Prevention or amelioration of acute mountain sickness
Adults: 500 to 1,000 mg P.O. in divided doses taken preferably 48 hours before ascent and continued for at least 48 hours after arrival at high altitude.

Myoclonic seizures, refractory generalized tonic-clonic or absence seizures, mixed seizures
Adults: 375 mg P.O. or I.V. daily up to 250 mg q.i.d. Initial dosage when used with other anticonvulsants usually is 250 mg daily.
Children: 8 to 30 mg/kg P.O. or I.V. daily, divided t.i.d. or q.i.d.

◊ *Diuresis and alkalization of urine in treatment of toxicity associated with weakly acidic drugs*
Adults: 5 mg/kg I.V., p.r.n.
Children: 5 mg/kg I.V. or 150 mg/m² I.V. once daily (in morning) for 1 to 2 days alternated with 1 drug-free day.

◊ *Prevention of cystine or uric acid nephrolithiasis*
Adults: 250 mg P.O. h.s.

◊ *Periodic paralysis*
Adults: 250 mg P.O. b.i.d. or t.i.d. Maximum dose, 1.5 g daily.

Pharmacodynamics

Antiglaucoma action: In open-angle glaucoma and perioperatively for acute angle-closure glaucoma, acetazolamide and acetazolamide sodium decrease the formation of aqueous humor, lowering intraocular pressure.

Anticonvulsant action: Inhibition of carbonic anhydrase in the CNS appears to slow abnormal paroxysmal discharge from the neurons.

Diuretic action: Acetazolamide and acetazolamide sodium act by noncompetitive reversible inhibition of the enzyme carbonic anhydrase, which is responsible for formation of hydrogen and bicarbonate ions from carbon dioxide and water. This inhibition results in decreased hydrogen concentration in the renal tubules, promoting excretion of bicarbonate, sodium, potassium, and water; because carbon dioxide isn't eliminated as rapidly, systemic acidosis may occur.

Altitude sickness action: Acetazolamide shortens the period of high-altitude acclimatization; by inhibiting conversion of carbon dioxide to bicarbonate, it may increase carbon dioxide tension in tissues and decrease it in the lungs. The resultant metabolic acidosis may also increase oxygenation during hypoxia.

Pharmacokinetics

- *Absorption:* Well absorbed from the GI tract after oral administration.
- *Distribution:* Distributed throughout body tissues.
- *Metabolism:* None.
- *Excretion:* Excreted primarily in urine via tubular secretion and passive reabsorption.

Contraindications and precautions

Contraindicated in patients with hypersensitivity to the drug and in those receiving long-term therapy for chronic noncongestive angle-closure glaucoma; also contraindicated in those with hyponatremia or hypokalemia, renal or hepatic disease or dysfunction, adrenal gland failure, and hyperchloremic acidosis.

Use cautiously in patients with respiratory acidosis, emphysema, diabetes, or COPD and in those receiving other diuretics.

Interactions

Drug-drug. *Amphetamines, flecainide, procainamide, quinidine:* Alkalinizes urine and thus may decrease excretion of these drugs. Monitor patient carefully.
Lithium, phenobarbital, salicylates: May increase excretion of these drugs, lowering plasma levels and possibly necessitating dosage adjustments. Monitor drug levels.

Adverse reactions

CNS: confusion, drowsiness, paresthesia.
EENT: hearing dysfunction, transient myopia, tinnitus.
GI: anorexia, altered taste, diarrhea, nausea, vomiting.
GU: hematuria, polyuria.
Hematologic: *aplastic anemia,* hemolytic anemia, leukopenia.
Metabolic: asymptomatic hyperuricemia, hyperchloremic acidosis, hypokalemia.
Skin: rash.

☑ Special considerations

- Suspensions containing 250 mg/5 ml of syrup are the most palatable and can be made by a pharmacist. These remain stable for about 1 week. Tablets won't dissolve in fruit juice.
- Reconstitute powder by adding at least 5 ml sterile water for injection.

Reactions may be *common*, uncommon, *life-threatening*, or COMMON AND LIFE-THREATENING.

• Direct I.V. administration is preferred if drug must be given parenterally.
• Because it alkalinizes urine, acetazolamide may cause false-positive proteinuria in Albustix or Albutest.
• Drug may also decrease thyroid iodine uptake.
• For toxicity, specific recommendations are unavailable.
• Treatment for toxicity is supportive and symptomatic. Acetazolamide increases bicarbonate excretion and may cause hypokalemia and hyperchloremic acidosis. Induce emesis or perform gastric lavage. Don't induce catharsis because this may exacerbate electrolyte disturbances. Monitor fluid and electrolyte levels.

Monitoring the patient
• Monitor patient for hematologic reactions common to all sulfonamides; a baseline CBC and platelet count is recommended before initiating therapy and at regular intervals during therapy.
• Periodic monitoring of serum electrolytes is recommended.

Information for the patient
• Warn patient to use caution while driving or performing tasks that require alertness, coordination, or physical dexterity because drug may cause drowsiness.

Geriatric patients
• Observe elderly and debilitated patients closely because they are more susceptible to drug-induced diuresis. Excessive diuresis promotes rapid dehydration, leading to hypovolemia, hypokalemia, and hyponatremia, and may cause circulatory collapse. Reduced dosages may be indicated in these patients.

Breast-feeding patients
• Safety of drug in breast-feeding women hasn't been established.

---

acetylcysteine
Mucomyst, Mucosil, Parvolex*

Pharmacologic classification: amino acid (L-cysteine) derivative
Therapeutic classification: mucolytic, antidote for acetaminophen overdose
Pregnancy risk category B

How supplied
Available by prescription only
Solution: 10%, 20%
Injection:* 200 mg/ml

Indications, route, and dosage
Acute and chronic bronchopulmonary disease, tracheostomy care, pulmonary complications of surgery, diagnostic bronchial studies
Administer by nebulization, direct application, or intratracheal instillation.
Adults and children: 1 to 2 ml of 10% or 20% solution by direct instillation into trachea as often as hourly; or 3 to 5 ml of 20% solution or 6 to 10 ml of 10% solution administered by nebulizer q 2 to 3 hours. For instillation via percutaneous intratracheal catheter, administer 1 to 2 ml of 20% solution or 2 to 4 ml of 10% solution q 1 to 4 hours; via tracheal catheter to treat a specific bronchopulmonary tree segment, administer 2 to 5 ml of 20% solution. For diagnostic bronchial studies (administered before procedure), administer 1 to 2 ml of 20% solution or 2 to 4 ml of 10% solution for 2 or 3 doses.
Acetaminophen toxicity
Adults and children: Initially, 140 mg/kg P.O.; then 70 mg/kg q 4 hours for 17 doses (a total of 1,330 mg/kg) or until acetaminophen assay reveals nontoxic level.
  Or I.V.: Loading dose 150 mg/kg I.V. in 200 ml D_5W over 15 minutes, then 50 mg/kg I.V. in 500 ml D_5W over 4 hours, then 100 mg/kg I.V. in 1,000 ml D_5W over 16 hours.

Pharmacodynamics
Mucolytic action: Produces its mucolytic effect by splitting the disulfide bonds of mucoprotein, the substance responsible for increased viscosity of mucus secretions in the lungs; thus, pulmonary secretions become less viscous and more liquid.
Acetaminophen antidote: Exact mechanism unknown. Thought that acetylcysteine restores hepatic stores of glutathione or inactivates the toxic metabolite of acetaminophen via a chemical interaction, thereby preventing hepatic damage.

Pharmacokinetics
• *Absorption:* Most inhaled acetylcysteine acts directly on the mucus in lungs; the remainder is absorbed by pulmonary epithelium. Action begins within 1 minute after inhalation and immediately upon direct intratracheal instillation; peak effect occurs in 5 to 10 minutes. After oral administration, drug is absorbed from the GI tract.
• *Distribution:* Unknown.
• *Metabolism:* Metabolized in the liver.
• *Excretion:* Unknown.

Contraindications and precautions
Contraindicated in patients with hypersensitivity to drug. Use cautiously in elderly or debilitated patients with severe respiratory insufficiency.

Interactions
Drug-drug. *Activated charcoal:* Adsorbs orally administered acetylcysteine. Use activated charcoal to prevent absorption of acetylcysteine.
Amphotericin B, ampicillin, chlortetracycline, chymotrypsin, erythromycin, hydrogen peroxide,

---

iodized oil, lactobionate, oxytetracycline, tetracycline, trypsin: Acetylcysteine is incompatible with these drugs. Drug should be administered separately.

Adverse reactions
CV: chest tightness, hypotension, hypertension, tachycardia.
EENT: *rhinorrhea.*
GI: *nausea, stomatitis, vomiting.*
Respiratory: *bronchospasm* (especially in asthmatic patients).
Other: clamminess, fever.

☑ Special considerations
• Acetylcysteine solutions release hydrogen sulfide and discolor on contact with rubber and some metals (especially iron, nickel, and copper); drug tarnishes silver (doesn't affect drug potency).
• Solution may turn light purple; this doesn't affect safety or efficacy. Use plastic, stainless steel, or other inert metal when administering drug by nebulization. Don't use hand-held bulb nebulizers; output is too small and particle size too large.
• After opening, store in refrigerator or use within 96 hours.
• When used orally for acetaminophen overdose, dilute with cola, fruit juice, or water to a 5% concentration and administer within 1 hour.
• Don't place directly in the chamber of a heated (hot pot) nebulizer.

Monitoring the patient
• Monitor cough type and frequency; for maximum effect, instruct patient to clear airway by coughing before aerosol administration. Many clinicians pretreat with bronchodilators before acetylcysteine administration. Keep suction equipment available; if patient has insufficient cough to clear increased secretions, suction will be needed to maintain open airway.

Information for the patient
• Warn patient of unpleasant odor (rotten egg odor of hydrogen sulfide), and explain that increased amounts of liquefied bronchial secretion plus unpleasant odor may cause nausea and vomiting. Have patient rinse mouth with water after nebulizer treatment.

Geriatric patients
• Elderly patients may have inadequate cough and be unable to clear airway completely of mucus. Keep suction equipment available and monitor patient closely.

Pediatric patients
• Drug may be given by tent or croupette. A sufficient volume (up to 300 ml) of a 10% or 20% solution should be used to maintain a heavy mist

in the tent for the time prescribed. Administration may be continuous or intermittent.

Breast-feeding patients
• It's unknown if drug appears in breast milk.

---

activated charcoal
Actidose-Aqua, CharcoAid,
CharcoCaps, Insta-Char Pediatric

Pharmacologic classification: adsorbent
Therapeutic classification: antidote, antidiarrheal, antiflatulent
Pregnancy risk category NR

How supplied
Available without a prescription
Tablets: 325 mg, 650 mg
Tablets with 40 mg simethicone: 200 mg
Tablets (delayed-release) with 80 mg simethicone: 250 mg
Capsules: 260 mg
Powder: 30 g, 50 g
Suspension: 0.625 g/5 ml, 0.7 g/5 ml (50 g), 1 g/5 ml, 1.25 g/5 ml

Indications, route, and dosage
Flatulence or dyspepsia
Adults: 600 mg to 5 g P.O. as a single dose, or 975 mg to 3.9 g t.i.d. after meals.
Poisoning
Adults and children: 5 to 10 times the estimated weight of drug or chemical ingested. Dose is 30 to 100 g in 250 ml water to make a slurry.
  Give orally, preferably within 30 minutes of ingestion. Larger doses are necessary if food is in stomach. Drug is used adjunctively in treating poisoning or overdose with acetaminophen, amphetamines, antimony, arsenic, aspirin, atropine, barbiturates, camphor, cardiac glycosides, cocaine, glutethimide, ipecac, malathion, morphine, opium, oxalic acid, parathion, phenol, phenothiazines, phenytoin, poisonous mushrooms, potassium permanganate, propoxyphene, quinine, strychnine, sulfonamides, or tricyclic antidepressants.
  Activated charcoal may be given 20 to 60 g q 4 to 12 hours (gastric dialysis) to enhance removal of some drugs from the bloodstream. Monitor serum drug level.
To relieve GI disturbances (halitosis, anorexia, nausea, vomiting) in uremic patients
Adults: 20 to 50 g daily.

Pharmacodynamics
Antidote action: Adsorbs ingested toxins, thereby inhibiting GI absorption.
Antidiarrheal action: Adsorbs toxic and nontoxic irritants that cause diarrhea or GI discomfort.
Antiflatulent action: Adsorbs intestinal gas to relieve discomfort.

Reactions may be *common*, uncommon, *life-threatening*, or COMMON AND LIFE-THREATENING.

Pharmacokinetics
- *Absorption:* Isn't absorbed from the GI tract.
- *Distribution:* None.
- *Metabolism:* None.
- *Excretion:* Excreted in feces.

Contraindications and precautions
None known.

Interactions
Drug-drug. *Acetylcysteine:* Inactivated by charcoal; remove charcoal by gastric lavage before administering acetylcysteine.
Syrup of ipecac, many oral drugs: Adsorbed and inactivated by activated charcoal when used together. May be used together for a therapeutic effect.
Drug-food. *Milk products:* Decreased effectiveness of activated charcoal. Don't use together.

Adverse reactions
GI: black stools, constipation, nausea.

☑ Special considerations
- Don't give activated charcoal by mouth to a semiconscious or unconscious patient; instead, administer the drug through a nasogastric tube.
- Because activated charcoal adsorbs and inactivates syrup of ipecac, give only after emesis is complete.
- Activated charcoal is most effective when used within 30 minutes of toxin ingestion; a cathartic is commonly administered with or after activated charcoal to speed removal of the toxin/charcoal complex.
- Powder form is most effective. Mix with tap water to form consistency of thick syrup. A small amount of fruit juice or flavoring may be added to make mixture more palatable.
- Dose may need to be repeated if patient vomits shortly after administration.
- Using drug for more than 72 hours may impair patient's nutritional status.
- If administering drug for indications other than poisoning, give other medications 1 hour before or 2 hours after activated charcoal.
- Activated charcoal may be used orally to decrease colostomy odor.

Monitoring the patient
- Monitor serum drug levels.
- If treatment is longer than 24 hours, monitor electrolytes.

Information for the patient
- Tell patient to call poison information center or hospital emergency department before taking activated charcoal as an antidote.
- If patient is using activated charcoal as an antidiarrheal or antiflatulent, instruct patient to take medications 1 hour before or 2 hours after acti-

vated charcoal. For antidiarrheal use, advise patient to report diarrhea that persists after 2 days of therapy, fever, or flatulence that persists after 7 days.
- Warn patient that activated charcoal turns stools black.
- Advise patient not to mix drug with milk products, which may lessen its effectiveness.

---

acyclovir (acycloguanosine)
acyclovir sodium
Zovirax

Pharmacologic classification: synthetic purine nucleoside
Therapeutic classification: antiviral
Pregnancy risk category B

How supplied
Available by prescription only
Tablets: 400 mg, 800 mg
Capsules: 200 mg
Oral suspension: 200 mg/5 ml
Injection: 500 mg/vial, 1 g/vial
Ointment: 5%

Indications, route, and dosage
Initial and recurrent mucocutaneous herpes simplex virus (HSV types 1 and 2) or severe initial genital herpes or herpes simplex in immunocompromised patients
Adults and children over age 12: 5 mg/kg, given at a constant rate over 1 hour by I.V. infusion q 8 hours for 7 days (5 days for genital herpes).
Children under age 12: 250 mg/m^2 given at a constant rate over 1 hour by I.V. infusion q 8 hours for 7 days (5 days for genital herpes).
◇ ***Disseminated herpes zoster***
Adults: 5 to 10 mg/kg I.V. q 8 hours for 7 to 10 days. Infuse over at least 1 hour.
Initial genital herpes
Adults: 200 mg P.O. q 4 hours while awake (a total of 5 capsules daily). Treatment should continue for 10 days.
Acute herpes zoster infections
Adults: 800 mg P.O. 5 times daily for 7 to 10 days. Initiate therapy within 48 hours of rash onset.
Intermittent therapy for recurrent genital herpes
Adults: 200 mg P.O. q 4 hours while awake (a total of 5 capsules daily). Treatment should continue for 5 days. Initiate therapy at first sign of recurrence.
Long-term suppressive therapy for recurrent genital herpes
Adults: 400 mg P.O. b.i.d. for up to 1 year; then reevaluation.

Genital herpes, non-life-threatening herpes simplex infection in immunocompromised patients
Adults and children: Apply sufficient quantity of ointment to adequately cover all lesions q 3 hours, 6 times daily for 7 days.
Acute varicella (chickenpox) infections
Adults and children ages 2 and older weighing over 40 kg (88 lb): 800 mg P.O. q.i.d. for 5 days. *Children ages 2 and older weighing below 40 kg:* 20 mg/kg P.O. q.i.d. for 5 days.
Immunocompromised patients
Adults and children over age 12: 10 mg/kg I.V. over 1 hour q 8 hours for 7 days.
Children under age 12: 500 mg/m² I.V. over 1 hour q 8 hours for 7 days.
Herpes simplex encephalitis
Adults and children over age 12: 10 mg/kg I.V. over 1 hour q 8 hours for 10 days.
Children ages 6 months to 12 years: 500 mg/m² I.V. over at least 1 hour for 10 days.
✦ *Dosage adjustment.* For patients with renal failure, adjust normal P.O. dosage (200 to 400 mg) to 200 mg q 12 hours if creatinine clearance drops below 10 ml/minute/1.73 m². For normal dosages exceeding 400 mg, refer to package insert.

For patients with renal failure, give 100% of the I.V. dose q 8 hours if creatinine clearance exceeds 50 ml/minute/1.73 m²; 100% of the dose q 12 hours if it's between 25 and 50 ml/minute/1.73 m²; 100% of the dose q 24 hours if it's between 10 and 25 ml/minute/1.73 m²; and 50% of the dose q 24 hours if it falls below 10 ml/minute/1.73 m².

Pharmacodynamics
Antiviral action: Converted by the viral cell into its active form (triphosphate) and inhibits viral DNA polymerase.

In vitro, is active against HSV types 1 and 2, varicella-zoster virus, Epstein-Barr virus, and cytomegalovirus. In vivo, may reduce the duration of acute infection and speed lesion healing in initial genital herpes episodes. Patients with frequent herpes recurrences (more than 6 episodes a year) may receive oral acyclovir prophylactically to prevent recurrences or reduce their frequency.

Pharmacokinetics
● *Absorption:* With oral administration, drug is absorbed slowly and incompletely (15% to 30%). Levels peak in 1¼ to 2 hours. Absorption isn't affected by food. With topical administration, absorption is minimal.
● *Distribution:* Distributed widely to organ tissues and body fluids. CSF levels equal about 50% of serum levels. About 9% to 33% of dose binds to plasma proteins.

● *Metabolism:* Metabolized inside the viral cell to its active form. About 10% of dose is metabolized extracellularly.
● *Excretion:* Up to 92% of systemically absorbed drug is excreted as unchanged drug by the kidneys by glomerular filtration and tubular secretion. In patients with normal renal function, half-life is 2 to 3¼ hours. Renal failure may extend half-life to 19 hours.

Contraindications and precautions
Contraindicated in patients with hypersensitivity to drug. Use cautiously in patients with underlying neurologic problems, renal disease, or dehydration and in those receiving nephrotoxic drugs.

Interactions
Drug-drug. *Probenecid:* May result in reduced renal tubular secretion of acyclovir, leading to increased drug half-life, reduced elimination rate, decreased urine excretion, and more sustained serum drug levels. Monitor drug levels.
Zidovudine: May result in increased levels of acyclovir, causing toxicity. Use together with extreme caution.

Adverse reactions
CNS: *encephalopathic changes (lethargy, obtundation, tremor, confusion, hallucinations, agitation, **seizures, coma**),* headache, malaise.
GI: diarrhea, *nausea, vomiting.*
GU: hematuria, *transient elevations of serum creatinine and BUN levels.*
Hematologic: bone marrow hypoplasia, leukopenia, megaloblastic hematopoiesis, thrombocytosis, thrombocytopenia.
Skin: itching, rash, transient burning and stinging, pruritus, urticaria, vulvitis.
Other: *inflammation, phlebitis at injection site.*

☑ Special considerations
● Drug shouldn't be administered S.C., I.M., by I.V. bolus, or ophthalmically.
● I.V. dose should be infused over at least 1 hour to prevent renal tubular damage.
● Solubility of acyclovir in urine is low. Ensure that patient taking the systemic form of drug is well hydrated to prevent nephrotoxicity.
● Encephalopathic signs are more likely in patients who have experienced neurologic reactions to cytotoxic drugs.
● Overdose has followed I.V. bolus administration in patients with unmonitored fluid status or in patients receiving inappropriately high parenteral dosages.
● Acute toxicity hasn't been reported after high oral dosage. Hemodialysis results in 60% decrease in plasma level of the drug.
● Effects of overdose include signs of nephrotoxicity, including elevated serum creatinine and BUN levels, progressing to renal failure.

Monitoring the patient
• Monitor serum creatinine level. If level doesn't return to normal within a few days after therapy begins, increase hydration, adjust dose, or discontinue drug.
• Monitor CBC.

Information for the patient
• Warn patient that although drug helps manage the disease, it doesn't cure it or prevent its spread to others.
• For best results, tell patient to begin taking drug when early infection symptoms (such as tingling, itching, or pain) occur.
• Instruct patient who is taking ointment to use a finger cot or rubber glove and to apply about a ¼-inch ribbon of ointment for every 4 square inches of area to be covered. Ointment should thoroughly cover each lesion. Warn patient to avoid getting ointment in eye.
• Instruct patient to avoid sexual intercourse during active genital infection.

Geriatric patients
• Administer drug cautiously to elderly patients; they may suffer from renal dysfunction or dehydration.

Pediatric patients
• Safety and effectiveness of oral and topical acyclovir in children haven't been established. I.V. acyclovir has been used with only a few children. To reconstitute acyclovir for children, don't use bacteriostatic water for injection containing benzyl alcohol.

Breast-feeding patients
• Drug appears in breast milk. Give drug to breast-feeding women with caution and only when indicated.

---

adenosine
Adenocard

Pharmacologic classification: nucleoside
Therapeutic classification: antiarrhythmic
Pregnancy risk category C

How supplied
Available by prescription only
Injection: 3 mg/ml in 2-ml and 5-ml vials

Indications, route, and dosage
Conversion of paroxysmal supraventricular tachycardia (PSVT) to sinus rhythm
Adults: 6 mg I.V. by rapid bolus injection (over 1 to 2 seconds). If PSVT isn't eliminated in 1 to 2 minutes, give 12 mg by rapid I.V. push. Repeat 12-mg dose if necessary. Single doses over 12 mg aren't recommended.

Pharmacodynamics
Antiarrhythmic action: A naturally occurring nucleoside. In the heart, it acts on the AV node to slow conduction and inhibit reentry pathways. Also is useful for the treatment of PSVT associated with accessory bypass tracts (Wolff-Parkinson-White syndrome).

Pharmacokinetics
• *Absorption:* Administered by rapid I.V. injection.
• *Distribution:* Rapidly taken up by erythrocytes and vascular endothelial cells.
• *Metabolism:* Metabolized within tissues to inosine and adenosine monophosphate.
• *Excretion:* Unknown; circulating plasma half-life is less than 10 seconds.

Contraindications and precautions
Contraindicated in patients with hypersensitivity to drug and in those with second- or third-degree heart block or sick sinus syndrome, unless an artificial pacemaker is present. Don't use in atrial fibrillation or atrial flutter. Don't use in patients with preexcitation syndromes. Use cautiously in patients with asthma because bronchoconstriction may occur.

Interactions
Drug-drug. *Carbamazepine:* Higher degrees of heart block may occur with concurrent use. Use together cautiously.
Dipyridamole: May potentiate effects of drug; smaller doses may be needed.
Methylxanthines: Antagonize effects of adenosine. Patients receiving theophylline may need higher doses or may not respond to adenosine therapy.
Drug-food. *Caffeine:* May antagonize effects of adenosine. Patient may need higher doses or may not respond to adenosine therapy.
Drug-herb. *Guarana:* May decrease response of adenosine. Monitor patient closely.

Adverse reactions
CNS: apprehension, back pain, blurred vision, burning sensation, dizziness, heaviness in arms, light-headedness, neck pain, numbness, tingling in arms.
CV: chest pain, *facial flushing,* headache, hypotension, palpitations, diaphoresis.
GI: metallic taste, nausea.
Respiratory: *chest pressure, dyspnea, shortness of breath,* hyperventilation.
Other: *throat tightness, groin pressure.*

☑ Special considerations
• Don't use drug in patients with second- or third-degree heart block or sick sinus syndrome, unless an artificial pacemaker is present, because adenosine decreases conduction through the AV node and may produce first-, second-, or third-degree heart block. These effects are usu-

---

ally transient; however, patients in whom significant heart block develops after a dose of adenosine shouldn't receive additional doses.

● Rapid I.V. injection is needed for drug action. Administer directly into a vein if possible; if an I.V. line is used, use the most proximal port and follow with a rapid sodium chloride flush to ensure that drug reaches the systemic circulation rapidly.

● Check solution for crystals, which may occur if solution is cold. If crystals are visible, gently warm solution to room temperature. Don't use solutions that aren't clear.

● Discard unused drug because it contains no preservatives.

● Treat lingering adverse effects symptomatically.

● Because half-life of adenosine is less than 10 seconds, adverse effects of overdose usually dissipate rapidly and are self-limiting.

Monitoring the patient
● Monitor heart rhythm and vital signs.
● Monitor patient for adverse effects.

Information for the patient
● Warn patient that adverse reactions may occur.

albumin, human (normal serum albumin, human)
Albuminar-5, Albuminar-25, Albutein 5%, Albutein 25%, Buminate 5%, Buminate 25%, Plasbumin-5, Plasbumin-25

Pharmacologic classification: blood derivative
Therapeutic classification: plasma protein
Pregnancy risk category C

How supplied
Injection: 5% (50 mg/ml) in 50-ml, 250-ml, 500-ml, 1,000-ml vials; 25% (250 mg/ml) in 20-ml, 50-ml, 100-ml vials

Indications, route, and dosage
Shock
Adults: Initially, 500 ml (5% solution) by I.V. infusion; may repeat after 30 minutes. Dosage varies with patient's condition and response. Don't exceed 250 g/48 hours.
Children: 10 to 20 ml/kg (5% solution) by I.V. infusion, at a rate up to 5 to 10 ml/minute.
Hypoproteinemia
Adults: 1,000 to 1,500 ml 5% solution by I.V. infusion daily, maximum rate 5 to 10 ml/minute; or 200 to 300 ml of 25% solution by I.V. infusion daily, maximum rate 3 ml/minute. Dosage varies with patient's condition and response.

Burns
Adults and children: Dosage varies based on extent of burn and patient's condition. Usually maintain plasma albumin level at 2 to 3 g/dl.
Hyperbilirubinemia
Infants: 1 g/kg albumin (4 ml/kg of 25% solution) 1 to 2 hours before transfusion.
◊ *High-risk neonates with low serum protein level:* 1.4 to 1.8 ml/kg of 25% solution.

Pharmacodynamics
Plasma volume-expanding action: Albumin 5% supplies colloid to the blood and expands plasma volume. Albumin 25% provides intravascular oncotic pressure at 5:1, causing fluid to shift from interstitial space to the circulation and slightly increasing plasma protein level.

Pharmacokinetics
● *Absorption:* Isn't adequately absorbed from the GI tract.
● *Distribution:* Accounts for about 50% of plasma proteins; it's distributed into the intravascular space and extravascular sites, including skin, muscle, and lungs. In patients with reduced circulating blood volume, hemodilution secondary to albumin administration persists for many hours; in patients with normal blood volume, excess fluid and protein are lost.
● *Metabolism:* Although drug is synthesized in the liver, liver isn't involved in clearance of albumin from plasma in healthy individuals.
● *Excretion:* Little is known about excretion in healthy individuals. Administration of albumin decreases hepatic albumin synthesis and increases albumin clearance if plasma oncotic pressure is high. In certain pathologic states, the liver, kidneys, or intestines may provide elimination mechanisms for albumin.

Contraindications and precautions
Contraindicated in patients with hypersensitivity to drug. Use with extreme caution in patients with hypertension, cardiac disease, severe pulmonary infection, severe chronic anemia, or hypoalbuminemia with peripheral edema.

Interactions
None reported.

Adverse reactions
CNS: headache.
CV: hypotension, tachycardia, ***vascular overload after rapid infusion.***
GI: increased salivation, nausea, vomiting.
Respiratory: altered respiration, dyspnea, pulmonary edema.
Skin: urticaria, rash.
Other: chills, fever, back pain.

☑ Special considerations
- Solution should be a clear amber color; don't use if cloudy or contains sediment. Store at room temperature; freezing may break bottle.
- Use opened solution promptly, discarding unused portion after 4 hours; solution contains no preservatives and becomes unstable.
- One volume of 25% albumin produces the same hemodilution and relative anemia as 5 volumes of 5% albumin; reference to "1 unit" albumin usually indicates 50 ml of the 25% concentration, containing 12.5 g of albumin.
- Dilute if necessary with normal saline solution or 5% dextrose injection. Use 5-micron or larger filter; don't give through 0.22-micron I.V. filter.
- Make sure patient is properly hydrated before starting infusion; product may be administered without regard to blood typing and crossmatching.
- Avoid rapid I.V. infusion; rate is individualized based on patient's age, condition, and diagnosis. In patients with hypovolemic shock, infuse 5% solution at rate not exceeding 2 to 4 ml/minute, and 25% solution (diluted or undiluted) at rate not exceeding 1 ml/minute. In patients with normal blood volume, infuse 5% solution at rate not exceeding 5 to 10 ml/minute, and 25% solution (diluted or undiluted), at rate not exceeding 2 to 3 ml/minute. Don't give more than 250 g in 48 hours.
- Each liter contains 130 to 160 mEq of sodium before dilution with other additional I.V. fluids; a 50-ml bottle of solution contains 7 to 8 mEq sodium. This preparation was once known as "salt-poor albumin."
- Symptoms of overdose include signs of circulatory overload (such as increased venous pressure and distended neck veins, or pulmonary edema); slow flow to a keep-vein-open rate and re-evaluate therapy.
- Preparations of albumin derived from placental tissue may increase serum alkaline phosphatase level; all products may slightly increase plasma albumin level.

Monitoring the patient
- Monitor vital signs carefully; observe patient for adverse reactions.
- Monitor intake and output, hematocrit, serum protein, hemoglobin, and electrolyte levels to help determine continuing dosage.

Information for the patient
- Tell patient to report adverse reactions promptly.

Pediatric patients
- Premature infants with low serum protein levels may receive 1.4 to 1.8 ml/kg of a 25% albumin solution/kg (350 to 450 mg albumin).

albuterol sulfate
Proventil, Proventil HFA, Proventil Repetabs, Proventil Syrup, Ventolin, Ventolin Syrup, Volmax

Pharmacologic classification: adrenergic
Therapeutic classification: bronchodilator
Pregnancy risk category C

How supplied
Available by prescription only
Tablets: 2 mg, 4 mg
Tablets (sustained-release): 4 mg, 8 mg
Syrup: 2 mg/5 ml
Aerosol inhaler: 90 mcg/metered spray
Solution for nebulization: 0.083%, 0.5%
Capsules for inhalation: 200 mcg microfine

Indications, route, and dosage
To prevent and treat bronchospasm in patients with reversible obstructive airway disease
Adults and children ages 12 and older: Tablets: 2 to 4 mg (immediate-release) P.O. t.i.d. or q.i.d.; maximum dose, 8 mg q.i.d. Sustained-release tablets: Usual starting dose is 4 mg q 12 hours. Increase to 8 mg q 12 hours if patient fails to respond. Cautiously increase stepwise as needed and tolerated to 16 mg q 12 hours.

Aerosol inhalation: 1 to 2 inhalations q 4 to 6 hours. More frequent administration or a greater number of inhalations isn't usually recommended. However, because deposition of inhaled medications is variable, higher doses are occasionally used, especially in patients with acute bronchospasm.

Solution for inhalation: 2.5 mg t.i.d. or q.i.d. by nebulizer.

Capsules for inhalation: 200 mcg inhaled q 4 to 6 hours using a Rotahaler inhalation device.
Children ages 6 to 11: Administer 2 mg P.O. t.i.d. or q.i.d.
Children ages 2 to 5: Administer 0.1 mg/kg P.O. t.i.d., not to exceed 2 mg t.i.d.
✚ *Dosage adjustment.* In adults over age 65, give 2 mg P.O. t.i.d. or q.i.d.
To prevent exercise-induced bronchospasm
Adults and children ages 12 and older: 2 inhalations 15 minutes before exercise.

Pharmacodynamics
Bronchodilator action: Selectively stimulates beta-adrenergic receptors of the lungs, uterus, and vascular smooth muscle. Bronchodilation results from relaxation of bronchial smooth muscles, which relieves bronchospasm and reduces airway resistance.

Pharmacokinetics

- *Absorption:* After oral inhalation, drug appears to be absorbed gradually (over several hours) from the respiratory tract; however, dose is mostly swallowed and absorbed through the GI tract. Onset of action occurs within 5 to 15 minutes, peaks in ¼ to 2 hours, and lasts 3 to 6 hours. After oral administration, drug is well-absorbed through the GI tract. Onset of action occurs within 30 minutes and peaks in 2 to 3 hours. Drug effect lasts 4 to 6 hours with immediate-release tablets and 12 hours with extended-release tablets.
- *Distribution:* Doesn't cross the blood-brain barrier.
- *Metabolism:* Extensively metabolized in the liver to inactive compounds.
- *Excretion:* Rapidly excreted in urine and feces. After oral inhalation, 70% of dose is excreted in urine unchanged and as metabolites within 24 hours; 10% in feces. Elimination half-life is about 4 hours. After oral administration, 75% of dose is excreted in urine within 72 hours as metabolites; 4% in feces.

Contraindications and precautions

Contraindicated in patients with hypersensitivity to drug or its components. Use cautiously in patients who are unusually responsive to adrenergics and in those with CV disorders, including coronary insufficiency and hypertension, and hyperthyroidism or diabetes mellitus.

Interactions

Drug-drug. *Digoxin:* May cause a decrease in serum digoxin levels. Monitor digoxin levels.
Epinephrine, other orally inhaled sympathomimetic amines: Concomitant use may increase sympathomimetic effects and risk of toxicity. Monitor patient carefully.
MAO inhibitors, tricyclic antidepressants: Serious CV effects may follow concomitant use. Don't use together.
Propranolol, other beta blockers: May antagonize effects of albuterol. Use together cautiously.

Adverse reactions

CNS: *tremor, nervousness,* dizziness, insomnia, *headache, hyperactivity,* weakness, CNS stimulation, malaise.
CV: *tachycardia, palpitations,* hypertension.
EENT: dry and irritated nose and throat (with inhaled form), nasal congestion, epistaxis, hoarseness, taste perversion.
GI: heartburn, *nausea, vomiting,* anorexia.
Respiratory: *bronchospasm,* cough, wheezing, dyspnea, bronchitis, increased sputum.
Other: muscle cramps, hypokalemia with high doses, increased appetite, hypersensitivity reactions.

☑ Special considerations

Besides the recommendations for all adrenergics, consider the following.
- Small, transient increases in blood glucose levels may occur after oral inhalation.
- Serum potassium levels may decrease after I.V. and inhalation therapy administration, but potassium supplementation is usually unnecessary.
- Albuterol may decrease the sensitivity of spirometry used for the diagnosis of asthma.
- Signs and symptoms of overdose include exaggeration of common adverse reactions, particularly angina, hypertension, hypokalemia, and seizures.
- To treat toxicity, use selective beta blockers such as metoprolol with extreme caution; they may induce asthmatic attack. Dialysis isn't appropriate. Monitor vital signs and electrolyte levels closely.

Monitoring the patient

- Effectiveness of treatment is measured by periodic monitoring of patient's pulmonary function.
- Carefully evaluate serum digoxin levels in patients who are concurrently receiving digoxin and albuterol.

Information for the patient

- Instruct patient in proper use of inhaler. Tell patient to read directions before use, that dryness of mouth and throat may occur, and that rinsing with water after each dose may help.
Administration by metered-dose nebulizers: Shake canister thoroughly to activate; place mouthpiece well into mouth, aimed at back of throat. Close lips and teeth around mouthpiece. Exhale through nose as completely as possible; then inhale through mouth slowly and deeply while actuating the nebulizer to release dose. Hold breath 10 seconds (count "1-100, 2-100, 3-100," until "10-100" is reached); remove mouthpiece, and exhale slowly.
Administration by metered powder inhaler: Caution patient not to take forced deep breath, but to breathe with normal force and depth. Observe patient closely for exaggerated systemic drug action.
Administration by oxygen aerosolization: Administer over 15- to 20-minute period, with oxygen flow rate adjusted to 4 L/minute. Turn on oxygen supply before patient places nebulizer in mouth. Lips need not be closed tightly around nebulizer opening. Placement of Y tube in rubber tubing permits patient to control administration. Advise patient to rinse mouth immediately after inhalation therapy to help prevent dryness and throat irritation. Rinse mouthpiece thoroughly with warm running water at least once daily to prevent clogging. (It is not dishwasher-safe.) After cleaning, wait until mouthpiece is completely dry before storing. Don't place near artificial heat (dishwasher or oven). Replace reservoir bag every

2 to 3 weeks or as needed; replace mouthpiece every 6 to 9 months or as needed.

Note: Replacement of bags or mouthpieces may require a prescription.
• Tell patient that repeated use may result in paradoxical bronchospasm. Patient should discontinue drug and call immediately.
• Tell patient to call if troubled breathing persists 1 hour after using medication, if symptoms return within 4 hours, if condition worsens, or if new (refill) canister is needed within 2 weeks.
• Tell patient to wait 15 minutes after using inhaled albuterol before using adrenocorticoids (beclomethasone, dexamethasone, flunisolide, or triamcinolone).
• Warn patient to use only as directed, and not to use more than prescribed amount or more often than prescribed.

Geriatric patients
• Lower dose may be required because elderly patients are more sensitive to sympathomimetic amines.

Pediatric patients
• Safety and efficacy of extended-release tablets in children under age 12 or immediate-release tablets in children under age 6 haven't been established.

Breast-feeding patients
• It's unknown if albuterol appears in breast milk, alternative feeding methods are recommended.

aldesleukin
(interleukin-2, IL-2)
Proleukin

Pharmacologic classification: lymphokine
Therapeutic classification: immunoregulatory drug
Pregnancy risk category C

How supplied
Available by prescription only
Injection: 22 million IU/vial

Indications, route, and dosage
Metastatic renal cell carcinoma; ◊ metastatic melanoma
Adults: 600,000 IU/kg (0.037 mg/kg) I.V. q 8 hours for 5 days (a total of 14 doses). After a 9-day rest, repeat the sequence for another 14 doses. Repeat courses may be administered after a rest period of at least 7 weeks from hospital discharge.
◊ *Adults:* Continuous I.V. infusion of 18 million IU/m² for 2 5-day cycles with a 5- to 8-day rest between cycles.
◊ *Adults:* 18 million IU S.C. daily for 5 days, then a 2-day rest period.

Pharmacodynamics
Immunoregulatory action: Aldesleukin is a lymphokine, a highly purified immunoregulatory protein synthesized using genetically engineered *Escherichia coli.* The drug produced is similar to human IL-2: it enhances lymphocyte mitogenesis, stimulates long-term growth of IL-2-dependent cell lines, enhances lymphocyte cytotoxicity, induces both lymphokine-activated and natural killer cell activity, and induces the production of interferon gamma.

Pharmacokinetics
• *Absorption:* Onset is rapid after I.V. administration.
• *Distribution:* Peak serum levels are proportional to dose. About 30% of drug rapidly is distributed to plasma; the balance is rapidly distributed to the liver, kidneys, and lungs. Initial studies indicate that the distribution half-life is 13 minutes after a 5-minute I.V. infusion.
• *Metabolism:* Metabolized by the kidneys to amino acids within the cells lining the proximal convoluted tubules.
• *Excretion:* Excreted through the kidneys by peritubular extraction and glomerular filtration. Peritubular extraction ensures drug clearance as renal function diminishes and serum creatinine increases. Elimination half-life is 85 minutes.

Contraindications and precautions
Contraindicated in patients with hypersensitivity to drug or its components and in those with abnormal cardiac (thallium) stress test or pulmonary function test results or organ allografts. Retreatment is contraindicated in patients who experience the following adverse reactions: pericardial tamponade; disturbances in cardiac rhythm uncontrolled or unresponsive to intervention; sustained ventricular tachycardia (5 beats or more); chest pain with ECG changes, indicating MI or angina pectoris; renal dysfunction requiring dialysis for 72 hours or more; coma or toxic psychosis lasting 48 hours or more; seizures repetitive or difficult to control; ischemia or perforation of the bowel; GI bleeding requiring surgery.

Use with extreme caution in patients with cardiac or pulmonary disease or seizure disorders.

Interactions
Drug-drug. *Antihypertensives:* Increased risk for hypotension. Use together cautiously.
Cardiotoxic, hepatotoxic, myelotoxic, nephrotoxic drugs: Concurrent use may enhance toxicity of these drugs. Use together with extreme caution.
Corticosteroids: May decrease antitumor effectiveness of aldesleukin. Avoid using together when possible.
Psychotropic drugs: May alter CNS function. Use together cautiously.

Adverse reactions

CNS: *malaise, headache, mental status changes, dizziness, sensory dysfunction, special senses disorders, syncope, motor dysfunction,* **coma,** fatigue.
CV: *hypotension, sinus tachycardia, arrhythmias,* **bradycardia, PVCs,** *premature atrial contractions,* **MI, heart failure, cardiac arrest,** myocarditis, endocarditis, **CVA,** pericardial effusion, thrombosis, **capillary leak syndrome (CLS).**
EENT: conjunctivitis.
GI: *nausea, vomiting, diarrhea, stomatitis, anorexia, bleeding, dyspepsia, constipation.*
GU: *elevated BUN and serum creatinine levels, oliguria, anuria, proteinuria, hematuria, dysuria,* urine retention, urinary frequency.
Hematologic: *anemia,* THROMBOCYTOPENIA, LEUKOPENIA, *coagulation disorders,* leukocytosis, eosinophilia.
Hepatic: *jaundice, ascites, hepatomegaly, elevated bilirubin, serum transaminase, and alkaline phosphatase levels.*
Metabolic: *hypomagnesemia, acidosis, hypocalcemia, hypophosphatemia, hypokalemia, hyperuricemia, hypoalbuminemia, hypoproteinemia, hyponatremia, hyperkalemia.*
Musculoskeletal: arthralgia, myalgia.
Respiratory: pulmonary congestion, dyspnea, pulmonary edema, **respiratory failure, pleural effusion, apnea, pneumothorax,** tachypnea.
Skin: pruritus, erythema, rash, dryness, exfoliative dermatitis, purpura, alopecia, petechiae.
Other: fever; chills; weakness; edema; infections of catheter tip, urinary tract, or injection site; phlebitis; SEPSIS; weight gain or loss; abdominal, chest, or back pain.

☑ Special considerations

• Discontinue drug if moderate to severe lethargy or somnolence develops because continued use can result in coma.
• Patients should be neurologically stable with a negative computed tomography scan for CNS metastases. Drug may exacerbate symptoms in patients with unrecognized or undiagnosed CNS metastases.
• Renal and hepatic impairment occur during treatment. Avoid administering other hepatotoxic or nephrotoxic drugs because toxicity may be additive. Be prepared to adjust dosage of other drugs to compensate for this impairment. Modify dosage because of toxicity by holding a dose or interrupting therapy rather than by reducing the dose to be administered.
• Severe anemia or thrombocytopenia may occur. Packed RBCs or platelets may be necessary.
• Treat CLS with careful monitoring of fluid status, pulse, mental status, urine output, and organ perfusion. Central venous pressure monitoring is necessary.
• Because fluid management or administration of pressor drugs may be essential to treat CLS,

use cautiously in patients who require large volumes of fluid (such as those with hypercalcemia).
• To avoid altering the pharmacologic properties of drug, reconstitute and dilute carefully, and follow manufacturer's recommendations. Don't mix with other drugs.
• Reconstitute vial containing 22 million IU (1.3 mg) with 1.2 ml sterile water for injection. Don't use bacteriostatic water or normal saline injection because these diluents cause increased aggregation of drug. Direct the stream at sides of vial and gently swirl to reconstitute; don't shake.
• Reconstituted solution will have a concentration of 18 million IU (1.1 mg)/ml. Reconstituted drug should be particle-free and colorless to slightly yellow.
• Add the correct dose of reconstituted drug to 50 ml D_5W and infuse over 15 minutes. Don't use an in-line filter. Plastic infusion bags are preferred; they provided consistent drug delivery in early clinical trials.
• Vials are for single use only and contain no preservatives. Discard unused drug.
• Powder for injection or reconstituted solutions must be stored in refrigerator. After reconstitution and dilution, drug must be administered within 48 hours. Be sure that solutions are returned to room temperature before administering drug to patient.
• Preliminary studies indicate that over 75% of patients develop nonneutralizing antibodies to aldesleukin when treated with the every-8-hour dosing regimen. Less than 1% develop neutralizing antibodies. Clinical significance of this finding is unknown.
• Aldesleukin has been investigated for various cancers, including Kaposi's sarcoma, metastatic melanoma, colorectal cancer, and malignant lymphoma.
• High doses produce rapid onset of expected adverse reactions, including cardiac, renal, and hepatic toxicity.
• Drug toxicity is dose-related. Treatment is supportive. Because of short serum half-life of drug, discontinuation may ameliorate many adverse effects. Dexamethasone may decrease toxicity but may also impair effectiveness.

Monitoring the patient

• Perform standard hematologic tests, including CBC, differential, and platelet counts; serum electrolytes; and renal and hepatic function tests before therapy. Also obtain chest X-ray. Repeat daily during drug administration.
• All patients should have baseline pulmonary function tests and arterial blood gases.
• All patients should be screened with a stress thallium study. Normal ejection fraction and unimpaired wall motion should be documented. If a thallium stress test suggests minor wall motion abnormalities, further testing is suggested to exclude significant coronary artery disease.

Reactions may be *common,* uncommon, **life-threatening,** or COMMON AND LIFE-THREATENING.

- Daily monitoring should include vital signs, weight, intake, and output.
- Monitor pulmonary function regularly during treatment by clinical examination, assessment of vital signs, and pulse oximetry.

Information for the patient
- Make sure patient understands the serious toxicity associated with drug. Adverse reactions are expected with normal doses, and serious toxicity may occur despite close clinical monitoring.

Pediatric patients
- Safety and effectiveness haven't been established in children under age 18.

Breast-feeding patients
- It's unknown if drug appears in breast milk; consider risk-benefit and decide whether to discontinue drug or breast-feeding because of risk of serious adverse effects to infant.

alendronate sodium
Fosamax

Pharmacologic classification: osteoclast-mediated bone resorption inhibitor
Therapeutic classification: anti-osteoporotic
Pregnancy risk category C

How supplied
Available by prescription only
Tablets: 5 mg, 10 mg, 40 mg

Indications, route, and dosage
Osteoporosis in postmenopausal women
Adults: 10 mg P.O. daily taken with water at least 30 minutes before first food, beverage, or medication of the day.
Prevention of osteoporosis in postmenopausal women
Adults: 5 mg P.O. daily taken with water at least 30 minutes before first food, beverage, or medication of the day.
Paget's disease of bone
Adults: 40 mg P.O. daily for 6 months taken with water at least 30 minutes before first food, beverage, or medication of the day.

Pharmacodynamics
Antiosteoporotic action: At the cellular level, suppresses osteoclast activity on newly formed resorption surfaces, which reduces bone turnover. Bone formation exceeds bone resorption at bone remodeling sites and thus leads to progressive gains in bone mass.

Pharmacokinetics
- *Absorption:* Absorbed from the GI tract. Food or beverages can decrease bioavailability significantly.
- *Distribution:* Distributed to soft tissues but is then rapidly redistributed to bone or excreted in urine. Protein-binding is about 78%.
- *Metabolism:* Doesn't appear to be metabolized.
- *Excretion:* Excreted in the urine.

Contraindications and precautions
Contraindicated in patients with hypersensitivity to drug or its components and in those with hypocalcemia or severe renal insufficiency (creatinine clearance below 35 ml/minute).

Use cautiously in patients with active upper GI problems, such as dysphagia, symptomatic esophageal diseases, gastritis, duodenitis, or ulcers, and in patients with mild to moderate renal insufficiency (creatinine clearance between 35 and 60 ml/minute).

Interactions
Drug-drug. *Antacids, calcium supplements:* Interfere with absorption of alendronate. Instruct patient to wait at least 30 minutes after taking alendronate before taking other drugs.
Aspirin, NSAIDs: Increased risk of upper GI adverse reactions with alendronate doses above 10 mg daily. Monitor patient closely.
Hormone replacement therapy: Effectiveness with alendronate when used in treatment of osteoporosis is unknown; concurrent use isn't recommended.

Adverse reactions
CNS: headache.
EENT: taste perversion.
GI: abdominal pain, nausea, dyspepsia, constipation, diarrhea, flatulence, acid regurgitation, esophageal ulcer, vomiting, dysphagia, abdominal distention, gastritis.
Musculoskeletal: musculoskeletal pain.

☑ Special considerations
- Hypocalcemia must be corrected before drug therapy begins. Other disturbances of mineral metabolism (such as vitamin D deficiency) should also be corrected before initiating therapy.
- When drug is used to treat osteoporosis in postmenopausal women, disease is confirmed by low bone mass findings on diagnostic studies or history of an osteoporotic fracture.
- Drug is indicated for patients with Paget's disease who have alkaline phosphatase levels at least twice the upper limit of normal, in those who are symptomatic, and in those at risk for future complications from the disease.
- Hypocalcemia, hypophosphatemia, and upper GI adverse reactions (upset stomach, heartburn, esophagitis, gastritis, or ulcer) may result from oral overdose.

- Although specific information is lacking regarding treatment of overdose, milk or antacids (to bind alendronate) should be considered; dialysis isn't beneficial.

Monitoring the patient
- Monitor patient's serum calcium and phosphate levels throughout therapy.
- Monitor patient for adverse GI reactions.

Information for the patient
- Stress importance of taking each tablet with glass of plain water (not mineral water or other beverage) first thing in the morning at least 30 minutes before food, beverages, or other medications. Tell patient that waiting longer than 30 minutes improves absorption of drug.
- Warn patient not to lie down for at least 30 minutes after taking drug to facilitate delivery to stomach and to reduce potential for esophageal irritation.
- Tell patient to take supplemental calcium and vitamin D if daily dietary intake is inadequate.
- Inform patient about the benefit of weight-bearing exercises in increasing bone mass and the importance of modifying excessive cigarette smoking and alcohol consumption, if applicable.

Geriatric patients
- Although there are no overall differences in efficacy or safety between elderly and younger patients, greater sensitivity of some older patients can't be ruled out. Use cautiously in this age group.

Pediatric patients
- Safety and effectiveness in children haven't been established.

Breast-feeding patients
- Because drug may appear in breast milk, don't give to breast-feeding women.

---

alitretinoin
Panretin

Pharmacologic classification: retinoid
Therapeutic classification: anti–Kaposi's sarcoma drug
Pregnancy risk category D

How supplied
Available by prescription only
Gel: 0.1%

Indications, route, and dosage
Topical treatment of cutaneous lesions in patients with Kaposi's sarcoma related to AIDS
Adults: Initially, apply generous coating of gel b.i.d. to lesions only. Frequency may be increased to t.i.d. or q.i.d. based on tolerance. If site toxici-

ty occurs, may need to reduce frequency. If severe irritation occurs, drug may be discontinued for a few days until symptoms subside.

Pharmacodynamics
Binds to and activates all known intracellular retinoid receptor subtypes. Once activated, these receptors function as transcription factors that regulate the expression of genes controlling cellular differentiation and proliferation in both normal and neoplastic cells. Inhibits growth of Kaposi's sarcoma cells in vitro.

Pharmacokinetics
No information available.

Contraindications and precautions
Contraindicated in patients with hypersensitivity to drug, its components, or retinoids and in women of childbearing potential.

Gel shouldn't be used on patients requiring systemic anti–Kaposi's sarcoma therapy, such as those with more than 10 new Kaposi's sarcoma lesions in the prior month, symptomatic lymphedema, symptomatic pulmonary Kaposi's sarcoma, or symptomatic visceral involvement.

Interactions
Drug-lifestyle. *DEET (N,N-diethyl-m-toluamide):* Concurrent use increases DEET toxicity; don't use insect repellent products containing DEET while applying this gel.
Sun exposure: Photosensitivity may result; minimize exposure of treated areas to sunlight and sunlamps.

Adverse reactions
CNS: paresthesia.
Skin: rash, burning pain at application site, pruritus, exfoliative dermatitis, skin disorder (excoriation, drainage, fissures, cracking, scabbing, crusting, oozing), edema.

☑ **Special considerations**
- If application site toxicity occurs, reduce frequency.
- Should severe irritation occur, discontinue drug for a few days until symptoms subside.
- Although effects of drug may be evident after 2 weeks, most patients require longer application time.
- Don't apply an occlusive dressing to site.
- There has been no experience with acute overdose of alitretinoin gel.
- Systemic toxicity following acute overdose with topical application of alitretinoin is unlikely because of limited systemic plasma levels observed with normal therapeutic doses.
- There is no specific antidote for overdose.

Monitoring the patient
• Observe patient for signs of skin changes and dermatitis.
• Monitor patient for edema.

Information for the patient
• Inform patient that response may be seen as soon as 2 weeks after starting treatment but most patients need longer application. Some patients have needed over 14 weeks to respond.
• Tell patient that drug should be continued as long as benefit is derived.
• Tell patient to use caution when exposed to sunlight and sunlamps because of photosensitivity reaction.
• Tell patient to allow gel to dry for 3 to 5 minutes before covering with clothing. Because unaffected skin may become irritated, avoid application of gel to normal skin surrounding lesions. Don't apply gel on or near mucosal surfaces of the body.

Geriatric patients
• Safety and effectiveness in patients ages 65 and older haven't been established.

Pediatric patients
• Safety and effectiveness in pediatric patients haven't been established.

Breast-feeding patients
• It's unknown if drug or its metabolites appear in breast milk. Because many drugs appear in breast milk and because of the potential for adverse reactions in breast-feeding infants, mothers should discontinue breast-feeding before taking drug.

allopurinol
Purinol*, Zyloprim

allopurinol sodium
Aloprim

Pharmacologic classification: xanthine oxidase inhibitor
Therapeutic classification: antigout drug
Pregnancy risk category C

How supplied
Available by prescription only
Tablets (scored): 100 mg, 200 mg*, 300 mg
Injection: 500 mg/30 ml

Indications, route, and dosage
Gout, primary or secondary hyperuricemia
Gout may be secondary to such diseases as acute or chronic leukemia, polycythemia vera, multiple myeloma, or psoriasis or may occur after administration of chemotherapeutic drugs. Dosage varies with severity of disease; can be

given as single dose or divided, but doses larger than 300 mg should be divided.
Adults: Mild gout, 200 to 300 mg P.O. daily; severe gout with large tophi, 400 to 600 mg P.O. daily. Same dose for maintenance in secondary hyperuricemia.
Hyperuricemia secondary to malignancies
Children ages 6 to 10: 300 mg P.O. daily (100 mg t.i.d.).
Children under age 6: 150 mg P.O. daily (50 mg t.i.d.).
To prevent acute gouty attacks
Adults: 100 mg P.O. daily; increase at weekly intervals by 100 mg without exceeding maximum dose (800 mg), until serum uric acid level falls to 6 mg/100 ml or less.
To prevent uric acid nephropathy during cancer chemotherapy
Adults: 600 to 800 mg P.O. daily for 2 to 3 days, with high fluid intake.
◊ *Adults:* 350 to 700 mg/m² (allopurinol sodium) I.V. over 24 hours or divided into 4- to 6-hour doses.
Recurrent calcium oxalate calculi
Adults: 200 to 300 mg P.O. daily in single dose or divided doses.
✦ *Dosage adjustment.* In adults with creatinine clearance up to 9 ml/minute, give 100 mg q 3 days; 10 to 19 ml/minute, give 100 mg every other day; 20 to 39 ml/minute, 100 mg daily; 40 to 59 ml/minute, 150 mg daily; 60 to 79 ml/minute, 200 mg daily; 80 ml/minute, 250 mg daily.
◊ *Stomatitis from fluorouracil*
Adults: Allopurinol mouthwash, 600 mg/day.

Pharmacodynamics
Antigout action: Inhibits xanthine oxidase, the enzyme catalyzing the conversion of hypoxanthine to xanthine, and the conversion of xanthine to uric acid. By blocking this enzyme, allopurinol and its metabolite, oxypurinol, prevent the conversion of oxypurines (xanthine and hypoxanthine) to uric acid, thus decreasing serum and urine levels of uric acid. Drug has no analgesic, anti-inflammatory, or uricosuric action.

Pharmacokinetics
• *Absorption:* After oral administration, about 80% to 90% is absorbed. Levels peak 2 to 6 hours after usual dose.
• *Distribution:* Distributed widely throughout the body except in the brain, where drug levels are 50% of those found in the rest of body. Allopurinol and oxypurinol aren't bound to plasma proteins.
• *Metabolism:* Metabolized to oxypurinol by xanthine oxidase. Half-life of allopurinol is 1 to 2 hours; of oxypurinol, about 15 hours.
• *Excretion:* 5% to 7% is excreted in urine unchanged within 6 hours of ingestion. It is then excreted by the kidneys as oxypurinol, allopurinol, and oxypurinol ribonucleosides. About 70% of

administered daily dose is excreted in urine as oxypurinol and an additional 2% appears in feces as unchanged drug within 48 to 72 hours.

Contraindications and precautions

Contraindicated in patients with hypersensitivity to drug and in those with idiopathic hemochromatosis.

Interactions

Drug-drug. *Amoxicillin, ampicillin:* Concomitant use may cause rash. Monitor patient.

Azathioprine, mercaptopurine: May increase toxic effects of these drugs, particularly bone marrow depression. Combined use of these drugs requires reduction of initial doses of azathioprine or mercaptopurine to 25% to 33% of usual dose, with subsequent doses adjusted according to patient response and toxic effects.

Chlorpropamide: Allopurinol or its metabolites may compete for renal tubular secretion. Watch for signs of excessive hypoglycemia.

Co-trimoxazole: Concomitant use has been associated with thrombocytopenia. Monitor patient carefully.

Cyclophosphamide: May cause bone marrow depression. Use together cautiously.

Dicumarol: Concurrent use inhibits hepatic microsomal metabolism of dicumarol, thus increasing its half-life. Watch for increased anticoagulant effects.

Theophylline: May increase plasma theophylline levels. Monitor theophylline levels.

Thiazide diuretic: May increase risk of allopurinol-induced hypersensitivity reactions in patients with decreased renal function. Use with caution.

Adverse reactions

CNS: drowsiness, headache, paresthesia, peripheral neuropathy, neuritis.

CV: hypersensitivity vasculitis, necrotizing angiitis.

EENT: epistaxis.

GI: nausea, vomiting, diarrhea, abdominal pain, gastritis, dyspepsia.

GU: *renal failure,* uremia.

Hematologic: *agranulocytosis,* anemia, *aplastic anemia, thrombocytopenia,* leukopenia, leukocytosis, eosinophilia.

Hepatic: altered liver function studies, *hepatitis, hepatic necrosis,* hepatomegaly, cholestatic jaundice.

Musculoskeletal: arthralgia, myopathy.

Skin: alopecia, ecchymoses, *rash (usually maculopapular); exfoliative, urticarial, and purpuric lesions; Stevens-Johnson syndrome (erythema multiforme);* severe furunculosis of nose; ichthyosis, *toxic epidermal necrolysis.*

Other: fever, taste loss or perversion, chills.

☑ Special considerations

● Rash occurs mostly in patients taking diuretics and in those with renal disorders.

● If renal insufficiency occurs during treatment, reduce allopurinol dose.

● Acute gout attacks may occur in first 6 weeks of therapy; concurrent use of colchicine or another anti-inflammatory drug may be prescribed prophylactically.

● Minimize GI adverse reactions by administering drug with meals or immediately after. Tablets may be crushed and administered with fluid or food.

● Allopurinol may predispose patient to ampicillin-induced rash if taken concomitantly.

● Allopurinol-induced rash may occur weeks after discontinuation of drug.

Monitoring the patient

● Monitor patient's intake and output. Daily urine output of at least 2 L and maintenance of neutral or slightly alkaline urine is desirable.

● Monitor CBC, serum uric acid levels, and hepatic and renal function at start of therapy and then periodically.

Information for the patient

● Encourage patient to drink plenty of fluids (10 to 12 8-oz [240-ml] glasses daily) while taking drug unless otherwise contraindicated.

● When using drug to treat recurrent calcium oxalate stones, advise patient to reduce dietary intake of animal protein, sodium, refined sugars, vitamin C, oxalate-rich foods, and calcium.

● Advise patient to avoid hazardous activities requiring alertness until CNS response to drug is known; drowsiness may occur.

● Advise patient to avoid alcohol because it decreases drug's effectiveness.

● Tell patient to report all adverse reactions immediately.

● Advise patient to take a missed dose when remembered unless it's time for next scheduled dose; don't double the dose.

● Inform patient to discontinue drug and call immediately if rash or other signs that may indicate allergic reaction occur.

Geriatric patients

● Follow dosage recommendations for adults. Watch for renal disorders or impaired renal function and treat according to dosage recommendations for patients with impaired renal function.

Pediatric patients

● Don't use drug in children except to treat hyperuricemia secondary to malignancies.

Breast-feeding patients

● Because oxypurinol and allopurinol appear in breast milk, use drug with extreme caution in breast-feeding women.

Reactions may be *common*, uncommon, *life-threatening*, or COMMON AND LIFE-THREATENING.

alprazolam
Alprazolam Intensol, Apo-Alpraz*,
Novo-Alprazol*, Xanax

Pharmacologic classification: benzodi-
azepine
Therapeutic classification: anxiolytic
Controlled substance schedule IV
Pregnancy risk category D

How supplied
Available by prescription only
Tablets: 0.25 mg, 0.5 mg, 1 mg, 2 mg
Oral solution: 0.1 mg/1 ml, 1 mg/1 ml

Indications, route, and dosage
Anxiety
Adults: Usual starting dose is 0.25 to 0.5 mg P.O.
t.i.d. Increase dose, p.r.n., q 3 to 4 days. Maximum total daily dose, 4 mg in divided doses.
+ Dosage adjustment. In elderly or debilitated
patients or those with hepatic impairment, initial
dose is 0.25 mg P.O. b.i.d. or t.i.d.
Panic disorder
Adults: Initially, 0.5 mg P.O. t.i.d. Increase as needed and tolerated at intervals of 3 or 4 days in increments of 1 mg daily. Most patients require
more than 4 mg daily; however, dosages from 1
to 10 mg daily have been reported.
◊ *Agoraphobia with social phobia*
Adults: 2 to 8 mg/day P.O.
◊ *Depression, premenstrual syndrome*
Adults: 0.25 mg P.O. t.i.d.

Pharmacodynamics
Anxiolytic action: Depresses the CNS at the limbic and subcortical levels of the brain. Produces
an antianxiety effect by enhancing the effect of
the neurotransmitter gamma-aminobutyric acid
on its receptor in the ascending reticular activating system, which increases inhibition and blocks
both cortical and limbic arousal.

Pharmacokinetics
• *Absorption:* When administered orally, alprazolam is well absorbed. Onset of action occurs
within 15 to 30 minutes, with peak action in 1 to
2 hours.
• *Distribution:* Distributed widely throughout the
body. About 80% to 90% of an administered dose
is bound to plasma protein.
• *Metabolism:* Metabolized in the liver equally to
alpha-hydroxyalprazolam and inactive metabolites.
• *Excretion:* Alpha-hydroxyalprazolam and other metabolites are excreted in urine. Drug half-
life is 12 to 15 hours.

Contraindications and precautions
Contraindicated in patients with hypersensitivity
to drug or other benzodiazepines and in those
with acute angle-closure glaucoma. Use cautiously in patients with hepatic, renal, or pulmonary
disease.

Interactions
Drug-drug. *Antidepressants, antihistamines, barbiturates, general anesthetics, MAO inhibitors,
narcotics, phenothiazines:* Potentiates CNS de-
pressant effects of these drugs. Use together cau-
tiously.
Cimetidine, disulfiram: Concomitant use diminishes hepatic metabolism of alprazolam, increasing
its plasma level. Monitor levels carefully.
Digoxin: Possible increase in plasma digoxin levels if used concurrently. Use together cautiously.
Haloperidol: Possible increase in serum levels.
Use together cautiously.
Rifampin: Possible decrease in drug's effects.
Use together cautiously.
Theophylline: Possible increase in drug's sedative effects. Use with caution.
Drug-herb. *Kava:* May induce coma if taken with
alprazolam. Avoid use together.
Drug-lifestyle. *Alcohol:* Potentiates CNS de-
pressant effects of alcohol. Discourage use to-
gether.
Heavy smoking: Accelerates alprazolam metab-
olism, thus lowering effectiveness. Avoid smok-
ing.

Adverse reactions
CNS: *drowsiness, light-headedness,* headache,
confusion, tremor, dizziness, syncope, *depres-
sion,* insomnia, nervousness.
CV: hypotension, tachycardia.
EENT: blurred vision, nasal congestion.
GI: *dry mouth,* nausea, vomiting, *diarrhea, con-
stipation,* elevated liver function test results.
Skin: dermatitis.
Other: muscle rigidity, weight gain or loss.

☑ Special considerations
Besides the recommendations for all benzodiazepines, consider the following.
• Wean patient receiving prolonged therapy with
high doses from drug gradually to prevent withdrawal symptoms. A 2- to 3-month withdrawal
may be necessary.
• Lower doses are effective in elderly patients
and patients with renal or hepatic dysfunction.
• Anxiety associated with depression is also responsive to drug but may require more frequent
dosing.
• Store drug in a cool, dry place away from direct light.
• As needed, use I.V. fluids and vasopressors,
such as dopamine and phenylephrine, to treat
hypotension.
• Signs and symptoms of overdose include somnolence, confusion, coma, hypoactive reflexes,
dyspnea, labored breathing, hypotension, brady-

cardia, slurred speech, unsteady gait, and impaired coordination.
• In overdose, support blood pressure and respiration until drug effects subside; monitor vital signs. Flumazenil may be useful. Mechanical ventilatory assistance via endotracheal tube may be needed.
• If patient is conscious, induce emesis. Use gastric lavage if ingestion was recent, but only if an endotracheal tube is in place to prevent aspiration. After emesis or lavage, administer activated charcoal with a cathartic as a single dose. Dialysis is of limited value. Don't use barbiturates if excitation occurs because of possible exacerbation of excitation or CNS depression.

Monitoring the patient
• When treatment is protracted, periodic blood counts, urinalysis, and blood chemistry analyses are advisable.
• Minor changes in EEG patterns (usually low-voltage, fast activity) may occur during and after alprazolam therapy.

Information for the patient
• Be sure patient understands potential for physical and psychological dependence with long-term use of alprazolam.
• Instruct patient not to alter drug regimen.
• Warn patient that sudden changes in position can cause dizziness. Dangle legs for a few minutes before getting out of bed to prevent falls and injury.

Geriatric patients
• Lower doses are usually effective in elderly patients because of decreased elimination.
• During initiation of therapy or after an increase in dose, elderly patients require supervision with ambulation and daily living activities.

Pediatric patients
• Closely observe neonate for withdrawal symptoms if mother took alprazolam during pregnancy. Administering alprazolam during labor may cause neonatal flaccidity.
• Safety hasn't been established in children or adolescents under age 18.

Breast-feeding patients
• The breast-fed infant of a woman taking alprazolam may become sedated, have feeding difficulties, or lose weight. Avoid use in breast-feeding women.

alprostadil
Prostin VR Pediatric

Pharmacologic classification: prostaglandin
Therapeutic classification: prostaglandin derivative
Pregnancy risk category NR

How supplied
Available by prescription only
Injection: 500 mcg/ml

Indications, route, and dosage
Temporary maintenance of patency of ductus arteriosus until surgery can be performed
Infants: Initial I.V. infusion of 0.05 to 0.1 mcg/kg/minute via infusion pump. After satisfactory response is achieved, reduce infusion rate to the lowest dosage that will maintain response. Maintenance dosages vary. Infusion rate should be the lowest possible dose and is usually achieved by progressively halving the initial dose. Rates as low as 0.002 to 0.005 mcg/kg/minute have been effective.

Pharmacodynamics
Ductus arteriosus patency adjunct action: Alprostadil, also known as prostaglandin E_1 or PGE_1, is a prostaglandin that relaxes or dilates the rings of smooth muscle of the ductus arteriosus and maintains patency in neonates when infused before natural closure.

Pharmacokinetics
• *Absorption:* Administered I.V.
• *Distribution:* Distributed rapidly throughout the body.
• *Metabolism:* 68% metabolized in 1 pass through the lung, primarily by oxidation; 100% metabolized within 24 hours.
• *Excretion:* All metabolites are excreted in urine within 24 hours.

Contraindications and precautions
Contraindicated in neonates with respiratory distress syndrome. Use cautiously in neonates with bleeding disorders.

Interactions
None reported.

Adverse reactions
CNS: *seizures.*
CV: *bradycardia,* hypotension, tachycardia, *cardiac arrest,* edema.
GI: diarrhea.
Hematologic: *DIC.*
Respiratory: APNEA.
Other: *flushing, fever, sepsis, hypokalemia.*

☑ Special considerations
● Adding a 500-mcg solution to 50 ml of D₅W or normal saline solution provides a concentration of 10 mcg/ml. At this concentration, a 0.01 ml/kg/minute infusion rate will deliver 0.1 mcg of alprostadil/kg/minute.
● Drug must be diluted before administration. Discard prepared solution after 24 hours.
● In infants with restricted pulmonary blood flow, measure drug effectiveness by monitoring blood oxygenation. In infants with restricted systemic blood flow, measure drug effectiveness by monitoring systemic blood pressure and blood pH.
● Apnea and bradycardia may reflect drug overdose. Stop infusion immediately if they occur.
● Peripheral arterial vasodilation (flushing) may respond to repositioning of the catheter.
● Drug should be administered only by personnel trained in pediatric intensive care.
● Store ampules in refrigerator.
● Signs and symptoms of overdose are similar to the adverse reactions and include apnea, bradycardia, pyrexia, hypotension, and flushing.
● Apnea most commonly occurs in neonates weighing below 4.4 lb (2 kg) at birth and usually develops during the first hour of drug therapy.
● Treatment of apnea or bradycardia requires discontinuance of the infusion and appropriate supportive therapy, including mechanical ventilation as needed. Pyrexia or hypotension may be treated by reducing the infusion rate. Flushing may be corrected by repositioning the intra-arterial catheter.

Monitoring the patient
● Assess all vital functions closely and frequently to prevent adverse effects.
● Monitor arterial pressure by umbilical artery catheter, auscultation, or Doppler transducer. Slow rate of infusion if arterial pressure decreases significantly.
● Monitor respiratory status during treatment; have ventilatory assistance immediately available.

alprostadil
Caverject, Muse

Pharmacologic classification: prostaglandin
Therapeutic classification: corrective drug for impotence
Pregnancy risk category NR

How supplied
Available by prescription only
Sterile powder for injection: 6.15-mcg, 11.9-mcg, 23.2-mcg vials
Urethral suppository pellet: 125 mcg, 250 mcg, 500 mcg, 1,000 mcg

Indications, route, and dosage
Erectile dysfunction due to vasculogenic, psychogenic, or mixed etiology
Adults: Dosages are highly individualized. For injection: initial dose is 2.5 mcg intracavernously. If partial response occurs, increase second dose by 2.5 to 5 mcg, and then increase dosage further in increments of 5 to 10 mcg until patient achieves an erection (suitable for intercourse but not lasting over 1 hour). If initial dose isn't effective, increase second dose to 7.5 mcg within 1 hour; then increase dosage further in 5- to 10-mcg increments until patient achieves an erection. Patient must remain in physician's office until complete detumescence occurs. If patient responds, don't repeat procedure for 24 hours. For pellet: start initially with lower doses (125 or 250 mcg). Increases or decreases should be made on separate occasions in a stepwise manner until patient achieves an erection that is sufficient for sexual intercourse.
Erectile dysfunction of pure neurologic etiology (spinal cord injury)
Adults: Dosages are highly individualized. Initial dose is 1.25 mcg intracavernously. If partial response occurs, give second dose of 1.25 mcg and then a third dose of 2.5 mcg; increase dosage further in 5-mcg increments until patient achieves an erection (suitable for intercourse but not lasting over 1 hour). If initial dose isn't effective, increase second dose to 2.5 mcg within 1 hour; then increase further in 5-mcg increments until patient achieves an erection. Patient must remain in physician's office until complete detumescence occurs. If patient responds, don't repeat procedure for 24 hours.

Pharmacodynamics
Corrective action of impotence: A prostaglandin derivative that induces erection by relaxation of trabecular smooth muscle and by dilation of cavernosal arteries. This leads to expansion of lacunar spaces and entrapment of blood by compressing the venules against the tunica albuginea (a process called the corporal veno-occlusive mechanism).

Pharmacokinetics
● Absorption: Absolute bioavailability hasn't been determined.
● Distribution: Bound in plasma protein primarily to albumin (81%).
● Metabolism: Rapidly converted to compounds that are further metabolized before excretion.
● Excretion: Metabolites are excreted primarily in urine; rest are excreted in the feces.

Contraindications and precautions
Contraindicated in patients with hypersensitivity to drug and in those with conditions associated with disposition to priapism (sickle cell anemia or trait, multiple myeloma, or leukemia) or penile

deformation (angulation, cavernosal fibrosis, or Peyronie's disease). Don't give to men with penile implants or when sexual activity is contraindicated. Avoid use in women, children, and newborns. Muse shouldn't be used for sexual intercourse with a pregnant woman unless a condom is used.

Interactions
Drug-drug. *Anticoagulants:* Increase risk of bleeding from intracavernosal injection site. Monitor patient closely.
Cyclosporine: May decrease serum level of cyclosporine. Monitor levels.
Vasoactive drugs: Because safety and efficacy of use with these drugs haven't been studied, drug isn't recommended.

Adverse reactions
CNS: headache, dizziness, fainting.
CV: hypertension, hypotension, swelling of leg veins.
GU: *penile pain,* prolonged erection, penile fibrosis, penis disorder, penile rash, penile edema, prostatic disorder, testicular and perineal aching, burning of urethra, minor urethral burning.
Respiratory: upper respiratory infection, flu syndrome, sinusitis, nasal congestion, cough.
Other: injection site hematoma, injection site ecchymosis, back pain, localized trauma, localized pain.

☑ Special considerations
● Underlying, treatable medical causes of erectile dysfunction must be diagnosed and treated before initiation of therapy.
● Regular follow-up, with careful examination of the penis, is strongly recommended to detect signs of penile fibrosis. Discontinue drug if penile angulation, cavernosal fibrosis, or Peyronie's disease develops.
● Female partners of Muse users may experience vaginal itching and burning.
● If intracavernous overdose of drug occurs, patient should be under medical supervision until systemic effects have resolved or penile detumescence has occurred. Symptomatic treatment of systemic symptoms is appropriate.

Monitoring the patient
● Monitor Muse users for hypotension; titrate drug to lowest effective dose.
● Monitor coagulation studies closely in patients receiving Muse concurrently with anticoagulant therapy.

Information for the patient
● To ensure safe and effective use, thoroughly instruct patient how to prepare and administer alprostadil before beginning intracavernosal treat-ment at home. Stress importance for following instructions carefully.
● Tell patient to discard vials with precipitates or discoloration. Reconstituted vial is designed for 1 use only and should be discarded after withdrawal of proper volume of the solution.
● Instruct patient not to shake contents of reconstituted vial.
● Stress importance of not sharing drug and not reusing or sharing needles or syringes.
● Make sure patient has manufacturer's instructions for administration of drug at home.
● Desirable dose is established in physician's office. Tell patient not to change dose without medical approval.
● Inform patient that he can expect an erection to occur within 5 to 20 minutes after drug administration and that standard treatment goal is to produce an erection not lasting over 1 hour.
● Inform patient that an erection lasting over 6 hours has been known to occur after alprostadil injection. If this occurs, patient should seek medical attention immediately.
● Tell patient that drug shouldn't be used more than 3 times weekly, with at least 24 hours between each use. Maximum frequency for Muse is 2 administrations per 24-hour period.
● Review possible adverse reactions with patient. Besides priapism, instruct patient to immediately report penile pain not present before or that has increased in intensity and nodules or hard tissue in penis.
● Instruct patient to inspect penis daily for signs or symptoms of infection (redness, swelling, tenderness, or curvature of the erect penis), and to report them immediately.
● Remind patient that regular follow-up visits are needed to evaluate effectiveness and safety of therapy.
● Inform patient that drug doesn't offer protection from transmission of sexually transmitted diseases and that protective measures continue to be necessary.
● Warn patient that a small amount of bleeding can occur at injection site, which can increase risk of transmitting blood-borne diseases (if present) to sexual partner.
● Caution patient using Muse to use condom when having sexual intercourse with a pregnant partner, and to prevent potential vaginal burning and itching in female partner.

Pediatric patients
● Drug isn't indicated for use with newborns or children.

Breast-feeding patients
● Drug isn't indicated for use in women.

---

alteplase (recombinant alteplase, tissue plasminogen activator)
Activase

Pharmacologic classification: enzyme
Therapeutic classification: thrombolytic enzyme
Pregnancy risk category C

How supplied
Available by prescription only
Injection: 20-mg (11.6 million IU), 50-mg (29 million IU), 100-mg (58 million IU) vials

Indications, route, and dosage
Lysis of thrombi obstructing coronary arteries in management of acute MI
Three-hour infusion:
Adults weighing over 65 kg (143 lb): 60 mg in first hour, with 6 to 10 mg I.V. bolus over first 1 to 2 minutes; then 20 mg/hour for an additional 2 hours. Total dose, 100 mg.
Adults weighing 65 kg or less: 1.25 mg/kg given over 3 hours as described above.
Accelerated infusion:
Adults weighing over 67 kg (148 lb): 15 mg I.V. push, 50 mg over 30 minutes; then 35 mg over 60 minutes.
Adults weighing 67 kg or less: 15 mg I.V. push, 0.75 mg/kg over 30 minutes (not to exceed 50 mg); then 0.50 mg/kg over 60 minutes (not to exceed 35 mg).
Pulmonary embolism
Adults: 100 mg by I.V. infusion over 2 hours. Heparin therapy should be initiated at the end of the infusion.
Acute ischemic stroke
Adults: 0.9 mg/kg (maximum dose, 90 mg). Administer 10% of dose as an I.V. bolus over 1 minute; remaining 90% over 1 hour.

Pharmacodynamics
Thrombolytic action: An enzyme that catalyzes the conversion of tissue plasminogen to plasmin in the presence of fibrin. This fibrin specificity produces local fibrinolysis in the area of recent clot formation, with limited systemic proteolysis. In patients with acute MI, this allows for reperfusion of ischemic cardiac muscle and improved left ventricular function with a decreased risk of heart failure after MI.

Pharmacokinetics
• *Absorption:* Must be given I.V.
• *Distribution:* Rapidly cleared from the plasma by the liver; 80% of dose is cleared within 10 minutes after infusion is discontinued.
• *Metabolism:* Primarily hepatic.
• *Excretion:* Over 85% is excreted in urine; 5% in feces. Plasma half-life is less than 10 minutes.

Contraindications and precautions
Contraindicated in patients with history or evidence of intracranial hemorrhage, suspected subarachnoid hemorrhage, seizure at the onset of stroke, active internal bleeding, intracranial neoplasm, arteriovenous malformation, aneurysm, and severe uncontrolled hypertension (more than 185 mm Hg systolic or 110 mm Hg diastolic). Also contraindicated in patients with a history of CVA, intraspinal or intracranial trauma or surgery within last 2 months, or known bleeding diathesis.

Use cautiously in patients with major surgery within last 10 days; organ biopsy; trauma (including cardiopulmonary resuscitation); GI or GU bleeding; cerebrovascular disease; hypertension; likelihood of left-sided heart thrombus; hemostatic defects, including those secondary to severe hepatic or renal disease; hepatic dysfunction; occluded AV cannula; severe neurologic deficit (NIH Stroke Scale over 22); signs of major early infarct on a computed tomographic (CT) scan; mitral stenosis; atrial fibrillation; acute pericarditis or subacute bacterial endocarditis; septic thrombophlebitis; diabetic hemorrhagic retinopathy or other hemorrhagic ophthalmic conditions. Also use cautiously in those receiving anticoagulants, in patients ages 75 and older, and in pregnancy and first 10 days postpartum.

Interactions
Drug-drug. *Drugs that antagonize platelet function (abciximab, aspirin, dipyridamole):* May increase risk of bleeding if given before, during, or after alteplase therapy. Avoid using together.

Adverse reactions
CNS: *cerebral hemorrhage,* fever.
CV: hypotension, *arrhythmias,* edema.
GI: nausea, vomiting.
Hematologic: *severe, spontaneous bleeding (cerebral, retroperitoneal, GU, GI).*
Other: bleeding at puncture sites, hypersensitivity reactions *(anaphylaxis).*

☑ Special considerations
• Expect to begin alteplase infusions as soon as possible after onset of MI symptoms (angina pain or equivalent, greater than 30 minutes duration; angina that is unresponsive to nitroglycerin; or ECG evidence of MI).
• Administer within 3 hours after onset of stroke symptoms after exclusion of intracranial hemorrhage by CT scan or other diagnostic imaging methods able to detect the presence of hemorrhage. Treatment should be performed only in facilities that can provide appropriate evaluation and management of intracranial hemorrhage.
• Heparin is usually administered during or after alteplase as part of treatment regimen for acute MI or pulmonary embolism. Use of anticoagulant or antiplatelet therapy for 24 hours is contraindi-

cated when alteplase is used for acute ischemic stroke.
• Drug therapy for acute ischemic stroke should be discontinued in patients who haven't recently used oral anticoagulants or heparin if pretreatment PT exceeds 15 seconds or if an elevated activated partial prothrombin time is identified.
• Avoid I.M. injections, venipuncture, and arterial puncture during therapy. Use pressure dressings or ice packs on recent puncture sites to prevent bleeding. If arterial puncture is needed, select a site on the arm and apply pressure for 30 minutes afterward.
• Prepare solution using supplied sterile water for injection. Don't use bacteriostatic water for injection.
• Don't mix other drugs with alteplase. Use 18G needle for preparing solution—aim water stream at lyophilized cake. Expect a slight foaming to occur. Don't use if vacuum isn't present.
• Drug may be further diluted with normal saline solution injection or D_5W to yield a concentration of 0.5 mg/ml. Reconstituted or diluted solutions are stable for up to 8 hours at room temperature.
• Altered results may be expected in coagulation and fibrinolytic tests. The use of aprotinin (150 to 200 U/ml) in the blood sample may attenuate this interference.
• Excessive I.V. dosage can lead to bleeding problems. Doses of 150 mg have been associated with intracranial bleeding.
• Discontinue infusion immediately if signs or symptoms of bleeding occur.
• Use in pregnancy increases risk of adverse reactions.

Monitoring the patient
• Monitor ECG for transient arrhythmias (sinus bradycardia, ventricular tachycardia, accelerated idioventricular rhythm, ventricular premature depolarizations) associated with reperfusion after coronary thrombolysis. Have antiarrhythmics available.
• Monitor potential bleeding sites (such as catheter insertion sites, venous and arterial puncture sites, sites of recent surgical intervention).

Information for the patient
• Teach patient signs and symptoms of internal bleeding and tell patient to report these immediately.
• Advise patient about proper dental care to avoid excessive gum trauma.

Geriatric patients
• Use in patients over age 75 increases the risks of Activase therapy.

aluminum carbonate
Basaljel

Pharmacologic classification: inorganic aluminum salt
Therapeutic classification: antacid, hypophosphatemic
Pregnancy risk category NR

How supplied
Available without a prescription
Tablets or capsules: aluminum hydroxide equivalent 500 mg
Suspension: aluminum hydroxide equivalent 400 mg/5 ml

Indications, route, and dosage
Antacid
Adults: 10 ml suspension P.O. q 2 hours, p.r.n., or 1 to 2 tablets or capsules q 2 hours, p.r.n.
Treatment of hyperphosphatemia and prevention of urinary phosphate stones formation (with low-phosphate diet)
Adults: 1 g P.O. t.i.d. or q.i.d.; adjust to lowest possible dosage after therapy is initiated, monitoring diet and serum levels.

Pharmacodynamics
Antacid action: Exerts its antacid effect by neutralizing gastric acid; this increases pH, thereby decreasing pepsin activity.
Hypophosphatemic action: Reduces serum phosphate levels by complexing with phosphate in the gut. This results in formation of insoluble, nonabsorbable aluminum phosphate, which is then excreted in feces. Calcium absorption increases secondary to reduced phosphate absorption.

Pharmacokinetics
• *Absorption:* Largely unabsorbed; small amounts may be absorbed systemically.
• *Distribution:* None.
• *Metabolism:* None.
• *Excretion:* Excreted in feces; some may appear in breast milk.

Contraindications and precautions
No known contraindications. Use cautiously in patients with chronic renal disease.

Interactions
Drug-drug. *Antimuscarinics, chenodiol, chlordiazepoxide, coumarin anticoagulants, diazepam, digoxin, indomethacin, iron salts, isoniazid, phenothiazines (especially chlorpromazine), quinolones, sodium or potassium phosphate, tetracycline, vitamin A:* May decrease absorption of these drugs, lessening their effectiveness. Separate administration by at least 2 hours. Avoid concurrent use.

Reactions may be *common,* uncommon, *life-threatening,* or COMMON AND LIFE-THREATENING.

Enterically coated drugs: Concomitant use causes premature drug release of enteric-coated drug. Separate doses by 1 hour.

Adverse reactions
CNS: encephalopathy.
GI: *constipation,* intestinal obstruction, increased serum gastrin levels.
Other: hypophosphatemia, osteomalacia.

☑ Special considerations
• Patients with impaired renal function are at a higher risk for aluminum toxicity to brain, bone, and parathyroid glands.
• When administering suspension, shake well and give with small amounts of water or fruit juice.
• After administration through a nasogastric tube, flush tube with water to prevent obstruction.
• When administering drug as an antiurolithic, encourage increased fluid intake to enhance drug effectiveness.
• Manage constipation with stool softeners or bulk laxatives, or administer alternately with antacids containing magnesium (unless patient has renal disease).
• Long-term aluminum carbonate use can lead to calcium resorption and subsequent bone demineralization.

Monitoring the patient
• Monitor serum calcium and phosphate levels periodically; reduced serum phosphate levels may increase serum calcium levels.
• Monitor patient for adverse effects.

Information for the patient
• Advise patient to take drug only as directed and not to take more than 24 capsules or tablets or 120 ml (24 tsp) of regular suspension in 24-hour period. Instruct patient to shake suspension well.
• As needed, advise patient to restrict sodium intake, drink plenty of fluids, and follow a low-phosphate diet.
• Advise patient not to switch antacids without medical approval.
• Aluminum carbonate may interfere with imaging techniques using sodium pertechnetate Tc99m and thus impair evaluation of Meckel's diverticulum.
• Aluminum carbonate may interfere with reticuloendothelial imaging of liver, spleen, or bone marrow using technetium Tc99m sulfur colloid.
• Aluminum carbonate may antagonize effect of pentagastrin during gastric acid secretion tests.

Geriatric patients
• Because elderly patients commonly have decreased GI motility, they may become constipated from drug.

Pediatric patients
• Use cautiously in children under age 6.

aluminum hydroxide
Alterna-GEL, Alu-Cap, Alu-Tab, Amphojel, Dialume, Nephrox

Pharmacologic classification: aluminum salt
Therapeutic classification: antacid, hypophosphatemic
Pregnancy risk category C

How supplied
Available without a prescription
Tablets: 300 mg, 500 mg, 600 mg
Capsules: 475 mg, 500 mg
Liquid: 600 mg/5 ml
Suspension: 320 mg/5 ml, 450 mg/5 ml, 675 mg/5 ml

Indications, route, and dosage
Antacid, hyperphosphatemia
Adults: 500 to 1,500 mg P.O. (tablet or capsule) 1 hour after meals and h.s.; or 5 to 30 ml of suspension, p.r.n., 1 hour after meals and h.s.

Pharmacodynamics
Antacid action: Neutralizes gastric acid, reducing the direct acid irritant effect. This increases pH, thereby decreasing pepsin activity.
Hypophosphatemic action: Reduces serum phosphate levels by complexing with phosphate in the gut, resulting in insoluble, nonabsorbable aluminum phosphate, which is then excreted in feces. Calcium absorption increases secondary to decreased phosphate absorption.

Pharmacokinetics
• *Absorption:* Absorbed minimally; small amounts may be absorbed systemically.
• *Distribution:* None.
• *Metabolism:* None.
• *Excretion:* Excreted in feces; some may appear in breast milk.

Contraindications and precautions
No known contraindications. Use cautiously in patients with renal disease.

Interactions
Drug-drug. *Antimuscarinics, chenodiol, chlordiazepoxide, coumarin anticoagulants, diazepam, digoxin, iron salts, isoniazid, phenothiazines (especially chlorpromazine), quinolones, sodium or potassium phosphate, tetracycline, vitamin A:* May decrease absorption of these drugs, decreasing their effectiveness. Separate drugs by at least 2 hours.
Enterically coated drugs: Causes premature release of enteric-coated drugs. Separate doses by 1 hour.

Adverse reactions
CNS: encephalopathy.
GI: *constipation*, intestinal obstruction, elevated serum gastrin levels.
Other: hypophosphatemia, osteomalacia.

☑ Special considerations
- Shake suspension well (especially extra-strength suspension) and give with small amounts of water or fruit juice.
- After administration through nasogastric tube, flush tube with water to prevent obstruction.
- When administering drug as an antiurolithic, encourage increased fluid intake to enhance drug effectiveness.
- Manage constipation with stool softeners or bulk laxatives. Also, alternate aluminum hydroxide with antacids containing magnesium (unless patient has renal disease).
- Patients with impaired renal function are at higher risk for aluminum toxicity to brain, bone, and parathyroid glands.
- Drug therapy may interfere with imaging techniques using sodium pertechnetate Tc99m and thus impair evaluation of Meckel's diverticulum.
- Drug may also interfere with reticuloendothelial imaging of liver, spleen, and bone marrow using technetium Tc99m sulfur colloid.
- Drug may antagonize pentagastrin's effect during gastric acid secretion tests.

Monitoring the patient
- Periodically monitor serum calcium and phosphate levels; decreased serum phosphate levels may lead to increased serum calcium levels.
- Observe patient for hypophosphatemia signs and symptoms (anorexia, muscle weakness, and malaise).

Information for the patient
- Caution patient to take drug only as directed; to shake suspension well or chew tablets thoroughly; and to follow with sips of water or juice.
- As indicated, instruct patient to restrict sodium intake, drink plenty of fluids, and follow a low-phosphate diet.
- Advise patient not to switch to another antacid without medical approval.

Geriatric patients
- Because elderly patients commonly have decreased GI motility, they may become constipated from this drug.

Pediatric patients
- Use with caution in children under age 6.

Breast-feeding patients
- Although drug may appear in breast milk, no problems have been associated with its use in breast-feeding women.

amantadine hydrochloride
Symmetrel

Pharmacologic classification: synthetic cyclic primary amine
Therapeutic classification: antiviral, antiparkinsonian
Pregnancy risk category C

How supplied
Available by prescription only
Capsules: 100 mg
Syrup: 50 mg/5 ml
Tablets: 100 mg

Indications, route, and dosage
Prophylaxis or symptomatic treatment of influenza type A virus, respiratory tract illnesses in elderly or debilitated patients
Adults up to age 64 and children ages 10 and older: 200 mg P.O. daily in a single dose or divided b.i.d.
Children ages 1 to 9: 4.4 to 8.8 mg/kg P.O. daily, divided b.i.d. or t.i.d. Don't exceed 150 mg/day.
Adults over age 64: 100 mg P.O. once daily.
   Treatment should continue for 24 to 48 hours after symptoms disappear. Prophylaxis should start as soon as possible after initial exposure and continue for at least 10 days after exposure. Prophylactic treatment may be continued up to 90 days for repeated or suspected exposures if influenza virus vaccine is unavailable. If used with influenza virus vaccine, continue dose for 2 to 4 weeks until protection from vaccine develops.
Drug-induced extrapyramidal reactions
Adults: 100 to 300 mg/day P.O. in divided doses.
Idiopathic parkinsonism, parkinsonian syndrome
Adults: 100 mg P.O. b.i.d.; in patients who are seriously ill or receiving other antiparkinsonians, 100 mg/day for at least 1 week; then 100 mg b.i.d., p.r.n. Patient may benefit from as much as 400 mg/day, but doses over 200 mg must be closely supervised.
✦ *Dosage adjustment.* For patients with renal dysfunction, base maintenance dose on creatinine clearance value, as follows:
   For syrup, give 200 mg on the first day; for capsules, give 200 mg the first day, then 100 mg daily if creatinine clearance is between 30 and 50 ml/minute/1.73 m^2; 200 mg on the first day and 100 mg q alternating day if it ranges between 15 and 29 ml/minute/1.73 m^2; and 200 mg q 7 days if it falls below 15 ml/minute/1.73 m^2.
   Note: Patients on long-term hemodialysis should receive 200 mg q 7 days.

Pharmacodynamics
Antiviral action: Interferes with viral uncoating of the RNA in lysosomes. In vitro, is active only against influenza type A virus. (However, spon-

taneous resistance commonly occurs.) In vivo, may protect against influenza type A virus in 70% to 90% of patients; when administered within 24 to 48 hours of onset of illness, reduces duration of fever and other systemic symptoms.
Antiparkinsonian action: Thought to cause release of dopamine in substantia nigra.

Pharmacokinetics
• *Absorption:* With oral administration, drug is well absorbed from the GI tract. Serum levels peak in 1 to 8 hours; usual serum level is 0.2 to 0.9 mcg/ml. (Neurotoxicity may occur at levels exceeding 1.5 mcg/ml.)
• *Distribution:* Distributed widely throughout body and crosses blood-brain barrier.
• *Metabolism:* About 10% is metabolized.
• *Excretion:* About 90% is excreted unchanged in urine, primarily by tubular secretion. Portion may be excreted in breast milk. Excretion rate depends on urine pH (acidic pH enhances excretion). Elimination half-life in patients with normal renal function is about 24 hours; in those with renal dysfunction, it may be prolonged to 10 days.

Contraindications and precautions
Contraindicated in patients with hypersensitivity to drug. Use cautiously in patients with seizure disorders, heart failure, peripheral edema, hepatic disease, mental illness, eczematoid rash, renal impairment, orthostatic hypotension, and CV disease, and in elderly patients.

Interactions
Drug-drug. *Benztropine, trihexyphenidyl:* May potentiate anticholinergic adverse effects of these drugs (when these drugs are given in high doses), possibly causing confusion and hallucinations. Use together cautiously.
CNS stimulants: May cause additive stimulation. Use together cautiously.
Hydrochlorothiazide, triamterene: May decrease urinary amantadine excretion, resulting in increased serum amantadine levels and possible toxicity. Monitor amantadine levels.
Drug-herb. *Jimsonweed:* May adversely affect function of cardiovascular system. Avoid use together.
Drug-lifestyle. *Alcohol:* May result in confusion, light-headedness, fainting, and hypotension. Discourage use together.

Adverse reactions
CNS: depression, fatigue, confusion, *dizziness,* hallucinations, anxiety, *irritability,* ataxia, *insomnia,* headache, *light-headedness.*
CV: peripheral edema, orthostatic hypotension, *heart failure.*
GI: anorexia, *nausea,* constipation, vomiting, dry mouth.
Skin: *livedo reticularis* (with prolonged use).

☑ Special considerations
• To prevent orthostatic hypotension, instruct patient to move slowly when changing position (especially when standing up).
• If patient experiences insomnia, administer dose several hours before bedtime.
• Prophylactic drug use is recommended for selected high-risk patients who can't receive influenza virus vaccine. Manufacturer recommends prophylactic therapy lasting up to 90 days with possible repeated or unknown exposure.
• Clinical effects of overdose include nausea, vomiting, anorexia, hyperexcitability, tremors, slurred speech, blurred vision, lethargy, anticholinergic symptoms, seizures, and possible ventricular arrhythmias, including torsades de pointes and ventricular fibrillation. CNS effects result from increased levels of dopamine in the brain.
• Treatment for overdose includes immediate gastric lavage or emesis induction along with supportive measures, forced fluids and, if necessary, I.V. fluids administration. Urine acidification may be used to increase drug excretion.
• In overdose, physostigmine may be given (1 to 2 mg by slow I.V. infusion at 1- to 2-hour intervals) to counteract CNS toxicity. Seizures or arrhythmias may be treated with conventional therapy.
• In overdose, monitor patient closely.

Monitoring the patient
• Monitor patient for CNS drug effects.
• Periodically evaluate patient for weight gain and edema.

Information for the patient
• Warn patient that drug may impair mental alertness.
• Advise patient to take drug after meals to ensure best absorption.
• Caution patient to avoid abrupt position changes; these may cause light-headedness or dizziness.
• If drug is being taken to treat parkinsonism, warn patient not to discontinue abruptly because that might precipitate a parkinsonian crisis.
• Warn patient to avoid alcohol while taking drug.
• Instruct patient to report adverse effects promptly, especially dizziness, depression, anxiety, nausea, and urine retention.

Geriatric patients
• Elderly patients are more susceptible to adverse neurologic effects; dividing daily dosage into 2 doses may reduce risk.

Pediatric patients
• Safety and effectiveness of drug in children under age 1 haven't been established.

Breast-feeding patients
• Drug appears in breast milk. Advise mothers to avoid breast-feeding during therapy.

amifostine
Ethyol

Pharmacologic classification: organic thiophosphate
Therapeutic classification: cytoprotective drug
Pregnancy risk category C

How supplied
Available by prescription only
Injection: 500 mg anhydrous basis and 500 mg mannitol/10 ml vial

Indications, route, and dosage
Reduction of cumulative renal toxicity associated with repeated administration of cisplatin in patients with advanced ovarian cancer
Adults: 910 mg/m² daily as a 15-minute I.V. infusion, starting within 30 minutes before chemotherapy. If hypotension occurs and blood pressure doesn't return to normal within 5 minutes of treatment, subsequent cycles should use 740 mg/m².

Pharmacodynamics
Cytoprotective action: Dephosphorylated by alkaline phosphatase in tissues to a pharmacologically active free thiol metabolite. The higher level of free thiol in normal tissues is available to bind to, and thereby detoxify, reactive metabolites of cisplatin, which can reduce the toxic effects of cisplatin on renal tissue. Free thiol can also act as a scavenger of free radicals that may be generated in tissues exposed to cisplatin.

Pharmacokinetics
• *Absorption:* Administered I.V.
• *Distribution:* Rapidly cleared from plasma with a distribution half-life of less than 1 minute. Found in bone marrow cells 5 to 8 minutes after administration.
• *Metabolism:* Rapidly metabolized to an active free thiol metabolite. A disulfide metabolite is produced subsequently and is less active than the free thiol.
• *Excretion:* Drug and its 2 metabolites are minimally excreted in the urine.

Contraindications and precautions
Contraindicated in patients with hypersensitivity to aminothiol compounds or mannitol. Shouldn't be used in patients receiving chemotherapy for malignancies that are potentially curable (certain malignancies of germ-cell origin). Also contraindicated in hypotensive or dehydrated patients and in those receiving antihypertensives that can't be stopped for 24 hours before amifostine administration.

Use cautiously in elderly patients and in patients with ischemic heart disease, arrhythmias, heart failure, or history of stroke or transient ischemic attacks. Use cautiously in patients in whom the common adverse effects of nausea, vomiting, and hypotension are likely to have serious consequences.

Interactions
Drug-drug. *Antihypertensives, other drugs that could potentiate hypotension:* Enhanced hypotensive effects. Special consideration should be given regarding concomitant use.

Adverse reactions
CNS: loss of consciousness, dizziness, somnolence.
CV: *hypotension.*
GI: hiccups, *nausea, vomiting.*
Other: flushing or feeling warm, chills or feeling cold, sneezing, hypocalcemia, allergic reactions ranging from rash to rigors.

☑ Special considerations
• Reconstitute each single-dose vial with 9.5 ml of sterile normal saline. Use of other solutions to reconstitute drug isn't recommended. Reconstituted solution (500 mg amifostine/10 ml) is chemically stable for up to 5 hours at room temperature (about 77° F [25° C]) or up to 24 hours under refrigeration (35° to 46° F [2° to 8° C]).
• Drug can be prepared in polyvinyl chloride bags at concentrations of 5 to 40 mg/ml and has the same stability as when reconstituted in the single-use vial.
• Inspect vial for particulate matter and discoloration before administration whenever solution and container permit. Don't use if cloudiness or precipitate is seen.
• If possible, stop antihypertensive therapy 24 hours before amifostine administration. If antihypertensive therapy can't be stopped, don't use drug because of severe hypotension risk.
• Patients receiving amifostine should be adequately hydrated before drug administration and be kept in a supine position during the infusion.
• Don't infuse for more than 15 minutes; longer infusion time has been associated with adverse reactions.
• Administer antiemetics, including dexamethasone 20 mg I.V. and a serotonin 5HT receptor antagonist, before and with amifostine. Additional antiemetics may be required based on the chemotherapy drugs administered.
• The most likely symptom of overdose is hypotension, which should be managed by infusion of normal saline solution and other supportive measures, as indicated.

Monitoring the patient
• Monitor serum calcium level in patients at risk for hypocalcemia, such as those with nephrotic syndrome. If necessary, administer calcium supplements.
• Monitor blood pressure every 5 minutes during infusion. If hypotension occurs, requiring interruption of therapy, place patient in Trendelenburg's position and give an infusion of normal saline solution using a separate I.V. line. If blood pressure returns to normal within 5 minutes and patient is asymptomatic, infusion may be restarted so that full dose of drug can be given. If full dose of amifostine can't be administered, drug dose for later cycles should be 740 mg/ m².
• When amifostine is used with highly emetogenic chemotherapy, monitor fluid balance of patient.

Information for the patient
• Instruct patient to remain in a supine position during infusion.

Geriatric patients
• Use drug with caution in elderly patients; safety hasn't been established in this age-group.

Pediatric patients
• Safety and effectiveness in children haven't been established.

Breast-feeding patients
• It's unknown if drug or its metabolites appear in breast milk. Patient shouldn't breast-feed if taking drug.

amikacin sulfate
Amikin

Pharmacologic classification: aminoglycoside
Therapeutic classification: antibiotic
Pregnancy risk category D

How supplied
Available by prescription only
Injection: 50 mg/ml, 250 mg/ml

Indications, route, and dosage
Serious infections caused by susceptible organisms
Adults and children with normal renal function: 15 mg/kg/day divided q 8 to 12 hours I.M. or I.V. (in 100 to 200 ml D₅W or normal saline administered over 30 to 60 minutes). Don't exceed 1.5 g/day.
◊ *Adults:* 4 to 20 mg given intrathecally or intraventricularly as a single dose in conjunction with I.M. or I.V. administration.
Neonates with normal renal function: Initially, 10 mg/kg I.M. or I.V. (in D₅W or normal saline administered over 1 to 2 hours); then 7.5 mg/kg q 12 hours.

Uncomplicated urinary tract infections
Adults: 250 mg I.M. or I.V. b.i.d.
✦ **Dosage adjustment.** In renal failure, initially, 7.5 mg/kg. Subsequent doses and frequency determined by blood amikacin levels and renal function studies. One method is to administer additional 7.5 mg/kg doses and alter dosing interval based on steady-state serum creatinine:

$$\frac{\text{Creatinine}}{\text{(mg/dl)}} \times 9 = \frac{\text{dosing interval}}{\text{(hours)}}$$

Keep peak serum levels between 15 and 30 mcg/ml; trough serum levels shouldn't exceed 5 to 10 mcg/ml.

Pharmacodynamics
Antibiotic action: Bactericidal; it binds directly to the 30S ribosomal subunit, thus inhibiting bacterial protein synthesis. Spectrum of activity includes many aerobic gram-negative organisms (including most strains of *Pseudomonas aeruginosa*) and some aerobic gram-positive organisms. May act against some organisms resistant to other aminoglycosides, such as *Proteus, Pseudomonas,* and *Serratia;* some strains of these may be resistant to amikacin. Is ineffective against anaerobes.

Pharmacokinetics
• *Absorption:* Poorly absorbed after oral administration and is given parenterally; after I.M. administration, serum levels peak in 45 minutes to 2 hours.
• *Distribution:* Distributed widely after parenteral administration; intraocular penetration is poor. Factors that increase volume of distribution (burns, peritonitis) may increase dosage requirements. CSF penetration is low, even in patients with inflamed meninges. Intraventricular administration produces high levels throughout the CNS. Protein-binding is minimal. Drug crosses the placenta.
• *Metabolism:* Isn't metabolized.
• *Excretion:* Excreted primarily in urine by glomerular filtration; small amounts may be excreted in bile and breast milk. Elimination half-life in adults is 2 to 3 hours. In patients with severe renal damage, half-life may extend to 30 to 86 hours. Over time, drug accumulates in inner ear and kidneys; urine levels approach 800 mcg/ml 6 hours after a 500-mg I.M. dose.

Contraindications and precautions
Contraindicated in patients with hypersensitivity to drug or other aminoglycosides. Use cautiously in patients with impaired renal function or neuromuscular disorders, in neonates and infants, and in elderly patients.

Interactions

Drug-drug. *Amphotericin B, capreomycin, cephalosporins, cisplatin, loop diuretics, methoxyflurane, polymyxin B, vancomycin, other aminoglycosides:* Concomitant use may increase hazard of nephrotoxicity, ototoxicity, and neurotoxicity. Use with extreme caution.

Antivertigo drugs, dimenhydrinate, other antiemetics: May mask amikacin-induced ototoxicity. Monitor patient carefully.

Bumetanide, ethacrynic acid, furosemide, mannitol, urea: Increased ototoxicity. Use together cautiously.

General anesthetics, neuromuscular blocking drugs such as succinylcholine, tubocurarine: May potentiate neuromuscular blockade. Use with caution.

Penicillins: Concomitant use results in a synergistic bactericidal effect against *Pseudomonas aeruginosa, Escherichia coli, Klebsiella, Citrobacter, Enterobacter, Serratia,* and *Proteus mirabilis.* However, the drugs are physically and chemically incompatible and are inactivated when mixed or given together. May be used for synergistic effect; don't mix or give at the same time.

Adverse reactions

CNS: *neuromuscular blockade.*
EENT: *ototoxicity.*
GU: *nephrotoxicity, azotemia.*
Musculoskeletal: arthralgia, acute muscular paralysis.

☑ Special considerations

Besides the recommendations for all aminoglycosides, consider the following.

● Because drug is dialyzable, patients undergoing hemodialysis need dosage adjustments.
● Clinical signs of overdose include ototoxicity, nephrotoxicity, and neuromuscular toxicity.
● Drug can be removed by hemodialysis or peritoneal dialysis. Treatment with calcium salts or anticholinesterases reverses neuromuscular blockade.

Monitoring the patient

● Monitor baseline renal function; reassess periodically.
● Observe patient closely for CNS effects.

Pediatric patients

● Because potential for ototoxicity is unknown, drug should be used in infants only when other drugs are ineffective or contraindicated. Patient should be closely monitored during therapy.

amiloride hydrochloride
Midamor

Pharmacologic classification: potassium-sparing diuretic
Therapeutic classification: diuretic, antihypertensive
Pregnancy risk category B

How supplied

Available by prescription only
Tablets: 5 mg

Indications, route, and dosage

Hypertension; edema associated with heart failure, usually in patients who are also taking thiazide or other potassium-wasting diuretics
Adults: Usually 5 mg P.O. daily. Dosage may be increased to 10 mg daily, if needed. Don't exceed 20 mg daily.

◊ **Lithium-induced polyuria**
Adults: 5 to 10 mg b.i.d.

◊ **Cystic fibrosis**
Adults: Aerosolized amiloride dissolved in 0.3% saline solution.

Pharmacodynamics

Diuretic action: Acts directly on the distal renal tubule to inhibit sodium reabsorption and potassium excretion, thereby reducing potassium loss.

Antihypertensive action: Commonly used with more effective diuretics to manage edema associated with heart failure, hepatic cirrhosis, and hyperaldosteronism. Mechanism of drug's hypotensive effect is unknown.

Pharmacokinetics

● *Absorption:* About 50% is absorbed from the GI tract. Food decreases absorption to 30%. Diuresis usually begins in 2 hours and peaks in 6 to 10 hours.
● *Distribution:* Has wide extravascular distribution.
● *Metabolism:* Insignificant.
● *Excretion:* Most is excreted in urine; half-life is 6 to 9 hours in patients with normal renal function.

Contraindications and precautions

Contraindicated in patients with hypersensitivity to drug and in those with serum potassium level over 5.5 mEq/L. Don't administer to patients receiving other potassium-sparing diuretics, such as spironolactone and triamterene. Also contraindicated in patients with anuria, acute or chronic renal insufficiency, or diabetic nephropathy.

   Use with extreme caution in patients with diabetes mellitus.

Interactions

Drug-drug. *Angiotensin-converting enzyme inhibitors, potassium-containing drugs (parenteral penicillin G), potassium-sparing diuretics, potassium supplements:* Increases risk of hyperkalemia when administered with these drugs. Use together with caution. Monitor potassium levels.
Antihypertensives: Enhanced hypotensive effects; this may be used to therapeutic advantage.
Digoxin: Decreased renal clearance of digoxin, along with inotropic effect. Monitor digoxin levels.
Lithium: May reduce renal clearance of lithium and increase lithium blood levels. Monitor lithium levels.
NSAIDs, such as ibuprofen, indomethacin: May alter renal function and thus affect potassium excretion. Monitor renal function.
Drug-food. *Salt substitutes containing potassium:* Increase risk of hyperkalemia. Avoid concurrent use.

Adverse reactions

CNS: *headache,* weakness, dizziness, encephalopathy.
CV: orthostatic hypotension.
GI: *nausea, anorexia, diarrhea, vomiting,* abdominal pain, constipation, appetite changes.
GU: impotence.
Hematologic: *aplastic anemia,* neutropenia.
Respiratory: dyspnea.
Other: hyperkalemia, fatigue, muscle cramps.

☑ Special considerations

● Recommendations for use of amiloride and for care and teaching of the patient during therapy are the same as those for all potassium-sparing diuretics.
● Amiloride therapy causes severe hyperkalemia in diabetic patients following I.V. glucose tolerance testing; discontinue amiloride at least 3 days before testing.
● Signs and symptoms of overdose are consistent with dehydration and electrolyte disturbance.
● Treatment of overdose is supportive and symptomatic. In acute ingestion, empty stomach by emesis or lavage. In severe hyperkalemia (6.5 mEq/L or more), reduce serum potassium levels with I.V. sodium bicarbonate or glucose with insulin. A cation exchange resin, sodium polystyrene sulfonate (Kayexalate), given orally or as a retention enema, may also reduce serum potassium levels. Monitor serum electrolytes.
● Transient abnormal renal and hepatic function tests have been noted in overdose.

Monitoring the patient

● Monitor patient for adverse effects.
● Perform periodic evaluations for electrolytes and blood count.

Information for the patient

● Tell patient to take drug with food to avoid stomach upset.
● Advise patient to avoid eating large quantities of foods that are high in potassium.
● Tell patient to notify physician if symptoms of dehydration occur.

Geriatric patients

● Elderly and debilitated patients require close observation; they are more susceptible to drug-induced diuresis and hyperkalemia. Reduced dosages may be indicated.

Pediatric patients

● Safety and efficacy in children haven't been established.

Breast-feeding patients

● Amiloride may appear in breast milk; use cautiously in breast-feeding women.

amino acid infusions

Aminosyn, Aminosyn with dextrose, Aminosyn with electrolytes, Aminosyn-PF, Aminosyn (pH6), Aminosyn II, Aminosyn II in dextrose, Aminosyn II with electrolytes, Aminosyn II with electrolytes in dextrose, FreAmine III, FreAmine III with electrolytes, Novamine, ProcalAmine, Travasol with electrolytes, Travasol, TrophAmine

amino acid infusions for renal failure

Aminess, Aminosyn-RF, NephrAmine, RenAmin

amino acid infusions for high metabolic stress

Aminosyn-HBC, BranchAmin, FreAmine HBC

amino acid infusions for hepatic failure or hepatic encephalopathy

HepatAmine

Pharmacologic classification: protein substrates
Therapeutic classification: parenteral nutritional therapy, caloric drug
Pregnancy risk category C

How supplied

Available by prescription only
Injection: without electrolytes—1,000 ml (3.5%, 5%, 8.5%, 10%; 10% with 60 mg potassium metabisulfite, 11.4%, 15%); 500 ml (5%, 5.5% with sodium bisulfite, 7%, 8.5%, 8.5% with sodium bisulfite, 10%, 10% with sodium bisulfite,

11.4%, 15%); 250 ml (5%, 10% with sodium bisul-fite, 11.4%)
Injection: with electrolytes—1,000 ml (3% with 50 mg potassium metabisulfite and 3 mEq cal-cium/L, 3% with potassium metabisulfite, 3.5%, 3.5% with 60 mg sodium hydrosulfite); 500 ml (3.5%, 5.5%, with 3 mEq sodium bisulfite/L, 7% with potassium bisulfite, 8% in 1,000-ml container with potassium metabisulfite, 8.5% with potassi-um metabisulfite, 8.5% with 3 mEq sodium bisul-fite/L)

Indications, route, and dosage
Hepatic encephalopathy in patients with cir-rhosis or hepatitis, nutritional support
Adults: 80 to 120 g of amino acids (12 to 18 g of nitrogen)/day. Use formulation specifically for he-patic failure or encephalopathy (HepatAmine). Typically, 500 ml amino acid injection is mixed with 500 ml dextrose 50% in water and adminis-tered over 8 to 12 hours. Add electrolytes, vita-mins, and trace elements.
Total supportive, or supplemental and pro-tein-sparing parenteral nutrition to maintain normal nutrition and metabolism (amino acid infusions)
Adults: 1 to 1.5 g/kg I.V. daily.
Children: 2 to 3 g/kg I.V. daily.
Note: Individualize dosage to metabolic and clinical response as determined by nitrogen bal-ance and body weight corrected for fluid balance. Add electrolytes, vitamins, trace elements, and nonprotein caloric drugs, p.r.n.

Pharmacodynamics
Nutritional action: Provide a substrate for protein synthesis in the protein-depleted patient or en-hance conservation of body protein.

Pharmacokinetics
• *Absorption:* Administered directly into vascu-lar system.
• *Distribution:* No information available.
• *Metabolism:* No information available.
• *Excretion:* No information available.

Contraindications and precautions
Contraindicated in patients with anuria and in those with inborn errors of amino acid metabo-lism, such as maple syrup urine disease and iso-valeric acidemia. Also contraindicated in patients with severe uncorrected electrolyte or acid-base imbalances, hyperammonemia, and decreased circulating blood volume.
Use cautiously in neonates (especially those with low birth weight), in pediatric patients, and in patients with impaired renal, hepatic, or car-diac function.

Interactions
Drug-drug. *Acidic I.V. solutions for total par-enteral nutrition (TPN):* May release bicarbonate as gas. Avoid using together.
Blood: Simultaneous administration with blood may cause pseudoagglutination. Don't give with blood.
Electrolytes, heparin, insulin, supplementary vi-tamins, trace minerals: May be added cautious-ly when needed; other drugs shouldn't be ad-ministered via the central venous catheter.
Folic acid: Concurrent use precipitates calcium salts as calcium folate. Avoid concurrent use.
Sodium bicarbonate: Concurrent use may pre-cipitate calcium and magnesium and decreases the activity of insulin and vitamin B complex with vitamin C. Avoid concurrent use.
Tetracycline: Concurrent administration may re-duce the protein-sparing effects of infused amino acids. Use together cautiously.
Vitamin K: Potential for incompatibility. Adminis-ter separately.
Other drugs: Shouldn't be mixed with amino acid solutions because of potential for incompatibility.

Adverse reactions
CV: thrombophlebitis, edema, thrombosis.
GI: nausea.
GU: glycosuria, osmotic diuresis.
Hepatic: elevated liver enzyme levels.
Skin: flushing.
Other: hypersensitivity reactions, tissue slough-ing at infusion site caused by extravasation, *catheter sepsis, rebound hypoglycemia* (when long-term infusions are abruptly stopped), hy-perglycemia, osteoporosis, metabolic acidosis, alkalosis, hypophosphatemia, *hyperosmolar hyperglycemic nonketotic syndrome,* hyper-ammonemia, *electrolyte imbalances,* fever, weight gain.

☑ Special considerations
• Consult pharmacist about compatibility before combining amino acid infusions with other sub-stances.
• Begin I.V. infusion slowly and increase over 1 to 2 days as tolerated to prevent hyperglycemia. Taper off over 1 to 2 days to prevent rebound hy-poglycemia.
• Replace all I.V. equipment (I.V. lines, filter, and bottle) every 24 hours.
• Observe infusion site for signs of infection, drainage, edema, and extravasation. Check for fever or other possible signs of infection or hy-persensitivity.
• Use TPN line solely for providing nutrition, not for collecting blood samples, transfusing blood, or administering drugs.
• High blood glucose levels may need supple-mentary insulin to prevent dehydration and coma.

Reactions may be *common,* uncommon, *life-threatening,* or COMMON AND LIFE-THREATENING.

- Essential fatty acid deficiency may result from long-term fat-free I.V. feedings. Fat emulsion (500 ml) weekly may be needed.
- If TPN must be interrupted, administer D_5W or $D_{10}W$ by peripheral vein to prevent rebound hypoglycemia.
- Frequent, meticulous mouth care is important to prevent parotitis.
- Administer 10 mg of phytonadione weekly to prevent vitamin K deficiency.

Monitoring the patient
- Check vital signs at least every 4 hours.
- Monitor intake, output, weight, and pattern as well as caloric intake for significant changes.
- Test patient's fingerstick blood glucose level every 6 hours until infusion rate is stabilized, then twice daily.
- Watch for signs of circulatory overload.
- Regularly monitor the following laboratory values throughout TPN therapy: CBC with differential and platelet count, serum electrolytes, blood glucose, urine glucose and ketones, PT, renal and hepatic function tests, trace elements, and plasma lipids.
- Carefully monitor BUN and creatinine ratios. A BUN-to-creatinine ratio exceeding 10:1 may indicate that patient is receiving too much protein per unit of glucose. Reportedly, 100 to 150 g carbohydrate calories per gram of nitrogen are required to use amino acids effectively.
- In patients receiving protein-sparing therapy, check BUN determinations daily. If BUN levels increase 10 to 15 mg/dl for more than 3 days, therapy adjustment is usually required.

Information for the patient
- Tell patient receiving TPN that he may imagine taste or smell of food. Explain that these sensations are common, and suggest some distracting activity during mealtimes.
- Encourage patient to take special care with oral hygiene. Advise patient to use a soft toothbrush and fluoride toothpaste and floss teeth daily.
- Inform patient that fewer bowel movements occur while receiving TPN.

Pediatric patients
- The effect of amino acid infusions without dextrose on the carbohydrate metabolism of children is unknown.
- Take special precautions in children with acute renal failure and especially in low-birth-weight infants. In these patients, laboratory and clinical monitoring must be extensive and frequent.
- Monitor serum calcium levels frequently to check for signs of bone demineralization.

aminocaproic acid
Amicar

Pharmacologic classification: carboxylic acid derivative
Therapeutic classification: fibrinolysis inhibitor
Pregnancy risk category C

How supplied
Available by prescription only
Tablets: 500 mg
Syrup: 250 mg/ml
Injection: 5 g/20 ml for dilution; 24 g/96 ml for infusion

Indications, route, and dosage
Excessive acute bleeding from hyperfibrinolysis; ◊ amegakaryocytic thrombocytopenia; ◊ missed abortion; ◊ allergic reaction; ◊ dermatitides; ◊ prophylaxis for blood transfusion reaction; ◊ connective tissue disease; ◊ rheumatoid arthritis; ◊ idiopathic thrombocytopenia; ◊ agranulocytosis
Adults: 4 to 5 g I.V. or P.O. over first hour; then constant infusion of 1 g/hour for about 8 hours or until bleeding is controlled. Maximum dosage, 30 g/24 hours.
Excessive acute bleeding from hyperfibrinolysis
Children: 100 mg/kg I.V., or 3 g/m^2 I.V. first hour; then constant infusion of 33.3 mg/kg/hour or 1 g/m^2/hour. Maximum dosage, 18 g/m^2 for 24 hours.
Chronic bleeding tendency
Adults: 5 to 30 g/day P.O. in divided doses at 3- to 6-hour intervals.
◊ **Antidote for excessive thrombolysis due to administration of streptokinase or urokinase**
Adults: 4 to 5 g I.V. in first hour; then continuous infusion of 1 g/hour. Continue treatment for 8 hours or until hemorrhage is controlled.
◊ **Secondary ocular hemorrhage in nonperforating traumatic hyphema**
Adults: 100 mg/kg P.O. q 4 hours for 5 days; maximum, 5 g/dose and 30 g/day.
◊ **Hereditary hemorrhagic telangiectasia**
Adults: 1 to 1.5 g P.O. b.i.d. for 1 to 2 months; then 1 to 2 g daily.

Pharmacodynamics
Hemostatic action: Inhibits plasminogen activators; to a lesser degree, blocks antiplasmin activity by inhibiting fibrinolysis.

Pharmacokinetics
- *Absorption:* Rapidly and completely absorbed from GI tract. Plasma levels peak in 2 hours; sustained plasma levels are achieved by repeated oral doses or continuous I.V. infusion.

- *Distribution:* Readily permeates human blood cells and other body cells; isn't protein-bound.
- *Metabolism:* Insignificant.
- *Excretion:* Duration of action of a single parenteral dose is less than 3 hours; 40% to 60% of a single oral dose is excreted unchanged in urine in 12 hours.

Contraindications and precautions
Contraindicated in patients with active intravascular clotting or presence of DIC unless heparin is used concomitantly. Injectable form is contraindicated in newborns. Use cautiously in patients with cardiac, renal, or hepatic disease.

Interactions
Drug-drug. *Estrogens, oral contraceptives containing estrogen:* Increased risk of hypercoagulability. Use with caution.

Adverse reactions
CNS: dizziness, malaise, headache, delirium, **seizures,** hallucinations, weakness.
CV: hypotension, **bradycardia, arrhythmias with rapid I.V. infusion,** generalized thrombosis.
EENT: tinnitus, nasal congestion, conjunctival suffusion.
GI: nausea, cramps, diarrhea.
GU: *acute renal failure.*
Hepatic: increased AST, ALT levels.
Metabolic: hyperkalemia.
Musculoskeletal: myopathy.
Skin: rash.

☑ Special considerations
- To prepare I.V. infusion, use normal saline injection, D_5W injection, or lactated Ringer's injection for dilution. Dilute doses up to 5 g with 250 ml of solution, doses of 5 g or greater with at least 500 ml.
- Avoid rapid I.V. infusion to minimize risk of CV adverse reactions; use infusion pump to ensure constancy of infusion.
- Signs and symptoms of overdose may include nausea, diarrhea, delirium, thrombotic episodes, and cardiac and hepatic necrosis. Discontinue drug immediately.

Monitoring the patient
- Monitor coagulation studies, heart rhythm, and blood pressure.
- Long-term use of drug requires routine CK determinations.
- Be alert for signs of phlebitis.

Information for the patient
- Tell patient to change positions slowly to minimize dizziness.
- With long-term use, tell patient that routine CK determinations will be necessary.

- Teach patient signs and symptoms of thrombophlebitis, and advise patient to report them promptly.

Pediatric patients
- Safety and effectiveness in children haven't been established.

Breast-feeding patients
- It's not known if drug appears in breast milk. Use caution when administrating drug to breast-feeding women.

aminophylline
Phyllocontin, Truphylline

Pharmacologic classification: xanthine derivative
Therapeutic classification: bronchodilator
Pregnancy risk category C

How supplied
Available by prescription only
Tablets: 100 mg, 200 mg
Tablets (controlled-release): 225 mg
Liquid: 105 mg/5 ml
Injection: 250-mg, 500-mg vials and ampules
Rectal suppositories: 250 mg, 500 mg

Indications, route, and dosage
Symptomatic relief of acute bronchospasm
Patients not currently receiving theophylline who require rapid relief of symptoms: Loading dose is 6 mg/kg (equivalent to 4.7 mg/kg anhydrous theophylline) I.V. slowly (25 mg/minute or less); then maintenance infusion.
Adults (nonsmokers): 0.7 mg/kg/hour I.V. for 12 hours, then 0.5 mg/kg/hour I.V.; or 3 mg/kg P.O. q 6 hours for 2 doses, then 3 mg/kg q 8 hours.
Otherwise healthy adult smokers: 1 mg/kg/hour I.V. for 12 hours, then 0.8 mg/kg/hour I.V.; or 3 mg/kg P.O. q 4 hours for 3 doses, then 3 mg/kg q 6 hours.
Older patients, adults with cor pulmonale: 0.6 mg/kg I.V. for 12 hours, then 0.3 mg/kg/hour I.V.; or 2 mg/kg P.O. q 6 hours for 2 doses, then 2 mg/kg q 8 hours.
Adults with heart failure or liver disease: 0.5 mg/kg/hour I.V. for 12 hours, then 0.1 to 0.2 mg/kg/hour I.V.; or 2 mg/kg P.O. q 8 hours for 2 doses, then 1 to 2 mg/kg q 12 hours.
Children ages 9 to 16: 1 mg/kg/hour I.V. for 12 hours, then 0.8 mg/kg/hour I.V.; or 3 mg/kg P.O. q 4 hours for 3 doses, then 3 mg/kg q 6 hours.
Children ages 6 months to 9 years: 1.2 mg/kg/hour I.V. for 12 hours, then 1 mg/kg/hour I.V.; or 4 mg/kg P.O. q 4 hours for 3 doses, then 4 mg/kg q 6 hours.
Patients currently receiving theophylline: Aminophylline loading infusions of 0.63 mg/kg (0.5 mg/kg anhydrous theophylline) will increase plasma lev-

els of theophylline by 1 mcg/ml, after serum levels have been evaluated. Some clinicians recommend a loading dose of 3.1 mg/kg I.V. (2.5 mg/kg anhydrous theophylline) if no obvious signs of theophylline toxicity are present; then maintenance infusion.

Chronic bronchial asthma
Adults: 400 mg P.O. daily divided t.i.d. or q.i.d.
Children: 16 mg/kg P.O. daily divided t.i.d. or q.i.d.
    Monitor serum levels to ensure that theophylline levels range from 10 to 20 mcg/ml.
◊ *Periodic apnea associated with Cheyne-Stokes respirations; left-sided heart failure*
Adults: 200 to 400 mg I.V. bolus.
◊ *Reduction of severe bronchospasm in infants with cystic fibrosis*
Infants: 10 to 12 mg/kg I.V.

Pharmacodynamics
Bronchodilating action: Acts at the cellular level after it's converted to theophylline. (Aminophylline [theophylline ethylenediamine] is 79% theophylline). Theophylline acts by either inhibiting phosphodiesterase or blocking adenosine receptors in the bronchi, resulting in relaxation of the smooth muscle. Also stimulates the respiratory center in the medulla and prevents diaphragmatic fatigue.

Pharmacokinetics
● *Absorption:* Most forms are absorbed well; absorption of the suppository, however, is unreliable and slow. Rate and onset of action also depend on form selected. Food may alter rate, but not extent, of absorption of oral doses.
● *Distribution:* Distributed in all tissues and extracellular fluids except fatty tissue.
● *Metabolism:* Converted to theophylline; then metabolized to inactive compounds.
● *Excretion:* Excreted in urine as theophylline (10%).

Contraindications and precautions
Contraindicated in patients with hypersensitivity to xanthine compounds (caffeine, theobromine) and ethylenediamine and in those with active peptic ulcer disease and seizure disorders (unless adequate anticonvulsant therapy is given). Rectal suppositories are also contraindicated in patients who have an irritation or infection of rectum or lower colon.
    Use cautiously in neonates and infants under age 1, young children, elderly patients, and in patients with heart failure, CV disorders, COPD, cor pulmonale, renal or hepatic disease, hyperthyroidism, diabetes mellitus, peptic ulcer, severe hypoxemia, or hypertension.

Interactions
Drug-drug. *Alkali-sensitive drugs:* Reduced activity of aminophylline. Don't add these drugs to I.V. fluids containing aminophylline.

Allopurinol (high dose), cimetidine, erythromycin, propranolol, quinolones, troleandomycin: May increase serum level of aminophylline by decreasing hepatic clearance. Use together cautiously.
Aminoglutethimide, carbamazepine, phenobarbital, phenytoin, rifampin: Decreased effects of aminophylline. Use together cautiously.
Lithium: Increased lithium excretion. Use together cautiously.
Drug-lifestyle. *Marijuana, tobacco:* Decreased effects of aminophylline. Discourage use.

Adverse reactions
CNS: *nervousness, restlessness,* headache, *insomnia,* **seizures,** muscle twitching, irritability.
CV: *palpitations, sinus tachycardia,* extrasystoles, flushing, marked hypotension, **arrhythmias.**
GI: *nausea, vomiting,* diarrhea, epigastric pain, hematemesis.
Respiratory: tachypnea, **respiratory arrest.**
Skin: urticaria.
Other: irritation from rectal suppositories, hyperglycemia, fever, increased plasma-free fatty acids and urinary catecholamines.

☑ **Special considerations**
● Before giving loading dose, check that patient hasn't had recent theophylline therapy.
● Don't combine in fluids for I.V. infusion with the following: ascorbic acid, chlorpromazine, codeine phosphate, dimenhydrinate, dobutamine, epinephrine, erythromycin gluceptate, hydralazine, insulin, levorphanol tartrate, meperidine, methadone, methicillin, morphine sulfate, norepinephrine bitartrate, oxytetracycline, penicillin G potassium, phenobarbital, phenytoin, prochlorperazine, promazine, promethazine, tetracycline, vancomycin, vitamin B complex with C.
● Don't crush controlled-release tablets.
● I.V. drug administration includes I.V. push at a very slow rate or an infusion with 100 to 200 ml of 5% dextrose or normal saline.
● GI symptoms may be relieved by taking oral drug with full glass of water at meals, although food in stomach delays absorption. Enteric-coated tablets may also delay absorption. There is no evidence that antacids reduce GI adverse reactions.
● Suppositories are slowly and erratically absorbed; retention enemas may be absorbed more rapidly. Rectally administered preparations can be given when patient can't take drug orally. Schedule after evacuation, if possible; may be retained better if given before meal. Advise patient to remain recumbent 15 to 20 minutes after insertion.
● Patients metabolize xanthines at different rates. Adjust dose by monitoring response, tolerance, pulmonary function, and theophylline blood levels. Therapeutic level is 10 to 20 mcg/ml, but some patients may respond at lower levels; toxicity occurs at levels over 20 mcg/ml.

• Plasma clearance may be decreased in patients with heart failure, hepatic dysfunction, or pulmonary edema. Smokers show accelerated clearance. Dosage adjustments necessary.

• Theophylline levels are falsely elevated in the presence of furosemide, phenylbutazone, probenecid, theobromine, caffeine, tea, chocolate, cola beverages, and acetaminophen, depending on type of assay used.

• Aminophylline may alter assay for uric acid, depending on method used.

• Signs and symptoms of overdose include nausea, vomiting, insomnia, irritability, tachycardia, extrasystoles, tachypnea, and tonic-clonic seizures. Onset of toxicity may be sudden and severe; arrhythmias and seizures are the first signs.

• If toxicity occurs, induce emesis, except in patients with seizures, then use activated charcoal and cathartics. Charcoal hemoperfusion may be beneficial. Treat arrhythmias with lidocaine and seizures with I.V. benzodiazepine; support respiratory and CV systems.

Monitoring the patient

• Monitor serum levels to ensure theophylline levels range from 10 to 20 mcg/ml.

• Monitor vital signs and ECG.

• Observe patient for CNS effects, which may range from restlessness to seizures.

Information for the patient

• Teach patient rationale for therapy and importance of compliance with prescribed regimen; if a dose is missed, patient should take it as soon as possible, but not double up on doses. Advise patient to avoid taking extra "breathing pills."

• Advise patient of adverse effects and possible signs of toxicity.

• Tell patient not to eat or drink large quantities of xanthine-containing foods and beverages.

• Warn patient that OTC remedies may contain ephedrine with theophylline salts; excessive CNS stimulation may result. Patient should seek medical approval before taking any other drugs.

Geriatric patients

• Use reduced doses and monitor the patient closely. Warn elderly patients of dizziness, a common adverse reaction at therapy start.

Pediatric patients

• Drug isn't recommended for use in infants under age 6 months.

Breast-feeding patients

• Drug appears in breast milk and may cause irritability, insomnia, or fretfulness in the breast-fed infant.

amiodarone hydrochloride
Cordarone

Pharmacologic classification: benzofuran derivative
Therapeutic classification: ventricular and supraventricular antiarrhythmic
Pregnancy risk category D

How supplied

Available by prescription only
Tablets: 100 mg*, 200 mg
Injection: 50 mg/ml

Indications, route, and dosage

Recurrent ventricular fibrillation and unstable ventricular tachycardia; ◊ *supraventricular arrhythmias;* ◊ *atrial fibrillation;* ◊ *angina;* ◊ *hypertrophic cardiomyopathy*

Adults: Loading dose of 800 to 1,600 mg P.O. daily for 1 to 3 weeks until initial therapeutic response occurs. Maintenance dosage, 200 to 600 mg P.O. daily. Or for first 24 hours 150 mg I.V. over 10 minutes (mixed in 100 ml D_5W); then 360 mg I.V. over 6 hours (mix 900 mg in 500 ml D_5W); then maintenance of 540 mg I.V. over 18 hours at a rate of 0.5 mg/minute. After first 24 hours, continue a maintenance infusion of 0.5 mg/minute in a 1- to 6-mg/ml concentration. For infusions greater than 1 hour, concentrations shouldn't exceed 2 mg/ml unless a central venous catheter is used. Don't use for more than 3 weeks.

◊ Children: 10 to 15 mg/kg P.O. daily or 600 to 800 mg/1.73 m^2 P.O. daily for 4 to 14 days or until response is seen. Then 5 mg/kg or 400 mg/1.73 m^2; usual maintenance dose is 2.5 mg/kg or 200 mg/1.73 m^2/day.

Conversion from I.V. to P.O.

Adults: Daily dose of 720 mg (rate 0.5 mg/minute): for 1 week, 800 to 1,600 mg daily; 1 to 3 weeks, 600 to 800 mg daily; more than 3 weeks, 400 mg daily.

Pharmacodynamics

Ventricular antiarrhythmic action: Although it has mixed class IC and III antiarrhythmic effects, amiodarone generally is considered a class III drug. It increases the action potential duration (repolarization inhibition). With prolonged therapy, the effective refractory period increases in the atria, ventricles, AV node, His-Purkinje system, and bypass tracts, and conduction slows in the atria, AV node, His-Purkinje system, and ventricles; sinus node automaticity decreases. Drug also noncompetitively blocks beta-adrenergic receptors. Clinically, it has little, if any, negative inotropic effect. Coronary and peripheral vasodilator effects may occur with long-term therapy. Amiodarone is among the most effective antiarrhythmics, but its therapeutic applications are somewhat limited by its severe adverse reactions.

Reactions may be *common*, uncommon, **life-threatening**, or COMMON AND LIFE-THREATENING.

Pharmacokinetics

• *Absorption:* Has slow, variable absorption. Bioavailability is about 22% to 86%. Plasma levels peak 3 to 7 hours after oral administration; however, onset of action may be delayed from 2 to 3 days to 2 to 3 months—even with loading doses.
• *Distribution:* Distributed widely because it accumulates in adipose tissue and in organs with marked perfusion, such as the lungs, liver, and spleen. 96% protein-bound. Therapeutic serum level isn't well defined but may range from 1 to 2.5 mcg/ml.
• *Metabolism:* Metabolized extensively in the liver to a pharmacologically active metabolite, desethyl amiodarone.
• *Excretion:* Main excretory route is hepatic, through the biliary tree (with enterohepatic recirculation). Because no renal excretion occurs, patients with impaired renal function don't require dosage reduction. Terminal elimination half-life—25 to 110 days—is the longest of any antiarrhythmic; in most patients, half-life ranges from 40 to 50 days.

Contraindications and precautions

Contraindicated in patients with hypersensitivity to drug and in those with severe SA node disease resulting in preexisting bradycardia. Unless an artificial pacemaker is present, drug is also contraindicated in patients with second- or third-degree AV block and in those in whom bradycardia has caused syncope. Use with caution in patients already receiving antiarrhythmics, beta blockers, and calcium channel blockers.

Interactions

Drug-drug. *Beta blockers, calcium channel blockers:* Concomitant use may cause sinus bradycardia, sinus arrest, and AV block. Use together cautiously.
Cholestyramine: Increases elimination of amiodarone. Use together cautiously.
Cimetidine: Increases amiodarone levels. Monitor amiodarone levels.
Cyclosporine, digoxin, flecainide, lidocaine, phenytoin, procainamide, quinidine, theophylline: May lead to increased serum levels of these drugs, resulting in enhanced effects. Use together cautiously.
Disopyramide, phenothiazines, quinidine, tricyclic antidepressants: Concurrent use may cause additive effects that lead to a prolonged QT interval, possibly resulting in torsades de pointes. Don't use together.
Phenytoin: Decreases amiodarone levels. Monitor amiodarone levels.
Warfarin: May cause prolonged PT as a result of enhanced drug displacement from protein-binding sites. Monitor PT.
Drug-herb. *Pennyroyal:* May change rate of formation of toxic metabolites of pennyroyal. Avoid concomitant use.

Drug-lifestyle. *Sunlight exposure:* Photosensitivity reactions may result. Take precautions.

Adverse reactions

CNS: peripheral neuropathy, ataxia, paresthesia, tremor, insomnia, sleep disturbances, headache, *malaise, fatigue.*
**CV: *bradycardia,* hypotension, *arrhythmias, heart failure, heart block, sinus arrest.*
EENT: *corneal microdeposits,* visual disturbances.
GI: *nausea, vomiting,* constipation, abdominal pain.
Hepatic: *altered liver enzymes,* hepatic dysfunction, *hepatic failure.*
Respiratory: SEVERE PULMONARY TOXICITY (PNEU-MONITIS, ALVEOLITIS).
Skin: *photosensitivity,* blue-gray skin pigmentation, solar dermatitis.
Other: hypothyroidism, hyperthyroidism, edema, coagulation abnormalities.

☑ Special considerations

• Drug is effective in treating arrhythmias resistant to other drug therapy. However, its many adverse effects limit its use.
• Divide loading dose into three equal doses, and give with meals to minimize GI intolerance. Maintenance dose may be given once daily but may be divided into 2 doses taken with meals if GI intolerance occurs.
• Digoxin, quinidine, phenytoin, and procainamide doses should be decreased during amiodarone therapy to avoid toxicity.
• Adverse effects are more prevalent with high doses but usually resolve within about 4 months after drug therapy stops.
• Amiodarone I.V. infusions exceeding 2 hours must be administered in glass or polyolefin bottles containing D_5W.
• Clinical effects of overdose include bradyarrhythmias.
• Treatment of overdose may require beta-adrenergic agonists (such as isoproterenol) or artificial pacing. To treat hypotension, positive inotropic drugs (such as dopamine or dobutamine) or vasopressors (such as epinephrine or norepinephrine) may be administered. Use general supportive measures as needed. Drug can't be removed by dialysis.

Monitoring the patient

• Monitor blood pressure and heart rate and rhythm frequently for significant change.
• Periodically monitor hepatic and thyroid function tests. Perform periodic ophthalmologic evaluations to assess corneal microdeposits.
• Monitor patient for signs and symptoms of pneumonitis, such as exertional dyspnea, nonproductive cough, and pleuritic chest pain. Also check pulmonary function tests and chest X-ray. (Pulmonary toxicity is more common with daily doses exceeding 600 mg.) Pulmonary complications

require discontinuation of amiodarone and possibly treatment with corticosteroids.

Information for the patient
• Advise patient to use sunscreen to prevent photosensitivity (sunlight and ultraviolet light), which may result in sunburn and blistering.
• Although corneal microdeposits typically appear 1 to 4 months after therapy begins, only 2% to 3% of patients have actual visual disturbances. To minimize this complication, recommend frequent instillation of methylcellulose ophthalmic solution.

Geriatric patients
• Use cautiously in elderly patients; ataxia may occur.

Pediatric patients
• Children receiving amiodarone with digoxin may experience more acute effects of interaction.
• Children may experience faster onset of action and shorter duration of effect than adults.

Breast-feeding patients
• Drug appears in breast milk and shouldn't be used in breast-feeding women.

---

amitriptyline hydrochloride
Amitriptyline, Elavil, Levate*, Novotriptyn*

Pharmacologic classification: tricyclic antidepressant
Therapeutic classification: antidepressant
Pregnancy risk category NR

How supplied
Available by prescription only
Tablets: 10 mg, 25 mg, 50 mg, 75 mg, 100 mg, 150 mg
Injection: 10 mg/ml

Indications, route, and dosage
Depression, ◊ anorexia or bulimia associated with depression, ◊ adjunctive treatment of neurogenic pain
Adults: Initial outpatient, 75 to 150 mg/day P.O. in divided doses or 50 to 150 mg h.s.; inpatient, 100 to 300 mg/day. I.M. dosage is 20 to 30 mg q.i.d., which should be changed to oral route as soon as possible. Maintenance dose is 50 to 100 mg/day.
✦ *Dosage adjustment.* In elderly or adolescent patients, 10 mg P.O. t.i.d. and 20 mg h.s.

Pharmacodynamics
Antidepressant action: Thought to exert its antidepressant effects by inhibiting reuptake of norepinephrine and serotonin in CNS nerve terminals (presynaptic neurons), resulting in increased concentrations and enhanced activity of these neurotransmitters in the synaptic cleft. More actively inhibits reuptake of serotonin than norepinephrine; carries a high risk of undesirable sedation, but tolerance to this effect usually develops within a few weeks.

Pharmacokinetics
• *Absorption:* Absorbed rapidly from the GI tract after oral administration and from muscle tissue after I.M. administration.
• *Distribution:* Distributed widely into the body, including the CNS and breast milk; 96% protein-bound. Peak effect occurs 2 to 12 hours after a given dose, and steady state is achieved within 4 to 10 days. Full therapeutic effect usually occurs in 2 to 4 weeks.
• *Metabolism:* Metabolized by the liver to the active metabolite nortriptyline; a significant first-pass effect may account for variability of serum levels in different patients taking the same dosage.
• *Excretion:* Excreted mostly in urine.

Contraindications and precautions
Contraindicated in patients with hypersensitivity to drug and in those who have received an MAO inhibitor within the past 14 days. Also contraindicated during acute recovery phase of MI.
Use cautiously in patients with recent history of MI and in those with unstable heart disease or renal or hepatic impairment.

Interactions
Drug-drug. *Antiarrhythmics (disopyramide, procainamide, quinidine), pimozide, thyroid hormones:* May increase arrhythmias and conduction defects. Monitor patient carefully.
Barbiturates: Induce amitriptyline metabolism and decrease therapeutic efficacy. Monitor patient carefully.
Beta blockers, cimetidine, methylphenidate, oral contraceptives, propoxyphene, selective serotonin reuptake inhibitors such as fluoxetine: May inhibit amitriptyline metabolism, increasing plasma levels and toxicity. Use together cautiously.
Centrally acting antihypertensives, such as clonidine, guanabenz, guanadrel, guanethidine, methyldopa, reserpine: Amitriptyline may decrease hypotensive effects. Use together cautiously.
CNS depressants (such as analgesics, anesthetics, barbiturates, narcotics, tranquilizers; atropine), other anticholinergic drugs (such as antihistamines, antiparkinsonians), meperidine, metrizamide, phenothiazines: Additive effects (such as oversedation, paralytic ileus, visual changes, severe constipation, increased risk of seizures) are likely after concomitant use. Use together cautiously.
Disulfiram, ethchlorvynol: May cause delirium and tachycardia. Use together cautiously.

Haloperidol, phenothiazines: Decrease amitriptyline's metabolism, decreasing therapeutic efficacy. Monitor patient for drug effect.

Sympathomimetics, such as ephedrine, epinephrine, phenylephrine, phenylpropanolamine: May increase blood pressure. Monitor blood pressure.

Warfarin: May increase PT and cause bleeding. Monitor patient for bleeding; monitor PT.

Drug-lifestyle. *Alcohol:* Additive effects are likely with concomitant use. Don't use together.

Heavy smoking: Induces amitriptyline metabolism and decreases therapeutic efficacy. Discourage use together.

Sun exposure: Photosensitivity reactions may result. Patient should take precautions.

Adverse reactions

CNS: *coma, seizures,* hallucinations, delusions, disorientation, ataxia, tremor, peripheral neuropathy, anxiety, insomnia, restlessness, drowsiness, dizziness, weakness, fatigue, headache, extrapyramidal reactions.

CV: *MI, stroke, arrhythmias,* heart block, *orthostatic hypotension, tachycardia, ECG changes,* hypertension.

EENT: *blurred vision,* tinnitus, mydriasis, increased intraocular pressure,

GI: *dry mouth,* nausea, vomiting, anorexia, epigastric distress, diarrhea, constipation, paralytic ileus.

GU: urine retention.

Hematologic: *agranulocytosis, thrombocytopenia,* leukopenia, eosinophilia.

Hepatic: elevated liver function test results.

Skin: rash, urticaria, photosensitivity.

Other: *diaphoresis,* hypersensitivity reaction, edema, decrease or increase in serum glucose levels.

After abrupt withdrawal of long-term therapy: nausea, headache, malaise (doesn't indicate addiction).

☑ Special considerations

Besides the recommendations for all tricyclic antidepressants, consider the following.

● Drug also may be used to prevent migraine and cluster headaches, intractable hiccups, and post-therapeutic neuralgia.

● Drug can cause sedative effects. Tolerance to sedative effects may develop over several weeks.

● Full dose may be given at bedtime to help offset daytime sedation.

● P.O. route should be substituted for parenteral route as soon as possible.

● I.M. administration may result in a more rapid onset of action than oral administration.

● Don't withdraw drug abruptly.

● Discontinue drug at least 48 hours before surgical procedures.

● Sugarless chewing gum, hard candy, or ice may alleviate dry mouth. Stress importance of regular dental hygiene because dry mouth can increase dental caries.

● Depressed patients, particularly those with known manic depressive illness, may experience a shift to mania or hypomania.

● The first 12 hours after acute ingestion are a stimulatory phase characterized by excessive anticholinergic activity (agitation, irritation, confusion, hallucinations, hyperthermia, parkinsonian symptoms, seizure, urine retention, dry mucous membranes, pupillary dilation, constipation, and ileus). This is followed by CNS depressant effects, including hypothermia, decreased or absent reflexes, sedation, hypotension, cyanosis, and cardiac irregularities, including tachycardia, conduction disturbances, and quinidine-like effects on the ECG.

● Severity of overdose is best indicated by widening of the QRS complex and usually represents a serum level in excess of 1,000 mg/ml; metabolic acidosis may follow hypotension, hypoventilation, and seizures. Delayed cardiac anomalies and death may occur.

● Treatment of overdose is symptomatic and supportive, including maintaining airway, stable body temperature, and fluid and electrolyte balance. Induce emesis with ipecac if gag reflex is intact; follow with gastric lavage and activated charcoal to prevent further absorption. Dialysis is of little use.

● Physostigmine may be cautiously used to reverse the symptoms of tricyclic antidepressant poisoning in life-threatening situations. Treatment of seizures may include parenteral diazepam or phenytoin; treatment of arrhythmias, parenteral phenytoin or lidocaine; and treatment of acidosis, sodium bicarbonate. Don't give barbiturates; these may enhance CNS and respiratory depressant effects.

Monitoring the patient

● Monitor blood pressure and ECG closely.

● Monitor CBC and liver function studies.

● Monitor patient for neurologic changes.

Information for the patient

● Tell patient to take drug exactly as prescribed; don't double dose for missed ones.

● Advise patient that full dose may be taken at bedtime to alleviate daytime sedation. It may be taken in the early evening to avoid morning hangover.

● Explain that full effects of drug may not become apparent for up to 4 weeks after drug start.

● Warn patient that drug may cause drowsiness or dizziness; avoid hazardous activities that require alertness until full effects of drug are known.

● Warn patient not to drink alcoholic beverages while taking drug.

● Suggest taking drug with food or milk if it causes stomach upset and using sugarless gum or candy to relieve dry mouth.

• After initial doses, advise patient to lie down for about 30 minutes and raise to upright position slowly to prevent dizziness or fainting.
• Warn patient not to stop taking drug suddenly.
• Encourage patient to report troublesome or unusual effects, especially confusion, movement disorders, rapid heartbeat, dizziness, fainting, or difficulty urinating.

Geriatric patients
• Elderly patients may be at greater risk for adverse cardiac effects.

Pediatric patients
• Drug isn't recommended for children under age 12.

Breast-feeding patients
• Drug appears in breast milk in levels equal to or greater than those in maternal serum. About 1% of ingested dose appears in the breast-fed infant's serum. The potential benefit to the mother should outweigh the possible adverse reactions in the infant.

amlodipine besylate
Norvasc

Pharmacologic classification: dihydropyridine calcium channel blocker
Therapeutic classification: antianginal, antihypertensive
Pregnancy risk category C

How supplied
Available by prescription only
Tablets: 2.5 mg, 5 mg, 10 mg

Indications, route, and dosage
Chronic stable angina, vasospastic angina (Prinzmetal's or variant angina)
Adults: Initially, 5 to 10 mg P.O. daily.
Hypertension
Adults: Initially, 5 mg P.O. daily. Adjust dosage based on patient response and tolerance. Maximum daily dose, 10 mg.
✦ *Dosage adjustment.* In small, frail, or elderly patients, those receiving other antihypertensives, or those with hepatic insufficiency, give 2.5 mg daily.

Pharmacodynamics
Antianginal and antihypertensive actions: Contractility of cardiac muscle and vascular smooth muscle depends on movement of extracellular calcium ions into cardiac and smooth-muscle cells through specific ion channels. Amlodipine inhibits the transmembrane influx of calcium ions into vascular smooth muscle and cardiac muscle, thus decreasing myocardial contractility and oxygen demand. As a peripheral arterial va-

sodilator, the drug acts directly on vascular smooth muscle to reduce peripheral vascular resistance and blood pressure. It also dilates coronary arteries and arterioles.

Pharmacokinetics
• *Absorption:* After oral administration of therapeutic doses, absorption produces peak plasma levels between 6 and 12 hours. Absolute bioavailability has been estimated between 64% and 90%.
• *Distribution:* About 93% of circulating drug is bound to plasma proteins in hypertensive patients.
• *Metabolism:* Extensively metabolized in the liver, with about 90% converted to inactive metabolites.
• *Excretion:* Excreted primarily in urine.

Contraindications and precautions
Contraindicated in patients with hypersensitivity to drug. Use cautiously in patients receiving other peripheral dilators and in those with aortic stenosis, heart failure, or severe hepatic disease.

Interactions
None reported.

Adverse reactions
CNS: *headache,* somnolence, fatigue, dizziness, light-headedness, paresthesia.
CV: *edema,* flushing, palpitations.
GI: nausea, abdominal pain.
Skin: rash, pruritus.
Other: dyspnea, muscle pain.

☑ Special considerations
• Some patients, especially those with severe obstructive coronary artery disease, develop increased frequency, duration, or severity of angina or even acute MI after initiation of calcium channel blocker therapy or when dosage is increased.
• Because vasodilation induced by the drug is gradual in onset, acute hypotension has rarely been reported after oral administration. However, exercise caution when administering drug, particularly in patients with severe aortic stenosis.
• Symptoms of overdose include nausea, weakness, dizziness, drowsiness, confusion, slurred speech, and excessive peripheral vasodilation with marked hypotension and bradycardia, resulting in reduced cardiac output. Junctional rhythms and second- or third-degree AV block also can occur.
• Massive overdose warrants active cardiac and respiratory monitoring and frequent blood pressure measurements.
• Treatment of hypotension consists of CV support, including elevation of the extremities and judicious administration of fluids. If hypotension

remains unresponsive to these conservative measures, consider administration of vasopressors such as phenylephrine, with attention to circulating volume and urine output. I.V. calcium gluconate may help reverse effects of calcium entry blockade. Because amlodipine is highly protein-bound, hemodialysis isn't likely to benefit patient.

Monitoring the patient
- Monitor blood pressure closely.
- Monitor response to drug therapy.

Information for the patient
- Tell patient to take nitroglycerin S.L. as needed for acute anginal symptoms. If patient continues nitrate therapy during titration of amlodipine dosage, urge continued compliance.
- Caution patient to continue taking amlodipine even when feeling better.
- Tell patient to report signs of heart failure, such as swelling of hands and feet or shortness of breath.

Geriatric patients
- Elderly patients may need a lower dosage.

Pediatric patients
- Safety and effectiveness in children haven't been established.

Breast-feeding patients
- It's unknown whether drug appears in breast milk. Breast-feeding isn't recommended during amlodipine therapy.

---

amobarbital
amobarbital sodium
Amytal

Pharmacologic classification: barbiturate
Therapeutic classification: sedative-hypnotic, anticonvulsant
Controlled substance schedule II
Pregnancy risk category D

How supplied
Available by prescription only
Tablets: 30 mg
Capsules: 200 mg
Powder for injection: 250-mg, 500-mg vials

Indications, route, and dosage
Sedation
Adults: Usually 30 to 50 mg P.O. b.i.d. or t.i.d. but may range from 15 to 120 mg b.i.d. to q.i.d.
Children: 2 mg/kg P.O. daily divided into four equal doses.

Insomnia
Adults: 65 to 200 mg P.O. or deep I.M. h.s.; I.M. injection not to exceed 5 ml in any one site. Maximum dose, 500 mg.
Children over age 6: 2 to 3 mg/kg deep I.M. h.s.
Preanesthetic sedation
Adults: 200 mg P.O. 1 to 2 hours before surgery.
Labor
Adults: 200 to 400 mg P.O.; may repeat at 1- to 3-hour intervals. Maximum dose, 1 g.
Anticonvulsant
Adults: 65 to 500 mg by slow I.V. injection (rate not exceeding 100 mg/minute). Maximum dose, 1 g.

Pharmacodynamics
Anticonvulsant action: Exact cellular site and mechanism of action unknown. Parenteral amobarbital suppresses the spread of seizure activity produced by epileptogenic foci in the cortex, thalamus, and limbic systems by enhancing the effect of gamma-aminobutyric acid (GABA). Both presynaptic and postsynaptic excitability are decreased.
Sedative-hypnotic action: Acts throughout the CNS as a nonselective depressant with an intermediate onset and duration of action. Particularly sensitive to this drug is the mesencephalic reticular activating system, which controls CNS arousal. Drug decreases both presynaptic and postsynaptic membrane excitability by facilitating the action of GABA.

Pharmacokinetics
- *Absorption:* Absorbed well after oral administration. Absorption after I.M. administration is 100%. Onset of action is 45 to 60 minutes.
- *Distribution:* Distributed well throughout body tissues and fluids.
- *Metabolism:* Metabolized in the liver by oxidation to a tertiary alcohol.
- *Excretion:* Less than 1% of dose is excreted unchanged in the urine; rest is excreted as metabolites. The half-life is biphasic, with a first phase half-life of about 40 minutes and a second phase of about 20 hours. Duration of action is 6 to 8 hours.

Contraindications and precautions
Contraindicated in patients with hypersensitivity to barbiturates and in those with bronchopneumonia or other severe pulmonary insufficiency, or porphyria.
Use cautiously in patients with suicidal tendencies, acute or chronic pain, history of drug abuse, hepatic or renal impairment, or pulmonary or CV disease.

Interactions
Drug-drug. *Antidepressants, antihistamines, MAO inhibitors, narcotics, sedative-hypnotics, tranquilizers:* May add to or potentiate CNS and

respiratory depressant effects of these drugs. Use together with caution.

Corticosteroids, digitoxin, doxycycline, oral contraceptives and other estrogens, theophylline and other xanthines: Enhanced hepatic metabolism of these drugs. Monitor patient carefully.

Disulfiram, MAO inhibitors, valproic acid: Decrease the metabolism of amobarbital and can increase its toxicity. Monitor patient carefully.

Griseofulvin: Impaired effectiveness of griseofulvin. Use cautiously.

Phenytoin: May cause unpredictable fluctuations in serum phenytoin levels. Monitor phenytoin levels.

Rifampin: May decrease amobarbital levels by increasing metabolism. Monitor patient for drug effect.

Warfarin, other oral anticoagulants: Enhanced enzymatic degradation of anticoagulants. Patient may need increased doses of anticoagulants.

Drug-food. *Food:* Decreases absorption of drug. Give on an empty stomach to enhance rate of absorption.

Drug-lifestyle. *Alcohol:* May add to or potentiate CNS and respiratory depressant effects. Don't use together.

Adverse reactions
CNS: *drowsiness, lethargy, hangover,* paradoxical excitement, somnolence.
CV: *bradycardia,* hypotension, syncope.
GI: nausea, vomiting.
Hematologic: exacerbation of porphyria.
Respiratory: *respiratory depression, apnea.*
Skin: rash; urticaria; *Stevens-Johnson syndrome;* pain, irritation, sterile abscess at injection site.
Other: *angioedema,* physical and psychological dependence.

☑ Special considerations
Besides the recommendations for all barbiturates, consider the following.
● Not commonly used as a sedative or aid to sleeping; barbiturates have been replaced by safer benzodiazepines for such use.
● Administer drug orally on an empty stomach to enhance rate of absorption.
● Reconstitute powder for injection with sterile water for injection. Roll vial in hands; don't shake. Use 2.5 or 5 ml (for 250 or 500 mg of amobarbital) to make 10% solution. For I.M. use, prepare 20% solution by using 1.25 or 2.5 ml of sterile water for injection.
● Administer reconstituted parenteral solution within 30 minutes after opening vial.
● Don't administer solution that is cloudy or forms a precipitate after 5 minutes of reconstitution.
● Administer I.V. dose at a rate no greater than 100 mg/minute in adults or 60 mg/m^2/minute in children to prevent possible hypotension and res-

piratory depression. Have emergency resuscitative equipment available.
● Administer I.M. dose deep into large muscle mass, giving no more than 5 ml in any one injection site. Sterile abscess or tissue damage may result from inadvertent superficial I.M. or S.C. injection.
● Administering full loading doses over short periods of time to treat status epilepticus may require ventilatory support in adults.
● Amobarbital may cause a false-positive phentolamine test.
● Physiologic effects of amobarbital may impair absorption of cyanocobalamin Co.
● Amobarbital may decrease serum bilirubin levels in neonates, epileptic patients, and patients with congenital nonhemolytic unconjugated hyperbilirubinemia.
● EEG patterns are altered, with a change in low-voltage, fast-activity; changes persist for a time after therapy is discontinued.
● Signs and symptoms of overdose include unsteady gait, slurred speech, sustained nystagmus, somnolence, confusion, respiratory depression, pulmonary edema, areflexia, and coma. Oliguria, jaundice, hypothermia, fever, and shock with tachycardia and hypotension may occur.
● In overdose, maintain and support ventilation as needed; support circulation with vasopressors and I.V. fluids as needed.
● Treatment of overdose aims to maintain and support ventilation and pulmonary function as needed; support cardiac function and circulation with vasopressors and I.V. fluids as needed. If patient is conscious with a functioning gag reflex and ingestion has been recent, induce emesis by administering ipecac syrup. Gastric lavage may be performed if a cuffed endotracheal tube is in place to prevent aspiration when emesis is inappropriate. Follow with administration of activated charcoal or sodium chloride cathartic. Measure fluid intake and output, vital signs, and laboratory parameters. Maintain body temperature.
● Alkalinization of urine may be helpful in removing amobarbital from the body; hemodialysis may be useful in severe overdose.
● In overdose, assess cardiopulmonary status frequently for possible alterations. Monitor blood counts for potential adverse reactions.
● Assess renal and hepatic laboratory studies to ensure adequate drug removal.

Monitoring the patient
● Monitor PT carefully when patient on amobarbital starts or ends anticoagulant therapy. Anticoagulant dosage may need to be adjusted.
● Monitor patient for adverse effects.

Information for the patient
● Warn patient of possible physical or psychological dependence with prolonged use.
● Tell patient to avoid alcohol while taking drug.

Reactions may be *common,* uncommon, **life-threatening**, or COMMON AND LIFE-THREATENING.

Geriatric patients
• Elderly patients usually require lower doses. Confusion, disorientation, and excitability may occur in elderly patients. Use with caution.

Pediatric patients
• Safe use in children under age 6 hasn't been established. Drug may cause paradoxical excitement in some children.

Breast-feeding patients
• Drug appears in breast milk and may cause drowsiness in infant. If so, dosage adjustment or discontinuation of drug or breast-feeding may be needed. Use with caution.

amoxapine
Asendin

Pharmacologic classification: dibenzoxazepine, tricyclic antidepressant
Therapeutic classification: antidepressant
Pregnancy risk category C

How supplied
Available by prescription only
Tablets: 25 mg, 50 mg, 100 mg, 150 mg

Indications, route, and dosage
Depression
Adults: Initial dosage is 50 mg P.O. b.i.d. or t.i.d.; may increase to 100 mg b.i.d. or t.i.d. by end of first week. Increases above 300 mg daily should be made only if this dosage has been ineffective during a trial period of at least 2 weeks. When effective dosage is established, entire dosage (not exceeding 300 mg) may be given h.s. Maximum dose in hospitalized patients, 600 mg.
    Note: Don't give more than 300 mg in a single dose.
✦ *Dosage adjustment.* In elderly patients, recommended starting dose is 25 mg P.O. b.i.d. or t.i.d.

Pharmacodynamics
Antidepressant action: Thought to exert its antidepressant effects by inhibiting reuptake of norepinephrine and serotonin in CNS nerve terminals (presynaptic neurons), which results in increased levels and enhanced activity of these neurotransmitters in the synaptic cleft. Has a greater inhibitory effect on norepinephrine reuptake than on serotonin. Also blocks CNS dopamine receptors, which may account for the higher risk of movement disorders during therapy.

Pharmacokinetics
• *Absorption:* Absorbed rapidly and completely from the GI tract after oral administration.

• *Distribution:* Distributed widely into the body, including the CNS and breast milk. Drug is 92% protein-bound. Peak effect occurs in 8 to 10 hours; steady state, within 2 to 7 days. Proposed therapeutic plasma levels (parent drug and metabolite) range from 200 to 500 ng/ml.
• *Metabolism:* Metabolized by the liver to the active metabolite 8-hydroxyamoxapine; a significant first-pass effect may explain variability of serum levels in different patients taking same dosage.
• *Excretion:* Excreted in urine and feces (7% to 18%); about 60% of dose is excreted as the conjugated form within 6 days.

Contraindications and precautions
Contraindicated in patients with hypersensitivity to drug, during acute recovery phase of MI, and in those who have received an MAO inhibitor within the past 14 days.
    Use cautiously in patients with history of urine retention, CV disease, angle-closure glaucoma, or increased intraocular pressure. Use with extreme caution in patients with history of seizures.

Interactions
Drug-drug. *Antiarrhythmics (disopyramide, procainamide, quinidine), pimozide, thyroid drugs:* May increase arrhythmias and conduction defects. Monitor ECG.
Barbiturates: Induce amoxapine metabolism and decrease therapeutic efficacy. Observe patient for drug effect.
Beta blockers, cimetidine, methylphenidate, oral contraceptives, propoxyphene: May inhibit amoxapine metabolism, increasing plasma levels and toxicity. Monitor amoxapine levels.
Centrally acting antihypertensives such as clonidine, guanabenz, guanadrel, guanethidine, methyldopa, reserpine: May decrease hypotensive effects. Monitor blood pressure.
CNS depressants (such as analgesics, anesthetics, alcohol, barbiturates, narcotics, tranquilizers), atropine or other anticholinergics (such as antihistamines, antiparkinsonians), meperidine, metrizamide, phenothiazines: Possible additive effects, such as oversedation, paralytic ileus, visual changes, severe constipation, increased risk of seizures. Monitor patient carefully.
Disulfiram, ethchlorvynol: May cause delirium and tachycardia. Monitor patient carefully.
Haloperidol, phenothiazines: Decreased drug metabolism, decreasing therapeutic efficacy. Monitor patient for drug effect.
Sympathomimetics, such as ephedrine, epinephrine, phenylephrine, phenylpropanolamine: May increase blood pressure. Use with caution.
Warfarin: May increase PT and cause bleeding. Monitor patient for bleeding; monitor PT.
Drug-lifestyle. *Heavy smoking:* Induces amoxapine metabolism and decreases therapeutic efficacy. Discourage concomitant use.

Sun exposure: Possible photosensitivity reactions. Patient should take precautions.

Adverse reactions
CNS: *drowsiness, dizziness,* excitation, tremor, weakness, confusion, anxiety, insomnia, restlessness, nightmares, ataxia, fatigue, headache, nervousness, *tardive dyskinesia, EEG changes,* **seizures, neuroleptic malignant syndrome** (high fever, tachycardia, tachypnea, profuse diaphoresis).
CV: *orthostatic hypotension, tachycardia,* hypertension, palpitations.
EENT: *blurred vision.*
GI: *dry mouth, constipation,* nausea, excessive appetite.
GU: *urine retention, acute renal failure* (with overdose).
Skin: rash, edema.
Other: *diaphoresis.*
    After abrupt withdrawal of long-term therapy: nausea, headache, malaise (doesn't indicate addiction).

☑ Special considerations
Besides the recommendations for all tricyclic antidepressants, consider the following.
• Amoxapine is associated with a high risk of seizures.
• Antidepressants can cause manic episodes during the depressed phase in patients with bipolar disorder.
• The full dose may be given at bedtime to help reduce daytime sedation.
• The full dose shouldn't be withdrawn abruptly.
• Tolerance to sedative effects usually develops over the first few weeks of therapy.
• Discontinue drug at least 48 hours before surgical procedures.
• Sugarless chewing gum, hard candy, or ice may alleviate dry mouth.
• Tardive dyskinesia and other extrapyramidal effects may occur because of the dopamine-blocking activity of amoxapine.
• Watch for gynecomastia in men and women; amoxapine may increase cellular division in breast tissue.
• Amoxapine may prolong conduction time (elongation of QT and PR intervals, flattened T waves on ECG).
• Drug may elevate liver function test results, decrease WBC counts, and decrease or increase serum glucose levels.
• The first 12 hours after acute ingestion are a stimulatory phase characterized by excessive anticholinergic activity (agitation, irritation, confusion, hallucinations, hyperthermia, parkinsonian symptoms, seizures, urine retention, dry mucous membranes, pupillary dilation, constipation, and ileus). This is followed by CNS depressant effects, including hypothermia, decreased or absent reflexes, sedation, hypotension, cyanosis,

and cardiac irregularities, including tachycardia, conduction disturbances, and quinidine-like effects on the ECG.
• Overdose produces a much higher risk of CNS toxicity than do other antidepressants. Acute deterioration of renal function (evidenced by myoglobin in urine) occurs in 5% of overdosed patients; this is most likely to occur in patients with repeated seizures after the overdose. Seizures may progress to status epilepticus within 12 hours
• Severity of overdose is best indicated by widening of the QRS complex, which generally represents a serum level in excess of 1,000 ng/ml; serum levels aren't usually helpful. Metabolic acidosis may follow hypotension, hypoventilation, and seizures.
• Treatment of overdose is symptomatic and supportive, including maintaining airway, stable body temperature, and fluid and electrolyte balance; monitor renal status because of the risk of renal failure. Induce emesis with ipecac if patient is conscious; follow with gastric lavage and activated charcoal to prevent further absorption. Dialysis is of little use. Treat seizures with parenteral diazepam or phenytoin (the value of physostigmine is less certain); arrhythmias, with parenteral phenytoin or lidocaine; and acidosis, with sodium bicarbonate. Don't give barbiturates; these may enhance CNS and respiratory depressant effects.

Monitoring the patient
• Monitor vital signs and ECG.
• Monitor patient for signs of seizures and neuroleptic malignant syndrome (high fever, tachycardia, tachypnea, profuse diaphoresis).

Information for the patient
• Explain that full effects of drug may not become apparent for at least 2 or more weeks after therapy begins, perhaps not for 4 to 6 weeks.
• Tell patient to take drug exactly as prescribed; however, full dose may be taken at bedtime to alleviate daytime sedation. Patient shouldn't double dose for missed ones.
• Warn patient that hazardous activities that require alertness should be avoided until drug's full effects are known.
• Tell patient not to drink alcoholic beverages while taking drug.
• Suggest that patient take drug with food or milk if it causes stomach upset; dry mouth can be relieved with sugarless gum or hard candy.
• After initial doses, tell patient to lie down for about 30 minutes and rise slowly to prevent dizziness.
• Warn patient not to discontinue drug suddenly.
• Encourage patient to report unusual or troublesome reactions immediately, especially confusion, movement disorders, rapid heartbeat, dizziness, fainting, or difficulty urinating.

Reactions may be *common,* uncommon, *life-threatening,* or COMMON AND LIFE-THREATENING.

• Inform patient that exposure to sunlight, sun-lamps, or tanning beds may cause burning of the skin or abnormal pigmentary changes.

Geriatric patients
• Lower doses are indicated because older patients are more sensitive to therapeutic and adverse effects of drug.
• Elderly patients are much more susceptible to tardive dyskinesia and extrapyramidal symptoms.

Pediatric patients
• Drug isn't recommended for patients under age 16.

Breast-feeding patients
• Amoxapine appears in breast milk (20% of maternal serum as parent drug and 30% as metabolites). Potential benefits to the mother should outweigh possible adverse reactions in the infant.

amoxicillin/clavulanate potassium
Augmentin, Clavulin*

Pharmacologic classification: amino-penicillin and beta-lactamase inhibitor
Therapeutic classification: antibiotic
Pregnancy risk category B

How supplied
Available by prescription only
Tablets (chewable): 125 mg amoxicillin trihydrate, 31.25 mg clavulanic acid; 200 mg amoxicillin trihydrate, 31.25 mg clavulanic acid; 250 mg amoxicillin trihydrate, 62.5 mg clavulanic acid; 400 mg amoxicillin trihydrate, 62.5 mg clavulanic acid
Tablets (film-coated): 250 mg amoxicillin trihydrate, 125 mg clavulanic acid; 500 mg amoxicillin trihydrate, 125 mg clavulanic acid; 875 mg amoxicillin trihydrate, 125 mg clavulanic acid
Oral suspension: 125 mg amoxicillin trihydrate and 31.25 mg clavulanic acid/5 ml (after reconstitution); 200 mg amoxicillin trihydrate and 28.5 mg clavulanic acid/5 ml (after reconstitution); 250 mg amoxicillin trihydrate and 62.5 mg clavulanic acid/5 ml (after reconstitution); 400 mg amoxicillin trihydrate and 57 mg clavulanic acid/5 ml (after reconstitution)

Indications, route, and dosage
Lower respiratory infections, otitis media, sinusitis, skin and skin-structure infections, and urinary tract infections caused by susceptible organisms
Adults and children weighing over 40 kg (88 lb): 250 mg (based on amoxicillin component) P.O. q 8 hours or 1 500-mg tablet q 12 hours. For more severe infections, 500 mg q 8 hours or 875 mg q 12 hours.

Children weighing under 40 kg: 20 to 40 mg/kg/day P.O. (based on amoxicillin component) given in divided doses q 8 hours.

Pharmacodynamics
Antibiotic action: Amoxicillin is bactericidal; it adheres to bacterial penicillin-binding proteins, thus inhibiting bacterial cell wall synthesis.

Clavulanate has only weak antibacterial activity and doesn't affect mechanism of action of amoxicillin. However, clavulanic acid has a beta-lactam ring and is structurally similar to penicillin and cephalosporins; it binds irreversibly with certain beta-lactamases and prevents them from inactivating amoxicillin, enhancing its bactericidal activity.

This combination acts against penicillinase-and non-penicillinase-producing gram-positive bacteria, *Neisseria gonorrhoeae, N. meningitidis, Haemophilus influenzae, Escherichia coli, Proteus mirabilis, Citrobacter diversus, Klebsiella pneumoniae, P. vulgaris, Salmonella,* and *Shigella.*

Pharmacokinetics
• *Absorption:* Amoxicillin and clavulanate potassium are well absorbed after oral administration; serum levels peak at 1 to 2½ hours.
• *Distribution:* Both amoxicillin and clavulanate potassium distribute into pleural fluid, lungs, and peritoneal fluid; high urine levels are attained. Amoxicillin also is distributed into synovial fluid, liver, prostate, muscle, and gallbladder; and penetrates into middle ear effusions, maxillary sinus secretions, tonsils, sputum, and bronchial secretions. Amoxicillin and clavulanate cross the placenta and low levels appear in breast milk. Amoxicillin and clavulanate potassium have minimal protein-binding of 17% to 20% and 22% to 30%, respectively.
• *Metabolism:* Amoxicillin is metabolized only partially. The metabolic fate of clavulanate potassium isn't completely identified, but it appears to undergo extensive metabolism.
• *Excretion:* Amoxicillin is excreted principally in urine by renal tubular secretion and glomerular filtration; drug is also excreted in breast milk.

Clavulanate potassium is excreted by glomerular filtration. Elimination half-life of amoxicillin in adults is 1 to 1½ hours; prolonged to 7½ hours in patients with severe renal impairment. Half-life of clavulanate in adults is about 1 to 1½ hours, prolonged to 4½ hours in patients with severe renal impairment.

Both drugs are removed readily by hemodialysis and minimally removed by peritoneal dialysis.

Contraindications and precautions
Contraindicated in patients with hypersensitivity to drug or other penicillins and in those with a previous history of amoxicillin-associated cholestatic jaundice or hepatic dysfunction. An oral peni-

cillin shouldn't be used in patients with severe pneumonia, empyema, bacteremia, pericarditis, meningitis, and purulent or septic arthritis. Use with caution in patients with mononucleosis.

Interactions

Drug-drug. *Allopurinol:* Appears to increase risk of rash from both drugs. Use together cautiously.

Methotrexate: Large doses of penicillins may interfere with renal tubular secretion of methotrexate, delaying elimination and prolonging elevated serum levels of methotrexate. Monitor levels.

Oral contraceptives: Concomitant use may reduce contraceptive effectiveness. Recommend alternative birth control method.

Probenecid: Blocks tubular secretion of amoxicillin, raising its serum levels; has no effect on clavulanate.

Adverse reactions

CNS: agitation, anxiety, insomnia, confusion, behavioral changes, dizziness.

GI: *nausea,* vomiting, *diarrhea,* indigestion, gastritis, stomatitis, glossitis, black "hairy" tongue, enterocolitis, pseudomembranous colitis.

Hematologic: anemia, *thrombocytopenia,* thrombocytopenic purpura, eosinophilia, leukopenia, *agranulocytosis.*

Other: hypersensitivity reactions (erythematous maculopapular rash, urticaria, *anaphylaxis*), overgrowth of nonsusceptible organisms, vaginitis.

☑ Special considerations

Besides the recommendations for all penicillins, consider the following.

● Oral dosage is maximally absorbed from an empty stomach, but food doesn't cause significant impairment of absorption.

● Suspension is stable for 10 days in refrigerator after reconstitution.

● When using film-coated tablets, be aware that both dosages contain different amounts of amoxicillin, but the same amount of clavulanate; therefore two 250-mg tablets aren't the equivalent of one 500-mg tablet.

● Because amoxicillin/clavulanate potassium is dialyzable, patients undergoing hemodialysis may need dosage adjustments.

● Amoxicillin/potassium clavulanate alters results of urine glucose tests that use cupric sulfate (Benedict's reagent or Clinitest). Make urine glucose determinations with glucose oxidase methods (Chemstrip uG or Diastix or glucose enzymatic test strip).

● Positive Coombs' tests have been reported with other clavulanate combinations.

● Amoxicillin/potassium clavulanate may produce a positive direct antiglobulin test (DAT).

● Clinical signs of overdose include neuromuscular sensitivity or seizures.

● After recent ingestion (4 hours or less), empty the stomach by induced emesis or gastric lavage; follow with activated charcoal to reduce absorption.

● Amoxicillin/clavulanate potassium can be removed by hemodialysis.

Monitoring the patient

● Monitor patient for signs of hypersensitivity to drug.

● Monitor patient for signs of internal bleeding.

Information for the patient

● Tell patient to chew chewable tablets thoroughly or crush before swallowing and wash down with liquid to ensure adequate absorption of drug; capsule may be emptied and contents swallowed with water.

● Instruct patient to report diarrhea promptly.

● Inform patient to complete full course of medication.

Geriatric patients

● In elderly patients, diminished renal tubular secretion may prolong half-life of amoxicillin.

Breast-feeding patients

● Both amoxicillin and potassium clavulanate appear in breast milk; use drug with caution in breast-feeding women.

amoxicillin trihydrate
Amoxil, Polymox, Trimox, Wymox

Pharmacologic classification: aminopenicillin
Therapeutic classification: antibiotic
Pregnancy risk category B

How supplied

Available by prescription only
Tablets (chewable): 125 mg, 250 mg
Capsules: 250 mg, 500 mg
Suspension: 125 mg/5 ml, 250 mg/5 ml
Pediatric drops: 50 mg/ml (after reconstitution)

Indications, route, and dosage

Systemic infections, acute and chronic urinary or respiratory tract infections caused by susceptible organisms, uncomplicated urinary tract infections caused by susceptible organisms

Adults: 250 mg P.O. q 8 hours. In adults and children weighing over 20 kg (44 lb) who have severe infections or those caused by susceptible organisms, 500 mg q 8 hours may be needed.

Children: 20 to 40 mg/kg P.O. daily, divided into doses given q 8 hours.

Pediatric drops: children under 6 kg (13 lb), 0.75 ml q 8 hours; 6 to 7 kg (13 to 15 lb), 1 ml q 8 hours; 7 to 8 kg (16 to 18 lb), 1.25 ml q 8 hours.

Children with lower respiratory tract infection only weighing under 6 kg, 1.25 ml q 8 hours; 6 to 7 kg, 1.75 ml q 8 hours; 7 to 8 kg, 2.25 ml q 8 hours.
Uncomplicated gonorrhea
Adults: 3 g P.O. as a single dose.
Children over age 2: 50 mg/kg given with 25 mg/kg probenecid as a single dose.
✦ **Dosage adjustment.** In renal failure, patients who require repeated doses may need adjustment of dosing interval. If creatinine clearance is 10 to 30 ml/minute, increase interval to q 12 hours; if creatinine clearance is less than 10 ml/minute, administer q 24 hours. Supplemental doses may be necessary after hemodialysis.
Oral prophylaxis of bacterial endocarditis
Consult current American Heart Association recommendations before administering drug.
Adults: 2 g 1 hour before procedure.
Children: 50 mg/kg 1 hour before procedure.

Pharmacodynamics
Antibacterial action: Bactericidal; adheres to bacterial penicillin-binding proteins, thus inhibiting bacterial cell-wall synthesis.

Spectrum of action includes non-penicillinase-producing gram-positive bacteria, *Streptococcus* group B, *Neisseria gonorrhoeae, Proteus mirabilis, Salmonella,* and *Haemophilus influenzae.* Also effective against non-penicillinase-producing *Staphylococcus aureus, S. pyogenes,* Streptococcus bovis, *S. pneumoniae, S. viridans, N. meningitidis, Escherichia coli, Salmonella typhi, Bordetella pertussis, Peptococcus,* and *Peptostreptococcus.*

Pharmacokinetics
● *Absorption:* About 80% absorbed after oral administration; serum levels peak at 1 to 2¼ hours after an oral dose.
● *Distribution:* Distributed into pleural peritoneal and synovial fluids and into the lungs, prostate, muscle, liver, and gallbladder; also penetrates middle ear, maxillary sinus and bronchial secretions, tonsils, and sputum. Readily crosses the placenta; about 17% to 20% is protein-bound.
● *Metabolism:* Metabolized only partially.
● *Excretion:* Excreted principally in urine by renal tubular secretion and glomerular filtration; also excreted in breast milk. Elimination half-life in adults is about 1 to 1¼ hours; severe renal impairment increases half-life to 7¼ hours.

Contraindications and precautions
Contraindicated in patients with hypersensitivity to drug or other penicillins. Use with caution in patients with mononucleosis.

Interactions
Drug-drug. *Allopurinol:* Appears to increase the risk of rash from both drugs. Monitor patient.

Clavulanate potassium: Enhances effect of amoxicillin against certain beta-lactamase-producing bacteria. Used for this therapeutic effect.
Methotrexate: Large doses of penicillins may interfere with renal tubular secretion of methotrexate, thus delaying elimination and prolonging elevated serum levels of methotrexate. Monitor patient and laboratory values for toxicity.
Oral contraceptives: Concomitant use may reduce contraceptive effectiveness. Recommend alternative birth control method.
Probenecid: Blocks renal tubular secretion of amoxicillin, raising its serum levels. Used for adjunctive antibiotic therapy.

Adverse reactions
CNS: lethargy, hallucinations, *seizures,* anxiety, confusion, agitation, depression, dizziness, fatigue.
GI: *nausea,* vomiting, *diarrhea,* glossitis, stomatitis, gastritis, abdominal pain, enterocolitis, pseudomembranous colitis, black "hairy" tongue.
GU: interstitial nephritis, nephropathy.
Hematologic: anemia, *thrombocytopenia,* thrombocytopenic purpura, eosinophilia, leukopenia, hemolytic anemia, *agranulocytosis.*
Other: hypersensitivity reactions (erythematous maculopapular rash, urticaria, *anaphylaxis*), overgrowth of nonsusceptible organisms, vaginitis.

☑ Special considerations
Besides the recommendations for all penicillins, consider the following.
● Oral dosage is maximally absorbed from an empty stomach, but food doesn't cause significant loss of potency.
● Pediatric drops may be placed on child's tongue or added to formula, milk, fruit juice, or soft drink. Be sure child ingests all of prepared dose.
● Suspension and drops are stable for 14 days in refrigerator after reconstitution.
● Amoxicillin may cause less diarrhea than ampicillin.
● Amoxicillin may alter results of urine glucose tests that use cupric sulfate (Benedict's reagent or Clinitest). Make urine glucose determinations with glucose oxidase methods (Chemstrip uG, Diastix, or glucose enzymatic test strip).
● Clinical signs of overdose include neuromuscular sensitivity or seizures.
● After recent ingestion (4 hours or less) in overdose, empty the stomach by induced emesis or gastric lavage; follow with activated charcoal to reduce absorption. Drug can be removed by hemodialysis.

Monitoring the patient
● Monitor renal, hepatic, and hematopoietic function periodically during prolonged therapy.
● Monitor patient for signs of allergic reaction.

Information for the patient
- Tell patient to chew tablets thoroughly or crush before swallowing and wash down with liquid to ensure adequate absorption of drug; capsule may be emptied and contents swallowed with water.
- Tell patient to report diarrhea promptly.
- Instruct patient to complete full course of drug.

Geriatric patients
- Because of diminished renal tubular secretion, half-life may be prolonged in elderly patients.

Breast-feeding patients
- Drug appears in breast milk; safe use in breast-feeding women hasn't been established. Alternative feeding method is recommended during therapy.

amphetamine sulfate

Pharmacologic classification: amphetamine
Therapeutic classification: CNS stimulant, short-term adjunctive anorexigenic, sympathomimetic amine
Controlled substance schedule II
Pregnancy risk category C

How supplied
Available by prescription only
Tablets: 5 mg, 10 mg

Indications, route, and dosage
Attention deficit disorder with hyperactivity
Children ages 6 and older: 5 mg P.O. daily. Increase at 5-mg increments weekly until desired response. Dosage rarely exceeds 40 mg/day. Give first dose upon awakening, and additional doses at 4- to 6-hour intervals.
Children ages 3 to 5: 2.5 mg P.O. daily; increase at 2.5-mg increments weekly until desired response is achieved.
Narcolepsy
Adults: 5 to 60 mg P.O. daily in divided doses or a single dose.
Children over age 12: 10 mg P.O. daily, with 10-mg increments weekly, p.r.n.
Children ages 6 to 12: 5 mg P.O. daily, with 5-mg increments weekly, p.r.n.
Short-term adjunct in exogenous obesity
Adults: 5 to 30 mg daily in divided doses of 5 to 10 mg.

Pharmacodynamics
CNS stimulant action: Amphetamines are sympathomimetic amines with CNS stimulant activity; in hyperactive children, they have a paradoxical calming effect. Used to treat narcolepsy and as adjuncts to psychosocial measures in attention deficit disorder (ADD) in children. The cerebral cortex and reticular activating system appear to be their primary sites of activity; amphetamines release nerve terminal stores of norepinephrine, promoting nerve impulse transmission. At high dosages, effects are mediated by dopamine.
Anorexigenic action: Anorexigenic effects are thought to occur in the hypothalamus, where decreased smell and taste acuity decreases the appetite. They may be tried for short-term control of refractory obesity, with caloric restriction and behavior modification.

Pharmacokinetics
- *Absorption:* Absorbed completely within 3 hours after oral administration; therapeutic effects persist for 4 to 24 hours.
- *Distribution:* Distributed widely throughout body, with high levels in the brain. Therapeutic plasma levels are 5 to 10 mcg/dl.
- *Metabolism:* Metabolized by hydroxylation and deamination in the liver.
- *Excretion:* Excreted in urine.

Contraindications and precautions
Contraindicated in patients with hypersensitivity or idiosyncrasy to sympathomimetic amines and in those with symptomatic CV disease, hyperthyroidism, moderate to severe hypertension, glaucoma, advanced arteriosclerosis, or history of drug abuse; within 14 days of MAO inhibitor therapy; and in agitated patients.
    Use cautiously in elderly, debilitated, or hyperexcitable patients and in those with suicidal or homicidal tendencies.

Interactions
Drug-drug. *Acetazolamide, antacids, sodium bicarbonate:* May enhance reabsorption of amphetamine and prolong its duration of action. Use together cautiously.
Ammonium chloride, ascorbic acid: Enhances amphetamine excretion or shortens duration of action. Observe for drug effects.
Antihypertensives: May antagonize their hypertensive effects. Avoid concomitant use.
Barbiturates: Counteract amphetamine by CNS depression. Monitor patient for drug effect.
Guanethidine: May decrease effectiveness of guanethidine. Use together cautiously.
Haloperidol, phenothiazines: Decreases amphetamine effects. Monitor patient carefully.
Insulin: May alter insulin requirements. Monitor glucose levels.
MAO inhibitors (or drugs with MAO-inhibiting effects such as furazolidone) or within 14 days of such therapy: May cause hypertensive crisis. Don't use concurrently or within this time period.
Other CNS stimulants: Produce additive effects. Monitor patient for cumulative effects.
Drug-food. *Caffeine:* Produces additive effects. Avoid using together.

Reactions may be *common*, uncommon, ***life-threatening***, or COMMON AND LIFE-THREATENING.

Adverse reactions

CNS: *restlessness,* tremor, *hyperactivity, talkativeness, insomnia,* irritability, dizziness, headache, chills, dysphoria, euphoria.
CV: *tachycardia, palpitations,* hypertension, ***arrhythmias.***
GI: dry mouth, metallic taste, diarrhea, constipation, anorexia, weight loss.
GU: impotence.
Skin: urticaria.
Other: altered libido, elevated plasma corticosteroid levels.

☑ Special considerations

● Recommendations for administration of amphetamine sulfate, for patient care and teaching during therapy, and for use in elderly or breastfeeding patients are the same as for all amphetamines.
● Avoid administration late in the day (after 4 p.m.) to prevent insomnia.
● Amphetamines may interfere with urinary corticosteroid determinations.
● Symptoms of acute overdose include increasing restlessness, irritability, insomnia, tremor, hyperreflexia, diaphoresis, mydriasis, flushing, confusion, hypertension, tachypnea, fever, delirium, self-injury, arrhythmias, seizures, coma, circulatory collapse, and death.
● Treat overdose symptomatically and supportively. If ingestion is recent (within 4 hours) use gastric lavage or emesis; activated charcoal, sodium chloride catharsis, and urinary acidification may enhance excretion. Forced fluid diuresis may help. In massive ingestion, hemodialysis or peritoneal dialysis may be needed. Keep patient in a cool room, monitor patient's temperature, and minimize external stimulation. Haloperidol may be used for psychotic symptoms; diazepam, for hyperactivity.

Monitoring the patient

● Monitor vital signs and ECG periodically during therapy.
● When used for ADD, interrupt drug administration occasionally to determine if there is a recurrence of behavioral symptoms sufficient to require continued therapy.

Information for the patient

● Instruct patient about the potential for drowsiness and tell patient to avoid activities that require alertness.

Pediatric patients

● Amphetamines aren't recommended for weight reduction in children under age 12; use of amphetamines for hyperactivity is contraindicated in children under age 3.

amphotericin B
Abelcet, Amphotec, Fungizone

Pharmacologic classification: polyene macrolide
Therapeutic classification: antifungal
Pregnancy risk category B

How supplied

Available by prescription only
Injection: 50-mg lyophilized cake; vials: 50 mg
Oral suspension: 100 mg/ml
Suspension for injection: 5 mg/ml
Cream: 3%
Lotion: 3%
Ointment: 3%

Indications, route, and dosage

Systemic (potentially fatal) fungal infections caused by susceptible organisms, ◊ *fungal endocarditis, fungal septicemia*
Adults and children: Some clinicians recommend an initial dose of 1 mg I.V. in 20 ml D_5W infused over 20 minutes. If test dose is tolerated, give daily doses of 0.25 to 0.30 mg/kg, gradually increasing by 5 to 10 mg/day until daily dose is 1 mg/kg/day or 1.5 mg/kg q alternate day. Duration of therapy depends upon severity and nature of infection.
Sporotrichosis: 0.4 to 0.5 mg/kg amphotericin B daily I.V. for up to 9 months. Total I.V. dosage of 2.5 g over 9 months.
Aspergillosis: Total I.V. dosage of 3.6 g over 11 months.
◊ **Fungal meningitis**
Adults: Intrathecal injection of 25 mcg/0.1 ml diluted with 10 to 20 ml of CSF and administered by barbotage 2 or 3 times weekly. Initial dose shouldn't exceed 50 mcg.
◊ **Candidal cystitis**
Adults: Bladder irrigations in concentrations of 5 to 50 mcg/ml instilled periodically or continuously for 5 to 7 days.
Oropharyngeal candidiasis
Adults and children: 100 mg/ml oral suspension q.i.d. swish and swallow.
Topical fungal infections (3% cream, lotion, ointment)
Adults and children: Apply liberally and rub well into affected area b.i.d. to q.i.d.
Cutaneous or mucocutaneous candidal infections
Adults and children: Apply topical product b.i.d., t.i.d., or q.i.d. for 1 to 3 weeks; apply up to several months for interdigital or paronychial lesions.
◊ **Sinus irrigation**
Adults: 1 mg/ml
◊ **Histoplasmal pulmonary and intrapleural effusion**
Adults: 15 to 20 mg with 25 mg hydrocortisone sodium succinate.

◇ *Pulmonary coccidioidomycosis*
Adults: Via intermittent positive pressure breathing device, 5 to 10 mg q.i.d.
◇ *Ophthalmic candidal infection*
Adults: 0.1 to 1 mg/ml drop suspension q 30 minutes.
Note: Intrathecal and intra-articular uses are unapproved.

Pharmacodynamics
Antifungal action: Fungistatic or *fungicidal,* depending on the levels available in body fluids and on the susceptibility of the fungus. Binds to sterols in the fungal cell membrane, increasing membrane permeability of fungal cells, causing subsequent leakage of intracellular components; also may interfere with some human cell membranes that contain sterols.

Spectrum of activity includes *Histoplasma capsulatum, Coccidioides immitis, Blastomyces dermatitidis, Cryptococcus neoformans, Candida* species, *Aspergillus fumigatus, Mucor* species, *Rhizopus* species, *Absidia* species, *Entomophthora* species, *Basidiobolus* species, *Paracoccidioides brasiliensis, Sporothrix schenckii,* and *Rhodotorula* species.

Pharmacokinetics
• *Absorption:* Absorbed poorly from the GI tract.
• *Distribution:* Distributed well into inflamed pleural cavities and joints; in low levels into aqueous humor, bronchial secretions, pancreas, bone, muscle, and parotids. CSF levels reach about 3% of serum levels. 90% to 95% bound to plasma proteins; reportedly crosses the placenta.
• *Metabolism:* Not well defined.
• *Excretion:* Elimination is biphasic: initial serum half-life of 24 hours, then a second phase half-life of about 15 days. About 2% to 5% excreted unchanged in urine. Isn't readily removed by hemodialysis.

Contraindications and precautions
Contraindicated in patients with hypersensitivity to drug. Use cautiously in patients with renal impairment.

Interactions
Drug-drug. *Aminoglycosides, cisplatin, other nephrotoxic drugs:* Added nephrotoxic effects. Avoid concomitant use when possible.
Corticosteroids: Added potassium depletion. Monitor serum electrolyte levels and cardiac function.
Digoxin: Increased risk of digitalis toxicity. Avoid concurrent use.
Flucytosine, other antibiotics: Concurrent use potentiates effects of these drugs. Use together cautiously.
Skeletal muscle relaxants: Amphotericin B–induced hypokalemia may enhance effects of skeletal muscle relaxants. Use together cautiously.

Drug-herb. *Gossypol:* May increase risk of renal toxicity. Avoid concomitant use.

Adverse reactions
CNS: *malaise, headache,* peripheral neuropathy, *seizures with systemic form.*
CV: hypotension, *arrhythmias, asystole,* hypertension with systemic form.
EENT: hearing loss, tinnitus, transient vertigo, blurred vision, diplopia with systemic form.
GI: *anorexia, weight loss, nausea, vomiting, dyspepsia, diarrhea, epigastric pain, cramping,* melena, *hemorrhagic gastroenteritis with systemic form,* increased alkaline phosphatase, and bilirubin levels.
GU: *abnormal renal function with hypokalemia, azotemia, hyposthenuria, renal tubular acidosis, nephrocalcinosis;* with large doses, *permanent renal impairment,* anuria, oliguria with systemic form.
Hematologic: *normochromic, normocytic anemia, thrombocytopenia,* leukopenia, *agranulocytosis,* eosinophilia, leukocytosis with systemic form.
Hepatic: hepatitis, jaundice, *acute liver failure with systemic form.*
Metabolic: hypokalemia, hypomagnesemia.
Musculoskeletal: arthralgia, myalgia.
Respiratory: dyspnea, tachypnea, bronchospasm, wheezing with systemic form.
Skin: maculopapular rash, pruritus without rash with systemic form; possible dryness, contact sensitivity, erythema, burning, pruritus with topical administration.
Other: tissue damage with extravasation, *phlebitis, thrombophlebitis, pain at injection site, fever, chills, generalized pain,* flushing, *anaphylactoid reactions with topical administration.*

☑ Special considerations
• There are differences in amphotericin B products. Don't use interchangeably.
• Cultures and histologic and sensitivity testing must be completed and diagnosis confirmed before starting therapy in nonimmunocompromised patient.
• Prepare infusion as manufacturer directs, with strict aseptic technique, using only 10 ml of sterile water to reconstitute. To avoid precipitation, don't mix with solutions containing sodium chloride, other electrolytes, or bacteriostatic drugs such as benzyl alcohol.
• Lyophilized cake contains no preservatives. Don't use if solution contains a precipitate or other foreign particles. Store cake at 35.6° to 46.4° F (2° to 8° C). Protect drug from light, and check expiration date.
• For I.V. infusion, use an in-line membrane with a mean pore diameter larger than 1 micron. Abelcet and Amphotec shouldn't be used with a filter.
• Infuse slowly; rapid infusion may cause CV collapse.

- Don't mix or piggyback antibiotics with amphotericin B infusion; the I.V. solution appears compatible with small amounts of heparin sodium, hydrocortisone sodium succinate, and methylprednisolone sodium succinate.
- Give in distal veins, and monitor site for discomfort or thrombosis. If thrombosis occurs, alternate-day therapy may be considered.
- Severity of some adverse reactions can be reduced by premedication with aspirin or acetaminophen, antihistamines, antiemetics, meperidine, or small doses of corticosteroids; by addition of phosphate buffer to the solution; and by alternate-day dosing. If reactions are severe, drug may have to be discontinued for varying periods.
- Use topical products for folds of groin, neck, or armpit; avoid occlusive dressing with ointment, and discontinue if signs of hypersensitivity develop.
- Store at room temperature. Solution is stable at room temperature and in indoor light for 24 hours or in the refrigerator for 1 week.
- Overdose may affect CV and respiratory function. Treatment is largely supportive.

Monitoring the patient
- Check vital signs every 30 minutes for at least 4 hours after start of I.V. infusion; fever may appear in 1 to 2 hours but should subside within 4 hours of discontinuing drug.
- Monitor intake and output and check for changes in urine appearance or volume; renal damage may be reversible if drug is stopped at earliest sign of dysfunction.
- Monitor potassium and magnesium levels closely; monitor calcium and magnesium levels twice weekly; perform liver and renal function studies and CBCs weekly

Information for the patient
- Teach patient signs and symptoms of hypersensitivity and other adverse reactions, especially those associated with I.V. therapy. Warn that fever and chills are likely to occur and can be quite severe when therapy is initiated. These symptoms usually subside with repeated doses. Encourage patient feedback during infusion.
- Warn patient that therapy may take several months; teach personal hygiene and other measures to prevent spread and recurrence of lesions.
- Urge patient to adhere to regimen and to return, as instructed, for follow-up.
- Tell patient that topical products may stain skin and clothing; cream or lotion may be removed from clothing with soap and water.

Breast-feeding patients
- Safety hasn't been established in breast-feeding patients.

amphotericin B cholesteryl sulfate complex
Amphotec

Pharmacologic classification: polyene macrolide
Therapeutic classification: antifungal
Pregnancy risk category B

How supplied
Available by prescription only
Injection: 50 mg/20 ml, 100 mg/50 ml

Indications, route, and dosage
Invasive aspergillosis in patients in whom renal impairment or unacceptable toxicity precludes use of amphotericin B deoxycholate in effective doses and in those with invasive aspergillosis in whom prior amphotericin B deoxycholate therapy has failed; ◊ *Candida and Cryptococcus infections not responsive or tolerable to conventional amphotericin B*
Adults and children: 3 to 4 mg/kg/day I.V.; may increase to 6 mg/kg/day if no improvement occurs or if fungal infection has progressed. Administer by continuous infusion at 1 mg/kg/hour.

Pharmacodynamics
Fungistatic/fungicidal action: Depends on level of drug and susceptibility of fungal organism. Binds to sterols in cell membranes of sensitive fungi, resulting in leakage of intracellular contents and causing cell death due to changes in membrane permeability. Also binds to sterols in mammalian cell membranes, which is believed to account for human toxicity.
    Spectrum of activity includes *Aspergillus fumigatus, Candida albicans, Coccidioides immitis,* and *Cryptococcus neoformans.*

Pharmacokinetics
- *Absorption:* For an infusion rate of 1 mg/kg/hour and dosage ranges from 3 to 6 mg/kg/day, maximum plasma level at the end of an infusion ranges from 2.6 to 3.4 mcg/ml.
- *Distribution:* Multicompartmental; steady-state volume increases with higher doses, possibly from uptake by tissues.
- *Metabolism:* No information available.
- *Excretion:* Unclear; elimination half-life, 27 to 29 hours; increasing doses increase the elimination half-life. Drug may not be removed by dialysis.

Contraindications and precautions
Contraindicated in patients with hypersensitivity to drug or its components unless benefits outweigh risk of hypersensitivity.

Interactions

No formal drug interaction studies completed; however, the following drugs are known to interact with amphotericin B.

Drug-drug. *Antineoplastics:* Enhanced renal toxicity, bronchospasm, hypotension. Use together cautiously.

Cardiac glycosides: Enhanced potassium excretion; increases risk of digitalis toxicity. Use together cautiously.

Corticosteroids: Enhanced potassium depletion; could predispose patient to cardiac dysfunction. Monitor patient.

Cyclosporine, tacrolimus: Possibly increased serum creatinine levels. Monitor creatinine levels.

Flucytosine: May cause synergistic effect and increased toxicity of flucytosine. Monitor patient carefully.

Imidazoles (clotrimazole, fluconazole, ketoconazole, miconazole): May cause antagonistic effects, although significance isn't determined. Use together cautiously.

Nephrotoxic drugs (such as aminoglycosides, pentamidine): May enhance renal toxicity. Monitor renal function closely.

Skeletal muscle relaxants such as tubocurarine: Amphotericin B–induced hypokalemia may enhance effects of skeletal muscle relaxants. Monitor serum potassium levels closely.

Drug-herb. *Gossypol:* Increases risk of renal toxicity. Avoid use together.

Adverse reactions

CNS: abnormal thoughts, anxiety, agitation, confusion, depression, dizziness, hallucinations, headache, hypertonia, neuropathy, paresthesia, *seizures,* somnolence, stupor.

CV: *arrhythmias, atrial fibrillation, bradycardia, cardiac arrest, heart failure, hemorrhage,* hypertension, *hypotension,* phlebitis, syncope, orthostatic hypotension, *shock, supraventricular tachycardia,* tachycardia, *ventricular extrasystoles.*

EENT: eye hemorrhage, tinnitus.

GI: anorexia, GI disorder, GI hemorrhage, hematemesis, melena, *nausea,* stomatitis, *vomiting.*

GU: abnormal renal function, hematuria, *renal failure.*

Hematologic: anemia, agranulocytosis, coagulation disorders, hypochromic anemia, increased PT, leukocytosis, *leukopenia, thrombocytopenia.*

Hepatic: jaundice, abnormal liver function test results, *hepatic failure.*

Metabolic: *hypokalemia,* hypocalcemia, hyperglycemia, hypervolemia, hypophosphatemia, hyponatremia, hyperkalemia, *increased creatinine, bilirubinemia,* hypomagnesemia, alkaline phosphatase, BUN, AST, ALT, LD levels.

Musculoskeletal: arthralgia, myalgia.

Respiratory: *apnea,* asthma, dyspnea, epistaxis, hemoptysis, hyperventilation, hypoxia, increased cough, lung or respiratory disorders, *pulmonary edema.*

Skin: pruritus, rash, sweating, skin disorder.

Other: *allergic reaction; anaphylaxis;* asthenia; *chills;* edema; *fever;* abdominal, chest, or back pain; peripheral or facial edema; infection; mucous membrane disorder; pain or reaction at injection site; sepsis.

☑ Special considerations

● Pretreatment with antihistamines and corticosteroids or reducing rate of infusion (or both) may reduce acute infusion-related reactions.

● Dilute in D_5W and administer by continuous infusion at 1 mg/kg/hour. Perform a test dose before commencing new courses of treatment; infuse a small amount of drug (10 ml of final preparation containing 1.6 to 8.3 mg of amphotericin B) over 15 to 30 minutes and Monitor patient for next 30 minutes. Can shorten infusion time to 2 hours or lengthen infusion time based on patient tolerance.

● Drug is incompatible with saline, electrolyte solutions, and bacteriostatic drugs.

● Infuse drug over at least 2 hours.

● Don't mix with other drugs. If administered through an existing I.V. line, flush line with D_5W before infusion or use a separate line.

● Store vials at room temperature. Reconstitute 50-mg vial with rapid addition of 10 ml of sterile water for injection, and 100-mg vial with rapid addition of 20 ml sterile water with a sterile syringe and 20G needle. Shake vial gently. Don't use diluent other than sterile water for injection.

● Reconstituted drug is clear or opalescent liquid and is stable for 24 hours refrigerated. Discard partially used vials.

● Don't filter or use an in-line filter; don't freeze.

● Amphotec isn't dialyzable. Amphotericin B deoxycholate overdose may result in cardiorespiratory arrest.

● If overdose is suspected, discontinue therapy, monitor clinical status, and administer supportive therapy.

Monitoring the patient

● Monitor vital signs every 30 minutes during initial therapy. Acute infusion-related reactions (fever, chills, hypotension, nausea, tachycardia) usually occur 1 to 3 hours after starting I.V. infusion. These reactions are usually more severe after initial doses and usually diminish with subsequent doses. If severe respiratory distress occurs, stop infusion immediately and don't treat further with drug.

● Monitor intake and output; report changes in urine appearance or volume.

● Monitor renal and hepatic function tests, serum electrolytes (especially potassium, magnesium, and calcium), CBCs, and PT.

Information for the patient

● Instruct patient to report symptoms of hypersensitivity immediately.

Reactions may be *common,* uncommon, *life-threatening,* or COMMON AND LIFE-THREATENING.

- Warn patient of possible discomfort at I.V. site.
- Advise patient of potential adverse effects, such as fever, chills, nausea, and vomiting. Tell patient that these can be severe with initial treatment but usually subside with repeated doses.

Breast-feeding patients
- It's unknown if drug appears in breast milk. Because of the potential for serious adverse reactions in breast-fed infants, a decision should be made to discontinue breast-feeding or to stop treatment, taking into account the importance of drug to the mother.

amphotericin B lipid complex
Abelcet

Pharmacologic classification: polyene antibiotic
Therapeutic classification: antifungal
Pregnancy risk category B

How supplied
Available by prescription only
Suspension for injection: 100 mg/20-ml vial

Indications, route, and dosage
Invasive fungal infections, including As-pergillus fumigatus, Candida albicans, C. guillermondii, C. stellatoidea, *and* C. tropi-calis, Cryptococcus sp., Coccidioidomyces sp., Histoplasma sp., *and* Blastomyces sp. *in patients who are refractory to or intolerant of conventional amphotericin B therapy
Adults and children: 5 mg/kg daily as a single I.V. infusion. Administer by continuous I.V. infusion at a rate of 2.5 mg/kg/hour.

Pharmacodynamics
Antifungal activity: Binds to sterols in fungal cell membranes, resulting in enhanced cellular permeability and cell damage. Has fungistatic or fungicidal effects depending on fungal susceptibility.

Pharmacokinetics
- *Absorption:* Given I.V.
- *Distribution:* Well distributed; distribution volume increases with increasing dose. Drug yields measurable amphotericin B levels in spleen, lung, liver, lymph nodes, kidney, heart, and brain.
- *Metabolism:* No information available.
- *Excretion:* Although rapidly cleared from blood, drug has long terminal half-life (173.4 hours), probably due to slow elimination from tissues.

Contraindications and precautions
Contraindicated in patients with a history of hy-persensitivity to amphotericin B or any of its components. Use cautiously in patients with renal impairment.

Interactions
Drug-drug. *Antineoplastics:* Increased risk of renal toxicity, bronchospasm, and hypotension. Use cautiously.
Cardiac glycosides: Increased risk of digitalis toxicity due to Amphotericin B–induced hypokalemia. Monitor serum potassium levels closely.
Corticosteroids, corticotropin: Enhanced hypokalemia, which may lead to cardiac toxicity. Monitor serum electrolytes and cardiac function.
Cyclosporine A: Increased renal toxicity. Monitor closely.
Flucytosine: Increased risk of flucytosine toxicity due to increased cellular uptake or impaired renal excretion. Use cautiously.
Imidazoles (clotrimazole, fluconazole, itracona-zole, ketoconazole, miconazole): Decreased efficacy of amphotericin B due to inhibition of ergosterol synthesis. Clinical significance is unknown.
Leukocyte transfusions: Acute pulmonary toxicity. Avoid concurrent use.
Nephrotoxic drugs (aminoglycosides, pentami-dine): Increased risk of renal toxicity. Use cautiously and monitor renal function closely.
Skeletal muscle relaxants: Enhanced effects of skeletal muscle relaxants due to amphotericin B–induced hypokalemia. Monitor serum potassium levels closely.
Zidovudine: Increased myelotoxicity and nephrotoxicity. Monitor renal and hematologic function.

Adverse reactions
CNS: headache, pain.
CV: chest pain, *cardiac arrest,* hypertension, hypotension.
GI: abdominal pain, diarrhea, *GI hemorrhage,* nausea, vomiting.
GU: *increased serum creatinine, kidney failure.*
Hematologic: anemia, *leukopenia, thrombo-cytopenia.*
Hepatic: bilirubinemia.
Metabolic: hypokalemia.
Respiratory: dyspnea, respiratory disorder, *res-piratory failure.*
Skin: rash.
Other: *chills, fever,* infection, MULTIPLE ORGAN FAILURE, *sepsis.*

☑ Special considerations
- Use cautiously in patients with renal impairment. Base dosage adjustment on overall status of patient. Renal toxicity is more common at higher doses.
- Different amphotericin B preparations aren't interchangeable and dosages vary.
- Premedicate with acetaminophen, antihistamines, and corticosteroids as ordered to prevent or lessen the severity of infusion-related reactions (fever, chills, nausea, and vomiting), which occur 1 to 2 hours after infusion start. These reactions are usually more common with the first

few doses of drug and generally diminish with subsequent doses.

• Slowing the infusion rate may also decrease infusion-related reactions. For infusions lasting more than 2 hours, shake the I.V. bag every 2 hours for even suspension.

• If severe respiratory distress occurs, discontinue infusion and provide supportive therapy for anaphylaxis. Drug shouldn't be reinstituted.

• Don't mix with saline or infuse in the same IV line as other medications. Don't use an in-line filter.

• If infusing through an existing I.V. line, flush first with D_5W.

• Infusions are stable for up to 48 hours under refrigeration 35.6° to 46.4° (2° to 8° C) and up to 6 hours at room temperature.

• Store under refrigeration 35.6° to 46.4° (2° to 8° C) and protect from light. Don't freeze.

• For patients with cardiovascular disease, recommended final concentration is 2 mg/ml.

• Overdose has been associated with cardio-respiratory arrest. Doses as high as 7 to 13 mg/kg haven't produced serious acute toxicity.

• If overdose is suspected, discontinue therapy, monitor patient's condition, and provide supportive treatment, as needed. Drug isn't removed by hemodialysis.

Monitoring the patient
• Monitor serum creatinine and electrolyte (especially magnesium and potassium) levels, liver function, and CBC during therapy.

• Monitor patient for adverse effects.

Information for the patient
• Inform patient that fever, chills, nausea, and vomiting may occur during infusion; these reactions usually subside with subsequent doses.

• Instruct patient to report any redness or pain at infusion site.

• Teach patient to recognize and report any symptoms of acute hypersensitivity such as respiratory distress.

• Warn patient that therapy may take several months.

• Tell patient to expect frequent laboratory testing to monitor kidney and liver function.

Geriatric patients
• No unexpected adverse reactions have been reported when patients are treated with 5 mg/kg/day.

Pediatric patients
• No unexpected adverse reactions have been reported in children age 16 and younger when treated with 5 mg/kg/day.

• For pediatric patients, recommended final concentration is 2 mg/ml.

Breast-feeding patients
• It's unknown if drug appears in breast milk. The decision to administer drug should be based on risk of adverse reactions in the infant compared to benefits of treatment for the mother.

amphotericin B liposomal
AmBisome

Pharmacologic classification: polyene antibiotic
Therapeutic classification: antifungal
Pregnancy risk category B

How supplied
Available by prescription only
Injection: 50-mg vial

Indications, route, and dosage
Empirical therapy for presumed fungal infection in febrile, neutropenic patients
Adults and children: 3 mg/kg I.V. infusion daily.
Systemic fungal infections caused by Aspergillus species, Candida species or Cryptococcus species refractory to amphotericin B deoxycholate or in patients where renal impairment or unacceptable toxicity precludes the use of amphotericin B deoxycholate
Adults and children: 3 to 5 mg/kg I.V. infusion daily.
Visceral leishmaniasis in immunocompetent patients
Adults and children: 3 mg/kg I.V. infusion daily on days 1 to 5, 14 and 21. A repeat course may be beneficial if initial treatment fails to achieve parasitic clearance.
Visceral leishmaniasis in immunocompromised patients
Adults and children: 4 mg/kg I.V. infusion daily on days 1 to 5, 10, 17, 24, 31 and 38. Expert advice regarding further treatment is recommended if initial therapy fails or patient experiences a relapse.

Pharmacodynamics
Antifungal activity: Amphotericin B, the active component of AmBisome, binds to the sterol component of a fungal cell membrane, leading to alterations in cell permeability and cell death. AmBisome, the liposomal preparation of amphotericin B, penetrates the cell wall of both extracellular and intracellular forms of susceptible fungi.

Pharmacokinetics
• *Absorption:* Given I.V.
• *Distribution:* No information available.
• *Metabolism:* No information available.
• *Excretion:* Initial half-life is 7 to 10 hours with 24-hour dosing; terminal elimination half-life is 100 to 153 hours.

Contraindications and precautions

Contraindicated in patients with hypersensitivity to drug or its components. Use cautiously in patients with impaired renal function, those receiving chemotherapy or bone marrow transplantation, elderly patients, and pregnant women.

Interactions

Drug-drug. *Antineoplastics:* May enhance potential for renal toxicity, bronchospasm, and hypotension. Use cautiously.
Cardiac glycosides: Increased risk of digitalis toxicity in potassium-depleted patients. Monitor serum potassium level closely.
Corticosteroids, corticotropin (ACTH): May potentiate potassium depletion, which could result in cardiac dysfunction. Monitor serum potassium level and cardiac function.
Flucytosine: May increase flucytosine toxicity by increasing cellular reuptake or impairing renal excretion of flucytosine. Use together cautiously.
Imidazole antifungals (clotrimazole, ketoconazole, miconazole): May induce fungal resistance to amphotericin B. Use together cautiously.
Leukocyte transfusions: Risk of acute pulmonary toxicity. Avoid concomitant use.
Other nephrotoxic drugs (antibiotics, antineoplastics): May cause additive nephrotoxicity. Administer cautiously. Monitor renal function closely.
Skeletal muscle relaxants: Enhanced effects of skeletal muscle relaxants due to amphotericin-induced hypokalemia. Monitor serum potassium levels.

Adverse reactions

CNS: anxiety, confusion, headache, insomnia, asthenia.
CV: chest pain, hypotension, tachycardia, hypertension, edema, vasodilation.
EENT: epistaxis, rhinitis.
GI: nausea, vomiting, abdominal pain, diarrhea, *GI hemorrhage.*
GU: hematuria, elevated creatinine and BUN.
Hepatic: *hepatocellular damage,* hepatomegaly, elevated ALT and AST levels, increased alkaline phosphatase, bilirubinemia.
Metabolic: hyperglycemia, hypernatremia, hypocalcemia, hypokalemia, hypomagnesemia.
Musculoskeletal: back pain.
Respiratory: cough increase, dyspnea, hypoxia, pleural effusion, lung disorder, hyperventilation.
Skin: pruritus, rash, sweating.
Other: chills, infection, *anaphylaxis,* pain, *sepsis,* fever, blood product infusion reaction.

☑ Special considerations

• Patients concomitantly receiving chemotherapy or bone marrow transplantation are at greater risk for additional adverse reactions, including seizures, arrhythmias, thrombocytopenia, and respiratory failure.
• To lessen the risk or severity of adverse reactions, premedicate patient with antipyretics, antihistamines, antiemetics, or corticosteroids.
• Therapy may take several weeks to months.
• Patients treated with AmBisome have a lower risk of chills, elevated BUN level, hypokalemia, and vomiting than patients treated with regular amphotericin B.
• Don't reconstitute with bacteriostatic water for injection; don't allow a bacteriostatic agent in the solution. Don't reconstitute with saline or add saline to reconstituted concentration or mix with other drugs.
• An existing I.V. line must be flushed with D_5W before drug infusion. If not feasible, drug should be administered through a separate line.
• Use a controlled infusion device and an in-line filter with a mean pore diameter larger than 1 micron. Initially, infuse drug over at least 2 hours. Infusion time may be reduced to 1 hour if the treatment is well tolerated. If patient experiences discomfort during infusion, duration may be increased.
• Observe patient closely for adverse reactions during infusion. If anaphylaxis occurs, stop infusion immediately, provide supportive therapy.
• Store unopened drug under refrigeration (36° to 46° F [2° to 8° C]). Once reconstituted, product may be refrigerated up to 24 hours. Don't freeze.
• Repeated daily doses of up to 7.5 mg/kg have been given without toxicity.
• If overdose occurs, stop drug immediately. Symptomatic supportive measures should be used. Monitor renal function. Drug isn't hemodialyzable.

Monitoring the patient
• Monitor serum creatinine, BUN, and serum electrolyte levels (particularly magnesium and potassium), liver function studies, and CBC.
• Monitor patient for signs of hypokalemia (ECG changes, muscle weakness, cramping, drowsiness).

Information for the patient
• Teach patient signs and symptoms of hypersensitivity; stress importance of reporting them immediately.
• Warn patient that therapy may take several months; teach personal hygiene and other measures to prevent spread and recurrence of lesions.
• Instruct patient to report any adverse reactions that occur while receiving drug.
• Instruct patient to watch for and report any signs of hypokalemia (muscle weakness, cramping, drowsiness).
• Advise patient that frequent laboratory testing will be performed.

Geriatric patients
• No dosage adjustment required; elderly patients should be carefully monitored.

Pediatric patients
• Safety and effectiveness in children below age 1 month haven't been established.

Breast-feeding patients
• It's unknown if drug appears in breast milk. Because of the potential for serious adverse reactions in breast-fed infants, discontinue breast-feeding or discontinue drug based on importance of drug to mother.

ampicillin
Apo-Ampi*, Novo-Ampicillin*, Omnipen, Penbritin*

ampicillin sodium
Ampicin*, Omnipen-N, Penbritin*

ampicillin trihydrate
Omnipen, Principen, Totacillin

Pharmacologic classification: aminopenicillin
Therapeutic classification: antibiotic
Pregnancy risk category B

How supplied
Available by prescription only
Capsules: 250 mg, 500 mg
Suspension: 125 mg/5 ml, 250 mg/5 ml, 500 mg/5 ml (after reconstitution)
Parenteral: 125 mg, 250 mg, 500 mg, 1 g, 2 g
Infusion: 500 mg, 1 g, 2 g

Indications, route, and dosage
Systemic infections, acute and chronic urinary tract infections caused by susceptible organisms
Adults: 250 to 500 mg P.O. q 6 hours.
Children: 50 to 100 mg/kg P.O. daily, divided into doses given q 6 hours; or 100 to 200 mg/kg I.M. or I.V. daily, divided into doses given q 6 to 8 hours.
Meningitis
Adults: 8 to 14 g I.V. divided q 3 to 4 hours for 3 days; then may give I.M. if desired.
Children ages 2 months to 12 years: Up to 400 mg/kg I.V. daily for 3 days; then up to 300 mg/kg I.M. divided q 4 hours. May be given concurrently with chloramphenicol, pending culture results.
Uncomplicated gonorrhea
Adults: 3.5 g P.O. with 1 g probenecid given as a single dose.
✦ Dosage adjustment. Dosing interval should be increased to q 12 hours in patients with severe renal impairment (creatinine clearance 10 ml/minute or less).

Prophylaxis for Salmonella in patients infected with HIV
Adults: 50 to 100 mg P.O. q.i.d. for several months.
Prophylaxis for bacterial endocarditis before dental or minor respiratory procedures
Adults: 2 g (I.V. or I.M.) 30 minutes before procedure.
Children: 50 mg/kg I.V. or I.M. 30 minutes before procedure.

Pharmacodynamics
Antibiotic action: Bactericidal; adheres to bacterial penicillin-binding proteins, inhibiting bacterial cell-wall synthesis.
  Spectrum of action includes non-penicillinase-producing gram-positive bacteria. Also effective against many gram-negative organisms, including *Neisseria gonorrhoeae, N. meningitidis, Haemophilus influenzae, Escherichia coli, Proteus mirabilis, Salmonella,* and *Shigella.* Should be used in gram-negative systemic infections only when organism sensitivity is known.

Pharmacokinetics
• *Absorption:* About 42% absorbed after an oral dose; serum levels peak at 1 to 2 hours. After I.M. administration, serum levels peak at 1 hour.
• *Distribution:* Distributed into pleural, peritoneal and synovial fluids, lungs, prostate, liver, and gallbladder; also penetrates middle ear effusions, maxillary sinus and bronchial secretions, tonsils, and sputum. Readily crosses the placenta; 15% to 25% protein-bound.
• *Metabolism:* Only partially metabolized.
• *Excretion:* Excreted in urine by renal tubular secretion and glomerular filtration; also excreted in breast milk. Elimination half-life is about 1 to 1½ hours; in patients with extensive renal impairment, half-life is extended to 10 to 24 hours.

Contraindications and precautions
Contraindicated in patients with hypersensitivity to drug or other penicillins. Use with caution in patients with mononucleosis.

Interactions
Drug-drug. *Allopurinol:* Appears to increase risk of rash from both drugs. Monitor patient carefully.
Aminoglycoside antibiotic: Concomitant use causes a synergistic bactericidal effect against some strains of *enterococci* and group B *streptococci.* Drugs are physically and chemically incompatible; inactivated if mixed or given together. Don't mix or give together.
Clavulanate: Results in increased bactericidal effects because clavulanic acid is beta-lactamase inhibitor. Used for this therapeutic purpose.
Methotrexate: Large doses of penicillins may interfere with renal tubular secretion of methotrexate, delaying elimination and elevating serum levels of methotrexate. Monitor methotrexate levels.

Reactions may be *common,* uncommon, *life-threatening,* or COMMON AND LIFE-THREATENING.

Oral contraceptives: Contraceptive effect may be decreased. Recommend alternate contraceptive method.

Probenecid: Inhibits renal tubular secretion of ampicillin, raising its serum levels. Use as adjunct to antibiotic therapy.

Adverse reactions

CNS: lethargy, hallucinations, *seizures,* anxiety, confusion, agitation, depression, dizziness, fatigue.

GI: *nausea,* vomiting, *diarrhea,* glossitis, stomatitis, gastritis, abdominal pain, enterocolitis, pseudomembranous colitis, black "hairy" tongue.

GU: interstitial nephritis, nephropathy.

Hematologic: anemia, *thrombocytopenia,* thrombocytopenic purpura, eosinophilia, leukopenia, hemolytic anemia, *agranulocytosis.*

Other: hypersensitivity reactions (erythematous maculopapular rash, urticaria, *anaphylaxis*), overgrowth of nonsusceptible organisms, pain at injection site, vein irritation, thrombophlebitis, vaginitis.

☑ Special considerations

Besides the recommendations for all penicillins, consider the following.

• Administer I.M. or I.V. only when patient is too ill to take oral drug.

• Alters results of urine glucose tests that use cupric sulfate (Benedict's reagent or Clinitest). Make urine glucose determinations with glucose oxidase methods (Chemstrip uG, Diastix, or glucose enzymatic test strip).

• Clinical signs of overdose include neuromuscular sensitivity or seizures.

• After recent ingestion (within 4 hours) in overdose, empty the stomach by induced emesis or gastric lavage; follow with activated charcoal to reduce absorption. Drug can be removed by hemodialysis.

Monitoring the patient

• Monitor patient for signs of hypersensitivity (erythematous maculopapular rash, urticaria, anaphylaxis).

• Observe patient for signs of internal bleeding.

Information for the patient

• Encourage patient to report diarrhea promptly.

• Instruct patient to complete all of prescribed drug.

Geriatric patients

• Because of diminished renal tubular secretion in elderly patients, half-life of drug may be prolonged.

Breast-feeding patients

• Use cautiously. Drug appears in breast milk; safety in breast-feeding women hasn't been established.

ampicillin sodium/sulbactam sodium
Unasyn

Pharmacologic classification: aminopenicillin/beta-lactamase inhibitor combination
Therapeutic classification: antibiotic
Pregnancy risk category B

How supplied

Available by prescription only

Injection: Vials and piggyback vials containing 1.5 g (1 g ampicillin sodium with 500 mg sulbactam sodium) and 3 g (2 g ampicillin sodium with 1 g sulbactam sodium)

Indications, route, and dosage

Skin and skin-structure infections, intra-abdominal and gynecologic infections caused by susceptible beta-lactamase-producing strains of Staphylococcus aureus, Escherichia coli, Klebsiella (including K. pneumoniae), Proteus mirabilis, Bacteroides (including B. fragilis), Enterobacter, and Acinetobacter calcoaceticus

Adults: 1.5 to 3 g I.M. or I.V. q 6 hours. Don't exceed 4 g/day sulbactam sodium.

✦ *Dosage adjustment.* For patients with renal failure, use these recommendations.

Creatinine clearance (ml/min/ 1.73 m^2)	Half-life (hours)	Recommended dosage
≥ 30	1	1.5 to 3 g q 6 to 8 hr
15 to 29	5	1.5 to 3 g q 12 hr
5 to 14	9	1.5 to 3 g q 24 hr

Pharmacodynamics

Antibiotic action: Ampicillin is bactericidal; adheres to bacterial penicillin-binding proteins, thus inhibiting bacterial cell-wall synthesis. Sulbactam inhibits beta-lactamase, an enzyme produced by ampicillin-resistant bacteria that degrades ampicillin.

Pharmacokinetics

• *Absorption:* Peak plasma levels occur immediately after I.V. infusion and within 1 hour after I.M. injection.

• *Distribution:* Both drugs distribute into pleural, peritoneal and synovial fluids, lungs, prostate, liver, and gallbladder; they also penetrate middle ear effusions, maxillary sinus and bronchial secretions, tonsils, and sputum. Ampicillin readily cross-

es the placenta; it is minimally protein-bound at 15% to 25%; sulbactam is about 38% bound.
• *Metabolism:* Only 15% to 25% of both drugs are metabolized.
• *Excretion:* Both ampicillin and sulbactam are excreted in the urine by renal tubular secretion and glomerular filtration. Also excreted in breast milk. Elimination half-life is 1 to 1¼ hours; in patients with extensive renal impairment, half-life can be as long as 10 to 24 hours.

Contraindications and precautions
Contraindicated in patients with hypersensitivity to drug or other penicillins. Use cautiously in patients with maculopapular rash.

Interactions
Drug-drug. *Allopurinol:* May lead to an increased risk of rash. Monitor patient.
Aminoglycosides: Ampicillin may cause in vitro inactivation of aminoglycosides if mixed in the same infusion container. Don't mix.
Anticoagulants: Prolongation of bleeding times with large doses of I.V. penicillins. Monitor bleeding times.
Probenecid: Decreases excretion of both ampicillin and sulbactam. Used as adjunct for antibiotic therapy.

Adverse reactions
GI: *nausea,* vomiting, *diarrhea,* glossitis, stomatitis, gastritis, black "hairy" tongue, enterocolitis, pseudomembranous colitis.
Hematologic: anemia, **thrombocytopenia,** thrombocytopenic purpura, eosinophilia, leukopenia, **agranulocytosis.**
Other: hypersensitivity reactions (erythematous maculopapular rash, urticaria, **anaphylaxis**), **overgrowth of nonsusceptible organisms,** pain at injection site, vein irritation, thrombophlebitis.

☑ Special considerations
• I.V. administration should be given by slow injection over at least 10 to 15 minutes or infused in greater dilutions with 50 to 100 ml of a compatible diluent over 15 to 30 minutes.
• For I.V. use, reconstitute powder in piggyback units to desired concentrations with sterile water for injection, normal saline injection, 5% dextrose injection, lactated Ringer's injection, 1/6 M sodium lactate injection, 5% dextrose in 0.45% saline, or 10% invert sugar.
• For I.M. injection, reconstitute with sterile water for injection, or 0.5% or 2% lidocaine hydrochloride injection. To obtain 375 mg/ml solutions (250 mg ampicillin/125 mg sulbactam/ml), add contents of the 1.5-g vial to 3.2 ml of diluent to produce 4 ml withdrawal volume; add 3-g vial to 6.4 ml of diluent to produce 8 ml withdrawal volume.
• Reconstituted solutions are stable for varying periods (from 2 hours to 72 hours) depending on diluent used. Check with pharmacist. For patients

on sodium restriction, note that a 1.5-g dose of ampicillin sodium/sulbactam sodium yields 5 mEq of sodium.
• Drug alters results of urine glucose tests that use cupric sulfate (Benedict's reagent or Clinitest). Make urine glucose determinations with glucose oxidase methods (Chemstrip uG, Diastix, or glucose enzymatic test strip).
• In pregnant women, transient decreases in serum estradiol, conjugated estrone, conjugated estriol, and estriol glucuronide may occur.
• Neurologic adverse reactions during overdose, including seizures, are likely. Treatment is supportive. Although confirming data are lacking, ampicillin and sulbactam are likely to be removed by hemodialysis.

Monitoring the patient
• Monitor renal function in patients with renal failure.
• Monitor patient for adverse effects.

Information for the patient
• Tell patient to report rash, fever, or chills. A rash is the most common allergic reaction.
• Advise patient to report discomfort at I.V. site.
• Warn patient that I.M. injection may cause pain at the injection site.

Geriatric patients
• Because of diminished renal tubular secretion in elderly patients, half-life of drug may be prolonged.

Pediatric patients
• Safe use in children under age 12 hasn't been established.

Breast-feeding patients
• Drug appears in breast milk; safety in breast-feeding women is unknown. Alternative feeding method is recommended during therapy.

amprenavir
Agenerase

Pharmacologic classification: protease inhibitor
Therapeutic classification: antiretroviral
Pregnancy risk category C

How supplied
Available by prescription only
Capsules: 50 mg, 150 mg
Oral solution: 15 mg/ml

Indications, route, and dosage
HIV-1 infection with other antiretrovirals
Adults and children ages 13 to 16 weighing over 50 kg (110 lb): 1,200 mg P.O. (8 150-mg capsules) b.i.d. with other antiretrovirals.

Children ages 4 to 12 or 13 to 16 weighing under 50 kg: Capsules: 20 mg/kg P.O. b.i.d. or 15 mg/kg P.O. t.i.d. (to maximum daily dose of 2,400 mg) with other antiretrovirals. Oral solution: 22.5 mg/kg P.O. (1.5 ml/kg) b.i.d. or 17 mg/kg P.O. (1.1 ml/kg) t.i.d. (to maximum daily dose of 2,800 mg) with other antiretrovirals.

✦ *Dosage adjustment.* Patients with moderate or severe hepatic impairment should receive reduced dosage.

Patients with Child-Pugh score of 5 to 8: 450 mg P.O. b.i.d.

Patients with Child-Pugh score of 9 to 12: 300 mg P.O. b.i.d.

Pharmacodynamics

Antiretroviral action: Binds to the active site of HIV-1 protease and thereby prevents the processing of viral *gag* and *gag-pol* polyprotein precursors, resulting in formation of immature noninfectious viral particles.

Pharmacokinetics

● *Absorption:* Rapidly absorbed.
● *Distribution:* About 90% bound to plasma proteins.
● *Metabolism:* Metabolized in the liver by the cytochrome P-450 CYP3A4 enzyme system.
● *Excretion:* Excretion of unchanged drug in urine and feces is minimal. Plasma elimination half-life ranges from 7.1 to 10.6 hours.

Contraindications and precautions

Contraindicated in patients with previously demonstrated significant hypersensitivity to drug or its components. Use cautiously in patients with sulfonamide allergy, with hepatic impairment, or hemophilia A and B.

Interactions

Drug-drug. *Antacids:* Possible interference with absorption. Separate administration times by at least 1 hour.

Antiarrhythmics (such as amiodarone, lidocaine [systemic], quinidine), anticoagulants (such as warfarin), tricyclic antidepressants: Coadministration affects serum levels of drug. Monitor closely.

Bepridil, cisapride, dihydroergotamine, midazolam, rifampin, triazolam: Serious and life-threatening interactions may occur. Avoid using together.

Rifabutin: Causes decrease in amprenavir levels and substantial increase in rifabutin levels. Reduce dosage.

Sildenafil: Substantially increases sildenafil levels and may cause an increase in sildenafil-associated effects, including hypotension, visual changes, and priapism. Use together cautiously.

Drug-food. *High-fat meal:* Reduces drug absorption. Drug shouldn't be taken with such meals.

Adverse reactions

CNS: *paresthesia,* depressive or mood disorders.
GI: *nausea, vomiting, diarrhea or loose stools,* taste disorders.
Metabolic: *hyperglycemia, hypertriglyceridemia,* hypercholesterolemia.
Skin: RASH (INCLUDING STEVENS-JOHNSON SYNDROME).

☑ Special considerations

● New onset diabetes mellitus, exacerbation of preexisting diabetes mellitus, and hyperglycemia have been reported. Some patients require either initiation or dose adjustments of insulin or oral hypoglycemic drugs for treatment of these events.
● Capsules and oral solution not interchangeable on mg per mg basis.
● To monitor maternal-fetal outcomes of pregnant women exposed to drug, an Antiretroviral Pregnancy Registry has been established. Physicians may call 1-800-258-4263 to register patients who have been exposed to drug during pregnancy.
● Store capsules and oral solution at room temperature.
● If overdose occurs, patient should be monitored for evidence of toxicity and given supportive treatment as needed.
● No known antidote. Not known if amprenavir can be removed by peritoneal or hemodialysis.

Monitoring the patient

● Monitor patient for adverse reactions. Drug may cause redistribution or accumulation of body fat including central obesity, dorsocervical fat enlargement (buffalo hump), peripheral wasting, breast enlargement or cushingoid appearance. Severe and life-threatening reactions, including Stevens-Johnson syndrome, have occurred in patients treated with drug.
● Perform CBC weekly and as clinically indicated to Monitor patient for neutropenia in patients also receiving rifabutin.

Information for the patient

● Inform patient that drug doesn't cure HIV infection, and patient may continue to develop opportunistic infections and other complications associated with the disease. Drug doesn't reduce risk of transmitting HIV to others through sexual contact.
● Tell patient drug may be taken without regard to meals but to avoid taking with high fat meals because this may decrease absorption.
● Advise patient to take drug each day as prescribed. It must always be taken with other antiretrovirals. Dose must not be altered or discontinued without consulting a physician.
● Tell patient if a dose is missed to take the dose as soon as possible and then return to the normal schedule. However, if a dose is skipped, don't double the next dose.

• Instruct patient taking hormonal contraceptives to use alternative contraceptive measures during drug therapy.

Geriatric patients
• Use cautiously in elderly patients because of greater frequency of decreased hepatic, renal, or cardiac function, and of concomitant disease or other drug therapy.

Pediatric patients
• Adverse event profile similar to adults is seen in children. Safety and effectiveness in children under age 4 haven't been evaluated.

Breast-feeding patients
• It's unknown if drug appears in breast milk. Mothers receiving drug shouldn't breast-feed. HIV-infected mothers shouldn't breast-feed to avoid risking postnatal transmission of HIV.

---

anastrozole
Arimidex

Pharmacologic classification: nonsteroidal aromatase inhibitor
Therapeutic classification: antineoplastic
Pregnancy risk category D

How supplied
Available by prescription only
Tablets: 1 mg

Indications, route, and dosage
Advanced breast cancer in postmenopausal women with disease progression following tamoxifen therapy
Adults: 1 mg P.O. daily.

Pharmacodynamics
Antineoplastic action: A potent and selective nonsteroidal aromatase inhibitor that significantly lowers serum estradiol levels. Estradiol is the principal estrogen circulating in postmenopausal women that has the ability to stimulate breast cancer cell growth.

Pharmacokinetics
• *Absorption:* Absorbed from the GI tract; food affects extent of absorption.
• *Distribution:* 40% bound to plasma proteins in the therapeutic range.
• *Metabolism:* Metabolized in the liver.
• *Excretion:* About 11% of drug is excreted in urine as parent drug; about 60% excreted as metabolites. Half-life is about 50 hours.

Contraindications and precautions
Contraindicated in pregnant women.

Interactions
None reported.

Adverse reactions
CNS: *asthenia, headache,* dizziness, depression, paresthesia.
CV: chest pain, edema, thromboembolic disease.
GI: dry mouth, *nausea,* vomiting, diarrhea, constipation, abdominal pain, anorexia.
GU: vaginal hemorrhage, vaginal dryness.
Musculoskeletal: *back pain,* bone pain, pelvic pain.
Respiratory: dyspnea, increased cough, pharyngitis.
Skin: *hot flashes,* rash, sweating.
Other: *pain,* peripheral edema, weight gain, increased appetite.

☑ Special considerations
• Pregnancy must be excluded before treatment begins.
• Drug should be administered by qualified staff experienced in the use of anticancer drugs.
• Patients treated with drug don't require glucocorticoid or mineralocorticoid therapy.
• There is no specific antidote to overdose, and treatment must be symptomatic.
• Vomiting may be induced if the patient is alert. Dialysis may be helpful. General supportive care is indicated.

Monitoring the patient
• Monitor patient for adverse drug effects.
• Perform pregnancy testing before starting drug.

Information for the patient
• Instruct patient to report adverse reactions.
• Stress importance of follow-up care.

Pediatric patients
• Safety and effectiveness in children haven't been established.

Breast-feeding patients
• It's unknown if drug appears in breast milk. Don't administer drug to breast-feeding women.

---

apraclonidine hydrochloride
Iopidine

Pharmacologic classification: alpha-adrenergic agonist
Therapeutic classification: ocular hypotensive
Pregnancy risk category C

How supplied
Available by prescription only
Ophthalmic solution: 0.5%, 1%

Indications, route, and dosage
Prevention or control of intraocular pressure elevations after argon laser trabeculoplasty or iridotomy
Adults: Instill 1 drop (1% solution) in the eye 1 hour before initiation of laser surgery on the anterior segment; then 1 drop immediately upon completion of surgery.
Short-term adjunctive therapy in patients on maximally tolerated medical therapy who require additional intraocular pressure reduction
Adults: Instill 1 to 2 drops (0.5% solution) in the eye t.i.d.
◊ *Open-angle glaucoma*
Adults: Instill 1 drop (0.5% solution) in the eye b.i.d. or t.i.d.

Pharmacodynamics
Ocular hypotensive action: An alpha-adrenergic agonist that reduces intraocular pressure, possibly by decreasing aqueous humor production.

Pharmacokinetics
• *Absorption:* No information available.
• *Distribution:* Onset of action is within 1 hour after instillation; maximum effect on intraocular pressure reduction occurs in 3 to 5 hours.
• *Metabolism:* No information available.
• *Excretion:* No information available.

Contraindications and precautions
Contraindicated in patients with hypersensitivity to apraclonidine or clonidine and in those on MAO inhibitor therapy. Use cautiously in patients with severe cardiac disease, including hypertension and vasovagal attacks.

Interactions
Drug-drug. *Pilocarpine, topical beta blockers:* May cause additive lowering of intraocular pressure. Avoid using together.

Adverse reactions
CNS: insomnia, irritability, dream disturbances, headache, irritability, paresthesia.
CV: *bradycardia,* vasovagal attack, palpitations, hypotension, orthostatic hypotension.
EENT: upper eyelid elevation, conjunctival blanching and microhemorrhage, mydriasis, eye burning or discomfort, foreign body sensation in eye, eye dryness and *itching, hyperemia,* conjunctivitis, blurred vision, nasal burning or dryness or increased pharyngeal secretions.
GI: abdominal pain, discomfort, diarrhea, vomiting, taste disturbances, dry mouth.
Skin: pruritus not associated with rash, sweaty palms.
Other: body heat sensation, decreased libido, extremity pain or numbness, allergic response.

☑ Special considerations
• Protect stored drug from light and freezing.

Monitoring the patient
• Monitor blood pressure, heart rate, and ECG as indicated in patients taking apraclonidine.
• Monitor patient for adverse effects.

Information for the patient
• Warn patient about potential for dizziness and drowsiness.
• If drug is used with other eyedrops, there should be a 5-minute interval between instillation of each drug to prevent washout of previous dose.

Pediatric patients
• Safety and efficacy in children haven't been established.

Breast-feeding patients
• It's unknown if drug appears in breast milk. Consider discontinuing breast-feeding on day of surgery.

ardeparin sodium
Normiflo

Pharmacologic classification: low-molecular-weight heparin
Therapeutic classification: anticoagulant
Pregnancy risk category C

How supplied
Available by prescription only
Injection: 5,000 anti-factor Xa U/0.5 ml, 10,000 anti-factor Xa U/0.5 ml

Indications, route, and dosage
Prevention of deep venous thrombosis that may lead to pulmonary embolism following knee replacement surgery
Adults: 50 anti-factor Xa units/kg S.C. q 12 hours for 14 days or until patient is ambulatory, whichever is shorter. Give initial dose the evening of day of surgery or the following morning.

Pharmacodynamics
Anticoagulant activity: A low-molecular-weight heparin that binds to and accelerates activity of antithrombin III. This results in an inactivation of factor Xa and thrombin, which prevents the formation of clots. Also inhibits thrombin by binding to heparin cofactor II.

Pharmacokinetics
• *Absorption:* Mean peak plasma anti-factor Xa and anti-factor IIa activity is obtained about 3 hours after S.C. injection. Mean absolute bioavailability based on anti-factor Xa activity is 92%.

- *Distribution:* Steady state volume of distribution based on anti-factor Xa activity is about 99 ml/kg.
- *Metabolism:* No information available.
- *Excretion:* Elimination half-life based on anti-factor Xa activity is about 3 hours.

Contraindications and precautions

Contraindicated in patients with known hypersensitivity to drug or pork products and in those with active bleeding or thrombocytopenia associated with antiplatelet antibodies in the presence of drug.

Use with extreme caution in patients with history of heparin-induced thrombocytopenia and in those with a hypersensitivity to methylparaben, propylparaben, and sulfites. Use cautiously in patients at increased risk for hemorrhage (bacterial endocarditis) and in those with congenital or acquired bleeding disorders; active ulcerative disease; angiodysplastic GI disease; hemorrhagic stroke; recent eye, spinal, or brain surgery or procedures; severe uncontrolled hypertension; or in patients treated concomitantly with platelet inhibitors. When epidural or spinal anesthesia or spinal puncture is used, patients who are anticoagulated or scheduled to be anticoagulated with low-molecular-weight heparins are at risk for developing epidural or spinal hematomas, which can result in long-term paralysis.

Interactions

Drug-drug. *Anticoagulants, antiplatelet drugs (such as aspirin, NSAIDs):* Increased risk of bleeding. Use cautiously and monitor coagulation studies.

Adverse reactions

CNS: dizziness, headache, *CVA,* insomnia.
CV: chest pain, peripheral edema.
GI: nausea, vomiting.
Hematologic: anemia, ecchymosis, *hemorrhage, thrombocytopenia,* hematoma at injection site
Skin: pruritus, rash, local reaction.
Other: arthralgia, fever, pain, increase transaminase and serum triglyceride levels.

☑ Special considerations

- Base dosing on actual body weight.
- Ardeparin can't be used interchangeably (unit for unit) with heparin sodium or other low-molecular-weight heparins.
- Don't mix with other injections or infusions.
- With patient sitting or lying down, administer drug with deep S.C. injection in the abdomen (avoiding the navel), outer aspect of upper arm, or anterior thigh. Extrude air and excess medication before administration. The full length of the needle should be introduced into the skin fold held between thumb and forefinger. Hold skin fold throughout the injection. Rotate injection site.

- Don't give drug I.M to avoid possible occurrence of hematoma at the injection site.
- Bleeding is the principal sign of ardeparin overdose.
- Most bleeding can be stopped by discontinuing the drug and applying pressure to the site and replacing hemostatic blood elements if necessary. Protamine sulfate can also be administered. Protamine dose should be equal to the dose of ardeparin administered (1 mg of protamine neutralizes 100 anti-factor Xa U of ardeparin).
- If bleeding persists after 2 hours, blood should be drawn and residual anti-factor Xa levels determined. Additional protamine can be administered if clinically important bleeding persists or anti-factor Xa levels remain high.
- Drug doesn't appear to be dialyzable.

Monitoring the patient
- Routinely monitor CBC, platelet counts, urinalysis, and occult blood in stools throughout therapy. Routine monitoring of coagulation parameters isn't required.
- Monitor patient for adverse effects.

Information for the patient
- Instruct patient to report abnormal bruising, bleeding, or dark stools.
- Instruct patient to observe for hematoma at injection site.
- Tell patient to avoid use of OTC products such as aspirin or NSAIDs.

Geriatric patients
- No significant difference was seen in patients over age 65 compared with those under age 65.

Pediatric patients
- Safety and effectiveness in children haven't been established.

Breast-feeding patients
- It's unknown if drug appears in breast milk. Use cautiously when administering to breast-feeding women.

ascorbic acid (vitamin C)
Ascorbicap, Cebid Timecelles, Cecon, Cevi-Bid, Dull-C, Flavorcee

Pharmacologic classification: water-soluble vitamin
Therapeutic classification: vitamin
Pregnancy risk category A (C if exceeds RDA)

How supplied
Available by prescription only
Injection: 250 mg/ml in 2-ml ampules and 2-ml and 30-ml vials; 500 mg/ml in 2-ml and 5-ml am-

pules and 50-ml vials; 500 mg/ml (with mono-thioglycerol) in 1-ml ampules
Available without a prescription
Tablets: 25 mg, 50 mg, 100 mg, 250 mg, 500 mg, 1,000 mg
Tablets (chewable): 100 mg, 250 mg, 500 mg
Tablets (timed-release): 500 mg, 1,000 mg, 1,500 mg
Capsules (timed-release): 500 mg
Crystals: 100 g (4 g/tsp), 1,000 g (4 g/tsp, sugar-free)
Lozenges: 60 mg
Powder: 100 g (4 g/tsp), 500 g (4 g/tsp)
Liquid: 50 ml (35 mg/0.6 ml)
Solution: 50 ml (100 mg/ml)
Syrup: 20 mg/ml in 120 ml and 480 ml; 500 mg/5 ml in 5 ml, 10 ml, 120 ml, and 473 ml

Indications, route, and dosage
Frank and subclinical scurvy
Adults: 100 to 250 mg, depending on severity, P.O., S.C., I.M., or I.V. daily or b.i.d.; then at least 50 mg/day for maintenance.
Children: 100 to 300 mg, depending on severity, P.O., S.C., I.M., or I.V. daily; then at least 35 mg/day for maintenance.
Infants: 50 to 100 mg P.O., I.M., I.V., or S.C. daily.
Prevention of ascorbic acid deficiency in patients with poor nutritional habits or increased requirements
Adults: 45 to 60 mg P.O., S.C., I.M., or I.V. daily.
Pregnant or breast-feeding women: At least 60 to 80 mg P.O., S.C., I.M., or I.V. daily.
Children and infants over age 2 weeks: At least 20 to 50 mg P.O., S.C., I.M., or I.V. daily.
◊ **Potentiation of methenamine in urine acidification**
Adults: 4 to 12 g daily in divided doses.
◊ **Adjunctive therapy in treatment of idiopathic methemoglobinemia**
Adults: 300 to 600 mg P.O. daily in divided doses.

Pharmacodynamics
Nutritional action: Ascorbic acid, an essential vitamin, is involved with the biologic oxidations and reductions used in cellular respiration. It is essential for the formation and maintenance of intracellular ground substance and collagen. In the body, ascorbic acid is reversibly oxidized to dehydroascorbic acid and influences tyrosine metabolism, conversion of folic acid to folinic acid, carbohydrate metabolism, resistance to infections, and cellular respiration. Ascorbic acid deficiency causes scurvy, a condition marked by degenerative changes in the capillaries, bone, and connective tissues. Restoring adequate ascorbic acid intake completely reverses symptoms of ascorbic acid deficiency. Data regarding use of ascorbic acid as a urinary acidifier are conflicting.

Pharmacokinetics
● *Absorption:* After oral administration, absorbed readily. After very large doses, absorption may be limited because absorption is an active process. Absorption also may be reduced in patients with diarrhea or GI diseases. Normal plasma levels of ascorbic acid are about 10 to 20 mcg/ml. Plasma levels below 1.5 mcg/ml are associated with scurvy. However, leukocyte levels (although not usually measured) may better reflect ascorbic acid tissue saturation. About 1.5 g of ascorbic acid is stored in the body. Within 3 to 5 months of ascorbic acid deficiency, signs of scurvy become evident.
● *Distribution:* Distributed widely in the body, with large concentrations found in the liver, leukocytes, platelets, glandular tissues, and lens of the eye. Ascorbic acid crosses the placenta; cord blood levels are usually 2 to 4 times the maternal blood levels. Ascorbic acid is distributed into breast milk.
● *Metabolism:* Metabolized in the liver.
● *Excretion:* Reversibly oxidized to dehydroascorbic acid. Some is metabolized to inactive compounds that are excreted in urine. The renal threshold is about 14 mcg/ml. When the body is saturated and blood levels exceed the threshold, unchanged ascorbic acid is excreted in urine. Renal excretion is directly proportional to blood levels. Ascorbic acid is also removed by hemodialysis.

Contraindications and precautions
No known contraindications. Use cautiously in patients with renal insufficiency.

Interactions
Drug-drug. *Acidic drugs:* In large doses (more than 2 g/day), may lower urine pH, causing renal tubular reabsorption of these drugs. Reduced dosage may be needed.
Basic drugs (such as amphetamines, tricyclic antidepressants): May cause decreased reabsorption and therapeutic effect. Dosage may need adjustment.
Dicumarol: Influences intensity and duration of anticoagulant effect. Monitor PT.
Ethinyl estradiol: May increase plasma levels of ethinyl estradiol. Monitor patient closely.
Iron: Concomitant use maintains drug in ferrous state and increases iron absorption in GI tract. A combination of 30 mg iron with 200 mg ascorbic acid is sometimes recommended.
Salicylates: Ascorbic acid uptake inhibited by leukocytes and platelets. Although no evidence exists that salicylates precipitate ascorbic acid deficiency, patients receiving high doses of salicylates with ascorbic acid supplements must be observed for symptoms of ascorbic acid deficiency.
Sulfonamides: Concurrent use may cause crystallization. Avoid using together.
Warfarin: May inhibit anticoagulant effect. Monitor PT.

Drug-lifestyle. *Smoking:* May decrease serum ascorbic acid levels, thus increasing dosage requirements of this vitamin. Monitor patient closely.

Adverse reactions
CNS: faintness, dizziness with too-rapid I.V. administration.
GI: diarrhea.
GU: acid urine, oxaluria, renal calculi.
Other: discomfort at injection site.

☑ Special considerations
• Administer large doses of ascorbic acid (1,000 mg/day) in divided amounts because the body uses only a limited amount and excretes the rest in urine. Large doses may increase small-intestine pH and impair vitamin B_{12} absorption. Recommended RDA of ascorbic acid is as follows:
Adults: 60 mg/day
Smokers: 100 mg/day
Pregnant women: 70 mg/day
Breast-feeding women: 90 to 95 mg/day
Infants and children: 30 to 60 mg/day
Patients on long-term hemodialysis: 100 to 200 mg/day
• Administer oral solutions of ascorbic acid directly into mouth or mix with food.
• Administer I.V. solution slowly.
• Conditions that elevate metabolic rate (hyperthyroidism, fever, infection, burns and other severe trauma, postoperative states, neoplastic disease, and chronic alcoholism) significantly increase ascorbic acid requirements.
• Reportedly, patients taking oral contraceptives require ascorbic acid supplements.
• Smokers appear to have increased need for ascorbic acid because the vitamin is oxidized and excreted more rapidly in smokers than in nonsmokers.
• Use ascorbic acid cautiously in patients with renal insufficiency because the vitamin is normally excreted in urine.
• Persons whose diets are chemically deficient in fruits and vegetables can develop subclinical ascorbic acid deficiency. Observe for such deficiency in elderly and indigent patients, patients on restricted diets, those receiving long-term treatment with I.V. fluids or hemodialysis, and drug addicts or alcoholics.
• Overt symptoms of ascorbic acid deficiency include irritability; emotional disturbances; general debility; pallor; anorexia; sensitivity to touch; limb and joint pain; follicular hyperkeratosis (particularly on thighs and buttocks); easy bruising; petechiae; bloody diarrhea; delayed healing; loosening of teeth; sensitive, swollen, and bleeding gums; and anemia.
• Protect ascorbic acid solutions from light.
• Ascorbic acid is a strong reducing drug; it alters results of tests that are based on oxidation-reduction reactions.

• Large doses of ascorbic acid (over 500 mg) may cause false-negative glucose determinations using the glucose oxidase method, or false-positive results using the copper reduction method or Benedict's reagent.
• Ascorbic acid shouldn't be used for 48 to 72 hours before an amine-dependent test for occult blood in the stool is conducted. A false-negative result may occur.
• Depending on the reagents used, ascorbic acid may also cause interactions with other diagnostic tests.
• Excessively high doses of parenteral ascorbic acid are excreted renally after tissue saturation and rarely accumulate.
• Serious adverse effects or toxicity are uncommon. Severe effects require discontinuation of therapy.

Monitoring the patient
• Monitor patient for severe adverse effects (rare).
• Observe patient for signs of ascorbic acid deficiency, especially elderly patients on several drug therapies.

Information for the patient
• Teach patient about good dietary sources of ascorbic acid, such as citrus fruits, leafy vegetables, tomatoes, green peppers, and potatoes.
• Inform patient to cover foods and fruit juices tightly and to use them promptly.
• Advise patient with ascorbic acid deficiency to decrease or stop smoking. Replacement ascorbic acid dosages are greater for the smoker.
• Tell patient who is prone to renal calculi, has diabetes, is undergoing tests for occult blood in stools, or is on sodium-restricted diet or anticoagulant therapy to avoid high doses of ascorbic acid.

Pediatric patients
• Infants fed on cow's milk alone require supplemental ascorbic acid.

Breast-feeding patients
• Drug appears in breast milk. Administer with caution to breast-feeding women.

---

asparaginase
Elspar

Pharmacologic classification: enzyme
(L-asparagine amidohydrolase; cell-cycle–phase specific, G1 phase)
Therapeutic classification: antineoplastic
Pregnancy risk category C

How supplied
Available by prescription only
Injection: 10,000-IU vials

Indications, route, and dosage
Dosage and indications may vary. Check current literature for recommended protocol.
Acute lymphocytic leukemia
Adults and children: When used alone, 200 IU/kg daily I.V. for 28 days. When used with other chemotherapeutic drugs, dosage is highly individualized.

Pharmacodynamics
Antineoplastic action: Exerts its cytotoxic activity by inactivating the amino acid asparagine, which is needed by tumor cells to synthesize proteins. Because the tumor cells can't synthesize their own asparagine, protein synthesis and eventually synthesis of DNA and RNA are inhibited.

Pharmacokinetics
• *Absorption:* Not absorbed across GI tract after oral administration; must be given I.V. or I.M.
• *Distribution:* Primarily distributed within the intravascular space, with detectable levels in the thoracic and cervical lymph. Crosses blood-brain barrier to a minimal extent.
• *Metabolism:* Metabolic fate of asparaginase is unclear; hepatic sequestration by the reticuloendothelial system may occur.
• *Excretion:* Plasma elimination half-life, which isn't related to dose, sex, age, or hepatic or renal function, ranges from 8 to 30 hours.

Contraindications and precautions
Contraindicated in patients with pancreatitis or history of pancreatitis and previous hypersensitivity unless desensitized. Use cautiously in patients with hepatic dysfunction.

Interactions
Drug-drug. *Methotrexate:* Decreased effectiveness of methotrexate because asparaginase destroys the actively replicating cells that methotrexate needs for its cytotoxic action. Use cautiously.
Prednisone: Hyperglycemia may result from an additive effect on the pancreas. Use cautiously.
Vincristine: Can cause additive neuropathy and disturbances of erythropoiesis. Use cautiously.

Adverse reactions
CNS: confusion, drowsiness, depression, hallucinations, *intracranial hemorrhage,* fatigue, *coma,* agitation, headache, lethargy, somnolence.
GI: HEMORRHAGIC PANCREATITIS, *vomiting, anorexia, nausea,* cramps, weight loss.
GU: *azotemia, renal failure,* glycosuria, polyuria.
Hematologic: *anemia, hypofibrinogenemia,* depression of other clotting factors, *leukopenia.*
Hepatic: elevated AST and ALT levels, *hepatotoxicity.*
Metabolic: *hyperglycemia.*
Skin: *rash, urticaria,* hypersensitivity reactions.
Other: ANAPHYLAXIS, chills, *death, fatal hyperthermia,* fever.

☑ Special considerations
• Reconstitute drug for I.M. administration with 2 ml unpreserved normal saline. Don't use if precipitate forms.
• I.M. injections shouldn't contain more than 2 ml per injection. Multiple injections may be used for each dose.
• For I.V. administration: Reconstitute with 5 ml of sterile water for injection or saline injection. Solution will be clear or slightly cloudy. May further dilute with saline injection or D$_5$W and administer I.V. over 30 minutes. Filtration through a 5-micron in-line filter during administration removes particulate matter that may develop on standing; filtration through a 0.22-micron filter results in a loss of potency. Don't use if precipitate forms.
• Shake vial gently when reconstituting; vigorous shaking results in a decrease of potency.
• Refrigerate unopened dry powder. Reconstituted solution should be used within 8 hours.
• Don't use as sole drug to induce remission unless combination therapy is inappropriate. Not recommended for maintenance therapy.
• Administer drug in hospital with close supervision.
• I.V. administration of asparaginase with or immediately before vincristine or prednisone may increase toxicity reactions.
• Conduct skin test before initial dose. Observe site for 1 hour. Erythema and wheal formation indicate a positive reaction.
• Risk of hypersensitivity increases with repeated doses. Patient may be desensitized, but this doesn't rule out risk of allergic reactions. Routine administration of 2-unit intradermal test dose may identify high-risk patients.
• Because of vomiting, patient may need parenteral fluids for 24 hours or until oral fluids are tolerated.
• Tumor lysis can result in uric acid nephropathy. Prevent occurrence by increasing fluid intake. Allopurinol should be started before therapy begins.
• Keep epinephrine, diphenhydramine, and I.V. corticosteroids available for treatment of anaphylaxis.
• Drug alters the results of thyroid function tests by decreasing levels of serum thyroxine-binding globulin.
• Signs and symptoms of overdose include nausea and diarrhea. Treatment is generally supportive and includes antiemetics and antidiarrheals.

Monitoring the patient
• Monitor CBC and bone marrow function. Bone marrow regeneration may take 5 to 6 weeks.
• Obtain frequent serum amylase determinations to check pancreatic status. If elevated, stop drug.
• Watch for signs of bleeding.
• Monitor blood glucose and test urine before and during therapy. Watch for signs of hyperglycemia, such as glycosuria and polyuria.

Information for the patient
● Encourage patient to maintain adequate intake of fluids to increase urine output and facilitate excretion of uric acid.
● Because drowsiness may occur during therapy or for several weeks after treatment has ended, tell patient to avoid hazardous activities requiring mental alertness.

Pediatric patients
● Drug toxicity appears to be less severe in children than in adults.

Breast-feeding patients
● It's unknown if drug appears in breast milk. Because of potential for serious adverse reactions and carcinogenicity in the infant, breast-feeding isn't recommended.

---

aspirin
A.S.A., Ascriptin, Aspergum, Bufferin, Ecotrin, Empirin, Halfprin, Novasen*, ZORprin

Pharmacologic classification: salicylate
Therapeutic classification: nonnarcotic analgesic, antipyretic, anti-inflammatory, antiplatelet
Pregnancy risk category D

How supplied
Available by prescription only
Tablets (enteric-coated): 975 mg
Tablets (extended-release): 800 mg
Available without a prescription
Tablets: 81 mg, 325 mg (5 grains), 500 mg, 650 mg
Tablets (enteric-coated): 81 mg, 162 mg, 165 mg, 325 mg, 500 mg, 650 mg
Tablets (extended-release): 650 mg
Chewing gum: 227.5 mg
Suppositories: 60 mg, 120 mg, 125 mg, 200 mg, 300 mg, 600 mg

Indications, route, and dosage
Arthritis
Adults: 3.6 to 5.4 g P.O. daily in divided doses.
Children: 80 to 130 mg/kg P.O. daily in divided doses.
Mild pain or fever
Adults: 325 to 650 mg P.O. or P.R. q 4 hours, p.r.n.
Mild pain
Children: 65 mg/kg P.O. or P.R. daily divided q 4 to 6 hours, p.r.n.
Transient ischemic attacks and thromboembolic disorders
Adults: 650 mg P.O. b.i.d. or 325 mg q.i.d.
Reduction of the risk of heart attack in patients with previous MI or unstable angina
Adults: 160 to 325 mg P.O once daily.

Kawasaki (mucocutaneous lymph node) syndrome
Adults: 80 to 100 mg/kg P.O. daily in 4 divided doses. Some patients may require up to 120 mg/kg daily to maintain acceptable serum salicylate levels of over 200 mcg/ml during the febrile phase. After fever subsides, reduce dosage to 3 to 5 mg/kg once daily. Therapy is usually continued for 6 to 8 weeks.
Rheumatic fever
Adults: 4.9 to 7.8 g P.O. daily divided q 4 to 6 hours for 1 to 2 weeks; then decrease to 60 to 70 mg/kg daily for 1 to 6 weeks; then gradually withdraw over 1 to 2 weeks.
Children: 90 to 130 mg/kg P.O. daily divided q 4 to 6 hours.

Pharmacodynamics
Analgesic action: Produces analgesia by an ill-defined effect on the hypothalamus (central action) and by blocking generation of pain impulses (peripheral action). The peripheral action may involve blocking of prostaglandin synthesis via inhibition of cyclo-oxygenase enzyme.
Anti-inflammatory effects: Exact mechanism unknown, but aspirin is believed to inhibit prostaglandin synthesis; may also inhibit synthesis or action of other inflammation mediators.
Antipyretic effect: Relieves fever by acting on hypothalamic heat-regulating center to produce peripheral vasodilation. This increases peripheral blood supply and promotes sweating, which leads to heat loss and cooling by evaporation.
Anticoagulant effects: At low doses, appears to impede clotting by blocking prostaglandin synthetase action, which prevents formation of platelet-aggregating substance thromboxane A_2. This interference with platelet activity is irreversible and can prolong bleeding time. However, at high doses, interferes with prostacyclin production, a potent vasoconstrictor and inhibitor of platelet aggregation, possibly negating its anticlotting properties.

Pharmacokinetics
● *Absorption:* Absorbed rapidly and completely from GI tract. Therapeutic blood salicylate levels for analgesia and anti-inflammatory effect are 150 to 300 mcg/ml; responses vary with patient.
● *Distribution:* Distributed widely into most body tissues and fluids. Protein-binding to albumin is level-dependent, ranges from 75% to 90%, and decreases as serum level increases. Severe toxic effects may occur at serum levels greater than 400 mcg/ml.
● *Metabolism:* Hydrolyzed partially in GI tract to salicylic acid with almost complete metabolism in the liver.
● *Excretion:* Excreted in urine as salicylate and its metabolites. Elimination half-life ranges from 15 to 20 minutes.

Reactions may be *common*, uncommon, **life-threatening**, or COMMON AND LIFE-THREATENING.

Contraindications and precautions

Contraindicated in patients with hypersensitivity to drug and in those with G6PD deficiency, bleeding disorders such as hemophilia, von Willebrand's disease, or telangiectasia. Also contraindicated in patients with NSAID-induced sensitivity reactions and in children with chickenpox or flulike symptoms.

Use cautiously in patients with GI lesions, impaired renal function, hypoprothrombinemia, vitamin K deficiency, thrombotic thrombocytopenic purpura, or hepatic impairment.

Interactions

Drug-drug. *Ammonium chloride, other urine acidifiers:* Increased aspirin blood levels. Watch for aspirin toxicity.

Antacids in high doses, other urine alkalizers: Decreased aspirin blood levels. Watch for decreased salicylate effect.

Anticoagulants, thrombolytics: May potentiate platelet-inhibiting effects of aspirin. Use together cautiously.

Corticosteroids: Enhances aspirin elimination. Avoid concomitant use.

Highly protein-bound drugs (phenytoin, sulfonylureas, warfarin): May cause displacement of either drug and adverse effects. Monitor therapy closely for both drugs.

Lithium carbonate: Decreases renal clearance of lithium carbonate, thus increasing serum lithium levels and risk of adverse effects. Avoid concurrent use.

Other GI irritant drugs (such as antibiotics, corticosteroids, other NSAIDs): May potentiate adverse GI effects of aspirin. Use together with caution.

Other ototoxic drugs (such as aminoglycosides, bumetanide, capreomycin, cisplatin, ethacrynic acid, erythromycin, furosemide, vancomycin): May potentiate ototoxic effects. Use together cautiously.

Phenylbutazone, probenecid, sulfinpyrazone: Antagonistic to uricosuric effects. Avoid concomitant use.

Drug-food. *Any food:* Delays and decreases absorption of aspirin. Advise patient to take without food to increase absorption.

Drug-herb. *Horse chestnut, kelpware, prickly ash, red clover:* May increase risk of bleeding. Avoid concomitant use.

Drug-lifestyle. *Alcohol:* May potentiate adverse GI effects of aspirin. Discourage use.

Adverse reactions

EENT: *tinnitus, hearing loss.*

GI: *nausea, GI distress, occult bleeding, dyspepsia,* **GI bleeding.**

Hematologic: leukopenia, **thrombocytopenia,** *prolonged bleeding time.*

Hepatic: abnormal liver function studies, hepatitis.

Skin: *rash, bruising, urticaria, angioedema.*

Other: hypersensitivity reactions (**anaphylaxis,** asthma, **Reye's syndrome.**

☑ Special considerations

Besides the recommendations for all salicylates, consider the following.

● Enteric-coated products are absorbed slowly and aren't suitable for acute therapy. They are ideal for long-term therapy, such as that for arthritis.

● There is no evidence that aspirin reduces risk of transient ischemic attacks in women.

● Stop aspirin therapy 1 week before elective surgery, if possible.

● Moisture may cause aspirin to lose potency. Store in cool, dry place; don't use if tablets smell like vinegar.

● Aspirin interferes with urinary glucose analysis performed with Diastix, Chemstrip uG, glucose enzymatic test strip, Clinitest, and Benedict's solution, and with urinary 5-hydroxyindoleacetic acid and vanillylmandelic acid tests.

● Serum uric acid levels may be falsely increased.

● Aspirin may interfere with the Gerhardt test for urine acetoacetic acid.

● Signs and symptoms of overdose include GI discomfort, oliguria, acute renal failure, hyperthermia, EEG abnormalities, and restlessness as well as metabolic acidosis with respiratory alkalosis, hyperpnea, and tachypnea because of increased CO_2 production and direct stimulation of the respiratory center.

● To treat aspirin overdose, empty the patient's stomach immediately by inducing emesis with ipecac syrup if patient is conscious, or by gastric lavage. Administer activated charcoal via nasogastric tube. Provide symptomatic and supportive measures (respiratory support and correction of fluid and electrolyte imbalances). Closely monitor laboratory parameters and vital signs. Enhance renal excretion by administering sodium bicarbonate to alkalinize urine. Use cooling blanket or sponging if patient's rectal temperature is more than 104° F (40° C). Hemodialysis is effective in removing aspirin, but is only used in severely poisoned individuals or those at risk for pulmonary edema.

Monitoring the patient

● Monitor patient for signs of overt or internal bleeding.

● Monitor patient for aspirin toxicity.

Information for the patient

● Tell parents to keep aspirin out of child's reach; encourage use of child-resistant closures because aspirin is a leading cause of poisoning.

● Advise patient receiving high-dose, long-term aspirin therapy to watch for petechiae, bleeding gums, and signs of GI bleeding.

● Instruct patient to avoid use of aspirin if allergic to tartrazine dye.

● Tell patient to take drug with food or after meals to avoid GI upset.

Geriatric patients
● Patients over age 60 may be more susceptible to toxic effects of aspirin. Use with caution.
● Effects of aspirin on renal prostaglandins may cause fluid retention and edema, a significant drawback for elderly patients and those with heart failure.

Pediatric patients
● Because of epidemiologic association with Reye's syndrome, the Centers for Disease Control and Prevention recommend that children with chickenpox or flulike symptoms not be given aspirin or other salicylates.
● Don't use long-term salicylate therapy in children under age 14; safety hasn't been established.

Breast-feeding patients
● Salicylates appear in breast milk. Avoid use during breast-feeding.

atenolol
Tenormin

Pharmacologic classification: beta blocker
Therapeutic classification: antihypertensive, antianginal
Pregnancy risk category C

How supplied
Available by prescription only
Tablets: 25 mg, 50 mg, 100 mg
Injection: 5 mg/10 ml

Indications, route, and dosage
Hypertension
Adults: Initially, 50 mg P.O. as a single daily dose. May increase dosage to 100 mg/day after 7 to 14 days. Higher dosages are unlikely to produce further benefit.
Chronic stable angina pectoris
Adults: 50 mg P.O. once daily; may be increased to 100 mg/day after 7 days for optimal effect. Maximum daily dose is 200 mg/day.
To reduce risk of CV mortality in patients with acute MI
Adults: 5 mg I.V. over 5 minutes; then another 5 mg I.V. 10 minutes later. Initiate oral therapy 10 minutes after final dose in patients who tolerate the full I.V. dose. Thereafter, 50 mg P.O. 12 hours later. Then, 100 mg P.O. daily or 50 mg P.O. b.i.d. for 6 to 9 days or until discharged from the hospital.
✦ *Dosage adjustment.* In patients with renal failure, adjust dosage if creatinine clearance is below 35 ml/minute. In patients with creatinine clearance of 15 to 35 ml/minute/1.73 m², give 50 mg/day; in patients with creatinine clearance below 15 ml/minute/1.73 m², give 25 mg/day; in patients undergoing hemodialysis, dosage is 25 to 50 mg after each treatment under close supervision.

Pharmacodynamics
Antihypertensive action: May reduce blood pressure by adrenergic receptor blockade, thereby decreasing cardiac output by decreasing the sympathetic outflow from the CNS and by suppressing renin release. At low doses, atenolol, like metoprolol, selectively inhibits cardiac beta₁-receptors; it has little effect on beta₂-receptors in bronchial and vascular smooth muscle.
Antianginal action: Aids in treating chronic stable angina by decreasing myocardial contractility and heart rate (negative inotropic and chronotropic effect), thus reducing myocardial oxygen consumption.
Cardioprotective action: The mechanism whereby atenolol improves survival in patients with MI is unknown. However, it does reduce frequency of PVCs, chest pain, and enzyme elevation.

Pharmacokinetics
● *Absorption:* About 50% to 60% is absorbed. An effect on heart rate usually occurs within 60 minutes, with peak effect at 2 to 4 hours. Antihypertensive effect persists for about 24 hours.
● *Distribution:* Distributed into most tissues and fluids except the brain and CSF; about 5% to 15% is protein-bound.
● *Metabolism:* Metabolized minimally.
● *Excretion:* About 40% to 50% of given dose is excreted unchanged in urine; remainder is excreted as unchanged drug and metabolites in feces. In patients with normal renal function, plasma half-life is 6 to 7 hours; half-life increases as renal function decreases.

Contraindications and precautions
Contraindicated in patients with sinus bradycardia, greater than first-degree heart block, overt cardiac failure, or cardiogenic shock. Use cautiously in patients at risk for heart failure and in those with bronchospastic disease, diabetes, and hyperthyroidism.

Interactions
Drug-drug. *Alpha-adrenergic drugs such as those found in OTC cold remedies, indomethacin, NSAIDs:* Antihypertensive effects of atenolol may be antagonized. Use together cautiously.
Antihypertensives: Enhanced antihypertensive effects. Use together cautiously.
Insulin, oral hypoglycemics: May alter dosage requirements in stable diabetic patients. Monitor glucose levels; adjust insulin dosage.

Adverse reactions
CNS: *fatigue,* lethargy, vertigo, drowsiness, *dizziness.*
CV: *bradycardia,* hypotension, **heart failure,** intermittent claudication.
GI: nausea, diarrhea.
GU: elevated BUN and creatinine.

Hepatic: elevated transaminase, alkaline phosphatase.
Metabolic: hyperkalemia, hyperglycemia, hypoglycemia.
Respiratory: dyspnea, *bronchospasm.*
Skin: rash.
Other: fever, leg pain.

☑ Special considerations
Besides the recommendations for all beta blockers, consider the following.
● Give oral single daily dose at same time each day.
● Drug may be taken without food.
● Dosage may need to be reduced in patients with renal insufficiency.
● I.V. atenolol affords a rapid onset of the protective effects of beta blockade against reinfarction.
● Patients who can't tolerate I.V. atenolol after an MI may be candidates for oral atenolol therapy. Some evidence suggests that gastric absorption of atenolol may be delayed in the early phase of MI. This may result from the physiologic changes that accompany MI or from the effects of morphine, which is commonly administered to treat chest pain. However, oral therapy alone may still provide benefits.
● Atenolol also may cause changes in exercise tolerance and ECG.
● Signs and symptoms of overdose include severe hypotension, bradycardia, heart failure, and bronchospasm. Empty stomach by emesis or gastric lavage; follow with activated charcoal to reduce absorption. Thereafter, treat symptomatically and supportively.

Monitoring the patient
● Monitor blood pressure response and frequency of angina episodes.
● Periodically perform ECG and determine platelet count and serum potassium, uric acid, transaminase, alkaline phosphatase, LD, creatinine, and BUN levels.

Information for the patient
● Stress importance of not missing doses, but tell patient not to double missed doses, especially if taking drug once daily.
● Advise patient to seek medical approval before taking OTC cold preparations.

Geriatric patients
● Elderly patients may require lower maintenance doses because of increased bioavailability or delayed metabolism; may also experience enhanced adverse effects.

Pediatric patients
● Safety and efficacy in children haven't been established. Use only if potential benefit outweighs risk.

Breast-feeding patients
● Safety hasn't been established. An alternative feeding method is recommended during therapy.

---

atorvastatin calcium
Lipitor

Pharmacologic classification: 3-hydroxy-3-methylglutaryl-coenzyme A (HMG-CoA) reductase inhibitor
Therapeutic classification: antilipemic
Pregnancy risk category X

How supplied
Available by prescription only
Tablets: 10 mg, 20 mg, 40 mg

Indications, route, and dosage
Adjunct to diet to reduce elevated low-density lipoprotein (LDL), total cholesterol, apo B, and triglyceride levels in patients with primary hypercholesterolemia and mixed dyslipidemia
Adults: Initially, 10 mg P.O. once daily. Increase dosage, p.r.n., to maximum of 80 mg daily as single dose. Dosage based on blood lipid levels drawn within 2 to 4 weeks after starting therapy.
Alone or as an adjunct to lipid-lowering treatments such as LDL apheresis in patients with homozygous familial hypercholesterolemia
Adults: 10 to 80 mg P.O. once daily.

Pharmacodynamics
Antilipemic action: Inhibits HMG-CoA reductase, an early (and rate-limiting) step in cholesterol biosynthesis.

Pharmacokinetics
● *Absorption:* Rapidly absorbed; plasma levels peak within 1 to 2 hours. Therapeutic response can be seen within 2 weeks; maximum response within 4 weeks and maintained during long-term therapy.
● *Distribution:* Mean volume of distribution is about 565 L. Drug is 98% or more bound to plasma proteins with poor drug penetration into RBCs. Drug is likely to be secreted in breast milk.
● *Metabolism:* Extensively metabolized to ortho-hydroxylated and parahydroxylated derivatives and various beta-oxidation products. In vitro inhibition of HMG-CoA reductase by orthohydroxylated and parahydroxylated metabolites is equivalent to that of atorvastatin. About 70% of circulating inhibitory activity for HMG-CoA reductase is attributed to active metabolites. In vitro studies suggest the importance of atorvastatin metabolism by cytochrome P-450 3A4.
● *Excretion:* Drug and its metabolites are eliminated primarily in bile following hepatic or extrahepatic metabolism; however, drug doesn't appear to undergo enterohepatic recirculation. Mean

plasma elimination half-life of atorvastatin is about 14 hours, but half-life of inhibitory activity for HMG-CoA reductase is 20 to 30 hours because of the contribution of active metabolites. Less than 2% is recovered in urine following oral administration.

Contraindications and precautions
Contraindicated in patients with hypersensitivity to drug or with active hepatic disease or conditions associated with unexplained persistent elevations of serum transaminase levels, in pregnant or breast-feeding women, and in women of childbearing age (except those not at risk for becoming pregnant).

Use cautiously in patients with history of hepatic disease or heavy alcohol use.

Interactions
Drug-drug. *Antacids:* May cause decreased levels of atorvastatin. LDL-cholesterol reduction not affected. Use together cautiously.
Azole antifungals, cyclosporine, erythromycin, fibric acid derivatives, niacin: May increase risk of rhabdomyolysis. Avoid use together.
Digoxin: May increase plasma digoxin levels. Monitor serum digoxin levels.
Erythromycin: Increases plasma level of drug. Use together cautiously.
Oral contraceptives: May increase levels of hormones. Monitor patient.

Adverse reactions
CNS: asthenia, *headache.*
GI: abdominal pain, constipation, diarrhea, dyspepsia, flatulence.
Hepatic: increased liver function tests.

Respiratory: pharyngitis, sinusitis.
Skin: rash.
Other: accidental injury, allergic reaction, flulike syndrome, *infection.*

☑ Special considerations
● Drug should be withheld or stopped in patients with serious, acute conditions that suggest myopathy or those at risk for renal failure secondary to rhabdomyolysis as a result of trauma; major surgery; severe metabolic, endocrine, and electrolyte disorders; severe acute infection; hypotension; or uncontrolled seizures.
● Use drug only after diet and other nonpharmacologic treatments prove ineffective. Patient should follow a standard low-cholesterol diet before and during therapy.
● Before initiating treatment, exclude secondary causes for hypercholesterolemia and perform a baseline lipid profile. Periodic liver function tests and lipid levels should be done before starting treatment, at 6 and 12 weeks after initiation, or after an increase in dosage and periodically thereafter.

● Drug may be given as a single dose at any time of day without regard for food.
● Watch for signs of myositis.
● There is no specific treatment for atorvastatin overdose. If overdose occurs, treat patient symptomatically, and provide supportive measures as required.
● Because of extensive drug binding to plasma proteins, hemodialysis isn't expected to significantly enhance drug clearance.

Monitoring the patient
● Liver function tests should be performed before and at 12 weeks following initiation of therapy, at any elevation of dose, and periodically thereafter.
● Monitor patient for adverse effects.

Information for the patient
● Teach patient proper dietary management, weight control, and exercise. Explain importance of controlling elevated serum lipid levels.
● Warn patient to avoid alcohol.
● Tell patient to report adverse reactions, such as muscle pain, malaise, and fever.
● Warn woman that drug is contraindicated during pregnancy because of potential danger to the fetus. Advise her to call immediately if pregnancy occurs.

Geriatric patients
● Safety and efficacy in patients ages 70 and older with drug doses up to 80 mg daily were similar to those of patients below age 70.

Pediatric patients
● Experience in children is limited to drug doses up to 80 mg daily for 1 year in 8 patients with homozygous familial hypercholesteremia. No abnormalities were reported in these patients. None of these patients was below age 9.

Breast-feeding patients
● Because of potential for adverse reactions in breast-fed infants, women taking drug shouldn't breast-feed.

---

atovaquone
Mepron

Pharmacologic classification: ubiquinone analogue
Therapeutic classification: antiprotozoal
Pregnancy risk category C

How supplied
Available by prescription only
Suspension: 750 mg/5 ml

Indications, route, and dosage
Mild to moderate Pneumocystis carinii *pneumonia (PCP) in patients who can't tolerate trimethoprim-sulfamethoxazole*
Adults: 750 mg P.O. b.i.d. for 21 days given with food.

Pharmacodynamics
Antiprotozoal action: Exact mechanism of action of atovaquone against *P. carinii* isn't known. In *Plasmodium* species, the site of action appears to be the cytochrome bc_1 complex (Complex III). Several metabolic enzymes are linked to the mitochondrial electron transport chain via ubiquinone. Inhibition of electron transport by atovaquone results in indirect inhibition of these enzymes. The ultimate metabolic effects of such a blockade may include inhibition of nucleic acid and ATP synthesis.

Pharmacokinetics
• *Absorption:* Limited absorption; however, drug bioavailability is increased about threefold when administered with meals. Fat significantly enhances absorption.
• *Distribution:* 99.9% bound to plasma proteins.
• *Metabolism:* Not metabolized.
• *Excretion:* Undergoes enterohepatic cycling and is primarily excreted in feces. Less than 0.6% is excreted in urine.

Contraindications and precautions
Contraindicated in patients with hypersensitivity to drug. Use cautiously in breast-feeding patients.

Interactions
Drug-drug. *Rifampin:* Significant decrease in plasma levels. Use together with caution.
Zidovudine: May increase zidovudine levels. Use together with caution.
Other highly plasma protein–bound drugs with narrow therapeutic indices (excluding phenytoin): Competition for binding sites may occur. Use together cautiously.
Drug-food. *Any food:* Increases absorption. Take drug with food.

Adverse reactions
CNS: *headache, insomnia,* asthenia, anxiety, dizziness.
EENT: *cough,* sinusitis, rhinitis, taste perversion.
GI: *nausea, diarrhea, vomiting,* constipation, *abdominal pain,* anorexia, dyspepsia.
Skin: *rash,* pruritus, *diaphoresis.*
Other: *fever, oral candidiasis, pain,* hypoglycemia, hypotension.

☑ Special considerations
• Drug hasn't been systematically studied for use in treating more severe episodes of PCP, nor has it been evaluated for PCP prophylaxis. Efficacy of atovaquone in patients who are failing therapy with trimethoprim-sulfamethoxazole hasn't been systematically studied.
• GI disorders may limit absorption of oral form; patients with these disorders may not achieve plasma drug levels associated with response to therapy.
• Drug is ineffective for concurrent pulmonary conditions, such as bacterial, viral, or fungal pneumonia or mycobacterial disease.
• Patients with acute PCP should be carefully evaluated for other possible causes of pulmonary disease and treated with additional drugs as appropriate.

Monitoring the patient
• Closely monitor patients with severe hepatic impairment.
• Monitor patient for adverse effects.

Information for the patient
• Instruct patient to take drug with meals because food significantly enhances absorption.

Geriatric patients
• Use cautiously in elderly patients; they have a greater frequency of decreased hepatic, renal, and cardiac function.

Pediatric patients
• Efficacy of drug hasn't been studied in children.

Breast-feeding patients
• It's unknown if drug appears in breast milk. Use caution when administering drug to breast-feeding women.

atracurium besylate
Tracrium

Pharmacologic classification: nondepolarizing neuromuscular blocker
Therapeutic classification: skeletal muscle relaxant
Pregnancy risk category C

How supplied
Available by prescription only
Injection: 10 mg/ml

Indications, route, and dosage
Adjunct to general anesthesia, to facilitate endotracheal intubation, and to provide skeletal muscle relaxation during surgery or mechanical ventilation
Dosage depends on anesthetic used, individual needs, and response. Doses are representative and must be adjusted.
Adults and children over age 2: Initially, 0.4 to 0.5 mg/kg by I.V. bolus. Maintenance dose of 0.08 to 0.10 mg/kg within 20 to 45 minutes of initial dose

should be administered during prolonged surgical procedures. Maintenance doses may be administered q 15 to 25 minutes in patients receiving balanced anesthesia. Maintenance infusion rate for intensive care unit (ICU) patients who require mechanical ventilation is 11 to 13 mcg/kg/minute.

Children ages 1 month to 2 years: Initially, 0.3 to 0.4 mg/kg by I.V. bolus when under halothane anesthesia. Frequent maintenance doses may be needed.

Pharmacodynamics

Skeletal muscle relaxant action: Produces skeletal muscle paralysis by causing a decreased response to acetylcholine (ACh) at the neuromuscular junction. Because of its high affinity to ACh receptor sites, atracurium competitively blocks access of ACh to the motor end-plate, thus blocking depolarization. At usual doses (0.45 mg/kg), atracurium produces minimal CV effects and doesn't affect intraocular pressure, lower esophageal sphincter pressure, barrier pressure, heart rate or rhythm, mean arterial pressure, systemic vascular resistance, cardiac output, or central venous pressure. CV effects such as decreased peripheral vascular resistance, usually seen at doses greater than 0.5 mg/kg, are caused by histamine release.

Pharmacokinetics

● *Absorption:* Onset of action within 2 minutes, with maximum neuromuscular blockade within 3 to 5 minutes. Maximum neuromuscular blockade increases with increasing dose. Repeated administration doesn't appear to be cumulative, nor is recovery time prolonged. Recovery from neuromuscular blockade under balanced anesthesia usually begins 20 to 35 minutes after dose is injected.

● *Distribution:* Distributed into the extracellular space after I.V. administration. Drug is about 82% protein-bound.

● *Metabolism:* In plasma, rapidly metabolized by Hofmann elimination and by nonspecific enzymatic ester hydrolysis. The liver doesn't appear to play a major role.

● *Excretion:* Drug and its metabolites are excreted in urine and feces by biliary elimination.

Contraindications and precautions

Contraindicated in patients with hypersensitivity to drug. Use cautiously in patients with CV disease; severe electrolyte disorder; bronchogenic carcinoma; hepatic, renal, or pulmonary impairment; neuromuscular disease; or myasthenia gravis; and in elderly or debilitated patients.

Interactions

Drug-drug. *Aminoglycoside antibiotics, beta blockers, clindamycin, depolarizing neuromuscular blocking drugs, furosemide, general anes-*thetics (particularly enflurane, isoflurane), lincomycin, lithium, parenteral magnesium salts, polymyxin antibiotics, potassium-depleting drugs, procainamide, quinidine, quinine, thiazide diuretics, other nondepolarizing neuromuscular blockers:* Neuromuscular blockade associated with atracurium may be enhanced. Use together cautiously.

Opioid analgesics: May cause additive respiratory depression. Use with extreme caution during surgery and immediately postoperatively.

Adverse reactions

CV: *bradycardia*, hypotension, tachycardia.
Respiratory: *prolonged dose-related apnea*, wheezing, increased bronchial secretions, dyspnea, *bronchospasm, laryngospasm.*
Skin: *flushing*, erythema, pruritus, urticaria, rash.
Other: *anaphylaxis.*

☑ Special considerations

● Administer drug by I.V. injection; I.M. injection causes tissue irritation.
● Reduce dose and administration rate in patients in whom histamine release may be hazardous.
● Prior administration of succinylcholine doesn't prolong duration of action of atracurium, but it quickens onset and may deepen neuromuscular blockade.
● Atracurium has a longer duration of action than succinylcholine and a shorter duration than tubocurarine or pancuronium.
● Drug has little or no effect on heart rate and doesn't counteract or reverse the bradycardia caused by anesthetics or vagal stimulation. Thus, bradycardia is seen more frequently with atracurium than with other neuromuscular blocking drugs. Pretreatment with anticholinergics (atropine or glycopyrrolate) is advised.
● If bradycardia occurs during drug administration, treat with I.V. atropine.
● Alkaline solutions such as barbiturates shouldn't be admixed in the same syringe or given through the same needle with atracurium.
● Use drug only if endotracheal intubation, administration of oxygen under positive pressure, artificial respiration, and assisted or controlled ventilation are immediately available.
● To evaluate patient for recovery from neuromuscular blocking effect, observe for ability to breathe, cough, protrude tongue, keep eyes open, lift head keeping mouth closed, and show adequate strength of hand-grip. Assess for adequate negative inspiratory force (-25 cm H_2O).
● Until head and neck muscles recover from blockade effects, patient may find speech difficult.
● If indicated, assess need for pain medication or sedation. Drug doesn't affect consciousness or relieve pain.
● Signs and symptoms of overdose include prolonged respiratory depression or apnea and CV

Reactions may be *common*, uncommon, *life-threatening*, or COMMON AND LIFE-THREATENING.

collapse. A sudden release of histamine may also occur.

• A peripheral nerve stimulator is recommended to monitor response and to determine the nature and degree of neuromuscular block. Maintain an adequate airway and manual or mechanical ventilation until patient can maintain respiration unassisted.

• For treatment, administer cholinesterase inhibitors, such as edrophonium, neostigmine, or pyridostigmine, to reverse neuromuscular blockade; and atropine or glycopyrrolate to counteract muscarinic adverse effects of cholinesterase inhibitors. Monitor vital signs at least every 15 minutes until patient is stable, then every 30 minutes for next 2 hours. Observe airway until patient has fully recovered from drug effects. Note rate, depth, and pattern of respirations.

Monitoring the patient
• Peripheral nerve stimulator should be used to monitor responses during ICU administration and may be used to detect residual paralysis during recovery and to avoid atracurium overdose.
• Monitor patient for adverse effects.

Geriatric patients
• Elderly patients may be more sensitive to drug's effects.

Pediatric patients
• Safety and efficacy haven't been established for children under age 1 month.

Breast-feeding patients
• It's unknown if drug appears in breast milk. Use cautiously in breast-feeding women.

---

atropine sulfate

Pharmacologic classification: anticholinergic, belladonna alkaloid
Therapeutic classification: antiarrhythmic, vagolytic
Pregnancy risk category C

How supplied
Available by prescription only
Tablets: 0.4 mg
Injection: 0.05 mg/ml, 0.1 mg/ml, 0.3 mg/ml, 0.4 mg/ml, 0.5 mg/ml, 0.8 mg/ml, and 1 mg/ml
Ophthalmic ointment: 1%
Ophthalmic solution: 0.5%, 1%, 2%

Indications, route, and dosage
Symptomatic bradycardia, bradyarrhythmia (junctional or escape rhythm)
Adults: Usually 0.5 to 1 mg by I.V. push; repeat q 3 to 5 minutes, to maximum of 2 mg. Lower doses (less than 0.5 mg) may cause bradycardia.

Children: 0.02 mg/kg I.V. up to maximum 1 mg; or 0.3 mg/m^2; may repeat q 5 minutes.
Preoperatively for diminishing secretions and blocking cardiac vagal reflexes
Adults and children weighing over 20 kg (44 lb): 0.4 mg I.M. or S.C. 30 to 60 minutes before anesthesia.
Children weighing less than 20 kg: 0.1 mg I.M. for 3 kg (6.6 lb), 0.2 mg I.M. for 4 to 9 kg (8.8 to 20 lb), 0.3 mg I.M. for 10 to 20 kg (22 to 44 lb) 30 to 60 minutes before anesthesia.
Antidote for anticholinesterase insecticide poisoning
Adults and children: 1 to 2 mg I.M. or I.V. repeated q 20 to 30 minutes until muscarinic symptoms disappear.
Hypotonic radiograph of the GI tract
Adults: 1 mg I.M.
Acute iritis, uveitis
Adults: 1 to 2 drops (0.5% or 1% solution) into the eye q.i.d. (in children use 0.5% solution) or a small amount of ointment in the conjunctival sac t.i.d.
Cycloplegic refraction
Adults: 1 to 2 drops (1% solution) 1 hour before refraction.
Children: 1 to 2 drops (0.5% solution) into each eye b.i.d. for 1 to 3 days before eye examination and 1 hour before examination.

Pharmacodynamics
Antiarrhythmic action: An anticholinergic (parasympatholytic) drug with many uses, atropine remains the mainstay of pharmacologic treatment for bradyarrhythmias. It blocks the effects of acetylcholine on the SA and AV nodes, thereby increasing SA and AV node conduction velocity. It also increases sinus node discharge rate and decreases the effective refractory period of the AV node. These changes result in an increased heart rate (both atrial and ventricular).

Atropine has variable—and clinically negligible—effects on the His-Purkinje system. Small doses (below 0.5 mg) and occasionally larger doses may lead to a paradoxical slowing of the heart rate, which may be followed by a more rapid rate.
Anticholinergic action: As a cholinergic blocker, atropine decreases the action of the parasympathetic nervous system on certain glands (bronchial, salivary, and sweat), resulting in decreased secretions. It also decreases cholinergic effects on the iris, ciliary body, and intestinal and bronchial smooth muscle.
Antidote for cholinesterase poisoning: Atropine blocks the cholinomimetic effects of these pesticides.

Pharmacokinetics
• *Absorption:* I.V. is most common route for bradyarrhythmia treatment. With endotracheal administration, atropine is well absorbed from the

bronchial tree (drug has been used in 1-mg doses in acute bradyarrhythmia when an I.V. line hasn't been established). Effects on heart rate peak within 2 to 4 minutes after I.V. administration. Drug is well absorbed after oral and I.M. administration; inhibitory effects on salivation peak in 30 minutes to 1 hour after either route.

• *Distribution:* Well distributed throughout the body, including CNS. Only 18% of drug binds with plasma protein.
• *Metabolism:* Metabolized in liver to several metabolites. About 30% to 50% of dose is excreted by kidneys as unchanged drug.
• *Excretion:* Excreted primarily through kidneys; however, small amounts may be excreted in feces and expired air. Elimination half-life is biphasic, with an initial 2-hour phase then a terminal half-life of about 12¼ hours.

Contraindications and precautions

Contraindicated in patients with hypersensitivity to drug or sodium metabisulfite and in those with acute angle-closure glaucoma, obstructive uropathy, obstructive disease of GI tract, paralytic ileus, toxic megacolon, intestinal atony, unstable CV status in acute hemorrhage, asthma, and myasthenia gravis.

Ophthalmic form is contraindicated in patients with hypersensitivity to drug or belladonna alkaloids, in those with glaucoma, and in those who have adhesions between the iris and lens. Drug shouldn't be used during the first 3 months of life because of the possible association between cycloplegia produced and development of amblyopia.

Use cautiously in patients with Down syndrome. Ophthalmic form should be used with caution in patients with increased intraocular pressure and in elderly patients.

Interactions

Drug-drug. *Amantadine:* May increase anticholinergic adverse effects. Avoid concurrent use.
Other anticholinergics, drugs with anticholinergic effects: Produce additive effects. Avoid concurrent use.
Drug-herb. *Betel palm:* May cause enhanced CNS effects. Avoid use together.
Jaborandi tree: May reduce effects of atropine. Monitor closely.
Jimsonweed: May adversely affect CV function. Avoid use together.
Pill-bearing spurge: May decrease effects of atropine. Use together cautiously.
Squaw vine: May decrease metabolic breakdown of atropine. Monitor patient.

Adverse reactions

CNS: *headache, restlessness,* ataxia, disorientation, hallucinations, delirium, *insomnia, dizziness,* excitement, agitation, confusion, especially in elderly patients (with systemic or oral form),

confusion, somnolence, headache (with ophthalmic form).
CV: palpitations and **bradycardia** following low-dose atropine, tachycardia after higher doses (with systemic or oral form), tachycardia (with ophthalmic form).
EENT: photophobia, increased intraocular pressure, *blurred vision, mydriasis,* cycloplegia (with systemic or oral form), ocular congestion with long-term use, conjunctivitis, contact dermatitis of eye, ocular edema, eye dryness, transient stinging and burning, eye irritation, hyperemia (with ophthalmic form).
GI: *dry mouth,* thirst, *constipation,* nausea, vomiting (with systemic or oral form); dry mouth, abdominal distention in infants (with ophthalmic form).
GU: urine retention, impotence (with systemic or oral form).
Hematologic: leukocytosis (with systemic or oral form).
Skin: dryness (with ophthalmic form).
Other: severe allergic reactions, including **anaphylaxis** and urticaria (systemic or oral form).

☑ Special considerations

• With I.V. administration, drug may cause paradoxical initial bradycardia, which usually disappears within 2 minutes.
• High doses may cause hyperpyrexia, urinary retention, and CNS effects, including hallucinations and confusion (anticholinergic delirium). Other anticholinergics may increase vagal blockage.
• Signs of overdose reflect excessive anticholinergic activity, especially CV and CNS stimulation.
• Treatment of overdose includes physostigmine administration, to reverse excessive anticholinergic activity, and general supportive measures, as needed.

Monitoring the patient

• If patient has cardiac disorder, observe for tachycardia.
• Monitor patient's fluid intake and output; drug causes urine retention and hesitancy. If possible, patient should void before taking drug.

Information for the patient

• Tell patient taking oral form how to handle distressing anticholinergic effects.
• Instruct patient to report serious or persistent adverse reactions promptly.
• Tell patient about potential photophobia; advise use of sunglasses.

Geriatric patients

• Monitor closely for urine retention in elderly men with benign prostatic hyperplasia.

attapulgite

Children's Kaopectate, Diasorb, Donnagel, Fowler's*, Kaopectate, Kaopectate Advanced Formula, Kaopectate Maximum Strength, K-Pek, Parepectolin, Rheaban, Rheaban Maximum Strength

Pharmacologic classification: hydrated magnesium aluminum silicate
Therapeutic classification: antidiarrheal
Pregnancy risk category NR

How supplied

Available without a prescription
Tablets: 300 mg, 600 mg*, 630 mg*, 750 mg
Tablets (chewable): 600 mg
Oral suspension: 600 mg/15 ml, 750 mg/5 ml, 750 mg/15 ml*, 900 mg/15 ml*

Indications, route, and dosage

Acute, nonspecific diarrhea
Adults and adolescents: 1.2 to 1.5 g (unless using Diasorb, in which case dosage can be as high as 3 g) P.O. after each loose bowel movement; don't exceed 9 g within 24 hours.
Children ages 6 to 12: 600 mg (suspension) or 750 mg (tablet) P.O. after each loose bowel movement; don't exceed 4.2 g (suspension and chewable tablets) or 4.5 g (tablet) within 24 hours.
Children ages 3 to 6: 300 mg P.O. after each loose bowel movement; don't exceed 2.1 g within 24 hours.

Pharmacodynamics

Antidiarrheal action: Exact mechanism unknown. Believed to absorb large numbers of bacteria and toxins and reduce water loss in GI tract.

Pharmacokinetics

• *Absorption:* Not absorbed.
• *Distribution:* Not applicable.
• *Metabolism:* Not applicable.
• *Excretion:* Drug is excreted unchanged in feces.

Contraindications and precautions

Contraindicated in patients with dysentery or suspected bowel obstruction. Use cautiously in dehydrated patients.

Interactions

Drug-drug. *Oral drugs:* May impair absorption if given together with attapulgite. Administer attapulgite not less than 2 hours before or 3 to 4 hours after these drugs; Monitor patient for decreased effectiveness.

Adverse reactions

GI: constipation.

☑ Special considerations

• Ensure that patient achieves adequate fluid intake to compensate for fluid loss from diarrhea.
• Drug shouldn't be used if diarrhea is accompanied by fever or blood or mucus in the stool. Discontinue drug if any of these signs occurs during treatment.
• Because attapulgite isn't absorbed, an overdose is unlikely to pose a significant health problem.

Monitoring the patient

• Monitor patient for constipation.
• Monitor fluid intake.

Information for the patient

• Tell patient to take drug after each loose bowel movement until diarrhea is controlled.
• Instruct patient to call if diarrhea isn't controlled within 48 hours or if fever develops.

Geriatric patients

• Drug should be used cautiously and only under medical supervision.

Pediatric patients

• Drug should be used only under medical supervision in children under age 3.

auranofin

Ridaura

Pharmacologic classification: gold salt
Therapeutic classification: antarthritic
Pregnancy risk category C

How supplied

Available by prescription only
Capsules: 3 mg

Indications, route, and dosage

Rheumatoid arthritis, ◊ **psoriatic arthritis,** ◊ **active systemic lupus erythematosus,** ◊ **Felty's syndrome**
Adults: 6 mg P.O. daily, administered either as 3 mg b.i.d. or 6 mg once daily. After 4 to 6 months, may be increased to 9 mg daily. If response remains inadequate after 3 months at 9 mg daily, discontinue drug.

Pharmacodynamics

Antarthritic action: Suppresses or prevents, but doesn't cure, adult or juvenile arthritis and synovitis. Is anti-inflammatory in active arthritis. Thought to reduce inflammation by altering the immune system. Auranofin has been shown to decrease high serum levels of immunoglobulins and rheumatoid factors in patients with arthritis. However, the exact mechanism of action remains unknown.

Pharmacokinetics
• *Absorption:* When administered P.O., 25% of the gold in auranofin is absorbed through the GI tract. Plasma level peaks in 1 to 2 hours.
• *Distribution:* 60% protein-bound and distributed widely in body tissues. Oral gold from auranofin is bound to a higher degree than gold from the injectable form. Synovial fluid levels are about 50% of blood levels. No correlation between blood-gold levels and safety or efficacy has been determined.
• *Metabolism:* Unknown, but it's believed that drug isn't broken down into elemental gold.
• *Excretion:* 60% of absorbed auranofin (15% of administered dose) is excreted in urine and the remainder in feces. Average plasma half-life is 26 days, compared with about 6 days for gold sodium thiomalate.

Contraindications and precautions
Contraindicated in patients with history of severe gold toxicity, necrotizing enterocolitis, pulmonary fibrosis, exfoliative dermatitis, bone marrow aplasia, severe hematologic disorders, or severe toxicity due to previous exposure to other heavy metals.

Use cautiously with other drugs that cause blood dyscrasias and in patients with renal, hepatic, or inflammatory bowel disease; rash; or bone marrow depression. Use of drug in pregnant women isn't recommended.

Interactions
Drug-drug. *Other drugs that may cause blood dyscrasias:* Possible additive hematologic toxicity. Use together cautiously.

Adverse reactions
CNS: confusion, hallucinations, *seizures.*
EENT: conjunctivitis.
GI: diarrhea, abdominal pain, nausea, stomatitis, glossitis, anorexia, metallic taste, dyspepsia, flatulence, constipation, dysgeusia, *ulcerative colitis.*
GU: proteinuria, hematuria, *nephrotic syndrome,* glomerulonephritis, *acute renal failure.*
Hematologic: *thrombocytopenia with or without purpura, aplastic anemia, agranulocytosis,* leukopenia, eosinophilia, anemia.
Hepatic: jaundice, elevated liver enzymes.
Respiratory: interstitial pneumonitis.
Skin: *rash, pruritus, dermatitis,* exfoliative dermatitis, urticaria, erythema, alopecia.

☑ Special considerations
• Discontinue drug if platelet count decreases to below 100,000/mm^3.
• When switching from injectable gold, start auranofin at 6 mg P.O. daily.
• Serum protein-bound iodine test, especially when done by the chloric acid digestion method, gives false readings during and for several weeks after gold therapy.
• In acute overdose, empty gastric contents by induced emesis or gastric lavage.
• When severe reactions to gold occur, corticosteroids, dimercaprol (a chelating drug), or penicillamine may be given to aid recovery. Prednisone 40 to 100 mg daily in divided doses is recommended to manage severe renal, hematologic, pulmonary, or enterocolitic reactions to gold.
• Dimercaprol may be used with corticosteroids to facilitate the removal of the gold when corticosteroid treatment alone is ineffective.
• Use of chelating drugs is controversial, and caution is recommended. Appropriate supportive therapy is indicated as necessary.

Monitoring the patient
• Monitor platelet count.
• Monitor patient for adverse effects.

Information for the patient
• Emphasize importance of monthly follow-up to monitor patient's platelet count.
• Reassure patient that beneficial drug effect may be delayed for 3 months. However, if response is inadequate after 6 to 9 months, auranofin probably will be discontinued.
• Encourage patient to take drug as prescribed and not to alter dosage schedule.
• Diarrhea is the most common adverse reaction. Tell patient to continue taking drug if he experiences mild diarrhea; however, tell patient to call immediately if blood appears in stool.
• Tell patient to continue taking concomitant drug therapy, such as NSAIDs, if prescribed.
• Dermatitis is a common adverse reaction. Advise patient to report rash or other skin problems immediately.
• Stomatitis is also a common adverse reaction. Tell patient that stomatitis is often preceded by a metallic taste and advise patient to call immediately if this occurs.

Geriatric patients
• Administer usual adult dose. Use cautiously in patients with decreased renal function.

Pediatric patients
• Safe dosage hasn't been established; use in children currently isn't recommended.

Breast-feeding patients
• Drug isn't recommended for use during breast-feeding.

azathioprine
Imuran

azathioprine sodium
Imuran

Pharmacologic classification: purine antagonist
Therapeutic classification: immunosuppressant
Pregnancy risk category D

How supplied
Available by prescription only
Tablets: 50 mg
Injection: 100 mg/vial

Indications, route, and dosage
Prevention of the rejection of kidney transplants
Adults and children: Initially, 3 to 5 mg/kg P.O. daily beginning on day of (or 1 to 3 days before) transplantation. After transplantation, dosage may be administered I.V., until patient is able to tolerate oral dosage. Usual maintenance dosage is 1 to 3 mg/kg daily. Dosage varies with patient response.
Severe, refractory rheumatoid arthritis
Adults: Initially, 1 mg/kg (about 50 to 100 mg) P.O. taken as a single dose or in divided doses. If patient response is unsatisfactory after 6 to 8 weeks, dosage may be increased by 0.5 mg/kg daily (up to a maximum of 2.5 mg/kg daily) at 4-week intervals.

Pharmacodynamics
Immunosuppressive action: Mechanism unknown. However, drug may inhibit RNA and DNA synthesis, mitosis, or (in patients undergoing renal transplantation) coenzyme formation and functioning. Suppresses cell-mediated hypersensitivity and alters antibody production.

Pharmacokinetics
• *Absorption:* Well absorbed orally.
• *Distribution:* Drug and its major metabolite, mercaptopurine, are distributed throughout the body; both are 30% protein-bound. Azathioprine and its metabolites cross the placenta.
• *Metabolism:* Metabolized primarily to mercaptopurine.
• *Excretion:* Small amounts of azathioprine and mercaptopurine are excreted in urine intact; most of a given dose is excreted in urine as secondary metabolites.

Contraindications and precautions
Contraindicated in patients with hypersensitivity to drug and during pregnancy. Use cautiously in patients with impaired renal or hepatic function.

Interactions
Drug-drug. *Allopurinol:* Impaired inactivation of azathioprine is inhibited by allopurinol. Reduce dose by one-third to one-fourth the usual dose.
Angiotensin-converting enzyme inhibitors: Can cause anemia and severe leukopenia. Avoid concomitant use.
Cyclosporine: Possible decrease in plasma levels. Monitor patient closely.
Methotrexate: Possible increase in metabolite 6-MP plasma levels. Monitor patient closely.
Pancuronium, tubocurarine: Drug may reverse neuromuscular blockade. Avoid concomitant use.

Adverse reactions
GI: *nausea, vomiting, **pancreatitis,** steatorrhea, diarrhea, abdominal pain.*
Hematologic: LEUKOPENIA, *bone marrow suppression,* anemia, *pancytopenia, thrombocytopenia, immunosuppression* (possibly profound).
Hepatic: *hepatotoxicity,* jaundice.
Skin: rash.
Other: arthralgia, alopecia, *infections,* fever, myalgia, *increased risk of neoplasia.*

☑ Special considerations
• If infection occurs, reduce drug dosage and treat infection.
• If nausea and vomiting occur, divide dose or give with or after meals.
• If used to treat rheumatoid arthritis, NSAIDs should be continued when azathioprine therapy is initiated.
• Chronic immunosuppression with azathioprine is associated with an increased risk of neoplasia.
• Imuran should not be given to pregnant women with rheumatoid arthritis.
• Signs of overdose include nausea, vomiting, diarrhea, and extension of hematologic effects.
• Supportive treatment for toxicity may include treatment with blood products, if necessary.

Monitoring the patient
• Monitor patient for unusual bleeding or bruising, fever, or sore throat.
• Hematologic status should be monitored while patient is receiving azathioprine. CBCs, including platelet counts, should be taken at least weekly during the first month, twice monthly for the second and third months, then monthly.
• Monitor patient for signs of hepatic damage: clay-colored stools, dark urine, jaundice, pruritus, and elevated liver enzyme levels.

Information for the patient
• Teach patient about disease and rationale for therapy; explain possible adverse effects and importance of reporting them, especially unusual bleeding or bruising, fever, sore throat, mouth sores, abdominal pain, pale stools, or dark urine.

- Encourage compliance with therapy and follow-up visits.
- Advise patient to avoid pregnancy during therapy and for 4 months after stopping therapy.
- Tell patient with rheumatoid arthritis that clinical response may not be apparent for up to 12 weeks.
- Suggest taking drug with or after meals or in divided doses to prevent nausea.

azithromycin
Zithromax

Pharmacologic classification: azalide macrolide
Therapeutic classification: antibiotic
Pregnancy risk category B

How supplied
Available by prescription only
Tablets: 250 mg
Powder for oral suspension: 100 mg/5 ml, 200 mg/5 ml; 300 mg*, 600 mg*, 900 mg*, 1,000 mg/packet
Injection: 500 mg

Indications, route, and dosage
Acute bacterial exacerbations of chronic obstructive pulmonary disease caused by Haemophilus influenzae, Moraxella (Branhamella) catarrhalis, *or* Streptococcus pneumoniae; uncomplicated skin and skin-structure infections caused by Staphylococcus aureus, Streptococcus pyogenes, *or* Streptococcus agalactiae; *and second-line therapy of pharyngitis or tonsillitis caused by* S. pyogenes
Adults and adolescents ages 16 and older: Initially, 500 mg P.O. as a single dose on day 1; then 250 mg daily on days 2 through 5. Total cumulative dose is 1.5 g.
Community-acquired pneumonia caused by Chlamydia pneumoniae, H. influenzae, Mycoplasma pneumoniae, S. pneumoniae; *I.V.* form can be used for above infections and those caused by Legionella pneumophila, M. catarrhalis, *and* S. aureus
Adults and adolescents ages 16 and over: 500 mg P.O. as a single dose on day 1; then 250 mg P.O. daily on days 2 through 5. Total dose is 1.5 g. For those who require initial I.V. therapy, 500 mg I.V. as a single daily dose for 2 days; then 500 mg P.O. as a single daily dose to complete a 7- to 10-day course of therapy. The timing of the change from I.V. to P.O. therapy is based on patient's clinical response.
Nongonococcal urethritis or cervicitis caused by Chlamydia trachomatis
Adults and adolescents ages 16: 1 g P.O. as a single dose.

Pelvic inflammatory disease caused by Chlamydia trachomatis, Neisseria gonorrhoeae, *or* Mycoplasma hominis *in patients requiring initial I.V. therapy*
Adults: 500 mg I.V. as a single daily dose for 1 to 2 days; then 250 mg P.O. daily to complete a 7-day course of therapy. The timing of the change from I.V. to P.O. therapy is based on patient's clinical response.
Otitis media
Children over age 6 months: 10 mg/kg P.O. on day 1; then 5 mg/kg on days 2 through 5.
Tonsillitis
Children over age 2: 12 mg/kg P.O. daily for 5 days.
Chancroid
Adults: 1 g P.O. as a single dose.
Disseminated Mycobacterium avium complex (MAC) in patients with advanced HIV infection
Adults: 1.2 g P.O. once weekly alone or with rifabutin.

Pharmacodynamics
Antibiotic action: A derivative of erythromycin that binds to the 50S subunit of bacterial ribosomes, blocking protein synthesis. Bacteriostatic or bactericidal, depending on concentration.

Pharmacokinetics
- *Absorption:* Rapidly absorbed from the GI tract; food decreases both maximum plasma levels and amount of drug absorbed.
- *Distribution:* Rapidly distributed throughout the body and readily penetrates cells; doesn't readily enter CNS. It concentrates in fibroblasts and phagocytes. Significantly higher levels of drug are reached in the tissues as compared with the plasma. Uptake and release of drug from tissues contributes to long half-life. With a loading dose, peak and trough blood levels are stable within 48 hours. Without a loading dose, 5 to 7 days are required before steady state is reached.
- *Metabolism:* Not metabolized.
- *Excretion:* Excreted mostly in feces after excretion into bile. Less than 10% excreted in urine. Terminal elimination half-life is 68 hours.

Contraindications and precautions
Contraindicated in patients with hypersensitivity to erythromycin or other macrolides. Use cautiously in patients with impaired hepatic function.

Interactions
Drug-drug. *Antacids containing aluminum and magnesium:* May result in lower peak plasma levels of azithromycin. Separate administration times by at least 2 hours.
Dihydroergotamine, ergotamine: Acute ergot toxicity may occur. Use cautiously.
Drugs metabolized by the hepatic cytochrome P-450 system (such as barbiturates, carba-

mazepine, cyclosporine, phenytoin): May result in impaired metabolism of these drugs and increased risk of toxicity. Monitor patient for signs of toxicity.
Theophyllines: Macrolides may increase plasma theophylline levels by decreasing theophylline clearance. Monitor theophylline levels.
Triazolam: Clearance may be decreased, increasing risk of triazolam toxicity. Monitor patient closely.
Warfarin: Other macrolides may increase PT; effect of azithromycin is unknown. Monitor PT carefully.

Adverse reactions
CNS: dizziness, vertigo, headache, fatigue, somnolence.
CV: palpitations, chest pain.
GI: *nausea, vomiting, diarrhea, abdominal pain,* dyspepsia, flatulence, melena, cholestatic jaundice, pseudomembranous colitis.
GU: candidiasis, vaginitis, nephritis.
Skin: rash, photosensitivity.
Other: angioedema.

☑ Special considerations
• Obtain culture and sensitivity tests before giving first dose. Therapy can begin before results are obtained.
• Drug may cause overgrowth of nonsusceptible bacteria or fungi. Watch for signs and symptoms of superinfection.
• Serologic tests for syphilis and cultures for gonorrhea should be taken from patients diagnosed with sexually transmitted urethritis or cervicitis. Drug shouldn't be used to treat gonorrhea or syphilis.
• Reconstitute 500-mg vial with 4.8 ml of sterile water for injection. Shake well until drug is dissolved (yields a concentration of 100 mg/ml). Dilute solution further in at least 250 ml of normal saline, 0.45% saline, D_5W, or lactated Ringer's solution to yield a concentration range of 1 to 2 mg/ml.
• Infuse 500-mg dose of azithromycin I.V. over 1 or more hours. Don't give as a bolus or I.M. injection.

Monitoring the patient
• Patients on warfarin will need close monitoring of INR because some macrolides have been shown to increase INR.
• Monitor patient for adverse drug effects.

Information for the patient
• Tell patient to take all of drug prescribed, even if feeling better.
• Remind patient that drug should always be taken on an empty stomach because food or antacids decrease absorption. Patient should take drug 1 hour before or 2 hours after a meal and shouldn't take antacids.

• Instruct patient to promptly report adverse reactions.

Geriatric patients
• In patients with normal hepatic and renal function, when using the 5-day dosage regimen, no significant pharmacokinetic differences were seen in those between ages 65 and 85.

Pediatric patients
• Safety and efficacy in children age 16 and younger haven't been established.

Breast-feeding patients
• It's unknown if drug appears in breast milk. Use cautiously in breast-feeding women.

aztreonam
Azactam

Pharmacologic classification: monobactam
Therapeutic classification: antibiotic
Pregnancy risk category B

How supplied
Available by prescription only
Injection: 500-mg, 1-g, 2-g vials

Indications, route, and dosage
Urinary tract, respiratory tract, intra-abdominal, gynecologic, or skin infections; septicemia caused by gram-negative bacteria; ◇ adjunct therapy in pelvic inflammatory disease; ◇ gonorrhea
Adults: 500 mg to 2 g I.V. or I.M. q 8 to 12 hours. For severe systemic or life-threatening infections, 2 g q 6 to 8 hours may be given. Maximum dose is 8 g daily. For gonorrhea, give 1 g I.M. single dose.
✦ Dosage adjustment. In patients with a creatinine clearance of 10 to 30 ml/minute/1.73 m^2, reduce dose by one-half after an initial dose of 1 to 2 g. In patients with a creatinine clearance below 10 ml/minute/1.73 m^2, an initial dose of 500 mg to 2 g should be followed by one-fourth of the usual dose at the usual intervals; give one-eighth the initial dose after each session of hemodialysis.

Pharmacodynamics
Antibacterial action: A monobactam that inhibits mucopeptide synthesis of the bacterial cell wall. It preferentially binds to penicillin-binding protein 3 (PBP3) of susceptible organisms and often causes cell lysis and cell death. Has a narrow spectrum of activity and is usually bactericidal in action. Effective against *Escherichia coli, Enterobacter, Klebsiella pneumoniae, Proteus mirabilis,* and *Pseudomonas aeruginosa.* Has limited activity against *Citrobacter, Haemophilus influen-*

zae, K. oxytoca, Hafnia, Serratia marcescens, E. aerogenes, Morganella morganii, Providencia, Branhamella catarrhalis, Proteus vulgaris, and Neisseria gonorrhoeae.

Pharmacokinetics

• *Absorption:* Absorbed poorly from GI tract after oral administration but absorbed rapidly and completely after I.M. or I.V. administration; levels peak in 60 minutes.

• *Distribution:* Distributed rapidly and widely to all body fluids and tissues, including bile, breast milk, and CSF. It crosses the placenta and is found in fetal circulation.

• *Metabolism:* From 6% to 16% is metabolized to inactive metabolites by nonspecific hydrolysis of the beta-lactam ring; 56% to 60% is protein-bound, less if renal impairment is present.

• *Excretion:* Excreted principally in urine as unchanged drug by glomerular filtration and tubular secretion; 1.5% to 3.5% is excreted in feces as unchanged drug. Half-life averages 1.7 hours. Excreted in breast milk; may be removed by hemodialysis and peritoneal dialysis.

Contraindications and precautions

Contraindicated in patients with hypersensitivity to drug. Use cautiously in patients with impaired renal function and in elderly patients.

Interactions

Drug-drug. *Aminoglycosides, other beta-lactam antibiotics (such as cefoperazone, cefotaxime, clindamycin, metronidazole, piperacillin):* Synergistic or additive effects occur. May be used for this therapeutic effect.

Chloramphenicol: Antagonistic effect. Give the 2 preparations several hours apart.

Clavulanic acid: May be synergistic or antagonistic, depending on organism involved. Use cautiously.

Potent inducers of beta-lactamase production (cefoxitin, imipenem): May inactivate aztreonam. Avoid concomitant use.

Probenecid: May prolong rate of tubular secretion of aztreonam. Avoid concomitant use.

Adverse reactions

CNS: *seizures,* headache, insomnia, confusion.
CV: hypotension.
GI: diarrhea, nausea, vomiting.
Hematologic: neutropenia, anemia, *pancytopenia, thrombocytopenia,* leukocytosis, thrombocytosis.
Other: hypersensitivity reactions (rash, *anaphylaxis*), transient elevation of LD, creatinine, ALT and AST; thrombophlebitis (at I.V. site); discomfort, swelling (at I.M. injection site).

☑ Special considerations

• Drug has been used to treat bone and joint infection caused by susceptible aerobic, gram-negative bacteria.

• To reconstitute for I.M. use, dilute with at least 3 ml of sterile water for injection, bacteriostatic water for injection, normal saline solution, or bacteriostatic normal saline solution for each gram of aztreonam (15-ml vial).

• To reconstitute for I.V. use, add 6 to 10 ml of sterile water for injection to each 15-ml vial; for I.V. infusion, prepare as for I.M. solution. May be further diluted by adding to normal saline, Ringer's solution, lactated Ringer's solution, 5% or 10% dextrose, or other electrolyte-containing solutions. For I.V. piggyback (100-ml bottles), add at least 50 ml of diluent for each gram of aztreonam. Final concentration shouldn't exceed 20 mg/ml.

• I.V. route is preferred for doses larger than 1 g or in patients with bacterial septicemia, localized parenchymal abscesses, peritonitis, or other life-threatening infections; administer by direct I.V. push over 3 to 5 minutes or by intermittent infusion over 20 to 60 minutes.

• Solutions may be colorless or light straw yellow. On standing, they may develop a slight pink tint; potency isn't affected.

• Reduced dose may be needed in patients with impaired renal function, cirrhosis, or other hepatic impairment.

• Drug may be stored at room temperature for 48 hours or in refrigerator for 7 days.

• Hemodialysis or peritoneal dialysis increases elimination of drug.

• Aztreonam therapy alters urinary glucose determinations using cupric sulfate (Clinitest or Benedict's solution) and gives false-positive Coombs' test results.

Monitoring the patient

• Careful monitoring is recommended during therapy in patients with impaired hepatic or renal function.

Information for the patient

• Tell patient to call immediately if rash, redness, or itching develops.

Geriatric patients

• The half-life of aztreonam may be prolonged in elderly patients because of their diminished renal function.

Breast-feeding patients

• Although drug appears in breast milk, it isn't absorbed from infant's GI tract and is unlikely to cause any serious problems.

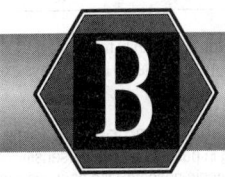

bacillus Calmette-Guérin (BCG) vaccine
TICE BCG

Pharmacologic classification: vaccine
Therapeutic classification: bacterial vaccine
Pregnancy risk category C

How supplied
Available by prescription only
Powder for injection: 1 to 8 × 10⁸ colony-forming units (CFU)/ml of Tice-University of Illinois strain BCG per ml, equivalent to about 50 mg

Indications, route, and dosage
Tuberculosis (TB) exposure
Adults and children over age 1 month: Apply 0.2 to 0.3 ml of prepared vaccine on the cleaned surface of skin; apply multiple-puncture disk through vaccine. The vaccine should flow into the wound and dry. Keep site dry for 24 hours.

Repeat dosage in all patients who have a negative tuberculin test reaction to 5 tuberculin units (TU) at 2- to 3-month follow-up. Advisory Committee on Immunization Practices (ACIP) and Advisory Committee for the Elimination of Tuberculosis (ACET) suggest revaccination with a full dose at age 1 if skin test reaction is negative to 5 TU.
Neonates under age 1 month: Reduce dosage to one-half by using 2 ml of sterile water when reconstituting.

Pharmacodynamics
Immunostimulant action: Promotes active immunity to tuberculosis. Immunity isn't permanent or entirely predictable.

Pharmacokinetics
No information available.

Contraindications and precautions
Contraindicated in patients with hypogamma-globulinemia, in the presence of a positive tuberculin reaction (when meant for use as immunoprophylactic after exposure to TB) in immunosuppressed patients, in those with fresh smallpox vaccinations, in those who have suffered burns, and in patients receiving corticosteroid therapy. Avoid use during pregnancy.

Interactions
Drug-drug. *Antituberculotics (isoniazid, rifampin, streptomycin):* Inhibits BCG multiplication and impairs vaccine efficacy. Use with caution.
Corticosteroids, immunosuppressants: May alter immune response to BCG vaccine. Avoid use.

Adverse reactions
Other: osteomyelitis, lymphadenopathy, allergic reaction.

☑ Special considerations
● Obtain thorough history of allergies and reactions to immunizations.
● Epinephrine solution 1:1,000 should be available to treat allergic reactions.
● Severe or prolonged reactions may be treated with antituberculotics.
● To prepare percutaneous injection, add 1 ml sterile water (without preservatives) to each vial of vaccine. Draw mixture into syringe and expel into ampule 3 times to ensure adequate mixing.
● If alcohol is used to swab the skin, allow it to evaporate before vaccination. Otherwise, it could inactivate the virus.
● Vaccinate patients with chronic skin diseases in area of healthy skin.
● BCG vaccine is of no value as an immunoprophylactic in patients with a positive purified protein derivative (PPD) test reaction.
● Articles contaminated with this live vaccine must be autoclaved or treated with formaldehyde before disposal.
● Store vaccine at 36° to 46° F (2° to 8° C). Avoid exposure to light.
● BCG vaccine has shown some value in treating various cancers, including malignant melanoma, multiple myeloma, leukemia, bladder cancer, some lung cancers, and some breast tumors. Consult other references and published protocols for appropriate dosage regimens.
● BCG vaccination may affect the interpretation of subsequent tuberculin skin test reactions.
● Treat overdose with antituberculosis drugs.

Monitoring the patient
● Monitor patient for signs of allergic reaction after administration.
● Monitor patient for adverse effects.

Information for the patient
● Tell patient to expect swollen lymph nodes or a body rash after vaccination. A lesion at the in-

jection site develops within 7 to 10 days of vaccination and may persist for up to 6 months.

● Tell patient to report distressing adverse reactions.

● Tell patient that a tuberculin skin test will be performed 2 to 3 months after vaccination to confirm development of delayed hypersensitivity.

bacitracin
AK-Tracin, Altracin, Baciguent, Baci-IM

Pharmacologic classification: polypeptide antibiotic
Therapeutic classification: antibiotic
Pregnancy risk category C

How supplied
Available by prescription only
Injection: 50,000-unit vials
Ophthalmic ointment: 500 units/g
Available without a prescription
Topical: ointment form (500 units/g) and in combination products containing neomycin, polymyxin B, and bacitracin

Indications, route, and dosage
Topical infections, impetigo, abrasions, cuts, minor wounds
Adults and children: Apply thin film to cleansed area once daily to t.i.d. for no more than 7 days.
Pneumonia and empyema caused by a staphylococcal infection
Children weighing under 2.5 kg (5.5 lb): Give 900 units/kg I.M. daily in 2 or 3 divided doses.
Children weighing over 2.5 kg: Give 1,000 units/kg I.M. daily in 2 or 3 divided doses.
Antibiotic-associated pseudomembranous colitis caused by Clostridium difficile
Adults: 20,000 to 25,000 units P.O. q 6 hours for 7 to 10 days.

Pharmacodynamics
Antibacterial action: Impairs bacterial cell-wall synthesis, damaging the bacterial plasma membrane and making the cell more vulnerable to osmotic pressure. Drug is effective against many gram-positive organisms, including *C. difficile.* Only minimally active against gram-negative organisms.

Pharmacokinetics
● *Absorption:* With I.M. administration, bacitracin is absorbed rapidly and completely; serum levels range from 0.2 to 2 mcg/ml. Drug isn't absorbed from GI tract, isn't significantly absorbed from intact or denuded skin wounds or mucous membranes.
● *Distribution:* Distributed widely throughout all body organs and fluids except CSF (unless meninges are inflamed). Binding to plasma protein is minimal.

● *Metabolism:* Not significantly metabolized.
● *Excretion:* When administered I.M., kidneys excrete 10% to 40% of dose.

Contraindications and precautions
Contraindicated in patients with hypersensitivity to drug and in atopic patients. Use cautiously in patients with myasthenia gravis or neuromuscular disease.

Interactions
Drug-drug. *Anesthetics, neuromuscular blockers:* May prolong or increase neuromuscular blockade. Use with caution.
Nephrotoxic drugs: Systemically administered bacitracin may induce additive damage when given with these drugs. Use with caution.

Adverse reactions
EENT: slowed corneal wound healing, temporary visual haze (with ophthalmic form), ototoxicity (when topical form is used over large areas for prolonged periods or with systemic use).
GU: *nephrotoxicity, renal failure.*
Skin: stinging, rash, other allergic reactions; pruritus, burning, swelling of lips or face (with topical form).
Other: *hypersensitivity reactions,* tightness in chest, hypotension, overgrowth of nonsusceptible organisms (with ophthalmic form).

☑ Special considerations
● Culture and sensitivity tests should be done before treatment starts.
● Patients allergic to neomycin may also be allergic to bacitracin.
● Injectable forms of drug may be used for I.M. administration only. I.V. administration may cause severe thrombophlebitis. Dilute injectable drug in solution containing sodium chloride and 2% procaine hydrochloride (if hospital policy permits). After reconstitution, bacitracin concentration should range from 5,000 to 10,000 units/ml. Inject deeply into upper outer quadrant of buttocks (may be painful). Don't give if patient is sensitive to procaine or para-aminobenzoic acid derivatives.
● Drug may be used orally with neomycin as bowel preparation or in solution as wound irrigating drug.
● With parenteral administration over several days, bacitracin may cause nephrotoxicity. Acute oral overdose may cause nausea, vomiting, and minor GI upset. Treatment is supportive.

Monitoring the patient
● Obtain baseline renal function studies before starting therapy, and monitor results daily for signs of deterioration.
● Monitor patient's urine pH. It should be kept above 6 with good hydration, and alkalinizing drugs (such as sodium bicarbonate) should be given, if needed, to limit nephrotoxicity.

- Ensure adequate fluid intake and monitor output closely.

Information for the patient
- Advise patient to discontinue topical use of drug and to call promptly if condition worsens or doesn't respond to treatment.
- Warn patient with a skin infection to avoid sharing washcloths and towels with family members.
- Instruct patient to wash hands before and after applying ointment.
- Advise patient using ophthalmic ointment to clean eye area of excess exudate before applying ointment. Warn patient not to touch tip of tube to any part of eye or surrounding tissue.
- Warn patient that ophthalmic ointment may cause blurred vision. Tell patient to stop drug immediately and report symptoms of sensitivity, such as itchy eyelids or constant burning.
- Instruct patient to store ophthalmic ointment in tightly closed, light-resistant container.
- Caution patient not to share eye medications with other persons.

---

baclofen
Lioresal

Pharmacologic classification: chlorophenyl derivative
Therapeutic classification: skeletal muscle relaxant
Pregnancy risk category C

How supplied
Available by prescription only
Tablets: 10 mg, 20 mg
Intrathecal kit: 500 mcg/ml, 2,000 mcg/ml

Indications, route, and dosage
Spasticity in multiple sclerosis and other spinal cord lesions
Adults: Initially, 5 mg P.O. t.i.d. for 3 days. Dosage may be increased (based on response) at 3-day intervals by 15 mg (5 mg/dose) daily up to maximum of 80 mg daily.
Intrathecal administration
Must be diluted with sterile preservative-free normal saline injection.
Adults: Initial intrathecal bolus of 50 mcg in 1 ml over not less than 1 minute. Observe patient for response over subsequent 4 to 8 hours. A positive response consists of a significant decrease in muscle tone or frequency or severity of spasm. If initial response is inadequate, repeat dose with 75 mcg in 1.5 ml 24 hours after last injection. Repeat observation of patient over 4 to 8 hours. If the response is still inadequate, repeat dosing at 100 mcg in 2 ml 24 hours later. If still no response, patient shouldn't be considered for an implantable pump for long-term baclofen administration.

Ranges for long-term doses are 12 to 2,003 mcg/day.
Postimplant dose titration
If the screening dose produced the desired effect for over 8 hours, the initial intrathecal dose is the same as the test dose; this dose is infused intrathecally for 24 hours. If the screening dose produced the desired effect for less than 8 hours, the initial intrathecal dose is twice the test dose, followed slowly by 10% to 30% increments at 24-hour intervals.

Pharmacodynamics
Skeletal muscle relaxant action: Exact mechanism unknown. Drug appears to act at the spinal cord level to inhibit transmission of monosynaptic and polysynaptic reflexes, possibly through hyperpolarization of afferent fiber terminals. It may also act at supraspinal sites because baclofen at high doses produces generalized CNS depression. Baclofen decreases the number and severity of spasms and relieves associated pain, clonus, and muscle rigidity and therefore improves mobility.

Pharmacokinetics
- *Absorption:* Rapidly and extensively absorbed from GI tract, but is subject to individual variation. Plasma levels peak at 2 to 3 hours. Also, as dose increases, rate and extent of absorption decreases. Onset of therapeutic effect may not be immediately evident; varies from hours to weeks. Peak effect is seen at 2 to 3 hours.
- *Distribution:* Studies indicate drug is widely distributed throughout body, with small amounts crossing the blood-brain barrier. About 30% is plasma protein-bound.
- *Metabolism:* About 15% metabolized in the liver via deamination.
- *Excretion:* 70% to 80% excreted in urine unchanged or as its metabolites; remainder, in feces.

Contraindications and precautions
Contraindicated in patients with hypersensitivity to drug. Use cautiously in patients with renal impairment or seizure disorders or when spasticity is used to maintain motor function.

Interactions
Drug-drug. *Antidiabetics, insulin:* Baclofen may increase blood glucose levels. Dosage adjustments may be needed.
CNS depressants, such as antipsychotics, anxiolytics, general anesthetics, narcotics: May add to the CNS effects of drug. Use cautiously.
MAO inhibitors, tricyclic antidepressants: May cause CNS depression, respiratory depression, and hypotension. Use with caution.
Drug-lifestyle. *Alcohol:* May add to the CNS effects of drug. Discourage use.

Adverse reactions
CNS: *CNS depression (potentially life-threatening with intrathecal administration),* drowsiness, dizziness, headache, *weakness, fatigue,* hypotonia, confusion, insomnia, dysarthria, SEIZURES.
CV: *CV collapse* (secondary to CNS depression), hypotension, hypertension.
EENT: blurred vision, nasal congestion, slurred speech.
GI: *nausea,* constipation, *vomiting.*
GU: urinary frequency.
Hepatic: increased AST and alkaline phosphatase levels.
Respiratory: *respiratory failure* (secondary to CNS depression).
Skin: rash, pruritus.
Other: excessive perspiration, hyperglycemia, weight gain, dyspnea.

☑ Special considerations
• Intrathecal administration should be performed only by qualified individuals familiar with administration techniques and patient management problems.
• Adverse reactions may be reduced by slowly decreasing the dosage. Abrupt withdrawal can result in hallucinations or seizures and acute exacerbation of spasticity.
• Drug is used investigationally to reduce choreiform movements in Huntington's chorea; to reduce rigidity in Parkinson's disease; to reduce spasticity in CVA, cerebral lesions, cerebral palsy, and rheumatic disorders; for analgesia in trigeminal neuralgia; and for treatment of unstable bladder.
• In some patients, smoother response may be obtained by giving daily dose in 4 divided doses.
• Patient may need supervision during walking. The initial loss of spasticity induced by baclofen may affect patient's ability to stand or walk. (In some patients, spasticity helps patient to maintain upright posture and balance.)
• Stop drug if signs of improvement don't occur within 1 to 2 months.
• Implantable pump or catheter failure can result in sudden loss of effectiveness of intrathecal baclofen.
• During prolonged intrathecal baclofen therapy for spasticity, about 10% of patients become refractory to baclofen therapy, requiring a "drug holiday" to regain sensitivity to its effects.
• Signs and symptoms of overdose include absence of reflexes, vomiting, muscular hypotonia, marked salivation, drowsiness, visual disorders, seizures, respiratory depression, and coma.
• Treatment of overdose requires supportive measures, including endotracheal intubation and positive-pressure ventilation. If patient is conscious, remove drug by inducing emesis then gastric lavage.

• If patient is comatose, don't induce emesis. Gastric lavage may be performed after endotracheal tube is in place with cuff inflated. Don't use respiratory stimulants. Monitor vital signs closely.

Monitoring the patient
• Watch for increased risk of seizures in patients with epilepsy.
• Watch for increased blood glucose levels in diabetic patients.
• Observe patient's response to drug. Signs of effective therapy may appear in a few hours to 1 week and may include diminished frequency of spasms and severity of foot and ankle clonus, increased ease and range of joint motion, and enhanced performance of daily activities.
• Closely monitor patients with epilepsy by EEG, clinical observation, and interview for possible loss of seizure control.

Information for the patient
• Advise patient to report adverse reactions promptly. Most can be reduced by decreasing dosage. Reportedly, drowsiness, dizziness, and ataxia are more common in patients over age 40.
• Warn patient of additive effects with use of other CNS depressants, including alcohol.
• Caution patient to avoid hazardous activities that require mental alertness.
• Tell diabetic patient that baclofen may elevate blood glucose levels and may require adjustment of insulin dosage during treatment with baclofen. Urge patient to promptly report changes in urine or blood glucose tests.
• Caution patient against taking OTC drugs without medical approval. Explain that hazardous drug interactions are possible.
• Inform patient that drug should be withdrawn gradually over 1 to 2 weeks. Abrupt withdrawal after prolonged use of drug may cause anxiety, agitated behavior, auditory and visual hallucinations, severe tachycardia, and acute spasticity.

Geriatric patients
• Elderly patients are especially sensitive to drug. Observe carefully for adverse reactions, such as mental confusion, depression, and hallucinations. Lower doses are usually indicated.

Pediatric patients
• Oral form isn't recommended for children under age 12.
• Safety of intrathecal administration in children under age 4 hasn't been established.

basiliximab
Simulect

Pharmacologic classification: recombinant chimeric human monoclonal antibody IgG
Therapeutic classification: immunosuppressant
Pregnancy risk category B

How supplied
Available by prescription only
Injection: 20-mg single dose vials

Indications, route, and dosage
Prophylaxis of acute organ rejection in patients receiving renal transplant when used as part of immunosuppressive regimen including cyclosporine and corticosteroids
Adults: 20 mg I.V. given within 2 hours before transplant surgery and 20 mg I.V. given 4 days after transplantation.
Children ages 2 to 15 years: 12 mg/m^2 (up to a maximum of 20 mg/dose) I.V. given within 2 hours of transplant surgery and 12 mg/m^2 (up to a maximum of 20 mg/dose) I.V. given 4 days after transplantation.

Pharmacodynamics
Immunosuppressant action: Basiliximab binds specifically to and blocks the interleukin-2 receptor alpha-chain (IL-2R a) on the surface of activated T-lymphocytes. This inhibits interleukin-2 mediated activation of lymphocytes, a critical pathway in the cellular immune response involved in allograft rejection.

Pharmacokinetics
- *Absorption:* Administered I.V.
- *Distribution:* No information available.
- *Metabolism:* No information available.
- *Excretion:* Half-life about 7.2 days in adults, 11.5 days in children.

Contraindications and precautions
Contraindicated in patients with known hypersensitivity to drug or its components. Anaphylactoid reactions may result following administration of proteins. Be sure that medications for treating severe hypersensitivity reactions are available for immediate use.

Interactions
None reported.

Adverse reactions
CNS: agitation, anxiety, *asthenia,* depression, *dizziness, headache,* hypoesthesia, *insomnia,* neuropathy, paresthesia, *tremor.*
CV: angina pectoris, **arrhythmias,** atrial fibrillation, **cardiac failure,** chest pain, abnormal heart sounds, aggravated hypertension, *hypertension,* hypotension, tachycardia.
EENT: abnormal vision, cataract, conjunctivitis, *rhinitis,* sinusitis.
GI: *abdominal pain,* candidiasis, *constipation, diarrhea, dyspepsia,* esophagitis, enlarged abdomen, flatulence, gastroenteritis, GI disorder, **GI hemorrhage,** gum hyperplasia, melena, *nausea,* ulcerative stomatitis, *vomiting.*
GU: abnormal renal function, albuminuria, bladder disorder, *dysuria,* frequent micturition, genital edema (male), hematuria, *increased nonprotein nitrogen,* oliguria, renal tubular necrosis, surgery, ureteral disorder, *urinary tract infection,* urinary retention, impotence.
Hematologic: *anemia,* hematoma, **hemorrhage,** polycythemia, purpura, **thrombocytopenia,** thrombosis.
Metabolic: *acidosis,* dehydration, diabetes mellitus, fluid overload, hypercalcemia, *hypercholesterolemia, hyperglycemia, hyperkalemia,* hyperlipemia, *hyperuricemia, hypocalcemia, hypokalemia, hypomagnesemia, hypophosphatemia,* hypoproteinemia, *weight increase, fever.*
Musculoskeletal: arthralgia, arthropathy, *back pain,* bone fracture, cramps, hernia, *leg pain,* myalgia.
Respiratory: abnormal chest sounds, bronchitis, bronchospasm, *cough, dyspnea, pharyngitis,* pneumonia, pulmonary disorder, **pulmonary edema,** upper respiratory tract infection.
Skin: *acne,* cyst, herpes simplex, herpes zoster, hypertrichosis, pruritus, rash, skin disorder or ulceration, *surgical wound complications.*
Other: accidental trauma, *viral infection, leg or peripheral edema,* fatigue, general edema, infection, **sepsis.**

☑ Special considerations
- Use cautiously and only under the supervision of a doctor experienced in immunosuppressive therapy and management of organ transplantation.
- Drug should be used only with cyclosporine and corticosteroids; data are lacking regarding use with other immunosuppressants.
- Not known if the response to vaccines will be altered with drug administration.
- Reconstitute with 5 ml sterile water for injection. Shake vial gently to dissolve powder. Dilute reconstituted solution to volume of 50 ml with normal saline or dextrose 5% for infusion. When mixing solution, gently invert bag to avoid foaming. Don't shake.
- Infuse over 20 to 30 minutes via a central or peripheral vein. Don't add or infuse other drugs simultaneously through same I.V. line.
- Use reconstituted solution immediately; otherwise, refrigerate at 36° to 46° F (2° to 8° C) for up to 24 hours or at room temperature for 4 hours.
- Single doses up to 60 mg have been given without significant adverse effects.

Monitoring the patient
• Monitor patient for electrolyte imbalances and acidosis during drug therapy.
• Monitor patient's intake and output, vital signs, hemoglobin, and hematocrit during therapy.
• Monitor patient for signs of opportunistic infections during drug therapy.

Information for the patient
• Inform patient of potential benefits of therapy and risks associated with immunosuppressive therapy, including a decreased risk of graft loss or acute rejection.
• Advise women of childbearing age to use effective contraception before beginning therapy and until 2 months after completion of therapy.
• Instruct patient to report adverse effects or any signs of infection immediately.
• Advise patient that immunosuppressive therapy increases risks of developing lymphoproliferative disorders and opportunistic infections.

Geriatric patients
• No significant difference seen between elderly and younger adults; however, caution should be used when prescribing immunosuppressive drugs to this population.

Pediatric patients
• Drug may be administered to children as young as age 2.

Breast-feeding patients
• It's unknown if drug appears in breast milk. Decision should be made to discontinue drug or to stop breast-feeding depending on importance of drug to the mother.

becaplermin
Regranex Gel

Pharmacologic classification: recombinant human platelet-derived growth factor (rhPDGF-BB)
Therapeutic classification: wound repair drug
Pregnancy risk category C

How supplied
Available by prescription only
Gel: 100 mcg/g in tubes of 2 g, 7.5 g, 15 g

Indications, route, and dosage
Lower extremity diabetic neuropathic ulcers that extend into the subcutaneous tissue and beyond and have an adequate blood supply
Adults: Apply daily in ⅟₁₆-inch even thickness to entire surface of wound. Cover site with a saline-moistened dressing. Remove after 12 hours. Rinse gel from wound with saline or water and cover

wound with moist dressing. Continue treatment until complete healing occurs.
    Length of gel to be applied varies with tube size and ulcer area.

Tube size (g)	Gel length (inches)	Gel length (cm)
2	ulcer length × ulcer width × 1.3	(ulcer length × ulcer width) ÷ 2
7.5, 15	ulcer length × ulcer width × 0.6	(ulcer length × ulcer width) ÷ 4

Pharmacodynamics
Wound repair action: Recombinant of human platelet-derived growth factor that promotes the chemotactic recruitment and proliferation of cells involved in wound repair and enhances the formation of new granulation tissue.

Pharmacokinetics
• *Absorption:* Minimal systemic absorption, less than 3% in rats.
• *Distribution:* No information available.
• *Metabolism:* No information available.
• *Excretion:* No information available.

Contraindications and precautions
Contraindicated in patients with hypersensitivity to drug or its components and in those with neoplasms at site of application. Gel is for external use only. If an application site reaction occurs, possibility of sensitization or irritation caused by parabens or m-cresol should be considered.

Interactions
None reported.

Adverse reactions
Skin: erythematous rash.

☑ Special considerations
• When used as an adjunct to, and not a substitute for, good ulcer care practices including initial sharp debridement, pressure relief, and infection control, gel increases complete healing of diabetic ulcers. Its efficacy in treating diabetic neuropathic ulcers that don't extend through the dermis into subcutaneous tissue or ischemic diabetic ulcers hasn't been evaluated.
• Don't use gel in wounds that close by primary intention.
• To apply gel, squeeze the calculated length of gel onto a clean measuring surface, such as wax paper. Then transfer the measured gel from the measuring surface using an application aid.
• Recalculate amount of gel to be applied weekly. If ulcer doesn't decrease in size by about one-third after 10 weeks or complete healing hasn't occurred by 20 weeks, reassess continued treatment.

Reactions may be *common,* uncommon, *life-threatening,* or COMMON AND LIFE-THREATENING.

- Use gel in addition to good ulcer care program, including a strict non–weight-bearing program.

Monitoring the patient
- Monitor patient's response to drug by measurement of ulcer.

Information for the patient
- Instruct patient to wash hands thoroughly before applying gel.
- Advise patient not to touch tip of tube against ulcer or other surfaces.
- Inform patient to use a cotton swab, tongue blade, or other application aid to apply gel evenly over surface of ulcer, producing a thin (1/16-inch) continuous layer.
- Tell patient to apply drug once daily in a carefully measured quantity. Quantity will change on a weekly basis.
- Tell patient to store gel in the refrigerator, and never to freeze it.
- Inform patient not to use gel after expiration date on the bottom, crimped end of tube.

Pediatric patients
- Safety and effectiveness in patients under age 16 haven't been established.

Breast-feeding patients
- It's unknown if drug appears in breast milk. Use drug with caution when administering to breast-feeding patients.

---

beclomethasone dipropionate

beclomethasone dipropionate monohydrate
Nasal inhalants
Beconase, Vancenase

Nasal sprays
Beconase AQ, Vancenase AQ, Vancenase AQ Double Strength, Vancenase AQ Pockethaler

Oral inhalants
Beclovent, Becloforte*, Vanceril, Vanceril Double Strength

Pharmacologic classification: glucocorticoid
Therapeutic classification: anti-inflammatory, antasthmatic
Pregnancy risk category C

How supplied
Available by prescription only
Nasal aerosol: 42 mcg/metered spray
Nasal spray: 42 mcg/metered spray, 84 mcg/metered spray

Oral inhalation aerosol: 42 mcg/metered spray, 84 mcg/metered spray

Indications, route, and dosage
Steroid-dependent asthma
Oral inhalation
Adults and children over age 12: For regular strength formulation: 2 inhalations t.i.d. or q.i.d. or 4 inhalations b.i.d. Maximum of 20 inhalations daily. Double strength: 2 inhalations b.i.d.; in severe asthma start with 4 to 8 inhalations and adjust down. Don't exceed 10 inhalations/day.
Children ages 6 to 12: For regular strength formulation: 1 to 2 inhalations t.i.d. or q.i.d. Maximum of 10 inhalations daily. Double strength: 2 inhalations b.i.d.; don't exceed 5 inhalations/day.
Perennial or seasonal rhinitis, prevention of recurrence of nasal polyps after surgical removal
Nasal inhalation
Adults and children over age 12: 1 spray (42 mcg) in each nostril b.i.d. to q.i.d. Usual total dosage is 168 to 336 mcg daily.
Children ages 6 to 12: 1 spray in each nostril t.i.d. (252 mcg daily).
Nasal spray
Adults and children over age 12: 1 or 2 sprays (42 to 84 mcg) in each nostril b.i.d. Usual total dosage is 168 to 336 mcg daily.
Children ages 6 to 12: Start with 1 spray in each nostril b.i.d. (168 mcg daily). If response is inadequate or symptoms more severe, dosage can be increased to 2 sprays per nostril b.i.d. (336 mcg daily).
Nonallergic (vasomotor) rhinitis
Nasal spray
Adults and children over age 12: 1 or 2 sprays (42 to 84 mcg) in each nostril b.i.d. Usual total dosage is 168 to 336 mcg daily.
Children ages 6 to 12: Start with 1 spray in each nostril b.i.d. (168 mcg daily). If response is inadequate or symptoms more severe, the dosage can be increased to 2 sprays per nostril b.i.d. (336 mcg daily).

Pharmacodynamics
Anti-inflammatory action: Stimulates the synthesis of enzymes needed to decrease the inflammatory response. The anti-inflammatory and vasoconstrictor potency of topically applied beclomethasone is, on a weight basis, about 5,000 times greater than that of hydrocortisone, 500 times greater than that of betamethasone or dexamethasone, and about 5 times greater than that of fluocinolone or triamcinolone.
Antiasthmatic action: Used as a nasal inhalant to treat symptoms of seasonal or perennial rhinitis and to prevent recurrence of nasal polyps after surgical removal, and as an oral inhalant to treat bronchial asthma in patients who require long-term administration of corticosteroids to control symptoms.

Pharmacokinetics

• *Absorption:* After nasal inhalation, is absorbed primarily through nasal mucosa, with minimal systemic absorption. After oral inhalation, is absorbed rapidly from lungs and GI tract. Greater systemic absorption is associated with oral inhalation, but systemic effects don't occur at usual doses because of rapid metabolism in liver and local metabolism of drug that reaches lungs. Onset of action usually occurs in a few days but may take as long as 3 weeks in some patients.

• *Distribution:* Distribution after intranasal administration hasn't been described. No evidence of tissue storage of drug or its metabolites. About 10% to 25% of a nasal spray or orally inhaled dose is deposited in respiratory tract. The remainder, deposited in mouth and oropharynx, is swallowed. When absorbed, drug is 87% bound to plasma proteins.

• *Metabolism:* Swallowed drug undergoes rapid metabolism in liver or GI tract to several metabolites, some of which have minor glucocorticoid activity. The portion inhaled into respiratory tract is partially metabolized before absorption into systemic circulation. Drug is mostly metabolized in liver.

• *Excretion:* Excretion of inhaled drug hasn't been described; however, when drug is administered systemically, its metabolites are excreted mainly in feces via biliary elimination and to a lesser extent in urine. Biological half-life of drug averages 15 hours.

Contraindications and precautions

Contraindicated in patients with hypersensitivity to drug and in those experiencing status asthmaticus or other acute episodes of asthma. Use cautiously in patients with tuberculosis, fungal or bacterial infection, herpes, or systemic viral infection.

Interactions

None reported.

Adverse reactions

CNS: headache.
EENT: *mild transient nasal burning and stinging,* nasal congestion, sneezing, burning, stinging, dryness, epistaxis, nasopharyngeal fungal infections, hoarseness, fungal infection of throat, throat irritation.
GI: dry mouth, fungal infection of mouth.
Skin: hypersensitivity reactions (urticaria, rash).
Other: *angioedema, bronchospasm,* suppression of hypothalamic-pituitary-adrenal function, **adrenal insufficiency,** facial edema, wheezing.

☑ Special considerations

• Use with extreme caution, if at all, in patients with tuberculosis, fungal or bacterial infections, ocular herpes simplex, or systemic viral infections.

• Don't use drug for patients with asthma controlled by bronchodilators or other noncorticosteroids alone or for those with nonasthmatic bronchial diseases.

• Use with caution in patients receiving systemic corticosteroid therapy.

• A spacer device may help ensure delivery of the proper dose and decrease local (oral) adverse effects.

• Remember that, during times of stress (trauma, surgery, or infection), systemic corticosteroids may be needed to prevent adrenal insufficiency in previously steroid-dependent patients.

• Taper oral glucocorticoid therapy slowly. Acute adrenal insufficiency and death have occurred in asthmatics who changed abruptly from oral corticosteroids to beclomethasone.

Monitoring the patient

• Periodic measurement of growth and development may be necessary during high-dose or prolonged therapy in children.

• To assess the risk of adrenal insufficiency in emergency situations, routine tests of adrenal cortical function, including measurement of early morning resting cortisol levels, should be performed periodically in all patients.

• Monitor mouth, pharynx, and larynx for localized infections with *C. albicans* or *Aspergillus niger.*

Information for the patient

• Inform patient that drug doesn't provide relief for acute asthma attacks.

• Tell patient requiring a bronchodilator to use it several minutes before beclomethasone.

• Instruct patient to carry a medical identification card indicating his need for supplemental systemic glucocorticoids during stress.

• If using a metered-dose inhaler, instruct patient to shake canister well before use.

• Advise patient to allow 1 minute to elapse before taking subsequent puffs of medication and to hold breath for a few seconds to enhance action of drug.

• Instruct patient to report decreased response to therapy or if symptoms don't improve within 3 weeks; dosage may need to be adjusted. Tell patient not to exceed recommended dose.

• Tell patient to keep inhaler clean and unobstructed. Patient should wash it with warm water and dry it thoroughly.

• Advise patient to prevent oral fungal infections by gargling or rinsing mouth with water after each use, but not to swallow the water.

• Tell patient to report symptoms associated with corticosteroid withdrawal, including fatigue, weakness, arthralgia, orthostatic hypotension, and dyspnea.

• Instruct patient to store medication between 59° and 86° F (15° and 30° C). Advise patient to ensure delivery of proper dose by gently warming canister to room temperature before using.

Pediatric patients
• Drug isn't recommended for children under age 6.

Breast-feeding patients
• It's unknown if drug appears in breast milk. Use with caution in breast-feeding women.

---

benazepril hydrochloride
Lotensin

Pharmacologic classification: ACE inhibitor
Therapeutic classification: antihypertensive
Pregnancy risk category C (D in second and third trimesters)

How supplied
Available by prescription only
Tablets: 5 mg, 10 mg, 20 mg, 40 mg

Indications, route, and dosage
Hypertension
Adults: Initially, 10 mg P.O. daily. Adjust dosage as needed and tolerated; maintenance dosage range is 20 to 40 mg daily in one or two equally divided doses.
✦ **Dosage adjustment.** In renal failure, if creatinine clearance is below 30 ml/minute/1.73 m², or serum creatinine levels exceed 3 mg/dl, initial dose is 5 mg P.O. daily. Don't exceed 40 mg daily.
Note: Although rare, angioedema has been reported in patients receiving ACE inhibitors. Angioedema associated with laryngeal edema or shock may be fatal. If angioedema of the face, extremities, lips, tongue, glottis, or larynx occurs, treatment with benazepril should be discontinued and appropriate therapy instituted immediately.

Pharmacodynamics
Antihypertensive action: Drug and its active metabolite, benazeprilat, inhibit ACE, preventing conversion of angiotensin I to angiotensin II, a potent vasoconstrictor. Reduced formation of angiotensin II decreases peripheral arterial resistance and aldosterone secretion, which reduces sodium and water retention and lowers blood pressure.

Although the primary mechanism through which benazepril lowers blood pressure is believed to be suppression of the renin-angiotensin-aldosterone system, benazepril has an antihypertensive effect even in patients with low renin levels.

Pharmacokinetics
• *Absorption:* At least 37% absorbed. After oral administration, plasma levels peak within 0.5 to 1 hour.
• *Distribution:* Serum protein-binding of about 96.7%; that of benazeprilat, 95.3%.
• *Metabolism:* Almost completely metabolized in liver to benazeprilat, which has much greater ACE inhibitory activity than benazepril, and to the glucuronide conjugates of benazepril and benazeprilat.
• *Excretion:* Primarily in urine.

Contraindications and precautions
Contraindicated in patients with hypersensitivity to ACE inhibitors. Use cautiously in patients with renal or hepatic impairment.

Interactions
Drug-drug. *Allopurinol:* May increase risk of hypersensitivity reaction. Use with caution.
Digoxin: May increase plasma digoxin levels. Monitor digoxin levels.
Diuretics, other antihypertensives: Increased risk of excessive hypotension. Diuretic may need to be stopped or benazepril dose lowered.
Lithium: Increases serum lithium levels and lithium toxicity. Avoid use together.
Potassium-sparing diuretics, potassium supplements, sodium substitutes containing potassium: Risk of hyperkalemia. Avoid concomitant use.

Adverse reactions
CNS: headache, dizziness, anxiety, fatigue, insomnia, nervousness, paresthesia.
CV: symptomatic hypotension, palpitations.
EENT: dysphagia, increased salivation.
GI: nausea, vomiting, abdominal pain, constipation.
Respiratory: dry, persistent, tickling, nonproductive cough; dyspnea.
Skin: hypersensitivity reactions (rash, pruritus), increased diaphoresis.
Other: *angioedema,* arthralgia, arthritis, impotence, myalgia, hyperkalemia.

☑ Special considerations
• Excessive hypotension can occur when drug is given with diuretics. If possible, diuretic therapy should be discontinued 2 to 3 days before starting benazepril to decrease potential for excessive hypotensive response. If benazepril doesn't adequately control blood pressure, diuretic therapy may be reinstituted with care. If the diuretic can't be discontinued, initiate benazepril therapy at 5 mg P.O. daily.
• Hypotension is the most common symptom of overdose. No data suggest physiologic maneuvers that might accelerate elimination of benazepril and its metabolite if an overdose occurs.

• Drug is only slightly dialyzable, but dialysis might be considered in overdosed patients with severely impaired renal function.

• Angiotensin II may serve as a specific antagonist-antidote, but angiotensin II is essentially unavailable outside of scattered research facilities.

• Because drug's hypotensive effect is achieved through vasodilation and effective hypovolemia, treatment of benazepril overdose by I.V. infusion of normal saline solution is reasonable.

Monitoring the patient

• Measure blood pressure when drug levels are at peak (2 to 6 hours after a dose) and at trough (just before a dose) to verify adequate blood pressure control.

• Assess renal and hepatic function before and periodically throughout therapy. Monitor serum potassium levels.

• Other ACE inhibitors have been associated with agranulocytosis and neutropenia. Monitor CBC with differential counts before therapy, every 2 weeks for first 3 months of therapy, and periodically thereafter.

Information for the patient

• Advise patient to report signs or symptoms of infection (such as fever and sore throat); easy bruising or bleeding; swelling of tongue, lips, face, eyes, mucous membranes, or extremities; difficulty swallowing or breathing; and hoarseness.

• Because light-headedness can occur, especially during the first few days of therapy, tell patient to rise slowly to minimize this effect and to report symptoms. Patients who experience syncope should stop taking drug and call immediately.

• Inadequate fluid intake, vomiting, diarrhea, and excessive perspiration can lead to light-headedness and syncope. Tell patient to use caution in hot weather and during exercise.

• Tell patient to avoid sodium substitutes; these products may contain potassium, which can cause hyperkalemia in patients on drug therapy.

• Tell woman of childbearing age about consequences of second- and third-trimester exposure to ACE inhibitors. Explain that these consequences don't appear to result from exposure during the first trimester. Advise her to report suspected pregnancy as soon as possible.

• A persistent dry cough may occur and usually doesn't subside unless drug is stopped. Advise patient to call if this effect becomes bothersome.

Pediatric patients

• Safety and effectiveness in children haven't been established.

Breast-feeding patients

• Minimal amounts of unchanged benazepril and benazeprilat appear in breast milk. Use cautiously when administering to breast-feeding women.

benzocaine
Americaine, Dermoplast, Hurricaine, Lanacane, Maximum Strength Anbesol, Orabase Gel, Orajel, Orajel Mouth Aid, Solarcaine

Pharmacologic classification: local anesthetic (ester)
Therapeutic classification: anesthetic
Pregnancy risk category C

How supplied
Available without a prescription
Gel: 20%
Ointment, cream, and dental paste: 1% to 20%
Topical solution: 20%
Topical spray: 20%
Lotion: 0.5% to 8%

Indications, route, and dosage
Local anesthetic for dental pain or dental procedures
Adults and children: Apply topical gel (20%) or dental paste to area, p.r.n.
Local anesthetic for pruritic dermatoses, pruritus, or other irritations
Adults: Apply topical preparation (1% to 20%) to affected area, p.r.n.
Relief of pain and pruritus in acute congestive and serous otitis media, acute swimmer's ear, and other forms of otitis externa
Adults: 4 to 5 drops (otic) in external auditory canal; insert cotton into meatus; repeat q 1 to 2 hours.

Pharmacodynamics
Analgesic action: Acts at sensory neurons to produce a local anesthetic effect.

Pharmacokinetics
No information available.

Contraindications and precautions
Contraindicated in patients with hypersensitivity to drug, its components, or related substances and in those with secondary infection in the area or serious burns. Don't use in eyes or in ears with a perforated tympanic membrane or discharge. Use cautiously in patients with severely traumatized mucosa or local sepsis.

Interactions
None significant.

Adverse reactions
Skin: urticaria, burning, stinging, tenderness, irritation, itching, erythema, rash.
Other: edema.
  Note: Discontinue drug if symptoms of hypersensitivity occur.

Reactions may be *common*, uncommon, **life-threatening**, or COMMON AND LIFE-THREATENING.

☑ Special considerations
• Use with antibiotic to treat underlying cause of pain because using alone may mask more serious condition.
• Keep container tightly closed and away from moisture.
• Maximum recommended dose is 5 g/day.
• Overdose is unlikely; however, methemoglobinemia has been reported after topical application for teething pain. Treat symptomatically; if necessary, administer methylene blue 1% 0.1 ml/kg I.V. over at least 10 minutes.

Monitoring the patient
• Watch for signs of hypersensitivity.

Information for the patient
• Tell patient to call if pain lasts longer than 48 hours, if burning or itching occurs, or if the condition persists.
• Instruct patient to keep container tightly closed and away from moisture.
• Advise patient not to eat or chew gum until effect of local anesthetic has worn off to avoid risk of bite trauma.

Pediatric patients
• Excessive use may cause methemoglobinemia in infants. Don't use in children under age 1.

benzonatate
Tessalon Perles

Pharmacologic classification: local anesthetic (ester)
Therapeutic classification: nonnarcotic antitussive
Pregnancy risk category C

How supplied
Available by prescription only
Capsules: 100 mg

Indications, route, and dosage
Cough suppression
Adults and children over age 10: 100 mg P.O. t.i.d.; up to 600 mg daily.
Children under age 10: 8 mg/kg daily P.O. in three to six divided doses.

Pharmacodynamics
Antitussive action: Suppresses the cough reflex at its source by anesthetizing peripheral stretch receptors located in the respiratory passages, lungs, and pleura.

Pharmacokinetics
• Absorption: Action begins within 15 to 20 minutes and lasts for 3 to 8 hours.
• Distribution: No information available.
• Metabolism: No information available.
• Excretion: No information available.

Contraindications and precautions
Contraindicated in patients with hypersensitivity to drug or para-aminobenzoic acid anesthetics (procaine, tetracaine).

Interactions
None reported.

Adverse reactions
CNS: dizziness, headache, sedation.
EENT: nasal congestion, burning sensation in eyes.
GI: nausea, constipation, GI upset.
Skin: hypersensitivity reactions (rash).
Other: chills.

☑ Special considerations
• CNS stimulation from overdose of drug may cause restlessness and tremors, which may lead to chronic seizures then profound CNS depression.
• In overdose, empty stomach by gastric lavage and follow with activated charcoal. Treat seizures with a short-acting barbiturate given I.V.; don't use CNS stimulants. Mechanical respiratory support may be necessary in severe cases.

Monitoring the patient
• Monitor cough type and frequency and volume and quality of sputum. Encourage fluid intake to help liquefy sputum.
• Monitor patient for adverse effects.

Information for the patient
• Instruct patient not to chew or dissolve capsules in the mouth because local anesthesia will result. Swallow whole.
• Teach patient comfort measures for a nonproductive cough: limit talking and smoking; use a cold mist or steam vaporizer; use sugarless hard candy to increase saliva flow.

Breast-feeding patients
• Safe use during breast-feeding hasn't been established.

benztropine mesylate
Cogentin

Pharmacologic classification: anticholinergic
Therapeutic classification: antiparkinsonian
Pregnancy risk category C

How supplied
Available by prescription only
Tablets: 0.5 mg, 1 mg, 2 mg
Injection: 1 mg/ml in 2-ml ampule

Indications, route, and dosage

Acute dystonic reaction
Adults: 1 to 2 mg I.M. or I.V.; then 1 to 2 mg P.O. b.i.d. to prevent recurrence.

Parkinsonism
Adults: 0.5 to 6 mg P.O. daily. Initially, 0.5 to 1 mg, increased 0.5 mg q 5 to 6 days. Adjust dose to meet individual requirements. Maximum dose, 6 mg/day.

Drug-induced extrapyramidal reactions
Adults: 1 to 4 mg P.O. or I.V. daily or b.i.d. Adjust dose to meet individual requirements. Maximum dose, 6 mg/day.

Pharmacodynamics
Antiparkinsonian action: Blocks central cholinergic receptors, helping to balance cholinergic activity in the basal ganglia. May also prolong effects of dopamine by blocking dopamine reuptake and storage at central receptor sites.

Pharmacokinetics
- *Absorption:* Absorbed from GI tract.
- *Distribution:* Largely unknown; however, drug crosses blood-brain barrier and may cross placenta.
- *Metabolism:* No known information.
- *Excretion:* Like other muscarinics, drug is excreted in urine as unchanged drug and metabolites. After oral therapy, small amounts are probably excreted in feces as unabsorbed drug.

Contraindications and precautions
Contraindicated in patients with hypersensitivity to drug or its components and in those with acute angle-closure glaucoma. Also contraindicated in children under age 3. Use cautiously in hot weather, in patients with mental disorders, and in children over age 3.

Interactions
Drug-drug. *Amantadine:* May amplify such adverse anticholinergic effects as confusion and hallucinations. Decrease benztropine dosage before giving amantadine.
Antacids, antidiarrheals: May decrease benztropine absorption. Administer benztropine at least 1 hour before administering these drugs.
CNS depressants: Increased sedative effects of benztropine. May require dosage adjustments.
Haloperidol, phenothiazines: May decrease effect of these drugs. Monitor patient for drug effect.
Phenothiazines: Drug increases risk of adverse anticholinergic effects of these drugs. Monitor patient carefully.
Drug-lifestyle. *Alcohol:* Increases sedative effects of benztropine. Discourage use.

Adverse reactions
CNS: disorientation, hallucinations, depression, toxic psychosis, confusion, memory impairment, nervousness.

CV: tachycardia.
EENT: dilated pupils, blurred vision.
GI: dry mouth, *constipation,* nausea, vomiting, paralytic ileus.
GU: urine retention, dysuria.
   Some adverse reactions may result from atropine-like toxicity and are dose-related.

☑ Special considerations
Besides the recommendations relevant to all anticholinergics, consider the following.
- To help prevent gastric irritation, administer drug after meals.
- Never discontinue drug abruptly.
- Signs and symptoms of overdose include central stimulation then depression and psychotic symptoms such as disorientation, confusion, hallucinations, delusions, anxiety, agitation, and restlessness. Peripheral effects may include dilated, nonreactive pupils; blurred vision; hot, flushed, dry skin; dryness of mucous membranes; dysphagia; decreased or absent bowel sounds; urine retention; hyperthermia; tachycardia; hypertension; and increased respiration.
- Treatment of overdose is primarily symptomatic and supportive, as necessary. If patient is alert, induce emesis (or use gastric lavage) and follow with a sodium chloride cathartic and activated charcoal to prevent further absorption.
- In severe overdose cases, physostigmine may be administered to block the antimuscarinic effects of benztropine. Give fluids as needed to treat shock, diazepam to control psychotic symptoms, and pilocarpine (instilled into the eyes) to relieve mydriasis. If urine retention occurs, catheterization may be necessary.

Monitoring the patient
- Monitor patient for intermittent constipation and abdominal distention and pain, which may indicate paralytic ileus.
- Monitor patient for adverse effects.

Information for the patient
- Explain to patient that drug's full effect may not occur for 2 to 3 days after therapy begins.
- Caution patient not to discontinue drug suddenly; dosage should be reduced gradually.
- Tell patient that drug may increase sensitivity of eyes to light.

Pediatric patients
- Drug isn't recommended for use in children under age 3.

Breast-feeding patients
- Drug may appear in breast milk, possibly causing infant toxicity. Avoid use of drug in breast-feeding women. Benztropine may decrease milk production.

Reactions may be *common,* uncommon, *life-threatening,* or COMMON AND LIFE-THREATENING.

bepridil hydrochloride
Vascor

Pharmacologic classification: calcium channel blocker
Therapeutic classification: antianginal
Pregnancy risk category C

How supplied
Available by prescription only
Tablets: 200 mg, 300 mg, 400 mg

Indications, route, and dosage
Chronic stable angina (classic effort-associated angina) in patients who are unresponsive or inadequately responsive to other antianginals
Adults: Initially, 200 mg P.O. daily; after 10 days, adjust dosage based on patient tolerance and response. Most common maintenance dosage is 300 mg daily. Maximum daily dose, 400 mg.

Pharmacodynamics
Antianginal action: Exact mechanism unknown. Inhibits calcium ion influx into cardiac and vascular smooth muscle and also inhibits the sodium inward influx, resulting in reductions in the maximal upstroke velocity and amplitude of the action potential. Believed to reduce heart rate and arterial pressure by dilating peripheral arterioles and reducing total peripheral resistance (afterload). The effects are dose-dependent. Has dose-related class I antiarrhythmic properties affecting electrophysiologic changes, such as prolongation of QT and QTc intervals.

Pharmacokinetics
• *Absorption:* Rapidly and completely absorbed after oral administration; levels peak in 2 to 3 hours.
• *Distribution:* More than 99% is plasma protein-bound.
• *Metabolism:* Metabolized in the liver.
• *Excretion:* Elimination is biphasic; distribution half-life of 2 hours. Over 10 days, 70% excreted in urine, 22% in feces as metabolites. Terminal half-life after multiple dosing averages 42 hours (range, 26 to 64 hours).

Contraindications and precautions
Contraindicated in patients with hypersensitivity to drug and in those with uncompensated cardiac insufficiency, sick sinus syndrome, or second- or third-degree AV block unless pacemaker is present; hypotension (below 90 mm Hg systolic); congenital QT interval prolongation; or history of serious ventricular arrhythmias. Also contraindicated in those receiving other drugs that prolong QT interval.
    Use cautiously in patients with left bundle-branch block, sinus bradycardia, impaired renal or hepatic function, or heart failure. Drug isn't recommended for use in patients within 3 months of an MI.

Interactions
Drug-drug. *Digoxin:* Modest increases in steady-state serum digoxin levels have been observed with concurrent use of bepridil. Significance in patients with cardiac conduction abnormalities isn't known.
Potassium-wasting diuretics: Potentiates hypokalemia, which increases risk of serious ventricular arrhythmias. Avoid use together.
Procainamide, quinidine, tricyclic antidepressants: Additive prolongation of QT interval. Avoid concomitant use.

Adverse reactions
CNS: *dizziness,* drowsiness, *nervousness, headache,* insomnia, paresthesia, *asthenia,* tremor.
CV: edema, flushing, palpitations, tachycardia, *ventricular arrhythmias, including torsades de pointes, ventricular tachycardia, ventricular fibrillation.*
EENT: tinnitus.
GI: *nausea, diarrhea,* constipation, abdominal discomfort, dry mouth, anorexia, increased ALT levels and abnormal liver function test.
Hematologic: *agranulocytosis.*
Respiratory: dyspnea, shortness of breath.
Skin: rash.
Other: flulike symptoms.

☑ Special considerations
• Careful patient selection and monitoring are essential. Use the following selection criteria: Diagnosis of chronic stable angina with failure to respond or inadequate response to other therapies, QTc interval less than 0.44 seconds, absence of hypokalemia, hypotension, severe left ventricular dysfunction, serious ventricular arrhythmias, unpacked sick sinus syndrome, second- or third-degree AV block, and no concomitant use of other drugs that prolong the QT interval.
• Beta blockers, nitrates, digoxin, insulin, and oral antidiabetics may be used with drug.
• Food doesn't interfere with absorption of drug. Food may alleviate or prevent nausea.
• Use cautiously in patients with renal or hepatic disorders.

Monitoring the patient
• Monitor serum potassium levels and correct hypokalemia before initiating therapy. Use potassium-sparing diuretics for patients who require diuretic therapy.
• Monitor QTc interval before and during therapy. Reduced dosage is required if QTc interval prolongation is greater than 0.52 seconds or increases more than 25%. If prolongation of QTc interval persists, discontinue bepridil.

• Exaggerated adverse reactions, especially significant hypotension, high-degree AV block, and ventricular tachycardia, have been observed. Treat with appropriate supportive measures, including gastric lavage, beta-adrenergic stimulation, parenteral calcium solutions, vasopressor drugs, and cardioversion, as necessary.
• Close observation in a cardiac care facility for a minimum of 48 hours is recommended for toxic reactions.

Information for the patient
• Instruct patient to recognize signs and symptoms of hypokalemia and the importance of compliance with prescribed potassium supplements.
• Tell patient to report signs or symptoms of infection, such as sore throat and fever.
• Instruct patient to take drug with food or at bedtime if nausea occurs.

Geriatric patients
• Recommended starting dose is same as in adult patients; however, more frequent monitoring may be required.

Pediatric patients
• Safety and efficacy in children haven't been established.

Breast-feeding patients
• Drug appears in breast milk; risk-benefit must be assessed.

---

betamethasone (systemic)
Celestone

betamethasone sodium phosphate
Betnesol*, Celestone Phosphate, Selestoject

betamethasone sodium phosphate and betamethasone acetate
Celestone Soluspan

Pharmacologic classification: glucocorticoid
Therapeutic classification: anti-inflammatory
Pregnancy risk category NR

How supplied
Available by prescription only
betamethasone
Tablets: 0.6 mg
Syrup: 0.6 mg/5 ml
betamethasone sodium phosphate
Tablets (effervescent): 500 mcg*
Injection: 4 mg (3 mg base)/ml in 5-ml vials
Enema:* 5 mg (base)

betamethasone sodium phosphate and betamethasone acetate suspension
Injection: betamethasone acetate 3 mg and betamethasone sodium phosphate (equivalent to 3 mg base) per ml (not for I.V. use)

Indications, route, and dosage
Note: Don't give betamethasone acetate suspension I.V.
Severe inflammation or immunosuppression
Adults: 0.6 to 7.2 mg P.O. daily.
betamethasone sodium phosphate
Adults: 0.5 to 9 mg I.M., I.V., or into joint or soft tissue daily.
betamethasone sodium phosphate and betamethasone acetate suspension
Adults: 0.5 to 2 ml into joint or soft tissue q 1 to 2 weeks, p.r.n.
Adrenocortical insufficiency
Adults: 0.6 to 7.2 mg P.O. daily, or up to 9 mg I.M. or I.V. daily.
Children: 17.5 mcg/kg P.O. daily or 500 mcg/m² P.O. daily in three or four divided doses; or 17.5 mcg/kg/day or 500 mcg/m²/day I.M. in three divided doses q 3 days.
◇ ***Hyaline membrane disease***
Adults: Give 2 ml I.M. daily to expectant mothers for 2 to 3 days before delivery.

Pharmacodynamics
Anti-inflammatory action: Stimulates synthesis of enzymes needed to decrease the inflammatory response. A long-acting corticosteroid with an anti-inflammatory potency 25 times that of an equal weight of hydrocortisone. Has essentially no mineralocorticoid activity. Betamethasone tablets and syrup are used as oral anti-inflammatories.
   Betamethasone sodium phosphate is highly soluble, has a prompt onset of action, and may be given I.V. Betamethasone sodium phosphate and betamethasone acetate (Celestone Soluspan) combine the rapid-acting phosphate salt and the slightly soluble, slowly released acetate salt to provide rapid anti-inflammatory effects with a sustained duration of action. It's a suspension and isn't to be given I.V. It's particularly useful as an anti-inflammatory in intra-articular, intradermal, and intralesional injections.

Pharmacokinetics
• *Absorption:* Absorbed readily after oral administration. After oral and I.V. administration, peak effects occur in 1 to 2 hours. Onset and duration of action of suspensions for injection vary, depending on their injection site (an intra-articular space or a muscle) and on local blood supply. Systemic absorption occurs slowly following intra-articular injections.
• *Distribution:* Removed rapidly from the blood and distributed to muscle, liver, skin, intestines, and kidneys. Betamethasone is bound weakly to

plasma proteins (transcortin and albumin). Only the unbound portion is active. Adrenocorticoids are distributed into breast milk and through the placenta.

• *Metabolism:* Metabolized in the liver to inactive glucuronide and sulfate metabolites.

• *Excretion:* Inactive metabolites and small amounts of unmetabolized drug are excreted by the kidneys. Insignificant quantities of drug are also excreted in feces. Biological half-life of drug is 36 to 54 hours.

Contraindications and precautions

Contraindicated in patients with hypersensitivity to drug and in those with viral or bacterial infections (except in life-threatening situations) or systemic fungal infections.

Use with caution in patients with renal disease, hypertension, osteoporosis, diabetes mellitus, hypothyroidism, cirrhosis, diverticulitis, non-specific ulcerative colitis, recent intestinal anastomoses, thromboembolic disorders, seizures, myasthenia gravis, heart failure, tuberculosis, ocular herpes simplex, emotional instability, and psychotic tendencies.

Interactions

Drug-drug. *Amphotericin B, diuretics:* May enhance hypokalemia. Monitor potassium levels.

Antacids, cholestyramine, colestipol: Decreased effect of betamethasone by adsorbing the corticosteroid, decreasing the amount absorbed. Avoid using together.

Barbiturates, phenytoin, rifampin: May cause decreased corticosteroid effects. Use cautiously; monitor patient.

Cardiac glycosides: Increased risk of toxicity from hypokalemia. Monitor potassium levels.

Estrogens: May reduce metabolism of corticosteroids by increasing transcortin levels. Half-life of the corticosteroid is then prolonged because of increased protein-binding. Use with caution.

Insulin, oral antidiabetics: May cause hyperglycemia. Dosage adjustment may be needed.

Isoniazid, salicylates: Increased metabolism of isoniazid and salicylates. Monitor patient for effects.

Oral anticoagulants: May decrease effects of oral anticoagulants (rarely). Monitor patient for effects.

Ulcerogenic drugs such as NSAIDs: May increase risk of GI ulceration. Avoid concomitant use.

Adverse reactions

Most adverse reactions to corticosteroids are dose- or duration-dependent.

CNS: *euphoria, insomnia,* psychotic behavior, pseudotumor cerebri, vertigo, headache, paresthesia, *seizures.*

CV: *heart failure,* hypertension, edema, *arrhythmias,* thrombophlebitis, *thromboembolism.*

EENT: cataracts, glaucoma.

Endocrine: menstrual irregularities, cushingoid state (moonface, buffalo hump, central obesity).

GI: *peptic ulceration,* GI irritation, increased appetite, pancreatitis, nausea, vomiting.

Skin: delayed wound healing, acne, various skin eruptions.

Other: muscle weakness, osteoporosis, hirsutism, susceptibility to infections; hypokalemia, hyperglycemia, and carbohydrate intolerance; increased thyroxine, and triiodothyronine levels growth suppression in children; *acute adrenal insufficiency may follow increased stress (infection, surgery, or trauma) or abrupt withdrawal after long-term therapy.*

After abrupt withdrawal: rebound inflammation, fatigue, weakness, arthralgia, fever, dizziness, lethargy, depression, fainting, orthostatic hypotension, dyspnea, anorexia, hypoglycemia. *After prolonged use, sudden withdrawal may be fatal.*

☑ Special considerations

• Recommendations for use of betamethasone and for care and teaching of patients during therapy are the same as those for all systemic adrenocorticoids.

• Drug has been used to prevent respiratory distress syndrome in premature infants (hyaline membrane disease). Give 6 mg (2 ml) of Celestone Soluspan I.M. once daily 24 to 36 hours before induced delivery.

• Adrenocorticoid therapy suppresses reactions to skin tests; causes false-negative results in the nitroblue tetrazolium tests for systemic bacterial infections; and decreases ^{131}I uptake and protein-bound iodine levels in thyroid function tests.

• Acute ingestion, even in massive doses, rarely occurs.

• Toxic signs and symptoms rarely occur if drug is used for less than 3 weeks, even at large doses.

• Long-term use causes adverse physiologic effects, including suppression of the hypothalamic-pituitary-adrenal axis, cushingoid appearance, muscle weakness, and osteoporosis.

Monitoring the patient

• Monitor serum electrolytes periodically during treatment.

• Monitor patient for adverse effects.

Pediatric patients

• Long-term use of drug in children and adolescents may delay growth and maturation.

Breast-feeding patients

• Information is incomplete. Risk versus benefits must be determined and reviewed with patient.

betamethasone dipropionate, augmented
Diprolene, Diprolene AF

betamethasone dipropionate
Alphatrex, Diprosone, Maxivate

betamethasone valerate
Betaderm*, Betatrex, Beta-Val, Betnovate*, Celestoderm-V*, Ectosone*, Metaderm*, Novobetamet*, Valisone

Pharmacologic classification: topical glucocorticoid
Therapeutic classification: anti-inflammatory
Pregnancy risk category C

How supplied
Available by prescription only
betamethasone dipropionate, augmented
Cream, gel, lotion, ointment: 0.05%
betamethasone dipropionate
Lotion, ointment, cream: 0.05%
Aerosol: 0.1%
betamethasone valerate
Lotion, ointment: 0.1%
Cream: 0.01%, 0.1%
Foam: 0.12%

Indications, route, and dosage
Inflammation of corticosteroid-responsive dermatoses
betamethasone valerate
Adults and children: Apply cream, lotion, ointment, or gel in a thin layer once daily to q.i.d.
Relief of inflammatory and pruritic manifestations of corticosteroid-responsive dermatoses of scalp
Adults: Gently massage small amounts of foam into affected scalp areas twice daily (apply once in the morning and once at night) until control is achieved. If no improvement is seen within 2 weeks, reassess diagnosis.
betamethasone dipropionate
Adults and children over age 12: Apply cream, lotion, or ointment sparingly daily or b.i.d. Dosage of augmented 0.05% gels or lotions shouldn't exceed 50 g or 50 ml per week. Dosage of Diprolene ointments or creams 0.05% shouldn't exceed 45 g per week. To apply aerosol, direct spray onto affected area from a distance of 6 in. (15 cm) for only 3 seconds t.i.d. or q.i.d.

Pharmacodynamics
Anti-inflammatory action: Stimulates synthesis of enzymes needed to decrease inflammatory response. Betamethasone, a fluorinated derivative, has the advantage of availability in various bases to vary the potency for individual conditions.

Pharmacokinetics
● *Absorption:* Amount absorbed depends on potency of preparation, amount applied, and nature of skin at application site. It ranges from about 1% in areas with a thick stratum corneum to as high as 36% in areas with a thin stratum corneum. Absorption increases in areas of skin damage, inflammation, or occlusion. Some systemic absorption of topical corticosteroids occurs.
● *Distribution:* After topical application, drug is distributed throughout the local skin. Drug absorbed into circulation is removed rapidly from the blood and distributed into muscle, liver, skin, intestines, and kidneys.
● *Metabolism:* After topical administration, drug is metabolized primarily in the skin. The small amount that is absorbed into systemic circulation is metabolized primarily in the liver to inactive compounds.
● *Excretion:* Inactive metabolites are excreted by the kidneys, primarily as glucuronides and sulfates, but also as unconjugated products. Small amounts of the metabolites are also excreted in feces.

Contraindications and precautions
Contraindicated in patients with hypersensitivity to corticosteroids.

Interactions
None reported.

Adverse reactions
Skin: burning, pruritus, irritation, dryness, erythema, folliculitis, acneiform eruptions, perioral dermatitis, hypopigmentation, hypertrichosis, allergic contact dermatitis; *secondary infection, maceration, atrophy, striae, miliaria* (with occlusive dressings).
Other: *hypothalamic-pituitary-adrenal (HPA) axis suppression,* Cushing's syndrome, hyperglycemia, glycosuria (with betamethasone dipropionate).

☑ Special considerations
Besides the recommendations relevant to all topical adrenocorticoids, consider the following.
● Diprolene ointment may suppress the hypothalamic-pituitary-adrenal axis at doses as low as 7 g daily. Patient shouldn't use more than 45 g weekly and shouldn't use occlusive dressings.

Monitoring the patient
● Monitor patient response to therapy. With betamethasone dipropionate, closely observe for HPA axis suppression, Cushing's syndrome, hyperglycemia, and glycosuria.
● Monitor patient for adverse effects.

Pediatric patients
● Treatment with Diprolene ointment isn't recommended in children under age 12.

• Pediatric patients may be more susceptible to HPA axis suppression.

betaxolol hydrochloride
Betoptic, Betoptic S, Kerlone

Pharmacologic classification: beta blocker
Therapeutic classification: antiglaucoma drug, antihypertensive
Pregnancy risk category C

How supplied
Available by prescription only
Tablets: 10 mg, 20 mg
Ophthalmic solution: 5 mg/ml (0.5%) in 2.5-ml, 5-ml, 10-ml, 15-ml dropper bottles
Ophthalmic suspension: 2.5 mg/ml (0.25%) in 2.5-ml, 5-ml, 10-ml, 15-ml dropper bottles

Indications, route, and dosage
Chronic open-angle glaucoma and ocular hypertension
Adults: Instill 1 to 2 drops in eyes b.i.d.
Management of hypertension (used alone or with other antihypertensives)
Adults: Initially, 10 mg P.O. once daily. After 7 to 14 days, full antihypertensive effect should be seen. If necessary, double dose to 20 mg P.O. once daily. (Doses up to 40 mg daily have also been used.)
✦ *Dosage adjustment.* In patients with renal impairment or in elderly patients, initial dose is 5 mg P.O. daily. Increase by 5-mg/day increments q 2 weeks to maximum of 20 mg/day.

Pharmacodynamics
Antihypertensive action: Cardioselective adrenergic blocking effects of betaxolol slow heart rate and decrease cardiac output.
Ocular hypotensive action: A cardioselective beta blocker that reduces intraocular pressure (IOP), possibly by reducing production of aqueous humor when administered as an ophthalmic solution.

Pharmacokinetics
• *Absorption:* Essentially complete after oral administration; minimal after ophthalmic use. A small first-pass effect reduces bioavailability by about 10%. Absorption isn't affected by food or alcohol.
• *Distribution:* Plasma levels peak about 3 hours (range, 1.5 to 6) after a single oral dose. Drug is about 50% bound to plasma proteins.
• *Metabolism:* Hepatic; about 85% is recovered in urine as metabolites. Elimination half-life is prolonged in patients with hepatic disease, but clearance isn't affected, so dosage adjustment is unnecessary.
• *Excretion:* Primarily renal (about 80%). Plasma half-life is 14 to 22 hours.

Contraindications and precautions
Contraindicated in patients with hypersensitivity to drug and in those with severe bradycardia, greater than first-degree heart block, cardiogenic shock, or uncontrolled heart failure.

Interactions
Drug-drug. *Calcium channel blockers:* Increased risk of hypotension, left-sided heart failure, and AV conduction disturbances. Monitor patient closely.
Carbonic anhydrase inhibitors, epinephrine, pilocarpine: Enhanced lowering of IOP. Monitor patient closely.
Catecholamine-depleting drugs, reserpine: May have an additive effect when administered with a beta blocker; enhanced hypotensive and bradycardiac effect. Use together cautiously.
General anesthetics: May cause increased hypotensive effects. Observe patient carefully for excessive hypotension, bradycardia, or orthostatic hypotension.
I.V. calcium antagonists: Enhanced effects. Use with caution.
Lidocaine: Increased effects of lidocaine. Use together cautiously.
Oral beta blockers: Ophthalmic betaxolol may increase systemic effect of oral beta blockers. Monitor patient carefully.

Adverse reactions
Ophthalmic form
CNS: insomnia, depressive neurosis.
EENT: *eye stinging on instillation causing brief discomfort,* photophobia, erythema, itching, keratitis, occasional tearing.
Systemic form
CNS: dizziness, fatigue, headache, insomnia, lethargy, anxiety.
CV: *bradycardia,* chest pain, *heart failure,* edema.
GI: nausea, diarrhea, dyspepsia.
Respiratory: dyspnea, pharyngitis, *bronchospasm.*
Skin: rash.
Other: impotence, arthralgia.

☑ Special considerations
Ophthalmic use
• Betaxolol is a cardioselective beta blocker. Its pulmonary and systemic effects are considerably milder than those of timolol or levobunolol.
• Ophthalmic betaxolol is intended for twice-daily dosage. Encourage patient to comply with this regimen.
• In some patients, a few weeks' treatment may be required to stabilize pressure-lowering response. Determine IOP during the first 4 weeks of drug therapy.
Systemic use
• Withdrawal of beta blocker therapy before surgery is controversial. Some clinicians advo-

cate withdrawal to prevent any impairment of cardiac responsiveness to reflex stimuli and to prevent any decreased responsiveness to exogenous catecholamines.
• To withdraw drug, gradually reduce dosage over at least 2 weeks.
• Oral beta blockers may alter results of glucose tolerance tests.
• Signs and symptoms of overdose, which are extremely rare with ophthalmic use, may include diplopia, bradycardia, heart block, hypotension, shock, increased airway resistance, cyanosis, fatigue, sleepiness, headache, sedation, coma, respiratory depression, seizures, nausea, vomiting, diarrhea, hypoglycemia, hallucinations, and nightmares.
• For toxic symptoms, discontinue drug and flush eye with normal saline solution or water.
• For treatment of accidental substantial ingestion, emesis is most effective if initiated within 30 minutes, provided the patient isn't obtunded, comatose, or having seizures. Activated charcoal may be used.
• Treat bradycardia, conduction defects, and hypotension with I.V. fluids, glucagon, atropine, or isoproterenol; refractory bradycardia may require a transvenous pacemaker.
• Treat bronchoconstriction with I.V. aminophylline; seizures with I.V. diazepam.

Monitoring the patient
• Patient receiving oral beta blockers and beta-blocking ophthalmic solution should be observed for potential additive effects either on the IOP or on the known systemic effects of beta blockade.
• Monitor patient for adverse effects.

Information for the patient
Ophthalmic use
• Tell patient to shake suspension well before use.
• Instruct patient to tilt head back and, while looking up, instill drug into the lower lid.
• Warn patient not to touch dropper to eye or surrounding tissue.
• Instruct patient not to close eyes tightly or blink more than usual after instillation.
• Remind patient to wait at least 5 minutes before using other eyedrops.
• Advise patient to wear sunglasses and avoid exposure to bright light.
Systemic use
• Advise patient to take drug exactly as prescribed and warn against discontinuing it suddenly.
• Advise patient to report shortness of breath or difficulty breathing, unusually fast heartbeat, cough, or fatigue with exertion.

Geriatric patients
• Use with caution in elderly patients with cardiac or pulmonary disease.

Breast-feeding patients
• Use with caution. After oral administration, drug appears in breast milk in sufficient amounts to exert an effect on breast-feeding infant.

bethanechol chloride
Duvoid, Myotonachol, Urecholine

Pharmacologic classification: cholinergic agonist
Therapeutic classification: urinary tract and GI tract stimulant
Pregnancy risk category C

How supplied
Available by prescription only
Tablets: 5 mg, 10 mg, 25 mg, 50 mg
Injection: 5 mg/ml

Indications, route, and dosage
Acute postoperative and postpartum nonobstructive (functional) urine retention, neurogenic atony of urinary bladder with retention
Adults: 10 to 50 mg P.O. t.i.d. or q.i.d. Or 2.5 to 5 mg S.C. (Use 10 mg S.C. with extreme caution.) *Never give I.M. or I.V.* When used for urine retention, some patients may require 50 to 100 mg P.O. per dose. Use such doses with extreme caution. Test dose: 2.5 mg S.C. repeated at 15- to 30-minute intervals to total of 4 doses to determine the minimal effective dose; then use minimal effective dose q 6 to 8 hours. Adjust dose to meet individual requirements.
◊ ***Bladder dysfunction caused by phenothiazines***
Adults: 50 to 100 mg P.O. q.i.d.
◊ ***To lessen the adverse effects of tricyclic antidepressants***
Adults: 25 mg P.O. t.i.d.
◊ ***Chronic gastric reflux***
Adults: 25 mg P.O. q.i.d.
◊ ***Familial dysautonomia***
Children: 0.2 to 0.4 mg/kg S.C. q.i.d. 30 minutes before meals with an oral antacid; then after 2 weeks, give 1 to 2 mg P.O. q.i.d.
◊ ***To diagnose flaccid or atonic neurogenic bladder***
Adults: 2.5 mg S.C.
◊ ***To diagnose cystic fibrosis***
Before administration, dilute 5 mg of drug in 3 ml of D_5W to yield a concentration of 1.25 mg/ml.
Children over age 1: 1 mg intradermally.
Children ages 2 months to 1 year: 0.5 mg intradermally.
Infants from birth to age 2 months: 0.25 mg intradermally.

Pharmacodynamics
Urinary tract stimulant action: Directly binds to and stimulates muscarinic receptors of the parasympathetic nervous system, which increases

---

tone of the bladder detrusor muscle, usually resulting in contraction, decreased bladder capacity, and subsequent urination.
GI tract stimulant action: Directly stimulates cholinergic receptors, leading to increased gastric tone and motility and peristalsis. Improves lower esophageal sphincter tone by directly stimulating cholinergic receptors, thereby alleviating gastric reflux.

Pharmacokinetics
● *Absorption:* Poorly absorbed from GI tract (absorption varies considerably among patients). After oral administration, action usually begins in 30 to 90 minutes; after S.C. administration, in 5 to 15 minutes.
● *Distribution:* Largely unknown; however, therapeutic doses don't penetrate blood-brain barrier.
● *Metabolism:* Unknown. Usual duration of effect after oral administration is 1 hour; after S.C. administration, up to 2 hours.
● *Excretion:* No information available.

Contraindications and precautions
Contraindicated for I.M. or I.V. use and in patients with hypersensitivity to drug or its components. Also contraindicated in those with uncertain strength or integrity of bladder wall; mechanical obstructions of GI or urinary tract; hyperthyroidism, peptic ulceration, latent or active bronchial asthma, pronounced bradycardia or hypotension, vasomotor instability, cardiac or coronary artery disease, seizure disorder, Parkinson's disease, spastic GI disturbances, acute inflammatory lesions of the GI tract, peritonitis, or marked vagotonia; or when increased muscular activity of GI or urinary tract is harmful. Use cautiously in pregnant women.

Interactions
Drug-drug. *Cholinergic drugs, especially cholinesterase inhibitors:* Additive effects may occur. Avoid concomitant use.
Ganglionic blockers such as mecamylamine: May cause critical blood pressure decrease, usually preceded by abdominal symptoms. Avoid concurrent use, if possible.
Procainamide, quinidine: May reverse cholinergic effect of bethanechol on muscle. Use cautiously.

Adverse reactions
CNS: headache, malaise.
CV: hypotension, reflex tachycardia.
EENT: lacrimation, miosis.
GI: *abdominal cramps, diarrhea,* excessive salivation, nausea, belching, borborygmus.
GU: urinary urgency.
Hepatic: increased serum levels of amylase, lipase, bilirubin, and AST.
Respiratory: **bronchoconstriction,** increased bronchial secretions.
Skin: flushing, diaphoresis.

☑ Special considerations
● Atropine sulfate should be readily available to counteract toxic reactions that may occur during treatment with bethanechol.
● Never give bethanechol I.M. or I.V. because that could cause circulatory collapse, hypotension, severe abdominal cramps, bloody diarrhea, shock, or cardiac arrest. Give only by S.C. route when giving parenterally.
● For treatment of urine retention, bedpan should be readily available.
● Give drug on an empty stomach; eating soon after drug administration may cause nausea and vomiting.
● Patients who have hypertension and are receiving bethanechol may experience precipitous decrease in blood pressure.
● Clinical signs and symptoms of overdose include nausea, vomiting, abdominal cramps, diarrhea, involuntary defecation, urinary urgency, excessive salivation, miosis, excessive tearing, bronchospasm, increased bronchial secretions, hypotension, excessive sweating, bradycardia or reflex tachycardia, and substernal pain.
● Treatment requires discontinuation of drug and administration of atropine by S.C., I.M., or I.V. route. Atropine must be administered cautiously; an overdose could cause bronchial plug formation.
● Contact local or regional poison control center for more information.

Monitoring the patient
● Monitor vital signs.
● With S.C. administration, watch for toxicity (nausea, vomiting, diarrhea, flushing, abdominal discomfort).

Breast-feeding patients
● It's unknown if drug appears in breast milk. A decision should be made to use drug based on importance of drug to the mother.

bexarotene
Targretin

Pharmacologic classification: retinoid (selective retinoid X receptor activator)
Therapeutic classification: tumor cell growth inhibitor
Pregnancy risk category X

How supplied
Available by prescription only
Capsules: 75 mg

Indications, route, and dosage
Cutaneous manifestations of cutaneous T-cell lymphoma in patients refractory to at least one prior systemic therapy
Adults: 300 mg/m²/day taken as a single oral dose with a meal.

✦ Dosage adjustment. For patients with hepatic insufficiency, expect drug clearance to be significantly decreased. Use drug only with great caution; lower doses may be necessary. In case of toxicity, dose level may be adjusted to 200 mg/m²/day, then to 100 mg/m²/day, or temporarily suspended. When toxicity is controlled, doses may be carefully readjusted upward. If lack of response after 8 weeks of treatment, dose may be escalated to 400 mg/m²/day if initial dose of 300 mg/m²/day was tolerated.

Pharmacodynamics

Tumor cell growth inhibitor action: Selectively binds and activates retinoid X receptor (RXR) subtypes. Once activated, these receptors function as transcription factors that regulate the expression of genes that control cellular differentiation and proliferation. Drug inhibits growth in vitro of some tumor cell lines of hematopoietic and squamous cell origin. Exact mechanism in treatment of cutaneous T-cell lymphoma is unknown.

Pharmacokinetics

• *Absorption:* Absorbed from GI tract; absorption appreciably higher if administered with a fat-containing meal.
• *Distribution:* More than 99% bound to plasma proteins.
• *Metabolism:* Metabolized through oxidative pathways, primarily by the cytochrome P-450 3A4 system, to 4 metabolites. Metabolites may maintain retinoid receptor activity. Terminal half-life is 7 hours.
• *Excretion:* Thought to be eliminated primarily through hepatobiliary system.

Contraindications and precautions

Contraindicated in patients with hypersensitivity to drug or its components and during pregnancy. Not recommended for patients who have risk factors for pancreatitis, such as prior pancreatitis, uncontrolled hyperlipidemia, excessive alcohol consumption, uncontrolled diabetes mellitus, and biliary tract disease, or for those who are taking drugs that increase triglyceride levels or are associated with pancreatic toxicity.

Use cautiously in women of childbearing potential. Use cautiously in patients with hepatic insufficiency.

Interactions

Drug-drug. *Erythromycin, gemfibrozil, itraconazole, ketoconazole, other inhibitors of cytochrome P-450 3A4:* Increased plasma levels of bexarotene. Avoid concomitant use.
Insulin, sulfonylureas, troglitazone: May enhance hypoglycemic action of these drugs, resulting in hypoglycemia in patients with diabetes mellitus. Monitor patient.

Phenobarbital, phenytoin, rifampin, other inducers of cytochrome P-450 3A4: Decreased plasma levels of bexarotene. Avoid concomitant use.
Vitamin A preparations: Increased potential for vitamin A toxicity. Avoid vitamin A supplements.
Drug-food. *Grapefruit juice:* May inhibit cytochrome P-450 3A4. Avoid concomitant use.

Adverse reactions

CNS: headache, insomnia, asthenia, fatigue, lethargy.
CV: peripheral edema.
EENT: cataracts, pharyngitis, rhinitis, hemoptysis, dry eyes, conjunctivitis, ear pain blepharitis, corneal lesion, keratitis, otitis externa, visual field defect.
GI: nausea, diarrhea, vomiting, anorexia, ***pancreatitis,*** abdominal pain, elevated amylase.
GU: elevated creatinine.
Hematologic: leukopenia, anemia, eosinophilia, thrombocythemia, lymphocytosis, ***thrombocytopenia.***
Hepatic: elevated LD, bilirubinemia, increased AST and ALT.
Metabolic: hyperlipemia, hypercholesteremia, hypothyroidism, hyperglycemia, hypoproteinemia.
Musculoskeletal: arthralgia, myalgia.
Respiratory: pneumonia.
Skin: rash, dry skin, ***exfoliative dermatitis,*** alopecia, photosensitivity, pruritus.
Other: infection, chills, fever, flulike symptoms, back pain.

☑ Special considerations

• Women of childbearing potential should use effective contraception at least 1 month before starting bexarotene therapy. While on therapy, patients should use 2 reliable forms of contraception simultaneously, unless abstinence is the chosen method. Pregnancy test should be negative before starting therapy and should be done monthly while on therapy.
• Male patients with sexual partners who are pregnant, possibly pregnant, or who could become pregnant must use condoms during sexual intercourse while taking drug.
• Give no more than a 1-month supply of drug to patient with childbearing potential so results of pregnancy testing can be assessed and counseling regarding avoidance of pregnancy and possibility of birth defects can be given.
• Overdose doesn't appear to produce acute toxic effects; treat symptomatically with supportive care.

Monitoring the patient

• Total cholesterol, HDL cholesterol, and triglyceride levels should be assessed at beginning of therapy and weekly thereafter until lipid response to drug is established (2 to 4 weeks); then at 8-week intervals. Treat elevated triglyceride levels

with antilipemic therapy; if necessary, reduce the dosage or stop the drug.
• Baseline thyroid function tests should be performed; patients should be monitored during treatment.
• Determination of WBC with differential should be obtained at baseline and periodically during treatment.
• Patients who experience visual difficulties should have an appropriate ophthalmologic evaluation for cataracts.
• Baseline liver function tests should be performed, then monitored carefully after 1, 2, and 4 weeks of treatment; then at least every 8 weeks thereafter if test results are stable.
• Drug therapy may increase CA 125 assay values in patients with ovarian cancer.

Information for the patient
• To avoid photosensitivity, advise patient to minimize exposure to sunlight and artificial ultraviolet light while taking drug.
• Tell patient that several capsules may be required for the necessary dose; all capsules should be taken at the same time with a meal.
• Inform patient not to take any vitamin A preparations.
• Teach woman of childbearing potential the dangers of becoming pregnant while taking drug and the need for monthly pregnancy tests.
• Explain the need for obtaining baseline laboratory test results and for periodic monitoring of these tests.
• Tell patient to report visual changes.

Geriatric patients
• Safety and effectiveness in elderly patients has been established, but greater sensitivity is possible in these patients.

Pediatric patients
• Safety and effectiveness in children haven't been established.

Breast-feeding patients
• Drug isn't recommended for breast-feeding patients. A decision should be made to discontinue breast-feeding or discontinue drug based on importance of drug to the mother.

bicalutamide
Casodex

Pharmacologic classification: nonsteroidal antiandrogen
Therapeutic classification: antineoplastic
Pregnancy risk category X

How supplied
Available by prescription only
Tablets: 50 mg

Indications, route, and dosage
Adjunct therapy for treatment of advanced prostate cancer
Adults: 50 mg P.O. once daily in morning or evening.

Pharmacodynamics
Antineoplastic action: Competitively inhibits action of androgens by binding to cytosol androgen receptors in target tissue. Prostatic carcinoma, known to be sensitive to androgens, responds to treatment that either counteracts the effect of androgen or removes its source.

Pharmacokinetics
• *Absorption:* Well absorbed from GI tract.
• *Distribution:* 96% of drug is protein-bound.
• *Metabolism:* Undergoes stereospecific metabolism. The S (inactive) isomer is metabolized primarily by glucuronidation. The R (active) isomer also undergoes glucuronidation but is predominantly oxidized to an inactive metabolite followed by glucuronidation.
• *Excretion:* Excreted in urine and feces.

Contraindications and precautions
Contraindicated in patients with hypersensitivity to drug or its components and during pregnancy. Use cautiously in patients with moderate to severe hepatic impairment. (Drug is extensively metabolized by the liver.)

Interactions
Drug-drug. *Coumarin anticoagulants:* Displaces coumarin anticoagulants from their protein-binding sites. Monitor PT and INR closely. Anticoagulant dose may need adjustment.

Adverse reactions
CNS: headache, dizziness, paresthesia, insomnia.
CV: *hot flashes, asthenia,* hypertension, chest pain, peripheral edema.
GI: *constipation, nausea, diarrhea,* abdominal pain, flatulence, increased liver enzymes, vomiting, weight loss.
GU: nocturia, hematuria, urinary tract infection, impotence, gynecomastia, urinary incontinence, increased BUN and creatinine levels.
Hematologic: iron-deficiency anemia, hypochromic anemia.
Metabolic: hyperglycemia.
Musculoskeletal: *back or pelvic pain,* bone pain.
Respiratory: dyspnea.
Skin: rash, sweating.
Other: *general pain, infection,* flulike symptoms.

☑ Special considerations
• Bicalutamide is used with a luteinizing hormone–releasing hormone (LHRH) analogue for the treatment of advanced prostate cancer. Treat-

ment should begin at the same time as that of the prescribed LHRH analogue.
● Administer bicalutamide at the same time each day.
● Drug isn't indicated for use in women.
● There is no specific antidote in the case of overdose; treatment is symptomatic. Vomiting may be induced if patient is alert. Dialysis isn't likely to be helpful because bicalutamide is highly protein-bound and is extensively metabolized.

Monitoring the patient
● Monitor serum prostate specific antigen (PSA) levels regularly. PSA levels help in assessing patient's response to therapy. Elevated levels require a reevaluation of patient to determine disease progression.
● Monitor liver function studies. Stop drug if patient develops jaundice or exhibits laboratory evidence of liver injury in the absence of liver metastases. Abnormalities are usually reversible on drug discontinuation.

Information for the patient
● Tell patient to take drug without regard to meals.
● Advise patient to take drug at the same time each day.
● Tell patient that bicalutamide is used with other drug therapy. Stress importance of not interrupting or stopping any of these drugs without medical consultation.

Pediatric patients
● Safety and effectiveness in children haven't been established.

Breast-feeding patients
● Drug isn't indicated for use in women.

---

biperiden hydrochloride
biperiden lactate
Akineton

Pharmacologic classification: anticholinergic
Therapeutic classification: antiparkinsonian
Pregnancy risk category C

How supplied
Available by prescription only
Tablets: 2 mg
Injection: 5 mg/ml in 1-ml ampule

Indications, route, and dosage
Extrapyramidal disorders
Adults: 2 mg P.O. daily, b.i.d. or t.i.d., depending on severity. Usual dose is 2 mg daily. For treatment of extrapyramidal symptoms induced by

drugs, give 2 mg I.M. or slow I.V. q 30 minutes, not to exceed 8 mg in a 24-hour period.
Parkinsonism
Adults: 2 mg P.O. t.i.d. or q.i.d. For prolonged therapy, adjust dose to maximum of 16 mg daily.

Pharmacodynamics
Antiparkinsonian action: Blocks central cholinergic receptors, helping to balance cholinergic activity in the basal ganglia. May also prolong effects of dopamine by blocking dopamine reuptake and storage at central receptor sites.

Pharmacokinetics
● *Absorption:* Well absorbed from GI tract.
● *Distribution:* Minimally absorbed; metabolized in the liver.
● *Metabolism:* Exact metabolic fate unknown.
● *Excretion:* Excreted in urine as unchanged drug and metabolites. After oral therapy, small amounts are probably excreted as unabsorbed drug.

Contraindications and precautions
Contraindicated in patients with hypersensitivity to drug and in those with angle-closure glaucoma, bowel obstruction, or megacolon. Use cautiously in patients with prostatic hyperplasia, arrhythmias, or seizure disorders.

Interactions
Drug-drug. *Amantadine:* May amplify anticholinergic adverse effects of biperiden, such as confusion and hallucinations. Decrease biperiden dose before giving amantadine.
Antacids, antidiarrheals: May decrease biperiden absorption. Administer biperiden at least 1 hour before these drugs.
CNS depressants: Increased sedative effects of biperiden. Use with caution.
Digoxin: Plasma levels of digoxin may be elevated. Monitor digoxin levels.
Haloperidol, phenothiazines: May decrease antipsychotic effectiveness of these drugs, possibly by direct CNS antagonism. Avoid concomitant use.
Phenothiazines: Increased risk of anticholinergic adverse effects. Avoid concomitant use.
Drug-lifestyle. *Alcohol:* Increased sedative effects of biperiden. Discourage use.

Adverse reactions
CNS: disorientation, euphoria, drowsiness, agitation.
CV: transient orthostatic hypotension (with parenteral use).
EENT: blurred vision.
GI: dry mouth, *constipation.*
GU: urine retention.
  Note: Adverse reactions are dose-related and may resemble atropine toxicity.

☑ Special considerations

Besides the recommendations relevant to all anticholinergics, consider the following.

• When giving drug parenterally, keep patient supine; parenteral administration may cause transient orthostatic hypotension and disturbed coordination.

• When giving biperiden I.V., inject drug slowly.

• Because biperiden may cause dizziness, patient may need assistance when walking.

• In patients with severe parkinsonism, tremors may increase when drug is administered to relieve spasticity.

• Clinical effects of overdose include central stimulation followed by depression and psychotic symptoms, such as disorientation, confusion, hallucinations, delusions, anxiety, agitation, and restlessness. Peripheral effects may include dilated, nonreactive pupils; blurred vision; hot, dry, flushed skin; dry mucous membranes; dysphagia; decreased or absent bowel sounds; urine retention; hyperthermia; headache; tachycardia; hypertension; and increased respiration.

• Treatment of overdose is primarily symptomatic and supportive, as necessary. Maintain patent airway. If the patient is alert, induce emesis (or use gastric lavage) and follow with a sodium chloride cathartic and activated charcoal to prevent further absorption of orally administered drug. In severe cases, physostigmine may be administered to block antimuscarinic effects of biperiden. Give fluids, as needed, to treat shock; diazepam to control psychotic symptoms; and pilocarpine (instilled into the eyes) to relieve mydriasis. If urine retention occurs, catheterization may be necessary.

Monitoring the patient

• Monitor patient for adverse effects; monitor patient response.

• Perform ECG in patients with history of arrhythmias.

Information for the patient

• Tell patient that tolerance to therapeutic and adverse effects can occur with chronic drug use.

• Tell patient that drug may increase sensitivity of the eyes to light.

• Instruct patient to take drug with food to avoid GI upset.

Geriatric patients

• Use cautiously in elderly patients. Lower doses are indicated.

Pediatric patients

• Drug isn't recommended for children.

Breast-feeding patients

• Drug may appear in breast milk, possibly resulting in infant toxicity. It may also decrease milk production. Avoid use of drug in breast-feeding women.

bisacodyl

Bisco-Lax, Dulcolax, Fleet Laxative

Pharmacologic classification: diphenylmethane derivative
Therapeutic classification: stimulant laxative
Pregnancy risk category B

How supplied

Available without a prescription
Tablets: 5 mg
Suppositories: 10 mg
Rectal suspension: 10mg/30 ml

Indications, route, and dosage

Constipation; preparation for delivery, surgery, or rectal or bowel examination
Adults: 10 to 15 mg P.O. daily. Up to 30 mg may be used for thorough evacuation needed for examinations or surgery. Or give 1 suppository (10 mg) or 30 ml of rectal suspension P.R. daily.
Children ages 6 to 12: 5 mg P.O. daily. Or give ½ of suppository (5 mg) or 15 ml of rectal suspension P.R. daily.

Pharmacodynamics

Laxative action: Has a direct stimulant effect on the colon, increasing peristalsis and enhancing bowel evacuation.

Pharmacokinetics

• *Absorption:* Absorption is minimal. Action begins 6 to 8 hours after oral administration; 15 to 60 minutes after P.R. administration.

• *Distribution:* Distributed locally.

• *Metabolism:* Absorbed minimally; metabolized in the liver.

• *Excretion:* Excreted primarily in feces; some in urine.

Contraindications and precautions

Contraindicated in patients with hypersensitivity to drug and in those with rectal bleeding, gastroenteritis, intestinal obstruction, abdominal pain, nausea, vomiting, or other symptoms of appendicitis or acute surgical abdomen.

Interactions

Drug-drug. *Antacids, drugs that increase gastric pH levels:* May cause premature dissolution of the enteric coating, resulting in intestinal or gastric irritation or cramping. Avoid concomitant use.

Drug-food. *Milk:* May cause premature dissolution of the enteric coating, resulting in intestinal or gastric irritation or cramping. Avoid concomitant use.

Adverse reactions
CNS: muscle weakness with excessive use, dizziness, faintness.
GI: *nausea, vomiting, abdominal cramps,* diarrhea (with high doses), *burning sensation in rectum* (with suppositories), laxative dependence with long-term or excessive use.
Metabolic: alkalosis, hypokalemia, tetany, protein-losing enteropathy in excessive use, fluid and electrolyte imbalance.

☑ Special considerations
● Patient should swallow tablets whole rather than crushing or chewing them to avoid GI irritation. Administer with 8 oz (240 ml) of fluid.

Monitoring the patient
● Evaluate patient's response to therapy.
● Monitor use; discourage excessive use.
● Check electrolyte levels as needed.

Information for the patient
● Instruct patient not to take drug within 1 hour of milk or antacid consumption.
● Tell patient to take only as directed to avoid laxative dependence.

Geriatric patients
● Use with caution because elderly patients are prone to dehydration.

Pediatric patients
● Dulcolax oral tablets shouldn't be given to children under age 6.

Breast-feeding patients
● Bisacodyl may be used by breast-feeding women.

bismuth subsalicylate
Pepto-Bismol

Pharmacologic classification: adsorbent
Therapeutic classification: antidiarrheal
Pregnancy risk category C (D in third trimester)

How supplied
Available without a prescription
Tablets (chewable): 262 mg
Suspension: 262 mg/15 ml, 524 mg/15 ml

Indications, route, and dosage
Mild, nonspecific diarrhea
Adults: 30 ml or 2 tablets q ½ to 1 hour to a maximum of eight doses and for no more than 2 days.
Children ages 9 to 12: 15 ml or 1 tablet.
Children ages 6 to 9: 10 ml or ⅔ tablet.
Children ages 3 to 6: 5 ml or ⅓ tablet.

Children's dosage given q ½ to 1 hour to a maximum of eight doses in 24 hours and for no more than 2 days.

Pharmacodynamics
Antidiarrheal action: Adsorbs extra water in the bowel during diarrhea. Also adsorbs toxins and forms a protective coating for the intestinal mucosa.

Pharmacokinetics
● *Absorption:* Absorbed poorly; significant salicylate absorption may occur after using bismuth subsalicylate.
● *Distribution:* Distributed locally in the gut.
● *Metabolism:* Metabolized minimally.
● *Excretion:* Excreted in urine.

Contraindications and precautions
Contraindicated in patients with hypersensitivity to salicylates. Use cautiously in patients already taking aspirin or aspirin-containing drugs.

Interactions
Drug-drug. *Aspirin:* Additive effect; may increase risk of aspirin toxicity. Avoid concomitant use.
Sulfinpyrazone: Impaired uricosuric effect. Avoid using together.
Tetracycline: May impair tetracycline absorption. Separate by 1 hour.

Adverse reactions
GI: temporary darkening of tongue and stools.
Other: salicylism (with high doses).

☑ Special considerations
● If drug is administered by tube, flush tube via nasogastric tube to clear it and ensure passage of drug to stomach.
● If patient is also receiving tetracycline, administer drugs at least 1 hour apart; to avoid decreased drug absorption, dosages or schedules of other drug administration may require adjustment.
● Drug has been used to treat peptic ulcer. Doses of 600 mg t.i.d. may be as effective as cimetidine 800 mg once daily.
● Drug is useful for indigestion without causing constipation, for nausea, and for relief of flatulence and abdominal cramps.
● Because drug is radiopaque, it may interfere with radiologic examination of the GI tract.
● Overdose hasn't been reported. However, overdose is more likely with bismuth subsalicylate; probable clinical effects include CNS effects, such as tinnitus, and fever.

Monitoring the patient
● Monitor hydration status and serum electrolyte levels; record number and consistency of stools.
● Monitor patient for adverse effects.

Information for the patient
• Advise patient taking anticoagulants or medication for diabetes or gout to seek medical approval before taking drug.
• Instruct patient to chew tablets well or to shake suspension well before using.
• Tell patient to report persistent diarrhea.
• Warn patient that drug may temporarily darken stools and tongue.

Geriatric patients
• Use cautiously because elderly patients are prone to dehydration.

Pediatric patients
• Children and teenagers who have or are recovering from flu or chickenpox shouldn't use this drug to treat nausea and vomiting, which could be an early sign of Reye syndrome.

Breast-feeding patients
• Small amounts of drug appear in breast milk. Patient should seek medical approval before use.

bisoprolol fumarate
Zebeta

Pharmacologic classification: beta blocker
Therapeutic classification: antihypertensive
Pregnancy risk category C

How supplied
Available by prescription only
Tablets: 5 mg, 10 mg

Indications, route, and dosage
Hypertension (used alone or with other antihypertensives)
Adults: Initially, 5 mg P.O. once daily. If response is inadequate, increase to 10 mg once daily. Maximum recommended dose is 20 mg daily.
✦ *Dosage adjustment.* In adults with renal impairment (creatinine clearance less than 40 ml/minute) or hepatic dysfunction, cirrhosis, or hepatitis, start at 2.5 mg P.O.; then increase with caution.

Pharmacodynamics
Antihypertensive action: Exact mechanism unknown. Possible antihypertensive factors include decreased cardiac output, inhibition of renin release by the kidneys, and diminution of tonic sympathetic outflow from the vasomotor centers in the brain.

Pharmacokinetics
• *Absorption:* Bioavailability after a 10-mg oral dose is about 80%. Absorption not affected by food.

• *Distribution:* About 30% binds to serum proteins.
• *Metabolism:* First-pass metabolism is about 20%.
• *Excretion:* Eliminated equally by renal and nonrenal pathways, with about 50% of dose appearing unchanged in urine and remainder appearing as inactive metabolites. Less than 2% of dose is excreted in feces. Plasma elimination half-life is 9 to 12 hours (slightly longer in elderly patients, in part because of decreased renal function in that population).

Contraindications and precautions
Contraindicated in patients with hypersensitivity to drug and in those with cardiogenic shock, overt cardiac failure, marked sinus bradycardia, or second- or third-degree AV block. Use cautiously in patients with bronchospastic disease.

Interactions
Drug-drug. *Catecholamine-depleting drugs such as reserpine, guanethidine:* Added beta-blocking action of bisoprolol may excessively reduce sympathetic activity. Monitor patient closely.
Clonidine: Hypertension may occur with concomitant withdrawal of therapy. Discontinue bisoprolol for several days before clonidine withdrawal.
Other beta blockers: Additive effect. Avoid concomitant use.

Adverse reactions
CNS: asthenia, fatigue, dizziness, *headache,* hypoesthesia, vivid dreams, depression, insomnia.
CV: *bradycardia,* peripheral edema, chest pain.
EENT: pharyngitis, rhinitis, sinusitis.
GI: nausea, vomiting, diarrhea, dry mouth.
Respiratory: cough, dyspnea.
Other: arthralgia.

☑ Special considerations
• Patients with renal or hepatic dysfunction or bronchospastic disease unresponsive to or intolerant of other antihypertensive therapies should start therapy at 2.5 mg daily. A beta$_2$-adrenergic agonist (bronchodilator) should be made available to patients with bronchospastic disease.
• Exacerbation of angina pectoris, MI, and ventricular arrhythmia has been observed in patients with coronary artery disease after abrupt cessation of therapy with beta blockers. It's advisable, even in patients without overt coronary artery disease, to taper therapy with bisoprolol over 1 week, with patient under careful observation. If withdrawal symptoms occur, bisoprolol therapy should be reinstituted, at least temporarily.
• Drug may produce hypoglycemia and interfere with glucose or insulin tolerance tests.
• The most common signs of overdose are bradycardia, hypotension, heart failure, bronchospasm, and hypoglycemia.

- If overdose occurs, drug therapy should be stopped; supportive and symptomatic treatment should be provided.

Monitoring the patient
- Monitor patient for adverse effects.
- Monitor serum glucose and renal and hepatic function as indicated.

Information for the patient
- Inform diabetic patients subject to spontaneous hypoglycemia or those requiring insulin or oral hypoglycemic drugs that bisoprolol may mask some signs of hypoglycemia, particularly tachycardia.
- Warn patient not to drive, operate machinery, or perform any other task requiring alertness until reaction to bisoprolol has been established.
- Stress importance of taking drug as prescribed, even when feeling well. Advise patient not to stop drug abruptly because serious consequences can occur.
- Instruct patient to call if adverse reactions occur.
- Tell patient to seek medical approval before taking OTC medications.

Pediatric patients
- Safety and effectiveness in children haven't been established.

Breast-feeding patients
- It's unknown if drug appears in breast milk. Use with caution when administering to breast-feeding women.

bitolterol mesylate
Tornalate

Pharmacologic classification: adrenergic, beta$_2$ agonist
Therapeutic classification: bronchodilator
Pregnancy risk category C

How supplied
Available by prescription only
Aerosol inhaler: 370 mcg/metered spray
Solution for nebulization: 0.2%

Indications, route, and dosage
To prevent and treat bronchial asthma and bronchospasm
Adults and children over age 12: For symptomatic relief of bronchospasm, 2 inhalations at an interval of at least 1 to 3 minutes then a third inhalation, if needed; to prevent bronchospasm, 2 inhalations q 8 hours. Usually, dose shouldn't exceed 3 inhalations q 6 hours or 2 inhalations q 4 hours. *Nebulizer:* For intermittent flow, 1 mg t.i.d. For continuous flow, 2.5 mg t.i.d. However, because deposition of inhaled medications is variable, higher doses are occasionally used, especially in patients with acute bronchospasm.

Pharmacodynamics
Bronchodilator action: Selectively stimulates beta$_2$-adrenergic receptors of the lungs. Bronchodilation results from relaxation of bronchial smooth muscles, which relieves bronchospasm and reduces airway resistance. Some CV stimulation may occur as a result of beta$_1$-adrenergic stimulation, including mild tachycardia, palpitations, and changes in blood pressure or heart rate.

Pharmacokinetics
- *Absorption:* After oral inhalation, bronchodilation results from local action on bronchial tree, with most of inhaled dose being swallowed. Onset of action occurs within 3 to 5 minutes, peaks in ½ to 2 hours and lasts 4 to 8 hours.
- *Distribution:* Widely distributed throughout body.
- *Metabolism:* Hydrolyzed by esterases to active metabolites.
- *Excretion:* After oral administration, drug and its metabolites are excreted primarily in urine.

Contraindications and precautions
Contraindicated in patients with hypersensitivity to drug. Use cautiously in patients with ischemic heart disease, hypertension, hyperthyroidism, diabetes mellitus, arrhythmias, seizure disorders, or history of unusual responsiveness to beta-adrenergic agonists.

Interactions
Drug-drug. *Orally inhaled beta-adrenergic agonists:* May produce additive sympathomimetic effects. Use with caution.
Propranolol, other beta blockers: May antagonize effects of bitolterol. Avoid concurrent use.
Theophylline salt such as aminophylline: May increase cardiotoxic effects. Avoid using together.

Adverse reactions
CNS: *tremor,* nervousness, headache, dizziness, light-headedness.
CV: palpitations, chest discomfort, tachycardia.
EENT: throat irritation, cough.
GI: nausea, vomiting, increased AST levels.
GU: proteinuria.
Hematologic: decreased platelet or leukocyte count.
Respiratory: dyspnea.
Other: hypersensitivity reactions.

☑ Special considerations
Besides the recommendations relevant to all adrenergics, consider the following.
- Repeated use may result in paradoxical bronchospasm. Discontinue immediately if this occurs.

• May render spirometry insensitive for the diagnosis of asthma.
• Signs and symptoms of overdose include exaggeration of common adverse reactions, especially arrhythmias, extreme tremor, nausea, and vomiting.
• Treatment of overdose requires supportive measures. To reverse effects, use selective beta$_1$-adrenergic blockers (acebutolol, atenolol, metoprolol) with extreme caution (may induce asthmatic attack).

Monitoring the patient
• Monitor vital signs and ECG closely, especially in cardiac patients.
• Monitor WBC, platelet count, and glucose and AST levels.

Information for the patient
• Tell patient to use drug only as directed and not to exceed the prescribed amount or shorten intervals between doses.
• Teach patient to use drug correctly. Tell patient to ensure proper delivery of dose by cleaning plastic mouthpiece with warm tap water and drying thoroughly at least once daily. Tell patient that dryness of mouth and throat may occur, but that rinsing with water after each dose may help.
• Tell patient to call promptly if troubled breathing persists 1 hour after using drug, if symptoms return within 4 hours, if condition worsens, or if new (refill) canister is needed within 2 weeks.
• Tell patient to wait 15 minutes after use of bitolterol before using adrenocorticoid inhaler.
• Give patient instructions on proper use of inhaler:
Metered-dose nebulizers. Shake canister to activate; place mouthpiece well into mouth, aimed at back of throat. Close lips and teeth around mouthpiece. Exhale through nose, then inhale through mouth slowly and deeply, while actuating the nebulizer, to release dose. Hold breath 10 seconds (count "1-100, 2-100, 3-100" to "10-100"), remove mouthpiece, then exhale slowly.
Metered powder inhaler. Caution patient not to take forced deep breaths, but to breathe normally. Observe patient closely for exaggerated systemic drug action. Patients requiring more than 3 aerosol treatments within 24 hours should be under close medical supervision.
Oxygen aerosolization. Administer over 15 to 20 minutes, with oxygen flow rate adjusted to 4 L/minute. Turn on oxygen supply before patient places nebulizer in mouth. (Patient need not close lips tightly around nebulizer opening.) Placement of Y tube in rubber tubing permits patient to control administration. Advise patient to rinse mouth immediately after inhalation therapy to help prevent dryness and throat irritation. Rinse mouthpiece with warm running water at least once daily to prevent clogging. (It isn't

dishwasher-safe.) Wait until mouthpiece is dry before storing. Don't place near artificial heat (dishwasher or oven). Replace reservoir bag every 2 to 3 weeks or as needed; replace mouthpiece every 6 to 9 months or as needed. Replacement of bags or mouthpieces may require a prescription.

Geriatric patients
• Lower doses are indicated in elderly patients who may be more sensitive to drug's effects.

Pediatric patients
• Drug isn't recommended for use in children under age 12.

Breast-feeding patients
• It's unknown whether drug appears in breast milk. Administer cautiously to breast-feeding women.

bleomycin sulfate
Blenoxane

Pharmacologic classification: antibiotic, antineoplastic (cell-cycle–phase specific, G$_2$ and M phase)
Therapeutic classification: antineoplastic
Pregnancy risk category D

How supplied
Available by prescription only
Injection: 15-unit, 30-unit vials

Indications, route, and dosage
Dosage and indications may vary. Check literature for current protocol.
Hodgkin's disease, squamous cell carcinoma, malignant lymphoma, testicular carcinoma
Adults: 10 to 20 units/m² (0.25 to 0.5 units/kg) I.V., I.M., or S.C. 1 or 2 times weekly. After 50% response, maintenance dose of 1 unit daily or 5 units weekly.
Malignant pleural effusion, prevention of recurrent pleural effusions
Adults: 60 units in 50 to 100 ml of normal saline solution by intracavitary administration.
◊ *Tumors of head and neck*
Adults: 10 to 20 units/m² daily by regional arterial administration for 5 to 14 days.

Pharmacodynamics
Antineoplastic action: Exact mechanism unknown. Its action may be through scission of single- and double-stranded DNA and inhibition of DNA, RNA, and protein synthesis. Drug also appears to inhibit cell progression out of the G$_2$ phase.

Pharmacokinetics
• *Absorption:* Poorly absorbed across GI tract after oral administration. I.M. administration results in lower serum levels than those occurring after equivalent I.V. doses.
• *Distribution:* Distributed widely into total body water, mainly in skin, lungs, kidneys, peritoneum, and lymphatic tissue.
• *Metabolism:* Metabolic fate undetermined; however, extensive tissue inactivation occurs in liver and kidney and much less in skin and lungs.
• *Excretion:* Drug and its metabolites excreted primarily in urine. Terminal plasma elimination phase half-life is reported at 2 hours.

Contraindications and precautions
Contraindicated in patients with hypersensitivity to drug. Use cautiously in patients with renal or pulmonary impairment.

Interactions
Drug-drug. *Digoxin, phenytoin:* Concomitant use may decrease serum levels of phenytoin and digoxin. Monitor serum levels of these drugs.

Adverse reactions
GI: stomatitis, anorexia, nausea, vomiting, diarrhea.
Respiratory: *pulmonary fibrosis,* pulmonary toxicity such as PNEUMONITIS.
Skin: *erythema, hyperpigmentation, acne, rash, reversible alopecia, striae, skin tenderness, pruritus.*
Other: *chills,* fever, weight loss; severe idiosyncratic reaction consisting of hypotension, mental confusion, fever, chills, wheezing has occurred in about 1% of patients with lymphoma.

☑ Special considerations
• To prepare solution for I.M. administration, reconstitute drug with 1 to 5 ml (15-unit vial) or 2 to 10 ml (30-unit vial) of normal saline solution, bacteriostatic water, or sterile water for injection. Don't use D_5W or dextrose containing diluents.
• For I.V. administration, dilute with a minimum of 5 ml of diluent and administer over 10 minutes as I.V. push injection.
• Use precautions in preparing and handling drug; wear gloves and wash hands after preparing and administering.
• Drug can be administered by intracavitary (see manufacturer's recommendation), intra-arterial, or intratumoral injection. It can also be instilled into bladder for bladder tumors.
• Cumulative lifetime dosage shouldn't exceed 400 units.
• Response to therapy may take 2 to 3 weeks.
• Administer a 1- to 2-unit test dose to lymphoma patients before the first 2 doses to assess hypersensitivity to bleomycin. If no reaction occurs, follow the dosing schedule. The test dose can be incorporated as part of total dose for regimen.

• Have epinephrine, diphenhydramine, I.V. corticosteroids, and oxygen available in case of anaphylactic reaction.
• Premedication with aspirin, corticosteroids, and diphenhydramine may reduce drug fever and risk of anaphylaxis.
• Reduce dosage in patients with renal or pulmonary impairment.
• Drug concentrates in keratin of squamous epithelium. To prevent linear streaking, don't use adhesive dressings on skin.
• Allergic reactions may be delayed especially in patients with lymphoma.
• Drug is stable for 24 hours at room temperature and 48 hours under refrigeration. Refrigerate unopened vials containing dry powder.
• Bleomycin therapy may increase blood and urine levels of uric acid.
• Signs and symptoms of overdose include pulmonary fibrosis, fever, chills, vesiculation, and hyperpigmentation. Treatment is usually supportive and includes antipyretics for fever.

Monitoring the patient
• Pulmonary function tests may be useful in predicting fibrosis; they should be performed to establish a baseline and then monitored periodically.
• Monitor chest X-rays and auscultate the lungs.

Information for the patient
• Explain to patient that hair should grow back after treatment ends.

Geriatric patients
• Use with caution in patients over age 70 because they are at increased risk for pulmonary toxicity.

Pediatric patients
• Safety and effectiveness in children haven't been established.

Breast-feeding patients
• It's unknown if drug appears in breast milk. However, because of risk of serious adverse reactions, mutagenicity, and carcinogenicity in infants, breast-feeding isn't recommended.

bretylium tosylate
Bretylate*, Bretylol

Pharmacologic classification: adrenergic blocker
Therapeutic classification: ventricular antiarrhythmic
Pregnancy risk category C

How supplied
Available by prescription only
Injection: 50 mg/ml

Reactions may be *common,* uncommon, *life-threatening,* or COMMON AND LIFE-THREATENING.

Indications, route, and dosage

Ventricular fibrillation and hemodynamically unstable ventricular tachycardia
Adults: 5 mg/kg undiluted by rapid I.V. injection. If ventricular fibrillation persists, increase dosage to 10 mg/kg and repeat, p.r.n. For continuous suppression, administer diluted solution by continuous I.V. infusion at 1 to 2 mg/minute, or infuse diluted solution at 5 to 10 mg/kg over more than 8 minutes q 6 hours.

Other ventricular arrhythmias
Adults: Initially, 5 to 10 mg/kg I.M., undiluted, or I.V. diluted. Repeat in 1 to 2 hours, if necessary. Maintenance dose is 5 to 10 mg/kg q 6 hours I.M. or I.V. or 1 to 2 mg/minute I.V. infusion.
◇*Children:* For acute ventricular fibrillation, initially 5 mg/kg I.V.; then 10 mg/kg q 15 to 30 minutes, with a maximum total dose of 30 mg/kg; maintenance dose is 5 to 10 mg/kg q 6 hours. For other ventricular arrhythmias, 5 to 10 mg/kg q 6 hours.

Pharmacodynamics

Ventricular antiarrhythmic action: A class III antiarrhythmic used to treat ventricular fibrillation and tachycardia. Like other class III antiarrhythmics, it widens the action potential duration (repolarization inhibition) and increases the effective refractory period (ERP); it doesn't affect conduction velocity. These actions follow a transient increase in conduction velocity and shortening of the action potential duration and ERP.

Initial effects stem from norepinephrine release from sympathetic ganglia and postganglionic adrenergic neurons immediately after drug administration. Norepinephrine release also accounts for an increased threshold for successful defibrillation, increased blood pressure, and increased heart rate. This initial phase of drug's action is brief (up to 1 hour).

Bretylium also alters the disparity in action potential duration between ischemic and nonischemic myocardial tissue; its antiarrhythmic action may result from this activity.

Hemodynamic drug effects include increased blood pressure, heart rate, and possible cardiac irritability (all resulting from initial norepinephrine release). Drug-induced adrenergic blockade ultimately predominates, leading to vasodilation and a subsequent blood pressure drop (primarily orthostatic). This effect has been referred to as chemical sympathectomy.

Pharmacokinetics

• *Absorption:* Incompletely and erratically absorbed from GI tract; well absorbed after I.M. administration. With I.M. administration, antiarrhythmic (ventricular tachycardia and ectopy) action begins within about 20 to 60 minutes but may not reach maximal level for 6 to 9 hours when given by this route (for this reason, I.M. administration isn't recommended for treating life-threatening ventricular fibrillation). With I.V. administration, antifibrillatory action begins within a few minutes. However, suppression of ventricular tachycardia and other ventricular arrhythmias occurs more slowly—usually within 20 minutes to 2 hours; peak antiarrhythmic effects may not occur for 6 to 9 hours.
• *Distribution:* Distributed widely throughout body; doesn't cross blood-brain barrier. Only about 1% to 10% is plasma protein-bound.
• *Metabolism:* No metabolites identified.
• *Excretion:* Excreted in urine mostly as unchanged drug. Half-life ranges from 5 to 10 hours (longer in patients with renal impairment). Duration of effect ranges from 6 to 24 hours; may increase with continued dosage increases. (Patients with ventricular fibrillation may need continuous infusion to maintain desired effect.)

Contraindications and precautions

Contraindicated in digitalized patients unless the arrhythmia is life-threatening, not caused by a cardiac glycoside, and unresponsive to other antiarrhythmics. Use with caution in patients with aortic stenosis and pulmonary hypertension.

Interactions

Drug-drug. *Cardiac glycosides:* May exacerbate ventricular tachycardia associated with digitalis toxicity. Monitor patient closely.
Pressor amines (sympathomimetics): May potentiate action of these drugs. Use together cautiously.
Other antiarrhythmics: May cause additive toxic effects and additive or antagonistic cardiac effects. Use cautiously.

Adverse reactions

CNS: *vertigo, dizziness, light-headedness, syncope* (usually secondary to hypotension).
CV: SEVERE HYPOTENSION (especially orthostatic), **bradycardia,** anginal pain, transient arrhythmias, transient hypertension, increased PVCs.
GI: severe nausea, vomiting (with rapid infusion).

☑ Special considerations

• Administer I.V. infusion at appropriate rate to avoid or minimize adverse reactions.
• For I.M. injection, don't exceed 5-ml volume in any 1 site and rotate sites.
• Patient should remain supine and avoid sudden postural changes until tolerance to hypotension develops.
• Avoid simultaneous initiation of therapy with a cardiac glycoside and bretylium.
• Because bretylium is excreted exclusively by the kidneys, patients with renal impairment require dosage modification. Increase dosage interval because the elimination half-life increases three- to sixfold.
• Subtherapeutic doses (less than 5 mg/kg) may cause hypotension.

• Drug isn't a first-line drug, according to American Heart Association advanced cardiac life-support guidelines. With ventricular fibrillation, drug should follow lidocaine; with ventricular tachycardia, drug should follow lidocaine and procainamide.
• Ventricular tachycardia and other ventricular arrhythmias respond to drug less rapidly than ventricular fibrillation.
• Drug is ineffective against atrial arrhythmias.
• Clinical effects of overdose primarily involve severe hypotension.
• Treatment of overdose includes administration of vasopressors (such as dopamine or norepinephrine) to support blood pressure and general supportive measures, as necessary. Volume expanders and positional changes also may be effective.

Monitoring the patient
• Monitor ECG and blood pressure throughout therapy for any significant change. If supine systolic pressure decreases to less than 75 mm Hg, norepinephrine, dopamine, or volume expanders may be prescribed to elevate blood pressure.
• If patient is receiving pressor amines (sympathomimetics) to correct hypotension, monitor closely; bretylium potentiates effects of these drugs.
• Observe susceptible patients for increased anginal pain.

Breast-feeding patients
• Safety in breast-feeding women hasn't been established.

---

bromocriptine mesylate
Parlodel

Pharmacologic classification: dopamine receptor agonist
Therapeutic classification: semisynthetic ergot alkaloid, dopaminergic agonist, antiparkinsonian, inhibitor of prolactin release, inhibitor of growth hormone release
Pregnancy risk category B

How supplied
Available by prescription only
Tablets: 2.5 mg
Capsules: 5 mg

Indications, route, and dosage
Amenorrhea and galactorrhea associated with hyperprolactinemia; female infertility
Adults: 0.5 to 2.5 mg daily, increased by 2.5 mg daily at 3- to 7-day intervals, as tolerated, until optimal therapeutic effects are achieved. Maintenance dose is usually 5 to 7.5 mg daily (range, 2.5 to 15 mg daily).

Acromegaly
Adults: Initially, 1.25 to 2.5 mg P.O. daily h.s. for 3 days. An additional 1.25 to 2.5 mg may be added q 3 to 7 days until patient receives therapeutic benefit. Therapeutic dose range varies from 20 to 30 mg daily in most patients. Maximum dose shouldn't exceed 100 mg daily. Dosages of 20 to 60 mg daily have been administered as divided doses.

Parkinson's disease
Adults: Initially, 1.25 to 2.5 mg P.O. b.i.d. with meals. Dosage may be increased by 2.5 mg daily q 14 to 28 days, up to 100 mg daily or until a maximal therapeutic response is achieved. Safety of dosages over 100 mg daily hasn't been established.
◇ **Premenstrual syndrome**
Adults: 2.5 to 7.5 mg P.O. b.i.d. from day 10 of menstrual cycle until onset of menstruation.
◇ **Cushing's syndrome**
Adults: 1.25 to 2.5 mg P.O. b.i.d. to q.i.d.
◇ **Hepatic encephalopathy**
Adults: 1.25 mg P.O. daily, increased by 1.25 mg q 3 days until 15 mg is reached.

Pharmacodynamics
Prolactin-inhibiting action: Reduces prolactin levels by inhibiting release of prolactin from the anterior pituitary gland, a direct action on the pituitary. May also stimulate postsynaptic dopamine receptors in the hypothalamus to release prolactin-inhibitory factor via a complicated catecholamine pathway. Reduces high serum prolactin levels and restores ovulation and ovarian function in amenorrheic women and suppresses puerperal or nonpuerperal lactation in women with adequate gonadotropin levels and ovarian function. The average time for reversing amenorrhea is 6 to 8 weeks, but it may take up to 24 weeks.
Antiparkinsonism action: Drug activates dopaminergic receptors in the neostriatum of the CNS, which may produce its antiparkinsonism activity. Dysregulation of brain serotonin activity also may occur. The precise role of bromocriptine in treating parkinsonian syndrome requires further study of its safety and efficacy in long-term therapy.

Pharmacokinetics
• *Absorption:* 28% absorbed when given orally and reaches peak levels in about 1 to 3 hours. Plasma levels for therapeutic effects are unknown. After an oral dose, serum prolactin decreases within 2 hours, is decreased maximally at 8 hours, and remains decreased at 24 hours.
• *Distribution:* About 90% to 96% is bound to serum albumin.
• *Metabolism:* First-pass metabolism occurs with over 90% of absorbed dose. Metabolized completely in the liver, principally by hydrolysis, before excretion. Metabolites aren't active or toxic.

Reactions may be *common*, uncommon, **life-threatening**, or COMMON AND LIFE-THREATENING.

• *Excretion:* Primarily excreted through bile. Only 2.5% to 5.5% excreted in urine. Almost all (85%) excreted in feces within 5 days.

Contraindications and precautions
Contraindicated in patients with hypersensitivity to ergot derivatives and in those with uncontrolled hypertension, or toxemia of pregnancy. Use cautiously in patients with renal or hepatic impairment and history of MI with residual arrhythmias.

Interactions
Drug-drug. *Amitriptyline, butyrophenones, imipramine, methyldopa, phenothiazines, reserpine:* Increased prolactin levels that may require increased dosage of bromocriptine. Monitor prolactin levels.
Antihypertensives: May potentiate antihypertensive action; dosage of these drugs may have to be reduced. Monitor blood pressure.
Drug-lifestyle. *Alcohol:* Intolerance may result when high doses of bromocriptine are administered. Limit concomitant use of alcohol.

Adverse reactions
CNS: *dizziness, headache,* fatigue, mania, lightheadedness, drowsiness, delusions, nervousness, insomnia, depression, **seizures.**
CV: *hypotension,* **stroke, acute MI.**
EENT: nasal congestion, blurred vision.
GI: *nausea,* vomiting, *abdominal cramps, constipation,* diarrhea, anorexia.
GU: urine retention, urinary frequency.
Skin: coolness and pallor of fingers and toes.

☑ Special considerations
• Examine patient carefully for pituitary tumor (Forbes-Albright syndrome). Use of bromocriptine doesn't affect tumor size, although it may alleviate amenorrhea or galactorrhea.
• First-dose phenomenon occurs in 1% of patients. Sensitive patients may experience syncope for 15 to 60 minutes but can usually tolerate subsequent treatment without ill effects. Patient should begin therapy with lowest dosage, taken at bedtime.
• Administer drug with meals, milk, or snacks to diminish GI distress.
• Alcohol intolerance may occur, especially when high doses of bromocriptine are administered; therefore, alcohol intake should be limited.
• As an antiparkinsonian, drug is usually given with either levodopa alone or levodopa-carbidopa combination.
• Adverse reactions are more common when drug is given in high doses, as in treating parkinsonism.
• Overdose of bromocriptine may cause nausea, vomiting, and severe hypotension.
• Treatment of overdose includes emptying the stomach by aspiration and lavage, and administering I.V. fluids to treat hypotension.

Monitoring the patient
• Monitor blood pressure.
• Monitor patient's response to drug therapy.

Information for the patient
• Advise patient that it may take 6 weeks or longer for menses to be reinstated and for galactorrhea to be suppressed.
• Tell patient to take first dose where and when she can lie down because drowsiness commonly occurs after initiation of therapy.
• Instruct patient to report visual problems, severe nausea and vomiting, or acute headaches.
• Tell patient to take drug with meals to avoid GI upset.
• Warn patient that CNS effects of drug may impair ability to perform tasks that require alertness and coordination.
• Advise patient to use a nonhormonal contraceptive during treatment because of potential amenorrheic adverse effects.
• Advise patient to limit use of alcohol during treatment.

Geriatric patients
• Use with caution, particularly in patients receiving long-term, high-dose therapy. Regular physical assessment is recommended, with particular attention toward changes in pulmonary function.
• Safety isn't established for long-term use at dosages required to treat Parkinson's disease.

Pediatric patients
• Drug isn't recommended for children under age 15.

Breast-feeding patients
• Drug inhibits lactation; don't use in women who intend to breast-feed.

brompheniramine maleate
Dimetapp Allergy

Pharmacologic classification: alkylamine antihistamine
Therapeutic classification: antihistamine (H_1-receptor antagonist)
Pregnancy risk category C

How supplied
Available with or without a prescription
Tablets: 4 mg
Elixir: 2 mg/5 ml
Injection: 10 mg/ml

Indications, route, and dosage
Rhinitis, allergies
Adults and children ages 12 and older: 4 mg P.O. q 4 to 6 hours. Don't exceed 24 mg in 24 hours.

Children ages 7 to 11: 2 mg P.O. q 4 to 6 hours. Don't exceed 12 mg in 24 hours.
Children ages 2 to 6: 1 mg P.O. q 4 to 6 hours. Don't exceed 6 mg in 24 hours.

Hypersensitivity
Adults and children ages 12 and older: 5 to 20 mg S.C., I.M., or I.V. b.i.d. Don't exceed 40 mg in 24 hours.
Children below age 12: 0.5 mg/kg/day or 15 mg/m²/day S.C., I.M., or I.V. in three or four divided doses.

Pharmacodynamics
Antihistamine action: Antihistamines compete with histamine for histamine$_1$ receptor sites on the smooth muscle of the bronchi, GI tract, uterus, and large blood vessels; by binding to cellular receptors, they prevent access of histamine and suppress histamine-induced allergic symptoms, even though they don't prevent its release.

Pharmacokinetics
- *Absorption:* Absorbed readily from GI tract; action begins within 15 to 30 minutes and peaks in 2 to 5 hours. A second lower peak effect apparently exists, possibly from drug reabsorption in the distal small intestine.
- *Distribution:* Distributed widely into body.
- *Metabolism:* About 90% to 95% metabolized by the liver.
- *Excretion:* Half-life ranges from about 12 to 34½ hours. Drug and its metabolites excreted primarily in urine; small amount excreted in feces. About 5% to 10% of oral dose excreted unchanged in urine.

Contraindications and precautions
Contraindicated in patients with hypersensitivity to drug or its components and in those with acute asthma, severe hypertension or coronary artery disease, angle-closure glaucoma, urine retention, and peptic ulcer; and within 14 days of MAO-inhibitor therapy. Use cautiously in patients with increased intraocular pressure, diabetes mellitus, ischemic heart disease, hyperthyroidism, hypertension, bronchial asthma, or prostatic hyperplasia, and in elderly patients.

Interactions
Drug-drug. *Heparin, sulfonylureas:* May diminish effects of these drugs. Use together cautiously; monitor PTT.
MAO inhibitors: Interfere with metabolism of brompheniramine, prolonging and intensifying their central depressant and anticholinergic effects. Use together cautiously.
Other CNS depressants such as anxiolytics, barbiturates, sleeping aids, tranquilizers: Possible additive CNS depression. Use together cautiously.
Drug-lifestyle. *Alcohol:* Possible additive CNS depression. Discourage use.

Adverse reactions
CNS: dizziness, tremors, irritability, insomnia, *drowsiness, stimulation.*
CV: hypotension, palpitations.
GI: anorexia, nausea, vomiting, *dry mouth and throat.*
GU: urine retention.
Hematologic: *thrombocytopenia, agranulocytosis.*
Skin: urticaria, rash.
Other: (after parenteral administration) local stinging, diaphoresis, syncope.

☑ Special considerations
Besides the recommendations relevant to all antihistamines, consider the following.
- Drug causes less drowsiness than some antihistamines.
- Store parenteral solutions and elixirs away from light and freezing temperatures; solution may crystallize if stored below 32° F (0° C). Crystals dissolve when warmed to 86° F (30° C).
- Discontinue drug 4 days before performing diagnostic skin tests; it can prevent, reduce, or mask positive skin test response.
- Signs and symptoms of overdose may include either those of CNS depression (sedation, reduced mental alertness, apnea, and CV collapse) or of CNS stimulation (insomnia, hallucinations, tremors, or seizures). Anticholinergic symptoms, such as dry mouth, flushed skin, fixed and dilated pupils, and GI symptoms, are common, especially in children.
- Treat overdose by inducing emesis with ipecac syrup (in conscious patients), then activated charcoal to reduce further drug absorption. Use gastric lavage if patient is unconscious or ipecac fails. Treat hypotension with vasopressors, and control seizures with diazepam or phenytoin I.V. Don't give stimulants.

Monitoring the patient
- Evaluate patient's response to drug therapy.
- Monitor patient for adverse reactions.

Information for the patient
- Instruct patient not to exceed 24 mg/day (for adults and children ages 12 and older) or 12 mg/day (for children ages 6 to 11).

Geriatric patients
- Elderly patients are usually more sensitive to adverse effects of antihistamines and are especially likely to experience a greater degree of dizziness, sedation, hyperexcitability, dry mouth, and urine retention than younger patients. Symptoms usually respond to a decrease in dosage.

Pediatric patients
- Drug isn't indicated for use in newborns; children, especially those under age 6, may experience paradoxical hyperexcitability.

Reactions may be *common,* uncommon, **life-threatening,** or COMMON AND LIFE-THREATENING.

Breast-feeding patients
• Antihistamines such as brompheniramine shouldn't be used during breast-feeding. Many of these drugs appear in breast milk, exposing the infant to risks of unusual excitability, especially premature infants and other neonates, who may experience seizures.

budesonide
Pulmicort Turbuhaler, Rhinocort

Pharmacologic classification: glucocorticosteroid
Therapeutic classification: anti-inflammatory
Pregnancy risk category C

How supplied
Available by prescription only
Nasal inhaler: 32 mcg/metered dose (200 doses per container)
Oral inhalation powder: 200 mcg/dose (200 doses per container)

Indications, route, and dosage
Management of symptoms of seasonal or perennial allergic rhinitis or nonallergic perennial rhinitis
Adults and children over age 6: 2 sprays in each nostril in the morning and evening or 4 sprays in each nostril in the morning. Maintenance dose should be the fewest number of sprays needed to control symptoms. Doses exceeding 256 mcg/day (4 sprays/nostril) aren't recommended.
Note: If improvement doesn't occur within 3 weeks, stop treatment.
Chronic asthma
Adults: 200 to 400 mcg oral inhalation b.i.d. when previously used bronchodilators alone or inhaled corticosteroids; 400 to 800 mcg oral inhalation b.i.d. when previously used oral corticosteroids.
Children ages 6 and older: Initially 200 mcg oral inhalation b.i.d. Maximum dose is 400 mg b.i.d.

Pharmacodynamics
Anti-inflammatory action: Exact mechanism of action against rhinitis unknown. Glucocorticosteroids show a wide range of inhibitory activities against multiple cell types (such as mast cells, eosinophils, neutrophils, macrophages, and lymphocytes) and mediators (such as histamine, eicosanoids, leukotrienes, and cytokines) involved in allergic and nonallergic, irritant-mediated inflammation.

Pharmacokinetics
• *Absorption:* Amount of intranasal dose that reaches systemic circulation is generally about 20%. Rapid onset of action with oral inhalation.
• *Distribution:* 88% protein-bound in plasma; volume of distribution is 200 L.

• *Metabolism:* Rapidly and extensively metabolized in the liver.
• *Excretion:* About 67% eliminated in urine and about 33% in feces.

Contraindications and precautions
Contraindicated in patients with hypersensitivity to drug or its components and in those who have had recent septal ulcers, nasal surgery, or nasal trauma, until total healing has occurred.
Use cautiously in patients with tuberculosis infections; untreated fungal, bacterial, or systemic viral infections; or ocular herpes simplex.

Interactions
Drug-drug. *Ketoconazole:* May increase plasma levels of budesonide. Monitor budesonide levels.
Other inhaled glucocorticosteroids, alternate-day prednisone therapy: May increase risk of hypothalamic-pituitary-adrenal suppression. Use together cautiously.

Adverse reactions
CNS: *headache,* nervousness.
EENT: *nasal irritation, epistaxis, pharyngitis, sinusitis,* reduced sense of smell, nasal pain, hoarseness.
GI: taste perversion, dry mouth, dyspepsia, nausea, vomiting.
Respiratory: *cough,* candidiasis, wheezing, dyspnea.
Skin: facial edema, rash, pruritus, contact dermatitis.
Other: myalgia, hypersensitivity reactions, weight gain.

☑ Special considerations
• Replacing a systemic glucocorticosteroid with a topical glucocorticosteroid can result in signs of adrenal insufficiency; in addition, some patients may experience symptoms of withdrawal, such as joint or muscular pain, lassitude, and depression.
• In patients with asthma or other clinical conditions requiring long-term systemic treatment, a too-rapid decrease in systemic glucocorticosteroids may severely exacerbate symptoms.
• Excessive doses of budesonide or use with other inhaled glucocorticosteroids may lead to signs or symptoms of hyperadrenocorticism.
• Acute overdose is unlikely due to the limited amount of product in each container.
• Chronic overdose may produce signs and symptoms of hyperadrenocorticism.

Monitoring the patient
• Carefully monitor patients previously treated for prolonged periods with systemic glucocorticosteroids who are subsequently given topical glucocorticosteroids for acute adrenal insufficiency in response to stress.

• Because glucocorticosteroids can affect growth, monitor children closely, weighing benefits of therapy against the possibility of growth suppression.
• Patients using budesonide for several months or longer should be examined periodically for evidence of *Candida* infection or other signs of adverse effects on the nasal mucosa.

Information for the patient
• Warn patient not to exceed prescribed dosage or to use for long periods because of risk of hypothalamic-pituitary-adrenal axis suppression.
• Have patient follow these instructions for the nasal inhaler: After opening aluminum pouch, use within 6 months. Shake canister well before using. Blow nose to clear nasal passages. Tilt head slightly forward; insert nozzle into nostril, pointing away from septum; hold other nostril closed; inspire gently; and spray. Shake canister again and repeat in other nostril. Store with valve downward. Don't store in area of high humidity. Don't break, incinerate, or store canister in extreme heat; contents under pressure.
• Instruct patient to hold the inhaler upright when loading Pulmicort Turbuhaler, not to blow or exhale into the inhaler nor shake it while loaded, and to hold inhaler upright while orally inhaling the dose. Place the mouthpiece between the lips and inhale forcefully and deeply.
• Assure patient that drug rarely causes nasal irritation or burning; advise patient to call if such symptoms occur.
• Warn patient to avoid exposure to chickenpox or measles, if at risk for contracting these diseases, and report exposure immediately.
• Teach patient good nasal and oral hygiene.
• Tell patient to call if condition worsens or if symptoms don't improve within 3 weeks.
• Inform patient that effects aren't immediate; response requires regular use.
• Inform patient that, with use of oral inhaler, improvement in asthma control can occur within 24 hours, with maximum benefit anticipated between 1 to 2 weeks and possibly taking longer.
• Advise patient that Pulmicort Turbuhaler isn't indicated for relief of acute bronchospasm.

Pediatric patients
• Safety and effectiveness of drug for treating seasonal or perennial allergic rhinitis in children under age 6 haven't been established. Drug isn't recommended for treatment of nonallergic rhinitis in children.

Breast-feeding patients
• Use cautiously when administering drug to breast-feeding women.

bumetanide
Bumex

Pharmacologic classification: loop diuretic
Therapeutic classification: diuretic
Pregnancy risk category C

How supplied
Available by prescription only
Tablets: 0.5 mg, 1 mg, 2 mg
Injection: 0.25 mg/ml

Indications, route, and dosage
Edema (heart failure, hepatic and renal disease), ◊ **postoperative edema,** ◊ **premenstrual syndrome,** ◊ **disseminated cancer**
Adults: 0.5 to 2 mg P.O. once daily. If diuretic response isn't adequate, give a second or third dose at 4- to 5-hour intervals. Maximum dose is 10 mg/day. Give parenterally when oral route isn't feasible. Usual initial dose is 0.5 to 1 mg I.V. over 1 to 2 minutes or I.M. If response isn't adequate, give a second or third dose at 2- to 3-hour intervals. Maximum dose is 10 mg/day.
◊ **Pediatric heart failure**
Children: 0.015 mg/kg every other day to 0.1 mg/kg daily. Use with extreme caution in neonates.

Pharmacodynamics
Diuretic action: Loop diuretics inhibit sodium and chloride reabsorption in the proximal part of the ascending loop of Henle, promoting excretion of sodium, water, chloride, and potassium; bumetanide produces renal and peripheral vasodilation and may temporarily increase glomerular filtration rate and decrease peripheral vascular resistance.

Pharmacokinetics
• *Absorption:* After oral administration, 85% to 95% of dose is absorbed; food delays oral absorption. I.M. bumetanide is completely absorbed. Diuresis usually begins 30 to 60 minutes after oral and 40 minutes after I.M. administration; peak diuresis occurs 1 to 2 hours after either. Diuresis begins a few minutes after I.V. administration and peaks in 15 to 30 minutes.
• *Distribution:* About 92% to 96% is protein-bound; unknown whether bumetanide enters CSF, breast milk, or crosses placenta.
• *Metabolism:* Metabolized by the liver to at least 5 metabolites.
• *Excretion:* 80% excreted in urine and 10% to 20% in feces. Half-life ranges from 1 to 1½ hours; duration of effect is about 2 to 4 hours.

Contraindications and precautions
Contraindicated in patients with hypersensitivity to drug or sulfonamides (possible cross-sensitivity), in those with anuria or hepatic coma, and

in patients in states of severe electrolyte depletion.

Use cautiously in patients with hepatic cirrhosis and ascites and in those with depressed renal function.

Interactions
Drug-drug. *Indomethacin, probenecid:* May reduce diuretic effect of bumetanide. Don't use together; however, if there is no therapeutic alternative, an increased dose of bumetanide may be needed.
Lithium: May reduce renal clearance of lithium and increase lithium levels. Monitor lithium levels; dosage adjustment may be needed.
Other antihypertensives, other diuretics: Potentiates hypotensive effect. Both actions are used to therapeutic advantage.
Other potassium-depleting drugs such as amphotericin B, corticosteroids: May cause severe potassium loss. Monitor serum potassium levels.
Ototoxic or nephrotoxic drugs: May result in enhanced toxicity. Use with caution.
Potassium-sparing diuretics (amiloride, spironolactone, triamterene): May decrease bumetanide-induced potassium loss. Monitor potassium levels.

Adverse reactions
CNS: dizziness, headache, vertigo.
CV: volume depletion and dehydration, orthostatic hypotension, ECG changes, chest pain.
EENT: transient deafness, tinnitus.
GI: nausea, vomiting, upset stomach, dry mouth, diarrhea, pain.
GU: *renal failure,* premature ejaculation, difficulty maintaining erection, oliguria.
Hematologic: azotemia, *thrombocytopenia.*
Metabolic: hypokalemia; hypochloremic alkalosis; asymptomatic hyperuricemia; fluid and electrolyte imbalances, including dilutional hyponatremia, hypocalcemia, hyperglycemia, and glucose intolerance impairment.
Musculoskeletal: weakness; arthritic pain; muscle pain and tenderness.
Skin: rash, pruritus, diaphoresis.

☑ Special considerations
Besides the recommendations relevant to all loop diuretics, consider the following.
● Give I.V. bumetanide slowly, over 1 to 2 minutes, for I.V. infusion; dilute bumetanide in D₅W, normal saline solution, or lactated Ringer's solution; use within 24 hours.
● Signs and symptoms of overdose include profound electrolyte and volume depletion, which may cause circulatory collapse.
● Treatment of drug overdose is primarily supportive; replace fluid and electrolytes as needed.

Monitoring the patient
● Monitor serum creatinine and electrolytes, especially in patients in states of severe electrolyte depletion or depressed renal function.
● Neutropenia has been observed in association with this therapy; monitor neutrophil counts during therapy.

Information for the patient
● To prevent nocturia, instruct patient to take drug in the morning. If second dose is necessary, patient should take it in early afternoon.
● Inform patient that intermittent doses may be taken on alternate days, or for 3 to 4 days with 1 or 2 days of rest periods.

Geriatric patients
● Elderly and debilitated patients require close observation; they are more susceptible to drug-induced diuresis. Excessive diuresis promotes rapid dehydration, hypovolemia, hypokalemia, and hyponatremia in these patients, and may cause circulatory collapse. Reduced dosages may be indicated.

Pediatric patients
● Safety and efficacy in children under age 18 haven't been established.

Breast-feeding patients
● Drug shouldn't be used by breast-feeding women.

buprenorphine hydrochloride
Buprenex

Pharmacologic classification: narcotic agonist-antagonist, opioid partial agonist
Therapeutic classification: analgesic
Controlled substance schedule V
Pregnancy risk category C

How supplied
Available by prescription only
Injection: 0.3 mg/ml in 1-ml ampules

Indications, route, and dosage
Moderate to severe pain
Adults and children over age 13: 0.3 mg I.M. or slow I.V. q 6 hours, p.r.n. May repeat 0.3 mg 30 to 60 minutes after initial dose or increase to 0.6 mg per dose if necessary. S.C. administration isn't recommended.
◊ *Adults:* 25 to 250 mcg/hour via I.V. infusion (over 48 hours for postoperative pain)
◊ *Adults:* 60 to 180 mcg via epidural injection.

◇ *Reverse fentanyl-induced anesthesia*
Adults: 0.3 to 0.8 mg, I.V. or I.M., 1 to 4 hours after the induction of anesthesia and about 30 minutes before the end of surgery.
◇ *Circumcision*
Children ages 9 months to 9 years: 3 mcg/kg I.M. along with surgical anesthesia.

Pharmacodynamics
Analgesic action: Exact mechanisms unknown. Believed to be a competitive antagonist at some and an agonist at other opiate receptors, thus relieving moderate to severe pain.

Pharmacokinetics
• *Absorption:* Absorbed rapidly after I.M. administration. Onset of action occurs in 15 minutes, with peak effect 1 hour after dosing.
• *Distribution:* About 96% of drug is protein-bound.
• *Metabolism:* Metabolized in the liver.
• *Excretion:* Duration of action is 6 hours. Excreted primarily in feces as unchanged drug with about 30% excreted in urine.

Contraindications and precautions
Contraindicated in patients with hypersensitivity to drug. Use cautiously in elderly or debilitated patients and in patients with head injuries, increased intracranial pressure, and intracranial lesions; respiratory, kidney, or hepatic impairment; CNS depression or coma; thyroid irregularities; adrenal insufficiency; prostatic hyperplasia; urethral stricture; acute alcoholism; delirium tremens; or kyphoscoliosis.

Interactions
Drug-drug. *Barbiturate anesthetics such as thiopental:* Drug may produce additive CNS and respiratory depressant effects and possibly apnea (if administered within a few hours of each other). Avoid concomitant use.
CNS depressants (antihistamines, barbiturates, benzodiazepines, narcotic analgesics, phenothiazines, sedative-hypnotics), muscle relaxants, tricyclic antidepressants: May potentiate respiratory and CNS depression, sedation, and hypotensive effects. Monitor patient. Reduced doses of buprenorphine are usually necessary.
Diazepam: May cause respiratory and CV collapse if used together. Avoid concomitant use.
General anesthetics: May cause severe CV depression. Avoid concomitant use.
MAO inhibitors: Enhanced CNS effects. Use together cautiously.
Narcotic antagonists: Physically dependent patients may experience acute withdrawal syndrome if given an antagonist. Use with caution and monitor closely.
Drug-lifestyle. *Alcohol:* May potentiate respiratory and CNS depression, sedation, and hypotensive effects of drug. Discourage use.

Adverse reactions
CNS: *dizziness, sedation, headache,* confusion, nervousness, euphoria, *vertigo,* **increased intracranial pressure.**
CV: *hypotension,* **bradycardia,** tachycardia, hypertension.
EENT: *miosis,* blurred vision.
GI: *nausea,* vomiting, constipation, dry mouth.
GU: urine retention.
Respiratory: *respiratory depression,* hypoventilation, dyspnea.
Skin: pruritus, *diaphoresis.*

☑ Special considerations
Besides the recommendations relevant to all opioid (narcotic) agonist-antagonists, consider the following.
• Adverse effects of drug may not be as readily reversed by naloxone as are those of pure agonists.
• Buprenorphine 0.3 mg is equal to 10 mg morphine or 75 to 100 mg meperidine in analgesic potency; duration of analgesia is longer than either.
• Safety of buprenorphine in acute overdose is expected to be better than that of other opioid analgesics because of its antagonist properties at high doses. Overdose may cause CNS depression, respiratory depression, and miosis (pinpoint pupils). Other acute toxic effects might include hypotension, bradycardia, hypothermia, shock, apnea, cardiopulmonary arrest, circulatory collapse, pulmonary edema, and seizures.
• To treat acute overdose, first establish a patent airway and ventilation as needed; administer a narcotic antagonist (naloxone) to reverse respiratory depression. The duration of buprenorphine is longer than that of naloxone, so repeated naloxone dosing is necessary. Naloxone shouldn't be given unless the patient has clinically significant respiratory or CV depression.
• Naloxone doesn't completely reverse buprenorphine-induced respiratory depression; mechanical ventilation and higher than usual doses of naloxone and doxapram may be indicated.
• In overdose, provide symptomatic and supportive treatment (continued respiratory support, correction of fluid or electrolyte imbalance).
• In overdose, closely monitor laboratory parameters, vital signs, and neurologic status.

Monitoring the patient
• Monitor patient for adverse effects.
• Monitor vital signs closely.

Information for the patient
• Teach patient to avoid activities that require full alertness.
• Instruct patient to avoid alcohol and other CNS depressants.

Reactions may be *common,* uncommon, *life-threatening,* or COMMON AND LIFE-THREATENING.

Geriatric patients
• Administer with caution; lower doses are usually indicated for elderly patients, who may be more sensitive to the therapeutic and adverse effects of these drugs.

Breast-feeding patients
• It's unknown if drug appears in breast milk. Use with caution in breast-feeding women.

bupropion hydrochloride
Wellbutrin, Wellbutrin SR

Pharmacologic classification: aminoketone
Therapeutic classification: antidepressant
Pregnancy risk category B

How supplied
Available by prescription only
Tablets: 75 mg, 100 mg
Tablets (sustained-release): 100 mg, 150 mg

Indications, route, and dosage
Depression
Adults: Initially, 100 mg P.O. b.i.d. If necessary, increase after 3 days to usual dosage of 100 mg P.O. t.i.d. If no response occurs after several weeks of therapy, consider increasing dosage to 150 mg t.i.d. For sustained-release tablets, start with 150 mg P.O. q morning; increase to target dose of 150 mg P.O. b.i.d. as tolerated as early as day 4 of dosing. Maximum dose is 400 mg/day.

Pharmacodynamics
Antidepressant action: Mechanism of action unknown. Doesn't inhibit MAO; weak inhibitor of norepinephrine, dopamine, and serotonin reuptake.

Pharmacokinetics
• *Absorption:* Only 5% to 20% of drug is bioavailable. Plasma levels peak within 2 to 3 hours.
• *Distribution:* At plasma levels up to 200 mcg/ml, drug appears to be about 80% bound to plasma proteins.
• *Metabolism:* Probably hepatic; several active metabolites identified. With prolonged use, active metabolites are expected to accumulate in plasma and their level may exceed that of parent compound. Bupropion appears to induce its own metabolism.
• *Excretion:* Primarily renal; elimination half-life of parent compound ranges from 8 to 24 hours for single dose.

Contraindications and precautions
Contraindicated in patients with hypersensitivity to drug, in those with seizure disorders, and in those who have taken MAO inhibitors within previous 14 days. Also contraindicated in patients

taking Zyban and in those with history of bulimia or anorexia nervosa because of higher risk of seizures. Use cautiously in patients with recent MI, unstable heart disease, and renal or hepatic impairment.

Interactions
Drug-drug. *Levodopa, MAO inhibitors, phenothiazines, tricyclic antidepressants, recent and rapid withdrawal of benzodiazepines:* May increase risk of adverse effects, including seizures. Monitor patient closely.

Adverse reactions
CNS: *headache, **seizures,*** anxiety, *confusion,* delusions, euphoria, hostility, impaired sleep quality, *insomnia, sedation, tremor,* akinesia, akathisia, *agitation, dizziness,* fatigue.
CV: ***arrhythmias,*** hypertension, hypotension, palpitations, syncope, *tachycardia.*
EENT: *auditory disturbances,* blurred vision.
GI: *dry mouth,* taste disturbance, increased appetite, *constipation,* dyspepsia, *nausea, vomiting, weight loss, anorexia, weight gain,* diarrhea.
GU: impotence, menstrual complaints, urinary frequency, decreased libido, urine retention.
Skin: pruritus, rash, cutaneous temperature disturbance, *excessive diaphoresis.*
Other: arthritis, fever, chills.

☑ Special considerations
• Consider the inherent risk of suicide until significant improvement of depressive state occurs. High-risk patients should have close supervision during initial drug therapy. To reduce risk of suicidal overdose, prescribe the smallest quantity of tablets consistent with good management.
• Many patients experience a period of increased restlessness, especially at initiation of therapy. This may include agitation, insomnia, and anxiety. In some patients, these symptoms require a sedative-hypnotic; drug may have to be discontinued in a few patients.
• Antidepressants can cause manic episodes during the depressed phase in patients with bipolar disorder.
• Signs of overdose include labored breathing, salivation, arched back, ptosis, ataxia, and seizures.
• If the ingestion was recent, empty the stomach using gastric lavage or induce emesis with ipecac, as appropriate; follow with activated charcoal. Treatment should be supportive.
• Control seizures with I.V. benzodiazepines; stuporous, comatose, or convulsing patients may need intubation. There are no data to evaluate the benefits of dialysis, hemoperfusion, or diuresis.

Monitoring the patient
• Monitor vital signs and ECG.

● Follow up with patient to determine adverse drug effects.

Information for the patient
● Advise patient to take drug regularly, as scheduled, and to take each day's dosage in three divided doses, preferably at 6-hour intervals, to minimize risk of seizures.
● Warn patient to avoid alcohol, which may contribute to the development of seizures.
● Advise patient to avoid activities that require alertness and coordination until CNS effects of drug are known.
● Tell patient not to chew, divide, or crush sustained-release tablets.
● Instruct patient not to take Zyban with Wellbutrin, nor should patient take other drugs, including OTC products, without medical approval.

Pediatric patients
● Safety in children under age 18 hasn't been established.

Breast-feeding patients
● Because of the potential for serious adverse reactions in the infant, breast-feeding during therapy isn't recommended.

bupropion hydrochloride
Zyban

Pharmacologic classification: aminoketone
Therapeutic classification: nonnicotine aid to smoking cessation
Pregnancy risk category B

How supplied
Available by prescription only
Tablets (sustained-release): 150 mg

Indications, route, and dosage
Aid to smoking cessation treatment
Adults: 150 mg daily P.O. for 3 days; increased to maximum of 300 mg daily P.O. given as two doses of 150 mg taken at least 8 hours apart.
   Note: Therapy is started while patient is still smoking; about 1 week is needed to achieve steady-state blood levels of drug. Patient should set target cessation date during second week of treatment. Course of treatment is usually 7 to 12 weeks.

Pharmacodynamics
Smoking cessation action: Mechanism unknown. Relatively weak inhibitor of the neuronal uptake of norepinephrine, serotonin, and dopamine, and doesn't inhibit MAO.

Pharmacokinetics
● *Absorption:* Following oral administration, plasma levels peak within 3 hours.
● *Distribution:* Volume of distribution from a single 150-mg dose is estimated to be 1,950 L. Drug is 84% bound to plasma proteins at levels up to 200 mcg/ml.
● *Metabolism:* Extensively metabolized in liver mainly by the P-450 2B6 isoenzyme system to 3 active metabolites.
● *Excretion:* Mean elimination half-life of drug is thought to be about 21 hours. Following oral administration, 87% of dose is recovered in urine and 10% in feces. Fraction of dose excreted unchanged is 0.5%.

Contraindications and precautions
Contraindicated in patients with seizure disorders or with a current or prior diagnosis of bulimia or anorexia nervosa because of potential for seizures.
   Concurrent administration of MAO inhibitors is contraindicated; at least 14 days must elapse between discontinuation of an MAO inhibitor and starting bupropion therapy. Concurrent administration of Wellbutrin, Wellbutrin SR, or other drugs containing bupropion is contraindicated because of potential for seizures. Also contraindicated in patients allergic to drug or its formulation.

Interactions
Drug-drug. *Antidepressants, antipsychotics, systemic steroids, theophylline, treatment regimens that lower seizure threshold (abrupt withdrawal of benzodiazepines):* May increase risk of seizures. Use together with extreme caution.
Carbamazepine, phenobarbital, phenytoin: May induce metabolism of bupropion. Use together cautiously.
Cimetidine: Inhibits metabolism of bupropion. Use together cautiously.
Drugs that affect enzyme metabolism, such as cyclophosphamide, orphenadrine: Increased risk of adverse effects. Use with caution.
Levodopa: May cause adverse reactions with concurrent use. If concurrent use is necessary, give small initial doses of bupropion and gradually increase dose.
MAO inhibitor, phenelzine: May cause acute toxicity of bupropion. Use cautiously.

Adverse reactions
CNS: agitation, dizziness, hot flashes, *insomnia,* somnolence, tremor.
CV: *complete AV block,* hypertension, hypotension, tachycardia.
EENT: *dry mouth,* taste perversion.
GI: anorexia, dyspepsia, increased appetite.
GU: impotence, polyuria, urinary frequency and urgency.
Metabolic: edema, weight gain.

Reactions may be *common,* uncommon, *life-threatening,* or COMMON AND LIFE-THREATENING.

Musculoskeletal: arthralgia, leg cramps and twitching, myalgia, neck pain.
Respiratory: bronchitis, ***bronchospasm.***
Skin: dry skin, pruritus, rash, urticaria.
Other: allergic reactions.

☑ Special considerations
● Because drug use is associated with a dose-dependent risk of seizures, don't exceed 300 mg daily for smoking cessation.
● If patient hasn't made progress toward abstinence by week 7 of therapy, stop therapy because it's unlikely that patient will quit smoking.
● Dose need not be tapered when stopping treatment.
● Hospitalization is recommended for overdoses. If patient is conscious, induce vomiting with syrup of ipecac. Activated charcoal may also be administered every 6 hours for first 12 hours. Perform ECG and EEG monitoring for first 48 hours. Provide adequate fluid intake and obtain baseline tests.
● If patient is stuporous, comatose, or experiencing seizures, airway intubation is recommended before undertaking gastric lavage. Gastric lavage may be beneficial within first 12 hours after ingestion because drug absorption may not be complete.
● Although diuresis, dialysis, or hemoperfusion is sometimes used to treat drug overdose, there is no experience with their use in managing bupropion overdose. Seizures can be treated with an I.V. benzodiazepine and other supportive measures.

Monitoring the patient
● Evaluate patient for effectiveness of drug.
● Monitor patient for adverse reactions.

Information for the patient
● Stress importance of combining behavioral interventions, counseling, and support services with drug therapy.
● Inform patient that risk of seizures is increased if he has a seizure or eating disorder (bulimia or anorexia nervosa), exceeds the recommended dose, or takes other drugs containing bupropion.
● Instruct patient to take doses at least 8 hours apart.
● Inform patient that drug is usually taken for 7 to 12 weeks.
● Advise patient that, although he may continue to smoke during drug therapy, it reduces his chance of breaking the smoking habit.
● Tell patient that drug and nicotine patch should only be used together under medical supervision because blood pressure may increase.

Geriatric patients
● Experience in patients ages 60 and older was similar to that in younger adult patients.

Pediatric patients
● Safety and efficacy in children haven't been established.

Breast-feeding patients
● Drug and its metabolites appear in breast milk. Because of the potential for serious adverse reactions in the infant, a choice must be made between breast-feeding and drug therapy.

buspirone hydrochloride
BuSpar

Pharmacologic classification: azaspirodecanedione derivative
Therapeutic classification: anxiolytic
Pregnancy risk category B

How supplied
Available by prescription only
Tablets: 5 mg, 10 mg, 15 mg

Indications, route, and dosage
Management of anxiety disorders
Adults: Initially, 5 mg P.O. t.i.d. Dosage may be increased at 3-day intervals. Usual maintenance dose is 20 to 30 mg daily in divided doses. Don't exceed 60 mg/day.

Pharmacodynamics
Anxiolytic action: An azaspirodecanedione derivative with anxiolytic activity. Suppresses conflict and aggressive behavior and inhibits conditioned avoidance responses. Exact mechanism unknown, but appears to depend on simultaneous effects on several neurotransmitters and receptor sites: decreasing serotonin neuronal activity, increasing norepinephrine metabolism, and partial action as a presynaptic dopamine antagonist.
   Not pharmacologically related to benzodiazepines, barbiturates, or other sedative and anxiolytic drugs. Exhibits a nontraditional clinical profile and is uniquely anxiolytic. Has no anticonvulsant or muscle relaxant activity and doesn't appear to cause physical dependence or significant sedation.

Pharmacokinetics
● *Absorption:* Absorbed rapidly and completely after oral administration, but extensive first-pass metabolism limits absolute bioavailability to 1% to 13% of oral dose. Food slows absorption but increases amount of unchanged drug in systemic circulation.
● *Distribution:* 95% protein-bound; it doesn't displace other highly protein-bound drugs such as warfarin. Onset of therapeutic effect may require 1 to 2 weeks.

● *Metabolism:* Metabolized in the liver by hydroxylation and oxidation, resulting in at least 1 pharmacologically active metabolite—1, pyrimidinylpiperazine (1-PP).
● *Excretion:* 29% to 63% excreted in urine in 24 hours, primarily as metabolites; 18% to 38% excreted in feces.

Contraindications and precautions
Contraindicated in patients with hypersensitivity to drug or within 14 days of MAO inhibitor therapy. Use cautiously in patients with renal or hepatic impairment.

Interactions
Drug-drug. *CNS depressants:* Sedation may result, especially with doses greater than 30 mg/day. Use together cautiously.
Digoxin: Buspirone may displace digoxin from serum-binding sites when drugs are used together. Avoid concomitant use.
Haloperidol: Serum haloperidol levels may increase. Monitor levels of haloperidol.
MAO inhibitors: Buspirone may elevate blood pressure. Avoid this combination.
Drug-lifestyle. *Alcohol:* Sedation may result. Discourage use.

Adverse reactions
CNS: *dizziness, drowsiness,* nervousness, insomnia, headache, light-headedness, fatigue, numbness.
EENT: blurred vision.
GI: dry mouth, nausea, diarrhea, abdominal distress.

☑ Special considerations
● Patients who have been treated with benzodiazepines previously may not show good response to this drug.
● Although buspirone doesn't appear to cause tolerance or physical or psychological dependence, the possibility exists that patients prone to drug abuse may experience these effects.
● Buspirone doesn't block the withdrawal syndrome associated with benzodiazepines or other common sedative and hypnotic drugs; therefore, these drugs should be withdrawn gradually before replacement with buspirone therapy.
● Signs of overdose include severe dizziness, drowsiness, unusual constriction of pupils, and stomach upset, including nausea and vomiting.
● Treatment of overdose is symptomatic and supportive; empty stomach with immediate gastric lavage. Monitor respiration, pulse, and blood pressure. No specific antidote is known.
● Effect of dialysis in overdose is unknown.

Monitoring the patient
● Monitor hepatic and renal function. Hepatic and renal impairment impedes metabolism and excretion of drug and may lead to toxic accumulation; dosage reduction may be necessary.
● Monitor patient for adverse effects.

Information for the patient
● Advise patient to take drug exactly as prescribed; explain that therapeutic effect may not occur for 2 weeks or more. Warn patient not to double the dose if one is missed, but to take a missed dose as soon as possible, unless it's almost time for next dose.
● Caution patient to avoid hazardous tasks requiring alertness until drug's effects are known. The effects of alcohol and other CNS depressants (such as antihistamines, sedatives, tranquilizers, sleeping aids, prescription pain medication, barbiturates, seizure medication, muscle relaxants, anesthetics, and medications for colds, coughs, hay fever, or allergies) may be enhanced by additive sedation and drowsiness caused by buspirone.
● Tell patient to store drug away from heat and light and out of children's reach.
● Explain importance of regular follow-up visits to check progress. Urge patient to report adverse reactions immediately.
● Inform patient that results may not be seen in 3 to 4 weeks; however, an improvement may be noted within 7 to 10 days.

Breast-feeding patients
● It's unknown if drug appears in breast milk. Avoid use in breast-feeding women.

---

busulfan
Myleran

Pharmacologic classification: alkylating drug (cell-cycle–phase nonspecific)
Therapeutic classification: antineoplastic
Pregnancy risk category D

How supplied
Available by prescription only
Tablets (scored): 2 mg

Indications, route, and dosage
Dosage and indications may vary. Check current literature for recommended protocol.
Chronic myelogenous leukemia
Adults: For remission induction, usual dosage is 4 to 8 mg P.O. daily; however, may range from 1 to 12 mg P.O. daily (0.06 mg/kg or 1.8 mg/m^2). For maintenance therapy, 1 to 3 mg P.O. daily.
Children: 0.06 to 0.12 mg/kg or 1.8 to 4.6 mg/m^2 P.O. daily. Adjust dose to maintain WBC count of about 20,000/mm^3.
◇ *Myelofibrosis*
Adults: 2 to 4 mg P.O. 2 to 3 times weekly.

Pharmacodynamics

Antineoplastic action: An alkylating drug that exerts its cytotoxic activity by interfering with DNA replication and RNA transcription, causing a disruption of nucleic acid function.

Pharmacokinetics

- *Absorption:* Well absorbed from GI tract.
- *Distribution:* Distribution into brain and CSF is unknown.
- *Metabolism:* Metabolized in the liver.
- *Excretion:* Cleared rapidly from plasma. Drug and its metabolites excreted in urine.

Contraindications and precautions

Contraindicated in patients whose chronic myelogenous leukemia has demonstrated prior resistance to drug. Also contraindicated in patients with chronic lymphocytic leukemia or acute leukemia and in those in blastic crisis of chronic myelogenous leukemia.

Use cautiously in patients recently given other myelosuppressants or radiation treatment; in those with depressed neutrophil or platelet counts, head trauma, and seizures; and in patients taking other drugs that reduce seizure threshold.

Interactions

None reported.

Adverse reactions

CNS: unusual tiredness or weakness, fatigue.
GI: cheilosis, dry mouth, anorexia.
Hematologic: leukopenia (WBC count decreasing after about 10 days and continuing to decrease for 2 weeks after stopping drug), *thrombocytopenia, anemia, severe pancytopenia.*
Respiratory: *irreversible pulmonary fibrosis (commonly called "busulfan lung").*
Skin: alopecia, *transient hyperpigmentation,* rash, urticaria, anhidrosis, jaundice.
Other: gynecomastia, Addison-like wasting syndrome, profound hyperuricemia caused by increased cell lysis, cataracts.

☑ Special considerations

- Avoid all I.M. injections when platelets are less than 100,000/mm³.
- Patient response (increased appetite, sense of well-being, decreased total leukocyte count, reduction in size of spleen) usually begins 1 to 2 weeks after initiating the drug.
- Pulmonary fibrosis may be delayed for 4 to 6 months.
- Persistent cough and progressive dyspnea with alveolar exudate may result from drug toxicity, not pneumonia. Instruct patient to report symptoms so dose adjustments can be made.
- Minimize hyperuricemia by adequate hydration, alkalinization of urine, and administration of allopurinol.

- Drug-induced cellular dysplasia may interfere with interpretation of cytologic studies.
- Signs and symptoms of overdose include hematologic manifestations, such as leukopenia and thrombocytopenia.
- Treatment of overdose is supportive and includes transfusion of blood components and antibiotics for infections that may develop.

Monitoring the patient

- Watch for signs or symptoms of infection (fever, sore throat).
- Monitor uric acid, CBC, and kidney function.
- Periodic measurement of serum transaminases, alkaline phosphatase, and bilirubin is indicated for early detection of hepatotoxicity.

Information for the patient

- Advise patient to use caution when taking aspirin-containing products and to promptly report any sign of bleeding.
- Tell patient to take drug at same time each day.
- Emphasize importance of continuing drug despite nausea and vomiting.
- Instruct patient about signs and symptoms of infection; tell patient to report them promptly if they occur.
- Advise patient to use contraceptive methods during therapy.

Breast-feeding patients

- It's unknown if drug appears in breast milk. However, potential for mutagenicity, carcinogenicity, and serious adverse reactions in the infant should be taken into consideration when a decision to breast-feed is made.

---

butoconazole nitrate
Femstat

Pharmacologic classification: synthetic imidazole derivative
Therapeutic classification: topical fungistat
Pregnancy risk category C

How supplied

Available by prescription only
Vaginal cream: 2% supplied with applicators

Indications, route, and dosage
Vulvovaginal candidiasis

Adults (nonpregnant): 1 applicator intravaginally h.s. for 3 days (may be extended to 6 days if necessary).

Adults (pregnant): 1 applicator intravaginally h.s. for 6 days. Use only during second or third trimester.

Pharmacodynamics

Antifungal action: Exact mechanism unknown. Thought to control or destroy fungi by disrupting the permeability of the cell membrane and reducing its osmotic pressure resistance. Active against many fungi, including dermatophytes and yeasts. Also active in vitro against some gram-positive bacteria.

Pharmacokinetics

- *Absorption:* About 5.5% absorbed through vaginal walls.
- *Distribution:* No information available.
- *Metabolism:* Systemically absorbed drug appears to be metabolized, probably in the liver.
- *Excretion:* Systemically absorbed drug appears to be excreted in urine and feces.

Contraindications and precautions

Contraindicated in patients with hypersensitivity to drug.

Interactions

None reported.

Adverse reactions

GU: vulvovaginal burning and itching, soreness, and swelling.
Skin: finger itching.

☑ Special considerations

- Ascertain that patient understands directions for use and length of therapy.
- Drug may be used with oral contraceptives and antibiotic therapy.

Monitoring the patient

- Monitor patient for adverse effects.
- Monitor therapeutic effect.

Information for the patient

- Instruct patient to follow directions enclosed in package and to insert applicator high into vagina; wash hands after use.
- Tell patient to complete full course of therapy, including through menstrual period. However, tell her to avoid using tampons during treatment.
- Advise patient to refrain from sexual contact or to have partner use a condom to avoid reinfection during therapy.
- Tell patient to use a sanitary napkin to prevent staining clothing and to absorb discharge.
- Tell patient to report symptoms that persist after full course of therapy.

Breast-feeding patients

- It's unknown if drug appears in breast milk. Use with caution in breast-feeding women.

---

butorphanol tartrate
Stadol, Stadol NS

Pharmacologic classification: narcotic agonist-antagonist; opioid partial agonist
Therapeutic classification: analgesic, adjunct to anesthesia
Controlled substance schedule IV
Pregnancy risk category C

How supplied

Available by prescription only
Injection: 1 mg/ml, 1-ml vials; 2 mg/ml, 1-ml, 2-ml, and 10-ml vials
Nasal spray: 10 mg/ml

Indications, route, and dosage

Moderate to severe pain
Adults: 1 to 4 mg I.M. q 3 to 4 hours, p.r.n.; or 0.5 to 2 mg I.V. q 3 to 4 hours, p.r.n., or around-the-clock. Or give 1 mg by nasal spray (1 spray in 1 nostril). Repeat if pain relief is inadequate after 1 to 1½ hours. Repeat q 3 to 4 hours, p.r.n.

Pain during labor
Adults: 1 to 2 mg I.M. or I.V. q 4 hours but not 4 hours before delivery.

Preoperative anesthesia
Adults: 2 mg I.M. 60 to 90 minutes before surgery or 2 mg I.V. shortly before induction.

✦ Dosage adjustment. Patients with hepatic or renal impairment and elderly patients should receive one-half of usual parenteral adult dose at 6-hour intervals, as needed.

Pharmacodynamics

Analgesic action: Exact mechanism unknown. Believed to be a competitive antagonist at some, and an agonist at other, opiate receptors, thus relieving moderate to severe pain. Like narcotic agonists, it causes respiratory depression, sedation, and miosis.

Pharmacokinetics

- *Absorption:* Well absorbed after I.M. administration. Onset of analgesia after parenteral administration is less than 10 minutes, with peak analgesic effect at ½ to 1 hour. Onset of analgesia usually occurs within 15 minutes after nasal administration.
- *Distribution:* Rapidly crosses placenta; neonatal serum levels are 0.4 to 1.4 times maternal levels.
- *Metabolism:* Metabolized extensively in the liver, primarily by hydroxylation, to inactive metabolites.
- *Excretion:* Duration of effect is 3 to 4 hours after parenteral administration; 4 to 5 hours after nasal administration. Drug is excreted in inactive form, mainly by kidneys. About 11% to 14% of parenteral dose is excreted in feces.

Contraindications and precautions

Contraindicated in patients with hypersensitivity to drug or to the preservative benzethonium chloride and in those receiving repeated doses of narcotics or with narcotic addiction; may precipitate withdrawal syndrome.

Use cautiously in emotionally unstable patients and in those with history of drug abuse, head injuries, increased intracranial pressure, acute MI, ventricular dysfunction, coronary insufficiency, respiratory disease or depression, and renal or hepatic dysfunction.

Interactions

Drug-drug. *Barbiturate anesthetics such as thiopental:* If administered within a few hours of barbiturate anesthetic, drug may produce additive CNS and respiratory depressant effects and possibly apnea. Avoid using together.

Cimetidine: May potentiate butorphanol toxicity, causing disorientation, respiratory depression, apnea, and seizures. Be prepared to administer a narcotic antagonist if toxicity occurs.

Drugs extensively metabolized in liver (digitoxin, phenytoin, rifampin): Drug accumulation and enhanced effects may result if drug is given concomitantly. Avoid concurrent use.

General anesthetics: May cause severe CV depression. Use with caution.

Narcotic antagonists: Patients physically dependent on opioids may experience acute withdrawal syndrome if given a narcotic antagonist. Use with caution and monitor patient closely.

Other CNS depressants (antihistamines, barbiturates, benzodiazepines, muscle relaxants, narcotic analgesics, phenothiazines, sedative-hypnotics, tricyclic antidepressants): May potentiate respiratory and CNS depression, sedation, and hypotensive effects of drug. Reduced doses of butorphanol are usually necessary when drug is used concomitantly.

Pancuronium: Use together may increase conjunctival changes. Avoid concomitant use.

Drug-lifestyle. *Alcohol:* May potentiate respiratory and CNS depression, sedation, and hypotensive effects of drug. Don't use together.

Adverse reactions

CNS: *confusion,* nervousness, lethargy, headache, *somnolence, dizziness, insomnia,* anxiety, paresthesia, euphoria, hallucinations, flushing, *increased intracranial pressure.*
CV: palpitations, vasodilation, hypotension.
EENT: blurred vision, *nasal congestion* (with nasal spray), tinnitus, taste perversion.
GI: *nausea, vomiting, constipation,* anorexia.
Respiratory: *respiratory depression.*
Skin: rash, hives, *clamminess, excessive diaphoresis.*
Other: sensation of heat.

☑ Special considerations

Besides the recommendations relevant to all opioid (narcotic) agonist-antagonists, consider the following.
● Patients who are using nasal formulation for severe pain may initiate therapy with 2 mg (one spray in each nostril) provided they remain recumbent. Dose isn't repeated for 3 to 4 hours.
● Drug has the potential to be abused. Closely supervise use in emotionally unstable patients and in those with history of drug abuse when long-term therapy is necessary.
● Mild withdrawal symptoms have been reported with long-term use of the injectable form.

Monitoring the patient
● Monitor patient for adverse effects.
● Monitor vital signs closely.

Information for the patient
● Teach patient how to use nasal spray. Patient should use 1 spray in 1 nostril unless otherwise directed.

Geriatric patients
● Lower doses are usually indicated for elderly patients because they may be more sensitive to drug's therapeutic and adverse effects. Plasma half-life is increased by 25% in patients over age 65.

Pediatric patients
● Safety and efficacy in children under age 18 haven't been established.

Breast-feeding patients
● Use of drug in breast-feeding women isn't recommended.

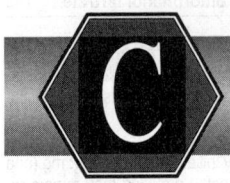

caffeine
Caffedrine, NoDoz, Quick Pep, Vivarin

Pharmacologic classification: methyl-xanthine
Therapeutic classification: CNS stimulant, analeptic, respiratory stimulant
Pregnancy risk category C

How supplied
Available without a prescription
Tablets: 150 mg, 200 mg
Chewable tablets: 100 mg
Available by prescription only
Injection: 250 mg/ml, caffeine (121.25 mg/ml) with sodium benzoate (128.75 mg/ml)

Indications, route, and dosage
CNS depression
Adults: 100 to 200 mg P.O. q 3 to 4 hours, p.r.n. For emergencies, 250 to 500 mg I.M. or I.V.
Infants and children: 4 mg/kg I.M., I.V., or S.C. q 4 hours, p.r.n.
   Note: This use is strongly discouraged by many clinicians.
◇ **Neonatal apnea**
Neonates: 5 to 10 mg/kg (base) I.V., I.M., or P.O. as loading dose; then 2.5 to 5 mg/kg I.V., I.M., or P.O. daily. Adjust dosage according to patient tolerance and plasma caffeine levels.

Pharmacodynamics
CNS stimulant action: Xanthine derivative; increases levels of cAMP by inhibiting phosphodiesterase. Caffeine stimulates all levels of the CNS; hastens and clarifies thinking and improves arousal and psychomotor coordination.
Respiratory stimulant action: In respiratory depression and in neonatal apnea (unlabeled use), larger doses of caffeine increase respiratory rate. Caffeine increases contractile force and decreases fatigue of skeletal muscle.

Pharmacokinetics
● *Absorption:* Well absorbed from GI tract; absorption after I.M. injection may be slower.
● *Distribution:* Distributed rapidly throughout body; crosses blood-brain barrier and placenta. About 17% protein-bound.
● *Metabolism:* Metabolized by the liver; in neonates, liver metabolism is much less evident and

half-life may approach 80 hours. Plasma half-life in adults is 3 to 4 hours.
● *Excretion:* Excreted in urine.

Contraindications and precautions
Contraindicated in patients with hypersensitivity to drug. Use cautiously in patients with history of peptic ulcer, symptomatic arrhythmias, or palpitations, and after an acute MI.

Interactions
Drug-drug. *Beta agonists (albuterol, metaproterenol, terbutaline):* Increased cardiac effects and tremors. Monitor patient closely.
Fluoroquinolones such as cimetidine, ciprofloxacin, disulfiram, enoxacin; oral contraceptives: Inhibits caffeine metabolism and increases its effects. Use together cautiously.
Xanthine derivatives (theophylline): May increase stimulant-induced adverse reactions, such as tremor, tachycardia, insomnia, and nervousness. Use together cautiously.
Drug-lifestyle. *Smoking:* May enhance elimination of caffeine. Discourage smoking.

Adverse reactions
CNS: *insomnia*, restlessness, nervousness, headache, excitement, agitation, muscle tremor, twitching.
CV: *tachycardia, palpitations,* extrasystoles.
GI: nausea, vomiting, diarrhea, stomach pain.
GU: *diuresis.*
Other: abrupt withdrawal symptoms (headache, irritability), tinnitus.

☑ Special considerations
● Restrict caffeine-containing beverages in patients with arrhythmic symptoms or in those who are taking aminophylline or theophylline.
● Caffeine content in beverages (mg/cup) is the following: cola drinks, 24 to 64; brewed tea, 20 to 110; instant coffee, 30 to 120; brewed coffee, 40 to 180; decaffeinated coffee, 3 to 5.
● Many OTC pain relievers contain caffeine, but evidence concerning its analgesic effects is conflicting. Caffeine (30%) may be used in a hydrophilic base or hydrocortisone cream to treat atopic dermatitis.
● Caffeine has been used to relieve headache after lumbar puncture and, in topical creams, to treat atopic dermatitis.
● Caffeine may increase blood glucose levels and cause false-positive urate levels.

Reactions may be *common*, uncommon, *life-threatening*, or COMMON AND LIFE-THREATENING.

• Caffeine may cause false-positive test results for pheochromocytoma or neuroblastoma by increasing certain urinary catecholamines.
• Signs and symptoms of overdose in adults may include insomnia, dyspnea, altered states of consciousness, muscle twitching, seizure, diuresis, arrhythmias, and fever.
• In infants, symptoms of overdose may include alternating hypotonicity and hypertonicity, opisthotonoid posture, tremors, bradycardia, hypotension, and severe acidosis.
• Treat overdose symptomatically and supportively; lavage and charcoal may help. Carefully monitor vital signs, ECG, and fluid and electrolyte balance.
• Seizures may be treated with diazepam or phenobarbital; diazepam can exacerbate respiratory depression.

Monitoring the patient
• Monitor patient for adverse effects.

Information for the patient
• Advise patient to avoid excessive caffeine consumption, and therefore CNS stimulation, by learning caffeine content of beverages and foods.
• Warn patient not to exceed recommended dosage, not to substitute caffeine for needed sleep, and to stop drug if dizziness or tachycardia occurs.

Pediatric patients
• Unlabeled uses include neonatal apnea. For control of neonatal apnea, maintain plasma caffeine level at 5 to 20 mcg/ml.
• Adverse CNS effects are usually more severe in children.
• In neonates, avoid using caffeine products containing sodium benzoate; they may cause kernicterus.

Geriatric patients
• Elderly patients are more sensitive to caffeine and should take lower doses.

Breast-feeding patients
• Caffeine appears in breast milk. Alternative feeding method is recommended during therapy with caffeine.

calcipotriene
Dovonex

Pharmacologic classification: synthetic vitamin D analogue
Therapeutic classification: topical antipsoriatic
Pregnancy risk category C

How supplied
Available by prescription only

Cream, lotion, ointment: 0.005%

Indications, route, and dosage
Moderate plaque psoriasis
Adults: Apply thin layer to affected skin b.i.d. Rub in gently and completely.

Pharmacodynamics
Antipsoriatic action: A synthetic vitamin D_3 analogue that binds to vitamin D_3 receptors in skin cells (keratinocytes), regulating skin cell production and development.

Pharmacokinetics
• *Absorption:* 6% of applied dose absorbed systemically when ointment is applied topically to psoriasis plaques; 5% when applied to normal skin.
• *Distribution:* Vitamin D and its metabolites are transported in blood, bound to specific plasma proteins, to many parts of the body containing keratinocytes. (The scaly red patches of psoriasis are caused by the abnormal growth and production of keratinocytes.)
• *Metabolism:* Rapid metabolism after systemic uptake; occurs via pathway similar to natural hormone. Primary metabolites are much less potent than parent compound.
• *Excretion:* Active form of the vitamin, 1,25-dihydroxy vitamin D_3 (calcitriol), is recycled via the liver and excreted in bile.

Contraindications and precautions
Contraindicated in patients with hypersensitivity to drug or its components. Also contraindicated in patients with hypercalcemia or evidence of vitamin D toxicity. Use cautiously in breast-feeding women and in elderly patients. Drug shouldn't be used on face.

Interactions
None reported.

Adverse reactions
Metabolic: hypercalcemia.
Skin: *burning, pruritus, irritation,* atrophy, dermatitis, dry skin, erythema, folliculitis, hyperpigmentation, peeling, rash, worsening of psoriasis.

☑ Special considerations
• Drug is for topical dermatologic use only; not intended for ophthalmic, oral, or intravaginal use.
• Improvement usually begins after 2 weeks of therapy. About 70% of patients show at least marked improvement after 8 weeks, but only about 10% show complete clearing.
• Safety and effectiveness of topical calcipotriene in dermatoses other than psoriasis haven't been established.
• May cause irritation of lesions and surrounding uninvolved skin. If irritation develops, stop drug.

• Transient, rapidly reversible elevation of serum calcium level has occurred with use. If serum calcium level rises outside normal range, stop treatment until normal calcium levels are restored.
• Topically applied calcipotriene can be absorbed in sufficient amounts to produce systemic effects.
• Serum calcium levels may rise with excessive use.

Monitoring the patient
• Monitor patient for adverse effects.
• Monitor calcium levels as indicated.

Information for the patient
• Tell patient that drug is for external use only, as directed, and to avoid contact with the face or eyes.
• Instruct patient to wash hands thoroughly after application.
• Tell patient to report signs of local adverse reactions.

Geriatric patients
• Adverse dermatologic effects of topical calcipotriene may be more severe in patients over age 65.

Pediatric patients
• Safety and effectiveness in children haven't been established.

Breast-feeding patients
• It's unknown if drug appears in breast milk. Use caution when administering ointment to breast-feeding woman.

calcitonin
Calcimar (salmon), Cibacalcin (human), Miacalcin (salmon), Osteocalcin (salmon), Salmonine (salmon)

Pharmacologic classification: thyroid hormone
Therapeutic classification: hypocalcemic
Pregnancy risk category C

How supplied
Available by prescription only
Injection: 200-IU/ml, 2-ml vials (salmon); 0.5 mg/vial (human)
Nasal spray: 200 IU/activation

Indications, route, and dosage
Paget's disease of bone (osteitis deformans)
Adults: Initially, 100 IU calcitonin (salmon) S.C. or I.M. daily or 0.5 mg calcitonin (human) S.C. Maintenance dosage is 50 to 100 IU calcitonin (salmon), three times weekly or 0.5 mg calcitonin (human) two or three times weekly or 0.25 mg calcitonin (human) daily.

Hypercalcemia
Adults: 4 IU/kg calcitonin (salmon) I.M. or S.C. q 12 hours; increase by 8 IU/kg q 12 hours.
Postmenopausal osteoporosis
Adults: 100 IU calcitonin (salmon) S.C. or I.M. daily, or 200 IU (1 spray) daily in alternating nostril.
◊ **Osteogenesis imperfecta**
Adults: 2 IU/kg calcitonin (salmon) 3 times weekly. With daily calcium supplementation.

Pharmacodynamics
Hypocalcemic action: Directly inhibits the bone resorption of calcium. Mediated by drug-induced increase of cAMP concentration in bone cells, which alters transport of calcium and phosphate across the plasma membrane of the osteoclast. A secondary effect occurs in the kidneys, where calcitonin directly inhibits tubular resorption of calcium, phosphate, and sodium, thereby increasing their excretion. A clinical effect may not be seen for several months in patients with Paget's disease. Calcitonin salmon and calcitonin human are pharmacologically the same, but calcitonin salmon is more potent and has a longer duration of action.

Pharmacokinetics
• *Absorption:* Administered parenterally or nasally. Plasma levels of 0.1 to 0.4 mg/ml achieved within 15 minutes of a 200-IU S.C. dose. Maximum effect seen in 2 to 4 hours; duration of action may be 8 to 24 hours for S.C. or I.M. doses, and ½ to 12 hours for I.V. doses. Plasma levels peak 31 to 39 minutes after using nasal form.
• *Distribution:* Not known if drug enters CNS or crosses placenta.
• *Metabolism:* Rapid metabolism occurs in kidney, with additional activity in blood and peripheral tissues. Calcitonin (salmon) has a longer half-life than calcitonin (human), which has a 1-hour half-life.
• *Excretion:* Excreted in urine as inactive metabolites.

Contraindications and precautions
Contraindicated in patients with hypersensitivity to calcitonin (salmon). Calcitonin (human) has no contraindications.

Interactions
None reported.

Adverse reactions
CNS: headache, weakness, dizziness, paresthesia.
CV: edema of feet, chills, chest pressure, shortness of breath.
EENT: eye pain, nasal congestion.
GI: *transient nausea,* unusual taste, diarrhea, anorexia, *vomiting,* epigastric discomfort, abdominal pain.
GU: *increased urinary frequency,* nocturia.

Reactions may be *common,* uncommon, **life-threatening**, or COMMON AND LIFE-THREATENING.

Skin: *facial flushing*, rash, pruritus of ear lobes, *inflammation at injection site*.
Other: hypersensitivity reactions *(anaphylaxis)*, tender palms and soles.

☑ Special considerations
● S.C. route is preferred method of administration.
● Before initiating therapy with calcitonin (salmon), a skin test using calcitonin (salmon) should be considered. If patient has allergic reactions to foreign proteins, test for hypersensitivity before therapy. Systemic allergic reactions are possible because hormone is a protein. Epinephrine should be readily available.
● Keep parenteral calcium available during the first doses in case of hypocalcemic tetany.
● Doses of calcitonin (salmon) are expressed in international units while calcitonin (human) are in milligrams. Don't confuse units of measurement.
● Refrigerate solution. Once activated, nasal spray should be stored upright at room temperature.
● Signs and symptoms of overdose include hypocalcemia and hypocalcemic tetany.
● Overdose occurs in patients at higher risk during the first few doses. Parenteral calcium should be readily available.

Monitoring the patient
● Periodically monitor serum calcium levels during therapy.
● Observe patient for signs of hypocalcemic tetany during therapy (muscle twitching, tetanic spasms, and convulsions if hypocalcemia is severe).
● Watch for signs of hypercalcemic relapse: bone pain, renal calculi, polyuria, anorexia, nausea, vomiting, thirst, constipation, lethargy, bradycardia, muscle hypotonicity, pathologic fracture, psychosis, and coma. Patients with good initial clinical response to calcitonin who suffer relapse should be evaluated for antibody formation response to the hormone protein.
● If using nasal spray, a periodic examination with visualization of nasal mucosa, turbinates, septum and mucosal blood vessel stratus is recommended.

Information for the patient
● Instruct patient on self-administration of drug and assist patient until proper technique is achieved.
● Tell patient to handle missed doses as follows: *Daily dosing:* Take as soon as possible; don't double up on doses. *Every other day dosing:* Take as soon as possible; then restart the alternate days from this dose.
● Stress importance of regular follow-up to assess progress.
● If given for postmenopausal osteoporosis, remind patient to take adequate calcium and vitamin D supplements.

● Instruct patient using the nasal spray to first activate pump.
● Tell patient to call if nasal irritation occurs; periodic nasal examination should be performed.

Pediatric patients
● No data to support use of nasal spray in pediatric patients.

Breast-feeding patients
● Breast-feeding should be discontinued during drug therapy.

calcitriol
Calcijex, Rocaltrol

Pharmacologic classification: vitamin D analogue
Therapeutic classification: antihypocalcemic
Pregnancy risk category C

How supplied
Available by prescription only
Capsules: 0.25 mcg, 0.5 mcg
Injection: 1 mcg/ml, 2 mcg/ml
Oral solution: 1 mcg/ml

Indications, route, and dosage
Management of hypocalcemia in patients undergoing long-term dialysis
Oral
Adults: Initially, 0.25 mcg P.O. daily. Dosage may be increased by 0.25 mcg daily at 4- to 8-week intervals. Maintenance dose is 0.25 mcg every other day up to 0.5 to 1 mcg daily.
Parenteral
Adults: 0.5 mcg I.V. three times weekly, about every other day. Dosage may be increased by 0.25 to 0.5 mcg at 2- to 4-week intervals. Maintenance dose is 0.5 to 3 mcg I.V. three times weekly.
Management of hypoparathyroidism and pseudohypoparathyroidism
Adults and children ages 6 and older: Initially, 0.25 mcg P.O. daily in morning. Dosage may be increased at 2- to 4-week intervals. Maintenance dose is 0.5 to 2 mcg daily.
Children ages 1 to 5: (hypoparathyroidism only) 0.25 to 0.75 mcg daily.
Management of secondary hyperparathyroidism and resultant metabolic bone disease in predialysis patients (moderate to severe chronic renal failure with creatinine clearance of 15 to 55 ml/minute)
Adults and children ages 3 and older: Initially, 0.25 mcg P.O. daily. Dosage may be increased to 0.5 mcg/day if necessary.
Children less than age 3: Initially, 10 to 15 ng/kg P.O. daily.

◇ *Psoriasis vulgaris*
Adults: 0.5 mcg/day P.O. for 6 months and topically (0.5 mcg/g petroleum) daily for 8 weeks.

Pharmacodynamics
Antihypocalcemic action: Vitamin D analogue (1,25-dihydroxycholecalciferol), or activated cholecalciferol. Promotes absorption of calcium from the intestine by forming a calcium-binding protein. Reverses the signs of rickets and osteomalacia in patients who can't activate or use ergocalciferol or cholecalciferol. In patients with renal failure it reduces bone pain, muscle weakness, and parathyroid serum levels.

Pharmacokinetics
• *Absorption:* Absorbed readily after oral administration.
• *Distribution:* Distributed widely; protein-bound.
• *Metabolism:* Metabolized in liver and kidney, with a half-life of 3 to 8 hours. No activation step is required.
• *Excretion:* Excreted primarily in feces.

Contraindications and precautions
Contraindicated in patients with hypercalcemia or vitamin D toxicity. Withhold all preparations containing vitamin D.

Interactions
Drug-drug. *Antacids, cholestyramine, colestipol, mineral oil:* May alter calcitriol absorption. Use together cautiously.
Barbiturates, phenytoin, primidone: May increase metabolism of calcitriol and reduce activity. Use together cautiously.
Cardiac glycosides: Concomitant use may potentiate effects of cardiac glycosides. Use together with caution.
Corticosteroids: May counteract effects of vitamin D analogues. Use together cautiously.
Thiazide diuretics: May result in hypercalcemia. Monitor serum calcium level.

Adverse reactions
Vitamin D intoxication associated with hypercalcemia:
CNS: headache, somnolence, weakness, irritability.
CV: hypertension, *arrhythmias.*
EENT: conjunctivitis, photophobia, rhinorrhea.
GI: nausea, vomiting, constipation, polydipsia, pancreatitis, metallic taste, dry mouth, anorexia.
GU: polyuria, nocturia.
Musculoskeletal: bone and muscle pain.
Skin: pruritus.
Other: weight loss, hyperthermia, nephrocalcinosis, decreased libido.

☑ **Special considerations**
• Protect drug from heat and light.

• Calcitriol therapy may falsely elevate cholesterol determinations made using the Zlatkis-Zak reaction.
• Calcitriol alters serum alkaline phosphatase levels and may alter electrolytes such as magnesium, phosphate, and calcium in serum and urine.
• A sign of overdose is hypercalcemia. Treatment requires discontinuation of drug, institution of a low-calcium diet, increased fluid intake, and supportive measures.
• Calcitonin administration may help reverse hypercalcemia.
• In severe cases of overdose, death has followed CV and renal failure.

Monitoring the patient
• Monitor serum calcium levels several times weekly after initiating therapy.
• There is some evidence that monitoring urine calcium and urine creatinine levels is very helpful in screening for hypercalciuria. The ratio of urine calcium to urine creatinine should be less than or equal to 0.18. A value above 0.2 suggests hypercalciuria, and the dose should be decreased regardless of serum calcium level. The product of serum calcium times phosphate shouldn't be allowed to exceed 70.

Information for the patient
• Instruct patient on importance of calcium-rich diet.
• Advise patient to report adverse reactions immediately.
• Tell patient to avoid magnesium-containing antacids and other self-prescribed drugs.

Pediatric patients
• Some infants may be hyperreactive to drug.

Breast-feeding patients
• Very little drug appears in breast milk; however, effect of vitamin D levels exceeding the RDA in infants isn't known. Therefore, large doses shouldn't be administered to breast-feeding women.

calcium polycarbophil
Equalactin, Fiberall, FiberCon, Fiber-Lax, Mitrolan

Pharmacologic classification: hydrophilic
Therapeutic classification: bulk laxative, antidiarrheal
Pregnancy risk category C

How supplied
Available without a prescription
Tablets: 500 mg (FiberCon), 625 mg (Fiber-Lax)
Tablets (chewable): 500 mg (Equalactin, Fiber-Lax, Mitrolan), 1,000 mg (Fiberall)

Reactions may be *common*, uncommon, **life-threatening**, or COMMON AND LIFE-THREATENING.

Indications, route, and dosage
Constipation; acute nonspecific diarrhea associated with irritable bowel syndrome
Adults: 1 g P.O. q.i.d. as required. Maximum dose is 6 g in 24-hour period.
Children ages 6 to 12: 500 mg P.O. once daily to t.i.d. as required. Maximum dose is 3 g in 24-hour period.
Children ages 3 to 6: 500 mg P.O. once daily to b.i.d. as required. Maximum dose is 1.5 g in 24-hour period.

Pharmacodynamics
Laxative action: Absorbs water and expands, thereby increasing stool bulk and moisture and promoting normal peristalsis and bowel motility.
Antidiarrheal action: Absorbs intestinal fluid, thereby restoring normal stool consistency and bulk.

Pharmacokinetics
- *Absorption:* None.
- *Distribution:* None.
- *Metabolism:* None.
- *Excretion:* Excreted in feces.

Contraindications and precautions
Contraindicated in patients with GI obstruction; drug may exacerbate condition.

Interactions
Drug-drug. *Tetracycline:* Calcium polycarbophil may impair absorption. Use together cautiously.

Adverse reactions
GI: abdominal fullness and increased flatus, intestinal obstruction.
Other: laxative dependence (with long-term or excessive use).

☑ Special considerations
- Patient must chew tablets (chewable) before swallowing; administer tablets with 8 oz (240 ml) of fluid. Administer less fluid for antidiarrheal effect.
- When using drug as an antidiarrheal, don't give if patient has high fever.

Monitoring the patient
- Before starting drug, be sure patient has adequate fluid intake, diet, and exercise.
- Evaluate response to drug therapy.
- Monitor patient for signs of drug dependence.

Information for the patient
- For chewable tablets: Instruct patient to chew tablets instead of swallowing them whole. If drug is being taken as a laxative, advise patient to drink a full glass (8 oz) of fluid after each tablet. Advise patient to take less water if drug is being used to treat diarrhea.
- Warn patient not to take more than 12 tablets in 24-hour period (6 tablets for child age 6 to 12;

three tablets for child age 3 to 6) and to take for length of time prescribed.
- If patient is taking drug as laxative, advise to call promptly and stop drug if constipation persists after 1 week or if fever, nausea, vomiting, or abdominal pain occurs.
- Instruct patient that dose may be taken every 30 minutes for acute diarrhea, but not to exceed maximum daily dosage.
- Tell patient that if abdominal discomfort or fullness occurs, smaller doses may be taken more frequently throughout the day, at regular intervals.

calcium salts

calcium acetate
Phos-Ex, PhosLo

calcium carbonate
Alka-Mints, Amitone, Calciday-667, Cal-Plus, Caltrate 600, Chooz, Os-Cal 500, Rolaids, Titralac, Tums, Tums E-X

calcium chloride

calcium citrate
Citracal

calcium glubionate
Neo-Calglucon

calcium gluceptate

calcium gluconate

calcium lactate

calcium phosphate, tribasic
Posture

Pharmacologic classification: calcium supplement
Therapeutic classification: therapeutic drug for electrolyte balance, cardiotonic
Pregnancy risk category C

How supplied
Available by prescription only
calcium chloride
Injection: 10% solution (1 g/10 ml; each ml of solution provides 27.2 mg or 1.36 mEq of calcium) in 10-ml ampules, vials, and syringes
calcium gluceptate
Injection: 1.1 g/5 ml ampules or 50-ml vials for preparation of I.V. admixtures (each ml of solution provides 18 mg or 0.9 mEq of calcium)
calcium gluconate
Injection: 10% solution (1 g/10 ml; each ml of solution provides 9.3 mg or 0.46 mEq of calcium) in 10-ml ampules and vials, or 20-ml vials

Available without a prescription
calcium acetate
Tablets: 250 mg (62.5 mg calcium), 668 mg (167 mg calcium), 1,000 mg (250 mg calcium)
Capsules: 500 mg
calcium carbonate
Tablets: 500 mg, 650 mg, 667 mg, 1.25 g, 1.5 g
Tablets (chewable): 350 mg, 420 mg, 500 mg, 750 mg, 835 mg, 850 mg, 1.25 g
Oral suspension: 1.25 g (500 mg of calcium) per 5 ml
Capsules: 1.25 g (500 mg of calcium), 1.5 g (600 mg of calcium)
Powder: 6.5 g
calcium citrate
Tablets: 950 mg (contains 200 mg of elemental calcium/g)
Tablets (effervescent): 2,376 mg (500 mg of calcium)
calcium glubionate
Syrup: 1.8 g/5 ml (contains 115 mg of elemental calcium/g)
calcium gluconate
Tablets: 500 mg, 650 mg, 975 mg, 1 g (contains 90 mg of elemental calcium/g)
calcium lactate
Tablets: 325 mg, 650 mg (contains 130 mg of elemental calcium/g)
calcium phosphate, tribasic
Tablets: 600 mg

Indications, route, and dosage
Emergency treatment of hypocalcemia
calcium chloride
Adults: 500 mg to 1 g I.V. slowly (don't exceed 1 ml/minute).
Children: 0.2 ml/kg I.V. slowly (don't exceed 1 ml/minute).
calcium gluconate
Adults: 7 to 14 mEq I.V. slowly (don't exceed 0.7 to 1.8 mEq/minute).
Children: 1 to 7 mEq I.V. slowly (don't exceed 0.7 to 1.8 mEq/minute).
Repeat above dosage based on clinical laboratory value.
Cardiotonic use
calcium chloride
Adults: 500 mg to 1 g I.V. slowly (don't exceed 1 ml/minute); or 200 to 800 mg intraventricularly as a single dose.
Hyperkalemia
calcium gluconate
Adults: 2.25 to 14 mEq I.V. slowly. Administration must be titrated based on ECG response.
Hypermagnesemia
calcium chloride
Adults: 500 mg I.V. initially, repeated based on clinical response.
calcium gluceptate
Adults: 2 to 5 ml I.M., or 5 to 20 ml I.V.
calcium gluconate
Adults: 4.5 to 9 mEq I.V. slowly.

During exchange transfusions
Adults: 1.35 mEq I.V. concurrently with each 100-ml citrated blood exchange.
Neonates: 0.45 mEq I.V. after every 100 ml of citrated blood exchange.
Hypocalcemia
calcium acetate
Adults: 2 to 4 tablets P.O. with meals.
calcium gluconate
Adults: For hypocalcemic tetany, 4.5 to 16 mEq I.V. until therapeutic response is obtained.
Children: For hypocalcemic tetany, 0.5 to 0.7 mEq/kg I.V. t.i.d. or q.i.d. or until tetany is controlled.
Neonates: 2.4 mEq/kg/day in divided doses until therapeutic response is obtained.
calcium lactate
Adults: 325 mg to 1.3 g P.O. t.i.d. with meals.
Osteoporosis prevention
Adults: 1 to 1.5 g P.O. daily of elemental calcium.
Hyperphosphatemia in end-stage renal failure
calcium acetate
Adults: 2 to 4 tablets with each meal.

Pharmacodynamics
Calcium replacement: Essential for maintaining the functional integrity of the nervous, muscular, and skeletal systems, and for cell membrane and capillary permeability. Calcium salts are used as a source of calcium cation to treat or prevent calcium depletion in patients in whom dietary measures are inadequate. Conditions associated with hypocalcemia are chronic diarrhea, vitamin D deficiency, steatorrhea, sprue, pregnancy and lactation, menopause, pancreatitis, renal failure, alkalosis, hyperphosphatemia, and hypoparathyroidism.

Pharmacokinetics
• *Absorption:* I.M. and I.V. calcium salts are absorbed directly into bloodstream. I.V. injection gives an immediate blood level, which will decrease to previous levels in about 30 to 120 minutes. Oral dose is absorbed actively in the duodenum and proximal jejunum and, to a lesser extent, in distal part of small intestine. Calcium is absorbed only in ionized form. Pregnancy and reduction of calcium intake may increase the efficiency of absorption. Vitamin D in its active form is required for calcium absorption.
• *Distribution:* Enters extracellular fluid; incorporated rapidly into skeletal tissue. Bone contains 99% of total calcium; 1% distributed equally between intracellular and extracellular fluids. CSF levels are about 50% of serum calcium levels.
• *Metabolism:* None significant.
• *Excretion:* Excreted mainly in feces as unabsorbed calcium secreted via bile and pancreatic juice into lumen of GI tract. Most calcium entering kidney is reabsorbed in loop of Henle and proximal and distal convoluted tubules. Only small amounts of calcium excreted in urine.

Reactions may be *common*, uncommon, *life-threatening*, or COMMON AND LIFE-THREATENING.

Contraindications and precautions

Contraindicated in patients with ventricular fibrillation, hypercalcemia, hypophosphatemia, or renal calculi. Use cautiously in patients with sarcoidosis, renal or cardiac disease, cor pulmonale, respiratory acidosis, or respiratory failure and in digitalized patients.

Interactions

Drug-drug. *Atenolol, iron salts, quinolones (such as norfloxacin):* Concurrent administration may decrease levels of these drugs. Use together cautiously; monitor drug levels.

Calcium channel blockers (verapamil): Calcium may antagonize the therapeutic effects of these drugs. Avoid concomitant use.

Calcium carbonates, phosphates, sulfates, tartrates: Progressive hypercalcemia may occur. Calcium shouldn't be physically mixed with these drugs, especially at high concentrations.

Cardiac glycoside, digitalis: Increases digitalis toxicity when used together. Administer calcium very cautiously, if at all, to digitalized patients.

Magnesium: Calcium competes with magnesium; may compete for absorption, thus decreasing amount of bioavailable magnesium. Use together cautiously.

Tetracycline: Concurrent administration of oral calcium decreases therapeutic effect of tetracycline. Use together cautiously.

Adverse reactions

CNS: tingling sensations, sense of oppression or heat waves, headache, irritability, weakness (with I.V. use); syncope (with rapid I.V. injection).

CV: mild fall in blood pressure; vasodilation, *bradycardia, arrhythmias, cardiac arrest* (with rapid I.V. injection).

GI: irritation, hemorrhage, *constipation* (with oral use); chalky taste, rebound hyperacidity, *nausea* (with I.V. use); hemorrhage, nausea, vomiting, thirst, abdominal pain (with oral calcium chloride).

GU: hypercalcemia, polyuria, renal calculi.

Skin: local reactions including burning, necrosis, tissue sloughing, cellulitis, soft tissue calcification (with I.M. use).

Other: pain and irritation (with S.C. injection); *vein irritation* (with I.V. use).

☑ Special considerations

● Give calcium chloride I.V. only.

● I.V. route is recommended in children, but not by scalp vein; may cause tissue necrosis.

● Give I.V. calcium slowly through small-bore needle into large vein to avoid extravasation and necrosis.

● After I.V. injection, patient should be recumbent for 15 minutes to prevent orthostasis.

● If perivascular infiltration occurs, stop I.V. immediately. Venospasm may be reduced by administering 1% procaine hydrochloride and hyaluronidase to the affected area.

● Use I.M. route only in emergencies when no I.V. route is available. Give I.M. injections in gluteal region in adults, lateral thigh in infants.

● Hypercalcemia may result when large doses are given to patients with chronic renal failure.

● Severe necrosis and sloughing of tissue may occur after extravasation. Calcium gluconate is less irritating to veins and tissue than calcium chloride.

● Crash carts usually contain both gluconate and chloride. Be sure to specify form to be administered.

● If GI upset occurs with oral calcium, give 2 to 3 hours after meals.

● Oxalic acid (found in rhubarb and spinach), phytic acid (in bran and whole-grain cereals), and phosphorus (in milk and dairy products) may interfere with calcium absorption.

● With oral product, patient may need laxatives or stool softeners to manage constipation.

● I.V. calcium may produce transient elevation of plasma 11-hydroxycorticosteroid levels (Glen-Nelson technique).

● I.V. calcium may produce false-negative values for serum and urine magnesium measured by Titan yellow method.

● Acute hypercalcemia syndrome is characterized by markedly elevated plasma calcium level, lethargy, weakness, nausea and vomiting, and coma, and may lead to sudden death.

● In case of overdose, stop calcium immediately.

● After oral ingestion of calcium overdose, treatment includes removal by emesis or gastric lavage then supportive therapy, as needed.

Monitoring the patient

● Monitor serum calcium levels frequently, especially in patients with renal impairment.

● Monitor ECG when giving calcium I.V. Injections should be given slowly at a rate dependent on salt form used. Stop injection if patient complains of discomfort.

● Assess Chvostek's and Trousseau's signs periodically to check for tetany.

● Monitor patient for symptoms of hypercalcemia (nausea, vomiting, headache, mental confusion, anorexia), and report them immediately. Calcium absorption of an oral dose is decreased in patients with certain disease states such as achlorhydria, renal osteodystrophy, steatorrhea, or uremia.

Information for the patient

● Tell patient not to exceed the manufacturer's recommended dose of calcium.

● Warn patient not to use bone meal or dolomite as a source of calcium; they may contain lead.

● Advise patient to avoid tobacco and to limit intake of alcohol and beverages containing caffeine.

Geriatric patients

● Calcium absorption (after oral administration) may be decreased in elderly patients.

Pediatric patients
● Calcium should be administered cautiously to children by I.V. route (usually not administered I.M.).

Breast-feeding patients
● Calcium appears in breast milk, but not in quantities large enough to affect infant.

---

candesartan cilexetil
Atacand

Pharmacologic classification: selective angiotensin II receptor antagonist
Therapeutic classification: antihypertensive
Pregnancy risk category C (D in second and third trimesters)

How supplied
Available by prescription only
Tablets: 4 mg, 8 mg, 16 mg, 32 mg

Indications, route, and dosage
Hypertension (used alone or with other antihypertensives)
Adults: Initially, 16 mg P.O. once daily when used as monotherapy; usual dosage range is 8 to 32 mg P.O. daily as a single dose or divided b.i.d.

Pharmacodynamics
Antihypertensive action: Inhibits vasoconstrictive action of angiotensin II by blocking the angiotensin II receptor on the surface of vascular smooth muscle and other tissue cells.

Pharmacokinetics
● *Absorption:* Rapidly and completely bioactivated during absorption from GI tract.
● *Distribution:* Highly bound to plasma proteins (about 99%).
● *Metabolism:* Undergoes minor hepatic metabolism.
● *Excretion:* Primarily recovered in urine and feces.

Contraindications and precautions
Contraindicated in patients with hypersensitivity to drug or its ingredients. Use cautiously in patients whose renal function depends on the renin-angiotensin-aldosterone system (such as patients with heart failure) because of potential for oliguria and progressive azotemia with acute renal failure or death. Also use cautiously in patients who are volume- or salt-depleted because of potential for symptomatic hypotension. Start therapy with a lower dosage range, and monitor blood pressure carefully.

Interactions
None reported.

Adverse reactions
CNS: dizziness, fatigue, headache.
CV: chest pain, peripheral edema.
EENT: pharyngitis, rhinitis, sinusitis.
GI: abdominal pain, diarrhea, nausea, vomiting.
GU: albuminuria.
Musculoskeletal: arthralgia, back pain.
Respiratory: coughing, bronchitis, upper respiratory tract infection.

☑ Special considerations
● Drugs that act directly on the renin-angiotensin system (such as candesartan) can cause fetal and neonatal morbidity and death when administered to pregnant women. These problems haven't been detected when exposure has been limited to first trimester. If pregnancy is suspected, stop drug immediately.
● If hypotension occurs after dose, place patient in supine position and, if necessary, give I.V. infusion of normal saline.
● Most of the antihypertensive effect is present within 2 weeks. Maximal antihypertensive effect is obtained within 4 to 6 weeks. Diuretic may be added if blood pressure isn't controlled by drug alone.
● Manifestation of overdose includes hypotension, dizziness, and tachycardia; bradycardia could occur from parasympathetic (vagal) stimulation. Treatment should be supportive.

Monitoring the patient
● Carefully monitor therapeutic response and occurrence of adverse reactions in elderly patients and in those with renal disease.
● Monitor patient for adverse effects.

Information for the patient
● Inform woman of childbearing age of the consequences of second and third trimester exposure to drug. Advise her to call immediately if pregnancy is suspected.
● Advise breast-feeding patient about risk of adverse drug effects on infant and need to either stop breast-feeding or discontinue drug.
● Instruct patient to store drug at room temperature and to keep container tightly sealed.
● Inform patient to report adverse reactions without delay.
● Inform patient that drug may be taken without regard to meals.

Geriatric patients
● Although serum levels of drug are higher in elderly patients as compared to younger adults, the drug and its inactive metabolite doesn't accumulate in the serum of patients over age 65 upon repeated, once-daily dosing.

Pediatric patients
● Safety and efficacy in children haven't been established.

Breast-feeding patients
• It's unknown if drug appears in breast milk; therefore, breast-feeding during drug therapy isn't recommended.

capecitabine
Xeloda

Pharmacologic classification: fluoropyrimidine carbamate
Therapeutic classification: antineoplastic
Pregnancy risk category D

How supplied
Available by prescription only
Tablets: 150 mg, 500 mg

Indications, route, and dosage
Treatment of patients with metastatic breast cancer resistant to both paclitaxel and an anthracycline-containing chemotherapy regimen or resistant to paclitaxel and for whom further anthracycline therapy isn't indicated
Adults: 2,500 mg/m² P.O. daily in two divided doses (about 12 hours apart) at end of a meal for 2 weeks; then a 1-week rest period given as 3-week cycles.
✦ *Dosage adjustment.* National Cancer Institute of Canada (NCIC) Common Toxicity Criteria:
NCIC grade 2: First appearance, interrupt treatment until resolved to grade 0 to 1, then restart at 100% of starting dose for next cycle; second appearance, interrupt treatment until resolved to grade 0 to 1 and use 75% of starting dose for next cycle; third appearance, interrupt treatment until resolved to grade 0 to 1 and use 50% of starting dose for next cycle; fourth appearance, stop treatment permanently.
NCIC grade 3: First appearance, interrupt treatment until resolved to grade 0 to 1 and use 75% of starting dose for next cycle; second appearance, interrupt treatment until resolved to grade 0 to 1 and use 50% of starting dose for next cycle; third appearance, stop treatment permanently.
NCIC grade 4: First appearance, stop treatment permanently or interrupt treatment until resolved to grade 0 to 1 and use 50% of starting dose for next cycle.
      Note: Toxicity criteria relate to degrees of severity of diarrhea, nausea, vomiting, stomatitis, and hand-foot syndrome. Refer to capecitabine package insert for specific toxicity definitions.

Pharmacodynamics
Antineoplastic action: Converted to the active drug 5-fluorouracil (5-FU). 5-FU is metabolized by both normal and tumor cells to metabolites that cause cellular injury via 2 different mechanisms: interference with DNA synthesis to inhibit cell division and interference with RNA processing and protein synthesis.

Pharmacokinetics
• *Absorption:* Readily absorbed from GI tract. Levels peak in 1½ hours for parent drug and 2 hours for active metabolite. Rate and extent of absorption decrease with food.
• *Distribution:* About 60% bound to plasma proteins.
• *Metabolism:* Extensively metabolized to 5-FU (an active metabolite).
• *Excretion:* Elimination half-life of parent drug and active moiety is about 45 minutes with 70% excreted in urine.

Contraindications and precautions
Contraindicated in patients with hypersensitivity to 5-FU. Use cautiously in patients with history of coronary artery disease, mild to moderate hepatic dysfunction due to liver metastases, hyperbilirubinemia, or renal insufficiency, and in elderly patients.

Interactions
Drug-drug. *Coumarin-derivative anticoagulants such as warfarin, phenprocoumon:* Altered coagulation parameters and bleeding have been reported in patients taking these drugs concomitantly with capecitabine. Monitor PT and INR closely.
Leucovorin: Has caused increased level of 5-FU with enhanced toxicity. Monitor patient carefully.

Adverse reactions
CNS: dizziness, *fatigue,* headache, insomnia, *paresthesia.*
CV: edema.
EENT: eye irritation.
GI: diarrhea, nausea, vomiting, stomatitis, abdominal pain, constipation, anorexia, intestinal obstruction, dyspepsia.
Hematologic: NEUTROPENIA, THROMBOCYTOPENIA, anemia, lymphopenia.
Hepatic: hyperbilirubinemia.
Musculoskeletal: myalgia, pain in limb.
Skin: hand-and-foot syndrome, dermatitis, nail disorder.
Other: pyrexia, dehydration.

☑ Special considerations
• Altered coagulation parameters and bleeding may occur within several days up to several months after initiating therapy and rarely within 1 month after stopping capecitabine therapy.
• Drug may need to be immediately interrupted until diarrhea resolves or decreases in intensity.
• Hyperbilirubinemia may require stopping drug.
• Manage overdose symptomatically. Dialysis may be of benefit in drug removal.

Monitoring the patient
• Severe diarrhea can occur, electrolytes and proper hydration should be monitored.

• Monitor patient for hand-foot syndrome (characterized by numbness, paresthesia, tingling, painless or painful swelling, erythema, desquamation, blistering and severe pain of hands or feet), hyperbilirubinemia, and severe nausea. Adjust drug therapy immediately if these occur.
• Monitor patient carefully for toxicity. Toxicity may be managed by symptomatic treatment, dose interruptions, and dosage adjustments.
• Watch for severe diarrhea. Give fluid and electrolyte replacement if patient becomes dehydrated.
• Patients taking coumadin-derivative anticoagulants concomitantly should be monitored regularly for alterations in coagulation parameters.

Information for the patient
• Inform patient and caregiver of expected adverse effects of drug, especially nausea, vomiting, diarrhea, and hand-and-foot syndrome (pain, swelling or redness of hands or feet). Tell them that patient-specific dose adaptations during therapy are expected and necessary.
• Instruct patient to stop taking drug and call immediately if the following adverse effects occur: diarrhea (over 4 bowel movements daily or diarrhea at night), vomiting (2 to 5 episodes in a 24-hour period), nausea, appetite loss or decrease in amount of food taken each day, stomatitis (pain, redness, swelling or sores in mouth), hand-foot syndrome, temperature of 100.5° F (38° C) or higher or other evidence of infection.
• Tell patient that most adverse effects improve within 2 to 3 days after stopping drug. If these don't improve, tell patient to call immediately.
• Tell patient the number of treatment cycles and how to take drug. Drug is usually taken for 14 days then a 7-day rest period (no drug) given as a 21-day cycle.
• Instruct patient to take drug with water within 30 minutes after end of a meal (breakfast and dinner).
• If a combination of tablets is prescribed, teach patient importance of correctly identifying tablets to avoid possible misdosing.
• For missed doses, instruct patient not to take missed dose and not to double the next one. Instead, patient should call and then continue with regular dosing schedule.
• Instruct patient to call if taking the vitamin folic acid.
• Advise woman of childbearing age to avoid becoming pregnant while receiving treatment.

Geriatric patients
• Patients older than age 80 may experience more GI adverse effects.

Pediatric patients
• Safety and efficacy in patients under age 18 haven't been established.

Breast-feeding patients
• Patients shouldn't breast-feed while on drug therapy.

---

capsaicin
Dolorac, Zostrix, Zostrix-HP

Pharmacologic classification: chemical derived from plants of the Solanaceae family
Therapeutic classification: topical analgesic
Pregnancy risk category NR

How supplied
Available without a prescription
Cream: 0.025% (Zostrix), 0.075% (Zostrix-HP), 0.25% (Dolorac)

Indications, route, and dosage
Temporary pain relief from rheumatoid arthritis, osteoarthritis, and certain neuralgias, such as pain associated with shingles (herpes zoster) or diabetic neuropathy
Zostrix
Adults and children over age 2: Apply to affected areas t.i.d. or q.i.d.
Dolorac
Adults and children over age 12: Apply thin film to affected areas b.i.d.

Pharmacodynamics
Analgesic action: Exact mechanism unknown. Current evidence suggests that drug renders skin and joints insensitive to pain by depleting and preventing reaccumulation of substance P in peripheral sensory neurons. Substance P is thought to be the principal chemomediator of pain impulses from the periphery to the CNS. In addition, substance P is released into joint tissues and activates inflammatory mediators involved with the pathogenesis of rheumatoid arthritis.

Pharmacokinetics
No information available.

Contraindications and precautions
Contraindicated in patients with hypersensitivity to drug.

Interactions
None reported.

Adverse reactions
Respiratory: cough, irritation.
Skin: redness, *stinging or burning on application.*

☑ Special considerations
• Transient burning or stinging with application is usually evident at initial therapy but will disappear in several days.

Reactions may be *common*, uncommon, ***life-threatening***, or COMMON AND LIFE-THREATENING.

- Application schedules of less than t.i.d. or q.i.d. may not provide optimum pain relief, and the burning sensation may persist.
- Capsaicin is for external use only. Avoid contact with eyes and broken or irritated skin.

Monitoring the patient
- Monitor patient for response to drug therapy.
- Monitor patient for signs of hypersensitivity.

Information for the patient
- Instruct patient how to apply cream, stressing importance of avoiding eyes and broken or irritated skin.
- Instruct patient to wash hands after applying cream, avoiding areas where drug was applied.
- Warn patient that transient burning or stinging with application may occur but will disappear with continued use after several days.
- Tell patient not to bandage areas tightly.
- Advise patient to stop drug and to call if condition worsens or doesn't improve after 28 days.

captopril
Capoten

Pharmacologic classification: ACE inhibitor
Therapeutic classification: antihypertensive, adjunctive treatment of heart failure
Pregnancy risk category C (D in second and third trimesters)

How supplied
Available by prescription only
Tablets: 12.5 mg, 25 mg, 50 mg, 100 mg

Indications, route, and dosage
Mild to severe hypertension, ◊ idiopathic edema, ◊ Raynaud's phenomenon
Adults: Initially, 25 mg P.O. b.i.d. or t.i.d.; if necessary, dosage may be increased to 50 mg b.i.d. or t.i.d. after 1 to 2 weeks; if control is still inadequate after 1 to 2 weeks more, a diuretic may be added. Dosage may be raised to a maximum of 150 mg t.i.d. (450 mg/day) while continuing the diuretic. Daily dose may be given b.i.d.
Heart failure
Adults: Initially, 25 mg P.O. t.i.d.; may be increased to 50 mg t.i.d., with maximum of 450 mg/day. In patients taking diuretics, initial dosage is 6.25 to 12.5 mg t.i.d.
Prevention of diabetic nephropathy
Adults: 25 mg P.O. t.i.d.
Left ventricular dysfunction after an MI
Adults: Give 6.25 mg P.O. as a single dose 3 days after an MI; then 12.5 mg t.i.d. increasing dosage to 25 mg t.i.d. Target dose is 50 mg t.i.d.
✦ **Dosage adjustment.** In patients with renal failure and in elderly patients, use lower initial daily doses and smaller increments for adjustment.

Pharmacodynamics
Antihypertensive action: Inhibits ACE, preventing conversion of angiotensin I to angiotensin II, a potent vasoconstrictor. Reduced formation of angiotensin II decreases peripheral arterial resistance, which results in decreased aldosterone secretion, thus reducing sodium and water retention and lowering blood pressure.
Cardiac load-reducing action: Decreases systemic vascular resistance (afterload) and pulmonary capillary wedge pressure (preload), thus increasing cardiac output in patients with heart failure.

Pharmacokinetics
- *Absorption:* 60% to 75% of oral dose is absorbed through GI tract; food may reduce absorption by up to 40%. Antihypertensive effect begins in 15 minutes; peak blood levels occur at 1 hour. Maximum therapeutic effect may require several weeks.
- *Distribution:* Distributed into most body tissues except CNS; drug is about 25% to 30% protein-bound.
- *Metabolism:* About 50% is metabolized in the liver.
- *Excretion:* Drug and its metabolites excreted primarily in urine; small amounts excreted in feces. Duration of effect is usually 2 to 6 hours; increases with higher doses. Elimination half-life is less than 3 hours. Duration of action may be increased in patients with renal dysfunction.

Contraindications and precautions
Contraindicated in patients with hypersensitivity to drug or other ACE inhibitors. Use cautiously in patients with impaired renal function, renal artery stenosis, or serious autoimmune diseases (especially lupus erythematosus) and in those taking drugs that affect WBC counts or immune response.

Interactions
Drug-drug. *Antacids:* Decreased effects of captopril. Separate administration times.
Aspirin, indomethacin, other NSAIDs: May decrease captopril's antihypertensive effect. Use together cautiously.
Digoxin: May increase serum digoxin levels. Monitor digoxin levels.
Diuretics, other antihypertensives: Enhanced antihypertensive effects. Monitor blood pressure closely.
Lithium: Increased lithium levels, which may lead to toxicity. Use together with caution; monitor lithium drug levels.
Phenothiazines: May lead to increased pharmacologic effects. Monitor patient closely.
Potassium-sparing diuretics, potassium supplements: Increased serum potassium levels. Monitor serum potassium level closely.

Probenecid: May increase captopril's plasma levels and decrease its clearance. Monitor patient.
Drug-food. *Salt substitutes:* May cause hyperkalemia during captopril therapy. Avoid use together.
Drug-herb. *Black catechu:* May cause additional hypotensive effects. Avoid use together.

Adverse reactions

CNS: dizziness, fainting, headache, malaise, fatigue.
CV: *tachycardia, hypotension,* angina pectoris.
GI: anorexia, *dysgeusia,* nausea, vomiting, abdominal pain, constipation, dry mouth.
Hematologic: *leukopenia, agranulocytosis, pancytopenia,* anemia, **thrombocytopenia.**
Hepatic: transient increase in hepatic enzymes.
Metabolic: hyperkalemia.
Respiratory: *dry, persistent, tickling, nonproductive cough,* dyspnea.
Skin: *urticarial rash, maculopapular rash,* pruritus, alopecia.
Other: fever, **angioedema of face and extremities.**

☑ Special considerations

● Diuretic therapy ends usually 2 to 3 days before beginning ACE inhibitor therapy, to reduce risk of hypotension; if drug doesn't adequately control blood pressure, diuretics may be reinstated.
● Lower dosage or reduced dosing frequency is necessary in patients with impaired renal function. Titrate dose to effective levels over a 1- to 2-week interval, then reduce dose to lowest effective level.
● Several weeks of therapy may be required before beneficial effects of captopril are seen.
● Proteinuria and nephrotic syndrome may occur.
● Because ACE inhibitors can cause fetal harm or death, drug should be stopped as soon as pregnancy is detected.
● Captopril may cause false-positive results for urinary acetone.
● Overdose is manifested primarily by severe hypotension. After acute ingestion, empty stomach by induced emesis or gastric lavage. Follow with activated charcoal to reduce absorption.
● Treatment of overdose is usually symptomatic and supportive.
● In severe cases of overdose, hemodialysis may be considered.

Monitoring the patient

● Perform WBC and differential counts before treatment, every 2 weeks for 3 months, and then periodically. Monitor serum potassium levels because potassium retention has been noted.
● Monitor patient for adverse effects.

Information for the patient

● Tell patient to report feelings of light-headedness, especially in first few days, so dose can be adjusted; signs of infection such as sore throat or fever because drug may decrease WBC count; facial swelling or difficulty breathing because drug may cause angioedema; and loss of taste, which may necessitate discontinuing drug.
● Instruct patient to take captopril 1 hour before meals to prevent decreased absorption.
● Advise patient to avoid sudden position changes to minimize orthostatic hypotension.
● Warn patient to seek medical approval before taking OTC cold preparations.
● Tell patient that a persistent, dry cough may occur and usually doesn't subside until drug is stopped. Tell patient to call if this effect becomes bothersome.
● Instruct patient to call immediately if pregnancy occurs.

Geriatric patients

● Elderly patients may need lower doses because of impaired drug clearance. They may be more sensitive to captopril's hypotensive effects.

Pediatric patients

● Safety and efficacy in children haven't been established; use only if potential benefit outweighs risk.

Breast-feeding patients

● Drug appears in breast milk, but its effect on infants is unknown; use drug with caution in breast-feeding women.

carbachol
Carboptic, Isopto Carbachol, Miostat

Pharmacologic classification: cholinergic agonist
Therapeutic classification: miotic
Pregnancy risk category C

How supplied

Available by prescription only
Intraocular injection: 0.01%
Ophthalmic solution: 0.75%, 1.5%, 2.25%, 3%

Indications, route, and dosage

Ocular surgery (to produce pupillary miosis)
Adults: Instill 0.5 ml of 0.01% (intraocular form) gently into the anterior chamber for production of satisfactory miosis. May be instilled before or after securing sutures.
Open-angle or narrow-angle glaucoma
Adults: Instill 2 drops of 0.75% to 3% solution up to t.i.d.

Pharmacodynamics

Miotic action: Cholinergic activity causes contraction of the sphincter muscles of the iris, producing miosis, and contraction of the ciliary muscle, resulting in accommodation. Acts to deepen the anterior chamber and dilates conjunctival vessels of the outflow tract.

Pharmacokinetics
- *Absorption:* Action begins within 10 to 20 minutes and peaks in less than 4 hours.
- *Distribution:* No information available.
- *Metabolism:* No information available.
- *Excretion:* Duration of effect is usually about 8 hours.

Contraindications and precautions
Contraindicated in patients with hypersensitivity to drug and in those in whom cholinergic effects, such as constriction, are undesirable (such as acute iritis, some forms of secondary glaucoma, pupillary block glaucoma, or acute inflammatory disease of the anterior chamber of the eye).

Use cautiously in patients with acute heart failure, bronchial asthma, peptic ulcer, hyperthyroidism, GI spasm, Parkinson's disease, and urinary tract obstruction.

Interactions
Drug-drug. *Cyclopentolate, ophthalmic belladonna alkaloids (atropine, homatropine):* May interfere with antiglaucoma actions of carbachol. Use together cautiously.

Adverse reactions
CNS: headache, syncope.
CV: *arrhythmias,* hypotension.
EENT: spasm of eye accommodation, conjunctival vasodilation, eye and brow pain, transient stinging and burning, corneal clouding, bullous keratopathy, salivation.
GI: abdominal cramps, diarrhea.
GU: urinary urgency.
Respiratory: asthma.
Other: diaphoresis, flushing.

☑ Special considerations
- Drug is especially useful in glaucoma patients resistant or allergic to pilocarpine hydrochloride or nitrate.
- Premixed drugs should be used for single-dose intraocular use only.
- Discard unused portions of injectable drug.
- Signs and symptoms of overdose include miosis, flushing, vomiting, bradycardia, bronchospasm, increased bronchial secretion, sweating, tearing, involuntary urination, hypotension, and seizures.
- With accidental oral ingestion, vomiting is usually spontaneous; if not, induce emesis and follow with activated charcoal or a cathartic.
- Treat dermal exposure by washing the area twice with water.
- Treat CV or blood pressure responses with epinephrine. Atropine has been suggested as a direct antagonist for toxicity.

Monitoring the patient
- Perform periodic tonometric readings.
- Monitor blood pressure and ECG as indicated.

Information for the patient
- Tell patient with glaucoma that long-term use may be necessary. Stress compliance, and explain importance of medical supervision for tonometric readings before and during therapy.
- Instruct patient to apply finger pressure on the lacrimal sac 1 to 2 minutes after topical instillation of drug.
- Reassure patient that blurred vision usually diminishes with continued use.
- Teach patient how to instill eyedrops correctly, and warn patient not to touch eye or surrounding area with dropper.
- Warn patient not to drive for 1 or 2 hours after administration until effect on vision is determined.

carbamazepine
Atretol, Carbatrol, Epitol, Tegretol

Pharmacologic classification: iminostilbene derivative; chemically related to tricyclic antidepressants
Therapeutic classification: anticonvulsant, analgesic
Pregnancy risk category D

How supplied
Available by prescription only
Tablets: 200 mg
Tablets (chewable): 100 mg
Tablets (extended-release): 100 mg, 200 mg, 400 mg
Capsules (extended-release): 200 mg, 300 mg
Oral suspension: 100 mg/5 ml

Indications, route, and dosage
Generalized tonic-clonic, complex-partial, mixed seizure patterns
Adults and children over age 12: 200 mg P.O. b.i.d. or 100 mg P.O. q.i.d. of suspension on day 1. May increase by 200 mg/day P.O. at weekly intervals, in divided doses at 6- to 8-hour intervals. Adjust to minimum effective level when control is achieved; don't exceed 1,000 mg/day in children ages 12 to 15 or 1,200 mg/day in those over age 15. In rare instances, dosages up to 1,600 mg/day have been used in adults.

For extended-release capsules, initial dosage 200 mg P.O. b.i.d. Increase at weekly intervals by up to 200 mg/day until optimal response obtained. Dosage shouldn't exceed 1,000 mg/day in children ages 12 to 15 and 1,200 mg/day in those over 15. Some doses may be up to 1,600 mg/day for adults. Maintenance dose is usually 800 to 1,200 mg/day.
Children ages 6 to 12: Initially, 100 mg P.O. b.i.d. or 50 mg P.O. q.i.d. of suspension. Increase at

weekly intervals by adding 100 mg P.O. daily, first using a t.i.d. schedule and then q.i.d., if necessary. Adjust dosage based on patient response. Generally, dose shouldn't exceed 1,000 mg/day. Children taking total daily dosage of immediate-release form of 400 mg or more may be converted to same total daily dosage of extended-release capsules using a b.i.d. regimen.

Children under age 6: Initially, 10 to 20 mg/kg/day P.O. b.i.d. or t.i.d. as tablets or q.i.d. as suspension. Increase weekly to achieve optimal clinical response administered t.i.d. or q.i.d. There is no recommendation for safe administration at doses above 35 mg/kg/day. If optimal clinical response hasn't been achieved at a dose less than 35 mg/kg/day, plasma levels should be checked to determine if they're within therapeutic range.

Oral loading dose for rapid seizure control
Adults and children over age 12: 8 mg/kg of oral suspension.

◊ ***Bipolar affective disorder, intermittent explosive disorder***
Adults: Initially, 200 mg P.O. b.i.d.; increase, p.r.n., q 3 to 4 days. Maintenance dose may range from 600 to 1,600 mg/day.

Trigeminal neuralgia
Adults: 100 mg P.O. b.i.d. with meals on day 1. Increase by 100 mg q 12 hours until pain is relieved. Don't exceed 1.2 g daily. Maintenance dose is 200 to 1,200 mg P.O. daily. For extended-release capsules, 200 mg P.O. day 1. Daily dose may be increased by up to 200 mg/day q 12 hours, p.r.n., to achieve freedom from pain. Maintenance dose is usually 400 to 800 mg/day.

◊ ***Chorea***
Children: 15 to 25 mg/kg/day.

◊ ***Restless leg syndrome***
Adults: 100 to 300 mg h.s.

Pharmacodynamics
Anticonvulsant action: Mechanism unknown. Chemically unrelated to other anticonvulsants. The anticonvulsant activity appears principally to involve limitations of seizure propagation by reduction of posttetanic potentiation (PTP) of synaptic transmissions.

Analgesic action: In trigeminal neuralgia, drug is a specific analgesic through its reduction of synaptic neurotransmission.

Pharmacokinetics
● *Absorption:* Absorbed slowly from GI tract; plasma levels peak at 1½ hours (suspension), 4 to 6 hours (tablets), and 6 hours (extended-release).
● *Distribution:* Distributed widely throughout body; crosses placenta and accumulates in fetal tissue. About 75% is protein-bound. Therapeutic serum levels in adults are 4 to 12 mcg/ml; nystagmus can occur above 4 mcg/ml and ataxia, dizziness, and anorexia at or above 10 mcg/ml. Serum levels may be misleading because an unmeasured active metabolite also can cause toxicity. Carba-

mazepine levels in breast milk approach 60% of serum levels. Poor correlation between plasma levels and dose in children.
● *Metabolism:* Metabolized by liver to an active metabolite. May also induce its own metabolism; over time, higher doses are needed to maintain plasma levels. Half-life is initially 25 to 65 hours and 12 to 17 hours with multiple dosing.
● *Excretion:* Excreted in urine (70%) and feces (30%).

Contraindications and precautions
Contraindicated in patients with hypersensitivity to drug or tricyclic antidepressants or history of previous bone marrow suppression and in those who have taken an MAO inhibitor within 14 days of therapy. Use cautiously in patients with mixed-type seizure disorders.

Interactions
Drug-drug. *Calcium channel blockers (verapamil, possibly diltiazem):* May increase serum levels of carbamazepine significantly; decrease carbamazepine dosage by 40% to 50% when given with verapamil.

Cimetidine, clarithromycin, erythromycin, isoniazid, propoxyphene, valproic acid: May increase serum carbamazepine levels. Use cautiously; monitor carbamazepine levels.

Ethosuximide, haloperidol, phenytoin, valproic acid, warfarin: Carbamazepine may increase metabolism of these drugs. Monitor patient carefully.

Felbamate: Concomitant use may result in lower serum levels of either drug. Monitor patient and drug levels.

Fluoxetine, fluvoxamine: May increase carbamazepine levels. Monitor carbamazepine levels.

MAO inhibitors: Concomitant use may cause hypertensive crisis. Avoid concomitant use or use drug within 14 days of MAOs.

Oral contraceptives, theophylline: Carbamazepine may decrease effectiveness of these drugs. Monitor patient; suggest alternate method of contraception.

Phenobarbital, phenytoin, primidone: Lowers serum carbamazepine levels. Monitor serum carbamazepine level.

Drug-herb. *Psyllium seed:* Inhibits GI absorption. Avoid use together.

Adverse reactions
CNS: *dizziness, vertigo, drowsiness,* fatigue, *ataxia,* ***worsening of seizures*** (usually in patients with mixed-type seizure disorders, including atypical absence seizures), confusion, headache, syncope.
CV: ***heart failure,*** hypertension, hypotension, aggravation of coronary artery disease, ***arrhythmias,*** AV block.
EENT: conjunctivitis, dry mouth and pharynx, blurred vision, diplopia, nystagmus.

GI: *nausea, vomiting,* abdominal pain, diarrhea, anorexia, stomatitis, glossitis.
GU: urinary frequency, urine retention, impotence, albuminuria, glycosuria, elevated BUN.
Hematologic: *aplastic anemia, agranulocytosis,* eosinophilia, leukocytosis, *thrombocytopenia.*
Hepatic: abnormal liver function test results, *hepatitis.*
Respiratory: pulmonary hypersensitivity.
Skin: rash, urticaria, erythema multiforme, *Stevens-Johnson syndrome.*
Other: excessive diaphoresis, fever, chills, SIADH, decreased values of thyroid function tests.

☑ Special considerations
• Adjust drug dosage based on individual response.
• Chewable tablets are available for children.
• Unlabeled uses of carbamazepine include hypophyseal diabetes insipidus, certain psychiatric disorders, and management of alcohol withdrawal.
• For administering via a nasogastric tube, mix with an equal volume of diluent (D_5W or normal saline solution) and administer; then flush with 100 ml of diluent.
• Diazepam may control seizures but can exacerbate respiratory depression.
• Symptoms of overdose may include irregular breathing, respiratory depression, tachycardia, blood pressure changes, shock, arrhythmias, impaired consciousness (ranging to deep coma), seizures, restlessness, drowsiness, psychomotor disturbances, nausea, vomiting, anuria, or oliguria.
• Treat overdose with repeated gastric lavage, especially if patient ingested alcohol concurrently. Oral charcoal and laxatives may hasten excretion.
• In overdose, carefully monitor vital signs, ECG, and fluid and electrolyte balance.

Monitoring the patient
• Hematologic toxicity is rare but serious. Routinely monitor hematologic and liver functions.
• Monitor patient for adverse effects.

Information for the patient
• Remind patient to store drug in a cool, dry place; not in medicine cabinet. Reduced bioavailability has been reported with use of improperly stored tablets.
• Tell patient that drug may cause GI distress. Patient should take drug with food at equally spaced intervals.
• Warn patient not to stop drug abruptly.
• Encourage patient to promptly report unusual bleeding, bruising, jaundice, dark urine, pale stools, abdominal pain, impotence, fever, chills, sore throat, mouth ulcers, edema, or disturbances in mood, alertness, or coordination.

• Emphasize importance of follow-up laboratory tests and continued medical supervision. Periodic eye examinations are recommended.
• Warn patient that drug may cause drowsiness, dizziness, and blurred vision. Patient should avoid hazardous activities that require alertness, especially during first week of therapy and when dosage is increased.
• Remind patient to shake suspension well before using.
• Tell patient, if necessary, that the Carbatrol capsule can be opened and its contents sprinkled over food (such as a teaspoon of applesauce), but the capsule or its contents should never be crushed or chewed.

Geriatric patients
• Drug may activate latent psychosis, confusion, or agitation in elderly patients; use with caution.

Pediatric patients
• Safety and efficacy haven't been established for children under age 6 in doses higher than 35 mg/kg/day.

Breast-feeding patients
• Significant amounts of drug appear in breast milk; alternative feeding method is recommended during therapy.

carbamide peroxide
Auro Ear Drops, Debrox, Gly-Oxide Liquid, Murine Ear, Orajel, Orajel Perioseptic, Proxigel

Pharmacologic classification: urea hydrogen peroxide
Therapeutic classification: ceruminolytic, topical antiseptic
Pregnancy risk category C

How supplied
Available without a prescription
Otic solution: 6.5% carbamide in glycerin or glycerin and propylene glycol
Oral solution: 10% carbamide with glycerin and propylene glycol; 15% with anhydrous glycerin, methylparaben, and propylene glycol
Oral gel: 10% carbamide in water-free gel base

Indications, route, and dosage
Impacted cerumen
Adults and children ages 12 and older: 5 to 10 drops otic solution into ear canal b.i.d. for 3 to 4 days.
Inflammation or irritation of lips, mouth, gums
Adults and children over age 3: Apply several drops of undiluted oral solution to affected area or place 10 drops on tongue (mix with saliva, swish for several minutes and expectorate after 1 to 3 minutes) after meals and h.s.

Children: Apply undiluted gel to affected area (massage into area with finger or swab) q.i.d.

Pharmacodynamics
Ceruminolytic action: Emulsifies and disperses accumulated cerumen.
Antiseptic action: Releases oxygen upon contact with oral mucosa, which results in a cleansing and mild anti-inflammatory action.

Pharmacokinetics
No information available.

Contraindications and precautions
Contraindicated in patients with a perforated eardrum.

Interactions
None reported.

Adverse reactions
GI: oral irritation or inflammation.

☑ Special considerations
• Don't use to treat swimmer's ear or itching of ear canal and if patient has perforated eardrum.
• Irrigation of ear may be necessary to aid removal of cerumen.
• Tip of dropper shouldn't touch ear or ear canal when using otic preparation.
• Remove cerumen remaining after instillation by using a soft rubber-bulb otic syringe to gently irrigate ear canal with warm water.
• Signs and symptoms of overdose include mild irritation to mucosal tissue or, if swallowed, irritation, inflammation, and burns in the mouth, throat, esophagus, or stomach. Gastric distention may result from liberation of oxygen.
• Accidental ocular exposure causes immediate pain and irritation, but severe injury is rare. Irrigate eyes with large amounts of warm water for at least 15 minutes.
• Accidental dermal exposure bleaches exposed area. Wash exposed skin twice with soap and water.
• Treat oral exposure by immediate dilution with water. Spontaneous vomiting may occur.

Monitoring the patient
• Evaluate patient for persistence of symptoms (redness, pain, swelling).
• Before using drug. ascertain that patient doesn't have a perforated eardrum.

Information for the patient
• Teach patient correct way to use product.
• Tell patient to call if inflammation or irritation persists.
• Warn patient not to use otic form for more than 4 consecutive days and to avoid contact with eyes.

• Instruct patient to keep otic solution in ear for at least 15 minutes by tilting head sideways or putting cotton in ear.
• Tell patient not to rinse mouth or drink for 5 minutes after use.

Pediatric patients
• Oral preparations shouldn't be self-administered by children under age 3; otic forms shouldn't be self-administered by children under age 12.

carboplatin
Paraplatin

Pharmacologic classification: alkylating drug (cell-cycle–phase nonspecific)
Therapeutic classification: antineoplastic
Pregnancy risk category D

How supplied
Available by prescription only
Injection: 50-mg, 150-mg, 450-mg vials

Indications, route, and dosage
Initial and secondary (palliative) treatment of ovarian carcinoma; ◊ retinoblastoma; ◊ advanced bladder cancer; ◊ lung cancer; ◊ head and neck cancer; ◊ Wilms' tumor; ◊ primary brain tumor; ◊ testicular neoplasm
Adults: Initial recommended dose for single-drug therapy is 360 mg/m² I.V. on day 1. Dose is repeated q 4 weeks. In combination therapy (with cyclophosphamide), give 300 mg/m² I.V. on day 1 q 4 weeks for 6 cycles.
✦ *Dosage adjustment.* Dosage adjustments are based on the lowest posttreatment platelet or neutrophil value obtained in weekly blood counts.
  In patients with impaired renal function, initial recommended dose is 250 mg/m² for creatinine clearance levels between 41 and 59 ml/minute; for creatinine clearance levels between 16 and 40 ml/minute, dose is 200 mg/m².

Lowest platelet count (per mm³)	Lowest neutrophil count (per mm³)	Adjusted dose
> 100,000	> 2,000	125%
50,000 to 100,000	500 to 2,000	No adjustment
< 50,000	< 500	75%

Pharmacodynamics
Antitumor action: Causes cross-linking of DNA strands.

Pharmacokinetics
• *Absorption:* Administered I.V.

• *Distribution:* Volume of distribution is about equal to total body water. Drug isn't protein-bound but degraded to platinum-containing products, which are 87% protein-bound at 24 hours.
• *Metabolism:* Hydrolyzed to form hydroxylated and aquated species. Half-life is 2 to 3 hours; terminal half-life for platinum is 4 to 6 days.
• *Excretion:* 65% excreted by kidneys within 12 hours, 71% within 24 hours. Enterohepatic recirculation may occur.

Contraindications and precautions
Contraindicated in patients with history of hypersensitivity to cisplatin, platinum-containing compounds, or mannitol and in those with severe bone marrow suppression or bleeding.

Interactions
Drug-drug. *Nephrotoxic drugs:* Concomitant use produces additive nephrotoxicity of carboplatin. Monitor patient closely.

Adverse reactions
CNS: dizziness, confusion, peripheral neuropathy, ototoxicity, central neurotoxicity, paresthesia, *CVA,* asthenia.
CV: *cardiac failure, embolism.*
EENT: visual disturbances, change in taste.
GI: constipation, diarrhea, *nausea, vomiting.*
GU: increased BUN and creatinine levels.
Hematologic: THROMBOCYTOPENIA, *leukopenia,* NEUTROPENIA, *anemia,* BONE MARROW SUPPRESSION.
Hepatic: increased AST or alkaline phosphatase levels.
Metabolic: decreased serum electrolyte levels.
Other: alopecia, hypersensitivity reactions, pain, *anaphylaxis.*

☑ Special considerations
• Reconstitute with D5W, normal saline solution, or sterile water for injection to make a concentration of 10 mg/ml.
• Drug can be further diluted to concentrations as low as 0.5 mg/ml using normal saline solution or D5W. Infuse over at least 15 minutes.
• Store unopened vials at room temperature. Once reconstituted and diluted as directed, solution is stable at room temperature for 8 hours. Because drug doesn't contain antibacterial preservatives, unused drug should be discarded after 8 hours.
• Don't use needles or I.V. administration sets containing aluminum because drug may precipitate and lose potency.
• Although drug is promoted as causing less nausea and vomiting than cisplatin, it can cause severe emesis. Administer antiemetic therapy.
• Carboplatin administration requires supervision of a physician experienced in using chemotherapeutic drugs.

• Symptoms of overdose result from bone marrow suppression or hepatotoxicity. There is no known antidote for carboplatin overdose.

Monitoring the patient
• Peripheral blood counts should be frequently monitored during therapy and when appropriate until recovery is achieved.
• Monitor BUN, creatinine, AST or alkaline phosphatase levels, and electrolytes.

Information for the patient
• Stress importance of adequate fluid intake and increase in urine output, to facilitate uric acid excretion.
• Tell patient to report tinnitus immediately to prevent permanent hearing loss. Patient should have audiometric testing before initial and subsequent course.
• Advise patient to avoid exposure to people with infections.
• Instruct patient to promptly report unusual bleeding or bruising.
• Advise woman to use contraception during therapy and to call if pregnancy is suspected.

Geriatric patients
• Patients over age 65 are at greater risk for neurotoxicity.

Pediatric patients
• Safety in children hasn't been established.

Breast-feeding patients
• It's unknown if carboplatin appears in breast milk; however, because of potential for toxicity to infant, breast-feeding should be discontinued.

carisoprodol
Soma

Pharmacologic classification: carbamate derivative
Therapeutic classification: skeletal muscle relaxant
Pregnancy risk category NR

How supplied
Available by prescription only
Tablets: 350 mg

Indications, route, and dosage
Adjunct for relief of discomfort in acute, painful musculoskeletal conditions
Adults and children over age 12: Administer 350 mg P.O. t.i.d. and h.s.

Pharmacodynamics
Skeletal muscle relaxant action: Exact mechanism unknown. Doesn't relax skeletal muscle directly but apparently as a result of its sedative ef-

fects. Drug possibly modifies central perception of pain without eliminating peripheral pain reflexes and has slight antipyretic activity.

Pharmacokinetics
• *Absorption:* With usual therapeutic doses, onset of action occurs within 30 minutes and persists 4 to 6 hours.
• *Distribution:* Widely distributed throughout body.
• *Metabolism:* Metabolized in liver. May induce microsomal enzymes in liver; half-life is 8 hours.
• *Excretion:* Excreted in urine mainly as its metabolites; less than 1% of dose is excreted unchanged. Drug may be removed by hemodialysis or peritoneal dialysis.

Contraindications and precautions
Contraindicated in patients with hypersensitivity to related compounds (such as meprobamate or tybamate) and in those with intermittent porphyria. Use cautiously in patients with impaired renal or hepatic function.

Interactions
Drug-drug. *Other CNS depressants (antipsychotics, anxiolytics, general anesthetics, opioid analgesics, tricyclic antidepressants):* Produces additive CNS depression. Exercise care to avoid overdose; dosage adjustments may be needed.
Drug-lifestyle. *Alcohol:* Produces additive CNS depression. Discourage use.

Adverse reactions
CNS: *drowsiness, dizziness,* vertigo, ataxia, tremor, agitation, irritability, headache, depressive reactions, insomnia.
CV: orthostatic hypotension, tachycardia, facial flushing.
GI: nausea, vomiting, hiccups, epigastric distress.
Hematologic: eosinophilia.
Respiratory: asthmatic episodes.
Skin: rash, *erythema multiforme,* pruritus.
Other: fever, angioedema, *anaphylaxis.*

☑ Special considerations
• Use with caution with other CNS depressants; effects may be cumulative.
• Initially, allergic or idiosyncratic reactions may occur (first to fourth dose). Symptoms usually subside after several hours; treat with supportive and symptomatic measures.
• Psychological dependence may follow long-term use.
• Withdrawal symptoms (abdominal cramps, insomnia, chills, headache, and nausea) may occur with abrupt termination of drug after prolonged use of higher-than-recommended doses.
• Commercially available formulations may contain sodium metabisulfite, which may cause an allergic reaction.

• Signs and symptoms of overdose include exaggerated CNS depression, stupor, coma, shock, and respiratory depression.
• Treatment of overdose in conscious patient requires emptying stomach by emesis or gastric lavage; activated charcoal may be used after gastric lavage to adsorb any remaining drug. If patient is comatose, secure endotracheal tube with cuff inflated before gastric lavage. Provide supportive therapy by maintaining adequate airway and assisted ventilation.
• In overdose, CNS stimulants and pressor drugs should be used cautiously. Monitor vital signs, fluid and electrolyte levels, and neurologic status closely.

Monitoring the patient
• Monitor urine output and avoid overhydration in overdose. Forced diuresis using mannitol, peritoneal dialysis, or hemodialysis may be beneficial. Continue to monitor patient for relapse from incomplete gastric emptying and delayed absorption.
• Monitor vital signs.
• Observe for adverse effects.

Information for the patient
• Inform patient that drug may cause dizziness and faintness. Symptoms may be controlled by making position changes slowly and in stages. Patient should report persistent symptoms.
• Tell patient to avoid alcoholic beverages and to use cough or cold preparations containing alcohol cautiously while taking this drug. Patient should also avoid other CNS depressants (effects may be additive) unless prescribed.
• Warn patient drug may cause drowsiness. Avoid hazardous activities that require alertness until CNS depressant effects can be determined.
• Advise patient to stop drug immediately and to call if rash, diplopia, dizziness, or other unusual signs or symptoms appear.
• Tell patient to store drug away from direct heat and light (not in bathroom medicine cabinet).
• Instruct patient to take missed dose only if remembered within 1 hour. If remembered later, patient should skip that dose and go back to regular schedule. Patient shouldn't double the dose.
• Tell patient that drug may be taken with food to avoid GI upset.

Geriatric patients
• Elderly patients may be more sensitive to drug's effects.

Pediatric patients
• Safety and efficacy haven't been established in children under age 12. However, some clinicians suggest a dosage of 25 mg/kg or 750 mg/m^2 divided q.i.d. for children ages 5 and older.

Breast-feeding patients
• Carisoprodol may appear in breast milk at two to four times maternal plasma levels.

carmustine (BCNU)
BiCNU, Gliadel

Pharmacologic classification: alkylating drug; nitrosourea (cell-cycle–phase nonspecific)
Therapeutic classification: antineoplastic
Pregnancy risk category D

How supplied
Available by prescription only
Injection: 100-mg vial (lyophilized), with a 3-ml vial of absolute alcohol supplied as a diluent
Implant: 7.7 mg wafer

Indications, route, and dosage
Dosage and indications may vary. Check current literature for recommended protocol.
◊ *Brain,* ◊ *breast,* ◊ *GI tract,* ◊ *lung,;* ◊ *hepatic cancer; Hodgkin's disease; malignant lymphomas;* ◊ *malignant melanomas; multiple myeloma*
Adults: 75 to 100 mg/m² I.V. by slow infusion daily for 2 consecutive days, repeated q 6 weeks if platelet count is above 100,000/mm³ and WBC count is above 4,000/mm³.
✦ *Dosage adjustment.* Reduce dosage, p.r.n., using the following guidelines.

Nadir after prior dose		Percentage of prior dose to be given
Leukocytes/mm³	Platelets/mm³	
> 4,000	>100,000	100%
3,000 to 3,999	75,000 to 99,999	100%
2,000 to 2,999	25,000 to 74,999	70%
< 2,000	< 25,000	50%

Alternative therapy: 150 to 200 mg/m² I.V. slow infusion as a single dose, repeated q 6 to 8 weeks.
Recurrent glioblastoma and metastatic brain tumors (adjunct to surgery to prolong survival)
Adults: Implant 8 wafers in the resection cavity if allowed by size and shape of cavity.

Pharmacodynamics
Antineoplastic action: Cytotoxic action of drug is mediated through its metabolites, which inhibit several enzymes involved with DNA formation. Drug can also cause cross-linking of DNA. Cross-linking interferes with DNA, RNA, and protein synthesis. Cross-resistance between carmustine and lomustine has occurred.

Pharmacokinetics
• *Absorption:* Not absorbed across GI tract. Implant wafers are biodegradable in the brain when implanted into tumor resection cavity.
• *Distribution:* Cleared rapidly from plasma. After I.V. administration, carmustine and its metabolites distribute rapidly into CSF.
• *Metabolism:* Metabolized extensively in liver.
• *Excretion:* About 60% to 70% of drug and its metabolites excreted in urine within 96 hours, 6% to 10% excreted as carbon dioxide by lungs, and 1% excreted in feces. Enterohepatic circulation and protein-binding can occur and may cause delayed hematologic toxicity.
Note: Absorption, distribution, metabolism, and excretion of copolymer in implant wafer is unknown.

Contraindications and precautions
Contraindicated in patients with hypersensitivity to drug. Use with caution in pregnant women due to risk to the fetus.

Interactions
Drug-drug. *Cimetidine:* Increases bone marrow toxicity of carmustine. Avoid use together.
Digoxin: Serum levels may decrease. Monitor serum digoxin level.
Phenytoin: Serum level may decrease. Monitor serum phenytoin level.

Adverse reactions
CNS: ataxia, drowsiness.
EENT: ocular toxicities.
GI: *nausea* beginning in 2 to 6 hours (can be severe), vomiting.
GU: nephrotoxicity, azotemia, *renal failure.*
Hematologic: *cumulative bone marrow suppression* (delayed 4 to 6 weeks, lasting 1 to 2 weeks); *leukopenia; thrombocytopenia; acute leukemia, bone marrow dysplasia* (after long-term use); anemia.
Hepatic: hepatotoxicity.
Respiratory: *pulmonary fibrosis.*
Skin: facial flushing, hyperpigmentation.
Other: *intense pain at infusion site from venous spasm;* possible hyperuricemia (in lymphoma patients when rapid cell lysis occurs).

☑ Special considerations
• Use double gloves and surgical instruments dedicated to the handling of implant wafers.
• Reconstitute 100-mg vial with the 3 ml of absolute alcohol provided by manufacturer; then dilute further with 27 ml sterile water for injection. Resultant solution contains 3.3 mg carmustine/ml in 10% ethanol. Dilute in normal saline or D₅W for I.V. infusion. Give at least 250 ml over 1 to 2 hours. Discard excess drug.

• Wear gloves to administer drug infusion and when changing I.V. tubing. Avoid contact with skin because carmustine will cause a brown stain. If drug comes into contact with skin, wash off thoroughly.

• Solution is unstable in plastic I.V. bags. Administer only in glass containers.

• Carmustine may decompose at temperatures above 80° F (26.6° C).

• If powder liquefies or appears oily, discard it because it's a sign of decomposition.

• Reconstituted solution may be stored in refrigerator for 24 hours (48 hours if reconstituted to 0.2 mg/ml in D_5W or normal saline solution).

• Don't mix with other drugs during administration.

• Avoid I.M. injections when platelet count is below 100,000/mm³.

• To reduce pain on infusion, dilute further or slow infusion rate.

• Intense flushing of skin may occur during I.V. infusion but usually disappears within 2 to 4 hours.

• To reduce nausea, give antiemetic before administering.

• Pulmonary toxicity is more likely in people who smoke.

• At first sign of extravasation, stop infusion and infiltrate area with liberal injections of 0.5 mEq/ml sodium bicarbonate solution.

• Drug has been applied topically in concentrations of 0.05% to 0.4% to treat mycosis fungoides.

• Because drug crosses blood-brain barrier, it may be used to treat primary brain tumors.

• Advise women of childbearing age to avoid pregnancy. Pregnant women should be informed of hazard to fetus.

• Signs and symptoms of overdose include leukopenia, thrombocytopenia, nausea, and vomiting.

• Treatment of overdose consists of supportive measures, including transfusion of blood components, antibiotics for infections that may develop, and antiemetics.

Monitoring the patient
• Monitor patient's CBC weekly for at least 6 weeks after a dose.

• Prescribe anticoagulants and aspirin products cautiously. Monitor patient closely for signs of bleeding.

• Liver and renal function tests should be monitored periodically.

• Baseline pulmonary function studies, along with frequent pulmonary function tests, should be conducted during treatment. Patients with a baseline below 70% of the predicted forced vital capacity or diffusing capacity for carbon monoxide (ml/min/mm Hg) are particularly at risk.

Information for the patient
• Warn patient to watch for signs of infection and bone marrow toxicity (fever, sore throat, anemia, fatigue, easy bruising, nose or gum bleeds, melena). Patient should take temperature daily.

• Remind patient to return for follow-up blood work weekly, or as needed, and to watch for signs and symptoms of infection.

• Advise patient to avoid exposure to people with infections.

• Tell patient to avoid OTC products containing aspirin because they may precipitate bleeding. Advise patient to report signs of bleeding promptly.

• Advise woman to avoid becoming pregnant and to call if pregnancy is suspected.

Pediatric patients
• Safety and effectiveness in children haven't been established.

Breast-feeding patients
• Active metabolites of drug appear in breast milk. It isn't advisable for women receiving drug to breast-feed their infants because of risk of serious adverse reactions, mutagenicity, and carcinogenicity in infant.

carteolol hydrochloride
Cartrol, Ocupress

Pharmacologic classification: beta blocker
Therapeutic classification: antihypertensive
Pregnancy risk category C

How supplied
Available by prescription only
Tablets: 2.5 mg, 5 mg
Ophthalmic solution: 1%

Indications, route, and dosage
Hypertension
Adults: Initially, 2.5 mg as a single daily dose. Gradually increase the dosage as required to 5 mg daily or 10 mg daily as a single dose.
◊ *Angina*
Adults: 10 mg/day.
✦ *Dosage adjustment.* Patients with substantial renal failure should receive the usual dose of carteolol scheduled at longer intervals as shown.

Creatinine clearance (ml/min)	Dosage interval (hours)
> 60	24
20 to 60	48
< 20	72

Open-angle glaucoma
Adults: 1 drop b.i.d. in eye.

Reactions may be *common*, uncommon, *life-threatening*, or COMMON AND LIFE-THREATENING.

Pharmacodynamics

Antihypertensive action: Nonselective beta blocker with intrinsic sympathomimetic activity (ISA). Its antihypertensive effects are probably caused by decreased sympathetic outflow from the brain and decreased cardiac output. Carteolol doesn't have a consistent effect on renin output.

Pharmacokinetics

• *Absorption:* Absorbed rapidly, achieving peak plasma levels in 1 to 3 hours. Bioavailability is about 85%.
• *Distribution:* 20% to 30% bound to plasma proteins.
• *Metabolism:* 30% to 50% of drug metabolized in liver to 8-hydroxycarteolol, an active metabolite, and the inactive metabolite glucuronoside.
• *Excretion:* Primarily renal. Plasma half-life is about 6 hours.

Contraindications and precautions

Contraindicated in patients with hypersensitivity to any component of drug and in those with bronchial asthma, severe COPD, sinus bradycardia, second- or third-degree AV block, overt cardiac failure, or cardiogenic shock.

Use cautiously in patients with nonallergic bronchospastic disease, diabetes mellitus, hyperthyroidism, or decreased pulmonary function and in breast-feeding women.

Interactions

Drug-drug. *Beta blockers, oral calcium antagonists:* Enhanced risk of hypotension, left-sided heart failure, and AV conduction disturbances. Avoid concurrent use.
Catecholamine-depleting drugs such as reserpine: May have an additive effect when given with a beta blocker. Monitor patient closely.
General anesthetics: Enhanced risk of hypotension. Observe carefully for excessive hypotension or bradycardia and for orthostatic hypotension.
Insulin, oral antidiabetics: Affect serum glucose level. Monitor serum glucose level; dosages may need adjustment.
I.V. calcium antagonists: Increased risk of hypotension. Use with caution.

Adverse reactions

CNS: lassitude, fatigue, somnolence, *asthenia, paresthesia.*
CV: *conduction disturbances.*
EENT: transient irritation, conjunctival hyperemia, *edema.*
GI: diarrhea, nausea, abdominal pain.
Musculoskeletal: *muscle cramps,* arthralgia.
Skin: rash.

☑ Special considerations

Besides the recommendations relevant to all beta blockers, consider the following.
• Dosage over 10 mg daily doesn't produce a greater response; it may actually decrease response.
• Food may slow the rate, but not the extent, of carteolol absorption.
• Steady-state levels are reached rapidly (within 1 to 2 days) in patients with normal renal function.
• No overdose information available. Probable symptoms are bradycardia, bronchospasm, heart failure, and hypotension.
• Atropine should be used to treat symptomatic bradycardia. If no response is seen, cautiously use isoproterenol. Bronchospasm should be treated with a beta$_2$-agonist, such as isoproterenol or theophylline. Cardiac glycosides or diuretics may be useful in treating heart failure. Vasopressors (epinephrine, dopamine, or norepinephrine) should be given to combat hypotension.

Monitoring the patient

• Monitor vital signs and ECG.
• Monitor patient for therapeutic response.

Information for the patient

• Advise patient to take drug exactly as prescribed and not to stop drug suddenly.
• Advise patient to report shortness of breath or difficulty breathing, unusually fast heartbeat, cough, or fatigue with exertion.
• Inform patient that transient stinging or discomfort may occur with ophthalmic use; if reaction is severe, tell patient to call immediately.

Pediatric patients

• Safety in children hasn't been established.

Breast-feeding patients

• Drug may appear in breast milk. Use with caution in breast-feeding women.

---

carvedilol
Coreg

Pharmacologic classification: alpha$_1$-nonselective beta blocker
Therapeutic classification: antihypertensive, adjunct treatment for heart failure
Pregnancy risk category C

How supplied

Available by prescription only
Tablets: 3.125 mg, 6.25 mg, 12.5 mg, 25 mg

Indications, route, and dosage

Hypertension

Adults: Dosage individualized. Initially, 6.25 mg P.O. b.i.d. with food; obtain standing systolic pressure 1 hour after initial dose. If tolerated, continue dosage for 7 to 14 days. Can increase to 12.5 mg P.O. b.i.d., repeating monitoring protocol as above. Maximum dosage is 25 mg P.O. b.i.d., as tolerated.

Heart failure
Adults: Dosage individualized and titrated carefully. Stabilize dosing of cardiac glycosides, diuretics, and ACE inhibitors before starting therapy. Initially, 3.125 mg P.O. b.i.d. with food for 2 weeks; if tolerated, can increase to 6.25 mg P.O. b.i.d. for 2 weeks. Dose can be doubled q 2 weeks to highest level tolerated by patient. At initiation of new dose, observe patient for dizziness or light-headedness for 1 hour. Maximum dosing for patients weighing less than 85 kg (187 lb) is 25 mg P.O. b.i.d.; for those weighing over 85 kg, give 50 mg P.O. b.i.d.

Pharmacodynamics
Antihypertensive action: Mechanism unknown. Beta blockade shown to reduce cardiac output and tachycardia. Alpha blockade is demonstrated by the attenuated pressor effects of phenylephrine, vasodilation, and decreases in peripheral vascular resistance.
Heart failure: Exact mechanism unknown. Has been shown to decrease systemic blood pressure, pulmonary artery pressure, right atrial pressure, systemic vascular resistance, and heart rate while increasing stroke volume index.

Pharmacokinetics
• *Absorption:* Rapidly and extensively metabolized following oral administration; absolute bioavailability of 25% to 35% due to significant first-pass metabolism. Mean terminal elimination half-life ranges from 7 to 10 hours.
• *Distribution:* Plasma levels proportional to oral dose administered. Absorption slowed when administered with food, as evidenced by delay in time to reach peak plasma levels with no significant difference in extent of bioavailability.
• *Metabolism:* Extensively metabolized, primarily by aromatic ring oxidation and glucuronidation. Oxidative metabolites further metabolized by conjugation via glucuronidation and sulfation. Demethylation and hydroxylation at phenol ring produce 3 active metabolites with beta-blocking activity.
• *Excretion:* Metabolites primarily excreted via bile into feces. Less than 2% of dose excreted unchanged in urine.

Contraindications and precautions
Contraindicated in patients with hypersensitivity to drug and in those with New York Heart Association (NYHA) class IV decompensated cardiac failure requiring I.V. inotropic therapy, bronchial asthma or related bronchospastic conditions, second- or third-degree AV block, sick sinus syndrome (unless a permanent pacemaker is in place), cardiogenic shock, severe bradycardia.

Drug isn't recommended for patients with hepatic impairment.
Use cautiously in hypertensive patients with left-sided heart failure, perioperative patients who receive anesthetics that depress myocardial function (such as ether, cyclopropane, trichloroethylene), diabetic patients receiving insulin or oral antidiabetics, and those subject to spontaneous hypoglycemia. Also use with caution in patients with thyroid disease (may mask hyperthyroidism, and drug withdrawal may precipitate thyroid storm or an exacerbation of hyperthyroidism), pheochromocytoma, Prinzmetal's variant angina, or peripheral vascular disease (may precipitate or aggravate symptoms of arterial insufficiency).

Interactions
Drug-drug. *Calcium channel blockers:* Can cause isolated conduction disturbances. Monitor ECG and blood pressure.
Catecholamine-depleting drugs (such as MAO inhibitors, reserpine): May cause severe bradycardia or hypotension. Use together cautiously.
Cimetidine: Increases bioavailability by 30%. Use together cautiously.
Clonidine: May potentiate blood pressure and heart rate–lowering effects. If patient is receiving beta blockers and clonidine, stop beta blocker first, then clonidine several days later by titration.
Digoxin: Serum digoxin levels increase about 15% with concurrent therapy. Monitor patient, especially digoxin levels.
Inhibitors of cytochrome P-2D6 (fluoxetine, paroxetine, propafenone, quinidine): Possible increased carvedilol levels. Monitor carvedilol levels.
Insulin, oral antidiabetics: May enhance hypoglycemic properties. Monitor blood glucose levels.
Rifampin: Reduces plasma levels of carvedilol by 70%. Monitor patient carefully.

Adverse reactions
CNS: malaise, *dizziness, fatigue,* headache, hypesthesia, insomnia, pain, paresthesia, somnolence, vertigo.
CV: aggravated angina pectoris, *AV block, bradycardia,* chest pain, fluid overload, hypertension, hypotension, orthostatic hypertension, syncope.
EENT: abnormal vision.
GI: abdominal pain, *diarrhea,* melena, nausea, periodontitis, vomiting.
GU: abnormal renal function, albuminuria, hematuria, impotence, urinary tract infection.
Hematologic: decreased PT, purpura, *thrombocytopenia.*
Hepatic: increased ALT, AST levels.
Metabolic: dehydration, glycosuria, gout, hypercholesterolemia, *hyperglycemia,* hypertriglyceridemia, hypervolemia, hyperuricemia, hypoglycemia, hyponatremia, weight gain, increased alkaline phosphatase, BUN, or nonprotein nitrogen levels.

Reactions may be *common,* uncommon, *life-threatening,* or COMMON AND LIFE-THREATENING.

Musculoskeletal: arthralgia, back pain, myalgia.
Respiratory: bronchitis, dyspnea, pharyngitis, rhinitis, sinusitis, *upper respiratory tract infection.*
Other: allergy, edema, fever, hypovolemia, peripheral edema, ***sudden death,*** viral infection.

☑ Special considerations
● Mild hepatocellular injury may occur during therapy. At first sign of hepatic dysfunction, perform tests for hepatic injury or jaundice; if present, stop drug.
● Discontinue drug gradually over 1 to 2 weeks. Decrease dosage if heart rate is below 55 beats/minute.
● Patients on beta blocker therapy with history of severe anaphylactic reaction to several allergens may be more reactive to repeated challenge, either accidental, diagnostic, or therapeutic. They may be unresponsive to the usual doses of epinephrine used to treat allergic reactions.
● Overdose may cause severe hypotension, bradycardia, cardiac insufficiency, cardiogenic shock, and cardiac arrest. Respiratory effects, bronchospasm, vomiting, lapses of consciousness, and generalized seizures may also occur.
● Gastric lavage or pharmacologically induced emesis may be effective shortly after ingestion. May use atropine 2 mg I.V. for bradycardia, glucagon 5 to 10 mg I.V. rapidly over 30 seconds, then continuous infusion at 5 mg/hour; sympathomimetics (dobutamine, isoprenaline, adrenaline) at doses based on body weight and effect.
● If peripheral vasodilation dominates, administer epinephrine or norepinephrine, if necessary, and continuously monitor circulatory conditions.
● For therapy-resistant bradycardia, perform pacemaker therapy.
● For bronchospasm, give beta-sympathomimetics by aerosol or I.V. or aminophylline I.V.
● If seizures occur, slow I.V. injection of diazepam or clonazepam may be effective.
● If severe intoxication and symptoms of shock occur, continue treatment with antidotes for a sufficiently long period of time consistent with the drug's 7- to 10-hour half-life.

Monitoring the patient
● Monitor heart failure patient for worsened condition, renal dysfunction, or fluid retention; diuretics may need to be increased. Also monitor diabetic patient because hyperglycemia may be worsened.
● In patients with low blood pressure (systolic blood pressure below 100 mm Hg), ischemic heart disease, diffuse vascular disease, or underlying renal insufficiency, it's recommended that renal function be monitored during up-titration of carvedilol.
● Monitor blood glucose level when carvedilol therapy is initiated, adjusted, or discontinued in congestive heart failure patients with diabetes.

Information for the patient
● Tell patient not to interrupt or stop drug without medical approval.
● Advise heart failure patient to call if weight gain or shortness of breath occurs.
● Inform patient that he may experience lowered blood pressure when standing. If dizziness and fainting (rare) occur, advise patient to sit or lie down.
● Caution patient against performing hazardous tasks during initiation of therapy. If dizziness or fatigue occur, tell patient to call for an adjustment in dosage.
● Tell patient to take drug with food.
● Advise diabetic patient to report changes in blood glucose level promptly.
● Inform patient who wears contact lenses that decreased lacrimation may occur.

Geriatric patients
● Monitor plasma levels carefully; drug levels are about 50% higher in elderly compared with younger adult patients.
● No significant difference between older and younger patients was found in adverse effects; dizziness was slightly more common in elderly patients.

Pediatric patients
● Safety of drug in patients under age 18 hasn't been established.

Breast-feeding patients
● It's unknown if drug appears in breast milk; use drug cautiously.

---

cascara sagrada
cascara sagrada aromatic fluidextract

Pharmacologic classification: anthraquinone glycoside mixture
Therapeutic classification: laxative
Pregnancy risk category C

How supplied
Available without a prescription
Tablets: 325 mg
Aromatic fluidextract: 1 g/ml with 18% alcohol

Indications, route, and dosage
Acute constipation, preparation for bowel or rectal examination
Adults: 1 tablet P.O. h.s.
Children ages 2 to 12: ½ of adult dose.
Children under age 2: ¼ of adult dose.

Pharmacodynamics
Laxative action: Obtained from the dried bark of the buckthorn tree *(Rhamnus purshiana),* con-

tains cascarosides A and B (barbaloin glycosides) and cascarosides C and D (chrysaloin glycosides). Exerts a direct irritant action on the colon that promotes peristalsis and bowel motility. Enhances colonic fluid accumulation, thus increasing laxative effect.

Pharmacokinetics
• *Absorption:* Minimal drug absorption in small intestine. Onset of action usually occurs in about 6 to 12 hours but may not occur for 3 or 4 days.
• *Distribution:* May be distributed in bile, saliva, and colonic mucosa.
• *Metabolism:* Metabolized in liver.
• *Excretion:* Excreted in feces via biliary elimination, in urine, or in both.

Contraindications and precautions
Contraindicated in patients with abdominal pain, nausea, vomiting, or other symptoms of appendicitis or acute surgical abdomen; acute surgical delirium; fecal impaction; or intestinal obstruction or perforation. Use cautiously in patients with rectal bleeding.

Interactions
None reported.

Adverse reactions
GI: *nausea;* vomiting; diarrhea; loss of normal bowel function with excessive use; *abdominal cramps,* especially in severe constipation; malabsorption of nutrients; "cathartic colon" (syndrome resembling ulcerative colitis radiologically and pathologically) with chronic misuse; discoloration of rectal mucosa after long-term use.
Metabolic: hypokalemia, protein enteropathy, electrolyte imbalance (with excessive use).
Other: laxative dependence (with long-term or excessive use).

☑ Special considerations
• Prescribe doses carefully; fluidextract preparation is five times as potent as aromatic fluidextract.
• Aromatic fluidextract tastes better than fluidextract.
• Drug may color urine reddish pink or brown, depending on urine pH.
• Cascara is a common ingredient in many so-called natural laxatives available without a prescription.
• Bulk-forming or surfactant laxatives are preferred during pregnancy.
• Cascara turns alkaline urine pink to red, red to violet, or red to brown and turns acidic urine yellow to brown in the phenolsulfonphthalein excretion test.

Monitoring the patient
• Evaluate response to therapy; monitor patient for overuse.

• With excessive use, monitor electrolyte levels.

Information for the patient
• Warn patient that drug may turn urine reddish pink or brown.

Geriatric patients
• Because many elderly people use laxatives, they have a particularly high risk of developing laxative dependence. Urge them to use laxatives only for short periods.

Pediatric patients
• Use with caution in children.

Breast-feeding patients
• Cascara may appear in breast milk, possibly causing diarrhea in infant.

castor oil
Emulsoil, Neoloid, Purge

Pharmacologic classification: glyceride, *Ricinus communis* derivative
Therapeutic classification: stimulant laxative
Pregnancy risk category X

How supplied
Available without a prescription
Liquid: 60 ml, 120 ml
Liquid (95%): 30 ml, 60 ml
Liquid emulsion: 60 ml (95%), 90 ml (67%)

Indications, route, and dosage
Preparation for rectal or bowel examination or surgery; acute constipation (rarely)
Liquid
Adults: 15 to 60 ml (or 30 to 60 ml, 95%) P.O.
Children ages 2 to 12: 5 to 15 ml P.O.
Liquid emulsion
Adults: 45 ml (67%) or 15 to 60 ml (95%) mixed with ½ to 1 glass liquid.
Children ages 2 to 12: 15 ml (67%) or 5 to 15 ml (95%) mixed with ½ to 1 glass liquid.

Pharmacodynamics
Laxative action: Acts primarily in small intestine, where it's metabolized to ricinoleic acid, which stimulates the intestine, promoting peristalsis and bowel motility.

Pharmacokinetics
• *Absorption:* No information available; action begins in 2 to 6 hours.
• *Distribution:* Distributed locally, primarily in small intestine.
• *Metabolism:* Like other fatty acids, castor oil is metabolized by intestinal enzymes into its active form, ricinoleic acid.
• *Excretion:* Excreted in feces.

Reactions may be *common,* uncommon, *life-threatening,* or COMMON AND LIFE-THREATENING.

Contraindications and precautions
Contraindicated in patients with ulcerative bowel lesions; abdominal pain, nausea, vomiting, or other symptoms of appendicitis or acute surgical abdomen; in those with anal or rectal fissures, fecal impaction, or intestinal obstruction or perforation; and during menstruation or pregnancy. Use cautiously in patients with rectal bleeding.

Interactions
Drug-drug. *Intestinally absorbed drugs:* May decrease absorption of intestinally absorbed drugs. Don't administer together.
Drug-herb. *Male fern:* May increase absorption and increase risk of toxicity. Avoid concomitant use.

Adverse reactions
GI: *nausea;* vomiting; diarrhea; loss of normal bowel function with excessive use; *abdominal cramps,* especially in severe constipation; malabsorption of nutrients; "cathartic colon" (syndrome resembling ulcerative colitis radiologically and pathologically) with chronic misuse; laxative dependence with long-term or excessive use. May cause constipation after catharsis.
Other: hypokalemia, protein-losing enteropathy, other electrolyte imbalances (with excessive use).

☑ Special considerations
• Castor oil isn't recommended for routine use in constipation; it's commonly used to evacuate bowels before diagnostic or surgical procedures.
• Don't administer at bedtime because of rapid onset of action.
• Shake well; drug is most effective when taken on empty stomach.
• Flavored preparations are available.

Monitoring the patient
• Observe patient for signs and symptoms of dehydration.
• Monitor patient for adverse effects.

Information for the patient
• Instruct patient not to take drug at bedtime.
• Recommend that drug be chilled or taken with juice or carbonated beverage for palatability.
• Instruct patient to shake emulsion well.
• Reassure patient that after response to drug he may not need to move bowels again for 1 or 2 days.

Geriatric patients
• With chronic use, elderly patients may experience electrolyte depletion, resulting in weakness, incoordination, and orthostatic hypotension.

Breast-feeding patients
• Breast-feeding women should seek medical approval before using castor oil.

cefaclor
Ceclor, Ceclor CD

Pharmacologic classification: second-generation cephalosporin
Therapeutic classification: antibiotic
Pregnancy risk category B

How supplied
Available by prescription only
Tablets (extended-release): 375 mg, 500 mg
Capsules: 250 mg, 500 mg
Suspension: 125 mg/5 ml, 187 mg/5 ml, 250 mg/5 ml, 375 mg/5 ml

Indications, route, and dosage
Infections of respiratory or urinary tract and skin; otitis media caused by susceptible organisms
Adults: 250 to 500 mg P.O. q 8 hours. Total daily dosage shouldn't exceed 4 g. For extended-release tablets, 375 to 500 mg P.O. q 12 hours for 7 to 10 days.
Children: 20 mg/kg P.O. daily (40 mg/kg for severe infections and otitis media) in divided doses q 8 hours; don't exceed 1 g/day.
◊ *Acute uncomplicated urinary tract infection*
Adults: 2 g as single dose.
✦ *Dosage adjustment.* Because drug is dialyzable, patients receiving hemodialysis or peritoneal dialysis may require dosage adjustment.

Pharmacodynamics
Antibacterial action: Primarily bactericidal; however, may be bacteriostatic. Activity depends on the organism, tissue penetration, drug dosage, and rate of organism multiplication. Acts by adhering to bacterial penicillin-binding proteins, thereby inhibiting cell-wall synthesis.
  Cefaclor has same bactericidal spectrum as other second-generation cephalosporins, except that it has increased activity against ampicillin- or amoxicillin-resistant *Haemophilus influenzae* and *Branhamella catarrhalis.*

Pharmacokinetics
• *Absorption:* Well absorbed from GI tract; serum levels peak 30 to 60 minutes after oral dose. Food will delay but not prevent complete GI tract absorption.
• *Distribution:* Distributed widely into most body tissues and fluids; poor CSF penetration. Crosses placenta; is 25% protein-bound.
• *Metabolism:* Not metabolized.
• *Excretion:* Excreted primarily in urine by renal tubular secretion and glomerular filtration; small amounts excreted in breast milk. Elimination half-life is ½ to 1 hour in patients with normal renal function; end-stage renal disease prolongs half-life to 3 to 5½ hours. Hemodialysis removes cefaclor.

Contraindications and precautions
Contraindicated in patients with hypersensitivity to other cephalosporins. Use cautiously in patients with impaired renal function or penicillin allergy and in breast-feeding women.

Interactions
Drug-drug. *Bacteriostatic drugs (chloramphenicol, erythromycin, tetracyclines):* May impair its bactericidal activity. Monitor patient for drug effect.
Loop diuretics, nephrotoxic drugs (aminoglycosides, colistin, polymyxin B, vancomycin): May increase risk of nephrotoxicity. Use together cautiously.
Probenecid: Competitively inhibits renal tubular secretion of cephalosporins, resulting in higher, prolonged serum levels of these drugs. Use together cautiously.

Adverse reactions
CNS: dizziness, headache, somnolence, malaise.
GI: *nausea,* vomiting, *diarrhea,* anorexia, dyspepsia, abdominal cramps, pseudomembranous colitis, oral candidiasis.
GU: vaginal candidiasis, vaginitis.
Hematologic: transient leukopenia, anemia, eosinophilia, **thrombocytopenia,** lymphocytosis.
Hepatic: transient increases in liver enzymes.
Skin: *maculopapular rash,* dermatitis, pruritus.
Other: hypersensitivity reactions (serum sickness, **anaphylaxis**), fever.

☑ Special considerations
Besides the recommendations relevant to all cephalosporins, consider the following.
● To prevent toxic accumulation, reduced dosage may be needed if patient's creatinine clearance is below 40 ml/minute.
● May be given with food to minimize GI distress.
● Total daily dosage may be administered b.i.d. rather than t.i.d. with similar therapeutic effect.
● Stock oral suspension is stable for 14 days if refrigerated.
● Cefaclor may cause false-positive Coombs' test results. Also causes false-positive results in urine glucose tests using cupric sulfate (Benedict's reagent or Clinitest); use glucose oxidase tests (Chemstrip uG, Diastix, or glucose enzymatic test strip) instead.
● Drug causes false elevations in serum or urine creatinine levels in tests using Jaffé's reaction.
● Clinical signs of overdose include neuromuscular hypersensitivity; seizure may follow high CNS concentrations.
● Remove cefaclor by hemodialysis or peritoneal dialysis.

Monitoring the patient
● Carefully observe patient for superinfection if prolonged use of drug is needed.

● Monitor renal patients carefully. Clinical observation and appropriate laboratory studies should be made before and during therapy.

Information for the patient
● Instruct patient to take extended-release tablets with food; tell patient not to cut, crush, or chew them.

Geriatric patients
● Dosage reduction may be needed in patients with reduced renal function.

Pediatric patients
● Drug can be used safely in children older than age 1 month. Extended release tablets should only be used in children ages 16 and older.

Breast-feeding patients
● Drug appears in breast milk; use with caution in breast-feeding women.

---

cefadroxil
Duricef

Pharmacologic classification: first-generation cephalosporin
Therapeutic classification: antibiotic
Pregnancy risk category B

How supplied
Available by prescription only
Tablets: 1 g
Capsules: 500 mg
Suspension: 125 mg/5 ml, 250 mg/5 ml, 500 mg/5 ml

Indications, route, and dosage
Urinary tract, skin, and soft-tissue infections caused by susceptible organisms; pharyngitis; tonsillitis
Adults: 1 to 2 g P.O. daily, depending on the infection treated. Usually given once or twice daily.
Children: 30 mg/kg daily in two divided doses.
✦ *Dosage adjustment.* In patients with creatinine clearance below 10 ml/minute, extend dosing interval to q 36 hours; if between 10 and 25 ml/minute, administer q 24 hours; if between 25 and 50 ml/minute, give q 12 hours.
    Because drug is dialyzable, patients receiving hemodialysis may require dosage adjustment.

Pharmacodynamics
Antibacterial action: Primarily bactericidal; however, may be bacteriostatic. Activity depends on the organism, tissue penetration, drug dosage, and rate of organism multiplication. Acts by adhering to bacterial penicillin-binding proteins, thereby inhibiting cell-wall synthesis.
    Cefadroxil is active against many gram-positive cocci, including penicillinase-producing

Staphylococcus aureus and *epidermidis; Streptococcus pneumoniae,* group B streptococci, and group A beta-hemolytic streptococci; and susceptible gram-negative organisms, including *Klebsiella pneumoniae, Escherichia coli,* and *Proteus mirabilis.*

Pharmacokinetics
• *Absorption:* Absorbed rapidly and completely from GI tract after oral administration; serum levels peak at 1 to 2 hours.
• *Distribution:* Distributed widely into most body tissues and fluids, including gallbladder, liver, kidneys, bone, bile, sputum, pleural and synovial fluids; poor CSF penetration. Crosses placenta; 20% protein-bound.
• *Metabolism:* Not metabolized.
• *Excretion:* Excreted primarily unchanged in urine via glomerular filtration and renal tubular secretion; small amounts may be excreted in breast milk. Elimination half-life is about 1 to 2 hours in patients with normal renal function; end-stage renal disease prolongs half-life to 25 hours. Can be removed by hemodialysis.

Contraindications and precautions
Contraindicated in patients with hypersensitivity to drug or other cephalosporins. Use cautiously in patients with impaired renal function or penicillin allergy and in breast-feeding women.

Interactions
Drug-drug. *Bacteriostatic drugs (chloramphenicol, erythromycin, tetracyclines):* May impair its bactericidal activity. Monitor patient for drug effect.
Loop diuretics, nephrotoxic drugs (aminoglycosides, colistin, polymyxin B, vancomycin): May increase risk of nephrotoxicity. Use together cautiously.
Probenecid: Competitively inhibits renal tubular secretion of cephalosporins, resulting in higher, prolonged serum levels of these drugs. Use with caution.

Adverse reactions
CNS: *seizures.*
GI: pseudomembranous colitis, *nausea,* vomiting, *diarrhea,* glossitis, abdominal cramps, oral candidiasis, transient increases in liver enzyme levels.
GU: genital pruritus, candidiasis, vaginitis, renal dysfunction.
Hematologic: transient neutropenia, eosinophilia, leukopenia, anemia, *agranulocytosis, thrombocytopenia.*
Skin: *maculopapular and erythematous rashes,* urticaria.
Other: hypersensitivity reactions (serum sickness, *anaphylaxis,* angioedema), dyspnea, fever.

☑ Special considerations
Besides the recommendations relevant to all cephalosporins, consider the following.
• Longer half-life of drug permits once- or twice-daily dosing.
• Cefadroxil causes false-positive results in urine glucose tests utilizing cupric sulfate (Benedict's reagent or Clinitest); use glucose oxidase test (Chemstrip uG, Diastix, or glucose enzymatic test strip) instead.
• Drug causes false elevations in serum or urine creatinine levels in tests using Jaffé's reaction.
• Positive Coombs' test results occur in about 3% of patients taking cephalosporins.
• Clinical signs of overdose include neuromuscular hypersensitivity; seizure may follow high CNS concentrations.
• Cefadroxil is removed by hemodialysis. Other treatment of overdose is supportive.

Monitoring the patient
• Carefully observe patient for superinfection if prolonged use of drug is needed.
• Monitor renal patients carefully. Clinical observation and appropriate laboratory studies should be made before and during therapy.

Information for the patient
• Inform patient of potential adverse reactions.

Geriatric patients
• Reduce dosage in elderly patients with diminished renal function.

Pediatric patients
• Serum half-life is prolonged in neonates and infants under age 1.

Breast-feeding patients
• Drug appears in breast milk; use with caution in breast-feeding women.

cefamandole nafate
Mandol

Pharmacologic classification: second-generation cephalosporin
Therapeutic classification: antibiotic
Pregnancy risk category B

How supplied
Available by prescription only
Injectable solution: 500 mg, 1 g, 2 g

Indications, route, and dosage
Serious respiratory, GU, skin and soft-tissue, and bone and joint infections; septicemia; peritonitis from susceptible organisms
Adults: 500 mg to 1 g q 4 to 8 hours. In life-threatening infections, up to 2 g q 4 hours may be needed.

Infants and children: 50 to 100 mg/kg daily in equally divided doses q 4 to 8 hours. May be increased to total daily dose of 150 mg/kg (not to exceed maximum adult dose) for severe infections.

Total daily dose is same for I.M. or I.V. administration and depends on susceptibility of organism and severity of infection. Drug should be injected deep I.M. into a large muscle mass, such as the gluteus or the lateral aspect of the thigh.

✦ *Dosage adjustment.* In patients with impaired renal function, doses or frequency of administration must be modified according to degree of renal impairment, severity of infection, and susceptibility of organism. The following table gives appropriate doses for adults.

Creatinine clearance (ml/min/1.73 m²)	Severe infections	Life-threatening infections (maximum dose)
> 80	1 to 2 g q 6 hr	2 g q 4 hr
50 to 80	750 mg to 1.5 g q 6 hr	1.5 g q 4 hr; or 2 g q 6 hr
25 to 50	750 mg to 1.5 g q 8 hr	1.5 g q 6 hr; or 2 g q 8 hr
10 to 25	500 mg to 1 g q 8 hr	1 g q 6 hr; or 1.25 g q 8 hr
2 to 10	500 to 750 mg q 12 hr	670 mg q 8 hr; or 1 g q 12 hr
< 2	250 to 500 mg q 12 hr	500 mg q 8 hr; or 750 mg q 12 hr

Pharmacodynamics

Antibacterial action: Primarily bactericidal; however, may be bacteriostatic. Activity depends on the organism, tissue penetration, drug dosage, and rate of organism multiplication. Acts by adhering to bacterial penicillin-binding proteins, thereby inhibiting cell-wall synthesis.

Cefamandole is active against *Escherichia coli* and other coliform bacteria, *Staphylococcus aureus* (penicillinase- and non–penicillinase-producing), *Staphylococcus epidermidis*, group A beta-hemolytic streptococci, *Klebsiella, Haemophilus influenzae, Proteus mirabilis,* and *Enterobacter* as the second-generation drugs. *Bacteroides fragilis* and *Acinetobacter* are resistant.

Pharmacokinetics

● *Absorption:* Not absorbed from GI tract and must be given parenterally; serum levels peak ½ to 2 hours after I.M. dose.
● *Distribution:* Distributed widely into most body tissues and fluids, including gallbladder, liver, kidneys, bone, sputum, bile, pleural and synovial fluids; poor CSF penetration. Crosses placenta; 65% to 75% protein-bound.
● *Metabolism:* Not metabolized.
● *Excretion:* Excreted primarily in urine by renal tubular secretion and glomerular filtration; small

amounts of drug excreted in breast milk. Elimination half-life is about ½ to 2 hours in patients with normal renal function; severe renal disease prolongs half-life to 12 to 18 hours. Hemodialysis removes some cefamandole.

Contraindications and precautions

Contraindicated in patients with hypersensitivity to drug or other cephalosporins. Use cautiously in patients with impaired renal function or penicillin allergy and in breast-feeding women.

Interactions

Drug-drug. *Anticoagulants:* May increase risk of bleeding. Avoid concomitant use.
Bacteriostatic drugs (chloramphenicol, erythromycin, tetracyclines): May impair its bactericidal activity. Monitor patient for drug effect.
Loop diuretics, nephrotoxic drugs (aminoglycosides, colistin, polymyxin B, vancomycin): May increase risk of nephrotoxicity. Use together cautiously.
Probenecid: Competitively inhibits renal tubular secretion of cephalosporins, resulting in higher, prolonged serum levels of these drugs. Use with caution.
Drug-lifestyle. *Alcohol:* May cause severe disulfiram-like reactions. Avoid concomitant use.

Adverse reactions

GI: pseudomembranous colitis, nausea, vomiting, *diarrhea,* oral candidiasis.
Hematologic: eosinophilia, coagulation abnormalities.
Skin: *maculopapular and erythematous rashes,* urticaria.
Other: hypersensitivity reactions (serum sickness, **anaphylaxis**); transient increases in liver enzymes; pain, induration, sterile abscesses, temperature elevation, tissue sloughing (at injection site); phlebitis, thrombophlebitis (with I.V. injection).

☑ Special considerations

● For most cephalosporin-sensitive organisms, cefamandole offers little advantage over others; it's less effective than cefoxitin against anaerobic infections. Some clinicians consider it inappropriate for pediatric use, especially for serious infections like *Haemophilus influenzae.*
● For I.V. use, reconstitute 1 g with 10 ml of sterile water for injection, 5% dextrose injection, or normal saline injection. Administer slowly, over 3 to 5 minutes, or by intermittent infusion or continuous infusion in compatible solutions. Check package insert.
● Don't mix with I.V. infusions containing magnesium or calcium ions, which are chemically incompatible and may cause irreversible effects.
● Cefamandole injection contains 3.3 mEq of sodium per g of drug.
● For I.M. use, dilute 1 g of cefamandole in 3 ml of sterile water for injection, bacteriostatic water

for injection, normal saline solution for injection, or 0.9% bacteriostatic saline for injection.
• Administer deeply into large muscle mass to ensure maximum absorption. Rotate injection sites.
• I.M. cefamandole is less painful than cefoxitin injection; it doesn't require addition of lidocaine.
• After reconstitution, solution remains stable for 24 hours at room temperature or 96 hours under refrigeration. Solution should be light yellow to amber. Don't use solution if discolored or contains a precipitate.
• Bleeding can be reversed by administering vitamin K or blood products.
• Use with alcohol will lead to disulfiram-like reaction. For patients who drink alcohol, consider alternative drugs if home I.V. antibiotic therapy is necessary.
• Cefamandole causes false-positive results in urine glucose tests using cupric sulfate (Benedict's reagent or Clinitest); use glucose oxidase tests (Chemstrip uG, Diastix, or glucose enzymatic test strip) instead.
• Drug causes false elevations in serum or urine creatinine levels in tests using Jaffé's reaction.
• Drug may cause positive Coombs' test results and may elevate liver function test results or PT.
• Clinical signs of overdose include neuromuscular hypersensitivity. Seizure may follow high CNS concentrations. Hypoprothrombinemia and bleeding may occur and may be treated with vitamin K or blood products.
• Some drug may be removed by hemodialysis.

Monitoring the patient
• Carefully observe patient for superinfection if prolonged use of drug is needed.
• Monitor renal patients carefully. Clinical observation and appropriate laboratory studies should be made before and during therapy.
• Monitor patient for signs or symptoms of bleeding. Monitor patient's PT and platelet level. Patient may require prophylactic use of vitamin K to prevent bleeding.

Information for the patient
• Inform patient of potential adverse reactions.

Geriatric patients
• Dosage reduction may be needed in patients with diminished renal function.
• Hypoprothrombinemia and bleeding occur most frequently in elderly, malnourished, and debilitated patients.

Pediatric patients
• Safe use in infants under age 1 month hasn't been established.

Breast-feeding patients
• Safe use hasn't been established. Drug appears in breast milk; use with caution in breast-feeding women.

cefazolin sodium
Ancef, Kefzol, Zolicef

Pharmacologic classification: first-generation cephalosporin
Therapeutic classification: antibiotic
Pregnancy risk category B

How supplied
Available by prescription only
Injection (parenteral): 250 mg, 500 mg, 1 g, 5 g, 10 g, 20 g
Infusion: 500 mg/50- or 100-ml vial, 1 g/50- or 100-ml vial, 500-mg or 1-g Redi Vials, Faspaks, or ADD-Vantage vials

Indications, route, and dosage
Serious respiratory, GU, skin and soft-tissue, and bone and joint infections; biliary tract infections; septicemia, endocarditis from susceptible organisms
Adults: 250 mg I.M. or I.V. q 8 hours to 1 g q 8 hours. Maximum dose is 12 g/day in life-threatening situations.
Children over age 1 month: 25 to 100 mg/kg/day I.M. or I.V. in divided doses q 8 hours.
  Total daily dose is same for I.M. or I.V. administration and depends on susceptibility of organism and severity of infection. Cefazolin should be injected deep I.M. into a large muscle mass, such as the gluteus or the lateral aspect of thigh.
✦ *Dosage adjustment.* Dose or frequency of administration must be modified according to degree of renal impairment, severity of infection, susceptibility of organism, and serum levels of drug. Because drug can be removed by hemodialysis, patients undergoing hemodialysis may require dosage adjustment.

Creatinine clearance (ml/min/1.73 m²)	Adult dosage
≥ 55	Usual adult dose
35 to 54	Full dose q 8 hr or less frequently
11 to 34	½ usual dose q 12 hr
≤ 10	½ usual dose q 18 to 24 hr

Creatinine clearance (ml/min/1.73 m²)	Dosage in children
> 70	Usual pediatric dose
40 to 70	60% of normal daily dose q 12 hr
20 to 40	25% of normal daily dose q 12 hr
5 to 20	10% of normal daily dose q 24 hr

Pharmacodynamics
Antibacterial action: Primarily bactericidal; however, may be bacteriostatic. Activity depends on the organism, tissue penetration, drug dosage, and rate of organism multiplication. Acts by adhering to bacterial penicillin-binding proteins, thereby inhibiting cell-wall synthesis.

Cefazolin is active against *Escherichia coli, Enterobacteriaceae, Haemophilus influenzae, Klebsiella, Proteus mirabilis, Staphylococcus aureus, Streptococcus pneumoniae,* and group A beta-hemolytic streptococci.

Pharmacokinetics
• *Absorption:* Not well absorbed from GI tract and must be given parenterally; serum levels peak 1 to 2 hours after an I.M. dose.
• *Distribution:* Distributed widely into most body tissues and fluids, including gallbladder, liver, kidneys, bone, sputum, bile, pleural and synovial fluids; poor CSF penetration. Crosses placenta; 74% to 86% protein-bound.
• *Metabolism:* Not metabolized.
• *Excretion:* Excreted primarily unchanged in urine by renal tubular secretion and glomerular filtration; small amounts of drug excreted in breast milk. Elimination half-life is about 1 to 2 hours in patients with normal renal function; end-stage renal disease prolongs half-life to 12 to 50 hours. Hemodialysis or peritoneal dialysis removes cefazolin.

Contraindications and precautions
Contraindicated in patients with hypersensitivity to other cephalosporins. Use cautiously in patients with impaired renal function or penicillin allergy and in breast-feeding women.

Interactions
Drug-drug. *Bacteriostatic drugs (chloramphenicol, erythromycin, tetracyclines):* May impair its bactericidal activity. Monitor patient for drug effect.
Loop diuretics, nephrotoxic drugs (aminoglycosides, colistin, polymyxin B, vancomycin): May increase risk of nephrotoxicity. Use together cautiously.
Probenecid: Competitively inhibits renal tubular secretion of cephalosporins, resulting in higher, prolonged serum levels of these drugs. Use with caution.

Adverse reactions
GI: pseudomembranous colitis, nausea, anorexia, vomiting, *diarrhea,* glossitis, dyspepsia, abdominal cramps, anal pruritus, oral candidiasis.
GU: genital pruritus, candidiasis, vaginitis.
Hematologic: *neutropenia,* leukopenia, eosinophilia, **thrombocytopenia.**
Hepatic: transient increases in liver enzymes.
Skin: *maculopapular and erythematous rashes,* urticaria, pruritus, **Stevens-Johnson syndrome.**
Other: hypersensitivity reactions (serum sickness, **anaphylaxis**); pain, induration, sterile abscesses, tissue sloughing (at injection site); *phlebitis, thrombophlebitis* (with I.V. injection).

☑ Special considerations
Besides the recommendations relevant to all cephalosporins, consider the following.
• For patients on sodium restrictions, note that cefazolin injection contains 2 mEq of sodium per gram of drug.
• For I.M. use, reconstitute with sterile water, bacteriostatic water, or normal saline solution: 2 ml to a 250-mg vial, 2 ml to a 500-mg vial, and 2.5 ml to a 1-g vial produce concentrations of 125 mg/ml, 225 mg/ml, and 330 mg/ml, respectively.
• Reconstituted solution is stable for 24 hours at room temperature; for 96 hours if refrigerated.
• I.M. cefazolin injection is less painful than that of other cephalosporins.
• Cephalosporins cause false-positive results in urine glucose tests utilizing cupric sulfate (Benedict's reagent or Clinitest); use glucose oxidase tests (Chemstrip uG, Diastix, or glucose enzymatic test strip) instead.
• Cefazolin causes false elevations in serum or urine creatinine levels in tests using Jaffé's reaction.
• Drug causes positive Coombs' test results.
• Signs and symptoms of overdose include neuromuscular hypersensitivity; seizure may follow high CNS concentrations. Remove cefazolin by hemodialysis.

Monitoring the patient
• Carefully observe patient for superinfection if prolonged use of drug is needed.
• Monitor renal patients carefully. Clinical observation and appropriate laboratory studies should be made before and during therapy.

Information for the patient
• Inform patient of potential adverse reactions.

Pediatric patients
• Drug has been used in children. However, safety in infants under age 1 month hasn't been established.

Breast-feeding patients
• Safety hasn't been established; use with caution in breast-feeding women.

---

cefdinir
Omnicef

Pharmacologic classification: third-generation cephalosporin
Therapeutic classification: antibiotic
Pregnancy risk category B

How supplied
Available by prescription only

Capsules: 300 mg
Suspension: 125 mg/5 ml

Indications, route, and dosage
Mild to moderate infections caused by susceptible strains of microorganisms for conditions of community-acquired pneumonia, acute exacerbations of chronic bronchitis, acute maxillary sinusitis, acute bacterial otitis media, and uncomplicated skin and skin-structure infections
Adults and adolescents ages 13 and older: 300 mg P.O. q 12 hours or 600 mg P.O. q 24 hours for 10 days. (Use q-12-hour dosages for pneumonia and skin infections.)
Children ages 6 months to 12 years: 7 mg/kg P.O. q 12 hours or 14 mg/kg P.O. q 24 hours for 10 days, to maximum dose of 600 mg daily. (Use q-12-hour dosages for skin infections.)
Pharyngitis, tonsillitis
Adults and adolescents ages 13 and older: 300 mg P.O. q 12 hours for 5 to 10 days or 600 mg P.O. q 24 hours for 10 days.
Children ages 6 months to 12 years: 7 mg/kg P.O. q 12 hours for 5 to 10 days or 14 mg/kg P.O. q 24 hours for 10 days.
✦ *Dosage adjustment.* If creatinine clearance is below 30 ml/minute, reduce dosage to 300 mg P.O. once daily for adults and 7 mg/kg P.O. (up to 300 mg) once daily for children.
In patients receiving long-term hemodialysis, give 300 mg or 7 mg/kg P.O. at end of each dialysis session and subsequently every other day.

Pharmacodynamics
Antibiotic action: Bactericidal activity results from inhibition of cell-wall synthesis. Stable in the presence of some beta-lactamase enzymes, causing some microorganisms resistant to penicillins and cephalosporins to be susceptible to cefdinir. Excluding *Pseudomonas, Enterobacter, Enterococcus,* and methicillin-resistant *Staphylococcus* species, cefdinir's spectrum of activity includes a broad range of gram-positive and gram-negative aerobic microorganisms.

Pharmacokinetics
● *Absorption:* Estimated bioavailability is 21% after 300-mg capsule dose, 16% after 600-mg capsule dose, and 25% for the suspension. After capsule or suspension, plasma levels peak in 2 to 4 hours; food doesn't affect absorption.
● *Distribution:* Mean volume of distribution for adults and children is 0.35 and 0.67 L/kg, respectively, and distribution to tonsil, sinus, lung, and middle ear tissue and fluid ranges from 15% to 35% of corresponding plasma levels. Drug is 60% to 70% bound to plasma proteins; binding is independent of concentration.
● *Metabolism:* Not appreciably metabolized; activity due mainly to parent drug.

● *Excretion:* Principally by renal excretion; mean plasma elimination half-life is 1.7 hours. Drug clearance reduced in patients with renal dysfunction.

Contraindications and precautions
Contraindicated in patients with allergy to cephalosporins. Use cautiously in patients with hypersensitivity to penicillin because of the possibility of cross-sensitivity with other beta-lactam antibiotics. Also use with caution in patients with history of colitis.

Interactions
Drug-drug. *Antacids (aluminum- and magnesium-containing), iron supplements:* Decrease cefdinir's rate of absorption and bioavailability. Administer such preparations 2 hours before or after cefdinir dose.
Probenecid: Inhibits renal excretion of cefdinir. Use together cautiously.
Drug-food. *Foods fortified with iron (such as infant formula):* Decrease cefdinir's rate of absorption and bioavailability. Use together with caution.

Adverse reactions
CNS: headache.
GI: abdominal pain, *diarrhea,* nausea, vomiting.
GU: vaginal candidiasis, vaginitis.
Skin: rash.

☑ Special considerations
● As with many antibiotics, prolonged drug treatment may result in possible emergence and overgrowth of resistant organisms. Alternative therapy should be considered if superinfection occurs.
● Pseudomembranous colitis has been reported with many antibiotics, including cefdinir, and should be considered in diagnosing patients who present with diarrhea subsequent to antibiotic therapy or in those with history of colitis.
● False-positive reactions for ketones (tests using nitroprusside only) and glucose (Clinitest, Benedict's solution, Fehling's solution) in the urine have been reported.
● Generally, cephalosporins can induce a positive direct Coombs' test.
● Toxic signs of overdose with other beta-lactam antibiotics include nausea, vomiting, epigastric distress, diarrhea, and seizures.
● Drug is removed by hemodialysis.

Monitoring the patient
● Monitor patient for severe diarrhea or diarrhea associated with abdominal pain.
● Monitor patient for therapeutic effect.

Information for the patient
● Instruct patient to take antacids, iron supplements, and iron-fortified foods 2 hours before or after cefdinir.

• Inform diabetic patient that each teaspoon of suspension contains 2.86 g of sucrose.
• Tell patient to take drug without regard to meals.
• Advise patient to report severe diarrhea or diarrhea accompanied by abdominal pain.
• Tell patient that mild diarrhea can be treated symptomatically.

Geriatric patients
• Cefdinir is well-tolerated in all age-groups. Safety and efficacy are comparable in elderly and younger patients. Dosage adjustment isn't necessary unless patient has renal impairment.

Pediatric patients
• Safety and efficacy in infants under age 6 months haven't been established. Pharmacokinetic data for pediatric population are comparable to those for adults.

Breast-feeding patients
• Drug doesn't appear in breast milk following 600-mg doses.

cefepime hydrochloride
Maxipime

Pharmacologic classification: semisynthetic third- or fourth-generation cephalosporin
Therapeutic classification: antibiotic
Pregnancy risk category B

How supplied
Available by prescription only
Injection: 500 mg/15-ml vial, 1 g/100-ml piggyback bottle, 1 g/ADD-Vantage vial, 1 g/15-ml vial, 2 g/100-ml piggyback bottle, 2 g/20-ml vial

Indications, route, and dosage
Mild to moderate urinary tract infections caused by Escherichia coli, Klebsiella pneumoniae, or Proteus mirabilis, including cases associated with concurrent bacteremia with these microorganisms
Adults and children ages 12 and older: 0.5 to 1 g I.M. (use I.M. route only for infections caused by *E. coli*), or I.V. infused over 30 minutes q 12 hours for 7 to 10 days.
Severe urinary tract infections including pyelonephritis caused by E. coli or K. pneumoniae
Adults and children ages 12 and older: 2 g I.V. infused over 30 minutes q 12 hours for 10 days.
Moderate to severe pneumonia caused by Streptococcus pneumoniae, Pseudomonas aeruginosa, K. pneumoniae, or Enterobacter species
Adults and children ages 12 and older: 1 to 2 g I.V. infused over 30 minutes q 12 hours for 10 days.

Moderate to severe uncomplicated skin and skin-structure infections caused by Staphylococcus aureus (methicillin-susceptible strains only) or Streptococcus pyogenes
Adults and children ages 12 and older: 2 g I.V. infused over 30 minutes q 12 hours for 10 days.
✦ *Dosage adjustment.* Adjust dosage in patients with impaired renal function. Consult manufacturer's recommendations. Patients receiving hemodialysis should receive a repeat dose at the end of dialysis. Patients undergoing continuous ambulatory peritoneal dialysis should receive the usual dose q 48 hours.

Pharmacodynamics
Antibiotic action: Exerts its bactericidal action by inhibition of cell-wall synthesis. Is usually active against gram-positive microorganisms such as *S. pneumoniae, S. aureus,* and *S. pyogenes* and gram-negative microorganisms such as *Enterobacter* species, *E. coli, K. pneumoniae, P. mirabilis,* and *P. aeruginosa.*

Pharmacokinetics
• *Absorption:* Completely absorbed after I.M. administration.
• *Distribution:* Widely distributed; about 20% bound to serum protein.
• *Metabolism:* Rapidly metabolized.
• *Excretion:* 85% excreted in urine as unchanged drug; less than 1% as metabolite, 6.8% as metabolite oxide, and 2.5% as epimer of cefepime.

Contraindications and precautions
Contraindicated in patients with hypersensitivity to drug, other cephalosporins, penicillins, or other beta-lactam antibiotics. Use cautiously in patients with history of GI disease (especially colitis), impaired renal function, or poor nutritional status and in those receiving a protracted course of antimicrobial therapy.

Interactions
Drug-drug. Aminoglycosides: May increase risk of nephrotoxicity and ototoxicity. Monitor patient's renal and hearing functions closely.
Potent diuretics such as furosemide: May increase risk of nephrotoxicity. Monitor patient's renal function closely.

Adverse reactions
CNS: headache.
GI: colitis, diarrhea, nausea, vomiting, oral candidiasis.
GU: vaginitis.
Skin: rash, pruritus, urticaria.
Other: phlebitis, pain, inflammation, fever.

☑ Special considerations
Besides the recommendations relevant to all cephalosporins, consider the following.

Reactions may be *common,* uncommon, *life-threatening,* or COMMON AND LIFE-THREATENING.

• Obtain culture and sensitivity tests before giving first dose, if appropriate. Therapy may begin pending results.

• For I.V. administration, follow manufacturer guidelines closely when reconstituting drug. Variations occur in constituting drug for administration and depend on concentration of drug required and how drug is packaged (piggyback vial, ADD-Vantage vial, or regular vial). Type of diluent used for constitution varies, depending on product used. Use only solutions recommended by manufacturer. The resulting solution should be administered over 30 minutes.

• Intermittent I.V. infusion with a Y-type administration set can be accomplished with compatible solutions. However, during infusion of a solution containing cefepime, discontinuing the other solution is recommended.

• For I.M. administration, constitute drug using sterile water for injection, normal saline solution, 5% dextrose injection, 5% or 1% lidocaine hydrochloride, or bacteriostatic water for injection with parabens or benzyl alcohol. Follow manufacturer guidelines for quantity of diluent to use.

• Inspect solution visually for particulate matter before administration. The powder and its solutions tend to darken depending on storage conditions. However, drug potency isn't adversely affected when stored as recommended.

• Cefepime may result in a false-positive reaction for glucose in the urine when using Clinitest tablets. Glucose tests based on enzymatic glucose oxidase reactions (such as Chemstrip uG, Diastix, or glucose enzymatic test strip) should be used instead.

• A positive direct Coombs' test may occur during treatment with drug.

• Overdose may result in seizures, encephalopathy, and neuromuscular excitability. Supportive treatment should be given. If renal insufficiency occurs, hemodialysis, not peritoneal dialysis, is recommended to aid in the removal of cefepime.

Monitoring the patient
• Carefully observe patient for superinfection if prolonged use of drug is needed.

• Monitor renal patients carefully. Clinical observation and appropriate laboratory studies should be made before and during therapy.

• Many cephalosporins may cause a fall in prothrombin activity; patients at risk include those with renal or hepatic impairment or poor nutritional status and those receiving prolonged cefepime therapy. Monitor PT in these patients. Administer exogenous vitamin K, if needed.

Information for the patient
• Warn patient receiving drug I.M. that pain may occur at injection site.

• Instruct patient to report adverse reactions promptly.

Geriatric patients
• Use caution when administering cefepime to elderly patients. Dosage adjustment may be needed in patients with impaired renal function.

Pediatric patients
• Safety and effectiveness in children under age 12 haven't been established.

Breast-feeding patients
• Drug appears in breast milk in very low levels; use caution when administering to breast-feeding women.

cefixime
Suprax

Pharmacologic classification: third-generation cephalosporin
Therapeutic classification: antibiotic
Pregnancy risk category B

How supplied
Available by prescription only
Tablets: 200 mg, 400 mg
Powder for oral suspension: 100 mg/5 ml

Indications, route, and dosage
Otitis media; acute bronchitis; acute exacerbations of chronic bronchitis, pharyngitis, tonsillitis; uncomplicated urinary tract infections caused by Escherichia coli *and* Proteus mirabilis; *uncomplicated gonorrhea*
Adults and children weighing over 50 kg (110 lb) or over age 12: 400 mg P.O. daily in one or two divided doses; for uncomplicated gonorrhea, 400 mg as a single dose.
Children over age 6 months weighing under 50 kg or under age 12: 8 mg/kg P.O. daily in one or two divided doses.
✦ *Dosage adjustment.* In renally impaired patients, dosage must be adjusted based on degree of renal impairment, severity of infection, and susceptibility of organism. To prevent toxic accumulation in patients with creatinine clearance below 60 ml/minute/1.73 m^2, reduced dosage may be needed.

Creatinine clearance (ml/min/1.73 m^2)	Adult dosage
> 60	Usual dose
20 to 60	75% of the usual dose
< 20 or patients receiving continuous ambulatory peritoneal dialysis	50% of the usual dose

Pharmacodynamics

Antibacterial action: Primarily bactericidal; acts by binding to penicillin-binding proteins in the bacterial cell wall, thereby inhibiting cell-wall synthesis.

Used in the treatment of otitis media caused by *Haemophilus influenzae* (penicillinase- and non–penicillinase-producing), *Moraxella (Branhamella) catarrhalis* (which is penicillinase-producing), and *Streptococcus pyogenes.* Substantial drug resistance has been noted. Cefixime is also active in the treatment of acute bronchitis and acute exacerbations of chronic bronchitis caused by *S. pneumoniae* and *H. influenzae* (penicillinase- and non–penicillinase-producing), pharyngitis and tonsillitis caused by *S. pyogenes,* and uncomplicated urinary tract infections caused by *E. coli* and *P. mirabilis.*

Pharmacokinetics

- *Absorption:* 30% to 50% absorbed following oral administration. Suspension form provides higher serum level than tablet form. Food delays absorption, but total amount absorbed isn't affected.
- *Distribution:* Widely distributed; about 65% bound to plasma proteins.
- *Metabolism:* 50% of drug is metabolized.
- *Excretion:* Excreted primarily in urine. Elimination half-life in patients with normal renal function is 3 to 4 hours. In patients with end-stage renal disease, half-life may be prolonged to 11½ hours.

Contraindications and precautions

Contraindicated in patients with hypersensitivity to drug or other cephalosporins. Use cautiously in patients with impaired renal function.

Interactions

Drug-drug. *Salicylates:* May increase serum level of cefixime. Monitor patient closely.

Adverse reactions

CNS: headache, dizziness.
GI: *diarrhea,* loose stools, abdominal pain, nausea, vomiting, dyspepsia, flatulence, pseudomembranous colitis.
GU: genital pruritus, vaginitis, genital candidiasis, transient increases in BUN and serum creatinine levels.
Hematologic: *thrombocytopenia,* leukopenia, eosinophilia.
Hepatic: transient increases in liver enzymes.
Skin: pruritus, rash, urticaria, erythema multiforme, *Stevens-Johnson syndrome.*
Other: drug fever, hypersensitivity reactions (serum sickness, *anaphylaxis*).

☑ Special considerations

Besides the recommendations relevant to all cephalosporins, consider the following.

- Cefixime is the first orally active, third-generation cephalosporin effective with once-daily dosage.
- Manufacturer advises not substituting tablets for suspension when treating otitis media.
- Patients with antibiotic-induced diarrhea should be evaluated for overgrowth of pseudomembranous colitis caused by *Clostridium difficile.* Mild cases usually respond to discontinuation of the drug; moderate to severe cases may require fluid, electrolyte, and protein supplementation. Oral vancomycin is drug of choice for treatment of antibiotic-associated *C. difficile* pseudomembranous colitis.
- Treat acute hypersensitivity reactions immediately. Emergency measures, such as airway management, pressor amines, epinephrine, oxygen, antihistamines, and corticosteroids, may be needed.
- Some cephalosporins may cause seizures, especially in patients with renal failure who receive full therapeutic dosages. If seizures occur, stop drug and initiate anticonvulsant therapy.
- Cefixime may cause false-positive results in urine glucose tests utilizing cupric sulfate (Benedict's reagent or Clinitest); use glucose oxidase tests (Chemstrip uG, Diastix, or glucose enzymatic test strip) instead.
- Cefixime may cause false-positive results in tests for urine ketones that utilize nitroprusside (but not nitroferricyanide).
- False-positive direct Coombs' test results have occurred with other cephalosporins.
- No specific antidote available. Gastric lavage and supportive treatment are recommended. Peritoneal dialysis and hemodialysis will remove substantial quantities of drug.

Monitoring the patient

- Carefully observe patient for superinfection if prolonged use of drug is needed.
- Monitor renal patients carefully. Clinical observation and appropriate laboratory studies should be made before and during therapy.

Information for the patient

- Instruct patient to report unpleasant effects, such as itching, rash, or severe diarrhea. Diarrhea is the most common adverse GI effect.
- Advise patient that oral suspension is stable for 14 days after reconstitution and doesn't require refrigeration.

Pediatric patients

- Adverse GI effects in children receiving oral suspension is similar to that in adults receiving tablets.

Breast-feeding patients

- It's unknown if drug appears in breast milk; breast-feeding during cefixime therapy isn't recommended.

Reactions may be *common*, uncommon, *life-threatening*, or COMMON AND LIFE-THREATENING.

cefoperazone sodium
Cefobid

Pharmacologic classification: third-generation cephalosporin
Therapeutic classification: antibiotic
Pregnancy risk category B

How supplied
Available by prescription only
Parenteral: 1 g, 2 g
Infusion: 1 g, 2 g piggyback

Indications, route, and dosage
Serious respiratory tract, intra-abdominal, gynecologic, skin and skin-structure, urinary tract, and enterococcal infections; bacterial septicemia caused by susceptible organisms
Adults: Usual dosage is 1 to 2 g q 12 hours I.M. or I.V. In severe infections or infections caused by less sensitive organisms, total daily dose or frequency may be increased up to 16 g/day in certain situations.
♦ **Dosage adjustment.** No dosage adjustment is usually needed in patients with renal impairment. However, give doses of 4 g/day cautiously to patients with hepatic disease. Adults with combined hepatic and renal function impairment shouldn't receive more than 1 g (base) daily without serum determinations. In patients who are receiving hemodialysis treatments, a dose should be scheduled after hemodialysis.

Pharmacodynamics
Antibacterial action: Primarily bactericidal; however, may be bacteriostatic. Activity depends on the organism, tissue penetration, drug dosage, and rate of organism multiplication. Acts by adhering to bacterial penicillin-binding proteins, thereby inhibiting cell-wall synthesis. Third-generation cephalosporins appear more active against some beta-lactamase-producing gram-negative organisms.

Cefoperazone is active against some gram-positive organisms and many enteric gram-negative bacilli, including *Streptococcus pneumoniae* and *Streptococcus pyogenes*, *Staphylococcus aureus* (penicillinase- and non–penicillinase-producing), *Staphylococcus epidermidis*, *Escherichia coli, Klebsiella, Haemophilus influenzae*, Enterobacter, Citrobacter, Proteus, some *Pseudomonas* species (including *Pseudomonas aeruginosa)*, and *Bacteroides fragilis*. *Acinetobacter* and *Listeria* usually are resistant. Cefoperazone is less effective than cefotaxime or ceftizoxime against *Enterobacteriaceae* but is slightly more active than those drugs against *Pseudomonas aeruginosa*.

Pharmacokinetics
● *Absorption:* Not absorbed from GI tract and must be given parenterally; serum levels peak 1 to 2 hours after an I.M. dose.
● *Distribution:* Distributed widely into most body tissues and fluids, including gallbladder, liver, kidneys, bone, sputum, bile, pleural and synovial fluids; CSF penetration in patients with inflamed meninges. Drug crosses placenta. Protein-binding is dose-dependent and decreases as serum levels rise; average is 82% to 93%.
● *Metabolism:* Not substantially metabolized.
● *Excretion:* Primarily in bile; some drug excreted in urine by renal tubular secretion and glomerular filtration; small amounts in breast milk. Elimination half-life is about 1½ to 2½ hours in patients with normal hepatorenal function; biliary obstruction or cirrhosis prolongs half-life to about 3½ to 7 hours. Hemodialysis removes cefoperazone.

Contraindications and precautions
Contraindicated in patients with hypersensitivity to drug or other cephalosporins. Use cautiously in patients with impaired renal or hepatic function or penicillin allergy and in breast-feeding women.

Interactions
Drug-drug. *Aminoglycosides, clavulanic acid:* Increased risk of nephrotoxicity. Use together cautiously; monitor patient closely.
Anticoagulants: May increase risk of bleeding. Monitor patient and coagulation studies.
Probenecid: Competitively inhibits renal tubular secretions of cephalosporins, causing prolonged serum levels of these drugs. Use together cautiously.
Drug-lifestyle. *Alcohol:* Possible disulfiram-like reaction (flushing, sweating, tachycardia, headache, and abdominal cramping). Discourage use.

Adverse reactions
GI: pseudomembranous colitis, nausea, vomiting, *diarrhea.*
Hematologic: transient neutropenia, *eosinophilia,* anemia, hypoprothrombinemia, bleeding.
Hepatic: mildly elevated liver enzyme levels.
Skin: *maculopapular and erythematous rashes, urticaria.*
Other: hypersensitivity reactions (serum sickness, **anaphylaxis**); *pain, induration, sterile abscesses, temperature elevation, tissue sloughing* (at injection site); *phlebitis, thrombophlebitis,* drug fever (with I.V. injection).

☑ Special considerations
Besides the recommendations relevant to all cephalosporins, consider the following.
● Diarrhea may be more common with drug than with other cephalosporins because of high degree of biliary excretion.

• Patients with biliary disease may need lower doses.
• For patients on sodium restriction, note that cefoperazone injection contains 1.5 mEq sodium per gram of drug.
• To prepare I.M. injection, use the appropriate diluent, including sterile water for injection or bacteriostatic water for injection. Follow manufacturer's recommendations for mixing drug with sterile water for injection and lidocaine 2% injection. Final solution for I.M. injection will contain 0.5% lidocaine and will be less painful upon administration (recommended for concentrations of 250 mg/ml or greater). Cefoperazone should be injected deep I.M. into a large muscle mass, such as the gluteus or the lateral aspect of the thigh.
• Store drug in refrigerator and away from light before reconstituting.
• Allow solution to stand after reconstituting to allow foam to dissipate and solution to clear. Solution can be shaken vigorously to ensure complete drug dissolution.
• After reconstitution, solution is stable for 24 hours at a controlled room temperature or 3 days if refrigerated. Protecting drug from light isn't required.
• Because cefoperazone is dialyzable, patients receiving hemodialysis may need dosage adjustment.
• Use with alcohol can lead to disulfiram-like reaction. Use drug cautiously in home antibiotic therapy patients who drink alcohol, or consider alternative drug therapy.
• Cephalosporins cause false-positive results in urine glucose tests using cupric sulfate (Benedict's reagent or Clinitest); use glucose oxidase (Chemstrip uG, Diastix, or glucose enzymatic test strip) instead.
• Cefoperazone may cause positive Coombs' test results.
• Clinical signs of overdose include neuromuscular hypersensitivity. Seizure may follow high CNS concentrations. Hypoprothrombinemia and bleeding may occur and may require treatment with vitamin K or blood products.
• Hemodialysis removes cefoperazone.

Monitoring the patient
• Carefully observe patient for superinfection if prolonged use of drug is needed.
• Monitor renal patients carefully. Clinical observation and appropriate laboratory studies should be made before and during therapy.
• Prothrombin time should be monitored and exogenous vitamin K given as indicated in patients with poor nutritional status, malabsorption states, or alcoholism, or those in prolonged therapy.

Information for the patient
• Inform patient of potential adverse reactions.
• Caution patient against alcohol use.

Geriatric patients
• Hypoprothrombinemia and bleeding occur more frequently in elderly patients. Use with caution; monitor PT and check for signs of abnormal bleeding.

Pediatric patients
• Safety and effectiveness in children under age 12 haven't been established.

Breast-feeding patients
• Drug appears in breast milk; use with caution in breast-feeding women.

cefotaxime sodium
Claforan

Pharmacologic classification: third-generation cephalosporin
Therapeutic classification: antibiotic
Pregnancy risk category B

How supplied
Available by prescription only
Injection: 500 mg, 1 g, 2 g
Pharmacy bulk package: 10-g vial
Infusion: 1 g, 2 g

Indications, route, and dosage
Serious lower respiratory, urinary, CNS, bone and joint, intra-abdominal, gynecologic, and skin infections; bacteremia; septicemia caused by susceptible organisms; ◊ pelvic inflammatory disease
Adults and children weighing over 50 kg (110 lb): Usual dosage is 1 g I.V. or I.M. q 6 to 12 hours. Up to 12 g daily can be administered in life-threatening infections.
Children ages 1 month to 12 years weighing under 50 kg: 50 to 180 mg/kg/day in four or six equally divided doses. Higher doses are reserved for serious infections (such as meningitis).
Neonates ages 1 to 4 weeks: 50 mg/kg I.V. q 8 hours.
Neonates up to age 1 week: 50 mg/kg I.V. q 12 hours.
    Total daily dose is same for I.M. or I.V. administration and depends on susceptibility of organism and severity of infection. Cefotaxime should be injected deep I.M. into a large muscle mass, such as gluteus or lateral aspect of thigh.
Uncomplicated gonorrhea
Adults and adolescents: 1 g I.M. as single dose.
Perioperative prophylaxis
Adults: 1 g I.V. or I.M. 30 to 90 minutes before surgery.
◊ Disseminated gonococcal infection
Adults: 1 g I.V. q 8 hours.
◊ Gonococcal ophthalmia
Adults: 500 mg I.V. q.i.d.

Neonates: 100 mg I.V. or I.M. for 1 dose; may continue until ocular cultures are negative at 48 to 72 hours.

◊ *Disseminated gonococcal infection*
Neonates and infants: 25 to 50 mg/kg I.V. q 8 to 12 hours for 7 days or 50 to 100 mg/kg I.M. or I.V. q 12 hours for 7 days.

◊ *Gonorrheal meningitis or arthritis*
Neonates and infants: 25 to 50 mg/kg I.V. q 8 to 12 hours for 10 to 14 days or 50 to 100 mg/kg I.M. or I.V. q 12 hours for 10 to 14 days.

✦ *Dosage adjustment.* In patients with impaired renal function, modify dose or frequency of administration based on degree of renal impairment, severity of infection, and susceptibility of organism. To prevent toxic accumulation, reduced dosage may be needed in patients with creatinine clearance below 20 ml/minute.

Pharmacodynamics
Antibacterial action: Primarily bactericidal; however, may be bacteriostatic. Activity depends on the organism, tissue penetration, drug dosage, and rate of organism multiplication. Acts by adhering to bacterial penicillin-binding proteins, thereby inhibiting cell-wall synthesis.

Third-generation cephalosporins appear more active against some beta-lactamase producing gram-negative organisms.

Cefotaxime is active against some gram-positive organisms and many enteric gram-negative bacilli, including streptococci (*Streptococcus pneumoniae* and *pyogenes*), *Staphylococcus aureus* (penicillinase- and non–penicillinase-producing), *Staphylococcus epidermidis*, *Escherichia coli*, *Klebsiella* species, *Haemophilus influenzae*, *Enterobacter* species, *Proteus* species, and *Peptostreptococcus* species, and some strains of *Pseudomonas aeruginosa*. *Listeria* and *Acinetobacter* are often resistant. The active metabolite of cefotaxime, desacetylcefotaxime, may act synergistically with parent drug against some bacterial strains.

Pharmacokinetics
● *Absorption:* Not absorbed from GI tract and must be given parenterally; serum levels peak 30 minutes after an I.M. dose.
● *Distribution:* Distributed widely into most body tissues and fluids, including gallbladder, liver, kidneys, bone, sputum, bile, pleural and synovial fluids. Unlike most other cephalosporins, drug has adequate CSF penetration when meninges are inflamed; crosses placenta; 13% to 38% protein-bound.
● *Metabolism:* Metabolized partially to an active metabolite, desacetylcefotaxime.
● *Excretion:* Drug and its metabolites excreted primarily in urine by renal tubular secretion; some drug may be excreted in breast milk. About 25% of cefotaxime is excreted in urine as the active

metabolite; elimination half-life in normal adults is about 1 to 1½ hours for cefotaxime and about 1½ to 2 hours for desacetylcefotaxime; severe renal impairment prolongs cefotaxime's half-life to 11½ hours and that of the metabolite to as much as 56 hours. Hemodialysis removes both drug and its metabolites.

Contraindications and precautions
Contraindicated in patients with hypersensitivity to drug or other cephalosporins. Use cautiously in patients with impaired renal function or penicillin allergies and in breast-feeding women.

Interactions
Drug-drug. Aminoglycosides: Increased risk of nephrotoxicity. Monitor patient closely.
Probenecid: May block renal tubular secretion of cefotaxime and prolong its half-life. Use with caution.

Adverse reactions
CNS: headache.
GI: pseudomembranous colitis, nausea, vomiting, *diarrhea.*
GU: vaginitis, moniliasis, interstitial nephritis.
Hematologic: transient neutropenia, eosinophilia, hemolytic anemia, **thrombocytopenia**, **agranulocytosis.**
Hepatic: transient increases in liver enzymes.
Skin: *maculopapular and erythematous rashes, urticaria.*
Other: hypersensitivity reactions (serum sickness, **anaphylaxis**); elevated temperature; *pain, induration, sterile abscesses, temperature elevation, tissue sloughing* (at injection site).

☑ Special considerations
Besides the recommendations relevant to all cephalosporins, consider the following.
● For patients on sodium restriction, note that cefotaxime contains 2.2 mEq sodium per gram of drug.
● For I.M. injection, add 2 ml, 3 ml, or 5 ml sterile or bacteriostatic water for injection to each 500-mg, 1-g, or 2-g vial. Shake well to dissolve drug completely. Check solution for particles and discoloration. Color ranges from light yellow to amber.
● Don't inject more than 1 g into a single I.M. site to prevent pain and tissue reaction.
● Don't mix with aminoglycosides or sodium bicarbonate or fluids with a pH above 7.5.
● For I.V. use, reconstitute all strengths of an I.V. dose with 10 ml of sterile water for injection. For infusion bottles, add 50 to 100 ml of normal saline solution injection or 5% dextrose injection. May be further reconstituted to 50 to 1,000 ml with fluids recommended by manufacturer.
● Administer drug by direct intermittent I.V. infusion over 3 to 5 minutes. Cefotaxime also may

be given more slowly into a flowing I.V. line of compatible solution.

• Solution is stable for 24 hours at room temperature or at least 10 days under refrigeration in the original container. Cefotaxime may be stored in disposable glass or plastic syringes for 24 hours at room temperature or 5 days in the refrigerator.

• Because drug is hemodialyzable, patients undergoing treatment with hemodialysis may require dosage adjustment.

• Cephalosporins cause false-positive results in urine glucose tests using cupric sulfate (Benedict's reagent or Clinitest); use glucose oxidase (Chemstrip uG, Diastix, or glucose enzymatic test strip) instead.

• Cefotaxime causes false elevations in urine creatinine levels in tests using Jaffé's reaction.

• Cefotaxime may cause positive Coombs' tests results.

• Clinical signs of overdose include neuromuscular hypersensitivity. Seizure may follow high CNS concentrations.

• Cefotaxime may be removed by hemodialysis.

Monitoring the patient
• Carefully observe patient for superinfection if prolonged use of drug is needed.
• Monitor renal patients carefully. Clinical observation and appropriate laboratory studies should be made before and during therapy.

Information for the patient
• Inform patient of potential adverse reactions.

Geriatric patients
• Use with caution in elderly patients with diminished renal function.

Pediatric patients
• Cefotaxime may be used in neonates, infants, and children.

Breast-feeding patients
• Drug appears in breast milk; use with caution in breast-feeding women.

cefotetan disodium
Cefotan

Pharmacologic classification: second-generation cephalosporin, cephamycin
Therapeutic classification: antibiotic
Pregnancy risk category B

How supplied
Available by prescription only
Injection: 1 g, 2 g
Infusion: 1 g, 2 g piggyback

Indications, route, and dosage
Serious urinary, lower respiratory, gynecologic, skin, intra-abdominal, and bone and joint infections caused by susceptible organisms
Adults: 500 mg to 3 g I.V. or I.M. q 12 hours for 5 to 10 days. Up to 6 g daily in life-threatening infections.
◇ *Children:* 40 to 60 mg/kg daily I.V. in equally divided doses q 12 hours.
Preoperative prophylaxis
Adults: 1 to 2 g I.V. 30 to 60 minutes before surgery.
Postcesarean
Adults: 1 to 2 g I.V. as soon as umbilical cord is clamped.

Total daily dose is same for I.M. or I.V. administration and depends on the susceptibility of the organism and severity of infection. Cefotetan should be injected deep I.M. into a large muscle mass, such as gluteus or lateral aspect of thigh.

✦ *Dosage adjustment.* In patients with impaired renal function, doses or frequency of administration must be modified based on degree of renal impairment, severity of infection, and susceptibility of organism. To prevent toxic accumulation, reduced dosage may be necessary in patients with creatinine clearance below 30 ml/minute. Because drug is hemodialyzable, hemodialysis patients may need dosage adjustment.

Creatinine clearance (ml/min/1.73 m²)	Adult dosage
> 30	Usual adult dose
10 to 30	Usual adult dose q 24 hours; or one-half the usual adult dose q 12 hours
< 10	Usual adult dose q 48 hours; or one-fourth the usual adult dose q 12 hours
Hemodialysis patients	One-fourth the usual adult dose q 24 hours on the days between hemodialysis sessions; and one-half the usual adult dose on the day of hemodialysis

Pharmacodynamics
Antibacterial action: Primarily bactericidal; however, may be bacteriostatic. Activity depends on the organism, tissue penetration, drug dosage, and rate of organism multiplication. Acts by adhering to bacterial penicillin-binding proteins, thereby inhibiting cell-wall synthesis.

Cefotetan is active against many gram-positive organisms and enteric gram-negative bacilli, including streptococci, *Staphylococcus aureus* (penicillinase- and non–penicillinase-producing), *Staphylococcus epidermidis, Escherichia coli, Klebsiella* species, *Enterobacter* species, *Proteus* species, *Haemophilus influenzae, Neisseria gonorrhoeae,* and *Bacteroides* species (including some strains of *B. fragilis*); however, some *B. fragilis* strains, *Pseudomonas,* and *Acinetobacter* are resistant to cefotetan. Most *Enterobacteriaceae* are more susceptible to cefotetan than to other second-generation cephalosporins.

Pharmacokinetics
• *Absorption:* Not absorbed from GI tract and must be given parenterally; serum levels peak 1½ to 3 hours after an I.M. dose.
• *Distribution:* Distributed widely into most body tissues and fluids, including gallbladder, liver, kidneys, bone, sputum, bile, pleural and synovial fluids; poor CSF penetration. Biliary serum levels of cefotetan can be 20 times higher than serum levels in patients with good gallbladder function. Crosses placenta; 75% to 90% protein-bound.
• *Metabolism:* Not metabolized.
• *Excretion:* Excreted primarily in urine by glomerular filtration and some renal tubular secretion; 20% is excreted in bile. Small amounts of drug excreted in breast milk. Elimination half-life is about 3 to 4½ hours in patients with normal renal function.

Contraindications and precautions
Contraindicated in patients with hypersensitivity to drug or other cephalosporins. Use cautiously in patients with impaired renal function or penicillin allergy and in breast-feeding women.

Interactions
Drug-drug. *Anticoagulants:* May increase risk of bleeding. Monitor PT and INR.
Loop diuretics, nephrotoxic drugs (aminoglycosides, colistin, polymyxin B, vancomycin): May increase risk of nephrotoxicity. Use with caution.
Drug-lifestyle. *Alcohol:* May cause disulfiram-like reactions (flushing, sweating, tachycardia, headache, and abdominal cramping). Discourage use.

Adverse reactions
CV: *phlebitis, thrombophlebitis* (with I.V. injection).
GI: pseudomembranous colitis, nausea, *diarrhea.*
GU: nephrotoxicity.
Hematologic: transient neutropenia, eosinophilia, hemolytic anemia, hypoprothrombinemia, bleeding, thrombocytosis, ***agranulocytosis, thrombocytopenia.***
Hepatic: transient increases in liver enzyme levels.

Skin: *maculopapular and erythematous rashes, urticaria.*
Other: hypersensitivity reactions (serum sickness, ***anaphylaxis***), elevated temperature, *pain, induration, sterile abscesses, tissue sloughing* (at injection site).

☑ Special considerations
Besides the recommendations relevant to all cephalosporins, consider the following.
• For I.V. use, reconstitute with sterile water for injection. Then mix with 50 to 100 ml D_5W or normal saline solution. Infuse intermittently over 30 to 60 minutes.
• For I.M. injection, reconstitute with sterile water or bacteriostatic water for injection or with normal saline or 0.5% or 1% lidocaine hydrochloride. Shake to dissolve and let solution stand until clear.
• Reconstituted solution remains stable for 24 hours at room temperature or for 96 hours when refrigerated.
• Bleeding can be reversed promptly by administering vitamin K.
• Use with alcohol may cause severe disulfiram-like reactions.
• Cefotetan causes false-positive results in urine glucose tests using cupric sulfate (Benedict's reagent or Clinitest); use glucose oxidase tests (Chemstrip uG, Diastix, or glucose enzymatic test strip) instead.
• Cefotetan causes false elevations in serum or urine creatinine levels in tests using Jaffé's reaction.
• Drug may cause positive Coombs' test results.
• Clinical signs of overdose include neuromuscular hypersensitivity. Seizure may follow high CNS concentrations. Hypoprothrombinemia and bleeding may occur.
• Treat overdose with vitamin K or blood products, if needed. Cefotetan can be removed by hemodialysis.

Monitoring the patient
• Carefully observe patient for superinfection if prolonged use of drug is needed.
• Monitor renal patients carefully. Clinical observation and appropriate laboratory studies should be made before and during therapy.
• Assess for signs and symptoms of overt and occult bleeding. Monitor vital signs. Check CBC with differential, platelet levels, and PT for abnormalities.

Information for the patient
• Inform patient of potential adverse reactions.
• Caution patient against alcohol use during therapy.
• Instruct patient to promptly report signs of bleeding.

Geriatric patients
• Hypoprothrombinemia and bleeding occur more frequently in elderly and debilitated patients.

Pediatric patients
• Safe use in children hasn't been established.

Breast-feeding patients
• Safe use hasn't been established. Cephalosporins appear in breast milk; use with caution in breast-feeding women.

cefoxitin sodium
Mefoxin

Pharmacologic classification: second-generation cephalosporin, cephamycin
Therapeutic classification: antibiotic
Pregnancy risk category B

How supplied
Available by prescription only
Injection: 1 g, 2 g
Pharmacy bulk package: 10 g
Infusion: 1 g, 2 g in 50-ml containers

Indications, route, and dosage
Serious respiratory, GU, gynecologic, skin, soft-tissue, bone and joint, blood, and intra-abdominal infections caused by susceptible organisms
Adults: 1 to 2 g q 6 to 8 hours for uncomplicated forms of infection. Up to 12 g daily in life-threatening infections.
Children over age 3 months: 80 to 160 mg/kg daily given in four to six equally divided doses. Don't exceed 12 g/day.
Total daily dose is same for I.M. or I.V. administration and depends on susceptibility of organism and severity of infection. Cefoxitin should be injected deep I.M. into a large muscle mass, such as the gluteus or lateral aspect of the thigh.
Preoperative prophylaxis
Adults: 2 g I.V. 30 to 60 minutes before surgery; then 2 g I.V. q 6 hours for 24 hours postoperatively.
Children over age 3 months: 30 to 40 mg/kg I.V. 30 to 60 minutes before surgery; then 30 mg/kg I.V. q 6 hours for 24 hours postoperatively.
Uncomplicated gonorrhea
Adults: Give 2 g I.M. as a single dose with 1 g probenecid P.O. at the same time or up to 30 minutes beforehand.
Pelvic inflammatory disease
Adults: 2 g I.V. q 6 hours. (If *Chlamydia trachomatis* is suspected, additional antichlamydial coverage should be given.)
✦ *Dosage adjustment.* In patients with impaired renal function, doses or frequency of administration must be modified based on degree of renal impairment, severity of infection, and sus-

ceptibility of organism. To prevent toxic accumulation, reduced dosage may be required in patients with creatinine clearance below 50 ml/minute/1.73 m².

Creatinine clearance (ml/min/1.73 m²)	Adult dosage
> 50	Usual adult dose
30 to 50	1 to 2 g q 8 to 12 hours
10 to 29	1 to 2 g q 12 to 24 hours
5 to 9	500 mg to 1 g q 12 to 24 hours
< 5	500 mg to 1 g q 24 to 48 hours

Pharmacodynamics
Antibacterial action: Primarily bactericidal; however, may be bacteriostatic. Activity depends on the organism, tissue penetration, drug dosage, and rate of organism multiplication. Acts by adhering to bacterial penicillin-binding proteins, thereby inhibiting cell-wall synthesis.
Cefoxitin is active against many gram-positive organisms and enteric gram-negative bacilli, including *Escherichia coli* and other coliform bacteria, *Staphylococcus aureus* (penicillinase- and non–penicillinase-producing), *Staphylococcus epidermidis*, streptococci, *Klebsiella*, *Haemophilus influenzae*, and *Bacteroides* species (including *B. fragilis*). *Enterobacter, Pseudomonas,* and *Acinetobacter* are resistant to cefoxitin.

Pharmacokinetics
• *Absorption:* Not absorbed from GI tract and must be given parenterally; serum levels peak 20 to 30 minutes after an I.M. dose.
• *Distribution:* Distributed widely into most body tissues and fluids, including gallbladder, liver, kidneys, bone, sputum, bile, pleural and synovial fluids; poor CSF. Crosses placenta; 50% to 80% protein-bound.
• *Metabolism:* About 2% of dose is metabolized.
• *Excretion:* Primarily in urine by renal tubular secretion and glomerular filtration; small amounts excreted in breast milk. Elimination half-life is about ½ to 1 hour in patients with normal renal function; half-life is prolonged in patients with severe renal dysfunction to 6½ to 21½ hours. Cefoxitin can be removed by hemodialysis but not by peritoneal dialysis.

Contraindications and precautions
Contraindicated in patients with hypersensitivity to drug or other cephalosporins. Use cautiously in patients with impaired renal function or penicillin allergy and in breast-feeding women.

Interactions

Drug-drug. *Bacteriostatic drugs (chloramphenicol, erythromycin, tetracyclines):* May impair cefoxitin's bactericidal activity. Monitor patient for drug effect.
Loop diuretics, nephrotoxic drugs (aminoglycosides, colistin, polymyxin B, vancomycin): May increase risk of nephrotoxicity. Use together with caution.
Probenecid: Competitively inhibits renal tubular secretion of cephalosporins, resulting in higher, prolonged serum levels of these drugs. Use together with caution.

Adverse reactions

CV: hypotension, *thrombophlebitis, phlebitis.*
GI: pseudomembranous colitis, nausea, transient increases in liver enzymes, vomiting, *diarrhea.*
GU: *acute renal failure.*
Hematologic: transient neutropenia, eosinophilia, **hemolytic anemia,** anemia, **thrombocytopenia.**
Respiratory: dyspnea (with I.V. injection).
Skin: *maculopapular and erythematous rash, urticaria,* exfoliative dermatitis.
Other: hypersensitivity reactions (serum sickness, **anaphylaxis**), elevated temperature; *pain, induration, sterile abscesses, tissue sloughing* (at injection site).

☑ Special considerations

Besides the recommendations relevant to all cephalosporins, consider the following.
• For I.V. use, reconstitute 1 g of cefoxitin with at least 10 ml sterile water for injection, or 2 g of cefoxitin with 10 to 20 ml sterile water for injection. Solutions of dextrose 5% and normal saline solution for injection can also be used.
• Cefoxitin has been associated with thrombophlebitis. Assess I.V. site frequently for signs of infiltration or phlebitis. Change I.V. site every 48 to 72 hours.
• For I.M. injection, reconstitute with 0.5% to 1% lidocaine hydrochloride (without epinephrine) to minimize pain at injection site; or with sterile water for injection.
• Administer I.M. dose deep into a large muscle mass. Aspirate before injecting to prevent inadvertent injection into a blood vessel. Rotate injection sites to prevent tissue damage.
• After reconstituting, shake vial and then let stand until clear to ensure complete drug dissolution. Solution is stable for 24 hours at room temperature, for 1 week if refrigerated, or 26 weeks if frozen.
• Solution may range from colorless to light amber and may darken during storage. Slight color change doesn't indicate loss of potency.
• Cefoxitin injection contains 2.3 mEq of sodium per gram of drug.
• Because drug is hemodialyzable, patients receiving hemodialysis may need dosage adjustments.

• Cefoxitin causes false-positive results in urine glucose tests using cupric sulfate (Benedict's reagent or Clinitest); use glucose oxidase tests (Chemstrip uG, Diastix, or glucose enzymatic test strip) instead.
• Cefoxitin causes false elevations in serum or urine creatinine levels in tests using Jaffé's reaction.
• May cause positive Coombs' test results.
• Signs and symptoms of overdose include neuromuscular hypersensitivity. Seizure may follow high CNS concentrations.
• Cefoxitin can be removed by hemodialysis.

Monitoring the patient
• Carefully observe patient for superinfection if prolonged use of drug is needed.
• Monitor renal patients carefully. Clinical observation and appropriate laboratory studies should be made before and during therapy.
• For course of treatment longer than 10 days, monitor blood counts.
• As with any potent antibacterial drug, periodic assessment of organ system functions, including renal, hepatic, and hematopoietic, is advisable during prolonged therapy.

Information for the patient
• Inform patient of potential adverse reactions.

Geriatric patients
• Dosage reduction may be necessary in patients with diminished renal function.

Pediatric patients
• Dosage may need to be reduced in infants under age 3 months. Safety hasn't been established.

Breast-feeding patients
• Drug appears in breast milk; use with caution in breast-feeding women.

cefpodoxime proxetil
Vantin

Pharmacologic classification: third-generation cephalosporin
Therapeutic classification: antibiotic
Pregnancy risk category B

How supplied
Available by prescription only
Tablets (film-coated): 100 mg, 200 mg
Oral suspension: 50 mg/5 ml, 100 mg/5 ml

Indications, route, and dosage
Acute, community-acquired pneumonia caused by non-beta-lactamase-producing strains of Haemophilus influenzae or Streptococcus pneumoniae
Adults: 200 mg P.O. q 12 hours for 14 days.

Acute bacterial exacerbations of chronic bronchitis caused by non-beta-lactamase-producing strains of H. influenzae, S. pneumoniae, *or* Moraxella catarrhalis
Adults: 200 mg P.O. q 12 hours for 10 days.

Uncomplicated gonorrhea in men and women, rectal gonococcal infections in women
Adults: 200 mg P.O. as a single dose. Follow with doxycycline 100 mg P.O. b.i.d. for 7 days.

Uncomplicated skin and skin-structure infections caused by Staphylococcus aureus *or* Streptococcus pyogenes
Adults: 400 mg P.O. q 12 hours for 7 to 14 days.

Acute otitis media caused by S. pneumoniae, H. influenzae, *or* M. catarrhalis
Children ages 5 months to 12 years: 5 mg/kg (don't exceed 200 mg) P.O. q 12 hours for 10 days.

Pharyngitis or tonsillitis caused by S. pyogenes
Adults: 100 mg P.O. q 12 hours for 7 to 10 days.
Children ages 5 months to 12 years: 5 mg/kg (don't exceed 100 mg) P.O. q 12 hours for 10 days.

Uncomplicated urinary tract infections caused by Escherichia coli, Klebsiella pneumoniae, Proteus mirabilis, *or* Staphylococcus saprophyticus
Adults: 100 mg P.O. q 12 hours for 7 days.

✦ *Dosage adjustment.* In patients with renal impairment whose creatinine clearance is below 30 ml/minute, dosage interval should be increased to q 24 hours. Patients receiving hemodialysis should get drug three times weekly, after dialysis.

Pharmacodynamics
Antibiotic action: A third-generation cephalosporin, cefpodoxime proxetil is a bactericidal drug that inhibits cell-wall synthesis. It's usually active against gram-positive aerobes, such as *S. aureus* (including penicillinase-producing strains), *S. saprophyticus, S. pneumoniae,* and *S. pyogenes,* and gram-negative aerobes, such as *E. coli, H. influenzae* (including beta-lactamase-producing strains), *K. pneumoniae, M. (Branhamella) catarrhalis, Neisseria gonorrhoeae* (including penicillinase-producing strains), and *P. mirabilis.*

Pharmacokinetics
• *Absorption:* Absorbed via GI tract. Absorption and mean peak plasma levels increase when administered with food.
• *Distribution:* Protein-binding ranges from 22% to 33% in serum and from 21% to 29% in plasma.
• *Metabolism:* De-esterified to its active metabolite, cefpodoxime.
• *Excretion:* Excreted primarily in urine.

Contraindications and precautions
Contraindicated in patients with hypersensitivity to drug or other cephalosporins. Use cautiously in patients with impaired renal function or penicillin allergy and in breast-feeding women.

Interactions
Drug-drug. Antacids, H_2 antagonists: Decreased absorption of cefpodoxime proxetil. Don't give concurrently.
Compounds of known nephrotoxic potential: Possible nephrotoxicity when administered together. Monitor renal function closely.
Probenecid: Decreased excretion of cefpodoxime proxetil. Monitor patient for cefpodoxime toxicity.

Adverse reactions
CNS: headache.
GI: *diarrhea,* nausea, vomiting, abdominal pain.
GU: vaginal fungal infections.
Skin: rash.
Other: hypersensitivity reactions *(anaphylaxis).*

☑ Special considerations
• Drug is highly stable in the presence of beta-lactamase enzymes. As a result, many organisms resistant to penicillins and some cephalosporins, because of presence of beta-lactamases, may be susceptible to cefpodoxime proxetil.
• Cefpodoxime is inactive against most strains of *Pseudomonas, Enterobacter,* and *Enterococcus.*
• Obtain specimen for culture and sensitivity tests before giving first dose. Therapy may begin pending test results.
• Store suspension in refrigerator (36° to 46° F [2 to 8° C]). Shake well before using. Discard unused portion after 14 days.
• Cefpodoxime proxetil may induce a positive direct Coombs' test.
• Toxic symptoms may include nausea, vomiting, epigastric distress, and diarrhea.
• For serious toxic reaction from overdose, hemodialysis or peritoneal dialysis may aid in removing drug from the body, particularly if renal function is compromised.

Monitoring the patient
• Prolonged use of cefpodoxime proxetil may result in overgrowth of nonsusceptible organisms. Repeated evaluation of the patient's condition is essential; take appropriate measures if superinfection occurs during therapy.
• Monitor patient for therapeutic effect.

Information for the patient
• Instruct patient to take drug with food to enhance absorption.
• Inform patient that oral suspension of cefpodoxime proxetil should be refrigerated. Instruct patient to shake container well before using and to discard unused portion after 14 days.

• Tell patient to continue taking drug for the prescribed course of therapy, even after feeling better.

Geriatric patients
• Elderly patients don't require dosage adjustment unless they have diminished renal function.

Pediatric patients
• Safety and efficacy in infants under age 6 months haven't been established.

Breast-feeding patients
• Drug appears in breast milk. Because of the potential for serious reactions in breast-fed infants, a decision must be made to discontinue breast-feeding or drug, taking into account importance of drug to the mother.

cefprozil
Cefzil

Pharmacologic classification: second-generation cephalosporin
Therapeutic classification: antibiotic
Pregnancy risk category B

How supplied
Available by prescription only
Tablets: 250 mg, 500 mg
Oral suspension: 125 mg/5 ml, 250 mg/5 ml

Indications, route, and dosage
Pharyngitis or tonsillitis caused by Streptococcus pyogenes
Adults and children ages 13 and older: 500 mg P.O. daily for at least 10 days.
Children ages 2 to 12: 7.5 mg/kg q 12 hours for 10 days.
Otitis media caused by Streptococcus pneumoniae, Haemophilus influenzae, and Moraxella (Branhamella) catarrhalis
Infants and children ages 6 months to 12 years: 15 mg/kg P.O. q 12 hours for 10 days.
Secondary bacterial infections of acute bronchitis and acute bacterial exacerbation of chronic bronchitis caused by S. pneumoniae, H. influenzae, and M. (B.) catarrhalis
Adults: 500 mg P.O. q 12 hours for 10 days.
Uncomplicated skin and skin-structure infections caused by Staphylococcus aureus and S. pyogenes
Adults and children ages 13 and older: 250 mg P.O. b.i.d., or 500 mg daily to b.i.d. for 10 days.
Children ages 2 to 12: 20 mg/kg q 24 hours for 10 days.
✦ **Dosage adjustment.** No adjustments are necessary for patients with creatinine clearance over 30 ml/minute. For patients with creatinine clearance of 30 ml/minute or less, dose should be reduced by 50%; however, dosing interval remains

unchanged. Because drug is partially removed by hemodialysis, it should be administered after the hemodialysis session.

Pharmacodynamics
Antibiotic action: Interferes with bacterial cell-wall synthesis during cell replication, leading to osmotic instability and cell lysis. Bactericidal or bacteriostatic, depending on concentration.

Pharmacokinetics
• *Absorption:* 95% absorbed from GI tract. Levels peak within 1½ hours of dose. Food doesn't interfere with capsule formulation; isn't known if food interferes with absorption of tablets or oral suspension.
• *Distribution:* 36% protein-bound.
• *Metabolism:* Probably metabolized by liver; plasma half-life increases only slightly in patients with impaired hepatic function.
• *Excretion:* 60% recovered unchanged in urine. Plasma half-life is 1.3 hours in patients with normal renal function; 2 hours, impaired hepatic function; and 5.2 to 5.9 hours, end-stage renal disease. Drug removed by hemodialysis.

Contraindications and precautions
Contraindicated in patients with hypersensitivity to drug or other cephalosporins. Use cautiously in patients with impaired renal function or penicillin allergy and in breast-feeding women.

Interactions
Drug-drug. *Aminoglycoside antibiotics:* May increase risk of nephrotoxicity of cephalosporins. Monitor patient closely.
Probenecid: May decrease excretion of cefprozil. Use together with caution.

Adverse reactions
CNS: dizziness, hyperactivity, headache, nervousness, insomnia, confusion, somnolence.
GI: *diarrhea, nausea,* vomiting, abdominal pain.
GU: elevated BUN and serum creatinine levels, genital pruritus, vaginitis.
Hematologic: decreased leukocyte count, eosinophilia.
Hepatic: elevated liver enzyme levels.
Skin: rash, urticaria, diaper rash.
Other: superinfection, hypersensitivity reactions (serum sickness, *anaphylaxis*).

☑ Special considerations
Besides the recommendations relevant to all cephalosporins, consider the following.
• Pseudomembranous colitis has been reported with nearly all antibacterial drugs. Consider this diagnosis in patients who develop diarrhea secondary to antibiotic therapy. Although most patients respond to withdrawal of drug therapy alone, it may be necessary to institute treatment with

an antibacterial drug effective against *Clostridium difficile*, an organism linked to this disorder.
• Obtain specimen for culture and sensitivity tests before giving first dose. Therapy may begin pending test results.
• Advise patients with phenylketonuria that oral suspension contains 28 mg/5 ml phenylalanine.
• Cephalosporins may produce a false-positive test for urine glucose with tests that use copper reduction method (Benedict's test, Fehling's solution, or Clinitest tablets). Instead, use enzymatic methods (such as glucose enzymatic test strip).
• A false-negative reaction may occur in the ferricyanide test for blood glucose.
• Because drug is eliminated primarily by the kidneys, hemodialysis may aid in removal of drug in cases of extreme overdose, especially in patients with decreased renal function.

Monitoring the patient
• Carefully observe patient for superinfection if prolonged use of drug is needed.
• Monitor renal patients carefully. Clinical observation and appropriate laboratory studies should be made before and during therapy.

Information for the patient
• Tell patient to take all of drug as prescribed, even if feeling better.

Geriatric patients
• Elderly volunteers (ages 65 and over) exhibited a higher area under the plasma concentration–versus-time curve and lower renal clearance compared with younger subjects.

Pediatric patients
• Oral suspensions contain drug in a bubble gum–flavored vehicle to improve palatability and compliance in children. Reconstituted suspension should be stored in the refrigerator, and unused drug should be discarded after 14 days. Shake suspension well before measuring dose.

Breast-feeding patients
• It's unknown if drug appears in breast milk. Use with caution in breast-feeding women.

---

ceftazidime
Ceptaz, Fortaz, Tazicef, Tazidime

Pharmacologic classification: third-generation cephalosporin
Therapeutic classification: antibiotic
Pregnancy risk category B

How supplied
Available by prescription only
Injection: 500 mg, 1 g, 2 g

Infusion: 1 g, 2 g in 20-, 50-, and 100-ml vials and bags

Indications, route, and dosage
Bacteremia, septicemia, and serious respiratory, urinary, gynecologic, bone and joint, intra-abdominal, CNS, and skin infections from susceptible organisms
Adults: 1 g I.V. or I.M. q 8 to 12 hours; up to 6 g daily in life-threatening infections.
Children ages 1 month to 12 years: 30 to 50 mg/kg I.V. q 8 hours to a maximum of 6 g/day (Fortaz, Tazicef, and Tazidime only).
Neonates up to 4 weeks: 30 mg/kg I.V. q 12 hours (Fortaz, Tazicef, and Tazidime only).
   Total daily dose is the same for I.M. or I.V. administration and depends on susceptibility of organism and severity of infection. Ceftazidime should be injected deep I.M. into a large muscle mass, such as the gluteus or lateral aspect of the thigh.
✦ **Dosage adjustment.** For patients with impaired renal function, doses or frequency of administration must be modified according to the degree of renal impairment, severity of infection, and susceptibility of organism. To prevent toxic accumulation, reduced dosage may be needed in patients with creatinine clearance below 50 ml/minute/1.73 m². In patients with creatinine clearance 50 ml/minute or less, initially give 1 g loading dose then follow below maintenance recommendations.

Creatinine clearance (ml/min/1.73 m²)	Adult dosage
> 50	Usual adult dose
31 to 50	1 g q 12 hours
16 to 30	1 g q 24 hours
6 to 15	500 mg q 24 hours
≤ 5	500 mg q 48 hours

For patients on hemodialysis, give 1 g after each hemodialysis period. For patients on peritoneal dialysis, give 500 mg q 24 hours.

Pharmacodynamics
Antibacterial action: Primarily bactericidal; however, may be bacteriostatic. Activity depends on the organism, tissue penetration, drug dosage, and rate of organism multiplication. Acts by adhering to bacterial penicillin-binding proteins, thereby inhibiting cell-wall synthesis. Third-generation cephalosporins appear more active against some beta-lactamase-producing gram-negative organisms.
   Ceftazidime is active against some gram-positive organisms and many enteric gram-negative bacilli as well as streptococci (*Streptococcus pneumoniae* and *S. pyogenes*); *Staph-*

ylococcus aureus (penicillinase- and non-penicillinase-producing); Escherichia coli; Klebsiella species; Proteus species; Enterobacter species; Haemophilus influenzae; Pseudomonas species; and some strains of Bacteroides species. It's more effective than any cephalosporin or penicillin derivative against Pseudomonas. Some other third-generation cephalosporins are more active against gram-positive organisms and anaerobes.

Pharmacokinetics
• Absorption: Not absorbed from GI tract and must be given parenterally; serum levels peak 1 hour after an I.M. dose.
• Distribution: Distributed widely into most body tissues and fluids, including gallbladder, liver, kidneys, bone, sputum, bile, pleural and synovial fluids; unlike most other cephalosporins, ceftazidime has good CSF penetration; crosses placenta. 5% to 24% protein-bound.
• Metabolism: Not metabolized.
• Excretion: Excreted primarily in urine by glomerular filtration; small amounts of drug excreted in breast milk. Elimination half-life is about 1½ to 2 hours in patients with normal renal function; up to 35 hours in patients with severe renal disease. Hemodialysis or peritoneal dialysis removes ceftazidime.

Contraindications and precautions
Contraindicated in patients with hypersensitivity to drug or other cephalosporins. Use cautiously in breast-feeding women and in patients with impaired renal function or penicillin allergy.

Interactions
Drug-drug. Aminoglycosides: Possible increased risk of nephrotoxicity. Monitor patient closely.
Clavulanic acid: Causes synergistic activity against some strains of Bacteroides fragilis. Use together cautiously.

Adverse reactions
CNS: headache, dizziness, paresthesia, *seizures.*
CV: phlebitis, thrombophlebitis (with I.V. injection).
GI: pseudomembranous colitis, nausea, vomiting, diarrhea, candidiasis, abdominal cramps.
GU: vaginitis.
Hematologic: eosinophilia, thrombocytosis, leukopenia, hemolytic anemia, *agranulocytosis, thrombocytopenia.*
Hepatic: transient elevation in liver enzyme levels.
Skin: maculopapular and erythematous rash, urticaria.
Other: hypersensitivity reactions (serum sickness, *anaphylaxis*), pain, induration, sterile abscesses, tissue sloughing (at injection site).

☑ Special considerations
Besides the recommendations relevant to all cephalosporins, consider the following.
• For patients on sodium restriction, note that ceftazidime contains 2.3 mEq sodium per gram of drug.
• Ceftazidime powders (excluding Ceptaz) for injection contain 118 mg sodium carbonate per gram of drug; ceftazidime sodium is more water-soluble and is formed in situ upon reconstitution.
• Vials are supplied under reduced pressure. When the antibiotic is dissolved, carbon dioxide is released and a positive pressure develops. Each brand of ceftazidime includes specific instructions for reconstitution. Read and follow these instructions carefully.
• Use separate I.V. sites for aminoglycosides and ceftazidime.
• Because drug is hemodialyzable, patients undergoing treatments with hemodialysis or peritoneal dialysis may require dosage adjustment.
• Ceftazidime causes false-positive results in urine glucose tests using cupric sulfate (Benedict's reagent or Clinitest); use glucose oxidase (Chemstrip uG, Diastix, or glucose enzymatic test strip) instead.
• Ceftazidime causes false elevations in urine creatinine levels in tests using Jaffé's reaction.
• Ceftazidime may cause positive Coombs' test results.
• Clinical signs of overdose include neuromuscular hypersensitivity. Seizure may follow high CNS concentrations.
• Drug may be removed by hemodialysis or peritoneal dialysis.

Monitoring the patient
• Carefully observe patient for superinfection if prolonged use of drug is needed.
• Monitor renal patients carefully. Clinical observation and appropriate laboratory studies should be made before and during therapy.
• PT should be monitored and exogenous vitamin K administered, as indicated, in patients with poor nutritional status, malabsorption states, or alcoholism and in those receiving prolonged therapy.

Information for the patient
• Inform patient of potential adverse reactions.

Geriatric patients
• Reduced dosage may be necessary in elderly patients with diminished renal function.

Pediatric patients
• Only Fortaz, Tazicef, and Tazidime may be used in infants and children. Ceptaz shouldn't be used in children under age 12 because of arginine component in product.

Breast-feeding patients
• Safe use hasn't been established. Drug appears in breast milk; use with caution in breast-feeding women.

ceftibuten
Cedax

Pharmacologic classification: third-generation cephalosporin
Therapeutic classification: antibiotic
Pregnancy risk category B

How supplied
Available by prescription only
Capsules: 400 mg
Oral suspension: 90 mg/5 ml, 180 mg/5 ml

Indications, route, and dosage
Acute bacterial exacerbations of chronic bronchitis caused by Haemophilus influenzae, Moraxella catarrhalis, or Streptococcus pneumoniae
Adults and children ages 12 and over: 400 mg P.O. daily for 10 days.
Pharyngitis and tonsillitis caused by Streptococcus pyogenes; acute bacterial otitis media caused by H. influenzae, M. catarrhalis, or S. pyogenes
Adults and children ages 12 and older: 400 mg P.O. daily for 10 days.
Children under age 12: 9 mg/kg P.O. daily for 10 days. Children weighing over 45 kg (99 lb) should receive the maximum daily dose of 400 mg.
✦ *Dosage adjustment.* No adjustments are necessary for patients with creatinine clearance over 50 ml/minute. Give 4.5 mg/kg (or 200 mg) daily to patients with creatinine clearance between 30 and 49 ml/minute and 2.25 mg/kg (or 100 mg) daily for those with creatinine clearance of 5 to 29 ml/minute. For patients undergoing hemodialysis two or three times weekly, give a single 400-mg dose (capsule form) or administer a single dose of 9 mg/kg (maximum dose, 400 mg) using oral suspension at the end of each hemodialysis session.

Pharmacodynamics
Antibiotic action: Exerts its bactericidal action by binding to essential target proteins of the bacterial cell wall. This binding leads to inhibition of cell-wall synthesis. Usually active against gram-positive aerobes (*S. pneumoniae, S. pyogenes*) and gram-negative aerobes (*H. influenzae, M. catarrhalis*).

Pharmacokinetics
• *Absorption:* Rapidly absorbed from GI tract. Food decreases drug bioavailability.
• *Distribution:* 65% bound to plasma proteins.

• *Metabolism:* Metabolized to its predominant component, cis-ceftibuten. About 10% of ceftibuten is converted to the transisomer.
• *Excretion:* Excreted in urine and feces.

Contraindications and precautions
Contraindicated in patients with hypersensitivity to cephalosporins. Use cautiously if administering to patients with history of hypersensitivity to penicillin because up to 10% of these patients will exhibit cross-sensitivity to a cephalosporin. Also use cautiously in patients with impaired renal function and GI disease (especially colitis).

Interactions
None reported.

Adverse reactions
CNS: headache, dizziness, fatigue, paresthesia, somnolence, taste perversion, agitation, hyperkinesia, insomnia, irritability, rigors.
EENT: nasal congestion.
GI: nausea, dyspepsia, abdominal pain, vomiting, anorexia, constipation, dry mouth, eructation, flatulence, loose stools.
GU: dysuria, hematuria, elevated BUN and serum creatinine levels, vaginitis. candidiasis.
Hematologic: elevated eosinophil count, decreased hemoglobin level, altered platelet count, decreased leukocyte count.
Hepatic: elevated liver enzyme, bilirubin, and alkaline phosphatase levels.
Respiratory: dyspnea.
Skin: rash, pruritus, diaper dermatitis, urticaria.
Other: dehydration, fever.

☑ Special considerations
Besides the recommendations relevant to all cephalosporins, consider the following.
• Pseudomembranous colitis has been reported with nearly all antibacterial drugs; consider this diagnosis in patients who develop diarrhea secondary to antibiotic therapy. Although most patients respond to withdrawal of drug therapy alone, it may be necessary to institute treatment with an antibacterial drug effective against *Clostridium difficile,* an organism linked to this disorder.
• Obtain specimen for culture and sensitivity tests before giving first dose. Therapy may begin pending test results.
• When preparing oral suspension, first tap bottle to loosen powder. Follow chart supplied by manufacturer for amount of water to add to powder when mixing oral suspension form. Add water in two portions, shaking well after each aliquot. After mixing, the suspension may be kept for 14 days and must be stored in the refrigerator.
• Although ceftibuten hasn't been known to affect the direct Coombs' test to date, other cephalosporins have caused a false-positive direct Coombs' test. A positive Coombs' test could be due to drug.

Reactions may be *common*, uncommon, **life-threatening**, or COMMON AND LIFE-THREATENING.

• Overdose of cephalosporins can cause cerebral irritation leading to seizures. Ceftibuten can be removed by hemodialysis.

Monitoring the patient
• Carefully observe patient for superinfection if prolonged use of drug is needed.
• Monitor renal patients carefully. Clinical observation and appropriate laboratory studies should be made before and during therapy.

Information for the patient
• Tell patient to take all of drug as prescribed, even if feeling better.
• Instruct patient using oral suspension to take it at least 2 hours before or 1 hour after a meal.
• Inform diabetic patient that oral suspension contains 1 g of sucrose per teaspoon of suspension.
• Instruct patient using oral suspension to shake bottle well before measuring dose.
• Tell patient to keep oral suspension in refrigerator with lid tightly closed and to discard unused drug after 14 days.

Geriatric patients
• Use with caution when administering drug to elderly patients. Dosage adjustment may be necessary if patient has impaired renal function.

Pediatric patients
• Safety and effectiveness in infants under age 6 months haven't been established.

Breast-feeding patients
• It's unknown if drug appears in breast milk; use cautiously in breast-feeding women.

ceftizoxime sodium
Cefizox

Pharmacologic classification: third-generation cephalosporin
Therapeutic classification: antibiotic
Pregnancy risk category B

How supplied
Available by prescription only
Injection: 500 mg, 1 g, 2 g, 10 g
Infusion: 1 g, 2 g in 100-ml vials; 50 ml in D_5W

Indications, route, and dosage
Bacteremia; septicemia; meningitis; pelvic inflammatory disease; serious respiratory, urinary, gynecologic, intra-abdominal, bone and joint, and skin infections from susceptible organisms
Adults: Usual dosage is 500 mg to 2 g I.V. or I.M. q 8 to 12 hours. In life-threatening infections, 3 to 4 g I.V. q 8 hours.
Children ages 6 months and older: 50 mg/kg q 6 to 8 hours.

Total daily dose is same for I.M. or I.V. administration and depends on susceptibility of organism and severity of infection. Ceftizoxime should be injected deep I.M. into a large muscle mass, such as the gluteus or lateral aspect of the thigh.
Uncomplicated gonorrhea
Adults: 1 g I.M. given as a single dose.
✦ *Dosage adjustment.* In patients with impaired renal function, modify doses or frequency of administration according to degree of renal impairment, severity of infection, and susceptibility of organism. To prevent toxic accumulation, reduced dosage may be needed in patients with creatinine clearance below 80 ml/minute. The following table gives appropriate doses for adults.

Creatinine clearance (ml/min/ 1.73 m²)	Less severe infections	Life-threatening infections
> 80	Usual adult dose	Usual adult dose
50 to 79	500 mg q 8 hours	750 mg to 1.5 g q 8 hours
5 to 49	250 to 500 mg q 12 hours	500 mg to 1 g q 12 hours
0 to 4	500 mg q 48 hours; or 250 mg q 24 hours	500 mg to 1 g q 48 hours; or 500 mg q 24 hours

Pharmacodynamics
Antibacterial action: Primarily bactericidal; however, may be bacteriostatic. Activity depends on the organism, tissue penetration, drug dosage, and rate of organism multiplication. It acts by adhering to bacterial penicillin-binding proteins, thereby inhibiting cell-wall synthesis. Third-generation cephalosporins appear more active against some beta-lactamase-producing gram-negative organisms.

Drug is active against some gram-positive organisms and many enteric gram-negative bacilli, as well as streptococci (*Streptococcus pneumoniae* and *pyogenes*); *Staphylococcus aureus* (penicillinase- and non–penicillinase-producing); *Staphylococcus epidermidis; Escherichia coli; Klebsiella* species; *Haemophilus influenzae; Enterobacter* species; *Proteus* species; *Bacteroides* species (including *Bacteroides fragilis*); *Peptostreptococcus* species; some strains of *Pseudomonas* and *Acinetobacter*. Cefotaxime and moxalactam are slightly more active than ceftizoxime against gram-positive organisms but are less active against gram-negative organisms.

Pharmacokinetics

• *Absorption:* Not absorbed from GI tract and must be given parenterally; serum levels peak at ½ to 1½ hours after I.M. dose.
• *Distribution:* Distributed widely into most body tissues and fluids, including gallbladder, liver, kidneys, bone, sputum, bile, pleural and synovial fluids; unlike most other cephalosporins, ceftizoxime has good CSF penetration and achieves adequate concentration in inflamed meninges; crosses placenta. 30% protein-bound.
• *Metabolism:* Not metabolized.
• *Excretion:* Excreted primarily in urine by renal tubular secretion and glomerular filtration; small amounts of drug excreted in breast milk. Elimination half-life is about 1½ to 2 hours in patients with normal renal function; severe renal disease prolongs half-life up to 30 hours. Hemodialysis or peritoneal dialysis removes minimal amounts of ceftizoxime.

Contraindications and precautions

Contraindicated in patients with hypersensitivity to ceftizoxime or other cephalosporins. Use cautiously in breast-feeding women and in patients with impaired renal function or penicillin allergy.

Interactions

Drug-drug. *Aminoglycosides:* May slightly increase risk of nephrotoxicity. Use together with caution.
Probenecid: Competitively inhibits renal tubular secretion of cephalosporins, causing higher, prolonged serum levels. Monitor patient closely.

Adverse reactions

CV: *phlebitis, thrombophlebitis.*
GI: pseudomembranous colitis, nausea, anorexia, vomiting, *diarrhea.*
GU: vaginitis.
Hematologic: transient neutropenia, eosinophilia, hemolytic anemia, thrombocytosis, anemia, **thrombocytopenia.**
Hepatic: transient elevation in liver enzymes (with I.V. injection).
Respiratory: dyspnea.
Skin: *maculopapular and erythematous rash, urticaria.*
Other: hypersensitivity reactions (serum sickness, **anaphylaxis**), elevated temperature, *pain, induration, sterile abscesses, tissue sloughing* (at injection site).

☑ Special considerations

Besides the recommendations relevant to all cephalosporins, consider the following.
• For patients on sodium restriction, note that ceftizoxime contains 2.6 mEq sodium per gram of drug.
• Drug may be supplied as frozen, sterile solution in plastic containers. Thaw at room temperature. Thawed solution is stable for 24 hours at room temperature or for 10 days if refrigerated. Don't refreeze.
• For I.M. use, reconstitute with sterile water for injection. Shake vial well to ensure complete dissolution of drug. To administer a dose that exceeds 1 g, divide dose and inject it into separate sites to prevent tissue injury.
• For I.V. use, reconstitute I.V. dose with sterile water for injection. Solution should clear after shaking well and range in color from yellow to amber. If particles are visible, discard solution. Reconstituted solution is stable for 24 hours at room temperature or 96 hours if refrigerated.
• Administer I.V. as a direct injection slowly over 3 to 5 minutes directly or through tubing of compatible infusion fluid. If given as intermittent infusion, dilute reconstituted drug in 50 to 100 ml of compatible fluid. Check package insert.
• Ceftizoxime causes false-positive results in urine glucose tests utilizing cupric sulfate (Benedict's reagent or Clinitest); use glucose oxidase (Chemstrip uG, Diastix, or glucose enzymatic test strip) instead.
• Ceftizoxime causes false elevations in urine creatinine levels using Jaffé's reaction.
• Ceftizoxime may cause positive Coombs' test results.
• Signs and symptoms of overdose include neuromuscular hypersensitivity. Seizure may follow high CNS concentrations.
• Ceftizoxime may be removed by hemodialysis.

Monitoring the patient

• Carefully observe patient for superinfection if prolonged use of drug is needed.
• Monitor renal patients carefully. Clinical observation and appropriate laboratory studies should be made before and during therapy.

Information for the patient

• Inform patient of potential adverse reactions.

Geriatric patients

• Reduced dosage may be necessary in elderly patients with diminished renal function.

Pediatric patients

• Safety and efficacy haven't been established in infants under age 6 months.

Breast-feeding patients

• Safe use hasn't been established. Drug appears in breast milk; use with caution in breast-feeding women.

---

ceftriaxone sodium
Rocephin

Pharmacologic classification: third-generation cephalosporin
Therapeutic classification: antibiotic
Pregnancy risk category B

How supplied
Available by prescription only
Injection: 250 mg, 500 mg, 1 g, 2 g
Infusion: 1 g, 2 g

Indications, route, and dosage
Bacteremia, septicemia, and serious respiratory, bone, joint, urinary, gynecologic, intra-abdominal, and skin infections from susceptible organisms
Adults and children ages 12 and older: 1 to 2 g I.M. or I.V. once daily or in equally divided doses b.i.d. Total daily dosage shouldn't exceed 4 g.
Children under age 12: Total daily dose is 50 to 75 mg/kg, given in divided doses q 12 hours. Maximum daily dose is 2 g.
Gonococcal meningitis, endocarditis
Adults: 1 to 2 g I.V. q 12 hours for 10 to 14 days for meningitis and 3 to 4 weeks for endocarditis.
Children: 50 to 100 mg/kg (maximum daily dose, 4 g) daily or divided q 12 hours for 7 to 14 days for meningitis and 28 days for endocarditis.
May give an initial dose of 100 mg/kg (not to exceed 4 g) to initiate therapy. Total daily dose is same for I.M. or I.V. administration and depends on susceptibility of organism and severity of infection. Ceftriaxone should be injected deep I.M. into a large muscle mass, such as the gluteus or lateral aspect of the thigh.
Preoperative prophylaxis
Adults: 1 g I.M. or I.V. 30 minutes to 2 hours before surgery.
Uncomplicated gonorrhea
Adults: 125 to 250 mg I.M. given as a single dose; ◊ 1 to 2 g I.M. or I.V. daily until improvement occurs.
◊ **Haemophilus ducreyi** *infection*
Adults: 250 mg I.M. as a single dose.
◊ **Sexually transmitted epididymitis, pelvic inflammatory disease**
Adults: 250 mg I.M. as a single dose; follow up with other antibiotics.
◊ **Anti-infectives for sexual assault victims**
Adults: 125 mg I.M. as a single dose with other antibiotics.
◊ **Lyme disease**
Adults: 1 to 2 g I.M. or I.V. q 12 to 24 hours.
✦ **Dosage adjustment.** In patients with impaired hepatic and renal function, dosage shouldn't exceed 2 g/day without monitoring serum drug levels.

Pharmacodynamics
Antibacterial action: Primarily bactericidal; however, may be bacteriostatic. Activity depends on organism, tissue penetration, and drug dosage and on rate of organism multiplication. Acts by adhering to bacterial penicillin-binding proteins, thereby inhibiting cell-wall synthesis. Third-generation cephalosporins appear more active against some beta-lactamase-producing gram-negative organisms.
Ceftriaxone is active against some gram-positive organisms and many enteric gram-negative bacilli, as well as streptococci; *Streptococcus pneumoniae* and *pyogenes; Staphylococcus aureus* (penicillinase- and non–penicillinase-producing); *Staphylococcus epidermidis; Escherichia coli; Klebsiella* species; *Haemophilus influenzae, Enterobacter; Proteus;* some strains of *Pseudomonas* and *Peptostreptococcus* and spirochetes such as *Borrelia burgdorferi* (the causative organism of Lyme disease). Most strains of *Listeria, Pseudomonas,* and *Acinetobacter* are resistant. Generally, ceftriaxone's activity is most like that of cefotaxime and ceftizoxime.

Pharmacokinetics
• *Absorption:* Not absorbed from GI tract and must be given parenterally; serum levels peak at 2 to 3 hours after I.M. dose.
• *Distribution:* Distributed widely into most body tissues and fluids, including gallbladder, liver, kidneys, bone, sputum, bile, pleural and synovial fluids; unlike most other cephalosporins, ceftriaxone has good CSF penetration. Crosses placenta. Protein-binding is dose-dependent and decreases as serum levels rise; average is 84% to 96%.
• *Metabolism:* Partially metabolized.
• *Excretion:* Excreted principally in urine; some drug excreted in bile by biliary mechanisms, and small amounts excreted in breast milk. Elimination half-life is 5½ to 11 hours in adults with normal renal function; severe renal disease prolongs half-life only moderately. Neither hemodialysis nor peritoneal dialysis will remove ceftriaxone.

Contraindications and precautions
Contraindicated in patients with hypersensitivity to ceftriaxone or other cephalosporins. Use cautiously in breast-feeding women and in patients with penicillin allergy.

Interactions
Drug-drug. *Aminoglycosides:* Produces synergistic antimicrobial activity against *Pseudomonas aeruginosa* and some strains of *Enterobacteriaceae.* Monitor patient closely.
Probenecid: May increase clearance by blocking biliary secretion and displacement of ceftriaxone from plasma proteins. Use together with caution.

Adverse reactions
CNS: headache, dizziness.
GI: pseudomembranous colitis, nausea, vomiting, diarrhea, urolithiasis.
GU: genital pruritus, moniliasis, elevated BUN levels.
Hematologic: eosinophilia, thrombocytosis, leukopenia.
Hepatic: increased liver function test results, jaundice.
Skin: pain, induration, tenderness (at injection site); phlebitis; *rash;* pruritus.
Other: hypersensitivity reactions (serum sickness, *anaphylaxis*), fever, chills.

☑ Special considerations
Besides the recommendations relevant to all cephalosporins, consider the following.
• For patients on sodium restriction, note that ceftriaxone injection contains 3.6 mEq sodium per gram of drug.
• Ceftriaxone causes false-positive results in urine glucose tests utilizing cupric sulfate (Benedict's reagent or Clinitest); use glucose oxidase (Chemstrip uG, Diastix, or glucose enzymatic test strip) instead.
• Ceftriaxone causes false elevations in urine creatinine levels in tests using Jaffé's reaction.
• Drug may cause positive Coombs' test results.
• Signs and symptoms of overdose include neuromuscular hypersensitivity. Seizure may follow high CNS concentrations. Treatment for overdose is supportive.

Monitoring the patient
• Carefully observe patient for superinfection if prolonged use of drug is needed.
• PT should be monitored and exogenous vitamin K administered, as indicated, in patients with poor nutritional status, malabsorption states, or alcoholism and in those on prolonged therapy.
• Dosage adjustment usually isn't necessary in patients with impaired renal function. However, blood levels should be monitored in patients with severe renal impairment (such as dialysis patients) and in those with both renal and hepatic dysfunction.
• Clinical observation and appropriate laboratory studies should be made before and during therapy.

Information for the patient
• Inform patient of potential adverse reactions.

Pediatric patients
• Ceftriaxone may be used in neonates and children. Use cautiously in hyperbilirubinemic neonates because of drug's ability to displace bilirubin.

Breast-feeding patients
• Drug appears in breast milk; use with caution in breast-feeding women.

cefuroxime axetil
Ceftin

cefuroxime sodium
Kefurox, Zinacef

Pharmacologic classification: second-generation cephalosporin
Therapeutic classification: antibiotic
Pregnancy risk category B

How supplied
Available by prescription only
cefuroxime axetil
Tablets: 125 mg, 250 mg, 500 mg
Suspension: 125 mg/5 ml, 250 mg/5ml
cefuroxime sodium
Injection: 750 mg, 1.5 g
Infusion: 750 mg, 1.5-g infusion packets

Indications, route, and dosage
Serious lower respiratory, urinary tract, skin and skin-structure infections; septicemia; meningitis caused by susceptible organisms
Adults: Usual dosage is 750 mg to 1.5 g I.M. or I.V. q 8 hours, usually for 5 to 10 days. For life-threatening infections and infections caused by less susceptible organisms, 1.5 g I.M. or I.V. q 6 hours; for bacterial meningitis, up to 3 g I.V. q 8 hours.
Children and infants over age 3 months: 50 to 100 mg/kg/day I.M. or I.V. in divided doses q 6 to 8 hours. Some clinicians give 100 to 150 mg/kg/day. For meningitis, the usual starting dose is 200 to 240 mg/kg/day I.V. in divided doses q 6 to 8 hours, reduced to 100 mg/kg/day when clinical improvement is seen. However, some clinicians prefer other drugs for meningitis.
    Total daily dose is same for I.M. or I.V. administration and depends on susceptibility of organism and severity of infection. Cefuroxime should be injected deep I.M. into a large muscle mass, such as the gluteus or lateral aspect of the thigh.
Pharyngitis, tonsillitis, lower respiratory infection, urinary tract infection
Adults and children over age 12: 125 to 500 mg P.O. b.i.d. for 10 days.
Children under age 12 who can swallow pills: 125 to 250 mg P.O. b.i.d. (tablets) for 10 days.
Children ages 3 months to 12 years: 20 mg/kg/day in divided doses b.i.d. (oral suspension) to maximum dose of 500 mg for 10 days.
Otitis media, impetigo
Children ages 3 months to 12 years: 30 mg/kg/day P.O. oral suspension divided into 2 doses (maximum dose is 1 g) for 10 days.

Children who can swallow pills: 250 mg P.O. b.i.d. for 10 days.

> *Note:* Compliance may be a problem when treating otitis media in children. Order suspension form if child is unable to swallow pills.

Preoperative prophylaxis
Adults: 1.5 g I.V. 30 to 60 minutes before surgery; then 750 mg I.M. or I.V. q 8 hours intraoperatively for a prolonged procedure.

◊ **Gonorrhea (urethral, endocervical, rectal)**
Adults: 1.5 g I.M. given as a single dose, alone or with other antibiotics.

Lyme disease (erythema migrans) caused by Borrelia burgdorferi
Adults and children ages 13 and older: 500 mg P.O. b.i.d. for 20 days.

✦ **Dosage adjustment.** Safety of drug in renal patients hasn't been established. In patients with impaired renal function, dose or frequency of administration must be modified based on degree of renal impairment, severity of infection, and susceptibility of organism. To prevent toxic accumulation, reduced I.M. or I.V. dosage may be required in patients with creatinine clearance below 20 ml/minute/1.73 m².

Creatinine clearance (ml/min/1.73 m²)	Adult dosage
> 20	750 mg to 1.5 g q 8 hours
10 to 20	750 mg q 12 hours
< 10	750 mg q 24 hours

For patients on hemodialysis, give 750 mg at the end of each dialysis period in addition to regular dose.

Pharmacodynamics
Antibacterial action: Primarily bactericidal; however, may be bacteriostatic. Activity depends on the organism, tissue penetration, drug dosage, and rate of organism multiplication. Acts by adhering to bacterial penicillin-binding proteins, thereby inhibiting cell-wall synthesis.

Cefuroxime is active against many gram-positive organisms and enteric gram-negative bacilli, including *Streptococcus pneumoniae* and *S. pyogenes, Haemophilus influenzae, Klebsiella* species, *Staphylococcus aureus, Escherichia coli, Enterobacter,* and *Neisseria gonorrhoeae; Bacteroides fragilis, Pseudomonas,* and *Acinetobacter* are resistant to cefuroxime.

Pharmacokinetics
• *Absorption:* Cefuroxime sodium isn't well absorbed from GI tract and must be given parenterally; serum levels peak 15 to 60 minutes after I.M. dose. Cefuroxime axetil is better absorbed orally, with between 37% to 52% of oral dose reaching systemic circulation. Serum levels after oral administration peak in about 2 hours. Food appears to enhance absorption. Tablets and suspension aren't bioequivalent.
• *Distribution:* Distributed widely into most body tissues and fluids, including gallbladder, liver, kidneys, bone, bile, pleural and synovial fluids; CSF penetration is greater than that of most first- and second-generation cephalosporins and achieves adequate therapeutic levels in inflamed meninges. Crosses placenta; 33% to 50% protein-bound.
• *Metabolism:* Not metabolized.
• *Excretion:* Primarily excreted in urine by renal tubular secretion and glomerular filtration; elimination half-life is 1 to 2 hours in patients with normal renal function; end-stage renal disease prolongs half-life 15 to 22 hours. Some drug excreted in breast milk. Hemodialysis removes drug.

Contraindications and precautions
Contraindicated in patients with hypersensitivity to cefuroxime or other cephalosporins. Use cautiously in breast-feeding women and in those with impaired renal function or penicillin allergy.

Interactions
Drug-drug. *Loop diuretics, nephrotoxic drugs (aminoglycosides, colistin, polymyxin B, vancomycin):* May increase risk of nephrotoxicity. Use together cautiously.
Probenecid: Competitively inhibits renal tubular secretion of cephalosporins, resulting in higher, prolonged serum levels of these drugs. Use together cautiously.

Adverse reactions
CV: *phlebitis, thrombophlebitis* (with I.V. injection).
GI: pseudomembranous colitis, nausea, anorexia, vomiting, *diarrhea.*
Hematologic: transient neutropenia, eosinophilia, **hemolytic anemia, thrombocytopenia,** decreased hemoglobin levels and hematocrit.
Hepatic: transient increases in liver enzyme levels.
Skin: *maculopapular and erythematous rash, urticaria.*
Other: hypersensitivity reactions (serum sickness, **anaphylaxis**); *pain, induration, sterile abscesses, temperature elevation, tissue sloughing* (at injection site).

☑ Special considerations
Besides the recommendations relevant to all cephalosporins, consider the following.
• Tablets and suspension aren't bioequivalent and can't be substituted on a mg/mg basis.
• For patients on sodium restriction, note that cefuroxime sodium contains 2.4 mEq sodium per gram of drug.

• Check solutions for particulate matter and discoloration. Solution may range in color from light yellow to amber without affecting potency.
• Shake I.M. solution gently before administration to ensure complete drug dissolution. Administer deep I.M. in a large muscle mass, preferably the gluteus area. Aspirate before injecting to prevent inadvertent injection into blood vessel. Rotate injection sites to prevent tissue damage. Apply ice to injection site to relieve pain.
• For direct intermittent I.V., inject solution slowly into vein over 3 to 5 minutes or slowly through tubing of free-running, compatible I.V. solution.
• Reconstituted solution retains potency for 24 hours at room temperature or for 48 hours if refrigerated.
• Reconstituted suspension can be stored at room temperature or in refrigerator. Unused portion should be discarded after 10 days. Shake well before each dose.
• Because drug is hemodialyzable, patients undergoing treatment with hemodialysis or peritoneal dialysis may require dosage adjustments.
• Drug causes false-positive results in urine glucose tests using cupric sulfate (Benedict's reagent or Clinitest); use glucose oxidase tests (Chemstrip uG, Diastix, or glucose enzymatic test strip) instead.
• Cefuroxime causes false elevations in serum or urine creatinine levels in tests using Jaffé's reaction.
• Cefuroxime may cause positive Coombs' test results.
• Signs and symptoms of overdose include neuromuscular hypersensitivity. Seizure may follow high CNS concentrations. Hemodialysis or peritoneal dialysis remove cefuroxime.

Monitoring the patient
• Carefully observe patient for superinfection if prolonged use of drug is needed.
• Monitor renal patients carefully. Clinical observation and appropriate laboratory studies should be made before and during therapy.

Information for the patient
• Inform patient of potential adverse reactions.

Geriatric patients
• Use with caution in elderly patients.

Pediatric patients
• Safe use in infants under age 3 months hasn't been established.

Breast-feeding patients
• Drug appears in breast milk; use with caution in breast-feeding women.

celecoxib
Celebrex

Pharmacologic classification: cyclooxygenase-2 (COX-2) inhibitor
Therapeutic classification: NSAID
Pregnancy risk category C

How supplied
Available by prescription only
Capsules: 100 mg, 200 mg

Indications, route, and dosage
Relief of signs and symptoms of osteoarthritis
Adults: 200 mg P.O. daily as a single dose or divided equally twice daily.
Relief of signs and symptoms of rheumatoid arthritis
Adults: 100 to 200 mg P.O. twice daily.
✦ *Dosage adjustment.* In patients weighing less than 50 kg (110 lb), start at lowest recommended dosage. In patients with moderate hepatic impairment (Child-Pugh Class II), start therapy with reduced dosage.

Pharmacodynamics
Anti-inflammatory, analgesic, and antipyretic action: Thought to act by selective inhibition of cyclooxygenase-2 (COX-2), resulting in decreased prostaglandin synthesis. Because celecoxib doesn't inhibit COX-1 at therapeutic levels, the reduction in symptoms of osteoarthritis and rheumatoid arthritis may be associated with fewer peripheral side effects.

Pharmacokinetics
• *Absorption:* Following oral administration, plasma levels peak in about 3 hours. Steady-state plasma levels expected within 5 days if celecoxib is given in several dosages.
• *Distribution:* Highly protein-bound, primarily to albumin.
• *Metabolism:* Primarily metabolized by cytochrome P-450 2C9.
• *Excretion:* Eliminated primarily by hepatic metabolism; 27% is excreted into urine. Elimination half-life under fasting conditions is about 11 hours.

Contraindications and precautions
Contraindicated in patients with severe hepatic impairment or hypersensitivity to celecoxib, sulfonamides, aspirin, or other NSAIDs and during the third trimester of pregnancy.
Use cautiously in patients with history of ulcers or GI bleeding, advanced renal disease, anemia, symptomatic liver disease, hypertension, edema, heart failure, or asthma. Also use cautiously in patients who smoke or use alcohol excessively, in those taking oral corticosteroids or anticoagulants, and in elderly or debilitated patients.

Interactions

Drug-drug. *Aluminum and magnesium antacids:* May decrease plasma levels of celecoxib. Administer these drugs at least 1 hour apart.

Angiotensin-converting enzyme inhibitors: Diminished antihypertensive effects. Monitor patient's blood pressure.

Aspirin: Can increase risk of ulcers; low aspirin dosages can be used safely for prevention of cardiovascular events. Monitor patient for signs and symptoms of GI bleeding.

Fluconazole: Can increase celecoxib levels. Reduce dosage of celecoxib to minimal effective dosage.

Furosemide: NSAIDs can reduce sodium excretion associated with diuretics, leading to sodium retention. Monitor patient for swelling and increase in blood pressure.

Lithium: Possible increased lithium level. Monitor lithium plasma levels closely during treatment.

Warfarin: Direct interaction hasn't been reported. Watch for signs and symptoms of bleeding because of increased risk with warfarin.

Drug-lifestyle. *Alcohol:* Possible increased risk of GI irritation or bleeding if being used excessively. Watch for signs and symptoms of bleeding.

Adverse reactions

CNS: dizziness, *headache,* insomnia.
EENT: pharyngitis, rhinitis, sinusitis.
GI: abdominal pain, diarrhea, dyspepsia, flatulence, nausea.
GU: elevated BUN level.
Hepatic: elevated liver enzyme levels.
Metabolic: hyperchloremia, hypophosphatemia.
Respiratory: upper respiratory tract infection.
Skin: rash.
Other: *back pain, peripheral edema, accidental injury.*

☑ Special considerations

● Patients may be allergic to celecoxib if they have an allergy to sulfonamides, aspirin, or other NSAIDs.

● Aluminum and magnesium antacids may decrease effect of celecoxib and should be administered at least 1 hour apart.

● Common signs and symptoms of overdose include lethargy, drowsiness, nausea, vomiting, epigastric pain, and GI bleeding. Other possible symptoms include hypertension, acute renal failure, respiratory depression, and coma.

● There is no antidote for overdose. Symptomatic and supportive care is usually sufficient. If patient is seen within 4 hours of overdose, emesis or activated charcoal or an osmotic cathartic can be used.

● Because of high protein-binding, dialysis is unlikely to be effective.

Monitoring the patient

● Patients with a history of ulcers or GI bleeding are at higher risk for GI bleeding. Watch for signs and symptoms of overt and occult bleeding. Other risk factors for GI bleeding include treatment with corticosteroids or anticoagulants, longer duration of NSAID treatment, smoking, alcoholism, older age, and poor overall health

● Watch for signs and symptoms of hepatic and renal toxicity, especially if patient is dehydrated.

● Patients on long-term treatment should have hemoglobin level and hematocrit checked if they exhibit any signs or symptoms of anemia or blood loss.

Information for the patient

● Inform patient that antacids containing aluminum or magnesium should be taken at least 1 hour apart.

● Inform patient that it may take several days before he feels consistent pain relief and to call if no relief is experienced.

● Advise patient to immediately report any signs of swelling, excessive fatigue, yellowing of skin, flulike symptoms, bleeding, or difficulty breathing.

● Instruct patient to take drug with food if stomach upset occurs.

Geriatric patients

● Dosage adjustment isn't necessary unless patient weighs less than 110 lb; however, elderly patients experience more adverse effects overall.

Pediatric patients

● Drug hasn't been studied in patients under age 18.

Breast-feeding patients

● It's unknown if drug appears in breast milk. Assess risks and benefits before using drug in breast-feeding women.

cephalexin hydrochloride
Keftab

cephalexin monohydrate
Biocef, Keflex, Novo-Lexin*

Pharmacologic classification: first-generation cephalosporin
Therapeutic classification: antibiotic
Pregnancy risk category B

How supplied

Available by prescription only
cephalexin hydrochloride
Tablets: 500 mg

cephalexin monohydrate
Tablets: 250 mg, 500 mg, 1 g
Capsules: 250 mg, 500 mg
Suspension: 125 mg/5 ml, 250 mg/5 ml

Indications, route, and dosage
Respiratory, GU, skin and soft-tissue, and bone and joint infections caused by susceptible organisms
Adults: 250 mg to 1 g P.O. q 6 hours.
Children: 25 to 50 mg/kg/day divided into four doses. In patients over age 1 with streptococcal pharyngitis or skin and skin-structure infections, dose may be administered q 12 hours.
Otitis media
Adults: 250 mg to 1 g P.O. q 6 hours.
Children: 75 to 100 mg/kg/day divided into four doses.
✦ *Dosage adjustment.* To prevent toxic accumulation in patients with impaired renal function whose creatinine clearance is below 40 ml/minute, give reduced dosage. If creatinine clearance is below 5 ml/minute, give 250 mg q 12 to 24 hours; between 5 and 10 ml/minute, give 250 mg q 12 hours; between 11 to 40 ml/minute, give 500 mg q 8 to 12 hours.

Pharmacodynamics
Antibacterial action: Primarily bactericidal; however, may be bacteriostatic. Activity depends on the organism, tissue penetration, drug dosage, and rate of organism multiplication. It acts by adhering to bacterial penicillin-binding proteins, thereby inhibiting cell-wall synthesis.

Drug is active against many gram-positive organisms, including penicillinase-producing *Staphylococcus aureus* and S. *epidermidis, Streptococcus pneumoniae,* group B streptococci, and group A beta-hemolytic streptococci; susceptible gram-negative organisms include *Klebsiella pneumoniae, Escherichia coli, Proteus mirabilis,* and *Shigella.*

Pharmacokinetics
● *Absorption:* Absorbed rapidly and completely from GI tract after oral administration; serum levels peak within 1 hour. Base monohydrate probably converted to the hydrochloride in stomach before absorption. Food delays but doesn't prevent complete absorption.
● *Distribution:* Distributed widely into most body tissues and fluids, including gallbladder, liver, kidneys, bone, sputum, bile, pleural and synovial fluids; poor CSF penetration. Crosses placenta; 6% to 15% protein-bound.
● *Metabolism:* Not metabolized.
● *Excretion:* Excreted primarily unchanged in urine by glomerular filtration and renal tubular secretion; small amounts may be excreted in breast milk. Elimination half-life is about ½ to 1 hour in patients with normal renal function; 7½ to

14 hours in patients with severe renal impairment. Hemodialysis or peritoneal dialysis removes cephalexin.

Contraindications and precautions
Contraindicated in patients with hypersensitivity to cephalosporins. Use cautiously in patients with impaired renal function or penicillin allergy and in breast-feeding women.

Interactions
Drug-drug. *Loop diuretics, nephrotoxic drugs (aminoglycosides, colistin, polymyxin B, vancomycin):* May increase risk of nephrotoxicity. Use together cautiously.
Probenecid: Competitively inhibits renal tubular secretion of cephalosporins, resulting in higher, prolonged serum levels of these drugs. Use together cautiously.

Adverse reactions
CNS: dizziness, headache, fatigue, agitation, confusion, hallucinations.
GI: pseudomembranous colitis, *nausea, anorexia,* vomiting, *diarrhea,* gastritis, glossitis, dyspepsia, abdominal pain, anal pruritus, tenesmus, oral candidiasis.
GU: genital pruritus and candidiasis, vaginitis, interstitial nephritis.
Hematologic: *neutropenia,* eosinophilia, anemia, *thrombocytopenia.*
Hepatic: transient increases in liver enzyme levels.
Musculoskeletal: arthritis, arthralgia, joint pain.
Skin: *maculopapular* and *erythematous rash, urticaria.*
Other: hypersensitivity reactions (serum sickness, **anaphylaxis**).

☑ Special considerations
Besides the recommendations relevant to all cephalosporins, consider the following.
● For oral suspension, add required amount of water to powder in two portions. Shake well after each addition. After mixing, store in refrigerator. Suspension is stable for 14 days without significant loss of potency. Store mixture in tightly closed container. Shake well before using.
● Because cephalexin is dialyzable, patients receiving hemodialysis or peritoneal dialysis may need dosage adjustment.
● Drug causes false-positive results in urine glucose tests utilizing cupric sulfate (Benedict's reagent or Clinitest); use glucose oxidase test (Chemstrip uG, Diastix, or glucose enzymatic test strip) instead.
● Cephalexin causes false elevations in serum or urine creatinine levels in tests using Jaffé's reaction.

Reactions may be *common,* uncommon, *life-threatening*, or COMMON AND LIFE-THREATENING.

● Positive Coombs' test results occur in about 3% of patients taking cephalexin.
● Signs and symptoms of overdose include neuromuscular hypersensitivity. Seizure may follow high CNS concentrations.
● Remove cephalexin by hemodialysis or peritoneal dialysis. Other treatment is supportive.

Monitoring the patient
● Carefully observe patient for superinfection if prolonged drug use is needed.
● Monitor renal patients carefully. Clinical observation and appropriate laboratory studies should be made before and during therapy.

Information for the patient
● Inform patient of potential adverse reactions.

Geriatric patients
● Reduce dosage in elderly patients with diminished renal function.

Pediatric patients
● Serum half-life is prolonged in neonates and in infants under age 1. Safety and effectiveness in children haven't been established.

Breast-feeding patients
● Drug appears in breast milk; use with caution in breast-feeding women.

cephradine
Velosef

Pharmacologic classification: first-generation cephalosporin
Therapeutic classification: antibiotic
Pregnancy risk category B

How supplied
Available by prescription only
Capsules: 250 mg, 500 mg
Suspension: 125 mg/5 ml, 250 mg/5 ml
Injection: 250 mg, 500 mg, 1 g, 2 g

Indications, route, and dosage
Serious respiratory, GU, skin and soft-tissue, bone and joint infections; septicemia; endocarditis; otitis media
Adults: 250 to 500 mg P.O. q 6 hours. Severe or chronic infections may need larger or more frequent doses (up to 1 g P.O. q 6 hours). Or 500 mg to 1 g I.M. or I.V. q 6 hours.
Children over age 9 months: 25 to 100 mg/kg P.O. daily in equally divided doses q 6 to 12 hours. Or 12.5 to 25 mg/kg I.M. or I.V. q 6 hours.
Larger doses (up to 1 g q.i.d.) may be given for severe or chronic infections in all patients regardless of age and weight.
✦ **Dosage adjustment.** To prevent toxic accumulation, reduced dosage may be required in patients with creatinine clearance below 20 ml/minute.

Creatinine clearance (ml/min/1.73 m²)	Adult dosage
> 20	500 mg q 6 hours
5 to 20	250 mg q 6 hours
< 5	250 mg q 12 hours

For patients on long-term intermittent dialysis, give 250 mg initially; repeat in 12 hours and after 36 to 48 hours. Children may need dose modifications proportional to weight and severity of infection.

Pharmacodynamics
Antibacterial action: Primarily bactericidal; however, may be bacteriostatic. Activity depends on the organism, tissue penetration, drug dosage, and rate of organism multiplication. It acts by adhering to bacterial penicillin-binding proteins, thereby inhibiting cell-wall synthesis.
Like other first-generation cephalosporins, cephradine is active against many gram-positive organisms and some gram-negative organisms. Susceptible organisms include *Escherichia coli* and other coliform bacteria, group A beta-hemolytic streptococci, *Hemophilus influenzae, Klebsiella, Proteus mirabilis, Staphylococcus aureus, Streptococcus pneumoniae,* staphylococci, and *Streptococcus viridans.*

Pharmacokinetics
● *Absorption:* Well absorbed from GI tract; serum levels peak within 1 hour after oral dose.
● *Distribution:* Distributed widely into most body tissues and fluids, including gallbladder, liver, kidneys, bone, sputum, bile, pleural and synovial fluids; poor CSF penetration. Crosses placenta; 6% to 20% protein-bound.
● *Metabolism:* Not metabolized.
● *Excretion:* Excreted primarily in urine by renal tubular and glomerular filtration; small amounts excreted in breast milk. Elimination half-life is about ½ to 2 hours in normal renal function; end-stage renal disease prolongs half-life to 8 to 15 hours. Hemodialysis or peritoneal dialysis removes drug.

Contraindications and precautions
Contraindicated in patients with hypersensitivity to drug and other cephalosporins. Use cautiously in patients with impaired renal function or penicillin allergy and in breast-feeding women.

Interactions
Drug-drug. *Bacteriostatic drugs (chloramphenicol, erythromycin, tetracyclines):* May in-

terfere with bactericidal activity. Monitor patient for drug effect.

Loop diuretics, nephrotoxic drugs (aminoglycosides, colistin, polymyxin B, vancomycin): May increase risk of nephrotoxicity. Use together cautiously.

Probenecid: Competitively inhibits renal tubular secretion of cephalosporins, resulting in higher, prolonged serum levels of these drugs. Use together cautiously.

Adverse reactions
CNS: dizziness, headache, malaise, paresthesia.
GI: pseudomembranous colitis, *nausea, anorexia,* vomiting, transient increases in liver enzymes, heartburn, abdominal cramps, *diarrhea,* oral candidiasis.
GU: genital pruritus and candidiasis, vaginitis.
Hematologic: transient neutropenia, eosinophilia, *thrombocytopenia.*
Skin: *maculopapular* and *erythematous rash, urticaria.*
Other: hypersensitivity reactions (serum sickness, *anaphylaxis*).

☑ Special considerations
Besides the recommendations relevant to all cephalosporins, consider the following.
• Reconstituted oral suspension may be stored for 7 days at room temperature or for 14 days in the refrigerator.
• Because drug is dialyzable, patients undergoing treatment with hemodialysis may require dosage adjustments.
• Drug causes false-positive results in urine glucose tests utilizing cupric sulfate (Benedict's reagent or Clinitest); use glucose oxidase tests (Chemstrip uG, Diastix, or glucose enzymatic test strip) instead.
• Cephradine causes false elevations in serum or urine creatinine levels in tests using Jaffé's reaction.
• Cephradine may cause positive Coombs' test results.
• Signs and symptoms of overdose include neuromuscular hypersensitivity. Seizure may follow high CNS concentrations.
• Remove cephradine by hemodialysis.

Monitoring the patient
• Carefully observe patient for superinfection if prolonged drug use is needed.
• Monitor renal patients carefully. Clinical observation and appropriate laboratory studies should be made before and during therapy.
• In patients with impaired hepatic or renal function, appropriate monitoring is recommended during therapy.

Information for the patient
• Inform patient of potential adverse reactions.

Geriatric patients
• Reduced dosage may be required in patients with reduced renal function. Use with caution.

Pediatric patients
• Serum half-life is prolonged in neonates and infants under age 1. Safe use hasn't been established.

Breast-feeding patients
• Safe use hasn't been established. Drug appears in breast milk; use with caution in breast-feeding women.

cerivastatin sodium
Baycol

Pharmacologic classification: 3-hydroxy-3-methylglutaryl-coenzyme A (HMG-CoA) reductase inhibitor
Therapeutic classification: antilipemic
Pregnancy risk category X

How supplied
Available by prescription only
Tablets: 0.2 mg, 0.3 mg

Indications, route, and dosage
Adjunct to diet for reducing elevated total and low-density lipoprotein (LDL) cholesterol levels in patients with primary hypercholesterolemia and mixed dyslipidemia when diet and other nonpharmacologic measures have been inadequate
Adults: 0.3 mg P.O. once daily in the evening.
✦ Dosage adjustment. In patients with significant renal impairment (creatinine clearance 60 ml/minute/1.73 m^2 or less), 0.2 mg P.O. once daily in the evening.

Pharmacodynamics
Antilipemic action: Competitive inhibitor of HMG-CoA reductase that's responsible for conversion of HMG-CoA to mevalonate, a precursor of sterols including cholesterol. Reducing the level of cholesterol in hepatic cells stimulates synthesis of LDL receptors, leading to an increase in uptake of LDL particles.

Pharmacokinetics
• *Absorption:* Absorbed in active form. Mean absolute bioavailability of 0.2-mg tablet is 60%, with levels peaking about 2½ hours after dose. Absorption is similar if taken with evening meal or 4 hours after evening meal.
• *Distribution:* Mean volume of distribution is 0.3 L/kg. Over 99% of circulating drug bound to plasma proteins (80% bound to albumin).
• *Metabolism:* Extensively metabolized to 2 active metabolites, M1 and M23. A demethylation reaction forms M1, a hydroxylation reaction forms

M23. Relative potencies of M1 and M23 are 50% and 80% of active compound, respectively. Relative concentrations of metabolites in comparison to parent compound are significantly less. Therefore, cholesterol-lowering effect of drug is due primarily to parent compound.
• *Excretion:* Doesn't occur in urine or feces; M1 and M23 are the major metabolites excreted by these routes. Following oral dose of 0.4 mg ^{14}C-cerivastatin to healthy volunteers, excretion of radioactivity is about 24% in urine and 70% in feces. Parent compound, cerivastatin, accounts for less than 2% of total radioactivity excreted.

Contraindications and precautions
Contraindicated in patients with hypersensitivity to drug and in those with active liver disease or unexplained persistent elevations of serum transaminase levels. Also contraindicated during pregnancy and in breast-feeding patients. Avoid use in women of childbearing age because of potential for fetal harm unless patient is highly unlikely to conceive. If patient becomes pregnant during therapy, stop drug. Use cautiously in patients with history of liver disease or long-term alcohol ingestion.

Interactions
Drug-drug. *Azole antifungals, cyclosporine, erythromycin, fibric acid derivatives, niacin:* May increase risk of myopathy. Use together cautiously.
Cholestyramine given within 4 hours of drug: Causes decreased absorption and decreased peak plasma levels of cerivastatin. However, administration of cerivastatin at bedtime and cholestyramine 1 hour before evening meal doesn't result in significant decrease in cerivastatin's effect. Monitor patient.
Erythromycin: Decreases hepatic metabolism of drug and increases serum levels of cerivastatin up to 50%. Use together cautiously.
Drug-lifestyle. *Alcohol:* May increase risk of liver toxicity. Don't use together.

Adverse reactions
CNS: asthenia, dizziness, *headache*, insomnia.
CV: chest pain, peripheral edema.
EENT: *pharyngitis, rhinitis,* sinusitis.
GI: abdominal pain, constipation, diarrhea, dyspepsia, flatulence, nausea.
GU: urinary tract infection.
Hepatic: elevated transaminase, CK, alkaline phosphatase, gamma glutamyl transpeptidase, and bilirubin levels.
Musculoskeletal: arthralgia, back or leg pain, myalgia.
Respiratory: increased cough.
Skin: rash.
Other: flulike symptoms.

☑ Special considerations
• Withhold drug temporarily in patients with acute or serious conditions (trauma; major surgery; severe metabolic, endocrine and electrolyte disorders; severe acute infection; hypotension; and uncontrolled seizures) predisposing them to renal failure secondary to rhabdomyolysis. Cases of rhabdomyolysis have occurred rarely with other HMG-CoA reductase inhibitors.
• Lipid-lowering drug therapy should be part of multiple risk factor intervention program; attempt to control cholesterol with appropriate diet, exercise, and weight reduction before starting drug therapy.
• Because maximal effect of drug is seen within 4 weeks, lipid determinations should be performed at this time.
• Give drug to women of childbearing age only if conception is highly unlikely and they have been warned of potential risks to fetus.
• For overdose, treat symptomatically and provide supportive measures.
• Because of extensive drug binding to plasma proteins, hemodialysis may not enhance drug clearance.

Monitoring the patient
• Before initiating treatment, exclude secondary causes for hypercholesterolemia and perform a baseline lipid profile. Periodic liver function tests and lipid levels should be done before starting treatment, at 6 and 12 weeks after initiation of treatment (or after an increase in dosage); then periodically.
• Monitor patient for adverse effects.

Information for the patient
• Teach patient proper dietary management, weight control, and exercise.
• Explain importance in controlling elevated serum lipid levels.
• Tell patient to take drug in evening with or without food.
• Warn patient to avoid alcohol.
• Inform patient that it may take up to 4 weeks for full therapeutic effect to occur.
• Caution woman that drug may cause fetal damage. Advise her to call immediately if pregnancy occurs or is suspected.
• Tell patient to immediately report unexplained muscle pain, tenderness, or weakness, especially if accompanied by fever or malaise.

Geriatric patients
• Plasma drug levels are similar in healthy men over age 65 and in men below age 40.

Pediatric patients
• Safety and efficacy in children haven't been established.

Breast-feeding patients
• Because of potential for adverse reactions in breast-fed infants, women taking cerivastatin shouldn't breast-feed.

cetirizine hydrochloride
Zyrtec

Pharmacologic classification: selective H_1-receptor antagonist
Therapeutic classification: antihistamine
Pregnancy risk category B

How supplied
Available by prescription only
Tablets: 5 mg, 10 mg
Syrup: 5 mg/ml

Indications, route, and dosage
Seasonal allergic rhinitis, perennial allergic rhinitis, chronic urticaria
Adults and children ages 6 and older: 5 or 10 mg P.O. daily.
✦ *Dosage adjustment.* In hemodialysis patients or those with hepatic impairment or creatinine clearance below 31 ml/minute, 5 mg P.O. daily.

Pharmacodynamics
Antihistaminic action: Principal effects are mediated via selective inhibition of peripheral H_1 receptors.

Pharmacokinetics
• *Absorption:* Rapidly absorbed.
• *Distribution:* 93% bound to plasma proteins.
• *Metabolism:* Metabolized to a very limited extent by oxidative O-dealkylation to a metabolite with negligible antihistaminic activity.
• *Excretion:* Primarily excreted in urine with 50% as unchanged drug; small amount excreted in feces.

Contraindications and precautions
Contraindicated in patients with hypersensitivity to drug or hydroxyzine. Use cautiously in patients with impaired renal function.

Interactions
Drug-drug. *Anticholinergics, CNS depressants:* Possible additive effect. Avoid use together.
Theophylline: Possible decreased clearance of cetirizine. Monitor patient closely.
Drug-lifestyle. *Alcohol:* Possible additive effect. Avoid use together.

Adverse reactions
CNS: somnolence, fatigue, dizziness.
EENT: pharyngitis.
GI: dry mouth.

☑ Special considerations
• Abuse or dependency isn't known to occur with cetirizine use.
• Overdose may result in somnolence. If overdose occurs, treatment should be symptomatic or supportive.
• No known specific antidote exists; drug isn't effectively removed by dialysis.

Monitoring the patient
• Monitor patient for adverse effects.
• For patients with impaired renal function, monitor BUN and creatinine closely.

Information for the patient
• Caution patient not to perform hazardous activities if somnolence occurs with drug use.
• Instruct patient not to consume alcohol or other CNS depressants while taking drug because of additive effect.

Geriatric patients
• A decrease in cetirizine clearance in elderly volunteers may be related to decreased renal function in this age group.

Pediatric patients
• Safety and effectiveness in children under age 6 haven't been established.

Breast-feeding patients
• Drug reportedly appears in breast milk; avoid use in breast-feeding women.

chloral hydrate
Aquachloral Supprettes, Noctec, Novo-Chlorhydrate*

Pharmacologic classification: general CNS depressant
Therapeutic classification: sedative-hypnotic
Controlled substance schedule IV
Pregnancy risk category C

How supplied
Available by prescription only
Capsules: 250 mg, 500 mg
Syrup: 250 mg/5 ml, 500 mg/5 ml
Suppositories: 325 mg, 500 mg, 650 mg

Indications, route, and dosage
Sedation
Adults: 250 mg P.O. t.i.d. after meals.
Children: 8 mg/kg P.O. t.i.d. Maximum dose is 500 mg t.i.d.
Management of alcohol withdrawal symptoms
Adults: 500 to 1,000 mg; may repeat q 6 hours, p.r.n.

Insomnia
Adults: 500 mg to 1 g P.O. or P.R. 15 to 30 minutes before bedtime.
Children: 50 mg/kg P.O. or P.R. single dose. Maximum dose is 1 g.

Premedication for EEG
Children: 20 to 25 mg/kg P.O. single dose. Maximum dose is 1 g.

Hypnosis
Children: 50 mg/kg P.O. or 1.5 g/m^2 as single dose. Maximum dose is 1 g.
✦ *Dosage adjustment.* Decrease dosage in elderly patients.

Pharmacodynamics
Sedative-hypnotic action: CNS depressant activities similar to those of barbiturates. Nonspecific CNS depression occurs at hypnotic doses; however, respiratory drive is only slightly affected. Drug's primary site of action is the reticular activating system, which controls arousal. The cellular site of action isn't known.

Pharmacokinetics
● *Absorption:* Well absorbed after oral and rectal administration. Sleep occurs 30 to 60 minutes after a 500-mg to 1-g dose.
● *Distribution:* Drug and active metabolite, trichloroethanol, distributed throughout body tissue and fluids. Trichloroethanol is 35% to 41% protein-bound.
● *Metabolism:* Metabolized rapidly and nearly completely in liver and erythrocytes to active metabolite trichloroethanol. Further metabolized in liver and kidneys to trichloroacetic acid and other inactive metabolites.
● *Excretion:* Inactive metabolites of drug hydrate excreted primarily in urine. Minor amounts excreted in bile. Trichloroethanol half-life is 8 to 10 hours.

Contraindications and precautions
Contraindicated in patients with hypersensitivity to drug and in those with impaired hepatic or renal function or severe cardiac disease. Oral administration contraindicated in patients with gastric disorders. Use with extreme caution in patients with mental depression, suicidal tendencies, or history of drug abuse.

Interactions
Drug-drug. *Antihistamines, narcotics, sedative-hypnotics, tranquilizers, tricyclic antidepressants, other CNS depressants:* Will add to or potentiate their effects. Monitor patient closely.
I.V. furosemide: May cause a hypermetabolic state by displacing thyroid hormone from binding sites, resulting in sweating, hot flashes, tachycardia, and variable blood pressure. Use together cautiously.
Oral anticoagulants: Possible increased hypoprothrombinemic effects. Monitor PT.

Phenytoin: Possible increased elimination of phenytoin. Monitor serum phenytoin levels.
Drug-lifestyle. *Alcohol:* May cause vasodilation, tachycardia, sweating, and flushing in some patients. Avoid use together.

Adverse reactions
CNS: drowsiness, nightmares, dizziness, ataxia, paradoxical excitement, hangover, somnolence, disorientation, delirium, light-headedness, hallucinations, confusion, vertigo, malaise.
GI: *nausea, vomiting, diarrhea,* flatulence.
Hematologic: eosinophilia, leukopenia.
Skin: hypersensitivity reactions (rash, urticaria).
Other: physical and psychological dependence.

☑ Special considerations
● Chloral hydrate isn't a first-line drug because of potential for adverse or toxic adverse effects.
● Some brands contain tartrazine, which may cause allergic reactions in susceptible individuals.
● Give drug capsules with 8 oz (240 ml) of water to lessen GI upset; dilute syrup in half glass of water or juice before administering to improve taste.
● Store in dark container away from heat and moisture to prevent breakdown of drug. Store suppositories in refrigerator.
● Assess level of consciousness before administering drug to ensure appropriate baseline level.
● Drug therapy may produce false-positive results for urine glucose with tests using cupric sulfate, such as Benedict's reagent and possibly Clinitest.
● Drug doesn't interfere with Chemstrip uG, Diastix, or glucose enzymatic test strip results.
● Drug will interfere with fluorometric tests for urine catecholamines; don't use drug for 48 hours before test.
● Drug may interfere with Reddy-Jenkins-Thorn test for urinary 17-hydroxycorticosteroids.
● Drug may cause a false-positive phentolamine test.
● Signs and symptoms of overdose include stupor, coma, respiratory depression, pinpoint pupils, hypotension, and hypothermia. Esophageal stricture may follow gastric necrosis and perforation; GI hemorrhage has been reported; hepatic damage and jaundice may occur.
● Treatment of overdose is supportive of respiration (including mechanical ventilation if needed), blood pressure, and body temperature. If patient is conscious, empty stomach by emesis or gastric lavage. Hemodialysis removes drug and its metabolite. Peritoneal dialysis may be effective.

Monitoring the patient
● Monitor vital signs frequently.
● Monitor patient for adverse effects.

Information for the patient
• Advise patient to take drug with 8 oz of water and to dilute syrup with juice or water before use.
• Instruct patient in proper administration of form prescribed.
• Warn patient not to attempt tasks that require mental alertness or physical coordination until the CNS effects of drug are known.
• Tell patient to avoid alcohol and other CNS depressants.
• Instruct patient to call before using OTC allergy or cold preparations.
• Warn patient not to increase dose or stop drug except as prescribed.

Geriatric patients
• Elderly patients may be more susceptible to drug's CNS depressant effects because of decreased elimination. Lower doses are indicated.

Pediatric patients
• Drug is safe and effective in children as a premedication for EEG and other procedures.

Breast-feeding patients
• Small amounts appear in breast milk and may cause drowsiness in breast-fed infants; avoid use in breast-feeding women.

---

chlorambucil
Leukeran

Pharmacologic classification: alkylating drug (cell-cycle–phase nonspecific)
Therapeutic classification: antineoplastic
Pregnancy risk category D

How supplied
Available by prescription only
Tablets (sugar-coated): 2 mg

Indications, route, and dosage
Dosage and indications may vary. Check current literature for recommended protocol.
Chronic lymphocytic leukemia, malignant lymphomas including lymphosarcoma, giant follicular lymphomas, Hodgkin's disease, ◇ autoimmune hemolytic anemias, ◇ nephrotic syndrome, ◇ polycythemia vera, ◇ macroglobulinemia, ◇ ovarian neoplasms
Adults: 100 to 200 mcg/kg P.O. daily or 3 to 6 mg/m² P.O. daily as a single dose or in divided doses, for 3 to 6 weeks. Usual dose is 4 to 10 mg daily. Reduce dose if within 4 weeks of a full course of radiation therapy.
◇ *Macroglobulinemia*
Adults: 2 to 10 mg P.O. daily.
◇ *Metastatic trophoblastic neoplasia*
Adults: 6 to 10 mg P.O. daily for 5 days; repeat q 1 to 2 weeks.

◇ *Idiopathic uveitis*
Adults: 6 to 12 mg P.O. daily for 1 year.
◇ *Rheumatoid arthritis*
Adults: 0.1 to 0.3 mg/kg P.O. daily.

Pharmacodynamics
Antineoplastic action: Exerts cytotoxic activity by cross-linking strands of cellular DNA and RNA, disrupting normal nucleic acid function.

Pharmacokinetics
• *Absorption:* Well absorbed from GI tract.
• *Distribution:* Not well understood; however, drug and metabolites have been shown to be highly bound to plasma and tissue proteins.
• *Metabolism:* Metabolized in liver. Primary metabolite, phenylacetic acid mustard, also possesses cytotoxic activity.
• *Excretion:* Drug's metabolites excreted in urine. Half-life of parent compound is 2 hours; the phenylacetic acid metabolite, 2½ hours. Drug probably isn't dialyzable.

Contraindications and precautions
Contraindicated in patients with hypersensitivity or resistance to previous therapy. Patients hypersensitive to other alkylating drugs also may be hypersensitive to drug.
   Use cautiously in patients with history of head trauma or seizures and in those receiving other drugs that lower seizure threshold.

Interactions
None reported.

Adverse reactions
CNS: *seizures,* peripheral neuropathy, tremor, muscle twitching, confusion, agitation, ataxia, flaccid paresis.
GI: *nausea, vomiting, stomatitis,* diarrhea.
GU: *azoospermia, infertility.*
Hematologic: *neutropenia,* delayed up to 3 weeks, lasting up to 10 days after last dose; *bone marrow suppression; thrombocytopenia; anemia.*
Hepatic: hepatotoxicity.
Respiratory: interstitial pneumonitis.
Skin: rash, hypersensitivity.
Other: allergic febrile reaction.

☑ Special considerations
• Prepare oral suspension in pharmacy by crushing tablets and mixing powder with a suspending drug and simple syrup.
• Avoid all I.M. injections when platelets are below 100,000/mm³.
• Drug-induced pancytopenia generally lasts 1 to 2 weeks but may persist for 3 to 4 weeks. It's reversible up to a cumulative dose of 6.5 mg/kg in a single course.

- Store tablets in a tightly closed, light-resistant container.
- Signs and symptoms of overdose include reversible pancytopenia in adults, and vomiting, ataxia, abdominal pain, muscle twitching, and major motor seizures in children.
- Treatment of overdose is usually supportive, with transfusion of blood components if necessary and appropriate anticonvulsant therapy if seizures occur. Induction of emesis, activated charcoal, and gastric lavage may be useful in removing unabsorbed drug.

Monitoring the patient
- Anticoagulants and aspirin products should be used cautiously. Watch closely for signs of bleeding.
- To prevent hyperuricemia with resulting uric acid nephropathy, allopurinol may be used with adequate hydration. Monitor uric acid.
- Examine blood weekly for hemoglobin levels, total and differential leukocyte counts, and quantitative platelet counts. During the first 3 to 6 weeks of therapy, it's recommended that WBC counts be made 3 or 4 days after each of the weekly complete blood counts.
- It's dangerous to allow patient to go more than 2 weeks without hematologic and clinical examinations during treatment.

Information for the patient
- Emphasize importance of continuing medication despite nausea and vomiting, and of keeping appointments for periodic blood work.
- Advise patient to call if vomiting occurs shortly after taking dose or if symptoms of infection or bleeding are present.
- Tell patient to avoid exposure to people with infections.
- Instruct patient to avoid OTC products containing aspirin.
- Advise patient to use contraceptive measures during therapy.

Pediatric patients
- Safety and efficacy in children haven't been established; evaluate benefits versus risks.

Breast-feeding patients
- It's unknown if drug appears in breast milk. Consider risk of potential serious adverse reactions, mutagenicity, and carcinogenicity in breast-fed infants and the mother's need for drug when deciding whether to stop drug or stop breast-feeding.

chloramphenicol
Chloromycetin, Chloroptic, Econochlor, Fenicol*, Ophthochlor, Pentamycetin*

chloramphenicol sodium succinate
Chloromycetin Sodium Succinate, Pentamycetin*

Pharmacologic classification: dichloroacetic acid derivative
Therapeutic classification: antibiotic
Pregnancy risk category C

How supplied
Available by prescription only
Powder for solution: 25 mg/vial
Injection: 1-g, 10-g vial
Ophthalmic solution: 0.5%
Ophthalmic ointment: 1%
Otic solution: 0.5%, 4.5%*

Indications, route, and dosage
Severe meningitis, brain abscesses, bacteremia, other serious infections
Adults and children: 50 to 100 mg/kg I.V. daily, divided q 6 hours. Maximum dose is 100 mg/kg daily.
Premature infants and neonates weighing less than 2 kg (4.4 lb) or under age 7 days: 25 mg/kg I.V. daily.
Neonates weighing more than 2 kg and age 7 days or older: 25 mg/kg I.V. q 12 hours. I.V. route must be used to treat meningitis.
Superficial infections of skin caused by susceptible bacteria
Adults and children: Rub into affected area b.i.d. or t.i.d.
External ear canal infection
Adults and children: Instill 2 to 3 drops into ear canal t.i.d or q.i.d.
Surface bacterial infection involving conjunctiva or cornea
Adults and children: Instill 2 drops of solution in eye q hour until condition improves, or instill q.i.d., depending on severity of infection. Apply small amount of ointment to lower conjunctival sac at bedtime as supplement to drops. To use ointment alone, apply small amount to lower conjunctival sac q 3 to 6 hours or more frequently if needed. Continue with treatment up to 48 hours after condition improves.

Pharmacodynamics
Antibacterial action: Chloramphenicol palmitate and chloramphenicol sodium succinate must be hydrolyzed to chloramphenicol before antimicrobial activity occurs. The active compound then inhibits bacterial protein synthesis by binding to the ribosome's 50S subunit, thus inhibiting peptide bond formation.

Drug usually produces bacteriostatic effects on susceptible bacteria, including *Rickettsia, Chlamydia, Mycoplasma,* and certain *Salmonella* strains, as well as most gram-positive and gram-negative organisms. Chloramphenicol is used to treat *Haemophilus influenzae,* Rocky Mountain spotted fever, meningitis, lymphogranuloma, psittacosis, severe meningitis, and bacteremia.

Pharmacokinetics

• *Absorption:* Serum levels vary greatly with I.V. administration depending on patient's metabolism.
• *Distribution:* Distributed widely to most body tissues and fluids, including CSF, liver, and kidneys; readily crosses placenta. About 50% to 60% binds to plasma proteins.
• *Metabolism:* Parent drug metabolized primarily by hepatic glucuronyl transferase to inactive metabolites.
• *Excretion:* 8% to 12% of dose excreted by kidneys as unchanged drug; remainder excreted as inactive metabolites. Some drug may be excreted in breast milk. Plasma half-life ranges from about 1½ to 4½ hours in adults with normal hepatic and renal function. Plasma half-life of parent drug is prolonged in patients with hepatic dysfunction. Peritoneal hemodialysis doesn't remove significant drug amounts. Plasma chloramphenicol levels may be elevated in patients with renal impairment after I.V. chloramphenicol administration.

Contraindications and precautions

Contraindicated in patients with hypersensitivity to drug. Use cautiously in patients with impaired renal or hepatic function, acute intermittent porphyria, or G6PD deficiency and in those taking drugs that suppress bone marrow function.

Interactions

Drug-drug. *Acetaminophen:* Causes elevated serum chloramphenicol level, possibly resulting in an enhanced pharmacologic effect. Use together cautiously.
Chlorpropamide, cyclophosphamide, dicumarol, phenobarbital, phenytoin, tolbutamide: Inhibits hepatic metabolism of these drugs, causing prolonged plasma half-life of these drugs and possible toxicity from increased serum drug levels. Use together cautiously.
Folic acid, iron salts, vitamin B: Reduces hematologic response to these substances. Use together cautiously.
Penicillin: Concomitant use may antagonize penicillin's bactericidal activity. Use with caution.

Adverse reactions

CNS: headache, mild depression, confusion, delirium, peripheral neuropathy with prolonged therapy.

EENT: optic neuritis (in patients with cystic fibrosis), glossitis, decreased visual acuity, optic atrophy in children, stinging or burning of eye after instillation, blurred vision (with ointment).
GI: nausea, vomiting, stomatitis, diarrhea, enterocolitis.
Hematologic: *aplastic anemia, hypoplastic anemia, agranulocytosis, thrombocytopenia.*
Skin: possible contact sensitivity; burning, urticaria, pruritus, angioedema in hypersensitive patients.
Other: hypersensitivity reactions (fever, rash, urticaria, *anaphylaxis*), hemoglobinuria, lactic acidosis, jaundice, *gray syndrome in neonates (abdominal distention, gray cyanosis, vasomotor collapse, respiratory distress, death within a few hours of onset of symptoms).*

☑ Special considerations

• Culture and sensitivity tests may be done concurrently with first dose and repeated as needed.
• Use drug only when clearly indicated for severe infection. Because of drug's potential for severe toxicity, it should be reserved for potentially life-threatening infections.
• Refrigerate ophthalmic solution.
• If administering drug with penicillin, give penicillin 1 hour or more before chloramphenicol to avoid reduction in penicillin's bactericidal activity.
• For I.V. administration, reconstitute 1-g vial of powder for injection with 10 ml of sterile water for injection; concentration will be 100 mg/ml. Solution remains stable for 30 days at room temperature; however, refrigeration is recommended. Don't use cloudy solutions. Administer I.V. infusion slowly, over at least 1 minute. Check injection site daily for phlebitis and irritation.
• Therapeutic range is 10 to 20 mcg/ml for peak levels and 5 to 10 mcg/ml for trough levels.
• False elevation of urinary para-aminobenzoic acid (PABA) levels will result if chloramphenicol is administered during a bentiromide test for pancreatic function.
• Drug therapy causes false-positive results on tests for urine glucose level using cupric sulfate (Clinitest).
• Adverse effects of parenterally administered overdose include anemia and metabolic acidosis; then hypotension, hypothermia, abdominal distention, and possible death.
• Initial treatment of overdose is symptomatic and supportive. Drug may be removed by charcoal hemoperfusion.

Monitoring the patient

• Monitor CBC, platelet count, reticulocyte count, and serum iron level before therapy begins and every 2 days during therapy. Stop drug immediately if test results indicate anemia, reticulocytopenia, leukopenia, or thrombocytopenia.

• Observe patient for signs and symptoms of superinfection by nonsusceptible organisms.

Information for the patient
• Instruct patient to report adverse reactions, especially nausea, vomiting, diarrhea, bleeding, fever, confusion, sore throat, or mouth sores.
• Tell patient to take drug for prescribed period and exactly as directed, even after feeling better.
• Instruct patient to wash hands before and after applying topical ointment or solution.
• Warn patient using otic solution not to touch ear with dropper.
• Caution patient using topical cream to avoid sharing washcloths and towels with family members.
• Tell patient using ophthalmic drug to clean eye area of excess exudate before applying drug, and show patient how to instill drug in eye. Warn patient not to touch applicator tip to eye or surrounding tissue. Instruct patient to observe for signs and symptoms of sensitivity, such as itchy eyelids or constant burning, and to stop drug and call immediately should any occur.

Geriatric patients
• Administer drug cautiously to elderly patients with impaired liver function.

Pediatric patients
• Use drug cautiously in children under age 2 because of risk of gray syndrome (although most cases occur in first 48 hours after birth). Drug has prolonged half-life in neonates, necessitating special dose.

Breast-feeding patients
• Drug appears in breast milk in low levels, posing risk of bone marrow depression and slight risk of gray syndrome. Alternative feeding method is recommended during drug therapy.

chlordiazepoxide
Libritabs

chlordiazepoxide hydrochloride
Librium, Mitran, Reposans-10

Pharmacologic classification: benzodiazepine
Therapeutic classification: anxiolytic, anticonvulsant, sedative-hypnotic
Controlled substance schedule IV
Pregnancy risk category D

How supplied
Available by prescription only
Tablets: 5 mg, 10 mg, 25 mg
Capsules: 5 mg, 10 mg, 25 mg
Powder for injection: 100 mg/ampule

Indications, route, and dosage
Mild to moderate anxiety and tension
Adults: 5 to 10 mg t.i.d. or q.i.d.
Children over age 6 and elderly or debilitated patients: 5 mg P.O. b.i.d. to q.i.d. Maximum dose is 10 mg P.O. b.i.d. or t.i.d.
Severe anxiety and tension
Adults: 20 to 25 mg P.O. t.i.d. or q.i.d.
Withdrawal symptoms of acute alcoholism
Adults: 50 to 100 mg P.O., I.M., or I.V. Maximum dose is 300 mg/day.
Preoperative apprehension and anxiety
Adults: 5 to 10 mg P.O. t.i.d. or q.i.d. on day before surgery; or 50 to 100 mg I.M. 1 hour before surgery.
Note: Parenteral form isn't recommended in children under age 12.

Pharmacodynamics
Anxiolytic action: Depresses the CNS at the limbic and subcortical levels of the brain. Produces an antianxiety effect by influencing the effect of the neurotransmitter gamma-aminobutyric acid (GABA) on its receptor in the ascending reticular activating system, which increases inhibition and blocks both cortical and limbic arousal after stimulation of the reticular formation.
Anticonvulsant action: Suppresses spread of seizure activity produced by the epileptogenic foci in the cortex, thalamus, and limbic structures by enhancing presynaptic inhibition.

Pharmacokinetics
• *Absorption:* Well absorbed through GI tract when given orally. Action begins within 30 to 45 minutes, with peak action in 1 to 3 hours. I.M. administration results in erratic drug absorption; onset of action usually occurs in 15 to 30 minutes. After I.V. administration, rapid onset of action occurs in 1 to 5 minutes after injection.
• *Distribution:* Distributed widely throughout body; 90% to 98% is protein-bound.
• *Metabolism:* Metabolized in liver to several active metabolites.
• *Excretion:* Most metabolites excreted in urine as glucuronide conjugates. Half-life is 5 to 30 hours.

Contraindications and precautions
Contraindicated in patients with hypersensitivity to drug. Use cautiously in patients with impaired renal or hepatic function, mental depression, or porphyria.

Interactions
Drug-drug. *Antacids:* May delay absorption of chlordiazepoxide. Don't give together.
Antihistamines, barbiturates, general anesthetics, MAO inhibitors, narcotics, phenothiazines: Enhances CNS depressant effects. Use together with caution.

Cimetidine, possibly disulfiram: Diminishes hepatic metabolism of chlordiazepoxide, which increases its plasma level. Use together cautiously.
Digoxin, phenytoin: Levels may be increased. Monitor serum levels of these drugs.
Haloperidol: Benzodiazepines may decrease serum levels of haloperidol. Use together cautiously.
Levodopa: May decrease therapeutic effects of levodopa. Monitor patient carefully.
Oral contraceptives: May impair metabolism of chlordiazepoxide. Suggest an alternative method of contraception.
Drug-lifestyle. *Alcohol:* Enhances CNS depressant effects. Discourage use together.
Heavy smoking: Accelerates chlordiazepoxide's metabolism, thus lowering clinical effectiveness. Discourage smoking.

Adverse reactions
CNS: *drowsiness, lethargy,* ataxia, confusion, extrapyramidal symptoms, EEG changes.
GI: nausea, constipation.
GU: increased or decreased libido, menstrual irregularities.
Hematologic: *agranulocytosis.*
Hepatic: jaundice.
Skin: *swelling, pain at injection site,* skin eruptions, edema.

☑ Special considerations
Besides the recommendations relevant to all benzodiazepines, consider the following.
• I.M. administration isn't recommended because of erratic and slow absorption. However, if I.M. route is used, reconstitute with special diluent only. Don't use diluent if hazy. Discard unused portion. Inject I.M. deep into large muscle mass.
• For I.V. administration, drug should be reconstituted with sterile water or normal saline solution and infused slowly, directly into a large vein, at a rate not exceeding 50 mg/minute for adults. Don't infuse into small veins. Avoid extravasation into subcutaneous tissue. Observe infusion site for phlebitis. Keep resuscitation equipment nearby in case of emergency.
• Prepare solutions for I.V. or I.M. use immediately before administration. Discard unused portions.
• Patients should remain in bed under observation for at least 3 hours after parenteral administration.
• Lower doses are effective in patients with renal or hepatic dysfunction. Closely monitor renal and hepatic studies for signs of dysfunction.
• Minor changes in EEG patterns, usually low-voltage, fast activity, may occur during and after therapy.
• Chlordiazepoxide may cause a false-positive pregnancy test, depending on method used.
• Drug may alter urinary 17-ketosteroids (Zimmerman reaction), urine alkaloid determination

(Frings thin layer chromatography method), and urinary glucose determinations (with Chemstrip uG and Diastix, but not glucose enzymatic test strip).
• Signs and symptoms of overdose include somnolence, confusion, coma, hypoactive reflexes, dyspnea, labored breathing, hypotension, bradycardia, slurred speech, and unsteady gait or impaired coordination.
• Flumazenil, a specific benzodiazepine antagonist, may be used in overdose. Supportive treatment should be given. Mechanical ventilatory assistance, I.V. fluids, and vasopressors may be indicated. Use gastric lavage for recent ingestion with endotracheal tube placement, or induce emesis if patient is conscious. Give activated charcoal after emesis or lavage. Dialysis is of limited value.

Monitoring the patient
• Monitor WBC as needed during prolonged therapy.
• Monitor patient for signs of excessive use.

Information for the patient
• Warn patient that sudden changes in position may cause dizziness. Advise patient to dangle legs a few minutes before getting out of bed to prevent falls and injury.
• Advise patient to avoid driving or performing other tasks that require alertness because drug may cause drowsiness.
• Tell patient to avoid alcohol consumption.

Geriatric patients
• Elderly patients demonstrate a greater sensitivity to CNS depressant effects of drug. Some may require supervision with ambulation and activities of daily living during initiation of therapy or after a dose increase.
• Lower doses are usually effective in elderly patients because of decreased elimination.
• Parenteral administration of drug is more likely to cause apnea, hypotension, and bradycardia in elderly patients.

Pediatric patients
• Safety of oral form hasn't been established in children under age 6. Safety of parenteral form hasn't been established in children under age 12.

Breast-feeding patients
• Don't administer drug to breast-feeding women. The breast-fed infant of a mother who uses chlordiazepoxide may become sedated, have feeding difficulties, or lose weight.

chloroquine hydrochloride
Aralen Hydrochloride

chloroquine phosphate
Aralen Phosphate

Pharmacologic classification: 4-amino-quinoline
Therapeutic classification: antimalarial, amebicide, anti-inflammatory
Pregnancy risk category C

How supplied
Available by prescription only
chloroquine hydrochloride
Injection: 50 mg/ml (40 mg/ml base)
chloroquine phosphate
Tablets: 250 mg (150-mg base), 500 mg (300-mg base)

Indications, route, and dosage
Suppressive prophylaxis of malaria
Adults: Give 500 mg (300-mg base) P.O. on same day once weekly beginning 2 weeks before exposure.
Children: 5 mg (base)/kg P.O. on same day once weekly (don't exceed adult dosage) beginning 2 weeks before exposure.
Acute attacks of malaria
Adults: 1 g (600-mg base) P.O. then 500 mg (300-mg base) P.O. after 6 to 8 hours; then a single dose of 500 mg (300-mg base) P.O. for next 2 days or 4 to 5 ml (160- to 200-mg base) I.M. repeated in 6 hours if needed; change to P.O. as soon as possible.
Children: Initial dose is 10 mg (base)/kg P.O.; then 5 mg (base)/kg after 6 hours. Third dose is 5 mg (base)/kg 18 hours after second dose; fourth dose is 5 mg (base)/kg 24 hours after third dose; or 5 mg (base)/kg I.M. May repeat in 6 hours and change to P.O. as soon as possible.
Extraintestinal amebiasis
Adults: 1 g (600-mg base) daily for 2 days, then 500 mg (300-mg base) daily for 2 to 3 weeks or 4 to 5 ml (160- to 200-mg base) I.M. for 10 to 12 days; change to P.O. as soon as possible.
◊ **Rheumatoid arthritis**
Adults: 250 mg daily (chloroquine phosphate) with evening meal.
◊ **Lupus erythematosus**
Adults: 250 mg daily (chloroquine phosphate) with evening meal; reduce dosage gradually over several months when lesions regress.

Pharmacodynamics
Antimalarial action: Binds to DNA, interfering with protein synthesis. Also inhibits both DNA and RNA polymerases.
Amebicidal action: Mechanism unknown.
Anti-inflammatory action: Mechanism unknown. May antagonize histamine and serotonin and in-hibit prostaglandin effects by inhibiting conversion of arachidonic acid to prostaglandin F_2; also may inhibit chemotaxis of polymorphonuclear leukocytes, macrophages, and eosinophils.
Chloroquine's spectrum of activity includes the asexual erythrocytic forms of *Plasmodium malariae, P. ovale, P. vivax,* many strains of *P. falciparum,* and *Entamoeba histolytica.*

Pharmacokinetics
• *Absorption:* Absorbed readily and almost completely, with plasma levels peaking at 1 to 2 hours.
• *Distribution:* 55% bound to plasma proteins. Concentrates in erythrocytes, liver, spleen, kidneys, heart, and brain; strongly bound in melanin-containing cells.
• *Metabolism:* 30% metabolized by liver to monodesethylchloroquine and bidesethylchloroquine.
• *Excretion:* 70% excreted unchanged in urine; unabsorbed drug excreted in feces. Small amounts may be present in urine for months after discontinuation. Renal excretion enhanced by urinary acidification. Drug excreted in breast milk.

Contraindications and precautions
Contraindicated in patients with hypersensitivity to drug and in those with retinal or visual field changes or porphyria. Use cautiously in patients with GI, neurologic, or blood disorders.

Interactions
Drug-drug. *Cimetidine:* May reduce oral clearance and metabolism. Use together cautiously.
Intradermal human diploid cell rabies vaccine: Chloroquine may interfere with antibody response to vaccine. Avoid concurrent use if possible.
Kaolin, magnesium trisilicate: May decrease absorption of chloroquine. Don't administer together.

Adverse reactions
CNS: mild and transient headache, psychic stimulation, **seizures,** dizziness, neuropathy.
CV: hypotension, ECG changes.
EENT: visual disturbances (blurred vision; difficulty in focusing; reversible corneal changes; typically irreversible, sometimes progressive or delayed retinal changes, such as narrowing of arterioles; macular lesions; pallor of optic disk; optic atrophy; patchy retinal pigmentation, typically leading to blindness); ototoxicity (nerve deafness, vertigo, tinnitus).
GI: anorexia, abdominal cramps, diarrhea, nausea, vomiting, stomatitis.
Hematologic: *agranulocytosis, aplastic anemia,* hemolytic anemia, *thrombocytopenia.*
Skin: pruritus, lichen planus eruptions, skin and mucosal pigmentary changes, pleomorphic skin eruptions.

☑ Special considerations

• Give immediately before or after meals on the same day each week to minimize gastric distress. Patients who can't tolerate drug because of GI distress may tolerate hydroxychloroquine.
• Resistance of *P. falciparum* to chloroquine has spread to most areas with malaria except the Dominican Republic, Haiti, Central America west of the Panama Canal, the Middle East, and Egypt.
• May also be advisable to provide travelers with sulfadoxine and pyrimethamine (Fansidar) to be taken with them. Patients should be instructed to take drug if a febrile illness occurs and professional medical care isn't available. (Recommended prescriptive dose for adults is 1,500 mg sulfadoxine and 75 mg pyrimethamine, or 3 tablets.) Self-treatment is a temporary measure, and patients must seek medical care as soon as possible. They should continue prophylaxis after treatment dose of Fansidar.
• Symptoms of overdose may appear within 30 minutes after ingestion and may include headache, drowsiness, visual changes, CV collapse, and seizures; then respiratory and cardiac arrest.
• Treatment of overdose is symptomatic. Empty stomach by emesis or lavage. Activated charcoal in an amount at least 5 times the estimated amount of drug ingested may be helpful if given within 30 minutes of ingestion. Ultra-short-acting barbiturates may help control seizures. Intubation may become necessary.
• Peritoneal dialysis and exchange transfusions also may be useful. Forced fluids and acidification of the urine are helpful after acute phase.

Monitoring the patient

• Baseline and periodic ophthalmologic examinations are necessary in prolonged or high-dosage therapy.
• Monitor patient for adverse effects.

Information for the patient

• Tell patient to report blurred vision, increased sensitivity to light, hearing loss, pronounced GI disturbances, or muscle weakness promptly.
• Warn patient to avoid excessive exposure to sun to prevent drug-induced dermatoses.

Pediatric patients

• Children are extremely susceptible to toxicity. Monitor closely for adverse effects.

Breast-feeding patients

• Safety hasn't been established. Use with caution in breast-feeding women.

chlorpheniramine maleate
Aller-Chlor, Chlo-Amine, Chlor-Trimeton, Chlor-Tripolon*, Novo-Pheniram*, Phenetron, Teldrin

Pharmacologic classification: propylamine-derivative antihistamine
Therapeutic classification: antihistamine (H₁-receptor antagonist)
Pregnancy risk category B

How supplied
Available with or without a prescription
Tablets: 4 mg, 8 mg, 12 mg
Tablets (chewable): 2 mg
Tablets (timed-release): 8 mg, 12 mg
Capsules (timed-release): 8 mg, 12 mg
Syrup: 2 mg/5 ml
Injection: 10 mg/ml, 100 mg/ml

Indications, route, and dosage
Rhinitis, allergy symptoms
Adults and children ages 12 and older: 4 mg (tablets or syrup) q 4 to 6 hours; or 8 to 12 mg (timed-release tablets) b.i.d. or t.i.d. Maximum dose is 24 mg/day; 10 to 20 mg S.C., I.V., or I.M. also may be used.
Children ages 6 to 11: 2 mg (tablets or syrup) q 4 to 6 hours; or 1 8-mg (timed-release) tablet in 24 hours. Maximum dose is 12 mg/day.
Children ages 2 to 5: 1 mg (syrup) q 4 to 6 hours. Maximum dose is 6 mg/day.

Pharmacodynamics
Antihistamine action: Antihistamines compete with histamine for H₁-receptor sites on smooth muscle of the bronchi, GI tract, uterus, and large blood vessels; they bind to cellular receptors, preventing access of histamine, thereby suppressing histamine-induced allergic symptoms. They don't directly alter histamine or its release.

Pharmacokinetics
• *Absorption:* Well absorbed from GI tract; action begins within 30 to 60 minutes, and peaks in 2 to 6 hours. Food in stomach delays absorption but doesn't affect bioavailability.
• *Distribution:* Distributed extensively into body; about 72% protein-bound.
• *Metabolism:* Metabolized largely in GI mucosal cells and liver (first-pass effect).
• *Excretion:* Half-life is 12 to 43 hours in adults and 10 to 13 hours in children; drug and metabolites excreted in urine.

Contraindications and precautions
Contraindicated in patients having acute asthmatic attacks. Antihistamines aren't recommended for breast-feeding women because small amounts of drug are excreted in breast milk.

Reactions may be *common*, uncommon, **life-threatening**, or COMMON AND LIFE-THREATENING.

Use cautiously in elderly patients and in patients with increased intraocular pressure, hyperthyroidism, CV or renal disease, hypertension, bronchial asthma, urine retention, prostatic hyperplasia, bladder neck obstruction, or stenosing peptic ulcers.

Interactions

Drug-drug. *Epinephrine:* Enhanced effects of epinephrine. Monitor patient closely.
Heparin: Partially counteracts anticoagulant action. Use together cautiously.
MAO inhibitors: Interfere with detoxification of chlorpheniramine and thus prolong and intensify its CNS depressant and anticholinergic effects. Use together cautiously.
Sulfonylureas: Diminished effects of sulfonylureas. Monitor patient closely.
Other CNS depressants, such as anxiolytics, barbiturates, sleeping aids, tranquilizers: Additive sedation may occur when used concomitantly. Use together cautiously.
Drug-lifestyle. *Alcohol:* Additive sedation may occur. Discourage use together.

Adverse reactions

CNS: *stimulation,* sedation, *drowsiness,* excitability (in children).
CV: hypotension, palpitations, weak pulse.
GI: epigastric distress, *dry mouth.*
GU: urine retention.
Respiratory: thick bronchial secretions.
Skin: rash, urticaria, local stinging, burning sensation (after parenteral administration), pallor.

☑ Special considerations

Besides the recommendations relevant to all antihistamines, consider the following.
● Give 100 mg/ml of injectable form S.C. or I.M. only. Don't give I.V.; I.V. preparation contains preservatives.
● Don't use parenteral solutions intradermally.
● Administer I.V. solution slowly, over 1 minute.
● Stop drug 4 days before diagnostic skin tests; antihistamines can prevent, reduce, or mask positive skin test response.
● Signs and symptoms of overdose may include either CNS depression (sedation, reduced mental alertness, apnea, and CV collapse) or CNS stimulation (insomnia, hallucinations, tremors, and seizures). Atropine-like symptoms, such as dry mouth, flushed skin, fixed and dilated pupils, and GI symptoms, are common, especially in children.
● Treat overdose by inducing emesis with ipecac syrup (in conscious patient), then activated charcoal to reduce further drug absorption. Use gastric lavage if patient is unconscious or ipecac fails.
● Treat hypotension with vasopressors, and control seizures with diazepam or phenytoin.

● In overdose, don't give stimulants. Administering ammonium chloride or vitamin C to acidify urine will promote drug excretion.

Monitoring the patient
● Monitor patient for adverse effects.
● Evaluate for hypotension with periodic blood pressure checks.

Information for the patient
● Instruct patient to swallow sustained-release tablets whole; don't crush or chew.
● Inform patient to store syrup and parenteral solution away from light.

Geriatric patients
● Elderly patients are usually more sensitive to adverse effects of antihistamines and are especially likely to experience a greater degree of dizziness, sedation, hyperexcitability, dry mouth, and urine retention than younger patients. Symptoms usually respond to a decrease in dosage.

Pediatric patients
● Drug isn't indicated for use in premature or newborn infants.
● Children, especially those under age 6, may experience paradoxical hyperexcitability.

Breast-feeding patients
● Antihistamines such as chlorpheniramine shouldn't be used during breast-feeding. Many of these drugs appear in breast milk, exposing infant to risks of unusual excitability; premature infants are at particular risk for seizures.

chlorpromazine hydrochloride
Chlorpromanyl-20*, Largactil*, Novo-Chlorpromazine*, Thorazine

Pharmacologic classification: aliphatic phenothiazine
Therapeutic classification: antipsychotic, antiemetic
Pregnancy risk category C

How supplied
Available by prescription only
Tablets: 10 mg, 25 mg, 50 mg, 100 mg, 200 mg
Capsules (sustained-release): 30 mg, 75 mg, 150 mg, 200 mg, 300 mg
Syrup: 10 mg/5 ml
Oral concentrate: 30 mg/ml, 100 mg/ml
Suppositories: 25 mg, 100 mg
Injection: 25 mg/ml

Indications, route, and dosage
Psychosis
Adults: 30 to 75 mg P.O. daily in two to four divided doses. Dosage may be increased twice

weekly by 20 to 50 mg until symptoms are controlled. Most patients respond to 200 mg daily, but doses up to 800 mg may be necessary.

Children age 6 months and over: 0.5 to 1 mg/kg P.O. q 4 to 6 hours; or 0.25 mg/lb I.M. q 6 to 8 hours; or 0.5 mg/lb P.R. q 6 to 8 hours. Maximum dose is 40 mg in children under age 5 and 75 mg in children ages 5 to 12.

Acute management of psychosis in severely agitated patients
Adults: 25 mg I.M.; may be repeated with 25 to 50 mg in 1 hour if necessary. A maximum dose of 400 mg q 4 to 6 hours may be gradually reached over several days.

Nausea, vomiting
Adults: 10 to 25 mg P.O. or 25 mg I.M. q 4 to 6 hours, p.r.n.; or 100 mg rectally q 6 to 8 hours, p.r.n.
Children and infants: 0.25 mg/lb P.O. q 4 to 6 hours; or 0.25 mg/lb I.M. q 6 to 8 hours; or 0.5 mg/lb P.R. q 6 to 8 hours.

Intractable hiccups
Adults: 25 to 50 mg P.O. or I.M. t.i.d. or q.i.d.
Mild alcohol withdrawal, acute intermittent porphyria, tetanus
Adults: 25 mg to 50 mg I.M. t.i.d. or q.i.d.

Pharmacodynamics
Antipsychotic action: Thought to exert its antipsychotic effects by postsynaptic blockade of CNS dopamine receptors, thereby inhibiting dopamine-mediated effects; antiemetic effects are attributed to dopamine receptor blockade in the medullary chemoreceptor trigger zone (CTZ). Drug has many other central and peripheral effects; it produces both alpha and ganglionic blockade and counteracts histamine- and serotonin-mediated activity. Its most prominent adverse reactions are antimuscarinic and sedative.

Pharmacokinetics
• *Absorption:* Rate and extent of absorption vary with route of administration. Oral tablet absorption is erratic and variable, with onset ranging from ½ to 1 hour; effects peak at 2 to 4 hours and duration of action is 4 to 6 hours. Sustained-release preparations have similar absorption, but action lasts for 10 to 12 hours. Suppositories act in 60 minutes and last 3 to 4 hours. Oral concentrates and syrups much more predictable; I.M. drug absorbed rapidly.
• *Distribution:* Distributed widely into body, including breast milk; level usually higher in CNS than plasma. Steady-state serum level achieved within 4 to 7 days. Drug is 91% to 99% protein-bound.
• *Metabolism:* Metabolized extensively by liver and forms 10 to 12 metabolites, some pharmacologically active.
• *Excretion:* Mostly excreted as metabolites in urine, some excreted in feces via biliary tract. May undergo enterohepatic circulation.

Contraindications and precautions
Contraindicated in patients with hypersensitivity to drug and in patients experiencing CNS depression, bone marrow suppression, subcortical damage, and coma.

Use cautiously in acutely ill or dehydrated children; elderly or debilitated patients; and in patients with impaired renal or hepatic function, severe CV disease, glaucoma, prostatic hyperplasia, respiratory or seizure disorders, hypocalcemia, reaction to insulin or electroconvulsive therapy, or exposure to heat, cold, or organophosphate insecticides.

Interactions
Drug-drug. *Antacids containing aluminum or magnesium, antidiarrheals, phenobarbital:* Possible pharmacokinetic alterations and subsequent decreased therapeutic response to chlorpromazine. Use together cautiously.
Antiarrhythmics, atropine, CNS depressants (such as analgesics; barbiturates; epidural, general, or spinal anesthetics; narcotics; tranquilizers), disopyramide, parenteral magnesium sulfate, procainamide, quinidine, other anticholinergics (such as antidepressants, MAO inhibitors): Additive effects likely. Avoid use together.
Beta blockers: May inhibit chlorpromazine metabolism, increasing plasma levels and toxicity. Use together cautiously.
Bromocriptine: Drug may antagonize therapeutic effect of bromocriptine on prolactin secretion. Monitor patient closely.
Centrally acting antihypertensives, such as clonidine, guanabenz, guanadrel, guanethidine, methyldopa, reserpine: Chlorpromazine may inhibit blood pressure response to these drugs. Monitor blood pressure.
Dopamine: Concomitant use may decrease vasoconstricting effects of high-dose dopamine; may decrease effectiveness and increase toxicity of levodopa (by dopamine blockade). Monitor patient closely.
Epinephrine: Drug may cause epinephrine reversal: the beta-adrenergic agonist activity of epinephrine is evident whereas its alpha effects are blocked, leading to decreased diastolic and increased systolic pressures and tachycardia. Use together cautiously.
Lithium: Possible severe neurologic toxicity with an encephalitis-like syndrome, and a decreased therapeutic response to chlorpromazine. Use together cautiously.
Phenytoin: Inhibited metabolism and increased toxicity of phenytoin. Use together cautiously. Monitor phenytoin levels.
Propylthiouracil: Increased risk of agranulocytosis. Monitor patient closely.
Sympathomimetics, such as appetite suppressants, ephedrine (often found in nasal sprays), epinephrine, phenylephrine, phenylpropanola-

---

Reactions may be *common*, uncommon, **life-threatening**, or COMMON AND LIFE-THREATENING.

mine: May decrease stimulatory and pressor effects of these drugs. Monitor patient closely.

Drug-food. *Caffeine:* Decreased therapeutic response. Avoid caffeinated foods and beverages.

Drug-lifestyle. *Alcohol:* Additive effects. Discourage use.

Heavy smoking: May reduce therapeutic response to chlorpromazine. Discourage use.

Sun exposure: Photosensitivity reactions may result. Advise patient to take precautions.

Adverse reactions

CNS: extrapyramidal reactions, drowsiness, sedation, *seizures,* tardive dyskinesia, pseudoparkinsonism, dizziness, *neuroleptic malignant syndrome.*

CV: *orthostatic hypotension,* tachycardia, ECG changes.

EENT: ocular changes, blurred vision, nasal congestion.

GI: *dry mouth, constipation,* nausea.

GU: *urine retention,* menstrual irregularities, gynecomastia, inhibited ejaculation, priapism.

Hematologic: leukopenia, *agranulocytosis,* eosinophilia, hemolytic anemia, *aplastic anemia, thrombocytopenia.*

Hepatic: jaundice, abnormal liver function test results.

Skin: *mild photosensitivity,* allergic reactions, *pain at I.M. injection site,* sterile abscess, skin pigmentation.

After abrupt withdrawal of long-term therapy: gastritis, nausea, vomiting, dizziness, tremor.

☑ Special considerations

Besides the recommendations relevant to all phenothiazines, consider the following.

• Urine may discolor to pink-brown.

• Chlorpromazine has a high risk of sedation, orthostatic hypotension, and photosensitivity reactions. Patient should avoid exposure to sunlight or heat lamps.

• Sustained-release preparations shouldn't be crushed or opened; swallow whole.

• Oral form may cause stomach upset and may be administered with food or fluid.

• Dilute concentrate in 2 to 4 oz (60 to 120 ml) of liquid, preferably water, carbonated drinks, fruit juice, tomato juice, milk, puddings, or applesauce.

• Store suppository form in a cool place.

• If tissue irritation occurs, chlorpromazine injection may be diluted with normal saline solution or 2% procaine.

• I.V. form should be used only during surgery or for severe hiccups. Dilute injection to 1 mg/ml with normal saline solution and administer at a rate of 1 mg/2 minutes for children and 1 mg/minute for adults.

• Give I.M. injection deep in upper outer quadrant of buttocks. Injection is usually painful; massaging area afterward may prevent abscess formation.

• Liquid and injectable forms may cause rash if skin contact occurs.

• Solution for injection may be slightly discolored. Don't use if drug is excessively discolored or if precipitate is evident. Monitor blood pressure before and after parenteral administration.

• Drug causes false-positive test results for urinary porphyrins, urobilinogen, amylase, and 5-hydroxyindoleacetic acid because of darkening of urine by metabolites; it also causes false-positive results in urine pregnancy tests using human chorionic gonadotropin.

• CNS depression is characterized by deep, unarousable sleep and possible coma, hypotension or hypertension, extrapyramidal symptoms, abnormal involuntary muscle movements, agitation, seizures, arrhythmias, ECG changes, hypothermia or hyperthermia, and autonomic nervous system dysfunction.

• Treatment of CNS depression is symptomatic and supportive, including maintaining vital signs, airway, stable body temperature, and fluid and electrolyte balance.

• Don't induce vomiting; drug inhibits cough reflex, and aspiration may occur. Use gastric lavage, then activated charcoal and sodium chloride cathartics; dialysis doesn't help. Regulate body temperature as needed.

• Treat hypotension with I.V. fluids; don't give epinephrine.

• Treat seizures with parenteral diazepam or barbiturates; arrhythmias with parenteral phenytoin (1 mg/kg with rate titrated to blood pressure); extrapyramidal reactions with benztropine 1 to 2 mg or parenteral diphenhydramine 10 to 50 mg.

Monitoring the patient

• Monitor patient for potentially fatal neuroleptic malignant syndrome (hyperpyrexia, muscle rigidity, altered mental status, and autonomic instability).

• Monitor vital signs closely.

• Perform periodic ECG during prolonged therapy.

• Monitor CBC and liver function.

Information for the patient

• Explain risks of dystonic reactions and tardive dyskinesia, and tell patient to report abnormal involuntary body movements or painful muscle contractions.

• Tell patient to avoid sun exposure and to wear sunscreen when going outdoors to prevent photosensitivity reactions. (Note that sunlamps and tanning beds also may cause burning or discoloration of skin.)

• Warn patient to avoid extremely hot or cold baths or exposure to temperature extremes. Drug may cause thermoregulatory changes.

• Tell patient not to spill the liquid preparation on skin because rash and irritation may result.

● Instruct patient to take drug exactly as prescribed; don't double dose to compensate for missed ones.

● Explain that many drug interactions are possible. Patient should seek medical approval before taking any self-prescribed drugs.

● Tell patient not to stop taking drug suddenly.

● Encourage patient to report difficulty urinating, sore throat, dizziness, fever, or fainting.

● Advise patient to avoid hazardous activities that require alertness until drug's effect is established. Excessive sedative effects tend to subside after several weeks.

● Tell patient to avoid alcohol and drugs that may cause excessive sedation.

● Explain what fluids are appropriate for diluting the concentrate and the dropper technique for measuring dose. Teach patient how to use suppository form.

● Inform patient that sugarless chewing gum or hard candy, ice chips, or artificial saliva may help to alleviate dry mouth.

Geriatric patients
● Older patients tend to require lower doses, titrated individually. They also are more likely to develop adverse reactions, especially tardive dyskinesia and other extrapyramidal effects.

Pediatric patients
● Drug isn't recommended for patients under age 6 months. Sudden infant death syndrome has been reported in children under age 1 receiving drug. Extrapyramidal effects may be more common in children.

Breast-feeding patients
● Drug appears in breast milk. Potential benefits to mother should outweigh potential harm to infant.

---

chlorpropamide
Diabinese, Novo-Propamide*

Pharmacologic classification: sulfonylurea
Therapeutic classification: antidiabetic
Pregnancy risk category C

How supplied
Available by prescription only
Tablets: 100 mg, 250 mg

Indications, route, and dosage
Adjunct to diet to lower blood glucose levels in patients with type 2 diabetes mellitus
Adults: 250 mg P.O. daily with breakfast or in divided doses if GI disturbances occur. First dosage increase may be made after 5 to 7 days because of extended duration of action; then dosage may be increased q 3 to 5 days by 50 to 125 mg, if needed, to a maximum of 750 mg daily.

✦ *Dosage adjustment.* In adults over age 65, initial dosage should be 100 to 125 mg daily.
To change from insulin to oral therapy
Adults: If insulin dosage is less than 40 units daily, insulin may be stopped and oral therapy started as above. If insulin dosage is 40 units or more daily, start oral therapy as above, with insulin dose reduced 50% the first few days. Further insulin reductions should be made based on patient response.

Pharmacodynamics
Antidiabetic action: Lowers blood glucose levels by stimulating insulin release from beta cells in the pancreas. After prolonged administration, it produces hypoglycemic effects through extrapancreatic mechanisms, including reduced basal hepatic glucose production and enhanced peripheral sensitivity to insulin; the latter may result from either an increased number of insulin receptors or changes in events that follow insulin binding.
Antidiuretic action: Appears to potentiate the effects of minimal levels of antidiuretic hormone.

Pharmacokinetics
● *Absorption:* Absorbed readily from GI tract. Onset of action occurs within 1 hour, with maximum decrease in serum glucose levels at 3 to 6 hours.
● *Distribution:* Distribution isn't fully understood; probably similar to other sulfonylureas. Highly protein-bound.
● *Metabolism:* 80% of drug metabolized by liver. Not known if metabolites have hypoglycemic activity.
● *Excretion:* Drug and metabolites excreted in urine. Rate of excretion depends on urinary pH; increases in alkaline urine and decreases in acidic urine. Duration of action up to 60 hours; half-life is 36 hours.

Contraindications and precautions
Contraindicated in patients with hypersensitivity to drug and in those with type 1 diabetes or diabetes that can be adequately controlled by diet; type 2 diabetes complicated by ketosis, acidosis, diabetic coma, major surgery, severe infections, or severe trauma; and during pregnancy or breast-feeding.

Use cautiously in elderly, debilitated, or malnourished patients and in those with porphyria or impaired renal or hepatic function.

Interactions
Drug-drug. *Acetazolamide, adrenocorticoids, amphetamines, baclofen, corticotropin, epinephrine, estrogens, ethacrynic acid, furosemide, glucocorticoids, oral contraceptives, phenytoin, thiazide diuretics, thyroid hormones, triamterene:* Increased glucose levels. Adjust dose as needed.

Anticoagulants: May increase plasma levels of both drugs; after continued therapy, may reduce plasma levels and anticoagulant effects. Monitor serum glucose level and coagulations studies.

Antidiuretic hormone: Enhanced effects of antidiuretic hormone. Monitor patient closely.

Beta blockers such as ophthalmics: May increase risk of hypoglycemia by masking symptoms such as rising pulse rate and blood pressure. Monitor patient and serum glucose level.

Chloramphenicol, guanethidine, insulin, MAO inhibitors, probenecid, salicylates, sulfonamides: May enhance hypoglycemic effects by displacing drug from its protein-binding sites. Monitor serum glucose level.

Drug-lifestyle. *Alcohol:* May produce a disulfiram-like reaction. Discourage use together.

Smoking: Increases corticosteroid release. Higher dosages may be needed.

Adverse reactions

CNS: paresthesia, fatigue, dizziness, vertigo, malaise, headache.
EENT: tinnitus.
GI: nausea, heartburn, epigastric distress.
GU: tea-colored urine.
Hematologic: leukopenia, *thrombocytopenia, aplastic anemia, agranulocytosis,* hemolytic anemia.
Metabolic: *prolonged hypoglycemia, dilutional hyponatremia,* alterations in cholesterol, alkaline phosphatase, bilirubin, urine phenyl ketone, porphyrins, protein levels, and cephalin flocculation.
Skin: rash, pruritus, erythema, urticaria.
Other: *hypersensitivity reactions.*

☑ Special considerations

Besides the recommendations relevant to all sulfonylureas, consider the following.

● To avoid GI intolerance in patients who require dosages of 250 mg/day or more and to improve control of hyperglycemia, use divided doses; give before morning and evening meals.

● Elderly, debilitated, or malnourished patients and those with impaired renal or hepatic function usually require lower initial dosage.

● Because of drug's long duration of action, adverse reactions, especially hypoglycemia, may be more frequent or severe than with some other sulfonylureas.

● Patients with severe diabetes who don't respond to 500 mg usually won't respond to higher doses.

● Oral hypoglycemics have been associated with increased risk of CV mortality compared with diet or diet and insulin treatments.

● Signs and symptoms of overdose include low blood glucose levels, tingling of lips and tongue, hunger, nausea, decreased cerebral function (lethargy, yawning, confusion, agitation, and nervousness), increased sympathetic activity (tachy-

cardia, sweating, and tremor), and ultimately seizures, stupor, and coma.

● Mild hypoglycemia (without loss of consciousness or neurologic findings) can be treated with oral glucose and dosage adjustments.

● If patient loses consciousness or experiences neurologic symptoms, he should receive rapid injection of dextrose 50%, then continuous infusion of dextrose 10% at a rate to maintain blood glucose levels greater than 100 mg/dl. Because of drug's long half-life, monitor patient for 3 to 5 days.

Monitoring the patient

● Patients switching from chlorpropamide to another sulfonylurea should be monitored closely for 1 week because of chlorpropamide's prolonged retention in body.

● Drug may accumulate in patients with renal insufficiency. Watch for such signs as dysuria, anuria, and hematuria.

● Drug may potentiate antidiuretic effects of vasopressin. Watch for drowsiness, muscle cramps, seizures, unconsciousness, water retention, and weakness.

● Blood and urine glucose should be monitored periodically. Measurement of glycosylated hemoglobin may be useful.

Information for the patient

● Emphasize importance of following prescribed diet as well as exercise and medical regimen.

● Instruct patient to take drug at same time each day. If a dose is missed, it should be taken immediately, unless it's almost time for next dose. Patient should never take double doses.

● Tell patient to avoid alcohol, and remind patient that many foods and OTC products contain alcohol. Alcohol may cause a disulfiram-like reaction.

● Encourage patient to wear medical identification bracelet or necklace.

● Instruct patient to take drug with food if it causes GI upset.

● Teach patient how to monitor blood glucose, urine glucose, and ketone levels, as needed.

● Teach patient to recognize signs and symptoms of hypoglycemia and hyperglycemia and what to do if they occur.

● Reassure patient that skin reactions are transient and usually subside with continued therapy.

Geriatric patients

● Elderly patients may be more sensitive to drug's effects because of reduced metabolism and elimination and are more likely to develop neurologic symptoms of hypoglycemia.

● Avoid using drug in elderly patients because of its longer duration of action.

● Elderly patients usually require a lower initial dosage.

Pediatric patients
● Drug is ineffective in type 1 diabetes mellitus.

Breast-feeding patients
● Drug appears in breast milk; don't use in breast-feeding women.

chlorthalidone
Apo-Chlorthalidone*, Hygroton, Novo-Thalidone*, Thalitone, Uridon*

Pharmacologic classification: thiazide-like diuretic
Therapeutic classification: diuretic, anti-hypertensive
Pregnancy risk category B

How supplied
Available by prescription only
Tablets: 15 mg, 25 mg, 50 mg, 100 mg

Indications, route, and dosage
Edema
Adults: 50 to 100 mg (Thalitone, 30 to 60 mg) P.O. daily or 100 mg (Thalitone, 60 mg) P.O. every other day.
Children: 2 mg/kg P.O. three times weekly.
Hypertension
Adults: 25 to 100 mg (Thalitone, 15 to 50 mg) P.O. daily.
Children: 2 mg/kg P.O. three times weekly.

Pharmacodynamics
Diuretic action: Increases urinary excretion of sodium and water by inhibiting sodium reabsorption in the cortical diluting tubule of the nephron, thus relieving edema.
Antihypertensive action: Exact mechanism unknown. This effect may partially result from direct arteriolar vasodilation and a decrease in total peripheral resistance.

Pharmacokinetics
● *Absorption:* Absorbed from GI tract; extent of absorption unknown.
● *Distribution:* 90% bound to erythrocytes.
● *Metabolism:* Limited data.
● *Excretion:* Between 30% and 60% of given dose excreted unchanged in urine; half-life is 54 hours. Duration of action is 24 to 72 hours.

Contraindications and precautions
Contraindicated in patients with hypersensitivity to thiazides or other sulfonamide-derived drugs and in those with anuria. Use cautiously in patients with impaired renal or hepatic function.

Interactions
Drug-drug. *Amphetamine, quinidine:* Makes urine slightly more alkaline and may decrease urinary excretion of some amines. Monitor patient closely.
Cholestyramine, colestipol: May bind to chlorthalidone, preventing its absorption. Give 1 hour apart.
Diazoxide: Enhanced hyperglycemic, hypotensive, and hyperuricemic effects of diazoxide. Monitor patient closely.
Lithium: May reduce renal clearance of lithium, elevating serum lithium levels. Lithium dose may need to be reduced by 50%.
Methenamine compounds such as methenamine mandelate: May decrease therapeutic efficacy of these drugs. Use together cautiously.
NSAIDs: Drug may increase risk of NSAID-induced renal failure. Use together cautiously.
Other antihypertensives: Enhanced hypotensive effects. Monitor patient closely.

Adverse reactions
CNS: dizziness, vertigo, headache, paresthesia, weakness, restlessness.
CV: volume depletion and dehydration, vasculitis.
GI: anorexia, nausea, pancreatitis, vomiting, abdominal pain, diarrhea, constipation.
GU: impotence.
Hematologic: *aplastic anemia, agranulocytosis,* leukopenia, thrombocytopenia.
Hepatic: jaundice.
Metabolic: hypokalemia; asymptomatic hyperuricemia; hyperglycemia and impairment of glucose tolerance, increased serum urate, glucose, cholesterol, and triglyceride levels; fluid and electrolyte imbalances, including dilutional hyponatremia and hypochloremia, metabolic alkalosis, hypercalcemia; gout.
Skin: dermatitis, photosensitivity, rash, purpura, urticaria.
Other: hypersensitivity reactions.

☑ Special considerations
Besides the recommendations relevant to all thiazide and thiazide-like diuretics, consider the following.
● Drug may interfere with tests for parathyroid function; discontinue before such tests.
● Signs of overdose include GI irritation and hypermotility, diuresis, and lethargy, which may progress to coma.
● Treatment of overdose is mainly supportive; monitor and assist respiratory, CV, and renal function as indicated. Monitor fluid and electrolyte balance.
● In overdose, induce vomiting with ipecac in conscious patient; otherwise, use gastric lavage to avoid aspiration. Don't give cathartics; these promote additional loss of fluids and electrolytes.

Monitoring the patient
● Serum electrolyte levels should be determined before initiating therapy and at periodic intervals during therapy.

Reactions may be *common*, uncommon, *life-threatening*, or COMMON AND LIFE-THREATENING.

- Monitor patient for adverse effects.

Geriatric patients
- Elderly and debilitated patients need close observation and may require reduced doses. They are more sensitive to excess diuresis because of age-related changes in CV and renal function. Excess diuresis promotes orthostatic hypotension, dehydration, hypovolemia, hyponatremia, hypomagnesemia, and hypokalemia.

Pediatric patients
- Safety and effectiveness in children haven't been established.

Breast-feeding patients
- Drug appears in breast milk; drug safety and effectiveness in breast-feeding women haven't been established.

chlorzoxazone
Paraflex, Parafon Forte DSC, Remular-S

Pharmacologic classification: benzoxazole derivative
Therapeutic classification: skeletal muscle relaxant
Pregnancy risk category C

How supplied
Available by prescription only
Tablets: 250 mg, 500 mg
Caplets (film-coated): 250 mg, 500 mg

Indications, route, and dosage
Adjunct in acute, painful musculoskeletal conditions
Adults: 250, 500, or 750 mg P.O. t.i.d. or q.i.d. Reduce to lowest effective dose after response is obtained.
Children: 20 mg/kg or 600 mg/m² P.O. daily divided t.i.d. or q.i.d., or 125 to 500 mg t.i.d. or q.i.d., depending on age and weight.

Pharmacodynamics
Skeletal muscle relaxant action: Exact mechanism unknown. Doesn't relax skeletal muscle directly, but apparently as a result of its sedative effects. Drug may modify central perception of pain without eliminating peripheral pain reflexes.

Pharmacokinetics
- *Absorption:* Rapidly and completely absorbed from GI tract. Onset of action occurs within 1 hour; duration of action is 3 to 4 hours.
- *Distribution:* Widely distributed in body.
- *Metabolism:* Metabolized in liver to inactive metabolites. Half-life of chlorzoxazone is 66 minutes.

- *Excretion:* Excreted in urine as glucuronide metabolite.

Contraindications and precautions
Contraindicated in patients with hypersensitivity to drug and in those with impaired hepatic function.

Interactions
Drug-drug. *CNS depressants:* Produces further CNS depression. Use together cautiously.
MAO inhibitors, tricyclic antidepressants: May result in increased CNS depression, respiratory depression, and hypotensive effects. Reduce dosage of one or both drugs.
Other depressant drugs (antipsychotics, anxiolytics, general anesthetics, opioid analgesics, tricyclic antidepressants): Enhanced depressant effects. Exercise care to avoid overdose.
Drug-lifestyle. *Alcohol:* Produces further CNS depression. Discourage alcohol use.

Adverse reactions
CNS: *drowsiness, dizziness, light-headedness,* malaise, headache, overstimulation, tremor.
GI: anorexia, nausea, vomiting, heartburn, abdominal distress, constipation, diarrhea.
GU: urine discoloration (orange or purple-red).
Hepatic: hepatic dysfunction.
Skin: urticaria, redness, pruritus, petechiae, bruising, angioneurotic edema, **anaphylaxis.**

☑ Special considerations
- Drug may cause drowsiness.
- Urine may turn orange or reddish purple.
- Determine what other CNS depressant drugs patient may be taking because of cumulative effects.
- Signs and symptoms of overdose include nausea, vomiting, diarrhea, drowsiness, dizziness, light-headedness, headache, malaise, or sluggishness; then loss of muscle tone, decreased or absent deep tendon reflexes, respiratory depression, and hypotension.
- To treat overdose, induce emesis or perform gastric lavage then activated charcoal. Closely monitor vital signs and neurologic status. Provide general supportive measures, including maintenance of adequate airway and assisted ventilation.
- Use caution if administering pressor drugs.

Monitoring the patient
- Monitor liver function tests in patients receiving long-term therapy.
- Monitor patient for adverse effects.

Information for the patient
- Caution patient to avoid hazardous activities that require alertness or physical coordination until CNS depression is determined.

• Warn patient to avoid alcoholic beverages and to use caution when taking cough and cold preparations because they may contain alcohol.
• Advise patient to store drug away from direct heat or light (not in bathroom medicine cabinet, where heat and humidity deteriorate drug).
• Tell patient to take missed dose only if remembered within 1 hour of scheduled time. If beyond 1 hour, patient should skip dose and resume regular schedule. Patient shouldn't double dose.
• Inform patient not to stop taking drug without calling for specific instructions.
• Tell patient urine may turn orange or reddish purple; effect is harmless.
• Warn athletic patient that skeletal muscle relaxants are banned in competition sponsored by the U.S. Olympics Committee and the National Collegiate Athletic Association. Use can lead to disqualification.

Geriatric patients
• Elderly patients may be more sensitive to drug's effects.

Pediatric patients
• Tablets may be crushed and mixed with food, milk, or fruit juice when giving to children.

Breast-feeding patients
• It's unknown if drug appears in breast milk. No clinical problems have been reported.

---

cholera vaccine

Pharmacologic classification: vaccine
Therapeutic classification: cholera prophylactic
Pregnancy risk category C

How supplied
Available by prescription only
Injection: suspension of killed *Vibrio cholerae* (each milliliter contains 8 units of Inaba and Ogawa serotypes) in 1.5-ml and 20-ml vials

Indications, route, and dosage
Primary immunization
Adults and children over age 10: 2 doses of 0.5 ml I.M. or S.C., 1 week to 1 month apart, before traveling in cholera area. Booster dosage is 0.5 ml q 6 months for as long as protection is needed.
Children ages 5 to 10: 0.3 ml I.M. or S.C. Boosters of same dose should be given q 6 months for as long as protection is needed.
Children ages 6 months to 4 years: 0.2 ml I.M. or S.C. Boosters of same dose should be given q 6 months for as long as protection is needed.

Pharmacodynamics
Cholera prophylaxis: Promotes active immunity to cholera in about 50% of those immunized.

Pharmacokinetics
• *Absorption:* No information available.
• *Distribution:* No information available. Virus-induced immunity begins to taper off within 3 to 6 months.
• *Metabolism:* No information available.
• *Excretion:* No information available.

Contraindications and precautions
Contraindicated in patients with acute illness or history of severe systemic reaction or allergic response to vaccine.

Interactions
Drug-drug. *Corticosteroids, immunosuppressants:* May impair immune response to cholera vaccine. Avoid use together.
Yellow fever vaccine: Simultaneous administration may decrease response to both. Avoid concurrent administration.

Adverse reactions
CNS: headache.
Skin: *erythema, swelling, pain, induration (at injection site).*
Other: malaise, fever.

☑ Special considerations
• Obtain a thorough history of allergies and reactions to immunizations.
• Epinephrine solution 1:1,000 should be available to treat allergic reactions.
• When possible, cholera and yellow fever vaccines should be administered at least 3 weeks apart; however, they may be administered simultaneously if time constraints make this necessary.
• Cholera vaccine may be given intradermally (0.2 ml) in persons over age 5, but higher levels of antibody may be achieved in children under age 5 by the S.C. or I.M. route.
• Shake vial well before removing a dose.
• Administer I.M. in deltoid muscle in adults and children over age 3 and in the anterolateral thigh in children under age 3.
• Don't use I.M. route in patients with thrombocytopenia or other coagulation disorders that would contraindicate I.M. injection. Cholera vaccine shouldn't be administered I.V. Aspirate before S.C. or I.M. injection.
• Store vaccine at 36° to 46° F (2° to 8° C). Don't freeze.

Monitoring the patient
• Monitor patient for adverse effects.
• Monitor therapeutic effect.

Information for the patient
• Tell patient to report skin changes, difficulty breathing, fever, or joint pain.
• Inform patient that acetaminophen may be taken to relieve minor adverse effects, such as pain and tenderness at injection site.
• Tell patient that use of vaccine doesn't prevent infection.
• Advise patient to avoid consumption of contaminated food or water.

Geriatric patients
• Elderly patients may be more sensitive to drug's effects.

Pediatric patients
• Drug isn't recommended for infants under age 6 months.

Breast-feeding patients
• It's unknown if cholera vaccine appears in breast milk or if transmission of cholera vaccine to a breast-fed infant presents any unusual risk.

---

cholestyramine
Questran, Questran Light

Pharmacologic classification: anion exchange resin
Therapeutic classification: antilipemic, bile acid sequestrant
Pregnancy risk category C

How supplied
Available by prescription only
Powder: 378-g cans, 9-g single-dose packets (Questran). 5-g single-dose packets (Questran Light). Each scoop of powder or single-dose packet contains 4 g of cholestyramine resin.

Indications, route, and dosage
Primary hyperlipidemia and hypercholesterolemia unresponsive to dietary measures alone; to reduce risks of atherosclerotic coronary artery disease and MI; to relieve pruritus associated with partial biliary obstruction; ◊ cardiac glycoside toxicity
Adults: 4 g before meals and h.s.; don't exceed 32 g daily. Can be given in one to six divided doses.
Children ages 6 to 12: 80 mg/kg, or 2.35 g/m² t.i.d.

Pharmacodynamics
Antilipemic action: Bile is normally excreted into the intestine to facilitate absorption of fat and other lipid materials. Cholestyramine binds with bile acid, forming an insoluble compound that is excreted in feces. With less bile available in the digestive system, less fat and lipid materials in food are absorbed, more cholesterol is used by the liver to replace its supply of bile acids, and the serum cholesterol level decreases. In partial biliary obstruction, excess bile acids accumulate in dermal tissue, resulting in pruritus; by reducing levels of dermal bile acids, cholestyramine combats pruritus.
    Drug can also act as an antidiarrheal in postoperative diarrhea caused by bile acids in the colon.

Pharmacokinetics
• *Absorption:* Not absorbed. Drug levels may begin to decrease 24 to 48 hours after start of therapy and may continue to fall for up to 12 months. In some patients, initial decrease is followed by a return to or above baseline drug levels on continued therapy. Relief of pruritus associated with cholestasis occurs 1 to 3 weeks after drug start. Diarrhea associated with bile acids may stop in 24 hours.
• *Distribution:* None.
• *Metabolism:* None.
• *Excretion:* Insoluble cholestyramine with bile acid complex excreted in feces.

Contraindications and precautions
Contraindicated in patients with hypersensitivity to bile acid–sequestering resins and in those with complete biliary obstruction. Use cautiously in patients with coronary artery disease or predisposition to constipation.

Interactions
Drug-drug. *Acetaminophen, cardiac glycosides, corticosteroids, thiazide diuretics, thyroid preparations:* May reduce absorption of these drugs, thus decreasing their therapeutic effects. Use together cautiously.
Oral drugs: May bind with cholestyramine. Dosage adjustment may be needed. Give other drugs at least 1 hour before or 4 to 6 hours or more after cholestyramine; readjustment must also be made when cholestyramine is withdrawn to prevent high-dose toxicity.
Warfarin: May decrease anticoagulant effects. Monitor PT and INR.

Adverse reactions
CNS: headache, anxiety, vertigo, dizziness, insomnia, fatigue, syncope, tinnitus.
GI: *constipation,* **fecal impaction,** hemorrhoids, *abdominal discomfort,* flatulence, *nausea,* vomiting, steatorrhea, GI bleeding, diarrhea, anorexia.
GU: hematuria, dysuria.
Hematologic: anemia; ecchymoses; bleeding tendencies.
Hepatic: alters serum concentrations of ALT, AST.
Metabolic: alters serum concentrations of chloride, phosphorus, potassium, calcium, and sodium; hyperchloremic acidosis (with long-term use or very high doses).

Musculoskeletal: backache, muscle and joint pain, osteoporosis.
Skin: *rash;* irritation of skin, tongue, and perianal area.
Other: *vitamin A, D, E, and K deficiencies from decreased absorption.*

☑ Special considerations
• To mix, sprinkle powder on surface of preferred beverage or wet food, let stand a few minutes and stir to obtain uniform suspension; avoid excess foaming by using large glass and mixing slowly. Use at least 90 ml of water or other fluid, soups, milk, or pulpy fruit; rinse container and have patient drink this liquid to be sure entire dose is ingested.
• Drug has been used to treat cardiac glycoside overdose because it binds these drugs and prevents enterohepatic recycling. When used as an adjunct to hyperlipidemia, monitor levels of cardiac glycosides and other drugs to ensure appropriate dosage during and after therapy with cholestyramine.
• Questran Light contains aspartame and provides 1.6 calories per packet or scoop.
• Cholecystography using iopanoic acid will yield abnormal results because iopanoic acid is also bound by cholestyramine.
• Drug overdose hasn't been reported. Chief potential risk is intestinal obstruction; treatment would depend on location and degree of obstruction and on amount of gut motility.

Monitoring the patient
• Determine serum cholesterol level frequently during first few months of therapy and then periodically.
• Monitor bowel function. Treat constipation promptly by decreasing dosage, adding a stool softener, or stopping drug.
• Monitor patient for signs of vitamin A, D, or K deficiency.

Information for the patient
• Explain disease process and rationale for therapy, and encourage patient to comply with continued blood testing and special diet; although therapy isn't curative, it helps control serum cholesterol level.
• Encourage patient to control weight and to stop smoking as part of attempt to increase awareness of other cardiac risk factors.
• Tell patient not to take the powder in dry form; teach patient to mix drug with fluids or pulpy fruits.

Geriatric patients
• Patients over age 60 are more likely to experience adverse GI effects as well as adverse nutritional effects.

Pediatric patients
• Children may be at greater risk of hyperchloremic acidosis during cholestyramine therapy.
• Safe dosage hasn't been established for children under age 6.

Breast-feeding patients
• Safety in breast-feeding women hasn't been established.

---

choline magnesium trisalicylates
Tricosal, Trilisate

choline salicylate
Arthropan

Pharmacologic classification: salicylate
Therapeutic classification: nonnarcotic analgesic, antipyretic, anti-inflammatory
Pregnancy risk category C

How supplied
Available by prescription only
Tablets: 500 mg, 750 mg, 1,000 mg of salicylate (as choline and magnesium salicylate)
Solution: 500 mg of salicylate/5 ml (as choline and magnesium salicylate); 870 mg/5 ml (as choline salicylate)

Indications, route, and dosage
Rheumatoid arthritis, osteoarthritis
Adults: 1,500 mg P.O. b.i.d. or 3,000 mg h.s.
✦ Dosage adjustment. In elderly patients, give 750 mg t.i.d.
Mild arthritis; antipyresis
Adults: 2,000 to 3,000 mg P.O. daily in divided doses b.i.d.
Mild to moderate pain and fever
Children: Based on weight, and the doses should be divided b.i.d.
Children weighing 12 to 13 kg (26 to 28.5 lb): 500 mg P.O. daily.
Children weighing 14 to 17 kg (30 to 37.5 lb): 750 mg P.O. daily.
Children weighing 18 to 22 kg (39 to 48.5 lb): 1,000 mg P.O. daily.
Children weighing 23 to 27 kg (50 to 59.5 lb): 1,250 mg P.O. daily.
Children weighing 28 to 32 kg (61 to 70.5 lb): 1,500 mg P.O. daily.
Children weighing 33 to 37 kg (73 to 81.5 lb): 1,750 mg P.O. daily.

Pharmacodynamics
Analgesic action: Produce analgesia by an ill-defined effect on the hypothalamus (central action) and by blocking generation of pain impulses (peripheral action). The peripheral action may involve inhibition of prostaglandin synthesis.

Anti-inflammatory action: Inhibit prostaglandin synthesis; may also inhibit synthesis or action of other inflammation mediators.

Antipyretic action: Act on the hypothalamic heat-regulating center to produce peripheral vasodilation. This increases peripheral blood supply and promotes sweating, which leads to loss of heat and to cooling by evaporation. Don't affect platelet aggregation and shouldn't be used to prevent thrombosis.

Pharmacokinetics

• *Absorption:* Absorbed rapidly and completely from GI tract. Therapeutic effect peaks in 2 hours.
• *Distribution:* Protein-binding depends on concentration and ranges from 75% to 90%, decreasing as serum level increases. Severe toxic effects may occur at serum levels greater than 400 mcg/ml.
• *Metabolism:* Hydrolyzed to salicylate in liver.
• *Excretion:* Metabolites excreted in urine.

Contraindications and precautions

Contraindicated in patients with hypersensitivity to drug. Also contraindicated in patients with hemophilia, bleeding ulcers, and hemorrhagic states, and for patients who consume three or more alcoholic beverages per day. Use cautiously in patients with impaired renal or hepatic function, peptic ulcer disease, or gastritis. Don't give to children or teenagers with chickenpox or influenza-like illnesses.

Interactions

Drug-drug. *Ammonium chloride, urine acidifiers:* Increase choline salicylate blood levels. Monitor drug blood levels and toxicity.

Antacids in high doses, other urine alkalizers: Decreased choline salicylate blood levels. Watch for decreased salicylate effect.

Corticosteroids: Enhanced salicylate elimination. Watch for decreased effect.

Lithium carbonate: Decreased renal clearance of lithium carbonate, thus increasing serum lithium levels and risk of adverse effects. Use together cautiously.

Methotrexate: May cause displacement of bound methotrexate and inhibition of renal excretion. Monitor patient closely.

Other GI irritant drugs (such as antibiotics, corticosteroids, other NSAIDs): May potentiate adverse GI effects of choline salicylates. Use together cautiously.

Phenytoin, sulfonylureas, warfarin: May cause adverse effects and displacement of these drugs. Monitor drug levels carefully.

Sulfonylureas: Hypoglycemic effects may be enhanced. Monitor serum glucose level.

Warfarin: Enhanced hypoprothrombinemic effects. Monitor PT and INR.

Drug-food. *Food:* Delays and decreases absorption of choline salicylates. Give on an empty stomach.

Adverse reactions

EENT: tinnitus, hearing loss.
GI: GI distress, nausea, vomiting.
GU: *acute tubular necrosis with renal failure.*
Skin: rash.
Other: elevated free T_4 levels, hypersensitivity reactions *(anaphylaxis), Reye's syndrome.*

☑ Special considerations

Besides the recommendations relevant to all salicylates, consider the following.
• Don't mix choline salicylates with antacids.
• Administer oral solution of choline salicylate mixed with fruit juice. Follow with 8-oz (240-ml) glass of water to ensure passage into stomach.
• Avoid choline salicylates in third trimester of pregnancy.
• Choline salicylates may interfere with urinary glucose analysis performed via Chemstrip uG, Diastix, glucose enzymatic test strip, Clinitest, and Benedict's solution.
• These drugs interfere with urinary 5-hydroxyindole acetic acid and vanillylmandelic acid.
• Signs and symptoms of overdose include metabolic acidosis with respiratory alkalosis, hyperpnea, and tachypnea from increased carbon dioxide production and direct stimulation of the respiratory center.
• To treat overdose, empty stomach immediately by inducing emesis with ipecac syrup, if patient is conscious, or by gastric lavage.
• In overdose, administer activated charcoal via nasogastric tube. Provide symptomatic and supportive measures (respiratory support and correction of fluid and electrolyte imbalances). Monitor laboratory parameters and vital signs closely.
• Hemodialysis is effective in removing choline salicylates but is used only in severe poisoning.
• Forced diuresis with alkalinizing drug accelerates salicylate excretion.

Monitoring the patient
• Monitor serum magnesium levels to prevent possible magnesium toxicity.
• Monitor patient for adverse effects.

Geriatric patients
• Patients over age 60 may be more susceptible to toxic effects of these drugs.

Pediatric patients
• Safety of long-term drug use in children under age 14 hasn't been established.
• Because of epidemiologic association with Reye's syndrome, the Centers for Disease Control and Prevention recommend that children with

---

chickenpox or flulike symptoms shouldn't be given salicylates.
• Febrile, dehydrated children can rapidly develop toxicity. Usually, children shouldn't receive more than five doses in 24 hours.

Breast-feeding patients
• Salicylates appear in breast milk. Avoid use in breast-feeding women.

---

chorionic gonadotropin, human (HCG)
A.P.L., Chorex 5, Chorex 10, Gonic, Pregnyl, Profasi, Profasi HP*

Pharmacologic classification: gonadotropin
Therapeutic classification: ovulation stimulant, spermatogenesis stimulant
Pregnancy risk category X

How supplied
Available by prescription only
Injection: 500 USP U/ml, 1,000 USP U/ml, 2,000 USP U/ml

Indications, route, and dosage
To induce ovulation and pregnancy
Adults: 5,000 to 10,000 USP U I.M. 1 day after last dose of menotropins.
Hypogonadotropic hypogonadism
Adults: 500 to 1,000 USP U I.M. three times weekly for 3 weeks, then twice weekly for 3 weeks; or 4,000 USP U I.M. three times weekly for 6 to 9 months, then 2,000 USP U three times weekly for 3 more months.
Nonobstructive prepubertal cryptorchidism
Children ages 4 to 9: 5,000 USP U I.M. every other day for four doses; or 4,000 USP U I.M. three times weekly for 3 weeks; or 15 doses of 500 to 1,000 USP U I.M. given over 6 weeks; or 500 USP U three times weekly for 4 to 6 weeks, which may be repeated if unsuccessful in 1 month, giving 1,000 USP U per injection.

Pharmacodynamics
Ovulation stimulant action: Mimics action of luteinizing hormone in stimulating ovulation of mature ovarian follicle.
Spermatogenesis stimulant action: Stimulates androgen production in Leydig's cells of testes and causes maturation of cells lining seminiferous tubules of testes.

Pharmacokinetics
• *Absorption:* Must administer I.M. Blood levels peak within 6 hours.
• *Distribution:* Distributed primarily into testes and ovaries.
• *Metabolism:* Initial half-life is 11 hours, with a terminal phase of 23 hours.

• *Excretion:* Excreted in urine.

Contraindications and precautions
Contraindicated in patients with hypersensitivity to HCG and in those with precocious puberty or androgen-responsive cancer (prostatic, testicular, male breast) because it stimulates androgen production. Use with caution in patients with asthma, seizure disorders, migraines, or cardiac or renal diseases because it may exacerbate these conditions.

Interactions
None reported.

Adverse reactions
CNS: headache, fatigue, irritability, restlessness, depression.
GU: early puberty (growth of testes, penis, pubic and axillary hair; voice change; down on upper lip; growth of body hair), hyperstimulation (ovarian enlargement), *rupture of ovarian cysts* (after use of gonadotropins).
Skin: pain at injection site.
Other: gynecomastia, edema.

☑ Special considerations
• Only those experienced in treating infertility disorders should administer drug.
• Pregnancies that occur after stimulation of ovulation with gonadotropins show a relatively high risk of multiple births.
• HCG is usually used only after failure of clomiphene in anovulatory patients.
• In infertility, encourage daily intercourse from day before HCG is given until ovulation occurs.
• Be alert to symptoms of ectopic pregnancy, usually evident between 8 and 12 weeks' gestation.
• May interfere with radioimmunoassays for gonadotropins.

Monitoring the patient
• Carefully observe young men receiving HCG for development of precocious puberty.
• Carefully monitor patients with disorders that may be aggravated by fluid retention.

Information for the patient
• Teach patient and family how to assess for edema and to report it promptly.
• Advise patient and family to report signs of precocious puberty promptly.
• Inform patient receiving HCG for infertility that multiple births are possible.

Geriatric patients
• Drug isn't indicated for use in elderly patients.

Pediatric patients
• Treating prepubertal cryptorchidism with HCG can help predict future need for orchidopexy. In-

---

Reactions may be *common*, uncommon, **life-threatening**, or COMMON AND LIFE-THREATENING.

duction of androgen secretion may induce precocious puberty in patients treated for cryptorchidism. Instruct parent to report the following: axillary, facial, or pubic hair; penile growth; acne; or deepening of voice.

Breast-feeding patients
• It's unknown whether chorionic gonadotropins appear in breast milk. Use caution when giving to breast-feeding women.

---

cidofovir
Vistide

Pharmacologic classification: nucleotide analogue
Therapeutic classification: antiviral
Pregnancy risk category C

How supplied
Available by prescription only
Injection: 75 mg/ml

Indications, route, and dosage
Cytomegalovirus (CMV) retinitis in patients with AIDS
Adults: Give 5 mg/kg I.V. infused over 1 hour once weekly for 2 consecutive weeks; then maintenance dose of 5 mg/kg I.V. infused over 1 hour once q 2 weeks. Probenecid must be administered concomitantly.
✦ *Dosage adjustment.* For patients with creatinine clearance of 41 to 55 ml/minute, induction and maintenance doses should be reduced to 2 mg/kg; for creatinine clearance 30 to 40 ml/minute, reduce to 1.5 mg/kg; for creatinine clearance 20 to 29 ml/minute, reduce to 1 mg/kg; and for creatinine clearance 19 ml/minute or less, reduce to 0.5 mg/kg.

Pharmacodynamics
Antiviral action: Suppresses CMV replication by selective inhibition of viral DNA synthesis.

Pharmacokinetics
• *Absorption:* Administered I.V. only.
• *Distribution:* No information available.
• *Metabolism:* Not metabolized.
• *Excretion:* 80% to 100% of drug excreted unchanged in urine.

Contraindications and precautions
Contraindicated in patients with hypersensitivity to drug or history of clinically severe hypersensitivity to probenecid or other sulfa-containing medications. Don't administer as a direct intraocular injection (direct injection may be associated with significant decreases in intraocular pressure and vision impairment). Use cautiously in patients with impaired renal function.

Interactions
Drug-drug. *Aminoglycosides, amphotericin B, foscarnet, I.V. pentamidine:* Increased nephrotoxic potential. Avoid concomitant use.
Zidovudine: Probenecid reduces metabolic clearance of zidovudine. Stop zidovudine therapy or reduce dosage by 50% in patients receiving zidovudine on the days cidofovir and probenecid are given.

Adverse reactions
CNS: malaise; *asthenia, headache,* amnesia, anxiety, confusion, **seizure,** depression, dizziness, abnormal gait, hallucinations, insomnia, neuropathy, paresthesia, somnolence, vasodilation.
CV: hypotension, orthostatic hypotension, pallor, syncope, tachycardia.
EENT: amblyopia, conjunctivitis, eye disorders, ocular hypotony, iritis, retinal detachment, taste perversion, uveitis, abnormal vision, pharyngitis, rhinitis, sinusitis.
GI: *nausea, vomiting, diarrhea, anorexia, abdominal pain,* dry mouth, colitis, constipation, tongue discoloration, dyspepsia, dysphagia, flatulence, gastritis, melena, oral candidiasis, rectal disorders, stomatitis, aphthous stomatitis, mouth ulceration.
GU: *elevated creatinine levels, nephrotoxicity, proteinuria,* decreased creatinine clearance levels, glycosuria, hematuria, urinary incontinence, urinary tract infection.
Hematologic: NEUTROPENIA, *anemia,* **thrombocytopenia.**
Hepatic: hepatomegaly, abnormal liver function tests, increased alkaline phosphatase levels.
Metabolic: fluid imbalances, hyperglycemia, hyperlipemia, hypocalcemia, hypokalemia, weight loss.
Musculoskeletal: arthralgia, myasthenia, myalgia.
Respiratory: asthma, bronchitis, coughing, dyspnea, hiccups, increased sputum, lung disorders, pneumonia.
Skin: *rash, alopecia,* acne, skin discoloration, dry skin, herpes simplex, pruritus, sweating, urticaria.
Other: *fever; infections; chills;* allergic reactions; facial edema; pain in back, chest, or neck; **sarcoma, sepsis.**

☑ Special considerations
• Renal impairment is the major adverse effect of cidofovir. To minimize possible nephrotoxicity, use I.V. prehydration with normal saline and administer probenecid with each cidofovir infusion.
• Administer 1 L of normal saline solution over a 1- to 2-hour period immediately before each cidofovir infusion. Administer a second liter in patients who can tolerate the additional fluid load. If second liter is given, administer either at the start of drug infusion or immediately after, and infuse it over a 1- to 3-hour period.

• Administer 2 g of probenecid P.O. 3 hours before cidofovir dose and 1 g at 2 hours, and again at 8 hours after completion of the 1-hour infusion (total 4 g).

• Because of the potential for increased nephrotoxicity, don't exceed recommended doses; don't exceed frequency or rate of administration.

• To prepare infusion, extract appropriate amount of cidofovir from vial with syringe and transfer dose to infusion bag containing 100 ml normal saline solution. Infuse entire volume I.V. at a constant rate over a 1-hour period. Use a standard infusion pump for administration.

• Because of the mutagenic properties of cidofovir, drug should be prepared in a class II laminar flow biological safety cabinet. Personnel preparing drug should wear surgical gloves and a closed front surgical-type gown with knit cuffs.

• If drug contacts skin, wash membranes and flush thoroughly with water. Place excess drug and all other materials used in the admixture preparation and administration in a leak-proof, puncture-proof container. Recommended disposal method is high temperature incineration.

• Administer cidofovir infusion admixtures within 24 hours of preparation; don't store in refrigerator or freezer to extend 24-hour period. If admixtures won't be used immediately, refrigerate at 36° to 46° F (2° to 8° C) for no more than 24 hours. Admixtures should be at room temperature before use.

• Don't add other drugs or supplements to cidofovir admixture for concurrent administration. Compatibility with Ringer's solution, lactated Ringer's solution, or bacteriostatic infusion fluids hasn't been evaluated.

• Drug is indicated only for CMV retinitis treatment in AIDS patients. Safety and efficacy of drug haven't been established for treating other CMV infections, congenital or neonatal CMV disease, and CMV disease in patients not infected with HIV.

• Cidofovir has been carcinogenic and teratogenic and has caused hypospermia.

• Don't initiate drug in patients with baseline serum creatinine exceeding 1.5 mg/dl or calculated creatinine clearances of 55 ml/minute or less unless potential benefits exceed potential risks.

• Fanconi's syndrome and decreased serum bicarbonate levels associated with evidence of renal tubular damage have been reported in patients receiving cidofovir. Monitor patient closely.

• Hemodialysis and hydration may reduce drug plasma levels in patients who receive an overdose of drug.

• Probenecid may reduce the potential for nephrotoxicity in patients who receive an overdose of drug through reduction of active tubular secretion.

Monitoring the patient
• Monitor WBC counts with differential before each dose.

• Monitor renal function (serum creatinine level and urine protein) before each dose; modify dosage for changes in renal function.

• Granulocytopenia has been associated with cidofovir treatment; monitor neutrophil counts during therapy.

• Monitor intraocular pressure, visual acuity, and ocular symptoms periodically.

Information for the patient
• Inform patient that drug isn't a cure for CMV retinitis and that regular ophthalmologic follow-up examinations are necessary.

• Alert patient on zidovudine therapy to obtain dosage guidelines on days that cidofovir is administered.

• Tell patient that close monitoring of renal function is needed during cidofovir therapy and that an abnormality may require a change in cidofovir therapy.

• Stress importance of completing a full course of probenecid with each cidofovir dose. Tell patient to take probenecid after a meal to decrease nausea.

• Advise patient that cidofovir is considered a potential carcinogen.

• Instruct woman of childbearing potential to use effective contraception during and for 1 month after treatment with cidofovir. Tell men to practice barrier contraceptive methods during and for 3 months after drug treatment.

Geriatric patients
• Use with caution when administering cidofovir to an elderly patient. Dosage adjustment will be necessary if patient is renally impaired.

Pediatric patients
• Safety and effectiveness in children haven't been established.

Breast-feeding patients
• It's unknown if drug appears in breast milk. Don't administer to breast-feeding women.

cilostazol
Pletal

Pharmacologic classification: quinolinone derivative
Therapeutic classification: phosphodiesterase inhibitor, antiplatelet drug, vasodilator
Pregnancy risk category C

How supplied
Available by prescription only
Tablets: 50-mg, 100-mg

Reactions may be *common*, uncommon, **life-threatening**, or COMMON AND LIFE-THREATENING.

Indications, route, and dosage
Intermittent claudication
Adults: 100 mg P.O. b.i.d., taken ½ hour before or 2 hours after breakfast and dinner.

Pharmacodynamics
Antiplatelet action: Exact mechanism unknown. Action believed to be due to inhibition of the enzyme phosphodiesterase (Type III), causing an increase of cAMP in platelets and blood vessels, resulting in inhibition of platelet aggregation and vasodilation. Cilostazol reversibly inhibits platelet aggregation induced by various stimuli, such as thrombin, adenosine diphosphate, collagen, arachidonic acid, epinephrine, and stress.

Pharmacokinetics
- *Absorption:* Absorbed following oral administration. A high-fat meal increases peak serum levels about 90% and bioavailability by 25%. Absolute bioavailability isn't known.
- *Distribution:* 95% to 98% protein-bound, primarily to albumin.
- *Metabolism:* Extensively metabolized by hepatic cytochrome P-450 enzyme system, primarily CYP3A4.
- *Excretion:* Excreted primarily in urine, mostly metabolites (about 74%). Remaining drug eliminated in feces (about 20%). Half-life of cilostazol and active metabolites is about 11 to 13 hours.

Contraindications and precautions
Contraindicated in patients with known or suspected hypersensitivity to drug or its components and in those with heart failure of any severity. Use cautiously in patients with severe underlying heart disease and with other drugs having antiplatelet activity.

Interactions
Drug-drug. *Diltiazem, erythromycin, omeprazole, other macrolides, strong inhibitors of CYP3A4 (such as fluconazole, fluoxetine, fluvoxamine, itraconazole, ketoconazole, miconazole, nefazodone, sertraline):* Increased peak serum levels of cilostazol or one of its metabolites. Use together cautiously.
Drug-food. *Grapefruit juice:* May increase cilostazol levels. Discourage concomitant use.
Drug-lifestyle. *Smoking:* Decreases drug exposure by about 20%. Discourage smoking.

Adverse reactions
CNS: *headache, dizziness,* vertigo.
CV: *palpitation,* tachycardia.
EENT: *pharyngitis, rhinitis.*
GI: *abnormal stools, diarrhea,* dyspepsia, abdominal pain, flatulence, nausea.
Musculoskeletal: back pain, myalgia.
Respiratory: cough aggravation.
Other: *infection,* peripheral edema.

☑ Special considerations
- Obtain a thorough medication history before initiating therapy.
- Administer drug at least ½ hour before or 2 hours after breakfast and dinner.
- Drug may take up to 12 weeks to produce beneficial effects.
- Several drugs that inhibit the enzyme phosphodiesterase have caused decreased survival in patients with class III-IV heart failure. Therefore, cilostazol is contraindicated in patients with congestive heart failure.
- There is uncertainty concerning cardiovascular risk in long-term use or in patients with severe underlying heart disease.
- Signs and symptoms of overdose include severe headache, diarrhea, hypotension, tachycardia, and, possibly, cardiac arrhythmias. Observe patient carefully and give supportive treatment.
- Because drug is highly protein-bound, it may not be efficiently removed by hemodialysis.

Monitoring the patient
- Monitor patient for adverse effects.
- Watch for signs of GI distress.

Information for the patient
- Advise patient that cilostazol should be taken at least ½ hour before or 2 hours after breakfast and dinner.
- Tell patient that a beneficial effect won't likely occur before 2 to 4 weeks; it may take as long as 12 weeks before a beneficial effect is experienced.
- To chart effects of drug therapy, advise patient to keep a log of how far he is able to walk without pain.
- Tell patient to avoid grapefruit juice while taking drug.
- Inform patient that there is currently no safety information on cardiovascular risk with long-term use or in those with severe underlying heart disease.

Geriatric patients
- No overall differences in safety, efficacy, or pharmacokinetics have been observed between elderly and younger patients.

Pediatric patients
- Safety and effectiveness in children haven't been established.

Breast-feeding patients
- Because drug appears in breast milk, a decision should be made to discontinue breast-feeding or discontinue cilostazol.

cimetidine
Tagamet, Tagamet HB

Pharmacologic classification: H_2-receptor antagonist
Therapeutic classification: antiulcerative
Pregnancy risk category B

How supplied
Available by prescription only
Tablets: 200 mg, 300 mg, 400 mg, 800 mg
Injection: 150 mg/ml, 300 mg/50 ml (premixed)
Liquid: 300 mg/5 ml
Available without a prescription
Tablets: 100 mg

Indications, route, and dosage
Duodenal ulcer (short-term treatment)
Adults: 800 mg h.s. for maximum of 8 weeks. Or 400 mg P.O. b.i.d. or 300 mg P.O. q.i.d. with meals and h.s. When healing occurs, stop treatment or give h.s. dose only to control nocturnal hypersecretion.
Parenteral
300 mg diluted to 20 ml with normal saline solution or other compatible I.V. solution by I.V. push over 5 minutes q 6 hours. Or 300 mg diluted in 50 ml dextrose 5% solution or other compatible I.V. solution by I.V. infusion over 15 to 20 minutes q 6 to 8 hours. Or 300 mg I.M. q 6 to 8 hours (no dilution necessary). To increase dose, give more frequently to maximum daily dose of 2,400 mg.
Duodenal ulcer prophylaxis
Adults: 400 mg h.s.
Active benign gastric ulcer
Adults: 800 mg h.s. or 300 mg q.i.d. with meals and h.s. for up to 8 weeks.
Pathologic hypersecretory conditions (such as Zollinger-Ellison syndrome, systemic mastocytosis, multiple endocrine adenomas); ◊ *short-bowel syndrome*
Adults: 300 mg P.O. q.i.d. with meals and h.s.; adjust to patient needs. Maximum daily dose is 2,400 mg.
Parenteral
300 mg diluted to 20 ml with normal saline solution or other compatible I.V. solution by I.V. push over 5 minutes q 6 to 8 hours. Or 300 mg diluted in 50 ml dextrose 5% solution or other compatible I.V. solution by I.V. infusion over 15 to 20 minutes q 6 to 8 hours. To increase dosage, give 300-mg doses more frequently to maximum daily dose of 2,400 mg.
Symptomatic relief of gastroesophageal reflux
Adults: 800 mg P.O. b.i.d. or 400 mg q.i.d., before meals and h.s.
◊ *Active upper GI bleeding, peptic esophagitis, stress ulcer*
Adults: 1 to 2 g I.V. or P.O. daily, in four divided doses.
Children: 20 to 40 mg/kg daily in divided doses.
Continuous infusion for patients unable to tolerate oral medication
Adults: 37.5 mg/hour (900 mg/day) by continuous I.V. infusion. Use an infusion pump if total volume is below 250 ml/day.
Heartburn, acid indigestion, sour stomach
Adults: 200 mg P.O. up to maximum of b.i.d. (400 mg).
✦ **Dosage adjustment.** In patients with renal failure, recommended dose is 300 mg P.O. or I.V. q 8 to 12 hours at end of dialysis. Dosage may be decreased further if hepatic failure is also present.

Pharmacodynamics
Antiulcer action: Competitively inhibits histamine's action at H_2 receptors in gastric parietal cells, inhibiting basal and nocturnal gastric acid secretion (such as from stimulation by food, caffeine, insulin, histamine, betazole, or pentagastrin). May also enhance gastromucosal defense and healing.
A 300-mg oral or parenteral dose inhibits about 80% of gastric acid secretion for 4 to 5 hours.

Pharmacokinetics
• *Absorption:* 60% to 75% of oral dose absorbed. Food may affect absorption rate (but not extent).
• *Distribution:* Distributed to many body tissues. About 15% to 20% is protein-bound. Apparently crosses placenta; distributed in breast milk.
• *Metabolism:* 30% to 40% metabolized in liver. Half-life is 2 hours in patients with normal renal function; half-life increases with decreasing renal function.
• *Excretion:* 48% of oral dose and 75% of parenteral dose excreted in urine; 10% of oral dose excreted in feces. Some drug excreted in breast milk.

Contraindications and precautions
Contraindicated in patients with hypersensitivity to drug. Use with caution in elderly or debilitated patients.

Interactions
Drug-drug. *Benzodiazepines, beta blockers (such as propranolol), carmustine, disulfiram, isoniazid, lidocaine, metronidazole, oral contraceptives, phenytoin, procainamide, quinidine, triamterene, tricyclic antidepressants, warfarin, xanthines:* Cimetidine decreases metabolism of these drugs, thus increasing potential toxicity. Dosage reduction may be needed.
Digoxin: Serum levels may be reduced. Monitor serum digoxin.
Ferrous salts, indomethacin, ketoconazole, tetracyclines: Concomitant use may affect absorption of these drugs by altering gastric pH. Use together cautiously.

Flecainide: May increase serum flecainide levels. Monitor serum flecainide levels.
Drug-herb. *Pennyroyal:* May change rate of formation of toxic metabolites of pennyroyal. Avoid using together.
Yerba maté methylxanthines: Decreased clearance of this herb and possible toxicity. Use together cautiously.
Drug-lifestyle. *Smoking:* May increase gastric acid secretion and worsen disease. Discourage use.

Adverse reactions
CNS: confusion, dizziness, headache, peripheral neuropathy, somnolence, hallucinations.
GI: *mild and transient diarrhea.*
GU: transient elevations in serum creatinine levels, impotence, mild gynecomastia if used for over 1 month.
Hematologic: *neutropenia.*
Musculoskeletal: muscle pain, arthralgia.
Other: hypersensitivity reactions.

☑ Special considerations
Besides the recommendations relevant to all H$_2$-receptor antagonists, consider the following.
• For I.V. use, cimetidine must be diluted before administration. Don't dilute drug with sterile water for injection; use normal saline solution or D$_5$W to a total volume of 20 ml.
• For I.M. administration, drug may be given undiluted. Injection may be painful.
• After administration of liquid via nasogastric tube, tube should be flushed to clear it and ensure drug's passage to stomach.
• Hemodialysis removes drug; schedule dose after dialysis session.
• Cimetidine may antagonize pentagastrin's effect during gastric acid secretion tests; it may cause false-negative results in skin tests using allergen extracts.
• Cimetidine therapy increases prolactin levels, serum alkaline phosphatase levels, and serum creatinine levels.
• FD and C blue dye #2 used in Tagamet tablets may impair interpretation of Hemoccult and Gastroccult tests on gastric content aspirate. Be sure to wait at least 15 minutes after tablet administration before drawing the sample, and follow test manufacturer's instructions closely.
• Effects of overdose include respiratory failure and tachycardia. Overdose is rare; intake of up to 10 g has caused no adverse effects. Support respiration and maintain a patent airway. Induce emesis or use gastric lavage; follow with activated charcoal to prevent further absorption. Treat tachycardia with propranolol if necessary.

Monitoring the patient
• Monitor patient for adverse effects.
• Evaluate patient's response to therapy.

Information for the patient
• Warn patient to take drug as directed and to continue taking it even after pain subsides to allow for adequate healing. Urge patient to avoid smoking; it may increase gastric acid secretion and worsen disease.

Geriatric patients
• Use caution when administering cimetidine to elderly patients because of potential for adverse reactions that affect CNS.

Breast-feeding patients
• Drug appears in breast milk; avoid use in breast-feeding women.

ciprofloxacin (systemic)
Cipro

Pharmacologic classification: fluoro-quinolone antibiotic
Therapeutic classification: antibiotic
Pregnancy risk category C

How supplied
Available by prescription only
Tablets: 250 mg, 500 mg, 750 mg
Injection: 200 mg/20-ml vial; 400 mg/40-ml vial; 200 mg in 100 ml D$_5$W; 400 mg in 200 ml D$_5$W

Indications, route, and dosage
Mild to moderate urinary tract infection caused by susceptible bacteria
Adults: 250 mg P.O. or 200 mg I.V. q 12 hours.
Infectious diarrhea, mild to moderate respiratory tract infections, bone and joint infections, severe or complicated urinary tract infections
Adults: 500 mg P.O. q 12 hours or 400 mg I.V. q 12 hours.
Severe or complicated infections of the respiratory tract, bones, joints, skin, or skin structures; ◊ *mycobacterial infections*
Adults: 750 mg P.O. q 12 hours or 400 mg I.V. q 12 hours.
Typhoid fever
Adults: 500 mg P.O. q 12 hours.
Intra-abdominal infections (with metronidazole)
Adults: 500 mg P.O. q 12 hours
Mild to moderate acute sinusitis caused by Haemophilus influenzae, Streptococcus pneumoniae, or Moraxella catarrhalis; mild to moderate chronic bacterial prostatitis caused by Escherichia coli or Proteus mirabilis
Adults: 400 mg I.V. infusion given over 60 minutes every 12 hours.
◊ *Uncomplicated gonorrhea*
Adults: 250 mg P.O. as a single dose.

◊ *Neisseria meningitidis in nasal passages*
Adults: 500 to 750 mg P.O. as a single dose, or 250 mg P.O. b.i.d. for 2 days, or 500 mg P.O. b.i.d. for 5 days.
✦ *Dosage adjustment.* For patients with renal failure, refer to the following tables.

ORAL CIPROFLOXACIN

Creatinine clearance (ml/min)	Adult dosage
> 50	No adjustment
30 to 50	250 to 500 mg q 12 hr
5 to 29	250 to 500 mg q 18 hr

For patients on hemodialysis or peritoneal dialysis, give 250 to 500 mg q 24 hours (after dialysis).

I.V. CIPROFLOXACIN

Creatinine clearance (ml/min)	Adult dosage
> 30	No adjustment
5 to 29	200 to 400 mg. I.V. q 18 to 24 hr

Pharmacodynamics
Antibiotic action: Inhibits DNA gyrase, preventing bacterial DNA replication. The following organisms have been reported to be susceptible (in-vitro) to ciprofloxacin: *Campylobacter jejuni, Citrobacter diversus, Citrobacter freundii, Enterobacter cloacae, Escherichia coli* (including enterotoxigenic strains), *Haemophilus parainfluenzae, Klebsiella pneumoniae, Morganella morganii, Proteus mirabilis, Proteus vulgaris, Providencia stuartii, Providencia rettgeri, Pseudomonas aeruginosa, Serratia marcescens, Shigella flexneri, Shigella sonnei, Staphylococcus aureus* (penicillinase- and non–penicillinase-producing strains), *Staphylococcus epidermidis, Streptococcus faecalis,* and *Streptococcus pyogenes.*

Pharmacokinetics
• *Absorption:* 70% absorbed after oral administration. Food delays rate but not extent of absorption.
• *Distribution:* Serum levels peak within 1 to 2 hours after oral dosing. Drug is 20% to 40% protein-bound; CSF levels are only about 10% of plasma levels.
• *Metabolism:* Metabolism is probably hepatic. Four metabolites identified; each has less antimicrobial activity than parent compound.
• *Excretion:* Primarily renal. Serum half-life about 4 hours in adults with normal renal function.

Contraindications and precautions
Contraindicated in patients sensitive to fluoroquinolone antibiotics. Use cautiously in patients with CNS disorders and in those at risk for seizures.

Interactions
Drug-drug. *Antacid supplements containing aluminum, calcium, magnesium:* May interfere with ciprofloxacin absorption. Give 2 hours before or 6 hours after ciprofloxacin.
Aminoglycosides, beta-lactams: Synergistic effects have occurred with concurrent use. Use together cautiously.
Iron, minerals, vitamins: May interfere with absorption of ciprofloxacin. Administer separately.
Probenecid: Interferes with renal tubular secretion, causing higher plasma levels of ciprofloxacin. Use together cautiously.
Sucralfate: Reduces absorption of ciprofloxacin by 50%. Monitor patient closely.
Theophylline: May increase risk of theophylline toxicity. Monitor theophylline levels.
Warfarin: Increased PT. Monitor PT.
Drug-herb. *Yerba maté methylxanthines:* May decrease clearance of this herb, causing toxicity. Use together cautiously.
Drug-lifestyle. *Caffeine:* Prolonged elimination half-life of caffeine. Use with caution.
Sun exposure: Photosensitivity reaction may occur. Encourage patient to take precautions.

Adverse reactions
CNS: headache, restlessness, tremor, dizziness, fatigue, drowsiness, insomnia, depression, lightheadedness, confusion, hallucinations, *seizures,* paresthesia.
CV: thrombophlebitis.
GI: *nausea, diarrhea,* vomiting, abdominal pain or discomfort, oral candidiasis, elevated liver enzymes, pseudomembranous colitis, dyspepsia, flatulence, constipation.
GU: crystalluria, increased serum creatinine and BUN levels, interstitial nephritis.
Musculoskeletal: arthralgia, joint or back pain, joint inflammation, joint stiffness, aching, neck or chest pain.
Skin: *rash,* photosensitivity, toxic epidermal necrolysis, exfoliative dermatitis.
Other: photosensitivity, ***Stevens-Johnson syndrome,*** hypersensitivity, burning, pruritus, erythema, edema (with I.V. administration).

☑ Special considerations
• Duration of therapy depends on type and severity of infection. Therapy should continue for 2 days after symptoms have abated. Most infections are well controlled in 1 to 2 weeks, but bone or joint infections may require therapy for 4 weeks or longer.
• To treat drug overdose, empty stomach by inducing vomiting or lavage. Use general support-

---

Reactions may be *common*, uncommon, ***life-threatening***, or COMMON AND LIFE-THREATENING.

ive measures. Peritoneal or hemodialysis may be helpful.

Monitoring the patient
• Closer monitoring of theophylline levels may be necessary because of increased risk of theophylline toxicity in patients receiving ciprofloxacin.
• Monitor patient for adverse effects.

Information for the patient
• Tell patient that drug may be taken without regard to meals. Preferred time is 2 hours after a meal.
• Advise patient to avoid taking drug with antacids, iron, or calcium and to drink plenty of fluids during therapy.
• Inform patient that because dizziness, light-headedness, or drowsiness may occur, hazardous activities that require mental alertness should be avoided until CNS effects of drug are determined.

Pediatric patients
• Avoid use in children.

Breast-feeding patients
• Drug may appear in breast milk. Consider discontinuing breast-feeding or drug to avoid serious infant toxicity.

---

ciprofloxacin hydrochloride (ophthalmic)
Ciloxan

Pharmacologic classification: fluoroquinolone
Therapeutic classification: antibacterial
Pregnancy risk category C

How supplied
Available by prescription only
Ophthalmic solution: 0.3% in 2.5- and 5-ml containers

Indications, route, and dosage
Corneal ulcers caused by Pseudomonas aeruginosa, Staphylococcus aureus, Staphylococcus epidermidis, Streptococcus pneumoniae, *and possibly* Serratia marcescens *and* Streptococcus viridans
Adults and children over age 12: Instill 2 drops in affected eye q 15 minutes for first 6 hours; then 2 drops q 30 minutes for remainder of first day. On day 2, instill 2 drops hourly. On days 3 through 14, instill 2 drops q 4 hours.
Bacterial conjunctivitis caused by S. aureus *and* S. epidermidis *and possibly* S. pneumoniae
Adults and children over age 12: Instill 1 or 2 drops into conjunctival sac of affected eye q 2 hours, while awake, for first 2 days. Then 1 or 2 drops q 4 hours while awake for next 5 days.

Pharmacodynamics
Antibacterial action: Inhibits bacterial DNA gyrase, an enzyme necessary for bacterial replication. Bacteriostatic or bactericidal, depending on concentration.

Pharmacokinetics
• *Absorption:* Limited systemic absorption. When drug is instilled 2 hours while awake for 2 days, then every 4 hours while awake for an additional 5 days, maximum plasma level is below 5 ng/ml, and mean plasma level is usually below 2.5 ng/ml.
• *Distribution:* No information available.
• *Metabolism:* No information available.
• *Excretion:* No information available.

Contraindications and precautions
Contraindicated in patients with hypersensitivity to drug or other fluoroquinolone antibiotics. Use with caution in breast-feeding women.

Interactions
None reported.

Adverse reactions
EENT: *local burning or discomfort, white crystalline precipitate* (in the superficial portion of the corneal defect in patients with corneal ulcers), *margin crusting, crystals or scales, foreign body sensation, itching, conjunctival hyperemia,* bad or bitter taste in mouth, corneal staining, allergic reactions, keratopathy, lid edema, tearing, photophobia, decreased vision.
GI: nausea.

✓ Special considerations
• If corneal epithelium is still compromised after 14 days of treatment, continue therapy.
• A topical overdose of drug may be flushed from the eye with warm tap water.

Monitoring the patient
• Monitor patient for adverse effects.

Information for the patient
• Teach patient how to instill drug correctly. Remind patient not to touch tip of bottle with hands and to avoid contact of tip with eye or surrounding tissue.
• Remind patient not to share washcloths or towels with other family members to avoid spreading infection.
• Advise patient to wash hands before and after instilling solution.

Pediatric patients
• Safety and efficacy in children under age 12 haven't been established.

Breast-feeding patients
• It's unknown if drug appears in breast milk after eye application; however, systemically ad-

ministered ciprofloxacin does appear in breast milk. Use caution.

---

cisatracurium besylate
Nimbex

Pharmacologic classification: nondepolarizing neuromuscular blocker
Therapeutic classification: skeletal muscle relaxant
Pregnancy risk category B

How supplied
Available by prescription only
Injection: 2 mg/ml, 10 mg/ml

Indications, route, and dosage
Adjunct to general anesthesia, to facilitate tracheal intubation, to provide skeletal muscle relaxation during surgery or mechanical ventilation in intensive care unit
Adults and children ages 12 and older: Initially, 0.15 or 0.20 mg/kg I.V.; then 0.03 mg/kg I.V. q 40 to 50 minutes after an initial dose of 0.15 mg/kg and q 50 to 60 minutes following an initial dose of 0.20 mg/kg for maintenance in prolonged surgical procedures. Or administer 3 mcg/kg/minute maintenance infusion after initial dose and then decrease to 1 to 2 mcg/kg/minute, p.r.n.
Children ages 2 to 12: 0.1 mg/kg I.V. over 5 to 10 seconds. Administer 3 mcg/kg/minute maintenance I.V. infusion after initial dose and then decrease to 1 to 2 mcg/kg/minute, p.r.n., in prolonged surgical procedures.
Maintenance of neuromuscular blockade in intensive care unit
Adults: 3 mcg/kg/minute I.V. infusion.
Note: There may be wide variability among patients in dosage requirements and these may increase or decrease over time.

Pharmacodynamics
Skeletal muscle relaxation action: Binds competitively to cholinergic receptors on the motor end-plate to antagonize action of acetylcholine, resulting in blockage of neuromuscular transmission.

Pharmacokinetics
• *Absorption:* Only administered I.V.
• *Distribution:* Volume of distribution limited by its large molecular weight and high polarity. Drug binding to plasma proteins hasn't been successfully studied because of its rapid degradation at physiologic pH.
• *Metabolism:* Degradation of cisatracurium largely independent of liver metabolism. Believed that drug undergoes Hofmann elimination (a pH- and temperature-dependent chemical process) to form laudanosine and the monoquaternary acrylate metabolite.

• *Excretion:* Metabolites excreted primarily in urine and feces. Elimination half-life is between 22 and 29 minutes.

Contraindications and precautions
Contraindicated in patients with hypersensitivity to drug, other bis-benzylisoquinolinium drugs, or benzyl alcohol. Use cautiously in pregnant women.

Interactions
Drug-drug. *Aminoglycosides, bacitracin, clindamycin, colistimethate sodium, colistin, lincomycin, lithium, local anesthetics, magnesium salts, polymyxins, procainamide, quinidine, tetracyclines:* May enhance neuromuscular blocking action of cisatracurium. Use together cautiously.
Carbamazepine, phenytoin: May cause slightly shorter duration of neuromuscular blockage, requiring higher infusion rates. Monitor patient closely.
Enflurane or isoflurane administered with nitrous oxide or oxygen: May prolong clinically effective duration of action of initial and maintenance doses of cisatracurium. In long surgical procedures, less frequent maintenance dosing, lower maintenance doses, or reduced infusion rates of cisatracurium may be needed.

Adverse reactions
CV: *bradycardia,* hypotension.
Respiratory: *bronchospasm.*
Skin: flushing, rash.

☑ Special considerations
• Drug isn't recommended for rapid sequence endotracheal intubation because of its intermediate onset of action.
• Drug has no known effect on consciousness, pain threshold, or cerebration. To avoid patient distress, neuromuscular block shouldn't be induced before patient is unconscious.
• For I.V. use, 20-ml vial is intended for use in intensive care unit only. Drug isn't compatible with propofol injection or ketorolac injection for Y-site administration. Drug is acidic and also may not be compatible with an alkaline solution having a pH greater than 8.5, such as barbiturate solutions for Y-site administration. Drug shouldn't be diluted in lactated Ringer's injection USP because of chemical instability.
• Drug is colorless to slightly yellow or greenish yellow solution. Inspect vial visually for particulate matter and discoloration before administration. Don't use solutions that aren't clear or contain visible particulates.
• To avoid inaccurate dosing, neuromuscular monitoring should be performed on a nonparetic limb in patients with hemiparesis or paraparesis.
• In patients with neuromuscular disease (myasthenia gravis and myasthenic syndrome), prolonged neuromuscular block may occur. The use

---

of a peripheral nerve stimulator and a dose not exceeding 0.02 mg/kg is recommended to assess the level of neuromuscular block and to monitor dosage requirements.
• Because patients with burns have been shown to develop resistance to nondepolarizing neuromuscular blocking drugs, these patients may require increased dosing requirements and exhibit shortened duration of action. Monitor closely.
• Administer pain medication, if necessary, regularly as patient will feel pain but not be able to exhibit signs of its presence.
• Overdose with neuromuscular blocking drugs may result in neuromuscular block beyond the time needed for surgery and anesthesia.
• Primary treatment of overdose is maintenance of a patent airway and controlled ventilation until recovery of normal neuromuscular function is assured. Once recovery from neuromuscular block begins, further recovery may be facilitated by administration of an anticholinesterase (neostigmine, edrophonium) and an appropriate anticholinergic.

Monitoring the patient
• Monitor neuromuscular function during drug administration with a nerve stimulator. Additional doses of drug shouldn't be given before there is a definite response to nerve stimulation. If no response occurs, stop infusion until a response returns.
• Monitor patient's acid-base balance and electrolyte levels. Acid-base or serum electrolyte abnormalities may potentiate or antagonize drug's action.
• Monitor patient for malignant hyperthermia.

Information for the patient
• Inform patient and family of need for drug and how it's administered.
• Reassure patient and family that patient will be monitored continuously throughout drug therapy.

Geriatric patients
• Use with caution when administering to elderly patients. The time to maximum block is about 1 minute slower in elderly patients.

Pediatric patients
• Safety and effectiveness in children under age 2 haven't been established.

Breast-feeding patients
• It's unknown if drug appears in breast milk; use caution when giving to breast-feeding women.

cisplatin (cis-platinum)
Platinol, Platinol AQ

Pharmacologic classification: alkylating drug (cell-cycle–phase nonspecific)
Therapeutic classification: antineoplastic
Pregnancy risk category D

How supplied
Available by prescription only
Injection: 10-mg, 50-mg vials (lyophilized); 50-mg, 100-mg vials (aqueous)

Indications, route, and dosage
Dosage and indications may vary. Check current literature for recommended protocol.
Adjunctive therapy in metastatic testicular cancer
Adults: 20 mg/m² I.V. daily for 5 days. Repeat q 3 weeks for three cycles or more. Frequently used in therapeutic regimen with bleomycin and vinblastine.
Adjunctive therapy in metastatic ovarian cancer
Adults: 75 to 100 mg/m² I.V. Repeat q 4 weeks or 50 mg/m² I.V. q 3 weeks with concurrent doxorubicin hydrochloride therapy.
Advanced bladder cancer
Adults: 50 to 70 mg/m² I.V. once q 3 to 4 weeks. Patients who have received other antineoplastics or radiation therapy should receive 50 mg/m² q 4 weeks.
◊ *Head and neck cancer*
Adults: 80 to 120 mg/m² I.V. once q 3 weeks.
◊ *Cervical cancer*
Adults: 50 mg/m² I.V. once q 3 weeks.
◊ *Non-small-cell lung cancer*
Adults: 70 to 120 mg/m² I.V. once q 3 to 6 weeks.
◊ *Brain tumor*
Children: 60 mg/m² I.V. for 2 days q 3 to 4 weeks.
◊ *Osteogenic sarcoma or neuroblastoma*
Children: 90 mg/m² I.V. q 3 weeks.
    Note: Prehydration and mannitol diuresis may significantly reduce renal toxicity and ototoxicity.

Pharmacodynamics
Antineoplastic action: Exerts its cytotoxic effects by binding with DNA and inhibiting DNA synthesis and, to a lesser extent, by inhibition of protein and RNA synthesis. Also acts as a bifunctional alkylating drug, causing intrastrand and interstrand cross-links of DNA. Interstrand cross-linking appears to correlate well with the cytotoxicity of drug.

Pharmacokinetics
• *Absorption:* Not administered orally or intramuscularly.
• *Distribution:* Distributed widely into tissues, with highest levels found in kidneys, liver, and prostate. Can accumulate in body tissues; detected up to

6 months after last dose. Doesn't readily cross blood-brain barrier. Extensively and irreversibly bound to plasma proteins and tissue proteins.
• *Metabolism:* Metabolic fate unclear.
• *Excretion:* Primarily unchanged in urine. In patients with normal renal function, half-life of initial elimination phase is 25 to 79 minutes and terminal phase 58 to 78 hours. Terminal half-life of total cisplatin is up to 10 days.

Contraindications and precautions
Contraindicated in patients with hypersensitivity to drug or to other platinum-containing compounds and in those with severe renal disease, hearing impairment, or myelosuppression.

Interactions
Drug-drug. *Aminoglycosides:* Potentiates cumulative nephrotoxicity caused by cisplatin. Don't give aminoglycosides within 2 weeks of cisplatin therapy.
Loop diuretics: Increased risk of ototoxicity. Closely monitor patient's audiologic status.
Phenytoin: May decrease serum phenytoin level. Monitor serum phenytoin level.

Adverse reactions
CNS: *peripheral neuritis,* loss of taste, *seizures.*
EENT: *tinnitus, hearing loss, ototoxicity,* vestibular toxicity.
GI: *nausea, vomiting* (beginning 1 to 4 hours after dose and lasting 24 hours).
GU: more prolonged and SEVERE RENAL TOXICITY with repeated courses of therapy.
Hematologic: MYELOSUPPRESSION; *leukopenia; thrombocytopenia; anemia;* nadirs in circulating platelet and WBC counts on days 18 to 23, with recovery by day 39.
Metabolism: *hypomagnesemia,* hypokalemia, hypocalcemia, hyponatremia, hypophosphatemia, hyperuricemia.
Other: *anaphylactoid reaction.*

☑ Special considerations
• Review hematologic status and creatinine clearance before therapy.
• Reconstitute 10-mg vial with 10 ml and 50-mg vial with 50 ml of sterile water for injection to yield a concentration of 1 mg/ml. Drug may be diluted further in a sodium chloride–containing solution for I.V. infusion.
• Don't use aluminum needles for reconstitution or administration of cisplatin; a black precipitate may form. Use stainless steel needles.
• Drug is stable for 24 hours in normal saline solution at room temperature. Don't refrigerate because precipitation may occur. Discard solution containing precipitate.
• Infusions are most stable in chloride-containing solutions, such as normal saline, 0.45% saline, or 0.225% saline.

• Mannitol may be given as a 12.5-g I.V. bolus before starting cisplatin infusion. Follow by infusion of mannitol at rate of up to 10 g/hour, as necessary, to maintain urine output during cisplatin infusion and for 6 to 24 hours after infusion.
• I.V. sodium thiosulfate may be administered with cisplatin infusion to decrease risk of nephrotoxicity.
• Hydrate patient with normal saline solution before giving drug. Maintain urine output of 100 ml/hour for 4 consecutive hours before and for 24 hours after infusion.
• Hydrate patient by encouraging oral fluid intake when possible.
• High-dose metoclopramide (2 mg/kg I.V.) has been used to prevent and treat nausea and vomiting. Dexamethasone 10 to 20 mg has been given I.V. with metoclopramide to help alleviate nausea and vomiting. Many patients respond favorably to treatment with ondansetron. Pretreatment with this 5-HT$_3$ antagonist should begin 30 minutes before cisplatin therapy is started.
• Treat extravasation with local injections of a 1/6 M sodium thiosulfate solution (prepared by mixing 4 ml of sodium thiosulfate 10% and 6 ml of sterile water for injection).
• Renal toxicity becomes more severe with repeated doses. Renal function must return to normal before next dose can be given.
• Anaphylactoid reaction usually responds to immediate treatment with epinephrine, corticosteroids, or antihistamines.
• Avoid contact with skin. If contact occurs, wash drug off immediately with soap and water.
• Signs and symptoms of overdose include leukopenia, thrombocytopenia, nausea, and vomiting. Treatment is generally supportive and includes transfusion of blood components, antibiotics for possible infections, and antiemetics.
• Cisplatin can be removed by dialysis, but only within 3 hours after administration.

Monitoring the patient
• Nausea and vomiting may be severe and protracted (up to 24 hours). Antiemetics can be started 24 hours before therapy. Monitor fluid intake and output. Continue I.V. hydration until patient can tolerate adequate oral intake.
• Monitor CBC, platelet count, and renal function studies before initial and subsequent doses. Don't repeat dose unless platelet count is over 100,000/mm^3, WBC count is over 4,000/mm^3, serum creatinine level is under 1.5 mg/dl, or BUN level is under 25 mg/dl.
• Monitor electrolytes extensively; aggressive supplementation is often required after a course of therapy.
• Liver function studies should be monitored periodically.
• Neurologic examinations should be performed regularly.

Information for the patient
- Stress importance of adequate fluid intake and increase in urine output to facilitate uric acid excretion.
- Tell patient to report tinnitus immediately to prevent permanent hearing loss. Patient should have audiometric tests before initial and subsequent courses.
- Advise patient to avoid exposure to people with infections.
- Inform patient to promptly report unusual bleeding or bruising.

Pediatric patients
- Pediatric dosage of cisplatin hasn't been fully established. Unlabeled uses of cisplatin include osteogenic sarcoma and neuroblastoma.
- Ototoxicity appears to be more severe in children.

Breast-feeding patients
- It's unknown if cisplatin appears in breast milk. Because of risk to infant of serious adverse reactions, mutagenicity, and carcinogenicity, breast-feeding isn't recommended during therapy.

citalopram hydrobromide
Celexa

Pharmacologic classification: selective serotonin reuptake inhibitor (SSRI)
Therapeutic classification: antidepressant
Pregnancy risk category C

How supplied
Available by prescription only
Tablets: 20 mg, 40 mg

Indications, route, and dosage
Depression
Adults: Initially, 20 mg P.O. once daily, increasing to 40 mg daily after no less than 1 week. Maximum recommended dose is 40 mg daily.
Elderly: 20 mg/day P.O. with increase to 40 mg/day for nonresponding patients.
✦ *Dosage adjustment.* For patients with hepatic impairment, use 20 mg/day P.O. with adjustment to 40 mg/day only for nonresponding patients.

Pharmacodynamics
An SSRI whose action is presumed to be linked to potentiation of serotonergic activity in CNS resulting from inhibition of neuronal reuptake of serotonin.

Pharmacokinetics
- *Absorption:* Absolute bioavailability is 80% following oral administration. Serum levels peak in 4 hours.
- *Distribution:* Highly bound to plasma proteins (80%).
- *Metabolism:* Extensively metabolized primarily by cytochrome P-450 3A4 and cytochrome P-450 2C19 to inactive metabolites.
- *Excretion:* 20% excreted in urine. Elimination half-life is about 35 hours. In patients over age 60, half-life is increased up to 30%.

Contraindications and precautions
Contraindicated in patients with hypersensitivity to drug or its inactive ingredients and in those also taking MAO inhibitors or within 14 days of MAO inhibitor therapy.

Interactions
Drug-drug. *Carbamazepine:* May increase citalopram clearance. Monitor patient for effects.
CNS drugs: Additive effects. Use together cautiously.
Drugs that inhibit cytochrome P-450 isoenzymes 3A4 and 2C19: Decreased clearance of citalopram. Monitor closely.
Imipramine, other tricyclic antidepressants: Concentration of imipramine metabolite desipramine increases by about 50%. Use together cautiously.
Lithium: May enhance serotonergic effect of citalopram. Use cautiously and monitor lithium levels.
MAO inhibitors: Serious, sometimes fatal, reactions may occur. Don't use drug within 14 days of MAO inhibitor therapy.
Warfarin: PT is increased by 5%. Monitor PT closely.
Drug-lifestyle. *Alcohol:* May increase CNS effects. Discourage use.

Adverse reactions
CNS: tremor, *somnolence, insomnia,* anxiety, agitation, dizziness, paresthesia, migraine, impaired concentration, amnesia, depression, apathy, *suicide attempt,* confusion, fatigue.
CV: tachycardia, orthostatic hypotension, hypotension.
EENT: rhinitis, sinusitis, abnormal accommodation.
GI: *dry mouth, nausea,* diarrhea, anorexia, dyspepsia, vomiting, abdominal pain, taste perversion, increased saliva, flatulence, decreased and increased weight, increased appetite.
GU: dysmenorrhea, amenorrhea, ejaculation disorder, impotence, polyuria, decreased libido.
Musculoskeletal: arthralgia, myalgia.
Respiratory: upper respiratory tract infection, coughing.
Skin: rash, pruritus.
Other: *increased sweating,* fever, yawning.

☑ Special considerations
- Use cautiously in patients with history of mania, seizures, suicidal ideation, or hepatic or renal impairment.

• Although drug hasn't been shown to impair psychomotor performance, any psychoactive drug has the potential to impair judgment, thinking, or motor skills.
• The possibility of a suicide attempt is inherent in depression and may persist until significant remission occurs. Closely supervise high-risk patients at start of drug therapy. Reduce risk of overdose by limiting amount of drug available per refill.
• At least 14 days should elapse between MAO inhibitor therapy and citalopram therapy.

Monitoring the patient
• Monitor patient for adverse effects.
• Close follow up with patient is needed during initiation of therapy to observe for suicidal tendencies.

Information for the patient
• Inform patient that, although improvement may occur within 1 to 4 weeks, therapy should be continued as prescribed.
• Instruct patient to exercise caution when operating hazardous machinery, including automobiles, because of the potential of psychoactive drugs to impair judgment, thinking, and motor skills.
• Advise patient to call before taking other prescription or OTC drugs.
• Warn patient to avoid concomitant use of alcohol.
• Caution patient against use of MAO inhibitors while taking citalopram.
• Tell patient that drug may be taken in the morning or evening without regard to meals.

Geriatric patients
• Use cautiously in elderly patients because greater sensitivity to drug hasn't been ruled out.

Pediatric patients
• Safety and effectiveness in children haven't been established.

Breast-feeding patients
• Drug appears in breast milk with subsequent effects in infant. A decision to discontinue drug or breast-feeding should be made during drug therapy.

---

cladribine
Leustatin

Pharmacologic classification: purine nucleoside analogue
Therapeutic classification: antineoplastic
Pregnancy risk category D

How supplied
Available by prescription only
Injection: 1 mg/ml

Indications, route, and dosage
Active hairy cell leukemia
Adults: 0.09 mg/kg daily by continuous I.V. infusion for 7 days.
◇ *Advanced cutaneous T-cell lymphomas, chronic lymphocytic leukemia, malignant lymphomas, acute myeloid leukemias, autoimmune hemolytic anemia, mycosis fungoides, or Sézary syndrome*
Adults: Usually 0.1 mg/kg/day by continuous I.V. infusion for 7 days.

Pharmacodynamics
Antineoplastic action: Enters tumor cells, where it's phosphorylated by deoxycytidine kinase and subsequently converted into an active triphosphate deoxynucleotide. This metabolite impairs synthesis of new DNA, inhibits repair of existing DNA, and disrupts cellular metabolism.

Pharmacokinetics
• *Absorption:* Not administered P.O. or I.M.
• *Distribution:* 20% bound to plasma proteins.
• *Metabolism:* No information available.
• *Excretion:* For patients with normal renal function, mean terminal half-life of cladribine is 5.4 hours.

Contraindications and precautions
Contraindicated in patients with hypersensitivity to drug. Use cautiously in patients with impaired renal or hepatic function.

Interactions
Drug-drug. *Amphotericin B:* May increase risk of nephrotoxicity, hypotension, and bronchospasm. Use together cautiously.
Other drugs known to cause myelosuppression: Cumulative effects. Use together cautiously.

Adverse reactions
CNS: *malaise, headache, fatigue,* dizziness, insomnia, asthenia.
CV: tachycardia, edema.
EENT: epistaxis.
GI: *nausea, decreased appetite, vomiting, diarrhea,* constipation, abdominal pain.
GU: acute renal insufficiency.
Hematologic: NEUTROPENIA, *anemia, thrombocytopenia.*
Musculoskeletal: *trunk pain, myalgia, arthralgia.*
Respiratory: *abnormal breath or chest sounds, cough,* shortness of breath.
Skin: *rash, pruritus, erythema, purpura,* petechiae, *local reaction at injection site.*
Other: *fever,* INFECTION, *chills, diaphoresis,* hyperuricemia.

☑ Special considerations
• Fever is commonly observed during the first month of therapy and frequently requires antibiotic therapy.

Reactions may be *common, uncommon, **life-threatening**,* OR COMMON AND LIFE-THREATENING.

- Because of risk of hyperuricemia from tumor lysis, allopurinol should be administered during therapy.
- For a 24-hour infusion, add the calculated dose to a 500-ml infusion bag of normal saline solution injection. Once diluted, administer promptly or store in the refrigerator for no more than 8 hours before administration. Don't use solutions that contain dextrose because increased drug degradation is possible. Because the product doesn't contain bacteriostatic drugs, use strict aseptic technique to prepare admixture. Solutions containing cladribine shouldn't be mixed with other I.V. drugs or infused simultaneously via a common I.V. line.
- Or prepare a 7-day infusion solution using bacteriostatic sodium chloride injection, which contains 0.9% benzyl alcohol. First, pass the calculated amount of drug through a disposable 0.22-micron hydrophilic syringe filter into a sterile infusion reservoir. Next, add sufficient bacteriostatic sodium chloride injection to bring the total volume to 100 ml. Clamp off line; then disconnect and discard filter. If necessary, aseptically aspirate air bubbles from reservoir, using new filter or sterile vent filter assembly.
- Pharmacia Deltec medication cassettes have shown acceptable physical and chemical stability.
- Refrigerate unopened vials at 36° to 46° F (2° to 8° C), and protect from light. Although freezing doesn't adversely affect drug, a precipitate may form; will disappear if drug is allowed to warm to room temperature gradually and vial is vigorously shaken. Don't heat, microwave, or refreeze.
- High doses of cladribine have been associated with irreversible neurologic toxicity (paraparesis/quadriparesis), acute nephrotoxicity, and severe bone marrow suppression that results in neutropenia, anemia, and thrombocytopenia. No antidote specific to cladribine overdose is known. Besides stopping drug, treatment consists of careful observation and appropriate supportive measures. It's unknown if drug can be removed from circulation by dialysis or hemofiltration.

Monitoring the patient
- Cladribine is a toxic drug; some toxicity expected during treatment. Monitor hematologic function closely, especially during first 4 to 8 weeks of therapy. Severe bone marrow suppression, including neutropenia, anemia, and thrombocytopenia, commonly has been observed in patients treated with drug; many patients also have preexisting hematologic impairment from their disease.
- Periodically assess renal and hepatic function as clinically indicated.

Information for the patient
- Tell woman of childbearing age to avoid pregnancy during drug therapy because of risk of fetal malformations.

Pediatric patients
- Safety and effectiveness in children haven't been established.

Breast-feeding patients
- It's unknown if drug appears in breast milk. A decision should be made to discontinue breast-feeding or discontinue drug, taking into account importance of drug to mother.

clarithromycin
Biaxin

Pharmacologic classification: macrolide
Therapeutic classification: antibiotic
Pregnancy risk category C

How supplied
Available by prescription only
Tablets: 250 mg, 500 mg
Suspension: 125 mg/5 ml, 250 mg/5 ml

Indications, route, and dosage
Pharyngitis or tonsillitis caused by Streptococcus pyogenes
Adults: 250 mg P.O. q 12 hours for 10 days.
Children: 15 mg/kg/day divided q 12 hours for 10 days.
Acute maxillary sinusitis caused by Streptococcus pneumoniae, Haemophilus influenzae, or Moraxella catarrhalis
Adults: 500 mg P.O. q 12 hours for 14 days.
Children: 15 mg/kg/day divided q 12 hours for 10 days.
Acute exacerbations of chronic bronchitis caused by M. (Branhamella) catarrhalis or S. pneumoniae; pneumonia caused by S. pneumoniae or Mycoplasma pneumoniae
Adults: 250 mg P.O. q 12 hours for 7 to 14 days.
Acute exacerbations of chronic bronchitis caused by H. influenzae
Adults: 500 mg P.O. q 12 hours for 7 to 14 days.
Uncomplicated skin and skin-structure infections caused by Staphylococcus aureus or S. pyogenes
Adults: 250 mg P.O. q 12 hours for 7 to 14 days.
Prophylaxis and treatment of disseminated infection caused by Mycobacterium avium complex
Adults: 500 mg P.O. b.i.d.
Children: 7.5 mg/kg b.i.d. up to 500 mg b.i.d.
Acute otitis media caused by H. influenzae, M. catarrhalis, or S. pneumoniae
Children: 7.5 mg/kg b.i.d. up to 500 mg b.i.d.

✦ Dosage adjustment. In patients with creatinine clearance of less than 30 ml/minute, dose should be halved or frequency interval doubled.

Pharmacodynamics
Antibiotic action: A macrolide antibiotic that is a derivative of erythromycin, binds to the 50S subunit of bacterial ribosomes, blocking protein synthesis. Bacteriostatic or bactericidal, depending on concentration.

Pharmacokinetics
• *Absorption:* Rapidly absorbed from GI tract; absolute bioavailability is about 50%. Serum levels peak within 2 hours. Food slightly delays onset of absorption and formation of active metabolite, but doesn't alter total amount absorbed.
• *Distribution:* Widely distributed; because it readily penetrates cells, tissue levels are higher than plasma levels. Plasma half-life is dose-dependent; half-life is 3 to 4 hours at doses of 250 mg q 12 hours and increases to 5 to 7 hours at doses of 500 mg q 12 hours.
• *Metabolism:* Major metabolite, 14-hydroxy clarithromycin, has significant antimicrobial activity; about twice as active against *H. influenzae* as parent drug.
• *Excretion:* In patients taking 250 mg q 12 hours, about 20% of dose eliminated in urine unchanged; increases to 30% in patients taking 500 mg q 12 hours. Major metabolite accounts for about 15% of drug in urine. Elimination half-life of active metabolite is dose-dependent: 5 to 6 hours with 250 mg q 12 hours; 7 hours with 500 mg q 12 hours.

Contraindications and precautions
Contraindicated in patients with hypersensitivity to erythromycin or other macrolides who have preexisting cardiac abnormalities or electrolyte disturbances. Use cautiously in patients with impaired renal or hepatic function.

Interactions
Drug-drug. *Carbamazepine, theophylline:* Increased serum levels of these drugs. Monitor plasma levels carefully.
Cyclosporine, phenytoin, triazolam: Decreased metabolism of these drugs. Monitor patient closely.
Digoxin: Increased digoxin levels. Monitor digoxin level.
Dihydroergotamine, ergotamine: Ergot toxicity. Monitor patient closely.
Warfarin: Increased PT. Monitor PT closely.

Adverse reactions
CNS: headache.
GI: *diarrhea, nausea, abnormal taste,* dyspepsia, abdominal pain or discomfort.

GU: elevated BUN and creatinine levels.
Hematologic: increased PT, decreased WBCs.
Hepatic: elevated liver function test results.

☑ Special considerations
• Obtain specimen for culture and sensitivity tests before giving first dose. Therapy may begin pending test results.
• Reconstituted suspension shouldn't be refrigerated; discard any unused portion after 14 days.

Monitoring the patient
• Drug may cause overgrowth of nonsusceptible bacteria or fungi. Monitor patient for signs and symptoms of superinfection.
• Monitor patient for adverse effects.

Information for the patient
• Tell patient to take all of drug as prescribed, even if feeling better.
• Inform patient that drug may be taken without regard to meals.
• Instruct patient to shake suspension well before use; don't refrigerate.

Pediatric patients
• Safety and efficacy in children under age 12 haven't been established.

Breast-feeding patients
• It's unknown if drug appears in breast milk; however, other macrolides have been found in breast milk. Use with caution.

clemastine fumarate
Tavist, Tavist-1

Pharmacologic classification: ethanolamine-derivative antihistamine
Therapeutic classification: antihistamine (H$_1$-receptor antagonist)
Pregnancy risk category C

How supplied
Available without a prescription
Tablets: 1.34 mg (Tavist-1), 2.68 mg (Tavist)
Syrup: 0.67 mg/5 ml (equivalent to 0.5 mg base/5 ml)

Indications, route, and dosage
Rhinitis, allergy symptoms
Adults and children ages 12 and older: 1.34 to 2.68 mg P.O. b.i.d. or t.i.d. Maximum recommended daily dose: 8.04 mg.
Children ages 6 to 11: 0.67 mg b.i.d.; don't exceed 4.02 mg/day.
Allergic skin manifestation of urticaria and angioedema
Adults and children ages 12 and older: 2.68 mg up to t.i.d. maximum.

Children ages 6 to 11: 1.34 mg b.i.d.; don't exceed 4.02 mg/day.

Pharmacodynamics
Antihistamine action: Antihistamines compete with histamine for histamine H_1-receptor sites on the smooth muscle of the bronchi, GI tract, uterus, and large blood vessels; by binding to cellular receptors, they prevent access of histamine and suppress histamine-induced allergic symptoms, even though they don't prevent its release.

Pharmacokinetics
● *Absorption:* Absorbed readily from GI tract; action begins in 15 to 30 minutes and peaks in 2 to 7 hours.
● *Distribution:* No information available.
● *Metabolism:* Extensively metabolized.
● *Excretion:* Excreted in urine.

Contraindications and precautions
Contraindicated in patients with hypersensitivity to drug or other antihistamines of similar chemical structure; in those with acute asthma; in neonates or premature infants; and in breast-feeding patients.

Use cautiously in elderly patients and in patients with increased intraocular pressure, glaucoma, hyperthyroidism, CV or renal disease, hypertension, bronchial asthma, pyloroduodenal obstruction, prostatic hyperplasia, bladder neck obstruction, and stenosing peptic ulcers.

Interactions
Drug-drug. *Heparin:* May partially counteract anticoagulant effects of heparin. Monitor patient, PTT, and INR.
MAO inhibitors: Interfere with detoxification of clemastine and thus prolong and intensify their central depressant and anticholinergic effects. Monitor patient closely.
Other CNS depressants such as anxiolytics, barbiturates, sleeping aids, tranquilizers: Additive CNS depression. Monitor patient carefully.
Sulfonylureas: Diminished effects of sulfonylureas. Monitor patient carefully.
Drug-lifestyle. *Alcohol:* Additive CNS depression. Discourage use together.

Adverse reactions
CNS: *sedation, drowsiness, seizures,* nervousness, tremor, confusion, restlessness, vertigo, headache, *sleepiness, dizziness, incoordination,* fatigue.
CV: hypotension, palpitations, tachycardia.
GI: *epigastric distress,* anorexia, diarrhea, nausea, vomiting, constipation, *dry mouth.*
GU: urine retention, urinary frequency.
Hematologic: hemolytic anemia, *thrombocytopenia, agranulocytosis.*
Respiratory: *thick bronchial secretions.*

Skin: rash, urticaria, photosensitivity, diaphoresis.
Other: *anaphylactic shock.*

☑ Special considerations
Besides the recommendations relevant to all antihistamines, consider the following.
● Drug is indicated for treatment of urticaria only at doses of 2.68 mg up to t.i.d.
● Stop drug 4 days before diagnostic skin tests; antihistamines can prevent, reduce, or mask positive skin test response.
● Signs and symptoms of overdose include either CNS depression (sedation, reduced mental alertness, apnea, and CV collapse) or CNS stimulation (insomnia, hallucinations, tremors, or seizures). Anticholinergic symptoms, such as dry mouth, flushed skin, fixed and dilated pupils, and GI symptoms, are common, especially in children.
● Treat overdose by inducing emesis with ipecac syrup (in conscious patient), then activated charcoal to reduce further drug absorption. Use gastric lavage if patient is unconscious or if ipecac fails.
● Treat hypotension with vasopressors, and control seizures with diazepam or phenytoin.

Monitoring the patient
● Monitor patient for adverse effects.
● Perform periodic CBC as needed.

Information for the patient
● Inform patient of potential adverse reactions.
● Instruct patient to avoid alcohol because of increased risk of CNS effects.

Geriatric patients
● Elderly patients are more susceptible to sedative effect of drug. Instruct older patient to change positions slowly and gradually. Elderly people may experience dizziness or hypotension more readily.

Pediatric patients
● Drug isn't indicated for use in premature infants or neonates. Children, especially those under age 6, may experience paradoxical hyperexcitability.

Breast-feeding patients
● Drug appears in breast milk. Don't use during breast-feeding because it exposes infant to risks of unusual excitability; premature infants are at particular risk for seizures.

clindamycin hydrochloride
Cleocin

clindamycin palmitate hydrochloride
Cleocin Pediatric

clindamycin phosphate
Cleocin Phosphate, Cleocin T

Pharmacologic classification: lincomycin derivative
Therapeutic classification: antibiotic
Pregnancy risk category NR (B vaginal and topical creams)

How supplied
Available by prescription only
Capsules: 75 mg, 150 mg, 300 mg
Solution (granules): 75 mg/5 ml
Injection: 150 mg/ml
Infusion for I.V. use: 300 mg, 600 mg, 900 mg
Gel, lotion, topical solution: 1%
Vaginal cream: 2%

Indications, route, and dosage
Infections caused by sensitive organisms
Adults: 150 to 450 mg P.O. q 6 hours; or 600 to 2,700 mg/day I.M. or I.V. divided into two to four equal doses.
Children over age 1 month: 8 to 20 mg/kg/day P.O. or 20 to 40 mg/kg/day I.V. divided into three or four equal doses.
Children under age 1 month: 15 to 20 mg/kg/day I.V. divided into three or four equal doses.
Bacterial vaginosis
Adults: 100 mg (1 applicator of clindamycin phosphate) intravaginally h.s. for 7 days.
Acne vulgaris
Adults: Apply thin film of topical solution, gel, or lotion to affected areas b.i.d.
◊ **Toxoplasmosis (cerebral or ocular) in immunocompromised patients**
Adults: 1,200 to 4,800 mg/day I.V. or P.O. Also administered with pyrimethamine in doses up to 75 mg/day P.O. and with folinic acid in a dose of 10 mg/day P.O.
◊ **Pneumocystis carinii pneumonia**
Adults: 600 mg I.V. q 6 hours or 300 to 450 mg P.O. q.i.d. With primaquine, give 15 to 30 mg P.O. daily.

Pharmacodynamics
Antibacterial action: Inhibits bacterial protein synthesis by binding to ribosome's 50S subunit. May produce bacteriostatic or bactericidal effects on susceptible bacteria, including most aerobic gram-positive cocci and anaerobic gram-negative and gram-positive organisms. Considered a first-line drug in treatment of *Bacteroides fragilis* and most other gram-positive and gram-negative anaer-

obes. Also effective against *Mycoplasma pneumoniae, Leptotrichia buccalis,* and some gram-positive cocci and bacilli.

Pharmacokinetics
● *Absorption:* When administered orally, absorbed rapidly and almost completely from GI tract, regardless of formulation. Levels of 1.9 to 3.9 mcg/ml peak in 45 to 60 minutes. May also be given I.M. with good absorption. Peak levels occur in about 3 hours. With 300-mg dose, peak levels are about 6 mcg/ml; with 600-mg dose, about 10 mcg/ml.
● *Distribution:* Distributed widely to most body tissues and fluids (except CSF) and crosses placenta. About 93% of drug bound to plasma proteins.
● *Metabolism:* Partially to inactive metabolites.
● *Excretion:* 10% excreted unchanged in urine; rest excreted as inactive metabolites (with some drug excreted in breast milk). Plasma half-life is 2½ to 3 hours in patients with normal renal function; 3½ to 5 hours in anephric patients; and 7 to 14 hours in patients with hepatic disease. Peritoneal dialysis and hemodialysis don't remove drug.

Contraindications and precautions
Contraindicated in patients with hypersensitivity to the antibiotic congener lincomycin; in those with a history of ulcerative colitis, regional enteritis, or antibiotic-associated colitis; and in those with a history of atopic reactions.
    Use cautiously in patients with asthma, impaired renal or hepatic function, or history of GI diseases or significant allergies.

Interactions
Drug-drug. *Acne preparations (such as benzoyl peroxide, tretinoin):* Cumulative irritant or drying effect. Use together cautiously.
Antidiarrheals (such as diphenoxylate, opiates): May prolong or worsen clindamycin-induced diarrhea by reducing excretion of bacterial toxins. Avoid concomitant use.
Erythromycin: May act as an antagonist, blocking clindamycin from reaching its site of action. Monitor patient for drug effect.
Kaolin products: May reduce GI absorption of clindamycin. Give at separate times.
Neuromuscular blockers (such as pancuronium, tubocurarine): May potentiate action of these drugs. Use together cautiously.

Adverse reactions
GI: nausea, vomiting, abdominal pain, *diarrhea, pseudomembranous colitis.*
GU: *cervicitis, vaginitis, Candida albicans* overgrowth, *vulvar irritation.*
Hematologic: transient leukopenia, eosinophilia, *thrombocytopenia.*
Hepatic: jaundice, abnormal liver function test results.

Reactions may be *common,* uncommon, *life-threatening,* or COMMON AND LIFE-THREATENING.

Skin: maculopapular rash, urticaria, dryness, *redness,* pruritus, swelling, irritation, contact dermatitis, burning.
Other: *anaphylaxis.*

☑ Special considerations
• Culture and sensitivity tests should be done before treatment starts and should be repeated as needed.
• Don't refrigerate reconstituted oral solution because it will thicken. Drug remains stable for 2 weeks at room temperature.
• I.M. preparation should be given deep I.M. Rotate sites. Doses exceeding 600 mg aren't recommended.
• I.M. injection may increase creatinine phosphokinase levels because of muscle irritation.
• For I.V. infusion, dilute each 300 mg in 50 ml of D₅W, normal saline, or lactated Ringer's solution and give no faster than 30 mg/minute. Don't administer more than 1.2 g/hour.
• Topical form may produce adverse systemic effects.
• Don't administer diphenoxylate compound (Lomotil) to treat drug-induced diarrhea because this may worsen and prolong diarrhea.

Monitoring the patient
• Monitor renal, hepatic, and hematopoietic functions during prolonged therapy.
• Monitor patient for therapeutic effect.

Information for the patient
• Warn patient that I.M. injection may be painful.
• Instruct patient to report adverse effects, especially diarrhea. Warn patient not to self-treat diarrhea.
• Advise patient to take capsules with 8 oz (240 ml) of water to prevent dysphagia.
• Instruct patient using topical solution to wash, rinse, and dry affected areas before application. Warn patient not to use topical solution near eyes, nose, mouth, or other mucous membranes, and caution about sharing washcloths and towels with family members.

Geriatric patients
• Elderly patients may tolerate drug-induced diarrhea poorly. Monitor closely for dehydration and change in bowel frequency.

Pediatric patients
• Administer drug cautiously, if at all, to neonates and infants. Monitor closely, especially for diarrhea.

Breast-feeding patients
• Drug appears in breast milk. Advise breast-feeding woman to use an alternative to breast-feeding during therapy.

clofazimine
Lamprene

Pharmacologic classification: substituted iminophenazine dye
Therapeutic classification: leprostatic
Pregnancy risk category C

How supplied
Available by prescription only
Capsules: 50 mg, 100 mg

Indications, route, and dosage
Dapsone-sensitive multibacillary leprosy
Adults: Combination therapy with two other drugs for at least 2 years until skin smears are negative; then monotherapy.
Dapsone-resistant leprosy
Adults: 100 mg P.O. once daily; usually given with one or more other antileprotics for at least 3 years; then monotherapy of 100 mg Lamprene daily.
Erythema nodosum leprosum
Adults: 100 to 200 mg P.O. daily for up to 3 months. Taper dosage to 100 mg daily as soon as possible. Dosages above 200 mg daily aren't recommended.
◇ *Atypical mycobacterial infections*
Adults: 100 mg P.O. q 8 hours. Usually given with several other antituberculotics.

Pharmacodynamics
Leprostatic action: A bright red iminophenazine dye, a relative of aniline dyes. Exerts a slow bactericidal effect on *Mycobacterium leprae* (Hansen's bacillus). Clinical benefit is usually noted in 1 to 3 months, with clearing observed by 6 months. Administration with dapsone produces a more rapid effect on leprosy lesions. No cross-resistance with dapsone or rifampin has been reported. Clofazimine inhibits mycobacterial growth and preferentially binds to mycobacterial DNA. Although exact mechanism is unknown, drug also exhibits anti-inflammatory properties in controlling erythema nodosum leprosum reactions.
Clofazimine also appears to have an important role in treatment of atypical mycobacterial infections, such as *Mycobacterium avium* infections, which have become prominent recently in patients with AIDS. Some efficacy has been demonstrated when used with ansamycin, ethionamide, or ethambutol. Further clinical information is required.

Pharmacokinetics
• *Absorption:* Variable absorption (45% to 62%) after oral administration.
• *Distribution:* Highly lipophilic; distributed widely into fatty tissues and taken up by macrophages into reticuloendothelial system. Little, if any, crosses blood-brain barrier or enters CNS.

• *Metabolism:* Not completely defined; some evidence exists of enterohepatic cycling. Serum half-lives of up to 70 days have been noted.
• *Excretion:* Mostly excreted in feces; some in sputum, sebum, and sweat; very little in urine. Drug appears in breast milk.

Contraindications and precautions
No known contraindications. Use cautiously in patients with GI dysfunction, such as abdominal pain or diarrhea.

Interactions
Drug-drug. *Dapsone:* May inhibit anti-inflammatory activity of clofazimine. Monitor patient closely.
Isoniazid: May increase plasma and urinary levels of clofazimine and decrease levels in skin. Monitor patient closely.

Adverse reactions
EENT: *conjunctival and corneal pigmentation, dryness, burning, itching, irritation.*
GI: *epigastric pain, diarrhea, nausea, vomiting, GI intolerance,* **bowel obstruction, GI bleeding.**
Hematologic: eosinophilia.
Hepatic: elevated albumin, serum bilirubin, and AST levels.
Metabolic: hypokalemia, elevated blood glucose levels.
Skin: *pink to brownish black pigmentation, ichthyosis, dryness,* rash, pruritus.
Other: **splenic infarction,** discolored body fluids and excrement.

☑ Special considerations
• Administer with meals. Use clofazimine with other antileprotics.
• Severe GI symptoms may require stopping drug if dosage reduction doesn't relieve symptoms.
• Pink to brownish black pigmentation of skin occurs in 75% to 100% of patients.
• In case of overdose, empty stomach by inducing vomiting or by gastric lavage. Treatment includes usual supportive measures.

Monitoring the patient
• Observe patient for signs of depression.
• Monitor patient for therapeutic effect.

Information for the patient
• Tell patient to take drug with meals to minimize GI problems.
• Advise patient to store drug away from heat and light and out of children's reach.
• Explain that pink to brownish black pigmentation of skin may occur. Although reversible, it may take several months or years to disappear after drug is stopped. Also explain that discoloration of eyes, urine, feces, sputum, sweat, and tears also may occur.

• Tell patient not to expect benefits for 1 to 3 months; observable benefits may take up to 6 months.
• Recommend use of skin oil or cream to help relieve dryness or ichthyosis.

Breast-feeding patients
• Drug appears in breast milk; don't use in breast-feeding women unless potential benefit to mother exceeds risk to infant.

clofibrate
Atromid-S

Pharmacologic classification: fibric acid derivative
Therapeutic classification: antilipemic
Pregnancy risk category C

How supplied
Available by prescription only
Capsules: 500 mg

Indications, route, and dosage
Hyperlipidemia and xanthoma tuberosum; type III hyperlipidemia that doesn't respond adequately to diet
Adults: 2 g P.O. daily in two to four divided doses. Some patients may respond to lower doses as assessed by serum lipid monitoring.
◇ **Diabetes insipidus**
Adults: 1.5 to 2 g P.O. daily in divided doses.
✦ **Dosage adjustment.** Patients with decreased renal function may need reduced dosage frequency (q 12 to 18 hours).

Pharmacodynamics
Antilipemic action: May lower serum triglyceride levels by accelerating catabolism of very low-density lipoproteins; lowers serum cholesterol levels (to a lesser degree) by inhibiting cholesterol biosynthesis. Both mechanisms are unknown. Closely related to gemfibrozil.

Pharmacokinetics
• *Absorption:* Absorbed slowly but completely from GI tract. Plasma level peak 2 to 6 hours after single dose. Serum triglyceride levels decrease in 2 to 5 days; peak effect at 21 days.
• *Distribution:* Distributed into extracellular space as active form, clofibric acid, which is up to 98% protein-bound. Fetal levels may exceed maternal levels.
• *Metabolism:* Hydrolyzed by serum enzymes to clofibric acid, which is metabolized by liver.
• *Excretion:* 20% of clofibric acid excreted unchanged in urine; 70% eliminated in urine as conjugated metabolite. Plasma half-life after single dose ranges from 6 to 25 hours; in patients with renal impairment and cirrhosis, half-life can be as long as 113 hours.

Contraindications and precautions

Contraindicated in patients with hypersensitivity to drug and in those with significant hepatic or renal dysfunction or primary biliary cirrhosis. Also contraindicated in pregnant or breast-feeding women. Use cautiously in patients with peptic ulcer or history of gallbladder disease.

Caution should be exercised when anticoagulants are given with this drug. Frequent PT determinations are advisable until it has been definitely determined that PT level has been stabilized.

Interactions

Drug-drug. *Cholestyramine:* Reduces absorption rate of clofibrate. Use together cautiously.
Furosemide: May cause increased diuresis because both drugs compete for albumin binding sites. Use cautiously.
Oral anticoagulants: Increased anticoagulant effects that may cause fatal hemorrhage. If combination is necessary, reduce oral anticoagulant dose by 50%, and evaluate PT and INR frequently.
Sulfonylureas: Enhanced effects of sulfonylureas, causing hypoglycemia. Dosage adjustment may be needed.

Adverse reactions

CNS: fatigue, weakness, drowsiness, dizziness, headache.
CV: *arrhythmias,* angina, *thromboembolic events,* intermittent claudication.
GI: *nausea, diarrhea, vomiting,* stomatitis, *dyspepsia,* flatulence, *cholelithiasis, cholecystitis.*
GU: impotence and decreased libido, renal dysfunction (dysuria, hematuria, proteinuria, decreased urine output).
Hematologic: leukopenia, anemia, eosinophilia.
Hepatic: gallstones, *transient and reversible elevations of liver function test results,* hepatomegaly.
Musculoskeletal: myalgia, arthralgia.
Skin: rash, urticaria, pruritus, dry skin and hair.
Other: *weight gain; polyphagia.*

☑ Special considerations

● Don't use clofibrate indiscriminately; it may pose an increased risk of gallstones, heart disease, and cancer.
● Studies suggest that clofibrate may increase risk of death from cancer, postcholecystectomy complications, and pancreatitis.

Monitoring the patient

● Monitor serum cholesterol and triglyceride levels regularly during therapy.
● Observe patient for the following serious adverse reactions: thrombophlebitis, pulmonary embolism, angina, and arrhythmias; monitor renal and hepatic function, blood counts, and serum electrolyte and blood glucose levels.

Information for the patient

● Warn patient to report flulike symptoms immediately.
● Stress importance of close medical supervision and of reporting adverse reactions; encourage patient to comply with prescribed regimen and diet.
● Warn patient not to exceed prescribed dose.
● Advise patient to take drug with food to minimize GI discomfort.
● Emphasize that drug therapy won't replace diet, exercise, and weight reduction for control of hyperlipidemia.

Pediatric patients

● Safety and efficacy in children under age 14 haven't been established.

Breast-feeding patients

● Drug may appear in breast milk; an alternative to breast-feeding is recommended during therapy.

clomiphene citrate
Clomid, Milophene, Serophene

Pharmacologic classification: chlorotrianisene derivative
Therapeutic classification: ovulation stimulant
Pregnancy risk category X

How supplied

Available by prescription only
Tablets: 50 mg

Indications, route, and dosage

To induce ovulation

Adults: 50 mg P.O. daily for 5 days, starting any time in patients without recent uterine bleeding; or 50 mg P.O. daily starting on day 5 of menstrual cycle (first day of menstrual flow is day 1). Dose may be increased to 100 mg if ovulation doesn't occur. Repeat 5-day course each ovulatory cycle until conception occurs or until 3 courses of therapy are completed.

◊ *Male infertility*

Adults: 50 to 400 mg P.O. daily for 2 to 12 months.

Pharmacodynamics

Ovulation stimulant action: Mechanism of action for inducing ovulation in anovulatory women is unknown. May stimulate release of pituitary gonadotropin, follicle-stimulating hormone (FSH), and luteinizing hormone (LH), which results in development and maturation of the ovarian follicle, ovulation, and subsequent development and function of corpus luteum.

Pharmacokinetics

● *Absorption:* Absorbed readily from GI tract.

• *Distribution:* May undergo enterohepatic recirculation or may be stored in body fat.
• *Metabolism:* Metabolized by liver.
• *Excretion:* Half-life is about 5 days. Excreted principally in feces via biliary elimination.

Contraindications and precautions
Contraindicated during pregnancy and in patients with undiagnosed abnormal genital bleeding, ovarian cyst not due to polycystic ovarian syndrome, hepatic disease or dysfunction, uncontrolled thyroid or adrenal dysfunction, or presence of organic intracranial lesion (such as a pituitary tumor).

Interactions
None reported.

Adverse reactions
CNS: headache, restlessness, insomnia, dizziness, light-headedness, depression, fatigue, aggressive behavior.
EENT: blurred vision, diplopia, scotoma, photophobia.
GI: nausea, vomiting, bloating, distention, weight gain.
GU: urinary frequency and polyuria; abnormal uterine bleeding; *ovarian enlargement* and cyst formation, which regress spontaneously when drug is stopped.
Hematologic: *thrombocytopenia,* leukopenia, anemia.
Respiratory: pharyngitis, rhinitis, sinusitis, coughing, epistaxis, dyspnea.
Skin: alopecia, urticaria, rash, dermatitis.
Other: *hot flashes,* reversible *breast discomfort;* increased levels of serum thyronine, thyroxine-binding globulin, sex hormone–binding globulin, sulfobromophthalein retention and FSH and LH secretion.

☑ Special considerations
• Human chorionic gonadotropin (5,000 to 10,000 units) may be administered 5 to 7 days after last dose of drug to stimulate ovulation.
• Drug is contraindicated during pregnancy.

Monitoring the patient
• Monitor patient for adverse effects.
• Monitor therapeutic effect.

Information for the patient
• Instruct patient on all aspects of infertility testing and therapy.
• Tell patient to report visual disturbances immediately.
• Advise patient of possibility of multiple births, which increases with higher doses.
• Teach patient to take basal body temperature every morning (starting on day 1 of menstrual period) and chart on a graph to detect ovulation.

• Instruct patient on importance of properly timed coitus.
• Advise patient to stop drug immediately if abdominal symptoms, weight gain, edema, or bloating occur because these may indicate ovarian enlargement or ovarian cysts.
• Warn patient to avoid hazardous tasks until response to drug is known because dizziness or visual disturbances may occur.
• Advise patient to stop drug and call immediately if she suspects she is pregnant; drug may have teratogenic effects.

Breast-feeding patients
• It's unknown if drug appears in breast milk. Use with caution in breast-feeding women. Drug may reduce lactation.

clomipramine hydrochloride
Anafranil

Pharmacologic classification: tricyclic antidepressant (TCA)
Therapeutic classification: anti-obsessional
Pregnancy risk category C

How supplied
Available by prescription only
Capsules: 25 mg, 50 mg, 75 mg

Indications, route, and dosage
Obsessive-compulsive disorder (OCD)
Adults: Initially, 25 mg P.O. daily, gradually increasing to 100 mg P.O. daily (in divided doses, with meals) during the first 2 weeks. Maximum dose is 250 mg daily. After adjustment, entire daily dose may be given h.s.
Children and adolescents: Initially, 25 mg P.O. daily, gradually increased to a maximum of 3 mg/kg or 100 mg P.O. daily, whichever is smaller (in divided doses, with meals) over the first 2 weeks. Maximum daily dose is 3 mg/kg or 200 mg, whichever is smaller. After adjustment, entire daily dose may be given h.s.

Pharmacodynamics
Antiobsessional action: A selective inhibitor of serotonin (5-HT) reuptake into neurons within the CNS. It may also have some blocking activity at postsynaptic dopamine receptors. The exact mechanism by which clomipramine treats OCD is unknown.

Pharmacokinetics
• *Absorption:* Well absorbed from GI tract, but extensive first-pass metabolism limits bioavailability to about 50%.
• *Distribution:* Distributed well into lipophilic tissues; volume of distribution is about 12 L/kg; 98% is bound to plasma proteins.

• *Metabolism:* Primarily hepatic. Several metabolites identified; primary active metabolite is desmethylclomipramine.

• *Excretion:* About 66% excreted in urine; remainder in feces. Mean elimination half-life of parent compound is about 36 hours; elimination half-life of desmethylclomipramine has a mean of 69 hours. After multiple dosing, half-life may increase.

Contraindications and precautions

Contraindicated in patients with hypersensitivity to drug or other TCAs; in those who have taken MAO inhibitors within the previous 14 days; and during acute recovery period after MI.

Use cautiously in patients with urine retention, suicidal tendencies, glaucoma, increased intraocular pressure, brain damage, or seizure disorders and in those taking drugs that may lower the seizure threshold. Also use cautiously in patients with impaired renal or hepatic function, hyperthyroidism, or tumors of the adrenal medulla and in those undergoing elective surgery or receiving thyroid medication or electroconvulsive treatment.

Interactions

Drug-drug. *Barbiturates:* Increases activity of hepatic microsomal enzymes with repeated doses; may decrease TCA blood levels. Monitor patient for decreased effectiveness.

Barbiturates, CNS depressants: May cause exaggerated depressant effect when used with TCAs. Use together cautiously.

Epinephrine, norepinephrine: May produce increased hypertensive effect in patients taking TCAs. Monitor blood pressure closely.

MAO inhibitors: May cause hyperpyretic crisis, seizures, coma, and death. Avoid use with TCAs.

Methylphenidate: May increase TCA blood levels. Monitor TCA levels.

Drug-lifestyle. *Alcohol:* May cause exaggerated depressant effect when used with TCAs. Discourage use together.

Adverse reactions

CNS: *somnolence, tremor, dizziness, headache, insomnia, nervousness, myoclonus, fatigue,* EEG changes, **seizures.**

CV: orthostatic hypotension, palpitations, tachycardia.

EENT: *pharyngitis, rhinitis, visual changes.*

GI: *dry mouth, constipation, nausea, dyspepsia, increased appetite,* diarrhea, *anorexia, abdominal pain.*

GU: *urinary hesitancy,* urinary tract infection, *dysmenorrhea, ejaculation failure, impotence.*

Hematologic: purpura, anemia.

Musculoskeletal: *myalgia.*

Skin: *diaphoresis,* rash, pruritus, dry skin.

Other: *weight gain, altered libido.*

☑ Special considerations

• To minimize risk of overdose, dispense drug in small quantities.

• Don't withdraw drug abruptly.

• Activation of mania or hypomania may occur with therapy.

• Signs and symptoms of overdose are similar to those of other TCAs and include sinus tachycardia, intraventricular block, hypotension, irritability, fixed and dilated pupils, drowsiness, delirium, stupor, hyperreflexia, and hyperpyrexia. Treatment should include gastric lavage with large quantities of fluid. Lavage should be continued for 12 hours because the anticholinergic effects of the drug slow gastric emptying.

• Hemodialysis, peritoneal dialysis, and forced diuresis are ineffective in overdose because of the high degree of plasma protein-binding. Support respirations and monitor cardiac function. Treat shock with plasma expanders or corticosteroids; treat seizures with diazepam.

Monitoring the patient

• Watch for urine retention and constipation. Suggest stool softener or high-fiber diet, as needed, and encourage adequate fluid intake.

• Monitor patient for adverse effects.

Information for the patient

• Warn patient to avoid hazardous activities that require alertness or good psychomotor coordination until adverse CNS effects are known. This is especially important during initial adjustment period when daytime sedation and dizziness may occur.

• Instruct patient to avoid alcohol and other depressants.

• Suggest that dry mouth may be relieved with saliva substitutes or sugarless candy or gum.

• Tell patient that adverse GI effects can be minimized by taking drug with meals during the adjustment period. Later, the entire daily dose may be taken at bedtime to limit daytime drowsiness.

• Inform patient to avoid using OTC products, particularly antihistamines and decongestants, without medical permission.

• Encourage patient to continue therapy, even if adverse reactions are troublesome. Advise him not to stop taking drug without medical permission.

Breast-feeding patients

• It's unknown if drug appears in breast milk. Use with caution in breast-feeding women.

clonazepam
Klonopin, Rivotril*

Pharmacologic classification: benzodiazepine
Therapeutic classification: anticonvulsant
Controlled substance schedule IV
Pregnancy risk category C

How supplied
Available by prescription only
Tablets: 0.5 mg, 1 mg, 2 mg

Indications, route, and dosage
Absence and atypical absence seizures; akinetic and myoclonic seizures; ◊ generalized tonic-clonic seizures
Adults: Initial dosage shouldn't exceed 1.5 mg P.O. daily, divided into three doses. May be increased by 0.5 to 1 mg q 3 days until seizures are controlled. Maximum recommended daily dose is 20 mg.
Children up to age 10 or weighing 30 kg (66 lb) or less: 0.01 to 0.03 mg/kg P.O. daily (don't exceed 0.05 mg/kg daily), divided q 8 hours. Increase dosage by 0.25 to 0.5 mg q third day to a maximum maintenance dose of 0.1 to 0.2 mg/kg daily.
◊ Leg movements during sleep; ◊ adjunct treatment in schizophrenia
Adults: 0.5 to 2 mg P.O. h.s.
◊ Parkinsonian dysarthria
Adults: 0.25 to 0.5 mg P.O. daily.
◊ Acute manic episodes
Adults: 0.75 to 16 mg P.O. daily.
◊ Multifocal tic disorders
Adults: 1.5 to 12 mg P.O. daily.
◊ Neuralgia
Adults: 2 to 4 mg P.O. daily.

Pharmacodynamics
Anticonvulsant action: Mechanism unknown; drug appears to act in the limbic system, thalamus, and hypothalamus. Drug is used to treat myoclonic, atonic, and absence seizures resistant to other anticonvulsants and to suppress or eliminate attacks of sleep-related nocturnal myoclonus (restless legs syndrome).

Pharmacokinetics
• *Absorption:* Well absorbed from GI tract. Action begins in 20 to 60 minutes; persists for 6 to 8 hours in infants and children; up to 12 hours in adults.
• *Distribution:* Distributed widely throughout body; about 85% protein-bound.
• *Metabolism:* Metabolized by liver to several metabolites. Half-life of 18 to 39 hours.
• *Excretion:* Excreted in urine.

Contraindications and precautions
Contraindicated in patients with significant hepatic disease, in those with sensitivity to benzodiazepines, and in patients with acute angle-closure glaucoma. Use cautiously in children, during pregnancy, and in patients with mixed-type seizures, respiratory disease, or glaucoma, and in pregnancy.

Interactions
Drug-drug. *Other anticonvulsants, other CNS depressants (anxiolytics, barbiturates, narcotics, tranquilizers):* Additive CNS depressant effects. Monitor patient closely.
Ritonavir: May significantly increase levels of clonazepam. Monitor clonazepam levels.
Valproic acid: May induce absence seizures. Use together cautiously.
Drug-lifestyle. *Alcohol:* Additive CNS depressant effects. Don't use together.

Adverse reactions
CNS: *drowsiness, ataxia, behavioral disturbances* (especially in children), slurred speech, tremor, confusion, psychosis, agitation.
CV: palpitations.
EENT: nystagmus, abnormal eye movements, sore gums.
GI: constipation, gastritis, change in appetite, nausea, anorexia, diarrhea.
GU: dysuria, enuresis, nocturia, urine retention.
Hepatic: increased liver function tests.
Hematologic: leukopenia, *thrombocytopenia,* eosinophilia.
Respiratory: *respiratory depression,* chest congestion, shortness of breath.
Skin: rash.

☑ Special considerations
• Abrupt withdrawal may precipitate status epilepticus; after long-term use, lower dosage gradually.
• Use with barbiturates or other CNS depressants may impair ability to perform tasks requiring mental alertness, such as driving a car. Warn patient to avoid such combined use.
• Drug should be used during pregnancy only if clinical situation warrants the risk to the fetus.
• Symptoms of overdose may include ataxia, confusion, coma, decreased reflexes, and hypotension. Treat overdose with gastric lavage and supportive therapy. Flumazenil, a specific benzodiazepine antagonist, may be useful. Vasopressors should be used to treat hypotension.
• In overdose, carefully monitor vital signs, ECG, and fluid and electrolyte balance. Clonazepam isn't dialyzable.

Monitoring the patient
• Monitor CBC and liver function tests periodically.

Reactions may be *common*, uncommon, *life-threatening*, or COMMON AND LIFE-THREATENING.

- Watch for oversedation, especially in elderly patients.

Information for the patient
- Explain rationale for therapy and risks and benefits that may be anticipated.
- Teach patient signs and symptoms of adverse reactions and the need to report them promptly.
- Tell patient to avoid alcohol and other sedatives to prevent added CNS depression.
- Warn patient not to stop drug or change dosage unless prescribed.
- Advise patient to avoid tasks that require mental alertness until degree of sedative effect is determined.

Geriatric patients
- Elderly patients may require lower doses because of diminished renal function; such patients also are at greater risk for oversedation from CNS depressants.

Pediatric patients
- Long-term safety in children hasn't been established.

Breast-feeding patients
- Alternative feeding method is recommended during clonazepam therapy.

clonidine hydrochloride
Catapres, Catapres-TTS, Dixarit*

Pharmacologic classification: centrally acting alpha-adrenergic agonist
Therapeutic classification: antihypertensive
Pregnancy risk category C

How supplied
Available by prescription only
Tablets: 0.1 mg, 0.2 mg, 0.3 mg
Transdermal: TTS-1 (releases 0.1 mg/24 hours), TTS-2 (releases 0.2 mg/24 hours), TTS-3 (releases 0.3 mg/24 hours)

Indications, route, and dosage
Hypertension
Adults: Initially, 0.1 mg P.O. b.i.d.; then increased by 0.1 to 0.2 mg daily or every few days until desired response is achieved. Usual dosage range is 0.2 to 0.6 mg daily in divided doses. Maximum effective dose is 2.4 mg/day. If transdermal patch is used, apply to area of hairless intact skin once q 7 days.
Children: No dosing recommendations for children.

◊ *Adjunctive therapy in nicotine withdrawal*
Adults: Initially, 0.15 mg P.O. daily, gradually increased to 0.4 mg P.O. daily as tolerated. Or apply transdermal patch (0.2 mg/24 hours) and re-

place weekly for the first 2 or 3 weeks after smoking cessation.
◊ *Prophylaxis for vascular headache*
Adults: 0.025 mg P.O. b.i.d. to q.i.d. up to 0.15 mg P.O. daily in divided doses.
◊ *Adjunctive treatment of menopausal symptoms*
Adults: 0.025 to 0.075 mg P.O. b.i.d.
◊ *Adjunctive therapy in opiate withdrawal*
Adults: 5 to 17 mcg/kg P.O. daily in divided doses for up to 10 days. Adjust dosage to avoid hypotension and excessive sedation, and slowly withdraw drug.
◊ *Ulcerative colitis*
Adults: 0.3 mg P.O. t.i.d.
◊ *Neuralgia*
Adults: 0.2 mg P.O. daily.
◊ *Tourette syndrome*
Adults: 0.15 to 0.2 mg P.O. daily.
◊ *Diabetic diarrhea*
Adults: 0.15 to 1.2 mg/day P.O. or 1 to 2 patches/week (0.3 mg/24 hours).
◊ *Growth delay in children*
Children: 0.0375 to 0.15 mg/m^2 P.O. daily.
◊ *To diagnose pheochromocytoma*
Adults: 0.3 mg given once.

Pharmacodynamics
Antihypertensive action: Decreases peripheral vascular resistance by stimulating central alpha-adrenergic receptors, thus decreasing cerebral sympathetic outflow; drug may also inhibit renin release. Initially, may stimulate peripheral alpha-adrenergic receptors, producing transient vasoconstriction.

Pharmacokinetics
- *Absorption:* Well absorbed from GI tract when administered orally; after oral administration, blood pressure begins to decline in 30 to 60 minutes, with maximal effect occurring in 2 to 4 hours. Well absorbed percutaneously after transdermal topical administration; transdermal therapeutic plasma levels achieved 2 to 3 days after initial application.
- *Distribution:* Distributed widely into body.
- *Metabolism:* Metabolized in liver, where nearly 50% transformed to inactive metabolites.
- *Excretion:* 65% excreted in urine; 20% excreted in feces. Half-life ranges from 6 to 20 hours in patients with normal renal function. After oral administration, antihypertensive effect lasts up to 8 hours; after transdermal application, antihypertensive effect persists up to 7 days.

Contraindications and precautions
Contraindicated in patients with hypersensitivity to drug. Transdermal form is contraindicated in patients with hypersensitivity to any component of the adhesive layer of the transdermal system. Use cautiously in patients with severe coronary

disease, recent MI, cerebrovascular disease, or impaired hepatic or renal function.

Interactions
Drug-drug. *Barbiturates, other sedatives:* Increased CNS depressant effects. Monitor patient closely.
MAO inhibitors, tolazoline, tricyclic antidepressants: May inhibit antihypertensive effects of clonidine. Use with caution.
Propranolol, other beta blockers: Additive effect, producing bradycardia; may increase rebound hypertension upon withdrawal. Monitor patient closely.
Drug-herb. *Capsicum:* May reduce antihypertensive effectiveness. Avoid use together.
Drug-lifestyle. *Alcohol:* Increased CNS depressant effects. Discourage use together.

Adverse reactions
CNS: *drowsiness, dizziness,* fatigue, *sedation, weakness,* malaise, agitation, depression.
CV: orthostatic hypotension, ***bradycardia, severe rebound hypertension.***
GI: *constipation, dry mouth,* nausea, vomiting, anorexia.
GU: urine retention, impotence, loss of libido.
Metabolic: possible slight increase in serum glucose levels.
Skin: *pruritus, dermatitis* (with transdermal patch), rash.
Other: weight gain.

☑ Special considerations
• Don't stop drug abruptly; reduce dosage gradually over 2 to 4 days to prevent severe rebound hypertension.
• Patients with renal impairment may respond to smaller drug doses.
• Give drug 4 to 6 hours before scheduled surgery.
• Clonidine may be used to lower blood pressure quickly in some hypertensive emergencies.
• Therapeutic plasma levels are achieved 2 or 3 days after applying transdermal form. Patient may need oral antihypertensive therapy during interim period.
• Remove transdermal systems when attempting defibrillation or synchronized cardioversion because of electrical conductivity.
• Drug may decrease urinary excretion of vanillylmandelic acid and catecholamines.
• Drug may slightly increase blood or serum glucose levels and may cause a weakly positive Coombs' test.
• Clinical signs of overdose include bradycardia, CNS depression, respiratory depression, hypothermia, apnea, seizures, lethargy, agitation, irritability, diarrhea, and hypotension; hypertension has also been reported.
• After overdose with oral clonidine, don't induce emesis because rapid onset of CNS depression

can lead to aspiration. After adequate airway is assured, empty stomach by gastric lavage then activated charcoal. If overdose occurs in patients receiving transdermal therapy, remove transdermal patch. Further treatment is usually symptomatic and supportive.

Monitoring the patient
• Monitor pulse and blood pressure frequently; dosage is usually adjusted to patient's response and tolerance.
• Monitor weight daily during initiation of therapy to monitor fluid retention.
• Monitor serum creatinine and electrolyte levels.

Information for the patient
• Explain disease and rationale for therapy; emphasize importance of follow-up visits in establishing therapeutic regimen.
• Teach patient signs and symptoms of adverse effects and need to report them; patient should also report excessive weight gain (more than 5 lb [2.27 kg] weekly).
• Warn patient to avoid hazardous activities that require mental alertness until tolerance develops to sedation, drowsiness, and other CNS effects.
• Advise patient to avoid sudden position changes to minimize orthostatic hypotension.
• Inform patient that ice chips, hard candy, or gum will relieve dry mouth.
• Warn patient to call for specific instructions before taking OTC cold preparations.
• Advise taking last dose at bedtime to ensure night-time blood pressure control.
• Tell patient not to stop drug suddenly; rebound hypertension may develop.
• Rotate transdermal patch site weekly.

Geriatric patients
• Elderly patients may require lower doses because they may be more sensitive to clonidine's hypotensive effects. Monitor renal function.

Pediatric patients
• Efficacy and safety in children haven't been established; use drug only if potential benefit outweighs risk.

Breast-feeding patients
• Clonidine appears in breast milk. An alternative to breast-feeding is recommended during treatment.

---

clopidogrel bisulfate
Plavix

Pharmacologic classification: inhibitor of ADP-induced platelet aggregation
Therapeutic classification: antiplatelet drug
Pregnancy risk category B

How supplied
Available by prescription only
Tablets: 75 mg

Indications, route, and dosage
To reduce atherosclerotic events (MI, CVA, vascular death) in patients with atherosclerosis documented by recent CVA, MI, or peripheral arterial disease
Adults: 75 mg P.O. once daily with or without food.

Pharmacodynamics
Antiplatelet action: Inhibits the binding of adenosine diphosphate (ADP) to its platelet receptor and the subsequent ADP-mediated activation of glycoprotein IIb/IIIa complex, thereby inhibiting platelet aggregation. Because clopidogrel acts by irreversibly modifying the platelet ADP receptor, platelets exposed to the drug are affected for their life span. Dose-dependent inhibition of platelet aggregation can be seen 2 hours after single doses and becomes maximal after 3 to 7 days of repeated dosing. After drug is stopped, platelet aggregation and bleeding time return to baseline in about 5 days.

Pharmacokinetics
• *Absorption:* After repeated oral doses, plasma levels of parent compound, which has no platelet-inhibiting effect, are very low and generally below quantification limit. Pharmacokinetic evaluations are generally stated in terms of the main circulating metabolite. Rapidly absorbed after oral dosing with peak plasma levels of the main circulating metabolite occurring about 1 hour after dosing. Following oral administration, about 50% of dose is absorbed.
• *Distribution:* Clopidogrel and main circulating metabolite binds reversibly to human plasma proteins (98% and 94%, respectively).
• *Metabolism:* Extensively metabolized by liver. Main circulating metabolite is carboxylic acid derivative with no effect on platelet aggregation; represents about 85% of circulating drug. Elimination half-life of main circulating metabolite is 8 hours after single and repeated doses.
• *Excretion:* Following oral administration, about 50% of drug excreted in urine and 46% in feces.

Contraindications and precautions
Contraindicated in patients with hypersensitivity to drug or its components and in those with patho-

logic bleeding, such as peptic ulcer or intracranial hemorrhage.
   Use with caution in patients at risk for increased bleeding from trauma, surgery, or other pathologic conditions and in those with hepatic impairment or severe hepatic disease.

Interactions
Drug-drug. *Aspirin:* May increase risk of GI bleeding. Monitor patient closely.
Heparin, warfarin: Safe use hasn't been established. Use together cautiously.
NSAIDs: Increased occult GI blood loss. Use cautiously.
Drug-herb. *Red clover:* May cause increased bleeding. Use cautiously.

Adverse reactions
CNS: asthenia, depression, dizziness, fatigue, headache, paresthesia, syncope.
CV: chest pain, edema, hypertension, palpitation.
EENT: epistaxis, rhinitis.
GI: abdominal pain, constipation, diarrhea, dyspepsia, gastritis, hemorrhage, nausea, vomiting.
GU: urinary tract infection.
Hematologic: purpura.
Respiratory: bronchitis, coughing, dyspnea, upper respiratory tract infection.
Skin: rash, pruritus.
Other: arthralgia, flulike symptoms, pain.

☑ Special considerations
• Drug is usually used in patients who are hypersensitive or intolerant to aspirin.
• If patient is to undergo surgery and an antiplatelet effect isn't desired, stop drug 7 days before surgery.
• No adverse effects were reported after single oral administration of 600 mg (equivalent to eight standard 75-mg tablets). The bleeding time was prolonged by a factor of 1.7, which is similar to that observed with the therapeutic dosage of 75 mg daily. Symptoms of acute toxicity included vomiting, prostration, GI hemorrhage, and difficulty breathing. Platelet transfusion may be appropriate to reverse drug effects if quick reversal is required.

Monitoring the patient
• Monitor patient for adverse effects.
• Carefully monitor patients on concurrent NSAID or aspirin therapy for signs of bleeding.

Information for the patient
• Inform patient that it may take longer than usual to stop bleeding; therefore, advise patient to refrain from activities in which trauma and bleeding may occur. Encourage use of seat belts.
• Instruct patient to report unusual bleeding or bruising.

- Tell patient to inform medical personnel of clopidogrel use before scheduling dental work or surgery or taking new drugs.
- Inform patient that drug may be taken without regard to meals.

Pediatric patients
- Safety and efficacy in children haven't been established.

Breast-feeding patients
- It's unknown if drug or its metabolite appears in breast milk. Assess risks and benefits before continuing drug in breast-feeding women.

clorazepate dipotassium
Novo-Clopate*, Tranxene*, Tranxene-SD, Tranxene-SD Half Strength

Pharmacologic classification: benzodiazepine
Therapeutic classification: anxiolytic, anticonvulsant, sedative-hypnotic
Controlled substance schedule IV
Pregnancy risk category NR

How supplied
Available by prescription only
Tablets: 3.75 mg, 7.5 mg, 11.25 mg, 15 mg, 22.5 mg
Capsules: 3.75 mg, 7.5 mg, 15 mg

Indications, route, and dosage
Acute alcohol withdrawal
Adults: Day 1—initially, 30 mg P.O., then 30 to 60 mg P.O. in divided doses; day 2—45 to 90 mg P.O. in divided doses; day 3—22.5 to 45 mg P.O. in divided doses; day 4—15 to 30 mg P.O. in divided doses; gradually reduce daily dose to 7.5 to 15 mg.
Anxiety
Adults: 15 to 60 mg P.O. daily.
Adjunct in treatment of partial seizures
Adults and children over age 12: Maximum recommended initial dose is 7.5 mg P.O. t.i.d. Dosage increases shouldn't exceed 7.5 mg/week. Maximum daily dose shouldn't exceed 90 mg.
Children ages 9 to 12: Maximum recommended initial dose is 7.5 mg P.O. b.i.d. Dosage increases shouldn't exceed 7.5 mg/week. Maximum daily dose shouldn't exceed 60 mg.

Pharmacodynamics
Anxiolytic and sedative actions: Depresses CNS at the limbic and subcortical levels of the brain. It produces an antianxiety effect by enhancing the effect of the neurotransmitter gamma-aminobutyric acid (GABA) on its receptor in the ascending reticular activating system, which increases inhibition and blocks both cortical and limbic arousal.

Anticonvulsant action: Suppresses spread of seizure activity produced by epileptogenic foci in the cortex, thalamus, and limbic structures by enhancing presynaptic inhibition.

Pharmacokinetics
- *Absorption:* After oral administration, drug is hydrolyzed in stomach to desmethyldiazepam, which is absorbed completely and rapidly. Serum levels peak at 1 to 2 hours.
- *Distribution:* Distributed widely throughout body. About 80% to 95% of dose bound to plasma protein.
- *Metabolism:* Desmethyldiazepam metabolized in liver to conjugated oxazepam.
- *Excretion:* Inactive glucuronide metabolites excreted in urine. Half-life of desmethyldiazepam ranges from 30 to 100 hours.

Contraindications and precautions
Contraindicated in patients with hypersensitivity to drug or other benzodiazepines and in those with acute angle-closure glaucoma. Avoid use in pregnant women, especially during first trimester. Use cautiously in patients with impaired renal or hepatic function, suicidal tendencies, or history of drug abuse.

Interactions
Drug-drug. *Antacids:* Delayed drug absorption and reduced total amount absorbed. Administer separately.
Antidepressants, antihistamines, barbiturates, general anesthetics, MAO inhibitors, narcotics, phenothiazines: Increased CNS depressant effects. Monitor patient closely.
Cimetidine, possibly disulfiram: Causes diminished hepatic metabolism of clorazepate, which increases its plasma level. Use cautiously together.
Haloperidol: Reduced serum levels of haloperidol. Use cautiously together.
Levodopa: May decrease therapeutic effectiveness of levodopa. Monitor patient closely.
Drug-lifestyle. *Alcohol:* Increased CNS depressant effects. Discourage use.
Heavy smoking: Accelerates clorazepate's metabolism, thus lowering clinical effectiveness. Discourage smoking.

Adverse reactions
CNS: *drowsiness,* dizziness, nervousness, confusion, headache, insomnia, depression, irritability, tremor.
CV: hypotension, minor changes in EEG patterns.
EENT: blurred vision, diplopia.
GI: nausea, vomiting, abdominal discomfort, dry mouth, elevated liver function test.
GU: urine retention, incontinence.
Skin: rash.

Reactions may be *common,* uncommon, **life-threatening**, or COMMON AND LIFE-THREATENING.

☑ Special considerations
Besides the recommendations relevant to all benzodiazepines, consider the following.
• Lower doses are effective in elderly patients and patients with renal or hepatic dysfunction.
• Store in a cool, dry place away from direct light.
• Signs and symptoms of overdose include somnolence, confusion, coma, hypoactive reflexes, dyspnea, labored breathing, hypotension, bradycardia, slurred speech, and unsteady gait or impaired coordination. Support blood pressure and respiration until drug effects subside; monitor vital signs.
• Flumazenil, a specific benzodiazepine antagonist, may be useful in overdose. Mechanical ventilatory assistance via endotracheal tube may be required to maintain a patent airway and support adequate oxygenation.
• Treat hypotension with I.V. fluids and vasopressors such as dopamine and phenylephrine as needed.
• Induce emesis if patient is conscious. Use gastric lavage if ingestion was recent, but only if endotracheal tube is present to prevent aspiration. After emesis or lavage, administer activated charcoal with a cathartic as a single dose. Dialysis is of limited value.
• Don't use barbiturates; they may worsen CNS adverse effects.

Monitoring the patient
• Monitor patient for adverse effects.
• Monitor patient for signs of drug dependence.

Information for the patient
• Advise patient of potential for physical and psychological dependence with long-term use of clorazepate.
• Instruct patient not to alter drug regimen without medical approval.
• Warn patient that sudden position changes may cause dizziness. Advise patient to dangle legs for a few minutes before getting out of bed to prevent falls and injury.
• Advise patient to take antacids 1 hour before or after clorazepate.
• Inform patient not to suddenly stop taking drug.

Geriatric patients
• Lower doses are usually effective in elderly patients because of decreased elimination. Use with caution.
• Elderly patients receiving this drug need supervision with ambulation and activities of daily living during initiation of therapy or after an increase in dose.

Pediatric patients
• Safety in children under age 9 hasn't been established.

Breast-feeding patients
• Drug appears in breast milk. The breast-fed infant of a mother who uses clorazepate may become sedated, have feeding difficulties, or lose weight. Avoid use in breast-feeding women.

clotrimazole
FemCare, Gyne-Lotrimin, Lotrimin, Lotrimin AF, Mycelex, Mycelex-G, Mycelex OTC, Mycelex-7

Pharmacologic classification: synthetic imidazole derivative
Therapeutic classification: topical antifungal
Pregnancy risk category B (C, oral form)

How supplied
Available by prescription only
Vaginal tablets: 500 mg
Topical cream: 1%
Topical lotion: 1%
Topical solution: 1%
Lozenges: 10 mg
Available without a prescription
Vaginal tablets: 100 mg
Vaginal cream: 1%
Combination pack: Vaginal tablets 500 mg/topical cream 1%

Indications, route, and dosage
Tinea pedis, tinea cruris, tinea versicolor, tinea corporis, cutaneous candidiasis
Adults and children: Apply thinly and massage into cleansed affected and surrounding area, morning and evening, for prescribed period (usually 1 to 4 weeks; however, therapy may take up to 8 weeks).
Vulvovaginal candidiasis
Adults: Insert 1 tablet intravaginally h.s. for 7 consecutive days. If vaginal cream is used, insert 1 applicator intravaginally h.s. for 7 to 14 consecutive days.
Oropharyngeal candidiasis
Adults and children: Administer orally and dissolve slowly (15 to 30 minutes) in mouth; usual dosage is one lozenge five times daily for 14 consecutive days.
◊ **Keratitis**
Adults: 1% ointment in sterile peanut oil q 2 to 4 hours for up to 6 weeks.

Pharmacodynamics
Antifungal action: Alters cell membrane permeability by binding with phospholipids in the fungal cell membrane. Inhibits or kills many fungi, including yeast and dermatophytes, and also is active against some gram-positive bacteria.

Pharmacokinetics
- *Absorption:* Limited absorption with topical administration. Absorption following dissolution of mouth lozenge not determined.
- *Distribution:* Distributed minimally with local application.
- *Metabolism:* No information available.
- *Excretion:* No information available.

Contraindications and precautions
Contraindicated in patients with hypersensitivity to drug. Also contraindicated for ophthalmic use.

Interactions
None reported.

Adverse reactions
GI: nausea, vomiting (with lozenges); lower abdominal cramps.
GU: *mild vaginal burning or irritation* (with vaginal use), cramping, urinary frequency.
Hepatic: abnormal liver function tests.
Skin: blistering, *erythema*, edema, blistering, pruritus, burning, stinging, peeling, urticaria, skin fissures, general irritation.

☑ Special considerations
- Patients treated with clotrimazole lozenges, especially those who have preexisting liver dysfunction, should have periodic liver function tests.

Monitoring the patient
- Monitor patient for adverse effects.
- Monitor therapeutic effect.

Information for the patient
- Advise patient that lozenges must dissolve slowly in mouth to achieve maximum effect; don't chew.
- Instruct patient using intravaginal application to insert drug high into vagina and to refrain from sexual contact during treatment period to avoid reinfection. Also tell patient to use a sanitary napkin to prevent staining of clothing and to absorb discharge.
- Tell patient to complete full course of therapy. Improvement usually will be noted within 1 week. Patient should call if no improvement occurs in 4 weeks or if condition worsens.
- Advise patient to watch for and report irritation or sensitivity and, if this occurs, to stop use.

Pediatric patients
- Drug isn't recommended for use in children under age 3.

Breast-feeding patients
- It's unknown if drug appears in breast milk. Use drug with caution in breast-feeding women.

cloxacillin sodium
Cloxapen, Tegopen

Pharmacologic classification: penicillinase-resistant penicillin
Therapeutic classification: antibiotic
Pregnancy risk category B

How supplied
Available by prescription only
Capsules: 250 mg, 500 mg
Oral solution: 125 mg/5 ml (after reconstitution)

Indications, route, and dosage
Systemic infections caused by penicillinase-producing staphylococci
Adults: 250 to 500 mg q 6 hours.
Children: 50 to 100 mg/kg P.O. daily, divided into doses given q 6 hours.

Pharmacodynamics
Antibiotic action: Bactericidal; adheres to bacterial penicillin-binding proteins, thereby inhibiting bacterial cell-wall synthesis. Resists the effects of penicillinases—enzymes that inactivate penicillin; therefore, is active against many strains of penicillinase-producing bacteria; this activity is most pronounced against penicillinase-producing staphylococci; some strains may remain resistant. Active against gram-positive aerobic and anaerobic bacilli but has no significant effect on gram-negative bacilli.

Pharmacokinetics
- *Absorption:* Absorbed rapidly but incompletely (37% to 60%) from GI tract; is relatively acid-stable. Plasma levels peak ½ to 2 hours after oral dose. Food may decrease both rate and extent of absorption.
- *Distribution:* Distributed widely. Poor CSF penetration but enhanced in meningeal inflammation. Drug crosses placenta; is 90% to 96% protein-bound.
- *Metabolism:* Only partially metabolized.
- *Excretion:* Cloxacillin and metabolites excreted in urine by renal tubular secretion and glomerular filtration; also excreted in breast milk. Elimination half-life in adults is ½ to 1 hour, extended minimally to 2½ hours in patients with renal impairment.

Contraindications and precautions
Contraindicated in patients with hypersensitivity to drug or other penicillins.

Interactions
Drug-drug. *Aminoglycosides:* Produces synergistic bactericidal effects. However, the drugs are physically and chemically incompatible and are inactivated when mixed or given together. Don't give together.

Probenecid: Blocks renal tubular secretion of carbenicillin, raising its serum levels. Monitor patient closely.

Drug-food. *Any food:* Decreased drug absorption. Give drug on empty stomach.

Carbonated beverages, fruit juices: May inactivate drug. Don't use during drug therapy.

Adverse reactions

CNS: lethargy, hallucinations, *seizures,* anxiety, confusion, agitation, depression, dizziness, fatigue.

GI: *nausea,* vomiting, *epigastric distress, diarrhea,* enterocolitis, pseudomembranous colitis, black "hairy" tongue, abdominal pain.

GU: interstitial nephritis, nephropathy.

Hematologic: eosinophilia, anemia, *thrombocytopenia,* leukopenia, hemolytic anemia, *agranulocytosis.*

Hepatic: intrahepatic cholestasis, transient elevations in liver function tests.

Other: hypersensitivity reactions (rash, urticaria, chills, fever, sneezing, wheezing, *anaphylaxis*), overgrowth of nonsusceptible organisms.

☑ Special considerations

Besides the recommendations relevant to all penicillins, consider the following.

• Give drug with water only; acid in fruit juice or carbonated beverage may inactivate drug.

• Give dose on empty stomach; food decreases absorption.

• Refrigerate oral suspension and discard any unused drug after 14 days. Unrefrigerated suspension is stable for 3 days.

• Cloxacillin alters test results for urine and serum proteins; it produces false-positive or elevated results in turbidimetric urine and serum protein tests using sulfosalicylic acid or trichloroacetic acid.

• Drug produces false results on Bradshaw screening test for Bence Jones protein.

• Drug may falsely decrease serum aminoglycoside levels.

• Signs and symptoms of overdose include neuromuscular irritability or seizures. Treatment is symptomatic. After recent ingestion (within 4 hours), empty stomach by induced emesis or gastric lavage; follow with activated charcoal to reduce absorption.

• Cloxacillin isn't appreciably removed by hemodialysis or peritoneal dialysis.

Monitoring the patient

• Monitor CBC.

• Monitor patient for adverse effects.

Information for the patient

• Inform patient of potential adverse reactions.

• Instruct patient to take on empty stomach and take with water only.

• Tell patient to refrigerate oral suspension and to discard any unused suspension after course of treatment.

Pediatric patients

• Elimination of cloxacillin is reduced in neonates. Safe use of drug in neonates hasn't been established.

Breast-feeding patients

• Drug appears in breast milk; use cautiously in breast-feeding women.

clozapine
Clozaril

Pharmacologic classification: tricyclic dibenzodiazepine derivative
Therapeutic classification: antipsychotic
Pregnancy risk category B

How supplied

Available by prescription only
Tablets: 25 mg, 100 mg

Indications, route, and dosage

Schizophrenia in severely ill patients unresponsive to other therapies

Adults: Initially, 12.5 mg P.O. once or twice daily, increased to 25 to 50 mg daily (if tolerated) to a daily dosage of 300 to 450 mg by end of 2 weeks. Individual dosage is based on clinical response, patient tolerance, and adverse reactions. Subsequent increases of dosage should occur no more than once or twice weekly and shouldn't exceed 100 mg. Many patients respond to dosages of 300 to 600 mg daily, but some patients require as much as 900 mg daily. Don't exceed 900 mg/day.

Pharmacodynamics

Antipsychotic action: Binds to dopamine receptors (D-1, D-2, D-3, D-4, and D-5) within the limbic system of the CNS. Also may interfere with adrenergic, cholinergic, histaminergic, and serotoninergic receptors.

Pharmacokinetics

• *Absorption:* Levels peak about 2½ hours after oral administration. Food doesn't appear to interfere with bioavailability. Only 27% to 50% of dose reaches systemic circulation.

• *Distribution:* 95% bound to serum proteins.

• *Metabolism:* Metabolism nearly complete; very little unchanged drug appears in urine.

• *Excretion:* 50% of drug appears in urine and 30% in feces, mostly as metabolites. Elimination half-life appears proportional to dose and may range from 4 to 66 hours.

Contraindications and precautions

Contraindicated in patients with uncontrolled epilepsy or history of clozapine-induced agranulocytosis, in patients with a WBC count below 3,500/mm³, in patients with severe CNS depression or coma, in patients taking other drugs that suppress bone marrow function, and in those with myelosuppressive disorders.

Use cautiously in patients with renal, hepatic, or cardiac disease; prostatic hyperplasia; or angle-closure glaucoma and in those receiving general anesthesia.

Interactions

Drug-drug. *Anticholinergics:* May potentiate anticholinergic effects of clozapine. Monitor patient closely.

Antihypertensives: Increased hypotensive effects. Monitor blood pressure carefully.

Benzodiazepines: May increase risk of respiratory arrest and severe hypotension. Avoid use together.

CNS-active drugs: Possible additive effects. Monitor patient closely.

Digoxin, warfarin, other highly protein-bound drugs: Possible increased serum levels of these drugs. Monitor closely for adverse reactions.

Drugs metabolized by cytochrome P-450 2D6 (such as antidepressants, carbamazepine, phenothiazines, type IC antiarrhythmics [encainide, flecainide, propafenone]); drugs that inhibit this enzyme (such as quinidine): Increased risk of abnormal drug metabolism. Use together cautiously.

Drugs that suppress bone marrow function: Risk of increased bone marrow toxicity. Monitor CBC.

Phenytoin: Possible decreased phenytoin levels; may lower seizure threshold. Avoid use with other drugs that have same effect.

Drug-herb. *Nutmeg:* May cause loss of symptom control. Avoid concurrent use.

Adverse reactions

CNS: *drowsiness, sedation, seizures,* dizziness, syncope, vertigo, headache, tremor, disturbed sleep or nightmares, restlessness, hypokinesia or akinesia, agitation, rigidity, akathisia, confusion, fatigue, insomnia, hyperkinesia, weakness, lethargy, ataxia, slurred speech, depression, myoclonus, anxiety, neuroleptic malignant syndrome.

CV: *tachycardia, hypotension,* hypertension, chest pain, ECG changes, orthostatic hypotension.

GI: dry mouth, *constipation,* nausea, vomiting, *excessive salivation,* heartburn, constipation, diarrhea.

GU: urinary abnormalities (urinary frequency or urgency, urine retention), incontinence, abnormal ejaculation.

Hematologic: *leukopenia, agranulocytosis.*

Musculoskeletal: muscle pain or spasm, muscle weakness.

Skin: rash.

Other: fever, weight gain, visual disturbances, diaphoresis.

After abrupt withdrawal of long-term therapy: possible abrupt recurrence of psychotic symptoms.

☑ Special considerations

● To discontinue clozapine therapy, withdraw drug gradually (over a 1- to 2-week period). However, changes in the patient's clinical status (including development of leukopenia) may require stopping drug abruptly. If so, monitor closely for recurrence of psychotic symptoms.

● To reinstate therapy in patients withdrawn from drug, follow usual guidelines for dosage buildup. However, reexposure of the patient may increase risk and severity of adverse reactions. If therapy ended for WBC counts below 2,000/mm³ or granulocyte counts below 1,000/mm³, don't reinstate drug.

● Some patients experience transient fevers (temperature above 100.4° F [38° C]), especially in the first 3 weeks of therapy. Monitor patients closely.

● Fatalities have occurred at doses exceeding 2.5 g. Symptoms include drowsiness, delirium, coma, hypotension, hypersalivation, tachycardia, respiratory depression, and, rarely, seizures. Treat symptomatically. Establish an airway and ensure adequate ventilation. Gastric lavage with activated charcoal and sorbitol may be effective.

● In overdose, monitor vital signs. Avoid epinephrine (and derivatives), quinidine, and procainamide when treating hypotension and arrhythmias.

Monitoring the patient

● For the first 6 months, clozapine therapy must be given with a monitoring program that ensures weekly testing of WBC counts. Blood tests must be performed weekly, and no more than a 1-week supply of drug can be distributed. Blood testing then can be done every other week.

● Assess patient periodically for abnormal body movement.

Information for the patient

● Warn patient about risk of developing agranulocytosis. Patient should know that safe use of drug requires blood tests weekly for the first 6 months, then every other week to monitor patient for agranulocytosis. Advise patient to promptly report flulike symptoms, fever, sore throat, lethargy, malaise, or other signs of infection.

● Advise patient to call before taking OTC drugs or alcohol.

● Tell patient that ice chips or sugarless candy or gum may help to relieve dry mouth.

● Warn patient to rise slowly to upright position to avoid orthostatic hypotension.

Geriatric patients
• Elderly patients may need reduced dosages because they may be more sensitive to adverse reactions, especially orthostatic hypotension, dry mouth, and constipation. Monitor closely.

Pediatric patients
• Safe use in children hasn't been established.

Breast-feeding patients
• Drug appears in breast milk. Women taking clozapine shouldn't breast-feed.

---

codeine phosphate
codeine sulfate

Pharmacologic classification: opioid
Therapeutic classification: analgesic, antitussive
Controlled substance schedule II
Pregnancy risk category C

How supplied
Available by prescription only
Tablets: 15 mg, 30 mg, 60 mg; 15 mg, 30 mg, 60 mg (soluble)
Oral solution: 15 mg/5 ml codeine phosphate
Injection: 15 mg/ml, 30 mg/ml, 60 mg/ml codeine phosphate

Indications, route, and dosage
Mild to moderate pain
Adults: 15 to 60 mg P.O. or 15 to 60 mg (phosphate) S.C. or I.M. q 4 to 6 hours, p.r.n., or around-the-clock.
Children: 0.5 mg/kg (or 15 mg/m²) q 4 to 6 hours. (Don't use I.V.)
Nonproductive cough
Adults and children ages 12 and older: 10 to 20 mg P.O. q 4 to 6 hours. Maximum dose is 120 mg/24 hours.
Children ages 6 to 11: 5 to 10 mg q 4 to 6 hours; don't exceed 60 mg daily.
Children ages 2 to 6: 1 mg/kg daily divided into four equal doses, administered q 4 to 6 hours; don't exceed 30 mg in 24 hours.

Pharmacodynamics
Analgesic action: Has analgesic properties that result from its agonist activity at the opiate receptors.
Antitussive action: Has a direct suppressant action on the cough reflex center.

Pharmacokinetics
• *Absorption:* Well absorbed after oral or parenteral administration. About two-thirds as potent orally as parenterally. After oral or subcutaneous administration, action occurs in less than 30 minutes. Peak analgesic effect seen at ½ to 1 hour, and duration of action 4 to 6 hours.
• *Distribution:* Distributed widely throughout body; crosses placenta and enters breast milk.
• *Metabolism:* Metabolized mainly in liver, by demethylation, or conjugation with glucuronic acid.
• *Excretion:* Excreted mainly in urine as norcodeine and free and conjugated morphine.

Contraindications and precautions
Contraindicated in patients with hypersensitivity to drug. Use cautiously in patients with impaired renal or hepatic function, head injuries, increased intracranial pressure, increased CSF pressure, hypothyroidism, Addison's disease, acute alcoholism, CNS depression, bronchial asthma, COPD, respiratory depression, or shock and in elderly or debilitated patients.

Interactions
Drug-drug. *Anticholinergics:* May cause paralytic ileus. Use together cautiously.
Cimetidine: May increase respiratory and CNS depression, causing confusion, disorientation, apnea, or seizures. Use together cautiously.
Drugs extensively metabolized in liver (digitoxin, phenytoin, rifampin): Drug accumulation and enhanced effects may result. Monitor patient closely.
Drugs that induce P-450 enzymes: Increased clearance and decreased effect of codeine. Monitor patient closely.
General anesthetics: Severe CV depression may result. Use together cautiously.
Narcotic antagonists: Patients physically dependent on drug may experience acute withdrawal syndrome. Use together cautiously.
Other CNS depressants (antihistamines, barbiturates, benzodiazepines, general anesthetics, MAO inhibitors, muscle relaxants, narcotic analgesics, phenothiazines, sedative-hypnotics, tricyclic antidepressants): Potentiate drug's respiratory and CNS depression, sedation, and hypotensive effects. Monitor patient closely.
Drug-lifestyle. *Alcohol:* Potentiates drug's respiratory and CNS depression, sedation, and hypotensive effects. Discourage use.

Adverse reactions
CNS: *sedation, clouded sensorium, euphoria, dizziness, light-headedness.*
CV: *hypotension, **bradycardia.***
GI: *nausea, vomiting, constipation, dry mouth,* ileus.
GU: *urine retention.*
Respiratory: ***respiratory depression.***
Skin: pruritus, flushing, *diaphoresis.*
Other: physical dependence.

☑ Special considerations
Besides the recommendations relevant to all opioids, consider the following.

- Codeine and aspirin have additive analgesic effects. Give together for maximum pain relief.
- Codeine has much less abuse potential than morphine.
- Drug may increase plasma amylase and lipase levels, delay gastric emptying, increase biliary tract pressure resulting from contraction of sphincter of Oddi, and may interfere with hepatobiliary imaging studies.
- Signs and symptoms of overdose are CNS depression, respiratory depression, and miosis (pinpoint pupils). Other acute toxic effects include hypotension, bradycardia, hypothermia, shock, apnea, cardiopulmonary arrest, circulatory collapse, pulmonary edema, and seizures.
- For acute overdose, establish adequate respiratory exchange via patent airway and ventilation as needed; administer narcotic antagonist (naloxone) to reverse respiratory depression. (Because the duration of action of codeine is longer than that of naloxone, repeated naloxone dosing is necessary.) Don't give naloxone unless patient has clinically significant respiratory or CV depression. Monitor vital signs closely.
- If within 2 hours of ingestion of oral overdose, empty stomach immediately by inducing emesis (ipecac syrup) or using gastric lavage. Use caution to avoid risk of aspiration. Administer activated charcoal via nasogastric tube for further drug removal. Provide symptomatic and supportive treatment. Monitor laboratory parameters, vital signs, and neurologic status closely.

Monitoring the patient
- When used in patients with renal or hepatic disease, monitor patient's renal and hepatic function.
- Closely monitor patients receiving concomitant CNS depressants for enhanced depressant effects.

Information for the patient
- Inform patient that codeine may cause drowsiness, dizziness, or blurring of vision; tell patient to use caution while driving or performing tasks that require mental alertness.
- Advise patient to avoid consumption of alcohol and other CNS depressants and to take drug with food if GI upset occurs.

Geriatric patients
- Lower doses are usually indicated for elderly patients, who may be more sensitive to the therapeutic and adverse effects of drug.

Pediatric patients
- Administer cautiously to children. Cough preparations containing codeine may be hazardous in young children. Use a calibrated measuring device and don't exceed recommended daily dose.

Breast-feeding patients
- Drug appears in breast milk; assess risk-to-benefit ratio before administering to a breast-feeding woman.

colchicine

Pharmacologic classification:
Colchicum autumnale alkaloid
Therapeutic classification: antigout drug
Pregnancy risk category C (oral), D (parenteral)

How supplied
Available by prescription only
Injection: 1 mg (1/60 grain)/2-ml ampule
Tablets: 0.6 mg (1/100 grain), 0.5 mg (1/120 grain) as sugar-coated granules

Indications, route, and dosage
To prevent acute attacks of gout as prophylactic or maintenance therapy
Adults: 0.5 or 0.6 mg P.O. one to four times weekly.
To prevent attacks of gout in patients undergoing surgery
Adults: 0.5 to 0.6 mg P.O. t.i.d. 3 days before and 3 days after surgery.
Acute gout, acute gouty arthritis
Adults: Initially, 0.5 to 1.3 mg P.O., then 0.5 to 0.65 mg P.O. q 1 to 2 hours or 1 to 1.3 mg P.O. q 2 hours; total daily dose is usually 4 to 8 mg P.O.; give until pain is relieved or until nausea, vomiting, or diarrhea ensues. Or 2 mg I.V.; then 0.5 mg I.V. q 6 hours if necessary. Total I.V. dose over 24 hours (one course of treatment) not to exceed 4 mg.
◊ *Familial Mediterranean fever*
Colchicine has been used effectively to treat familial Mediterranean fever (hereditary disorder characterized by acute episodes of fever, peritonitis, and pleuritis).
Adults: 1 to 2 mg/day in divided doses.
◊ *Amyloidosis suppressant*
Adults: 500 to 600 mcg P.O. once daily to b.i.d.
◊ *Dermatitis herpetiformis suppressant*
Adults: 600 mcg P.O. b.i.d. or t.i.d.
◊ *Hepatic cirrhosis*
Adults: 1 mg 5 days weekly.
◊ *Primary biliary cirrhosis*
Adults: 0.6 mg b.i.d.

Pharmacodynamics
Antigout action: Exact mechanism unknown. It's involved in leukocyte migration inhibition; reduction of lactic acid production by leukocytes, resulting in decreased deposits of uric acid; and interference with kinin formation.
Anti-inflammatory action: Reduces inflammatory response to deposited uric acid crystals and diminishes phagocytosis.

Reactions may be *common*, uncommon, **life-threatening**, or COMMON AND LIFE-THREATENING.

Pharmacokinetics
• *Absorption:* When administered P.O., rapidly absorbed from GI tract. Unchanged drug may be reabsorbed from intestine by biliary processes.
• *Distribution:* Distributed rapidly into various tissues after reabsorption from intestine. Concentrated in leukocytes and distributed into kidneys, liver, spleen, and intestinal tract but is absent in heart, skeletal muscle, and brain.
• *Metabolism:* Metabolized partially in liver and also slowly metabolized in other tissues.
• *Excretion:* Drug and its metabolites excreted primarily in feces, with lesser amounts excreted in urine.

Contraindications and precautions
Contraindicated in patients with hypersensitivity to drug and in those with blood dyscrasias or serious CV, renal, or GI disease. Use cautiously in elderly or debilitated patients and in those with early signs of CV, renal, or GI disease.

Interactions
Drug-drug. *Acidifying drugs:* Inhibits colchicine. Use together cautiously.
Alkalinizing drugs: Increased action of alkalinizing drugs. Use together cautiously.
CNS depressants: Enhanced CNS effects. Monitor patient closely.
Cyclosporine: May cause GI dysfunction, hepatonephropathy, and neuromyopathy. Use together cautiously.
Sympathomimetics: Enhanced sympathomimetic response. Monitor patient and vital signs closely.
Vitamin B₁₂: Colchicine induces reversible malabsorption of vitamin B₁₂. Monitor patient carefully.
Drug-lifestyle. *Alcohol:* May inhibit drug action. Discourage use together.

Adverse reactions
CNS: peripheral neuritis.
GI: *nausea, vomiting, abdominal pain, diarrhea.*
GU: reversible azoospermia.
Hematologic: *aplastic anemia, thrombocytopenia, and agranulocytosis* (with long-term use); nonthrombocytopenic purpura.
Hepatic: increased alkaline phosphatase, AST, and ALT levels.
Skin: alopecia, urticaria, dermatitis, hypersensitivity reactions.
Other: severe local irritation if extravasation occurs, myopathy.

☑ Special considerations
• To avoid cumulative toxicity, don't repeat a course of oral colchicine for at least 3 days; don't repeat a course of I.V. colchicine for several weeks.
• Don't administer I.M. or S.C.; severe local irritation occurs.

• Give I.V. by slow I.V. push over 2 to 5 minutes by direct I.V. injection or into tubing of a free-flowing I.V. with compatible I.V. fluid. Avoid extravasation. Don't dilute colchicine injection with bacteriostatic normal saline solution, dextrose 5% injection, or any other fluid that might change pH of colchicine solution. If lower concentration of colchicine injection is needed, dilute with sterile water or normal saline solution. However, if diluted solution becomes turbid, don't inject.
• Stop drug if weakness, anorexia, nausea, vomiting, or diarrhea appears. First sign of acute overdose may be GI symptoms, then vascular damage, muscle weakness, and ascending paralysis. Delirium and convulsions may occur without loss of consciousness.
• Store drug in a tightly closed, light-resistant container, away from moisture and high temperatures.
• Colchicine may cause false-positive results of urine tests for RBCs or hemoglobin.
• Signs and symptoms of overdose include nausea, vomiting, abdominal pain, and diarrhea. Diarrhea may be severe and bloody from hemorrhagic gastroenteritis. Burning sensations in throat, stomach, and skin also may occur. Extensive vascular damage may result in shock, hematuria, and oliguria, indicating kidney damage. Patient develops severe dehydration, hypotension, and muscle weakness with an ascending paralysis of CNS. Patient usually remains conscious, but delirium and convulsions may occur. Death may result from respiratory depression.
• There is no known specific antidote. Treat overdose with gastric lavage and preventive measures for shock. Hemodialysis and peritoneal dialysis may be used.
• Atropine and morphine may relieve abdominal pain; paregoric usually is administered to control diarrhea and cramps.

Monitoring the patient
• Obtain baseline laboratory studies, including CBC, before initiating therapy and periodically thereafter.
• Monitor patient for adverse effects.

Information for the patient
• Advise patient to report rash, sore throat, fever, unusual bleeding, bruising, tiredness, weakness, numbness, or tingling.
• Tell patient to stop drug as soon as gout pain is relieved or at the first sign of nausea, vomiting, stomach pain, or diarrhea. Advise patient to report persistent symptoms.
• Instruct patient to avoid alcohol during drug therapy because alcohol may inhibit drug action.

Geriatric patients
• Administer with caution to elderly or debilitated patients, especially those with renal, GI, or heart disease or hematologic disorders. Reduce

dosage if weakness, anorexia, nausea, vomiting, or diarrhea occurs.

Pediatric patients
• Safety and efficacy in children haven't been established.

Breast-feeding patients
• It's unknown if drug appears in breast milk. Safe use hasn't been established.

colestipol hydrochloride
Colestid

Pharmacologic classification: anion exchange resin
Therapeutic classification: antilipemic
Pregnancy risk category C

How supplied
Available by prescription only
Tablets: 1 g
Granules: 300-g and 500-g multidose bottles, 5-g packets

Indications, route, and dosage
Primary hypercholesterolemia and xanthomas
Adults: Tablets: Initially, 2 g P.O. once daily or b.i.d.; then increase in 2-g increments at 1- to 2-month intervals. Usual dosage is 2 to 16 g P.O. daily given as a single dose or in divided doses. Granules: Initially, 5 g P.O. once daily or b.i.d.; then increase in 5-g increments at 1- to 2-month intervals. Usual dosage is 5 to 30 g P.O. daily given as a single dose or in divided doses.
◊ *Children:* 10 to 20 g or 500 mg/kg daily in two to four divided doses (lower dosages of 125 to 250 mg/kg used when serum cholesterol levels are 15% to 20% above normal after only dietary management).
◊ **Digitoxin overdose**
Adults: Initially, 10 g P.O.; then 5 g P.O. q 6 to 8 hours.

Pharmacodynamics
Antilipemic action: Bile is normally excreted into the intestine to facilitate absorption of fat and other lipid materials. Colestipol binds with bile acid, forming an insoluble compound that is excreted in feces. With less bile available in the digestive system, less fat and lipid materials in food are absorbed, more cholesterol is used by the liver to replace its supply of bile acids, and the serum cholesterol level decreases.

Pharmacokinetics
• *Absorption:* Not absorbed. Cholesterol levels may decrease in 24 to 48 hours, with peak effect at 1 month. In some patients, initial decrease is followed by a return to or above baseline cholesterol levels on continued therapy.

• *Distribution:* None.
• *Metabolism:* None.
• *Excretion:* Excreted in feces; cholesterol levels return to baseline within 1 month after therapy stops.

Contraindications and precautions
Contraindicated in patients with hypersensitivity reactions to bile-acid sequestering resins. Use cautiously in patients prone to constipation and in those with conditions aggravated by constipation, such as symptomatic coronary artery disease.

Interactions
Drug-drug. *Cardiac glycosides (such as digitoxin, digoxin), chenodiol, penicillin G, tetracycline, thiazide diuretics:* Impaired absorption of these drugs, decreasing their therapeutic effect. Use together cautiously.
Oral drugs: Possible binding with colestipol. Dosage may need adjustment; give other drugs at least 1 hour before or 4 to 6 hours after colestipol (longer if possible); readjustment must also be made when colestipol is withdrawn to prevent high-dose toxicity.
Oral phosphate supplements: Interference with phosphate action. Use together cautiously.
Propranolol: Decreased GI absorption of propranolol. Use together cautiously.

Adverse reactions
CNS: headache, dizziness, anxiety, vertigo, insomnia, fatigue, syncope, tinnitus.
GI: *constipation, fecal impaction,* hemorrhoids, abdominal discomfort, flatulence, nausea, vomiting, steatorrhea, **GI bleeding,** diarrhea, anorexia.
GU: dysuria, hematuria.
Hematologic: anemia, ecchymoses, bleeding tendencies.
Hepatic: alterations in serum alkaline phosphatase, ALT, and AST levels.
Metabolic: alterations in serum chloride, phosphorus, potassium, and sodium levels.
Musculoskeletal: backache, muscle and joint pain, osteoporosis.
Skin: rash, irritation of tongue and perianal area.
Other: vitamin A, D, E, and K deficiencies from decreased absorption; hyperchloremic acidosis with long-term use or high dosage.

☑ Special considerations
• To mix, sprinkle granules on surface of preferred beverage or wet food, let stand a few minutes, and stir to obtain uniform suspension; avoid excess foaming by using large glass and mixing slowly. Use at least 90 ml of water or other fluid, soups, milk, or pulpy fruit; rinse container and have patient drink this to be sure entire dose is ingested. Tablets should be swallowed whole.

Reactions may be *common*, uncommon, *life-threatening*, or COMMON AND LIFE-THREATENING.

• Drug effects are most successful if used with a diet and exercise program.
• Overdose hasn't been reported. Chief potential risk is intestinal obstruction. Treatment would depend on location and degree of obstruction and on amount of gut motility.

Monitoring the patient
• Monitor levels of cardiac glycosides and other drugs to ensure appropriate dosage during and after therapy with colestipol.
• Determine serum cholesterol level frequently during first few months of therapy and periodically thereafter.
• Monitor bowel habits; treat constipation promptly by decreasing dosage, increasing fluid intake, adding a stool softener, or stopping drug.
• Monitor patient for signs of vitamin A, D, or K deficiency.

Information for the patient
• Explain disease process and rationale for therapy and encourage patient to comply with continued blood testing and special diet; although therapy isn't curative, it helps control serum cholesterol level.
• Teach patient how to administer drug. Other drugs should be taken at least 1 hour before or 4 hours after colestipol.

Geriatric patients
• Elderly patients are more likely to experience adverse GI and nutritional effects.

Pediatric patients
• Safety in children hasn't been established. Drug isn't usually recommended; however, it has been used in a limited number of children with hypercholesteremia.

Breast-feeding patients
• Safety in breast-feeding women hasn't been established.

---

corticotropin (adrenocorticotropic hormone, ACTH)
ACTH, Acthar, H.P. Acthar Gel

Pharmacologic classification: anterior pituitary hormone
Therapeutic classification: diagnostic aid, replacement hormone, multiple sclerosis and nonsuppurative thyroiditis treatment
Pregnancy risk category C

How supplied
Available by prescription only
Injection: 25 units/vial, 40 units/vial
Repository injection: 40 units/ml, 80 units/ml

Indications, route, and dosage
Diagnostic test of adrenocortical function
Adults: Up to 80 units I.M. or S.C. in divided doses; or a single dose of repository form; or 10 to 25 units (aqueous form) in 500 ml of D_5W I.V. over 8 hours, between blood samplings.
   Individual dosages vary with adrenal glands' sensitivity to stimulation and with the specific disease. Infants and younger children require larger doses per kilogram than do older children and adults.
Replacement hormone
Adults: 20 units S.C. or I.M. q.i.d.
Exacerbations of multiple sclerosis
Adults: 80 to 120 units I.M. daily for 2 to 3 weeks.
Severe allergic reactions, collagen disorders, dermatologic disorders, inflammation
Adults: 40 to 80 units/day I.M. or S.C. Adjust dosage based upon patient response.
Infantile spasms
Infants: 20 to 40 units I.M. (of repository injection) daily or 80 units I.M. every other day for 3 months or 1 month after spasm ceases.

Pharmacodynamics
Diagnostic action: Used to test adrenocortical function. Binds with a specific receptor in the adrenal cell plasma membrane, stimulating the synthesis of the entire spectrum of adrenal steroids, one of which is cortisol. The effect of corticotropin is measured by analyzing plasma cortisol before and after drug administration. In patients with primary adrenocortical insufficiency, corticotropin doesn't increase plasma cortisol levels significantly.
Anti-inflammatory action: In nonsuppurative thyroiditis and acute exacerbations of multiple sclerosis, stimulates release of adrenal cortex hormones, which combat tissue responses to inflammatory processes.

Pharmacokinetics
• *Absorption:* Absorbed rapidly after I.M. administration; occurs over 8 to 16 hours after I.M. administration of zinc or repository form. Maximum stimulation occurs after infusing 1 to 6 units of corticotropin over 8 hours. Peak cortisol levels achieved within 1 hour of I.M. or rapid I.V. administration of corticotropin. Peak 17-hydroxycorticosteroid levels within 7 to 24 hours with zinc and 3 to 12 hours with repository form.
• *Distribution:* Exact distribution unknown, but is removed rapidly from plasma by many tissues.
• *Metabolism:* No information available.
• *Excretion:* Probably excreted by kidneys. Drug's duration of action is about 2 hours with zinc form and up to 3 days with repository form. Half-life is about 15 minutes.

Contraindications and precautions
Contraindicated in patients with peptic ulcer, scleroderma, osteoporosis, systemic fungal infec-

tions, ocular herpes simplex, heart failure, hypertension, sensitivity to pork and pork products, adrenocortical hyperfunction or primary insufficiency, or Cushing's syndrome. Also contraindicated in those who have had surgery recently.

Use cautiously in pregnant women and in women of childbearing age. Also use cautiously in patients being immunized and in those with latent tuberculosis, hypothyroidism, cirrhosis, acute gouty arthritis, psychotic tendencies, renal insufficiency, diverticulitis, ulcerative colitis, thromboembolic disorders, seizures, uncontrolled hypertension, or myasthenia gravis.

Use with caution if surgery or emergency treatment is required.

Interactions
Drug-drug. *Amphotericin B, carbonic anhydrase inhibitors:* May cause severe hypokalemia. Monitor potassium levels.
Amphotericin B: Also decreases adrenal responsiveness to corticotropin. Monitor patient closely.
Cardiac glycosides: May increase the risk of arrhythmias or digitalis toxicity associated with hypokalemia; monitor patient and serum potassium.
Cortisone, estrogens, hydrocortisone: May elevate plasma cortisol levels abnormally. Monitor patient closely.
Diuretics: May accentuate electrolyte loss; monitor serum electrolytes.
Hepatic enzyme-inducing drugs: May increase corticotropin metabolism resulting from induction of hepatic microsomal enzymes; use with caution.
Indomethacin, NSAIDs, salicylates: Ulcerogenic effects; use together cautiously.
Insulin, oral antidiabetic drugs: May require increased dosage of antidiabetic drug; monitor serum glucose.

Adverse reactions
CNS: *seizures,* dizziness, vertigo, *increased intracranial pressure with papilledema,* pseudotumor cerebri.
CV: hypertension, *heart failure,* necrotizing vasculitis, *shock.*
EENT: cataracts, glaucoma.
GI: *peptic ulceration with perforation and hemorrhage,* pancreatitis, abdominal distention, ulcerative esophagitis, nausea, vomiting.
GU: menstrual irregularities.
Metabolic: activation of latent diabetes mellitus, *sodium and fluid retention,* calcium and potassium loss, hypokalemic alkalosis, negative nitrogen balance.
Musculoskeletal: muscle weakness, steroid myopathy, loss of muscle mass, osteoporosis, suppression of growth in children, vertebral compression fractures.
Respiratory: pneumonia.

Skin: impaired wound healing; thin, fragile skin; petechiae; ecchymoses; facial erythema; diaphoresis; acne; hyperpigmentation; allergic reactions; hirsutism.
Other: abscess and septic infection, cushingoid symptoms, progressive increase in antibodies, loss of corticotropin stimulatory effect, hypersensitivity reactions (rash, *bronchospasm*).

☑ Special considerations
● Cosyntropin is less antigenic and less likely to cause allergic reactions than corticotropin. However, allergic reactions occur rarely with corticotropin.
● In patient with suspected sensitivity to porcine proteins, skin testing should be performed. To decrease risk of anaphylactic reaction in patient with limited adrenal reserves, 1 mg of dexamethasone may be given at midnight before corticotropin test and 0.5 mg at start of test.
● Observe neonates of corticotropin-treated women for signs of hypoadrenalism.
● Counteract edema by low-sodium, high-potassium intake; nitrogen loss by high-protein diet; and psychotic symptoms by reducing corticotropin dosage or administering sedatives.
● Drug may mask signs of chronic disease and decrease host resistance and ability to localize infection.
● Insulin or oral antidiabetic dosages may need to be increased during corticotropin therapy.
● Refrigerate reconstituted product and use within 24 hours.
● If administering gel, warm it to room temperature, draw into large needle, and give slowly, deep I.M. with 22G needle.
● Don't stop drug abruptly, especially after prolonged therapy. An Addisonian crisis may occur.
● Corticotropin therapy alters protein-bound iodine levels; radioactive iodine (^{131}I) uptake and T_3 uptake; total protein values; serum amylase, urine amino acid, serotonin, uric acid and 17-ketosteroid levels; and leukocyte counts.
● High plasma cortisol levels may be reported erroneously in patients receiving spironolactone, cortisone, or hydrocortisone when fluorometric analysis is used. This doesn't occur with radioimmunoassay or competitive protein-binding method. However, therapy can be maintained with prednisone, dexamethasone, or betamethasone because they aren't detectable by fluorometric method.
● Treatment of overdose is supportive.

Monitoring the patient
● Monitor weight, fluid exchange, and resting blood pressure levels until minimal effective dosage is achieved.
● Monitor patient for adverse effects.

Information for the patient
● Warn patient that injection is painful.

Reactions may be *common,* uncommon, *life-threatening,* or COMMON AND LIFE-THREATENING.

- Tell patient to report marked fluid retention, muscle weakness, abdominal pain, seizures, or headache.
- Instruct patient not to be vaccinated during corticotropin therapy.
- Teach patient how to monitor patient for edema and explain the need for fluid and salt restriction as appropriate.
- Warn patient not to stop drug except as prescribed. Tell patient that stopping drug suddenly may provoke severe adverse reactions.

Geriatric patients
- Use with caution in elderly patients because they are more likely to develop osteoporosis.

Pediatric patients
- Use with caution because prolonged use of drug will inhibit skeletal growth. Intermittent administration is recommended.

Breast-feeding patients
- Safety hasn't been established. Because the potential for severe adverse reactions exists, benefits and risks must be weighed.

cortisone acetate
Cortone

Pharmacologic classification: glucocorticoid, mineralocorticoid
Therapeutic classification: anti-inflammatory, replacement therapy
Pregnancy risk category NR

How supplied
Available by prescription only
Tablets: 5 mg, 10 mg, 25 mg
Injection (I.M. use): 50 mg/ml suspension

Indications, route, and dosage
Adrenal insufficiency, allergy, inflammation
Adults: 25 to 300 mg P.O. or 20 to 300 mg I.M. daily or on alternate days. Dosage highly individualized, depending on severity of disease.
Children: 20 to 300 mg/m² P.O. daily in four divided doses or 7 to 37.5 mg/m² I.M. once or twice daily. Dosage must be highly individualized.

Pharmacodynamics
Adrenocorticoid replacement: Adrenocorticoid with both glucocorticoid and mineralocorticoid properties. A weak anti-inflammatory drug, it has only about 80% of the anti-inflammatory activity of an equal weight of hydrocortisone. It's a potent mineralocorticoid, however, having twice the potency of prednisone. Cortisone (or hydrocortisone) is usually the drug of choice for replacement therapy in patients with adrenal insufficiency. It usually isn't used for inflammatory or immunosuppressant activity because of the extremely large doses that must be used and because of the unwanted mineralocorticoid effects. Injectable form has a slow onset but a long duration of action. It's usually used only when the oral form can't be used.

Pharmacokinetics
- *Absorption:* Absorbed readily after oral administration, with peak effects in about 1 to 2 hours. Suspension for injection has variable onset of 24 to 48 hours.
- *Distribution:* Distributed rapidly to muscle, liver, skin, intestines, and kidneys. Cortisone is extensively bound to plasma proteins (transcortin and albumin). Only unbound portion is active. Cortisone is distributed into breast milk and through placenta.
- *Metabolism:* Metabolized in liver to active metabolite hydrocortisone, which is metabolized to inactive glucuronide and sulfate metabolites. Duration of hypothalamic-pituitary-adrenal (HPA) axis suppression is 1¼ to 1½ days.
- *Excretion:* Inactive metabolites and small amounts of unmetabolized drug excreted by kidneys. Insignificant quantities of drug also excreted in feces. Biological half-life is 8 to 12 hours.

Contraindications and precautions
Contraindicated in patients with hypersensitivity to drug or its ingredients or systemic fungal infections. Use cautiously in patients with renal disease, recent MI, GI ulcer, hypertension, osteoporosis, diabetes mellitus, hypothyroidism, cirrhosis, diverticulitis, ulcerative colitis, recent intestinal anastomosis, thromboembolic disorders, seizures, myasthenia gravis, heart failure, tuberculosis, ocular herpes, emotional instability, or psychotic tendencies.

Interactions
Drug-drug. *Amphotericin B, diuretics:* Enhanced risk of hypokalemia. Monitor serum glucose.
Antacids, cholestyramine, colestipol: Decreases cortisone's effect by adsorbing the corticosteroid, decreasing amount absorbed. Separate administration times.
Barbiturates, phenytoin, rifampin: May cause decreased corticosteroid effects because of increased hepatic metabolism. Monitor patient closely.
Cardiac glycosides: If hypokalemia occurs, may increase the risk of toxicity. Use together cautiously.
Estrogens: May reduce the metabolism of cortisone; monitor patient closely.
Inactivated vaccines, toxoids: Diminished response. Avoid concurrent use if possible.
Isoniazid, salicylates: May increase metabolism and cause hyperglycemia, requiring dosage adjustment of insulin or oral antidiabetic drugs in diabetic patients.

Oral anticoagulants: Decreased anticoagulant effects. Monitor PT, INR.
Ulcerogenic drugs such as NSAIDs: Increased risk of GI ulceration. Monitor patient for bleeding.

Adverse reactions

Most adverse reactions to corticosteroids are dose- or duration-dependent.
CNS: euphoria, insomnia, psychotic behavior, pseudotumor cerebri, vertigo, headache, paresthesia, *seizures.*
CV: *heart failure,* hypertension, edema, *arrhythmias,* thrombophlebitis, *thromboembolism.*
EENT: cataracts, glaucoma.
GI: *peptic ulcer,* GI irritation, increased appetite, pancreatitis, nausea, vomiting.
Musculoskeletal: muscle weakness, osteoporosis.
Skin: delayed wound healing, acne, various skin eruptions, atrophy at I.M. injection sites.
Other: hirsutism; susceptibility to infections; possible hypokalemia, hyperglycemia, and carbohydrate intolerance; growth suppression in children; *acute adrenal insufficiency* may follow increased stress (infection, surgery, trauma) or abrupt withdrawal after long-term therapy; increased glucose and cholesterol levels; decreased serum potassium, calcium, thyroxine, and triiodothyronine levels; increased urine glucose and calcium levels; menstrual irregularities, cushingoid symptoms (moonface, buffalo hump, central obesity).
After abrupt withdrawal: rebound inflammation, fatigue, weakness, arthralgia, fever, dizziness, lethargy, depression, fainting, orthostatic hypotension, dyspnea, anorexia, hypoglycemia. *After prolonged use, sudden withdrawal may be fatal.*

☑ Special considerations

● Recommendations for use of cortisone and for care and teaching of patients during therapy are the same as those for all systemic adrenocorticoids.
● Drug therapy suppresses reactions to skin tests.
● Cortisone causes false-negative results in nitroblue tetrazolium test for systemic bacterial infections.
● Cortisone decreases ^{131}I uptake and protein-bound iodine concentrations in thyroid function tests.
● Acute ingestion is rarely a clinical problem. Toxic signs and symptoms rarely occur if drug is used for less than 3 weeks, even at large doses.
● Long-term use causes adverse physiologic effects, including suppression of the HPA axis, cushingoid appearance, muscle weakness, and osteoporosis.

Monitoring the patient

● PT should be checked frequently in patients on concurrent corticosteroids and coumarin anticoagulants.
● In cardiac patients, monitor intake, output, and daily weight; also check electrolytes.
● Closely monitor glucose levels in diabetic patients.

Information for the patient

● Inform patient of potential adverse reactions.

Geriatric patients

● Use with caution in elderly patients because they are more likely to develop osteoporosis.

Pediatric patients

● Long-term use of cortisone in children and adolescents may delay growth and maturation.

co-trimoxazole (trimethoprim-sulfamethoxazole)

Apo-Sulfatrim*, Bactrim, Bactrim DS, Bactrim I.V., Cotrim, Cotrim D.S., Novo-Trimel*, Roubac*, Septra, Septra DS, Septra I.V., SMZ-TMP, Sulfatrim

Pharmacologic classification: sulfonamide and folate antagonist
Therapeutic classification: antibiotic
Pregnancy risk category C

How supplied

Available by prescription only
Tablets: trimethoprim 80 mg and sulfamethoxazole 400 mg; trimethoprim 160 mg and sulfamethoxazole 800 mg
Suspension: trimethoprim 40 mg and sulfamethoxazole 200 mg/5 ml
Injectable: trimethoprim 80 mg and sulfamethoxazole 400 mg/5 ml

Indications, route, and dosage

Urinary tract infections and shigellosis
Adults: 1 double-strength or 2 regular-strength tablets P.O. q 12 hours for 10 to 14 days or 5 days for shigellosis. Or 8 to 10 mg/kg (based on trimethoprim) I.V. daily given in two to four equally divided doses for up to 14 days (5 days for shigellosis). Maximum daily dose, 960 mg.
Children over age 2 months: 8 mg/kg trimethoprim and 40 mg/kg sulfamethoxazole P.O. daily in two divided doses q 12 hours for 10 days (5 days for shigellosis).
Otitis media
Children over age 2 months: 8 mg/kg trimethoprim and 40 mg/kg sulfamethoxazole P.O. daily, in two divided doses q 12 hours for 10 days.

Reactions may be *common*, uncommon, **life-threatening**, or COMMON AND LIFE-THREATENING.

Pneumocystis carinii pneumonitis
Adults and children over age 2 months: 15 to 20 mg/kg trimethoprim and 75 to 100 mg/kg sulfamethoxazole P.O. daily, in equally divided doses, q 6 to 8 hours for 14 to 21 days.
Chronic bronchitis
Adults: 1 double-strength or 2 regular-strength tablets q 12 hours for 14 days.
Traveler's diarrhea
Adults: 1 double-strength or 2 regular-strength tablets q 12 hours for 5 days.
Note: For the following unlabeled uses, dosages refer to oral trimethoprim (as co-trimoxazole).
◇ *Septic agranulocytosis*
Adults: 2.5 mg/kg I.V. q.i.d.; for prophylaxis, 80 to 160 mg b.i.d.
◇ *Nocardia infection*
Adults: 640 mg P.O. daily for 7 months.
◇ *Pharyngeal gonococcal infections*
Adults: 720 mg P.O. daily for 5 days.
◇ *Chancroid*
Adults: 160 mg P.O. b.i.d for 7 days.
◇ *Pertussis*
Adults: 320 mg P.O. daily in two divided doses.
Children: 40 mg/kg/day P.O. in two divided doses.
◇ *Cholera*
Adults: 160 mg P.O. b.i.d for 3 days.
Children: 5 mg/kg P.O. b.i.d for 3 days.
◇ *Isosporiasis*
Adults: 160 mg P.O. q.i.d. for 10 days, then 160 mg b.i.d. for 3 weeks.
✚ *Dosage adjustment.* In patients with impaired renal function, adjust dose or frequency of administration of parenteral form according to degree of renal impairment, severity of infection, and susceptibility of organism.

Creatinine clearance (ml/min/1.73 m²)	Adult dosage
> 30	Usual regimen
15 to 30	One-half the usual regimen
< 15	Use isn't recommended

Pharmacodynamics
Antibacterial action: Generally bactericidal; it acts by sequential blockade of folic acid enzymes in the synthesis pathway. The sulfamethoxazole component inhibits formation of dihydrofolic acid from para-aminobenzoic acid (PABA), whereas trimethoprim inhibits dihydrofolate reductase. Both drugs block folic acid synthesis, preventing bacterial cell synthesis of essential nucleic acids.
Effective against *Escherichia coli, Klebsiella, Enterobacter, Proteus mirabilis, Haemophilus influenzae, Streptococcus pneumoniae, Staphy-*

lococcus aureus, Acinetobacter, Salmonella, Shigella, and *Pneumocystis carinii.*

Pharmacokinetics
• *Absorption:* Well absorbed from GI tract after oral administration; peak serum levels occur at 1 to 4 hours.
• *Distribution:* Distributed widely into body tissues and fluids, including middle ear fluid, prostatic fluid, bile, aqueous humor, and CSF. Protein binding is 44% for trimethoprim, 70% for sulfamethoxazole. Co-trimoxazole crosses placenta.
• *Metabolism:* Metabolized by liver.
• *Excretion:* Both drug components excreted primarily in urine by glomerular filtration and renal tubular secretion; some drug excreted in breast milk. Trimethoprim's plasma half-life in patients with normal renal function is 8 to 11 hours, extended to 26 hours in severe renal dysfunction; sulfamethoxazole's plasma half-life is normally 10 to 13 hours, extended to 30 to 40 hours in severe renal dysfunction. Hemodialysis removes some co-trimoxazole.

Contraindications and precautions
Contraindicated in patients with hypersensitivity to trimethoprim or sulfonamides, severe renal impairment (creatinine clearance below 15 ml/minute), or porphyria; in those with megaloblastic anemia caused by folate deficiency; in pregnant women at term; in breast-feeding women; and in children under 2 months.
Use cautiously in patients with impaired renal or hepatic function, severe allergies, severe bronchial asthma, G6PD deficiency, or blood dyscrasia.

Interactions
Drug-drug. *Cyclosporine:* Decreased therapeutic effect; increased risk of nephrotoxicity. Monitor patient and cyclosporine levels.
Methotrexate: Increases levels. Monitor methotrexate levels.
Oral anticoagulants: Inhibited hepatic metabolism of anticoagulants, enhancing anticoagulant effects. Monitor PT, INR.
Oral sulfonylureas: Enhances their hypoglycemic effects; monitor serum glucose.
PABA: Antagonizes sulfonamide effects; monitor serum glucose.
Phenytoin: Hepatic clearance may be decreased and half-life prolonged. Monitor patient closely; monitor phenytoin level.
Zidovudine: Serum levels may be increased due to reduced renal clearance. Monitor serum zidovudine level.
Drug-lifestyle. *Sun exposure:* Photosensitivity reaction may occur. Advise patient to take precautions.

Adverse reactions
CNS: headache, mental depression, aseptic meningitis, tinnitus, apathy, *seizures,* hallucinations, ataxia, nervousness, fatigue, muscle weakness, vertigo, insomnia.
CV: thrombophlebitis.
GI: *nausea, vomiting, diarrhea,* abdominal pain, anorexia, stomatitis, *pancreatitis,* pseudomembranous colitis.
GU: *toxic nephrosis with oliguria and anuria,* crystalluria, hematuria, interstitial nephritis.
Hematologic: *agranulocytosis, aplastic anemia,* megaloblastic anemia, *thrombocytopenia,* leukopenia, *hemolytic anemia.*
Hepatic: jaundice, *hepatic necrosis.*
Respiratory: pulmonary infiltrates.
Skin: *erythema multiforme (Stevens-Johnson syndrome),* generalized skin eruptions, *epidermal necrolysis, exfoliative dermatitis,* photosensitivity, urticaria, pruritus.
Other: hypersensitivity reactions (*serum sickness, drug fever, anaphylaxis*), arthralgia, myalgia.

☑ Special considerations
Besides the recommendations relevant to all sulfonamides, consider the following.
• Co-trimoxazole has been used effectively to treat chronic bacterial prostatitis and as prophylaxis against recurrent urinary tract infection in women and traveler's diarrhea.
• For I.V. use, dilute infusion in D₅W. Don't mix with other drugs. Don't administer by rapid infusion or bolus injection. Infuse slowly over 60 to 90 minutes. Change infusion site every 48 to 72 hours.
• I.V. infusion must be diluted before use. Each 5 ml should be added to 125 ml D₅W. Don't refrigerate solution; diluted solutions must be used within 6 hours. A dilution of 5 ml per 75 ml D₅W may be prepared for patients requiring fluid restriction, but these solutions should be used within 2 hours.
• Check solution carefully for precipitate before starting infusion. Don't use solution containing precipitate.
• Assess I.V. site for signs of phlebitis or infiltration.
• Shake oral suspension thoroughly before administering.
• Note that DS means double-strength.
• Trimethoprim can interfere with serum methotrexate assay as determined by the competitive binding protein technique. No interference occurs if radioimmunoassay is used.
• Clinical signs of overdose include mental depression, drowsiness, anorexia, jaundice, confusion, headache, nausea, vomiting, diarrhea, facial swelling, slight elevations in liver function test results, and bone marrow depression.

• Treat overdose by emesis or gastric lavage, then supportive care (correction of acidosis, forced oral fluid, and I.V. fluids).
• Treatment of renal failure may be required; transfuse appropriate blood products in severe hematologic toxicity; use folinic acid to rescue bone marrow.
• Hemodialysis has limited ability to remove co-trimoxazole. Peritoneal dialysis isn't effective.

Monitoring the patient
• CBC should be done frequently in patients receiving Bactrim. If a significant reduction in count of any formed blood element occurs, stop Bactrim.
• Urinalyses with careful microscopic examination and renal function tests should be performed during therapy, particularly for patients with impaired renal function.

Information for the patient
• Inform patient of potential adverse reactions.

Geriatric patients
• In elderly patients, diminished renal function may prolong half-life. Such patients also have an increased risk of adverse reactions.

Pediatric patients
• Drug isn't recommended for infants under age 2 months.

Breast-feeding patients
• Drug isn't recommended in breast-feeding women because sulfonamides appear in breast milk and may cause kernicterus.

cromolyn sodium
Gastrocrom, Intal, Intal Inhaler, Intal Syncroner, Intal Nebulizer Solution, Nasalcrom, Opticrom

Pharmacologic classification: chromone derivative
Therapeutic classification: mast cell stabilizer, antasthmatic
Pregnancy risk category B

How supplied
Available by prescription only
Capsules: 100 mg
Aerosol: 800 mcg/metered spray
Solution: 20 mg/2 ml for nebulization
Ophthalmic solution: 4%
Nasal solution: 5.2 mg/metered spray (40 mg/ml)
Powder for inhalation: 20 mg (in capsules)

Indications, route, and dosage
Adjunct in treatment of severe perennial bronchial asthma
Adults and children over age 5: 2 inhalations q.i.d. at regular intervals; aqueous solution adminis-

tered through a nebulizer, 1 ampule q.i.d; or 1 capsule (20 mg) of powder for inhalation q.i.d.

Prevention and treatment of allergic rhinitis
Adults and children age 6 and over: 1 spray (5.2 mg) of nasal solution in each nostril t.i.d or q.i.d. May give up to six times daily.

Prevention of exercise-induced broncho-spasm
Adults and children over age 5: 2 metered sprays using inhaler or 1 capsule (20 mg) of powder for inhalation no more than 1 hour before anticipated exercise.

Inhalation of 20 mg of oral inhalation solution may be used in adults or children age 2 and over. Repeat inhalation as required for protection during long exercise.

Allergic ocular disorders (giant papillary conjunctivitis, vernal keratoconjunctivitis, vernal keratitis, allergic keratoconjunctivitis)
Adults and children over age 4: Instill 1 to 2 drops in each eye four to six times daily at regular intervals. One drop contains about 1.6 mg cromolyn sodium.

Systemic mastocytosis
Adults: 200 mg P.O. q.i.d.
Children age 2 to 12: 100 mg P.O. q.i.d.
Children under age 2: 20 mg/kg daily P.O. divided in four equal doses.

◇ **Food allergy, inflammatory bowel disease**
Adults: 200 mg P.O. q.i.d. 15 to 20 minutes before meals.

Pharmacodynamics

Antiasthmatic action: Prevents release of mediators of Type I allergic reactions, including histamine and slow-reacting substance of anaphylaxis (SRS-A), from sensitized mast cells after the antigen-antibody union has taken place. Doesn't inhibit binding of immunoglobulin E (IgE) to mast cells nor the interaction between cell-bound IgE and the specific antigen. It does inhibit the release of substances (such as histamine and SRS-A) in response to IgE binding to mast cells. Main site of action occurs locally on the lung mucosa, nasal mucosa, and eyes.

Bronchodilating action: Besides mast cell stabilization, recent evidence suggests that drug may have a bronchodilating effect by an unknown mechanism. Comparative studies have shown cromolyn and theophylline to be equally efficacious but less effective than orally inhaled beta$_2$-adrenergic agonists in preventing this bronchospasm.

Ocular antiallergy action: Inhibits degranulation of sensitized mast cells that occurs after exposure to specific antigens, preventing release of histamine and SRS-A.

Cromolyn has no direct anti-inflammatory, vasoconstrictor, antihistamine, antiserotonin, or corticosteroid-like properties.

Cromolyn dissolved in water and given orally has been found to be effective in managing food allergy, inflammatory bowel disease (Crohn's disease, ulcerative colitis), and systemic mastocytosis.

Pharmacokinetics

● *Absorption:* Only 0.5% to 2% of oral dose absorbed. Amount reaching lungs depends on patient's ability to use inhaler correctly, amount of bronchoconstriction, and size or presence of mucous plugs. Degree of absorption depends on method of administration; most absorption occurs with aerosol via metered-dose inhaler, and least occurs with administration of solution via power-operated nebulizer. Less than 7% of intranasal dose as a solution is absorbed systemically. Only minimal absorption (0.03%) of ophthalmic dose occurs after eye instillation. Absorption half-life from lung is 1 hour. Plasma concentration of 9 ng/ml can be achieved 15 minutes after 20-mg dose.

● *Distribution:* Doesn't cross most biological membranes; is ionized and lipid-insoluble at body's pH. Less than 0.1% of dose crosses placenta; not known if drug is distributed into breast milk.

● *Metabolism:* None significant.

● *Excretion:* Excreted unchanged in urine (50%) and bile (about 50%). Small amounts may be excreted in feces or exhaled. Elimination half-life is 81 minutes.

Contraindications and precautions

Contraindicated in patients experiencing acute asthma attacks or status asthmaticus and in patients with hypersensitivity to drug. Use inhalation form cautiously in patients with cardiac disease or arrhythmias.

Interactions

Drug-drug. *Isoproterenol:* Adverse fetal effects when administered parenterally in high doses. Avoid concomitant use.

Adverse reactions

CNS: dizziness, headache.
EENT: *irritated throat and trachea,* nasal congestion, pharyngeal irritation, *sneezing,* nasal burning and irritation, epistaxis, lacrimation, swollen parotid gland, bad taste in mouth.
GI: nausea, esophagitis, abdominal pain.
GU: dysuria, urinary frequency.
Musculoskeletal: joint swelling and pain.
Respiratory: *bronchospasm* (after inhalation of dry powder), *cough,* wheezing, *eosinophilic pneumonia.*
Skin: rash, urticaria.
Other: *angioedema.*

☑ Special considerations

● Bronchospasm or cough occasionally occurs after inhalation and may require stopping therapy. Prior bronchodilation may help but it still may be necessary to stop cromolyn therapy.

- Asthma symptoms may recur if cromolyn dosage is reduced below recommended dosage.
- Use reduced dosage in patients with impaired renal or hepatic function.
- Eosinophilic pneumonia or pulmonary infiltrates with eosinophilia requires stopping drug.
- Nasal solution may cause nasal stinging or sneezing immediately after instillation of drug but this reaction rarely requires stopping drug.
- Watch for recurrence of asthmatic symptoms when corticosteroids are also used. Use only when acute episode has been controlled, airway is cleared, and patient is able to inhale.
- Protect oral solution and ophthalmic solution from direct sunlight.
- Therapeutic effects may not be seen for 2 to 4 weeks after drug start.

Monitoring the patient
- Monitor pulmonary status before and immediately after therapy.
- Perform pulmonary function tests to confirm significant bronchodilator-reversible component of airway obstruction in patients considered for cromolyn therapy.

Information for the patient
- Teach correct use of metered-dose inhaler: exhale completely before placing mouthpiece between lips, then inhale deeply and slowly with steady, even breath; remove inhaler from mouth, hold breath for 5 to 10 seconds, and exhale.
- Urge patient to call if drug causes wheezing or coughing.
- Instruct patient with asthma or seasonal or perennial allergic rhinitis to administer drug at regular intervals to ensure clinical effectiveness.
- Advise patient that gargling and rinsing mouth after administration can help reduce mouth dryness.
- Tell patient taking prescribed adrenocorticoids to continue taking them during therapy, if appropriate.
- Instruct patient who uses bronchodilator inhaler to administer dose about 5 minutes before taking cromolyn (unless otherwise indicated); explain that this step helps reduce adverse reactions.

Pediatric patients
- Cromolyn use in children under age 5 is limited to inhalation route of administration. Safety of nebulizer solution in children under age 2 hasn't been established. Safety of nasal solution in children under age 6 hasn't been established.

cyanocobalamin (vitamin B$_{12}$)
Bedoz,* Cobex, Crystamine, Cyanoject, Cyomin, Rubesol-1000, Rubramin PC, Vibal

hydroxocobalamin (vitamin B$_{12}$)
Hydrobexan, Hydro-Cobex, LA-12

Pharmacologic classification: water-soluble vitamin
Therapeutic classification: vitamin, nutrition supplement
Pregnancy risk category C (parenteral)

How supplied
Available by prescription only
Injection: 30-ml vials (30 mcg/ml, 100 mcg/ml, 120 mcg/ml with benzyl alcohol, 1,000 mcg/ml, 1,000 mcg/ml with benzyl alcohol), 10-ml vials (100 mcg/ml, 100 mcg/ml with benzyl alcohol, 1,000 mcg/ml, 1,000 mcg/ml with benzyl alcohol, 1,000 mcg/ml with methyl and propyl parabens), 5-ml vials (1,000 mcg/ml with benzyl alcohol), 1-ml vials (1,000 mcg/ml with benzyl alcohol), 1-ml unimatic (1,000 mcg/ml with benzyl alcohol)
Tablets: 25 mcg, 50 mcg, 100 mcg, 250 mcg, 500 mcg, 1,000 mcg

Indications, route, and dosage
Vitamin from any cause except malabsorption related to pernicious anemia or other GI disease
Adults: 25 mcg P.O. daily as dietary supplement, or 30 to 100 mcg S.C. or I.M. daily for 5 to 10 days, depending on severity of deficiency. (I.M. route recommended for pernicious anemia.)
   Maintenance dosage is 100 to 200 mcg I.M. monthly. For subsequent prophylaxis, advise adequate nutrition and daily RDA vitamin B$_{12}$ supplements.
Children: 100 mcg I.M. or S.C. over the course of 2 or more weeks to maximum dose of 1 to 5 mg. Maintenance dosage, 60 mcg/month I.M. or S.C.
Diagnostic test for vitamin B$_{12}$ deficiency without concealing folate deficiency in patients with megaloblastic anemias
Adults and children: 1 mcg I.M. daily for 10 days with diet low in vitamin B$_{12}$ and folate. Reticulocytosis between days 3 and 10 confirms diagnosis of vitamin B$_{12}$ deficiency.
Schilling test flushing dose
Adults and children: 1,000 mcg I.M. in a single dose.

Pharmacodynamics
Nutritional action: Can be converted to coenzyme B$_{12}$ in tissues and, as such, is essential for conversion of methyl-malonate to succinate and synthesis of methionine from homocystine, a reaction that also requires folate. Without coenzyme

B_{12}, folate deficiency occurs. Associated with fat and carbohydrate metabolism and protein synthesis. Cells characterized by rapid division (epithelial cells, bone marrow, and myeloid cells) appear to have the greatest requirement for vitamin B_{12}.

Vitamin B_{12} deficiency may cause megaloblastic anemia, GI lesions, and neurologic damage; it begins with an inability to produce myelin then gradual degeneration of the axon and nerve. Parenteral administration of vitamin B_{12} completely reverses the megaloblastic anemia and GI symptoms of vitamin B_{12} deficiency.

Pharmacokinetics
● *Absorption:* After oral administration, absorbed irregularly from distal small intestine. Is protein-bound; bond must be split by proteolysis and gastric acid before absorption. Absorption depends on sufficient intrinsic factor and calcium. Inadequate in malabsorptive states and in pernicious anemia. Absorbed rapidly from I.M. and S.C. injection sites; plasma level peaks within 1 hour. After oral administration below 3 mcg, peak plasma levels aren't reached for 8 to 12 hours.
● *Distribution:* Distributed into liver, bone marrow, other tissues, and placenta. At birth, concentration in neonates is three to five times that in mother. Distributed into breast milk in concentrations about equal to maternal vitamin B_{12} concentration. Unlike cyanocobalamin, hydroxocobalamin is absorbed more slowly parenterally and may be taken up by liver in larger quantities; also produces greater increase in serum cobalamin levels and less urinary excretion.
● *Metabolism:* Cyanocobalamin and hydroxocobalamin metabolized in liver.
● *Excretion:* In healthy persons receiving only dietary vitamin B_{12}, about 3 to 8 mcg of vitamin secreted into GI tract daily, mainly from bile, and all but about 1 mcg reabsorbed; less than 0.25 mcg is usually excreted in urine daily. When administered in amounts that exceed binding capacity of plasma, liver, and other tissues, it's free in blood for urinary excretion.

Contraindications and precautions
Contraindicated in patients hypersensitive to vitamin B_{12} or cobalt and in patients with early Leber's disease. Use cautiously in anemic patients with coexisting cardiac, pulmonary, or hypertensive disease and in those with severe vitamin B_{12}-dependent deficiencies.

Interactions
Drug-drug. *Aminoglycosides, aminosalicylic acid and its salts, anticonvulsants, cobalt irradiation of small bowel, colchicine, extended-release potassium preparations:* Decreases vitamin B_{12} absorption from GI tract. Use together cautiously.
Chloramphenicol: May cause antagonized hematopoietic response; don't give concurrently.

Colchicine: May increase neomycin-induced malabsorption of vitamin B_{12}. Use together cautiously.
Large amounts of ascorbic acid: May destroy vitamin B_{12}; don't administer within 1 hour of taking vitamin.

Adverse reactions
CV: peripheral vascular thrombosis, pulmonary edema, heart failure.
GI: transient diarrhea.
Skin: itching, transitory exanthema, urticaria.
Other: *anaphylaxis, anaphylactoid reactions* (with parenteral administration); pain, burning (at S.C. or I.M. injection sites).

☑ Special considerations
● RDA for vitamin B_{12} is 0.3 mcg in infants to 2 mcg in adults, as follows:
Infants up to age 6 months: 0.3 mcg
Children ages 6 months to 1 year: 0.5 mcg
Children ages 1 to 3: 0.7 mcg
Children ages 4 to 6: 1 mcg
Children ages 7 to 10: 1.4 mcg
Children age 11 to adult: 2 mcg
Pregnant women: 2.2 mcg
Breast-feeding women: 2.6 mcg
● Determine patient's diet and drug history, including patterns of alcohol use, to identify poor nutritional habits.
● Administer oral solution promptly after mixing with fruit juice. Ascorbic acid causes instability of vitamin B_{12}. Protect oral solution from light.
● Administer oral vitamin B_{12} with meals to increase absorption.
● Don't mix parenteral form with dextrose solutions, alkaline or strongly acidic solutions, or oxidizing and reducing drugs because anaphylactic reactions may occur with I.V. use. Check compatibility with pharmacist.
● Parenteral therapy is preferred for patients with pernicious anemia because oral administration may be unreliable. In patients with neurologic complications, prolonged inadequate oral therapy may lead to permanent spinal cord damage. Oral therapy is appropriate for mild conditions without neurologic signs and for those patients who refuse or are sensitive to parenteral form.
● Patients with a history of sensitivities and those suspected of being sensitive to vitamin B_{12} should receive an intradermal test dose before therapy begins. Sensitization to vitamin B_{12} may develop after as many as 8 years of treatment.
● Expect therapeutic response to occur within 48 hours; is measured by laboratory values and effect on fatigue, GI symptoms, anorexia, pallid or yellow complexion, glossitis, distaste for meat, dyspnea on exertion, palpitation, neurologic degeneration (paresthesia, loss of vibratory and position sense and deep reflexes, incoordination), psychotic behavior, anosmia, and visual disturbances.
● Therapeutic response to vitamin B_{12} may be impaired by concurrent infection, uremia, folic

acid or iron deficiency, or drugs having bone marrow suppressant effects. Large doses of vitamin B_{12} may improve folate-deficient megaloblastic anemia.

• Expect reticulocyte level to rise in 3 to 4 days, peak in 5 to 8 days, and then gradually decline as erythrocyte count and hemoglobin rise to normal levels (in 4 to 6 weeks).

• Patients with mild peripheral neurologic defects may respond to concomitant physical therapy. Usually, neurologic damage that doesn't improve after 12 to 18 months of therapy is considered irreversible. Severe vitamin B_{12} deficiency that persists for 3 months or longer may cause permanent spinal cord degeneration.

• Vitamin B_{12} therapy may cause false-positive results for intrinsic factor antibodies, which are present in blood of half of all patients with pernicious anemia.

• Methotrexate, pyrimethamine, and most anti-infectives invalidate diagnostic blood assays for vitamin B_{12}.

• Even in large doses, vitamin B_{12} is usually nontoxic.

Monitoring the patient

• Monitor bowel function because regularity is essential for consistent absorption of oral preparations.

• Monitor vital signs in patients with cardiac disease and those receiving parenteral vitamin B_{12}. Watch for symptoms of pulmonary edema, which tend to develop early in therapy.

• Monitor potassium levels during first 48 hours, especially in patients with pernicious anemia or megaloblastic anemia. Potassium supplements may be required. Conversion to normal erythropoiesis increases erythrocyte potassium requirement and can result in fatal hypokalemia in these patients.

• Continue periodic hematologic evaluations throughout patient's lifetime.

Information for the patient

• Emphasize importance of a well-balanced diet. To prevent progression of subacute combined degeneration, don't use folic acid instead of vitamin B_{12} to prevent anemia.

• Tell patient to avoid smoking, which appears to increase requirement for vitamin B_{12}.

• Instruct patient to report infection or disease in case condition requires more vitamin B_{12}.

• Tell patient with pernicious anemia that lifelong treatment with vitamin B_{12} is necessary to prevent recurring symptoms and risk of incapacitating and irreversible spinal cord damage.

• Inform patient to store tablets in a tightly closed container at room temperature.

Pediatric patients

• Safety and efficacy of vitamin B_{12} for use in children haven't been established. Intake for children should be 0.5 to 2 mcg daily, as recommended by the Food and Nutrition Board of the National Academy of Sciences–National Research Council.

• Some of these products contain benzyl alcohol, which has been associated with a fatal "gasping syndrome" in premature infants.

Breast-feeding patients

• Vitamin B_{12} appears in breast milk in levels that approximate maternal vitamin B_{12} level. The Food and Nutrition Board of the National Academy of Sciences–National Research Council recommends that breast-feeding women consume 2.6 mcg/day of vitamin B_{12}.

cyclizine hydrochloride
Marezine

cyclizine lactate
Marezine, Marzine*

Pharmacologic classification: piperazine-derivative antihistamine
Therapeutic classification: antiemetic, antivertigo drug
Pregnancy risk category B

How supplied
Available with or without a prescription
cyclizine hydrochloride
Tablets: 50 mg
cyclizine lactate
Injection: 50 mg/ml

Indications, route, and dosage
Motion sickness (prophylaxis and treatment)
Adults and children over age 12: 50 mg P.O. (hydrochloride) 30 minutes before travel, then q 4 to 6 hours, p.r.n., to maximum of 200 mg daily; or 50 mg I.M. (lactate) q 4 to 6 hours, p.r.n.
Children ages 6 to 12: 25 mg P.O. up to t.i.d. under medical supervision.

Pharmacodynamics
Antiemetic action: Probably inhibits nausea and vomiting by centrally depressing sensitivity of the labyrinth apparatus that relays stimuli to the chemoreceptor trigger zone and thus stimulates the vomiting center in the brain.
Antivertigo action: Depresses conduction in vestibular-cerebellar pathways and reduces labyrinth excitability.

Pharmacokinetics
• *Absorption:* Not well characterized; onset of action between 30 and 60 minutes.
• *Distribution:* Well distributed throughout body.
• *Metabolism:* Metabolized in liver.
• *Excretion:* No information available; drug effect lasts 4 to 6 hours.

Reactions may be *common*, uncommon, **life-threatening**, or COMMON AND LIFE-THREATENING.

Contraindications and precautions

Contraindicated in patients hypersensitive to drug. Use cautiously in patients with heart failure and who have recently had surgery, benign prostatic hypertrophy, or asthma.

Interactions

Drug-drug. *Aminoglycosides, cisplatin, loop diuretics, salicylates, vancomycin:* May mask signs of ototoxicity. Don't give concurrently.
CNS depressants such as antianxiety drugs, barbiturates, sleeping drugs, tranquilizers: Additive sedative and CNS depressant effects. Monitor patient closely.
Drug-lifestyle. *Alcohol:* Additive sedative and CNS depressant effects. Discourage use of alcohol.

Adverse reactions

CNS: *drowsiness,* auditory and visual hallucinations, restlessness, excitation, nervousness.
CV: hypotension, palpitations, tachycardia.
EENT: blurred vision, diplopia, tinnitus, dry nose and throat.
GI: constipation, dry mouth, anorexia, nausea, vomiting, diarrhea, cholestatic jaundice.
GU: urine retention, urinary frequency.
Skin: urticaria, rash.

☑ Special considerations

Besides the recommendations relevant to all antihistamines, consider the following.
● Injectable cyclizine is for I.M. use only. When giving I.M., aspirate and check carefully for blood return; inadvertent I.V. administration can cause anaphylactic reaction.
● Injectable solution is incompatible with many drugs; check compatibility before mixing in same syringe.
● Store in a cool place; at room temperature, injection may turn slightly yellow but doesn't indicate loss of potency.
● Stop cyclizine 4 days before diagnostic skin testing to avoid preventing, reducing, or masking test response.
● Signs and symptoms of overdose may include either CNS depression (sedation, reduced mental alertness, apnea, and CV collapse) or CNS stimulation (insomnia, hallucinations, tremors, or seizures). Anticholinergic symptoms, such as dry mouth, flushed skin, fixed and dilated pupils, and GI symptoms, are common, especially in children.
● Treat overdose with gastric lavage to empty stomach contents; inducing emesis with ipecac syrup may be ineffective.
● Treat hypotension with vasopressors and control seizures with diazepam or phenytoin. Don't give stimulants.

Monitoring the patient

● Monitor patient for adverse effects.

● Closely monitor patients with history of heart failure when using this drug.

Information for the patient

● Instruct patient to stay in places of minimal motion (such as in middle, not front or back, of ship), avoid excessive intake of food or drink, and not to read while in motion.
● Tell patient to avoid hazardous activities requiring mental alertness until CNS reaction is determined.

Geriatric patients

● Elderly patients are usually more sensitive to adverse effects of antihistamines and are especially likely to experience a greater degree of dizziness, sedation, hyperexcitability, dry mouth, and urine retention than younger patients.

Pediatric patients

● Drug isn't indicated for use in children under age 6; they may experience paradoxical hyperexcitability. Safety and efficacy of I.M. administration in children haven't been established and use isn't recommended.

Breast-feeding patients

● Antihistamines such as cyclizine shouldn't be used during breast-feeding. Most appear in breast milk, exposing infant to risks of unusual excitability; premature infants are at particular risk for seizures. Cyclizine also may inhibit lactation.

cyclobenzaprine hydrochloride
Flexeril

Pharmacologic classification: tricyclic antidepressant derivative
Therapeutic classification: skeletal muscle relaxant
Pregnancy risk category B

How supplied

Available by prescription only
Tablets: 10 mg

Indications, route, and dosage
Adjunct in acute, painful musculoskeletal conditions
Adults: 20 to 40 mg P.O. divided b.i.d. to q.i.d.; maximum dosage, 60 mg daily. Don't administer for more than 2 weeks.
◊ *Fibrositis*
Adults: 10 to 40 mg P.O. daily.

Pharmacodynamics
Skeletal muscle relaxant action: Relaxes skeletal muscles through an unknown mechanism of action. Cyclobenzaprine is a CNS depressant.

Drug also potentiates the effects of norepinephrine and exhibits anticholinergic effects similar to those of tricyclic antidepressants, including central and peripheral antimuscarinic actions, sedation, and an increase in heart rate.

Pharmacokinetics
• *Absorption:* Almost completely absorbed during first pass through GI tract. Onset of action occurs within 1 hour, with peak levels in 3 to 8 hours. Duration of action 12 to 24 hours.
• *Distribution:* 93% plasma protein-bound.
• *Metabolism:* During first pass through GI tract and liver, drug and metabolites undergo enterohepatic recycling. Half-life is 1 to 3 days.
• *Excretion:* Excreted primarily in urine as conjugated metabolites; also in feces via bile as unchanged drug.

Contraindications and precautions
Contraindicated in patients who have received MAO inhibitors within 14 days; during acute recovery phase of MI; and in patients with hyperthyroidism, hypersensitivity to drug, heart block, arrhythmias, conduction disturbances, or heart failure. Use cautiously in elderly or debilitated patients and in those with increased intraocular pressure, glaucoma, or urine retention.

Interactions
Drug-drug. *Antidyskinetics, antimuscarinics (especially atropine and related compounds):* Antimuscarinic effects may be potentiated. Use together cautiously.
CNS depressants such as antipsychotics, anxiolytics, narcotics, parenteral magnesium salts, tricyclic antidepressants: May enhance CNS depressant effects. Use together cautiously.
Guanadrel, guanethidine: Decreased or blocked antihypertensive effects. Monitor blood pressure carefully.
MAO inhibitors: Hyperpyretic crisis, severe seizures, and death have resulted from tricyclic antidepressant-like effect of cyclobenzaprine. Concurrent use isn't recommended for outpatients. Allow 14 days after stopping MAO inhibitor before starting cyclobenzaprine, and 5 to 7 days after stopping cyclobenzaprine before start of MAO inhibitor.
Drug-lifestyle. *Alcohol:* May potentiate CNS depressant effects; discourage alcohol use.

Adverse reactions
CNS: *drowsiness,* headache, insomnia, fatigue, asthenia, nervousness, confusion, paresthesia, *dizziness,* depression, visual disturbances, *seizures.*
CV: tachycardia, syncope, *arrhythmias,* palpitations, hypotension, vasodilation.
EENT: blurred vision, *dry mouth.*
GI: dyspepsia, abnormal taste, constipation, nausea.

GU: urine retention, urinary frequency.
Skin: rash, urticaria, pruritus.
Other: with high doses, watch for adverse reactions similar to those of other tricyclic antidepressants.

☑ Special considerations
• Drug may cause effects and adverse reactions similar to those of tricyclic antidepressants.
• Note that drug's antimuscarinic effect may inhibit salivary flow, resulting in development of dental caries, periodontal disease, oral candidiasis, and mouth discomfort.
• Allow 14 days to elapse after stopping MAO inhibitors before starting cyclobenzaprine; 5 to 7 days after stopping cyclobenzaprine before starting MAO inhibitors.
• Drug is intended for short-term (2 or 3 weeks) treatment because risk-benefit ratio associated with prolonged use isn't known. Additionally, muscle spasm accompanying acute musculoskeletal conditions is usually transient.
• Spasmolytic effect usually begins within 1 or 2 days and may be manifested by reduction of pain and tenderness, increase range of motion, and ability to perform activities of daily living.
• Signs and symptoms of overdose include severe drowsiness, troubled breathing, syncope, seizures, tachycardia, arrhythmias, hallucinations, increase or decrease in body temperature, and vomiting.
• To treat overdose, induce emesis or perform gastric lavage. As ordered, give 20 to 30 g activated charcoal every 4 to 6 hours for 24 to 48 hours.
• Monitor ECG and cardiac functions for arrhythmias. Monitor vital signs, especially body temperature and ECG.
• Maintain adequate airway and fluid intake. If needed, 1 to 3 mg I.V. physostigmine may be given to combat severe life-threatening antimuscarinic effects. Provide supportive therapy for arrhythmias, cardiac failure, circulatory shock, seizures, and metabolic acidosis as necessary.

Monitoring the patient
• Monitor patient for GI problems.
• Closely monitor elderly patient for excessive CNS effects.

Information for the patient
• Warn patient about possible drowsiness and dizziness. Tell patient to avoid hazardous activities that require alertness until reaction to drug is known.
• Instruct patient to avoid alcohol and other CNS depressants (unless prescribed) because combined use with drug will cause additive effects.
• Advise patient to relieve dry mouth (anticholinergic effect) with frequent clear water rinses, extra fluid intake, or with sugarless gum or candy.
• Tell patient to report discomfort immediately.

Reactions may be common, uncommon, **life-threatening**, or COMMON AND LIFE-THREATENING.

- Inform patient to use cough and cold preparations cautiously because some products contain alcohol.
- Instruct patient to check with dentist to minimize risk of dental disease (tooth decay, fungal infections, or gum disease) if treatment lasts longer than 2 weeks.

Geriatric patients
- Elderly patients are more sensitive to drug's effects.

Pediatric patients
- Drug isn't recommended for children under age 15.

Breast-feeding patients
- It's unknown whether drug appears in breast milk. Use with caution in breast-feeding women.

cyclopentolate hydrochloride
AK-Pentolate, Cyclogyl, Minims Cyclopentolate*, Pentolair

Pharmacologic classification: anticholinergic
Therapeutic classification: cycloplegic, mydriatic
Pregnancy risk category C

How supplied
Available by prescription only
Ophthalmic solution: 0.5%, 1%, 2%

Indications, route, and dosage
Diagnostic procedures requiring mydriasis and cycloplegia
Adults: Instill 1 drop of 1% solution in eye, then another drop in 5 minutes, 40 to 50 minutes before procedure. Use 2% solution in heavily pigmented irises.
Children: Instill 1 drop of 0.5%, 1%, or 2% solution in each eye, then 1 drop of 0.5% or 1% solution in 5 minutes, if necessary, 40 to 50 minutes before procedure.

Pharmacodynamics
Cycloplegic and mydriatic action: Anticholinergic action prevents the sphincter muscle of the iris and the muscle of the ciliary body from responding to cholinergic stimulation. This results in unopposed adrenergic influence, producing pupillary dilation (mydriasis) and paralysis of accommodation (cycloplegia).

Pharmacokinetics
- *Absorption:* Peak mydriatic effect occurs within 15 to 60 minutes and cycloplegic effect within 15 to 60 minutes.
- *Distribution:* No information available.
- *Metabolism:* No information available.

- *Excretion:* Recovery from mydriasis usually occurs in about 24 hours; recovery from cycloplegia may occur in 6 to 24 hours.

Contraindications and precautions
Contraindicated in patients with glaucoma, hypersensitivity to drug or belladonna alkaloids, or adhesions between the iris and lens. Use cautiously in children, elderly patients, and in patients with increased intraocular pressure.

Interactions
Drug-drug. *Carbachol, cholinesterase inhibitors, pilocarpine:* Cyclopentolate may interfere with the antiglaucoma action. Use together cautiously.

Adverse reactions
CNS: irritability, confusion, somnolence, hallucinations, ataxia, *seizures,* behavioral disturbances in children.
CV: tachycardia.
EENT: eye burning on instillation, blurred vision, eye dryness, *photophobia,* ocular congestion, contact dermatitis in eye, conjunctivitis, increased intraocular pressure, transient stinging and burning, irritation, hyperemia.
GU: urine retention.
Skin: dryness.

☑ Special considerations
- Superior to homatropine hydrobromide, cyclopentolate has a shorter duration of action.
- Recovery usually occurs within 24 hours; however, 1 to 2 drops of a 1% or 2% pilocarpine solution instilled into eye may reduce recovery time to 3 to 6 hours.
- To minimize systemic absorption, physician should apply light finger-pressure to lacrimal sac during and for 1 to 2 minutes following topical instillation especially in children and when 2% solution is used.
- Signs and symptoms of overdose include flushing, warm dry skin, dry mouth, dilated pupils, delirium, hallucinations, tachycardia, bladder distention, ataxia, hypotension, respiratory depression, coma, and death.
- Induce emesis or give activated charcoal.
- Use physostigmine to antagonize cyclopentolate's anticholinergic activity, and in severe toxicity; propranolol may be used to treat symptomatic tachyarrhythmias unresponsive to physostigmine.

Monitoring the patient
- Monitor patient for adverse effects.
- Carefully observe elderly patient for enhanced CNS effects.

Information for the patient
- Warn patient that drug will cause burning sensation when instilled.
- Advise patient to protect eyes from bright illumination; dark glasses may reduce sensitivity.

• Tell patient to use care to avoid contamination of dropper tip.

Geriatric patients
• Use drug with caution in elderly patients because undiagnosed narrow-angle glaucoma may be present.

Pediatric patients
• Avoid getting preparation in child's mouth while administering.
• Infants and young children may experience an increased sensitivity to cardiopulmonary and CNS effects of drug.
• Young infants shouldn't be given solution more concentrated than 0.5%.

Breast-feeding patients
• No data are available; however, use drug with extreme caution in breast-feeding women because of potential for CNS and cardiopulmonary effects in infants.

---

cyclophosphamide
Cytoxan, Neosar

Pharmacologic classification: alkylating drug (cell-cycle–phase nonspecific)
Therapeutic classification: antineoplastic
Pregnancy risk category D

How supplied
Available by prescription only
Tablets: 25 mg, 50 mg
Injection: 100-mg, 200-mg, 500-mg, 1-g, 2-g vials

Indications, route, and dosage
Dosage and indications may vary. Check literature for recommended protocols.
Breast, head, neck, lung, and ovarian carcinoma; Hodgkin's disease; chronic lymphocytic or myelocytic and acute lymphoblastic leukemia; neuroblastoma; retinoblastoma; malignant lymphomas; multiple myeloma; mycosis fungoides; sarcomas; severe rheumatoid disorders; glomerular and nephrotic syndrome (in children); immunosuppression after transplants
Adults: 40 to 50 mg/kg I.V. in divided doses over 2 to 5 days. Oral dosing for initial and maintenance dosage is 1 to 5 mg/kg P.O. daily.
◇ **Polymyositis**
Adults: 1 to 2 mg/kg P.O. daily.
◇ **Rheumatoid arthritis**
Adults: 1.5 to 3 mg/kg P.O. daily.
◇ **Wegener's granulomatosis**
Adults: 1 to 2 mg/kg P.O. daily (usually administered with prednisone).
◇ **Nephrotic syndrome in children**
Children: 2.5 to 3 mg/kg P.O. daily for 60 to 90 days.

✦ *Dosage adjustment.* Adjust dosage of cyclophosphamide in patients with renal impairment.

Pharmacodynamics
Antineoplastic action: Cytotoxic action is mediated by its two active metabolites. These metabolites have alkylating functions, preventing cell division by cross-linking DNA strands. This results in an imbalance of growth within the cell, leading to cell death. Also has significant immunosuppressive activity.

Pharmacokinetics
• *Absorption:* Almost completely absorbed from GI tract at doses of 100 mg or less. Higher doses (300 mg) about 75% absorbed.
• *Distribution:* Distributed throughout body, although only minimal amounts have been found in saliva, sweat, and synovial fluid. CSF concentration too low for treatment of meningeal leukemia. Active metabolites about 50% bound to plasma proteins.
• *Metabolism:* Metabolized to active form by hepatic microsomal enzymes. Metabolites' activity terminated by metabolism to inactive forms.
• *Excretion:* Drug and its metabolites eliminated primarily in urine, with 15% to 30% excreted as unchanged drug. Elimination half-life ranges from 3 to 12 hours.

Contraindications and precautions
Contraindicated in patients with hypersensitivity to drug or with severe bone marrow suppression. Use cautiously in patients with impaired renal or hepatic function, leukopenia, thrombocytopenia, or malignant cell infiltration of bone marrow and in those who have recently undergone radiation therapy or chemotherapy.

Interactions
Drug-drug. *Allopurinol, chloramphenicol, chloroquine, imipramine, phenothiazines, potassium iodide, vitamin A:* May inhibit cyclophosphamide metabolism. Use together cautiously.
Barbiturates, chloral hydrate, phenytoin: Increases rate of metabolism of cyclophosphamide. These drugs are known to be inducers of hepatic microsomal enzymes. Use together with caution.
Corticosteroids: Initially inhibit metabolism of cyclophosphamide, reducing its effect. Eventual reduction of dose or discontinuation of corticosteroids may increase metabolism of cyclophosphamide to a toxic level. Use together cautiously.
Doxorubicin: May potentiate cardiotoxic effects. Use with caution.
Succinylcholine: Prolonged respiratory distress and apnea. This may occur up to several days after stopping cyclophosphamide. Cyclophosphamide depresses the activity of pseudocholinesterases, the enzyme responsible for inactivation of succinylcholine. Use succinylcholine with caution or not at all.

Reactions may be *common*, uncommon, **life-threatening**, or COMMON AND LIFE-THREATENING.

Adverse reactions
CV: *cardiotoxicity* (with very high doses and with doxorubicin).
GI: anorexia, *nausea, vomiting* (within 6 hours); abdominal pain; stomatitis; mucositis, **hepatotoxicity.**
GU: HEMORRHAGIC CYSTITIS, fertility impairment.
Hematologic: *leukopenia,* nadir between days 8 to 15, recovery in 17 to 28 days; **thrombocytopenia; anemia.**
Respiratory: *pulmonary fibrosis* (with high doses).
Other: *reversible alopecia,* **secondary malignant disease, anaphylaxis,** hypersensitivity reactions; increased serum uric acid levels and decreased serum pseudocholinesterase levels.

☑ Special considerations
• Follow institutional guidelines for safe preparation, administration, and disposal of chemotherapeutic drugs.
• Reconstitute vials with appropriate volume of bacteriostatic or sterile water for injection to give a concentration of 20 mg/ml.
• Reconstituted solution is stable 6 days if refrigerated or 24 hours at room temperature.
• Drug can be given by direct I.V. push into a running I.V. line or by infusion in normal saline solution or D₅W.
• Avoid all I.M. injections when platelet counts are low.
• Oral medication should be taken with or after a meal. Higher oral doses (400 mg) may be tolerated better if divided into smaller doses.
• Administration with cold foods such as ice cream may improve toleration of oral dose.
• Push fluid (3 L daily) to prevent hemorrhagic cystitis. Some clinicians use uroprotectant drugs such as mesna. Drug shouldn't be given at bedtime because voiding afterward is too infrequent to avoid cystitis. If hemorrhagic cystitis occurs, stop drug. Cystitis can occur months after therapy has ended.
• Reduce drug dosage if patient is also receiving corticosteroid therapy and develops viral or bacterial infections.
• Nausea and vomiting are most common with high doses of I.V. cyclophosphamide.
• Drug has been used successfully to treat many nonmalignant conditions (such as multiple sclerosis) because of its immunosuppressive activity.
• Drug may suppress positive reaction to *Candida,* mumps, trichophytin, and tuberculin TB skin tests.
• A false-positive result for the Papanicolaou test may occur.
• Signs and symptoms of overdose include myelosuppression, alopecia, nausea, vomiting, and anorexia.
• Treatment of overdose is supportive and includes transfusion of blood components and antiemetics.

• Drug is dialyzable.

Monitoring the patient
• Monitor patient for cyclophosphamide toxicity if patient's corticosteroid therapy ends.
• Monitor uric acid, CBC, and renal and hepatic functions.
• Urine should be examined regularly for red cells which may recede hemorrhagic cystitis.

Information for the patient
• Advise both men and women to practice contraception while taking drug and for 4 months after because drug has teratogenic properties.
• Emphasize importance of continuing drug despite nausea and vomiting.
• Advise patient to report vomiting that occurs shortly after an oral dose.
• Warn patient that alopecia is likely to occur, but is reversible.
• Encourage adequate fluid intake to prevent hemorrhagic cystitis and to facilitate uric acid excretion.
• Tell patient to promptly report unusual bleeding or bruising.
• Advise patient to avoid individuals with infections and to call immediately if fever, chills, or signs of infection occur.

Breast-feeding patients
• Drug appears in breast milk; discontinue breast-feeding because of risk of serious adverse reactions, mutagenicity, and carcinogenicity in infant.

cycloserine
Seromycin

Pharmacologic classification: isoxizolidone, d-alanine analogue
Therapeutic classification: antituberculotic
Pregnancy risk category C

How supplied
Available by prescription only
Capsules: 250 mg

Indications, route, and dosage
Adjunctive treatment in pulmonary or extrapulmonary tuberculosis
Adults: Initially, 250 mg P.O. q 12 hours for 2 weeks; then, if blood levels are below 25 to 30 mcg/ml and there are no clinical signs of toxicity, increase to 250 mg P.O. q 8 hours for 2 weeks. If optimum blood levels still aren't achieved and there are no signs of clinical toxicity, then increase to 250 mg P.O. q 6 hours. Maximum dosage is 1 g/day. If CNS toxicity occurs, stop drug for 1 week, then resume at 250 mg/ day for 2 weeks. If no serious toxic effects occur, increase by 250-mg increments q 10 days until blood levels reach 25 to 30 mcg/ml.

◇ *Children:* 10 to 20 mg/kg (maximum, 750 to 1,000 mg) daily administered in two equally divided doses.
Urinary tract infections
Adults: 250 mg P.O. q 12 hours for 2 weeks.

Pharmacodynamics

Antibiotic action: Inhibits bacterial cell utilization of amino acids, thereby inhibiting cell-wall synthesis. Its action is bacteriostatic or bactericidal, depending on organism susceptibility and drug concentration at infection site. Active against *Mycobacterium tuberculosis, M. bovis,* and some strains of *M. kansasii, M. marinum, M. ulcerans, M. avium, M. smegmatis,* and *M. intracellulare.* It's also active against some gram-negative and gram-positive bacteria, including *Staphylococcus aureus, Enterobacter,* and *Escherichia coli.* Considered adjunctive therapy in tuberculosis and is combined with other antituberculosis drugs to prevent or delay development of drug resistance by *Mycobacterium tuberculosis.*

Pharmacokinetics

● *Absorption:* 80% of oral dose absorbed from GI tract; peak serum levels occur 3 to 4 hours after ingestion.
● *Distribution:* Distributed widely into body tissues and fluids, including CSF. Drug crosses placenta; doesn't bind to plasma proteins.
● *Metabolism:* May be metabolized partially.
● *Excretion:* Excreted primarily in urine by glomerular filtration. Small amounts of drug excreted in feces and breast milk. Elimination plasma half-life in adults is 10 hours. Drug is hemodialyzable.

Contraindications and precautions

Contraindicated in patients with hypersensitivity to drug and in those with seizure disorders, depression or severe anxiety, psychosis, severe renal insufficiency, or excessive concurrent use of alcohol. Use cautiously in patients with impaired renal function.

Interactions

Drug-drug. *Ethionamide, isoniazid:* Increases hazard of CNS toxicity, drowsiness, and dizziness. Monitor patient carefully.
Phenytoin: Inhibited metabolism, producing toxic blood levels of phenytoin. Dosage adjustment may be required.
Drug-lifestyle. *Alcohol:* May increase risk of seizures. Don't use together.

Adverse reactions

CNS: *seizures,* drowsiness, somnolence, headache, tremor, dysarthria, vertigo, confusion, loss of memory, *possible suicidal tendencies,* psychosis, hyper-irritability, character changes, aggression, paresthesia, paresis, hyperreflexia, **coma.**

CV: *sudden-onset heart failure.*
Skin: hypersensitivity reactions (allergic dermatitis), rash.
Other: elevated transaminase level.

☑ Special considerations

● Give drug after meals to avoid gastric irritation.
● Obtain specimens for culture and sensitivity testing before first dose. Therapy may begin pending test results. Repeat periodically to detect drug resistance.
● Pyridoxine (200 to 300 mg daily) may be used to treat or prevent neurotoxic effects.
● Anticonvulsants, tranquilizers, or sedatives may be prescribed to relieve adverse reactions.
● Signs of overdose include CNS depression accompanied by dizziness, hyperreflexia, confusion, or seizures.
● Treat overdose with gastric lavage and supportive care, including oxygen, I.V. fluids, pressor drugs (for circulatory shock), and body temperature stabilization.
● Treat seizures with anticonvulsants and pyridoxine.

Monitoring the patient

● Monitor hematologic, renal, and liver function studies before and periodically during therapy to minimize toxicity; toxic reactions may occur at blood levels in excess of 30 mcg/ml.
● Assess level of consciousness and neurologic function; monitor patient for personality changes and other early signs of CNS toxicity.

Information for the patient

● Explain disease process and rationale for long-term therapy.
● Teach signs and symptoms of hypersensitivity and other adverse reactions, and emphasize need to report any unusual effects and rash promptly.
● Warn patient to avoid hazardous tasks that require mental alertness because drug may cause patient to become drowsy or dizzy.
● Warn patient not to use alcohol; explain hazard of serious CNS toxicity.
● Advise patient to take drug after meals to avoid gastric irritation.
● Urge patient to complete entire prescribed regimen, to comply with instructions for around-the-clock dosage, and not to stop drug without medical approval.
● Explain importance of follow-up appointments.

Geriatric patients

● Because elderly patients commonly have renal impairment, which decreases excretion of drugs, use drug with caution.

Pediatric patients

● Safety and effectiveness in children haven't been established.

Reactions may be *common,* uncommon, *life-threatening,* or COMMON AND LIFE-THREATENING.

Breast-feeding patients
● Drug appears in breast milk; use cautiously in breast-feeding women.

cyclosporine
Neoral, Sandimmune

Pharmacologic classification: polypeptide antibiotic
Therapeutic classification: immunosuppressant
Pregnancy risk category C

How supplied
Available by prescription only
Capsules: 25 mg, 50 mg, 100 mg
Oral solution: 100 mg/ml
Capsules for microemulsion: 25 mg, 100 mg
Injection: 50 mg/ml

Indications, route, and dosage
Prophylaxis of organ rejection in kidney, liver, heart, bone marrow, ◊ pancreas, ◊ cornea transplants
Adults and children: 15 mg/kg P.O. daily 4 to 12 hours before transplantation. Continue daily dose postoperatively for 1 to 2 weeks. Then gradually reduce dosage by 5% weekly to maintenance level of 5 to 10 mg/kg/day. Or administer an I.V. concentrate of 5 to 6 mg/kg 4 to 12 hours before transplantation.

Postoperatively, administer 5 to 6 mg/kg daily as an I.V. dilute solution infusion (50 mg per 20 to 100 ml infused over 2 to 6 hours) until patient can tolerate oral forms.

Note: Sandimmune and Neoral aren't bioequivalent and can't be used interchangeably without physician supervision. When converting to Neoral from Sandimmune, start with same daily dose (1:1) and follow serum trough levels frequently.

Pharmacodynamics
Immunosuppressant action: Exact mechanism is unknown; purportedly, its action is related to the inhibition of induction of interleukin II, which plays a role in both cellular and humoral immune responses.

Pharmacokinetics
● *Absorption:* Varies widely between patients and in same individual after oral administration. Only 30% of oral dose reaches systemic circulation; peak levels occur at 3 to 4 hours. Neoral has a greater bioavailability than Sandimmune.
● *Distribution:* Distributed widely outside blood volume. About 33% to 47% found in plasma; 4% to 9% in leukocytes; 5% to 12% in granulocytes; and 41% to 58% bound in erythrocytes. In plasma, about 90% is bound to proteins, primarily lipoproteins. Drug crosses placenta; cord blood levels are about 60% those of maternal blood. Drug enters breast milk.

● *Metabolism:* Metabolized extensively in liver.
● *Excretion:* Drug is primarily excreted in feces (biliary excretion) with only 6% of drug found in urine.

Contraindications and precautions
Contraindicated in patients hypersensitive to drug or to polyoxyethylated castor oil (found in injectable form).

Interactions
Drug-drug. *Aminoglycosides, amphotericin B:* Increased nephrotoxicity. Monitor patient carefully.

Co-trimoxazole, phenobarbital, phenytoin, rifampin: Increased hepatic metabolism; may lower plasma levels of cyclosporine. Monitor cyclosporine levels.

Diltiazem, erythromycin, fluconazole, itraconazole, ketoconazole, verapamil, possibly corticosteroids: Impaired hepatic enzyme metabolism and increased plasma cyclosporine levels; reduced dosage of cyclosporine may be needed.

Immunosuppressants (except for corticosteroids): Increased risk of malignancy (lymphoma) and susceptibility to infection. Don't use concomitantly.

Drug-food. *Food, grapefruit juice:* Decreased cyclosporine levels. Don't take with food or grapefruit juice.

Drug-herb. *Pill-bearing spurge:* May inhibit enzyme affecting drug metabolism. Use together cautiously.

Adverse reactions
CNS: *tremor, headache, **seizures,** confusion,* paresthesia.
CV: *hypertension.*
EENT: *gum hyperplasia,* oral candidiasis, sinusitis.
GI: *nausea, vomiting,* diarrhea, abdominal discomfort.
GU: NEPHROTOXICITY.
Hematologic: anemia, ***leukopenia, thrombocytopenia,*** hemolytic anemia.
Hepatic: *hepatotoxicity.*
Skin: acne, flushing.
Other: increased low-density lipoprotein levels, ***infections,*** hirsutism, ***anaphylaxis,*** gynecomastia.

☑ Special considerations
● Cyclosporine usually is prescribed with corticosteroids.
● Possible kidney rejection should be considered before stopping drug for suspected nephrotoxicity.
● Give dose at same time each day. Measure oral solution carefully in oral syringe and mix with plain or chocolate milk or fruit juice to increase palatability; serve in a glass to minimize drug adherence to container walls. Drug can be taken with food to minimize nausea.
● Neoral capsules and oral solution are bioequivalent. Sandimmune capsules and oral solution have decreased bioavailability compared with Neoral.

• Signs and symptoms of overdose include extensions of common adverse effects. Hepatotoxicity and nephrotoxicity often accompany nausea and vomiting; tremor and seizures may occur.
• Up to 2 hours after toxic ingestion, empty stomach by induced emesis or lavage; then treat supportively.
• Monitor vital signs and fluid and electrolyte levels closely. Drug isn't removed by hemodialysis or charcoal hemoperfusion.

Monitoring the patient
• Monitor hepatic and renal function tests routinely; hepatotoxicity may occur in first month after transplantation, but renal toxicity may be delayed for 2 to 3 months.
• Monitor patient for therapeutic drug levels periodically.

Information for the patient
• Teach patient about rationale for therapy; explain possible adverse effects and importance of reporting them, especially fever, sore throat, mouth sores, abdominal pain, unusual bleeding or bruising, pale stools, or dark urine.
• Encourage compliance with therapy and follow-up visits.
• Teach patient how and when to take medication for optimal benefit and minimal discomfort; caution against stopping drug without medical approval.
• Advise patient to make oral solution more palatable by diluting with room temperature milk, chocolate milk, or orange juice. Don't take Neoral with grapefruit juice or food.
• Tell patient not to rinse syringe with water.

Pediatric patients
• Safety and efficacy haven't been established; however, drug has been used in children as young as 6 months. Use with caution.

Breast-feeding patients
• Safety hasn't been established; breast-feeding women should avoid drug.

cyproheptadine hydrochloride
Periactin

Pharmacologic classification: piperidine-derivative antihistamine
Therapeutic classification: antihistamine (H₁-receptor antagonist), antipruritic
Pregnancy risk category B

How supplied
Available by prescription only
Tablets: 4 mg
Syrup: 2 mg/5 ml

Indications, route, and dosage
Allergy symptoms, pruritus, cold urticaria, allergic conjunctivitis, appetite stimulant, vascular cluster headaches
Adults: 4 mg P.O. t.i.d. or q.i.d. Maximum dosage, 0.5 mg/kg daily.
Children ages 7 to 14: 4 mg P.O. b.i.d. or t.i.d. Maximum dosage, 16 mg daily.
Children ages 2 to 6: 2 mg P.O. b.i.d. or t.i.d. Maximum dosage, 12 mg daily.
◇ *Cushing's syndrome*
Adults: 8 to 24 mg P.O. daily in divided doses.

Pharmacodynamics
Antihistamine action: Antihistamines compete with histamine for histamine H₁-receptor sites on smooth muscle of the bronchi, GI tract, uterus, and large blood vessels; they bind to cellular receptors, preventing access of histamine, thereby suppressing histamine-induced allergic symptoms. They don't directly alter histamine or its release.
Drug also displays significant anticholinergic and antiserotonin activity.

Pharmacokinetics
• *Absorption:* Well absorbed from GI tract; peak action occurs in 6 to 9 hours.
• *Distribution:* No information available.
• *Metabolism:* Drug appears to be almost completely metabolized in liver.
• *Excretion:* Metabolites excreted primarily in urine; unchanged drug isn't excreted in urine. Small amounts of unchanged cyproheptadine and metabolites excreted in feces.

Contraindications and precautions
Contraindicated in patients with hypersensitivity to drug or other drugs of similar chemical structure; in those with acute asthma, angle-closure glaucoma, stenosing peptic ulcer, symptomatic prostatic hyperplasia, bladder neck obstruction, and pyloroduodenal obstruction; in concurrent therapy with MAO inhibitors; in neonates or premature infants; in elderly or debilitated patients; and in breast-feeding patients.
Use cautiously in patients with increased intraocular pressure, hyperthyroidism, CV disease, hypertension, or bronchial asthma.

Interactions
Drug-drug. *CNS depressants such as antianxiety drugs, barbiturates, sleeping aids, tranquilizers:* Additive sedative effects. Monitor patient closely.
MAO inhibitors: Prolonged central depressant and anticholinergic effects; monitor patient closely.
Thyrotropin-releasing hormone: Serum amylase and prolactin levels may be increased. Monitor drug levels.

Drug-lifestyle. *Alcohol:* Additive sedative effects. Discourage alcohol use.

Adverse reactions
CNS: *drowsiness,* dizziness, headache, fatigue, sedation, sleepiness, incoordination, confusion, restlessness, insomnia, nervousness, tremor, *seizures.*
CV: hypotension, palpitations, tachycardia.
GI: nausea, vomiting, epigastric distress, *dry mouth,* diarrhea, constipation.
GU: urine retention, urinary frequency.
Hematologic: hemolytic anemia, leukopenia, *agranulocytosis, thrombocytopenia.*
Skin: rash, urticaria, photosensitivity.
Other: weight gain, *anaphylactic shock.*

☑ Special considerations
Besides the recommendations relevant to all antihistamines, consider the following.
• Drug also has been used experimentally to stimulate appetite and increase weight gain in children.
• In some patients, sedative effect disappears within 3 or 4 days.
• Stop drug 4 days before diagnostic skin tests. Antihistamines can prevent, reduce, or mask positive skin test response.
• Signs and symptoms of overdose may include either CNS depression (sedation, reduced mental alertness, apnea, and CV collapse) or CNS stimulation (insomnia, hallucinations, tremors, or seizures). Anticholinergic symptoms, such as dry mouth, flushed skin, fixed and dilated pupils, and GI symptoms, are common, especially in children.
• Treat overdose by inducing emesis with ipecac syrup (in conscious patient), then activated charcoal to reduce further drug absorption. Use gastric lavage if patient is unconscious or ipecac fails.
• Treat hypotension with vasopressors, and control seizures with diazepam or phenytoin. Don't give stimulants.

Monitoring the patient
• Drug can cause weight gain. Monitor weight.
• Monitor CBC, as needed, to assess hematologic effects.

Information for the patient
• Inform patient about potential adverse reactions.

Geriatric patients
• Elderly patients are more susceptible to sedative effect of drug. Instruct patient to change positions slowly and gradually. Elderly patients may experience dizziness or hypotension more readily than younger patients.

Pediatric patients
• CNS stimulation (agitation, confusion, tremors, hallucinations) is more common in children and may require dosage reduction. Drug isn't indicated for use in newborn or premature infants.

Breast-feeding patients
• Antihistamines such as cyproheptadine shouldn't be used during breast-feeding. Many of these drugs appear in breast milk, exposing infant to risks of unusual excitability; premature infants are at particular risk for seizures.

cytarabine (ara-C, cytosine arabinoside)
Cytosar-U

Pharmacologic classification: antimetabolite (cell-cycle–phase specific, S phase)
Therapeutic classification: antineoplastic
Pregnancy risk category D

How supplied
Available by prescription only
Injection: 100-mg, 500-mg, 1-g, 2-g vials

Indications, route, and dosage
Dosage and indications may vary. Check literature for recommended protocols.
Acute myelocytic and other acute leukemias
Adults and children: 100 mg/m^2 I.V. once daily or q 12 hours by continuous I.V. infusion or rapid I.V. injection in divided doses for 5 days at 2-week intervals for remission induction; or 30 mg/m^2 intrathecally (range, 5 to 75 mg/m^2) q 4 days until CSF findings are normal, then one additional dose. Dosages up to 3 g/m^2 q 12 hours for up to 12 doses have been given by continuous infusion for refractory acute leukemias.

Pharmacodynamics
Antineoplastic action: Requires conversion to its active metabolite within the cell. This metabolite acts as a competitive inhibitor of the enzyme DNA polymerase, disrupting the normal synthesis of DNA.

Pharmacokinetics
• *Absorption:* Poorly absorbed (less than 20%) across GI tract because of rapid deactivation in gut lumen. After I.M. or subcutaneous administration, peak plasma levels are less than after I.V. administration.
• *Distribution:* Rapidly distributed widely through body. About 13% of drug is bound to plasma proteins. Drug penetrates blood-brain barrier only slightly after rapid I.V. dose; however, when administered by continuous I.V. infusion, CSF levels achieve a concentration 40% to 60% of that of plasma levels.
• *Metabolism:* Metabolized primarily in liver but also in kidneys, GI mucosa, and granulocytes.

• *Excretion:* Biphasic elimination of drug, with initial half-life of 8 minutes and terminal phase half-life of 1 to 3 hours. Cytarabine and its metabolites excreted in urine. Less than 10% of dose excreted as unchanged drug in urine.

Contraindications and precautions
Contraindicated in patients hypersensitive to drug. Use cautiously in patients with impaired hepatic function.

Interactions
Drug-drug. *Combination chemotherapy (including cytarabine):* May decrease digoxin absorption even several days after stopping chemotherapy. Digoxin capsules and digitoxin don't appear to be affected.
Gentamicin: May antagonize gentamicin effect. Use together cautiously.
Methotrexate: Reduced effectiveness. Use together cautiously.

Adverse reactions
CNS: neurotoxicity, malaise, dizziness, headache.
EENT: conjunctivitis.
GI: *nausea, vomiting,* diarrhea, anorexia, anal ulcer, abdominal pain, oral ulcers in 5 to 10 days, high dose given rapidly I.V. may cause projectile vomiting.
GU: renal dysfunction.
Hematologic: *leukopenia,* with initial WBC count nadir 7 to 9 days after drug is stopped and a second (more severe) nadir 15 to 24 days after drug is stopped; anemia; reticulocytopenia; *thrombocytopenia,* with platelet count nadir occurring between days 12 and 15; *megaloblastosis.*
Hepatic: hepatotoxicity (usually mild and reversible), jaundice.
Musculoskeletal: myalgia, bone pain.
Skin: rash, pruritus.
Other: flulike symptoms, hyperuricemia, infection, fever, thrombophlebitis, *anaphylaxis,* edema.

☑ Special considerations
• To reconstitute 100-mg vial for I.V. administration use 5 ml bacteriostatic water for injection (20 mg/ml); for 500-mg vial use 10 ml bacteriostatic water for injection (50 mg/ml).
• Drug may be further diluted with D_5W or normal saline solution for continuous I.V. infusion.
• For intrathecal injection, dilute drug in 5 to 15 ml of lactated Ringer's solution, Elliot's B solution, or normal saline solution with no preservative, and administer after withdrawing an equivalent volume of CSF.
• Don't reconstitute drug with bacteriostatic diluent for intrathecal administration because the preservative, benzyl alcohol, has been associated with a higher risk of neurologic toxicity.

• Reconstituted solutions are stable for 48 hours at room temperature. Infusion solutions up to a concentration of 5 mg/ml are stable for 7 days at room temperature. Discard cloudy reconstituted solution.
• Dose modification may be required in thrombocytopenia, leukopenia, renal or hepatic disease, and after other chemotherapy or radiation therapy.
• Excellent mouth care can help prevent adverse oral reactions.
• Nausea and vomiting are more frequent when large doses are administered rapidly by I.V. push. These reactions are less frequent with infusion. To reduce nausea, give antiemetic before administering.
• Prescribe steroid eyedrops (dexamethasone) to prevent drug-induced keratitis.
• Avoid I.M. injections of any drugs in patients with severely depressed platelet count (thrombocytopenia) to prevent bleeding.
• Pyridoxine supplements may be administered to prevent neuropathies; reportedly, however, prophylactic use of pyridoxine doesn't prevent cytarabine neurotoxicity.
• Signs and symptoms of overdose include myelosuppression, nausea, vomiting, and megaloblastosis.
• Treatment is usually supportive and includes transfusion of blood components and antiemetics.

Monitoring the patient
• Watch for signs of infection (cough, fever, sore throat). Monitor CBC.
• Monitor intake and output carefully. Maintain high fluid intake and give allopurinol, if ordered, to avoid urate nephropathy in leukemia induction therapy. Monitor uric acid and plasma digoxin levels.
• Monitor hepatic function.
• Monitor patients receiving high doses for cerebellar dysfunction.

Information for the patient
• Encourage adequate fluid intake to increase urine output and facilitate excretion of uric acid.
• Advise patient to avoid exposure to people with infections. Tell patient to call immediately if signs of infection or unusual bleeding occurs.

Breast-feeding patients
• It isn't known if drug appears in breast milk. However, because of risk of serious adverse reactions, mutagenicity, and carcinogenicity in infant, breast-feeding isn't recommended.

Reactions may be *common,* uncommon, *life-threatening,* or COMMON AND LIFE-THREATENING.

dacarbazine (DTIC)
DTIC-Dome

Pharmacologic classification: alkylating
drug (cell cycle–phase nonspecific)
Therapeutic classification: antineoplastic
Pregnancy risk category C

How supplied
Available by prescription only
Injection: 10 mg/ml

Indications, route, and dosage
Dosage and indications may vary. Check current
literature for recommended protocols.
Metastatic malignant melanoma
Adults: 2 to 4.5 mg/kg I.V. daily for 10 days; then
repeat q 4 weeks as tolerated. Or 250 mg/m² I.V.
daily for 5 days, repeated at 3-week intervals.
Hodgkin's disease
Adults: 150 mg/m² I.V. (with other drugs) for 5
days, repeated q 4 weeks; or 375 mg/m² on day
1 of a combination regimen, repeated q 15 days.
✦ Dosage adjustment. Reduce dosage when
giving repeated doses to patients with severely
impaired renal function. Use lower dose if renal
function or bone marrow is impaired.

Pharmacodynamics
Antineoplastic action: Three mechanisms have
been proposed to explain the cytotoxicity of dacarbazine: alkylation, in which DNA and RNA synthesis are inhibited; antimetabolite activity as a
false precursor for purine synthesis; and binding
with protein sulfhydryl groups.

Pharmacokinetics
• *Absorption:* Not administered orally because
of poor absorption from GI tract.
• *Distribution:* Believed to localize in body tissues, especially liver. Crosses blood-brain barrier to limited extent; minimally bound to plasma
proteins.
• *Metabolism:* Rapidly metabolized in liver to several compounds, some of which may be active.
• *Excretion:* Eliminated in biphasic manner; initial phase half-life of 19 minutes and terminal
phase of 5 hours in patients with normal renal
and hepatic function. About 30% to 45% excreted unchanged in urine.

Contraindications and precautions
Contraindicated in patients with hypersensitivity
to drug. Use cautiously in patients with impaired
bone marrow function.

Interactions
Drug-drug. *Allopurinol:* May potentiate activity
of allopurinol because of inhibition of xanthine
oxidase. Avoid concomitant use.
Amphotericin B: May increase risk of nephrotoxicity. Avoid concomitant use.
Anticoagulants, aspirin: May cause increased risk
of bleeding. Monitor closely.
Bone marrow suppressants: May cause additive
toxicity. Monitor closely.
*Phenobarbital, phenytoin, other drugs that in-
duce hepatic metabolism:* May enhance dacarbazine activation and increase risk of toxicity. Use
cautiously and monitor patient closely.
Drug-lifestyle. *Sun exposure:* Photosensitivity
reactions may occur, especially during first 2 days
of therapy. Tell patient to take precautions in sun.

Adverse reactions
CNS: facial paresthesia.
GI: *severe nausea and vomiting, anorexia.*
GU: increased serum BUN level.
Hematologic: *leukopenia, thrombocytopenia.*
Hepatic: transient increase in liver enzyme lev-
els.
Skin: phototoxicity, rash, facial flushing.
Other: *flulike syndrome* (fever, malaise, and myal-
gia beginning 7 days after treatment ends and
lasting possibly 7 to 21 days), alopecia, severe
pain (if I.V. solution infiltrates or if solution is too
concentrated); tissue damage, *anaphylaxis.*

☑ Special considerations
• Follow all procedures for safe handling, administration, and disposal of chemotherapeutic drugs.
• To reconstitute drug for I.V. administration, use
a volume of sterile water for injection that gives
a concentration of 10 mg/ml (9.9 ml for 100-mg
vial, 19.7 ml for 200-mg vial).
• Drug may be diluted further with D₅W or normal saline solution to a volume of 100 to 200 ml
for I.V. infusion over 30 minutes. Increase volume
or slow the rate of infusion to decrease pain at
infusion site.
• Drug may be administered by I.V. push over 1
to 2 minutes.
• A change in solution color from ivory to pink indicates some drug degradation. During infusion,

protect solution from light to avoid possible drug breakdown.
• Discard refrigerated solution after 72 hours; room temperature solution after 8 hours.
• Minimize nausea and vomiting by administering dacarbazine by I.V. infusion and by hydrating patient 4 to 6 hours before therapy.
• Monitor daily temperature. Observe for signs of infection.
• Avoid all I.M. injections when platelet count is below 100,000/mm³.
• Use anticoagulants and aspirin products with caution. Watch closely for signs of bleeding.
• Signs and symptoms of overdose include myelosuppression and diarrhea. Treatment is supportive and includes transfusion of blood components and monitoring of hematologic parameters.

Monitoring the patient
• Monitor uric acid levels.
• Stop drug if WBC count falls to 3,000/mm³ or platelet count drops to 100,000/mm³. Monitor CBC.
• Treatment of extravasation with application of hot packs may relieve burning sensation, local pain, and irritation.

Information for the patient
• Advise patient to avoid sunlight and sunlamps for first 2 days after treatment.
• Instruct patient to avoid contact with people who have infections and to report signs of infection or unusual bleeding immediately.
• Reassure patient that hair should start growing 4 to 8 weeks after treatment has ended, but is usually of a different texture, and its color will be lost as therapy continues.
• Reassure patient that flulike syndrome may be treated with mild antipyretics such as acetaminophen.
• Tell patient to avoid aspirin and products containing aspirin. Teach patient signs and symptoms of bleeding; urge him to report them promptly.

Breast-feeding patients
• It's unknown if drug appears in breast milk. Because of risk of serious adverse reactions, mutagenicity, and carcinogenicity in infant, breast-feeding isn't recommended during therapy.

daclizumab
Zenapax

Pharmacologic classification: humanized immunoglobulin G1 monoclonal antibody
Therapeutic classification: immunosuppressant
Pregnancy risk category C

How supplied
Available by prescription only
Injection (for I.V. use): 25 mg/5 ml

Indications, route, and dosage
Prophylaxis of acute organ rejection in patients receiving renal transplants
Adults: 1.0 mg/kg in 50 ml normal saline solution I.V., given over 15 minutes via a central or peripheral line. Standard course of therapy is five doses. Administer first dose no more than 24 hours before transplantation; remaining four doses are given at 14-day intervals.

Drug is used as part of an immunosuppressive regimen that includes corticosteroids and cyclosporine.

Pharmacodynamics
Immunosuppressive action: An interleukin (IL)-2 receptor antagonist that binds to the 1-alpha Tac subunit of the IL-2 receptor complex and inhibits IL-2 binding. This effect prevents IL-2 mediated activation of lymphocytes, a critical pathway in the cellular immune response against allografts. Once in circulation, drug impairs the response of the immune system to antigenic challenges. Following drug administration, the Tac subunit of the IL-2 receptor is saturated for about 120 days post-transplant.

Pharmacokinetics
• *Absorption:* Serum levels increase between first and fifth doses.
• *Distribution:* No information available.
• *Metabolism:* No information available, but given a known relationship between body weight and systemic clearance, dosing is based on mg/kg.
• *Excretion:* Estimated terminal elimination half-life is 20 days (480 hours).

Contraindications and precautions
Contraindicated in patients with hypersensitivity to drug or its components.

It's unknown if drug has a long-term effect on the immune response to antigens first encountered during therapy. Readministration of drug after initial course of treatment hasn't been studied. The possible risks of prolonged immunosuppression, anaphylaxis, or anaphylactoid reactions haven't been identified.

Interactions
None reported.

Adverse reactions
CNS: *tremor, headache, dizziness, insomnia,* generalized weakness, prickly sensation, *fever, pain, fatigue,* depression, anxiety.
CV: tachycardia, hypertension, **pulmonary edema,** hypotension, aggravated hypertension, *edema,* fluid overload, chest pain.
EENT: blurred vision, pharyngitis, rhinitis.
GI: constipation, nausea, diarrhea, vomiting, abdominal pain, dyspepsia, pyrosis, abdominal distention, epigastric pain, flatulence, gastritis, hemorrhoids.

Reactions may be *common*, uncommon, ***life-threatening***, or COMMON AND LIFE-THREATENING.

GU: *oliguria, dysuria, **renal tubular necrosis,
renal damage,*** urinary retention, hydronephrosis, urinary tract bleeding, urinary tract disorder, ***renal insufficiency.***
Hematologic: *lymphocele.*
Metabolic: diabetes mellitus, dehydration.
Musculoskeletal: *musculoskeletal or back pain,* arthralgia, myalgia, leg cramps.
Respiratory: *dyspnea, coughing,* atelectasis, congestion, ***hypoxia,*** rales, abnormal breath sounds, pleural effusion.
Skin: *acne, impaired wound healing without infection,* pruritus, hirsutism, rash, night sweats, increased sweating.
Other: *posttraumatic pain,* shivering, extremity edema.

☑ Special considerations
● Only clinicians experienced in immunosuppressive therapy, management, and follow-up of organ transplant patients should administer drug. Patients receiving drug should be managed in facilities equipped and staffed with adequate laboratory and supportive medical care.
● Risk of lipoproliferative disorders and opportunistic infections was no greater when compared with placebo. However, patients undergoing immunosuppressive therapy are at increased risk; monitor patient carefully.
● Drug isn't for direct injection.
● Other drugs shouldn't be added or infused simultaneously through same I.V. line.
● No information on overdose available. Maximum tolerated dosage hasn't been determined.

Monitoring the patient
● Monitor patient for signs of infection.
● Monitor patient for weight gain and edema.

Information for the patient
● Tell patient to call before taking other drugs during drug therapy.
● Advise patient to practice infection prevention precautions.
● Inform patient that neither he nor any household member should receive vaccinations unless medically approved.
● Tell patient to immediately report wounds that fail to heal, unusual bruising or bleeding, or fever.
● Advise patient to drink plenty of fluids during drug therapy and to report painful urination, blood in urine, or decrease in urine amount.

Geriatric patients
● Use drug cautiously in elderly patients.

Pediatric patients
● No data on safety and efficacy in children exist. The immune response to vaccines, infection, or other antigenic stimuli during or after therapy isn't known. Ongoing studies are being conducted.

Breast-feeding patients
● It's unknown if drug appears in breast milk. Because of potential risks, discontinue either drug or breast-feeding.

---

dactinomycin (actinomycin D)
Cosmegen

Pharmacologic classification: antibiotic antineoplastic (cell cycle–phase nonspecific)
Therapeutic classification: antineoplastic
Pregnancy risk category C

How supplied
Available by prescription only
Injectable: 500-mcg vial

Indications, route, and dosage
Dosage and indications may vary. Check current literature for recommended protocols.
Uterine cancer, testicular cancer, Wilms' tumor, rhabdomyosarcoma, Ewing's sarcoma, sarcoma botryoides, ◇ Kaposi's sarcoma, ◇ acute organ (kidney or heart) rejection, ◇ malignant melanoma, ◇ acute lymphocytic leukemia, ◇ advanced tumors of breast or ovary, ◇ Paget's disease of bone
Adults: 500 mcg (0.5 mg) I.V. daily for a maximum of 5 days. Maximum dosage is 15 mcg/kg/day or 400 to 600 mcg/m²/day for 5 days. After bone marrow recovery, course may be repeated.
Children: 15 mcg/kg (0.015 mg/kg) I.V. daily for a maximum of 5 days. Or give a total dosage of 2,500 mcg/m² I.V. over a 1-week period. Maximum dosage is 15 mcg/kg/day or 400 to 600 mcg/m²/day. After bone marrow recovery, course may be repeated.
     For isolation-perfusion, use 50 mcg/kg for lower extremity or pelvis; 35 mcg/kg for upper extremity.
     Dose should be based on body surface area in obese or edematous patients.

Pharmacodynamics
Antineoplastic action: Exerts its cytotoxic activity by intercalating between DNA base pairs and uncoiling the DNA helix. The result is inhibition of DNA synthesis and DNA-dependent RNA synthesis.

Pharmacokinetics
● *Absorption:* Because of its vesicant properties, drug must be administered I.V.
● *Distribution:* Widely distributed into body tissues, with highest levels found in bone marrow and nucleated cells. Doesn't cross blood-brain barrier significantly.
● *Metabolism:* Only minimally metabolized in liver.

• *Excretion:* Drug and its metabolites excreted in urine and bile. Plasma elimination half-life is 36 hours.

Contraindications and precautions
Contraindicated in patients with chickenpox or herpes zoster.

Interactions
Drug-drug. *Bone marrow suppressants:* May cause additive toxicity. Monitor patient closely.
Vitamin K derivatives: Decreased effectiveness of drug. Monitor patient closely.

Adverse reactions
CNS: malaise, fatigue, lethargy.
GI: *anorexia, nausea, vomiting,* abdominal pain, diarrhea, *stomatitis,* ulceration, proctitis.
Hematologic: *anemia, leukopenia, thrombocytopenia, pancytopenia, aplastic anemia, agranulocytosis.*
Hepatic: *hepatotoxicity.*
Metabolic: increased blood and urine levels of uric acid, hypocalcemia.
Musculoskeletal: myalgia.
Skin: *erythema;* desquamation; *hyperpigmentation of skin, especially in previously irradiated areas; acnelike eruptions* (reversible).
Other: phlebitis, severe damage to soft tissue (at injection site); reversible alopecia, fever, ***death.***

☑ Special considerations
• To reconstitute for I.V. administration, add 1.1 ml of preservative-free sterile water for injection to drug to give a concentration of 0.5 mg/ml. Don't use preserved diluent; precipitation may occur.
• Use gloves when preparing and administering drug.
• Drug may be diluted further with D_5W or normal saline solution for administration by I.V. infusion.
• Discard unused solution because it doesn't contain preservatives.
• Drug may be administered by I.V. push injection into tubing of freely flowing I.V. infusion. Don't administer through in-line I.V. filter.
• Use body surface area calculation in obese or edematous patients.
• To reduce nausea, give antiemetic before drug. Nausea usually occurs within 30 minutes of dose.
• Patients who have received other cytotoxic drugs or radiation within 6 weeks of dactinomycin may exhibit erythema, then hyperpigmentation or edema, or both; desquamation; vesiculation; and, rarely, necrosis.
• May interfere with bioassay procedures for determination of antibacterial drug levels.
• Signs and symptoms of overdose include myelosuppression, nausea, vomiting, glossitis, and oral ulceration. Treatment is generally supportive and includes antiemetics and transfusion of blood components.

Monitoring the patient
• Monitor CBC daily and platelet counts every third day. Leukocyte and platelet nadirs usually occur 14 to 21 days after completion of course of therapy. Observe for signs of bleeding.
• Monitor renal and hepatic functions.
• Monitor patient for extravasation. Treatment includes topical dimethyl sulfoxide and cold compresses.

Information for the patient
• Advise patient to avoid exposure to people with infections.
• Warn patient that alopecia may occur but is usually reversible.
• Tell patient to report sore throat, fever, or signs of bleeding promptly.

Pediatric patients
• Restrict use of drug in infants ages 6 months and older; adverse reactions are more frequent in infants under age 6 months.

Breast-feeding patients
• It's unknown if drug appears in breast milk. Because of risks of serious adverse reactions, mutagenicity, and carcinogenicity in infants, breast-feeding isn't recommended.

dalteparin sodium
Fragmin

Pharmacologic classification: low-molecular-weight heparin derivative
Therapeutic classification: anticoagulant
Pregnancy risk category B

How supplied
Available by prescription only
Injection: 2,500 anti-factor Xa IU/0.2 ml, 5,000 anti-factor Xa IU/0.2 ml, 10,000 IU anti-factor Xa/ml.

Indications, route, and dosage
Prophylaxis against deep vein thrombosis (DVT) in patients undergoing abdominal surgery who are at risk for thromboembolic complications (including those who are over age 40, obese, undergoing general anesthesia lasting longer than 30 minutes, and with history of DVT or pulmonary embolism)
Adults: 2,500 IU S.C. daily, starting 1 to 2 hours before surgery and repeated once daily for 5 to 10 days postoperatively.
Prophylaxis against DVT in patients undergoing hip replacement surgery
Adults: 2,500 IU S.C. within 2 hours before surgery and second dose 2,500 IU S.C. in the evening of surgery (at least 6 hours after first dose). If surgery is performed in the evening, omit second dose on day of surgery. Starting on first postoperative

day, administer 5,000 IU S.C. once daily for 5 to 10 days. Or administer 5,000 IU S.C. on the evening before surgery, then 5,000 IU S.C. once daily starting in the evening of surgery for 5 to 10 days postoperatively. Patients receiving dalteparin who require neuraxial anesthesia or spinal puncture may be at increased risk for developing an epidural or spinal hematoma, which can result in long-term or permanent paralysis.

Pharmacodynamics
Anticoagulant action: Enhances inhibition of factor Xa and thrombin by antithrombin.

Pharmacokinetics
• *Absorption:* Absolute bioavailability measured in anti-factor Xa activity is about 87%.
• *Distribution:* Volume of distribution for dalteparin anti-factor Xa activity is 40 to 60 ml/kg.
• *Metabolism:* No information available.
• *Excretion:* No information available.

Contraindications and precautions
Contraindicated in patients with hypersensitivity to drug, heparin, or pork products and in those with active major bleeding or thrombocytopenia associated with positive in vitro tests for antiplatelet antibody in the presence of drug.

Use with extreme caution in patients with history of heparin-induced thrombocytopenia and in those with increased risk of hemorrhage, such as those with severe uncontrolled hypertension, bacterial endocarditis, congenital or acquired bleeding disorders, active ulceration and angiodysplastic GI disease, or hemorrhagic stroke; or shortly after brain, spinal, or ophthalmic surgery. Use cautiously in patients with bleeding diathesis, thrombocytopenia, or platelet defects; severe liver or kidney insufficiency; hypertensive or diabetic retinopathy; or recent GI bleeding.

Interactions
Drug-drug. *Oral anticoagulants, platelet inhibitors:* May increase risk of bleeding. Use together cautiously.

Adverse reactions
Hematologic: *thrombocytopenia,* hemorrhage, ecchymoses, bleeding complications.
Hepatic: elevated AST and ALT levels.
Skin: pruritus, rash, *hematoma.*
Other: fever.

☑ Special considerations
• Patient should sit or lie down when drug is administered. Inject drug S.C. deeply. Injection sites include U-shaped area around navel, upper outer side of thigh, or upper outer quadrangle of buttock. Rotate sites daily. When area around navel or thigh is used, thumb and forefinger should be used to lift up fold of skin while giving injection.

Insert entire length of needle at a 45- to 90-degree angle.
• Never administer drug I.M.
• Don't mix drug with other injections or infusions unless specific compatibility data are available supporting such mixing.
• Drug isn't interchangeable (unit for unit) with unfractionated heparin or other low-molecular-weight heparins.
• Stop drug if thromboembolic event occurs despite dalteparin prophylaxis.
• Overdose may cause hemorrhagic complications. These generally may be stopped by the slow I.V. injection of protamine sulfate (1% solution), at a dose of 1 mg protamine for every 100 anti-factor Xa IU of dalteparin given.
• A second infusion of 0.5 mg protamine sulfate per 100 anti-factor Xa IU of dalteparin may be administered if activated partial thromboplastin time (APTT) measured 2 to 4 hours after the first infusion remains prolonged. Even with these additional doses of protamine sulfate, APTT may remain more prolonged than would usually be found after conventional heparin.

Monitoring the patient
• Periodic routine CBC, including platelet count, and stool occult blood tests are recommended in patients receiving dalteparin. Patients don't require regular monitoring of PT, INR, or APTT.
• Monitor patient closely for thrombocytopenia.

Information for the patient
• Instruct patient and family to watch for signs of bleeding and to report immediately.
• Tell patient to avoid OTC products containing aspirin or other salicylates.

Pediatric patients
• Safety and effectiveness in children haven't been established.

Breast-feeding patients
• It's unknown if drug appears in breast milk; use with caution in breast-feeding women.

danaparoid sodium
Orgaran

Pharmacologic classification: glycosaminoglycuronan
Therapeutic classification: antithrombotic
Pregnancy risk category B

How supplied
Available by prescription only
Ampule: 750 anti-Xa units/0.6 ml
Syringe: 750 anti-Xa units/0.6 ml

Indications, route, and dosage
Prophylaxis against postoperative deep vein thrombosis (DVT) that may lead to pulmonary embolism in patients undergoing elective hip replacement surgery
Adults: 750 anti-Xa units S.C. b.i.d. beginning 1 to 4 hours preoperatively; then no sooner than 2 hours after surgery. Continue for 7 to 10 days postoperatively or until risk of DVT has diminished.

Pharmacodynamics
Antithrombotic action: Prevents fibrin formation by inhibiting generation of thrombin by anti-Xa and anti-IIa. Because of its predominant anti-Xa activity, danaparoid injection has little effect on clotting assays such as PT, INR, and partial thromboplastin time (PTT). Drug has only minor effect on platelet function and platelet aggregability.

Pharmacokinetics
Drug pharmacokinetics have been described by monitoring biologic activity (plasma anti-Xa activity) because no specific chemical assay methods are currently available.
• *Absorption:* S.C. administration about 100% bioavailable, compared with same dose administered I.V. Onset and duration unknown. Peak anti-Xa activity occurs in 2 to 5 hours.
• *Distribution:* No information available.
• *Metabolism:* No information available.
• *Excretion:* Mainly eliminated through kidneys. Mean value for terminal half-life is about 24 hours. In patients with severely impaired renal function, elimination half-life of plasma anti-Xa activity may be prolonged.

Contraindications and precautions
Contraindicated in patients with hypersensitivity to drug or to pork products, severe hemorrhagic diathesis (such as hemophilia or idiopathic thrombocytopenic purpura), active major bleeding (including hemorrhagic stroke in the acute phase), or type II thrombocytopenia associated with positive in vitro tests for antiplatelet antibody in the presence of drug.
 Use with extreme caution in patients at increased risk of hemorrhage, such as in severe uncontrolled hypertension, acute bacterial endocarditis, congenital or acquired bleeding disorders, active ulcerative and angiodysplastic GI disease, nonhemorrhagic stroke, postoperative use of indwelling epidural catheter; or shortly after brain, spinal, or ophthalmic surgery.
 Use cautiously in patients with impaired renal function and in those receiving oral anticoagulants or platelet inhibitors.

Interactions
Drug-drug. *Oral anticoagulants, platelet inhibitors:* May increase risk of bleeding. Use together cautiously.

Adverse reactions
CNS: insomnia, headache, asthenia, dizziness.
CV: peripheral edema, *hemorrhage.*
GI: *nausea, constipation,* vomiting.
GU: urinary tract infection, urine retention.
Hematologic: anemia.
Musculoskeletal: joint disorder, pain.
Skin: rash, pruritus.
Other: *fever,* pain at injection site, infection.

☑ Special considerations
• Carefully consider drug's risks and benefits before giving to patients with severely impaired renal function or hemorrhagic disorders.
• Don't give drug I.M. To administer drug, have patient lie down. Give S.C. injection deeply, using a 25G to 26G needle. Alternate injection sites between left and right anterolateral and posterolateral abdominal wall. Gently pull up a skin fold with thumb and forefinger and insert entire length of needle into tissue. Don't rub or pinch afterward.
• Drug isn't interchangeable (unit for unit) with heparin or low-molecular-weight heparin.
• Danaparoid overdose may lead to bleeding complications. Effects of danaparoid on anti-Xa activity can't be currently antagonized with other known drugs. Although protamine sulfate partially neutralizes the anti-Xa activity of danaparoid and can be safely coadministered, there's no evidence that protamine sulfate is capable of reducing severe nonsurgical bleeding during treatment with danaparoid.
• If serious bleeding occurs, stop drug and administer blood or blood products as needed.
• Signs and symptoms of acute toxicity after I.V. administration include respiratory depression, prostration, and twitching.

Monitoring the patient
• Drug contains sodium sulfite, which may cause allergic-type reactions, including anaphylactic symptoms and life-threatening or less severe asthmatic episodes in certain patients. Overall prevalence of sulfite allergy in general population is unknown and probably low. Sulfite sensitivity is seen more frequently in asthmatic than in nonasthmatic patients.
• Periodic, routine CBCs (including platelet count) and fecal occult blood tests recommended during therapy. Patients don't require regular monitoring of PT, INR, and PTT. Drug has little effect on PT, INR, PTT, fibrinolytic activity, and bleeding time.
• Monitor patient's hematocrit and blood pressure closely; a decrease in either may signal hemorrhage. If serious bleeding occurs, stop drug and transfuse blood products if needed.
• Carefully monitor patients with serum creatinine level of 2 mg/dl or more.

Reactions may be *common*, uncommon, *life-threatening*, or COMMON AND LIFE-THREATENING.

- Monitoring of anticoagulant activity of oral anticoagulants by PT and Thrombotest is unreliable within 5 hours after danaparoid administration.

Information for the patient
- Instruct patient and family to watch for and report signs of bleeding.
- Tell patient to avoid OTC drugs containing aspirin or other salicylates.

Pediatric patients
- Safety and effectiveness in pediatric patients haven't been established.

Breast-feeding patients
- It's unknown if drug appears in breast milk; use cautiously in breast-feeding women.

danazol
Cyclomen*, Danocrine

Pharmacologic classification: androgen
Therapeutic classification: antiestrogen, androgen
Pregnancy risk category X

How supplied
Available by prescription only
Capsules: 50 mg, 100 mg, 200 mg

Indications, route, and dosage
Mild endometriosis
Adults: Initially, 200 to 400 mg P.O. b.i.d. uninterrupted for 3 to 6 months; may continue for 9 months. Subsequent dosage based on patient response.
Moderate to severe endometriosis
Adults: 800 mg P.O. b.i.d. uninterrupted for 3 to 6 months; may continue for 9 months.
Fibrocystic breast disease
Adults: 100 to 400 mg P.O. daily in two divided doses uninterrupted for 2 to 6 months.
Prevention of hereditary angioedema
Adults: 200 mg P.O. b.i.d. or t.i.d., continued until favorable response is achieved. Then dosage should be decreased by half at 1- to 3-month intervals.

Pharmacodynamics
Antiestrogenic action: Causes regression and atrophy of normal and ectopic endometrial tissue. Also decreases rate of growth and nodularity of abnormal breast tissue in fibrocystic breast disease.
Androgenic action: Increases levels of the C1 and C4 components of complement, which reduces frequency and severity of attacks associated with hereditary angioedema.

Pharmacokinetics
- *Absorption:* Amount absorbed by body isn't proportional to administered dose; doubling drug dose increases absorption only 35% to 40%.
- *Distribution:* No information available.
- *Metabolism:* Metabolized to 2-hydroxymethylethisterone.
- *Excretion:* No information available.

Contraindications and precautions
Contraindicated in patients with undiagnosed abnormal genital bleeding; porphyria; or impaired renal, cardiac, or hepatic function; during pregnancy; and in breast-feeding women.
    Use cautiously in patients with seizure disorders or migraine headaches.

Interactions
Drug-drug. *Carbamazepine:* May increase plasma levels of carbamazepine. Avoid concomitant use.
Cyclosporine: May increase cyclosporine levels and chance of nephrotoxicity. Monitor renal function.
Insulin: May increase insulin requirements in diabetes. Monitor patient closely.
Warfarin-type anticoagulants: May potentiate action of anticoagulants, prolonging PT and INR. Avoid concomitant use.

Adverse reactions
CNS: dizziness, headache, sleep disorders, fatigue, tremor, irritability, excitation, lethargy, mental depression, chills, paresthesia.
CV: elevated blood pressure.
EENT: visual disturbances.
GI: gastric irritation, nausea, vomiting, diarrhea, constipation, change in appetite.
GU: hematuria, *hypoestrogenic effects (flushing, diaphoresis, vaginitis [including itching, dryness, and burning]; vaginal bleeding, nervousness, emotional lability, menstrual irregularities).*
Hematologic: prolonged PT and INR (especially in patients on anticoagulant therapy).
Hepatic: reversible jaundice, elevated liver enzyme levels, hepatic dysfunction.
Metabolic: androgenic effects in women *(weight gain, hirsutism,* hoarseness, clitoral enlargement, *decreased breast size,* acne, edema, changes in libido, *oily skin or hair,* voice deepening).
Musculoskeletal: muscle cramps or spasms.

☑ Special considerations
Besides the recommendations relevant to all androgens, consider the following.
- To treat endometriosis and fibrocystic breast disease, therapy should begin during menstruation.
- Glucose tolerance test results may be abnormal. Total serum T_4 may decrease; T_3 may increase.

- Drug provides alternative therapy for patients who can't tolerate or fail to respond to other means of therapy. (Isn't indicated in cases in which surgery is best choice.)
- No information available on overdose. Empty stomach by induced emesis or gastric lavage; follow with activated charcoal to reduce absorption. Treatment is supportive.

Monitoring the patient

- Because drug may cause hepatic dysfunction, perform periodic liver function studies.
- In men, periodically evaluate semen.
- In children, monitor X-rays every 6 months to assess skeletal maturation and avoid precocious puberty and premature closure of epiphyses.

Information for the patient

- Tell woman desiring birth control to use a non-hormonal contraceptive; during danazol treatment, ovulation may not be suppressed by hormonal contraceptives.
- Advise woman to report voice changes or other signs of virilization promptly. Some androgenic effects such as deepening of voice may not be reversible after therapy ends.
- Instruct patient to immediately report nausea, vomiting, headache, and visual disturbances, which may suggest pseudotumor cerebri.
- Advise patient who is taking danazol for fibrocystic disease to examine breasts regularly. If breast nodule enlarges during treatment, she should call immediately.
- Advise woman that amenorrhea usually occurs after 6 to 8 weeks of therapy.
- Advise man that periodic evaluation of semen may be indicated.

Geriatric patients

- Use with caution. Observe elderly men for possible prostatic hypertrophy; stop drug if symptomatic prostatic hypertrophy or prostatic carcinoma occurs.

Pediatric patients

- Use with caution because of possible androgenic effects. Use danazol with extreme caution in children to avoid precocious puberty and premature closure of epiphyses. Conduct X-ray examinations every 6 months to assess skeletal maturation.

Breast-feeding patients

- Because of the potential for serious adverse reactions in the infant, a decision should be made to discontinue breast-feeding or drug, depending on drug's importance to mother.

dantrolene sodium
Dantrium

Pharmacologic classification: hydantoin derivative
Therapeutic classification: skeletal muscle relaxant
Pregnancy risk category C

How supplied
Available by prescription only
Capsules: 25 mg, 50 mg, 100 mg
Injection: 20 mg parenteral (contains 3 g mannitol)

Indications, route, and dosage
Spasticity resulting from upper motor neuron disorders
Adults: 25 mg P.O. daily, increased gradually in increments of 25 mg at 4- to 7-day intervals, up to 100 mg b.i.d. to q.i.d., to maximum of 400 mg daily.
Children over age 5: 0.5 mg/kg P.O. b.i.d., increased to t.i.d., then q.i.d. Increase dosage further, p.r.n., by 0.5 mg/kg up to 3 mg/kg b.i.d. to q.i.d. Maximum dosage is 100 mg q.i.d.
Prevention of malignant hyperthermia in susceptible patients who require surgery
Adults: 4 to 8 mg/kg/day P.O. given in three or four divided doses for 1 to 2 days before procedure; administer last dose 3 to 4 hours before procedure. Or give 2.5 mg/kg I.V. over 1 hour about 75 minutes before anesthesia.
Management of malignant hyperthermia crisis
Adults and children: Initially, 1 mg/kg I.V.; then continue until symptoms subside or maximum cumulative dose of 10 mg/kg has been reached.
Prevention of recurrence of malignant hyperthermia after crisis
Adults: 4 to 8 mg/kg/day P.O. given in four divided doses for up to 3 days after crisis. Or give 1 mg/kg or more I.V. based on situation.
◇ *To reduce succinylcholine-induced muscle fasciculations and postoperative muscle pain*
Adults under 45 kg (99 lb): 100 mg P.O. 2 hours before succinylcholine.
Adults over 45 kg: 150 mg P.O. 2 hours before succinylcholine.

Pharmacodynamics
Skeletal muscle relaxant action: A hydantoin derivative that is chemically and pharmacologically unrelated to other skeletal muscle relaxants. It directly affects skeletal muscle, reducing muscle tension. It interferes with the release of calcium ions from the sarcoplasmic reticulum, resulting in decreased muscle contraction. This mechanism is of particular importance in malignant hyperthermia when increased myoplasmic calcium ion concentrations activate acute catabolism in

---

the skeletal muscle cell. Drug prevents or reduces the increase in myoplasmic calcium levels associated with malignant hyperthermia crises.

Pharmacokinetics

- *Absorption:* 35% of oral dose absorbed through GI tract, with serum half-life reached within 8 to 9 hours after oral administration and 5 hours after I.V. administration. Therapeutic effect in patients with upper motor neuron disorders may take 1 week or more.
- *Distribution:* Substantially plasma protein-bound, mainly to albumin.
- *Metabolism:* Metabolized in liver to less active 5-hydroxy derivatives and to amino derivative by reductive pathways.
- *Excretion:* Excreted in urine as metabolites.

Contraindications and precautions

Contraindicated when spasticity is used to maintain motor function in patients with upper motor neuron disorders, for spasms in rheumatic disorders, in patients with active hepatic disease, and in breast-feeding women. Contraindicated with verapamil in management of malignant hyperthermia.

Use cautiously in women (especially those taking estrogen), in patients over age 35, and in patients with severely impaired cardiac or pulmonary function or preexisting hepatic disease.

Interactions

Drug-drug. *Antipsychotics, anxiolytics, CNS depressant drugs, narcotics, tricyclic antidepressants:* May increase CNS depression. Reduce dosage of one or both if used concurrently.

Estrogen therapy: May increase risk of hepatotoxicity with concomitant use in women over age 35. Use cautiously and monitor patient closely.

Verapamil: Cardiac collapse has occurred rarely when administered with dantrolene. Monitor patient closely.

Drug-lifestyle. *Alcohol:* May increase CNS depression. Avoid use together.

Sun exposure: May evoke a photosensitivity reaction. Patient should take precautions.

Adverse reactions

CNS: *muscle weakness, drowsiness, dizziness, light-headedness, malaise, fatigue, headache, confusion, nervousness, insomnia, seizures.*

CV: tachycardia, blood pressure changes.

EENT: excessive lacrimation, speech disturbance, altered taste, diplopia, visual disturbances.

GI: anorexia, constipation, cramping, dysphagia, metallic taste, severe diarrhea, GI bleeding.

GU: urinary frequency, hematuria, incontinence, nocturia, dysuria, crystalluria, difficult erection, urine retention.

Hepatic: altered liver function test results, *hepatitis.*

Musculoskeletal: myalgia, back pain.

Respiratory: pleural effusion with pericarditis.

Skin: eczematous eruption, pruritus, urticaria.

Other: abnormal hair growth, diaphoresis, chills, fever.

☑ Special considerations

- To prepare suspension for single oral dose, dissolve contents of appropriate number of capsules in fruit juice or other suitable liquid.
- Before therapy begins, check patient's baseline neuromuscular functions (posture, gait, coordination, range of motion, muscle strength and tone, presence of abnormal muscle movements, reflexes) for later comparisons.
- Drug may cause muscle weakness and impaired walking ability. Use with caution and carefully supervise patients receiving drug for prophylactic treatment for malignant hyperthermia.
- Walking should be supervised until patient's reaction to drug is known. With relief of spasticity, patient may lose ability to maintain balance.
- Improvement may require 1 week or more of drug therapy.
- In malignant hyperthermia crisis, give drug by rapid I.V. injection as soon as reaction is recognized.
- To reconstitute, add 60 ml sterile water for injection to 20-mg vial. Don't use bacteriostatic water, D₅W, or normal saline for injection. Store reconstituted solution away from direct sunlight at room temperature and discard after 6 hours.
- Signs and symptoms of overdose include exaggeration of adverse reactions, particularly CNS depression, and nausea and vomiting.
- Treatment of overdose includes supportive measures, gastric lavage, and observation of symptoms. Maintain adequate airway, have emergency ventilation equipment on hand, monitor ECG, and administer large quantities of I.V. solutions to prevent crystalluria. Monitor vital signs closely. Benefit of dialysis isn't known.

Monitoring the patient

- Perform baseline and regularly scheduled liver function tests (alkaline phosphatase, ALT, AST, and total bilirubin), blood cell counts, and renal function tests. Risk of hepatotoxicity may be greater in women, patients over age 35, and in those taking other drugs (especially estrogen) or high dantrolene doses (400 mg or more daily) for prolonged periods.
- Because of risk of hepatic injury, stop drug if improvement isn't evident within 45 days.
- Treating malignant hyperthermia requires continual monitoring of body temperature, management of fever, correction of acidosis, maintenance of fluid and electrolyte balance, monitoring of intake and output, adequate oxygenation, and seizure precautions.
- Signs and symptoms of malignant hyperthermia include skeletal muscle rigidity (often first sign), sudden tachycardia, cardiac arrhythmias,

cyanosis, tachypnea, severe hypercarbia, unstable blood pressure, rapidly rising temperature, acidosis, and shock.

Information for the patient
● Instruct patient to report promptly the onset of jaundice: yellow skin or sclerae, dark urine, clay-colored stools, itching, and abdominal discomfort. Hepatotoxicity occurs more frequently between the third and twelfth months of therapy.
● Advise patient susceptible to malignant hyperthermia to wear medical identification indicating diagnosis, physician's name and telephone number, drug causing reaction, and treatment used.
● Warn patient to avoid OTC drugs, alcoholic beverages, and other CNS depressants except as prescribed because hepatotoxicity occurs more commonly after use of other drugs with dantrolene.
● Advise patient to avoid excessive or unnecessary exposure to sunlight and to use protective clothing and sunscreen; photosensitivity reactions may occur.
● Drug may cause drowsiness. Warn patient to avoid hazardous activities that require alertness until CNS depressant effects are determined.
● Advise patient to report adverse reactions immediately.
● Tell patient to store drug away from heat and direct light (not in bathroom medicine cabinet). Keep out of reach of children.
● Tell patient who misses a dose to take it within 1 hour; otherwise, he should omit dose and return to regular dosing schedule. Tell him not to take double doses.

Geriatric patients
● Administer drug with extreme caution to elderly patients.

Pediatric patients
● Drug isn't recommended for long-term use in children under age 5.

Breast-feeding patients
● Contraindicated for use in breast-feeding women.

dapsone

Pharmacologic classification: synthetic sulfone
Therapeutic classification: antileprotic, antimalarial
Pregnancy risk category C

How supplied
Available by prescription only
Tablets: 25 mg, 100 mg

Indications, route, and dosage
All forms of leprosy (Hansen's disease) except in cases of proven dapsone resistance
Adults: 100 mg P.O. daily for at least 2 years, plus rifampin 600 mg daily for 6 months.
Children: 1 to 1.5 mg/kg P.O. daily.
Prophylaxis for leprosy patient's close contacts
Adults and children ages 12 and older: 50 mg P.O. daily.
Children ages 6 to 12: 25 mg P.O. daily.
Children ages 2 to 5: 25 mg P.O. three times weekly.
Infants ages 6 to 23 months: 12 mg P.O. three times weekly.
Infants under age 6 months: 6 mg P.O. three times weekly.
Dermatitis herpetiformis
Adults: Initially, 50 mg P.O. daily; may increase dose, p.r.n., to obtain full control.
✦ **Dosage adjustment.** Dapsone levels are influenced by acetylation rates. Patients with high acetylation rates may need dose adjustments.
◇ **Malaria suppression or prophylaxis**
Adults: 100 mg P.O. weekly, with pyrimethamine 12.5 mg P.O. weekly.
Children: 2 mg/kg P.O. weekly, with pyrimethamine 0.25 mg/kg weekly.
    Continue prophylaxis throughout exposure and 6 months postexposure.
◇ **Pneumocystis carinii pneumonia**
Adults: 100 mg P.O. daily. Usually administered with trimethoprim, 20 mg/kg daily, for 21 days.

Pharmacodynamics
Antibiotic action: Bacteriostatic and bactericidal; like sulfonamides, thought to act principally by inhibition of folic acid. Acts against *Mycobacterium leprae* and *M. tuberculosis* and has some activity against *P. carinii* and *Plasmodium.*

Pharmacokinetics
● *Absorption:* Given orally, rapid and almost complete absorption. Serum levels peak in 2 to 8 hours.
● *Distribution:* Distributed widely into most body tissues and fluids; 50% to 90% protein-bound.
● *Metabolism:* Undergoes acetylation by liver enzymes; rate varies and is genetically determined. Almost 50% of blacks and whites are slow acetylators; over 80% of Chinese, Japanese, and Inuits are fast acetylators.
● *Excretion:* Drug and metabolites excreted primarily in urine; small amounts of drug excreted in feces; substantial amounts in breast milk. Drug undergoes enterohepatic circulation; half-life in adults ranges from 10 to 50 hours (average 28 hours). Orally administered charcoal may enhance excretion. Dapsone is dialyzable.

Contraindications and precautions

Contraindicated in patients with hypersensitivity to drug. Use cautiously in patients with impaired renal, hepatic, or CV disease; refractory types of anemia; and G6PD deficiency.

Interactions

Drug-drug. *Barbiturates, rifampin:* May be associated with increased hepatic metabolism of dapsone. Monitor patient for lack of efficacy.
Didanosine: May produce possible therapeutic failure of dapsone, leading to increase in infection. Avoid use together.
Folic acid antagonists (methotrexate): May be associated with increased risk of adverse hematologic reactions. Avoid use together.
PABA: May antagonize effect of dapsone by interfering with primary mechanism of action. Monitor patient for lack of efficacy.
Probenecid: Reduced urinary excretion of dapsone metabolites, increasing plasma levels. Monitor patient closely.
Trimethoprim: Increased serum levels of dapsone and trimethoprim may occur when used together, possibly increasing pharmacologic and toxic effects of each. Monitor patient closely.

Adverse reactions

CNS: insomnia, psychosis, headache, paresthesia, peripheral neuropathy, vertigo.
CV: tachycardia.
EENT: tinnitus, blurred vision.
GI: anorexia, abdominal pain, nausea, vomiting, *pancreatitis.*
GU: albuminuria, nephrotic syndrome, renal papillary necrosis, male infertility.
Hematologic: *agranulocytosis, hemolytic anemia* (dose-related), *aplastic anemia.*
Respiratory: pulmonary eosinophilia.
Skin: lupus erythematosus, phototoxicity, *exfoliative dermatitis, toxic erythema, erythema multiforme, toxic epidermal necrolysis, morbilliform and scarlatiniform reactions, urticaria, erythema nodosum.*
Other: fever, infectious mononucleosis-like syndrome, *sulfone syndrome (fever, malaise, jaundice [with hepatic necrosis], exfoliative dermatitis, lymphadenopathy, methemoglobinemia, hemolytic anemia).*
Leprosy reactional states
When treating leprosy with dapsone, it's essential to recognize two types of leprosy reactional states that are related to effectiveness of dapsone therapy.
  Type I, reversal reaction, includes erythema, then swelling of skin and nerve lesions in tuberculoid patients; skin lesions may ulcerate and multiply, and acute neuritis may cause neural dysfunction. Severe cases need hospitalization, analgesics, corticosteroids, and nerve trunk decompression while dapsone therapy is continued.

  Type II, erythema nodosum leprosum, occurs primarily in lepromatous leprosy, with an incidence of about 50% during the first year of therapy. Signs and symptoms include tender erythematous skin nodules, fever, malaise, orchitis, neuritis, albuminuria, iritis, joint swelling, epistaxis, and depression; skin lesions may ulcerate. Treatment includes corticosteroids and analgesics while dapsone is continued.
  Additional treatment guidelines are available from National Hansen's Disease Center at the U.S. Public Health Service at Carville, LA, (800) 642-2477.

☑ Special considerations

● Give drug with or after meals to avoid gastric irritation. Ensure adequate fluid intake.
● Observe skin and mucous membranes for early signs of allergic reactions or leprosy reactional states.
● Isolation of patient with inactive leprosy isn't needed; however, surfaces in contact with discharge from nose or skin lesions should be disinfected.
● Therapeutic effect on leprosy may not be evident until 3 to 6 months after start of therapy.
● Because drug is dialyzable, patients undergoing hemodialysis may need dosage adjustments.
● Signs and symptoms of overdose include nausea, vomiting, and hyperexcitability, occurring within minutes or up to 24 hours after ingestion; methemoglobin-induced depression, cyanosis, and seizures may occur. Hemolysis is a late complication (up to 14 days after ingestion).
● Use gastric lavage to treat overdose, then activated charcoal; dapsone-induced methemoglobinemia (in patients without G6PD-deficiency) can be treated with methylene blue. Hemodialysis may also be used to enhance elimination.
● New mothers need not be separated from infant during therapy.

Monitoring the patient

● Obtain specimens for culture and sensitivity testing before giving first dose, but therapy may begin before test results are complete; repeat periodically to detect drug resistance.
● Observe patient for adverse effects and monitor hematologic and liver function studies to minimize toxicity.
● Monitor dapsone serum levels periodically to maintain effective levels. Levels of 0.1 to 7 mcg/ml (average 2.3 mcg/ml) are usually effective and safe.
● Monitor vital signs frequently during early weeks of drug therapy. Frequent or high fever may require reducing dosage or stopping drug.

Information for the patient

● Explain disease process and rationale for long-term therapy to patient and family; emphasize that improvement may not occur for 3 to 6 months

---

◇ Unlabeled clinical use

and that treatment must continue for at least 1 to 2 years.
• Teach signs and symptoms of hypersensitivity and other adverse reactions, and emphasize need to report these promptly; explain possibility of cumulative effects; urge patient to report any unusual effects or reactions and to report promptly loss of appetite, nausea, or vomiting.
• Teach patient how to take drug and the need to comply with prescribed regimen. Encourage patient to report no improvement or worsening of symptoms after 3 months of treatment. Urge patient not to stop drug without medical approval.
• Explain importance of follow-up visits and need to monitor close contacts at 6- to 12-month intervals for 10 years.
• Teach sanitary disposal of secretions from nose or skin lesions.
• Assure patient and family that inactive leprosy isn't a barrier to employment or school attendance.
• Teach new mothers signs of cyanosis and methemoglobinemia that may occur in infants.
• Tell patient to avoid prolonged exposure to sunlight.

Geriatric patients
• Elderly patients often have decreased renal function, which decreases drug excretion. Use with caution in elderly patients.

Pediatric patients
• Use drug with caution in children.

Breast-feeding patients
• Dapsone appears in breast milk and may be tumorigenic. An alternative to breast-feeding is recommended during therapy.

daunorubicin citrate liposomal
DaunoXome

Pharmacologic classification: anthracycline
Therapeutic classification: antineoplastic
Pregnancy risk category D

How supplied
Available by prescription only
Injection: 2 mg/ml (equivalent to 50 mg daunorubicin base)

Indications, route, and dosage
First-line cytotoxic therapy for advanced HIV-associated Kaposi's sarcoma
Adults: 40 mg/m² I.V. over 60 minutes once every 2 weeks. Continue treatment until there is evidence of progressive disease or until other complications of HIV preclude continuation of therapy.

✦ *Dosage adjustment.* In patients with impaired hepatic and renal function, reduce dosage as follows: If serum bilirubin is 1.2 to 3 mg/dl, give three-quarters normal dose; if serum bilirubin or creatinine is greater than 3 mg/dl, give one-half normal dose.

Pharmacodynamics
Antineoplastic action: Exerts cytotoxic activity by intercalating between DNA base pairs and uncoiling the DNA helix. This inhibits DNA synthesis and DNA-dependent RNA synthesis. May also inhibit polymerase activity. The liposomal preparation of daunorubicin maximizes selectivity of daunorubicin for solid tumors in situ. After penetrating the tumor, daunorubicin is released over time to exert its antineoplastic activity.

Pharmacokinetics
• *Absorption:* Must be administered I.V. because of its vesicant nature.
• *Distribution:* Thought to be distributed primarily in vascular fluid volume.
• *Metabolism:* Metabolized by liver into active metabolites.
• *Excretion:* Apparent elimination half-life is 4.4 hours.

Contraindications and precautions
Contraindicated in patients who have experienced a severe hypersensitivity reaction to daunorubicin citrate liposomal or its components. Use cautiously in patients with myelosuppression, preexisting cardiac disease, previous radiotherapy encompassing the heart, previous anthracycline use (doxorubicin greater than 300 mg/m² or equivalent), and hepatic or renal dysfunction.

Interactions
None reported.

Adverse reactions
CNS: *headache, neuropathy,* depression, dizziness, insomnia, amnesia, anxiety, ataxia, confusion, **seizures,** hallucination, tremor, hypertonia, meningitis, *fatigue,* malaise, emotional lability, abnormal gait, hyperkinesia, somnolence, abnormal thinking.
CV: ***cardiomyopathy*** (dose-related), chest pain, hypertension, palpitation, syncope, ***arrhythmias, pericardial effusion, pericardial tamponade, cardiac arrest,*** angina pectoris, ***pulmonary hypertension,*** flushing, edema, tachycardia, ***MI.***
EENT: *rhinitis,* stomatitis, sinusitis, abnormal vision, conjunctivitis, tinnitus, eye pain, deafness, taste disturbances, earache, gingival bleeding, tooth caries, dry mouth.
GI: *nausea, diarrhea, abdominal pain, vomiting, anorexia,* constipation, ***GI hemorrhage,*** gastritis, dysphagia, stomatitis, increased appetite, melena, hemorrhoids, tenesmus.
GU: dysuria, nocturia, polyuria.

Hematologic: NEUTROPENIA.
Hepatic: hepatomegaly.
Musculoskeletal: *rigors, back pain,* arthralgia, myalgia.
Respiratory: *cough, dyspnea,* hemoptysis, hiccups, pulmonary infiltration, increased sputum.
Skin: alopecia, pruritus, *increased sweating,* dry skin, seborrhea, folliculitis.
Other: *fever,* splenomegaly, lymphadenopathy, *opportunistic infections, allergic reactions,* flulike symptoms, dehydration, thirst, injection site inflammation.

☑ Special considerations

● For I.V. administration, drug should be diluted with D₅W before administration. Withdraw calculated volume of drug from vial and transfer into an equivalent amount of D₅W. Recommended concentration after dilution should be 1 mg/ml.
● Don't mix daunorubicin citrate liposomal with other drugs, saline, bacteriostatic products, or any other solution.
● After dilution, immediately administer I.V. over 60 minutes. If unable to use immediately, refrigerate at 2° to 8° C (36° to 46° F) for a maximum of 6 hours.
● Don't use in-line filters for I.V. infusion.
● A triad of back pain, flushing, and chest tightness may occur within first 5 minutes of infusion. Triad subsides after stopping infusion and generally doesn't recur when infusion is administered at slower rate.
● Because local tissue necrosis is possible, monitor I.V. site closely to avoid extravasation.
● Follow procedures for proper handling and disposal of antineoplastics.
● Acute overdose symptoms include increased severity of adverse effects, such as myelosuppression, fatigue, nausea and vomiting. Treatment is usually supportive.

Monitoring the patient

● Monitor cardiac function regularly and assess before administering each dose because of potential risk of cardiac toxicity and heart failure. Determination of left ventricular ejection fraction should be performed at total cumulative doses of 320 mg/m² and every 160 mg/m² thereafter.
● Careful hematologic monitoring is needed because severe myelosuppression may occur. Blood counts should be repeated and evaluated before each dose. Withhold treatment if absolute granulocyte count is less than 750 cells/mm³.
● Monitor patient closely for signs of opportunistic infections, especially because patients with HIV infection are immunocompromised.

Information for the patient

● Inform patient that alopecia may occur but is usually reversible.

● Instruct patient to call if sore throat, fever, or any other signs of infection occur. Tell patient to avoid exposure to people with infections.
● Advise woman receiving drug to report suspected or confirmed pregnancy.
● Tell patient to report back pain, flushing, and chest tightness during infusion.

Geriatric patients

● Safety and efficacy in elderly patients haven't been established.

Pediatric patients

● Safety and efficacy in children haven't been established.

Breast-feeding patients

● Safety during breast-feeding hasn't been established. Because of potential for serious adverse reactions in infant, patient should avoid breast-feeding.

daunorubicin hydrochloride
Cerubidine

Pharmacologic classification: antibiotic antineoplastic (cell cycle–phase nonspecific)
Therapeutic classification: antineoplastic
Pregnancy risk category D

How supplied

Available by prescription only
Injection: 20-mg vials (with 100 mg of mannitol)

Indications, route, and dosage

Dosage and indications may vary. Check current literature for recommended protocols.
Remission induction in acute nonlymphocytic leukemia (myelogenous, monocytic, erythroid)
Adults under age 60: 45 mg/m² I.V. daily on days 1 to 3 of first course and on days 1 and 2 of subsequent courses. Give all courses with cytosine arabinoside infusions.
Adults ages 60 and over: 30 mg/m² on days 1 to 3 of first course and on days 1 and 2 of subsequent courses. Give all courses with cytosine arabinoside infusions.
Remission induction in acute lymphocytic leukemia
Adults: 45 mg/m²/day I.V. on days 1 to 3; give with vincristine, prednisone, and l-asparaginase.
Children ages 2 and over: 25 mg/m² I.V. on day 1 weekly for up to 6 weeks, if needed; give with vincristine and prednisone.
Children under age 2 or with a body surface area under 0.5 m²: Dose should be calculated based on body weight (1 mg/kg) rather than body surface area

✦ *Dosage adjustment.* Use reduced dosage if patient has hepatic or renal impairment. In patients with serum bilirubin of 1.2 to 3 mg/dl, reduce dosage by 25%; with serum bilirubin or creatinine levels over 3 mg/dl, reduce dosage by 50%.

Pharmacodynamics

Antineoplastic action: Exerts cytotoxic activity by intercalating between DNA base pairs and uncoiling the DNA helix. Inhibition of DNA synthesis and DNA-dependent RNA synthesis results. May also inhibit polymerase activity.

Pharmacokinetics

● *Absorption:* Drug must be given I.V. because of its vesicant nature.
● *Distribution:* Widely distributed into body tissues, with highest levels found in spleen, kidneys, liver, lungs, and heart. Doesn't cross blood-brain barrier.
● *Metabolism:* Extensively metabolized in liver by microsomal enzymes. One metabolite has cytotoxic activity.
● *Excretion:* Drug and metabolites primarily excreted in bile; small portion excreted in urine. Plasma elimination biphasic, with initial phase half-life of 45 minutes and terminal phase half-life of 18½ hours.

Contraindications and precautions

No known contraindications. Use cautiously in patients with myelosuppression or impaired cardiac, renal, or hepatic function.

Interactions

Drug-drug. *Dexamethasone phosphate, heparin sodium:* Admixture of these with daunorubicin results in precipitate formation. Don't mix together.
Doxorubicin: May cause additive cardiotoxicity. Monitor patient closely.
Hepatotoxic drugs: May increase risk of hepatotoxicity. Avoid concomitant use.

Adverse reactions

CV: ECG changes, *irreversible cardiomyopathy* (dose-related).
GI: *nausea, vomiting,* diarrhea, *mucositis* (may occur 3 to 7 days after administration).
GU: red urine (transient).
Hematologic: *bone marrow suppression* (lowest blood counts 10 to 14 days after administration).
Hepatic: *hepatotoxicity.*
Metabolic: hyperuricemia.
Skin: rash.
Other: *severe cellulitis, tissue sloughing* (if drug extravasates), *alopecia,* fever, chills.

☑ Special considerations

● To reconstitute drug for I.V. administration, add 4 ml of sterile water for injection to 20-mg vial to give concentration of 5 mg/ml.
● Drug may be diluted further into 100 ml of D_5W or normal saline solution and infused over 30 to 45 minutes.
● For I.V. push, withdraw reconstituted drug into syringe containing 10 to 15 ml normal saline or D_5W and inject over 2 to 3 minutes into tubing of free flowing I.V. infusion. Reconstituted solution is stable for 24 hours at room temperature and 48 hours refrigerated.
● Drug's reddish color looks similar to doxorubicin (Adriamycin). Don't confuse the two drugs.
● Erythematous streaking along vein or flushing in face indicates that drug is being administered too rapidly.
● Antiemetics may be used to prevent or treat nausea and vomiting.
● Darkening or redness of skin may occur in prior radiation fields.
● Don't use scalp tourniquet or apply ice to prevent alopecia; may compromise drug effectiveness.
● Signs and symptoms of overdose include myelosuppression, nausea, vomiting, and stomatitis. Treatment is usually supportive and includes transfusion of blood components and antiemetics.

Monitoring the patient

● Watch for extravasation. May be treated with topical application of dimethyl sulfoxide and ice packs to site.
● ECG monitoring or monitoring of systolic injection fraction may help to identify early changes associated with drug-induced cardiomyopathy. An ECG or determination of systolic injection fraction should be performed before each course of therapy.
● To prevent cardiomyopathy, limit cumulative dose in adults to 500 to 600 mg/m² (400 to 450 mg/m² when patient has been receiving other cardiotoxic drugs, such as cyclophosphamide, or radiation therapy that encompasses heart).
● Monitor CBC and hepatic function.
● Monitor resting pulse rate. If high, it may be a sign of cardiac adverse reactions.

Information for the patient

● Warn patient that urine may be red for 1 to 2 days and that it's a drug effect, not bleeding.
● Advise patient that alopecia may occur but is usually reversible.
● Tell patient to avoid exposure to people with infections.
● Encourage adequate fluid intake to increase urine output and facilitate excretion of uric acid.
● Warn patient that nausea and vomiting may be severe and may last for 24 to 48 hours.

Reactions may be *common*, uncommon, *life-threatening*, or COMMON AND LIFE-THREATENING.

• Instruct patient to call if a sore throat, fever, or signs of bleeding occur.

Geriatric patients
• Elderly patients have an increased risk of drug-induced cardiotoxicity.
• Watch for hematologic toxicity because some elderly patients have poor bone marrow reserve.

Pediatric patients
• Children have an increased risk of drug-induced cardiotoxicity, which may occur at lower doses. Total lifetime dosage for children over age 2 is 300 mg/m^2; for children under age 2, 10 mg/kg.

Breast-feeding patients
• It's unknown if drug appears in breast milk. Because of potential for serious adverse reactions, mutagenicity, and carcinogenicity in infant, breast-feeding isn't recommended.

deferoxamine mesylate
Desferal

Pharmacologic classification: chelating drug
Therapeutic classification: heavy metal antagonist
Pregnancy risk category C

How supplied
Available by prescription only
Powder for injection: 500-mg vial

Indications, route, and dosage
Acute iron intoxication
Adults and children: 1 g I.M. or I.V. (I.M. injection is preferred route for all patients in shock), then 500 mg I.M. or I.V. q 4 hours for two doses; then 500 mg I.M. or I.V. q 4 to 12 hours, if needed. I.V. infusion rate shouldn't exceed 15 mg/kg/hour. Don't exceed 6 g in 24 hours. (I.V. infusion should be reserved for patients in CV collapse.)
Chronic iron overload resulting from multiple transfusions
Adults and children: 500 mg to 1 g I.M. daily and 2 g slow I.V. infusion in separate solution along with each unit of blood transfused. I.V. infusion rate shouldn't exceed 15 mg/kg/hour. Or give 1 to 2 g via S.C. infusion pump over 8 to 24 hours.

Pharmacodynamics
Chelating action: Chelates iron by binding ferric ions to the 3 hydroxamic groups of the molecule, preventing it from entering into further chemical reactions. Also chelates aluminum to a lesser extent.

Pharmacokinetics
• *Absorption:* Absorbed poorly after oral administration; however, absorption may occur in patients with acute iron toxicity.

• *Distribution:* Distributed widely into body after parenteral administration.
• *Metabolism:* Small amounts metabolized by plasma enzymes.
• *Excretion:* Excreted in urine as unchanged drug or as ferrioxamine, the deferoxamine-iron complex.

Contraindications and precautions
Contraindicated in patients with severe renal disease or anuria. Use cautiously in patients with impaired renal function.

Interactions
None reported.

Adverse reactions
CV: tachycardia with long-term use, *hypotension,* **shock** (after too-rapid I.V. administration).
EENT: blurred vision, cataracts, hearing loss.
GI: diarrhea, abdominal discomfort with long-term use.
GU: dysuria with long-term use.
Musculoskeletal: leg cramps.
Skin: *erythema, urticaria.*
Other: hypersensitivity reactions (cutaneous wheal formation, pruritus, rash, **anaphylaxis**), pain and induration at injection site, fever.

☑ Special considerations
• Use I.M. route for acute iron intoxication if patient isn't in shock. If patient is in shock, administer I.V. slowly; avoid S.C. route.
• Drug has been used to treat iron overload from congenital anemias and in diagnosis and treatment of primary hemochromatosis. Has also been applied topically to remove corneal rust rings and has been used I.V. or intraperitoneally to promote aluminum excretion or removal.
• Drug has been used experimentally as a chelator to reduce aluminum levels in bones of patients with renal failure and in patients with dialysis-induced encephalopathy. Has slowed cognitive deterioration by 50% in long-term clinical trials.
• Acute intoxication may include extension and exacerbation of adverse reactions. Treat symptomatically. Drug can be removed by hemodialysis.

Monitoring the patient
• Monitor renal, vision, and hearing function throughout therapy. Observe closely and be prepared to treat hypersensitivity reactions.
• Monitor renal function before initiating treatment and periodically throughout.
• Perform ophthalmic and, possibly, audiometric examinations every 3 to 6 months during continuous therapy.

Information for the patient
• Stress importance of reporting changes in vision or hearing.
• Explain that drug may turn urine red.

Geriatric patients
• Use drug with caution because elderly patients are more likely than younger patients to have visual or hearing impairment and renal dysfunction.

Pediatric patients
• Drug is safe and effective in children over age 3.

delavirdine mesylate
Rescriptor

Pharmacologic classification: nonnucleoside reverse-transcriptase (RT) inhibitor of HIV-1
Therapeutic classification: antiviral
Pregnancy risk category C

How supplied
Available by prescription only
Tablets: 100 mg

Indications, route, and dosage
HIV infection
Adults: 400 mg P.O. t.i.d.; use with other antiretrovirals as appropriate.

Pharmacodynamics
Antiviral action: Binds directly to RT and blocks RNA- and DNA-dependent DNA polymerase activities.

Pharmacokinetics
• *Absorption:* Rapidly absorbed following oral administration with peak occurring at about 1 hour.
• *Distribution:* 98% bound to plasma proteins, primarily albumin. Distribution into CSF, saliva, and semen is about 0.4%, 6%, and 2%, respectively, of corresponding plasma levels.
• *Metabolism:* Converted to several inactive metabolites; primarily metabolized in liver by cytochrome P-450 3A (CYP3A) enzyme system. In vitro data also suggest CYP2D6 may also be involved. Drug can reduce CYP3A activity and can inhibit its own metabolism; this is usually reversed within 1 week after stopping drug. In vitro data also suggest drug reduces CYP2C9 and CYP2C19 activity.
• *Excretion:* After multiple doses, 44% of dose excreted in feces and 51% excreted in urine. Less than 5% recovered unchanged in urine. Mean elimination half-life is 5.8 hours.

Contraindications and precautions
Contraindicated in patients with hypersensitivity to drug or its components. Use caution when administering to patients with impaired hepatic function. Nonnucleoside RT inhibitors, when used alone or in combination, may confer cross-resistance to other drugs in that class.

Interactions
Drug-drug. *Amphetamines, benzodiazepines, calcium channel blockers, clarithromycin, dapsone, ergot alkaloid preparations, indinavir, nonsedating antihistamines, quinidine, rifabutin, saquinavir, sedative hypnotics, warfarin:* Concomitant use may result in increased plasma levels of these drugs, possibly increasing or prolonging both therapeutic and adverse effects. Dose reduction of drugs may be necessary.
Antacids: Reduced absorption of delavirdine when coadministered. Separate doses by at least 1 hour.
Carbamazepine, phenobarbital, phenytoin, rifabutin, rifampin: Decreased delavirdine plasma levels. Use with caution.
Clarithromycin, fluoxetine, ketoconazole: 50% increase in delavirdine bioavailability. Monitor patient closely.
Didanosine: Bioavailability of both drugs reduced by 20% when coadministered. Separate doses by at least 1 hour.
Enzyme-inducing or inhibiting drugs (phenobarbital, rifampin): Use together cautiously.
H_2 receptor antagonists: Increased gastric pH; may reduce absorption of delavirdine. Long-term use of these drugs with delavirdine isn't recommended.
Indinavir: Increased plasma levels of indinavir. Consider lower dose of indinavir when administered with delavirdine.
Saquinavir: Fivefold increase in bioavailability when used concurrently; possible increase in liver enzymes. Monitor AST and ALT levels frequently when using together.

Adverse reactions
CNS: asthenia, *fatigue,* headache, abnormal coordination, agitation, amnesia, anxiety, change in dreams, lethargy, malaise, cognitive impairment, confusion, depression, disorientation, emotional lability, hallucinations, hyperesthesia, hyperreflexia, hypesthesia, impaired concentration, insomnia, manic symptoms, muscle cramps, nervousness, neuropathy, nightmares, nystagmus, paralysis, paranoid symptoms, paresthesia, restlessness, somnolence, tingling, tremor, vertigo, weakness, pallor.
CV: *bradycardia,* palpitation, orthostatic hypotension, syncope, tachycardia, vasodilation, chest pain.
EENT: blepharitis, conjunctivitis, diplopia, dry eyes, ear pain, photophobia, taste perversion, tinnitus.
GI: *nausea,* vomiting, diarrhea, anorexia, aphthous stomatitis, bloody stools, colitis, constipation, decreased appetite, diverticulitis, duodenitis, dry mouth, dyspepsia, dysphagia, enteritis, esophagitis, fecal incontinence, flatulence, gagging, gastritis, gastroesophageal reflux, *GI bleeding,* gingivitis, gum hemorrhage, increased thirst and appetite, increased saliva, mouth ulcer, *pan-*

creatitis, sialadenitis, stomatitis, tongue edema or ulceration, abdominal cramps, distention, pain (generalized or localized).

GU: breast enlargement, renal calculi, epididymitis, hematuria, hemospermia, impotence, renal pain, metrorrhagia, nocturia, polyuria, proteinuria, vaginal moniliasis, decreased libido.

Hematologic: bruise, *anemia,* ecchymosis, eosinophilia, *granulocytosis, neutropenia, pancytopenia,* petechia, prolonged PTT, purpura, spleen disorder, *thrombocytopenia.*

Hepatic: *nonspecific hepatitis, increased ALT and AST levels.*

Metabolic: alcohol intolerance; bilirubinemia; hyperkalemia; hyperuricemia; hypocalcemia; hyponatremia; hypophosphatemia; increased GTT, lipase, serum alkaline phosphatase, serum amylase, and serum CK; peripheral edema; weight gain or loss.

Musculoskeletal: flank pain, back pain, pain (generalized or localized), neck rigidity, arthralgia or arthritis of single and multiple joints, bone pain, leg cramps, muscular weakness, myalgia, tendon disorder, tenosynovitis, tetany.

Respiratory: upper respiratory infection, bronchitis, chest congestion, cough, dyspnea, epistaxis, laryngismus, pharyngitis, rhinitis, sinusitis.

Skin: epidermal cyst, *rash, pruritus, angioedema,* dermal leukocytoblastic vasculitis, dermatitis, desquamation, diaphoresis, dry skin, *erythema multiforme,* folliculitis, fungal dermatitis, alopecia, nail disorder, petechial rash, seborrhea, skin nodule, *Stevens-Johnson syndrome,* urticaria.

Other: *allergic reaction,* chills, edema (generalized or localized), fever, flu syndrome, lip edema, sebaceous cyst, trauma.

☑ Special considerations

• Drug-induced rash (typically diffuse, maculopapular, erythematous, and often pruritic) occurs commonly; doesn't appear to be significantly reduced by adjusted drug doses.

• Rash is more common in patients with lower CD4+ cell counts and usually occurs within first 3 weeks of treatment. Severe rash occurred in 3.6% of patients. In most cases, rash lasted less than 2 weeks and didn't require reducing dose or discontinuing therapy. Most patients were able to resume therapy after treatment interruption caused by rash.

• Rash occurred mainly on upper body and proximal arms, with decreasing lesion intensity on neck and face and less on rest of trunk and limbs. Erythema multiforme and Stevens-Johnson syndrome were rarely seen, and resolved after drug was stopped. Occurrence of drug-related rash after 1 month of therapy is uncommon unless prolonged interruption of drug treatment occurs.

• Symptomatic relief may been obtained by using diphenhydramine, hydroxyzine, or topical corticosteroids.

• For overdose, provide supportive treatment. Remove drug by gastric lavage or emesis if needed. Dialysis is unlikely to be effective because drug is highly protein-bound.

Monitoring the patient

• Monitor carefully patients with hepatic or renal impairment because effect of drug hasn't been studied. Elevated ALT and AST (over five times upper limit of normal), bilirubin (over 2½ times upper limit of normal) and amylase (over twice upper limit of normal) levels may occur while taking drug.

• Monitor CBC. Neutropenia (absolute neutrophil count below 750/mm³), anemia (hemoglobin less than 7 g/dl), and thrombocytopenia (platelet count under 50,000/mm³) may occur. Monitor patient carefully.

Information for the patient

• Instruct patient to stop drug and call if severe rash or such symptoms as fever, blistering, oral lesions, conjunctivitis, swelling, or muscle or joint aches occur.

• Tell patient that drug isn't a cure for HIV-1 infection. Patient may continue to acquire illnesses associated with HIV-1 infection, including opportunistic infections. Therapy hasn't been shown to reduce risk or frequency of such illnesses.

• Advise patient to remain under medical supervision when taking drug because long-term effects aren't known.

• Inform patient to take drug as prescribed; don't alter doses without medical approval. If dose is missed, tell him to take next dose as soon as possible; don't double the next dose.

• Inform patient that drug may be dispersed in water before ingestion. Add tablets to at least 3 oz (90 ml) of water, allow to stand for a few minutes, and stir until a uniform dispersion occurs. Tell him to drink dispersion promptly, rinse glass, and swallow the rinse to ensure that entire dose is consumed.

• Tell patient that drug may be taken with or without food.

• Advise patient with achlorhydria to take drug with an acidic beverage such as orange or cranberry juice.

• Instruct patient to take drug and antacids at least 1 hour apart.

• Advise patient to report use of other prescriptions or OTC products.

Geriatric patients

• Safety and effectiveness in patients over age 65 haven't been studied.

Pediatric patients

• Safety and effectiveness in patients under age 16 haven't been studied.

Breast-feeding patients
• Women infected with HIV are advised not to breast-feed.

---

demeclocycline hydrochloride
Declomycin

Pharmacologic classification: tetracycline antibiotic
Therapeutic classification: antibiotic
Pregnancy risk category D

How supplied
Available by prescription only
Tablets: 150 mg, 300 mg
Capsules: 150 mg

Indications, route, and dosage
Infections caused by susceptible organisms
Adults: 150 mg P.O. q 6 hours, or 300 mg P.O. q 12 hours.
Children over age 8: 6.6 to 13.2 mg/kg P.O. daily, divided q 6 to 12 hours.
Gonorrhea
Adults: 600 mg P.O. initially; then 300 mg P.O. q 12 hours for 4 days (total 3 g).
◇ *SIADH secretion (a hyposmolar state)*
Adults: 600 to 1,200 mg P.O. daily in three or four divided doses.

Pharmacodynamics
Antibacterial action: Bacteriostatic. Tetracyclines bind reversibly to ribosomal subunits, thereby inhibiting bacterial protein synthesis. Drug is active against many gram-negative and gram-positive organisms, *Mycoplasma, Rickettsia, Chlamydia,* and spirochetes.

Pharmacokinetics
• *Absorption:* About 60% to 80% absorbed from GI tract after oral administration; serum levels peak at 3 to 4 hours. Food or milk reduces absorption by 50%; antacids chelate with tetracyclines and further reduce absorption. Drug has greatest affinity of all tetracyclines for calcium ions.
• *Distribution:* Distributed widely into body tissues and fluids, including synovial, pleural, prostatic, and seminal fluids; bronchial secretions; saliva; and aqueous humor. Poor CSF penetration. Crosses placenta; about 36% to 91% is protein-bound.
• *Metabolism:* Not metabolized.
• *Excretion:* Excreted primarily unchanged in urine by glomerular filtration; some drug may be excreted in breast milk. Plasma half-life is 10 to 17 hours in adults with normal renal function. Hemodialysis and peritoneal dialysis remove only minimal amounts of drug.

Contraindications and precautions
Contraindicated in patients with hypersensitivity to drug or other tetracyclines. Use cautiously in women during second half of pregnancy, in children under age 8, and in patients with impaired renal or hepatic function.

Interactions
Drug-drug. *Antacids containing aluminum, calcium, magnesium; antidiarrheals; laxatives containing aluminum, magnesium, calcium:* Oral absorption of tetracyclines impaired by concomitant use because of chelation. Monitor patient for desired effects.
Digoxin: Increased bioavailability. Lower dosages of digoxin may be needed when used concomitantly.
Iron products, sodium bicarbonate, zinc: Impaired absorption of tetracyclines. Monitor patient for desired effects.
Methoxyflurane: Increased risk of nephrotoxicity. Monitor renal function.
Oral anticoagulants: Enhanced effects. Lower dosages of oral anticoagulants may be needed.
Oral contraceptives: May render oral contraceptives less effective; breakthrough bleeding possible. Avoid concomitant use; tell patient to use alternative birth control methods.
Penicillin: May inhibit cell growth because of bacteriostatic action and may interfere with bactericidal action of penicillins. Administer penicillin 2 to 3 hours before tetracycline.
Drug-food. *Any food, milk, other dairy products:* May impair absorption of tetracyclines. Tell patient to avoid these foods.
Drug-lifestyle. *Sun exposure:* May potentiate photosensitivity reactions. Tell patient to take precautions.

Adverse reactions
CNS: *intracranial hypertension (pseudotumor cerebri),* dizziness.
CV: pericarditis.
EENT: dysphagia, glossitis, tinnitus, visual disturbances.
GI: anorexia, *nausea, vomiting, diarrhea,* enterocolitis, anogenital inflammation, **pancreatitis.**
GU: *increased BUN level.*
Hematologic: *neutropenia,* eosinophilia, **thrombocytopenia, hemolytic anemia.**
Hepatic: elevated liver enzyme levels.
Musculoskeletal: bone growth retardation (in children under age 8).
Skin: *maculopapular and erythematous rash, photosensitivity, increased pigmentation, urticaria.*
Other: Systemic hypersensitivity reactions *(anaphylaxis),* diabetes insipidus syndrome (polyuria, polydipsia, weakness), permanent tooth discoloration.

☑ Special considerations
Besides the recommendations relevant to all tetracyclines, consider the following.
- As an anti-infective, drug is usually reserved for patients intolerant of other antibiotics.
- A reversible diabetes insipidus syndrome has been reported with long-term use of demeclocycline; monitor patient for disorder (weakness, polyuria, polydipsia).
- Drug causes false-negative results in urine tests using glucose oxidase reagent (Diastix, Chemstrip uG, or glucose enzymatic test strip) and false elevations in fluorometric tests for urinary catecholamines.
- Signs and symptoms of overdose are usually limited to GI tract. Treatment may include antacids or gastric lavage if ingestion occurred within 4 hours.

Monitoring the patient
- Monitor renal and hepatic function before starting drug and periodically during therapy.
- Monitor urine output.

Information for the patient
- Advise patient to take drug at least 1 hour before or 2 hours after meals. Drug shouldn't be taken with dairy products.
- Tell patient to avoid prolonged exposure to sunlight.
- Advise woman taking oral contraceptives to use barrier contraceptives for duration of treatment.

Pediatric patients
- Don't use drug in children under age 8.

Breast-feeding patients
- Because drug appears in breast milk, avoid use of drug in breast-feeding women.

---

desipramine hydrochloride
Norpramin

Pharmacologic classification: dibenzazepine tricyclic antidepressant
Therapeutic classification: antidepressant
Pregnancy risk category NR

How supplied
Available by prescription only
Tablets: 10 mg, 25 mg, 50 mg, 75 mg, 100 mg, 150 mg

Indications, route, and dosage
Depression
Adults: 100 to 200 mg P.O. daily in divided doses, increasing to maximum of 300 mg daily. Or entire dosage can be given once daily, usually h.s.

Elderly patients and adolescents: 25 to 100 mg P.O. daily, increasing gradually to a maximum of 100 mg daily (maximum 150 mg/daily only for the severely ill in these age-groups).

Pharmacodynamics
Antidepressant action: Thought to exert antidepressant effects by inhibiting reuptake of norepinephrine and serotonin in CNS nerve terminals (presynaptic neurons), which results in increased levels and enhanced activity of these neurotransmitters in the synaptic cleft. Drug more strongly inhibits reuptake of norepinephrine than serotonin; causes fewer sedative effects and less anticholinergic and hypotensive activity than its parent compound, imipramine.

Pharmacokinetics
- *Absorption:* Absorbed rapidly from GI tract after oral administration.
- *Distribution:* Distributed widely into body, including CNS and breast milk. 90% protein-bound. Peak effect occurs in 4 to 6 hours; steady state, within 2 to 11 days, with full therapeutic effect in 2 to 4 weeks. Proposed therapeutic plasma levels (parent drug and metabolite) range from 125 to 300 ng/ml.
- *Metabolism:* Metabolized by liver; a significant first-pass effect may explain variability of serum levels in different patients taking same dosage.
- *Excretion:* Excreted primarily in urine.

Contraindications and precautions
Contraindicated in patients with hypersensitivity to drug, in those who have taken MAO inhibitors within previous 14 days, and in patients during acute recovery phase of MI. Use with extreme caution in patients with history of seizure disorders or urine retention, CV or thyroid disease, or glaucoma, and in those taking thyroid drugs.

Interactions
Drug-drug. *Antiarrhythmics (disopyramide, procainamide, quinidine), pimozide, thyroid drugs:* May increase risk of cardiac arrhythmias and conduction defects. Monitor patient closely.
Atropine, other anticholinergics (such as antihistamines, antiparkinsonians, meperidine, phenothiazines): Oversedation, paralytic ileus, visual changes, and severe constipation. Use cautiously.
Barbiturates: Induced desipramine metabolism and decreased therapeutic efficacy. Monitor patient closely for drug effect.
Beta blockers, cimetidine, methylphenidate, oral contraceptives, propoxyphene: May inhibit desipramine metabolism, increasing plasma levels and toxicity. Monitor drug levels closely.
Centrally acting antihypertensives (such as clonidine, guanabenz, guanadrel, guanethidine, meth-

yldopa, reserpine): Concomitant use may decrease hypotensive effects. Monitor blood pressure closely.

Cimetidine, fluoxetine, fluvoxamine, paroxetine, sertraline: May increase serum desipramine levels. Monitor patient closely.

Clonidine, ephedrine, epinephrine, norepinephrine, phenylephrine, phenylpropanolamine: May increase blood pressure. Monitor blood pressure closely.

CNS depressants (such as analgesics, anesthetics, barbiturates, narcotics, tranquilizers): Additive effects are likely. Avoid concomitant use.

Disulfiram, ethchlorvynol: May cause delirium and tachycardia. Monitor patient closely.

Haloperidol, phenothiazines: Decreased desipramine metabolism, decreasing therapeutic efficacy. Monitor patient for drug effects.

MAO inhibitors: May cause severe excitation, hyperpyrexia, or seizures, usually with high dosage. Use cautiously together.

Metrizamide: Increased risk of seizures. Monitor patient closely.

Selective serotonin-reuptake inhibiting drugs: Concomitant use may cause patient toxicity to tricyclic antidepressant at much lower dosages. Use together cautiously.

Warfarin: May increase PT and cause bleeding. Monitor INR.

Drug-lifestyle. *Alcohol:* May enhance CNS depression. Discourage concomitant use.

Heavy smoking: May lower plasma levels of desipramine. Discourage smoking.

Sun exposure: May increase risk of photosensitivity. Tell patient to take precautions.

Adverse reactions

CNS: *drowsiness, dizziness,* excitation, tremor, weakness, confusion, anxiety, restlessness, agitation, headache, nervousness, EEG changes, **seizures,** extrapyramidal reactions.
CV: orthostatic hypotension, *tachycardia, ECG changes,* hypertension, **sudden death** (in children).
EENT: *blurred vision,* tinnitus, mydriasis.
GI: *dry mouth, constipation,* nausea, vomiting, anorexia, paralytic ileus.
GU: *urine retention.*
Hematologic: decreased WBC counts.
Hepatic: elevated liver function tests.
Metabolic: hyperglycemia, hypoglycemia.
Skin: rash, urticaria, photosensitivity.
Other: *diaphoresis,* **hypersensitivity reaction.**
    After abrupt withdrawal of long-term therapy: nausea, headache, malaise (doesn't indicate addiction).

☑ Special considerations
Besides the recommendations relevant to all tricyclic antidepressants, consider the following.

• Dispense drug in smallest possible quantities to depressed outpatients to avoid suicide with drug.
• Drug causes fewer sedative, anticholinergic, and hypotensive effects than parent compound imipramine.
• Tolerance usually develops to sedative effects of drug during initial weeks of therapy.
• Don't withdraw drug abruptly; taper gradually over 3 to 6 weeks.
• Stop drug at least 48 hours before surgical procedures.
• Drug therapy in patients with bipolar illness may induce a hypomanic state.
• With overdose, the first 12 hours after ingestion are stimulatory; excessive anticholinergic activity (agitation, irritation, confusion, hallucinations, parkinsonian symptoms, hyperthermia, seizures, urine retention, dry mucous membranes, pupillary dilatation, constipation, and ileus). Then CNS depressant effects, including hypothermia, decreased or absent reflexes, sedation, hypotension, cyanosis; and cardiac irregularities, including tachycardia, conduction disturbances, and quinidine-like effects on ECG.
• Overdose severity indicated by widening of QRS complex, which usually represents serum level over 1,000 ng/ml; serum levels aren't generally helpful. Metabolic acidosis may follow hypotension, hypoventilation, and seizures.
• Treatment of overdose is symptomatic and supportive, including maintaining airway, stable body temperature, and fluid and electrolyte balance. Induce emesis with ipecac if patient is conscious; then gastric lavage and activated charcoal to prevent further absorption.
• Dialysis is of little use. Use physostigmine with caution to reverse CV abnormalities or coma; too rapid administration may cause seizures.
• Treat seizures with parenteral diazepam or phenytoin, arrhythmias with parenteral phenytoin or lidocaine, and acidosis with sodium bicarbonate. Don't give barbiturates; may enhance CNS and respiratory depressant effects.

Monitoring the patient
• Monitor standing and sitting blood pressure to assess orthostasis before administering desipramine.
• Monitor coagulation studies if patient takes oral anticoagulants.

Information for the patient
• Tell patient to take full dose at bedtime to reduce daytime sedation.
• Explain that full effects of drug may not become apparent for 4 weeks or more after drug start.
• Tell patient to take drug exactly as prescribed; don't double dose if a dose is missed.
• To prevent dizziness, advise patient to lie down for about 30 minutes after each dose at start of

therapy and to avoid sudden postural changes, especially when rising.
• Warn patient not to stop taking drug suddenly.
• Encourage patient to report unusual or troublesome effects, especially confusion, movement disorders, rapid heartbeat, dizziness, fainting, or difficulty urinating.
• Tell patient that sugarless chewing gum, hard candy, or ice may alleviate dry mouth.
• Stress importance of regular dental hygiene to avoid caries.
• Tell patient to store drug safely away from children.

Geriatric patients
• Elderly patients may be more susceptible to adverse cardiovascular and anticholinergic effects.

Pediatric patients
• Drug isn't recommended for patients under age 12.

Breast-feeding patients
• Drug appears in breast milk in levels equal to those in maternal serum. Benefit to mother should outweigh possible adverse reactions in infant.

desmopressin acetate
DDAVP, Stimate

Pharmacologic classification: posterior pituitary hormone
Therapeutic classification: antidiuretic, hemostatic
Pregnancy risk category B

How supplied
Available by prescription only
Tablets: 0.1 mg, 0.2 mg
Nasal solution: 0.1 mg/ml, 1.5 mg/ml
Injection: 4 mcg/ml in 1-ml single-dose ampules and 10-ml multiple-dose vials; 15 mcg/ml in 1-ml and 2-ml ampules

Indications, route, and dosage
Central cranial diabetes insipidus, temporary polyuria, polydipsia associated with pituitary trauma
Adults: 0.1 to 0.4 ml (10 to 40 mcg) intranasally in one to three divided doses daily. Adjust morning and evening doses separately for adequate diurnal rhythm of water turnover. Or 0.05 mg P.O. b.i.d. initially. Adjust individual dosage in increments of 0.1 mg to 1.2 mg daily, divided into two or three doses. Optimal dosage range is 0.1 to 0.8 mg daily in divided doses. Or give 0.5 ml (2 mcg) to 1 ml (4 mcg) I.V. or S.C. daily, usually in two divided doses.

Children ages 3 months to 12 years: 0.05 to 0.3 ml (5 to 30 mcg) intranasally daily in one or two doses.
Hemophilia A, von Willebrand's disease
Adults and children: 0.3 mcg/kg diluted in normal saline solution and infused I.V. slowly over 15 to 30 minutes. May repeat dosage, if necessary, as indicated by laboratory response and patient's condition. Or give one spray per nostril.
Primary nocturnal enuresis
Children ages 6 and older: 20 mcg (two to four metered sprays), intranasally h.s. Dosage adjusted according to response. Maximum recommended dose is 40 mcg daily.

Pharmacodynamics
Antidiuretic action: Used to control or prevent signs and complications of neurogenic diabetes insipidus. Site of action is primarily at the renal tubular level. Drug increases water permeability at the renal tubule and collecting duct, resulting in increased urine osmolality and decreased urinary flow rate.
Hemostatic action: Drug increases factor VIII activity by releasing endogenous factor VIII from plasma storage sites.

Pharmacokinetics
• *Absorption:* Destroyed in GI tract. After intranasal administration, 10% to 20% of dose absorbed through nasal mucosa; antidiuretic action occurs within 1 hour and peaks in 1 to 5 hours. After I.V. infusion, plasma factor VIII activity increases within 15 to 30 minutes and peaks between 1½ and 3 hours.
• *Distribution:* Not fully understood.
• *Metabolism:* No information available.
• *Excretion:* Plasma levels decline in two phases: half-life of fast phase about 8 minutes; slow phase, 75 minutes. Duration of action after intranasal administration, 8 to 20 hours; after I.V. administration, 12 to 24 hours for mild hemophilia and about 3 hours for von Willebrand's disease.

Contraindications and precautions
Contraindicated in patients with hypersensitivity to drug and in those with type IIB von Willebrand's disease.
    Use cautiously in patients with coronary artery insufficiency or hypertensive CV disease and in those with conditions associated with fluid and electrolyte imbalances, such as cystic fibrosis, because these patients are prone to hyponatremia.

Interactions
Drug-drug. Carbamazepine, chlorpropamide, clofibrate: May potentiate desmopressin's antidiuretic action. Avoid concomitant use.

Demeclocycline, epinephrine, heparin, lithium, norepinephrine: May decrease antidiuretic effect. Monitor patient's intake and output closely.
Drug-lifestyle. *Alcohol:* May increase risk of adverse effects. Avoid use.

Adverse reactions
CNS: headache.
CV: slight rise in blood pressure (at high doses).
EENT: rhinitis, epistaxis, sore throat, cough.
GI: nausea, abdominal cramps.
GU: vulval pain.
Other: flushing, local erythema, swelling, burning after injection.

☑ Special considerations
Besides the recommendations relevant to all posterior pituitary hormones, consider the following.
• May be administered intranasally through flexible catheter called a rhinyle. A measured quantity is drawn up into catheter, one end is inserted into patient's nose, and patient blows on other end to deposit drug into nasal cavity. Or drug is newly available in nasal spray, which may be easier for some patients.
• Patients may be switched from intranasal to S.C. desmopressin (for example, during episodes of rhinorrhea). They should receive one-tenth of their usual dosage parenterally.
• Adjust patient's fluid intake to reduce risk of water intoxication and sodium depletion, especially in young or elderly patients.
• Desmopressin isn't indicated for hemophilia A patients with factor VIII levels up to 5% or in patients with severe von Willebrand's disease.
• Drug therapy may enable some patients to avoid hazards of contaminated blood products.
• Check drug expiration date.
• Signs and symptoms of overdose include drowsiness, listlessness, headache, confusion, anuria, and weight gain (water intoxication). Treatment requires water restriction and temporary withdrawal of drug until polyuria occurs.
• Severe water intoxication may require osmotic diuresis with mannitol, hypertonic dextrose, or urea—alone or with furosemide.

Monitoring the patient
• Watch for early signs of water intoxication (drowsiness, listlessness, headache, confusion, anuria, and weight gain) to prevent seizures, coma, and death.
• Weigh patient daily and watch for edema.
• Monitor serum electrolytes periodically.

Information for the patient
• Teach patient correct administration technique, then evaluate proficiency at drug administration and accurate measurement on return visits; some patients may have difficulty measuring and inhaling drug into nostrils.

• Emphasize that patient shouldn't increase or decrease dosage unless prescribed.
• Assist patient in planning schedule for fluid intake if oral fluids must be reduced to decrease possibility of water intoxication and hyponatremia. A diuretic may be administered if excessive fluid retention occurs.
• Tell patient to store drug away from heat and direct light, not in bathroom where heat and moisture can cause drug to deteriorate.

Geriatric patients
• Elderly patients have an increased risk of hyponatremia and water intoxication; restriction of fluid intake is recommended.
• Because elderly patients are more sensitive to drug's effects, they may need a lower dosage.

Pediatric patients
• Drug isn't recommended in infants under age 3 months because of increased tendency to develop fluid imbalance.
• Use with caution in infants because of risk of hyponatremia and water intoxication.
• Safety and efficacy of parenteral desmopressin haven't been established for management of diabetes insipidus in children under age 12.

desonide
DesOwen, Tridesilon

Pharmacologic classification: topical adrenocorticoid
Therapeutic classification: anti-inflammatory
Pregnancy risk category C

How supplied
Available by prescription only
Cream, lotion, ointment: 0.05%

Indications, route, and dosage
Adjunctive therapy for inflammation in acute and chronic corticosteroid-responsive dermatoses
Adults and children: Apply sparingly to affected area b.i.d. to q.i.d.

Pharmacodynamics
Anti-inflammatory action: Stimulates synthesis of enzymes needed to decrease the inflammatory response. A group IV nonfluorinated glucocorticoid with a potency similar to that of alclometasone dipropionate 0.05% and fluocinolone acetonide 0.01%.

Pharmacokinetics
• *Absorption:* Amount absorbed depends on amount applied and on nature and condition of skin at application site. Ranges from about 1% in areas with thick stratum corneum (palms, soles,

elbows, and knees) to as much as 36% in areas of thinnest stratum corneum (face, eyelids, genitals). Absorption increases in areas of skin damage, inflammation, or occlusion. Some systemic absorption of topical steroids occurs, especially through oral mucosa.

• *Distribution:* After topical application, is distributed throughout local skin layer. Any drug absorbed into circulation is removed rapidly from blood and distributed into muscle, liver, skin, intestines, and kidneys.

• *Metabolism:* After topical administration, metabolized primarily in skin. Small amount absorbed into systemic circulation is metabolized primarily in liver to inactive compounds.

• *Excretion:* Inactive metabolites excreted by kidneys, primarily as glucuronides and sulfates, but also as unconjugated products. Small amounts of metabolites also excreted in feces.

Contraindications and precautions
Contraindicated in patients with hypersensitivity to drug.

Interactions
None reported.

Adverse reactions
Metabolic: hyperglycemia, glucosuria, *hypothalamic-pituitary-adrenal axis suppression,* Cushing's syndrome.
Skin: burning, pruritus, irritation, dryness, erythema, folliculitis, perioral dermatitis, allergic contact dermatitis, hypertrichosis, hypopigmentation, acneiform eruptions, *maceration of skin, secondary infection, atrophy, striae, miliaria* (with occlusive dressings).

☑ Special considerations
• Recommendations for use of desonide, for care and teaching of patients during therapy, and for use in elderly patients, children, and breastfeeding women are the same as those for all topical adrenocorticoids.

Monitoring the patient
• Monitor patient's response to treatment.
• Watch for adverse reactions.

Information for the patient
• Instruct patient to use drug only as directed.
• Tell patient to report worsening of condition.

Pediatric patients
• Children may be more susceptible to systemic absorption leading to HPA-axis suppression.

dexamethasone (ophthalmic suspension)
Maxidex

dexamethasone sodium phosphate
AK-Dex, Decadron, Dexair, Ocu-Dex

Pharmacologic classification: corticosteroid
Therapeutic classification: ophthalmic anti-inflammatory
Pregnancy risk category C

How supplied
Available by prescription only
dexamethasone
Ophthalmic suspension: 0.1%
dexamethasone sodium phosphate
Ophthalmic ointment: 0.05%
Ophthalmic solution: 0.1%

Indications, route, and dosage
Uveitis; iridocyclitis; inflammation of eyelids, conjunctiva, cornea, anterior segment of globe; corneal injury from burns or penetration by foreign bodies; allergic conjunctivitis; suppression of graft rejection after keratoplasty
Adults and children: Instill 1 to 2 drops of suspension or solution or apply 1.25 to 2.5 cm of ointment into conjunctival sac. For initial therapy in severe cases, instill solution or suspension into conjunctival sac every hour, gradually taper dose as patient's condition improves. In mild condition, use drops up to four to six times daily or apply ointment t.i.d. or q.i.d. As patient's condition improves, taper dose to b.i.d. then once daily. Treatment may extend from a few days to several weeks.

Pharmacodynamics
Anti-inflammatory action: Corticosteroids stimulate synthesis of enzymes needed to decrease inflammatory response. Dexamethasone, a long-acting fluorinated synthetic adrenocorticoid with strong anti-inflammatory activity and minimal mineralocorticoid activity, is 25 to 30 times more potent than an equal weight of hydrocortisone.
　　Drug is poorly soluble and therefore has a slower onset of action but a longer duration of action when applied in a liquid suspension. The sodium phosphate salt is highly soluble and has a rapid onset but short duration of action.

Pharmacokinetics
• *Absorption:* After ophthalmic administration, absorbed through aqueous humor. Because only low doses are administered, little if any systemic absorption occurs.

• *Distribution:* Distributed throughout local tissue layers. Absorbed into circulation, rapidly removed from blood and distributed into muscle, liver, skin, intestines, and kidneys.
• *Metabolism:* Primarily metabolized locally. Small amount absorbed into systemic circulation is metabolized primarily in liver to inactive compounds.
• *Excretion:* Inactive metabolites excreted by kidneys, primarily as glucuronides and sulfates, but also as unconjugated products. Small amounts of metabolites excreted in feces.

Contraindications and precautions
Contraindicated in patients with acute superficial herpes simplex (dendritic keratitis), vaccinia, varicella, or other fungal or viral diseases of cornea and conjunctiva; ocular tuberculosis; or acute, purulent, untreated infections of the eye.
   Use cautiously in patients with corneal abrasions that may be infected (especially with herpes). Also use cautiously in patients with glaucoma because intraocular pressure may increase. Glaucoma drugs may need to be increased to compensate.

Interactions
None reported.

Adverse reactions
EENT: increased intraocular pressure; thinning of cornea; interference with corneal wound healing; increased susceptibility to viral or fungal corneal infection; corneal ulceration; glaucoma exacerbation; cataracts; defects in visual acuity and visual field; optic nerve damage; mild blurred vision; burning, stinging, or redness of eyes; watery eyes; discharge; discomfort; ocular pain; foreign body sensation (with excessive or long-term use).
Metabolic: adrenal suppression (with excessive or long-term use).

☑ Special considerations
• Shake suspension well before use.
• Drug isn't recommended for long-term use.

Monitoring the patient
• Monitor patient's response to treatment.
• Watch for corneal ulceration; may require stopping drug.

Information for the patient
• Teach patient how to apply.
• Tell patient to avoid touching tip of container to eye.

dexamethasone (systemic)
Decadron, Deronil*, Dexasone*, Dexone, Hexadrol

dexamethasone acetate
Dalalone D.P., Decadron-LA, Decaject-L.A., Dexasone-L.A., Dexone L.A., Solurex LA

dexamethasone sodium phosphate
AK-Dex, Dalalone, Decadrol, Decadron, Decaject, Dexameth, Dexasone, Dexone, Hexadrol Phosphate, Oradexon*, Solurex

Pharmacologic classification: glucocorticoid
Therapeutic classification: anti-inflammatory, immunosuppressant
Pregnancy risk category NR

How supplied
Available by prescription only
dexamethasone
Tablets: 0.25 mg, 0.5 mg, 0.75 mg, 1 mg, 1.5 mg, 2 mg, 4 mg, 6 mg
Elixir: 0.5 mg/5 ml
Oral solution: 0.5 mg/0.5 ml, 0.5 mg/5 ml
dexamethasone acetate
Injection: 8 mg/ml, 16 mg/ml suspension
dexamethasone sodium phosphate
Injection: 4 mg/ml, 10 mg/ml, 20 mg/ml, 24 mg/ml

Indications, route, and dosage
Cerebral edema
dexamethasone sodium phosphate
Adults: Initially, 10 mg I.V., then 4 mg I.M. q 6 hours for 2 to 4 days, then taper over 5 to 7 days.
Inflammatory conditions, allergic reactions, neoplasias
Adults: 0.75 to 9 mg P.O. daily divided b.i.d., t.i.d., or q.i.d.
Children: 0.024 to 0.34 mg/kg P.O. daily in four divided doses.
dexamethasone acetate
Adults: 4 to 16 mg intra-articularly or into soft tissue q 1 to 3 weeks; 0.8 to 1.6 mg into lesions q 1 to 3 weeks; or 8 to 16 mg I.M. q 1 to 3 weeks, p.r.n.
dexamethasone sodium phosphate
Adults: 0.2 to 6 mg intra-articularly, intralesionally, or into soft tissue; or 0.5 to 9 mg I.M.
Shock (other than adrenal crisis)
dexamethasone sodium phosphate
Adults: 1 to 6 mg/kg I.V. daily as a single dose; or 40 mg I.V. q 2 to 6 hours, p.r.n.
Dexamethasone suppression test
Adults: 0.5 mg P.O. q 6 hours for 48 hours.

Adrenal insufficiency
Adults: 0.75 to 9 mg P.O. daily in divided doses.
Children: 0.024 to 0.34 mg/kg P.O. daily in four divided doses.
dexamethasone sodium phosphate
Adults: 0.5 to 9 mg I.M. or I.V. daily.
Children: 0.235 to 1.25 mg/m² I.M. or I.V. once daily or b.i.d.
◊ *Prevention of hyaline membrane disease in premature infants*
Adults: 5 mg (phosphate) I.M. t.i.d. to mother for 2 days before delivery.
◊ *Prevention of cancer chemotherapy–induced nausea and vomiting*
Adults: 10 to 20 mg I.V. before administration of chemotherapy. Additional doses (individualized for each patient and usually lower than initial dose) may be administered I.V. or P.O. for 24 to 72 hours following cancer chemotherapy, if needed.

Pharmacodynamics
Anti-inflammatory action: Dexamethasone stimulates synthesis of enzymes needed to decrease inflammatory response. Causes suppression of the immune system by reducing activity and volume of the lymphatic system, producing lymphocytopenia (primarily T-lymphocytes), decreasing passage of immune complexes through basement membranes and possibly by depressing reactivity of tissue to antigen-antibody interactions.

Drug is a long-acting synthetic adrenocorticoid with strong anti-inflammatory activity and minimal mineralocorticoid properties. It's 25 to 30 times more potent than an equal weight of hydrocortisone.

Because the acetate salt is a suspension, it shouldn't be used I.V. It's particularly useful as an anti-inflammatory drug in intra-articular, intradermal, and intralesional injections.

The sodium phosphate salt is highly soluble and has a more rapid onset and a shorter duration of action than does the acetate salt. It's most commonly used for cerebral edema and unresponsive shock. It can also be used in intra-articular, intralesional, or soft tissue inflammation. Other uses for dexamethasone are chemotherapy-induced nausea, symptomatic treatment of bronchial asthma, and as a diagnostic test for Cushing's syndrome.

Pharmacokinetics
• *Absorption:* After oral administration, absorbed readily; peak effects in about 1 to 2 hours. Suspension for injection has variable onset and duration of action (ranging from 2 days to 3 weeks), depending on if injected into intra-articular space, muscle, or blood supply to muscle. After I.V. injection, is rapidly and completely absorbed into tissues.
• *Distribution:* Removed rapidly from blood and distributed to muscle, liver, skin, intestines, and kidneys. Bound weakly to plasma proteins (transcortin and albumin). Only unbound portion is active. Adrenocorticoids distributed into breast milk and through placenta.
• *Metabolism:* Metabolized in liver to inactive glucuronide and sulfate metabolites.
• *Excretion:* Inactive metabolites and small amounts of unmetabolized drug excreted by kidneys. Insignificant quantities also excreted in feces; biologic half-life 36 to 54 hours.

Contraindications and precautions
Contraindicated in patients with hypersensitivity to drug or its components and in those with systemic fungal infections.

Use cautiously in patients with recent MI, GI ulcer, renal disease, hypertension, osteoporosis, diabetes mellitus, hypothyroidism, cirrhosis, diverticulitis, nonspecific ulcerative colitis, recent intestinal anastomoses, thromboembolic disorders, seizures, myasthenia gravis, heart failure, tuberculosis, ocular herpes simplex, emotional instability, and psychotic tendencies. Because some formulations contain sulfite preservatives, also use cautiously in patients sensitive to sulfites.

Interactions
Drug-drug. *Amphotericin B, diuretics:* May enhance hypokalemia. Monitor potassium levels.
Antacids, cholestyramine, colestipol: Decreased corticosteroid effect due to decreased amount of corticosteroid absorbed. Monitor patient closely.
Barbiturates, phenytoin, rifampin: May cause decreased corticosteroid effects because of increased hepatic metabolism. Monitor patient closely.
Cardiac glycosides: In patients with hypokalemia, toxicity with cardiac glycosides can occur. Monitor glycoside levels.
Estrogens: May reduce metabolism of dexamethasone by increasing transcortin level. Half-life of corticosteroid is prolonged because of increased protein-binding. Monitor patient closely.
Insulin, oral antidiabetics: Dexamethasone causes hyperglycemia. Monitor serum glucose levels.
Isoniazid, salicylates: Possible increased metabolism of these drugs. Avoid concomitant use.
Oral anticoagulants: Concomitant use may decrease effects of oral anticoagulants by unknown mechanisms. Monitor INR.
Toxoids, vaccines: Decreased antibody response; increased risk of neurologic complications. Defer until therapy ends.
Ulcerogenic drugs (such as aspirin, NSAIDs): May increase risk of GI ulceration. Monitor patient closely.
Drug-lifestyle. *Alcohol:* Increases risk of gastric irritation and GI ulceration. Avoid use.

Adverse reactions
Most adverse reactions to corticosteroids are dose-dependent or duration-dependent.
CNS: *euphoria, insomnia,* psychotic behavior, pseudotumor cerebri, vertigo, headache, paresthesia, *seizures.*
CV: *heart failure,* hypertension, edema, *arrhythmias,* thrombophlebitis, *thromboembolism.*
EENT: cataracts, glaucoma.
GI: *peptic ulceration,* GI irritation, increased appetite, *pancreatitis,* nausea, vomiting.
GU: menstrual irregularities.
Metabolic: hypokalemia, hypocalcemia, hyperglycemia, carbohydrate intolerance, decreased levels of thyroxine, and triiodothyronine, and increased urine glucose and calcium levels, *acute adrenal insufficiency* may follow increased stress (infection, surgery, or trauma) or abrupt withdrawal after long-term therapy.
Musculoskeletal: muscle weakness, osteoporosis, growth suppression in children.
Skin: delayed wound healing, acne, various skin eruptions, atrophy (at I.M. injection sites).
Other: hirsutism, susceptibility to infections, cushingoid state (moonface, buffalo hump, central obesity).
   After abrupt withdrawal: rebound inflammation, fatigue, weakness, arthralgia, fever, dizziness, lethargy, depression, fainting, orthostatic hypotension, dyspnea, anorexia, hypoglycemia. *After prolonged use, sudden withdrawal may be fatal.*

☑ Special considerations
• Recommendations for use of dexamethasone, for care and teaching of patients during therapy, and for use in elderly patients and breast-feeding women are the same as those for all systemic adrenocorticoids.
• Drug is being used for investigational purposes to prevent hyaline membrane disease (respiratory distress syndrome) in premature infants. The suspension (phosphate salt) is administered I.M. to mother b.i.d. or t.i.d. for 2 days before delivery.
• Drug causes false-negative results in the nitroblue tetrazolium test for systemic bacterial infections and decreases ^{131}I uptake and protein-bound iodine levels in thyroid function tests.
• Acute ingestion, even in massive doses, rarely poses a clinical problem for less than 3 weeks, even at large dosage ranges.
• Long-term use causes adverse physiologic effects, including suppression of the hypothalamic-pituitary-adrenal axis, cushingoid appearance, muscle weakness, and osteoporosis.

Monitoring the patient
• Monitor coagulation studies if patient is taking oral anticoagulants.
• Monitor serum glucose level if patient is diabetic.
• Monitor serum electrolyte levels if patient is taking diuretics or antifungals.

Information for the patient
• Tell patient not to discontinue drug abruptly or without physician's consent.
• Instruct patient to take drug with food or milk.
• Teach patient the signs of early adrenal insufficiency, namely fatigue, muscular weakness, joint pain, fever, anorexia, nausea, dyspnea, dizziness, and fainting.

Pediatric patients
• Long-term use of drug in children and adolescents may delay growth and maturation.

dexamethasone (topical)
Aeroseb-Dex, Decaspray

dexamethasone sodium phosphate
Decadron Phosphate

Pharmacologic classification: corticosteroid
Therapeutic classification: anti-inflammatory
Pregnancy risk category C

How supplied
Available by prescription only
dexamethasone
Aerosol: 0.01%, 0.04%
dexamethasone sodium phosphate
Cream: 0.1%

Indications, route, and dosage
Inflammation of corticosteroid-responsive dermatoses
Adults and children: Apply sparingly t.i.d. or q.i.d. For aerosol use on scalp, shake can well and apply to dry scalp after shampooing. Hold can upright. Slide applicator tube under hair so that it touches scalp. Spray while moving tube to all affected areas, keeping tube under hair and in contact with scalp throughout spraying, which should take about 2 seconds. Inadequately covered areas may be spot sprayed. Slide applicator tube through hair to touch scalp; press and immediately release spray button. Don't massage drug into scalp or spray forehead or eyes.

Pharmacodynamics
Anti-inflammatory action: A synthetic fluorinated corticosteroid. It's usually classed as a group VII potency anti-inflammatory. Occlusive dressings may be used in severe cases. The aerosol spray is usually used for dermatologic conditions of the scalp.

Pharmacokinetics
- *Absorption:* Depends on preparation potency, amount applied, vehicle used, and nature and condition of skin at application site. Ranges from about 1% in areas with thick stratum corneum (palms, soles, elbows, and knees) to 25% in areas of thinnest stratum corneum (face, eyelids, genitals). Inflamed or damaged skin may absorb more than 33%. Absorption increases in areas of skin damage, inflammation, or occlusion. Some systemic absorption occurs, especially through oral mucosa.
- *Distribution:* After topical applications, is distributed throughout local skin layer. If absorbed into circulation, is distributed rapidly into muscle, liver, skin, intestines, and kidneys.
- *Metabolism:* After topical administration, is metabolized primarily in skin. Small amount absorbed into systemic circulation is primarily metabolized in liver to inactive compounds.
- *Excretion:* Inactive metabolites excreted by kidneys, primarily as glucuronides and sulfates, but also as unconjugated products. Small amounts of metabolites also excreted in feces.

Contraindications and precautions
Contraindicated in patients with hypersensitivity to drug.

Interactions
None reported.

Adverse reactions
Metabolic: hyperglycemia, glucosuria, ***hypothalamic-pituitary-adrenal axis suppression,*** Cushing's syndrome.
Skin: burning, pruritus, irritation, dryness, erythema, folliculitis, hypertrichosis, acneiform eruptions, perioral dermatitis, hypopigmentation, allergic contact dermatitis, *maceration, secondary infection, atrophy, striae, miliaria* (with occlusive dressings).

☑ Special considerations
- Recommendations for use of dexamethasone, for care and teaching of patients during therapy, and for use in elderly patients, children, and breast-feeding women are the same as those for all topical adrenocorticoids.

Monitoring the patient
- Monitor patient's response to treatment.
- Topical corticosteroids can be absorbed in sufficient amounts to produce systemic effects.

Information for the patient
- Tell patient to report any signs of allergy (burning, itching, redness).

dexmedetomidine hydrochloride
Precedex

Pharmacologic classification: selective alpha$_2$-adrenoceptor agonist with sedative properties
Therapeutic classification: sedative
Pregnancy risk category C

How supplied
Injection: 100 mcg/ml 2-ml vials and 2-ml ampules

Indication, route, and dosage
Sedation of initially intubated and mechanically ventilated patients in ICU setting
Adults: Loading infusion of 1 mcg/kg over 10 minutes; then maintenance infusion of 0.2 to 0.7 mcg/kg/hr adjusted to achieve desired level of sedation. Not indicated for infusions lasting longer than 24 hours.
✦ ***Dosage adjustment.*** For elderly patients and for those with renal or hepatic failure, dosage reductions may be needed.

Pharmacodynamics
Sedative action: Produces sedation by selective stimulation of alpha$_2$-adrenoceptor in the CNS.

Pharmacokinetics
- *Absorption:* Must be given parenterally.
- *Distribution:* After I.V. administration, is rapidly and widely distributed; 94% protein-bound.
- *Metabolism:* Almost completely hepatically metabolized to inactive metabolites.
- *Excretion:* Inactive metabolites 95% renally eliminated and 4% fecally eliminated. Elimination half-life is about 2 hours.

Contraindications and precautions
Use cautiously in breast-feeding women, patients with heart block, elderly patients, and those with hepatic impairment.
    Not recommended for use during labor and delivery

Interactions
Drug-drug. *Anesthetics, hypnotics, opioids, sedatives:* Possible enhanced effects. Dose reduction of dexmedetomidine may be needed.

Adverse reactions
CV: *hypotension,* hypertension, ***bradycardia,*** tachycardia, ***arrhythmias.***
GI: nausea, vomiting, thirst.
GU: oliguria.
Hematologic: anemia, leukocytosis.
Respiratory: hypoxia, pleural effusion, pulmonary edema.
Other: pain, infection.

☑ Special considerations

- Drug should only be administered by those skilled in patient management in intensive care setting where patient's cardiac status can be continuously monitored.
- Administer drug using a controlled infusion device at rate calculated for body weight.
- Drug has been continuously infused in mechanically ventilated patients before extubation, during extubation, and after extubation. It's not necessary to stop drug before extubation.
- Dilute drug in 0.9% sodium chloride solution before administration. To prepare infusion, withdraw 2 ml of drug and add to 48 ml of 0.9% sodium chloride injection to total 50 ml. Shake gently to mix well.
- Don't coadminister with blood or plasma through same I.V. catheter; physical compatibility hasn't been established. Dexmedetomidine infusion is compatible with lactated Ringer's, 5% dextrose in water, 0.9% sodium chloride in water, and 20% mannitol. Also compatible with thiopental sodium, etomidate, vecuronium bromide, pancuronium bromide, succinylcholine, atracurium besylate, mivacurium chloride, glycopyrrolate bromide, phenylephrine hydrochloride, atropine sulfate, midazolam, porphin sulfate, fentanyl citrate, and plasma-substitute.
- Don't infuse for more than 24 hours because safety and efficacy haven't been established for longer periods.
- If administered long-term and stopped abruptly, withdrawal symptoms similar to those reported for clonidine may result, including nervousness, agitation, and headaches, with or followed by rapid rise in blood pressure and elevated plasma catecholamine levels.
- Store at controlled room temperature (59° to 86° F [15° to 30° C]).
- Bradycardia, hypotension, and first- and second-degree AV block have been reported in patients receiving doses substantially higher than those recommended. These conditions resolved spontaneously.
- In case of overdose, stop infusion and give supportive care and resuscitation, if needed. Increasing rate of I.V. fluid administration, elevating lower extremities, and using pressor drugs may be needed for hypotension and bradycardia.
- Because bradycardia is associated with dexmedetomidine-induced increase in vagal tone, consider I.V. administration of anticholinergics such as atropine to modify vagal tone.
- It's unlikely that drug can be removed by hemodialysis or peritoneal dialysis because of its high protein-binding.

Monitoring the patient

- Monitor cardiac status continuously during infusion.

- Monitor renal and hepatic function before treatment, particularly in elderly patients.
- Some patients receiving drug are arousable and alert when stimulated. This alone shouldn't be considered evidence of lack of efficacy in the absence of other signs and symptoms.

Information for the patient

- Explain to patient and family that he will be sedated; assure patient that he will be closely monitored.
- Explain to patient and family that, while sedated, patient may be arousable when stimulated.

Geriatric patients

- There is a higher risk of bradycardia and hypotension in patients over age 65. Dose reduction may be needed for this age-group.
- Carefully select dose in elderly patients; it may be useful to monitor renal function.

Pediatric patients

- Safety and efficacy in children haven't been established; drug isn't recommended.

Breast-feeding patients

- It's unknown if drug appears in breast milk. Use with caution in breast-feeding women.

dexrazoxane
Zinecard

Pharmacologic classification: intracellular chelating drug
Therapeutic classification: cardioprotective
Pregnancy risk category C

How supplied

Available by prescription only
Injection: 250 mg, 500 mg in single-dose vials

Indications, route, and dosage

Reduction of incidence and severity of doxorubicin-induced cardiomyopathy in women with metastatic breast cancer who have received a cumulative doxorubicin dose of 300 mg/m² but would benefit from continued therapy with doxorubicin

Adults: Dosage ratio of dexrazoxane to doxorubicin must be 10:1, such as 500 mg/m² dexrazoxane:50 mg/m² doxorubicin. After reconstitution, administer dexrazoxane by slow I.V. push or rapid drip I.V. infusion. After completion of dexrazoxane administration and before a total elapsed time of 30 minutes from the beginning of dexrazoxane administration, give the I.V. injection of doxorubicin dose.

Pharmacodynamics

Cardioprotective action: Exact mechanism unknown. A cyclic derivative of ethylenediamine-tetra-acetic acid (EDTA) that readily penetrates cell membranes. Studies suggest that drug is converted intracellularly to a ring-opened chelating drug that interferes with iron-mediated free radical generation believed to be responsible, in part, for anthracycline-induced cardiomyopathy.

Pharmacokinetics

- *Absorption:* Given I.V.
- *Distribution:* No information available. Drug isn't bound to plasma proteins.
- *Metabolism:* Not believed to be metabolized.
- *Excretion:* Excreted primarily in urine.

Contraindications and precautions

Contraindicated in patients who aren't receiving doxorubicin as part of the chemotherapy regimen. Use cautiously in all patients because additive effects of immunosuppression may occur from concomitant administration of cytotoxic drugs.

Interactions

None reported.

Adverse reactions

The following reactions (except for pain on injection) may be attributed to the FAC regimen (fluorouracil, doxorubicin [Adriamycin], cyclophosphamide) given shortly after dexrazoxane.

CNS: *fatigue, malaise,* **neurotoxicity.**
GI: *nausea, vomiting, anorexia, stomatitis, diarrhea,* esophagitis, dysphagia.
Hematologic: *hemorrhage.*
Skin: urticaria, *alopecia,* erythema.
Other: *fever, infection, pain on injection,* **sepsis,** streaking at I.V. insertion site, phlebitis, extravasation.

☑ Special considerations

- Don't give doxorubicin before dexrazoxane. Dexrazoxane isn't recommended for use with initiation of doxorubicin therapy but only after an accumulate dosage of doxorubicin of 300 mg/m^2 has been reached and continuation of doxorubicin is desired.
- Dilute with diluent supplied with drug (0.167 M sodium lactate injection) to give a concentration of 10 mg dexrazoxane for each ml of sodium lactate. Reconstituted solution should be given by slow I.V. push or rapid drip I.V. infusion from bag.
- Reconstituted solution, when transferred to an empty infusion bag, is stable for 6 hours from time of reconstitution when stored at controlled room temperature (36° to 46° F [2° to 8° C]) or under refrigeration. Discard unused solution.

- Reconstituted drug may be diluted with either normal saline solution or D$_5$W injection to a concentration of 1.3 to 5.0 mg/ml in I.V. infusion bags. The resultant solution is stable for 6 hours under same storage conditions as for diluted drug.
- Dexrazoxane shouldn't be mixed with other drugs because of possible incompatibility.
- Use caution when handling and preparing reconstituted solution; follow same precautions as for handling antineoplastics. Use gloves; if powder or solution contacts skin or mucosa, immediately wash thoroughly with soap and water.
- There are no reports of overdose, although myelosuppression is most likely to occur.
- Because dexrazoxane isn't bound to plasma protein, peritoneal dialysis or hemodialysis may be effective in removing drug from body. Suspected overdose should be managed with supportive care until resolution of myelosuppression and related conditions is complete. Management of overdose should include treatment of infections, fluid regulation, and maintenance of nutritional requirements.

Monitoring the patient

- Monitor CBC closely.
- Drug is always used with other cytotoxic drugs and giving drug with doxorubicin doesn't eliminate possibility of cardiac toxicity. Carefully monitor cardiac function. May add to myelosuppressive effects of these drugs.

Information for the patient

- Inform patient of need for drug during continued doxorubicin therapy.
- Warn patient to watch for signs of infection (fever, sore throat, fatigue) and bleeding (easy bruising, nose bleeds, bleeding gums, melena). Tell patient to take temperature daily and teach patient infection control and bleeding precautions.
- Inform patient that alopecia may occur but is usually reversible.

Pediatric patients

- Safety and effectiveness in children haven't been established.

Breast-feeding patients

- Because of potential for serious adverse effects in breast-fed infants, breast-feeding isn't recommended. It's unknown whether drug appears in breast milk.

dextran 1
Promit

dextran, low-molecular-weight (dextran 40)
Gentran 40, LMD 10%, Rheomacrodex

dextran, high-molecular-weight (dextran 70, dextran 75)
Gendex 75, Gentran 70, Macrodex

Pharmacologic classification: glucose polymer
Therapeutic classification: plasma volume expander
Pregnancy risk category C

How supplied
Available by prescription only
dextran 1
Injection: 150 mg/ml in 20-ml vials
low-molecular-weight dextran
Injection: 10% dextran 40 in D_5W or normal saline solution
high-molecular-weight dextran
Injection: 6% dextran 70 in normal saline solution or D_5W; 6% dextran 75 in normal saline solution or D_5W

Indications, route, and dosage
Prevention of severe anaphylactic reaction caused by low- or high-molecular-weight dextran
Adults: 20 ml dextran 1 by rapid I.V. push 1 to 2 minutes before dextran infusion.
Children: 0.3 ml/kg dextran 1 by rapid I.V. push 1 to 2 minutes before dextran infusion.
Plasma volume expansion
Dosage depends on amount of fluid loss.
Adults: Initially, 500 ml of dextran 40 with central venous pressure (CVP) monitoring. Infuse remaining dose slowly. Total daily dose shouldn't exceed 2 g/kg (20 ml/kg) body weight. If therapy continues past 24 hours, don't exceed 1 g/kg daily. Continue for no more than 5 days.
   Usual dose of dextran 70 or 75 solution is 30 g (500 ml of 6% solution) I.V. In emergencies, may be administered at a rate of 1.2 to 2.4 g/minute (20 to 40 ml/minute). Total dose during the first 24 hours isn't to exceed 1.2 g/kg; actual dose depends on amount of fluid loss and resultant hemoconcentration and must be determined individually. In normovolemic patients, the rate of administration shouldn't exceed 240 mg/minute (4 ml/minute).
Children: Total dosage of dextran 70 or 75 shouldn't exceed 1.2 g/kg (20 ml/kg), with the dose based on body weight or surface area. If therapy is continued, dosage shouldn't exceed 0.6 g/kg (10 ml/kg) daily.

Priming pump oxygenators
Adults: Dextran 40 can be used as the only priming fluid or as an additive to other primers in pump oxygenators. Dextran 40 is added to the perfusion circuit as the 10% solution in a dose of 1 to 2 g/kg (10 to 20 ml/kg); total dose shouldn't exceed 2 g/kg (20 ml/kg).
Prophylaxis of venous thrombosis and pulmonary embolism
Adults: Dextran 40 therapy usually should be given during the surgical procedure. On the day of surgery, dextran 40 (10% solution) is given at the dose of 50 to 100 g (500 to 1,000 ml or about 10 ml/kg). Treatment is continued for 2 to 3 days at a dose of 50 g (500 ml) daily. Then, if needed, 50 g (500 ml) may be given q 2 or 3 days for up to 2 weeks to reduce the risk of thromboembolism (deep venous thrombosis) or pulmonary embolism.

Pharmacodynamics
Plasma-expanding action: Dextran 40 (10%) has an average molecular weight of 40,000, the osmotic equivalent of twice the volume of plasma. Dextran 40 has a duration of action of 2 to 4 hours. Dextran 70 has an average molecular weight of 70,000; the I.V. infusion results in an expansion of the plasma volume slightly in excess of the volume infused. This effect, useful in treating shock, lasts for about 12 hours.
   Dextran 40, 70, and 75 enhance blood flow, particularly in the microcirculation.
Prophylaxis of venous thrombosis and pulmonary embolism: Dextran 40 inhibits vascular stasis and platelet adhesiveness and alters the structure and lysability of fibrin clots. Dextran 40 increases cardiac output and arterial, venous, and microcirculatory flow and reduces mean transit time, mainly by expanding plasma volume and by reducing blood viscosity through hemodilution and reducing red cell aggregation.

Pharmacokinetics
- *Absorption:* Dextran 40 and 70 given by I.V. infusion. Plasma level depends on rate of infusion and rate of disappearance of drug from plasma.
- *Distribution:* Distributed throughout vascular system.
- *Metabolism:* Dextran molecules with molecular weights above 50,000 are enzymatically degraded by dextrinase to glucose at a rate of about 70 to 90 mg/kg/day. Process is variable.
- *Excretion:* Dextran molecules with molecular weights below 50,000 are eliminated by renal excretion, with 40% of dextran 70 appearing in urine within 24 hours. About 50% of dextran 40 excreted in urine within 3 hours, 60% within 6 hours, and 75% within 24 hours. Remaining 25% is hydrolyzed partially and excreted in urine, excreted partially in feces, and partially oxidized.

Contraindications and precautions

Low-molecular-weight dextran is contraindicated in patients with hypersensitivity to drug and in those with marked hemostatic defects, marked cardiac decompensation, and renal disease with severe oliguria or anuria. High-molecular-weight dextran is also contraindicated in patients with hypervolemic conditions and severe bleeding disorders.

Use low-molecular-weight dextran cautiously in patients with active hemorrhage, thrombocytopenia, or diabetes mellitus. High-molecular-weight dextran should be used cautiously in patients with active hemorrhage, thrombocytopenia, impaired renal clearance, chronic liver disease, and abdominal conditions or in those undergoing bowel surgery.

Interactions

Drug-drug. *Anticoagulants, antiplatelet drugs:* Abnormally prolonged bleeding times can occur if either high-molecular-weight dextran or low-molecular-weight dextran is given concomitantly. Monitor patient closely.

Adverse reactions

CV: *thrombophlebitis.*
EENT: nasal congestion (with high-molecular-weight dextran).
GI: nausea, vomiting.
GU: tubular stasis and blocking, increased urine viscosity; oliguria, anuria, increased specific gravity of urine (with high-molecular-weight dextran).
Hematologic: *decreased hemoglobin level and hematocrit;* increased bleeding time (with higher doses of low-molecular-weight dextran); increased bleeding time and significant suppression of platelet function (with high-molecular-weight dextran in doses of 15 ml/kg body weight).
Hepatic: increased AST and ALT levels.
Metabolic: arthralgia.
Other: hypersensitivity reactions (urticaria, *anaphylaxis*), fever.

☑ Special considerations

• Dehydrated patients should be well hydrated before dextran infusions.
• Dextran in saline solution is hazardous when given to patients with heart failure, severe renal failure, and clinical states in which edema exists with sodium restriction. Use D_5W solution.
• Drug works as plasma expander via colloidal osmotic effect, drawing fluid from interstitial to intravascular space. Provides plasma expansion slightly greater than volume infused. Observe for circulatory overload or rise in CVP readings.
• Dextran 1 should be given just before infusing low- or high-molecular-weight dextran. Repeat dosage of dextran 1 if more than 15 minutes elapses during infusion.
• Avoid doses that exceed recommendations because dose-related increases in wound hema-

toma, wound seroma, wound bleeding, distant bleeding (such as hematuria and melena), and pulmonary edema have been observed.
• Store at constant temperature of 77° F (25° C). Solution may precipitate in storage. Discard any solution that isn't clear.
• Falsely elevated blood glucose levels may occur in patients receiving dextran 40 or 70 if test uses high levels of acid.
• Dextran may cause turbidity, which interferes with bilirubin assays that use alcohol, total protein levels using biuret reagent, and blood glucose levels using orthotoluidine method.
• Blood typing and cross-matching using enzyme techniques may give unreliable readings if samples are taken after dextran infusion.

Monitoring the patient

• Monitor urine output during administration. If oliguria or anuria occurs or isn't reversed by initial infusion (500 ml), stop administration.
• Monitor urine or serum osmolarity; urine specific gravity will be increased by urine dextran concentration.
• Monitor CVP when dextran is given by rapid I.V. infusion. A precipitous rise in CVP or other signs of fluid overload indicate need to stop infusion.
• Monitor hemoglobin level and hematocrit; don't allow to fall below 30% by volume.
• Monitor patient closely during early phase of infusion; check for infiltration, phlebitis, and anaphylactic reactions.

Information for the patient

• Explain use and administration of dextran to patient and family.
• Tell patient to report adverse effects.

Geriatric patients

• Use dextran with caution in elderly patients; they may be at increased risk for fluid overload.

Breast-feeding patients

• It's unknown if dextran appears in breast milk. A decision should be made to stop either breast-feeding or drug.

dextroamphetamine sulfate
Dexedrine

Pharmacologic classification: amphetamine
Therapeutic classification: CNS stimulant, short-term adjunctive anorexigenic drug, sympathomimetic amine
Controlled substance schedule II
Pregnancy risk category C

How supplied

Available by prescription only
Tablets: 5 mg, 10 mg, 20 mg

Capsules (sustained-release): 5 mg, 10 mg, 15 mg
Elixir: 5 mg/5 ml

Indications, route, and dosage
Narcolepsy
Adults: 5 to 60 mg P.O. daily in divided doses. Long-acting dosage forms allow once-daily dosing.
Children over age 12: 10 mg P.O. daily, with 10-mg increments weekly, as indicated.
Children ages 6 to 12: 5 mg P.O. daily, with 5-mg increments weekly, as indicated.
◇ *Short-term adjunct in exogenous obesity*
Adults: 5 to 30 mg P.O. daily 30 to 60 minutes before meals in divided doses of 5 to 10 mg. Or give one 10- or 15-mg sustained-release capsule daily as a single dose in the morning.
Attention deficit hyperactivity disorder
Children ages 6 and older: 5 mg once daily or b.i.d., with 5-mg increments weekly, p.r.n. Total daily dose should rarely exceed 40 mg.
Children ages 3 to 5: 2.5 mg P.O. daily, with 2.5-mg increments weekly, as necessary; not recommended for children under age 3.

Pharmacodynamics
CNS stimulant action: Amphetamines are sympathomimetic amines with CNS stimulant activity; in hyperactive children, they have a paradoxical calming effect.
Anorexigenic action: Anorexigenic effects are thought to occur in the hypothalamus, where decreased smell and taste acuity decreases appetite. They may be tried for short-term control of refractory obesity, with caloric restriction and behavior modification.

The cerebral cortex and reticular activating system appear to be the primary sites of activity; amphetamines release nerve terminal stores of norepinephrine, promoting nerve impulse transmission. At high dosages, effects are mediated by dopamine.

Amphetamines are used to treat narcolepsy and as adjuncts to psychosocial measures in attention deficit disorder in children. Their precise mechanism of action in these conditions is unknown.

Pharmacokinetics
● *Absorption:* Rapidly absorbed from GI tract; serum levels peak 2 to 4 hours after oral administration; long-acting capsules absorbed more slowly and have longer duration of action.
● *Distribution:* Distributed widely throughout body.
● *Metabolism:* No information available.
● *Excretion:* Excreted in urine.

Contraindications and precautions
Contraindicated in patients with hypersensitivity or idiosyncrasy to the sympathomimetic amines, within 14 days of MAO inhibitor therapy, and in those with hyperthyroidism, moderate to severe hypertension, symptomatic CV disease, glaucoma, advanced arteriosclerosis, and history of drug abuse. Use cautiously in patients with motor and phonic tics, Tourette syndrome, and agitated states.

Interactions
Drug-drug. *Acetazolamide, alkalizing drugs, antacids, sodium bicarbonate:* Enhanced reabsorption of dextroamphetamine and prolonged duration of action. Monitor patient for desired effects.
Acidifying drugs, ammonium chloride, ascorbic acid: Enhanced dextroamphetamine excretion and shortened duration of action. Monitor patient for desired effects.
Adrenergic blockers: Inhibited by amphetamines. Monitor patient closely.
Antihypertensives: May antagonize antihypertensive effects. Monitor blood pressure closely.
Barbiturates: Antagonize dextroamphetamine by CNS depression. Monitor patient closely.
Chlorpromazine: Inhibited central stimulant effects of amphetamines. Can be used to treat amphetamine poisoning. Monitor patient closely.
CNS stimulants, haloperidol, phenothiazines, theophylline, tricyclic antidepressants: Increased CNS effects. Monitor patient closely.
Insulin, oral antidiabetics: May alter actions of these drugs. Monitor serum glucose levels.
Lithium carbonate: May inhibit antiobesity and stimulating effects of amphetamines. Monitor effects.
MAO inhibitors (or drugs with MAO-inhibiting activity such as furazolidone): Concomitant use or use within 14 days of such therapy may cause hypertensive crisis. Don't administer within 2 weeks of MAO therapy.
Meperidine: Amphetamines potentiate analgesic effect. Monitor patient closely.
Methenamine therapy: Increased urinary excretion of amphetamines and reduced efficacy. Monitor patient closely.
Norepinephrine: Enhanced adrenergic effect. Monitor patient closely.
Phenobarbital, phenytoin: May produce synergistic anticonvulsant action. Use together cautiously; monitor patient.
Drug-food. *Caffeine:* May increase amphetamine and related amine effects. Avoid concomitant use.

Adverse reactions
CNS: *restlessness,* tremor, *insomnia,* dizziness, headache, chills, overstimulation, dysphoria, euphoria.
CV: *tachycardia, palpitations,* hypertension, **arrhythmias.**
GI: dry mouth, unpleasant taste, diarrhea, constipation, anorexia, weight loss, other GI disturbances.

Reactions may be common, uncommon, **life-threatening**, or COMMON AND LIFE-THREATENING.

GU: impotence, altered libido.
Skin: urticaria.

☑ Special considerations
Besides the recommendations relevant to all amphetamines, consider the following.
● Administer dextroamphetamine 30 to 60 minutes before meals when using as anorexigenic drug. To minimize insomnia, avoid giving within 6 hours of bedtime.
● When tolerance to anorexigenic effect develops, dosage should be discontinued, not increased.
● For narcolepsy, patient should take first dose on awakening.
● Drug may elevate plasma corticosteroid levels and may interfere with urinary steroid determinations.
● Individual responses to overdose vary widely. Toxic symptoms may occur at 15 mg and 30 mg and can cause severe reactions; however, doses of 400 mg or more haven't always proved fatal.
● Overdose symptoms include restlessness, tremor, hyperreflexia, tachypnea, confusion, aggressiveness, hallucinations, and panic; fatigue and depression usually follow excitement stage. Other symptoms may include arrhythmias, shock, alterations in blood pressure, nausea, vomiting, diarrhea, and abdominal cramps; death is usually preceded by seizures and coma.
● Treat overdose symptomatically and supportively: if ingestion is recent (within 4 hours), use gastric lavage or emesis and sedate with a barbiturate; monitor vital signs and fluid and electrolyte balance.
● Urinary acidification may enhance excretion. Saline catharsis (magnesium citrate) may hasten GI evacuation of unabsorbed sustained-release drug.

Monitoring the patient
● Monitor vital signs regularly. Observe patient for signs of excessive stimulation.
● Monitor blood and urine glucose levels. Drug may alter daily insulin requirement in patients with diabetes.

Information for the patient
● Warn patient to avoid hazardous activities that require alertness until CNS response is determined.
● Instruct patient to take drug early in day to minimize insomnia.
● Tell patient not to crush sustained-release forms or to increase dosage.
● Teach parents to provide drug-free periods for children with attention deficit disorder, especially during times of reduced stress.

Geriatric patients
● Use lower doses in elderly patients. Avoid using drug in elderly patients with cardiovascular, CNS, or GI disturbances.

Pediatric patients
● Drug isn't recommended for treatment of obesity in children under age 12.

Breast-feeding patients
● Safety hasn't been established. An alternative to breast-feeding is recommended during therapy. Amphetamines appear in breast milk.

dextromethorphan hydrobromide
Balminil D.M.*, Benylin DM, Broncho-Grippol-DM*, Delsym, DM Syrup*, Hold DM, Koffex DM*, St. Joseph Cough Suppressant, Sucrets Cough Control, Suppress, Trocal, Vicks Formula 44

Pharmacologic classification: levorphanol derivative (dextrorotatory methyl ether)
Therapeutic classification: antitussive (nonnarcotic)
Pregnancy risk category C

How supplied
Available without a prescription
Syrup: 10 mg/5 ml, 15 mg/15 ml
Liquid (sustained-action): 30 mg/5 ml
Liquid: 3.5 mg/5 ml, 7.5 mg/5 ml, 15 mg/5 ml
Lozenges: 2.5 mg, 5 mg, 7.5 mg
Chewable pieces: 15 mg

Indications, route, and dosage
Nonproductive cough (chronic)
Adults and children ages 12 and older: 10 to 20 mg q 4 hours, or 30 mg q 6 to 8 hours. Or the controlled-release liquid b.i.d. (60 mg b.i.d.). Maximum dose is 120 mg daily.
Children ages 6 to 12: 5 to 10 mg q 4 hours, or 15 mg q 6 to 8 hours. Or the controlled-release liquid b.i.d. (30 mg b.i.d.). Maximum dose is 60 mg daily.
Children ages 2 to 6: 2.5 to 5 mg q 4 hours, or 7.5 mg q 6 to 8 hours. Or the sustained-action liquid 15 mg b.i.d. Maximum dose is 30 mg daily.

Pharmacodynamics
Antitussive action: Suppresses the cough reflex by direct action on the cough center in the medulla. Almost equal in antitussive potency to codeine, but causes no analgesia or addiction and little or no CNS depression and has no expectorant action; also produces fewer subjective and GI adverse effects than codeine. Treatment is intended to relieve cough frequency without abolish‐

protective cough reflex. In therapeutic doses, drug doesn't inhibit ciliary activity.

Pharmacokinetics
● *Absorption:* Absorbed readily from GI tract; action begins within 15 to 30 minutes.
● *Distribution:* No information available.
● *Metabolism:* Metabolized extensively by liver. Plasma half-life is about 11 hours.
● *Excretion:* Little drug excreted unchanged. Metabolites excreted primarily in urine; about 7% to 10% excreted in feces. Antitussive effect persists for 5 to 6 hours.

Contraindications and precautions
Contraindicated in patients currently taking MAO inhibitors or within 2 weeks of discontinuing MAO inhibitors. Use cautiously in atopic children, sedated or debilitated patients, and those patients confined to the supine position. Also use cautiously in patients with a sensitivity to aspirin.

Interactions
Drug-drug. *MAO inhibitors:* Possible nausea, hypotension, excitation, hyperpyrexia, and coma. Don't give drug until at least 2 weeks after MAO inhibitors are discontinued.
Selegiline: Possible confusion, coma, or hyperpyrexia. Monitor patient closely.
Drug-herb. *Parsley:* Possibly promotes or produces serotonin syndrome. Avoid concomitant use.

Adverse reactions
CNS: drowsiness, dizziness.
GI: nausea, vomiting, stomach pain.

☑ Special considerations
● Treatment is intended to relieve cough intensity and frequency without completely abolishing protective cough reflex.
● Use with percussion and chest vibration.
● Signs and symptoms of overdose may include nausea, vomiting, drowsiness, dizziness, blurred vision, nystagmus, shallow respirations, urine retention, toxic psychosis, stupor, and coma.
● Treat overdose with activated charcoal to reduce drug absorption and I.V. naloxone to support respiration. Treat other symptoms supportively.

Monitoring the patient
● Monitor nature and frequency of coughing.
● Watch for signs of overdose.

Information for the patient
● Tell patient to call if cough persists more than 7 days.
● Instruct patient to use sugarless throat lozenges for throat irritation and resulting cough.
● Recommend a humidifier to filter out dust, smoke, and air pollutants.

Pediatric patients
● Don't use syrup, tablets, or lozenges in children under age 2. Sustained-action liquid may be used in children under age 2, but dosage must be individualized.

Breast-feeding patients
● Safety in breast-feeding infants hasn't been established. It's unknown if drug appears in breast milk.

dextrose (d-glucose)
$D_{2.5}W$, D_5W, $D_{10}W$, $D_{20}W$, $D_{25}W$, $D_{30}W$, $D_{38}W$, $D_{40}W$, $D_{50}W$, $D_{60}W$, $D_{70}W$

Pharmacologic classification: carbohydrate
Therapeutic classification: total parenteral nutrition (TPN) component, caloric product, fluid volume replacement
Pregnancy risk category C

How supplied
Available by prescription only
Injection: 1,000 ml (2.5%, 5%, 10%, 20%, 30%, 40%, 50%, 60%, 70%); 500 ml (5%, 10%, 20%, 30%, 40%, 50%, 60%, 70%); 400 ml (5%); 250 ml (5%, 10%); 100 ml (5%); 70-ml pin-top vial (70% for additive use only); 50 ml (5% and 50% available in vial, ampule, and Bristoject); 10 ml (25%); 5-ml ampule (10%); 3-ml ampule (10%)

Indications, route, and dosage
Fluid replacement and caloric supplementation in patients who can't maintain adequate oral intake or who are restricted from doing so
Adults and children: Dosage depends on fluid and caloric requirements. Use peripheral I.V. infusion of 2.5% or 5% solution or central I.V. infusion of 10% or 20% solution for minimal fluid needs. Use 50% solution to treat insulin-induced hypoglycemia. Solutions from 10% to 70% are used diluted in admixtures, normally with amino acid solutions, and administered via a central vein.

Pharmacodynamics
Metabolic action: A rapidly metabolized source of calories and fluids in patients with inadequate oral intake. While increasing blood glucose levels, dextrose may decrease body protein and nitrogen losses, promote glycogen deposition, and decrease or prevent ketosis if sufficient doses are given. Dextrose also may induce diuresis. Parenterally injected doses of dextrose undergo oxidation to carbon dioxide and water. A 5% solution is isotonic and is administered peripherally. Concentrated dextrose infusions provide in-

creased caloric intake with less fluid volume; they may be irritating if given by peripheral infusions. Concentrated solutions (above 10%) should be administered only by central venous catheters.

Pharmacokinetics
• *Absorption:* After oral administration, dextrose (a monosaccharide) is absorbed rapidly by small intestine, principally by an active mechanism. In patients with hypoglycemia, blood glucose levels increase within 10 to 20 minutes after oral administration. Blood levels may peak 40 minutes after oral administration.
• *Distribution:* As a source of calories and water for hydration, dextrose solutions expand plasma volume.
• *Metabolism:* Metabolized to carbon dioxide and water.
• *Excretion:* In some patients, dextrose solutions may produce diuresis.

Contraindications and precautions
Contraindicated in patients in diabetic coma while blood glucose level remains excessively high. Concentrated solutions are contraindicated in patients with intracranial or intraspinal hemorrhage, in dehydrated patients with alcohol withdrawal syndrome, and in patients with severe dehydration, anuria, hepatic coma, or glucose-galactose malabsorption syndrome.

Use cautiously in patients with cardiac or pulmonary disease, hypertension, renal insufficiency, urinary obstruction, or hypovolemia.

Interactions
Drug-drug. *Additives:* Possible incompatibility. Must be introduced aseptically, mixed thoroughly, and not stored.
Blood: Possible pseudoagglutination of RBC. Don't give with blood through same infusion set.
Corticosteroids, corticotropin: May cause increased serum glucose levels. Administer cautiously; monitor patient closely.
Insulin, oral hypoglycemics: May alter drug requirements and cause vitamin B complex deficiency. Monitor serum glucose levels.

Adverse reactions
CNS: confusion, *unconsciousness in hyperosmolar hyperglycemic nonketotic syndrome.*
CV: *pulmonary edema, exacerbated hypertension, heart failure* in susceptible patients (with fluid overload); *phlebitis, venous sclerosis,* tissue necrosis (with prolonged or concentrated infusions, especially when administered peripherally).
GU: glycosuria, osmotic diuresis.
Metabolic: hyperglycemia, hypervolemia, hypovolemia, dehydration, hyperosmolarity (with rapid infusion of concentrated solution or prolonged infusion); hypoglycemia from rebound hyperinsulinemia.

Skin: sloughing and tissue necrosis, if extravasation occurs with concentrated solutions.
Other: fever, vitamin B complex deficiency (with rapid termination of long-term infusion).

☑ Special considerations
• Monitor infusion rate for maximum dextrose infusion of 0.5 g/kg/hour, using largest available peripheral vein and well-placed needle or catheter. However, hypertonic dextrose solutions may cause thrombosis if infused via peripheral vein; therefore, administer via central venous catheter.
• Avoid rapid administration, which may cause hyperglycemia, hyperosmolar syndrome, or glycosuria.
• Infuse concentrated solutions slowly; rapid infusion can cause hyperglycemia and fluid shifts.
• Hypertonic solutions are more likely than isotonic or hypotonic solutions to cause irritation; they should be administered into larger central veins.
• Depletion of pancreatic insulin production and secretion can occur. To avoid an adverse effect on insulin production, patient may need to have insulin added to infusions.
• Excessive administration of potassium-free solutions may result in hypokalemia. Potassium should be added to dextrose solutions and administered to fasting patients with good renal function; special precautions should be taken with patients receiving a cardiac glycoside.
• Infuse concentrated solutions via central venous catheter with meticulous aseptic technique, as bacterial contamination thrives in high glucose environments.
• Dextrose 5% or 10% solution is advisable upon discontinuation of concentrated dextrose infusions to avoid rebound hypoglycemia.

Monitoring the patient
• Monitor serum glucose levels during long-term treatment.
• Monitor fluid imbalance or changes in electrolyte levels and acid-base balance by periodic laboratory determinations during prolonged therapy. Additional electrolyte supplementation may be needed.
• Carefully monitor patient's intake, output, and body weight, especially in patients with renal dysfunction.
• If fluid or solute overload occurs during I.V. therapy, reevaluate patient's condition and institute appropriate corrective treatment. Decrease infusion rate or adjust insulin dosage as needed.

Information for the patient
• Explain need for drug.
• Tell patient to report adverse effects promptly.

Pediatric patients
• Use with caution in infants of diabetic women, except as may be indicated for newborn infants who are hypoglycemic.

---

diazepam
Apo-Diazepam*, Diastat, Novo-Dipam*, Valium, Vivol*

Pharmacologic classification: benzodi-azepine
Therapeutic classification: anxiolytic; skeletal muscle relaxant; amnesic drug; anticonvulsant; sedative-hypnotic
Controlled substance schedule IV
Pregnancy risk category D

How supplied
Available by prescription only
Tablets: 2 mg, 5 mg, 10 mg
Capsules (extended-release): 15 mg
Oral solution: 5 mg/ml; 5 mg/5 ml
Oral suspension: 5 mg/5 ml
Injection: 5 mg/ml in 2-ml ampules or 10-ml vials
Disposable syringe: 2-ml Tel-E-Ject
Rectal gel: 2.5 mg, 5 mg, 10 mg, 15 mg, 20 mg Twin Packs

Indications, route, and dosage
Anxiety
Adults: Depending on severity, 2 to 10 mg P.O. b.i.d. to q.i.d. or 15 to 30 mg extended-release capsules P.O. once daily. Or 2 to 10 mg I.M. or I.V. q 3 to 4 hours, p.r.n.
Children ages 6 months and older: 1 to 2.5 mg P.O. t.i.d. or q.i.d.; increase dose gradually, as needed and tolerated.
Acute alcohol withdrawal
Adults: 10 mg P.O. t.i.d. or q.i.d. for the first 24 hours; reduce to 5 mg t.i.d. or q.i.d., p.r.n.; or 10 mg I.M. or I.V. initially, then 5 to 10 mg q 3 to 4 hours, p.r.n.
Muscle spasm
Adults: 2 to 10 mg P.O. b.i.d. to q.i.d.; or 15 to 30 mg extended-release capsules once daily. Or 5 to 10 mg I.M. or I.V. q 3 to 4 hours, p.r.n.
Tetanus
Infants over age 30 days to children age 5: 1 to 2 mg I.M. or I.V. slowly, repeated q 3 to 4 hours.
Children ages 5 and older: 5 to 10 mg I.M. or I.V. slowly q 3 to 4 hours, p.r.n.
Adjunct to convulsive disorders
Adults: 2 to 10 mg P.O. b.i.d. to q.i.d.
Children ages 6 months and older: Initially, 1 to 2.5 mg P.O. t.i.d. or q.i.d.; increase dose as tolerated and needed.
Adjunct to anesthesia; endoscopic procedures
Adults: 5 to 10 mg I.M. before surgery; or administer I.V. slowly just before procedure, titrat-

ing dose to effect. Usually, less than 10 mg is used, but up to 20 mg may be given.
Status epilepticus
Adults: 5 to 10 mg I.V. (preferred) or I.M. initially, repeated at 10- to 15-minute intervals up to a maximum dose of 30 mg. Repeat q 2 to 4 hours, p.r.n.
Children ages 5 and older: 1 mg I.V. q 2 to 5 minutes up to a maximum dose of 10 mg; repeat in 2 to 4 hours, p.r.n.
Infants over age 30 days to children age 5: 0.2 to 0.5 mg I.V. q 2 to 5 minutes up to a maximum dose of 5 mg.
Cardioversion
Adults: Administer 5 to 15 mg I.V. 5 to 10 minutes before procedure.
Control of acute repetitive seizure activity in patients already taking antiepileptics
Children ages 12 years and older: 0.2 mg/kg P.R. using applicator. A second dose may be given 4 to 12 hours after first dose, if needed.
Children ages 6 to 11: 0.3 mg/kg P.R. using applicator. A second dose may be given 4 to 12 hours after first dose, if needed.
Children ages 2 to 5: 0.5 mg/kg P.R. using applicator. A second dose may be given 4 to 12 hours after first dose, if needed.

Pharmacodynamics
Anxiolytic and sedative-hypnotic actions: Depresses the CNS at the limbic and subcortical levels of the brain. Produces an anti-anxiety effect by influencing the effect of the neurotransmitter gamma-aminobutyric acid on its receptor in the ascending reticular activating system, which increases inhibition and blocks cortical and limbic arousal.
Anticonvulsant action: Suppresses spread of seizure activity produced by epileptogenic foci in the cortex, thalamus, and limbic structures by enhancing presynaptic inhibition.
Amnesic action: Exact mechanism unknown.
Skeletal muscle relaxant action: Exact mechanism unknown; believed to involve inhibiting polysynaptic afferent pathways.

Pharmacokinetics
• *Absorption:* When administered orally, absorbed through GI tract. Onset of action occurs within 30 to 60 minutes, with peak action in 1 to 2 hours. I.M. administration results in erratic drug absorption; onset of action usually occurs in 15 to 30 minutes. After I.V. administration, rapid onset of action occurs 1 to 5 minutes after injection. Well absorbed rectally and reaches peak plasma levels in 1½ hours.
• *Distribution:* Widely distributed throughout body. About 85% to 95% of dose is bound to plasma protein.
• *Metabolism:* Metabolized in liver to active metabolite desmethyldiazepam.
• *Excretion:* Most metabolites excreted in urine, with only small amounts excreted in feces. Half-

tal signs. Mechanical ventilatory assistance via endotracheal tube may be required to maintain patent airway and support adequate oxygenation.
• Flumazenil, a specific benzodiazepine antagonist, may be useful in overdose but shouldn't be administered during status epilepticus. Use I.V. fluids and vasopressors such as dopamine and phenylephrine to treat hypotension, as needed.
• In overdose, if patient is conscious, induce emesis; use gastric lavage if ingestion was recent, but only if endotracheal tube is present to prevent aspiration. After emesis or lavage, administer activated charcoal with a cathartic as a single dose. Dialysis is of limited value.

Monitoring the patient
• Patient should remain in bed under observation for at least 3 hours after parenteral administration to prevent potential hazards; keep resuscitation equipment nearby.
• Assess gag reflex postendoscopy and before resuming oral intake to prevent aspiration.
• During prolonged therapy, periodically monitor blood counts and liver function studies. Lower doses are effective in patients with renal or hepatic dysfunction.
• Monitor serum digoxin levels if patient is taking digoxin.

Information for the patient
• Advise patient of potential for physical and psychological dependence with long-term use.
• Warn patient that sudden changes of position can cause dizziness. Advise patient to dangle legs for a few minutes before getting out of bed to prevent falls and injury.
• Encourage patient to avoid or limit smoking to prevent increased diazepam metabolism.
• Warn woman to call immediately if she becomes pregnant.
• Caution patient to avoid alcohol while taking diazepam.
• Advise patient not to suddenly stop drug.
• Teach patient's caregiver when to use rectal gel (to control bouts of increased seizure activity) and how to monitor and record patient's clinical response.
• Teach patient's caregiver how to administer rectal gel.

Geriatric patients
• Elderly patients are more sensitive to the CNS depressant effects of diazepam. Use with caution.
• Lower doses are usually effective in elderly patients because of decreased elimination.
• Elderly patients who receive this drug need assistance with walking and activities of daily living during initiation of therapy or after an increase in dosage.

• Parenteral administration of drug is more likely to cause apnea, hypotension, and bradycardia in elderly patients.

Pediatric patients
• Safe use of oral diazepam in infants under age 6 months hasn't been established. Safe use of parenteral diazepam in infants under age 30 days hasn't been established.
• Closely observe neonates whose mothers took diazepam for a prolonged period during pregnancy; infants may show withdrawal symptoms. Diazepam use during labor may cause neonatal flaccidity.

Breast-feeding patients
• Diazepam appears in breast milk. The breast-fed infant of a mother who uses diazepam may become sedated, have feeding difficulties, or lose weight. Avoid use of drug in breast-feeding women.

diazoxide
Hyperstat IV, Proglycem

Pharmacologic classification: peripheral vasodilator
Therapeutic classification: antihypertensive, antihypoglycemic
Pregnancy risk category C

How supplied
Available by prescription only
Capsules: 50 mg
Oral suspension: 50 mg/ml in 30-ml bottle
Injection: 300 mg/20 ml ampule

Indications, route, and dosage
Hypertensive crisis
Adults and children: 1 to 3 mg/kg I.V. (up to maximum of 150 mg) q 5 to 15 minutes until an adequate reduction in blood pressure is achieved.
Note: The use of 300-mg I.V. bolus push is no longer recommended. Switch to therapy with oral antihypertensives as soon as possible.
Hypoglycemia from hyperinsulinism
Adults and children: Usual daily dose is 3 to 8 mg/kg/day P.O. divided in two or three equal doses.
Infants and newborns: Usual daily dose is 8 to 15 mg/kg/day P.O. divided in two or three equal doses.

Pharmacodynamics
Antihypertensive action: Directly relaxes arteriolar smooth muscle, causing vasodilation and reducing peripheral vascular resistance, thus reducing blood pressure.
Antihypoglycemic action: Increases blood glucose levels by inhibiting pancreatic secretion of insulin, stimulating catecholamine release, or increasing hepatic release of glucose.

Reactions may be *common*, uncommon, *life-threatening*, or COMMON AND LIFE-THREATENING.

Diazoxide is a nondiuretic congener of thiazide diuretics.

Pharmacokinetics

• *Absorption:* After I.V. administration, blood pressure should decrease promptly, with maximum decrease in under 5 minutes. After oral administration, hyperglycemic effect begins in 1 hour.

• *Distribution:* Distributed throughout body; highest level found in kidneys, liver, and adrenal glands; diazoxide crosses placenta and blood-brain barrier. Drug is about 90% protein-bound.

• *Metabolism:* Metabolized partially in liver.

• *Excretion:* Drug and metabolites excreted slowly by kidneys. Duration of antihypertensive effect varies widely, from 30 minutes to 72 hours (average 3 to 12 hours) after I.V. administration; after oral administration, antihypoglycemic effect persists for about 8 hours. Antihypertensive and antihypoglycemic effects may be prolonged in patients with renal dysfunction.

Contraindications and precautions

Parenteral form is contraindicated in patients with hypersensitivity to drug, other thiazides, or sulfonamide-derived drugs and in treatment of compensatory hypertension (such as that associated with coarctation of the aorta or arteriovenous shunt). Oral form is contraindicated in patients with functional hypoglycemia.

Use cautiously in patients with uremia or impaired cerebral or cardiac function.

Interactions

Drug-drug. *Antihypertensives:* May potentiate antihypertensive effects, especially if I.V. diazoxide is administered within 6 hours after patient has received another antihypertensive. Avoid concomitant use.

Diuretics: May potentiate antihypoglycemic, hyperuricemic, or antihypertensive effects of diazoxide. Avoid concomitant use.

Insulin, oral antidiabetics: Concomitant use may alter requirements in previously stable diabetic patients. Monitor serum glucose levels.

Phenytoin: May increase metabolism and decrease plasma protein-binding of phenytoin. Avoid concomitant use.

Thiazides: May enhance effects of diazoxide. Monitor patient's intake and output closely.

Warfarin (also bilirubin or other highly protein-bound substances from protein-binding sites): May be displaced by diazoxide. Monitor patient closely.

Adverse reactions

CNS: dizziness, weakness, headache, malaise, anxiety, insomnia, paresthesia (with oral form); headache, *seizures, paralysis, cerebral ischemia,* light-headedness, euphoria (with parenteral form).

CV: *arrhythmias,* tachycardia, hypotension, hypertension (with oral form); *sodium and water retention, orthostatic hypotension,* diaphoresis, flushing, warmth, angina, myocardial ischemia, ECG changes, *shock, MI* (with parenteral form).

EENT: diplopia, transient cataracts, blurred vision, lacrimation (with oral administration); optic nerve infarction (with parenteral form).

GI: abdominal discomfort, diarrhea, nausea, vomiting, anorexia, taste alteration (with oral form); *nausea, vomiting,* dry mouth, constipation (with parenteral form).

GU: azotemia, reversible nephrotic syndrome, decreased urine output, hematuria, albuminuria (with oral administration).

Hematologic: *leukopenia, thrombocytopenia,* anemia, eosinophilia, excessive bleeding (with oral administration).

Metabolic: *sodium and fluid retention, ketoacidosis and hyperosmolar nonketotic syndrome, hyperuricemia, hyperglycemia.*

Skin: rash, pruritus (with oral administration).

Other: hirsutism, fever (with oral administration), inflammation and pain resulting from extravasation.

☑ Special considerations

• Diazoxide is used to treat only hypoglycemia resulting from hyperinsulinism; isn't used to treat functional hypoglycemia. May be used temporarily to control preoperative or postoperative hypoglycemia in patients with hyperinsulinism.

• I.V. use of diazoxide is seldom necessary for more than 4 or 5 days.

• Drug may be given by constant I.V. infusion (7.5 to 30 mg/minute) until adequate blood pressure reduction occurs.

• Diazoxide inhibits glucose-stimulated insulin release and may cause false-negative insulin response to glucagon.

• Overdose is manifested primarily by hyperglycemia; ketoacidosis and hypotension may occur. Treat acute overdose supportively and symptomatically. If hyperglycemia develops, give insulin and replace fluid and electrolyte losses; use vasopressors if hypotension fails to respond to conservative treatment.

• Prolonged monitoring may be necessary with overdose because of diazoxide's long half-life.

Monitoring the patient

• After I.V. injection, monitor blood pressure every 5 minutes for 15 to 30 minutes, then hourly when patient is stable. Stop drug if severe hypotension develops or if blood pressure continues to fall 30 minutes after infusion; keep patient recumbent during this time and have norepinephrine available. Monitor I.V. site for infiltration or extravasation.

• Monitor patient's intake, output, and weight carefully. If fluid or sodium retention develops, diuretics may be given 30 to 60 minutes after diazox-

ide. Keep patient recumbent for 8 to 10 hours after diuretic administration.
• Monitor daily blood glucose and electrolyte levels, watching diabetic patients closely for severe hyperglycemia or hyperglycemic hyperosmolar nonketotic coma; also monitor daily urine glucose and ketone levels. Significant hypotension doesn't occur after oral administration in doses used to treat hypoglycemia.
• Check serum uric acid levels frequently.
• Monitor serum phenytoin levels if patient is taking phenytoin.
• Monitor coagulation studies if patient is taking oral anticoagulants.

Information for the patient
• Explain that orthostatic hypotension can be minimized by rising slowly and avoiding sudden position changes.
• Tell patient to report adverse effects immediately, including pain and redness at injection site, which may indicate infiltration.
• Instruct patient to check weight daily and report gains of over 5 lb (2.3 kg)/week; diazoxide causes sodium and water retention.
• Reassure patient that excessive hair growth is common and subsides when treatment ends.

Geriatric patients
• Elderly patients may have a more pronounced hypotensive response.

Pediatric patients
• Use with caution in children.

Breast-feeding patients
• It's unknown if drug appears in breast milk; an alternative to breast-feeding is recommended during therapy.

dibucaine
Nupercainal

Pharmacologic classification: local anesthetic (amine)
Therapeutic classification: local amide anesthetic
Pregnancy risk category B

How supplied
Available without a prescription
Ointment: 1%
Cream: 0.5%

Indications, route, and dosage
Temporary relief of pain and itching associated with abrasions, sunburn, minor burns, insect bites, and other minor skin conditions
Adults and children: Apply to affected areas, p.r.n. Maximum daily dose of 1% ointment is 30 g for adults and 7.5 g for children.

Temporary relief of pain, itching, and burning caused by hemorrhoids
Adults: Instill 1% ointment into rectum using a rectal applicator each morning and evening and after each bowel movement, p.r.n. Apply additional ointment topically to anal tissues. Maximum daily dose is 30 g.

Pharmacodynamics
Anesthetic action: Inhibits conduction of nerve impulses and decreases cell membrane permeability to ions, anesthetizing local nerve endings.

Pharmacokinetics
• *Absorption:* Limited absorption.
• *Distribution:* None.
• *Metabolism:* None.
• *Excretion:* None.

Contraindications and precautions
Contraindicated in patients with hypersensitivity to drug, sulfites, or other amide-type local anesthetics and for use on large skin areas, on broken skin or mucous membranes, and in eyes.

Interactions
None reported.

Adverse reactions
Skin: irritation, inflammation, contact dermatitis, cutaneous lesions.
Other: *hypersensitivity reactions* (urticaria, edema, burning, stinging, tenderness).

☑ Special considerations
• Use dibucaine topically only and for short periods.
• Stop drug if sensitization occurs or if condition worsens.
• For overdose, clean area thoroughly with mild soap and water.

Monitoring the patient
• Monitor patient for worsened symptoms lasting longer than 7 days.
• Monitor patient for adverse effects.

Information for the patient
• Advise patient to call if condition worsens or if symptoms persist for more than 7 days after use.
• Explain correct use of drug.
• Emphasize need to wash hands thoroughly after use.
• Caution patient to apply drug sparingly to minimize adverse effects.
• Tell patient to keep drug out of reach of children.

Geriatric patients
• Dosage should be adjusted to patient's age, size, and physical condition.

Reactions may be *common*, uncommon, *life-threatening*, or COMMON AND LIFE-THREATENING.

Pediatric patients
● Adjust dosage to patient's age, size, and physical condition.

Breast-feeding patients
● Because it's unknown if drug appears in breast milk, it shouldn't be used in breast-feeding women.

diclofenac potassium
Cataflam

diclofenac sodium
Voltaren, Voltaren Ophthalmic, Voltaren-XR

Pharmacologic classification: NSAID
Therapeutic classification: antarthritic, anti-inflammatory
Pregnancy risk category B

How supplied
Available by prescription only
Tablets: 25 mg*, 50 mg
Tablets (enteric-coated): 25 mg, 50 mg, 75 mg, 100 mg
Ophthalmic solution: 0.1%

Indications, route, and dosage
Osteoarthritis
Adults: 50 mg P.O. b.i.d. or t.i.d., or 75 mg P.O. b.i.d. (diclofenac sodium only).
Ankylosing spondylitis
Adults: 25 mg P.O. q.i.d. An additional 25 mg dose may be needed h.s.
Rheumatoid arthritis
Adults: 50 mg P.O. t.i.d. or q.i.d. Or 75 mg P.O. b.i.d. (diclofenac sodium only).
Analgesia and primary dysmenorrhea
Adults: 50 mg (diclofenac potassium only) P.O. t.i.d. Or 100 mg (diclofenac potassium only) P.O. initially, then 50 mg doses, up to a maximum dose of 200 mg in first 24 hours; subsequent dosing should follow 50 mg t.i.d. regimen.
Postoperative inflammation following cataract removal
Adults: 1 drop in the conjunctival sac q.i.d., beginning 24 hours after surgery and continuing throughout the first 2 weeks of postoperative period.

Pharmacodynamics
Anti-inflammatory action: Exerts its anti-inflammatory and antipyretic actions through an unknown mechanism that may involve inhibition of prostaglandin synthesis.

Pharmacokinetics
● *Absorption:* After oral administration, is rapidly and almost completely absorbed, with peak plasma levels occurring in 10 to 30 minutes. Absorption delayed by food, with peak plasma lev-

els occurring in 2½ to 12 hours; doesn't alter bioavailability.
● *Distribution:* Highly (nearly 100%) protein-bound.
● *Metabolism:* Undergoes first-pass metabolism, with 60% unchanged drug reaching systemic circulation. Principal active metabolite, 48-hydroxydiclofenac, has about 3% of activity of parent compound. Mean terminal half-life is about 1¼ to 1¾ hours after an oral dose.
● *Excretion:* About 40% to 60% excreted in urine; balance excreted in bile. 4'-hydroxy metabolite accounts for 20% to 30% of dose excreted in urine; other metabolites account for 10% to 20%; 5% to 10% excreted unchanged in urine. More than 90% excreted within 72 hours. Moderate renal impairment doesn't alter elimination rate of unchanged diclofenac but may reduce elimination rate of metabolites. Hepatic impairment doesn't appear to affect pharmacokinetics.

Contraindications and precautions
Oral form is contraindicated in patients with hypersensitivity to drug and in those with hepatic porphyria or a history of asthma, urticaria, or other allergic reactions after taking aspirin or other NSAIDs. Avoid use during late pregnancy and in breast-feeding women. Ophthalmic solution is contraindicated in patients with hypersensitivity to any component of drug and in those wearing soft contact lenses.

Use oral form cautiously in patients with history of peptic ulcer disease, hepatic or renal dysfunction, cardiac disease, hypertension, or conditions associated with fluid retention.

Use ophthalmic solution cautiously in patients with hypersensitivity to aspirin, phenyl-acetic acid derivatives, and other NSAIDs, in surgical patients with known bleeding tendencies, and in those receiving drugs that may prolong bleeding time.

Interactions
Drug-drug. *Aspirin:* May lower plasma levels of diclofenac. Don't use together.
Beta blockers: May blunt antihypertensive effects. Monitor blood pressure closely.
Cyclosporine, digoxin, methotrexate: Concurrent use may increase toxicity of these drugs. Use cautiously together.
Diuretics: Concurrent use may inhibit action of diuretics. Monitor patient closely.
Insulin, oral antidiabetics: Concomitant use may alter patient's response to these drugs. Monitor serum glucose levels.
Lithium: Decreased renal clearance of lithium, increased plasma levels with concomitant use. Lithium toxicity may occur. Monitor patient.
Phenytoin: May increase serum levels. Monitor phenytoin levels closely.
Potassium-sparing diuretics: May increase serum potassium levels. Monitor potassium levels.

Warfarin: Affects platelet function. Monitor anticoagulant dosage closely.
Drug-lifestyle. *Sun exposure:* May cause photosensitivity reactions. Tell patient to take precautions.

Adverse reactions
Unless otherwise noted, the following adverse reactions refer to oral administration of drug.
CNS: anxiety, depression, dizziness, drowsiness, insomnia, irritability, headache.
CV: *heart failure,* hypertension, edema.
EENT: *tinnitus,* laryngeal edema, swelling of the lips and tongue, blurred vision, eye pain, night blindness, epistaxis, taste disorder, reversible hearing loss; *transient stinging and burning, increased intraocular pressure, keratitis,* anterior chamber reaction, ocular allergy (with ophthalmic solution).
GI: *abdominal pain or cramps, constipation, diarrhea, indigestion, nausea,* vomiting, abdominal distention, flatulence, peptic ulceration, *bleeding,* melena, bloody diarrhea, appetite change, colitis.
GU: proteinuria, *acute renal failure,* oliguria, interstitial nephritis, papillary necrosis, *nephrotic syndrome,* fluid retention.
Hematologic: increased platelet aggregation time.
Hepatic: elevated liver enzymes, jaundice, *hepatitis, hepatotoxicity.*
Metabolic: hypoglycemia, hyperglycemia.
Musculoskeletal: back, leg, or joint pain.
Respiratory: asthma.
Skin: rash, pruritus, urticaria, eczema, dermatitis, alopecia, photosensitivity, bullous eruption, allergic purpura.
Other: *angioedema,* viral infection (with ophthalmic solution); *anaphylaxis, anaphylactoid reactions.*

☑ Special considerations
● Administration with other drugs, such as glucocorticoids, that produce adverse GI effects may aggravate such effects.
● Because anti-inflammatory, antipyretic, and analgesic effects of diclofenac may mask usual signs of infection, monitor carefully for infection.
● No special antidote for overdose. Supportive and symptomatic treatment may include induction of vomiting or gastric lavage.
● Treatment with activated charcoal or dialysis may also be appropriate.

Monitoring the patient
● Monitor renal function during treatment. Use with caution and at reduced dosage in patients with renal impairment.
● Monitor liver function during therapy. Abnormal liver function test results and severe hepatic reactions may occur.

● Periodic evaluation of hematopoietic function is recommended because bone marrow abnormalities have occurred. Check hemoglobin level regularly to detect toxic effects on GI tract.
● Periodic ophthalmologic examinations are recommended during prolonged therapy.
● Monitor coagulation studies if patient is taking anticoagulants.
● Monitor serum glucose level if patient is diabetic.
● Monitor serum potassium level if patient is taking potassium-sparing diuretics.
● Monitor serum digoxin level if patient is taking digoxin.

Information for the patient
● Advise patient to take drug with meals or milk to avoid GI upset.
● Teach patient to restrict salt intake; drug may cause edema, especially if patient is hypertensive.
● Instruct patient to report symptoms that may be related to GI ulceration, such as epigastric pain and black or tarry stools, as well as other unusual symptoms, such as skin rash, pruritus, or significant edema or weight gain.

Geriatric patients
● Use with caution in elderly patients. Elderly patients may be more susceptible to adverse reactions, especially GI toxicity and nephrotoxicity. Reduce dosage to lowest level that controls symptoms.

Pediatric patients
● Drug isn't recommended for use in children.

Breast-feeding patients
● Low levels of drug appear in breast milk; consider risk-to-benefit ratio.

dicloxacillin sodium
Dycill, Dynapen, Pathocil

Pharmacologic classification: penicillinase-resistant penicillin
Therapeutic classification: antibiotic
Pregnancy risk category NR

How supplied
Available by prescription only
Capsules: 125 mg, 250 mg, 500 mg
Oral suspension: 62.5 mg/5 ml (after reconstitution)

Indications, route, and dosage
Systemic infections caused by penicillinase-producing staphylococci
Adults and children weighing 40 kg (88 lb) or more: 125 to 250 mg P.O. q 6 hours.

Infants and children over age 1 month weighing under 40 kg: 12.5 to 50 mg/kg P.O. daily, divided into doses given q 6 hours. Serious infection may require higher dosage (75 to 100 mg/kg/day in divided doses q 6 hours).

Pharmacodynamics
Antibiotic action: Bactericidal; adheres to bacterial penicillin-binding proteins, thus inhibiting bacterial cell wall synthesis. Resists effects of penicillinases—enzymes that inactivate penicillin—and is thus active against many strains of penicillinase-producing bacteria; this activity is most important against penicillinase-producing staphylococci; some strains may remain resistant. Drug is also active against a few gram-positive aerobic and anaerobic bacilli but has no significant effect on gram-negative bacilli.

Pharmacokinetics
• *Absorption:* Absorbed rapidly but incompletely (35% to 76%) from GI tract; relatively acid stable. Plasma levels peak ½ to 2 hours after oral dose. Food may decrease both rate and extent of absorption.
• *Distribution:* Distributed widely into bone, bile, and pleural and synovial fluids. Poor CSF penetration but is enhanced by meningeal inflammation. Drug crosses placenta; 95% to 99% protein-bound.
• *Metabolism:* Metabolized only partially.
• *Excretion:* Drug and metabolites excreted in urine by renal tubular secretion and glomerular filtration; also excreted in breast milk. Elimination half-life in adults is ½ to 1 hour, extended minimally to 2¼ hours in patients with renal impairment.

Contraindications and precautions
Contraindicated in patients with hypersensitivity to drug or other penicillins. Use cautiously in patients with other drug allergies, especially to cephalosporins, and in those with mononucleosis.

Interactions
Drug-drug. *Aminoglycosides:* Synergistic bactericidal effects against *Staphylococcus aureus.* However, drugs are physically and chemically incompatible and are inactivated when mixed or given together. Don't administer together.
Oral contraceptives: May decrease efficacy of these drugs. Tell patient to use an alternative method of birth control.
Probenecid: Blocked renal tubular secretion of dicloxacillin, raising its serum levels. Monitor patient for desired effects.

Adverse reactions
CNS: neuromuscular irritability, *seizures,* lethargy, hallucinations, anxiety, confusion, agitation, depression, dizziness, fatigue.

GI: *nausea,* vomiting, *epigastric distress,* flatulence, *diarrhea,* enterocolitis, pseudomembranous colitis, black "hairy" tongue, abdominal pain.
GU: interstitial nephritis, nephropathy.
Hematologic: eosinophilia, anemia, **thrombocytopenia, leukopenia,** hemolytic anemia, **agranulocytosis.**
Hepatic: transient elevations in liver function study results, cholestasis, hepatitis.
Other: hypersensitivity reactions (pruritus, urticaria, rash, **anaphylaxis**), overgrowth of non-susceptible organisms.

☑ Special considerations
Besides the recommendations relevant to all penicillins, consider the following.
• Give drug with water only; acid in fruit juice or carbonated beverage may inactivate drug.
• Give dose on empty stomach; food decreases absorption.
• Drug alters test results for urine and serum proteins; produces false-positive or elevated results in turbidimetric urine and serum protein tests using sulfosalicylic acid or trichloroacetic acid; also reportedly produces false results on Bradshaw screening test for Bence Jones protein.
• Drug may falsely decrease serum aminoglycoside levels.
• Signs and symptoms of overdose include neuromuscular irritability or seizures. Treatment is supportive. After recent ingestion (4 hours or less), empty stomach by induced emesis or gastric lavage; then use activated charcoal to reduce absorption. Drug isn't appreciably dialyzable.

Monitoring the patient
• Regularly assess renal, hepatic, and hematopoietic function during prolonged therapy.
• Monitor patient for adverse effects.

Information for the patient
• Tell patient to report severe diarrhea promptly.
• Tell patient to report rash or itching.
• Instruct patient to complete full course of therapy.

Geriatric patients
• Half-life may be prolonged in elderly patients because of impaired renal function.

Pediatric patients
• Elimination of dicloxacillin is reduced in neonates; safe use of drug in neonates hasn't been established.

Breast-feeding patients
• Drug appears in breast milk; use with caution in breast-feeding women.

dicyclomine hydrochloride
Antispas, A-Spas, Bentyl, Bentylol*,
Byclomine, Dibent, Formulex*,
Lomine*, Or-Tyl, Spasmoban

Pharmacologic classification: anticholinergic
Therapeutic classification: antimuscarinic, GI antispasmodic
Pregnancy risk category B

How supplied
Available by prescription only
Tablets: 20 mg
Capsules: 10 mg, 20 mg
Syrup: 10 mg/5 ml
Injection: 10 mg/ml in 2-ml vials, 10-ml vials, 2-ml ampules

Indications, route, and dosage
Irritable bowel syndrome and other functional GI disorders
Adults: Initially, 20 mg P.O. q.i.d.; then increase to 40 mg P.O. q.i.d. during first week of therapy unless precluded by adverse reactions. Or give 20 mg I.M. q 4 to 6 hours.
Children ages 2 and older: 10 mg P.O. t.i.d. or q.i.d.
Infants ages 6 to 23 months: 5 to 10 mg P.O. t.i.d. or q.i.d.
◊ *Infant colic*
Infants age 6 months and over: 5 to 10 mg P.O. t.i.d. or q.i.d. Adjust dosage according to patient's needs and response.
Note: High environmental temperatures may induce heatstroke during drug use. If symptoms occur, stop drug.

Pharmacodynamics
Antispasmodic action: Exerts a nonspecific, direct spasmolytic action on smooth muscle. It also has some local anesthetic properties that may contribute to spasmolysis in the GI and biliary tracts.

Pharmacokinetics
• *Absorption:* About 67% of oral dose absorbed from GI tract.
• *Distribution:* Largely unknown.
• *Metabolism:* No information available.
• *Excretion:* After oral administration, 80% of dose excreted in urine and 10% in feces.

Contraindications and precautions
Contraindicated in patients with hypersensitivity to anticholinergics and in those with obstructive uropathy, obstructive disease of the GI tract, reflux esophagitis, severe ulcerative colitis, myasthenia gravis, unstable CV status in acute hemorrhage, or glaucoma. Also contraindicated in breast-feeding women and in children under age 6 months.
Use cautiously in patients with autonomic neuropathy, hyperthyroidism, coronary artery disease, arrhythmias, heart failure, hypertension, hiatal hernia, hepatic or renal disease, prostatic hyperplasia, and ulcerative colitis.

Interactions
Drug-drug. *Amantadine, antihistamines, antiparkinsonians, disopyramide, glutethimide, meperidine, phenothiazines, procainamide, quinidine, tricyclic antidepressants:* May cause additive adverse effects. Monitor patient closely.
Antacids: Decreased oral absorption of anticholinergics. Administer dicyclomine at least 1 hour before antacids.
Anticholinergics (such as ketoconazole, levodopa): Possible decreased GI absorption. Monitor patient for desired effects.
Digoxin (slowly dissolving digoxin tablets): May yield higher serum digoxin levels. Monitor digoxin levels.
Methotrimeprazine: May enhance risk of extrapyramidal reactions. Watch for development of symptoms.
Oral potassium supplements (especially wax-matrix formulations): Possible increased risk of potassium-induced GI ulcerations. Monitor patient closely.

Adverse reactions
CNS: *headache; dizziness;* light-headedness; insomnia; drowsiness; nervousness, confusion, excitement (in elderly patients).
CV: *palpitations,* tachycardia.
EENT: blurred vision, increased intraocular pressure, mydriasis.
GI: nausea, vomiting, *constipation, dry mouth,* abdominal distention, heartburn, paralytic ileus.
GU: *urinary hesitancy, urine retention,* impotence.
Skin: urticaria, decreased sweating or possible anhidrosis, other dermal manifestations, local irritation.
Other: fever, *allergic reactions.*
Note: Dicyclomine is a synthetic tertiary derivative that may have atropine-like adverse reactions.

☑ Special considerations
Besides the recommendations relevant to all anticholinergics, consider the following.
• Never give dicyclomine I.V. or S.C.
• Signs and symptoms of overdose include curare-like symptoms of CNS stimulation then depression, and psychotic symptoms such as disorientation, confusion, hallucinations, delusions, anxiety, agitation, and restlessness. Peripheral effects may include dilated, nonreactive pupils; hot, flushed, dry skin; tachycardia; hypertension; and increased respiration.

Reactions may be *common,* uncommon, **life-threatening**, or COMMON AND LIFE-THREATENING.

- Treatment of overdose is primarily symptomatic and supportive, as necessary. Maintain patent airway. If patient is alert, induce emesis (or use gastric lavage) and follow with a saline cathartic and activated charcoal to prevent further drug absorption.
- In severe overdose cases, physostigmine may be administered to block dicyclomine's antimuscarinic effects. Give fluids, as needed, to treat shock; diazepam to control psychotic symptoms; and pilocarpine (instilled into eyes) to relieve mydriasis. If urine retention occurs, catheterization may be necessary.

Monitoring the patient
- Monitor changes in mental status with elderly patients.
- Monitor patient for adverse effects.

Information for the patient
- Tell patient that syrup formulation may be diluted with water.
- Warn patient that high environmental temperatures may induce heatstroke while drug is being used; tell patient to avoid exposure to such temperatures.

Geriatric patients
- Administer drug cautiously to elderly patients. Lower doses are indicated.

Pediatric patients
- Safety and effectiveness in children haven't been established. Administer cautiously to infants age 6 months or over; seizures have been reported. Drug is contraindicated in infants under age 6 months.

Breast-feeding patients
- Drug may appear in breast milk and may decrease milk production. Breast-feeding women shouldn't use drug.

didanosine (ddI)
Videx

Pharmacologic classification: purine analogue
Therapeutic classification: antiviral
Pregnancy risk category B

How supplied
Available by prescription only
Tablets (chewable): 25 mg, 50 mg, 100 mg, 150 mg
Powder for solution (buffered): 100 mg/packet, 167 mg/packet, 250 mg/packet, 375 mg/packet
Powder for oral solution (pediatric): 10 mg/ml in 2-g and 4-g bottles

Indications, route, and dosage
HIV infection when antiretroviral therapy is warranted
Adults weighing 60 kg (132 lb) and over: 200 mg (tablets) P.O. q 12 hours, or 250 mg buffered powder P.O. q 12 hours.
Adults weighing less than 60 kg: 125 mg (tablets) P.O. q 12 hours, or 167 mg buffered powder P.O. q 12 hours.
Children: 120 mg/m² P.O. q 12 hours. To prevent gastric acid degradation, children over age 1 should receive a 2-tablet dose, and children under age 1 should receive a 1-tablet dose.
✦ *Dosage adjustment.* Patients with renal or hepatic impairment may need dosage adjustment; however, insufficient data exist to provide specific recommendations.

Pharmacodynamics
Antiviral action: A synthetic purine analogue of deoxyadenosine. After didanosine enters the cell, it's converted to its active form, dideoxyadenosine triphosphate (ddATP), which inhibits replication of HIV by preventing DNA replication. In addition, ddATP inhibits the enzyme HIV-RNA dependent DNA polymerase (reverse transcriptase).

Pharmacokinetics
- *Absorption:* Degrades rapidly in gastric acid. Commercially available preparations contain buffers to raise stomach pH. Bioavailability averages about 33%; tablets may exhibit better bioavailability than buffered powder for oral solution. Food can decrease absorption by 50%.
- *Distribution:* Widely distributed; CNS penetration varies, but CSF levels average 46% of concurrent plasma levels.
- *Metabolism:* Not fully understood; probably similar to endogenous purines.
- *Excretion:* Excreted in urine as allantoin, hypoxanthine, xanthine, and uric acid. Serum half-life averages 0.8 hours.

Contraindications and precautions
Contraindicated in patients with hypersensitivity to drug or its components. Use cautiously in patients with history of pancreatitis and in those with peripheral neuropathy, impaired renal or hepatic function, or hyperuricemia.

Interactions
Drug-drug. *Antacids containing magnesium or aluminum hydroxides:* May produce enhanced adverse effects, such as diarrhea or constipation. Monitor patient for adverse effects.
Dapsone, ketoconazole, other drugs that require gastric acid for adequate absorption: May be rendered ineffective because of buffering action of didanosine formulations on gastric acid. Administer such drugs 2 hours before didanosine.

Fluoroquinolones, tetracyclines: May show decreased absorption because of buffering ingredients in didanosine tablets or antacids in pediatric suspension. Monitor patient for drug effects.
Itraconazole: May decrease serum levels of itraconazole. Monitor drug levels closely.

Adverse reactions
CNS: *headache, seizures,* confusion, anxiety, nervousness, asthenia, abnormal thinking, twitching, depression, *peripheral neuropathy.*
GI: *diarrhea, nausea, vomiting, abdominal pain, pancreatitis,* dry mouth, anorexia.
Hematologic: *leukopenia,* granulocytosis, *thrombocytopenia,* anemia.
Hepatic: *hepatic failure,* elevated liver enzymes.
Metabolic: increased serum uric acid levels.
Musculoskeletal: myopathy.
Respiratory: pneumonia, dyspnea.
Skin: rash, pruritus, sarcoma.
Other: pain, infection, *allergic reactions,* chills, *fever.*

☑ Special considerations
• Give drug on empty stomach, regardless of dosage form. Giving drug with meals can result in a 50% decrease in absorption.
• Most patients over age 1 should receive two tablets per dose. Tablets contain buffers that raise stomach pH to levels that prevent degradation of active drug. Tablets should be thoroughly chewed before swallowing, and patient should drink at least 1 oz (30 ml) water with each dose. If tablets are manually crushed, mix drug in 1 oz water, stir to disperse uniformly, then have patient drink immediately. Single-dose packets containing buffered powder for oral solution are available.
• To administer buffered powder for oral solution, carefully open packet and pour contents into 4 oz (120 ml) water. Don't use fruit juice or other acidic beverages. Stir for 2 or 3 minutes until powder dissolves completely. Administer immediately.
• Reports indicate that about one-third of patients taking buffered powder for oral solution develop diarrhea. Although there's no evidence that other formulations are less likely to cause diarrhea, consider substituting chewable tablets if diarrhea occurs.
• When preparing powder or crushing tablets, avoid excessive dispersal of drug particles into air.
• Pediatric powder for oral solution must be prepared by a pharmacist before dispensing. It must be constituted with water, then diluted with antacid (manufacturer recommends either Mylanta Double Strength Liquid or Maalox TC) to final concentration of 10 mg/ml. Admixture is stable for 30 days if refrigerated (36° to 46° F [2° to 8° C]). Be sure to shake well before measuring dose.
• Patients who received doses 10 times greater than currently recommended dosage developed

diarrhea, pancreatitis, peripheral neuropathy, hyperuricemia, and hepatic dysfunction. Treatment is supportive. No specific antidote known; unknown if drug is dialyzable.

Monitoring the patient
• Monitor patient for pancreatitis, which must be considered when patient develops abdominal pain, nausea, and vomiting, or biochemical markers are elevated. Stop drug until pancreatitis is excluded.
• For pediatric patients, give retinal examination every 6 months or sooner if vision changes.

Information for the patient
• Tell patient to take drug on empty stomach to ensure adequate absorption, to chew tablets thoroughly before swallowing, and to drink at least 1 oz water with each dose.
• Remind patient using buffered powder for oral solution not to use fruit juice or other acidic beverages. He should allow 3 minutes for powder to dissolve completely, and take immediately. Be sure patient understands how to mix solution.

Pediatric patients
• Retinal depigmentation has occurred in some children receiving drug. Children should receive dilated retinal examinations at least every 6 months or sooner if vision changes.

Breast-feeding patients
• It's unknown if drug appears in breast milk. Because of risk of serious adverse effects in infant, breast-feeding isn't recommended.

diflorasone diacetate
Florone, Florone E, Maxiflor, Psorcon

Pharmacologic classification: topical adrenocorticoid
Therapeutic classification: anti-inflammatory
Pregnancy risk category C

How supplied
Available by prescription only
Cream, ointment: 0.05%

Indications, route, and dosage
Inflammation of corticosteroid-responsive dermatoses
Adults and children: Apply sparingly in a thin film once daily to q.i.d., as determined by severity of condition.

Pharmacodynamics
Anti-inflammatory action: Stimulates synthesis of enzymes needed to decrease the inflammatory response. A group I-II potency anti-inflammatory.

Pharmacokinetics

- *Absorption:* Amount of drug absorbed depends on amount applied and on nature and condition of skin at application site. Ranges from about 1% in areas with thick stratum corneum (palms, soles, elbows, knees) to as high as 36% in areas of thinnest stratum corneum (face, eyelids, genitals). Absorption increases in areas of skin damage, inflammation, or occlusion. Some systemic absorption of topical steroids occurs, especially through oral mucosa.
- *Distribution:* After topical application, is distributed throughout local skin. Absorbed into circulation, is distributed rapidly into muscle, liver, skin, intestines, and kidneys.
- *Metabolism:* After topical administration, metabolized primarily in skin. Small amount absorbed into systemic circulation is metabolized primarily in liver into inactive compounds.
- *Excretion:* Inactive metabolites excreted by kidneys, primarily as glucuronides and sulfates, but also as unconjugated products. Small amounts of metabolites also excreted in feces.

Contraindications and precautions

Contraindicated in patients with hypersensitivity to drug.

Interactions

None reported.

Adverse reactions

Metabolic: hyperglycemia, glycosuria, ***hypothalamic-pituitary-adrenal axis suppression,*** Cushing's syndrome.
Skin: burning, pruritus, irritation, dryness, erythema, folliculitis, perioral dermatitis, hypertrichosis, hypopigmentation, acneiform eruptions; *maceration, secondary infection, atrophy, striae, miliaria* (with occlusive dressings).

☑ Special considerations

- Recommendations for use of diflorasone, for care and teaching of patients during therapy, and for use in elderly patients, children, and breastfeeding women are the same as those for all topical adrenocorticoids.

Monitoring the patient

- Monitor patient's response to treatment.
- Monitor patient for adverse effects.

Information for the patient

- Tell patient to use drug only as instructed, to use externally only, and to keep away from eyes.
- Instruct patient not to bandage or wrap treated area without medical approval.
- Tell parents not to put tight clothes or diapers over treated areas in infants.

diflunisal
Dolobid

Pharmacologic classification: NSAID, salicylic acid derivative
Therapeutic classification: nonnarcotic analgesic, antipyretic, anti-inflammatory
Pregnancy risk category C

How supplied

Available by prescription only
Tablets: 250 mg, 500 mg

Indications, route, and dosage

Mild to moderate pain
Adults: Initiate therapy with 1 g, then 500 mg daily in two or three divided doses, usually q 8 to 12 hours. Maximum dose is 1,500 mg daily.
✦ Dosage adjustment. In adults over age 65, start with one-half usual adult dose.
Rheumatoid arthritis and osteoarthritis
Adults: 500 to 1,000 mg P.O. daily in two divided doses, usually q 12 hours. Maximum dose is 1,500 mg daily.
✦ Dosage adjustment. In adults over age 65, start with one-half usual dose.

Pharmacodynamics

Analgesic, antipyretic, and anti-inflammatory actions: Mechanisms unknown. Are probably related to inhibition of prostaglandin synthesis. Drug is a salicylic acid derivative but isn't hydrolyzed to free salicylate in vivo.

Pharmacokinetics

- *Absorption:* Absorbed rapidly and completely via GI tract. Plasma levels peak in 2 to 3 hours. Analgesia achieved within 1 hour; peaks within 2 to 3 hours.
- *Distribution:* Highly protein-bound.
- *Metabolism:* Metabolized in liver; isn't metabolized to salicylic acid.
- *Excretion:* Excreted in urine. Half-life is 8 to 12 hours.

Contraindications and precautions

Contraindicated in patients with hypersensitivity to drug and in those in whom acute asthmatic attacks, urticaria, or rhinitis are precipitated by aspirin or other NSAIDs. Use cautiously in patients with GI bleeding, history of peptic ulcer disease, renal impairment, and compromised cardiac function, hypertension, or other conditions predisposing patient to fluid retention.

Because of epidemiologic association with Reye's syndrome, the Centers for Disease Control and Prevention recommend not giving salicylates to children and teenagers with chickenpox or flulike illness.

Interactions

Drug-drug. *Acetaminophen:* May increase serum acetaminophen levels as much as 50%, leading to potential hepatotoxicity and, possibly, nephrotoxicity. Monitor renal and hepatic function closely.

Antacids: Cause delays and decreases in absorption of diflunisal. Monitor patient for effects.

Anticoagulants, thrombolytics: May potentiate anticoagulant effects by platelet-inhibiting effect of diflunisal. Avoid concomitant use.

Antihypertensives: May decrease effect on blood pressure. Monitor closely.

Aspirin: May decrease bioavailability of diflunisal. Monitor patient for effects.

Cyclosporine: Concomitant use may enhance nephrotoxicity. Monitor renal function.

Diuretics: May increase nephrotoxic potential. Monitor renal function.

Furosemide: May decrease furosemide's hyperuricemic effect. Monitor patient for effects.

GI-irritating drugs, such as antibiotics, corticosteroids, other NSAIDs: Concomitant use may potentiate adverse GI effects of diflunisal. Use together cautiously.

Gold compounds: May increase nephrotoxicity. Monitor renal function.

Highly protein-bound drugs (phenytoin, sulfonylureas, warfarin): Concomitant use may cause displacement of either drug and adverse effects. Monitor patient closely.

Hydrochlorothiazide: May increase plasma level of hydrochlorothiazide but decrease hyperuricemic, diuretic, antihypertensive, and natriuretic effects. Monitor patient closely.

Indomethacin: Concomitant use has been associated with decreased renal clearance of indomethacin. Fatal GI hemorrhage has also been reported. Monitor patient closely.

Lithium: May result in increased lithium serum levels. Monitor patient for effects.

Methotrexate, nifedipine, verapamil: May decrease renal excretion of these drugs with concomitant use. Monitor renal function.

Probenecid: May decrease renal clearance of diflunisal. Monitor patient for adverse effects.

Sulindac: Decreases blood levels of active metabolite. Monitor patient closely.

Drug-food. *Any food:* Delays and decreases absorption of diflunisal. Instruct patient to take on empty stomach.

Drug-lifestyle. *Alcohol:* May potentiate adverse GI effects of diflunisal. Discourage use.

Adverse reactions

CNS: *dizziness,* somnolence, insomnia, *headache,* fatigue.
EENT: *tinnitus.*
GI: *nausea, dyspepsia, GI pain, diarrhea,* vomiting, constipation, flatulence.
GU: increased serum BUN and creatinine, renal impairment, hematuria, interstitial nephritis.

Hematologic: prolonged bleeding time.
Hepatic: increased liver function tests.
Metabolic: hyperkalemia, hypouricemia.
Skin: *rash,* pruritus, sweating, stomatitis, ***erythema multiforme, Stevens-Johnson syndrome.***

☑ Special considerations

Besides the recommendations relevant to all NSAIDs, consider the following.
● Diflunisal is recommended for twice-daily dosing for added patient convenience and compliance.
● Don't break, crush, or allow patient to chew diflunisal. Patient should swallow tablet whole.
● Administer with water, milk, or meals to minimize GI upset.
● Don't administer with aspirin or acetaminophen.
● Institute safety measures to prevent injury if patient experiences CNS effects.
● Signs and symptoms of overdose include drowsiness, nausea, vomiting, hyperventilation, tachycardia, sweating, tinnitus, disorientation, stupor, and coma.
● To treat overdose, empty stomach immediately by inducing emesis with ipecac syrup if patient is conscious or by gastric lavage. Administer activated charcoal via nasogastric tube. Provide symptomatic and supportive measures (respiratory support and correction of fluid and electrolyte imbalances). Monitor laboratory parameters and vital signs closely. Hemodialysis has little effect.

Monitoring the patient
● Make sure teenagers don't have chickenpox virus or influenza-like illness before treatment.
● Evaluate patient's response to diflunisal therapy as evidenced by reduced pain or inflammation. Monitor vital signs frequently, especially temperature.
● Assess patient for signs and symptoms of potential hemorrhage, such as bruising, petechiae, coffee-ground emesis, and black, tarry stools.
● Monitor serum coagulation studies if patient is taking anticoagulants.
● Monitor serum glucose level if patient is taking sulfonylureas.
● Monitor serum phenytoin level if patient is taking phenytoin.
● Monitor results of laboratory tests, especially renal and liver function studies.
● Monitor patient for presence and amount of peripheral edema.
● Monitor weight frequently.

Information for the patient
● Instruct patient in diflunisal regimen and need for compliance. Advise him to report adverse reactions.
● Tell patient to take diflunisal with food to minimize GI upset and to swallow tablet whole.

- Caution patient to avoid activities requiring alertness or concentration, such as driving, until CNS effects are known.
- Instruct patient in safety measures to prevent injury.

Geriatric patients
- Patients over age 60 may be more susceptible to toxic effects (particularly GI toxicity) of drug.
- Drug effects on renal prostaglandins may cause fluid retention and edema, a significant drawback for elderly patients, especially those with heart failure or hypertension.

Pediatric patients
- Don't use long-term diflunisal therapy in children under age 14; safe use hasn't been established.

Breast-feeding patients
- Because drug appears in breast milk, breast-feeding isn't recommended.

digoxin
Lanoxicaps, Lanoxin, Novo-Digoxin

Pharmacologic classification: cardiac glycoside
Therapeutic classification: antiarrhythmic, inotropic
Pregnancy risk category C

How supplied
Available by prescription only
Tablets: 0.125 mg, 0.25 mg, 0.5 mg
Capsules: 0.05 mg, 0.10 mg, 0.20 mg
Elixir: 0.05 mg/ml
Injection: 0.05 mg/ml, 0.1 mg/ml (pediatric), 0.25 mg/ml

Indications, route, and dosage
Heart failure, atrial fibrillation and flutter, paroxysmal atrial tachycardia
Tablets, elixir
Adults: For rapid digitalization, give 0.75 to 1.25 mg P.O. over 24 hours in two or more divided doses q 6 to 8 hours. For slow digitalization, give 0.125 to 0.5 mg daily for 5 to 7 days. Maintenance dose is 0.125 to 0.5 mg daily.
Children ages 10 and older: 10 to 15 mcg/kg P.O. over 24 hours in two or more divided doses q 6 to 8 hours. Maintenance dose is 25% to 35% of total digitalizing dose.
Children ages 5 to 10: 20 to 35 mcg/kg P.O. over 24 hours in two or more divided doses q 6 to 8 hours. Maintenance dose is 25% to 35% of total digitalizing dose.
Children ages 2 to 5: 30 to 40 mcg/kg P.O. over 24 hours in two or more divided doses q 6 to 8 hours. Maintenance dose is 25% to 35% of total digitalizing dose.

Infants ages 1 month to 2 years: 35 to 60 mcg/kg P.O. over 24 hours in two or more divided doses q 6 to 8 hours. Maintenance dose is 25% to 35% of total digitalizing dose.
Neonates: 25 to 35 mcg/kg P.O. over 24 hours in two or more divided doses q 6 to 8 hours. Maintenance dose is 25% to 35% of total digitalizing dose.
Premature infants: 20 to 30 mcg/kg P.O. over 24 hours in two or more divided doses q 6 to 8 hours. Maintenance dose is 20% to 30% of total digitalizing dose.
Capsules
Adults: For rapid digitalization, give 0.4 to 0.6 mg P.O. initially, then 0.1 to 0.3 mg q 6 to 8 hours, as needed and tolerated, for 24 hours. For slow digitalization, give 0.05 to 0.35 mg daily in two divided doses for 7 to 22 days, as needed, until therapeutic serum levels are reached. Maintenance dose is 0.05 to 0.35 mg daily in one or two divided doses.
Children: Digitalizing dose is based on child's age and is administered in three or more divided doses over the first 24 hours. Initial dose should be 50% of the total dose; subsequent doses are given q 4 to 8 hours as needed and tolerated.
Children ages 10 and over: For rapid digitalization, give 8 to 12 mcg/kg P.O. over 24 hours, divided as above. Maintenance dose is 25% to 35% of total digitalizing dose, given daily as a single dose.
Children ages 5 to 10: For rapid digitalization, give 15 to 30 mcg/kg P.O. over 24 hours, divided as above. Maintenance dose is 25% to 35% of total digitalizing dose, divided and given in two or three equal doses daily.
Children ages 2 to 5: For rapid digitalization, give 25 to 35 mcg/kg P.O. over 24 hours, divided as above. Maintenance dose is 25% to 35% of total digitalizing dose, divided and given in two or three equal doses daily.
Injection
Adults: For rapid digitalization, give 0.4 to 0.6 mg I.V. initially, then 0.1 to 0.3 mg I.V. q 4 to 8 hours, as needed and tolerated, for 24 hours. For slow digitalization, give appropriate daily maintenance dosage for 7 to 22 days as needed until therapeutic serum levels are reached. Maintenance dose is 0.125 to 0.5 mg I.V. daily in one or two divided doses.
Children: Digitalizing dose is based on child's age and is administered in three or more divided doses over the first 24 hours. Initial dose should be 50% of total dose; subsequent doses are given q 4 to 8 hours as needed and tolerated.
Children ages 10 and over: For rapid digitalization, give 8 to 12 mcg/kg I.V. over 24 hours, divided as above. Maintenance dosage is 25% to 35% of total digitalizing dose, given daily as a single dose.
Children ages 5 to 10: For rapid digitalization, give 15 to 30 mcg/kg I.V. over 24 hours, di-

as above. Maintenance dose is 25% to 35% of total digitalizing dose, divided and given in two or three equal doses daily.

Children ages 2 to 5: For rapid digitalization, give 25 to 35 mcg/kg I.V. over 24 hours, divided as above. Maintenance dose is 25% to 35% of total digitalizing dose, divided and given in two or three equal doses daily.

Infants ages 1 month to 2 years: For rapid digitalization, give 30 to 50 mcg/kg I.V. over 24 hours, divided as above. Maintenance dose is 25% to 35% of total digitalizing dose, divided and given in two or three equal doses daily.

Neonates: For rapid digitalization, give 20 to 30 mcg/kg I.V. over 24 hours, divided as above. Maintenance dose is 25% to 35% of the total digitalizing dose, divided and given in two or three equal doses daily.

Premature infants: For rapid digitalization, give 15 to 25 mcg/kg I.V. over 24 hours, divided as above. Maintenance dose is 20% to 30% of the total digitalizing dose, divided and given in two or three equal doses daily.

✦ **Dosage adjustment.** Reduce dosage in patients with impaired renal function. Hypothyroid patients are highly sensitive to glycosides; hyperthyroid patients may need larger doses.

Pharmacodynamics

Digoxin is the most widely used cardiac glycoside. Several oral forms and a parenteral form are available, facilitating drug's use in both acute and chronic clinical settings.

Inotropic action: Digoxin's effect on myocardium is dose-related and involves both direct and indirect mechanisms. It directly increases force and velocity of myocardial contraction, AV node refractory period, and total peripheral resistance; at higher doses, it also increases sympathetic outflow. It indirectly depresses the SA node and prolongs conduction to the AV node. In patients with heart failure, increased contractile force boosts cardiac output, improves systolic emptying, and decreases heart size. It also reduces ventricular end-diastolic pressure and, consequently, pulmonary and systemic venous pressures. Increased myocardial contractility and cardiac output reflexively reduce sympathetic tone in patients with heart failure. This compensates for drug's direct vasoconstrictive action, thereby reducing total peripheral resistance. It also slows increased heart rate and causes diuresis in edematous patients.

Antiarrhythmic action: Digoxin-induced slowing of heart rate in patients without heart failure is negligible and stems mainly from vagal (cholinergic) and sympatholytic effects on the SA node; however, with toxic doses, slowing of heart rate results from direct depression of SA node automaticity. Therapeutic doses produce little effect on the action potential, but toxic doses increase the automaticity (spontaneous diastolic depolarization) of all cardiac regions except the SA node.

Pharmacokinetics

● *Absorption:* With tablet or elixir, 60% to 85% of dose is absorbed. With capsule, bioavailability increases. About 90% to 100% of dose is absorbed. With I.M. administration, about 80% of dose is absorbed. With oral administration, onset of action occurs in 30 minutes to 2 hours, with peak effects occurring in 6 to 8 hours. With I.M. administration, onset of action occurs in 30 minutes, with peak effects in 4 to 6 hours. With I.V. administration, action occurs in 5 to 30 minutes, with peak effects in 1 to 5 hours.

● *Distribution:* Distributed widely in body tissues; highest levels occur in heart, kidneys, intestine, stomach, liver, and skeletal muscle; lowest levels in plasma and brain. Crosses blood-brain barrier and placenta; fetal and maternal digoxin levels are equivalent at birth. About 20% to 30% of drug is bound to plasma proteins. Usual therapeutic range for steady-state serum levels is 0.5 to 2 ng/ml. In treatment of atrial tachyarrhythmias, higher serum levels (such as 2 to 4 ng/ml) may be needed. Because of drug's long half-life, achievement of steady-state levels may take 7 days or longer, depending on patient's renal function. Toxic symptoms may appear within usual therapeutic range; however, these are more frequent and serious with levels above 2.5 ng/ml.

● *Metabolism:* In most patients, a small amount metabolized in liver and gut by bacteria. Metabolism varies and may be substantial in some patients. Drug undergoes some enterohepatic recirculation (also variable). Metabolites have minimal cardiac activity.

● *Excretion:* Most of dose excreted by kidneys as unchanged drug. Some patients excrete a substantial amount of metabolized or reduced drug. In patients with renal failure, biliary excretion is a more important excretion route. In healthy patients, terminal half-life is 30 to 40 hours. In patients lacking functioning kidneys, half-life increases to at least 4 days.

Contraindications and precautions

Contraindicated in patients with hypersensitivity to drug and in those with digitalis-induced toxicity, ventricular fibrillation, or ventricular tachycardia unless caused by heart failure.

Use cautiously in elderly patients and in patients with acute MI, incomplete AV block, sinus bradycardia, PVCs, chronic constrictive pericarditis, hypertrophic cardiomyopathy, renal insufficiency, severe pulmonary disease, or hypothyroidism.

Interactions

Drug-drug. *Amiloride:* Inhibited digoxin effect and increased digoxin excretion. Monitor patient for arrhythmias.

Aminosalicylic acid, antacids containing aluminum or magnesium hydroxide, kaolin-pectin, magnesium trisilicate, sulfasalazine: Decreased absorption of orally administered digoxin with concomitant use. Use cautiously if administered together and monitor patient for arrhythmias.

Amiodarone, diltiazem, nifedipine, quinidine, verapamil: May cause increased serum digoxin levels, predisposing patient to toxicity. Watch for cardiac effects.

Amphotericin B, carbenicillin, corticosteroids, corticotropin, edetate disodium, laxatives, sodium polystyrene sulfonate, ticarcillin: Depleted total body potassium, possibly causing digoxin toxicity. Monitor potassium levels and cardiac effects.

Antibiotics: When used together, certain antibiotics may interfere with bacterial flora that allow formation of inactive reduction products in GI tract, possibly causing significant increase in digoxin bioavailability and increased serum digoxin levels. Monitor patient closely.

Anticholinergics: May increase digoxin absorption of oral digoxin tablets. Monitor patient closely.

Cardiac drugs affecting AV conduction (such as procainamide, propranolol, verapamil): May cause additive cardiac effects. Monitor patient closely.

Cholestyramine, colestipol, metoclopramide: May bind digoxin in GI tract and impair absorption. Monitor patient for arrhythmias.

Cytotoxic drugs, radiation therapy: May decrease digoxin absorption if intestinal mucosa is damaged. Use digoxin elixir or capsules instead. Monitor patient closely.

Dextrose-insulin infusions, glucagon, large dextrose doses: Reduced extracellular potassium, possibly leading to digitalis toxicity. Watch for arrhythmias.

Electrolyte-altering drugs such as bumetanide, ethacrynic acid, furosemide, and thiazides: May increase or decrease serum electrolyte levels, predisposing patient to digoxin toxicity. Monitor electrolyte levels; monitor cardiac effects closely.

I.V. calcium preparations: May cause synergistic effects that precipitate arrhythmias. Monitor patient closely.

Rauwolfia alkaloids, sympathomimetics (such as ephedrine, epinephrine, isoproterenol): May increase risk of arrhythmias. Monitor patient closely.

Succinylcholine: May precipitate arrhythmias by potentiating digoxin's effects. Monitor patient closely.

Drug-herb. *Betel palm, fumitory, goldenseal, lily-of-the-valley, motherwort, rue, shepherd's purse:* Enhanced cardiac effects. Discourage concomitant use.

Licorice, oleander, Siberian ginseng, squill: May enhance toxicity. Discourage concomitant use.

Adverse reactions
The following signs of toxicity may occur with all cardiac glycosides.
CNS: *fatigue, generalized muscle weakness, agitation, hallucinations,* headache, malaise, dizziness, vertigo, stupor, paresthesia.
CV: *arrhythmias* (most commonly, conduction disturbances with or without AV block, PVCs, and supraventricular arrhythmias) that may lead to increased severity of *heart failure* and hypotension. *Toxic effects on the heart may be life-threatening and require immediate attention.*
EENT: *yellow-green halos around visual images, blurred vision,* light flashes, photophobia, diplopia.
GI: *anorexia, nausea,* vomiting, diarrhea.

☑ Special considerations
● Question patient about use of cardiac glycosides within previous 2 to 3 weeks before administering loading dose. Always divide loading dose over first 24 hours unless situation indicates otherwise.
● GI absorption may be reduced in patients with heart failure, especially right-sided heart failure.
● Because digoxin may predispose patients to postcardioversion asystole, most clinicians withhold digoxin 1 or 2 days before elective cardioversion in patients with atrial fibrillation. (However, consider consequences of increased ventricular response to atrial fibrillation if drug is withheld.)
● Don't administer calcium rapidly by I.V. route to patient receiving digoxin. Calcium affects cardiac contractility and excitability in much the same way that digoxin does and may lead to serious arrhythmias.
● Because Lanoxicaps (soft capsules containing digoxin solution) are better absorbed than tablets, dose is usually slightly smaller.
● Effects of overdose are primarily GI, CNS, and cardiac reactions.
● Severe intoxication may cause hyperkalemia, which may develop rapidly and result in life-threatening cardiac manifestations. Cardiac signs of digoxin toxicity may occur with or without other toxicity signs and commonly precede other toxic effects. Because toxic cardiac effects also can occur as manifestations of heart disease, determining whether these effects result from underlying heart disease or digoxin toxicity may be difficult.
● Digoxin has caused almost every kind of arrhythmia; various combinations of arrhythmias may occur in same patient.
● Patients with chronic digoxin toxicity commonly have ventricular arrhythmias or AV conduction disturbances. Patients with digoxin-induced ventricular tachycardia have a high risk of mortality because ventricular fibrillation or asystole may result. If toxicity is suspected, stop drug and obtain serum drug levels. Usually, drug takes at least

6 hours to distribute between plasma and tissue and reach equilibrium; plasma levels drawn earlier may show higher digoxin levels than those present after drug appears in tissues.
• Other treatment measures for overdose include immediate emesis induction, gastric lavage, and activated charcoal to reduce absorption of remaining drug. Multiple doses of activated charcoal (such as 50 g q 6 hours) may help reduce further absorption, especially of any drug undergoing enterohepatic recirculation. Some clinicians advocate cholestyramine administration if digoxin was recently ingested; however, it may not be useful if the ingestion is life-threatening. Interacting drugs probably should be stopped.
• Ventricular arrhythmias may be treated with I.V. potassium (replacement dose; but not in patients with significant AV block), I.V. phenytoin, I.V. lidocaine, or I.V. propranolol.
• Refractory ventricular tachyarrhythmias may be controlled with overdrive pacing. Procainamide may be used for ventricular arrhythmias that don't respond to above treatments. In severe AV block, asystole, and hemodynamically significant sinus bradycardia, atropine restores normal rate.
• Administration of digoxin-specific antibody fragments (digoxin immune Fab [Digibind]) is a treatment for life-threatening digoxin toxicity. Each 40 mg of digoxin immune Fab binds about 0.6 mg of digoxin in bloodstream. Complex is then excreted in urine, rapidly decreasing serum levels of cardiac drug.

Monitoring the patient
• Obtain baseline heart rate and rhythm, blood pressure, and serum electrolyte levels before giving first dose.
• Adjust dose to patient's clinical condition and renal function; monitor ECG and serum levels of digoxin, calcium, potassium, and magnesium as well as serum creatinine. Therapeutic serum digoxin levels range from 0.5 to 2 ng/ml. Take corrective action before hypokalemia occurs.
• Monitor clinical status. Take apical-radial pulse for a full minute. Watch for significant changes (sudden rate increase or decrease, pulse deficit, irregular beats, and especially regularization of a previously irregular rhythm). Check blood pressure and obtain 12-lead ECG if these changes occur.

Information for the patient
• Inform patient and responsible family member about drug action, drug regimen, how to take pulse, reportable signs, and follow-up plans. Patient must understand importance of follow-up laboratory tests, and have access to outpatient laboratory facilities.
• Instruct patient not to take an extra dose of digoxin if dose is missed.

• Tell patient to call if severe nausea, vomiting, or diarrhea occurs because these conditions may make patient more prone to toxicity.
• Advise patient to use the same brand consistently.
• Tell patient to call before using OTC preparations, especially those high in sodium.

Geriatric patients
• Use digoxin with caution in elderly patients (especially if renally compromised); adjust dosage to prevent systemic accumulation.

Pediatric patients
• Children have a poorly defined range of serum levels; however, toxicity apparently doesn't occur at same levels considered toxic in adults. Divided daily dosing is recommended for infants and children under age 10; older children require adult doses proportional to body weight.

---

digoxin immune Fab (ovine)
Digibind

Pharmacologic classification: antibody fragment
Therapeutic classification: cardiac glycoside antidote
Pregnancy risk category C

How supplied
Available by prescription only
Injection: 38-mg vial

Indications, route, and dosage
Potentially life-threatening digoxin or digitoxin intoxication
Adults and children: Administered I.V. through a 0.22-micron membrane filter over 15 to 30 minutes or as a bolus if cardiac arrest is imminent. Dosage varies based on amount of drug to be neutralized; average dose for adults is 6 vials (228 mg). However, if toxicity resulted from acute digoxin ingestion, and neither a serum digoxin level nor an estimated ingestion amount is known, 10 to 20 vials (380 to 760 mg) should be administered. See package insert for complete, specific dosage instructions.

Pharmacodynamics
Cardiac glycoside antidote: Specific antigen-binding fragments bind to free digoxin in extracellular fluid and intravascularly to prevent and reverse pharmacologic and toxic effects of the cardiac glycoside. This binding is preferential for digoxin and digitoxin; preliminary evidence suggests some binding to other digoxin derivatives and cardioactive metabolites.
    Once free digoxin is bound and removed from serum, tissue-bound digoxin is released into the serum to maintain efflux-influx balance. As digox-

---

in is released, it, too, is bound and removed by digoxin immune Fab, resulting in a reduction of serum and tissue digoxin. Cardiac glycoside toxicity begins to subside within 30 minutes after completion of a 15- to 30-minute I.V. infusion of digoxin immune Fab. The onset of action and response is variable and appears to depend on rate of infusion, dose administered relative to body load of glycoside, and possibly other, as yet unidentified factors. Reversal of toxicity, including hyperkalemia, is usually complete within 2 to 6 hours after administration of digoxin immune Fab.

Pharmacokinetics

• *Absorption:* Serum levels peak at completion of I.V. infusion. Drug has a serum half-life of 15 to 20 hours. Association reaction between Fab fragments and glycoside molecules appears to occur rapidly; data are limited.

• *Distribution:* Not fully characterized. After I.V. administration, appears to distribute rapidly throughout extracellular space, into both plasma and interstitial fluid. Not known if drug crosses placental barrier or is distributed into breast milk.

• *Metabolism:* No information available.

• *Excretion:* Excreted in urine via glomerular filtration.

Contraindications and precautions

No known contraindications. Use cautiously in patients known to be allergic to ovine proteins. In these high-risk patients, skin testing is recommended because the drug is derived from digoxin-specific antibody fragments obtained from immunized sheep.

Interactions

Drug-drug. *Cardiac glycosides (such as digitoxin, digoxin, lanatoside C):* Binding of cardiac glycosides if used concomitantly. This will also occur if redigitalization is attempted before elimination of digoxin immune Fab is complete (several days with normal renal function; 1 week or longer with renal impairment). Use cautiously and monitor patient closely.

Adverse reactions

CV: *heart failure,* rapid ventricular rate (both caused by reversal of cardiac glycoside's therapeutic effects).

Metabolic: hypokalemia.

Other: hypersensitivity reactions *(anaphylaxis).*

☑ Special considerations

• Give I.V. using 0.22-micron filter needle over 30 minutes or as bolus injection when cardiac arrest is imminent. Dose depends on amount of digoxin to be neutralized. Each 38-mg vial binds about 0.5 mg of digoxin or digitoxin. Reconstitute vial with 4 ml of sterile water for injection, mix gently, and use immediately. May be stored in refrigerator up to 4 hours.

• To determine appropriate dose, divide the total digitalis body load by 0.5; the resultant number is an estimate of the number of vials required for appropriate dose. Or in cases of acute ingestion of known quantity of digitalis, multiply amount of digitalis ingested in milligrams by 0.8 (to account for incomplete absorption).

• Skin testing may be appropriate for high-risk patients. One of two methods may be used:

Intradermal test—dilute 0.1 ml of reconstituted solution in 9.9 ml of sterile saline for injection; then withdraw and inject 0.1 ml of this solution intradermally. Inspect site after 20 minutes for signs of erythema or urticaria.

Scratch test—dilute as for intradermal test. Place one drop of diluted solution on skin and make a one-quarter inch scratch through drop with sterile needle. Inspect site after 20 minutes for signs of erythema or urticaria. If results are positive, avoid use of digoxin immune Fab unless necessary. If systemic reaction occurs, treat symptomatically.

• Pretreat patients with sensitivity or allergy to sheep or ovine products, or when skin test results are positive, with an antihistamine such as diphenhydramine and a corticosteroid before administering digoxin immune Fab.

• Digoxin immune Fab therapy alters standard cardiac glycoside determinations by radioimmunoassay procedures. Results may be falsely increased or decreased, depending on separation method used. Serum potassium levels may decrease rapidly.

• Administration of doses larger than needed for neutralizing cardiac glycoside may subject patient to increased risk of allergic or febrile reaction or delayed serum sickness. Large doses may also prolong time required before redigitalization.

Monitoring the patient

• Keep drugs and equipment for cardiopulmonary resuscitation readily available during administration of digoxin immune Fab for patients who respond poorly to withdrawal of digoxin's inotropic effects. Dopamine or dobutamine, or other cardiac load-reducing drugs, may be used. Catecholamines may aggravate arrhythmias induced by digitalis toxicity and should be used with caution.

• Measure serum digoxin or digitoxin levels before giving antidote because serum levels may be difficult to interpret after therapy with antidote.

• Closely monitor temperature, blood pressure, ECG, and potassium level before, during, and after administration of antidote.

• Potassium levels must be checked repeatedly because severe digitalis intoxication can cause life-threatening hyperkalemia, and reversal by digoxin immune Fab may lead to rapid hypolemia.

Information for the patient
• Explain use and administration of drug to patient and family.
• Instruct patient to report adverse effects promptly.

Pediatric patients
• Consider risk-to-benefit ratio. Adverse effects haven't occurred in infants and small children.
• Monitor patient for volume overload in small children.
• Very small doses may require diluting reconstituted solution with 36 ml of sterile saline for injection to produce a 1 mg/ml solution.
• Infants may need smaller doses; manufacturer recommends reconstituting as directed and administering with a tuberculin syringe.

Breast-feeding patients
• It's unknown if drug appears in breast milk; use cautiously in breast-feeding women.

dihydroergotamine mesylate
D.H.E. 45, Migranal

Pharmacologic classification: ergot alkaloid
Therapeutic classification: vasoconstrictor
Pregnancy risk category X

How supplied
Available by prescription only
Injection: 1 mg/ml
Nasal spray: 4 mg/ml

Indications, route, and dosage
To prevent or abort vascular headaches, including migraine headaches
Adults: 1 mg I.M. or I.V., repeated at 1-hour intervals, up to total of 3 mg I.M. or 2 mg I.V. Maximum weekly dose is 6 mg.
To acutely treat migraine headaches with or without aura
Adults: 1 spray (0.5 mg) administered in each nostril, then another spray in each nostril in 15 minutes for a total of 4 sprays (2 mg).

Pharmacodynamics
Vasoconstrictor action: By stimulating alpha-adrenergic receptors, drug causes peripheral vasoconstriction (if vascular tone is low). However, it causes vasodilation in hypertonic blood vessels. At high doses, it's a competitive alpha-adrenergic blocker. In therapeutic doses, drug inhibits the reuptake of norepinephrine. A weak antagonist of serotonin, drug reduces the increased rate of platelet aggregation caused by serotonin.

In treatment of vascular headaches, drug probably causes direct vasoconstriction of the dilated carotid artery bed while decreasing the amplitude of pulsations. Its serotoninergic and catecholamine effects also appear to be involved.

Effects on blood pressure are minimal. The vasoconstrictor effect is more pronounced on veins and venules than on arteries and arterioles.

Pharmacokinetics
• *Absorption:* Incompletely and irregularly absorbed from GI tract. Onset of action depends on how quickly after headache drug is given. After I.M. injection or intranasal administration, onset of action occurs within 15 to 30 minutes, and after I.V. injection, within a few minutes. Duration of action persists 3 to 4 hours after I.M. injection.
• *Distribution:* 90% of dose is plasma protein-bound.
• *Metabolism:* Extensively metabolized, probably in liver.
• *Excretion:* 10% of dose excreted in urine within 72 hours as metabolites; rest in feces.

Contraindications and precautions
Contraindicated in patients with hypersensitivity to drug, in pregnant or breast-feeding women, and in those with peripheral and occlusive vascular disease, coronary artery disease, uncontrolled hypertension, sepsis, hemiplegic or basilar migraine, and severe hepatic or renal dysfunction. Avoid use of drug in patients with uncontrolled hypertension or within 24 hours of 5-HT$_1$ agonists, ergotamine-containing or ergot-type drugs, or methysergide.

Interactions
Drug-drug. *Antihypertensives:* May antagonize their antihypertensive effects. Monitor blood pressure closely.
Erythromycin, other macrolides: May cause ergot toxicity. Monitor patient for drug effects.
Propranolol, other beta blockers: Blocked natural pathway for vasodilation in patients receiving ergot alkaloids; may result in excessive vasoconstriction and cold extremities. Monitor patient closely.
Vasodilators: May result in pressor effects and dangerous hypertension. Monitor blood pressure closely.

Adverse reactions
CV: numbness and tingling in fingers and toes, transient tachycardia or **bradycardia,** precordial distress and pain, increased arterial pressure, localized edema.
GI: *nausea, vomiting.*
Musculoskeletal: weakness in legs, muscle pain in extremities.
Skin: itching.

☑ Special considerations

Besides the recommendations relevant to all ergot alkaloids, consider the following.

• Drug is most effective when used at first sign of migraine, or as soon after onset as possible.

• If severe vasospasm occurs, keep extremities warm. Provide supportive treatment to prevent tissue damage. Give vasodilators if needed.

• Protect ampules from heat and light. Don't use if discolored.

• For short-term use only. Don't exceed recommended dose.

• Ergotamine rebound or an increase in frequency or duration of headaches may occur when drug is stopped.

• Signs and symptoms of overdose include symptoms of ergot toxicity: peripheral ischemia, paresthesia, headache, nausea, and vomiting. Treatment requires prolonged and careful monitoring. Provide respiratory support, treat seizures, if necessary, and apply warmth (not direct heat) to ischemic extremities if vasospasm occurs. Administer vasodilators, if needed.

Monitoring the patient

• If patient is of childbearing age, rule out pregnancy before therapy.

• Monitor blood pressure if drug is used for orthostatic hypotension.

• Monitor patient for signs of illness or infection.

Information for the patient

• Advise patient to lie down and relax in a quiet, darkened room after dose is administered.

• Urge patient to report immediately feelings of numbness or tingling in fingers and toes or red or violet blisters on hands or feet.

• Warn patient to avoid alcoholic beverages during drug therapy.

• Caution patient to avoid smoking during therapy because the adverse effects of drug may be increased.

• Tell patient to avoid prolonged exposure to very cold temperatures while taking drug. Cold may increase adverse reactions.

• Advise patient to report illness or infection, which may increase sensitivity to drug reactions.

• Instruct patient to prime the pump before using nasal spray.

• Instruct patient to discard nasal spray applicator once it has been prepared and unused drug after 8 hours.

Geriatric patients

• Use drug cautiously in elderly patients. Safety and efficacy haven't been established.

Breast-feeding patients

• Because it's likely that drug appears in breast milk, breast-feeding isn't recommended while patient is taking drug.

dihydrotachysterol
DHT, DHT Intensol, Hytakerol

Pharmacologic classification: vitamin D analogue
Therapeutic classification: antihypocalcemic
Pregnancy risk category C

How supplied

Available by prescription only
Tablets: 0.125 mg, 0.2 mg, 0.4 mg
Capsules: 0.125 mg
Solution: 0.2 mg/ml (Intensol), 0.2 mg/5 ml (in 4% alcohol), 0.25 mg/ml (in sesame oil)

Indications, route, and dosage

Hypocalcemia associated with hypoparathyroidism and pseudohypoparathyroidism
Adults: Initially, 0.8 to 2.4 mg P.O. daily for several days. Maintenance dose is 0.2 to 1 mg daily, as needed for normal serum calcium levels. Average dose is 0.6 mg daily.
Children: Initially, 1 to 5 mg P.O. daily for 4 days, then continue dosage or reduce to one-fourth the initial amount. Usual maintenance dosage is 0.5 to 1.5 mg daily, as needed for normal serum calcium levels.
Prevention of thyroidectomy-induced hypocalcemia
Adults: 0.25 mg P.O. daily given with calcium supplements until danger of hypocalcemic tetany has passed.
◇ **Familial hypophosphatemia**
Adults and children: 0.5 to 2 mg P.O. daily (until healing of bones occurs). Maintenance dose is 0.2 to 1.5 mg daily.
◇ **Renal osteodystrophy in chronic uremia**
Adults: 0.1 to 0.6 mg P.O. daily.
Children: 0.1 to 0.5 mg P.O. daily.
◇ **Osteoporosis**
Adults: 0.6 mg P.O. daily given with calcium and fluoride.

Pharmacodynamics

Antihypocalcemic action: Once activated to its 25-hydroxy form, drug works with parathyroid hormone to regulate levels of calcium. Appears to have little activity as the parent compound.

Pharmacokinetics

• *Absorption:* Absorbed readily from small intestine.
• *Distribution:* Distributed widely; largely protein-bound.
• *Metabolism:* Metabolized in liver; duration of action up to 9 weeks.
• *Excretion:* Excreted in urine and bile.

Contraindications and precautions
Contraindicated in patients with hypercalcemia or vitamin D toxicity. Use cautiously in those with a history of renal calculi.

Interactions
Drug-drug. *Antacids containing magnesium:* May alter absorption of dihydrotachysterol. Monitor patient for effects.
Barbiturates, phenytoin, primidone: May increase metabolism and reduce activity of dihydrotachysterol. Increases in calcium may potentiate effects of cardiac glycosides. Monitor glycoside levels closely.
Cardiac glycosides: Increased risk of arrhythmias. Monitor patient closely.
Cholestyramine, colestipol: Concomitant use may result in decreased absorption of vitamin D analogues. Monitor patient for effects.
Corticosteroids: Counteract vitamin D analogue effects. Monitor patient for effects.
Mineral oil: Excessive use may interfere with intestinal absorption of vitamin D analogues. Monitor patient for effects.
Thiazide diuretics: May cause hypercalcemia. Monitor calcium levels and patient effects.
Vitamin D analogues: Increased toxicity. Monitor patient.

Adverse reactions
CNS: headache, somnolence, irritability.
CV: hypertension, *arrhythmias.*
EENT: conjunctivitis, photophobia, rhinorrhea.
GI: nausea, vomiting, constipation, polydipsia, pancreatitis, metallic taste, dry mouth, anorexia, diarrhea.
GU: polyuria, nocturia, decreased libido, nephrocalcinosis.
Hepatic: altered serum alkaline phosphatase.
Metabolic: weight loss; alterations in cholesterol levels and electrolytes, such as magnesium, phosphate, and calcium, in serum and urine; thirst; hyperthermia.
Musculoskeletal: weakness, bone and muscle pain.

☑ Special considerations
● Adequate dietary calcium intake is necessary; usually supplemented with 10 to 15 g oral calcium lactate or gluconate daily.
● 1 mg of dihydrotachysterol is equivalent to 120,000 units ergocalciferol (vitamin D₂).
● Hypercalcemia is only sign of overdose. Treatment involves stopping therapy, instituting low-calcium diet, increasing fluid intake, and providing supportive measures.
● Calcitonin administration may help reverse hypercalcemia.
● In severe overdose, death from cardiac and renal failure has occurred.

Monitoring the patient
● Monitor serum and urine calcium levels. Observe patient for signs and symptoms of hypercalcemia.
● Monitoring urine calcium and urine creatinine levels may be helpful in hypercalciuria screening. Ratio of urine calcium to urine creatinine should be less than or equal to 0.18. A value over 0.2 suggests hypercalciuria; decrease dose regardless of serum calcium level.

Information for the patient
● Explain importance of calcium-rich diet.

Pediatric patients
● Some infants may be hyperreactive to drug.

Breast-feeding patients
● Because drug appears in small amounts in breast milk, don't use in breast-feeding women.

---

diltiazem hydrochloride
Cardizem, Cardizem CD,
Cardizem SR, Dilacor XR, Tiazac

Pharmacologic classification: calcium channel blocker
Therapeutic classification: antianginal
Pregnancy risk category C

How supplied
Available by prescription only
Tablets: 30 mg, 60 mg, 90 mg, 120 mg
Capsules (extended-release): 120 mg, 180 mg, 240 mg, 300 mg (extended-release Cardizem CD only); 360 mg (extended-release Tiazac only)
Capsules (sustained-release): 60 mg, 90 mg, 120 mg (Cardizem SR)
Injection: 5 mg/ml 5-ml vials, Lyo-Ject 25-mg syringe

Indications, route, and dosage
Management of Prinzmetal's or variant angina or chronic stable angina pectoris
Adults: 30 mg P.O. q.i.d. before meals and h.s. Increase dose gradually to maximum of 360 mg/day divided into three to four doses, as indicated. Or give 120 or 180 mg (extended-release) P.O. once daily. Adjust over a 7- to 14-day period, as needed and tolerated, to a maximum dose of 480 mg daily.
Hypertension
Adults: 60 to 120 mg P.O. b.i.d. (sustained-release). Adjust to maximum dose of 360 mg/day, as necessary. Or give 180 to 240 mg (extended-release) P.O. once daily. Adjust dose, based on patient response, to a maximum dose of 480 mg/day.

Atrial fibrillation or flutter; paroxysmal supraventricular tachycardia
Adults: 0.25 mg/kg I.V. as a bolus injection over 2 minutes. Repeat after 15 minutes if response isn't adequate with a dosage of 0.35 mg/kg I.V. over 2 minutes. Follow bolus with continuous I.V. infusion at 5 to 15 mg/hour (for up to 24 hours).

Pharmacodynamics
Antianginal or antihypertensive action: By dilating systemic arteries, diltiazem decreases total peripheral resistance and afterload, slightly reduces blood pressure, and increases cardiac index when given in high doses (over 200 mg). Afterload reduction, which occurs at rest and with exercise, and the resulting decrease in myocardial oxygen consumption account for diltiazem's effectiveness in controlling chronic stable angina.

Diltiazem also decreases myocardial oxygen demand and cardiac work by reducing heart rate, relieving coronary artery spasm (through coronary artery vasodilation), and dilating peripheral vessels. These effects relieve ischemia and pain. In patients with Prinzmetal's angina, diltiazem inhibits coronary artery spasm, increasing myocardial oxygen delivery.

Antiarrhythmic action: By impeding the slow inward influx of calcium at the AV node, diltiazem decreases conduction velocity and increases refractory period, thereby decreasing the impulses transmitted to the ventricles in atrial fibrillation or flutter. The result is a decreased ventricular rate.

Pharmacokinetics
● *Absorption:* About 80% of dose absorbed rapidly from GI tract. However, only about 40% enters systemic circulation because of significant first-pass effect in liver. Serum levels peak in about 2 to 3 hours.
● *Distribution:* About 70% to 85% of circulating drug bound to plasma proteins.
● *Metabolism:* Metabolized in liver.
● *Excretion:* About 35% excreted in urine; about 65% in bile as unchanged drug, inactive and active metabolites. Elimination half-life is 3 to 9 hours. Half-life may increase in elderly patients; however, renal dysfunction doesn't appear to affect half-life.

Contraindications and precautions
Contraindicated in patients with hypersensitivity to drug and in those with sick sinus syndrome or second- or third-degree AV block in the absence of an artificial pacemaker, supraventricular tachycardias associated with a bypass tract such as in Wolfe-Parkinson-White syndrome or Lown-Ganong-Levine syndrome, left-sided heart failure, hypotension (systolic blood pressure below 90 mm Hg), acute MI, or pulmonary congestion (documented by X-ray).

Use cautiously in elderly patients and in patients with heart failure or impaired hepatic or renal function.

Interactions
Drug-drug. *Anesthetics:* Anesthetic effects may be potentiated. Use together cautiously.
Beta blockers: Concomitant use may cause combined effects that result in heart failure, conduction disturbances, arrhythmias, and hypotension. Monitor patient closely.
Cimetidine: May increase diltiazem plasma level. Monitor patient carefully for change in diltiazem effects when initiating and discontinuing therapy with cimetidine.
Cyclosporine: May cause increased serum cyclosporine levels and subsequent cyclosporine-induced nephrotoxicity. Monitor renal function.
Digoxin: May increase serum levels of digoxin. Monitor digoxin levels closely.
Furosemide: Forms precipitate when mixed with diltiazem injection. Don't administer together.

Adverse reactions
CNS: *headache,* dizziness, asthenia, somnolence.
CV: *edema,* **arrhythmias,** flushing, **bradycardia,** hypotension, conduction abnormalities, **heart failure,** AV block, abnormal ECG.
GI: *nausea, constipation,* abdominal discomfort.
Hepatic: acute hepatic injury.
Skin: *rash.*

☑ Special considerations
Besides the recommendations relevant to all calcium channel blockers, consider the following.
● Sublingual nitroglycerin may be administered concomitantly, as needed, if patient has acute angina symptoms.
● Diltiazem has been used for investigational purposes to prevent reinfarction after non-Q-wave MI; as an adjunct in treatment of peripheral vascular disorders; and in treatment of several spastic smooth muscle disorders, including esophageal spasm.
● Effects of overdose primarily are extensions of drug's adverse reactions. Heart block, asystole, and hypotension are the most serious effects and need immediate attention.
● Treatment of overdose may involve I.V. isoproterenol, norepinephrine, epinephrine, atropine, or calcium gluconate administered in usual doses. Ensure adequate hydration. Inotropic drugs, such as dobutamine and dopamine, may be used, if necessary. If patient develops severe conduction disturbances (such as heart block and asystole) with hypotension that don't respond to drug therapy, initiate cardiac pacing immediately with cardiopulmonary resuscitation measures, as indicated.

Monitoring the patient
- Evaluate ECG before treatment.
- If diltiazem is added to therapy of patient receiving digoxin, monitor serum digoxin levels and observe closely for signs of toxicity, especially in elderly patients, those with unstable renal function, and those with serum digoxin levels in the upper therapeutic range.
- Monitor serum digoxin level if patient is taking digoxin.

Information for the patient
- Tell patient that nitrate therapy prescribed during adjustment of diltiazem dosage may cause dizziness. Urge patient to continue compliance.
- Inform patient of proper use, dose, and adverse effects associated with diltiazem use.
- Instruct patient to continue taking drug even when feeling better.
- Tell patient to report feelings of dizziness or light-headedness and to avoid sudden position changes.

Geriatric patients
- Use drug with caution in elderly patients because the half-life may be prolonged.

Breast-feeding patients
- Drug appears in breast milk; women shouldn't breast-feed during therapy.

---

dimenhydrinate
Apo-Dimenhydrinate*, Calm-X, Dimetabs, Dinate, Dramamine, Dymenate, Gravol*, Hydrate, PMS-Dimenhydrinate*

Pharmacologic classification: ethanol-amine-derivative antihistamine
Therapeutic classification: antihistamine (H_1-receptor antagonist), antiemetic, antivertigo drug
Pregnancy risk category B

How supplied
Available with or without a prescription
Tablets: 50 mg
Liquid: 12.5 mg/4 ml, 15 mg/5 ml*
Injection: 50 mg/ml

Indications, route, and dosage
Prophylaxis and treatment of nausea, vomiting, dizziness associated with motion sickness
Adults and children ages 12 and older: 50 to 100 mg q 4 to 6 hours P.O., I.V., or I.M. For I.V. administration, dilute each 50-mg dose in 10 ml of normal saline solution and inject slowly over 2 minutes.

Children: 1.25 mg/kg/day or 37.5 mg/m²/day P.O. or I.M. q.i.d. not to exceed 300 mg/day, or according to the following schedule:
Children ages 6 to 12: 25 to 50 mg P.O. q 6 to 8 hours; maximum dose is 150 mg/day.
Children ages 2 to 6: 12.5 to 25 mg P.O. q 6 to 8 hours; maximum dose is 75 mg/day.
◇ **Ménière's disease**
Adults: 50 mg I.M. for acute attack; maintenance dose is 25 to 50 mg P.O. t.i.d.

Pharmacodynamics
Antiemetic and antivertigo actions: Probably inhibits nausea and vomiting by centrally depressing sensitivity of the labyrinth apparatus that relays stimuli to the chemoreceptor trigger zone and stimulates the vomiting center in the brain.

Pharmacokinetics
- *Absorption:* Well absorbed. Action begins within 15 to 30 minutes after oral administration, 20 to 30 minutes after I.M. administration, and almost immediately after I.V. administration. Duration of action 3 to 6 hours.
- *Distribution:* Well distributed throughout body; crosses placenta.
- *Metabolism:* Metabolized in liver.
- *Excretion:* Metabolites excreted in urine.

Contraindications and precautions
Contraindicated in patients with hypersensitivity to drug or its components. I.V. product contains benzyl alcohol, which has been associated with a fatal "gasping syndrome" in premature infants and low birth weight infants.
Use cautiously in patients with seizures, acute angle-closure glaucoma, or enlarged prostate gland and in those receiving ototoxic drugs.

Interactions
Drug-drug. *CNS depressants (such as anxiolytics, barbiturates, sleeping aids, tranquilizers):* Additive CNS sedation and depression may occur. Avoid concomitant use.
Ototoxic drugs (such as aminoglycosides, cisplatin, loop diuretics, salicylates, vancomycin): Concomitant use may mask signs of ototoxicity. Use cautiously and monitor patient closely.
Drug-lifestyle. *Alcohol:* May cause additive CNS depression. Discourage use.

Adverse reactions
CNS: drowsiness, headache, dizziness, confusion, nervousness, insomnia (especially in children), vertigo, tingling and weakness of hands, lassitude, excitation.
CV: palpitations, hypotension, tachycardia, tightness of chest.
EENT: blurred vision, dry respiratory passages, diplopia, nasal congestion.
GI: dry mouth, nausea, vomiting, diarrhea, epigastric distress, constipation, anorexia.

Respiratory: wheezing, thickened bronchial secretions.
Skin: photosensitivity, urticaria, rash.
Other: *anaphylaxis.*

☑ **Special considerations**
Besides the recommendations relevant to all antihistamines, consider the following.
• Incorrectly administered or undiluted I.V. solution is irritating to veins and may cause sclerosis.
• Parenteral solution is incompatible with many drugs; don't mix other drugs in same syringe.
• Advise safety measures for all patients; dimenhydrinate can cause drowsiness. Tolerance to CNS depressant effects usually develops within a few days.
• To prevent motion sickness, patient should take drug 30 minutes before traveling and again before meals and at bedtime.
• Antiemetic effect may diminish with prolonged use.
• Drug may alter or confuse test results for xanthines (caffeine, aminophylline) because of its 8-chlorotheophylline content; stop dimenhydrinate 4 days before diagnostic skin tests to avoid preventing, reducing, or masking test response.
• Signs and symptoms of overdose may include either CNS depression (sedation, reduced mental alertness, apnea, and CV collapse) or CNS stimulation (insomnia, hallucinations, tremors, or seizures). Anticholinergic symptoms (dry mouth, flushed skin, fixed and dilated pupils, and GI symptoms) are likely to occur, especially in children.
• In overdose, use gastric lavage to empty stomach contents; emetics may be ineffective. Diazepam or phenytoin may be used to control seizures. Provide supportive treatment.

Monitoring the patient
• Monitor patient for ototoxicity.
• Monitor patient for adverse effects.

Information for the patient
• Tell patient to avoid hazardous activities, such as driving or operating heavy machinery, until adverse CNS effects of drug are known.
• Tell patient to take drug for motion sickness 30 minutes before departure.

Geriatric patients
• Elderly patients are usually more sensitive to adverse effects of antihistamines than younger patients and are likely to experience a greater degree of dizziness, sedation, hyperexcitability, dry mouth, and urine retention.

Pediatric patients
• Safety in neonates hasn't been established. Infants and children under age 6 may experience paradoxical hyperexcitability. I.V. dosage for children hasn't been established.

Breast-feeding patients
• Avoid use of antihistamines in breast-feeding women. Many of these drugs, including dimenhydrinate, appear in breast milk, exposing infant to risks of unusual excitability; premature infants are at particular risk for seizures.

dimercaprol
BAL in Oil

Pharmacologic classification: chelating
Therapeutic classification: heavy metal antagonist
Pregnancy risk category NR

How supplied
Available by prescription only
Injection: 100 mg/ml

Indications, route, and dosage
Severe arsenic or gold poisoning
Adults and children: 3 mg/kg deep I.M. q 4 hours for 2 days, then q.i.d. on day 3, then b.i.d. for 10 days.
Mild arsenic or gold poisoning
Adults and children: 2.5 mg/kg deep I.M. q.i.d. for 2 days, then b.i.d. on day 3, then once daily for 10 days.
Severe gold dermatitis
Adults and children: 2.5 mg/kg deep I.M. q 4 hours for 2 days, then b.i.d. for 7 days.
Gold-induced thrombocytopenia
Adults and children: 100 mg deep I.M. b.i.d. for 15 days.
Mercury poisoning
Adults and children: Initially, 5 mg/kg deep I.M., then 2.5 mg/kg daily or b.i.d. for 10 days.
Acute lead encephalopathy or blood lead level greater than 100 mcg/dl
Adults and children: 4 mg/kg (or 75 to 83 mg/m²) deep I.M. injection, then give simultaneously with edetate calcium disodium (250 mg/m²) q 4 hours for 3 to 5 days. Use separate injection sites.

Pharmacodynamics
Chelating action: The sulfhydryl groups of dimercaprol form heterocyclic ring complexes with heavy metals, particularly arsenic, mercury, and gold, preventing or reversing their binding to body ligands.

Pharmacokinetics
• *Absorption:* Absorbed slowly through skin. After I.M. injection, serum levels peak in 30 to 60 minutes.
• *Distribution:* Distributed to all tissues, mainly the intracellular space, with highest levels occurring in liver and kidneys.
• *Metabolism:* Uncomplexed dimercaprol is metabolized rapidly to inactive products.

• *Excretion:* Most dimercaprol-metal complexes and inactive metabolites are excreted in urine and feces.

Contraindications and precautions
Contraindicated in patients with hepatic dysfunction (except postarsenical jaundice). Use cautiously in patients with hypertension or oliguria. Avoid use in pregnant women unless needed to treat a life-threatening acute poisoning.

Interactions
Drug-drug. *Cadmium, iron, selenium, uranium:* Form toxic complexes with dimercaprol. Delay iron therapy for 24 hours after stopping dimercaprol.

Adverse reactions
CNS: pain or tightness in throat, chest, or hands; headache; paresthesia; muscle pain or weakness; anxiety.
CV: *transient increase in blood pressure* (returns to normal in 2 hours), *tachycardia.*
EENT: blepharospasm, conjunctivitis, lacrimation, rhinorrhea, excessive salivation.
GI: *nausea; vomiting; burning sensation in lips, mouth, and throat; abdominal pain.*
Other: *fever* (especially in children).

☑ Special considerations
• Treat patient as soon as possible after poisoning for optimal therapeutic effect; administer drug by deep I.M. injection only.
• Adverse effects of dimercaprol are usually mild and transitory and occur in about one-half of patients who receive I.M. dose of 5 mg/kg. In patients who receive doses in excess of 5 mg/kg, adverse effects usually occur within 30 minutes after injection and subside in 1 to 6 hours.
• Drug has strong garlic odor.
• Dimercaprol therapy blocks thyroid uptake of ^{131}I, causing decreased values.
• Signs and symptoms of overdose include vomiting, seizures, stupor, coma, hypertension, and tachycardia; effects subside in 1 to 6 hours.
• Support CV and respiratory status; control seizures with diazepam.

Monitoring the patient
• Monitor vital signs and intake and output during therapy, and keep urine alkaline to prevent renal failure.

Information for the patient
• Advise patient that drug may cause bad taste in mouth or bad breath. It also may cause burning sensation of lips, mouth, throat, eyes, and penis and pain in teeth.
• Monitor patient for adverse effects.

Geriatric patients
› Use drug with caution in elderly patients.

Pediatric patients
• Fever is common, usually appearing after second or third dose, and may persist throughout therapy. Acrodynia in infants and children has been treated with 3 mg/kg of dimercaprol I.M. every 4 hours for 2 days, then every 6 hours for 1 day, then every 12 hours for 7 to 8 days.

---

dinoprostone (prostaglandin E₂)
Cervidil, Prepidil, Prostin E$_2$

Pharmacologic classification: prostaglandin
Therapeutic classification: oxytocic
Pregnancy risk category C

How supplied
Available by prescription only
Vaginal suppositories: 20 mg
Vaginal gel: 0.5 mg
Vaginal insert: 10 mg

Indications, route, and dosage
Abort second-trimester pregnancy, evacuate uterus in cases of missed abortion, intrauterine fetal deaths up to 28 weeks of gestation, benign hydatidiform mole
Adults: Insert 20-mg suppository high into posterior vaginal fornix. Repeat q 3 to 5 hours until abortion is complete. Don't exceed 240 mg.
Ripening of an unfavorable cervix in pregnant patients at or near term (gel or insert)
Adults: Insert one applicator (0.5 mg) of gel into vagina. May repeat dose in 6 hours if no response. Maximum recommended dose in 24 hours is 1.5 mg. Or one 10-mg insert into posterior vaginal fornix. Have patient remain supine for 2 hours. Remove insert upon onset of active labor or 12 hours after insertion.

Pharmacodynamics
Oxytocic action: Exact mechanism unknown. Stimulates myometrial contractions in the gravid uterus similar to the contractions of term labor. Its action may result from one or more of the following: direct stimulation, regulation of cellular calcium transport, or regulation of intracellular levels of cyclic 3,5-adenosine monophosphate. Reductions in plasma estrogen and progesterone levels play a role in drug's uterine action, but this effect doesn't occur consistently. Drug facilitates cervical dilations by directly softening the cervix.

Pharmacokinetics
• *Absorption:* Following vaginal insertion, is diffused slowly into maternal blood. Some local absorption into uterus through cervix or local vascular and lymphatic channels, but accounts for only small portion of dose. Contractions appear within 10 minutes of dosing, with peak effect in

17 hours. No correlation of activity with plasma levels.
- *Distribution:* Distributed widely in mother.
- *Metabolism:* Metabolized in lungs, liver, kidneys, spleen, and other maternal tissues. At least nine inactive metabolites.
- *Excretion:* Drug and metabolites excreted primarily in urine, with small amounts in feces.

Contraindications and precautions

Gel form is contraindicated when prolonged contractions of the uterus are considered inappropriate and in patients with hypersensitivity to prostaglandins or constituents of the gel. Also contraindicated in patients with placenta previa or unexplained vaginal bleeding during this pregnancy and in whom vaginal delivery isn't indicated (because of vasa previa or active herpes genitalia).

Suppository form is contraindicated in patients with hypersensitivity to the drug and in those with acute pelvic inflammatory disease or active cardiac, pulmonary, renal, or hepatic disease.

Vaginal insert is contraindicated in patients with hypersensitivity to prostaglandins or when there is suspicion or definite evidence of marked cephalopelvic disproportion or fetal distress where delivery isn't imminent. The insert is also contraindicated in patients with unexplained vaginal bleeding during pregnancy, multiparity with six or more previous term pregnancies, and when oxytocics are contraindicated or the patient is already receiving I.V. oxytocic drugs.

Use suppository form cautiously in patients with asthma, seizure disorders, anemia, diabetes, hypertension or hypotension, jaundice, scarred uterus, cervicitis, acute vaginitis, and CV, renal, or hepatic disease. Use gel form cautiously in patients with asthma or history of asthma, glaucoma or raised intraocular pressure, or renal or hepatic dysfunction and in those with ruptured membranes. Insert should be used cautiously in patients with nonvertex presentation and in those with ruptured membranes or history of previous uterine hypertonia, glaucoma, or childhood asthma.

Interactions

Drug-drug. *Oxytocics (oxytocin):* Enhances effects of oxytocin and other oxytocics. Cervical laceration and trauma have been reported when oxytocin is used concurrently. When using gel for cervical ripening, concomitant use isn't recommended. Dosing interval of 6 to 12 hours should be allowed before starting oxytocin treatment.
Drug-lifestyle. *Alcohol:* Inhibits effectiveness of drug with high doses. Discourage use.

Adverse reactions

CNS: *headache, dizziness,* anxiety, hot flashes, paresthesia, weakness, syncope.
CV: chest pain, ***arrhythmias.***
EENT: blurred vision, eye pain.

GI: *nausea, vomiting, diarrhea.*
GU: vaginal pain, vaginitis, endometritis, breast tenderness.
Musculoskeletal: *nocturnal leg cramps,* backache, muscle cramps.
Respiratory: coughing, dyspnea.
Skin: diaphoresis, rash.
Other: *fever, shivering, chills.*

☑ Special considerations

- Store suppositories in freezer at –4° F (–20°C); warm to room temperature (in foil) just before use.
- To prevent absorption through skin, use gloves and keep drug handling to a minimum.
- Premedicate patient with an antiemetic and antidiarrheal to minimize GI effects.
- Abortion should be complete within 30 hours.
- Drug-induced fever is self-limiting and transient. Sponge baths or increased fluid intake usually corrects problem.
- Signs and symptoms of overdose are extensions of adverse reactions. Because drug is rapidly metabolized, stop drug and provide supportive treatment.

Monitoring the patient

- Confirmation of fetal death is imperative before administration when used for missed abortion or intrauterine fetal death.
- Monitor patient adverse effects.

Information for the patient

- Advise patient of expected adverse reactions, especially fever, nausea, vomiting (occurs in two-thirds of all patients), or diarrhea (occurs in about half of all patients), all of which are self-limiting.
- Instruct patient to remain in prone position for 10 minutes after insertion of drug.

diphenhydramine hydrochloride

Benadryl, Benadryl Allergy, Benylin, Compoz, Diphen AF, Diphen Cough, Diphenadryl, Hydramine, Nervine Nighttime Sleep-Aid, Nytol, Sleep-Eze 3, Sominex, Tusstat, Twilite

Pharmacologic classification: ethanolamine-derivative antihistamine
Therapeutic classification: antihistamine (H_1-receptor antagonist), antiemetic, antivertigo drug, antitussive, sedative-hypnotic, topical anesthetic, antidyskinetic (anticholinergic)
Pregnancy risk category B

How supplied

Available with or without a prescription
Tablets: 25 mg, 50 mg
Capsules: 25 mg, 50 mg

Capsules (chewable): 12.5 mg
Elixir: 12.5 mg/5 ml (14% alcohol)
Syrup: 12.5 mg/5 ml (5% alcohol)
Injection: 50 mg/ml
Cream: 1%, 2%
Gel: 1%, 2%
Spray: 1%, 2%

Indications, route, and dosage
Rhinitis, allergy symptoms, motion sickness, Parkinson's disease
Adults and children ages 12 and older: 25 to 50 mg P.O. t.i.d. or q.i.d.; or 10 to 50 mg I.V. or deep I.M. Maximum I.M. or I.V. dose is 400 mg daily.
Children under age 12: 5 mg/kg daily P.O., deep I.M., or I.V. in divided doses q.i.d. Maximum dose is 300 mg daily.
Nonproductive cough
Adults and children ages 12 and older: 25 mg P.O. q 4 to 6 hours. Maximum dose is 150 mg daily.
Children ages 6 to 12: 12.5 mg P.O. q 4 to 6 hours. Maximum dose is 75 mg daily.
Children ages 2 to 6: 6.25 mg P.O. q 4 to 6 hours. Maximum dose is 25 mg daily.
Insomnia
Adults: 50 mg P.O. h.s.
Sedation
Adults: 25 to 50 mg P.O., or deep I.M., p.r.n.

Pharmacodynamics
Antihistamine action: Antihistamines compete for H$_1$-receptor sites on the smooth muscle of the bronchi, GI tract, uterus, and large blood vessels; by binding to cellular receptors, they prevent access of histamine and suppress histamine-induced allergic symptoms, even though they don't prevent its release.
Antivertigo, antiemetic, and antidyskinetic actions: Central antimuscarinic actions of antihistamines probably are responsible for these effects.
Antitussive action: Suppresses the cough reflex by a direct effect on the cough center.
Sedative action: Mechanism unknown.
Anesthetic action: Structurally related to local anesthetics, which prevent initiation and transmission of nerve impulses; this is the probable source of its topical and local anesthetic effects.

Pharmacokinetics
- *Absorption:* Well absorbed from GI tract. Action begins within 15 to 30 minutes; peaks in 1 to 4 hours.
- *Distribution:* Distributed widely throughout body, including CNS; crosses placenta; excreted in breast milk. About 82% protein-bound.
- *Metabolism:* About 50% to 60% of oral dose metabolized by liver before reaching systemic circulation (first-pass effect); virtually all available drug is metabolized by liver within 24 to 48 hours.

- *Excretion:* Plasma elimination half-life of drug is about 2½ to 9 hours; drug and metabolites excreted primarily in urine.

Contraindications and precautions
Contraindicated in patients with hypersensitivity to drug, during acute asthmatic attacks, and in newborns, premature neonates, and breast-feeding women.
    Use with extreme caution in patients with angle-closure glaucoma, prostatic hyperplasia, pyloroduodenal and bladder neck obstruction, asthma or COPD, increased intraocular pressure, hyperthyroidism, CV disease, hypertension, and stenosing peptic ulcer.

Interactions
Drug-drug. *CNS depressants (anxiolytics, barbiturates, sleeping aids, tranquilizers):* Additive CNS depression may occur. Avoid concomitant use.
Epinephrine: Enhanced effects. Monitor patient closely.
Heparin: Partially counteracts anticoagulant effects. Monitor partial thromboplastin time.
MAO inhibitors: Interference with detoxification of drug, prolonging their central depressant and anticholinergic effects. Avoid concomitant use or use cautiously if necessary. Monitor patient closely.
Sulfonylureas: Diminished effects. Monitor serum glucose levels.
Drug-lifestyle. *Alcohol:* May cause additive CNS depression. Discourage use.
Sun exposure: May cause photosensitivity reactions. Tell patient to take precautions.

Adverse reactions
CNS: *drowsiness,* confusion, insomnia, headache, vertigo, *sedation, sleepiness, dizziness, incoordination,* fatigue, restlessness, tremor, nervousness, *seizures.*
CV: palpitations, hypotension, tachycardia.
EENT: diplopia, blurred vision, tinnitus.
GI: *nausea,* vomiting, diarrhea, *dry mouth,* constipation, *epigastric distress,* anorexia.
GU: dysuria, urine retention, urinary frequency.
Hematologic: hemolytic anemia, *thrombocytopenia, agranulocytosis.*
Respiratory: nasal congestion, *thickening of bronchial secretions.*
Skin: urticaria, photosensitivity, rash.
Other: *anaphylactic shock.*

☑ Special considerations
Besides the recommendations relevant to all antihistamines, consider the following.
- Diphenhydramine injection is compatible with most I.V. solutions but is incompatible with some drugs; check compatibility before mixing in same I.V. line.

• Alternate injection sites to prevent irritation. Administer deep I.M. into large muscle.
• Drowsiness is most common adverse effect during initial therapy but usually disappears with continued use.
• Injectable and elixir solutions are light-sensitive; protect from light.
• Stop drug 4 days before diagnostic skin tests; antihistamines can prevent, reduce, or mask positive skin test response.
• Drowsiness is usual symptom of overdose. Seizures, coma, and respiratory depression may occur with profound overdose. Anticholinergic symptoms, such as dry mouth, flushed skin, fixed and dilated pupils, and GI symptoms, are common, especially in children.
• Treat overdose by inducing emesis with ipecac syrup (in conscious patient), then activated charcoal to reduce further drug absorption. Use gastric lavage if patient is unconscious or ipecac fails. Treat hypotension with vasopressors, and control seizures with diazepam or phenytoin. Don't give stimulants.

Monitoring the patient
• Monitor serum coagulation studies if patient takes heparin.
• Monitor serum glucose level if patient takes sulfonylureas.
• Monitor CBC.

Information for the patient
• Advise patient that drowsiness is very common initially, but may be reduced with continued therapy.
• Warn patient to avoid alcohol during therapy.
• Advise patient undergoing skin testing for allergies to notify health care personnel of current drug therapy.

Geriatric patients
• Elderly patients are usually more sensitive to adverse effects of antihistamines than younger patients and are especially likely to experience a greater degree of dizziness, sedation, hyperexcitability, dry mouth, and urine retention. Symptoms usually respond to a decrease in dosage.

Pediatric patients
• Drug shouldn't be used in premature infants or neonates. Infants and children, especially those under age 6, may experience paradoxical hyperexcitability.

Breast-feeding patients
• Avoid use of antihistamines during breast-feeding. Many of these drugs appear in breast milk, exposing infant to risks of unusual excitability; premature infants are at particular risk for seizures.

diphenoxylate hydrochloride and atropine sulfate
Logen, Lomanate, Lomotil, Lonox

Pharmacologic classification: opiate
Therapeutic classification: antidiarrheal
Controlled substance schedule V
Pregnancy risk category C

How supplied
Available by prescription only
Tablets: 2.5 mg diphenoxylate hydrochloride and 0.025 mg atropine sulfate per tablet
Liquid: 2.5 mg diphenoxylate hydrochloride and 0.025 mg atropine sulfate/5 ml

Indications, route, and dosage
Acute, nonspecific diarrhea
Adults: 5 mg diphenoxylate component P.O. q.i.d., then adjust, p.r.n.
Children ages 2 and over: 0.3 to 0.4 mg/kg/day diphenoxylate component in divided doses; or administer according to diphenoxylate component, as follows:
Children ages 9 to 12: 3.5 to 5 ml.
Children ages 6 to 8: 2.5 to 5 ml.
Children age 5: 2.5 to 4.5 ml.
Children age 4: 2 to 4 ml.
Children age 3: 2 to 3 ml.
Children age 2: 1.5 to 3 ml.

Pharmacodynamics
Antidiarrheal action: A meperidine analogue that inhibits GI motility locally and centrally. In high doses, may produce an opiate effect. Atropine is added in subtherapeutic doses to prevent abuse by deliberate overdose.

Pharmacokinetics
• *Absorption:* About 90% of oral dose absorbed. Action begins in 45 to 60 minutes.
• *Distribution:* Distributed in breast milk.
• *Metabolism:* Metabolized extensively by liver.
• *Excretion:* Metabolites excreted mainly in feces via biliary tract, with lesser amounts excreted in urine. Duration of effect is 3 to 4 hours.

Contraindications and precautions
Contraindicated in patients with hypersensitivity to diphenoxylate or atropine and in those with acute diarrhea resulting from poison until toxic material is eliminated from GI tract, acute diarrhea caused by organisms that penetrate intestinal mucosa, or diarrhea resulting from antibiotic-induced pseudomembranous enterocolitis or enterotoxin-producing bacteria. Also contraindicated in patients with obstructive jaundice and in children under age 2.
    Use cautiously in children ages 2 and older, in patients with hepatic disease, narcotic dependence, or acute ulcerative colitis; and '

nant women. Stop drug immediately if abdominal distention or other signs of toxic megacolon develop.

Interactions
Drug-drug. *CNS depressants (such as barbiturates, CNS depressants, narcotics, tranquilizers):* May result in increased depressant effect. Avoid concomitant use.
MAO inhibitors: Hypertensive crisis may be precipitated. Avoid concomitant use.
Drug-lifestyle. *Alcohol:* May enhance CNS depression. Discourage use.

Adverse reactions
CNS: *sedation, dizziness,* headache, drowsiness, lethargy, restlessness, depression, euphoria, malaise, confusion, numbness in extremities.
CV: tachycardia.
EENT: mydriasis.
GI: *dry mouth,* nausea, vomiting, abdominal discomfort or distention, *paralytic ileus,* anorexia, fluid retention in bowel or megacolon (may mask depletion of extracellular fluid and electrolytes, especially in young children treated for acute gastroenteritis), increased serum amylase, *pancreatitis,* swollen gums.
GU: urine retention.
Respiratory: *respiratory depression.*
Skin: pruritus, rash, dry skin.
Other: *angioedema, anaphylaxis,* possible physical dependence with long-term use.

☑ Special considerations
• Drug is usually ineffective in treating antibiotic-induced diarrhea.
• Reduce dosage as soon as symptoms are controlled.
• Drug may decrease urinary excretion of phenolsulfonphthalein (PSP) during PSP excretion test.
• Effects of overdose include drowsiness, low blood pressure, marked seizures, apnea, blurred vision, miosis, flushing, dry mouth and mucous membranes, and psychotic episodes. Treatment is supportive; maintain airway and support vital functions. A narcotic antagonist, such as naloxone, may be given. Gastric lavage may be performed.
• After overdose, monitor patient for 48 to 72 hours.

Monitoring the patient
• Monitor vital signs and intake and output; observe patient for adverse reactions, especially CNS reactions.
• Monitor bowel function.
• Monitor respiratory status of elderly patients.

Information for the patient
• Warn patient to take drug exactly as ordered and not to exceed recommended dose.

• Advise patient to maintain adequate fluid intake during course of diarrhea; inform about diet and fluid replacement.
• Caution patient to avoid driving during drug therapy because drowsiness and dizziness may occur; warn patient to avoid alcohol while taking drug because additive depressant effect may occur.
• Advise patient to call if drug isn't effective within 48 hours.
• Warn patient that prolonged use may result in tolerance; larger-than-recommended doses may result in drug dependence.

Geriatric patients
• Elderly patients may be more susceptible to respiratory depression and to exacerbation of preexisting glaucoma.

Pediatric patients
• Drug is contraindicated in children under age 2; some children may experience respiratory depression. Children, especially those with Down syndrome, appear to be particularly sensitive to atropine content of drug.

Breast-feeding patients
• Drug appears in breast milk; drug effects have been reported in breast-fed infants of patients taking drug.

diphtheria and tetanus toxoids, adsorbed (Td, DT)

Pharmacologic classification: toxoid
Therapeutic classification: diphtheria and tetanus prophylaxis
Pregnancy risk category C

How supplied
Available by prescription only
Available in pediatric (DT) and adult (Td) strengths
Injection: pediatric—6.6 to 15 Lf (limit flocculation) units of inactivated diphtheria and 5 to 10 Lf units of inactivated tetanus per 0.5 ml, in 5-ml vials; adult—2 Lf units of inactivated diphtheria and 2 to 10 Lf units of inactivated tetanus per 0.5 ml, in 5-ml vials

Indications, route, and dosage
Primary immunization
Adults and children ages 7 and older: Use adult strength. Give 0.5 ml I.M. 4 to 8 weeks apart for two doses and a third dose 6 to 12 months later. Booster dose is 0.5 ml I.M. q 10 years.
Children ages 1 to 7: Use pediatric strength. Give two 0.5-ml doses I.M. 4 to 8 weeks apart. Give a third dose 6 to 12 months after second injection. If final immunizing dose is given after 7th birthday, use adult strength.

Infants ages 6 weeks to 1 year: Use pediatric strength. Give three 0.5-ml doses I.M. 4 to 8 weeks apart. Give a fourth dose 6 to 12 months after third injection.

Pharmacodynamics
Diphtheria and tetanus prophylaxis: Promote active immunization to diphtheria and tetanus by inducing production of antitoxins.

Pharmacokinetics
No information available.

Contraindications and precautions
Contraindicated in immunosuppressed patients and in those receiving radiation or corticosteroid therapy. Vaccination should be deferred in patients with respiratory illness and during polio outbreaks; also defer in those with acute illness except during emergency. When polio is a risk, a single antigen is used. In children under age 6, use only when diphtheria, tetanus, and pertussis combination is contraindicated because of pertussis component. DT shouldn't be used in children age 7 or older because of an increased risk of adverse reactions. Also contraindicated in patients with history of adverse reactions to components of drug.

Interactions
Drug-drug. *Corticosteroids, immunosuppressants:* May impair immune response to diphtheria and tetanus toxoids. Avoid elective immunization if patient is taking these drugs.

Adverse reactions
CNS: malaise, headache.
CV: flushing, tachycardia, hypotension, *shock.*
Skin: *pain, stinging, edema, erythema, induration at injection site,* urticaria, pruritus.
Other: chills, fever, **anaphylaxis.**

☑ Special considerations
• Obtain thorough history of allergies and reactions to immunizations.
• Epinephrine solution 1:1,000 should be available to treat allergic reactions.
• Diphtheria and tetanus toxoids are used primarily when pertussis vaccine is contraindicated or used separately.
• These toxoids aren't used to treat active tetanus or diphtheria infections.
• Teratogenicity hasn't been reported. Immunization during pregnancy is recommended when needed.
• To prevent sciatic nerve damage, avoid administration in gluteal muscle. During primary immunization, don't inject same site more than once.

Monitoring the patient
• Monitor patient's response to treatment.
• Monitor patient for adverse effects.

Information for the patient
• Inform patient that he may experience discomfort at injection site and that a nodule may develop at site and persist for several weeks after immunization. Patient also may develop fever, headache, upset stomach, general malaise, or body aches and pains. Tell patient to take acetaminophen for relief.
• Tell patient to report adverse reactions.
• Stress importance of keeping all scheduled appointments for subsequent doses because full immunization requires a series of injections.

diphtheria and tetanus toxoids and pertussis vaccine, adsorbed (DTP)
Acel-Imune, diphtheria and tetanus toxoids and acellular pertussis vaccine adsorbed (DTaP), Certiva, DTwP, Infantrix, Tri-Immunol, Tripedia

Pharmacologic classification: combination toxoid and vaccine
Therapeutic classification: diphtheria, tetanus, and pertussis prophylaxis
Pregnancy risk category C

How supplied
Available by prescription only
Whole-cell vaccine
Injection: 6.5 Lf (limit flocculation) units inactivated diphtheria, 5 Lf units inactivated tetanus, and 4 protective units pertussis per 0.5 ml, in 2.5-, 5-, and 7.5-ml vials; 10 Lf units inactivated diphtheria, 5.5 Lf units inactivated tetanus, and 4 protective units pertussis per 0.5 ml in 5-ml vials (DTwP); 12.5 Lf units inactivated diphtheria, 5 Lf units inactivated tetanus, and 4 protective units pertussis per 0.5 ml, in 7.5-ml vials (Tri-Immunol)
Acellular vaccine
Injection: 5 Lf units inactivated diphtheria, 5 Lf units inactivated tetanus, and 300 hemagglutinin units of acellular pertussis vaccine per 0.5 ml; 66.7 Lf units inactivated diphtheria, 5 Lf units inactivated tetanus, and 46.8 pertussis antigens per 0.5 ml

Indications, route, and dosage
Primary immunization
Children ages 6 weeks to 7 years: Give 0.5 ml I.M. 4 to 8 weeks apart for three doses and a fourth dose 6 to 12 months after the third dose.
Booster immunization
Booster dosage is 0.5 ml I.M. when starting school at age 4 to 6 unless fourth dose in series was administered after child's fourth birthday; then a booster isn't necessary at time of school entrance. Not advised for adults or for children age 7 or older.
 Note: The acellular vaccine may be used for the fourth or fifth dose in children

months (Tripedia) or 17 months (Acel-Imune) to 7 years who have been immunized with three or four doses of the whole-cell vaccine.

Pharmacodynamics
Diphtheria, tetanus, and pertussis (whooping cough) prophylaxis: Vaccine promotes active immunity to diphtheria, tetanus, and pertussis by inducing production of antitoxin and antibodies.

Pharmacokinetics
No information available.

Contraindications and precautions
Contraindicated in immunosuppressed patients and in those on corticosteroid therapy or with history of seizures. Vaccination should be deferred in patients with acute febrile illness. Children with preexisting neurologic disorders shouldn't receive pertussis component. Also, children who exhibit neurologic signs after injection shouldn't receive pertussis component in any succeeding injections. Diphtheria and tetanus toxoids (called DT) should be given instead.

Interactions
Drug-drug. *Corticosteroids, immunosuppressants:* May impair immune response to toxoids and vaccine. Avoid elective immunization while patient is taking these drugs.

Adverse reactions
CNS: *encephalopathy, seizures,* peripheral neuropathy.
Hematologic: thrombocytopenic purpura.
Skin: soreness, redness, expected nodule remaining several weeks at injection site, urticaria.
Other: fever, *hypersensitivity reactions, anaphylaxis, shock.*

☑ Special considerations
• Obtain history of allergies and reactions to immunizations, especially to pertussis vaccine.
• Epinephrine solution 1:1,000 should be available to treat allergic reactions.
• Vaccine may be given at same time as trivalent oral polio vaccine and, if indicated, when patient receives vaccines against *Haemophilus influenzae* type b, measles, mumps, and rubella.
• Don't use to treat active tetanus, diphtheria, or pertussis infections.

Monitoring the patient
• Monitor patient's response to treatment.
• Monitor patient for adverse effects.

Information for the patient
• Explain to parents that child may experience discomfort at injection site and that a nodule may develop at site and persist for several weeks. Fever, upset stomach, or general malaise may also develop. Recommend acetaminophen liquid to relieve discomfort.
• Tell parents to report worrisome or intolerable reactions promptly.
• Stress importance of keeping scheduled appointments for subsequent doses. Full immunization requires a series of injections.

dipivefrin hydrochloride
Propine

Pharmacologic classification: sympathomimetic
Therapeutic classification: antiglaucoma drug
Pregnancy risk category B

How supplied
Available by prescription only
Ophthalmic solution: 0.1%

Indications, route, and dosage
To reduce intraocular pressure in chronic open-angle glaucoma
Adults: For initial glaucoma therapy, 1 drop in eye q 12 hours; then adjust dose based on patient response as determined by tonometric readings.

Pharmacodynamics
Antiglaucoma action: A prodrug converted to epinephrine in the eye. Decreases aqueous humor production and enhances outflow. Often used with a miotic drug.

Pharmacokinetics
• *Absorption:* Action begins in about 30 minutes, with peak effect in 1 hour.
• *Distribution:* No information available.
• *Metabolism:* No information available.
• *Excretion:* No information available.

Contraindications and precautions
Contraindicated in patients with angle-closure glaucoma or hypersensitivity to drug. Use cautiously in patients with asthma, hypersensitivity to epinephrine, or aphakia or CV disease.

Interactions
Drug-drug. *Anesthetics, digoxin, tricyclic antidepressants:* Possible additive toxic effects and increased risk of cardiac arrhythmias. Monitor patient closely.
Carbonic anhydrase inhibitors, ophthalmic beta blockers, osmotic drugs: Concomitant use may enhance lowering of intraocular pressure. Monitor patient for drug effect.
Sympathomimetics: Additive effects if significant systemic absorption occurs. Monitor patient.

Adverse reactions
CV: tachycardia, hypertension, *arrhythmias.*

EENT: eye burning or stinging, conjunctival injection, conjunctivitis, mydriasis, allergic reaction, photophobia.

☑ Special considerations

● Drug may cause fewer adverse reactions than with conventional epinephrine therapy; it's often used with other antiglaucoma drugs.
● Store away from heat and light.
● Overdose is quite rare with ophthalmic use but may cause hypertension with tachycardia or bradycardia, arrhythmias, precordial pain, anxiety, nervousness, insomnia, muscle tremor, cerebral hemorrhage, seizures, altered mental status, anorexia, nausea and vomiting, and acute renal failure.
● To treat oral overdose, dilute immediately and initiate emesis; then use activated charcoal and a cathartic unless patient is comatose or obtunded.

Monitoring the patient

● Monitor patient's response to treatment.
● Monitor ECG if patient reports chest pain, dizziness, or palpitations.
● Monitor urine output. Treat seizures with I.V. diazepam, and hypertension with nitroprusside; treat arrhythmias.
● Preparations containing sulfites may cause GI or cardiac toxicities and hypotension.

Information for the patient

● Teach patient correct way to instill drops and warn patient not to touch eye with dropper.
● Teach patient that if also using other eye drops, dipivefrin should be instilled first, then wait at least 5 minutes before using other drops.
● Instruct patient not to blink more than usual and not to close eyes tightly after instillation.
● Tell patient instillation may cause transient burning or stinging.

Geriatric patients

● Drug should be used with caution in elderly patients to avoid precipitating narrow-angle glaucoma.

---

dipyridamole
Persantine

Pharmacologic classification: pyrimidine analogue
Therapeutic classification: coronary vasodilator, platelet aggregation inhibitor
Pregnancy risk category B

How supplied

Available by prescription only
Tablets: 25 mg, 50 mg, 75 mg
Injection: 10 mg/ampule

Indications, route, and dosage

Alternative to exercise in thallium myocardial perfusion imaging
Adults: 0.142 mg/kg/minute infused over 4 minutes (0.57 mg/kg total).
Inhibition of platelet adhesion in patients with prosthetic heart valves, with warfarin or aspirin
Adults: 75 to 100 mg P.O. q.i.d.
◇ *Chronic angina pectoris*
Adults: 50 mg P.O. t.i.d. at least 1 hour before meals; 2 to 3 months of therapy may be required to achieve a response.
◇ *Prevention of thromboembolic complications in patients with various thromboembolic disorders other than prosthetic heart valves*
Adults: 150 to 400 mg P.O. daily (with warfarin or aspirin).

Pharmacodynamics

Coronary vasodilating action: Increases coronary blood flow by selectively dilating the coronary arteries. Coronary vasodilator effect follows inhibition of serum adenosine deaminase, which allows accumulation of adenosine, a potent vasodilator. Drug inhibits platelet adhesion by increasing effects of prostacyclin or by inhibiting phosphodiesterase.

Pharmacokinetics

● *Absorption:* Variable and slow; bioavailability ranges from 27% to 59%. Serum levels peak 45 minutes to 2½ hours after oral administration.
● *Distribution:* Widely distributed in body tissues; small amounts cross placenta. Protein-binding ranges from 91% to 97%.
● *Metabolism:* Metabolized by liver.
● *Excretion:* Elimination occurs via biliary excretion of glucuronide conjugates. Some dipyridamole and conjugates may undergo enterohepatic circulation and fecal excretion; small amount excreted in urine. Half-life varies from 1 to 12 hours.

Contraindications and precautions

No known contraindications. Use cautiously in patients with hypotension.

Interactions

Drug-drug. *Aminophylline:* Inhibited action of dipyridamole. Monitor patient for effects.
Heparin, oral anticoagulants: Enhanced effects. Monitor PT, INR closely.

Adverse reactions

CNS: *headache, dizziness.*
CV: flushing, fainting, *hypotension;* angina, chest pain, *blood pressure lability, hypertension* (with I.V. infusion).
GI: *nausea,* vomiting, diarrhea, abdominal distress.
Hematologic: increased bleeding time.

Skin: rash, irritation (with undiluted injection), pruritus.

☑ Special considerations
- Give drug at least 1 hour before meals.
- When used as a pharmacologic "stress test," total doses beyond 60 mg appear to be unnecessary.
- Dilute I.V. form to at least a 1:2 ratio with 0.45% saline injection, normal saline injection, or D_5W to a total volume of 20 to 50 ml. Inject thallium within 5 minutes of dipyridamole.
- Signs and symptoms of overdose include peripheral vasodilation and hypotension. Maintain blood pressure and treat symptomatically.

Monitoring the patient
- Monitor serum coagulation studies if patient takes oral anticoagulants.
- Watch for adverse reactions, including signs of bleeding and prolonged bleeding time, especially at high doses and during long-term therapy.
- Monitor blood pressure.

Information for the patient
- Explain that clinical response may require 2 to 3 months of continuous therapy; encourage patient compliance.
- Discuss adverse reactions and how to manage therapy.

Pediatric patients
- Dosage hasn't been established in children.

Breast-feeding patients
- Drug appears in breast milk; caution should be used when giving drug to breast-feeding women.

---

dirithromycin
Dynabac

Pharmacologic classification: macrolide
Therapeutic classification: antibiotic
Pregnancy risk category C

How supplied
Available by prescription only
Tablets: 250 mg

Indications, route, and dosage
Acute bacterial exacerbations of chronic bronchitis due to Moraxella catarrhalis or Streptococcus pneumoniae; secondary bacterial infection of acute bronchitis due to M. catarrhalis or S. pneumoniae; uncomplicated skin and skin-structure infections due to Staphylococcus aureus (methicillin-susceptible)
Adults and children ages 12 and older: 500 mg P.O. daily with food for 7 days.

Community-acquired pneumonia due to Legionella pneumophila, Mycoplasma pneumoniae, or S. pneumoniae
Adults and children ages 12 and older: 500 mg P.O. daily with food for 14 days.
Pharyngitis or tonsillitis due to Streptococcus pyogenes
Adults and children ages 12 and older: 500 mg P.O. daily with food for 10 days.

Pharmacodynamics
Antibiotic action: Inhibits bacterial RNA-dependent protein synthesis by binding to the 50S subunit of the ribosome. Its spectrum of activity includes gram-positive aerobes such as *S. aureus* (methicillin-susceptible strains only), *S. pneumoniae*, *S. pyogenes;* gram-negative aerobes such as *L. pneumophila* and *M. catarrhalis;* and other bacteria such as *M. pneumoniae.*

Pharmacokinetics
- *Absorption:* Rapidly absorbed from GI tract; converted by nonenzymatic hydrolysis to microbiologically active compound erythromycylamine. Food slightly increases bioavailability.
- *Distribution:* Widely distributed throughout body. Protein-binding ranges from 15% to 30%.
- *Metabolism:* Little to no hepatic metabolism.
- *Excretion:* Primarily eliminated in bile or feces with small amount in urine. Mean half-life is about 8 hours.

Contraindications and precautions
Contraindicated in patients with hypersensitivity to dirithromycin, erythromycin, or other macrolide antibiotics. Use cautiously in patients with hepatic insufficiency and in pregnant women.

Interactions
Drug-drug. *Alfentanil, anticoagulants, bromocriptine, carbamazepine, cyclosporine, digoxin, disopyramide, ergotamine, hexobarbital, lovastatin, phenytoin, triazolam, valproate:* May increase or decrease serum levels of these drugs. Not known if same interactions occur with dirithromycin. Use together cautiously.
Antacids, H_2 antagonists: Absorption slightly enhanced when dirithromycin is administered immediately after these drugs. Monitor patient for effects.
Theophylline: May alter steady-state plasma level of theophylline. Monitor theophylline plasma level. Dosage adjustments may be needed.
Drug-food. *Any food:* Increased absorption. Give drug with food.

Adverse reactions
CNS: headache, dizziness, vertigo, insomnia, asthenia.
GI: abdominal pain, nausea, diarrhea, vomiting, dyspepsia, GI disorder, flatulence.

Hematologic: increased platelet, eosinophil, and neutrophil counts.
Metabolic: hyperkalemia, decreased bicarbonate levels, increased CK levels.
Respiratory: increased cough, dyspnea.
Skin: rash, pruritus, urticaria.
Other: pain (nonspecific).

☑ Special considerations
● Don't use drug in patients with known, suspected, or potential bacteremias; serum levels are inadequate to provide antibacterial coverage of bloodstream.
● Give drug with food or within 1 hour of eating.
● Symptoms of a macrolide antibiotic overdose include nausea, vomiting, epigastric distress, and diarrhea. Treatment should be supportive; forced diuresis, dialysis, or hemoperfusion haven't been established as helpful for overdose.

Monitoring the patient
● Monitor hepatic function before drug start.
● Obtain culture and sensitivity tests before therapy begins; therapy may begin pending results.
● Monitor patient for superinfection. Drug may cause overgrowth of nonsusceptible bacteria or fungi.

Information for the patient
● Tell patient to take all of drug as prescribed, even after feeling better.
● Instruct patient to take drug with food or within 1 hour of having eaten. Tell patient not to cut, chew, or crush tablet.

Pediatric patients
● Safety and effectiveness in children under age 12 haven't been established.

Breast-feeding patients
● It's unknown if drug appears in breast milk; use cautiously in breast-feeding women.

disopyramide phosphate
Norpace, Norpace CR, Rythmodan*, Rythmodan-LA*

Pharmacologic classification: pyridine derivative antiarrhythmic, group IA antiarrhythmic
Therapeutic classification: ventricular antiarrhythmic, supraventricular antiarrhythmic, atrial antitachyarrhythmic
Pregnancy risk category C

How supplied
Available by prescription only
Capsules: 100 mg, 150 mg
Capsules (extended-release): 100 mg, 150 mg

Indications, route, and dosage
PVCs (unifocal, multifocal, or coupled); ventricular tachycardia; ◊ conversion of atrial fibrillation, atrial flutter, and paroxysmal atrial tachycardia to normal sinus rhythm
Adults: Initially, 200 to 300 mg loading dose. Usual maintenance dosage is 150 mg P.O. q 6 hours or 300 mg (extended-release) P.O. q 12 hours; for patients weighing below 50 kg (110 lb), give 100 mg P.O. q 6 hours or 200 mg (extended-release) P.O. q 12 hours; and for patients with cardiomyopathy or possible cardiac decompensation, give 100 mg P.O. q 6 to 8 hours initially and then adjust as indicated.
Children ages 12 to 18: 6 to 15 mg/kg/day.
Children ages 4 to 12: 10 to 15 mg/kg/day.
Children ages 1 to 4: 10 to 20 mg/kg/day.
Children under age 1: 10 to 30 mg/kg/day.
    All children's doses should be divided into equal amounts and given q 6 hours. Extended-release capsules aren't recommended for use in children.
✦ **Dosage adjustment.** Elderly patients may need dosage reduction. Adults with hepatic insufficiency or moderately impaired renal function should receive 100 mg P.O. q 6 hours or 200 mg (extended-release) q 12 hours. Patients with severely impaired renal function should receive only 100 mg (regular-release) at the following intervals.

Creatinine clearance (ml/minute)	Dosage interval
30 to 40	q 8 hr
15 to 30	q 12 hr
< 15	q 24 hr

Pharmacodynamics
Antiarrhythmic action: A class IA antiarrhythmic drug that depresses phase O of the action potential. Considered a myocardial depressant because it decreases myocardial excitability and conduction velocity and may depress myocardial contractility. Also possesses anticholinergic activity that may modify the drug's direct myocardial effects. In therapeutic doses, reduces conduction velocity in the atria, ventricles, and His-Purkinje system. By prolonging the effective refractory period (ERP), it helps control atrial tachyarrhythmias (however, this indication is unapproved in the United States). Its anticholinergic action, which is much greater than quinidine's, may increase AV node conductivity.
    Also has a greater myocardial depressant (negative inotropic) effect than quinidine. Helps manage premature ventricular beats by suppressing automaticity in the His-Purkinje system and ectopic pacemakers. At therapeutic doses usually doesn't prolong the QRS complex

ment duration and PR interval but may prolong the QT interval.

Pharmacokinetics

• *Absorption:* Rapidly and well absorbed from GI tract; about 60% to 80% reaches systemic circulation. Onset of action usually occurs in 30 minutes; blood levels peak about 2 hours after administration of conventional capsules, 5 hours after extended-release capsules.

• *Distribution:* Well distributed throughout extracellular fluid but isn't extensively tissue bound. Plasma protein-binding varies, depending on drug levels, but generally ranges from about 50% to 65%. Usual therapeutic serum level ranges from 2 to 4 mcg/ml, although some patients may need up to 7 mcg/ml. Levels above 9 mcg/ml considered toxic.

• *Metabolism:* Metabolized in liver to one major metabolite that possesses little antiarrhythmic activity but greater anticholinergic activity than parent compound.

• *Excretion:* About 30% of an orally administered dose excreted in urine as metabolites; 40% to 60% excreted as unchanged drug. Usual elimination half-life is about 7 hours but lengthens in patients with renal or hepatic insufficiency. Duration of effect is usually 6 to 7 hours.

Contraindications and precautions

Contraindicated in patients with hypersensitivity to drug and in those with cardiogenic shock or second- or third-degree heart block in the absence of an artificial pacemaker.

Use cautiously and avoid, if possible, in patients with heart failure. Use cautiously in patients with underlying conduction abnormalities, urinary tract diseases (especially prostatic hyperplasia), hepatic or renal impairment, myasthenia gravis, or acute angle-closure glaucoma.

Interactions

Drug-drug. *Antiarrhythmics:* May cause additive or antagonistic cardiac effects and additive toxicity. Monitor patient closely; avoid concomitant use.

Anticholinergics: May cause additive anticholinergic effects. Monitor patient closely.

Enzyme inducers such as rifampin: May impair disopyramide's antiarrhythmic activity. Monitor patient closely.

Erythromycin: May increase disopyramide levels, causing arrhythmias and increased QT intervals. Monitor patient closely.

Insulin, oral antidiabetics: May cause additive hypoglycemia. Monitor serum glucose levels.

Warfarin: May potentiate anticoagulant effects. Monitor INR.

Drug-herb. *Jimsonweed:* May adversely affect cardiovascular system function. Discourage concomitant use.

Adverse reactions

CNS: dizziness, agitation, depression, fatigue, muscle weakness, syncope.
CV: *hypotension, **heart failure, heart block**,* edema, ***arrhythmias,*** shortness of breath, chest pain.
EENT: *blurred vision, dry eyes or nose.*
GI: nausea, vomiting, anorexia, bloating, abdominal pain, diarrhea.
Hepatic: cholestatic jaundice.
Metabolic: weight gain.
Musculoskeletal: aches, pain, muscle weakness.
Skin: rash, pruritus, dermatosis.

☑ Special considerations

• Don't give sustained-release capsules for rapid control of ventricular arrhythmias if therapeutic blood drug levels must be attained rapidly or if patient has cardiomyopathy, possible cardiac decompensation, or severe renal impairment.

• If drug causes constipation, administer laxatives and ensure proper diet.

• Drug is commonly prescribed for patients who can't tolerate quinidine or procainamide.

• Pharmacist may prepare disopyramide suspension; 100-mg capsules are used with cherry syrup to prepare suspension (may be best form for young children).

• Drug is removed by hemodialysis. Dosage adjustments may be necessary in patients undergoing dialysis.

• Signs and symptoms of overdose include anticholinergic effects, severe hypotension, widening of QRS complex and QT interval, ventricular arrhythmias, cardiac conduction disturbances, bradycardia, heart failure, asystole, loss of consciousness, seizures, apnea episodes, and respiratory arrest.

• Treatment of overdose is generally supportive, including respiratory and CV support and hemodynamic and ECG monitoring. If ingestion was recent, gastric lavage, emesis induction, and activated charcoal may decrease absorption.

• Isoproterenol or dopamine may be administered to correct hypotension after ensuring adequate hydration.

• Digoxin and diuretics may be administered to treat heart failure. Hemodialysis and charcoal hemoperfusion may effectively remove disopyramide. Some patients may require intra-aortic balloon counterpulsation, mechanically assisted respiration, or endocardial pacing.

Monitoring the patient

• Correct underlying electrolyte abnormalities, especially hypokalemia, before giving drug because disopyramide may be ineffective in patients with these problems.

• Watch for signs of developing heart block, such as QRS complex widening by more than 25% or

QT interval lengthening by more than 25% above baseline.
• Patients with atrial flutter or fibrillation should be digitalized before drug administration to ensure that enhanced AV conduction doesn't lead to ventricular tachycardia.

Information for the patient
• When changing from immediate-release to sustained-release capsules, advise patient to begin taking sustained-release capsule 6 hours after last immediate-release capsule.
• Teach patient importance of taking drug on time, exactly as prescribed. To do this, patient may have to use an alarm clock for night doses.
• Advise patient to use sugarless gum or hard candy to relieve dry mouth.

Geriatric patients
• Monitor closely for signs of toxicity; also monitor serum electrolyte and drug levels.

Pediatric patients
• Although drug's safety and effectiveness in children haven't been established, current recommendations call for total daily dose given in equally divided doses every 6 hours or at intervals based on individual needs.
• Monitor pediatric patients during initial adjustment period; dosage adjustment should begin at lower end of recommended ranges. Monitor serum drug levels and therapeutic response carefully.

Breast-feeding patients
• Drug appears in breast milk; recommend an alternative to breast-feeding during therapy.

disulfiram
Antabuse

Pharmacologic classification: aldehyde dehydrogenase inhibitor
Therapeutic classification: alcoholic deterrent
Pregnancy risk category NR

How supplied
Available by prescription only
Tablets: 250 mg, 500 mg

Indications, route, and dosage
Adjunct in management of chronic alcoholism
Adults: Give maximum dose of 500 mg P.O. as a single dose in the morning for 1 to 2 weeks. Can be taken in evening if drowsiness occurs. Maintenance dose is 125 to 500 mg daily (average dose 250 mg) until permanent self-control is established. Treatment may continue for months or years.

Pharmacodynamics
Antialcoholic action: Irreversibly inhibits aldehyde dehydrogenase, which prevents the oxidation of alcohol after the acetaldehyde stage. Interacts with ingested alcohol to produce acetaldehyde levels five to ten times higher than are produced by normal alcohol metabolism. Excess acetaldehyde produces a highly unpleasant reaction (nausea and vomiting) to even a small quantity of alcohol. Tolerance to disulfiram doesn't occur; rather, sensitivity to alcohol increases with longer duration of therapy.

Pharmacokinetics
• *Absorption:* Absorbed completely after oral administration, but 3 to 12 hours may be required before effects occur. Toxic reactions to alcohol may occur up to 2 weeks after last dose.
• *Distribution:* Highly lipid-soluble; initially localized in adipose tissue.
• *Metabolism:* Mostly oxidized in liver and excreted in urine as free drug and metabolites (such as diethyldithiocarbamate, diethylamine, carbon disulfide).
• *Excretion:* 5% to 20% of drug unabsorbed and eliminated in feces. Small amount eliminated through lungs, but most excreted in urine. Several days may be required for total elimination.

Contraindications and precautions
Contraindicated in patients intoxicated by alcohol and within 12 hours of alcohol ingestion; in those with psychoses, myocardial disease, coronary occlusion, or hypersensitivity to disulfiram or other thiuram derivatives used in pesticides and rubber vulcanization; and in patients receiving metronidazole, paraldehyde, alcohol, or alcohol-containing preparations.
    Use with extreme caution in patients with diabetes mellitus, hypothyroidism, seizure disorder, cerebral damage, or nephritis or hepatic cirrhosis or insufficiency, and in those receiving phenytoin therapy. Drug shouldn't be administered during pregnancy.

Interactions
Drug-drug. *Alfentanil:* May prolong duration of effect. Use cautiously and monitor patient closely.
Bacampicillin: May precipitate disulfiram reaction. Avoid concomitant use.
Barbiturates, chlordiazepoxide, CNS depressants, coumarin anticoagulants, diazepam, midazolam, paraldehyde, phenytoin: Interference with metabolism of these drugs; possible increased blood levels of these drugs. Monitor patient closely.
Isoniazid: May produce ataxia, unsteady gait, or marked behavioral changes. Avoid concomitant use.
Metronidazole: May produce psychosis or confusion. Avoid concomitant use.

Tricyclic antidepressants (especially amitriptyline): May cause transient delirium. Monitor patient closely.

Drug-herb. *Passion flower, pill-bearing spurge, pokeweed, squaw vine, squill, sundew, sweet flag, tormentil, valerian, yarrow:* May cause disulfiram reaction if herbal form contains alcohol. Discourage concomitant use.

Drug-food. *Caffeine:* Metabolism of caffeine inhibited, greatly increasing its half-life; exaggerated or prolonged effects of caffeine may occur. Discourage concomitant use.

Drug-lifestyle. *Alcohol (all sources, such as cough syrups, liniments, shaving lotions, backrub preparations):* May precipitate disulfiram reaction. Discourage concomitant use.
Marijuana: Synergistic CNS stimulation when used with marijuana. Discourage concomitant use.

Adverse reactions
CNS: drowsiness, headache, fatigue, delirium, depression, neuritis, peripheral neuritis, polyneuritis, restlessness, psychotic reactions.
EENT: optic neuritis.
GI: metallic or garlic aftertaste.
GU: impotence.
Metabolic: elevated serum cholesterol.
Skin: acneiform or allergic dermatitis, occasional eruptions.
Other: disulfiram reaction (precipitated by ethanol use), which may include flushing, throbbing headache, dyspnea, nausea, copious vomiting, diaphoresis, thirst, chest pain, palpitations, hyperventilation, hypotension, syncope, anxiety, weakness, blurred vision, confusion, arthropathy.

In severe reactions: *respiratory depression, CV collapse, arrhythmias, MI, acute heart failure, seizures, unconsciousness, death.*

☑ Special considerations
● Drug use requires close medical supervision. Patients should clearly understand consequences of therapy and give informed consent before use.
● Use drug only in patients who are cooperative and well motivated and who are receiving supportive psychiatric therapy.
● Alcohol reaction may occur as long as 2 weeks after single disulfiram dose; the longer patient remains on drug, the more sensitive he becomes to alcohol.
● Don't administer for at least 12 hours after alcohol ingestion.
● May decrease urinary vanillylmandelic acid excretion and increase urinary levels of homovanillic acid. Decrease of uptake or protein-bound iodine levels may occur rarely.
● Overdose symptoms include GI upset and vomiting, abnormal EEG findings, drowsiness, altered consciousness, hallucinations, speech impairment, incoordination, and coma. Treat overdose

by gastric aspiration or lavage along with supportive therapy.
● Treatment of alcohol-induced disulfiram reaction is supportive and symptomatic. Reactions aren't usually life-threatening. Emergency equipment and drugs should be available because arrhythmias and severe hypotension may occur.
● Treat severe reactions such as shock by administering plasma or electrolyte solutions, as needed. Large I.V. doses of ascorbic acid, iron, and antihistamines have been used but are of questionable value.
● Hypokalemia has been reported and requires careful monitoring and potassium supplements.

Monitoring the patient
● A complete physical examination and laboratory studies (CBC, electrolytes, transaminases) should be done before therapy; repeat regularly.
● Ascertain that patient hasn't ingested alcohol for 12 hours before treatment.

Information for the patient
● Explain that, although disulfiram can help discourage use of alcohol, it isn't a cure for alcoholism.
● Inform patient of seriousness of disulfiram-alcohol reaction and the consequences of alcohol use.
● Warn patient to avoid all sources of alcohol, including sauces or soups made with sherry or other wines or alcohol (even cooking alcohol), some herbal preparations, and cough syrups. External applications of aftershave lotion, liniments, or other topical preparations may cause disulfiram reaction (because of products' alcohol content).
● Tell patient that alcohol reaction may occur for up to 2 weeks after a single dose of disulfiram. The longer the disulfiram therapy, the more sensitive patient will be to alcohol.
● Warn patient that drug may cause drowsiness.
● Instruct patient to carry identification card stating that he is using disulfiram. Card should include phone number of physician or clinic to contact if reaction occurs.

dobutamine hydrochloride
Dobutrex

Pharmacologic classification: adrenergic, beta$_1$ agonist
Therapeutic classification: inotropic drug
Pregnancy risk category B

How supplied
Available by prescription only
Injection: 12.5 mg/ml in 20-ml vials (parenteral)

Indications, route, and dosage
To increase cardiac output in short-term treatment of cardiac decompensation caused by depressed contractility
Adults: 2.5 to 15 mcg/kg/minute as an I.V. infusion. Rarely, infusion rates up to 40 mcg/kg/minute may be needed. Titrate dosage carefully to patient response.
✦ *Dosage adjustment.* Elderly patients require lower doses because they may be more sensitive to the drug's effects.

Pharmacodynamics
Inotropic action: Selectively stimulates beta$_1$-adrenergic receptors to increase myocardial contractility and stroke volume, resulting in increased cardiac output (a positive inotropic effect in patients with normal hearts or in heart failure). At therapeutic doses, drug decreases peripheral resistance (afterload), reduces ventricular filling pressure (preload), and may facilitate AV node conduction. Systolic blood pressure and pulse pressure may remain unchanged or increased from increased cardiac output. Increased myocardial contractility results in increased coronary blood flow and myocardial oxygen consumption. Heart rate usually remains unchanged; however, excessive doses do have chronotropic effects. Drug doesn't appear to affect dopaminergic receptors, nor does it cause renal or mesenteric vasodilation; however, urine flow may increase because of increased cardiac output.

Pharmacokinetics
- *Absorption:* After I.V. administration, onset of action occurs within 2 minutes; levels peak within 10 minutes. Effects persist a few minutes after I.V. stops.
- *Distribution:* Widely distributed throughout body.
- *Metabolism:* Metabolized by liver and by conjugation to inactive metabolites.
- *Excretion:* Excreted mainly in urine (with minor amounts in feces) as its metabolites and conjugates.

Contraindications and precautions
Contraindicated in patients with hypersensitivity to drug or its components and in those with idiopathic hypertrophic subaortic stenosis. Use cautiously in patients with a history of hypertension or after recent MI. Drug may precipitate an exaggerated pressor response.

Interactions
Drug-drug. *Beta blockers:* May antagonize cardiac effects of dobutamine, resulting in increased peripheral resistance and predominance of alpha-adrenergic effects. Monitor patient closely.
Bretylium: May potentiate actions of vasopressors on adrenergic receptors, resulting in arrhythmias. Monitor patient closely.

Guanadrel, guanethidine: May decrease hypotensive effects of these drugs; however, these drugs may potentiate pressor effects of dobutamine, possibly resulting in hypertension and cardiac arrhythmias. Monitor patient closely.
Inhalation hydrocarbon anesthetics (especially cyclopropane, halothane): May trigger ventricular arrhythmias. Use cautiously and monitor patient closely.
Nitroprusside: May cause higher cardiac output and lower pulmonary artery wedge pressure. Monitor patient for effects.
Tricyclic antidepressants: May potentiate pressor response. Monitor patient closely.
Drug-herb. *Rue:* May increase inotropic potential. Use cautiously; monitor patient closely.

Adverse reactions
CNS: headache.
CV: *increased heart rate,* **hypertension, PVCs,** angina, nonspecific chest pain, palpitations, hypotension.
GI: nausea, vomiting.
Respiratory: shortness of breath, *asthmatic episodes.*
Other: phlebitis, hypersensitivity reactions *(anaphylaxis).*

☑ Special considerations
Besides the recommendations relevant to all adrenergics, consider the following.
- Most patients experience an increase of 10 to 20 mm Hg in systolic blood pressure; some show an increase of 50 mm Hg or more. Most also experience an increase in heart rate of 5 to 15 beats/minute; some show increases of 30 or more beats/minute. Premature ventricular arrhythmias may also occur in about 5% of patients. Dosage reduction may be needed when these occur.
- Dose should be adjusted to meet individual needs and achieve desired response. Drug must be administered by I.V. infusion using an infusion pump or other device to control flow rate.
- Concentration of infusion solution shouldn't exceed 5,000 mcg/ml; use solution within 24 hours. Rate and duration of infusion depend on patient response.
- Dobutamine is incompatible with alkaline solution (sodium bicarbonate). Also, don't mix with or give through same I.V. line as heparin, hydrocortisone, cefazolin, or penicillin.
- Signs and symptoms of overdose include nervousness and fatigue. No treatment is necessary beyond dosage reduction or withdrawal of drug.

Monitoring the patient
- Monitor blood pressure throughout treatment.
- Before drug therapy, correct hypovolemia with appropriate plasma volume expanders.

- Monitor ECG, blood pressure, cardiac output, and pulmonary artery wedge pressure.
- Before therapy, administer a cardiac glycoside if patient has atrial fibrillation (dobutamine increases AV conduction).

Information for the patient
- Advise patient to report adverse reactions.
- Inform patient that vital signs will need frequent monitoring.

Geriatric patients
- Use with caution in elderly patients.

Pediatric patients
- Safety and efficacy haven't been established. Drug isn't recommended for use in children.

Breast-feeding patients
- It's unknown if drug appears in breast milk. Administer cautiously to breast-feeding women.

docetaxel
Taxotere

Pharmacologic classification: taxoid
Therapeutic classification: antineoplastic
Pregnancy risk category D

How supplied
Available by prescription only
Injection: 20 mg, 80 mg

Indications, route, and dosage
Treatment of patients with locally advanced or metastatic breast cancer who have progressed during anthracycline-based therapy or have relapsed during anthracycline-based adjuvant therapy
Adults: 60 to 100 mg/m^2 I.V. over 1 hour q 3 weeks.

Pharmacodynamics
Antineoplastic action: Acts by disrupting the microtubular network in cells that is essential for mitotic and interphase cellular functions.

Pharmacokinetics
- *Absorption:* Administered I.V.
- *Distribution:* About 94% protein-bound.
- *Metabolism:* Undergoes oxidative metabolism.
- *Excretion:* Eliminated primarily in feces; small amount eliminated in urine.

Contraindications and precautions
Contraindicated in patients with history of severe hypersensitivity to drug or other drugs formulated with polysorbate 80. Docetaxel shouldn't be used in patients with neutrophil counts below 1,500 cells/mm^3.

Interactions
Drug-drug. *Cyclosporine, erythromycin, ketoconazole, troleandomycin:* Metabolism of docetaxel may be modified by drugs that induce, inhibit, or are metabolized by cytochrome P-450 3A4. Use together cautiously.

Adverse reactions
CNS: paresthesia, dysesthesia, pain (including burning sensation), weakness.
CV: fluid retention, hypotension, chest tightness.
GI: *stomatitis,* nausea, vomiting, diarrhea.
Hematologic: *anemia,* NEUTROPENIA, FEBRILE NEUTROPENIA, LEUKOPENIA, *myelosuppression* (dose-limiting), *thrombocytopenia.*
Hepatic: *increased liver function tests.*
Musculoskeletal: *myalgia,* arthralgia, back pain.
Respiratory: dyspnea.
Skin: *alopecia,* maculopapular eruptions, desquamation, nail pigmentation alteration, onycholysis, nail pain, flushing, rash.
Other: *hypersensitivity reactions,* infections, drug fever, chills.

☑ Special considerations
- Premedicate all patients with oral corticosteroids such as dexamethasone 16 mg daily for 5 days starting 1 day before docetaxel to reduce incidence and severity of fluid retention and hypersensitivity reactions.
- Drug requires dilution before administration using the diluent supplied with drug. Allow drug and diluent to stand at room temperature for about 5 minutes before mixing. After adding entire contents of diluent to vial of docetaxel, gently rotate vial for about 15 seconds. Then allow solution to stand for a few minutes to allow any foam to dissipate. It isn't required that all foam dissipate before continuing preparation.
- To prepare docetaxel infusion solution, aseptically withdraw required amount of premix solution from vial and inject into a 250-ml infusion bag or bottle of normal saline solution or D$_5$W solution to produce a final concentration of 0.3 to 0.9 mg/ml. Doses exceeding 240 mg require a larger volume of infusion solution so that a concentration of 0.9 mg/ml of docetaxel isn't exceeded. Thoroughly mix infusion by manual rotation.
- Use caution during preparation and administration; gloves are recommended. If solution contacts skin, wash skin immediately and thoroughly with soap and water. If docetaxel contacts mucous membranes, flush membranes thoroughly with water. Mark all waste materials with CHEMOTHERAPY HAZARD labels.
- Contact of undiluted concentrate with plasticized polyvinyl chloride equipment or devices used to prepare solutions for infusion isn't recommended. Prepare and store infusion solutions in bottles (glass, polypropylene) or plastic bags (polypropylene, polyolefin) and administer through polyethylene-lined administration sets.

Reactions may be *common*, uncommon, **life-threatening**, or COMMON AND LIFE-THREATENING.

• Patient who is initially given 100 mg/m² and who experiences either febrile neutropenia, a neutrophil count under 500 cells/mm³ for more than 1 week, severe or cumulative cutaneous reactions, or severe peripheral neuropathy during docetaxel therapy should have dosage adjusted from 100 to 75 mg/m². If patient continues to experience these reactions, either decrease dosage from 75 to 55 mg/m² or stop drug.

• Patient who is initially given 60 mg/m² and who doesn't experience febrile neutropenia, a neutrophil count below 500 cells/mm³ for more than 1 week, severe or cumulative cutaneous reactions, or severe peripheral neuropathy during docetaxel therapy may tolerate higher doses.

• Signs and symptoms of overdose include bone marrow suppression, peripheral neurotoxicity, and mucositis. There is no known antidote. Patient should be kept in a specialized unit where vital functions can be closely monitored.

Monitoring the patient
• Patients with bilirubin values greater than the upper limits of normal (ULN) generally shouldn't receive docetaxel. Also, patients with ALT or AST levels that exceed 1.5 times ULN, with alkaline phosphatase level greater than 2.5 times ULN, generally shouldn't receive drug.
• Bone marrow toxicity is the most frequent and dose-limiting toxicity. Frequent monitoring of blood count is necessary during therapy.
• Monitor patient closely for hypersensitivity reactions, especially during first and second infusions. If minor reactions such as flushing or localized skin reactions occur, interruption of therapy isn't required. More severe reactions require stopping drug immediately and treating reaction aggressively.

Information for the patient
• Advise patient of childbearing age to avoid becoming pregnant during therapy with docetaxel because of potential harm to fetus.
• Warn patient that alopecia occurs in almost 80% of patients.
• Tell patient to promptly report sore throat, fever, unusual bruising, or bleeding.

Pediatric patients
• Safety and effectiveness in children under age 16 haven't been established.

Breast-feeding patients
• Because of potential for serious adverse reactions in breast-fed infants, it's recommended that breast-feeding be stopped during therapy.

docusate calcium
Pro-Cal-Sof, Surfak
docusate potassium
Dialose, Diocto-K, Kasof
docusate sodium
Colace, Diocto, DOK, D.O.S., D-S-S, Modane Soft, Pro-Sof, Regulax SS, Regulex*

Pharmacologic classification: surfactant
Therapeutic classification: emollient laxative
Pregnancy risk category C

How supplied
Available without a prescription
Tablets: 100 mg
Capsules: 50 mg, 100 mg, 250 mg
Syrup: 50 mg/15 ml, 60 mg/15 ml
Liquid: 150 mg/15 ml

Indications, route, and dosage
Stool softener
docusate sodium
Adults and children ages 12 and older: 50 to 200 mg P.O. daily until bowel movements are normal. Or add 50 to 100 mg to saline or oil retention enema to treat fecal impaction.
Children ages 6 to 12: 40 to 120 mg P.O. daily.
Children ages 3 to 6: 20 to 60 mg P.O. daily.
Children under age 3: 10 to 40 mg P.O. daily.
docusate calcium or potassium
Adults: 240 mg (calcium) or 100 to 300 mg (potassium) P.O. daily until bowel movements are normal. Higher doses are for initial therapy. Adjust dose to individual response.
Children ages 6 and older: 50 to 150 mg (calcium) or 100 mg (potassium) P.O. daily.

Pharmacodynamics
Laxative action: Docusate salts act as detergents in the intestine, reducing surface tension of interfacing liquids; this promotes incorporation of fat and additional liquid, softening the stool.

Pharmacokinetics
• *Absorption:* Absorbed minimally in duodenum and jejunum; acts in 1 to 3 days.
• *Distribution:* Distributed primarily locally, in gut.
• *Metabolism:* None.
• *Excretion:* Excreted in feces.

Contraindications and precautions
Contraindicated in patients with hypersensitivity to drug and in those with intestinal obstruction, undiagnosed abdominal pain, vomiting or other signs of appendicitis, fecal impaction, or acute surgical abdomen.

Interactions
Drug-drug. *Mineral oil:* May increase absorption of mineral oil. Monitor patient for effects.

Adverse reactions
GI: bitter taste, mild abdominal cramping, diarrhea, laxative dependence (with long-term or excessive use).

☑ Special considerations
● Liquid or syrup must be given in 6 to 8 oz (180 to 240 ml) of milk or fruit juice or in infant's formula to prevent throat irritation.
● Avoid using docusate sodium in sodium-restricted patients.
● Available with casanthranol (Peri-Colace), senna (Senokot, Gentlax), and phenolphthalein (Ex-Lax, Feen-A-Mint, Correctol).
● Docusate salts are preferred laxative for most patients who must avoid straining at stool, such as those recovering from MI or rectal surgery. Used commonly to treat patients with postpartum constipation.

Monitoring the patient
● Monitor patient's response to treatment.
● Monitor patient for adverse effects.

Information for the patient
● Docusate salts lose effectiveness over time; advise patient to report failure of drug.

Geriatric patients
● Docusate salts are good choices for elderly patients because they rarely cause laxative dependence, cause fewer adverse effects, and are gentler than other laxatives.

Breast-feeding patients
● Because absorption is minimal, drug should pose no risk to breast-feeding infants.

dofetilide
Tikosyn

Pharmacologic classification: antiarrhythmic
Therapeutic classification: class III antiarrhythmic
Pregnancy risk category C

How supplied
Available by prescription only
Capsules: 125 mcg (0.125 mg), 250 mcg (0.25 mg), 500 mcg (0.5 mg)

Indications, route, and dosage
Maintenance of normal sinus rhythm in patients with symptomatic atrial fibrillation or atrial flutter for more than 1 week; conversion of atrial fibrillation and atrial flutter to normal sinus rhythm
Adults: Dosage is individualized and is based on creatinine clearance and QT interval, which must be determined before first dose. Usual recommended dose is 500 mcg P.O. b.i.d. for patients with creatinine clearance greater than 60 ml/minute.
+ Dosage adjustment. If creatinine clearance is 40 to 60 ml/minute, starting dose is 250 mcg P.O. b.i.d.; 20 to 39 ml/minute, 125 mcg P.O. b.i.d.
   At 2 to 3 hours after first dose, determine QT interval. If it has increased by more than 15% over baseline or if it's more than 500 msec (550 msec in patients with ventricular conduction abnormalities), adjust dosage as follows: If starting dose based on creatinine clearance was 500 mcg P.O. b.i.d., give 250 mcg P.O. b.i.d. If starting dose based on creatinine clearance was 250 mcg P.O. b.i.d., give 125 mcg P.O. b.i.d. If starting dose based on creatinine clearance was 125 mcg P.O. b.i.d., give 125 mcg P.O. once daily.
   Determine QT interval 2 to 3 hours after each subsequent dose while patient is in hospital. If at any time after second dose QT interval is more than 500 msec (550 msec in patients with ventricular conduction abnormalities), stop drug.

Pharmacodynamics
Antiarrhythmic action: Prolongs repolarization without affecting conduction velocity by blocking the cardiac ion channel carrying potassium current. No affect is seen on sodium channels, adrenergic alpha-adrenergic receptors, or adrenergic-beta receptors.

Pharmacokinetics
● *Absorption:* Bioavailability after oral administration is greater than 90% with plasma levels peaking in 2 to 3 hours. Steady-state plasma levels are achieved in 2 to 3 days. Absorption unaffected by food or antacid.
● *Distribution:* Widely distributed throughout body; has a distribution volume of 3 L/kg. Plasma protein-binding is 60% to 70%.
● *Metabolism:* Metabolized to a small extent by CYP3A4 isoenzyme of cytochrome P-450 system of the liver.
● *Excretion:* About 80% is excreted in urine, of which 80% is excreted as unchanged drug with remaining 20% as inactive or minimally active metabolites.

Contraindications and precautions
Contraindicated in patients with creatinine clearance less than 20 ml/minute and in those with congenital or acquired long QT interval syndrome. Don't use drug in patients with baseline QT interval greater than 440 msec (500 msec in patients with ventricular conduction abnormalities).

Use with caution in patients with severe hepatic impairment.

Drug is distributed only to hospitals and other institutions confirmed to have received applicable dosing and treatment initiation programs. Such confirmation is also needed for inpatient and subsequent outpatient discharge and refill prescriptions.

Interactions

Drug-drug. *Amiloride, amiodarone, diltiazem, macrolide antibiotics, metformin, nefazodone, norfloxacin, protease inhibitors, quinine, serotonin reuptake inhibitors, triamterene, zafirlukast:* Possible increased plasma dofetilide levels. Use together cautiously.

Class I, Class III antiarrhythmics: Effect hasn't been studied; concomitant use not recommended. Hold antiarrhythmics for at least three half-lives before giving dofetilide.

Drugs that prolong QT interval (bepridil, oral macrolides, phenothiazines, tricyclic antidepressants): May enhance QT interval prolongation. Don't use concomitantly.

Potassium-wasting diuretics: Increased risk of torsades de pointes. Maintain potassium levels within normal range before and throughout drug therapy.

Verapamil, drugs that inhibit renal cation transport system (cimetidine, ketoconazole, megestrol, prochlorperazine, sulfamethoxazole, trimethoprim): Decreased dofetilide metabolism and excretion and increased plasma levels with concomitant use. Don't use together.

Drug-food. *Grapefruit juice:* Possible decreased hepatic metabolism and increased plasma levels. Don't give together.

Adverse reactions

CNS: *headache,* dizziness, syncope, paresthesia, insomnia, anxiety, migraine, cerebral ischemia, facial paralysis, CVA.
CV: *ventricular fibrillation, ventricular tachycardia, torsades de pointes, AV block,* chest pain, **bradycardia,** edema, **cardiac arrest, MI.**
GI: nausea, diarrhea, abdominal pain.
GU: urinary tract infection.
Hepatic: liver damage.
Musculoskeletal: back pain, arthralgia, flaccid paralysis.
Respiratory: respiratory tract infection, dyspnea, increased cough.
Skin: rash.
Other: flulike syndrome, accidental injury, *sudden death, angioedema.*

☑ Special considerations
● Patients in atrial fibrillation should be anticoagulated according to usual practice before electrical or pharmacologic cardioversion. Anticoagulation therapy may be continued after cardioversion according to usual medical practice.
● Dofetilide can be taken without regard to meals because food won't interfere with absorption.
● If a dose is missed, patient shouldn't double next dose. Instead, patient should skip that dose and wait until the next administration time for regularly scheduled dose.
● The most prominent symptom of overdose is likely to be excessive prolongation of QT interval. There is no known antidote. Treatment is symptomatic and supportive.
● In case of overdose, start cardiac monitoring. Charcoal slurry may be given and is useful especially within first 15 minutes after administration.
● Treatment of torsades de pointes or overdose may include isoproterenol, with or without cardiac pacing. Magnesium sulfate also may be effective.

Monitoring the patient
● Monitor patient for prolonged diarrhea, sweating, or vomiting. These symptoms may indicate an electrolyte imbalance that may increase potential for arrhythmia.
● Monitor renal function routinely (at least every 3 months) and creatinine clearance.
● Withhold Class I or III antiarrhythmics for at least 3 half-lives before starting drug.

Information for the patient
● Inform patient to report any change in OTC, prescription, or supplement/herb use.
● Tell patient not to use OTC Tagamet-HB for ulcers or heartburn. Antacids, Zantac 75 mg, and other acid-reduction drugs, such as Pepcid, Prilosec, Axid, Pilosec, and Prevacid, can be used.
● Inform patient that dofetilide can be taken without regard to meals or antacid administration.
● Inform patient that grapefruit juice can decrease metabolism of drug and lead to toxicity.
● Instruct woman to call if she becomes pregnant.
● Advise woman not to breast-feed while taking drug.

Geriatric patients
● There is no change in elimination based on age when dosage is adjusted for renal function.

Pediatric patients
● Safety and effectiveness in patients under age 18 haven't been established.

Breast-feeding patients
● Because there is no information on dofetilide use in breast-feeding mothers, advise women not to breast-feed while taking drug.

dolasetron mesylate
Anzemet

Pharmacologic classification: selective
serotonin 5-HT$_3$ receptor antagonist
Therapeutic classification: antinauseant,
antiemetic
Pregnancy risk category B

How supplied
Available by prescription only
Tablets: 50 mg, 100 mg
Injection: 20 mg/ml as 12.5 mg/0.625-ml ampules
or 100 mg/5-ml vials

Indications, route, and dosage
Prevention of nausea and vomiting associated with cancer chemotherapy
Adults: 100 mg P.O. given as a single dose 1 hour
before chemotherapy, or 1.8 mg/kg as a single
I.V. dose given 30 minutes before chemotherapy,
or a fixed dose of 100 mg I.V. given 30 minutes
before chemotherapy.
Children ages 2 to 16: 1.8 mg/kg P.O. given 1
hour before chemotherapy, or 1.8 mg/kg as a
single I.V. dose given 30 minutes before chemotherapy. Injectable form can be mixed with apple
or apple-grape juice and administered P.O. 1 hour
before chemotherapy. Maximum daily dose is
100 mg.
Prevention of postoperative nausea and vomiting
Adults: 100 mg P.O. within 2 hours before surgery;
12.5 mg as a single I.V. dose about 15 minutes
before cessation of anesthesia.
Children ages 2 to 16: 1.2 mg/kg P.O. given within 2 hours before surgery, to maximum of 100
mg; or 0.35 mg/kg (up to 12.5 mg) given as a single I.V. dose about 15 minutes before the cessation of anesthesia. Injectable form (1.2 mg/kg
up to 100-mg dose) can be mixed with apple or
apple-grape juice and administered P.O. 2 hours
before surgery.
Treatment of postoperative nausea and vomiting (I.V. form only)
Adults: 12.5 mg as a single I.V. dose as soon as
nausea or vomiting occurs.
Children ages 2 to 16: 0.35 mg/kg, to maximum
dose of 12.5 mg, given as a single I.V. dose as
soon as nausea or vomiting occurs.

Pharmacodynamics
Antinauseant and antiemetic actions: A selective
serotonin 5-HT$_3$ receptor antagonist that blocks
the action of serotonin. 5HT$_3$ receptors are located on the nerve terminals of the vagus nerve
in the periphery and in the central chemoreceptor trigger zone. Blocking the activity of the serotonin receptors prevents serotonin from stimulating the vomiting reflex.

Pharmacokinetics
• *Absorption:* Orally administered drug, injection,
I.V. solution, and tablets are bioequivalent. Oral
dolasetron is well absorbed, although parent drug
is rarely detected in plasma because of rapid and
complete metabolism to most clinically relevant
metabolite, hydrodolasetron.
• *Distribution:* Widely distributed in body, with
mean apparent distribution volume of 5.8 L/kg;
69% to 77% of hydrodolasetron bound to plasma protein.
• *Metabolism:* A ubiquitous enzyme, carbonyl reductase, mediates reduction to hydrodolasetron.
Cytochrome P-450 (CYP) 2D6 and CYP3A are
responsible for subsequent hydroxylation and
N-oxidation of hydrodolasetron, respectively.
• *Excretion:* Two-thirds of dose excreted in urine
and one-third in feces. Mean elimination half-life
is 8.1 hours.

Contraindications and precautions
Contraindicated in patients with hypersensitivity
to drug.
   Use cautiously in patients with or at risk for
developing prolonged cardiac conduction intervals, particularly QTc. These include patients taking antiarrhythmics or other drugs that lead to QT
interval prolongation and those with hypokalemia or hypomagnesemia; a potential for electrolyte abnormalities, including those receiving
diuretics; or congenital QT syndrome; and those
who have received cumulative high-dose anthracycline therapy.

Interactions
Drug-drug. *Antiarrhythmics:* Administration with
drugs that prolong ECG intervals can increase
risk of arrhythmias. Monitor patient closely.
Cimetidine: Drugs that inhibit P-450 enzymes
can increase hydrodolasetron levels. Monitor patient for adverse effects.
Rifampin: Drugs that induce P-450 enzymes may
decrease hydrodolasetron levels. Monitor patient
for decreased efficacy of antiemetic.

Adverse reactions
CNS: *headache,* dizziness, drowsiness, fatigue.
CV: *arrhythmias,* ECG changes, hypotension,
hypertension**,** tachycardia, *bradycardia.*
GI: *diarrhea,* dyspepsia, abdominal pain, consti-
pation, anorexia.
GU: oliguria, urine retention.
Hepatic: elevation of liver function test results.
Skin: pruritus, rash.
Other: fever, chills, pain at injection site.

☑ Special considerations
• Safety and efficacy of multiple doses haven't
been evaluated.
• Injection can be infused as rapidly as 100 mg/30
seconds or diluted in 50 ml compatible solution
and infused over 15 minutes.

Reactions may be *common*, uncommon, **life-threatening**, or COMMON AND LIFE-THREATENING.

• Injection for oral administration is stable in apple or apple-grape juice for 2 hours at room temperature.
• There is no specific antidote for overdose. Provide supportive care. It's not known if drug is removed by hemodialysis or peritoneal dialysis.

Monitoring the patient
• Monitor patient for signs or symptoms of arrhythmias.
• Monitor therapeutic effect.

Information for the patient
• Inform patient that oral doses of drug must be taken 1 to 2 hours before surgery or 1 hour before chemotherapy to be effective.
• Inform patient of potential adverse effects.
• Instruct patient not to mix injection in juice for oral administration until just before dosing.
• Tell patient to report nausea or vomiting.

Geriatric patients
• Dosage adjustment isn't needed in patients over age 65.
• Effectiveness in prevention of nausea and vomiting in elderly patients is no different from that in younger age-groups.

Pediatric patients
• There is no information on drug use in children under age 2.
• Efficacy in children ages 2 to 17 who are receiving cancer chemotherapy is consistent with that seen in adults.
$ Efficacy in postoperative nausea and vomiting in children is unknown.

Breast-feeding patients
• It's unknown if drug appears in breast milk. Use with caution in breast-feeding women.

donepezil hydrochloride
Aricept

Pharmacologic classification: acetylcholinesterase inhibitor
Therapeutic classification: cholinomimetic
Pregnancy risk category C

How supplied
Available by prescription only
Tablets: 5 mg, 10 mg

Indications, route, and dosage
Mild to moderate dementia of the Alzheimer's type
Adults: Initially, 5 mg P.O. daily h.s. After 4 to 6 weeks, dosage may be increased to 10 mg daily.

Pharmacodynamics
Anticholinesterase action: Believed to inhibit the enzyme acetylcholinesterase in the CNS, increasing level of acetylcholine and temporarily improving cognitive function in patients with Alzheimer's disease. Doesn't alter the course of the underlying disease process.

Pharmacokinetics
• *Absorption:* Well absorbed with relative bioavailability of 100%; reaches peak plasma levels in 3 to 4 hours. Steady-state reached within 15 days.
• *Distribution:* Steady-state volume of distribution is 12 L/kg. About 96% bound to plasma proteins, mainly to albumins (about 75%) and alpha$_1$-acid glycoprotein (about 21%) over concentration range of 2 to 1,000 ng/ml.
• *Metabolism:* Extensively metabolized to four major metabolites (two are known to be active) and several minor metabolites (not all identified). Metabolized by CYP 450 isoenzymes 2D6 and 3A4; undergoes glucuronidation.
• *Excretion:* Excreted intact in urine and extensively metabolized by liver. Elimination half-life is about 70 hours; mean apparent plasma clearance is 0.13 L/hour/kg. About 17% eliminated unchanged by kidneys.

Contraindications and precautions
Contraindicated in patients with hypersensitivity to drug or piperidine derivatives. Use cautiously in patients with "sick sinus syndrome" or other supraventricular cardiac conduction conditions because drug may cause bradycardia. Also use cautiously in patients with CV disease, asthma, or history of ulcer disease and in those taking NSAIDs.

Interactions
Drug-drug. *Anticholinergics:* May interfere with anticholinergic activity. Avoid concomitant use.
Bethanechol, succinylcholine: May produce additive effects. Monitor patient closely.
Carbamazepine, dexamethasone, phenobarbital, phenytoin, rifampin: May increase rate of elimination of donepezil. Monitor patient.
Cholinesterase inhibitors, cholinomimetics: May produce synergistic effect. Monitor patient closely.
Drug-herb. *Jaborandi tree, pill-bearing spurge:* Concomitant use may cause additive effect; may increase risk of toxicity. Use together cautiously.

Adverse reactions
CNS: abnormal dreams or crying, aggression, aphasia, ataxia, dizziness, fatigue, depression, *headache, insomnia,* irritability, nervousness, paresthesia, restlessness, somnolence, **seizures,** tremor, vertigo.
CV: atrial fibrillation, chest pain, hypertens' vasodilation, hypotension, syncope.

EENT: blurred vision, cataract, eye irritation.
GI: anorexia, bloating, *diarrhea,* epigastric pain, fecal incontinence, GI bleeding, *nausea,* vomiting.
GU: frequent urination, hot flashes, nocturia, increased libido.
Hematologic: ecchymosis.
Metabolic: dehydration, weight loss.
Musculoskeletal: arthritis, bone fracture, muscle cramps, toothache.
Respiratory: bronchitis, dyspnea, sore throat.
Skin: diaphoresis, pruritus, urticaria.
Other: influenza, pain.

☑ Special considerations
● Diarrhea, nausea, and vomiting occur more frequently with 10-mg dose than with 5-mg dose. These effects are mostly mild and transient, sometimes lasting 1 to 3 weeks, and resolve during continued therapy.
● Drug may cause bladder outflow obstruction.
● Cholinomimetics have potential to cause generalized seizures. However, seizure activity also may be due to Alzheimer's disease.
● Overdose can result in cholinergic crisis characterized by severe nausea, vomiting, salivation, sweating, bradycardia, hypotension, respiratory depression, collapse, and seizures. Increasing muscle weakness also may occur and may result in death if respiratory muscles are involved.
● Tertiary anticholinergics such as atropine may be used as an antidote for drug overdose. I.V. atropine sulfate adjusted to effect is recommended; give initial dose of 1 to 2 mg I.V. and base subsequent doses on response.
● Atypical responses in blood pressure and heart rate have been reported with other cholinomimetics when administered with quaternary anticholinergics such as glycopyrrolate.
● It's unknown if donepezil or its metabolites can be removed by dialysis.

Monitoring the patient
● Monitor heart rate.
● Monitor patient for syncopal episodes, which have been reported with drug use.
● Drug may increase gastric acid secretion owing to increased cholinergic activity. Closely monitor patients at increased risk for developing ulcers (such as those with history of ulcer disease or those receiving NSAIDs) for symptoms of active or occult GI bleeding.

Information for the patient
● Explain to patient and caregiver that drug doesn't alter disease but can stabilize or alleviate symptoms. Effects of therapy depend on drug administration at regular intervals.
● Tell caregiver to give drug in evening, just before bedtime.

● Advise patient and caregiver to immediately report significant adverse effects or changes in overall health status.
● Tell patient and caregiver to report donepezil use before patient receives anesthesia.

Geriatric patients
● Mean plasma drug levels of elderly patients with Alzheimer's disease are comparable with those observed in young, healthy volunteers.

Pediatric patients
● Safety and efficacy in children haven't been established.

Breast-feeding patients
● It's unknown if drug appears in breast milk. Avoid use in breast-feeding women.

dopamine hydrochloride
Intropin

Pharmacologic classification: adrenergic
Therapeutic classification: inotropic drug, vasopressor
Pregnancy risk category C

How supplied
Available by prescription only
Injection: 40 mg/ml, 80 mg/ml, and 160 mg/ml parenteral concentrate for injection for I.V. infusion; 0.8 mg/ml (200 or 400 mg) in D_5W, 1.6 mg/ml (400 or 800 mg) in D_5W, and 3.2 mg/ml (800 mg) in D_5W parenteral injection for I.V. infusion

Indications, route, and dosage
Adjunct in shock to increase cardiac output, blood pressure, and urine flow
Adults: 1 to 5 mcg/kg/minute I.V. infusion, up to 20 to 50 mcg/kg/minute. Infusion rate may be increased by 1 to 4 mcg/kg/minute at 10- to 30-minute intervals until optimum response is achieved. In severely ill patient, infusion may begin at 5 mcg/kg/minute and gradually increase by increments of 5 to 10 mcg/kg/minute until optimum response is achieved.
Short-term treatment of severe, refractory, chronic heart failure
Adults: Initially, 0.5 to 2 mcg/kg/minute I.V. infusion. Dosage may be increased until desired renal response occurs. Average dose is 1 to 3 mcg/kg/minute.

Pharmacodynamics
Vasopressor action: An immediate precursor of norepinephrine, dopamine stimulates dopaminergic, beta-adrenergic, and alpha-adrenergic receptors of the sympathetic nervous system. The main effects produced are dose-dependent. It has a direct stimulating effect on $beta_1$ receptors (in I.V. doses of 2 to 10 mcg/kg/minute) and little

---

tions may be *common*, uncommon, ***life-threatening***, or COMMON AND LIFE-THREATENING.

or no effect on beta$_2$ receptors. In I.V. doses of 0.5 to 2 mcg/kg/minute, it acts on dopaminergic receptors, causing vasodilation in the renal, mesenteric, coronary, and intracerebral vascular beds; in I.V. doses above 10 mcg/kg/minute, it stimulates alpha receptors.

Low to moderate doses result in cardiac stimulation (positive inotropic effects) and renal and mesenteric vasodilation (dopaminergic response). High doses result in increased peripheral resistance and renal vasoconstriction.

Pharmacokinetics
• *Absorption:* Onset of action after I.V. administration occurs within 5 minutes; lasts for less than 10 minutes.
• *Distribution:* Widely distributed throughout body; doesn't cross blood-brain barrier.
• *Metabolism:* Metabolized to inactive compounds in liver, kidneys, and plasma by MAO and catechol-O-methyltransferase. About 25% is metabolized to norepinephrine within adrenergic nerve terminals.
• *Excretion:* Excreted in urine, mainly as metabolites.

Contraindications and precautions
Contraindicated in patients with uncorrected tachyarrhythmias, pheochromocytoma, or ventricular fibrillation. Use cautiously in patients with occlusive vascular disease, cold injuries, diabetic endarteritis, or arterial embolism; in those taking MAO inhibitors; and in pregnant women.

Interactions
Drug-drug. *Alpha blockers:* May antagonize peripheral vasoconstriction caused by high doses of dopamine. Use cautiously; monitor patient closely.
Beta blockers: Antagonized cardiac effects of dopamine. Use cautiously and monitor patient closely.
Diuretics: Increased diuretic effects of both drugs. Monitor patient closely.
Ergot alkaloids: May cause extreme elevations in blood pressure. Monitor blood pressure closely.
General anesthetics (especially cyclopropane, halothane): Combined use may cause ventricular arrhythmias and hypertension. Monitor patient closely.
MAO inhibitors: May prolong and intensify effects of dopamine. Use cautiously; monitor patient closely.
Oxytocics: May cause advanced vasoconstriction. Dosage adjustments may be needed.
Phenytoin: May cause hypotension and bradycardia. Monitor patient closely.

Adverse reactions
CNS: headache.

CV: ectopic beats, tachycardia, anginal pain, palpitations, *hypotension;* **bradycardia,** conduction disturbances, hypertension, vasoconstriction, widening of QRS complex (less frequently).
GI: nausea, vomiting.
GU: azotemia.
Metabolic: hyperglycemia.
Respiratory: dyspnea, *asthmatic episodes.*
Other: necrosis and tissue sloughing with extravasation, piloerection, *anaphylactic reactions.*

☑ Special considerations
Besides the recommendations relevant to all adrenergics, consider the following.
• Dopamine is administered by I.V. infusion using an infusion device to control rate of flow.
• Administer drug into large vein to prevent possibility of extravasation. If necessary to administer in hand or ankle veins, change injection site to larger vein as soon as possible. Monitor continuously for free flow. Central venous access is recommended.
• Adjust dose to meet individual needs of patient and to achieve desired response. If dose required to obtain desired systolic blood pressure exceeds optimum rate of renal response, reduce dose as soon as hemodynamic condition is stabilized.
• Severe hypotension may result with abrupt withdrawal of infusion; therefore, reduce dose gradually.
• Don't mix other drugs in dopamine solutions. Discard solutions after 24 hours.
• Dopamine may cause elevated urinary catecholamine levels.
• Signs and symptoms of overdose include excessive, severe hypertension. No treatment is necessary beyond dosage reduction or withdrawal of drug. If blood pressure isn't lowered, a short-acting alpha blocker may be helpful.

Monitoring the patient
• Monitor blood pressure, cardiac output, ECG, and intake and output during infusion, especially if dose exceeds 20 mcg/kg/minute. Watch for cold extremities.
• Hypovolemia should be corrected with appropriate plasma volume expanders before starting dopamine therapy.
• If extravasation occurs, stop infusion and infiltrate site promptly with 10 to 15 ml saline injection containing 5 to 10 mg phentolamine. Use syringe with a fine needle, and infiltrate area liberally with phentolamine solution.

Information for the patient
• Advise patient to report adverse reactions.
• Inform patient of need for frequent monitoring of vital signs and condition.

Geriatric patients
• Lower doses are indicated because elderly patients may be more sensitive to drug's effects.

dornase alfa
Pulmozyme

Pharmacologic classification: recombinant human deoxyribonuclease I, mucolytic enzyme
Therapeutic classification: respiratory inhalant
Pregnancy risk category B

How supplied
Available by prescription only
Inhalation solution: 2.5-ml ampule containing 1 mg/ml dornase alfa

Indications, route, and dosage
To improve pulmonary function and reduce frequency of moderate to severe respiratory infections in patients with cystic fibrosis (CF)
Adults and children ages 5 and over: One ampule (2.5 mg/2.5 ml) inhaled once daily. Treatment usually takes 10 to 15 minutes. Use drug only with an approved nebulizer. Patients over age 21 and those with a baseline forced vital capacity greater than 85% may need twice-daily dosing.

Pharmacodynamics
Respiratory inhalant action: A purified solution of recombinant human deoxyribonuclease I, an enzyme that selectively breaks down DNA. Patients with CF retain thick, purulent pulmonary secretions rich in extracellular DNA. Dornase alfa hydrolyzes the excess DNA, reducing sputum viscosity.

Pharmacokinetics
• *Absorption:* After inhalation, drug achieves mean sputum level of 3 mcg/ml within 15 minutes, declining to an average of 0.6 mcg/ml within 2 hours.
• *Distribution:* No information available.
• *Metabolism:* No information available.
• *Excretion:* No information available.

Contraindications and precautions
Contraindicated in patients with hypersensitivity to drug or Chinese hamster ovary cell-derived products.

Interactions
None reported.

Adverse reactions
CV: *chest pain.*
EENT: *pharyngitis, voice alteration,* laryngitis, conjunctivitis.
Skin: *rash,* urticaria.

☑ Special considerations
• Mixing dornase alfa with another drug in nebulizer could cause adverse changes in one or both drugs.
• Drug should be used with standard therapies prescribed for CF.
• Safety and efficacy of daily administration haven't been demonstrated in patients with forced vital capacity less than 40% of predicted value or for longer than 12 months.

Monitoring the patient
• Monitor patient's response to treatment.
• CF patients have received up to 20 mg twice daily for up to 6 days and 10 mg twice daily intermittently (2 weeks on, 2 weeks off) for 168 days. These doses were well tolerated.

Information for the patient
• Inform patient to store drug in refrigerator at 36° to 46° F (2° to 8° C) and protect from strong light. Refrigerate during transport and don't expose to room temperatures for more than 24 hours.
• Tell patient to discard solution if cloudy or discolored.
• Inform patient that drug contains no preservative, and once opened entire ampule must be used or discarded.
• Instruct patient in proper use and maintenance of nebulizer and compressor system.

Pediatric patients
• Safety and efficacy of daily administration haven't been demonstrated in patients under age 5.

Breast-feeding patients
• It's unknown if drug appears in breast milk. Use cautiously when administering to breast-feeding women.

dorzolamide hydrochloride
Trusopt

Pharmacologic classification: sulfonamide
Therapeutic classification: antiglaucoma drug
Pregnancy risk category C

How supplied
Available by prescription only
Ophthalmic solution: 2%

Indications, route, and dosage
Increased intraocular pressure in patients with ocular hypertension or open-angle glaucoma
Adults: Instill 1 drop in conjunctival sac of affected eye t.i.d.

Reactions may be *common,* uncommon, **life-threatening,** or COMMON AND LIFE-THREATENING.

Pharmacodynamics

Antiglaucoma action: Inhibits carbonic anhydrase in the ciliary processes of the eye, which decreases aqueous humor secretion, presumably by slowing the formation of bicarbonate ions with subsequent reduction in sodium and fluid transport. The result is a reduction in intraocular pressure.

Pharmacokinetics

• *Absorption:* Reaches systemic circulation when applied topically.
• *Distribution:* Accumulates in RBCs during long-term dosing as a result of binding to carbonic anhydrase II.
• *Metabolism:* No information available.
• *Excretion:* Primarily excreted unchanged in urine.

Contraindications and precautions

Contraindicated in patients with hypersensitivity to drug or its components and in those with impaired renal function. Use cautiously in patients with impaired hepatic function.

Interactions

Drug-drug. *Oral carbonic anhydrase inhibitors:* Potential for additive effects. Don't administer together.

Adverse reactions

CNS: asthenia, headache, fatigue.
EENT: *ocular burning, stinging, discomfort; superficial punctate keratitis; ocular allergic reactions; blurred vision; lacrimation; dryness; photophobia;* iridocyclitis.
GI: *bitter taste,* nausea.
GU: urolithiasis.
Skin: rash.

☑ Special considerations

• Because dorzolamide is a sulfonamide and is absorbed systemically, the same types of adverse reactions that are attributable to sulfonamides may occur with topical administration of drug.
• If signs of serious adverse reactions or hypersensitivity occur, stop drug.
• Overdose may result in electrolyte imbalance, acidosis, and possible CNS effects. Serum electrolyte levels (especially potassium) and blood pH levels should be monitored. Treatment is supportive.

Monitoring the patient

• Monitor patient's response to treatment.
• Monitor patient for ocular reactions.

Information for the patient

• Instruct patient that if more than one topical ophthalmic drug is being used, they should be administered at least 10 minutes apart.

• Teach patient how to instill drops. Advise patient to wash hands before and after instilling solution and not to touch dropper or tip to eye or surrounding tissue.
• Advise patient to apply light finger pressure on lacrimal sac for 1 minute after instillation to minimize systemic absorption of drug.
• Inform patient to report ocular reactions, particularly conjunctivitis and lid reactions, and stop drug.
• Tell patient not to wear soft contact lenses while using drug.
• Stress importance of compliance with recommended therapy.

Geriatric patients

• Use with caution because greater sensitivity to drug may occur in older adults.

Pediatric patients

• Safety and effectiveness in children haven't been established.

Breast-feeding patients

• It's unknown if drug appears in breast milk. Because of risk of serious adverse reactions in breast-fed infants, use in breast-feeding women isn't recommended.

doxacurium chloride
Nuromax

Pharmacologic classification: nondepolarizing neuromuscular blocker
Therapeutic classification: skeletal muscle relaxant
Pregnancy risk category C

How supplied

Available by prescription only
Injection: 1 mg/ml

Indications, route, and dosage

To provide skeletal muscle relaxation for endotracheal intubation and during surgery as an adjunct to general anesthesia
Adults: Dosage is highly individualized; 0.05 mg/kg rapid I.V. produces adequate conditions for endotracheal intubation in 5 minutes in about 90% of patients when used as part of a thiopental-narcotic induction technique. Lower doses may require longer delay before intubation is possible. Neuromuscular blockade at this dose lasts an average of 100 minutes.
Children over age 2: Dosage is highly individualized; an initial dose of 0.03 mg/kg I.V. administered during halothane anesthesia produces effective blockade in 7 minutes and has a duration of 30 minutes. Under the same conditions, 0.05 mg/kg produces a blockade in 4 minutes and lasts 45 minutes.

Maintenance of neuromuscular blockade during long procedures

Adults and children over age 2: After initial dose of 0.05 mg/kg I.V., maintenance dosages of 0.005 and 0.01 mg/kg will prolong neuromuscular blockade for an average of 30 minutes and 45 minutes, respectively. Children usually require more frequent administration of maintenance dosages.

✦ *Dosage adjustment.* Adjust dosage to ideal body weight in obese patients (patients whose weight is 30% or more above their ideal weight) to avoid prolonged neuromuscular blockade.

Pharmacodynamics

Skeletal muscle relaxant action: Binds competitively to cholinergic receptors on the motor endplate to antagonize action of acetylcholine, resulting in a block of neuromuscular transmission.

Pharmacokinetics

- *Absorption:* First signs of neuromuscular blockade occur within about 2 minutes after I.V. administration. Maximum effects occur in about 3 to 6 minutes.
- *Distribution:* Plasma protein-binding is about 30% in plasma.
- *Metabolism:* Not thought to be metabolized.
- *Excretion:* Primarily eliminated as unchanged drug in urine and bile.

Contraindications and precautions

Contraindicated in patients with hypersensitivity to drug and in neonates. Drug contains benzyl ethanol, which has been associated with death in newborns.

Use cautiously, perhaps at reduced dose, in debilitated patients; in patients with metastatic cancer, severe electrolyte disturbances, or neuromuscular diseases; and in those in whom potentiation or difficulty in reversal of neuromuscular blockade is anticipated. Patients with myasthenia gravis or myasthenic syndrome (Eaton-Lambert syndrome) are particularly sensitive to the effects of nondepolarizing relaxants. Shorter-acting drugs are recommended for such patients.

Interactions

Drug-drug. *Alkaline solutions:* Precipitate may form because drug is physically incompatible with solution. Don't administer together.

Antibiotics (such as aminoglycosides, bacitracin, clindamycin, colistimethate sodium, colistin, gentamycin, kanamycin, lincomycin, neomycin, polymyxins, streptomycin, tetracyclines), lithium, local anesthetics, magnesium salts, procainamide, quinidine: Enhanced neuromuscular blocking action. Use cautiously and monitor patient closely.

Carbamazepine, phenytoin: Delayed onset of neuromuscular blockade induced by doxacurium and shortens its duration. Monitor patient.

Enflurane, halothane, isoflurane: Decreased ED_{50} (effective dose required to produce a 50% suppression of response to ulnar nerve stimulation) of doxacurium by 30% to 45%. May also prolong clinically effective duration of action of doxacurium by up to 25%. Use cautiously.

Adverse reactions

Musculoskeletal: prolonged muscle weakness.
Respiratory: dyspnea, *respiratory depression, respiratory insufficiency or apnea.*

☑ Special considerations

- All times of onset and duration of neuromuscular blockade are averages; considerable individual variation in dosage needs is normal.
- Drug may prolong neuromuscular block in patients undergoing renal transplantation, and onset and duration of the block may vary with patients undergoing liver transplantation.
- Drug should be used only under direct medical supervision by those familiar with use of neuromuscular blocking drugs and in airway management. Don't use unless facilities and equipment for mechanical ventilation, oxygen therapy, and intubation and an antagonist are within reach.
- Use of a peripheral nerve stimulator will permit most advantageous use of drug, minimize possibility of overdose or underdose, and assist in evaluation of recovery.
- Doxacurium is acidic (pH 3.9 to 5.0) and may not be compatible with alkaline solutions having a pH above 8.5 (such as barbiturate solutions).
- Doxacurium diluted up to 1:10 in D_5W injection, USP, or normal saline injection, USP; is physically and chemically stable when stored in polypropylene syringes at 41° to 77° F (5° to 25° C) for up to 24 hours. Because dilution reduces preservative effectiveness of benzyl alcohol, aseptic technique should be used to prepare diluted product. Use diluted product immediately; discard any unused portion after 8 hours.
- Overdose with neuromuscular blockers such as doxacurium may result in neuromuscular block beyond the time needed for surgery and anesthesia.
- Primary treatment of overdose is maintenance of patent airway and controlled ventilation until recovery of normal neuromuscular function is assured. Once initial evidence of recovery is observed, further recovery may be facilitated by using an anticholinesterase (such as neostigmine or edrophonium) with an appropriate anticholinergic.

Monitoring the patient

- As with other nondepolarizing neuromuscular blockers, a reduction in dosage of doxacurium must be considered in cachectic or debilitated patients; in patients with neuromuscular diseases, severe electrolyte abnormalities, or carcinomatosis; and in other patients in whom potentiation of neuromuscular block or difficulty with reversal is anticipated. Increased doses of doxacurium may be required in burn patients.

• Drug has no effect on consciousness or pain threshold. To avoid distress to patient, administer after general anesthetic.

Geriatric patients
• Elderly patients may be more sensitive to the drug's effects. They may experience a slower onset of the blockade and a longer duration.

Pediatric patients
• Drug use hasn't been studied in children younger than age 2.

Breast-feeding patients
• It's unknown if drug appears in breast milk. Use cautiously in breast-feeding women.

doxapram hydrochloride
Dopram

Pharmacologic classification: analeptic
Therapeutic classification: CNS and respiratory stimulant
Pregnancy risk category B

How supplied
Available by prescription only
Injection: 20 mg/ml (benzyl alcohol 0.9%)

Indications, route, and dosage
Postanesthesia respiratory stimulation
Adults: 0.5 to 1 mg/kg of body weight as a single I.V. injection (not to exceed 1.5 mg/kg) or as multiple injections q 5 minutes, not to exceed 2 mg/kg total dosage. Or 250 mg in 250 ml of normal saline solution or D_5W infused at an initial rate of 5 mg/minute I.V. until a satisfactory response is achieved. Maintain at 1 to 3 mg/minute. Recommended total dose for infusion shouldn't exceed 4 mg/kg.
Drug-induced CNS depression
Adults: For injection, priming dose of 2 mg/kg I.V. repeated in 5 minutes and again q 1 to 2 hours until patient awakens (and if relapse occurs). Maximum daily dose is 3 g.

For infusion, priming dose of 2 mg/kg I.V., repeated in 5 minutes and again in 1 to 2 hours if needed. If response occurs, give I.V. infusion (1 mg/ml) at 1 to 3 mg/minute until patient awakens. Don't infuse for longer than 2 hours or administer more than 3 g/day. May resume I.V. infusion after a rest period of 30 minutes to 2 hours, if needed.
Chronic pulmonary disease associated with acute hypercapnia
Adults: Infusion of 1 to 2 mg/minute (using 2 mg/ml solution). Maximum dosage is 3 mg/minute for a maximum duration of 2 hours. Don't use drug

with mechanical ventilation. Use infusion pump to regulate rate.

Pharmacodynamics
Respiratory stimulant action: Increases respiratory rate by direct stimulation of the medullary respiratory center and possibly by indirect action on chemoreceptors in the carotid artery and aortic arch. Causes increased release of catecholamines.

Pharmacokinetics
• *Absorption:* After I.V. administration, action begins within 20 to 40 seconds; peak effect occurs in 1 to 2 minutes. Pharmacologic action persists for 5 to 12 minutes.
• *Distribution:* Distributed throughout body.
• *Metabolism:* 99% metabolized by liver.
• *Excretion:* Excreted in urine.

Contraindications and precautions
Contraindicated in patients with seizure disorders; head injury; CV disorders; frank, uncompensated heart failure; severe hypertension; CVA; respiratory failure or incompetence secondary to neuromuscular disorders, muscle paresis, flail chest, obstructed airway, pulmonary embolism, pneumothorax, restrictive respiratory disease, acute bronchial asthma, or extreme dyspnea; or hypoxia not associated with hypercapnia. Also contraindicated in newborns because product contains benzyl alcohol.

Use cautiously in patients with bronchial asthma, severe tachycardia or arrhythmias, cerebral edema or increased CSF pressure, hyperthyroidism, pheochromocytoma, or metabolic disorders.

Interactions
Drug-drug. *Anesthetics (such as cyclopropane, enflurane, halothane):* These drugs sensitize myocardium to catecholamines. Stop at least 10 minutes before giving doxapram.
MAO inhibitors, sympathomimetics: May produce added pressor effects. Monitor patient closely.
Neuromuscular blockers: Effects may be temporarily masked after anesthesia due to doxapram. Monitor patient closely.

Adverse reactions
CNS: *seizures,* headache, dizziness, apprehension, disorientation, hyperactivity, bilateral Babinski's signs, paresthesia.
CV: *chest pain and tightness, variations in heart rate, hypertension,* lowered T waves, **arrhythmias.**
EENT: sneezing, *laryngospasm.*
GI: nausea, vomiting, diarrhea.
GU: urine retention, bladder stimulation with incontinence, increased BUN levels, albuminuria

Hematologic: decreased erythrocyte and leuko-cyte counts, reduced hemoglobin levels and hematocrit.
Musculoskeletal: muscle spasms.
Respiratory: cough, *bronchospasm,* dyspnea, rebound hypoventilation.
Skin: pruritus.
Other: hiccups, diaphoresis, flushing.

☑ Special considerations
• Doxapram's use as an analeptic is strongly dis-couraged; drug should be used only in surgery or emergency room.
• For I.V. infusion, dilute to 1 mg/ml. Don't infuse faster than recommended rate because hemo-lysis may occur. Drug should be used only on an intermittent basis; maximum infusion period is 2 hours.
• Avoid repeated injections in the site for long pe-riods because of risk of thrombophlebitis or lo-cal skin irritation.
• Don't combine doxapram, which is acidic, with alkaline solutions, such as thiopental sodium; so-lution is compatible with D_5W or $D_{10}W$ and nor-mal saline solution.
• Give oxygen cautiously to patients with COPD who are narcotized or those who have just un-dergone surgery; doxapram-stimulated respira-tion increases oxygen demand.
• Signs of overdose include hypertension, tachy-cardia, arrhythmias, skeletal muscle hyperactiv-ity, and dyspnea. Treatment is supportive. Keep oxygen and resuscitative equipment available, but use oxygen with caution because rapid in-crease in partial pressure of oxygen can sup-press carotid chemoreceptor activity. Keep I.V. anticonvulsants available to treat seizures.

Monitoring the patient
• Establish adequate airway before administer-ing drug; prevent aspiration of vomitus by plac-ing patient on his side.
• Monitor blood pressure, heart rate, deep ten-don reflexes, and arterial blood gas (ABG) lev-els before giving drug and every 30 minutes af-terward. Stop drug if ABG levels deteriorate or mechanical ventilation is started.

Geriatric patients
• No specific recommendations exist for drug use in elderly patients. However, elderly patients may be predisposed to one of several illnesses that preclude use.

Pediatric patients
• Safety in children under age 12 hasn't been es-tablished.

Breast-feeding patients
• It's unknown if drug appears in breast milk. Safe use in breast-feeding women hasn't been es-tablished.

---

doxazosin mesylate
Cardura

Pharmacologic classification: alpha blocker
Therapeutic classification: antihyperten-sive
Pregnancy risk category C

How supplied
Available by prescription only
Tablets: 1 mg, 2 mg, 4 mg, 8 mg

Indications, route, and dosage
Essential hypertension
Adult: Dosage must be individualized. Initially, ad-minister 1 mg P.O. daily and determine effect on standing and supine blood pressure at 2 to 6 hours and 24 hours after dosing. If necessary, in-crease dose to 2 mg daily. To minimize adverse reactions, adjust dose slowly (dosage typically increased only q 2 weeks). If necessary, increase dose to 4 mg daily, then 8 mg. Maximum daily dose is 16 mg, but doses exceeding 4 mg daily are associated with more adverse reactions.
Benign prostatic hyperplasia
Adults: Initially, 1 mg P.O. once daily in the morn-ing or evening; increase to 2 mg and, thereafter, to 4 mg and 8 mg once daily. Recommended ad-justment interval is 1 to 2 weeks.

Pharmacodynamics
Hypotensive action: Selectively blocks post-synaptic $alpha_1$-adrenergic receptors, dilating both resistance (arterioles) and capacitance (veins) vessels. It lowers both supine and stand-ing blood pressure, producing more pronounced effects on diastolic pressure. Maximum reduc-tions occur 2 to 6 hours after dosing and are as-sociated with a small increase in standing heart rate. Has a greater effect on blood pressure and heart rate in the standing position.
Benign prostatic hyperplasia: Improves urine flow related to relaxation of smooth muscles produced by blockade of alpha adrenoreceptors in the blad-der neck and prostate.

Pharmacokinetics
• *Absorption:* Readily absorbed from GI tract af-ter oral administration. Plasma levels peak in 2 to 3 hours.
• *Distribution:* 98% protein-bound. Distributed in breast milk in levels about 20 times greater than in maternal plasma.
• *Metabolism:* Extensively metabolized in liver by O-demethylation or hydroxylation. Secondary peaking of plasma levels suggests enterohepat-ic recycling.
• *Excretion:* 63% excreted in bile and feces (4.8% as unchanged drug); 9% excreted in urine.

---

ctions may be *common,* uncommon, *life-threatening,* or COMMON AND LIFE-THREATENING.

Contraindications and precautions
Contraindicated in patients with hypersensitivity to drug and quinazoline derivatives (including prazosin and terazosin). Use cautiously in patients with impaired hepatic function.

Interactions
Drug-drug. *Clonidine:* Decreased antihypertensive effects. Monitor blood pressure closely.
Drug-herb. *Butcher's broom:* May reduce effects. Discourage use.

Adverse reactions
CNS: *dizziness,* vertigo, somnolence, drowsiness, *asthenia, headache.*
CV: *orthostatic hypotension,* hypotension, edema, palpitations, **arrhythmias,** tachycardia.
EENT: rhinitis, pharyngitis, abnormal vision.
GI: nausea, vomiting, diarrhea, constipation.
Hematologic: mean WBC and neutrophil counts may be decreased.
Musculoskeletal: arthralgia, myalgia, pain.
Respiratory: dyspnea.
Skin: rash, pruritus.

☑ Special considerations
• Tolerance to doxazosin's antihypertensive effects hasn't been observed.
• No apparent differences exist in hypotensive response of whites and blacks or of elderly patients.
• In overdose, keep patient supine to restore blood pressure and heart rate. If necessary, treat shock with volume expanders. Administer vasopressors and monitor patient; support renal function.

Monitoring the patient
• Monitor hepatic function before treatment.
• Orthostatic effects are most likely to occur 2 to 6 hours after dose. Monitor blood pressure during this time after first dose and after subsequent increases in dosage. Daily doses above 4 mg increase potential of excessive orthostatic effects.
• First-dose effect (orthostatic hypotension) occurs with doxazosin but is less pronounced than with prazosin or terazosin.

Information for the patient
• Tell patient that orthostatic hypotension and syncope may occur, especially after first few doses and with dosage changes. Patient should rise slowly to prevent orthostatic hypertension.
• Caution patient that drug may cause drowsiness and somnolence. Patient should avoid driving and other hazardous tasks that require alertness for 12 to 24 hours after first dose, after dosage increases, and after resumption of interrupted therapy.
• Tell patient to report bothersome palpitations or dizziness.
• Tell patient drug may be taken with food if nausea occurs. Inform patient that nausea should improve as therapy continues.

Geriatric patients
• Use drug with caution in elderly patients with underlying autonomic dysfunction or arrhythmias.

Pediatric patients
• Safety and efficacy in children haven't been established.

Breast-feeding patients
• Because it's unknown if drug appears in breast milk, caution should be used if giving the drug to breast-feeding women.

doxepin hydrochloride
Sinequan, Triadapin*

Pharmacologic classification: tricyclic antidepressant
Therapeutic classification: antidepressant
Pregnancy risk category NR

How supplied
Available by prescription only
Capsules: 10 mg, 25 mg, 50 mg, 75 mg, 100 mg, 150 mg
Oral concentrate: 10 mg/ml

Indications, route, and dosage
Depression or anxiety
Adults: Initially, 25 to 75 mg P.O. daily in divided doses, to a maximum of 300 mg daily. Or give entire maintenance dosage once daily with a maximum dose of 150 mg P.O.
✦ **Dosage adjustment.** Reduce dosage in elderly, debilitated, and adolescent patients and in those receiving other drugs (especially anticholinergics).

Pharmacodynamics
Antidepressant action: Thought to exert its antidepressant effects by inhibiting reuptake of norepinephrine and serotonin in CNS nerve terminals (presynaptic neurons), which results in increased levels and enhanced activity of these neurotransmitters in the synaptic cleft. More actively inhibits reuptake of serotonin than norepinephrine. Anxiolytic effects of this drug usually precede antidepressant effects. Also may be used as an anxiolytic. It has the greatest sedative effect of all tricyclic antidepressants; tolerance to this effect usually develops in a few weeks.

Pharmacokinetics
• *Absorption:* Absorbed rapidly from GI tract after oral administration.
• *Distribution:* Distributed widely into body, including CNS and breast milk. 90% protein-bound. Peak effect occurs in 2 to 4 hours; steady-state achieved within 7 days. Therapeutic levels (par-

ent drug and metabolite) range from 150 to 250 ng/ml.
• *Metabolism:* Metabolized by liver to active metabolite desmethyldoxepin. A significant first-pass effect may explain variability of serum levels in different patients taking same dosage.
• *Excretion:* Mostly excreted in urine.

Contraindications and precautions
Contraindicated in patients with hypersensitivity to drug and in those with glaucoma or tendency to retain urine.

Interactions
Drug-drug. *Antiarrhythmics (disopyramide, procainamide, quinidine), pimozide, thyroid drugs:* May increase risk of cardiac arrhythmias and conduction defects. Monitor patient closely.
Antihistamines, antiparkinsonians, atropine, meperidine, other anticholinergics (such as phenothiazines): May cause oversedation, paralytic ileus, visual changes, and severe constipation. Monitor patient for effects.
Barbiturates: Induced doxepin metabolism and decreased therapeutic efficacy. Observe for effects. Dosage adjustments may be needed.
Beta blockers, cimetidine, fluoxetine, methylphenidate, oral contraceptives, propoxyphene, sertraline: May inhibit doxepin metabolism, increasing plasma levels and toxicity. Monitor patient for effects. Dosage adjustments may be needed.
Centrally acting antihypertensives (such as clonidine, guanabenz, guanadrel, guanethidine, methyldopa, reserpine): May decrease hypotensive effects. Monitor blood pressure closely.
Clonidine: Increased hypertensive effect. Monitor blood pressure closely.
CNS depressants (such as analgesics, anesthetics, barbiturates, narcotics, tranquilizers): Possible additive effects. Use cautiously and monitor patient closely.
Disulfiram, ethchlorvynol: May cause delirium and tachycardia. Monitor patient closely.
Haloperidol, phenothiazines: Decreased metabolism of drug, decreasing therapeutic efficacy. Observe for effects. Dosage adjustments may be needed.
MAO inhibitors: May cause severe excitation, hyperpyrexia, or seizures, usually with high dose. Monitor patient closely.
Metrizamide: May cause increased risk of seizures. Monitor patient closely.
Sympathomimetics (such as ephedrine [often found in nasal sprays], epinephrine, norepinephrine, phenylephrine, phenylpropanolamine): May increase blood pressure. Monitor blood pressure.
Warfarin: Additive effects may cause bleeding. Monitor INR.
Drug-lifestyle. *Alcohol:* Induced doxepin metabolism, decreased therapeutic efficacy, and enhanced CNS depression. Discourage use.

Heavy smoking: Induces doxepin metabolism and decreases therapeutic efficacy. Discourage use.
Sun exposure: Increases risk of photosensitivity reactions. Tell patient to take precautions.

Adverse reactions
CNS: *drowsiness, dizziness,* confusion, numbness, hallucinations, paresthesia, ataxia, weakness, headache, **seizures,** extrapyramidal reactions.
CV: *orthostatic hypotension, tachycardia,* ECG changes.
EENT: *blurred vision,* tinnitus.
GI: dry mouth, constipation, nausea, vomiting, anorexia.
GU: urine retention.
Hematologic: *eosinophilia, bone marrow depression.*
Hepatic: elevated liver function tests.
Metabolic: hyperglycemia, hypoglycemia.
Skin: *diaphoresis,* rash, urticaria, photosensitivity.
Other: *hypersensitivity reaction.*
    After abrupt withdrawal of long-term therapy: nausea, headache, malaise (doesn't indicate addiction).

☑ Special considerations
• Recommendations for administration of doxepin, care of patients during therapy, and use in pediatric patients are the same as those for all tricyclic antidepressants.
• Doxepin may prolong conduction time (elongation of QT and PR intervals, flattened T waves on ECG); it also may elevate liver function test results, decrease WBC counts, and decrease or increase serum glucose levels.
• The first 12 hours after acute ingestion are a stimulatory phase characterized by excessive anticholinergic activity (agitation, irritation, confusion, hallucinations, hyperthermia, parkinsonian symptoms, seizures, urine retention, dry mucous membranes, pupillary dilatation, constipation, and ileus). Then CNS depressant effects, including hypothermia, decreased or absent reflexes, sedation, hypotension, cyanosis, and cardiac irregularities, including tachycardia, conduction disturbances, and quinidine-like effects on the ECG.
• Severity of overdose is best indicated by widening of QRS complex. Usually, this represents a serum level in excess of 1,000 ng/ml. Serum levels usually aren't helpful. Metabolic acidosis may follow hypotension, hypoventilation, and seizures.
• Treatment of overdose is symptomatic and supportive, including maintaining airway, stable body temperature, and fluid and electrolyte balance. Induce emesis with ipecac if patient is conscious; follow with gastric lavage and activated charcoal to prevent further absorption. Dialysis is of little use.

Reactions may be *common*, uncommon, **life-threatening**, or COMMON AND LIFE-THREATENING.

• Physostigmine may be cautiously used to reverse central anticholinergic effects.
• Treat seizures with parenteral diazepam or phenytoin, arrhythmias with parenteral phenytoin or lidocaine, and acidosis with sodium bicarbonate. Don't give barbiturates; these may enhance CNS and respiratory depressant effects.

Monitoring the patient
• Monitor serum coagulation studies if patient is taking oral anticoagulants.
• Monitor serum glucose level if patient is a diabetic.
• Monitor patient for signs and symptoms of arrhythmias.

Information for the patient
• Teach patient to dilute oral concentrate with 4 oz (120 ml) water, milk, or juice (grapefruit, orange, pineapple, prune, or tomato). Drug is incompatible with carbonated beverages.
• Tell patient to use ice chips, sugarless gum or hard candy, or saliva substitutes to treat dry mouth.
• Warn patient to avoid taking other drugs while taking doxepin unless they have been prescribed.
• Instruct patient to take full dose at bedtime.

Geriatric patients
• Elderly patients are more likely to develop adverse CNS reactions, orthostatic hypotension, and GI and GU disturbances.

Pediatric patients
• Doxepin is rarely used for treatment of anxiety in children.

Breast-feeding patients
• Drug appears in breast milk. Avoid use in breast-feeding women, especially if high doses are used.

---

doxercalciferol
Hectorol

Pharmacologic classification: synthetic vitamin D analogue
Therapeutic classification: parathyroid hormone antagonist
Pregnancy risk category B

How supplied
Available by prescription only
Capsules: 2.5 mcg

Indication, route, and dosage
Reduction of elevated intact parathyroid hormone (PTH) levels in the management of secondary hyperparathyroidism in patients undergoing long-term renal dialysis
Adults: Initially, 10 mcg P.O. three times weekly at dialysis. Dosage adjusted as needed to lower intact PTH levels to 150 to 300 pg/ml. Dosage

may be increased by 2.5 mcg at 8-week intervals if the intact PTH level isn't decreased by 50% and fails to reach target range. Maximum dose is 20 mcg P.O. three times weekly. If intact PTH levels fall below 100 pg/ml, drug should be suspended for 1 week, then resumed at a dose that's at least 2.5 mcg lower than the last administered dose.

Pharmacodynamics
PTH antagonist action: Once activated, drug and other biologically active vitamin D metabolites regulate blood calcium levels required for essential body functions. Doxercalciferol acts directly on the parathyroid glands to suppress PTH synthesis and secretion. Also acts directly on bone cells (osteoblasts) to stimulate skeletal growth.

Pharmacokinetics
• *Absorption:* Absorbed from GI tract and peaks within 11 to 12 hours. Major metabolite attains peak blood levels at 11 to 12 hours after repeated oral doses.
• *Distribution:* No information available.
• *Metabolism:* Metabolized to active forms in the liver.
• *Excretion:* Elimination half-life is 32 to 37 hours, with a range of up to 96 hours.

Contraindications and precautions
Contraindicated in patients with recent history of hypercalcemia, hyperphosphatemia, or vitamin D toxicity. Use cautiously in patients with hepatic insufficiency.

Interactions
Drug-drug. *Antacids containing magnesium:* May cause hypermagnesemia. Avoid concomitant use.
Cholestyramine, mineral oil: Reduced intestinal absorption of doxercalciferol. Avoid concomitant use.
Glutethimide, phenobarbital, phenytoin, other enzyme inducers, other enzyme inhibitors: May affect metabolism of doxercalciferol. Adjust dosage as needed.
Phosphate binders containing calcium or non-aluminum: May cause hypercalcemia or hyperphosphatemia and decrease effectiveness of doxercalciferol. Use cautiously together; adjust dose of phosphate binders as needed.
Vitamin D supplements: May cause additive effects and hypercalcemia. Avoid concomitant use.

Adverse reactions
CNS: *dizziness, headache, malaise,* sleep disorder.
CV: *bradycardia, edema.*
GI: anorexia, dyspepsia, *nausea, vomiting,* constipation.
Metabolic: weight gain.
Musculoskeletal: arthralgia.

Respiratory: *dyspnea.*
Skin: pruritus.
Other: abscess.

☑ Special considerations
• Doxercalciferol is administered about every other day with dialysis. Dosing must be individualized and based on intact PTH levels, with monitoring of serum calcium and phosphorus levels before doxercalciferol therapy and weekly thereafter.
• Management of secondary hyperparathyroidism may prevent bone disease in patients with renal failure.
• Calcium-based or nonaluminum-containing phosphate binders and a low-phosphate diet are used to control serum phosphorus levels in patients undergoing dialysis. Expect that adjustments in doses of doxercalciferol and concurrent therapies will be needed in order to sustain PTH suppression and maintain serum calcium and phosphorus levels within acceptable ranges.
• Excessive doses can cause hypercalcemia, hypercalciuria, hyperphosphatemia, and oversuppression of PTH secretion.
• Progressive hypercalcemia secondary to vitamin D overdose may need emergency attention. Acute hypercalcemia may exacerbate arrhythmias and seizures and affects the action of digoxin. Chronic hypercalcemia can lead to vascular and soft-tissue calcification.
• If hypercalcemia, hyperphosphatemia, or a product of serum calcium × serum phosphorus (Ca × P) greater than 70 is noted, administration of doxercalciferol should be stopped immediately until these parameters are lowered.
• For hypercalcemia of greater than 1 mg/dl above the upper limit of normal, suspend doxercalciferol therapy immediately, institute a low-calcium diet, and withdraw calcium supplements.
• Check serum calcium levels weekly until levels return to normal, usually in 2 to 7 days. Dialysis, using a low-calcium or calcium-free dialysate, may correct persistently or markedly elevated serum calcium levels.
• When serum calcium levels have returned to within normal limits, drug can be restarted at a dose at least 2.5 mcg lower than previous therapy.
• For acute overdose, treatment should consist of general supportive measures. Within 10 minutes of ingestion, induce vomiting or perform gastric lavage to prevent further absorption. If postingestion time is more than 10 minutes, administer mineral oil to promote fecal elimination.
• Monitor serum calcium levels, the rate of urinary calcium excretion, and ECG findings. If serum calcium levels are persistently and markedly elevated, consider such drugs as corticosteroids or phosphates or such therapeutic measures as dialysis or forced diuresis.

Monitoring the patient
• Monitor calcium, phosphorus, and intact PTH levels. Monitor more frequently in patients with hepatic insufficiency.
• Monitor patient for adverse effects.

Information for the patient
• Inform patient that dose must be adjusted over several months to achieve satisfactory PTH suppression.
• Tell patient to adhere to a low-phosphorus diet and to follow instructions regarding calcium supplementation.
• Tell patient to obtain medical approval before using OTC drugs, including antacids and vitamin preparations containing calcium or vitamin D.
• Inform patient that early signs and symptoms of hypercalcemia include weakness, headache, somnolence, nausea, vomiting, dry mouth, constipation, muscle pain, bone pain, and metallic taste. Late signs and symptoms include polyuria, polydipsia, anorexia, weight loss, nocturia, conjunctivitis, pancreatitis, and photophobia.

Geriatric patients
• Safety and efficacy in elderly patients are unknown.

Pediatric patients
• Safety and efficacy in children haven't been established.

Breast-feeding patients
• It's unknown if drug appears in breast milk. Because other vitamin D derivatives appear in breast milk and because of the potential for serious adverse reactions in breast-feeding infants, a decision should be made to discontinue either drug or breast-feeding.

doxorubicin hydrochloride
Adriamycin PFS, Adriamycin RDF, Doxil, Rubex

Pharmacologic classification: antineoplastic antibiotic (cell cycle–phase nonspecific)
Therapeutic classification: antineoplastic
Pregnancy risk category D

How supplied
Available by prescription only
Injection: 10-mg, 20-mg, 50-mg, 100-mg, 150-mg vials
Injection (preservative-free): 2 mg/ml

Indications, route, and dosage
Dosage and indications may vary. Check current literature for recommended protocol.
Bladder, breast, lung, ovarian, stomach, and thyroid cancers; Hodgkin's disease; acute

lymphoblastic and myeloblastic leukemia; Wilms' tumor; neuroblastoma; lymphoma; sarcoma
Adults: 60 to 75 mg/m^2 I.V. as a single dose q 21 days; or 25 to 30 mg/m^2 I.V. as a single daily dose on days 1 to 3 of 4-week cycle. Or 20 mg/m^2 I.V. once weekly. Maximum cumulative dose is 550 mg/m^2 (450 mg/m^2 in patients who have received chest irradiation).

Pharmacodynamics
Antineoplastic action: Exerts cytotoxic activity by intercalating between DNA base pairs and un-coiling the DNA helix. The result is inhibition of DNA synthesis and DNA-dependent RNA synthesis. Also inhibits protein synthesis.

Pharmacokinetics
• *Absorption:* Because of its vesicant effects, must be administered I.V.
• *Distribution:* Distributed widely into body tissues, with highest levels found in liver, heart, and kidneys. Doesn't cross blood-brain barrier.
• *Metabolism:* Extensively metabolized by hepatic microsomal enzymes to several metabolites, one of which possesses cytotoxic activity.
• *Excretion:* Drug and metabolites excreted primarily in bile; minute amount eliminated in urine. Plasma elimination described as biphasic; half-life of about 15 to 30 minutes in initial phase and 16½ hours in terminal phase.

Contraindications and precautions
Contraindicated in patients with marked myelosuppression induced by previous treatment with other antitumor drugs or by radiotherapy and in those who have received lifetime cumulative dosage of 550 mg/m^2.

Interactions
Drug-drug. *Aminophylline, cephalosporins, dexamethasone phosphate, fluorouracil, heparin sodium, hydrocortisone, sodium phosphate:* Mixing with doxorubicin will result in precipitate. Don't administer together.
Cyclophosphamide, daunorubicin: May potentiate cardiotoxicity of doxorubicin through additive effects on heart. Monitor cardiac function closely.
Cyclophosphamide, mercaptopurine: May worsen cyclophosphamide-induced hemorrhagic cystitis and mercaptopurine-induced hepatotoxicity. Monitor patient closely.
Digoxin: Serum levels may be decreased if used with doxorubicin. Monitor digoxin levels.
Streptozocin: May increase plasma half-life of doxorubicin, increasing activity of doxorubicin. Monitor effects.
Drug-herb. *Green tea:* May enhance antitumor activity of doxorubicin. May be used for therapeutic effect.

Adverse reactions
CV: cardiac depression, seen in such ECG changes as sinus tachycardia, T-wave flattening, ST-segment depression, voltage reduction; *arrhythmias; acute left ventricular failure; irreversible cardiomyopathy.*
EENT: conjunctivitis.
GI: *nausea, vomiting,* diarrhea, *stomatitis,* esophagitis, anorexia.
GU: red urine (transient).
Hematologic: *leukopenia* during days 10 to 15 with recovery by day 21, *thrombocytopenia,* MYELOSUPPRESSION.
Metabolic: hyperuricemia.
Skin: urticaria, facial flushing.
Other: *severe cellulitis or tissue sloughing* (if drug extravasates); *complete alopecia within 3 to 4 weeks* (hair may regrow 2 to 5 months after drug is stopped); fever; chills, *anaphylaxis.*

☑ Special considerations
• To reconstitute, add 5 ml of normal saline injection, USP, to the 10-mg vial, 10 ml to the 20-mg vial, and 25 ml to the 50-mg vial to yield a concentration of 2 mg/ml.
• Drug may be further diluted with normal saline solution or D$_5$W and administered by I.V. infusion.
• Drug may be administered by I.V. push injection over 5 to 10 minutes into tubing of a free-flowing I.V. infusion.
• Alternative dosage schedule (once-weekly dosing) reduces risk of cardiomyopathy.
• If cumulative dose exceeds 550 mg/m^2 body surface area, 30% of patients develop cardiac adverse reactions, which begin 2 weeks to 6 months after stopping drug. With high doses of doxorubicin, consider concomitant dosing with the cardioprotective drug dexrazoxane.
• Streaking along a vein or facial flushing indicates that drug is being administered too rapidly.
• Applying a scalp tourniquet or ice may decrease alopecia. However, don't use these if treating leukemias or other neoplasms where tumor stem cells may be present in scalp.
• Esophagitis is common in patients who have also received radiation therapy.
• Signs and symptoms of overdose include myelosuppression, nausea, vomiting, mucositis, and irreversible myocardial toxicity. Treatment is usually supportive and includes transfusion of blood components, antiemetics, antibiotics for infections which may develop, symptomatic treatment of mucositis, and cardiac glycoside preparations.

Monitoring the patient
• Monitor CBC before treatment and periodically throughout.
• Monitor serum digoxin levels if patient is taking digoxin.
• Stop drug or slow rate of infusion if tachycardia develops.

• Monitor patient for extravasation. Treat with topical application of dimethyl sulfoxide and ice packs.
• Monitor hepatic function.
• Decrease dosage as follows if serum bilirubin level increases: 50% of dose when bilirubin level is 1.2 to 3 mg/100 ml; 25% of dose when bilirubin level exceeds 3 mg/100 ml.

Information for the patient
• Encourage adequate fluid intake to increase urine output and facilitate excretion of uric acid.
• Advise patient to avoid exposure to people with infections.
• Warn patient that alopecia will occur. Explain that hair growth should resume 2 to 5 months after drug is stopped.
• Advise patient that urine will appear red for 1 to 2 days after dose and doesn't indicate bleeding. Urine may stain clothes.
• Tell patient not to receive immunizations during therapy and for several weeks afterward. Other members of patient's household also should not receive immunizations during same period.
• Tell patient to call if unusual bruising or bleeding or signs of infection occur.

Geriatric patients
• Patients over age 70 have an increased risk of drug-induced cardiotoxicity. Use caution in elderly patients with low bone marrow reserve to prevent serious hematologic toxicity.

Pediatric patients
• Children under age 2 have a greater risk of drug-induced cardiotoxicity.

Breast-feeding patients
• It's unknown if drug appears in breast milk. Because of risk of serious adverse reactions, mutagenicity, and carcinogenicity in infant, breast-feeding isn't recommended.

---

doxorubicin hydrochloride liposomal
Doxil

Pharmacologic classification: anthracycline
Therapeutic classification: antineoplastic
Pregnancy risk category D

How supplied
Available by prescription only
Injection: 2 mg/ml

Indications, route, and dosage
Metastatic carcinoma of ovary in patients with disease refractory to both paclitaxel- and platinum-based chemotherapy regimens
Adults: 50 mg/m² (doxorubicin hydrochloride equivalent) I.V. at initial infusion rate of 1 mg/minute

once every 4 weeks for minimum of four courses. Continue as long as condition doesn't progress and patient shows no evidence of cardiotoxicity and continues to tolerate treatment. If no infusion-related adverse effects are observed, increase infusion rate to complete administration over 1 hour.
AIDS-related Kaposi's sarcoma in patients with disease that has progressed on previous combination chemotherapy and in patients intolerant to such therapy
Adults: 20 mg/m² (doxorubicin hydrochloride equivalent) I.V. over 30 minutes once every 3 weeks. Continue as long as patient responds satisfactorily and tolerates treatment.
✦ *Dosage adjustment.* For patients with impaired hepatic function, reduce dosage as follows: If serum bilirubin is 1.2 to 3 mg/dl, give one-half normal dose. If serum bilirubin is more than 3 mg/dl, give one-quarter normal dose.

The dosage adjustments on page 369 are recommended for palmar-plantar erythrodysesthesia, hematologic toxicity, and stomatitis.

Pharmacodynamics
Antineoplastic action: Drug is doxorubicin hydrochloride encapsulated in liposomes that, because of their small size and persistence in the circulation, are able to penetrate the altered vasculature of tumors. Mechanism of action is thought to be related to drug's ability to bind DNA and inhibit nucleic acid synthesis.

Pharmacokinetics
• *Absorption:* No information available.
• *Distribution:* Distributed mostly to vascular fluid. Plasma protein-binding not yet determined; however, plasma protein-binding of doxorubicin is about 70%.
• *Metabolism:* Doxorubicinol, major metabolite of doxorubicin, is detected at very low levels in plasma.
• *Excretion:* Plasma elimination is slow and biphasic; half-life of about 5 hours in first phase and 55 hours in second phase at doses of 10 to 20 mg/m².

Contraindications and precautions
Contraindicated in patients with hypersensitivity to drug or its components or any component in the liposomal formulation and in those with marked myelosuppression. Also contraindicated in patients who have received a lifetime cumulative dose of 550 mg/m², or 400 mg/m² in patients who have received radiotherapy to the mediastinal area or therapy with other cardiotoxic drugs such as cyclophosphamide. Use in patients with history of cardiovascular disease only when benefit of drug outweighs risk to patient.

Use cautiously in patients who have received other anthracyclines. For total dose, also take into account any previous or concomitant therapy with related compounds such as daunorubicin. Heart

---

...tions may be *common*, uncommon, **life-threatening**, or COMMON AND LIFE-THREATENING.

DOSAGE ADJUSTMENTS

Palmer-plantar erythrodysesthesia

Grade	Symptoms	Dosage adjustment
1	Mild erythema, swelling, or desquamation not interfering with daily activities	Redose unless patient has experienced a previous grade 3 or 4 skin toxicity. If so, delay dose up to 2 weeks and decrease by 25%. Return to original dosing interval.
2	Erythema, desquamation, or swelling interfering with but not precluding normal physical activities; small blisters or ulcerations less than 2 cm in diameter	Delay dosing up to 2 weeks or until resolved to grade 0 to 1. If no resolution after 2 weeks, discontinue drug.
3	Blistering, ulceration, or swelling interfering with walking or normal daily activities; patient can't wear regular clothing	Delay dosing up to 2 weeks or until resolved to grade 0 to 1. Decrease dose by 25% and return to original dosing interval. If no resolution after 2 weeks, discontinue drug.
4	Diffuse or local process causing infectious complications, a bedridden state, or hospitalization	Delay dosing up to 2 weeks or until resolved to grade 0 to 1. Decrease dose by 25% and return to original dosing interval. If no resolution after 2 weeks, discontinue drug.

Hematologic toxicity

Grade	ANC (cells/mm³)	Platelets (cells/mm³)	Dosage adjustment
1	1,500 to 1,900	75,000 to 150,000	Resume treatment with no dose reduction.
2	1,000 to < 1,500	50,000 to < 75,000	Wait until ANC > 1,500 and platelets > 75,000; redose with no dose reduction.
3	500 to 999	25,000 to < 50,000	Wait until ANC ≥ 1,500 and platelets ≥ 75,000; redose with no dose reduction.
4	< 500	< 25,000	Wait until ANC ≥ 1,500 and platelets ≥ 75,000; redose at 25% dose reduction or continue full dose with cytokine support.

Stomatitis

Grade	Symptoms	Dosage adjustment
1	Painless ulcers, erythema, or mild soreness	Redose unless patient has experienced previous grade 3 or 4 toxicity. If so, delay dose up to 2 weeks and decrease dosage by 25%. Return to original dosing interval.
2	Painful erythema, edema, or ulcers; patient can eat	Delay dosing up to 2 weeks or until resolved to grade 0 or 1. If no resolution after 2 weeks, discontinue drug.
3	Painful erythema, edema, or ulcers; patient can't eat	Delay dosing up to 2 weeks or until resolved to grade 0 or 1. Decrease dose by 25% and return to original dosing interval. If no resolution after 2 weeks, discontinue drug.
4	Patient needs parenteral or enteral support	Delay dosing up to 2 weeks or until resolved to grade 0 or 1. Decrease dose by 25% and return to original dosing interval. If no resolution after 2 weeks, discontinue drug.

failure and cardiomyopathy may occur after stopping drug.

Interactions

None reported. However, drug may interact with drugs known to affect conventional formulation of doxorubicin hydrochloride.

Adverse reactions

CNS: *asthenia,* paresthesia, headache, somnolence, dizziness, depression, insomnia, anxiety, malaise, emotional lability, fatigue.
CV: chest pain, hypotension, tachycardia, peripheral edema, cardiomyopathy, ***heart failure, arrhythmias,*** pericardial effusion.

EENT: *mucous membrane disorder,* mouth ulceration, pharyngitis, rhinitis, conjunctivitis, retinitis, optic neuritis.
GI: *nausea, vomiting, constipation, anorexia, diarrhea,* abdominal pain, dyspepsia, oral candidiasis, enlarged abdomen, esophagitis, dysphagia, *stomatitis,* taste perversion, glossitis.
GU: albuminuria.
Hematologic: LEUKOPENIA, NEUTROPENIA, THROMBOCYTOPENIA, *anemia,* increased PT.
Hepatic: hyperbilirubinemia.
Metabolic: dehydration, weight loss, hypocalcemia, hyperglycemia.
Musculoskeletal: myalgia, back pain.
Respiratory: dyspnea, increased cough, pneumonia.
Skin: *rash, alopecia,* dry skin, pruritus, skin discoloration, skin disorder, exfoliative dermatitis, herpes zoster, sweating, *palmar-plantar erythrodysesthesia,* alopecia.
Other: fever, allergic reaction, chills, infection, infusion-related reactions.

☑ Special considerations
● Drug exhibits unique pharmacokinetic properties compared to conventional doxorubicin hydrochloride and shouldn't be substituted on a mg per mg basis.
● Drug may potentiate toxicity of other antineoplastic therapies.
● Evaluate patient's hepatic function before therapy and adjust dosage accordingly.
● Leukopenia is usually transient. Hematologic toxicity may require dose reduction or suspension or delay of therapy. Persistent severe myelosuppression may result in superinfection or hemorrhage. Patient may require granulocyte-colony stimulating factor (G-CSF or granulocyte macrophage [GM]-CSF) to support blood counts.
● Acute overdose causes increases in mucositis, leukopenia, and thrombocytopenia.
● Treat acute overdose (severely myelosuppressed patient) with hospitalization, antibiotics, platelet and granulocyte transfusions, and symptomatic treatment of mucositis.

Monitoring the patient
● Monitor cardiac function closely by endomyocardial biopsy, echocardiography, or gated radionuclide scans. If results indicate possible cardiac injury, benefits of continued therapy must be weighed against risk of myocardial injury.
● Monitor CBC, including platelets, before each dose and frequently throughout therapy.

Information for the patient
● Tell patient to report any symptoms of hand-foot syndrome, such as tingling or burning, redness, flaking, bothersome swelling, small blisters, or small sores on palms of hands or soles of feet.

● Advise patient to report symptoms of stomatitis, such as painful redness, swelling, or sores in mouth.
● Advise patient to avoid exposure to people with infections. Tell patient to report temperature of 100.5° F (38° C) or higher.
● Inform patient to report nausea, vomiting, tiredness, weakness, rash, or mild hair loss.
● Advise woman of childbearing age to avoid pregnancy during therapy.

Geriatric patients
● No overall differences were observed between elderly and younger patients, but greater sensitivity in some elderly patients can't be ruled out.

Pediatric patients
● Safety and effectiveness in children haven't been established.

Breast-feeding patients
● It's unknown if drug appears in breast milk. Because many drugs appear in breast milk and because of potential for serious adverse reactions in breast-feeding infants, mothers should stop breast-feeding before taking drug.

doxycycline
Vibramycin

doxycycline calcium
Vibramycin

doxycycline hyclate
Doryx, Doxy 100, Doxy 200, Doxy Caps, Vibramycin, Vibra-Tabs

doxycycline monohydrate
Monodox, Vibramycin

Pharmacologic classification: tetracycline
Therapeutic classification: antibiotic
Pregnancy risk category D

How supplied
Available by prescription only
doxycycline
Oral suspension: 25 mg/5 ml
doxycycline calcium
Syrup: 50 mg/5 ml
doxycycline hyclate
Tablets: 50mg, 100 mg
Capsules: 50 mg, 100 mg
Injection: 100 mg, 200 mg
doxycycline monohydrate
Capsules: 50 mg, 100 mg
Oral suspension: 25 mg/5 ml

Indications, route, and dosage

Infections caused by sensitive organisms
Adults and children weighing 45 kg (99 lb) and over: 100 mg P.O. q 12 hours on day 1, then 100 mg P.O. daily; or 200 mg I.V. on day 1 in one or two infusions, then 100 to 200 mg I.V. daily.
Children over age 8 weighing less than 45 kg: 4.4 mg/kg P.O. or I.V. daily, divided q 12 hours day 1, then 2.2 to 4.4 mg/kg daily.
Give I.V. infusion slowly (minimum 1 hour). Infusion must be completed within 12 hours (within 6 hours in lactated Ringer's solution or D₅W in lactated Ringer's solution).

Gonorrhea in patients allergic to penicillin
Adults: 100 mg P.O. b.i.d. for 7 days; or 300 mg P.O. initially and repeat dose in 1 hour.

◊ *Syphilis in patients allergic to penicillin*
Adults: 100 mg P.O. b.i.d. for 2 weeks (early detection) or 4 weeks (if more than 1 year's duration).

Chlamydia trachomatis, nongonococcal urethritis, and uncomplicated urethral, endocervical, or rectal infections
Adults: 100 mg P.O. b.i.d. for at least 7 days.

Acute pelvic inflammatory disease (PID)
Adults: 250 mg I.M. ceftriaxone, then 100 mg doxycycline P.O. b.i.d. for 10 to 14 days.

Acute epididymoorchitis caused by C. trachomatis or Neisseria gonorrhoeae
Adults: 100 mg P.O. b.i.d for at least 10 days.

◊ *To prevent traveler's diarrhea commonly caused by enterotoxigenic Escherichia coli*
Adults: 100 mg P.O. daily for up to 3 days.

◊ *Prophylaxis for rape victims*
Adults and adolescents: 100 mg P.O. b.i.d. for 7 days after a single 2-g oral dose of metronidazole is given in conjunction with a single 125-mg I.M. dose of ceftriaxone.

Chemoprophylaxis for malaria in travelers to areas where chloroquine-resistant Plasmodium falciparum is endemic and mefloquine is contraindicated
Adults: 100 mg P.O. once daily. Begin prophylaxis 1 to 2 days before travel to malarious areas; continue daily while in affected area, and continue for 4 weeks after return from malarious area.
Children over age 8: Give 2 mg/kg P.O. daily as a single dose; don't exceed 100 mg daily. Use the same dosage schedule as for adults.

◊ *Lyme disease*
Adults and children ages 9 and older: 100 mg P.O. b.i.d. or t.i.d. for 10 to 30 days.

◊ *Pleural effusions associated with cancer*
Adults: 500 mg of doxycycline diluted in 250 ml of normal saline and instilled into pleural space via a chest tube.

Pharmacodynamics
Antibacterial action: Bacteriostatic; binds reversibly to ribosomal units, thereby inhibiting bacterial protein synthesis.

Drug's spectrum of activity includes many gram-negative and gram-positive organisms, *Mycoplasma, Rickettsia, Chlamydia,* and spirochetes.

Pharmacokinetics
● *Absorption:* 90% to 100% absorbed after oral administration; serum levels peak at 1½ to 4 hours. Drug has least affinity for calcium of all tetracyclines; absorption is insignificantly altered by milk or other dairy products.
● *Distribution:* Distributed widely into body tissues and fluids, including synovial, pleural, prostatic, seminal fluids; bronchial secretions; saliva; aqueous humor. Poor CSF penetration. Readily crosses placenta; 25% to 93% protein-bound.
● *Metabolism:* Insignificantly metabolized; some hepatic degradation occurs.
● *Excretion:* Excreted primarily unchanged in urine by glomerular filtration; some may be excreted in breast milk. Plasma half-life 22 to 24 hours after multiple dosing in adults with normal renal function; 20 to 30 hours in patients with severe renal impairment. Some drug excreted in feces.

Contraindications and precautions
Contraindicated in patients with hypersensitivity to drug or other tetracyclines. Use cautiously in patients with impaired renal or hepatic function. Use during last half of pregnancy and in children under age 8 may cause permanent discoloration of teeth, enamel defects, and bone growth retardation.

Interactions
Drug-drug. *Antacids containing aluminum, calcium, magnesium; laxatives containing magnesium:* Decreased oral absorption of doxycycline because of chelation. Monitor patient for effects.
Carbamazepine, phenobarbital: May cause decreased antibiotic effect. Monitor patient for effects.
Digoxin: Increased bioavailability. Concomitant use requires lowered dosages of digoxin.
Methoxyflurane: May cause nephrotoxicity with tetracyclines. Use cautiously together; monitor renal function.
Oral anticoagulants: Enhanced effects. Concomitant use requires lowered dosage of oral anticoagulants.
Oral contraceptives: May cause decreased contraceptive effectiveness and increase risk of breakthrough bleeding. Tell patient to use alternative means of birth control.
Oral iron products, sodium bicarbonate, zinc: Impaired absorption of tetracyclines. Use cautiously and monitor patient for effects.
Penicillin: May antagonize bactericidal effects of penicillin, inhibiting cell growth. Administer penicillin 2 to 3 hours before doxycycline.
Drug-lifestyle. *Alcohol:* May decrease antibiotic effect. Discourage use.

Sun exposure: May cause photosensitivity reactions. Tell patient to take precautions.

Adverse reactions
CNS: *intracranial hypertension (pseudotumor cerebri).*
CV: pericarditis.
EENT: glossitis, dysphagia.
GI: anorexia, *epigastric distress, nausea,* vomiting, *diarrhea,* oral candidiasis, enterocolitis, anogenital inflammation.
Hematologic: *neutropenia,* eosinophilia, *thrombocytopenia,* hemolytic anemia.
Hepatic: elevated liver enzymes.
Skin: *maculopapular and erythematous rashes, photosensitivity, increased pigmentation, urticaria.*
Other: hypersensitivity reactions *(anaphylaxis);* permanent discoloration of teeth, enamel defects, bone growth retardation if used in children under age 8; superinfection; thrombophlebitis.

☑ Special considerations
Besides the recommendations relevant to all tetracyclines, consider the following.
• Reconstitute powder for injection with sterile water for injection. Use 10 ml in a 100-mg vial and 20 ml in a 200-mg vial. Dilute solution to 100 to 1,000 ml for I.V. infusion. Don't infuse solutions more concentrated than 1 mg/ml.
• Reconstituted solution is stable for 72 hours if refrigerated and protected from light.
• Don't inject S.C. or I.M.
• Drug may be used in patients with impaired renal function; it doesn't accumulate or cause a significant rise in BUN levels.
• Drug causes false elevations in fluorometric tests for urinary catecholamines.
• Drug causes false-negative results in urine tests using glucose oxidase reagent (Diastix, Chemstrip uG, or glucose enzymatic test strip); parenteral dosage form may cause false-negative Clinitest results.
• Signs and symptoms of overdose are usually limited to GI tract; give antacids or empty stomach by gastric lavage if ingestion occurred within preceding 4 hours.

Monitoring the patient
• Monitor renal and hepatic function.
• Monitor serum coagulation studies if patient is taking oral anticoagulants.

Information for the patient
• Avoid drug in children under age 8 unless other drugs prove ineffective or are contraindicated.

Breast-feeding patients
• Avoid use in breast-feeding women.

dronabinol
Marinol

Pharmacologic classification: cannabinoid
Therapeutic classification: antiemetic, appetite stimulant
Controlled substance schedule III
Pregnancy risk category C

How supplied
Available by prescription only
Capsules: 2.5 mg, 5 mg, 10 mg

Indications, route, and dosage
Nausea and vomiting associated with cancer chemotherapy
Adults and children: 5 mg/m² P.O. 1 to 3 hours before chemotherapy; then same dose q 2 to 4 hours after chemotherapy for a total of 4 to 6 doses daily. Dose may be increased in increments of 2.5 mg/m² to maximum of 15 mg/m² per dose.
Appetite stimulation in treatment of anorexia associated with AIDS-related weight loss
Adults: 2.5 mg P.O. b.i.d. before lunch and supper, increased, if necessary, to a maximum of 20 mg daily.

Pharmacodynamics
Antiemetic action: A synthetic cannabinoid that inhibits vomiting centers in the brain and possibly in the chemoreceptor trigger zone and other sites.

Pharmacokinetics
• *Absorption:* 90% to 95% of dose absorbed; action begins in 30 to 60 minutes, with peak action in 1 to 3 hours.
• *Distribution:* Distributed rapidly into many tissue sites. 97% to 99% protein-bound.
• *Metabolism:* Extensive metabolism in liver. Metabolite activity unknown.
• *Excretion:* Excreted primarily in feces via biliary tract. Drug effect may persist for several days after treatment ends; duration varies considerably among patients.

Contraindications and precautions
Contraindicated in patients with hypersensitivity to sesame oil or cannabinoids. Use cautiously in elderly, pregnant, or breast-feeding patients and in those with heart disease, psychiatric illness, or history of drug abuse.

Interactions
Drug-drug. *Anticholinergics:* May cause tachycardia. Monitor patient closely.
Psychotomimetic drugs, sedatives: Concomitant use may have additive sedative effect. Use cautiously; monitor patient closely.

Drug-lifestyle. *Alcohol:* May cause additive sedative effect. Discourage use.

Adverse reactions
CNS: *dizziness, drowsiness, euphoria, ataxia,* depersonalization, hallucinations, somnolence, headache, muddled thinking, asthenia, amnesia, confusion, *paranoia.*
CV: tachycardia, orthostatic hypotension, palpitations, vasodilation.
EENT: visual disturbances.
GI: *dry mouth, nausea, vomiting,* diarrhea.

☑ Special considerations
• Drug is used only in patients with nausea and vomiting resulting from cancer chemotherapy who don't respond to other treatment; give drug before chemotherapy infusion.
• Drug is major active ingredient of *Cannabis sativa* (marijuana); has potential for abuse.
• Treat overdose with symptomatic and supportive therapy. Observe patient in quiet environment and provide supportive measures.

Monitoring the patient
• Monitor frequency and degree of vomiting.
• Monitor pulse, blood pressure, and fluid intake and output to help prevent dehydration; observe for signs of confusion.

Information for the patient
• Warn patient to avoid driving and other activities requiring sound judgment until extent of CNS depressant effects are known.
• Urge family to ensure that patient is supervised by a responsible person during and immediately after treatment.
• Caution patient and family to anticipate drug's mood-altering effects.

Geriatric patients
• Elderly patients may be more susceptible to adverse reactions. Use with caution.

Breast-feeding patients
• Because drug appears in breast milk and is absorbed by breast-feeding infants, it shouldn't be given to breast-feeding women.

---

droperidol
Inapsine

Pharmacologic classification: butyrophenone derivative
Therapeutic classification: tranquilizer
Pregnancy risk category C

How supplied
Available by prescription only
Injection: 2.5 mg/ml

Indications, route, and dosage
Anesthetic premedication
Adults: 2.5 to 10 mg I.M. 30 to 60 minutes before induction of general anesthesia.
Children ages 2 to 12: 0.088 to 0.165 mg/kg I.V. or I.M.
Adjunct for induction of general anesthesia
Adults: 0.22 to 0.275 mg/kg I.V. (preferably) or I.M. with an analgesic or general anesthetic.
Children: 0.088 to 0.165 mg/kg I.V. or I.M.
Adjunct for maintenance of general anesthesia
Adults: 1.25 to 2.5 mg I.V.
For use without a general anesthetic during diagnostic procedures
Adults: 2.5 to 10 mg I.M. 30 to 60 minutes before the procedure. Additional doses of 1.25 to 2.5 mg I.V., p.r.n.
Adjunct to regional anesthesia
Adults: 2.5 to 5 mg I.M. or slow I.V. injection.
◇ **Antiemetic with cancer chemotherapy**
Adults: 6.25 mg I.M. or by slow I.V. injection.

Pharmacodynamics
Tranquilizer action: Produces marked sedation by directly blocking subcortical receptors. Also blocks CNS receptors at chemoreceptor trigger zone, producing an antiemetic effect.

Pharmacokinetics
• *Absorption:* Well absorbed after I.M. injection. Sedation begins in 3 to 10 minutes, peaks at 30 minutes, and lasts for 2 to 4 hours; some alteration of consciousness may persist for 12 hours.
• *Distribution:* Not well understood; crosses blood-brain barrier and is distributed in CSF. Also crosses placenta.
• *Metabolism:* Metabolized by liver to p-fluorophenylacetic acid and p-hydroxypiperidine.
• *Excretion:* Drug and metabolites excreted in urine and feces.

Contraindications and precautions
Contraindicated in patients with hypersensitivity or intolerance to drug. Use cautiously in patients with hypotension and other CV disease because of its vasodilatory effects, in patients with hepatic or renal disease in whom drug clearance may be impaired, and in patients taking other CNS depressants, including alcohol, opiates, and sedatives because droperidol may potentiate effects of these drugs.

Interactions
Drug-drug. *Analgesics, opiates:* Potentiated CNS depressant effects. Avoid concomitant use.
CNS depressants, such as barbiturates, sedative-hypnotics, tranquilizers: Possible additive or potentiating effect when used concomitantly. When used concurrently, reduce dosage of both drugs.

Fentanyl citrate: May cause hypertension and respiratory depression. Avoid concomitant use; if both drugs are necessary, use cautiously and monitor patient closely.
Drug-lifestyle. *Alcohol:* Potentiated CNS depressant effects. Discourage use.

Adverse reactions
CNS: *sedation,* altered consciousness, respiratory depression, postoperative hallucinations, extrapyramidal reactions (dystonia [extended tongue, stiff rotated neck, upward rotation of eyes], akathisia [restlessness], fine tremors of limbs), temporarily altered EEG pattern.
CV: *hypotension* with rebound tachycardia, **bradycardia** (occasional), decreased pulmonary artery pressure.

☑ Special considerations
● If opiates are needed during recovery from anesthesia to prevent potentiation of respiratory depression, use initially in reduced dosages (as low as one-fourth to one-third of usual recommended dosage).
● Drug has been used for its antiemetic effects in preventing or treating cancer chemotherapy–induced nausea and vomiting, especially that produced by cisplatin.
● Stop drug if patient shows signs of hypersensitivity, severe persistent hypotension, respiratory depression, paradoxical hypertension, or dystonia.
● Signs and symptoms of overdose include extension of drug's pharmacologic actions. Treat overdose symptomatically and supportively.

Monitoring the patient
● Monitor hepatic and renal function.
● Monitor blood pressure.
● Monitor vital signs and watch carefully for extrapyramidal reactions. Drug is related to haloperidol and is more likely than other antipsychotics to cause extrapyramidal symptoms.
● Observe patient for postoperative hallucinations or emergence delirium and drowsiness.
● Be prepared to treat severe hypotension.

Information for the patient
● Advise patient of possible postoperative effects.

Geriatric patients
● Use drug with caution in elderly patients because they are more prone to extrapyramidal reactions, CNS disturbances, and CV side effects than are younger patients.

Pediatric patients
● Safety and efficacy in children under age 2 haven't been established.

Breast-feeding patients
● It's unknown if drug appears in breast milk. Avoid use in breast-feeding women.

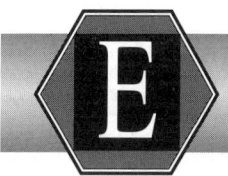

econazole nitrate
Spectazole

Pharmacologic classification: synthetic imidazole derivative
Therapeutic classification: antifungal
Pregnancy risk category C

How supplied
Available by prescription only
Cream: 1% (water-soluble base)

Indications, route, and dosage
Cutaneous candidiasis
Adults and children: Gently rub sufficient quantity into affected areas b.i.d. in morning and evening.
Tinea pedis, tinea cruris, tinea corporis, tinea versicolor
Adults and children: Gently rub into affected area once daily.

Pharmacodynamics
Antifungal action: Exact mechanism unknown. Thought to exert its effects by altering cellular membranes and interfering with intracellular enzymes. Active against many fungi, including dermatophytes and yeasts, as well as some gram-positive bacteria.

Pharmacokinetics
• *Absorption:* Minimal but rapid percutaneous absorption.
• *Distribution:* Minimal.
• *Metabolism:* No information available.
• *Excretion:* No information available.

Contraindications and precautions
Contraindicated in patients with hypersensitivity to drug.

Interactions
None reported.

Adverse reactions
Skin: burning, pruritus, stinging, erythema.

☑ Special considerations
• Wash affected area with soap and water; dry thoroughly before applying drug.
• Don't apply drug to eye or administer intravaginally.

• If a reaction suggesting sensitivity or chemical irritation occurs, discontinue therapy.

Monitoring the patient
• Monitor patient for adverse effects.
• Monitor therapeutic effect.

Information for the patient
• Instruct patient to wash hands well after application.
• Advise patient to use medication for entire treatment period, even though symptoms lessen. Relief of symptoms usually occurs within 1 to 2 weeks of therapy.
• Inform patient with tinea pedis (athlete's foot) to wear well-fitting, well-ventilated shoes and to change shoes and all-cotton socks daily.

Breast-feeding patients
• It's unknown if drug appears breast milk; use with caution in breast-feeding women.

edetate calcium disodium (calcium EDTA)
Calcium Disodium Versenate

Pharmacologic classification: chelating drug
Therapeutic classification: heavy metal antagonist
Pregnancy risk category NR

How supplied
Available by prescription only
Injection: 200 mg/ml

Indications, route, and dosage
Acute lead encephalopathy or blood lead levels above 70 mcg/dl
Adults and children: 1.5 g/m² I.V. or I.M. daily in divided doses at 12-hour intervals for 3 to 5 days, usually given with dimercaprol. Administer second course in 5 to 7 days, if necessary.
Lead poisoning without encephalopathy or asymptomatic with blood levels below 70 mcg/dl
Children: 1 g/m² I.V. or I.M. daily in divided doses.
◇ **Other heavy metal poisonings**
Adults: 1 g in 500 ml of D_5W or normal saline injection infused I.V. over a 5-hour period once daily for 3 days.

Pharmacodynamics
Chelating action: Calcium in edetate calcium disodium is displaced by divalent and trivalent heavy metals, forming a soluble complex, which is then excreted in urine, removing the heavy metal.

Pharmacokinetics
• *Absorption:* Well absorbed after I.M. or S.C. injection. After I.V. administration, chelated lead appears in urine within 1 hour; excretion of lead peaks in 24 to 48 hours.
• *Distribution:* Distributed primarily in extracellular fluid.
• *Metabolism:* None.
• *Excretion:* Excreted rapidly in urine. After I.V. administration, 50% of drug excreted in urine unchanged or as a metal chelate in 1 hour; 95% of drug excreted in 24 hours.

Contraindications and precautions
Contraindicated in patients with anuria, hepatitis, and acute renal disease. Use with extreme caution in patients with mild renal disease.

Interactions
Drug-drug. *Zinc insulin:* Interference with action of insulin by binding with zinc. Monitor glucose levels; insulin dose may need adjustment.

Adverse reactions
CNS: tremor, headache, numbness, tingling, malaise, fatigue.
CV: hypotension, cardiac rhythm irregularities.
GI: cheilosis, nausea, vomiting, anorexia, thirst.
GU: proteinuria, hematuria, ***nephrotoxicity with renal tubular necrosis leading to fatal nephrosis.***
Hematologic: transient bone marrow depression.
Hepatic: *mild increases in ALT and AST levels.*
Musculoskeletal: myalgia, arthralgia.
Other: pain at I.M. injection site, fever, chills.

☑ Special considerations
• Add 1% procaine or lidocaine to solution before I.M. injection to decrease pain at site.
• Avoid rapid I.V. infusion and infusions of large fluid volumes in patients with lead encephalopathy.
• Hydrate patients before giving drug to ensure adequate urine flow; monitor renal status frequently.
• Parenterally administered edetate calcium disodium has been used in poisoning by radioactive and nuclear fusion products and other heavy metals except mercury, gold, or arsenic poisoning. Has also been used to aid diagnosis of lead poisoning.
• For I.V. infusion, dilute drug with D_5W solution or normal saline; administer one-half the daily dose over at least 1 hour in asymptomatic pa-

tients, 2 hours in symptomatic patients. The second daily infusion should be given 6 or more hours after the first infusion. If administered as a single dose, infuse over 12 to 24 hours.
• If drug is administered as a continuous I.V. infusion, interrupt infusion for at least 1 hour before a blood lead level reading to avoid a falsely elevated value.
• Signs and symptoms of overdose include acute renal failure with anuria and altered consciousness consistent with increased intracranial pressure, in patients with lead encephalopathy. Reduce intracranial pressure with hyperventilation and furosemide or mannitol; monitor vital signs and ECG closely.
• Barbiturate infusion may be needed in severe cases; hemodialysis may be needed in acute renal failure.

Monitoring the patient
• Monitor infusion site closely. Extravasation severely irritates tissue; rotate infusion sites with multiple doses or long-term therapy.
• Monitor calcium levels, and observe patient for seizures or altered vital signs and ECG during infusion. Administer infusion over at least 3 hours; have patient remain supine for 20 to 30 minutes after infusion because of possible orthostatic hypotension. Drug also exerts a negative inotropic effect on the heart.
• Monitor hepatic and renal function before treatment and periodically throughout.
• Monitor intake and output, urinalysis, BUN level, and ECG throughout treatment; interrupt I.V. for 1 hour before drawing blood.

Information for the patient
• Explain measures as needed to avoid future heavy metal poisoning.

Pediatric patients
• I.M. route is recommended for children.

edetate disodium (EDTA)
Disotate, Endrate

Pharmacologic classification: chelating drug
Therapeutic classification: heavy metal antagonist
Pregnancy risk category NR

How supplied
Available by prescription only
Injection: 150 mg/ml

Indications, route, and dosage
Hypercalcemia
Adults: 50 mg/kg daily by slow I.V. infusion to a maximum of 3 g in 24 hours. Dilute in 500 ml of

D_5W or normal saline solution. Give over 3 or more hours.

Children: 40 mg/kg by slow I.V. infusion, diluted to a maximum concentration of 30 mg/ml in D_5W or normal saline solution administered over 3 or more hours. Maximum daily dose is 70 mg/kg.

Cardiac glycoside–induced ventricular arrhythmias
Adults and children: I.V. infusion of 15 mg/kg/hour; maximum dose is 60 mg/kg daily. Dilute in D_5W.

Pharmacodynamics
Chelating action: Binds many divalent and trivalent ions but has the strongest affinity for calcium, with which it forms a stable complex readily excreted by the kidneys. Also chelates magnesium, zinc, and other trace metals, increasing their excretion in urine; doesn't decrease CSF calcium levels.

Pharmacokinetics
• *Absorption:* Absorbed poorly from GI tract.
• *Distribution:* Doesn't enter CSF in significant amounts but is distributed widely throughout rest of body.
• *Metabolism:* None.
• *Excretion:* After I.V. administration, is excreted rapidly in urine; 95% of dose excreted within 24 hours.

Contraindications and precautions
Contraindicated in patients with hypersensitivity to drug and in those with anuria, known or suspected hypocalcemia, significant renal disease, active or healed tubercular lesions, or history of seizures or intracranial lesions.

Use cautiously in patients with limited cardiac reserve, heart failure, or hypokalemia.

Interactions
Drug-drug. *Cardiac glycosides:* Drug indirectly interferes with cardiac effects of cardiac glycosides by decreasing intracellular calcium via chelation and urinary excretion of extracellular calcium. Monitor patient.
Insulin: Requirements may be decreased by chelation of zinc in exogenous insulin. Monitor serum glucose levels.

Adverse reactions
CNS: circumoral paresthesia, numbness, headache, *seizures.*
CV: hypotension, thrombophlebitis.
GI: nausea, vomiting, diarrhea.
GU: *nephrotoxicity* with urinary urgency, nocturia, dysuria, polyuria, proteinuria, renal insufficiency; *acute renal failure, acute tubular necrosis in excessive doses.*
Hepatic: decreased serum alkaline phosphatase levels.

Metabolic: *severe hypocalcemia,* decreased magnesium level, hypoglycemia.
Skin: exfoliative dermatitis, erythema.
Other: pain at infusion site, extravasation.

☑ Special considerations
• Don't exceed recommended rate of infusion or dosage; rapid infusion or high levels of edetate disodium may precipitously decrease serum calcium levels, causing seizures and death. Have I.V. calcium replacement readily available whenever drug is administered.
• Drug has also been used topically or by iontophoresis to treat corneal calcium deposits.
• Drug lowers serum calcium levels when measured by oxalate or other precipitation methods and by colorimetry.
• Signs and symptoms of overdose include hypotension, arrhythmias, and cardiac arrest. Treat hypotension with fluids, if necessary. Treat arrhythmias with lidocaine; seizures and tetany with calcium replacement. Use I.V. diazepam for refractory seizures.
• Replace magnesium and potassium as necessary.

Monitoring the patient
• Monitor serum calcium and potassium levels before treatment.
• Monitor infusion site closely. Extravasation severely irritates tissue; rotate infusion sites with multiple doses or long-term therapy.
• Monitor infusion rate. Don't exceed recommended rate of infusion or dosage.
• Monitor serum calcium level, ECG, and vital signs continuously throughout therapy.
• Monitor serum glucose level if patient is diabetic.

Information for the patient
• Explain possible adverse reactions; stress importance of reporting signs and symptoms promptly.
• Tell diabetic patient that insulin dosage may need adjustment.

Geriatric patients
• Elderly patients with renal or cardiac failure are at increased risk; lower doses are recommended.

Pediatric patients
• Give recommended dose slowly, over at least 3 hours.

edrophonium chloride
Enlon, Reversol, Tensilon

Pharmacologic classification: cholinesterase inhibitor
Therapeutic classification: cholinergic agonist, diagnostic
Pregnancy risk category NR

How supplied
Available by prescription only
Injection: 10 mg/ml in 1-ml ampule, 10-ml vial, 15-ml vial

Indications, route, and dosage
Curare antagonist (to reverse neuromuscular blocking action)
Adults: 10 mg I.V. given over 30 to 45 seconds, repeated, p.r.n., to 40 mg maximum dose. Larger doses may potentiate rather than antagonize effect of curare.
Diagnostic aid in myasthenia gravis
Adults: 2 mg I.V. within 15 to 30 seconds, then 8 mg if no response (increase in muscular strength) occurs. Or 10 mg I.M. If cholinergic reaction occurs, 2 mg I.M. 30 minutes later to rule out false-negative response.
Children weighing over 34 kg (75 lb): 2 mg I.V. If no response within 45 seconds, give 1 mg q 45 seconds to maximum dose of 10 mg; or 5 mg I.M.
Children weighing 34 kg or less: 1 mg I.V. If no response within 45 seconds, give 1 mg q 45 seconds to maximum dose of 5 mg; or 2 mg I.M.
Infants: 0.5 mg I.V.
To differentiate myasthenic crisis from cholinergic crisis
Adults: 1 mg I.V. If no response occurs in 1 minute, repeat dose once. Increased muscular strength confirms myasthenic crisis; no increase or exaggerated weakness confirms cholinergic crisis.
Tensilon test for evaluating treatment requirements in myasthenia gravis
Adults: 1 to 2 mg I.V. administered 1 hour after oral intake of drug being used in treatment. Response will be myasthenic in the undertreated patient, adequate in the controlled patient, and cholinergic in the overtreated patient.
◊ **To terminate paroxysmal atrial tachycardia or as an aid in diagnosing supraventricular tachyarrhythmias and evaluating the function of demand pacemakers**
Adults: 10 mg I.V. over 5 minutes.
✦ **Dosage adjustment.** In elderly patients or digitalized adults, 5 to 7 mg I.V. over 5 minutes.
To slow supraventricular tachyarrhythmias unresponsive to cardiac glycoside
Adults: 2 mg/minute I.V. test dose, then 2 mg q minute until a total dose of 10 mg is given. If heart rate decreases in response to this dose, infusion of 0.25 mg/minute may be started; rate of infu-

sion may be increased to 2 mg/minute if necessary.

Pharmacodynamics
Cholinergic action: Blocks acetylcholine's hydrolysis by cholinesterase, resulting in acetylcholine accumulation at cholinergic synapses, leading to increased cholinergic receptor stimulation at the neuromuscular junction and vagal sites. A short-acting drug, which makes it particularly useful for the diagnosis of myasthenia gravis.

Pharmacokinetics
● *Absorption:* Action begins 30 to 60 seconds after I.V. administration and 2 to 10 minutes after I.M. administration.
● *Distribution:* Not clearly identified.
● *Metabolism:* Exact metabolic fate unknown; isn't hydrolyzed by cholinesterases. Duration of effect ranges from 5 to 10 minutes after I.V. administration; 5 to 30 minutes after I.M. administration.
● *Excretion:* No information available.

Contraindications and precautions
Contraindicated in patients with hypersensitivity to anticholinesterases and in those with mechanical obstruction of the intestine or urinary tract. Use cautiously in patients with bronchial asthma or arrhythmias.

Interactions
Drug-drug. *Aminoglycosides, anesthetics:* May potentiate prolonged or enhanced muscle weakness. Monitor patient closely.
Cardiac glycosides: May increase heart's sensitivity to drug. Use together cautiously.
Corticosteroids: May decrease drug's cholinergic effects; when corticosteroids are stopped, cholinergic effects may increase, possibly affecting muscle strength. Monitor drug effects.
Ganglionic blockers (such as mecamylamine): Concurrent use may lead to critical blood pressure decrease, usually preceded by abdominal symptoms. Monitor blood pressure carefully.
Magnesium: Concomitant use may antagonize drug's anticholinesterase effect. Use together cautiously.
Other cholinergics: May lead to additive toxicity. Monitor patient for drug effects.
Procainamide, quinidine: May reverse drug's cholinergic effect on muscle. Use together cautiously and monitor drug effects.
Succinylcholine: May cause prolonged respiratory depression from plasma esterase inhibition, leading to delayed succinylcholine hydrolysis. Monitor patient closely.
Drug-herb. *Jaborandi tree, pill-bearing spurge:* May cause additive effect when used together; possible increased risk of toxicity. Avoid concomitant use.

Adverse reactions
CNS: *seizures,* weakness.
CV: hypotension, ***bradycardia,*** AV block.
EENT: excessive lacrimation, diplopia, miosis, conjunctival hyperemia.
GI: nausea, vomiting, *diarrhea, abdominal cramps,* dysphagia, excessive salivation.
GU: urinary frequency, incontinence.
Musculoskeletal: dysarthria, muscle cramps, muscle fasciculation.
Respiratory: *paralysis of muscles of respiration, central respiratory paralysis, bronchospasm, laryngospasm,* increased bronchial secretions.
Skin: diaphoresis.

☑ Special considerations
Besides the recommendations relevant to all cholinesterase inhibitors, consider the following.
● Of all cholinergics, edrophonium has most rapid onset of action but shortest duration of effect; isn't used to treat myasthenia gravis.
● When giving edrophonium to differentiate myasthenic crisis from cholinergic crisis, closely evaluate patient's muscle strength.
● For easier administration, use a tuberculin syringe with an I.V. needle.
● Atropine sulfate injection should always be readily available as an antagonist for drug's muscarinic effects.
● Signs and symptoms of overdose include muscle weakness, nausea, vomiting, diarrhea, blurred vision, miosis, excessive tearing, bronchospasm, increased bronchial secretions, hypotension, incoordination, excessive sweating, cramps, fasciculations, paralysis, bradycardia or tachycardia, excessive salivation, and restlessness or agitation. Muscles first weakened by overdose include neck, jaw, and pharyngeal muscles, then shoulder, upper extremities, pelvis, outer eye, and legs.
● In case of overdose, stop drug immediately. Support respiration; bronchial suctioning may be performed. Atropine may be given to block muscarinic effects but won't counter drug's paralytic effects on skeletal muscle. Avoid atropine overdose; it may lead to bronchial plug formation.

Monitoring the patient
● Monitor patient for muscarinic effects; be prepared to administer atropine.
● Monitor therapeutic effect.

Information for the patient
● Tell patient that, because of drug's short duration of action, adverse effects are transient.

Geriatric patients
● Elderly patients may be more sensitive to effects. Use with caution.

Pediatric patients
● Children may need I.M. administration; with this route, drug effects may be delayed for 2 to 10 minutes.

Breast-feeding patients
● Safety hasn't been established. Avoid drug in breast-feeding women.

efavirenz
Sustiva

Pharmacologic classification: nonnucleoside reverse transcriptase inhibitor (NNRTI)
Therapeutic classification: antiretroviral
Pregnancy risk category C

How supplied
Available by prescription only
Capsules: 50 mg, 100 mg, 200 mg

Indications, route, and dosage
HIV-1 infection
Adults: 600 mg P.O. once daily with a protease inhibitor or nucleoside analogue reverse transcriptase inhibitors.
Children ages 3 and older weighing 40 kg (88 lb) or more: 600 mg P.O. once daily with a protease inhibitor or nucleoside analogue reverse transcriptase inhibitors.
Children ages 3 and older weighing 10 to under 40 kg (22 to under 88 lb):
 Children weighing 10 to under 15 kg (22 to under 33 lb): 200 mg P.O. once daily.
 Children weighing 15 to under 20 kg (33 to under 44 lb): 250 mg P.O. once daily.
 Children weighing 20 to under 25 kg (44 to under 55 lb): 300 mg P.O. once daily.
 Children weighing 25 to under 32.5 kg (55 to under 72 lb): 350 mg P.O. once daily.
 Children weighing 32.5 to under 40 kg (72 to under 88 lb): 400 mg P.O. once daily.
 Give above doses with a protease inhibitor or nucleoside analogue reverse transcriptase inhibitors.

Pharmacodynamics
Antiretroviral action: Inhibits transcription of HIV-1 RNA to DNA, a critical step in the viral replication process. Therefore, lowers amount of HIV in the blood (the viral load) and increases CD4 lymphocytes.

Pharmacokinetics
● *Absorption:* Relative bioavailability increased by about 50% when taken with high-fat meal. Plasma levels peak after 5 hours.
● *Distribution:* About 99.5% to 99.75% bound to plasma proteins. Also distributed into CSF.

- *Metabolism:* Metabolized primarily by cytochrome P-450 3A4 and cytochrome P-450 2B6 to hydroxylated inactive metabolites.
- *Excretion:* 14% to 34% excreted in urine (less than 1% excreted unchanged), and 16% to 61% excreted in feces. Terminal elimination half-life is 52 to 76 hours.

Contraindications and precautions
Contraindicated in patients with hypersensitivity to drug or its components. Use cautiously in patients with hepatic impairment and in those concurrently receiving hepatotoxic drugs.

Interactions
Drug-drug. *Clarithromycin, indinavir:* May decrease plasma levels. Consider alternative therapy or dosage adjustment.

Drugs that induce cytochrome P-450 enzyme system (such as phenobarbital, rifabutin, rifampin): Increased clearance of efavirenz, resulting in lower plasma levels. Avoid use together.

Ergot derivatives, midazolam, triazolam: Competition for cytochrome P-450 enzyme system may result in inhibition of metabolism and cause serious or life-threatening adverse events (such as arrhythmias, prolonged sedation, or respiratory depression). Avoid use together.

Estrogens, ritonavir: Increased plasma levels. Monitor patient.

Oral contraceptives: Potential interaction hasn't been determined. Advise use of reliable barrier contraception in addition to oral contraceptives.

Psychoactive drugs: May cause additive CNS effects. Avoid use together.

Saquinavir: Significant decrease in plasma levels. Don't use with saquinavir as sole protease inhibitor.

Warfarin: Plasma levels and effects are potentially increased or decreased. Monitor INR.

Drug-food. *High-fat meals:* May increase absorption of drug. Patient should maintain proper low-fat diet.

Drug-lifestyle. *Alcohol:* Enhances CNS effects. Avoid use together.

Adverse reactions
CNS: abnormal dreams or thinking, agitation, amnesia, confusion, depersonalization, depression, *dizziness*, euphoria, fatigue, hallucinations, headache, hypoesthesia, impaired concentration, insomnia, somnolence, nervousness.

GI: abdominal pain, anorexia, *diarrhea,* dyspepsia, flatulence, *nausea,* vomiting.

GU: hematuria, kidney stones.

Hepatic: increased AST, ALT, and total cholesterol.

Skin: increased sweating, **erythema multiforme, Stevens-Johnson syndrome, toxic epidermal necrolysis,** *rash,* pruritus.

Other: fever.

☑ Special considerations
- Use drug with other antiretrovirals; resistant viruses emerge rapidly when used alone. Drug shouldn't be used as monotherapy or added on as a single drug to a failing regimen.
- Combination with ritonavir is associated with higher frequency of adverse effects (such as dizziness, nausea, paresthesia) and laboratory abnormalities (elevated liver enzyme levels).
- Drug therapy may cause false-positive urine cannabinoid test results.
- Overdose has caused nervous system symptoms and involuntary muscle contractions. Treatment should involve supportive care, including frequent monitoring of vital signs and observation of clinical status. Activated charcoal may be given to aid in the removal of unabsorbed drug. Drug is unlikely to be removed by hemodialysis.

Monitoring the patient
- Monitor cholesterol levels.
- Rule out pregnancy before starting therapy in women of childbearing age.
- Monitor hepatic function before treatment and periodically throughout.

Information for the patient
- Instruct patient to take drug with water, juice, milk, or soda. May be taken without regard to meals.
- Inform patient about need for scheduled blood tests to monitor liver function and cholesterol levels.
- Advise patient to use reliable method of barrier contraception in addition to oral contraceptives. Tell her to call immediately if pregnancy is suspected.
- Inform patient that drug isn't a cure for HIV infection; it won't affect development of opportunistic infections and other complications associated with HIV disease or transmission of HIV to others through sexual contact or blood contamination.
- Instruct patient to take drug at same time daily, always with other antiretrovirals.
- Tell patient to take drug exactly as prescribed and not to stop without medical approval. Also instruct patient to report if adverse reactions occur.
- Inform patient that rash is the most common adverse effect. If this occurs, tell patient to report it immediately because it may be serious in rare cases.
- Advise patient to report use of other drugs.
- Advise patient that dizziness, difficulty sleeping or concentrating, drowsiness, or unusual dreams may occur the first few days of therapy. Reassure patient that these symptoms generally resolve after 2 to 4 weeks and may be less problematic if drug is taken at bedtime.

Reactions may be *common,* uncommon, **life-threatening,** or COMMON AND LIFE-THREATENING.

• Tell patient to avoid alcoholic beverages, driving, or operating machinery until drug's effects are known.

Geriatric patients
• Elderly patients may be more susceptible to CNS effects of drug.

Pediatric patients
• Children may be more prone to adverse reactions, especially diarrhea, nausea, vomiting, and rash.

Breast-feeding patients
• Drug appears in breast milk. To avoid risk of transmitting infection, HIV-infected mothers shouldn't breast-feed.

enalaprilat
Vasotec I.V.

enalapril maleate
Vasotec

Pharmacologic classification: ACE inhibitor
Therapeutic classification: antihypertensive
Pregnancy risk category C (D in second and third trimesters)

How supplied
Available by prescription only
Tablets: 2.5 mg, 5 mg, 10 mg, 20 mg
Injection: 1.25 mg/ml in 2-ml vials

Indications, route, and dosage
Hypertension
Adults: For patient not receiving diuretics, initially 5 mg P.O. once daily, then adjusted according to response. Usual dosage range is 10 to 40 mg daily as a single dose or two divided doses. Or 1.25 mg I.V. infusion q 6 hours over 5 minutes. For patient on diuretics, initially 2.5 mg P.O. once daily. Or administer 0.625 mg I.V. over 5 minutes, repeat in 1 hour, if needed, then 1.25 mg I.V. q 6 hours.
To convert from I.V. therapy to oral therapy
Adults: If patient wasn't treated with diuretics and was receiving 1.25 mg q 6 hours, then initially 5 mg P.O. once daily. If patient is being treated with diuretics and was receiving 0.625 mg I.V. q 6 hours, then 2.5 mg P.O. once daily. Adjust dose according to response.
To convert from oral therapy to I.V. therapy
Adults: 1.25 mg I.V. over 5 minutes q 6 hours. Higher doses haven't demonstrated greater efficacy.
✦ *Dosage adjustment.* In hypertensive patients with renal failure who have a creatinine clearance below 30 ml/minute, begin therapy at 2.5 mg/day.

Gradually titrate dosage according to response. Patients undergoing hemodialysis should receive a supplemental dose of 2.5 mg on days of dialysis.
Heart failure
Adults: Initially, 2.5 mg P.O. Recommended dosing range is 2.5 to 20 mg b.i.d. Adjust dosage upward, as tolerated, over a period of a few days or weeks. Maximum daily dose is 40 mg P.O. daily in divided doses.
Asymptomatic left ventricular dysfunction
Adults: Initially, 2.5 mg P.O. b.i.d.; titrate dosage to targeted daily dose of 20 mg (in divided doses) as tolerated.
✦ *Dosage adjustment.* In patients with heart failure and renal impairment or hyponatremia (serum sodium less than 130 mEq/L or serum creatinine above 1.6 mg/dl), begin therapy with 2.5 mg P.O. daily. Increase dosage to 2.5 mg b.i.d., then 5 mg b.i.d. and higher as indicated, usually at intervals of 4 days or more.

Pharmacodynamics
Antihypertensive action: Enalapril inhibits ACE, preventing conversion of angiotensin I to angiotensin II, a potent vasoconstrictor. Reduced angiotensin II levels decrease peripheral arterial resistance, lowering blood pressure, and decrease aldosterone secretion, thus reducing sodium and water retention.

Pharmacokinetics
• *Absorption:* About 60% of dose absorbed from GI tract; blood pressure decreases within 1 hour, with peak antihypertensive effect at 4 to 6 hours.
• *Distribution:* No information available; doesn't appear to cross blood-brain barrier.
• *Metabolism:* Metabolized extensively to active metabolite enalaprilat.
• *Excretion:* About 94% of dose excreted in urine and feces as enalaprilat and enalapril.

Contraindications and precautions
Contraindicated in patients with hypersensitivity to drug or history of angioedema related to previous treatment with an ACE inhibitor. Use cautiously in patients with impaired renal function.

Interactions
Drug-drug. *Aspirin, NSAIDs:* May decrease enalapril's antihypertensive effect. Monitor blood pressure closely.
Diuretics, phenothiazines, other antihypertensives: Enalapril may increase antihypertensive effects. Monitor blood pressure closely.
Insulin, oral antidiabetics: May potentiate risk of hypoglycemia, especially at start of enalapril therapy. Monitor serum glucose level.
Lithium: May decrease renal clearance of lithium. Monitor lithium levels.

Potassium-sparing diuretics, potassium supplements: Enalapril may enhance effects, causing hyperkalemia. Use together cautiously.
Rifampin: May decrease pharmacologic effects of rifampin. Monitor patient.
Drug-food. *Salt substitutes:* May enhance effects, causing hyperkalemia. Monitor patient closely.

Adverse reactions
CNS: *headache, dizziness, fatigue,* vertigo, asthenia, syncope.
CV: *hypotension,* chest pain.
GI: diarrhea, nausea, abdominal pain, vomiting.
GU: elevated BUN and serum creatinine levels, decreased renal function (in patients with bilateral renal artery stenosis or heart failure).
Hematologic: *neutropenia, thrombocytopenia, agranulocytosis.*
Hepatic: increased liver enzyme and bilirubin levels.
Respiratory: *dry, persistent, tickling, nonproductive cough;* dyspnea.
Skin: rash.
Other: *angioedema.*

☑ Special considerations
● Stop diuretic therapy 2 to 3 days before beginning enalapril therapy to reduce risk of hypotension; if drug doesn't adequately control blood pressure, diuretics should be reinstated.
● Proteinuria and nephrotic syndrome may occur in patients who are on enalapril therapy.
● Packaging and labeling may be similar to those of pancuronium. Examine label carefully.
● With overdose, hypotension will probably occur.
● After acute ingestion, empty stomach by induced emesis or gastric lavage. Follow with activated charcoal to reduce absorption. Consider hemodialysis in severe cases. Subsequent treatment is usually symptomatic and supportive.

Monitoring the patient
● Perform WBC and differential counts before treatment, every 2 weeks for 3 months, and periodically thereafter.
● Monitor renal function before treatment and periodically throughout.
● Monitor blood pressure.
● If patient is on potassium supplements or potassium-sparing diuretics, monitor serum potassium levels.

Information for the patient
● Tell patient to report light-headedness, especially in first few days, so dosage can be adjusted; signs of infection, such as sore throat and fever, because drug may decrease WBC count; facial swelling or difficulty breathing because drug

may cause angioedema; and loss of taste, which may require stopping drug.
● Advise patient not to change position suddenly to minimize orthostatic hypotension.
● Warn patient to seek medical approval before taking OTC cold preparations, particularly cough medications.

Geriatric patients
● Elderly patients may need lower doses because of impaired drug clearance.

Pediatric patients
● Safety and efficacy in children haven't been established; use only if potential benefit outweighs risk.

Breast-feeding patients
● It's unknown if drug appears in breast milk; an alternative to breast-feeding is recommended during therapy.

enoxacin
Penetrex

Pharmacologic classification: fluoroquinolone, antibacterial
Therapeutic classification: antibiotic
Pregnancy risk category C

How supplied
Available by prescription only
Tablets (film-coated): 200 mg, 400 mg

Indications, route, and dosage
Uncomplicated urinary tract infections (cystitis) caused by Escherichia coli, Staphylococcus epidermidis, *or* Staphylococcus saprophyticus
Adults: 200 mg P.O. q 12 hours for 7 days.
Complicated urinary tract infections caused by E. coli, Klebsiella pneumoniae, Proteus mirabilis, Pseudomonas aeruginosa, Staphylococcus epidermidis, *or* Enterobacter cloacae
Adults: 400 mg P.O. q 12 hours for 14 days.
Uncomplicated urethral or endocervical gonorrhea caused by Neisseria gonorrhoeae
Adults: 400 mg P.O. as a single dose.
✦ *Dosage adjustment.* In patients with renal impairment, if creatinine clearance is 30 ml/minute/$1.73 m^2$ or less, start therapy with the usual initial dose. Subsequent doses should be decreased by 50%.
Note: Stop therapy if hypersensitivity or phototoxicity occurs.

Pharmacodynamics
Antibiotic action: Bactericidal. Inhibits the bacterial enzyme DNA gyrase, which is necessary for DNA replication. Active against most strains of

gram-positive aerobes, such as *Staphylococcus epidermidis* and *S. saprophyticus,* and against many gram-negative aerobes, such as *E. cloacae, E. coli, K. pneumoniae, N. gonorrhoeae, P. mirabilis,* and *P. aeruginosa.*

Pharmacokinetics
● *Absorption:* After oral administration, plasma levels may peak within 1 to 3 hours. Absolute oral bioavailability is about 90%.
● *Distribution:* About 40% bound to plasma proteins in healthy individuals and 14% bound to plasma proteins in patients with impaired renal function.
● *Metabolism:* Five metabolites identified in urine; account for 15% to 20% of administered dose.
● *Excretion:* Excreted primarily by kidneys. Plasma half-life is 3 to 6 hours.

Contraindications and precautions
Contraindicated in patients with hypersensitivity to drug or other fluoroquinolone antibiotics. Use cautiously in patients with CNS disorders, such as severe cerebral arteriosclerosis or seizure disorders, and in those at increased risk for seizures. Drug may cause CNS stimulation. Use with caution and with dosage adjustments in patients with impaired renal or hepatic function.

Interactions
Drug-drug. *Aminophylline, cyclosporine, theophylline:* Possible increased levels of these drugs because of decreased metabolism. Use together cautiously.
Bismuth subsalicylate: Decreased enoxacin bioavailability (by about 25%) when given within 60 minutes after enoxacin. Avoid concomitant use.
Digoxin: May raise serum digoxin levels. If signs and symptoms of digoxin toxicity occur, obtain serum digoxin levels and adjust digoxin doses appropriately.
Oral anticoagulants: Increased anticoagulant effect. Monitor PT and INR.
Quinolones with antacids containing aluminum, calcium, magnesium; with divalent or trivalent cations (such as iron); with multivitamins containing zinc; with sucralfate: May substantially interfere with drug absorption and result in insufficient plasma and tissue quinolone levels. Give 8 hours before or 2 hours after enoxacin.
Ranitidine: Oral bioavailability of enoxacin is reduced by 60% with coadministration. Give ranitidine 8 hours before or 2 hours after enoxacin.
Drug-food. *Any food:* Affects absorption. Give drug on an empty stomach.
Caffeine: Drug interferes with metabolism of caffeine, resulting in decrease in caffeine clearance of up to 80%; increases caffeine-related adverse effects. Discourage use.

Adverse reactions
CNS: headache, restlessness, light-headedness, tremor, confusion, hallucinations, *seizures.*
GI: *nausea, diarrhea,* vomiting, abdominal pain or discomfort, oral candidiasis.
GU: crystalluria.
Hematologic: eosinophilia.
Hepatic: elevated liver enzymes.
Musculoskeletal: tendon pain, tendon rupture.
Respiratory: dyspnea, cough.
Skin: *rash,* pruritus, photosensitivity.
Other: *hypersensitivity.*

☑ Special considerations
● Safety and efficacy in pregnant women haven't been established.
● Moderate to severe phototoxicity reactions have been observed in patients exposed to direct sunlight while on drug.
● For acute overdose, empty stomach by inducing vomiting or by gastric lavage; observe patient carefully and give supportive treatment. Enoxacin is poorly removed (less than 5% over 4 hours) by hemodialysis.

Monitoring the patient
● Obtain specimen for culture and sensitivity tests before giving first dose. Therapy may begin pending results.
● Monitor patient for diarrhea. Pseudomembranous colitis has been reported and may range in severity from mild to life-threatening. Consider this diagnosis in patients who have diarrhea after drug administration.

Information for the patient
● Advise patient to avoid excessive sunlight and to take other precautions as necessary to prevent phototoxicity.
● Instruct patient to call immediately if pregnancy is suspected.
● Tell patient to avoid antacids containing aluminum, calcium, or magnesium; bismuth subsalicylate; products containing iron; or multivitamins that contain zinc for 8 hours before taking enoxacin.
● Instruct patient to drink fluids liberally but to avoid consumption of products containing caffeine during enoxacin therapy.
● Caution patient that enoxacin may cause dizziness and light-headedness; advise patient not to operate an automobile or other hazardous machinery or to engage in activities requiring mental alertness and coordination until response to therapy is known.
● Advise patient that enoxacin may be associated with hypersensitivity reaction, even after first dose. Tell patient to stop drug and call at first sign of rash or other allergic reactions.
● Instruct patient to take enoxacin at least 1 hour before or 2 hours after a meal.

Pediatric patients
● Safety and effectiveness in children haven't been established.

Breast-feeding patients
● Safety and effectiveness in breast-feeding patients haven't been established.

enoxaparin sodium
Lovenox

Pharmacologic classification: low-molecular-weight heparin
Therapeutic classification: anticoagulant
Pregnancy risk category B

How supplied
Available by prescription only
Ampules: 30 mg/0.3 ml
Syringes (prefilled): 30 mg/0.3 ml, 40 mg/0.4 ml
Syringes (graduated prefilled): 60 mg/0.6 ml, 80 mg/0.8 ml, 100 mg/1 ml

Indications, route, and dosage
Prevention of deep vein thrombosis (DVT), which may lead to pulmonary embolism, following hip or knee replacement surgery
Adults: 30 mg S.C. q 12 hours for 7 to 10 days. Give initial dose between 12 and 24 hours postoperatively provided hemostasis has been established.
Prevention of DVT, which may lead to pulmonary embolism, following abdominal surgery
Adults: 40 mg S.C. once daily for 7 to 10 days. Give initial dose 2 hours before surgery.
Prevention of ischemic complications of unstable angina and non-Q-wave MI, when concurrently administered with aspirin
Adults: 1 mg/kg S.C. q 12 hours for 2 to 8 days with oral aspirin therapy (100 to 325 mg once daily).
   Note: To minimize risk of bleeding following vascular instrumentation during treatment of unstable angina, adhere precisely to recommended intervals between enoxaparin doses.
Inpatient treatment of acute DVT with and without pulmonary embolism when administered with warfarin sodium
Adults: 1 mg/kg S.C. q 12 hours; or 1.5 mg/kg S.C. once daily (at same time daily) for 5 to 7 days until therapeutic oral anticoagulant effect (INR 2 to 3) has been achieved. Warfarin sodium therapy is usually initiated within 72 hours of enoxaparin injection.
Outpatient treatment of acute DVT without pulmonary embolism when administered with warfarin sodium
Adults: 1 mg/kg S.C. q 12 hours for 5 to 7 days until therapeutic oral anticoagulant effect (INR 2 to 3) has been achieved. Warfarin sodium therapy is usually initiated within 72 hours of enoxaparin injection.

Pharmacodynamics
Anticoagulant action: Low-molecular-weight heparin that accelerates formation of antithrombin III-thrombin complex and deactivates thrombin, preventing conversion of fibrinogen to fibrin. Has a higher anti-factor Xa to anti-factor IIa activity than unfractionated heparin.

Pharmacokinetics
● *Absorption:* Maximum anti-factor Xa and anti-factor IIa (antithrombin) activities occur 3 to 5 hours after S.C. injection.
● *Distribution:* Volume of distribution of anti-factor Xa activity is about 6 L.
● *Metabolism:* No information available.
● *Excretion:* Elimination half-life based on anti-factor Xa activity is about 4½ hours after S.C. administration.

Contraindications and precautions
Contraindicated in patients with hypersensitivity to drug or heparin or pork products; in patients with active, major bleeding or thrombocytopenia; and in those who demonstrate antiplatelet antibodies in the presence of drug.
   Use with extreme caution in patients with history of heparin-induced thrombocytopenia. Use cautiously in patients with conditions that put them at increased risk for hemorrhage, such as bacterial endocarditis, congenital or acquired bleeding disorders, ulcer disease, angiodysplastic GI disease, hemorrhagic stroke, or recent spinal, eye, or brain surgery; and in those treated concomitantly with NSAIDs, platelet inhibitors, or other anticoagulants that affect hemostasis. Also use cautiously in patients with a bleeding diathesis, uncontrolled arterial hypertension, or history of recent GI ulceration, diabetic retinopathy, and hemorrhage. Use with care in elderly patients and in those with renal insufficiency who may show delayed elimination of enoxaparin.
   Use with extreme caution in patients with postoperative indwelling epidural catheters. Epidural or spinal hematomas have been reported with the use of enoxaparin and spinal or epidural anesthesia or spinal puncture, resulting in long-term or permanent paralysis.

Interactions
Drug-drug. *Anticoagulants, antiplatelet drugs, NSAIDs:* Increased risk of bleeding. May also lead to spinal or epidural hematomas in patients with spinal punctures or epidural or spinal anesthesia. Avoid concomitant use.
Plicamycin, valproic acid: May cause hypoprothrombinemia and inhibit platelet aggregation. Monitor CBC, coagulation studies.

Adverse reactions
CNS: confusion, *neurologic injury* when used with spinal or epidural puncture.
CV: edema, peripheral edema, CV toxicity (chest pain, dizziness, irregular heartbeat).
GI: nausea.
Hematologic: hypochromic anemia, *thrombocytopenia, hemorrhage,* ecchymoses, bleeding complications.
Hepatic: elevated liver enzyme levels.
Skin: *rash, hives.*
Other: irritation, pain, hematoma, erythema at injection site, fever, *angioedema.*

☑ Special considerations
• Enoxaparin isn't intended for I.M. administration.
• Drug can't be used interchangeably (unit for unit) with unfractionated heparin or other low-molecular-weight heparins.
• Don't mix drug with other injections or infusions.
• Screen all patients before prophylactic administration of enoxaparin to rule out a bleeding disorder.
• Administer drug by deep S.C. injection with patient lying down. Full length of needle should be introduced into skin fold held between thumb and forefinger; hold skin fold throughout injection. Other sites exist between left and right anterolateral and left and right posterolateral abdominal wall.
• Don't expel air bubble from syringe before injection; drug may be lost.
• Accidental overdose after drug administration may lead to hemorrhagic complications. Use slow I.V. injection of protamine sulfate (1%) solution. Dose of protamine sulfate should be equal to dose of enoxaparin injection (1 mg of protamine neutralizes 1 mg of enoxaparin).

Monitoring the patient
• Monitor CBC and coagulation studies throughout treatment.
• Monitor patient for adverse effects.

Information for the patient
• Instruct patient on self-administration as necessary.
• Instruct patient to report any easy bruising or bleeding.

Pediatric patients
• Safety and effectiveness in children haven't been established.

Breast-feeding patients
• It's unknown if drug appears in breast milk. Use cautiously when administering to breast-feeding women.

entacapone
Comtan

Pharmacologic classification: catechol-O-methyltransferase (COMT) inhibitor
Therapeutic classification: antiparkinsonian
Pregnancy risk category C

How supplied
Available by prescription only
Tablets: 200 mg

Indications, route, and dosage
Adjunct to levodopa and carbidopa for treatment of idiopathic Parkinson's disease in patients who experience signs and symptoms of end-of-dose wearing off
Adults: 200 mg P.O. with each dose of levodopa and carbidopa to maximum of eight times daily. Maximum recommended daily dose of entacapone is 1,600 mg/day. Reductions in daily levodopa dose or extending the interval between doses may be necessary to optimize patient's response.

Pharmacodynamics
Antiparkinsonian action: A reversible inhibitor of peripheral COMT, which is responsible for elimination of various catecholamines, including dopamine. Blocking this pathway when administering levodopa and carbidopa should result in higher serum levels of levodopa, thereby allowing greater dopaminergic stimulation in the CNS with greater effect in treating parkinsonian symptoms.

Pharmacokinetics
• *Absorption:* Rapid, with serum levels peaking in about 1 hour. Food doesn't affect absorption.
• *Distribution:* About 98% protein-bound, mainly to albumin; isn't distributed widely into tissues. Duration is about 6 hours.
• *Metabolism:* Almost completely metabolized by glucuronidation before elimination. No active metabolites identified.
• *Excretion:* About 10% excreted in urine; remainder excreted in bile and feces. Biphasic half-life: 0.4 to 0.7 hours for first phase; 2.4 hours for second phase.

Contraindications and precautions
Contraindicated in patients with hypersensitivity to drug. Use cautiously in patients with hepatic impairment, biliary obstruction, or orthostatic hypotension.

Interactions
Drug-drug. *Ampicillin, chloramphenicol, cholestyramine, erythromycin, probenecid:* May block bil-

iary excretion, resulting in higher serum levels of entacapone. Use cautiously.

CNS depressants: Additive effect. Use cautiously.

Drugs metabolized by COMT (bitolterol, dobutamine, dopamine, epinephrine, isoetharine, isoproterenol, norepinephrine): May cause higher serum levels of these drugs, resulting in increased heart rate, changes in blood pressure or, possibly, arrhythmias. Use cautiously.

Nonselective MAO inhibitors (such as phenelzine, tranylcypromine): May inhibit normal catecholamine metabolism. Avoid concomitant use.

Drug-lifestyle. *Alcohol:* May cause additive CNS effects. Discourage use.

Adverse reactions

CNS: *dyskinesia, hyperkinesia,* hypokinesia, dizziness, anxiety, somnolence, agitation, fatigue, asthenia, hallucinations.

GI: *nausea, diarrhea,* abdominal pain, constipation, vomiting, dry mouth, dyspepsia, flatulence, gastritis, taste perversion.

GU: *urine discoloration.*

Hematologic: purpura.

Musculoskeletal: back pain.

Respiratory: dyspnea.

Skin: sweating.

Other: bacterial infection.

☑ Special considerations

• Drug should only be used with levodopa and carbidopa; no antiparkinsonian effects will occur when drug is given as monotherapy.

• Levodopa and carbidopa dosage requirements are usually lower when given with entacapone; the levodopa and carbidopa dose should be lowered or dosing interval increased to avoid adverse effects.

• Drug may cause or exacerbate preexisting dyskinesia, despite reduction of levodopa dose.

• Hallucinations may occur or worsen when taking this drug.

• Diarrhea most commonly begins within 4 to 12 weeks of starting therapy, but may begin as early as first week or as late as many months after starting treatment.

• Drug may cause urine discoloration.

• Rarely, rhabdomyolysis has occurred with drug use.

• Rapid withdrawal or abrupt reduction in drug dose could lead to signs and symptoms of Parkinson's disease; it may also lead to hyperpyrexia and confusion, a symptom complex resembling neuroleptic malignant syndrome. Discontinue drug slowly and monitor patient closely. Adjust other dopaminergic treatment, as needed.

• Drug can be given with immediate or sustained-release levodopa and carbidopa and can be taken with or without food.

• Management of overdose is symptomatic; hemodialysis isn't effective because of high protein-binding. In acute stages of overdose, gastric lavage or activated charcoal may be helpful to limit absorption in GI tract.

Monitoring the patient

• Monitor blood pressure closely. Observe for orthostatic hypotension.

• Monitor patient for adverse effects.

Information for the patient

• Instruct patient not to crush or break tablet and to take it at same time as levodopa and carbidopa.

• Warn patient to avoid potentially hazardous activities, such as driving or operating heavy machinery, until CNS effects of drug are known.

• Advise patient to avoid alcohol during treatment.

• Instruct patient to use caution when standing after prolonged period of sitting or lying down because dizziness may occur. This effect is more common during initial therapy.

• Warn patient that hallucinations, increased dyskinesia, nausea, and diarrhea may occur.

• Inform patient that drug may cause urine to turn brownish orange.

• Advise patient to report if she is pregnant or breast-feeding or if she plans to become pregnant.

Pediatric patients

• No identified potential use in children.

Breast-feeding patients

• It's unknown if drug appears in breast milk. Because many drugs appear in breast milk, use caution when administering to breast-feeding women.

---

ephedrine

ephedrine hydrochloride

ephedrine sulfate
Kondon's Nasal, Pretz-D

Pharmacologic classification: adrenergic
Therapeutic classification: bronchodilator, vasopressor (parenteral form), nasal decongestant
Pregnancy risk category C

How supplied
Available with and without a prescription
Capsules: 25 mg, 50 mg
Nasal spray: 0.25%
Injection: 25 mg/ml, 50 mg/ml (parenteral)

Indications, route, and dosage
To correct hypotensive states
Adults: 25 to 50 mg I.M. or S.C., or 10 to 25 mg slow I.V. bolus. If necessary, a second I.M. dose of 50 mg or I.V. dose of 25 mg may be adminis-

tered. Additional I.V. doses may be given in 5 to 10 minutes. Maximum dose is 150 mg daily.
Children: 3 mg/kg or 16.7 mg/m² S.C. or I.M. daily, divided into four to six doses.

Orthostatic hypotension
Adults: 25 mg P.O. once daily to q.i.d.
Children: 3 mg/kg P.O. daily, divided into four to six doses.

Bronchodilator or nasal decongestant
Adults and children over age 12: 12.5 to 50 mg P.O. q 3 to 4 hours, p.r.n., not to exceed 150 mg in 24 hours. As nasal decongestant, 2 to 3 sprays in each nostril not more often than q 4 hours.
Children ages 6 to 12: 6.25 to 12.5 mg P.O. q 4 hours, not to exceed 75 mg in 24 hours. As nasal decongestant, 1 to 2 sprays in each nostril, not more often than q 4 hours. Or children ages 2 and older may receive 2 to 3 mg/kg or 100 mg/m² P.O. daily in four to six divided doses.

Severe, acute bronchospasm
Adults: 12.5 to 25 mg I.M., S.C., or I.V.

Enuresis
Adults: 25 to 50 mg P.O. h.s.

Myasthenia gravis
Adults: 25 mg t.i.d. or q.i.d.

Pharmacodynamics
Ephedrine is both a direct- and indirect-acting sympathomimetic that stimulates alpha- and beta-adrenergic receptors. Release of norepinephrine from its storage sites is one of its indirect effects. In therapeutic doses, ephedrine relaxes bronchial smooth muscle and produces cardiac stimulation with increased systolic and diastolic blood pressure when norepinephrine stores aren't depleted.

Bronchodilator action: Ephedrine relaxes bronchial smooth muscle by stimulating beta$_2$-adrenergic receptors, resulting in increased vital capacity, relief of mild bronchospasm, improved air exchange, and decreased residual volume.

Vasopressor action: Drug produces positive inotropic effects with low doses by action on beta$_1$-receptors in the heart. Vasodilation results from its effect on beta$_2$-adrenergic receptors; vasoconstriction from its alpha-adrenergic effects. Pressor effects may result from vasoconstriction or cardiac stimulation; however, when peripheral vascular resistance is decreased, blood pressure elevation results from increased cardiac output.

Nasal decongestant action: Ephedrine stimulates alpha-adrenergic receptors in blood vessels of nasal mucosa, producing vasoconstriction and nasal decongestion.

Pharmacokinetics
• *Absorption:* Rapidly and completely absorbed after oral, S.C., or I.M. administration. After oral administration, onset of action occurs within 15 to 60 minutes and persists 2 to 4 hours. Pressor and cardiac effects last 1 hour after I.V. dose of

10 to 25 mg or I.M. or S.C. dose of 25 to 50 mg; they last up to 4 hours after oral dose of 15 to 50 mg.
• *Distribution:* Widely distributed throughout body.
• *Metabolism:* Slowly metabolized in liver by oxidative deamination, demethylation, aromatic hydroxylation, and conjugation.
• *Excretion:* Mostly excreted unchanged in urine; rate of excretion depends on urine pH.

Contraindications and precautions
Contraindicated in patients with hypersensitivity to drug and other sympathomimetics; in those with porphyria, severe coronary artery disease, arrhythmias, angle-closure glaucoma, psychoneurosis, angina pectoris, substantial organic heart disease, and CV disease; and in those taking MAO inhibitors.

Nasal solution is contraindicated in patients with hypersensitivity to drug or other sympathomimetics and in those with angle-closure glaucoma, psychoneurosis, angina pectoris, substantial organic heart disease, or CV disease.

Use with extreme caution in elderly men and in those with hypertension, hyperthyroidism, nervous or excitable states, diabetes, and prostatic hyperplasia. Use nasal solution cautiously in patients with hyperthyroidism, hypertension, diabetes mellitus, or prostatic hyperplasia.

Interactions
Drug-drug. *Acetazolamide:* May increase serum ephedrine levels. Avoid concomitant use.
Alpha blockers, guanadrel, guanethidine: May decrease vasopressor effects of ephedrine. Monitor patient closely.
Antihypertensives: May decrease effects. Monitor blood pressure.
Atropine: Blocked reflex bradycardia and enhanced pressor effects. Monitor patient closely.
Beta blockers: May block CV and bronchodilating effects of ephedrine. Monitor patient.
Cardiac glycosides, general anesthetics (especially cyclopropane, halothane): May sensitize myocardium to effects of ephedrine, causing arrhythmias. Monitor patient closely.
Diuretics, methyldopa, reserpine: May decrease ephedrine's pressor effects. Monitor patient.
Ergot alkaloids: May enhance vasoconstrictor activity. Avoid concomitant use.
Levodopa: May enhance risk of ventricular arrhythmias. Monitor patient closely.
MAO inhibitors, tricyclic antidepressants: May potentiate pressor effects of ephedrine, possibly resulting in hypertensive crisis. Allow 14 days to lapse after withdrawal of MAO inhibitor before using ephedrine.
Sympathomimetics: May add to their effects and toxicity. Avoid concomitant use.
Theophylline derivatives: Coadministration reportedly causes more adverse reactions than

with either drug used alone. Avoid concomitant use.

Adverse reactions
CNS: *insomnia, nervousness,* dizziness, headache, euphoria, confusion, delirium; nervousness, excitation (with nasal solution).
CV: *palpitations,* tachycardia, hypertension, precordial pain; *tachycardia* (with nasal solution).
EENT: dry nose and throat; rebound nasal congestion with long-term or excessive use, mucosal irritation (with nasal solution).
GI: nausea, vomiting, anorexia.
GU: urine retention, painful urination due to visceral sphincter spasm.
Musculoskeletal: muscle weakness.
Skin: diaphoresis.

☑ Special considerations
Besides the recommendations relevant to all adrenergics, consider the following.
• Tolerance may develop after prolonged or excessive use; increased dose may be needed. Also, if drug is stopped for a few days and re-administered, effectiveness may be restored.
• To prevent insomnia, last dose should be taken at least 2 hours before bedtime.
• Signs and symptoms of overdose include exaggeration of common adverse reactions, especially arrhythmias, extreme tremor or seizures, nausea and vomiting, fever, and CNS and respiratory depression.
• Treatment requires supportive and symptomatic measures. If patient is conscious, induce emesis with ipecac then activated charcoal. If patient is depressed or hyperactive, perform gastric lavage. Maintain airway and blood pressure. Don't administer vasopressors. Monitor vital signs closely.
• A beta blocker (such as propranolol) may be used to treat arrhythmias. A cardioselective beta blocker is recommended in asthmatic patients. Phentolamine may be used for hypertension, paraldehyde or diazepam for seizures, and dexamethasone for pyrexia.

Monitoring the patient
• With parenteral dosing, monitor vital signs closely during infusion. Tachycardia is common.
• As a pressor drug, ephedrine isn't a substitute for blood, plasma, fluids, or electrolytes. Correct fluid volume depletion before administration.

Information for the patient
• Tell patient using OTC product to follow directions on label, to take last dose a few hours before bedtime to reduce possibility of insomnia, to take only as directed, and not to increase dose or frequency.
• Advise patient to store drug away from heat and light (not in bathroom medicine cabinet) and to keep out of reach of children.

• Instruct patient who misses a dose to take it as soon as remembered if within 1 hour. If beyond 1 hour, patient should skip dose and return to regular schedule.
• Teach patient to be aware of palpitations and significant pulse rate changes.
• Instruct patient to clear nose before instillation of nasal solutions.

Geriatric patients
• Administer cautiously because elderly patients may be more sensitive to drug's effects. Lower dose may be recommended.

Pediatric patients
• Use cautiously in children.

Breast-feeding patients
• Because it's unknown if drug appears in breast milk, avoid breast-feeding during treatment with ephedrine.

epinephrine
Bronkaid Mist, Bronkaid Mistometer*, EpiPen, EpiPen Jr., Primatene Mist, Sus-Phrine

epinephrine bitartrate
AsthmaHaler Mist

epinephrine hydrochloride
Adrenalin Chloride, AsthmaNefrin, Epifrin, Glaucon, microNefrin, Vaponefrin

epinephryl borate
Epinal

Pharmacologic classification: adrenergic
Therapeutic classification: bronchodilator, vasopressor, cardiac stimulant, local anesthetic (adjunct), topical antihemorrhagic, antiglaucoma drug
Pregnancy risk category C

How supplied
Available by prescription only
Injection: 0.01 mg/ml (1:100,000), 0.1 mg/ml (1:10,000), 0.5 mg/ml (1:2,000), 1 mg/ml (1:1,000) parenteral; 5 mg/ml (1:200) parenteral suspension
Ophthalmic: 0.1%, 0.25%, 0.5%, 1%, 2% solution
Available without a prescription
Nebulizer inhaler: 1% (1:100), 1.25%, 2.25%
Aerosol inhaler: 160 mcg, 200 mcg, 250 mcg/metered spray
Nasal solution: 0.1%

Indications, route, and dosage

Bronchospasm, hypersensitivity reactions, anaphylaxis

Adults: Initially, 0.1 to 0.5 mg (0.1 to 0.5 ml of a 1:1,000 solution) S.C. or I.M.; may be repeated at 10- to 15-minute intervals, p.r.n. Or 0.1 to 0.25 mg (1 to 2.5 ml of a 1:10,000 solution) I.V. slowly over 5 to 10 minutes. May be repeated q 5 to 15 minutes if needed or then a 1 to 4 mcg/minute I.V. infusion.

Children: 0.01 mg/kg (0.01 ml/kg of a 1:1,000 solution) or 0.3 mg/m^2 (0.3 ml/m^2 of a 1:1,000 solution) S.C. Dose not to exceed 0.5 mg. May be repeated at 20-minute to 4-hour intervals, p.r.n. Or 0.02 to 0.025 mg/kg (0.004 to 0.005 ml/kg) or 0.625 mg/m^2 (0.125 ml/m^2) of a 1:200 solution. May be repeated but not more often than q 6 hours. Or 0.1 mg (10 ml of a 1:100,000 dilution) I.V. slowly over 5 to 10 minutes, then a 0.1 to 1.5 mcg/kg/minute I.V. infusion.

Bronchodilator

Adults and children: 1 inhalation via metered aerosol, repeated once if needed after 1 minute; subsequent doses shouldn't be repeated for at least 3 hours. Or 1 or 2 deep inhalations via hand-bulb nebulizer of a 1% (1:100) solution; may be repeated at 1- to 2-minute intervals. Or 0.03 ml (0.3 mg) of a 1% solution via intermittent positive pressure breathing.

To restore cardiac rhythm in cardiac arrest

Adults: Initially, 0.5 to 1 mg (range, 0.1 to 1 mg to 10 ml of a 1:10,000 solution) I.V. bolus; may be repeated q 3 to 5 minutes, p.r.n. Or initial dose, then 0.3 mg S.C. or 1 to 4 mcg/minute I.V. infusion. Or 1 mg (10 ml of a 1:10,000 solution) intratracheally, or 0.1 to 1 mg (1 to 10 ml of a 1:10,000 solution) by intracardiac injection.

Children: Initially, 0.01 mg/kg (0.1 ml/kg of a 1:10,000 solution) I.V. bolus or intratracheally; may be repeated q 5 minutes, p.r.n.

Or, initially, 0.1 mcg/kg/minute; may increase in increments of 0.1 mcg/kg/minute to a maximum of 1 mcg/kg/minute. Or 0.005 to 0.01 mg/kg (0.05 to 0.1 ml/kg of a 1:10,000 solution) by intracardiac injection.

Infants: Initially, 0.01 to 0.03 mg/kg (0.1 to 0.3 ml/kg of a 1:10,000 solution) I.V. bolus or by intratracheal injection. May be repeated q 5 minutes, p.r.n.

Hemostatic use

Adults: 1:50,000 to 1:1,000, applied topically.

To prolong local anesthetic effect

Adults and children: 1:500,000 to 1:50,000 mixed with local anesthetic.

Open-angle glaucoma

Adults: 1 or 2 drops of 1% to 2% solution instilled daily or b.i.d.

Nasal congestion, local superficial bleeding

Adults and children: Instill 1 or 2 drops of solution.

Pharmacodynamics

Epinephrine acts directly by stimulating alpha- and beta-adrenergic receptors in the sympathetic nervous system. Its main therapeutic effects include relaxation of bronchial smooth muscle, cardiac stimulation, and dilation of skeletal muscle vasculature.

Bronchodilator action: Epinephrine relaxes bronchial smooth muscle by stimulating beta$_2$-adrenergic receptors. Epinephrine constricts bronchial arterioles by stimulating alpha-adrenergic receptors, resulting in relief of bronchospasm, reduced congestion and edema, and increased tidal volume and vital capacity. By inhibiting histamine release, it may reverse bronchiolar constriction, vasodilation, and edema.

CV and vasopressor actions: As a cardiac stimulant, epinephrine produces positive chronotropic and inotropic effects by action on beta$_1$-receptors in the heart, increasing cardiac output, myocardial oxygen consumption, and force of contraction and decreasing cardiac efficiency. Vasodilation results from its effect on beta$_2$-receptors; vasoconstriction results from alpha-adrenergic effects.

Local anesthetic (adjunct) action: Epinephrine acts on alpha receptors in skin, mucous membranes, and viscera; it produces vasoconstriction, which reduces absorption of local anesthetic, thus prolonging its duration of action, localizing anesthesia, and decreasing risk of anesthetic's toxicity.

Local vasoconstriction action: Epinephrine's effect results from action on alpha receptors in skin, mucous membranes, and viscera, which produces vasoconstriction and hemostasis in small vessels.

Antiglaucoma action: Epinephrine's exact mechanism of lowering intraocular pressure is unknown. When applied topically to the conjunctiva or injected into the interior chamber of the eye, epinephrine constricts conjunctival blood vessels, contracts the dilator muscle of the pupil, and may dilate the pupil.

Pharmacokinetics

- *Absorption:* Well absorbed after S.C. or I.M. injection; rapid onset of action; short duration of action. Bronchodilation occurs within 5 to 10 minutes and peaks in 20 minutes after S.C. injection; onset after oral inhalation is within 1 minute. Topical administration or intraocular injection usually produces local vasoconstriction within 5 minutes; lasts less than 1 hour. After topical application to conjunctiva, reduction of intraocular pressure occurs within 1 hour, peaks in 4 to 8 hours, and persists up to 24 hours.
- *Distribution:* Distributed widely throughout body.
- *Metabolism:* Metabolized at sympathetic nerve endings, liver, and other tissues to inactive metabolites.

• *Excretion:* Excreted in urine, mainly as metabolites and conjugates.

Contraindications and precautions

Contraindicated in patients with angle-closure glaucoma, shock (other than anaphylactic shock), organic brain damage, cardiac dilation, arrhythmias, coronary insufficiency, or cerebral arteriosclerosis. Also contraindicated in patients during general anesthesia with halogenated hydrocarbons or cyclopropane and in patients in labor (may delay second stage).

Some commercial products contain sulfites and are contraindicated in patients with sulfite allergies except when epinephrine is being used for treatment of serious allergic reactions or other emergencies.

With local anesthetics, epinephrine is contraindicated for use in fingers, toes, ears, nose, or genitalia.

Ophthalmic preparation is contraindicated in patients with hypersensitivity to drug, in those with angle-closure glaucoma or when nature of the glaucoma hasn't been established, and in patients with organic mental syndrome or cardiac dilation and coronary insufficiency. Nasal solution is contraindicated in patients with hypersensitivity to drug.

Use with extreme caution in patients with long-standing bronchial asthma and emphysema who have developed degenerative heart disease. Also use cautiously in elderly patients and in those with hyperthyroidism, CV disease, hypertension, psychoneurosis, or diabetes.

Use ophthalmic preparation cautiously in elderly patients and in those with diabetes, hypertension, Parkinson's disease, hyperthyroidism, aphakia (eye without lens), cardiac disease, cerebral arteriosclerosis, or bronchial asthma.

Interactions

Drug-drug. *Alpha blockers:* Antagonized vasoconstriction and hypertension. Monitor patient closely.
Antidiabetics: May decrease effects. Dosage adjustments may be necessary. Monitor serum glucose levels.
Antihistamines, thyroid hormones, tricyclic antidepressants: May potentiate adverse cardiac effects of epinephrine. Avoid concomitant use.
Beta blockers such as propranolol: Antagonized cardiac and bronchodilating effects of epinephrine. Monitor patient closely.
Cardiac glycosides, general anesthetics (especially cyclopropane, halothane): May sensitize myocardium to epinephrine's effects, causing arrhythmias. Monitor patient closely.
Doxapram, mazindol, methylphenidate: May enhance CNS stimulation or pressor effects. Monitor patient closely.

Ergot alkaloids, oxytocics: May cause severe hypertension. Monitor blood pressure; avoid concomitant use.
Guanadrel, guanethidine: May decrease drug's hypotensive effects while potentiating epinephrine's effects, resulting in hypertension and arrhythmias. Monitor patient closely.
Levodopa: May enhance risk of cardiac arrhythmias. Monitor patient closely.
MAO inhibitors: Increased risk of hypertensive crisis. Monitor blood pressure; avoid concomitant use.
Miotics: Reduced ciliary spasm, mydriasis, blurred vision, and increased intraocular pressure that may occur with miotics or epinephrine alone. Use for therapeutic effect.
Ophthalmic epinephrine with carbonic anhydrase inhibitors, osmotic drugs, topical beta blockers, topical miotics: May cause additive lowering of intraocular pressure. Monitor patient.
Phenothiazines: May cause reversal of epinephrine's pressor effects; don't use epinephrine for circulatory collapse or hypotension caused by phenothiazines; such use may cause further lowering of blood pressure. Monitor blood pressure closely.
Sympathomimetics: May produce additive effects and toxicity. Avoid concomitant use.

Adverse reactions

CNS: *nervousness, tremor,* vertigo, *headache,* disorientation, agitation, *drowsiness,* fear, pallor, dizziness, weakness, *cerebral hemorrhage, CVA.* In patients with Parkinson's disease, drug increases rigidity, tremor; brow ache, headache, light-headedness (with ophthalmic preparation); nervousness, excitation (with nasal solution).
CV: *palpitations;* widened pulse pressure; *hypertension; tachycardia; ventricular fibrillation; shock;* anginal pain; ECG changes, including a decreased T-wave amplitude; palpitations, tachycardia, *arrhythmias,* hypertension (with ophthalmic preparation); *tachycardia* (with nasal solution).
EENT: corneal or conjunctival pigmentation or corneal edema in long-term use, follicular hypertrophy, chemosis, conjunctivitis, iritis, hyperemic conjunctiva, maculopapular rash, eye pain, allergic lid reaction, ocular irritation, eye stinging, burning, and tearing on instillation (with ophthalmic preparation); rebound nasal congestion, slight sting upon application (with nasal solution).
GI: *nausea, vomiting.*
GU: increased BUN levels.
Metabolic: increased blood glucose and serum lactic acid levels.
Respiratory: dyspnea.
Skin: urticaria, pain, hemorrhage at injection site.

☑ Special considerations

Besides the recommendations relevant to all adrenergics, consider the following.

Reactions may be *common,* uncommon, *life-threatening,* or COMMON AND LIFE-THREATENING.

• After S.C. or I.M. injection, massaging site may hasten absorption.

• Epinephrine is destroyed by oxidizing drugs, alkalis (including sodium bicarbonate), halogens, permanganates, chromates, nitrates, and salts of easily reducible metals, such as iron, copper, and zinc.

• A tuberculin syringe may assure greater accuracy in measurement of parenteral doses.

• Repeated injections may cause tissue necrosis from vascular constriction. Rotate injection sites, and observe for signs of blanching.

• Avoid I.M. injection into buttocks. Epinephrine-induced vasoconstriction favors growth of *Clostridium perfringens.*

• Intracardiac administration requires external cardiac massage to move drug into coronary circulation.

• Drying effect on bronchial secretions may make mucus plugs more difficult to dislodge. Bronchial hygiene program, including postural drainage, breathing exercises, and adequate hydration, may be necessary.

Inhalation
• Treatment should start with first symptoms of bronchospasm. Patient should use fewest number of inhalations that provide relief. To prevent excessive dosage, at least 1 or 2 minutes should elapse before taking additional inhalations of epinephrine. Dosage requirements vary.

Nasal Use
• Instill nose drops with patient's head in lateral, head-low position to prevent entry of drug into throat.

Ophthalmic Use
• Ophthalmic preparation may cause mydriasis with blurred vision and sensitivity to light in some patients being treated for glaucoma. Drug is usually administered at bedtime or after prescribed miotic to minimize these symptoms.

• Patients, especially elderly patients, should have regular tonometer readings during continuous therapy.

• When using separate solutions of epinephrine and a topical miotic, instill the miotic 2 to 10 minutes before epinephrine.

• Epinephrine interferes with tests for urinary catecholamines.

• Signs and symptoms of overdose include a sharp increase in systolic and diastolic blood pressure, rise in venous pressure, severe anxiety, irregular heartbeat, severe nausea or vomiting, severe respiratory distress, unusually large pupils, unusual paleness and coldness of skin, pulmonary edema, renal failure, and metabolic acidosis. Treatment is symptomatic and supportive because epinephrine is rapidly inactivated in the body. Monitor vital signs closely.

• Trimethaphan or phentolamine may be needed for hypotension; beta blockers (such as propranolol) for arrhythmias.

Monitoring the patient
• Monitor blood pressure, pulse, respirations, and urine output, and observe patient closely. Epinephrine may widen pulse pressure. If arrhythmias occur, stop drug immediately. Watch for changes in intake and output ratio.

• When drug is administered I.V., check patient's blood pressure repeatedly during first 5 minutes, then every 3 to 5 minutes until patient is stable.

Information for the patient
• Urge patient to report diminishing effect. Repeated or prolonged use of epinephrine can cause tolerance to drug's effects. Continuing to take epinephrine despite tolerance can be hazardous. Interrupting drug therapy for 12 hours to several days may restore responsiveness to drug.

Inhalation
• Instruct patient in correct use of inhaler.

• Tell patient to avoid contact with eyes and to take no more than 2 inhalations at a time with 1- to 2-minute intervals between them.

• Instruct patient to rinse mouth and throat with water immediately after inhalation to avoid swallowing residual drug (propellant in aerosol preparation may cause epigastric pain and systemic effects) and to prevent dryness of oropharyngeal membranes.

• Warn patient that overuse or too-frequent use can cause severe adverse reactions.

• Tell patient to save applicator; refills may be available.

• Advise patient to call immediately if no relief is experienced within 20 minutes or if condition worsens.

Nasal Use
• Warn patient that intranasal applications may sting slightly and cause rebound congestion or drug-induced rhinitis after prolonged use. Nose drops should be used for 3 or 4 days only. Encourage patient to use drug exactly as prescribed.

• Tell patient to rinse nose dropper or spray tip with hot water after each use to avoid contaminating solution.

• Instruct patient to gently press finger against nasolacrimal duct for at least 1 or 2 minutes immediately after drug instillation to avoid excessive systemic absorption.

• Tell patient to call if symptoms aren't relieved in 20 minutes or if they become worse and to report bronchial irritation, nervousness, or sleeplessness, which require reduction of dosage.

Ophthalmic Use
• To minimize systemic absorption, tell patient to press finger to lacrimal sac during and for 1 to 2 minutes after instillation of eyedrops.

• To prevent contamination, tell patient not to touch applicator tip to any surface and to keep container tightly closed.

• Tell patient not to use if epinephrine solution is discolored or contains a precipitate.

● Advise patient to remove soft contact lenses before instilling eyedrops to avoid staining or damaging them.
● Tell patient to apply a missed dose as soon as possible. If too close to time for next dose, patient should wait and apply at regularly scheduled time.
● Tell patient to store drug away from heat and light (not in bathroom medicine cabinet where heat and moisture can cause drug to deteriorate) and out of children's reach.

Geriatric patients
● Elderly patients may be more sensitive to effects of epinephrine; lower doses are indicated.

Pediatric patients
● Safety and efficacy of ophthalmic epinephrine in children haven't been established. Use with caution.

Breast-feeding patients
● Drug appears in breast milk. Patient should avoid breast-feeding during therapy.

epirubicin hydrochloride
Ellence

Pharmacologic classification: anthracycline
Therapeutic classification: antineoplastic
Pregnancy risk category D

How supplied
Available by prescription only
Injection: 2 mg/ml; available in 50 mg/25-ml vial or 200 mg/100-ml vial

Indications, route, and dosage
Adjuvant therapy in patients with evidence of axillary node tumor involvement following resection of primary breast cancer
Adults: 100 to 120 mg/m^2 I.V. infusion over 3 to 5 minutes via a free-flowing I.V. solution on day 1 of each cycle q 3 to 4 weeks; or divided equally in two doses on days 1 and 8 of each cycle. Maximum cumulative (lifetime) dose is 900 mg/m^2.
  Dosage modification after the first cycle is based on toxicity. For patients experiencing platelet counts below 50,000/mm^3, absolute neutrophil count (ANC) below 250/mm^3, neutropenic fever or grade 3 or 4 nonhematologic toxicity, the day 1 dose in subsequent cycles should be reduced to 75% of the day 1 dose given in the current cycle. Day 1 therapy in subsequent cycles should be delayed until platelets are 100,000/mm^3 or more, ANC is 1,500/mm^3 or more, and nonhematologic toxicities recover to grade 1.
  For patients receiving divided doses (days 1 and 8), the day 8 dose should be 75% of the day 1 dose if platelet counts are 75,000 to

100,000/mm^3 and ANC is 1,000 to 1,499/mm^3. If day 8 platelet counts are below 75,000/mm^3, ANC is below 1,000/mm^3, or grade 3 or 4 nonhematologic toxicity has occurred, the day 8 dose should be omitted.
✦ *Dosage adjustment.* In patients with bone marrow dysfunction (heavily pretreated patients, patients with bone marrow depression, or those with neoplastic bone marrow infiltration), start at lower doses of 75 to 90 mg/m^2. In hepatic dysfunction, if bilirubin is 1.2 to 3 mg/dl or AST is two to four times upper limit of normal, give one-half of recommended starting dose. If bilirubin is above 3 mg/dl or AST is above 4 times upper limit of normal, give one-quarter of recommended starting dose. In patients with severe renal dysfunction (serum creatinine above 5 mg/dl), consider lower dosages.

Pharmacodynamics
Antineoplastic action: Exact mechanism unknown. Thought to form a complex with DNA by intercalation between nucleotide base pairs, thereby inhibiting DNA, RNA, and protein synthesis. DNA cleavage occurs, resulting in cytocidal activity. May also interfere with replication and transcription of DNA and generate cytotoxic free radicals.

Pharmacokinetics
● *Absorption:* Vesicant and must be given I.V.
● *Distribution:* Rapidly and widely distributed into tissues. Binds to plasma proteins, predominantly albumin, and appears to concentrate in RBC.
● *Metabolism:* Extensively and rapidly metabolized by liver. Several metabolites form with little to no cytotoxic activity.
● *Excretion:* Eliminated mostly by biliary excretion and, to lesser extent, urinary excretion.

Contraindications and precautions
Contraindicated in those with hypersensitivity to drug, other anthracyclines, or anthracenediones. Also contraindicated in patients with baseline neutrophil counts below 1,500 cells/mm^3, in those with severe myocardial insufficiency or recent myocardial infarction, in patients who have had previous treatment with anthracyclines to total cumulative doses, and in those with severe hepatic dysfunction.
  Use cautiously in patients with active or dormant cardiac disease, previous or concomitant radiotherapy to the mediastinal and pericardial area, or previous therapy with other anthracyclines or anthracenediones; also use cautiously when other cardiotoxic drugs are used concomitantly.

Interactions
Drug-drug. *Calcium channel blockers, other cardioactive compounds:* May increase risk of heart failure. Monitor cardiac function closely.

Reactions may be *common*, uncommon, **life-threatening**, or COMMON AND LIFE-THREATENING.

Cimetidine: Increased levels of epirubicin by 50%. Avoid concomitant use.
Cytotoxic drugs: Additive toxicities (especially hematologic and gastrointestinal) may occur. Monitor patient closely.
Radiation therapy: Enhanced effects. Monitor patient closely.

Adverse reactions
CNS: *lethargy.*
CV: ***cardiomyopathy, heart failure.***
EENT: *conjunctivitis, keratitis.*
GI: *nausea, vomiting, diarrhea,* anorexia, mucositis.
GU: *amenorrhea.*
Hematologic: LEUKOPENIA, NEUTROPENIA, *febrile neutropenia,* anemia, THROMBOCYTOPENIA.
Skin: *alopecia,* rash, itch, skin changes.
Other: *infection,* fever, *hot flashes, local toxicity.*

☑ Special considerations
● It may be necessary to give antiemetics before epirubicin to reduce nausea and vomiting.
● Epirubicin should be administered under the supervision of medical personnel experienced in the use of cancer chemotherapy.
● Wear protective clothing (goggles, gown, disposable gloves) when handling drug.
● Signs and symptoms of overdose are similar to known toxicities of drug. If overdose occurs, provide supportive treatment, as needed, until recovery of toxicities. Watch for signs of heart failure, which may occur months after therapy, and provide supportive measures as appropriate.

Monitoring the patient
● Monitor patient's total dose. Patients receiving 120 mg/m^2 of epirubicin should also receive prophylactic antibiotic therapy with trimethoprim-sulfamethoxazole or a fluoroquinolone.
● Evaluate baseline total bilirubin, AST, and creatinine levels; CBC, including ANC; and cardiac function by measuring left ventricular ejection fraction (LVEF) before therapy.
● Monitor LVEF regularly during therapy; stop drug at first sign of impaired cardiac function. Early signs of cardiac toxicity may include sinus tachycardia, ECG abnormalities, tachyarrhythmias, bradycardia, AV block, and bundle branch block.
● Delayed cardiac toxicity may occur 2 to 3 months after completion of treatment and causes reduced LVEF and signs and symptoms of heart failure (tachycardia, dyspnea, pulmonary edema, dependent edema, hepatomegaly, ascites, pleural effusion, and gallop rhythm). Delayed cardiac toxicity is dependent upon the cumulative dose of epirubicin. Don't exceed a cumulative dose of 900 mg/m^2.
● Monitor total and differential WBC, RBC, and platelet counts before and during each cycle of therapy. Anthracycline-induced leukemia may occur.

● The WBC nadir is usually reached 10 to 14 days after drug administration and returns to normal by day 21.
● Monitor serum uric acid, potassium, calcium phosphate, and creatinine levels immediately after initial chemotherapy in patients susceptible to tumor lysis syndrome. Hydration, urine alkalinization, and prophylaxis with allopurinol may prevent hyperuricemia and minimize potential complications of tumor lysis syndrome.
● Monitor patient for inflammatory cell reaction at site of irradiation, which may occur with drug administration after previous radiation therapy.

Information for the patient
● Advise patient to report nausea, vomiting, stomatitis, dehydration, fever, evidence of infection, or symptoms of heart failure (tachycardia, dyspnea, edema).
● Inform patient of risk of cardiac damage and treatment-related leukemia with drug use.
● Advise men to use effective contraception during treatment.
● Advise women that irreversible amenorrhea or premature menopause may occur.
● Tell patient that hair regrowth usually occurs within 2 to 3 months after therapy stops.

Geriatric patients
● Plasma clearance is decreased in elderly women. Monitor closely for toxicity in elderly patients, especially women over age 70.

Pediatric patients
● Safety and effectiveness in children haven't been established. These patients may be at greater risk for anthracycline-induced cardiotoxicity and heart failure.

Breast-feeding patients
● It's unknown if drug appears in breast milk. Because many drugs, including anthracyclines, appear in breast milk and because of potential for serious adverse reactions from drug in breast-feeding infants, patient should stop breast-feeding before therapy.

epoetin alfa (erythropoietin)
Epogen, Procrit

Pharmacologic classification: glycoprotein
Therapeutic classification: antianemic
Pregnancy risk category C

How supplied
Available by prescription only
Injection: 2,000 units, 3,000 units, 4,000 units, 10,000 units, 20,000 units

Indications, route, and dosage

Anemia associated with chronic renal failure
Adults: Initiate therapy at 50 to 100 units/kg three times weekly. Patients receiving dialysis should receive drug I.V.; chronic renal failure patients not on dialysis may receive drug S.C. or I.V.

Reduce dosage when target hematocrit is reached or if hematocrit rises more than four points within a 2-week period. Increase dosage if hematocrit doesn't rise by five to six points after 8 weeks of therapy and hematocrit is below target range. Maintenance dose is highly individualized.

Anemia related to zidovudine therapy in patients infected with HIV
Adults: Before therapy, determine endogenous serum epoetin alfa levels. Patients with levels of 500 milliunits/ml or more are unlikely to respond to therapy.

Initial dose for patients with levels of under 500 milliunits/ml who are receiving 4,200 mg weekly or less of zidovudine is 100 units/kg I.V. or S.C. three times weekly for 8 weeks. If response is inadequate after 8 weeks, increase dose by increments of 50 to 100 units/kg three times weekly and reevaluate response q 4 to 8 weeks. Individualize maintenance dose to maintain response, which may be influenced by zidovudine dose or infection or inflammation.

Anemia secondary to cancer chemotherapy
Adults: 150 units/kg S.C. three times weekly for 8 weeks or until target hemoglobin level is reached. If response isn't satisfactory after 8 weeks, increase dose up to 300 units/kg S.C. three times weekly.

Reduction of need for allogeneic blood transfusion in anemic patients scheduled to undergo elective, noncardiac, nonvascular surgery
Adults: 300 units/kg/day S.C. daily for 10 days before surgery, on day of surgery, and for 4 days after surgery. Or 600 units/kg S.C. in once-weekly doses (21, 14, and 7 days before surgery), plus a fourth dose on day of surgery. Before treatment, establish that hemoglobin level is above 10 g/dl and less than or equal to 13 g/dl.

Pharmacodynamics

Antianemic action: Glycoprotein consisting of 165 amino acids synthesized using recombinant DNA technology. Mimics naturally occurring erythropoietin, which is produced by the kidneys. Stimulates the division and differentiation of cells within bone marrow to produce RBCs.

Pharmacokinetics

• *Absorption:* May be given S.C. or I.V. After S.C. administration, peak serum levels occur within 5 to 24 hours.
• *Distribution:* No information available.
• *Metabolism:* No information available.
• *Excretion:* No information available.

Contraindications and precautions

Contraindicated in patients with hypersensitivity to mammalian cell-derived products or albumin (human) or uncontrolled hypertension.

Interactions

None reported.

Adverse reactions

CNS: *headache, seizures, paresthesia, fatigue, asthenia,* dizziness.
CV: *hypertension, edema.*
GI: *nausea, vomiting, diarrhea.*
GU: increased BUN and creatinine levels.
Hematologic: increased clotting of arteriovenous grafts.
Metabolic: increased uric acid, phosphorus, and potassium levels.
Musculoskeletal: *arthralgia.*
Respiratory: *cough, shortness of breath.*
Skin: *rash,* urticaria.
Other: *pyrexia, injection site reactions.*

☑ Special considerations

• For HIV-infected patients treated with zidovudine, measure hematocrit once weekly until stabilized; then periodically.
• If a patient fails to respond to epoetin alfa therapy, consider the following possible causes: vitamin deficiency, iron deficiency, underlying infection, occult blood loss, underlying hematologic disease, hemolysis, aluminum intoxication, osteitis fibrosa cystica, or increased dosage of zidovudine.
• Maximum safe dose hasn't been established. Doses up to 1,500 units/kg have been administered three times weekly for 3 weeks without direct toxic effects.
• With overdose, polycythemia may occur; phlebotomy may be used to bring hematocrit within appropriate levels.

Monitoring the patient

• Monitor hematocrit at least twice weekly during initiation of therapy and during dosage adjustments.
• In patients with chronic renal failure, measure hematocrit twice weekly until stabilized and during adjustment to maintenance dose. An interval of 2 to 6 weeks may elapse before a dosage change is reflected in hematocrit.
• Most patients eventually require supplemental iron therapy. Before and during therapy, monitor patient's iron stores, including serum ferritin and transferrin saturation.
• Monitor blood pressure closely.
• Monitor CBC with differential and platelet counts routinely.

Information for the patient

• Explain importance of regularly monitoring blood pressure because of potential drug effects.

- Advise patient to adhere to dietary restrictions during therapy. Make sure patient understands that drug won't influence disease process.

Pediatric patients
- Safety and efficacy in children haven't been established.

Breast-feeding patients
- It's unknown if drug appears in breast milk. Use with caution in breast-feeding women.

epoprostenol sodium
Flolan

Pharmacologic classification: naturally occurring prostaglandin
Therapeutic classification: vasodilator, antiplatelet aggregator
Pregnancy risk category B

How supplied
Available by prescription only
Injection: 0.5 mg/17-ml vial, 1.5 mg/17-ml vial

Indications, route, and dosage
Long-term I.V. treatment of primary pulmonary hypertension in New York Heart Association (NYHA) class III and class IV patients
Adults: Initially, 2 ng/kg/minute as an I.V. infusion; increase in increments of 2 ng/kg/minute q 15 minutes or longer until dose-limiting pharmacologic effects are elicited. Begin maintenance (long-term) dosing with 4 ng/kg/minute less than the maximum tolerated infusion rate as determined during initial dosing. If maximum tolerated infusion rate is below 5 ng/kg/minute, begin maintenance infusion at one-half maximum tolerated infusion rate. Base subsequent dosage adjustments on persistence, recurrence, or worsening of patient's symptoms of primary pulmonary hypertension and the occurrence of adverse events because of excessive doses of drug. Increases in dose from initial maintenance dose can generally be expected and are done in increments of 1 to 2 ng/kg/minute at intervals of at least 15 minutes.

Pharmacodynamics
Vasodilator and antiplatelet actions: Causes direct vasodilation of pulmonary and systemic arterial vascular beds and inhibits platelet aggregation.

Pharmacokinetics
- *Absorption:* Administered I.V.
- *Distribution:* No information available.
- *Metabolism:* Extensively metabolized.
- *Excretion:* Excreted primarily in urine with small amount excreted in feces.

Contraindications and precautions
Contraindicated in patients with hypersensitivity to drug or structurally related compounds. Long-term use of drug is also contraindicated in patients with heart failure because of severe left ventricular systolic dysfunction and in those who develop pulmonary edema during initial dosing.

Interactions
Drug-drug. *Anticoagulants, antiplatelet drugs:* May increase risk of bleeding. Monitor closely for bleeding.
Antihypertensives, diuretics, other vasodilators: May cause additional reduction in blood pressure. Monitor blood pressure closely.

Adverse reactions
CNS: *headache, anxiety, nervousness, agitation, dizziness, hyperesthesia, paresthesia.*
CV: *tachycardia; hypotension, chest pain,* **bradycardia** (during initial dosing).
GI: *nausea, vomiting;* abdominal pain, dyspepsia (during initial dosing); *diarrhea* (during maintenance dosing).
Hematologic: **thrombocytopenia.**
Musculoskeletal: musculoskeletal pain, back pain, *jaw pain, myalgia, nonspecific musculoskeletal pain* (during maintenance dosing).
Respiratory: dyspnea.
Skin: *flushing,* sweating (during initial dosing).
Other: *flulike symptoms, chills, fever,* **sepsis.**

☑ Special considerations
- Drug should be used only by staff experienced in diagnosis and treatment of primary pulmonary hypertension. Determining appropriate dose for patient (dose ranging) must be done in setting with personnel and equipment adequate for physiologic monitoring and emergency care.
- Reconstitute drug only as directed using sterile diluent for Flolan. Don't reconstitute or mix with other parenteral drugs or solutions before or during administration.
- Follow manufacturer guidelines for reconstituting drug to achieve concentration needed. Concentration selected should be compatible with infusion pump being used with respect to minimum and maximum flow rates, reservoir capacity, and infusion pump criteria recommended by manufacturer. When used for maintenance infusion, drug should be prepared in drug delivery reservoir appropriate for infusion pump with a total reservoir volume of at least 100 ml. Drug should be prepared using two vials of sterile diluent for epoprostenol for use during a 24-hour period.
- Before use, reconstituted solutions of drug must be protected from light and must be refrigerated at 36° to 46° F (2° to 8° C) if not used immediately. Don't freeze reconstituted drug solutions. Discard reconstituted solution that has been

frozen. Discard reconstituted solution if refrigerated for more than 48 hours.
• Maintenance dosing should be administered by continuous I.V. infusion via a permanent indwelling central venous catheter using an ambulatory infusion pump. During establishment of dosing range, drug may be administered peripherally.
• To facilitate extended use at ambient temperatures exceeding 77° F (25° C), use a cold pouch with frozen gel packs. A cold pouch must be capable of maintaining temperature of reconstituted drug between 36° and 46° F for 12 hours. If such a cold pouch is used during infusion, reconstituted solution should be used for no longer than 24 hours.
• Following establishment of a new maintenance infusion rate, observe patient closely and monitor patient's standing and supine blood pressure and heart rate for several hours to ensure that new dose is tolerated.
• During maintenance infusion, dose-related pharmacologic events similar to those seen during initial dosing may occur and require a decrease in infusion rate; however, the adverse event may occasionally resolve without dosage adjustment.
• Avoid abrupt withdrawal or sudden large reductions in infusion rates. Ensure that patient has access to backup infusion pump and I.V. infusion sets to avoid potential interruptions in drug delivery. A multilumen catheter should be considered if other I.V. therapies are routinely administered.
• To reduce risk of infection, use aseptic technique in drug reconstitution and administration as well as in routine catheter care.
• Overdose may result in flushing, headache, hypotension, tachycardia, nausea, vomiting, and diarrhea. Treatment usually requires dose reduction of epoprostenol.

Monitoring the patient
• Administer anticoagulant therapy during longterm use of drug, unless contraindicated. Monitor PT and INR closely.
• Monitor CBC regularly.
• Monitor standing and supine blood pressure and heart rate for several hours.

Information for the patient
• Before therapy starts, ensure that patient and family understand that there's a high likelihood that I.V. therapy with epoprostenol will be needed for prolonged periods, possibly years, and that patient or family has the ability to accept and care for a permanent I.V. catheter and infusion pump.
• Show patient and family how to reconstitute drug and administer drug via infusion pump using aseptic technique. Explain how to use infusion pump. Stress importance of maintaining continuous drug therapy. Provide patient and family with instructions on how to switch to a new infusion pump in the event of pump failure. Also instruct patient and family on drug storage.
• Instruct patient to report adverse reactions regarding drug therapy immediately because dosage adjustments may be necessary.
• Provide patient with telephone number to obtain assistance for 24-hour support.

Geriatric patients
• In general, dose selection for an elderly patient should be cautious, reflecting the greater frequency of decreased hepatic, renal, or cardiac function and concomitant disease or other drug therapy.

Pediatric patients
• Safety and effectiveness in children haven't been established.

Breast-feeding patients
• It's unknown if drug appears in breast milk. Use cautiously in breast-feeding women.

eprosartan mesylate
Teveten

Pharmacologic classification:
angiotensin II receptor antagonist
Therapeutic classification: antihypertensive
Pregnancy risk category C (D in second and third trimesters)

How supplied
Available by prescription only
Tablets: 400 mg, 600 mg

Indications, route, and dosage
Hypertension, alone or with other antihypertensives
Adults: Initially, 600 mg P.O. daily. Daily dose ranges from 400 to 800 mg given as single daily dose or two divided doses.

Pharmacodynamics
Antihypertensive action: An angiotensin II receptor that blocks vasoconstrictor and aldosterone-secreting effects of angiotensin II by selectively blocking binding of angiotensin II to its receptor sites found in many tissues, such as vascular smooth muscle and the adrenal gland.

Pharmacokinetics
• *Absorption:* Absolute bioavailability of single oral dose is about 13%. Onset of action occurs in about 1 to 2 hours, with plasma levels peaking in 1 to 3 hours.
• *Distribution:* Plasma protein-binding about 98%. Duration about 24 hours.
• *Metabolism:* No active metabolites.

• *Excretion:* Eliminated by biliary and renal excretion, primarily as unchanged drug. Following oral administration, about 90% recovered in feces and about 7% in urine. Terminal elimination half-life typically 5 to 9 hours.

Contraindications and precautions
Contraindicated in patients with hypersensitivity to drug or its components. Use cautiously in patients with an activated renin-angiotensin system, such as volume- or salt-depleted patients, and in patients whose renal function may depend on the activity of the renin-angiotensin-aldosterone system, such as patients with severe heart failure. Also use cautiously in patients with renal artery stenosis.

Interactions
None reported.

Adverse reactions
CNS: depression, fatigue, headache, dizziness.
CV: chest pain.
EENT: pharyngitis, rhinitis, sinusitis.
GI: abdominal pain, dyspepsia, diarrhea.
GU: urinary tract infection, increased BUN level.
Hematologic: *neutropenia.*
Metabolic: hypertriglyceridemia.
Musculoskeletal: arthralgia, myalgia.
Respiratory: cough, upper respiratory tract infection, bronchitis.
Other: injury, viral infection, dependent edema, facial edema, *angioedema.*

☑ Special considerations
• Drugs that act directly on the renin-angiotensin system can cause fetal and neonatal morbidity and death when administered to pregnant women. If pregnancy is detected, stop drug as soon as possible. These adverse effects haven't occurred when intrauterine drug exposure has been limited to first trimester.
• Correct hypovolemia and hyponatremia before therapy to reduce risk of symptomatic hypotension.
• A transient episode of hypotension isn't a contraindication to continued treatment. Drug may be restarted once patient's blood pressure has stabilized.
• Use drug alone or with other antihypertensives, such as diuretics and calcium channel blockers. Maximal blood pressure response may take 2 to 3 weeks.
• In case of overdose, give symptomatic and supportive therapy. Drug is poorly removed by hemodialysis.

Monitoring the patient
• Monitor blood pressure closely for 2 hours during start of therapy. If hypotension occurs, place patient in supine position and, if necessary, give intravenous infusion of normal saline.

• Monitor patient for facial or lip swelling; angioedema has occurred with other angiotensin II antagonists.
• Closely observe neonates exposed to eprosartan in utero for hypotension, oliguria, and hyperkalemia.
• Monitor renal function before treatment and periodically throughout.

Information for the patient
• Advise woman of childbearing age to use reliable form of contraception and to call immediately if pregnancy is suspected. Drug may need to be stopped under medical supervision.
• Advise patient to report facial or lip swelling and signs and symptoms of infection, such as fever or sore throat.
• Tell patient to obtain medical approval before taking OTC product for dry cough.
• Inform patient that drug may be taken without regard to meals.
• Tell patient to store drug at a controlled room temperature (68° to 77° F [20 to 25° C]).

Geriatric patients
• There is a slightly decreased response to drug in elderly patients. No initial dose adjustment necessary.

Pediatric patients
• Safety and effectiveness in children haven't been established.

Breast-feeding patients
• It's unknown if drug appears in breast milk. Because of potential for serious adverse reactions in breast-feeding infants, a decision should be made to stop drug or breast-feeding.

eptifibatide
Integrilin

Pharmacologic classification: glycoprotein IIb/IIIa (GP IIb/IIIa) inhibitor
Therapeutic classification: antiplatelet drug
Pregnancy risk category B

How supplied
Available by prescription only.
Injection: 2 mg/ml, 10-ml vial, 0.75 mg/ml, 100-ml vials.

Indications, route, and dosage
Treatment of patients with acute coronary syndrome (unstable angina or non-Q-wave MI), including patients who are to be managed medically and those undergoing percutaneous coronary intervention
Adults: 180 mcg/kg (up to maximum dose of 22.6 mg) I.V. bolus as soon as possible following di-

agnosis; then a continuous I.V. infusion of 2 mcg/kg/minute (up to maximum infusion rate of 15 mg/hour) for up to 72 hours. Infusion rate may be decreased to 0.5 mcg/kg/minute during percutaneous coronary intervention. Continue infusion for an additional 20 to 24 hours after procedure for up to 96 hours of therapy.

Treatment of patients not presenting with an acute coronary syndrome who are undergoing percutaneous coronary intervention
Adults: I.V. bolus of 135 mcg/kg administered immediately before procedure; then a continuous infusion of 0.5 mcg/kg/minute for 20 to 24 hours.

Pharmacodynamics
Antiplatelet action: Reversibly inhibits platelet aggregation by preventing the binding of fibrinogen, von Willebrand factor, and other adhesion molecules to the GP IIb/IIIa receptor on platelets.

Pharmacokinetics
• *Absorption:* Not applicable with I.V. administration.
• *Distribution:* 25% bound to plasma proteins.
• *Metabolism:* No information available. No major metabolites detected in plasma.
• *Excretion:* Elimination half-life is 2.5 hours. Most drug excreted in urine.

Contraindications and precautions
Contraindicated in patients with hypersensitivity to drug or its components.

Contraindicated in patients with a history of bleeding diathesis or evidence of active abnormal bleeding within previous 30 days; severe hypertension (systolic blood pressure exceeding 200 mm Hg or diastolic blood pressure over 110 mm Hg) not adequately controlled on antihypertensive therapy; major surgery within previous 6 weeks; history of stroke within 30 days or hemorrhagic stroke; current or planned use of another parenteral GP IIb/IIIa inhibitor; or a platelet count below 100,000/mm³.

Contraindicated in patients with serum creatinine level of 2 mg/dl or higher (for the 180 mcg/kg bolus and 2 mcg/kg/minute infusion) or 4 mg/dl or higher (for the 135 mcg/kg bolus and 0.5 mcg/kg/minute infusion); and in patients who are dependent on renal dialysis.

Use cautiously in patients at increased risk for bleeding and in those weighing over 315 lb (143 kg).

Interactions
Drug-drug. *Clopidogrel, dipyridamole, NSAIDs, oral anticoagulants (warfarin), thrombolytics, ticlopidine:* May increase risk of bleeding. Monitor patient closely.
Other inhibitors of platelet receptor GP IIb/IIIa: May potentiate serious bleeding. Don't administer together.

Adverse reactions
CV: hypotension.
GU: hematuria.
Hematologic: *bleeding, thrombocytopenia,* bleeding at femoral artery access site.

☑ Special considerations
• Withdraw bolus dose from 10-ml vial into a syringe and administer by I.V. push over 1 to 2 minutes.
• Administer I.V. infusion undiluted directly from 100-ml vial using an infusion pump.
• Inspect solution for particulate before administration. If visible particles occur, then sterility is suspect; discard solution.
• Drug may be administered in same I.V. line as alteplase, atropine, dobutamine, heparin, lidocaine, meperidine, metoprolol, midazolam, morphine, nitroglycerin, or verapamil.
• Drug may be administered in same I.V. line with normal saline or normal saline solution and 5% dextrose and may also contain up to 60 mEq/L of potassium chloride.
• Don't administer drug in same I.V. line as furosemide.
• Drug should be used with heparin and aspirin.
• Discontinue eptifibatide and heparin and achieve sheath hemostasis by standard compressive techniques at least 4 hours before hospital discharge. Arterial access site is most common site of bleeding.
• If patient is to undergo coronary artery bypass graft surgery, infusion should be stopped before surgery.
• Minimize use of arterial and venous punctures, I.M. injections, urinary catheters, and nasotracheal and nasogastric tubes.
• When obtaining I.V. access, avoid noncompressible sites (such as subclavian or jugular veins).
• Store vials in refrigerator at 36° to 46° F (2° to 8° C).
• Protect from light until administration.

Monitoring the patient
• Perform baseline laboratory tests before start of drug therapy; determine hematocrit, hemoglobin level, platelet count, serum creatinine level, PT, INR, and PTT.
• If patient's platelet count is below 100,000/mm³, stop eptifibatide and heparin.
• Monitor patient for bleeding.
• Monitor serum creatinine level before starting treatment and regularly throughout infusion.

Information for the patient
• Explain that drug works by making platelets less sticky and may prevent chest pain, heart attack, and death.
• Instruct patient to report chest discomfort or other adverse effects immediately.

- Caution patient to avoid activities that might cause bleeding or bruising.

Geriatric patients
- Drug has been used in patients up to age 94; effects of drug are same in this group as in younger population.

Pediatric patients
- Safety and efficacy in children haven't been established.

Breast-feeding patients
- It's unknown if drug appears in breast milk. Administer cautiously to breast-feeding women.

ergocalciferol (vitamin D₂)
Calciferol, Drisdol, Vitamin D

Pharmacologic classification: vitamin
Therapeutic classification: antihypocalcemic
Pregnancy risk category C

How supplied
Available by prescription only
Capsules: 1.25 mg (50,000 units)
Injection: 12.5 mg (500,000 units)/ml
Available without a prescription
Liquid: 8,000 units/ml in 60-ml dropper bottle

Indications, route, and dosage
Nutritional rickets or osteomalacia
Adults: 25 to 125 mcg P.O. daily if patient has normal GI absorption. With severe malabsorption, 250 mcg to 7.5 mg P.O. or 250 mcg I.M. daily.
Children: 25 to 125 mcg P.O. daily if patient has normal GI absorption. With malabsorption, 250 to 625 mcg P.O. daily.
Familial hypophosphatemia
Adults: 250 mcg to 1.5 mg P.O. daily with phosphate supplements.
Children: 1 to 2 mg P.O. daily with phosphate supplements. Increase daily dose in 250- to 500-mcg increments at 3- to 4-month intervals until adequate response is obtained.
Vitamin D–dependent rickets
Adults: 250 mcg to 1.5 mg P.O. daily.
Children: 75 to 125 mcg P.O. daily.
Anticonvulsant-induced rickets and osteomalacia
Adults: 50 mcg to 1.25 mg P.O. daily.
Hypoparathyroidism and pseudohypoparathyroidism
Adults: 625 mcg to 5 mg P.O. daily with calcium supplements.
Children: 1.25 to 5 mg P.O. daily with calcium supplements.
◇ Fanconi's syndrome
Adults: 1.25 to 5 mg P.O. daily.
Children: 625 mcg to 1.25 mg P.O. daily.

◇ Osteoporosis
Adults: 25 to 250 mcg P.O. daily or 1.25 mg P.O. weekly with calcium and fluoride supplements.

Pharmacodynamics
Antihypocalcemic action: Once activated, ergocalciferol acts to regulate the serum levels of calcium by regulating absorption from the GI tract and resorption from bone.

Pharmacokinetics
- *Absorption:* Absorbed readily from small intestine. Onset of action is 10 to 24 hours.
- *Distribution:* Distributed widely; bound to proteins stored in liver.
- *Metabolism:* Metabolized in liver and kidneys. Average half-life of 24 hours; duration of up to 6 months.
- *Excretion:* Bile (feces) is primary excretion route; small percentage excreted in urine.

Contraindications and precautions
Contraindicated in patients with hypercalcemia, hypervitaminosis A, or renal osteodystrophy with hyperphosphatemia. Use with extreme caution, if at all, in patients with impaired renal function, heart disease, renal stones, or arteriosclerosis.

Interactions
Drug-drug. *Antacids containing magnesium:* May lead to hypermagnesemia. Monitor magnesium level.
Cardiac glycosides: May cause additive effects, resulting in arrhythmias. Avoid concomitant use.
Cholestyramine, colestipol, excessive use of mineral oil: May interfere with ergocalciferol absorption. Monitor patient for effects.
Corticosteroids: Counteract drug's effects. Monitor patient.
Phenobarbital, phenytoin: May increase drug's metabolism to inactive metabolites. Observe for drug's effects.
Thiazide diuretics: May cause hypercalcemia in patients with hypoparathyroidism. Monitor serum calcium levels.
Verapamil: May induce recurrence of atrial fibrillation when supplemental calcium and ergocalciferol have induced hypercalcemia. Avoid concomitant use.

Adverse reactions
Adverse reactions listed usually occur only in vitamin D toxicity.
CNS: headache, weakness, somnolence, decreased libido, overt psychosis, irritability.
CV: *calcifications of soft tissues, including the heart,* hypertension, **arrhythmias.**
EENT: rhinorrhea, conjunctivitis (calcific), photophobia.
GI: anorexia, nausea, vomiting, constipation, dry mouth, metallic taste, polydipsia.

GU: polyuria, albuminuria, hypercalciuria, nocturia, *impaired renal function,* reversible azotemia.
Hepatic: elevated liver enzymes (falsely or actually).
Metabolic: *hypercalcemia,* hyperthermia, increased serum cholesterol levels, weight loss.
Musculoskeletal: bone and muscle pain, bone demineralization.
Skin: pruritus.

☑ Special considerations
● I.M. injection of ergocalciferol dispersed in oil is preferable in patients who are unable to absorb oral form.
● If I.V. route is necessary, use only water-miscible solutions intended for dilution in large-volume parenterals. Use cautiously in cardiac patients, especially if they are receiving cardiotonic glycosides. In such patients, hypercalcemia may precipitate arrhythmias.
● Patients with hyperphosphatemia need dietary phosphate restrictions and binding drugs to avoid metastatic calcifications and renal calculi.
● When high therapeutic doses are used, frequent serum and urine calcium, potassium, and urea determinations should be made.
● Patients with malabsorption due to inadequate bile or hepatic dysfunction may require addition of exogenous bile salts.
● Doses of 60,000 IU daily can cause hypercalcemia.
● Signs and symptoms of overdose include hypercalcemia, hypercalciuria, and hyperphosphatemia, which may be treated by stopping therapy, starting a low-calcium diet, and increasing fluid intake.
● After overdose, a loop diuretic, such as furosemide, may be given with saline I.V. infusion to increase calcium excretion. Provide supportive measures. In severe cases, death from cardiac or renal failure may occur. Calcitonin may decrease hypercalcemia.

Monitoring the patient
● Determine baseline serum calcium and phosphorus levels and renal function.
● Monitor serum and urine calcium, potassium, and urea levels frequently.
● Monitor eating and bowel habits; dry mouth, nausea, vomiting, metallic taste, and constipation can be early signs of toxicity.

Information for the patient
● Explain importance of a calcium-rich diet.
● Caution patient not to increase daily dose on own initiative. Vitamin D is a fat-soluble vitamin; vitamin D toxicity is thus more likely to occur.
● Tell patient to avoid mineral oil and antacids containing magnesium.
● Instruct patient to swallow tablets whole without crushing or chewing.

Pediatric patients
● Some infants may be hyperreactive to drug.

Breast-feeding patients
● Very little drug appears in breast milk; however, effect on infants of amounts exceeding RDA levels is unknown.

ergonovine maleate
Ergotrate Maleate

Pharmacologic classification: ergot alkaloid
Therapeutic classification: oxytocic
Pregnancy risk category NR

How supplied
Available by prescription only
Injection: 0.2-mg/ml ampules

Indications, route, and dosage
Prevention or treatment of postpartum and postabortion hemorrhage due to uterine atony or subinvolution
Adults: 0.2 mg I.M. q 2 to 4 hours, maximum five doses; or 0.2 mg I.V. (only for severe uterine bleeding or other life-threatening emergency) over 1 minute while blood pressure and uterine contractions are monitored. I.V. dose may be diluted to 5 ml with normal saline injection.
◇ *To diagnose coronary artery spasm (Prinzmetal's angina)*
Adults: 0.1 to 0.4 mg I.V. for one dose.

Pharmacodynamics
Oxytocic action: Stimulates contractions of uterine and vascular smooth muscle, producing intense uterine contractions, then periods of relaxation. Produces vasoconstriction of primarily capacitance blood vessels, causing an increased CVP and elevated blood pressure.
    The clinical effect is secondary to contraction of the uterine wall around bleeding vessels, producing hemostasis.

Pharmacokinetics
● *Absorption:* Rapid following I.M. administration. Immediate onset of action for I.V., 2 to 5 minutes for I.M.
● *Distribution:* No information available.
● *Metabolism:* Metabolized in liver.
● *Excretion:* Primarily nonrenal elimination in feces suggested.

Contraindications and precautions
Contraindicated in patients sensitive to ergot preparations; in threatened spontaneous abortion, induction of labor, or before delivery of placenta because captivation of placenta may occur; and in those with history of allergic or idiosyncratic reactions to drug.

Reactions may be *common,* uncommon, *life-threatening,* or COMMON AND LIFE-THREATENING.

Because of the potential for adverse CV effects, use cautiously in patients with hypertension, toxemia, sepsis, occlusive vascular disease, or hepatic, renal, or cardiac disease.

Interactions
Drug-drug. *Calcium gluconate:* If patient isn't also taking a cardiac glycoside, cautious administration of calcium gluconate I.V. may produce desired oxytocic action in calcium-deficient patients. Monitor patient for desired effects.
Local anesthetics with vasoconstrictors (lidocaine with epinephrine): Enhanced vasoconstriction. Avoid concomitant use.
Sympathomimetic amines, ergot alkaloids: Enhanced vasoconstrictor potential. Avoid concomitant use.
Drug-lifestyle. *Smoking:* Enhanced vasoconstriction. Educate patient about concomitant use.

Adverse reactions
CNS: headache, confusion, dizziness, ringing in ears.
CV: chest pain, weakness in legs (peripheral vasospasm), hypertension, thrombophlebitis, *signs of shock.*
GI: nausea, vomiting, diarrhea, cramping.
Metabolic: decreased serum prolactin.
Musculoskeletal: pain in arms, legs, or lower back.
Respiratory: shortness of breath.
Other: itching; sweating; *hypersensitivity reactions.*
Note: Stop drug if hypertension or allergic reactions occur.

☑ Special considerations
• Contractions begin immediately after I.V. injection and may continue for 45 minutes.
• Hypocalcemia may decrease patient response; I.V. administration of calcium salts is necessary.
• High doses during delivery may cause uterine tetany and possible infant hypoxia or intracranial hemorrhage.
• Drug has been used as a diagnostic for angina pectoris.
• Signs and symptoms of overdose include seizures, with nausea, vomiting, diarrhea, dizziness, fluctuations in blood pressure, weak pulse, chest pain, tingling, and numbness and coldness in the extremities. Rarely, gangrene has occurred.
• Treat seizures with anticonvulsants and hypercoagulability with heparin; give vasodilators to improve blood flow. Gangrene may require amputation.

Monitoring the patient
• Monitor hepatic and renal function before starting treatment.
• Monitor blood pressure, pulse rate, uterine response, and character and amount of vaginal bleeding. Watch for sudden changes in vital signs and frequent periods of uterine relaxation.

Information for the patient
• Tell patient not to smoke while taking drug.
• Advise patient of possible adverse reactions.

Breast-feeding patients
• Drug appears in breast milk, and ergotism has occurred in breast-fed infants of mothers treated with other ergot alkaloids. Use with caution. Ergot alkaloids inhibit lactation.

ergotamine tartrate
Cafergot, Ergomar, Ergostat, Gynergen, Wigraine

Pharmacologic classification: ergot alkaloid
Therapeutic classification: vasoconstrictor
Pregnancy risk category X

How supplied
Available by prescription only
Tablets (S.L.): 2 mg
Tablets: 1 mg* (with or without caffeine 100 mg)
Suppositories: 2 mg (with caffeine 100 mg)

Indications, route, and dosage
To prevent or abort vascular headache, including migraine and cluster headaches
Adults: Initially, 2 mg S.L. or P.O., then 1 to 2 mg S.L. or P.O. q 30 minutes, to maximum 6 mg per attack or in 24 hours, and 10 mg weekly. Or, initially, 1 inhalation; if not relieved in 5 minutes, repeat 1 inhalation. May repeat inhalations at least 5 minutes apart up to maximum of 6 inhalations per 24 hours or 15 inhalations weekly. Patient may also use rectal suppositories. Initially, 2 mg P.R. at onset of attack; repeat in 1 hour, p.r.n. Maximum dose is 2 suppositories per attack or 5 suppositories weekly.
◊ *Children:* 1 mg S.L. in older children and adolescents; if no improvement, additional 1-mg dose may be given in 30 minutes.

Pharmacodynamics
Vasoconstricting action: By stimulating alpha-adrenergic receptors, ergotamine in therapeutic doses causes peripheral vasoconstriction (if vascular tone is low); however, if vascular tone is high, it produces vasodilation. In high doses, it's a competitive alpha-adrenergic blocker. In therapeutic doses, it inhibits the reuptake of norepinephrine, which increases the vasoconstricting activity of ergotamine. A weaker serotonin antagonist, it reduces the increased rate of platelet aggregation caused by serotonin.
In treatment of vascular headaches, ergotamine probably causes direct vasoconstri

of dilated carotid artery beds while decreasing the amplitude of pulsations. Its serotoninergic and catecholamine effects also seem to be involved.

Pharmacokinetics
• *Absorption:* Rapidly absorbed after inhalation; variably absorbed after oral administration. Plasma levels peak in ½ to 3 hours. Caffeine may increase rate and extent of absorption. Undergoes first-pass metabolism after oral administration.
• *Distribution:* Widely distributed throughout body.
• *Metabolism:* Extensively metabolized in liver.
• *Excretion:* 4% of dose excreted in urine within 96 hours; remainder presumed excreted in feces; is dialyzable. Onset of action depends on how promptly drug is given after headache onset.

Contraindications and precautions
Contraindicated in patients with hypersensitivity to ergot alkaloids and in those with peripheral and occlusive vascular diseases, coronary artery disease, hypertension, hepatic or renal dysfunction, severe pruritus, or sepsis; also contraindicated during pregnancy.

Interactions
Drug-drug. *Erythromycin, other macrolides:* May cause symptoms of ergot toxicity. Monitor patient closely.
Propranolol, other beta blockers: Blocked natural pathway for vasodilation in patients receiving ergot alkaloids; may result in excessive vasoconstriction. Monitor patient closely.
Drug-lifestyle. *Caffeine:* May increase rate and extent of absorption. Discourage concomitant use.
Smoking: May increase adverse drug effects. Discourage patient from smoking.
Cold temperatures: May increase adverse drug effects. Caution patient to avoid extreme cold.

Adverse reactions
CNS: numbness and tingling in fingers and toes.
CV: transient tachycardia or bradycardia, precordial distress and pain, increased arterial pressure, angina pectoris, peripheral vasoconstriction.
GI: nausea, vomiting.
Musculoskeletal: weakness in legs, muscle pain in extremities.
Skin: pruritus, localized edema.

☑ Special considerations
Besides the recommendations relevant to all alpha blockers, consider the following.
• Drug is most effective when used in prodromal stage of headache or as soon as possible after onset. Provide quiet, low-light environment to relax patient after dose is administered.

• Store drug in light-resistant container.
• Sublingual tablet is preferred during early stage of attack because of rapid absorption.
• Obtain an accurate dietary history to determine possible relationship between certain foods and onset of headache.
• Rebound headache or an increase in duration or frequency of headache may occur when drug is stopped.
• If patient experiences severe vasoconstriction with tissue necrosis, administer I.V. sodium nitroprusside or intra-arterial tolazoline. I.V. heparin and 10% dextran 40 in D_5W injection also may be administered to prevent vascular stasis and thrombosis.
• Drug isn't effective for muscle contraction headaches.
• Vasodilators such as nifedipine, nitroprusside, or prazosin may be used to treat ergot toxicity.
• Signs and symptoms of overdose include adverse vasospastic effects, nausea, vomiting, lassitude, impaired mental function, delirium, severe dyspnea, hypotension or hypertension, rapid or weak pulse, unconsciousness, spasms of the limbs, seizures, and shock.
• Treatment of overdose is supportive and symptomatic and requires prolonged and careful monitoring. If patient is conscious and ingestion is recent, empty stomach by emesis or gastric lavage; if comatose, perform gastric lavage after placement of endotracheal tube with cuff inflated. Activated charcoal and a saline (magnesium sulfate) cathartic may be used. Provide respiratory support.
• In overdose, apply warmth (not direct heat) to ischemic extremities if vasospasm occurs. Administer vasodilators (nitroprusside, prazosin, or tolazoline) as needed and, if necessary, I.V. diazepam to treat convulsions. Dialysis may be helpful.

Monitoring the patient
• Monitor hepatic and renal function and blood pressure before therapy starts and periodically throughout.
• Monitor patient for adverse effects.

Information for the patient
• Instruct patient in correct use of inhaler.
• Urge patient to immediately report feelings of numbness or tingling in fingers or toes, or red or violet blisters on hands or feet.
• Caution patient to avoid alcoholic beverages, which may worsen headache. Also avoid smoking, which may increase adverse effects of drug.
• Warn patient to avoid prolonged exposure to very cold temperatures, which may increase adverse effects of drug.
• Advise patient who uses inhaler to call promptly if mouth, throat, or lung infection occurs or if condition worsens. Cough, hoarseness, or throat irritation may occur. The patient should gargle

and rinse mouth after each dose to help prevent hoarseness and irritation.
- Instruct patient to call promptly if persistent numbness or tingling of fingers or toes and chest, muscle, or abdominal pain occur.
- Advise patient not to exceed recommended dose.
- Tell patient not to eat, drink, or smoke while sublingual tablet is dissolving.

Geriatric patients
- Administer cautiously to elderly patients.

Pediatric patients
- Safety and efficacy in children haven't been established.

Breast-feeding patients
- Drug appears in breast milk; use with caution in breast-feeding women. Excessive dosage or prolonged use of drug may inhibit lactation.

erythromycin base
E-Base, E-Mycin, ERYC, Ery-Tab, PCE

erythromycin estolate
Ilosone

erythromycin ethylsuccinate
E.E.S., EryPed, Pediazole

erythromycin gluceptate
Ilotycin Gluceptate

erythromycin lactobionate
Erythrocin

erythromycin stearate
Apo-Erythro-S*, Erythrocin Stearate Filmtab, Novo-Rythro*

erythromycin (topical)
Akne-Mycin, A/T/S, Del-Mycin, Erycette, EryDerm, Erymax, Ery-Sol, Erythra-Derm, Staticin, Theramycin Z, T-Stat

Pharmacologic classification: erythromycin
Therapeutic classification: antibiotic
Pregnancy risk category B

How supplied
Available by prescription only
Oral suspension: 125 mg/5 ml, 200 mg/5 ml, 400 mg/5 ml
erythromycin base
Tablets (enteric-coated): 250 mg, 333 mg, 500 mg
Pellets (enteric-coated): 250 mg
erythromycin estolate
Tablets: 500 mg

Capsules: 250 mg
Suspension: 125 mg/5 ml, 250 mg/5 ml
erythromycin ethylsuccinate
Tablets (chewable): 200 mg
Topical solution: 1.5%, 2%
Topical gel: 2%
Topical ointment: 2%
Oral suspension: 400 mg/5 ml
Powder for oral suspension: 200 mg/5 ml (after reconstitution)
Granules for oral suspension: 400 mg/5 ml (after reconstitution)
Ophthalmic ointment: 5 mg/g
erythromycin gluceptate
Injection: 1-g vials
erythromycin lactobionate
Injection: 500-mg, 1-g vials
erythromycin stearate
Tablets (film-coated): 250 mg, 500 mg

Indications, route, and dosage
Acute pelvic inflammatory disease caused by Neisseria gonorrhoeae
Adults: 500 mg I.V. (gluceptate, lactobionate) q 6 hours for 3 days; then 250 mg (base, estolate, stearate) or 400 mg (ethylsuccinate) P.O. q 6 hours for 7 days.
Endocarditis prophylaxis for dental procedures in patients allergic to penicillin
Adults: Initially, 800 mg (ethylsuccinate) or 1 g (stearate) P.O. 2 hours before procedure; then 400 mg (ethylsuccinate) or 500 mg (stearate) P.O. 6 hours later.
Children: Initially, 20 mg/kg (ethylsuccinate or stearate) P.O. 2 hours before procedure; then 10 mg/kg 6 hours later.
Intestinal amebiasis in patients who can't receive metronidazole
Adults: 250 mg (base, estolate, stearate) or 400 mg (ethylsuccinate) P.O. q 6 hours for 10 to 14 days.
Children: 30 to 50 mg/kg (base, estolate, ethylsuccinate, stearate) P.O. q 6 hours for 10 to 14 days. (*Note:* Base and stearate forms not available in liquid form).
Mild to moderately severe respiratory tract, skin, and soft-tissue infections caused by susceptible organisms
Adults: 250 to 500 mg (base, estolate, stearate) P.O. q 6 hours; or 400 to 800 mg (ethylsuccinate) P.O. q 6 hours; or 15 to 20 mg/kg (gluceptate, lactobionate) I.V. daily, in divided doses q 6 hours.
Children: 30 mg/kg to 50 mg/kg (oral erythromycin salts) P.O. daily, in divided doses q 6 hours; or 15 to 20 mg/kg I.V. daily, in divided doses q 4 to 6 hours.
Syphilis
Adults: 500 mg (base, estolate, stearate) P.O. q.i.d. for 14 days.

Legionnaire's disease
Adults: 500 mg to 1 g I.V. or P.O. (base, estolate, stearate) or 800 mg to 1,600 mg (ethylsuccinate) P.O. q 6 hours for 21 days.
Uncomplicated urethral, endocervical, or rectal infections when tetracyclines are contraindicated
Adults: 500 mg (base, estolate, stearate) or 800 mg (ethylsuccinate) P.O. q.i.d. for at least 7 days.
Urogenital Chlamydia trachomatis *infections during pregnancy*
Adults: 500 mg (base, estolate, stearate) P.O. q.i.d. for at least 7 days or 250 mg (base, estolate, stearate) or 400 mg (ethylsuccinate) P.O. q.i.d. for at least 14 days.
Conjunctivitis caused by C. trachomatis *in neonates*
Neonates: 50 mg/kg/day P.O. in four divided doses for at least 2 weeks.
Pneumonia of infancy caused by C. trachomatis
Infants: 50 mg/kg/day P.O. in four divided doses for at least 3 weeks.
Topical treatment of acne vulgaris
Adults and children: Apply to the affected area b.i.d.
Prophylaxis of ophthalmia neonatorum
Neonates: Apply 1-cm ribbon of ointment in lower conjunctival sac of each eye no later than 1 hour after birth. Use new tube for each infant and don't flush after instillation.
Acute and chronic conjunctivitis, trachoma, other eye infections
Adults and children: Apply 1-cm ribbon of ointment directly into infected eye up to six times daily, depending on severity of infection.

Pharmacodynamics
Antibacterial action: Inhibits bacterial protein synthesis by binding to the ribosomal 50S subunit. Used to treat *Haemophilus influenzae, Entamoeba histolytica, Mycoplasma pneumoniae, Corynebacterium diphtheriae, C. minutissimum, Legionella pneumophila,* and *Bordetella pertussis.* May be used as an alternative to penicillins or tetracycline in treatment of *Streptococcus pneumoniae, S. viridans, Listeria monocytogenes, Staphylococcus aureus, C. trachomatis, N. gonorrhoeae,* and *Treponema pallidum.*

Pharmacokinetics
- *Absorption:* Base salt is acid-sensitive; must be buffered or have enteric coating to prevent destruction by gastric acids. Acid salts and esters (estolate, ethylsuccinate, and stearate) not affected by gastric acidity and are well absorbed. Give base and stearate preparations on empty stomach. Absorption of estolate and ethylsuccinate preparations is unaffected or possibly enhanced by food. Topical route absorbed minimally.

- *Distribution:* Distributed widely to most body tissues and fluids except CSF, where it appears only in low levels. Drug crosses placenta. About 80% of base and 96% of erythromycin estolate protein-bound.
- *Metabolism:* Metabolized partially in liver to inactive metabolites.
- *Excretion:* Excreted mainly unchanged in bile. Less than 5% excreted in urine; some drug excreted in breast milk. In patients with normal renal function, plasma half-life is about 1½ hours. Drug isn't dialyzable.

Contraindications and precautions
Contraindicated in patients with hypersensitivity to drug or other macrolides. Erythromycin estolate is contraindicated in patients with hepatic disease. Use erythromycin salts cautiously in patients with impaired hepatic function.

Interactions
Drug-drug. *Carbamazepine:* May increase carbamazepine blood levels and risk of toxicity. Monitor carbamazepine levels.
Clindamycin, lincomycin: May be antagonistic. Monitor patient for drug effects.
Cyclosporine: May increase serum cyclosporine levels and increase risk of subsequent nephrotoxicity. Monitor renal function.
Digoxin: May cause increased serum digoxin levels. Monitor patient for arrhythmias.
Disopyramide: May increase disopyramide plasma levels, resulting in arrhythmias and increased QT intervals. Monitor cardiac function.
Isotretinoin: May cause cumulative dryness, resulting in excessive skin irritation. Observe for skin changes.
Midazolam, triazolam: May increase effects of these drugs. Monitor patient.
Oral anticoagulants: May cause excessive anticoagulant effect. Monitor INR.
Theophylline: May cause increased serum theophylline levels and decreased erythromycin blood level. Monitor patient for effect of erythromycin and observe for theophylline toxicity.
Drug-herb. *Pill-bearing spurge:* May inhibit CYP3A enzymes, affecting drug metabolism. Discourage concomitant use.
Drug-lifestyle. *Abrasive or medicated soaps or cleansers; acne preparations or other preparations containing peeling drugs (benzoyl peroxide, resorcinol, salicylic acid, sulfur, tretinoin); astringent soaps or cosmetics; medicated cosmetics or cover-ups); products containing alcohol (aftershave, cosmetics, perfumed toiletries, shaving creams, lotions):* May cause cumulative dryness, resulting in excessive skin irritation. Instruct patient to watch for skin changes.

Adverse reactions
CV: *ventricular arrhythmias.*

EENT: bilateral reversible hearing loss (with high systemic or oral doses in patients with renal or hepatic insufficiency); slowed corneal wound healing, blurred vision (with ophthalmic administration).

GI: *abdominal pain, cramping, nausea, vomiting, diarrhea* (with oral or systemic administration).

Hepatic: cholestatic jaundice (with estolate).

Skin: urticaria, rash, eczema (with oral or systemic administration); urticaria, dermatitis (with ophthalmic administration); sensitivity reactions, erythema, burning, *dryness, pruritus,* irritation, peeling, oily skin (with topical application).

Other: overgrowth of nonsusceptible bacteria or fungi; **anaphylaxis,** fever (with oral or systemic administration); *venous irritation, thrombophlebitis* (after I.V. injection); overgrowth of nonsusceptible organisms (with long-term use); **hypersensitivity reactions,** including itching and burning eyes (with ophthalmic administration).

☑ Special considerations
• Administer base and stearate preparations on empty stomach. Absorption of estolate and ethylsuccinate preparations is unaffected or possibly even enhanced by presence of food. When administered topically, drug is minimally absorbed.

• Reconstitute injectable form (lactobionate) based on manufacturer's instructions and dilute every 250 mg in at least 100 ml of normal saline solution. Continuous infusions are preferred, but drug may be given by intermittent infusion at a maximum concentration of 5 mg/ml infused over 20 to 60 minutes.

• Don't administer erythromycin lactobionate with other drugs because of chemical instability. Reconstituted solutions are acidic and should be completely administered within 8 hours of preparation.

• Drug may cause overgrowth of nonsusceptible bacteria or fungi.

• Although drug is bacteriostatic, it may be bactericidal in high levels or against highly susceptible organisms.

• Erythromycin may interfere with fluorometric determination of urinary catecholamines.

• False elevation of liver function tests using colorimetric assays may occur (rare).

Monitoring the patient
• Monitor hepatic function before treatment.

• Erythromycin estolate may cause serious hepatotoxicity (reversible cholestatic jaundice) in adults. Monitor liver function tests for increased serum bilirubin, AST, and alkaline phosphatase levels. Other erythromycin salts can cause less severe hepatotoxicity. (Patients who develop hepatotoxicity from erythromycin estolate may react similarly to any erythromycin preparation.)

• Perform culture and sensitivity tests before treatment starts and then as needed.

Information for the patient
• For best absorption, instruct patient to take oral form with full glass of water 1 hour before or 2 hours after meals. (However, patient receiving enteric-coated tablets may take them with meals.) Advise him not to take drug with fruit juice. Instruct patient taking chewable tablets not to swallow whole.

• If using topical solution, instruct patient to wash, rinse, and dry affected areas before applying. Warn him not to apply solution near eyes, nose, mouth, or other mucous membranes. Caution patient to avoid sharing washcloths and towels with family members.

• Instruct patient applying ophthalmic ointment to wash hands before and after applying ointment. Instruct him to cleanse eye area of excess exudate before applying ointment. Warn patient not to allow tube to touch the eye or surrounding tissue. Instruct him to promptly report signs of sensitivity, such as itching eyelids and constant burning.

• Tell patient to take drug exactly as directed and to continue taking it for prescribed period, even after feeling better.

• Instruct patient to report adverse reactions promptly.

Breast-feeding patients
• Although drug appears in breast milk, no adverse reactions have been reported. Use cautiously in breast-feeding women.

esmolol hydrochloride
Brevibloc

Pharmacologic classification: beta blocker
Therapeutic classification: antiarrhythmic
Pregnancy risk category C

How supplied
Available by prescription only
Injection: 10 mg/ml in 10-ml vials; 250 mg/ml in 10-ml ampules

Indications, route, and dosage
Supraventricular tachycardia
Adults: Dosage range is 50 to 200 mcg/kg/minute; average dose is 100 mcg/kg/minute. Individual dosage adjustment requires stepwise titration in which each step consists of a loading dose then a maintenance dose.

To begin treatment, administer a loading infusion of 500 mcg/kg/minute for 1 minute, then a 4-minute maintenance infusion of 50 mcg/kg/minute. If tachycardia doesn't subside within 5 m̃ utes, repeat loading dose and follow with maintenance infusion increased to 100 mcg/kg/minute. Continue titration, repeating loading infusion and increasing each maintenance infusion by 50 mcg/kg/minute. As patient's heart rate or blood pressure reaches a safety endpoint, omit loading infusion and reduce the increase in maintenance infusion from 50 to 25 mcg/kg/minute or less; also, increase the interval between titration steps from 5 to 10 minutes.

Intraoperative and postoperative tachycardia and hypertension

Adults: For immediate control, 80 mg (about 1 mg/kg) I.V. bolus dose over 30 seconds then a 150 mcg/kg/minute infusion, if necessary; for gradual control, a loading I.V. infusion of 500 mcg/kg/minute for 1 minute, then a 4-minute maintenance infusion of 50 mcg/kg/minute. If an adequate therapeutic effect isn't observed within 5 minutes, repeat the same loading dose and follow with a maintenance infusion increased to 100 mcg/kg/minute (see supraventricular tachycardia, above).

Pharmacodynamics

Antiarrhythmic action: A beta blocker with rapid onset and very short duration of action that decreases blood pressure and heart rate in a dose-related, titratable manner. Hemodynamic effects are similar to those of propranolol, but doesn't increase vascular resistance.

Pharmacokinetics

• *Absorption:* Immediate absorption after I.V. infusion.
• *Distribution:* Distributed rapidly throughout plasma. Half-life is about 2 minutes. Drug is 55% protein-bound.
• *Metabolism:* Hydrolyzed rapidly by plasma esterases.
• *Excretion:* Excreted by kidneys as metabolites. Elimination half-life is about 9 minutes.

Contraindications and precautions

Contraindicated in patients with sinus bradycardia, heart block greater than first-degree, cardiogenic shock, or overt heart failure. Use cautiously in patients with impaired renal function, diabetes, or bronchospasm.

Interactions

Drug-drug. *Antihypertensives:* May potentiate their hypotensive effects. May require dosage adjustments based on blood pressure measurements. Monitor blood pressure.
Digoxin: I.V. administration with digoxin may increase digoxin blood levels 10% to 20%. Observe closely for cardiac arrhythmias.
Insulin, oral antidiabetics: May mask symptoms of developing hypoglycemia. Monitor blood glucose levels regularly.

Morphine: I.V. administration of morphine increases esmolol steady-state levels by 46%. Monitor patient closely if concomitant use is necessary.
Nondepolarizing neuromuscular blockers (such as gallamine, metocurine, pancuronium, succinylcholine, tubocurarine): May potentiate and prolong action of these drugs. Careful postoperative monitoring of patient may be necessary after concurrent or sequential use, especially if there is possibility of incomplete reversal of neuromuscular blockade.
Phenytoin: I.V. phenytoin may produce additive cardiac depressant effects. Monitor patient closely.
Reserpine, other catecholamine-depleting drugs: May result in additive and possibly excessive beta-adrenergic blockade, with bradycardia and hypotension. Monitor patient closely.
Sympathomimetic amines with beta-adrenergic stimulant activity: Additive effects may cause mutual but transient inhibition of therapeutic effects. Avoid concomitant use.
Xanthines (especially aminophylline, theophylline): May cause mutual inhibition of therapeutic effects and (except for dyphylline) may decrease theophylline clearance, especially in patients with increased theophylline clearance induced by smoking. Monitor patient carefully to prevent toxic theophylline accumulation.

Adverse reactions

CNS: dizziness, somnolence, headache, agitation, fatigue, confusion.
CV: HYPOTENSION (sometimes with diaphoresis), peripheral ischemia.
GI: *nausea,* vomiting.
Respiratory: *bronchospasm,* wheezing, dyspnea, nasal congestion.
Other: inflammation, induration at infusion site.

☑ Special considerations

• Dilute drug injection and administer by I.V. infusion. Concentrations exceeding 10 mg of esmolol per ml may produce irritation.
• To prepare esmolol hydrochloride injection for administration by I.V. infusion, aseptically remove 20 ml from a 500-ml bottle of I.V. fluid (D_5W injection USP, 5% dextrose in Ringer's injection, 5% dextrose and 0.45% saline injection USP, 5% dextrose and normal saline injection USP, lactated Ringer's injection USP, 0.45% saline injection USP, or normal saline injection USP) and then add 5-g esmolol hydrochloride injection to the bottle to produce a solution containing 10 mg of esmolol hydrochloride per ml.
• Drug isn't compatible with 5% sodium bicarbonate injection USP.
• Diluted solutions of drug are stable for at least 24 hours at room temperature.

• If irritation occurs at infusion site, stop infusion and resume at another site. Don't use butterfly needles for I.V. administration.

• To convert to other antiarrhythmic therapy after control has been achieved with esmolol, reduce infusion rate of esmolol by 50% 30 minutes after first dose of other drug. If a satisfactory response is maintained for 1 hour after the second dose of other drug, stop esmolol.

• Symptoms of overdose (most likely hypotension) usually disappear quickly after drug is withdrawn. In addition to immediately stopping drug infusion, treatment is supportive and symptomatic.

• Glucagon effectively combats CV effects (bradycardia, hypotension) of overdose with beta blockers. An I.V. dose of 2 to 3 mg is administered over 30 seconds and repeated, if necessary; then infusion at 5 mg/hour until patient's condition has stabilized.

Monitoring the patient
• Monitor patient's pulse, blood pressure, and cardiac rhythm before and during treatment.
• Monitor renal function.
• Monitor serum glucose levels if patient is diabetic.
• Monitor serum digoxin levels if patient is on digoxin (expect an increased level of 10% to 20%).

Information for the patient
• Advise patient to report pain at I.V. site.
• Inform patient that vital signs will be frequently monitored.
• Because drug may mask signs of hypoglycemia, tell patient to be alert for possible hypoglycemia.

Geriatric patients
• Elderly patients may be less sensitive to some effects of beta blockers. Reduced metabolic and excretory capabilities in many elderly patients may lead to increased myocardial depression and require dosage reduction of beta blockers. Dosage adjustment should be based on response.

Pediatric patients
• Safety and efficacy in children haven't been established.

Breast-feeding patients
• It's unknown if drug appears in breast milk; however, no problems associated with breast-feeding have been reported.

estazolam
ProSom

Pharmacologic classification: benzodiazepine
Therapeutic classification: hypnotic
Controlled substance schedule IV
Pregnancy risk category X

How supplied
Available by prescription only
Tablets: 1 mg, 2 mg

Indications, route, and dosage
Short-term management of insomnia characterized by difficulty in falling asleep, frequent nocturnal awakenings, or early-morning awakenings
Adults: Initially, 1 mg P.O. h.s.; may increase to 2 mg as needed and tolerated.
✦ *Dosage adjustment.* In small or debilitated older adults, initially, 0.5 mg P.O. h.s.; may increase with care to 1 mg if needed.

Pharmacodynamics
Hypnotic action: Depresses the CNS at the limbic and subcortical levels of the brain. Produces a sedative-hypnotic effect by potentiating the effect of the neurotransmitter gamma-aminobutyric acid on its receptor in the ascending reticular activating system, which increases inhibition and blocks both cortical and limbic arousal.

Pharmacokinetics
• *Absorption:* Rapidly and completely absorbed through GI tract in 1 to 3 hours. Levels peak within 2 hours (range is ½ to 6 hours).
• *Distribution:* 93% protein-bound.
• *Metabolism:* Extensively metabolized in liver.
• *Excretion:* Metabolites excreted primarily in urine. Less than 5% excreted in urine as unchanged drug; 4% of a 2-mg dose excreted in feces. Elimination half-life ranges from 10 to 24 hours; clearance is accelerated in smokers.

Contraindications and precautions
Contraindicated in patients with hypersensitivity to drug and in pregnant women. Use cautiously in patients with depression, suicidal tendencies, and hepatic, renal, or pulmonary disease.

Interactions
Drug-drug. *Antihistamines, barbiturates, general anesthetics, MAO inhibitors, narcotics, phenothiazines, tricyclic antidepressants:* CNS depressant effects potentiated. Monitor patient closely.
Cimetidine, disulfiram, isoniazid, oral contraceptives: Possible diminished hepatic metabolism, resulting in increased plasma levels of estazo-

lam and increased CNS depressant effects. Avoid concomitant use.

Digoxin, phenytoin: Increased serum levels, possibly resulting in toxicity. Monitor patient closely.

Probenecid: More rapid onset and more prolonged benzodiazepine effect. Monitor patient closely.

Rifampin: Increased clearance and decreased half-life of estazolam. Observe for desired effects.

Theophylline: Antagonized pharmacologic effects of estazolam. Observe for desired effects.

Drug-lifestyle. *Alcohol:* May cause excessive respiratory and CNS depression. Discourage concomitant use.

Heavy smoking: Accelerated estazolam metabolism, resulting in diminished efficacy. Discourage use.

Adverse reactions

CNS: fatigue, dizziness, *daytime drowsiness, somnolence, asthenia, hypokinesia, abnormal thinking.*
GI: dyspepsia, abdominal pain.
Hepatic: possible increased AST levels.
Musculoskeletal: back pain, stiffness.

☑ Special considerations

Besides the recommendations relevant to all benzodiazepines, consider the following.

• Remove all potential safety hazards such as cigarettes from patient's reach.
• Ask patient about other drugs he is taking and his usual alcohol consumption.
• Withdraw drug slowly after prolonged use.
• Encourage good sleep habits and regular exercise. Stress avoidance of caffeine or other stimulants, especially late in day.
• Signs and symptoms of benzodiazepine overdose include somnolence, confusion with reduced or absent reflexes, respiratory depression, apnea, hypotension, impaired coordination, slurred speech, seizures, or coma. If excitation occurs, don't use barbiturates.
• Remember that in overdose many drugs may have been ingested. Gastric evacuation and lavage should be performed immediately. Monitor respiration, pulse rate, and blood pressure. Use symptomatic and supportive measures. Maintain airway and administer fluids. Flumazenil, a specific benzodiazepine antagonist, may be useful.

Monitoring the patient

• Monitor patient for presence of hepatic, renal, and pulmonary disease.
• Monitor serum phenytoin and digoxin levels if patient is taking these drugs.
• Monitor CBC, urinalysis, and chemistry panels regularly.

Information for the patient

• Tell patient to avoid alcohol and other CNS depressants while taking this drug. After taking drug in evening, patient should avoid alcohol the following day.
• Advise woman of childbearing age to call immediately if she suspects pregnancy or plans to become pregnant during therapy.
• Warn patient that drug may cause drowsiness. Advise special caution and avoidance of driving or operating hazardous machinery until adverse CNS effects of drug are known.
• Inform patient that sleep may be disturbed for 1 or 2 nights after drug is stopped.
• Caution patient not to stop drug abruptly after taking daily for prolonged period and not to vary dosage or increase dose unless prescribed. Drug should be taken until sleep pattern is established and then slowly tapered as prescribed.
• Advise patient that rebound insomnia may occur after stopping drug.

Geriatric patients

• Elderly patients may be more susceptible to CNS depressant effects of estazolam. Use with caution. Lower dosage may be needed. To prevent injury from dizziness and falls, elderly patients should be supervised during activities of daily living, especially at start of treatment and after dosage adjustments.

Pediatric patients

• Safety and efficacy in children haven't been established.

Breast-feeding patients

• Drug appears in breast milk; avoid use in breast-feeding women.

---

esterified estrogens
Estratab, Menest

Pharmacologic classification: estrogen
Therapeutic classification: estrogen replacement, antineoplastic
Pregnancy risk category X

How supplied

Available by prescription only
Tablets: 0.3 mg, 0.625 mg, 1.25 mg, 2.5 mg

Indications, route, and dosage

Palliative treatment of advanced inoperable prostatic cancer
Adults: 1.25 to 2.5 mg P.O. t.i.d.
Breast cancer
Men and postmenopausal women: 10 mg P.O. t.i.d. for 3 or more months.
Female hypogonadism
Adults: 2.5 mg P.O. daily to t.i.d. in cycles of 20 days on, 10 days off.

Castration, primary ovarian failure
Adults: 2.5 mg daily to t.i.d. in cycles of 3 weeks on, 1 week off.
Vasomotor menopausal symptoms
Adults: 0.3 to 1.25 mg P.O. daily in cycles of 3 weeks on, 1 week off; dosage may be increased to 2.5 or 3.75 mg P.O. daily, if necessary.
Atrophic vaginitis and atrophic urethritis
Adults: 0.3 to 1.25 mg P.O. daily in cycles of 3 weeks on, 1 week off.

Pharmacodynamics
Estrogenic action: Mimics action of endogenous estrogen in treating female hypogonadism, menopausal symptoms, and atrophic vaginitis. Inhibits growth of hormone-sensitive tissue in advanced, inoperable prostatic cancer and in certain carefully selected cases of breast cancer in men and postmenopausal women.

Pharmacokinetics
• *Absorption:* After oral administration, well absorbed from GI tract.
• *Distribution:* About 50% to 80% plasma protein-bound, particularly estradiol-binding globulin. Distribution occurs throughout body with highest levels appearing in fat.
• *Metabolism:* Metabolized primarily in liver, where conjugated with sulfate and glucuronide.
• *Excretion:* Eliminated through kidneys as sulfate or glucuronide conjugates.

Contraindications and precautions
Contraindicated in patients with hypersensitivity to drug and in those with breast cancer (except metastatic disease), estrogen-dependent neoplasia, active thrombophlebitis or thromboembolic disorders, undiagnosed abnormal genital bleeding, history of thromboembolic disease, and during pregnancy.
    Use cautiously in patients with history of hypertension, mental depression, liver impairment, or cardiac or renal dysfunction and in those with bone diseases, migraine, seizures, or diabetes mellitus.

Interactions
Drug-drug. *Anticoagulants:* May decrease effects of warfarin-type anticoagulants. Monitor INR.
Corticosteroids: May cause possible enhanced effects. Monitor patient closely.
Cyclosporine: May increase risk of toxicity. Monitor patient closely.
Dantrolene, other hepatotoxic drugs: May increase risk of hepatotoxicity. Monitor liver function.
Drugs that induce hepatic metabolism (such as barbiturates, carbamazepine, phenytoin, primidone, rifampin): May result in decreased estrogenic effects from given dose. Monitor patient closely.

Insulin, oral antidiabetics: Esterified estrogens may increase blood glucose levels, necessitating dosage adjustment. Monitor serum glucose levels. Avoid concomitant use.
Tamoxifen: Effects may be altered with estrogen use. Avoid concomitant use.
Drug-food. *Caffeine:* May increase serum caffeine levels. Discourage concomitant use.
Drug-lifestyle. *Smoking:* Increased risk of CV adverse effects. Discourage concomitant use.

Adverse reactions
CNS: headache, dizziness, chorea, depression, *seizures.*
CV: thrombophlebitis; *thromboembolism;* hypertension; edema; *increased risk of CVA, pulmonary embolism, MI.*
EENT: worsening of myopia or astigmatism, intolerance of contact lenses.
GI: *nausea,* vomiting, abdominal cramps, bloating, anorexia, increased appetite, weight changes, *pancreatitis,* gallbladder disease.
GU: in women—breakthrough bleeding, altered menstrual flow, dysmenorrhea, amenorrhea, *increased risk of endometrial cancer, possibility of increased risk of breast cancer,* cervical erosion, altered cervical secretions, enlargement of uterine fibromas, vaginal candidiasis; breast changes (tenderness, enlargement, secretion); in men—gynecomastia, testicular atrophy, impotence.
Hematologic: increased PT and INR and clotting factors VII to X and norepinephrine-induced platelet aggregability.
Hepatic: cholestatic jaundice, *hepatic adenoma.*
Metabolic: decreased serum folate, pyridoxine, and antithrombin III levels; increased triglyceride, glucose, and phospholipid levels; hypercalcemia.
Skin: melasma, rash, hirsutism or hair loss, erythema nodosum, dermatitis.

☑ Special considerations
• Recommendations for administration of esterified estrogens and for care and teaching of patient during therapy are the same as for all estrogens.
• Glucose tolerance may be impaired. Pregnanediol excretion may decrease.
• Esterified estrogens increase sulfobromophthalein retention. Increases in thyroid-binding globulin level may occur, resulting in increased total thyroid levels (measured by protein-bound iodine or total T_4) and decreased uptake of free T_3 resin.
• Serious toxicity after overdose hasn't been reported. Nausea may occur. Appropriate supportive care should be provided.

Monitoring the patient
- If patient is of childbearing age, rule out pregnancy before therapy.
- Monitor blood pressure regularly.

Information for the patient
- Emphasize importance of regular physical examinations. Drug therapy may require adjustment.
- Instruct patient to immediately report abdominal pain; pain, numbness, or stiffness of legs or buttocks; pressure or pain in chest; shortness of breath; severe headaches; visual disturbances; vaginal bleeding or discharge; breast lumps; swelling of hands or feet; yellow skin or sclera; or dark urine and light-colored stools.

Breast-feeding patients
- Because they appear in breast milk, esterified estrogens are contraindicated in breast-feeding women.

estradiol
Climara, Estrace, Estrace Vaginal Cream, Estraderm, Vivelle

estradiol cypionate
depGynogen, Depo-Estradiol Cypionate, Depogen, Estro-Cyp, Estrofem

estradiol valerate
Delestrogen*, Dioval 40, Dioval XX, Estra-L 40, Gynogen L.A. 20, Valergen-20

polyestradiol phosphate
Estradurin

Pharmacologic classification: estrogen
Therapeutic classification: estrogen replacement, antineoplastic
Pregnancy risk category X

How supplied
Available by prescription only
estradiol
Tablets: 0.5 mg, 1 mg, 2 mg
Vaginal: 0.1 mg/g cream (in nonliquefying base)
Transdermal: 4 mg/10 cm² (delivers 0.05 mg/ 24 hours); 8 mg/20 cm² (delivers 0.1 mg/24 hours)
estradiol cypionate
Injection: 5 mg/ml (in oil)
estradiol valerate
Injection: 10 mg/ml, 20 mg/ml, 40 mg/ml (in oil)
polyestradiol phosphate
Injection: 40 mg/2 ml

Indications, route, and dosage
Atrophic vaginitis, atrophic dystrophy of the vulva, vasomotor menopausal symptoms, hypogonadism, female castration, primary ovarian failure
estradiol (tablets)
Adults: 1 to 2 mg P.O. daily, in cycles of 21 days on and 7 days off or cycles of 5 days on and 2 days off; or 0.2 to 1 mg I.M. weekly.
estradiol valerate
Adults: 10 to 20 mg I.M. once monthly.
estradiol (transdermal)
Adults: Place one Estraderm transdermal patch on trunk of the body, preferably the abdomen, twice weekly. Administer on an intermittent cyclic schedule (3 weeks on and 1 week off).
Atrophic vaginitis
estradiol (vaginal cream)
Adults: 2 to 4 g daily for 1 to 2 weeks. When vaginal mucosa is restored, begin maintenance dosage of 1 g one to three times weekly.
Female hypogonadism
estradiol cypionate
Adults: 1.5 to 2 mg I.M. at monthly intervals.
Inoperable breast cancer
estradiol (tablets)
Adults: 10 mg P.O. t.i.d. for 3 months.
Inoperable prostatic cancer
estradiol valerate
Adults: 30 mg I.M. q 1 to 2 weeks.
estradiol (tablets)
Adults: 1 to 2 mg P.O. t.i.d.
polyestradiol phosphate
Adults: 40 mg I.M. q 2 to 4 weeks.

Pharmacodynamics
Estrogenic action: Estradiol mimics the action of endogenous estrogen in treating female hypogonadism, menopausal symptoms, and atrophic vaginitis. It inhibits growth of hormone-sensitive tissue in advanced, inoperable prostatic cancer and in certain carefully selected cases of breast cancer in men and postmenopausal women.

Pharmacokinetics
- *Absorption:* After oral administration, estradiol and other natural unconjugated estrogens are well absorbed but substantially inactivated by the liver. Therefore, unconjugated estrogens are usually administered parenterally. After I.M. administration, absorption begins rapidly and continues for days. Cypionate and valerate esters administered in oil have prolonged durations of action because of their slow absorption characteristics. Topically applied estradiol is absorbed readily into systemic circulation.
- *Distribution:* Estradiol and other natural estrogens are about 50% to 80% plasma protein–bound, particularly estradiol-binding globulin. Distribution occurs throughout body, with highest levels appearing in fat.

• *Metabolism:* Steroidal estrogens, including estradiol, are metabolized primarily in liver, where they are conjugated with sulfate and glucuronide. Because of rapid metabolism rate, nonesterified forms of estrogen, including estradiol, usually must be administered daily.

• *Excretion:* Majority of elimination occurs through kidneys as sulfate or glucuronide conjugates.

Contraindications and precautions

Contraindicated in patients with thrombophlebitis or thromboembolic disorders, estrogen-dependent neoplasia, breast or reproductive organ cancer (except for palliative treatment), or undiagnosed abnormal genital bleeding and during pregnancy. Also contraindicated in patients with history of thrombophlebitis or thromboembolic disorders associated with previous estrogen use (except for palliative treatment of breast and prostate cancer).

Use cautiously in patients with cerebrovascular or coronary artery disease, asthma, bone diseases, migraine, seizures, or cardiac, hepatic, or renal dysfunction and in women with a strong family history of breast cancer or who have breast nodules, fibrocystic disease, or abnormal mammographic findings.

Interactions

Drug-drug. *Anticoagulants:* May decrease effects of warfarin-type anticoagulants. Monitor INR.

Corticosteroids: May cause enhanced effects. Monitor patient closely.

Cyclosporine: May increase risk of toxicity. Monitor patient closely.

Dantrolene, other hepatotoxic drugs: May increase risk of hepatotoxicity. Monitor liver function closely.

Drugs that induce hepatic metabolism (such as barbiturates, carbamazepine, phenytoin, primidone, rifampin): May result in decreased estrogenic effects from given dose. Monitor patient closely.

Insulin, oral antidiabetics: Esterified estrogens may increase blood glucose levels, requiring dosage adjustment. Monitor serum glucose levels.

Tamoxifen: May interfere with effectiveness. Avoid concomitant use.

Drug-food. *Caffeine:* May increase serum caffeine levels. Discourage concomitant use.

Drug-lifestyle. *Smoking:* Increased risk of adverse CV effects. Discourage concomitant use.

Adverse reactions

CNS: headache, dizziness, chorea, depression, *seizures.*

CV: thrombophlebitis; *thromboembolism;* hypertension; edema; *increased risk of CVA, pulmonary embolism, MI.*

EENT: worsening of myopia or astigmatism, intolerance of contact lenses.

GI: *nausea,* vomiting, abdominal cramps, bloating, anorexia, increased appetite, weight changes, *pancreatitis,* gallbladder disease.

GU: in women—breakthrough bleeding, altered menstrual flow, dysmenorrhea, amenorrhea, *increased risk of endometrial cancer, possibility of increased risk of breast cancer,* cervical erosion, altered cervical secretions, enlargement of uterine fibromas, vaginal candidiasis; breast changes (tenderness, enlargement, secretion); in men—gynecomastia, testicular atrophy, impotence.

Hematologic: increased PT and INR and clotting factors VII to X and norepinephrine-induced platelet aggregability.

Hepatic: cholestatic jaundice, *hepatic adenoma.*

Metabolic: decreased serum folate, pyridoxine, and antithrombin III levels; increased triglyceride, glucose, and phospholipid levels; hypercalcemia.

Skin: melasma, rash, hirsutism or hair loss, erythema nodosum, dermatitis.

☑ Special considerations

Besides the recommendations relevant to all estrogens, consider the following.

• Before injection, make sure drug is well dispersed in solution by rolling the reconstituted vial between the palms.

• Administer by deep I.M. injection into large muscles.

• Therapy with estradiol increases sulfobromophthalein retention. Increases in the thyroid-binding globulin level may occur, resulting in increased total thyroid levels (measured by protein-bound iodine or total T_4) and decreased uptake of free T_3 resin. Glucose tolerance may be impaired. Pregnanediol excretion may decrease.

• Serious toxicity after overdose hasn't been reported. Nausea may occur. Provide appropriate supportive care.

Monitoring the patient

• If patient is of childbearing age, rule out pregnancy before therapy.

• Monitor blood pressure regularly.

Information for the patient

• Tell patient not to apply patch to breast areas.

• Remind patient not to use same skin site for at least 1 week after removal of transdermal system.

Geriatric patients

• Frequent physical examinations are recommended in postmenopausal women taking estrogen.

Breast-feeding patients

• Drug is contraindicated in breast-feeding women.

estradiol/norethindrone acetate transdermal system
CombiPatch

Pharmacologic classification: estrogen/progesterone
Therapeutic classification: postmenopausal drug
Pregnancy risk category X

How supplied
Available by prescription only
Transdermal: 9-cm² system (0.05 mg estradiol and 0.14 mg norethindrone); 16-cm² system (0.05 mg estradiol and 0.25 mg norethindrone)

Indications, route and dosage
Moderate to severe vasomotor symptoms associated with menopause, vulvar and vaginal atrophy, and hypoestrogenemia due to hypogonadism, castration, or primary ovarian failure in women with an intact uterus
Adults: Continuous combined regimen—9-cm² patch worn continuously on the lower abdomen. Old system should be removed and new system applied twice weekly during a 28-day cycle. May increase to 16-cm² patch if more progestin is desired.
Continuous sequential regimen—patch can be applied as a sequential regimen in combination with an estradiol-only transdermal system (such as Alora, Esclim, Estraderm, Vivelle). A 0.05-mg estradiol-only transdermal patch is worn for first 14 days of a 28-day cycle; replace system twice weekly according to product directions. For remainder of 28-day cycle, apply the 9-cm² patch system to the lower abdomen. May increase to 16-cm² patch if more progestin is desired.
    Women not currently receiving continuous estrogen or estrogen and progestin therapy may start therapy at any time.
    Women currently receiving continuous hormone replacement therapy should complete the current cycle of therapy before initiating therapy. Women often experience withdrawal bleeding at the completion of the cycle; first day of withdrawal bleeding is an appropriate time to initiate therapy.

Pharmacodynamics
Hormone action: Estrogen replacement therapy can reduce frequency of menopausal symptoms by replacing the naturally declining levels that occur in postmenopausal women.

Pharmacokinetics
• *Absorption:* Estradiol and norethindrone well absorbed transdermally.
• *Distribution:* Estradiol primarily bound to sex hormone–binding protein (SHBG); norethindrone primarily bound to albumin and SHBG.

• *Metabolism:* Estradiol minimally metabolized; norethindrone metabolized primarily by liver.
• *Excretion:* Elimination half-life of estradiol is 2 to 3 hours; of norethindrone, 6 to 8 hours.

Contraindications and precautions
Contraindicated in women with known hypersensitivity to estrogen, progestin, or any component of the patch. Also contraindicated in those who may be pregnant or have known or suspected breast cancer, known or suspected estrogen-dependent neoplasia, undiagnosed abnormal genital bleeding, active thrombophlebitis, thromboembolic disorders, or stroke.
    Use cautiously in patients with impaired liver function, asthma, epilepsy, migraine, or cardiac or renal dysfunction.

Interactions
None reported.

Adverse reactions
CNS: *asthenia,* depression, insomnia, nervousness, dizziness, *headache.*
EENT: tooth disorder, *pharyngitis, rhinitis, sinusitis.*
GI: *abdominal pain, diarrhea,* dyspepsia, flatulence, *nausea,* constipation.
GU: *dysmenorrhea, leukorrhea, menstrual disorder,* suspicious Papanicolaou smear, *vaginitis,* menorrhagia, vaginal hemorrhage.
Musculoskeletal: arthralgia, *back pain.*
Respiratory: *respiratory disorder,* bronchitis.
Skin: application site reactions, acne.
Other: *accidental injury, flu syndrome, pain, breast pain,* peripheral edema, breast enlargement, infection.

☑ Special considerations
• Reevaluate hormonal therapy every 3 to 6 months.
• Combination estrogen and progestin regimens are indicated for women with an intact uterus.
• Progestins taken with estrogen significantly reduce, but don't eliminate, risk of endometrial cancer associated with estrogen use.
• Treatment of postmenopausal symptoms is usually initiated during menopausal stage when vasomotor symptoms occur.
• Store norethindrone patches in refrigerator before dispensing.
• Drug may cause a reduced response to the metyrapone test and sulfobromophthalein retention. Increased thyroid-binding globulin may lead to increased total T_3 and T_4 levels and decreased T_3 resin uptake. Free T_4 and T_3 levels are unaffected.
• The most common consequences of overdose are nausea and withdrawal bleeding. Treatment should involve discontinuation or removal of patch. Medical treatment may be initiated.

• INR, activated partial thromboplastin time, and platelet aggregation times may be altered; platelet count and fibrinogen activity may increase. Monitor accordingly if patient is on any drugs that possess these actions.

Monitoring the patient
• If patient is of childbearing age, rule out pregnancy before treatment.
• Blood pressure increases have been associated with estrogen use. Monitor patient's blood pressure regularly.

Information for the patient
• Teach patient how to apply system properly. Only one system should be worn at any time during dosing intervals.
• Instruct patient to apply patch system to a smooth (fold-free), clean, dry, nonirritated area of skin on lower abdomen, avoiding waistline. Application sites should be rotated, with an interval of at least 1 week between applications to same site.
• Don't apply patch on or near breasts.
• Reapply system, if necessary, to another area of lower abdomen. If the system fails to adhere, replace with a new one.
• Tell patient an oil-based cream or lotion may help remove adhesive from skin once a system has been removed and the area allowed to dry for 15 minutes.
• Advise patient not to use patch if pregnancy occurs or is being planned.
• Instruct patient that, for the continuous combined regimen, irregular bleeding may occur, particularly in the first 6 months, but generally decreases with time, often to an amenorrheic state.
• Tell patient that, for the continuous sequential regimen, monthly withdrawal bleeding often occurs.
• Advise patient to alert prescriber and remove patch at first sign of thrombotic disorders (thrombophlebitis, cerebrovascular disorders, and pulmonary embolism).
• Instruct patient to remove patch and call if a partial or complete loss of vision, sudden onset of proptosis (a downward displacement of the eyeball), double vision, or migraine occurs.
• Tell patient to store patches at room temperature for up to 3 months.
• Advise patient not to store patches where extreme temperatures can occur.
• Tell patient to avoid application to areas that may get prolonged sun exposure.

Breast-feeding patients
• Estrogen and progestin appear in breast milk. Don't use patch during breast-feeding.

estramustine phosphate sodium
Emcyt

Pharmacologic classification: estrogen, alkylating drug
Therapeutic classification: antineoplastic
Pregnancy risk category NR

How supplied
Available by prescription only
Capsules: 140 mg

Indications, route, and dosage
Dosage and indications may vary. Check literature for recommended protocols.
Palliative treatment of metastatic or progressive cancer of the prostate
Adults: 10 to 16 mg/kg P.O. in three or four divided doses. Usual dosage is 14 mg/kg daily. Therapy should continue for up to 3 months and, if successful, be maintained as long as patient responds.

Pharmacodynamics
Antineoplastic action: Exact mechanism unknown. However, the estrogenic portion of the molecule may act as a carrier of the drug to facilitate selective uptake by tumor cells with estradiol hormone receptors, such as those in the prostate gland. At that point, the nitrogen mustard portion of the drug acts as an alkylating drug.

Pharmacokinetics
• *Absorption:* After oral administration, about 75% of dose absorbed across GI tract.
• *Distribution:* Distributed widely into body tissues.
• *Metabolism:* Extensively metabolized in liver.
• *Excretion:* Drug and metabolites eliminated primarily in feces, with a small amount excreted in urine. Terminal phase of plasma elimination has a half-life of 20 hours.

Contraindications and precautions
Contraindicated in patients with hypersensitivity to estradiol and nitrogen mustard and in those with active thrombophlebitis or thromboembolic disorders, except when the actual tumor mass is the cause of the thromboembolic phenomenon.
    Use cautiously in patients with history of thrombophlebitis or thromboembolic disorders and cerebrovascular or coronary artery disease.

Interactions
Drug-drug. *Anticoagulants:* Concomitant use may decrease anticoagulant effect and require increased dosage of anticoagulants. Monitor INR.

Drugs containing calcium (such as antacids): May impair absorption of estramustine. Monitor patient for desired effects.

Drug-food. *Calcium-rich foods (dairy products, milk):* May impair absorption of estramustine. Discourage consumption of calcium-rich foods.

Adverse reactions
CNS: lethargy, insomnia, headache, anxiety.
CV: chest pain, *MI,* sodium and fluid retention, thrombophlebitis, **heart failure, stroke.**
GI: *nausea, vomiting,* diarrhea, anorexia, flatulence, GI bleeding, thirst.
GU: *painful gynecomastia and breast tenderness.*
Hematologic: *leukopenia, thrombocytopenia,* increased norepinephrine-induced platelet aggregability.
Hepatic: elevated liver enzyme levels.
Metabolic: decreased serum folate, pyridoxine, phosphate, and pregnanediol levels; increased ceruloplasmin, cortisol, prolactin PT, sodium, triglyceride, and phospholipid levels.
Musculoskeletal: leg cramps.
Respiratory: *edema, pulmonary embolism,* dyspnea.
Skin: rash, pruritus, dry skin, flushing.
Other: thinning of hair.

☑ Special considerations
Besides the recommendations relevant to all alkylating drugs, consider the following.
• Store capsules in refrigerator.
• Phenothiazines can be used to treat nausea and vomiting.
• Patients may continue estramustine as long as they are responding favorably. Some patients have taken drug for more than 3 years.
• Estramustine therapy may cause a reduced response to the metyrapone test. Glucose tolerance may be decreased.
• Signs and symptoms of overdose include headache, nausea, vomiting, and myelosuppression. Treatment is usually supportive and includes induction of emesis, gastric lavage, transfusion of blood components, and appropriate symptomatic therapy. Hematologic monitoring should continue for at least 6 weeks after ingestion.

Monitoring the patient
• Monitor blood pressure at baseline and routinely during therapy. Estramustine may cause hypertension.
• Drug may exaggerate preexisting peripheral edema or heart failure. Weight gain should be monitored regularly in these patients.
• Monitor glucose tolerance periodically during therapy.

Information for the patient
• Emphasize importance of continuing therapy despite nausea and vomiting.

• Advise patient to call immediately if vomiting occurs shortly after a dose is taken.
• Because of possibility of mutagenic effects, advise patients of childbearing age to use birth control.

Geriatric patients
• Use with caution in elderly patients, who are more likely to have vascular disorders; estrogen use is associated with vascular complications.

estrogen and progestin
Alesse-21, Alesse-28, Brevicon-21, Brevicon-28, Demulen 1/35, Demulen 1/35-21, Demulen 1/35-28, Demulen 1/50-21, Demulen 1/50-28, Loestrin 21 1/20, Loestrin 21 1.5/30, Loestrin Fe 1/20, Loestrin Fe 1.5/30, Lo/Ovral, Lo/Ovral-28, ModiCon 21, ModiCon 28, Nordette-21, Nordette-28, Norinyl 1+35 21-Day, Norinyl 1+35 28-Day, Norinyl 1+50 21-Day, Ortho-Novum 1/35 21, Ortho-Novum 1/35 28, Ortho-Novum 7/7/7-21, Ortho-Novum 7/7/7-28, Ortho-Novum 10/11-21, Ortho-Novum 10/11-28, Ovcon-35, Ovcon-50, Ovral, Ovral-28, Tri-Norinyl-21, Tri-Norinyl-28, Triphasil-21, Triphasil-28

Pharmacologic classification: estrogen with progestin
Therapeutic classification: contraceptive (hormonal)
Pregnancy risk category X

How supplied
Available by prescription only
Tablets—monophasic type
Mestranol 0.1 mg and norethynodrel 2.5 mg
Mestranol 0.1 mg and norethindrone 2 mg
Mestranol 0.1 mg and ethynodiol diacetate 1 mg
Mestranol 0.08 mg and norethindrone 1 mg
Mestranol 0.05 mg and norethindrone 1 mg
Ethinyl estradiol 0.02 mg and levonorgestrel 0.1 mg
Ethinyl estradiol 0.05 mg and norethindrone 1 mg
Ethinyl estradiol 0.05 mg and norethindrone acetate 1 mg
Ethinyl estradiol 0.05 mg and ethynodiol diacetate 1 mg
Ethinyl estradiol 0.05 mg and norethindrone acetate 2.5 mg
Ethinyl estradiol 0.05 mg and norgestrel 0.5 mg
Ethinyl estradiol 0.035 mg and norethindrone 1 mg
Ethinyl estradiol 0.035 mg and norethindrone 0.5 mg
Ethinyl estradiol 0.035 mg and norethindrone 0.4 mg

Ethinyl estradiol 0.035 mg and ethynodiol diacetate 1 mg
Ethinyl estradiol 0.03 mg and norethindrone acetate 1.5 mg
Ethinyl estradiol 0.03 mg and norgestrel 0.3 mg
Ethinyl estradiol 0.03 mg and levonorgestrel 0.15 mg
Ethinyl estradiol 0.02 mg and norethindrone 1 mg
Tablets—biphasic type
10 tablets ethinyl estradiol 0.035 mg and norethindrone 0.5 mg; 11 tablets ethinyl estradiol 0.035 mg and norethindrone 1 mg
Tablets—triphasic type
7 tablets ethinyl estradiol 0.035 mg and norethindrone 0.5 mg; 9 tablets ethinyl estradiol 0.035 mg and norethindrone 1 mg; 5 tablets ethinyl estradiol 0.035 mg and norethindrone 0.5 mg
7 tablets ethinyl estradiol 0.035 mg and norethindrone 0.5 mg; 7 tablets ethinyl estradiol 0.035 mg and norethindrone 0.75 mg; 7 tablets ethinyl estradiol 0.035 mg and norethindrone 1 mg
6 tablets ethinyl estradiol 0.03 and levonorgestrel 0.05 mg; 5 tablets ethinyl estradiol 0.04 mg and levonorgestrel 0.075 mg; 10 tablets ethinyl estradiol 0.03 mg and levonorgestrel 0.125 mg

Indications, route, and dosage
Contraception
Monophasic
Adults: One tablet P.O. daily, beginning on day 5 of menstrual cycle (first day of menstrual flow is day 1), or on the first Sunday after onset of menstruation, or on day 1 of menstrual cycle depending on specific contraceptive. With 20- and 21-tablet packages, new dosing cycle begins 7 days after last tablet taken. With 28-tablet packages, dosage is one tablet daily without interruption; extra tablets are placebos or contain iron. If next menstrual period doesn't begin on schedule, rule out pregnancy before starting new dosing cycle. If menstrual period begins, start new dosing cycle 7 days after last tablet was taken. If all doses have been taken on schedule and one menstrual period is missed, continue dosing cycle. If two consecutive menstrual periods are missed, pregnancy test is required before new dosing cycle is started.
Biphasic
Adults: One color tablet P.O. daily (Ortho-Novum 10/11) for 10 days, then next color tablet for 11 days.
Triphasic
Adults: One tablet P.O. daily (Ortho-Novum 7/7/7, Tri-Norinyl, Triphasil) in the sequence specified by the manufacturer.
Hypermenorrhea
Adults: Use high-dose combinations only. Dosage is same as for contraception.
Endometriosis
Adults: cyclic therapy: One 10-mg tablet P.O. daily (Ortho-Novum) for 20 days from day 5 to day 24 of menstrual cycle. Suppressive therapy: One

5- or 10-mg tablet P.O. daily for 2 weeks, starting on day 5 of menstrual cycle. Continue without interruption for 6 to 9 months, increasing dose by 5 to 10 mg q 2 weeks, up to 20 mg daily. Up to 40 mg daily may be needed if breakthrough bleeding occurs.

Pharmacodynamics
Contraceptive action: Estrogen components of oral contraceptives inhibit release of follicle-stimulating hormone, thereby stopping follicular development and suppressing ovulation.

Progestin components of oral contraceptives inhibit release of luteinizing hormone, preventing ovulation even in the event of incomplete suppression of follicular development. Progestins also change the endometrial environment to inhibit nidation (implantation of the fertilized egg into the endometrium) and cause thickening of the cervical mucus, blocking the upward migration of sperm.

Pharmacokinetics
- *Absorption:* Most components absorbed relatively well from GI tract. Bioavailabilities range from 40% to 70%; considerable individual variation exists in extent of absorption. Levels peak 1 to 2 hours after dosing.
- *Distribution:* Protein-binding of various drugs used in oral contraceptives ranges from 80% to 98%. Distributed extensively into virtually all body tissues.
- *Metabolism:* Undergo metabolic transformation before excretion; rates of metabolism may be affected by drugs that induce or inhibit metabolism.
- *Excretion:* Very little, if any, excreted unchanged in urine or feces. Appear primarily as sulfate and glucuronide conjugates.

Contraindications and precautions
Oral contraceptives are contraindicated in patients with thromboembolic disorders, cerebrovascular or coronary artery disease, or MI because of their association with thromboembolic disease; in patients with known or suspected cancer of the breast or reproductive organs or with benign or malignant liver tumors because of their association with tumorigenesis; in patients with undiagnosed abnormal vaginal bleeding; in women known or believed to be pregnant or breast-feeding; in adolescents with incomplete epiphyseal closure; and in women smokers over age 35.

Oral contraceptives should be used cautiously in patients with systemic lupus erythematosus, hypertension, mental depression, migraine, epilepsy, asthma, diabetes mellitus, amenorrhea, scanty or irregular periods, fibrocystic breast disease, family history (mother, grandmother, sister) of breast or genital tract cancer, or renal or gallbladder disease. Development or worsening of any of these conditions should be reported. Prolonged therapy may be inadvisable in women who plan to become pregnant.

Interactions

Drug-drug. *Aminoglutethimide, ampicillin, antihistamines, barbiturates, carbamazepine, chloramphenicol, griseofulvin, isoniazid, neomycin, nitrofurantoin, penicillin V, phenylbutazone, phenytoin, primidone, rifampin, sulfonamides, tetracycline:* Increased metabolism of oral contraceptives, resulting in reduced efficacy, breakthrough bleeding, and occasionally contraceptive failure. Advise patient to use alternative method of birth control.

Anticonvulsants, antihypertensives, oral warfarin-type anticoagulants, tricyclic antidepressants: Concomitant use may decrease effectiveness of these drugs. Monitor PT and INR.

Insulin, oral antidiabetics: Concomitant use may require adjustment of insulin or oral antidiabetics. Monitor serum glucose levels.

Drug-food. *Caffeine:* May increase serum caffeine levels. Discourage concomitant use.

Drug-lifestyle. *Smoking:* Increased risk of CV adverse effects. Discourage concomitant use.

Adverse reactions

CNS: headache, dizziness, depression, lethargy, migraine.

CV: *thromboembolism,* hypertension, edema, increase in varicosities.

EENT: worsening of myopia or astigmatism, intolerance of contact lenses, unexplained loss of vision, optic neuritis, diplopia, retinal thrombosis, papilledema.

GI: *nausea, vomiting,* abdominal cramps, bloating, diarrhea, constipation, changes in appetite, weight gain, bowel ischemia.

GU: breakthrough bleeding, granulomatous colitis, dysmenorrhea, amenorrhea, cervical erosion or abnormal secretions, enlargement of uterine fibromas, vaginal candidiasis, urinary tract infections, breast tenderness, enlargement, or secretion.

Hematologic: increased prothrombin and clotting factors VII to X, norepinephrine-induced platelet aggregation, plasminogen, fibrinogen; decreased antithrombin III.

Hepatic: gallbladder disease, cholestatic jaundice, *liver tumors.*

Metabolic: hyperglycemia, hypercalcemia, folic acid deficiency; increased sulfobromophthalein retention, thyroid-binding globulin, triglycerides, phospholipids, transcortin and corticosteroids, transferrin, prolactin, renin, and vitamin A; decreased metyrapone, pregnanediol excretion, free T_3 resin uptake, glucose tolerance, zinc, and vitamin B_{12}.

Skin: rash, acne, seborrhea, oily skin, *erythema multiforme,* hyperpigmentation.

Other: libido changes, possible increased risk of congenital anomalies.

Adverse effects may be more serious, frequent, and rapid in onset with high-dose than with low-dose combinations.

Note: Stop drug if patient becomes hypertensive during therapy.

☑ Special considerations

Besides the recommendations relevant to all estrogens and progestins, consider the following for oral contraceptives.

● Astigmatic error and myopic refractive error may be increased twofold to threefold, usually after 6 months of oral contraceptive therapy. Changes in ocular contour and lubricant quality of tears may necessitate change in size and shape of contact lenses.

● Serious toxicity after drug overdose hasn't been reported. Nausea, vomiting, and withdrawal bleeding may occur.

Monitoring the patient

● If patient is of childbearing age, rule out pregnancy before starting therapy.

● Monitor weight gain and development of edema.

● Monitor serum glucose levels during initial phases of treatment if patient is diabetic.

Information for the patient

● Warn patient that headache, nausea, dizziness, breast tenderness, spotting, and breakthrough bleeding are common initially. These should diminish after three to six dosing cycles (months). However, breakthrough bleeding in patients taking high-dose estrogen-progestin combinations for menstrual disorders may necessitate dosage adjustment.

● Advise patient to use additional method of birth control for the first week of administration in initial cycle (unless using day-1 start).

● If one menstrual period is missed and tablets have been taken on schedule, tell patient to continue taking them. If two consecutive menstrual periods are missed, tell patient to stop drug and have pregnancy test.

● Teach patient to take drug at the same time each day at 24-hour intervals for efficacy of medication, to keep tablets in original container, and to take them in correct (color-coded) sequence.

● Tell patient that night-time dosing may reduce nausea and headaches.

● Suggest taking drug with or immediately after food to reduce nausea.

● Stress importance of annual Papanicolaou smears and gynecologic examinations while taking estrogen-progestin combinations.

● Warn patient of possible delay in achieving pregnancy when drug is stopped.

● Advise patient of increased risks associated with simultaneous use of cigarettes and oral con-

---

traceptives, especially risk of serious cardiovascular side effects. Women who use oral contraceptives should be strongly advised not to smoke.
• Instruct patient to weigh herself at least twice weekly and to report sudden weight gain or edema.
• Warn patient to avoid exposure to ultraviolet light or prolonged exposure to sunlight; chloasma seems to be aggravated by sunlight. With anticipated sunlight exposure (as in summer), taking pill at bedtime will reduce daytime levels of circulating hormone.
• Advise patient to avoid pregnancy for 2 months after stopping drug and to seek medical advice about how soon pregnancy may be safely attempted after drug is stopped.
• Instruct patient as follows regarding missed doses.

Monophasic or biphasic cycles
For 20-, 21-, or 24-day dosing schedule:
• If one regular dose is missed, take tablet as soon as possible; if remembered on the next day, take two tablets, then continue regular dosing schedule.
• If 2 consecutive days are missed, take two tablets daily for next 2 days, then resume regular dosing schedule.
• If 3 consecutive days are missed, stop drug and substitute other contraceptive method until period begins or pregnancy is ruled out. Then start new cycle of tablets.
For 28-day dosing schedule:
• Follow instructions for 21-day dosing schedule; if 1 of the last 7 tablets is missed, be sure to take first tablet of next month's cycle on regularly scheduled day.

Triphasic cycle
For 21-day dosing schedule:
• If 1 day is missed, take dose as soon as possible; if remembered on the next day, take two tablets, then continue regular dosing schedule while using additional method of contraception for remainder of cycle.
• If 2 consecutive days are missed, take two tablets daily for next 2 days, then continue regular schedule while using additional contraceptive method for remainder of cycle.
• If 3 consecutive days are missed, stop drug and use other contraceptive method until period begins or pregnancy is ruled out. Then start new cycle of tablets.
For 28-day dosing schedule:
• Follow instructions for 21-day dosing schedule; if one of the last seven tablets was missed, be sure to take first tablet of next month's cycle on regularly scheduled day.

Pediatric patients
• To avoid later fertility and menstrual problems, hormonal contraception isn't advised for adolescent until after at least 2 years of well-established menstrual cycles and completion of physiologic maturation.
• An estrogen-dominant product is best choice for adolescent with scanty menses, moderate or severe acne, or candidiasis. A progestin-dominant product is best choice for the adolescent with dysmenorrhea, hypermenorrhea, fibrocystic breast disease, or cyclic premenstrual weight gain.

Breast-feeding patients
• Because oral contraceptives appear in breast milk, they are contraindicated in breast-feeding women.

estrogens, conjugated
Premarin

Pharmacologic classification: estrogen
Therapeutic classification: estrogen replacement, antineoplastic, anti-osteoporotic
Pregnancy risk category X

How supplied
Available by prescription only
Tablets: 0.3 mg, 0.625 mg, 0.9 mg, 1.25 mg, 2.5 mg
Injection: 25 mg/5 ml
Vaginal cream: 0.0625%

Indications, route, and dosage
Abnormal uterine bleeding (hormonal imbalance)
Adults: 25 mg I.V. or I.M. Repeat in 6 to 12 hours.
Castration and primary ovarian failure
Adults: 1.25 mg P.O. daily in cycles of 3 weeks on, 1 week off.
Osteoporosis
Adults: 0.625 mg P.O. daily in cycles of 3 weeks on, 1 week off.
Female hypogonadism
Adults: 2.5 to 7.5 mg P.O. daily in divided doses for 20 consecutive days, then 10 days without drug.
Vasomotor menopausal symptoms
Adults: 1.25 mg P.O. daily in cycles of 3 weeks on, 1 week off.
Atrophic vaginitis or kraurosis vulvae
Adults: 0.3 mg to 1.25 mg or more P.O. daily. Or 2 to 4 g intravaginally or topically once daily in cycles of 3 weeks on, 1 week off.
Palliative treatment of inoperable prostatic cancer
Adults: 1.25 to 2.5 mg P.O. t.i.d.
Palliative treatment of breast cancer
Adults: 10 mg P.O. t.i.d. for 3 months or more.

Pharmacodynamics
Estrogenic action: Conjugated estrogenic substances mimic the action of endogenous estro-

418	estrogens, conjugated

gen in treating female hypogonadism, menopausal symptoms, and atrophic vaginitis. They inhibit growth of hormone-sensitive tissue in advanced, inoperable prostatic cancer and in certain carefully selected cases of breast cancer in men and postmenopausal women; they also retard progression of osteoporosis by enhancing calcium and phosphate retention and limiting bone decalcification.

Pharmacokinetics

• *Absorption:* Not well characterized. After I.M. administration, absorption begins rapidly and continues for days.
• *Distribution:* About 50% to 80% plasma protein-bound, particularly estradiol-binding globulin. Distribution occurs throughout body, with highest levels appearing in fat.
• *Metabolism:* Metabolized primarily in liver, where drug is conjugated with sulfate and glucuronide. Because of rapid rate of metabolism, nonesterified forms of estrogen, including estradiol, must usually be administered daily.
• *Excretion:* Majority of estrogen elimination occurs through kidneys, as sulfate or glucuronide conjugates, or both.

Contraindications and precautions

Contraindicated in patients with thrombophlebitis or thromboembolic disorders, estrogen-dependent neoplasia, breast or reproductive organ cancer (except for palliative treatment), or undiagnosed abnormal genital bleeding. Also contraindicated during pregnancy.

Use cautiously in patients with cerebrovascular or coronary artery disease, asthma, bone disease, migraine, seizures, or cardiac, hepatic, or renal dysfunction and in women with family history (mother, grandmother, sister) of breast or genital tract cancer or who have breast nodules, fibrocystic disease, or abnormal mammographic findings.

Interactions

Drug-drug. *Anticoagulants:* May decrease effects of warfarin-type anticoagulants. Monitor PT and INR.
Corticosteroids: May cause possible enhanced effects. Monitor patient closely.
Cyclosporine: May increase risk of toxicity. Monitor patient closely.
Dantrolene, other hepatotoxic drugs: May increase risk of hepatotoxicity. Monitor liver function.
Drugs that induce hepatic metabolism (such as barbiturates, carbamazepine, phenytoin, primidone, rifampin): May result in decreased estrogenic effects from a given dose. Advise patient to use alternative methods of birth control.
Insulin, oral antidiabetics: Dosage adjustment may be needed because esterified estrogens

may increase blood glucose levels. Monitor serum glucose levels.
Tamoxifen: Effectiveness may be altered with estrogens. Avoid concomitant use.
Drug-food. *Caffeine:* May increase serum caffeine levels. Discourage concomitant use.
Drug-lifestyle. *Smoking:* Increased risk of adverse CV effects. Discourage concomitant use.

Adverse reactions

CNS: headache, dizziness, chorea, depression, *seizures.*
CV: thrombophlebitis; *thromboembolism;* hypertension; edema; *increased risk of CVA, pulmonary embolism, MI.*
EENT: worsening of myopia or astigmatism, intolerance of contact lenses.
GI: *nausea,* vomiting, abdominal cramps, bloating, anorexia, increased appetite, *pancreatitis,* gallbladder disease.
GU: in women—breakthrough bleeding, altered menstrual flow, dysmenorrhea, amenorrhea, *increased risk of endometrial cancer, possibility of increased risk of breast cancer,* cervical erosion, altered cervical secretions, enlargement of uterine fibromas, vaginal candidiasis; breast changes (tenderness, enlargement, secretion); in men—gynecomastia, testicular atrophy, impotence.
Hematologic: increased PT and INR and clotting factors VII to X and norepinephrine-induced platelet aggregability.
Hepatic: cholestatic jaundice, *hepatic adenoma.*
Metabolic: decreased serum folate, pyridoxine, and antithrombin III levels; increased triglyceride, glucose, and phospholipid levels; hypercalcemia, weight changes.
Skin: melasma, urticaria, flushing (with rapid I.V. administration), hirsutism or hair loss, erythema nodosum, dermatitis.

☑ Special considerations

Besides the recommendations relevant to all estrogens, consider the following.
• For rapid treatment of dysfunctional uterine bleeding or reduction of surgical bleeding, parenteral administration is preferred.
• Refrigerate before reconstitution. After adding diluent, agitate gently until drug is in solution; use within a few hours. Reconstituted drug may be safely stored in refrigerator for 60 days.
• Increases in the thyroid-binding globulin concentration may occur, resulting in increased total thyroid levels (measured by protein-bound iodine or total T_4) and decreased uptake of free T_3 resin.
• Therapy with estrogens increases sulfobromophthalein retention.
• Glucose tolerance may be impaired.
• Pregnanediol excretion may decrease.

Reactions may be *common*, uncommon, *life-threatening*, or COMMON AND LIFE-THREATENING.

• Serious toxicity after overdose hasn't been reported. Nausea may occur. Give supportive care.

Monitoring the patient
• Monitor serum glucose level if patient is a diabetic.
• Monitor patient for adverse effects.

Geriatric patients
• Long-term use for menopausal symptoms may be associated with increased risk of certain types of cancer. Frequent physical examinations are recommended.

Breast-feeding patients
• Because estrogens appear in breast milk, they are contraindicated in breast-feeding women.

---

estropipate
Ogen, Ortho-Est

Pharmacologic classification: estrogen
Therapeutic classification: estrogen replacement
Pregnancy risk category X

How supplied
Estropipate is available as estrone sodium sulfate. Available by prescription only.
Tablets: 0.625 mg, 1.25 mg, 2.5 mg

Indications, route, and dosage
Atrophic vaginitis, kraurosis vulvae, and vasomotor menopausal symptoms
Adults: 0.625 to 5 mg P.O. daily for 21 days, then 7 days off therapy.
Female hypogonadism, primary ovarian failure, or after castration
Adults: 1.25 to 7.5 mg P.O. daily for 3 weeks, then 8 to 10 days off therapy. Cycle may be repeated if no withdrawal bleeding occurs within 10 days of discontinuing therapy.
Prevention of osteoporosis
Adults: 0.625 mg P.O. daily for 25 days of a 31-day cycle.

Pharmacodynamics
Estrogenic action: Mimics action of endogenous estrogen in treating female hypogonadism, menopausal symptoms, and atrophic vaginitis.

Pharmacokinetics
• *Absorption:* After oral administration, estropipate, and other synthetic derivatives of natural estrogens, are rapidly absorbed.
• *Distribution:* About 50% to 80% plasma protein–bound. Distribution occurs throughout body, with highest levels appearing in fat.
• *Metabolism:* Steroidal estrogens are metabolized primarily in liver, where they are conjugated with sulfate and glucuronide. Because of the rapid rate of metabolism, many forms of estrogen must usually be administered daily.
• *Excretion:* Mostly eliminated through kidneys as sulfate or glucuronide conjugates.

Contraindications and precautions
Contraindicated in patients with thrombophlebitis or thromboembolic disorders, estrogen-dependent neoplasia, breast or reproductive organ cancer (except for palliative treatment), or undiagnosed abnormal genital bleeding. Also contraindicated during pregnancy.
Use cautiously in patients with cerebrovascular or coronary artery disease, asthma, bone diseases, mental depression, migraine, seizures, or cardiac, hepatic, or renal dysfunction and in women with family history (mother, grandmother, sister) of breast or genital tract cancer or who have breast nodules, fibrocystic disease, or abnormal mammographic findings.

Interactions
Drug-drug. *Anticoagulants:* May decrease effects of warfarin-type anticoagulants. Monitor INR.
Corticosteroids: May enhance effects. Monitor patient closely.
Cyclosporine: May increase risk of toxicity. Monitor patient closely.
Dantrolene, other hepatotoxic medications: May increase risk of hepatotoxicity. Monitor liver function.
Drugs that induce hepatic metabolism (barbiturates, carbamazepine, phenytoin, primidone, rifampin): May result in decreased estrogenic effects from a given dose. Instruct patient to use alternative method of birth control.
Insulin, oral antidiabetics: Dosage adjustment may be needed because esterified estrogens may increase blood glucose levels. Monitor serum glucose levels.
Tamoxifen: Effectiveness may be altered with estrogens. Avoid concomitant use.
Drug-food. *Caffeine:* May increase serum caffeine levels. Discourage concomitant use.
Drug-lifestyle. *Smoking:* May increase risk of CV adverse effects. Discourage concomitant use.

Adverse reactions
CNS: headache, dizziness, depression, migraine, **seizures.**
CV: ***increased risk of CVA, pulmonary embolism, MI, thromboembolism,*** thrombophlebitis, edema.
EENT: worsening of myopia or astigmatism, intolerance of contact lenses.
GI: vomiting, abdominal cramps, bloating, gallbladder disease.
GU: in women—breakthrough bleeding, increased size of uterine fibromas, dysmenorrhea, amenorrhea, vaginal candidiasis, ***increased risk of endometrial cancer, possibility of increased risk of breast cancer,*** altered menstrual flow,

---

cervical erosion, altered cervical secretions, breast changes (tenderness, enlargement, secretion); in men—gynecomastia, testicular atrophy; cystitis-like syndrome, condition resembling premenstrual syndrome; libido changes.

Hematologic: increased PT and clotting factors VII to X and norepinephrine-induced platelet aggregability, aggravation of porphyria.

Hepatic: cholestatic jaundice, *hepatic adenoma.*

Metabolic: decreased serum folate, pyridoxine, and antithrombin III levels; increased triglyceride, glucose, and phospholipid levels; hypercalcemia, weight changes.

Skin: *erythema multiforme,* erythema nodosum, hair loss, hemorrhagic eruption, hirsutism, melasma.

☑ Special considerations

Besides the recommendations relevant to all estrogens, consider the following.

● When used for progressive, inoperable prostate cancer, remission should be apparent within 3 weeks of therapy.

● When submitting specimens to pathologist for evaluation, be sure to note that patient is taking estrogens.

● Therapy with estrogens increases sulfobromophthalein retention.

● Increases in the thyroid-binding globulin concentration may occur, resulting in increased total thyroid levels (measured by protein-bound iodine or total T_4) and decreased uptake of free T_3 resin.

● Glucose tolerance may be impaired.

● Pregnanediol excretion may decrease.

● Serious toxicity after overdose hasn't been reported. Nausea may occur. Provide appropriate supportive care.

Monitoring the patient

● If patient is of childbearing age, rule out pregnancy before initiating treatment.

● Monitor serum glucose level if patient is a diabetic.

● Monitor coagulation studies if patient is taking oral anticoagulants.

Information for the patient

● Emphasize importance of regular physical examinations.

● Tell patient on therapy for postmenopausal symptoms that, although withdrawal bleeding may occur during the week off the drug, fertility is not restored.

● Instruct patient to report adverse effects immediately.

● Tell diabetic patient to report elevated glucose levels so medication can be adjusted.

Geriatric patients

● Frequent physical examinations are recommended for postmenopausal women taking estrogens.

Breast-feeding patients

● Because drug appears in breast milk, its use is contraindicated in breast-feeding women.

etanercept
Enbrel

Pharmacologic classification: tumor necrosis factor (TNF) blocker
Therapeutic classification: antirheumatic
Pregnancy risk category B

How supplied

Available by prescription only
Injection: 25 mg single-use vial

Indications, route, and dosage

Reduction in signs and symptoms of moderately to severely active rheumatoid arthritis in patients with demonstrated inadequate response to one or more disease-modifying antirheumatic drugs; or with methotrexate in patients who don't respond adequately to methotrexate alone

Adults: 25 mg S.C. twice weekly.
Children ages 4 to 17: 0.4 mg/kg (maximum dose 25 mg) S.C. twice weekly for 3 months.

Pharmacodynamics

Antirheumatic action: Binds specifically to TNF and blocks its action with cell surface TNF receptors, reducing inflammatory and immune responses found in rheumatoid arthritis.

Pharmacokinetics

● *Absorption:* Serum levels peak in 72 hours.
● *Distribution:* No information available.
● *Metabolism:* No information available.
● *Excretion:* Elimination half-life is 115 hours.

Contraindications and precautions

Contraindicated in patients with hypersensitivity to etanercept or any of its components and in those with sepsis. Use cautiously in patients with underlying diseases which could predispose them to infection (diabetes, heart failure, history of active or chronic infections).

Interactions

None reported.

Adverse reactions

CNS: asthenia, *headache,* dizziness.
EENT: *rhinitis,* pharyngitis, sinusitis.
GI: abdominal pain, dyspepsia.

Respiratory: *upper respiratory tract infections,* cough, respiratory disorder.
Skin: *injection site reaction,* rash.
Other: *infections,* malignancies.

☑ Special considerations
• Anti-TNF therapies, including etanercept, may affect defenses against infection. Stop therapy if serious infection occurs.
• Live vaccines shouldn't be given concurrently during drug therapy.
• Patients with juvenile rheumatoid arthritis should, if possible, be brought up-to-date with all immunizations in compliance with current immunization guidelines before treatment.
• Reconstitute aseptically with 1 ml of supplied sterile bacteriostatic water for injection, USP (0.9% benzyl alcohol). Don't filter reconstituted solution during preparation or administration. Inject diluent slowly into vial. Minimize foaming by gently swirling during dissolution rather than shaking. Dissolution takes less than 5 minutes.
• Visually inspect solution for particulates and discoloration before use. Reconstituted solution should be clear and colorless. Don't use if solution is discolored, cloudy, or if particulates remain.
• Don't add other drugs or diluents to reconstituted solution.
• Use reconstituted solution as soon as possible; may be refrigerated in vial for up to 6 hours at 36° to 46° F (2° to 8° C).
• Injection sites should be at least 1 inch apart; areas where skin is tender, bruised, red, or hard should never be used. Recommended sites include thigh, abdomen, and upper arm. Rotate sites regularly.
• Patient may develop positive antinuclear antibodies (ANA) or positive anti-double-stranded DNA antibodies measured by radioimmunoassay and *Crithidia lucilae* assay.
• Needle cover of diluent syringe contains dry natural rubber (latex) and shouldn't be handled by persons sensitive to latex.

Monitoring the patient
• Monitor patient for development of infection.
• Monitor therapeutic effect.

Information for the patient
• Instruct patient who will be self-administering about mixing and injection techniques, including rotation of injection sites.
• Instruct patient to use puncture-resistant container for disposal of needles and syringes.
• Tell patient injection site reactions generally occur within first month of therapy and decrease thereafter.
• Tell patient to avoid live vaccine administration while receiving drug. Stress importance of alerting other health care providers of drug use.
• Instruct patient to promptly report signs and symptoms of infection.

Geriatric patients
• Differences in safety and effectiveness haven't been noted between elderly patients and younger adults; however, greater sensitivity to drug effects may occur in this age-group.

Pediatric patients
• Safety and effectiveness are unknown in children under age 4. Children with juvenile rheumatoid arthritis are more prone to abdominal pain and vomiting than are adults with rheumatoid arthritis.

Breast-feeding patients
• Because of potential serious reactions in the infant, a decision should be made either to discontinue breast-feeding or the drug.

---

ethacrynate sodium
ethacrynic acid
Edecrin

Pharmacologic classification: loop diuretic
Therapeutic classification: diuretic
Pregnancy risk category B

How supplied
Available by prescription only
Tablets: 25 mg, 50 mg
Injectable: 50 mg (with 62.5 mg of mannitol and 0.1 mg of thimerosal)

Indications, route, and dosage
Acute pulmonary edema
Adults: 50 mg or 0.5 to 1 mg/kg I.V. to maximum dose of 100 mg of ethacrynate sodium I.V. slowly over several minutes.
Edema
Adults: 50 to 200 mg P.O. daily. Refractory cases may require up to 200 mg b.i.d.
Children: Initially, 25 mg P.O., given cautiously and increased in 25-mg increments daily until desired effect is achieved.
◊ **Hypertension**
Adults: Initially, 25 mg P.O. daily. Adjust dose, as necessary. Maximum maintenance dose is 200 mg P.O. daily in two divided doses.

Pharmacodynamics
Diuretic action: Ethacrynic acid inhibits sodium and chloride reabsorption in the proximal part of the ascending loop of Henle, promoting the excretion of sodium, water, chloride, and potassium.

Pharmacokinetics
• *Absorption:* Absorbed rapidly from GI tract; diuresis occurs in 30 minutes and peaks in 2 hours. After I.V. administration, diuresis occurs in 5 minutes and peaks in 15 to 30 minutes.

- *Distribution:* Accumulates in liver. Doesn't enter CSF; unknown distribution into breast milk or placenta.
- *Metabolism:* Metabolized by liver to potentially active metabolite.
- *Excretion:* 30% to 65% of drug excreted in urine; 35% to 40% excreted in bile as metabolite. Duration of action 6 to 8 hours after oral administration; about 2 hours after I.V. administration.

Contraindications and precautions
Contraindicated in infants and in patients with anuria or hypersensitivity to drug. Use cautiously in patients with electrolyte abnormalities or impaired hepatic function.

Interactions
Drug-drug. *Aminoglycosides, other ototoxic drugs (such as cisplatin):* May increase risk of deafness. Avoid use of such combinations.
Antihypertensives: May potentiate hypotensive effects. Monitor blood pressure.
Cardiac glycosides: May increase risk of digitalis toxicity from ethacrynic acid-induced hypokalemia. Monitor patient for arrhythmias.
Diuretics (such as metolazone): May enhance diuretic effect of other drugs. Reduce dosage when adding ethacrynic acid to diuretic regimen.
Insulin, oral antidiabetics: May increase serum glucose. May need increased dosages when taking ethacrynic acid. Monitor serum glucose levels.
Lithium: Ethacrynic acid may reduce renal clearance of lithium, elevating serum lithium levels. Monitor lithium levels and adjust dosage.
NSAIDs: May decrease diuretic effectiveness. Monitor patient's intake and output.
Potassium-depleting drugs (amphotericin B, corticosteroids): May cause severe potassium loss. Avoid concomitant use.
Potassium-sparing diuretics (amiloride, spironolactone, triamterene): May decrease potassium loss induced by ethacrynic acid. May be a therapeutic advantage.
Warfarin: May potentiate anticoagulant effects. Monitor PT and INR.

Adverse reactions
CNS: confusion, fatigue, vertigo, headache, malaise.
CV: volume depletion and dehydration, orthostatic hypotension.
EENT: transient deafness (with too-rapid I.V. injection), blurred vision, tinnitus, hearing loss.
GI: diarrhea, anorexia, nausea, vomiting, GI bleeding, *pancreatitis.*
GU: oliguria, hematuria, nocturia, polyuria, frequent urination, azotemia.
Hematologic: *agranulocytosis, neutropenia, thrombocytopenia.*
Metabolic: hypokalemia; hypochloremic alkalosis; asymptomatic hyperuricemia; fluid and electrolyte imbalances, including dilutional hyponatremia, hypocalcemia, hypomagnesemia; hyperglycemia; impaired glucose tolerance.
Other: fever, chills.

☑ Special considerations
Besides the recommendations relevant to all loop diuretics, consider the following.
- Don't give drug either I.M. or S.C. because it may cause severe local pain and irritation. When giving I.V., check infusion site frequently for infiltration (edema or skin blanching).
- Infuse drug slowly over 20 to 30 minutes, by I.V. infusion or by direct I.V. injection over a period of several minutes; rapid injection may cause hypotension.
- Don't administer drug simultaneously with whole blood or blood products; hemolysis may occur.
- I.V. ethacrynate sodium has been used to treat hypercalcemia and to manage ethylene glycol poisoning and bromide intoxication.
- Signs and symptoms of overdose include profound electrolyte and volume depletion, which may precipitate circulatory collapse. Treatment is primarily supportive; replace fluid and electrolytes as needed.

Monitoring the patient
- Periodically assess hearing function in patients receiving high-dose therapy. Drug may potentiate ototoxicity of other drugs.
- Determine hepatic function before therapy starts.
- Monitor electrolyte values before treatment starts and regularly throughout.
- Monitor CBC periodically.

Information for the patient
- Advise patient receiving I.V. form of drug to report pain or irritation at I.V. site immediately.
- Notify diabetic patient that antidiabetic dosage may need to be increased.

Geriatric patients
- Elderly and debilitated patients need close observation because they are more susceptible to drug-induced diuresis. Excessive diuresis promotes rapid dehydration, leading to hypovolemia, hypokalemia, hyponatremia, and circulatory collapse. Reduced dosages may be indicated.

Pediatric patients
- Ethacrynate sodium and ethacrynic acid are contraindicated in infants. Don't use I.V. form in children.

Breast-feeding patients
- Because it's unknown if drug appears in breast milk, it shouldn't be used in breast-feeding women.

ethambutol hydrochloride
Myambutol

Pharmacologic classification: semi-synthetic antituberculotic
Therapeutic classification: anti-tuberculotic
Pregnancy risk category NR

How supplied
Available by prescription only
Tablets: 100 mg, 400 mg

Indications, route, and dosage
Adjunctive treatment in pulmonary tuberculosis
Adults and children ages 13 and older: Initial treatment for patients who haven't received previous antitubercular therapy, 15 mg/kg P.O. daily single dose. Retreatment: 25 mg/kg P.O. daily single dose for 60 days with at least one other antituberculotic; then decrease to 15 mg/kg P.O. daily single dose.

Pharmacodynamics
Antitubercular action: Bacteriostatic; interferes with mycolic acid incorporation into the mycobacterial cell wall. Active against *Mycobacterium tuberculosis, M. bovis,* and *M. marinum,* some strains of *M. kansasii, M. avium, M. fortuitum,* and *M. intracellulare,* and the combined strain of *M. avium* and *M. intracellulare* (MAC). Considered adjunctive therapy in tuberculosis and is combined with other antituberculotics to prevent or delay development of drug resistance by *M. tuberculosis.*

Pharmacokinetics
• *Absorption:* Absorbed rapidly from GI tract; serum levels peak 2 to 4 hours after ingestion.
• *Distribution:* Distributed widely into body tissues and fluids, especially into lungs, erythrocytes, saliva, and kidneys; lesser amounts into brain, ascitic, pleural, and cerebrospinal fluids. 8% to 22% protein-bound.
• *Metabolism:* Undergoes partial hepatic metabolism.
• *Excretion:* After 24 hours, about 50% of unchanged drug and 8% to 15% of its metabolites excreted in urine; 20% to 25% excreted in feces. Small amounts of drug may be excreted in breast milk. Plasma half-life in adults is about 3¼ hours; half-life is prolonged in patients with decreased renal or hepatic function. Drug can be removed by peritoneal dialysis and, to a lesser extent, by hemodialysis.

Contraindications and precautions
Contraindicated in children under age 13 and in patients with optic neuritis or hypersensitivity to drug. Use cautiously in patients with impaired renal function, cataracts, recurrent eye inflammations, gout, and diabetic retinopathy.

Interactions
Drug-drug. *Aluminum salts:* May delay and reduce absorption of ethambutol. Separate administration times by several hours.
Drugs that produce neurotoxicity: May potentiate adverse effects of these drugs. Avoid concomitant use.

Adverse reactions
CNS: headache, malaise, dizziness, mental confusion, possible hallucinations, peripheral neuritis (numbness and tingling of extremities).
EENT: optic neuritis (related to dose and duration of treatment).
GI: anorexia, nausea, vomiting, abdominal pain, GI upset.
Hematologic: *thrombocytopenia.*
Hepatic: abnormal liver function tests.
Metabolic: elevated uric acid level.
Musculoskeletal: joint pain, precipitation of acute gout.
Respiratory: bloody sputum, *anaphylactoid reactions.*
Skin: dermatitis, pruritus, toxic epidermal necrolysis.
Other: fever.

☑ Special considerations
• Give drug with food if necessary to prevent gastric irritation; food doesn't interfere with absorption.
• No specific recommendation on overdose available. Treatment is supportive. After recent ingestion (4 hours or less), empty stomach by induced emesis or gastric lavage. Follow with activated charcoal to decrease absorption.

Monitoring the patient
• Obtain specimens for culture and sensitivity testing before first dose, but therapy can begin before test results are complete; repeat testing periodically to detect drug resistance.
• Assess visual status before therapy; test visual acuity and color discrimination monthly in patients taking more than 15 mg/kg/day. Visual disturbances are dose-related and reversible if detected in time.
• Monitor blood (including serum uric acid), renal, and liver function studies, CBC before and periodically during therapy to minimize toxicity.
• Watch for change in renal function. Dosage reduction may be necessary.

Information for the patient
• Explain disease process and rationale for long-term therapy.
• Teach signs and symptoms of hypersensitivity and other adverse reactions, and emphasize need to call if these occur; urge patient to report ↗

unusual adverse effects, especially blurred vision, red-green color blindness, or changes in urine elimination.
● Assure patient that visual alterations will disappear within several weeks or months after therapy ends.
● Urge patient to complete entire prescribed regimen, to comply with instructions for daily dose, to avoid missing doses, and not to stop drug without medical approval. Explain importance of keeping follow-up appointments.

Pediatric patients
● Drug isn't recommended for use in children under age 13.

Breast-feeding patients
● Drug appears in breast milk. Use with caution in breast-feeding women.

ethinyl estradiol
Estinyl

Pharmacologic classification: estrogen
Therapeutic classification: estrogen replacement, antineoplastic
Pregnancy risk category X

How supplied
Available by prescription only
Tablets: 0.02 mg, 0.05 mg, 0.5 mg

Indications, route, and dosage
Palliative treatment of metastatic breast cancer (at least 5 years after menopause)
Adults: 1 mg P.O. t.i.d. for at least 3 months.
Female hypogonadism
Adults: 0.05 mg daily to t.i.d. for 2 weeks monthly, then 2 weeks progesterone therapy; continue for three to six monthly dosing cycles, then 2 months off.
Vasomotor menopausal symptoms
Adults: 0.02 to 0.05 mg P.O. daily for cycles of 3 weeks on, 1 week off.
Palliative treatment of metastatic inoperable prostatic cancer
Adults: 0.15 to 2 mg P.O. daily.

Pharmacodynamics
Estrogenic action: Mimics action of endogenous estrogen in treating female hypogonadism and menopausal symptoms. It inhibits growth of hormone-sensitive tissue in advanced, inoperable prostatic cancer and in certain carefully selected cases of breast cancer in men and postmenopausal women.

Pharmacokinetics
● *Absorption:* After oral administration, is well absorbed but substantially inactivated by liver.

● *Distribution:* Estradiol and other natural estrogens are about 50% to 80% plasma protein–bound, particularly estradiol-binding globulin. Distribution occurs throughout body, with highest levels appearing in fat.
● *Metabolism:* Steroidal estrogens, including estradiol, are metabolized primarily in liver, where they are conjugated with sulfate and glucuronide. Because of rapid metabolism, nonesterified forms of estrogen, including estradiol, usually must be administered daily.
● *Excretion:* Majority of elimination occurs through kidneys as sulfate or glucuronide conjugates.

Contraindications and precautions
Contraindicated in patients with thrombophlebitis or thromboembolic disorders, estrogen-dependent neoplasia, breast or reproductive organ cancer (except for palliative treatment), or undiagnosed abnormal genital bleeding. Also contraindicated during pregnancy.
Use cautiously in patients with cerebrovascular or coronary artery disease, asthma, mental depression, bone disease, or cardiac, hepatic, or renal dysfunction and in women with a family history (mother, grandmother, sister) of breast or genital tract cancer or who have breast nodules, fibrocystic disease, or abnormal mammographic findings.

Interactions
Drug-drug. *Anticoagulants:* May decrease effects of warfarin-type anticoagulants. Monitor INR.
Corticosteroids: Possible enhanced effects. Monitor patient closely.
Cyclosporine: May increase risk of toxicity. Monitor patient closely.
Dantrolene, other hepatotoxic medications: May increase risk of hepatotoxicity. Monitor liver function closely.
Drugs that induce hepatic metabolism (barbiturates, carbamazepine, phenytoin, primidone, rifampin): May result in decreased estrogenic effects from given dose. Tell patient to use alternative method of birth control.
Insulin, oral antidiabetics: Esterified estrogens may increase blood glucose levels. Monitor serum glucose levels.
Tamoxifen: Estrogens may interfere with effectiveness. Avoid concomitant use.
Drug-food. *Caffeine:* May increase serum caffeine levels. Discourage concomitant use.
Drug-lifestyle. *Smoking:* May increase risk of CV adverse effects. Discourage concomitant use.

Adverse reactions
CNS: headache, dizziness, chorea, depression, *seizures.*
CV: thrombophlebitis; *thromboembolism;* hypertension; edema; *increased risk of CVA, pulmonary embolism, MI.*

EENT: worsening of myopia or astigmatism, intolerance of contact lenses.
GI: *nausea,* vomiting, abdominal cramps, bloating, anorexia, increased appetite, gallbladder disease.
GU: in women—breakthrough bleeding, altered menstrual flow, dysmenorrhea, amenorrhea, *increased risk of endometrial cancer, possibility of increased risk of breast cancer,* cervical erosion, altered cervical secretions, enlargement of uterine fibromas, vaginal candidiasis; breast changes (tenderness, enlargement, secretion); in men—gynecomastia, testicular atrophy, impotence.
Hematologic: increased PT and INR and clotting factors VII to X and norepinephrine-induced platelet aggregability.
Hepatic: cholestatic jaundice, *hepatic adenoma.*
Metabolic: decreased serum folate, pyridoxine, and antithrombin III levels; increased triglyceride, glucose, and phospholipid levels; hypercalcemia, weight changes.
Skin: melasma, urticaria, flushing (with rapid I.V. administration), hirsutism or hair loss, erythema nodosum, dermatitis.

☑ Special considerations
• Because of risk of thromboembolism, discontinue drug therapy at least 1 month before procedures associated with prolonged immobilization or thromboembolism.
• Notify pathologist of patient receiving estrogen therapy when specimens are obtained and sent to pathology for evaluation.
• Therapy with ethinyl estradiol increases sulfobromophthalein retention. Increases in the thyroid-binding globulin level may occur, resulting in increased total thyroid levels (measured by protein-bound iodine or total T_4) and decreased uptake of free T_3 resin.
• Glucose tolerance may be impaired.
• Pregnanediol excretion may decrease.
• Serious toxicity after overdose hasn't been reported. Nausea may occur. Provide appropriate supportive care.

Monitoring the patient
• If patient is of childbearing age, rule out pregnancy before treatment.
• Give patient thorough physical examination before estrogen therapy. Patients receiving long-term therapy should have examinations yearly.
• Monitor serum glucose level if patient is a diabetic.
• Monitor coagulation studies if patient is taking anticoagulants.
• Periodically monitor serum lipid levels, blood pressure, body weight, and hepatic function.

Information for the patient
• Provide patient with package insert (and verbal explanation) describing estrogen's adverse reactions.
• Emphasize importance of regular physical examinations. Studies suggest that postmenopausal women who use estrogen replacement for over 5 years to treat menopausal symptoms may be at increased risk for endometrial cancer. This risk is reduced by using cyclic rather than continuous therapy and the lowest possible dosages of estrogen. Adding progestins to regimen decreases the risk of endometrial hyperplasia; however, it's unknown if progestins affect occurrence of endometrial cancer. Most studies show no increased risk of breast cancer.
• Explain to patient on cyclic therapy for postmenopausal symptoms that, although withdrawal bleeding may occur during week off drug, fertility isn't restored. Pregnancy can't occur because patient doesn't ovulate.
• Warn patient to immediately report abdominal pain; pain, numbness, or stiffness in legs or buttocks; pressure or pain in chest; shortness of breath; severe headaches; visual disturbances such as blind spots, flashing lights, or blurriness; vaginal bleeding or discharge; breast lumps; swelling of hands or feet; yellow skin or sclera; dark urine; or light-colored stools.
• Tell diabetic patient to report elevated blood glucose test results; antidiabetic dosage may be adjusted.
• Teach woman how to perform routine breast self-examination.
• Teach patient methods to decrease risk of thromboembolism.

Geriatric patients
• Use with caution in patients whose condition may be aggravated by fluid retention.

Breast-feeding patients
• Drug appears in breast milk; its use is contraindicated in breast-feeding women.

ethosuximide
Zarontin

Pharmacologic classification: succinimide derivative
Therapeutic classification: anticonvulsant
Pregnancy risk category NR

How supplied
Available by prescription only
Capsules: 250 mg
Syrup: 250 mg/5 ml

Indications, route, and dosage
Absence seizures
Adults and children ages 6 and older: Initially, 250 mg P.O. b.i.d. May increase by 250 mg q 4 to 7 days up to 1.5 g daily.
Children ages 3 to 6: 250 mg P.O. daily. Optimal dose is 20 mg/kg/day.

Pharmacodynamics
Anticonvulsant action: Raises seizure threshold; suppresses characteristic spike-and-wave pattern by depressing neuronal transmission in the motor cortex and basal ganglia. Indicated for absence seizures refractory to other drugs.

Pharmacokinetics
• *Absorption:* Absorbed from GI tract; steady-state plasma levels occur in 4 to 7 days.
• *Distribution:* Distributed widely throughout body; minimal protein binding.
• *Metabolism:* Metabolized extensively in liver to several inactive metabolites.
• *Excretion:* Excreted in urine, with small amounts in bile and feces. Plasma half-life is about 60 hours in adults; about 30 hours in children.

Contraindications and precautions
Contraindicated in patients with hypersensitivity to succinimide derivatives. Use with extreme caution in patients with hepatic or renal disease.

Interactions
Drug-drug. *CNS depressants (antidepressants, antipsychotics, anxiolytics, narcotics, other anticonvulsants):* May cause additive CNS depression and sedation. Monitor patient closely.
Phenytoin: May increase serum phenytoin levels. Monitor serum phenytoin levels.
Valproic acid: May increase or decrease serum ethosuximide levels. Monitor serum ethosuximide levels.
Drug-lifestyle. *Alcohol:* May cause additive CNS depression and sedation. Discourage concomitant use.

Adverse reactions
CNS: *drowsiness, headache, fatigue, dizziness, ataxia, irritability, hiccups, euphoria, lethargy, depression, psychosis.*
EENT: myopia, tongue swelling, gingival hyperplasia.
GI: *nausea, vomiting, diarrhea, weight loss, cramps, anorexia, epigastric and abdominal pain.*
GU: vaginal bleeding, urinary frequency, abnormal renal function tests.
Hematologic: *leukopenia,* eosinophilia, ***agranulocytosis, pancytopenia.***
Hepatic: elevated liver enzyme levels.
Skin: urticaria, pruritic and erythematous rash, hirsutism, ***Stevens-Johnson syndrome.***

☑ Special considerations
Besides the recommendations relevant to all succinimide derivatives, consider the following.
• Administer ethosuximide with food to minimize GI distress.
• Avoid stopping drug abruptly; may precipitate absence seizures.
• Therapeutic plasma levels range from 40 to 100 mcg/ml.
• Ethosuximide may cause false-positive Coombs' test results.
• Symptoms of overdose, when drug is used alone or with other anticonvulsants, include CNS depression, ataxia, stupor, and coma. Treatment is symptomatic and supportive. Carefully monitor vital signs and fluid and electrolyte balance.

Monitoring the patient
• Monitor hepatic and renal function before starting therapy.
• Perform CBC, liver function tests, and urinalysis periodically.
• Observe patient for dermatologic reactions, joint pain, unexplained fever, or unusual bruising or bleeding (which may signal hematologic or other severe adverse reactions).

Information for the patient
• Tell patient to take drug with food or milk to prevent GI distress, to avoid alcoholic beverages, and to avoid hazardous tasks that require alertness if drug causes drowsiness, dizziness, or blurred vision.
• Inform patient that drug may color urine pink to reddish-brown.
• Encourage patient to wear medical identification bracelet or necklace.
• Tell patient to report rash, joint pain, fever, sore throat, or unusual bleeding or bruising.
• Advise patient to call immediately if pregnancy is suspected.

Geriatric patients
• Use with caution in elderly patients.

Pediatric patients
• Don't use drug in children under age 3.

Breast-feeding patients
• It's unknown if drug appears in breast milk. Because safety hasn't been established, advise breast-feeding mothers to use an alternative to breast-feeding during therapy.

ethyl chloride (chloroethane)
Ethyl Chloride

Pharmacologic classification: halogenated hydrocarbon
Therapeutic classification: local anesthetic, counterirritant
Pregnancy risk category C

How supplied
Available by prescription only
Topical liquid spray: 3-oz., 3.5-oz. bottles

Indications, route, and dosage
Local anesthetic in minor operative procedures; relief of pain caused by insect stings, burns, bruises, contusions, abrasions, swelling, and minor sprains associated with sports injuries; tinea lesions and creeping eruption
Adults and children: Dosage varies with different procedures. Use smallest dosage needed to produce desired effect. For local anesthesia, use the fine-spray nozzle; hold container about 12 inches (30 cm) from area and spray downward until a light frosting appears.
Infants: Hold a cotton ball saturated with ethyl chloride to area for a few seconds.
Counterirritant to relieve myofascial and visceral pain syndromes
Adults, children, and infants: Dosage varies with use. Use smallest dosage needed to produce desired effect. Use the large-sized nozzle; hold container 24 inches (60 cm) from skin and spray at an acute angle in one direction in a sweeping motion until area has been covered.

Pharmacodynamics
Anesthetic action: Rapid vaporization of ethyl chloride freezes superficial tissues, producing insensitivity of peripheral nerve endings and local anesthesia. Anesthesia lasts for up to 1 minute.

Pharmacokinetics
- *Absorption:* Limited with topical use.
- *Distribution:* None.
- *Metabolism:* None.
- *Excretion:* None.

Contraindications and precautions
Contraindicated for use near eyes or on broken skin or mucous membranes; don't inhale. Freezing and thawing process may damage epithelial cells; avoid repeated use over long periods. Drug is highly flammable and explosive; don't use near open fire and store away from heat or open flame.

Interactions
None reported.

Adverse reactions
Skin: skin lesions, rash, urticaria, burning, stinging, tenderness, inflammation, frostbite, tissue necrosis with prolonged use, pain and muscle spasm from excessive cooling.

☑ Special considerations
- Don't apply to broken skin or mucous membranes.
- Protect adjacent skin with petroleum jelly.
- When using as a counterirritant, avoid frosting the skin because excessive cooling may increase spasms and pain.
- Stop drug if sensitization develops.
- If overdose occurs, stop drug and clean area thoroughly.

Monitoring the patient
- Monitor environment because drug is highly flammable.
- Monitor patient for adverse effects.

Information for the patient
- Tell patient drug will cause temporary numbness.

Pediatric patients
- Use smaller amounts of drug in children.

Breast-feeding patients
- Patient should clean drug from breast area before breast-feeding.

etidronate disodium
Didronel

Pharmacologic classification: pyrophosphate analogue
Therapeutic classification: antihypercalcemic
Pregnancy risk category C

How supplied
Available by prescription only
Tablets: 200 mg, 400 mg
Injection: 50 mg/ml (300-mg ampule)

Indications, route, and dosage
Symptomatic Paget's disease
Adults: 5 mg/kg P.O. daily as a single dose 2 hours before a meal with water or juice. Patient shouldn't eat, consume milk or milk products, or take antacids or vitamins with mineral supplements for 2 hours after dose. May give up to 10 mg/kg/day in severe cases, not to exceed 6 months. Maximum dose is 20 mg/kg/day, not to exceed 3 months.
Heterotopic ossification in spinal cord injuries
Adults: 20 mg/kg/day P.O. for 2 weeks, then 10 mg/kg/day for 10 weeks. Total treatment period is 12 weeks.

Heterotopic ossification after total hip replacement
Adults: 20 mg/kg/day P.O. for 1 month before total hip replacement and for 3 months afterward.
Hypercalcemia associated with malignancy
Adults: 7.5 mg/kg I.V. daily for 3 days. May repeat up to 7 days. Then wait 7 days before beginning a second course of treatment.

Pharmacodynamics
Bone-metabolism inhibitor action: Exact mechanism unknown. Acts on bone by adsorbing to hydroxyapatite crystals in the bone, thereby inhibiting their growth and dissolution. Also decreases the number of osteoclasts in bone, thereby slowing excessive remodeling of pagetic or heterotopic bone.

Pharmacokinetics
• *Absorption:* Variable following oral dose, and is decreased in presence of food. May also be dose-related.
• *Distribution:* About half of dose distributed to bone.
• *Metabolism:* Not metabolized.
• *Excretion:* About 50% excreted in urine within 24 hours.

Contraindications and precautions
Contraindicated in patients with hypersensitivity to drug and in those with overt osteomalacia. Use cautiously in patients with impaired renal function.

Interactions
Drug-drug. *Antacids containing aluminum, calcium, magnesium; mineral supplements containing aluminum, calcium, iron, magnesium:* May inhibit absorption. Avoid use within 2 hours of dose.
Drug-food. *Foods containing large amounts of calcium (such as dairy products, milk):* May prevent oral absorption. Avoid use within 2 hours of dose.

Adverse reactions
CNS: *seizures.*
CV: fluid overload.
GI: reactions occur most frequently at dose of 20 mg/kg daily—diarrhea, increased frequency of bowel movements, nausea, constipation, stomatitis.
Hepatic: abnormal hepatic function.
Metabolic: *elevated serum phosphate level.*
Musculoskeletal: increased or recurrent bone pain, pain at previously asymptomatic sites, increased risk of fracture.
Respiratory: dyspnea.
Other: fever, *hypersensitivity reactions.*

☑ Special considerations
• Drug should be taken in a single dose. However, if nausea occurs, dosage may be divided.
• Signs and symptoms of overdose include diarrhea, nausea, and hypocalcemia. Treat with gastric lavage and emesis. Administer calcium if needed.

Monitoring the patient
• Monitor renal function before therapy starts.
• Determine drug effect by monitoring serum alkaline phosphate and urinary hydroxyproline excretion; both are lowered by effective therapy.

Information for the patient
• Instruct patient to take drug on empty stomach with water or juice and to avoid food, milk or milk products, antacids, and vitamins with mineral supplements for 2 hours.
• Remind patient that improvement may take at least 3 months and may continue even after drug is stopped.

etodolac
Lodine, Lodine XL

Pharmacologic classification: NSAID
Therapeutic classification: antarthritic
Pregnancy risk category C

How supplied
Available by prescription only
Capsules: 200 mg, 300 mg
Tablets: 400 mg
Tablets (extended-release): 400 mg, 600 mg

Indications, route, and dosage
Acute and long-term management of osteoarthritis, rheumatoid arthritis, and pain
Adults: For acute pain, give 200 to 400 mg P.O. q 6 to 8 hours, p.r.n., not to exceed 1,200 mg daily. For patients weighing 60 kg (132 lb) or less, total daily dose shouldn't exceed 20 mg/kg.

For osteoarthritis or rheumatoid arthritis, give 800 to 1,200 mg P.O. daily in divided doses initially, then adjustments of 600 to 1,200 mg in divided doses: 200 mg P.O. t.i.d. or q.i.d.; 300 mg P.O. b.i.d., t.i.d., or q.i.d.; 400 mg P.O. b.i.d. or t.i.d. Total daily dose isn't to exceed 1,200 mg. For patients weighing 60 kg or less, total daily dose shouldn't exceed 20 mg/kg, or 400 to 1,000 mg P.O. daily (extended-release form). Adjust dosage to lowest effective dose based on patient response. Don't exceed maximum dose of 1,000 mg daily.

Pharmacodynamics
Antarthritic action: Mechanism of action unknown; presumed to be associated with inhibition of prostaglandin biosynthesis.

Pharmacokinetics
• *Absorption:* Well absorbed from GI tract, with peak levels reached in 1 to 2 hours. Onset of analgesic activity occurs within 30 minutes, lasting 4 to 6 hours. Antacids don't appear to affect absorption; can decrease peak levels reached by 15% to 20% but have no effect on when peak levels are reached.
• *Distribution:* Drug found in liver, lungs, heart, and kidneys.
• *Metabolism:* Extensively metabolized in liver.
• *Excretion:* Excreted in urine primarily as metabolites; 16% excreted in feces.

Contraindications and precautions
Contraindicated in patients with hypersensitivity to drug and in those with history of aspirin- or NSAID-induced asthma, rhinitis, urticaria, or other allergic reactions.

Use cautiously in patients with impaired renal or hepatic function, history of peptic ulcer disease, cardiac disease, hypertension, or conditions associated with fluid retention.

Interactions
Drug-drug. *Antacids:* May decrease peak levels of drug. Observe for desired effects.
Aspirin: Concurrent use reduces etodolac's protein-binding without altering its clearance; may increase GI toxicity. Monitor patient closely.
Beta blockers, diuretics: May blunt drug's effects. Observe for desired effects.
Cyclosporine: Concomitant use may enhance nephrotoxicity. Avoid concomitant use.
Cyclosporine, digoxin, lithium, methotrexate: Additive effects may change in elimination, resulting in increased levels of these drugs. Monitor drug levels.
Phenytoin: May increase serum phenytoin levels. Monitor serum phenytoin levels.
Warfarin: Concomitant use may result in decreased protein-binding of warfarin but doesn't change its clearance. No dosage adjustment is necessary, but monitor PT and INR and watch for bleeding.
Drug-lifestyle. *Alcohol:* May increase risk of adverse effects. Discourage concomitant use.
Sun exposure: May result in photosensitivity reactions. Tell patient to take precautions.

Adverse reactions
CNS: *asthenia, malaise, dizziness,* depression, drowsiness, nervousness, insomnia.
CV: hypertension, **heart failure,** syncope, flushing, palpitations, edema, fluid retention.
EENT: blurred vision, tinnitus, photophobia, dry mouth.
GI: *dyspepsia, flatulence, abdominal pain, diarrhea, nausea,* constipation, gastritis, melena, vomiting, anorexia, peptic ulceration with or without **GI bleeding** or perforation, ulcerative stomatitis, thirst.
GU: dysuria, urinary frequency, *renal failure.*
Hematologic: *leukopenia, thrombocytopenia,* hemolytic anemia, **agranulocytosis.**
Hepatic: elevated liver function tests, **hepatitis.**
Metabolic: decreased serum uric acid levels, weight gain.
Respiratory: asthma.
Skin: pruritus, rash, **Stevens-Johnson syndrome.**
Other: chills, fever.

✓ Special considerations
• Use caution with concurrent use of diuretics in patients with cardiac, renal, or hepatic failure.
• Etodolac 1,200 mg was shown to cause less GI bleeding than ibuprofen 2,400 mg daily, indomethacin 200 mg daily, naproxen 750 mg daily, or piroxicam 20 mg daily.
• In chronic conditions, a therapeutic response to therapy is most often seen within 2 weeks.
• A false-positive test for urinary bilirubin may be caused by phenolic metabolites.
• Signs and symptoms of overdose include lethargy, drowsiness, nausea, vomiting, and epigastric pain. Rare symptoms include GI bleeding, coma, renal failure, hypertension, and anaphylaxis. Treatment is symptomatic and supportive, including stomach decontamination.

Monitoring the patient
• Monitor renal and hepatic function before starting treatment and periodically throughout.
• Watch for signs and symptoms of GI ulceration and bleeding.
• Monitor CBC periodically.
• Monitor blood pressure and weight, and watch for development of edema periodically throughout treatment.

Information for the patient
• Instruct patient to report GI effects of drug.
• Advise patient to avoid use during pregnancy.
• Tell patient that drug may be taken with food.

Geriatric patients
• Drug is well tolerated in older and younger adults; generally, dosage adjustments aren't needed. No age-related differences have been reported.

Pediatric patients
• Safety and efficacy haven't been established in children under age 18.

Breast-feeding patients
• It's unknown if drug appears in breast milk. Use cautiously in breast-feeding women.

etoposide
Etopophos, Toposar, VePesid

Pharmacologic classification: podophyllotoxin (cell cycle–phase specific, G2 and late S phases)
Therapeutic classification: antineoplastic
Pregnancy risk category D

How supplied
Available by prescription only
Capsules: 50 mg
Injection: 100 mg single, 20 mg/ml

Indications, route, and dosage
Dosage and indications may vary. Check literature for current protocol.
Small-cell carcinoma of the lung
Adults: 70 mg/m²/day P.O. (rounded to the nearest 50 mg) for 4 days; or 100 mg/m² P.O. (rounded to the nearest 50 mg) daily for 5 days. Repeat q 3 to 4 weeks. Or 35 mg/m² I.V. daily for 4 days or 50 mg/m² I.V. daily for 5 days. Repeat q 3 to 4 weeks.
Testicular carcinoma
Adults: 50 to 100 mg/m² I.V. daily on days 1 to 5; or 100 mg/m²/day on days 1, 3, and 5 of a regimen repeated q 3 or 4 weeks.
✦ *Dosage adjustment.* Dosage reduction may be needed in patients with impaired renal function.

Pharmacodynamics
Antineoplastic action: Exerts cytotoxic action by arresting cells in the metaphase portion of cell division. Also inhibits cells from entering mitosis and depresses DNA and RNA synthesis.

Pharmacokinetics
• *Absorption:* Only moderately absorbed across GI tract after oral administration. Bioavailability ranges from 25% to 75%; average of 50% of dose absorbed.
• *Distribution:* Distributed widely into body tissues; highest levels found in liver, spleen, kidneys, healthy brain tissue, and brain tumor tissue. Crosses blood-brain barrier to limited and variable extent. About 94% bound to serum albumin.
• *Metabolism:* Only small portion of dose metabolized. Metabolism occurs in liver.
• *Excretion:* Excreted primarily in urine as unchanged drug. Smaller portion of dose excreted in feces. Plasma elimination is biphasic; initial phase half-life of about ½ to 2 hours and terminal phase of about 5¼ to 11 hours.

Contraindications and precautions
Contraindicated in patients with hypersensitivity to drug. Use cautiously in patients who have had cytotoxic or radiation therapy.

Interactions
Drug-drug. Cisplatin: Concurrent use increases cytotoxicity against certain tumors. Monitor patient closely.
Warfarin: Concomitant administration may cause additive effects. Monitor INR.

Adverse reactions
CNS: peripheral neuropathy.
CV: hypotension (from too-rapid infusion).
GI: *nausea, vomiting, anorexia, diarrhea,* abdominal pain, *stomatitis.*
Hematologic: *anemia,* **myelosuppression** (dose-limiting), LEUKOPENIA, THROMBOCYTOPENIA.
Other: *reversible alopecia,* phlebitis at injection site (infrequent).

☑ Special considerations
• To prepare solution, dilute prescribed dose to a level of 0.2 to 0.4 mg/ml with normal saline solution or D₅W. Higher levels may crystallize. Discard solution if cloudy.
• Solutions diluted to 0.2 mg/ml are stable for 96 hours at room temperature in plastic or glass unprotected from light; solutions diluted to 0.4 mg/ml are stable for 48 hours under the same conditions.
• Administer infusion over 30 to 60 minutes to avoid hypotensive reactions.
• Pretreatment with antiemetics may reduce frequency and duration of nausea and vomiting.
• At doses below 200 mg, extent of absorption after oral administration isn't affected by food.
• Intrapleural and intrathecal administration of drug is contraindicated because of severe toxicity.
• Store capsules in refrigerator.
• Etoposide has produced complete remissions in small-cell lung cancer and testicular cancer.
• Signs and symptoms of overdose include myelosuppression, nausea, and vomiting. Treatment is usually supportive and includes transfusion of blood components, antiemetics, and appropriate symptomatic therapy.

Monitoring the patient
• Monitor patient for anaphylaxis, which can occur rarely. Have diphenhydramine, hydrocortisone, epinephrine, and emergency equipment available to establish an airway in case of anaphylactic reaction.
• Monitor blood pressure before infusion and at 30-minute intervals during infusion. If systolic blood pressure falls below 90 mm Hg, stop infusion.
• Monitor CBC. Observe patient for signs of bone marrow depression. Withhold drug if platelet count is below 50,000/mm³ or absolute neutrophil count is below 500/mm³ until blood counts have sufficiently recovered.
• Watch for GI toxicity, which occurs more frequently after oral administration.

---

actions may be *common*, uncommon, **life-threatening**, or COMMON AND LIFE-THREATENING.

- Watch for extravasation. Treatment includes local injections of hyaluronidase, which aids in systemic reabsorption of etoposide.

Information for the patient
- Emphasize importance of continuing therapy despite nausea and vomiting.
- Tell patient to call immediately if vomiting occurs shortly after dose is taken.
- Advise patient to avoid exposure to people with infections.
- Tell patient not to receive immunizations during therapy with etoposide; other family members also shouldn't receive immunizations during duration of therapy.
- Instruct patient to promptly report sore throat, fever, or unusual bruising or bleeding.
- Reassure patient that hair should grow back after therapy ends.
- Advise patient to use contraceptive measures during therapy.

Geriatric patients
- Elderly patients may be particularly susceptible to hypotensive effects of etoposide.

Pediatric patients
- Safety and effectiveness in children haven't been established.

Breast-feeding patients
- Because drug appears in breast milk, use in breast-feeding women isn't recommended.

etoposide phosphate
Etopophos

Pharmacologic classification: semisynthetic derivative of podophyllotoxin
Therapeutic classification: antineoplastic
Pregnancy risk category D

How supplied
Available by prescription only
Injection: Single-dose vial containing etoposide phosphate that is equivalent to 100 mg etoposide (20 mg etoposide = 22.7 mg etoposide phosphate)

Indications, route, and dosage
Adjunct treatment of refractory testicular cancer
Adults: Etoposide phosphate doses that are equivalent to 50 to 100 mg/m^2/day of etoposide I.V. on days 1 through 5 of each cycle and given in conjunction with other approved chemotherapeutic drugs. Cycle is repeated when adequate recovery from drug toxicity has occurred (usually at 3- to 4-week intervals). Or etoposide phosphate doses that are equivalent to 100 mg/m^2/day of etoposide I.V. on days 1, 3, and 5 of each cycle and

given in conjunction with other approved chemotherapeutic drugs. Cycle is repeated at 3- to 4-week intervals if adequate recovery from drug toxicity has occurred. Infusion rate may range from 5 minutes to 210 minutes.
Adjunct treatment of small-cell lung cancer
Adults: Dosage is individualized but may range from etoposide phosphate doses that are equivalent to 35 mg/m^2/day etoposide I.V. for 4 days to etoposide phosphate doses that are equivalent to 50 mg/m^2/day etoposide I.V. for 5 days and given in conjunction with other approved chemotherapeutic drugs. Cycle is repeated when adequate recovery from drug toxicity has occurred (usually at 3- to 4-week intervals). Infusion rate may range from 5 minutes to 210 minutes.
✦ *Dosage adjustment.* For patients with renal impairment who have creatinine clearance above 50 ml/minute, give usual dosage; for creatinine clearance between 15 and 50 ml/minute, give 75% of usual dosage.

Pharmacodynamics
Antineoplastic action: Exact mechanism unknown. Believed to exert cytotoxicity by arresting cells in the metaphase portion of cell division. May also inhibit cells from entering mitosis and depressing DNA and RNA synthesis.

Pharmacokinetics
- *Absorption:* Only administered as I.V. infusion.
- *Distribution:* Distribution believed to be similar to etoposide. Etoposide crosses blood-brain barrier to limited and variable extent and is about 97% bound to serum albumin.
- *Metabolism:* Rapidly and completely converted to etoposide in plasma.
- *Excretion:* After etoposide phosphate is converted to etoposide, etoposide is excreted primarily in urine as unchanged drug. Smaller portion of dose is excreted in feces. Plasma elimination of etoposide is biphasic; initial phase half-life of about ½ to 2 hours and terminal phase of about 5¼ to 11 hours.

Contraindications and precautions
Contraindicated in patients with hypersensitivity to etoposide phosphate, etoposide, or components of drugs.

Interactions
Drug-drug. *Drugs that inhibit phosphatase activities (such as levamisole hydrochloride):* May alter effects of drug. Use together cautiously.
High-dose cyclosporine: May increase toxic effects of etoposide phosphate because of delayed drug excretion. Monitor patient closely.
Warfarin: May cause additive effects. Monitor PT and INR.

Adverse reactions
CNS: *asthenia, malaise,* dizziness, peripheral neurotoxicity.
CV: hypertension, hypotension.
GI: *nausea, vomiting, anorexia, mucositis,* constipation, abdominal pain, diarrhea, taste alteration.
Hematologic: *anemia, myelosuppression* (dose-limiting), LEUKOPENIA, THROMBOCYTOPENIA, NEUTROPENIA.
Skin: facial flushing, rash, *reversible alopecia.*
Other: *chills, fever,* phlebitis, **anaphylaxis.**

☑ Special considerations
● To prepare solution, reconstitute each vial with either 5 or 10 ml sterile water for injection, D$_5$W, normal saline solution, bacteriostatic water for injection with benzyl alcohol, or bacteriostatic saline for injection with benzyl alcohol to a level equivalent to 20 mg/ml or 10 mg/ml etoposide (22.7 mg/ml or 11.4 mg/ml etoposide phosphate), respectively.
● Use gloves when handling etoposide phosphate. If solution comes into contact with skin or mucosa, immediately and thoroughly wash skin with soap and water; flush mucosa with water.
● After reconstitution, solution may be administered without further dilution or can be further diluted to levels as low as 0.1 mg/ml etoposide with either D$_5$W injection or normal saline solution.
● Unopened drug vials are stable until date indicated on package when stored under refrigeration in original package. When reconstituted or diluted as directed, drug can be stored in glass or plastic containers at room temperature or under refrigeration for 24 hours. Refrigerated solutions should be used immediately upon return to room temperature.
● I.V. infusions may be administered at rates from 5 to 210 minutes.
● Modify dosage to take into account the myelosuppressive effect of other drugs in combination therapy or effects of previous radiation or chemotherapy.
● Patients with low serum albumin may be at increased risk for etoposide-associated toxicities.
● Because drug is rapidly converted to etoposide, signs and symptoms of overdose would be expected to be similar. Signs of etoposide overdose include myelosuppression, nausea, and vomiting. Treatment is usually supportive and includes transfusion of blood components, antiemetics, and appropriate symptomatic therapy.

Monitoring the patient
● Monitor CBC. Observe patient for signs of bone marrow depression. Withhold drug if platelet count is below 50,000/mm^3 or absolute neutrophil count is below 500/mm^3 until the blood counts have sufficiently recovered.
● If an anaphylactic reaction occurs, stop infusion immediately and administer pressor drugs, corticosteroids, antihistamines, or volume expanders as needed.

Information for the patient
● Warn woman of childbearing age to avoid becoming pregnant. If pregnancy is suspected, tell patient to promptly report it.
● Advise patient to avoid exposure to people with infections.
● Tell patient to promptly report sore throat, fever, unusual bruising, or bleeding.
● Reassure patient that hair should grow back after therapy ends.

Pediatric patients
● Safety and effectiveness in children haven't been established. Anaphylactic reactions have been reported in children who received etoposide.

Breast-feeding patients
● It's unknown if drug appears breast milk. Because of potential risk of serious adverse reactions, mutagenicity, and carcinogenicity in infant, breast-feeding isn't recommended.

exemestane
Aromasin

Pharmacologic classification: aromatase inactivator
Therapeutic classification: antineoplastic
Pregnancy risk category D

How supplied
Available by prescription only
Tablets: 25 mg

Indications, route, and dosage
Advanced breast cancer in postmenopausal women whose disease has progressed following treatment with tamoxifen
Adults: 25 mg P.O. once daily after a meal.

Pharmacodynamics
Antineoplastic action: An irreversible, steroidal aromatase inactivator that acts as a false substrate for the aromatase enzyme, the principal enzyme that converts androgens to estrogens in premenopausal and postmenopausal women. Drug is then processed to an intermediate that binds irreversibly to the enzyme's active site, causing inactivation. This effect is known as "suicide inhibition," and results in lower levels of circulating estrogens. Deprivation of estrogen is an effective and selective way to treat estrogen-dependent breast cancer in postmenopausal women.

Pharmacokinetics
• *Absorption:* Rapidly absorbed, with about 42% of dose absorbed from GI tract following oral administration. Peak actions occur in 1 to 2 hours.
• *Distribution:* Extensively distributed in tissues; is 90% bound to plasma proteins. Duration is about 24 hours.
• *Metabolism:* Extensively metabolized by liver. Isoenzyme involved is cytochrome P-450 A4 (CYP3A4).
• *Excretion:* Excreted equally in both urine and feces. Less than 1% excreted unchanged in urine. Elimination half-life is about 24 hours.

Contraindications and precautions
Contraindicated in patients with hypersensitivity to drug or its components. Ingestion may cause fetal harm if patient is pregnant.

Interactions
Drug-drug. *Drugs that induce CYP3A4:* May decrease exemestane plasma levels. Monitor patient closely.
Estrogens: May inactivate exemestane. Avoid concomitant use.

Adverse reactions
CNS: *depression, insomnia, anxiety, fatigue, pain,* dizziness, headache, paresthesia, generalized weakness, asthenia, confusion, hypoesthesia.
CV: hypertension, edema, chest pain.
EENT: sinusitis, rhinitis, pharyngitis.
GI: *nausea,* vomiting, abdominal pain, anorexia, constipation, diarrhea, increased appetite, dyspepsia.
GU: urinary tract infection.
Musculoskeletal: pathologic fractures, arthritis, arthralgia, back pain, skeletal pain.
Respiratory: *dyspnea,* bronchitis, coughing, upper respiratory tract infection.
Skin: rash, increased sweating, alopecia, itching.
Other: fever, infection, flulike syndrome, *hot flashes,* lymphedema.

☑ Special considerations
• Don't administer with estrogen-containing drugs because this could interfere with intended action.
• Drug should be used only in postmenopausal women.
• Treatment should continue until tumor progression is apparent.
• No known antidote for overdose. Treatment is supportive, with frequent monitoring of vital signs and close observation.

Monitoring the patient
• Monitor hepatic and renal function before therapy starts and periodically throughout.
• Monitor CBC periodically.

Information for the patient
• Advise patient to take drug after a meal.
• Tell patient that she may need to take drug for a long period of time.
• Advise patient to report adverse effects.

Geriatric patients
• No special adjustments are needed in elderly patients.

Pediatric patients
• Safety and effectiveness in children haven't been studied.

Breast-feeding patients
• Exemestane shouldn't be administered to premenopausal women. Because many drugs appear in breast milk, use caution if a breast-feeding woman is inadvertently exposed to drug.

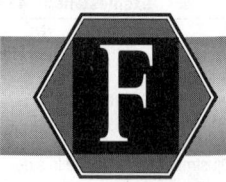

famciclovir
Famvir

Pharmacologic classification: synthetic acyclic guanine derivative
Therapeutic classification: antiviral
Pregnancy risk category B

How supplied
Available by prescription only
Tablets: 125 mg, 250 mg, 500 mg

Indications, route, and dosage
Management of acute herpes zoster
Adults: 500 mg P.O. q 8 hours for 7 days.
✦ **Dosage adjustment.** Dosage in adult patients with reduced renal function.

Creatinine clearance (ml/min)	Dosage regimen
≥ 60	500 mg q 8 hr
40 to 59	500 mg q 12 hr
20 to 39	500 mg q 24 hr
< 20	250 mg q 48 hr

Recurrent genital herpes
Adults: 125 mg P.O. b.i.d. for 5 days.
✦ **Dosage adjustment.** Dosage in adult patients with reduced renal function.

Creatinine clearance (ml/min)	Dosage regimen
≥ 40	125 mg q 12 hr
20 to 39	125 mg q 24 hr
< 20	125 mg q 48 hr

Pharmacodynamics
Antiviral action: A prodrug that undergoes rapid biotransformation to the active antiviral compound penciclovir. Enters viral cells (herpes simplex types 1 and 2, varicella zoster), where it inhibits DNA polymerase, viral DNA synthesis and, therefore, viral replication.

Pharmacokinetics
• *Absorption:* Absolute bioavailability is 77%. Bioavailability not affected by food; drug can be taken without regard to meals.
• *Distribution:* Less than 20% bound to plasma proteins.
• *Metabolism:* 98.5% metabolized in liver to active drug penciclovir and other inactive metabolites.
• *Excretion:* Penciclovir primarily eliminated in urine.

Contraindications and precautions
Contraindicated in patients with hypersensitivity to drug. Use cautiously in patients with impaired renal or hepatic function.

Interactions
Drug-drug. *Digoxin:* May increase digoxin levels; potential for toxicity. Monitor serum digoxin levels. *Probenecid, other drugs significantly eliminated by active renal tubular secretion:* Concurrent use may result in increased plasma levels of penciclovir. Monitor patient for increased adverse effects.

Adverse reactions
CNS: *headache*, fatigue, dizziness, paresthesia, somnolence.
EENT: pharyngitis, sinusitis.
GI: diarrhea, *nausea*, vomiting, constipation, anorexia, abdominal pain.
Musculoskeletal: back pain, arthralgia.
Skin: pruritus; zoster-related signs, symptoms, and complications; injury; pain.
Other: fever, rigors.

☑ Special considerations
• Drug may be given without regard to meals.
• No acute overdose reported. Treatment is symptomatic and supportive.
• Not known if hemodialysis removes famciclovir from blood. Hemodialysis enhances elimination of acyclovir, a related nucleoside analogue.

Monitoring the patient
• Monitor renal and liver function tests.
• Monitor serum digoxin levels in patients taking digoxin.

Information for the patient
• Teach patient to recognize early symptoms of herpes zoster infection, such as tingling, itching,

and pain. Explain that treatment is more effective when started within 48 hours of rash onset.
• Inform patient that drug isn't a cure for genital herpes but can decrease duration and severity of symptoms.

Pediatric patients
• Safety and effectiveness haven't been established in children under age 18.

Breast-feeding patients
• It's unknown if drug appears in breast milk. A decision should be made to either stop drug or breast-feeding, taking into account importance of drug to mother.

---

famotidine
Pepcid, Pepcid AC, Pepcid RPD

Pharmacologic classification: H$_2$-receptor antagonist
Therapeutic classification: antiulcerative
Pregnancy risk category B

How supplied
Available by prescription only
Tablets: 10 mg, 20 mg, 40 mg
Injection: 10 mg/ml
Injection, premixed: 20 mg/50 ml normal saline solution (premixed)
Suspension: 40 mg/5 ml
Available without a prescription (Pepcid AC)
Tablets (orally disintegrating): 20 mg, 40 mg

Indications, route, and dosage
Duodenal and gastric ulcer
Adults: For acute therapy, 40 mg P.O. h.s. for 4 to 8 weeks; for maintenance therapy, 20 mg P.O. h.s.
Pathologic hypersecretory conditions (such as Zollinger-Ellison syndrome)
Adults: 20 mg P.O. q 6 hours. As much as 160 mg q 6 hours may be administered.
Short-term treatment of gastroesophageal reflux disease (GERD)
Adults: 20 to 40 mg P.O. b.i.d. for up to 12 weeks.
Hospitalized patients with intractable ulcers or hypersecretory conditions or patients who can't take oral medication; ◊ patients with GI bleeding; ◊ to control gastric pH in critically ill patients
Adults: 20 mg I.V. q 12 hours.
Prevention or treatment of heartburn
Adults: 10 mg P.O. (Pepcid AC) when symptoms occur; or 10 mg P.O. 1 hour before meals for prevention of symptoms. Drug can be used b.i.d. if needed.
✦ Dosage adjustment. In patients with severe renal insufficiency (creatinine clearance below 10 ml/minute), dosage may be reduced to 20 mg h.s. or the dosing interval may be prolonged to 36 to 48 hours to avoid excess accumulation of drug.

Pharmacodynamics
Antiulcer action: Competitively inhibits histamine's action at H$_2$ receptors in gastric parietal cells. This inhibits basal and nocturnal gastric acid secretion from stimulation by such factors as caffeine, food, and pentagastrin.

Pharmacokinetics
• *Absorption:* When administered orally, about 40% to 45% of dose is absorbed; onset of action occurs in 1 hour, with peak action in 1 to 3 hours. After parenteral administration, action peaks in 30 minutes.
• *Distribution:* Distributed widely to many body tissues.
• *Metabolism:* About 30% to 35% of dose metabolized by liver.
• *Excretion:* Most drug excreted unchanged in urine; has a longer duration of effect than its 2½- to 4-hour half-life suggests.

Contraindications and precautions
Contraindicated in patients with hypersensitivity to drug.

Interactions
Drug-drug. *Drugs with enteric coatings:* May cause these drugs to dissolve too rapidly because of increased gastric pH. Monitor patient closely.
Ketoconazole: May decrease absorption. Increased ketoconazole dose may be needed.

Adverse reactions
CNS: *headache,* dizziness, vertigo, malaise, paresthesia.
CV: palpitations.
EENT: tinnitus, taste disorder, orbital edema.
GI: diarrhea, constipation, anorexia, dry mouth.
GU: increased BUN and creatinine levels.
Hepatic: elevated liver enzyme levels.
Musculoskeletal: musculoskeletal pain.
Skin: acne, dry skin, flushing, transient irritation at I.V. site.
Other: fever.

☑ Special considerations
Besides the recommendations relevant to all H$_2$-receptor antagonists, consider the following.
• Drug isn't recommended for use longer than 8 weeks in patients with uncomplicated duodenal ulcer.
• After administration via nasogastric tube, tube should be flushed to clear it and ensure drug's passage to stomach.
• For I.V. push administration, dilute with normal saline solution to total volume of 5 to 10 ml; administer over period exceeding 2 minutes. For I.V. infusion, dilute in 100 ml of D$_5$W, administer over 15 to 30 minutes. Drug is stable at room temperature for 48 hours. Don't use drug if discolored or contains precipitate.
• Antacids may be administered concurrentl⸜

• Drug appears to cause fewer adverse reactions and drug interactions than cimetidine.
• Drug may antagonize pentagastrin in gastric acid secretion tests. In skin tests using allergen extracts, drug may cause false-negative results.
• Overdose hasn't been reported. Treatment should be supportive and symptomatic and include gastric lavage or induced emesis, then activated charcoal to prevent further absorption. Hemodialysis doesn't remove drug.

Monitoring the patient
• Watch for adverse CNS effects in elderly patients.
• Monitor patient for therapeutic effect

Information for the patient
• Caution patient to take drug only as directed and to continue taking doses even after pain subsides to ensure adequate healing.
• Instruct patient to take dose at bedtime.

Geriatric patients
• Use drug cautiously in elderly patients because of increased risk of adverse reactions, particularly those affecting CNS.

Breast-feeding patients
• Drug may appear in breast milk; use with caution in breast-feeding women.

fat emulsions
Intralipid 10%, Intralipid 20%, Intralipid 30%, Liposyn II 10%, Liposyn II 20%, Liposyn III 10% and 20%

Pharmacologic classification: lipid
Therapeutic classification: total parenteral nutrition (TPN)
Pregnancy risk category C

How supplied
Available by prescription only
Injection: 50 ml (10%, 20%), 100 ml (10%, 20%, 30%), 200 ml (10%, 20%), 250 ml (10%, 20%), 500 ml (10%, 20%)

Indications, route, and dosage
Source of calories adjunctive to TPN
Intralipid
Adults: 1 ml/minute I.V. for 15 to 30 minutes (10% emulsion); or 0.5 ml/minute I.V. for 15 to 30 minutes (20% emulsion). If no adverse reactions occur, increase rate to deliver 500 ml over 4 to 8 hours. Total daily dose shouldn't exceed 2.5 g/kg (10% emulsion) and 3 g/kg (20% emulsion).
Children: 0.1 ml/minute for 10 to 15 minutes (10% emulsion); or 0.05 ml/minute I.V. for 10 to 15 minutes (20% emulsion). If no adverse reactions occur, increase rate to deliver 1 g/kg over 4 hours. Daily dose shouldn't exceed 4 g/kg, which equals

60% of daily caloric intake. Protein-carbohydrate TPN should supply remaining 40%.
Fatty acid deficiency
Intralipid
Adults and children: 8% to 10% of total caloric intake I.V.

Pharmacodynamics
Metabolic action: I.V. fat emulsions are prepared from soybean or safflower oil and provide a mixture of neutral triglycerides, predominantly fatty acids. Besides fatty acids (linoleic, oleic, palmitic, stearic, and linolenic), these preparations also contain 1.2% egg yolk phospholipids (an emulsifier) and glycerol (to adjust tonicity). I.V. fat emulsions are isotonic and may be given centrally or peripherally.
   Linoleic, linolenic, and arachidonic acids are essential in humans. Signs of essential fatty acid deficiency (EFAD) include scaly dermatitis, alopecia, growth retardation, poor wound healing, thrombocytopenia, and fatty liver. I.V. fat emulsions prevent or reverse the biochemical and clinical signs of EFAD and provide 1.1 kcal/ml (10%) or 2 kcal/ml (20%).

Pharmacokinetics
• *Absorption:* Administered as I.V. infusion through either peripheral or central vein.
• *Distribution:* Distributed through plasma compartment.
• *Metabolism:* Metabolized and used as energy source, causing increased heat production, decreased respiratory quotient, and increased oxygen consumption.
• *Excretion:* Infused fat particles cleared from bloodstream in manner similar to chylomicrons.

Contraindications and precautions
Contraindicated in patients with hyperlipidemia, lipid nephrosis, acute pancreatitis accompanied by hyperlipidemia, or severe egg allergies. Use cautiously in patients with severe hepatic disease, pulmonary disease, anemia, or blood coagulation disorders (especially thrombocytopenia) and in those at risk for fat embolism.

Interactions
None reported.

Adverse reactions
Early reactions to fat overload:
CNS: headache, sleepiness, dizziness.
EENT: pressure over eyes.
GI: nausea, vomiting.
Hematologic: *hypercoagulability.*
Hepatic: transient abnormalities in liver function tests, altered results of serum bilirubin tests (especially in infants).
Metabolic: hyperlipidemia.
Musculoskeletal: chest and back pain.
Respiratory: dyspnea, cyanosis.

eactions may be *common*, uncommon, **life-threatening**, or COMMON AND LIFE-THREATENING.

Skin: flushing, diaphoresis, irritation (at infusion site).
Other: fever, splenomegaly, *hypersensitivity reactions.*
Delayed reactions to fat overload:
CNS: *focal seizures.*
Hematologic: *thrombocytopenia, leukopenia,* leukocytosis.
Hepatic: transient increases in liver function test values, altered results of serum bilirubin tests (especially in infants), hepatomegaly.

☑ **Special considerations**
● Some brands of fat emulsion can be mixed with amino acid solution and dextrose in the same I.V. container. The order of mixing is important; see package insert for further information.
● Don't use an in-line filter when administering drug; fat particles (0.5 mcg) are larger than 0.22-mcg cellulose filter.
● Fat emulsions may extract small amounts of plasticizers from I.V. administration sets made of polyvinyl chloride. Nonphthalate administration sets are available; however, phthalate extraction can be minimized from regular I.V. tubing by not storing primed administration sets.
● Discard fat emulsion if it separates or becomes oily.
● Change all I.V. tubing at each infusion because lipids support bacterial growth.
● Avoid rapid infusion by using infusion pump to regulate rate.
● Abnormally high mean corpuscular hemoglobin and mean corpuscular hemoglobin concentration values may be found in blood samples drawn during or shortly after fat emulsion infusion.
● Signs and symptoms of overdose or "overloading syndrome" include focal seizures, splenomegaly, leukocytosis, fever, and shock. Stop infusion until visual inspection of plasma, determination of triglyceride levels, or nephelometric measurement of plasma light-scattering activity confirms lipid clearance. Reevaluate patient and institute appropriate corrective measures.

Monitoring the patient
● Monitor lipid levels before and during treatment.
● Monitor hepatic function with long-term use.
● Check injection site daily for signs of inflammation or infection.
● Watch closely for adverse effects, especially during the first half hour of infusion.
● Monitor patient for allergic reactions.
● *Neonates:* Monitor platelet count frequently; these patients tend to develop thrombocytopenia.
● *Jaundiced infants:* Monitor bilirubin levels.
● *Premature infants:* Monitor bilirubin level and triglycerides or serum free fatty acid levels daily; free fatty acids displace bilirubin bound to albumin.

Pediatric patients
● Because premature and small-for-gestational-age infants have poor clearance of I.V. fat emulsions, lower doses are needed to reduce likelihood of fat overload.
● Cautiously administer fat emulsions to jaundiced or premature infants. Deaths in preterm infants have been reported from intravascular fat accumulation in lungs.

felodipine
Plendil

Pharmacologic classification: calcium channel blocker
Therapeutic classification: antihypertensive
Pregnancy risk category C

How supplied
Available by prescription only
Tablets (extended-release): 2.5 mg, 5 mg, 10 mg

Indications, route, and dosage
Hypertension
Adults: 5 mg P.O. daily. Adjust dosage based on patient response, generally at intervals not less than 2 weeks. Usual dose is 2.5 to 10 mg daily; doses exceeding 10 mg daily increase rate of peripheral edema and vasodilatory adverse effects.
✦ *Dosage adjustment.* Elderly patients or patients with impaired hepatic function should receive a starting dose of 2.5 mg daily. Doses above 10 mg shouldn't be considered.

Pharmacodynamics
Antihypertensive action: A dihydropyridine-derivative calcium channel blocker that blocks entry of calcium ions into vascular smooth muscle and cardiac cells. This type of calcium channel blocker shows some selectivity for smooth muscle as compared with cardiac muscle. Effects on vascular smooth muscle are relaxation and vasodilation.

Pharmacokinetics
● *Absorption:* Almost completely absorbed, but extensive first-pass metabolism reduces absolute bioavailability to about 20%. Plasma levels peak within 2½ to 5 hours after dose.
● *Distribution:* Over 99% bound to plasma proteins.
● *Metabolism:* Probably hepatic; at least six inactive metabolites identified.
● *Excretion:* Over 70% of dose appears in urine; 10% appears in feces as metabolites.

Contraindications and precautions
Contraindicated in patients with hypersensitivity to drug. Use cautiously in patients with impaired

hepatic function or heart failure, especially those receiving beta blockers.

Interactions

Drug-drug. *Anticonvulsants:* May decrease plasma level of felodipine. Monitor felodipine levels.
Cimetidine: Decreased clearance of felodipine. Use lower doses of felodipine.
Digoxin: Decreased peak serum levels of digoxin but total absorbed drug is unchanged. Monitor digoxin levels.
Metoprolol: Concomitant use may alter pharmacokinetics of metoprolol. No dosage adjustment is necessary, but monitor patient for adverse effects.
Theophylline: May slightly decrease theophylline levels. Monitor theophylline levels.
Drug-food. *Grapefruit juice:* May increase drug's bioavailability and effect when taken together. Discourage use together.

Adverse reactions

CNS: *headache,* dizziness, paresthesia, asthenia.
CV: *flushing, peripheral edema,* chest pain, palpitations.
EENT: rhinorrhea, pharyngitis, gingival hyperplasia.
GI: abdominal pain, nausea, constipation, diarrhea.
Musculoskeletal: muscle cramps, back pain.
Respiratory: upper respiratory tract infection, cough.
Skin: rash.

☑ Special considerations

Besides the recommendations relevant to all calcium channel blockers, consider the following.
• Peripheral edema appears to be both dose- and age-dependent. It's more common in patients taking higher doses, especially those age 60 and over.
• Drug may be taken without regard to meals. However, there may be a more than twofold increase of bioavailability when drug is taken with doubly concentrated grapefruit juice compared with water or orange juice.
• Expected symptoms of overdose include peripheral vasodilation, bradycardia, and hypotension. Provide supportive care. I.V. fluids or sympathomimetics may be useful in treating hypotension, and atropine (0.5 to 1 mg I.V.) may treat bradycardia. It's unknown if drug is removed by dialysis.

Monitoring the patient
• Monitor hepatic and renal function before starting treatment.
• Monitor patient for edema.

Information for the patient
• Tell patient to practice good oral hygiene and to see a dentist regularly because drug has been associated with mild gingival hyperplasia.

• Remind patient to swallow tablet whole and not to crush or chew tablet.
• Inform patient that he should continue taking drug, even when feeling better. He should watch his diet and call before taking other drugs, including OTC products.

Geriatric patients
• Higher blood levels of drug are seen in elderly patients. Mean clearance of drug from elderly hypertensive patients (average age 74) was less than half of that observed in young patients (average age 26). Check blood pressure closely during dosage adjustment. Maximum daily dose is 10 mg.

Pediatric patients
• Safety and efficacy in children haven't been established.

Breast-feeding patients
• It's unknown if drug appears in breast milk. Because of risk of serious adverse effects to infant, breast-feeding isn't recommended.

fenofibrate (micronized)
Tricor

Pharmacologic classification: fibric acid derivative
Therapeutic classification: antihyperlipidemic
Pregnancy risk category C

How supplied
Available by prescription only
Capsules: 67 mg

Indications, route, and dosage
Adjunct to diet for treatment of patients with very high serum triglyceride levels (type IV and V hyperlipidemia) who are at high risk of pancreatitis and who don't respond adequately to diet alone
Adults: Initiate therapy with one (67-mg) capsule P.O. once daily. Based on response, increase dose, if necessary, following repeat triglyceride levels at 4- to 8-week intervals to maximum dose of three capsules daily (201 mg).
✦ *Dosage adjustment.* Minimize dose in renally impaired patients. Initiate therapy at dose of 67 mg/day and increase only after effects on renal function and triglyceride levels have been evaluated at this dose.

Pharmacodynamics
Antihyperlipidemic action: Exact mechanism unknown. Thought to lower triglyceride levels by inhibiting triglyceride synthesis, resulting in a decrease in the amount of very-low-density lipoprotein released into the circulation. Fenofibrate

may stimulate the breakdown of triglyceride-rich protein.

Pharmacokinetics
• *Absorption:* Well absorbed; plasma levels peak within 6 to 8 hours. Food increases absorption by 35%.
• *Distribution:* Steady-state plasma levels achieved within 5 days after drug start. Almost entirely bound to plasma protein.
• *Metabolism:* Rapidly hydrolyzed by esterases to fenofibric acid, an active metabolite. Fenofibric acid is primarily conjugated with glucuronic acid and excreted in urine.
• *Excretion:* Primarily excreted in urine; 25% excreted in feces; elimination half-life is 20 hours.

Contraindications and precautions
Contraindicated in patients with hypersensitivity to drug and in those with preexisting gallbladder disease, hepatic dysfunction (including primary biliary cirrhosis), severe renal dysfunction, or unexplained persistent liver function abnormalities.

Interactions
Drug-drug. *Bile acid resins:* May bind and inhibit absorption of fenofibrate. Fenofibrate should be taken 1 hour before or 4 to 6 hours after taking these products.
Coumarin-type anticoagulants: Concomitant administration requires extreme caution due to protein-binding displacement of anticoagulant and potentiation of its effects. Reduce anticoagulant dose to maintain PT and INR within desired range.
Cyclosporine: May cause renal dysfunction that may compromise elimination of fenofibrate. Use together cautiously.
Gemfibrozil, HMG-CoA inhibitors (statins): Although no data are available on use with fenofibrate, risk of myopathy, rhabdomyolysis, and acute renal failure reported when statins are used with gemfibrozil (another fibrate derivative). Avoid concomitant use.

Adverse reactions
CNS: dizziness, miscellaneous pain, asthenia, fatigue, paresthesia, insomnia, headache.
CV: *arrhythmias.*
EENT: eye irritation, eye floaters, earache, conjunctivitis, blurred vision, rhinitis, sinusitis.
GI: dyspepsia, eructation, flatulence, increased appetite, nausea, vomiting, abdominal pain, constipation, diarrhea.
GU: polyuria, vaginitis, increased creatinine and BUN levels.
Hematologic: decreased hemoglobin.
Hepatic: elevated liver enzyme levels.
Metabolic: decreased uric acid levels, decreased libido.
Musculoskeletal: arthralgia.

Respiratory: cough.
Skin: urticaria, pruritus, rash.
Other: *infections,* flu syndrome.

☑ Special considerations
• Stop therapy in patients who don't achieve an adequate response after 2 months of treatment with maximum daily dose.
• Fenofibrate lowers serum uric acid levels in normal patients as well as hyperuricemic patients by increasing uric acid excretion.
• Drug shouldn't be used for primary or secondary prevention of coronary artery disease.
• If possible, change or stop use of beta blockers, estrogens, and thiazide diuretics because they may increase plasma triglyceride levels.
• Drug may cause excretion of cholesterol into bile leading to cholelithiasis. If suspected, perform appropriate tests and stop drug.
• Mild to moderate decreases in hemoglobin level, hematocrit, and WBC count may occur at drug start, but should stabilize on long-term administration.
• Pancreatitis may occur in patients receiving fenofibrate; myositis and rhabdomyolysis may occur in those with renal failure. Assess CK levels in patients with myalgia, muscle tenderness, or weakness.
• No cases of overdose have been reported. If overdose does occur, use supportive measures.
• Because drug is highly protein-bound, hemodialysis is unlikely to be of value.

Monitoring the patient
• Evaluate for presence of gallbladder disease before treatment and periodically throughout treatment.
• Monitor hepatic and renal function before and during treatment.
• Monitor serum coagulation studies for patients on oral anticoagulants.
• Monitor serum CK levels in patients who develop myalgia, muscle tenderness, or weakness.

Information for the patient
• Advise patient to promptly report symptoms of unexplained muscle weakness, pain, or tenderness, especially if accompanied by malaise or fever.
• Instruct patient to follow triglyceride-lowering diet during treatment.
• Inform patient to take drug with meals to optimize drug absorption.
• Advise patient to continue weight-control measures, including diet and exercise, and to reduce alcohol intake before starting drug therapy.

Geriatric patients
• Drug acts similarly in elderly patients (ages 77 to 87) as in younger adults; similar dosing regimens can be used.

Pediatric patients
• Drug isn't indicated for use in children. Safety and efficacy haven't been established.

Breast-feeding patients
• Because it's unknown if drug appears in breast milk, don't give to breast-feeding patients; either stop drug or discontinue breast-feeding.

fenoldopam mesylate
Corlopam

Pharmacologic classification: dopamine D_1-like receptor agonist
Therapeutic classification: antihypertensive
Pregnancy risk category B

How supplied
Available by prescription only
Ampules: 10 mg/ml in single-dose 1-ml, 2-ml, 5-ml ampules

Indications, route, and dosage
Short-term (up to 48 hours) in-hospital management of severe hypertension when rapid but quickly reversible reduction of blood pressure is indicated, including malignant hypertension with deteriorating end-organ function
Adults: Administer by continuous I.V. infusion. Infusion rate is initiated at 0.1 to 0.3 mcg/kg/minute and titrated upward or downward at a frequency not exceeding q 15 minutes to achieve desired blood pressure. Recommended increments for titration are 0.05 to 0.1 mcg/kg/minute. Doses less than 0.1 mcg/kg/min have very modest effects and appear to be only marginally useful.

Pharmacodynamics
Antihypertensive action: Rapid-acting vasodilator. An agonist for D_1-like dopamine receptors; binds with moderate affinity to alpha$_2$-adrenoreceptors. No significant affinity for D_2-like receptors, alpha$_1$ or beta adrenoreceptors, 5HT, 5HT$_2$, or muscarinic receptors has been noted. Drug has no effect on ACE activity, although it may increase norepinephrine plasma levels.

Pharmacokinetics
• *Absorption:* Given by I.V. infusion only.
• *Distribution:* Steady-state plasma levels of 3.2 to 4 ng/ml reported with infusion rates of 0.1 mcg/kg/minute.
• *Metabolism:* Principal routes of conjugation are methylation, glucuronidation, and sulfation.
• *Excretion:* Eliminated largely by conjugation, without participation of cytochrome P-450 enzymes. Elimination half-life about 5 minutes. Following I.V. administration, 90% of drug excreted in urine, 10% in feces. Only 4% of drug excreted unchanged.

Contraindications and precautions
No known contraindications. Use cautiously because drug is a rapid-acting, potent vasodilator that may precipitate severe hypotension.

Use cautiously in patients with glaucoma or ocular hypertension because dose-dependent increases in intraocular pressure may occur. Drug may cause symptomatic hypotension; use particular caution when administering to patients who have sustained an acute cerebral infarction or hemorrhage.

Fenoldopam contains sodium metabisulfite, which may cause allergic-type reactions (including anaphylactic symptoms and severe asthmatic episodes in certain susceptible individuals). Sulfite sensitivity is more frequent in asthmatic than in nonasthmatic people.

Interactions
Drug-drug. *Beta blockers:* Unexpected hypotension may result from beta-blocker inhibition of reflex response to fenoldopam. Avoid concurrent use.

Adverse reactions
CNS: dizziness, headache, insomnia.
CV: hypotension, orthostatic hypotension, palpitations, **bradycardia,** tachycardia, angina, *MI,* **heart failure,** T-wave inversion, flushing, nonspecific chest pain.
EENT: nasal congestion.
GI: nausea, vomiting, abdominal pain, constipation, diarrhea.
GU: oliguria, urinary tract infection, increased BUN and creatinine levels.
Hematologic: leukocytosis, bleeding.
Metabolic: increased serum glucose, LD, and transaminase levels; hypokalemia.
Musculoskeletal: limb cramp, back pain.
Respiratory: dyspnea.
Skin: injection site reaction.
Other: pyrexia.

☑ Special considerations
• Use during pregnancy only if clearly needed.
• Drug causes a dose-related tachycardia, which diminishes over time but remains substantial at higher doses.
• Follow manufacturer's instructions for diluting drug before I.V. use. Diluted solution is stable at room temperature for at least 24 hours.
• Infuse drug with a calibrated mechanical infusion pump.
• Don't use a bolus dose.
• Drug may be abruptly stopped or infusion gradually tapered. Oral antihypertensives can be added once blood pressure is stable during infusion or after infusion is stopped.

- Intentional overdose hasn't been reported. Excessive hypotension expected; stop drug and use supportive measures.

Monitoring the patient
- Monitor blood pressure frequently during infusions. Check blood pressure and heart rate every 15 minutes until patient is stable.
- Monitor serum electrolytes and watch for hypokalemia.

Information for the patient
- Tell patient that drug causes dose-related decreases in blood pressure and increases in heart rate. Advise patient to change positions slowly to avoid orthostatic symptoms.
- Inform patient that drug must be given by controlled infusion, which should last no more than 48 hours.
- Encourage patient to report adverse reactions promptly.

Pediatric patients
- Safety and effectiveness in children haven't been established.

Breast-feeding patients
- Drug may appear in breast milk; use caution in administering to breast-feeding women.

fenoprofen calcium
Nalfon

Pharmacologic classification: NSAID
Therapeutic classification: nonnarcotic analgesic, antipyretic, anti-inflammatory
Pregnancy risk category NR

How supplied
Available by prescription only
Tablets: 600 mg
Capsules: 200 mg, 300 mg

Indications, route, and dosage
Rheumatoid arthritis and osteoarthritis
Adults: 300 to 600 mg P.O. t.i.d. or q.i.d. Maximum dose is 3.2 g daily.
Mild to moderate pain
Adults: 200 mg P.O. q 4 to 6 hours, p.r.n.
◇ **Fever**
Adults: Single oral doses up to 400 mg.
◇ **Acute gouty arthritis**
Adults: 200 mg P.O. q 6 hours; decrease dose based on patient response.

Pharmacodynamics
Analgesic, anti-inflammatory, and antipyretic actions: Mechanisms unknown. Thought to inhibit prostaglandin synthesis. Decreases platelet aggregation and may prolong bleeding time.

Pharmacokinetics
- Absorption: Absorbed rapidly and completely from GI tract. Onset of analgesic activity occurs within 15 to 30 minutes, with plasma levels peaking in 2 hours. Duration of action about 4 to 6 hours.
- Distribution: About 99% protein-bound.
- Metabolism: Metabolized in liver.
- Excretion: Excreted chiefly in urine with a serum half-life of 2½ to 3 hours. Small amount excreted in feces.

Contraindications and precautions
Contraindicated in patients with hypersensitivity to drug and in those with significantly impaired renal function or history of aspirin- or NSAID-induced asthma, rhinitis, or urticaria. Also contraindicated during pregnancy.
    Use cautiously in elderly patients and in those with history of GI events, peptic ulcer disease, compromised cardiac function, or hypertension.

Interactions
Drug-drug. Acetaminophen, gold compounds, other anti-inflammatory drugs: Increased nephrotoxicity may occur. Monitor renal function.
Anticoagulants, thrombolytics (coumarin derivatives, heparin, streptokinase, urokinase): May potentiate anticoagulant effects. Monitor PT, PTT, INR as necessary.
Antihypertensives, diuretics: May decrease effectiveness of these drugs. Monitor patient for drug effect.
Anti-inflammatories, corticosteroids, corticotropin, salicylates: May cause increased GI adverse reactions, including ulceration and hemorrhage. Monitor patient closely.
Aspirin: May decrease bioavailability of fenoprofen. Use together cautiously.
Coumarin derivatives, nifedipine, phenytoin, verapamil: Toxicity may occur. Monitor drug levels and patient closely.
Diuretics: May increase nephrotoxic potential. Monitor renal function.
Drugs that inhibit platelet aggregation (such as aspirin, cefamandole, cefoperazone, dextran, dipyridamole, mezlocillin, piperacillin, plicamycin, salicylates, sulfinpyrazone, ticarcillin, valproic acid, other anti-inflammatories): Bleeding problems may occur with concomitant use. Monitor patient closely.
Highly protein-bound drugs: May displace these drugs from binding sites. Monitor patient.
Insulin, oral antidiabetics: Because of prostaglandins' influence on glucose metabolism, concomitant use may potentiate hypoglycemic effects. Monitor serum glucose levels.
Lithium, methotrexate: May decrease renal clearance of these drugs. Monitor renal function.
Drug-lifestyle. Alcohol: May increase risk of adverse GI reactions. Discourage concomitant use.

Adverse reactions
CNS: *headache,* dizziness, *somnolence,* fatigue, nervousness, asthenia, tremor, confusion.
CV: peripheral edema, palpitations.
EENT: tinnitus, blurred vision, decreased hearing.
GI: *epigastric distress, nausea,* **GI bleeding,** vomiting, occult blood loss, peptic ulceration, constipation, anorexia, *dyspepsia,* flatulence.
GU: oliguria, interstitial nephritis, proteinuria, reversible **renal failure,** papillary necrosis, cystitis, hematuria, increased BUN and creatinine.
Hematologic: prolonged bleeding time, anemia, **aplastic anemia, agranulocytosis, thrombocytopenia, hemorrhage,** bruising, hemolytic anemia.
Hepatic: elevated enzymes, **hepatitis.**
Metabolic: hyperkalemia.
Respiratory: dyspnea, upper respiratory tract infections, nasopharyngitis.
Skin: *pruritus,* rash, urticaria, increased diaphoresis.
Other: angioedema, **anaphylaxis.**

☑ Special considerations
Besides the recommendations relevant to all NSAIDs, consider the following.
• Fenoprofen has been used to treat fever, acute gouty arthritis, and juvenile arthritis.
• Drug may cause false elevations in both free and total serum T_3, but thyroid-stimulating hormone and T_4 are unaffected.
• Elevations in serum creatinine and BUN levels have been reported.
• Little is known about acute toxicity of fenoprofen. Nonoliguric renal failure, tachycardia, and hypotension have been observed. Other symptoms include drowsiness, dizziness, confusion, lethargy, nausea, vomiting, headache, tinnitus, and blurred vision. Empty stomach immediately by inducing emesis with ipecac syrup or by gastric lavage. Administer activated charcoal via nasogastric tube.
• In overdose, provide symptomatic and supportive measures (respiratory support and correction of fluid and electrolyte imbalances). Monitor laboratory parameters and vital signs closely. Dialysis is of little value.

Monitoring the patient
• If patient is of childbearing age, test for pregnancy.
• Watch for potential CNS effects. Institute safety measures to prevent injury.
• Monitor renal, hepatic, and auditory function in patients on long-term therapy. Stop drug if abnormalities occur.

Information for the patient
• Tell patient to avoid activities that require alertness or concentration until CNS effects of drug are known.

• Instruct patient in safety measures to prevent injury.
• Advise patient to call for specific instruction before taking OTC analgesics.

Geriatric patients
• Patients over age 60 may be more susceptible to toxic effects of fenoprofen, especially adverse GI reactions. Use with caution.
• Effects of drug on renal prostaglandins may cause fluid retention and edema, a significant drawback for elderly patients and those with heart failure.

Pediatric patients
• Safe use in children hasn't been established. Drug isn't recommended for children under age 14.

Breast-feeding patients
• Drug appears in breast milk; avoid use in breast-feeding women.

fentanyl citrate
Sublimaze

fentanyl transdermal system
Duragesic-25, Duragesic-50, Duragesic-75, Duragesic-100

fentanyl transmucosal
Actiq, Fentanyl Oralet

Pharmacologic classification: opioid agonist
Therapeutic classification: analgesic, adjunct to anesthesia, anesthetic
Controlled substance schedule II
Pregnancy risk category C

How supplied
Available by prescription only
Injection: 50 mcg/ml
Transdermal system: patches designed to release 25 mcg, 50 mcg, 75 mcg, or 100 mcg of fentanyl/hour.
Transmucosal: 100 mcg, 200 mcg, 300 mcg, 400 mcg, 600 mcg, 800 mcg, 1,200 mcg, 1,600 mcg

Indications, route, and dosage
Preoperatively
Adults: 50 to 100 mcg I.M. 30 to 60 minutes before surgery. Or one Oralet unit consisting of 100 mcg, 200 mcg, 300 mcg, or 400 mcg P.O. for patient to suck until dissolved, 20 to 40 minutes before surgery.
Adjunct to general anesthetic
Low-dose regimen for minor procedures
Adults: 2 mcg/kg I.V.

Reactions may be common, uncommon, *life-threatening*, or COMMON AND LIFE-THREATENING.

Moderate-dose regimen for major procedures
Adults: Initial dose is 2 to 20 mcg/kg I.V.; may give additional doses of 25 to 100 mcg I.V. or I.M., p.r.n.
High-dose regimen for complicated procedures
Adults: Initial dose is 20 to 50 mcg/kg; additional doses of 25 mcg to one-half the initial dose may be administered, p.r.n.
Adjunct to regional anesthesia
Adults: 50 to 100 mcg I.M. or slow I.V. over 1 to 2 minutes.
Induction and maintenance of anesthesia
Children ages 2 to 12: Reduced dose as low as 2 to 3 mcg/kg.
Postoperative analgesic
Adults: 50 to 100 mcg I.M. q 1 to 2 hours, p.r.n.
Management of chronic pain in patients who can't be managed by lesser means
Adults: Apply one transdermal system to a portion of the upper torso on an area of skin that isn't irritated and hasn't been irradiated. Initiate therapy with the 25-mcg/hour system; adjust dosage as needed and tolerated. Each system may be worn for 72 hours.
✦ *Dosage adjustment.* Lower doses are usually indicated for elderly patients who may be more sensitive to therapeutic and adverse effects of drug.

Pharmacodynamics
Analgesic action: Binds to the opiate receptors as an agonist to alter the patient's perception of painful stimuli, thus providing analgesia for moderate to severe pain. Its CNS and respiratory depressant effects are similar to those of morphine. Has little hypnotic activity and rarely causes histamine release.

Pharmacokinetics
• *Absorption:* Immediate onset of action after I.V. route; within 7 to 8 minutes of I.M. injection; within 5 to 15 minutes of transmucosal use; onset after transdermal use may take several hours as it's absorbed through skin. Effect after I.V. use peaks in 3 to 5 minutes; after I.M. or transmucosal use, 20 to 30 minutes; after transdermal use, 1 to 3 days.
• *Distribution:* Redistribution suggested as main cause of brief analgesic effect.
• *Metabolism:* Metabolized in liver.
• *Excretion:* Excreted in urine as metabolites and unchanged drug. Elimination half-life is about 7 hours after parenteral use, 5 to 15 hours after transmucosal use, and 18 hours after transdermal use.

Contraindications and precautions
Contraindicated in patients with known intolerance of drug. Use cautiously in elderly or debilitated patients and in those with head injuries, increased CSF pressure, COPD, decreased respiratory reserve, compromised respirations, arrhythmias, or hepatic, renal, or cardiac disease.

Interactions
Drug-drug. *Anticholinergics, drugs extensively metabolized in liver (digitoxin, phenytoin, rifampin):* Paralytic ileus may result from drug accumulation. Use together cautiously.
Cimetidine: May increase respiratory and CNS depression, causing confusion, disorientation, apnea, or seizures. Reduce fentanyl dosage by one-quarter to one-third.
CNS depressants (antihistamines, barbiturates, benzodiazepines, general anesthetics, muscle relaxants, narcotic analgesics, phenothiazines, sedative-hypnotics, tricyclic antidepressants): May potentiate drug's respiratory and CNS depression, sedation, and hypotensive effects. Avoid concomitant use.
Diazepam: May produce CV depression when given with high doses of fentanyl. Monitor patient closely.
Droperidol: May cause hypotension and decrease in pulmonary artery pressure. (A droperidol-fentanyl combination, Innovar, is available.) Use very cautiously together.
General anesthetics: May result in severe CV depression. Monitor patient closely.
MAO inhibitors: Concomitant use may cause additive CNS depressant effects, including hypoventilation, hypotension, profound sedation or coma. Avoid using within a 2-week period of MAO administration.
Narcotic antagonists: Acute withdrawal may occur in patients who become physically dependent on drug. Withdraw cautiously.
Some peridural anesthetics, spinal anesthesia: May alter respiration by blocking intercostal nerves. Monitor patient.
Drug-lifestyle. *Alcohol:* May cause additive effects. Discourage concomitant use.

Adverse reactions
CNS: *sedation, somnolence, clouded sensorium, euphoria,* dizziness, headache, *confusion, asthenia,* nervousness, hallucinations, anxiety, depression, physical dependence.
CV: *hypotension,* hypertension, **arrhythmias,** chest pain.
GI: *nausea, vomiting, constipation,* ileus, abdominal pain, *dry mouth,* anorexia, diarrhea, dyspepsia, increased plasma amylase and lipase levels.
GU: *urine retention.*
Respiratory: *respiratory depression,* hypoventilation, dyspnea, *apnea.*
Skin: reaction at application site (erythema, papules, edema), *pruritus, diaphoresis.*

☑ Special considerations
Besides the recommendations relevant to all opioid (narcotic) agonists, consider the following.

- High doses can produce muscle rigidity. This effect can be reversed by naloxone.
- Many anesthesiologists use epidural and intrathecal fentanyl as a potent adjunct to epidural anesthesia.

Transdermal form

- Transdermal fentanyl isn't recommended for postoperative pain.
- Dosage equivalent charts are available to calculate fentanyl transdermal dose based on daily morphine intake—for example, for every 90 mg of oral morphine or 15 mg of I.M. morphine per 24 hours, 25 mcg/hour of transdermal fentanyl is needed. Some patients will need other means of opiate administration when dose exceeds 300 mcg/hour.
- Dosage adjustments in patients using transdermal system should be made gradually. Reaching steady-state levels of a new dose may take up to 6 days; delay dosage adjustment until after at least two applications.
- Most patients experience good control of pain for 3 days while wearing transdermal system, although a few may need new application after 48 hours. Because serum fentanyl level rises for the first 24 hours after application, analgesic effect can't be evaluated for the first day. Be sure patient has adequate supplemental analgesic to prevent breakthrough pain.
- When reducing opiate therapy or switching to another analgesic, withdraw transdermal system gradually. Because fentanyl's serum level drops very gradually after removal, give half of the equianalgesic dose of new analgesic 12 to 18 hours after removal.
- Common signs and symptoms of fentanyl overdose are extensions of drug's actions. They include CNS depression, respiratory depression, and miosis (pinpoint pupils). Other acute toxic effects include hypotension, bradycardia, hypothermia, shock, apnea, cardiopulmonary arrest, circulatory collapse, pulmonary edema, and seizures.
- For overdose, first establish adequate respiratory exchange via a patent airway and ventilation as needed; administer a narcotic antagonist (naloxone) to reverse respiratory depression. Repeated dosing may be necessary. Naloxone shouldn't be given unless patient has clinically significant respiratory or CV depression. Provide symptomatic and supportive treatment (continued respiratory support, correction of fluid or electrolyte imbalance). Monitor laboratory values, vital signs, and neurologic status closely.

Monitoring the patient

- Monitor respiratory rate, respiratory effort, and heart rate before, during, and immediately after treatment.
- Monitor patient for delayed onset of respiratory depression. The high lipid solubility of fentanyl may contribute to this potential adverse effect.

- Monitor patient's heart rate. Fentanyl may cause bradycardia. Pretreatment with an anticholinergic (such as atropine or glycopyrrolate) may minimize this effect.
- Monitor patients who develop adverse reactions to transdermal system for at least 12 hours after removal. Serum levels of fentanyl drop very gradually and may take as long as 17 hours to decline by 50%.

Information for the patient

- Teach patient proper application of transdermal patch. Clip hair at application site; don't use razor, which may irritate skin. Wash area with clear water if necessary, but not with soaps, oils, lotions, alcohol, or other substances that may irritate skin or prevent adhesion. Dry area completely before applying patch.
- Tell patient to remove transdermal system from package just before applying. Hold in place for 10 to 20 seconds, and be sure edges of patch adhere to patient's skin.
- Teach patient to dispose of transdermal patch by folding so adhesive side adheres to itself and then flushing it down toilet.
- If another patch is needed after 72 hours, tell patient to apply to new site.

Geriatric patients

- Use with caution in elderly patients.

Pediatric patients

- Safe use in children under age 2 hasn't been established for parenteral use. Safe use in children of all ages for transdermal system hasn't been established.

Breast-feeding patients

- Drug appears in breast milk; use cautiously in breast-feeding women.

ferrous fumarate
Femiron, Feostat, Fumasorb, Fumerin, Hemocyte, Ircon, Ircon-FA, Neo-Fer*, Nephro-Fer, Novofumar*, Palafer*, Span-FF

Pharmacologic classification: oral iron supplement
Therapeutic classification: hematinic
Pregnancy risk category A

How supplied
Available without a prescription. Ferrous fumarate is 33% elemental iron.
Tablets: 63 mg, 195 mg, 200 mg, 324 mg, 325 mg, 350 mg
Tablets (chewable): 100 mg
Capsules (extended-release): 325 mg
Suspension: 100 mg/5 ml
Drops: 45 mg/0.6 ml

Reactions may be *common*, uncommon, **life-threatening**, or COMMON AND LIFE-THREATENING.

Indications, route, and dosage
Iron-deficiency states
Adults: 50 to 100 mg P.O. of elemental iron, t.i.d. Adjust dose gradually, as needed and tolerated.
Children: 4 to 6 mg/kg P.O. daily divided into three doses.
✦ *Dosage adjustment.* Elderly patients may need higher doses because reduced gastric secretions and achlorhydria may lower capacity for iron absorption.

Pharmacodynamics
Hematinic action: Replaces iron, an essential component in the formation of hemoglobin.

Pharmacokinetics
• *Absorption:* Absorbed from entire length of GI tract, but primary absorption sites are duodenum and proximal jejunum. Up to 10% of iron is absorbed by healthy individuals; patients with iron-deficiency anemia may absorb up to 60%. Enteric coating and some extended-release formulas have decreased absorption because they are designed to release iron past points of highest absorption; food may decrease absorption by 33% to 50%.
• *Distribution:* Transported through GI mucosal cells directly into blood; there it's immediately bound to a carrier protein, transferrin, and transported to bone marrow for incorporation into hemoglobin. Iron is highly protein-bound.
• *Metabolism:* Liberated by destruction of hemoglobin, but is conserved and reused by body.
• *Excretion:* Healthy individuals lose only small amounts of iron daily. Men and postmenopausal women lose about 1 mg/day; premenopausal women about 1.5 mg/day. Loss usually occurs in nails, hair, feces, and urine; trace amounts lost in bile and sweat.

Contraindications and precautions
Contraindicated in patients with primary hemochromatosis or hemosiderosis, hemolytic anemia unless iron-deficiency anemia is also present, peptic ulcer disease, regional enteritis, or ulcerative colitis and in those receiving repeated blood transfusions. Use cautiously on long-term basis.

Interactions
Drug-drug. *Antacids, cholestyramine, cimetidine, vitamin E:* May decrease ferrous fumarate absorption. Separate doses by 1 to 2 hours.
Chloramphenicol: Delayed response to iron therapy. Monitor patient for desired effects.
Doxycycline: May interfere with ferrous fumarate absorption even when doses are separated. Watch for desired effects.
Levodopa, methyldopa: May decrease absorption and efficacy of these drugs. Avoid concomitant use.

L-thyroxine: May decrease L-thyroxine absorption. Separate doses by at least 2 hours; monitor thyroid function.
Penicillamine: Decreased absorption. Separate doses by at least 2 hours.
Quinolones: May decrease absorption of quinolones. Monitor patient closely.
Tetracycline: Inhibited absorption of both drugs. Avoid concomitant use and give tetracycline 3 hours after or 2 hours before iron.
Vitamin C: May increase iron absorption. Beneficial drug interaction.
Drug-food. *Cereals, cheese, coffee, eggs, milk, tea, whole-grain breads, yogurt:* May impair oral iron absorption. Don't administer together. Tell patient to avoid these foods.

Adverse reactions
GI: *nausea,* epigastric pain, vomiting, *constipation,* diarrhea, black stools, anorexia.
Other: temporary staining of teeth (with suspension and drops).

☑ Special considerations
• Ferrous fumarate may cause dark-colored feces; may interfere with tests for occult blood in stool.
• Drug may stain teeth.
• Guaiac test and orthotoluidine test may yield false-positive results, but benzidine test usually isn't affected.
• Iron overload may decrease uptake of technetium 99m and interfere with skeletal imaging.
• The lethal dose of iron is between 200 to 250 mg/kg; fatalities have occurred with lower doses. Symptoms may follow ingestion of 20 to 60 mg/kg.
• Signs and symptoms of acute overdose at 30 minutes to 8 hours after ingestion include lethargy, nausea and vomiting, green then tarry stools, weak and rapid pulse, hypotension, dehydration, acidosis, and coma. If death doesn't immediately ensue, symptoms may clear for about 24 hours.
• At 12 to 48 hours, symptoms may return, accompanied by diffuse vascular congestion, pulmonary edema, shock, seizures, anuria, and hyperthermia. Death may follow.
• Treatment of overdose requires immediate support of airway, respiration, and circulation. In conscious patient with intact gag reflex, induce emesis with ipecac; in unconscious patient, empty stomach by gastric lavage. Follow emesis with lavage, using a 1% sodium bicarbonate solution, to convert iron to less irritating, poorly absorbed form. (Phosphate solutions have been used, but carry hazard of other adverse effects.)
• X-ray abdomen to determine continued presence of excess iron; if serum iron levels exceed 350 mg/dl, deferoxamine may be used for systemic chelation. Survivors are likely to sustain organ damage, including pyloric or antral stenosis, hepatic cirrhosis, CNS damage, and intestinal obstruction.

Monitoring the patient
• Monitor patient for adverse effects.
• Monitor therapeutic response.

Information for the patient
• Instruct patient to take tablets with orange juice or water, but not with milk or antacids.
• Tell patient to take suspension with straw and place drops at back of throat.

Geriatric patients
• Iron-induced constipation is common in elderly patients; stress proper diet.

Pediatric patients
• Iron overdose may be fatal in children; treat immediately.

Breast-feeding patients
• Iron supplements are often recommended for breast-feeding women; no adverse effects have been documented.

ferrous gluconate
Apo-Ferrous Gluconate*, Fergon, Ferralet, Fertinic*, Novoferrogluc*, Simron

Pharmacologic classification: oral iron supplement
Therapeutic classification: hematinic
Pregnancy risk category A

How supplied
Available without a prescription. Ferrous gluconate is 11.6% elemental iron.
Tablets: 240 mg (27 mg Fe), 300 mg (contains 35 mg Fe+), 320 mg, 325 mg (320-mg tablet contains 37 mg Fe+)
Capsules: 86 mg (contains 10 mg Fe+), 325 mg (contains 38 mg Fe+)
Elixir: 300 mg/5 ml (contains 35 mg Fe+)

Indications, route, and dosage
Iron deficiency
Adults: 325 mg P.O. q.i.d., dosage increased as needed and tolerated, up to 650 mg q.i.d.
Children ages 2 to 12: 3 mg/kg/day P.O. in three or four divided doses.
Children ages 6 months to 2 years: up to 6 mg/kg/day P.O. in three or four divided doses.
Infants: 10 to 25 mg/day P.O. divided into three or four doses.
✦ *Dosage adjustment.* Elderly patients may need higher doses because reduced gastric secretions and achlorhydria may lower capacity for iron absorption.

Pharmacodynamics
Hematinic action: Replaces iron, an essential component in the formation of hemoglobin.

Pharmacokinetics
• *Absorption:* Absorbed from entire length of GI tract, but primary absorption sites are duodenum and proximal jejunum. Up to 10% of iron is absorbed by healthy individuals; patients with iron-deficiency anemia may absorb up to 60%. Food may decrease absorption by 33% to 50%.
• *Distribution:* Transported through GI mucosal cells directly into blood; there it's immediately bound to a carrier protein, transferrin, and transported to bone marrow for incorporation into hemoglobin. Iron is highly protein-bound.
• *Metabolism:* Liberated by destruction of hemoglobin, but is conserved and reused by body.
• *Excretion:* Healthy individuals lose only small amounts of iron daily. Men and postmenopausal women lose about 1 mg/day, premenopausal women about 1.5 mg/day. Loss usually occurs in nails, hair, feces, and urine; trace amounts lost in bile and sweat.

Contraindications and precautions
Contraindicated in patients with peptic ulceration, regional enteritis, ulcerative colitis, hemosiderosis, primary hemochromatosis, or hemolytic anemia unless iron deficiency anemia is also present and in those receiving repeated blood transfusions. Use cautiously on long-term basis.

Interactions
Drug-drug. *Antacids, cholestyramine, cimetidine, vitamin E:* May decrease iron absorption. Separate doses by 1 to 2 hours.
Chloramphenicol: Delayed response to iron therapy. Watch for desired effects.
Doxycycline: May interfere with iron absorption even when doses are separated. Watch for desired effects.
Levodopa, methyldopa: May decrease absorption and efficacy of these drugs. Avoid concomitant use.
L-thyroxine: May decrease L-thyroxine absorption. Separate doses by at least 2 hours; monitor thyroid function.
Penicillamine: Decreased absorption. Separate doses by at least 2 hours.
Quinolones: May decrease absorption of quinolones. Avoid concomitant use.
Tetracycline: Inhibited absorption of both drugs. Avoid concomitant use. Give tetracycline 3 hours after or 2 hours before iron.
Vitamin C: May increase iron absorption. Beneficial drug interaction.
Drug-food. *Cereals, cheese, coffee, eggs, milk, tea, whole-grain breads, yogurt:* May impair oral iron absorption. Don't administer together. Tell patient to avoid these foods.

Adverse reactions
EENT: temporary staining of teeth (with elixir).
GI: *nausea,* epigastric pain, vomiting, *constipation,* diarrhea, *black stools,* anorexia.

☑ Special considerations
- Drug can be given between meals or with some food, but absorption may be decreased.
- Ferrous gluconate blackens feces; may interfere with test for occult blood in the stools.
- Guaiac test and orthotoluidine test may yield false-positive results, but the benzidine test usually isn't affected.
- Iron overload may decrease uptake of technetium 99m and interfere with skeletal imaging.
- The lethal dose of iron is between 200 to 250 mg/kg; fatalities have occurred with lower doses. Symptoms may follow ingestion of 20 to 60 mg/kg.
- Signs and symptoms of acute overdose at 30 minutes to 8 hours after ingestion include lethargy, nausea and vomiting, green then tarry stools, weak and rapid pulse, hypotension, dehydration, acidosis, and coma. If death doesn't immediately ensue, symptoms may clear for about 24 hours.
- At 12 to 48 hours, symptoms may return, accompanied by diffuse vascular congestion, pulmonary edema, shock, seizures, anuria, and hyperthermia. Death may follow.
- Treatment of overdose requires immediate support of airway, respiration, and circulation. In conscious patient with intact gag reflex, induce emesis with ipecac; in unconscious patient, empty stomach by gastric lavage. Follow emesis with lavage, using a 1% sodium bicarbonate solution, to convert iron to less irritating, poorly absorbed form. (Phosphate solutions have been used, but carry hazard of other adverse effects.)
- X-ray abdomen to determine continued presence of excess iron; if serum iron levels exceed 350 mg/dl, deferoxamine may be used for systemic chelation. Survivors are likely to sustain organ damage, including pyloric or antral stenosis, hepatic cirrhosis, CNS damage, and intestinal obstruction.

Monitoring the patient
- Monitor patient for adverse effects.
- Monitor therapeutic rsponse.

Information for the patient
- Tell patient to take elixir with straw and place drops in back of throat.
- Warn patient to exercise, eat properly, and drink plenty of fluids to avoid constipation.

Geriatric patients
- Iron-induced constipation is common in elderly patients; stress proper diet.

Pediatric patients
- Overdose may be fatal in children; treat immediately.

Breast-feeding patients
- Iron supplements are often recommended for breast-feeding women; no adverse effects have been documented.

ferrous sulfate
Apo-Ferrous Sulfate*, Feosol, Feratab, Fer-In-Sol, Fer-Iron, Fero-Grad-500*, Fero-Gradumet, Ferospace, Ferralyn Lanacaps, Ferra-TD, Mol-Iron, Novoferrosulfa*, PMS Ferrous Sulfate*, Slow FE

Pharmacologic classification: oral iron supplement
Therapeutic classification: hematinic
Pregnancy risk category A

How supplied
Available without a prescription. Ferrous sulfate is 20% elemental iron; dried and powdered (exsiccated), it's about 32% elemental iron.
Tablets: 195 mg, 300 mg, 324 mg, 325 mg; 200 mg (exsiccated); 160 mg (exsiccated, extended-release); 525 mg (timed-release)
Capsules: 150 mg, 190 mg, 250 mg
Capsules (extended-release): 150 mg, 159 mg, 250 mg
Syrup: 90 mg/5 ml
Elixir: 220 mg/5 ml
Liquid: 75 mg/0.6 ml, 125 mg/ml

Indications, route, and dosage
Iron deficiency
Adults: 300 mg P.O. b.i.d.; dosage gradually increased to 300 mg q.i.d. as needed and tolerated. For extended-release capsule, 150 to 250 mg P.O. once or twice daily; for extended-release tablets, 160 to 525 mg once or twice daily.
Children ages 2 to 12: 3 mg/kg/day P.O. in three or four divided doses.
Children ages 6 months to 2 years: Up to 6 mg/kg/day P.O. in three or four divided doses.
Infants: 10 to 25 mg/day P.O. in three or four divided doses.
✦ *Dosage adjustment.* Elderly patients may need higher doses because reduced gastric secretions and achlorhydria may lower capacity for iron absorption.

Pharmacodynamics
Hematinic action: Replaces iron, an essential component in the formation of hemoglobin.

Pharmacokinetics
- *Absorption:* Absorbed from entire length of GI tract, but primary absorption sites are duodenum and proximal jejunum. Up to 10% of iron is absorbed by healthy individuals; patients with iron-deficiency anemia may absorb up to 60%. Enteric coating and some extended-release formulas have decreased absorption because they are designed to release iron past points of highest absorption; food may decrease absorption by 33% to 50%.

• *Distribution:* Transported through GI mucosal cells directly into blood, where it's immediately bound to a carrier protein, transferrin, and transported to bone marrow for incorporation into hemoglobin. Iron is highly protein-bound.
• *Metabolism:* Liberated by destruction of hemoglobin, but is conserved and reused by body.
• *Excretion:* Healthy individuals lose very little iron each day. Men and postmenopausal women lose about 1 mg/day, and premenopausal women about 1.5 mg/day. Loss usually occurs in nails, hair, feces, and urine; trace amounts lost in bile and sweat.

Contraindications and precautions
Contraindicated in patients with hemosiderosis, primary hemochromatosis, hemolytic anemia unless iron deficiency anemia is also present, peptic ulceration, ulcerative colitis, or regional enteritis and in those receiving repeated blood transfusions. Use cautiously on long-term basis.

Interactions
Drug-drug. *Antacids, cholestyramine, cimetidine, vitamin E:* May decrease iron absorption. Separate doses by 1 to 2 hours.
Chloramphenicol: Delayed response to iron therapy. Monitor patient for desired effects.
Doxycycline: May interfere with iron absorption even when doses are separated. Monitor patient for desired effects.
Levodopa, methyldopa: May decrease absorption and efficacy of these drugs. Avoid concomitant use.
L-thyroxine: May decrease L-thyroxine absorption. Separate doses by at least 2 hours. Monitor thyroid function.
Penicillamine: Decreased absorption. Separate doses by at least 2 hours.
Quinolones: May decrease absorption of quinolones. Avoid concomitant use.
Tetracycline: Inhibited absorption of both drugs. Avoid concomitant use. Give tetracycline 3 hours after or 2 hours before iron.
Vitamin C: May increase iron absorption. Beneficial drug interaction.
Drug-food. *Cereals, cheese, coffee, eggs, milk, tea, whole-grain breads, yogurt:* May impair oral iron absorption. Don't administer together. Tell patient to avoid these foods.

Adverse reactions
GI: *nausea*, epigastric pain, vomiting, *constipation, black stools*, diarrhea, anorexia.
Other: temporary staining of teeth (with liquid forms).

☑ Special considerations
• Drug may cause dark-colored feces; may interfere with tests for occult blood in stool.
• Drug may stain teeth.

• Guaiac test and orthotoluidine test may yield false-positive results, but the benzidine test usually isn't affected.
• Iron overload may decrease uptake of technetium 99m and interfere with skeletal imaging.
• The lethal dose of iron is 200 to 250 mg/kg; fatalities have occurred with lower doses. Symptoms may follow ingestion of 20 to 60 mg/kg.
• Signs and symptoms of acute overdose at 30 minutes to 8 hours after ingestion include lethargy, nausea and vomiting, green then tarry stools, weak and rapid pulse, hypotension, dehydration, acidosis, and coma. If death doesn't immediately ensue, symptoms may clear for about 24 hours.
• At 12 to 48 hours, symptoms may return, accompanied by diffuse vascular congestion, pulmonary edema, shock, seizures, anuria, and hyperthermia. Death may follow.
• Treatment of overdose requires immediate support of airway, respiration, and circulation. In conscious patient with intact gag reflex, induce emesis with ipecac; in unconscious patient, empty stomach by gastric lavage. Follow emesis with lavage, using a 1% sodium bicarbonate solution, to convert iron to less irritating, poorly absorbed form. (Phosphate solutions have been used, but carry hazard of other adverse effects.)
• X-ray abdomen to determine continued presence of excess iron; if serum iron levels exceed 350 mg/dl, deferoxamine may be used for systemic chelation. Survivors are likely to sustain organ damage, including pyloric or antral stenosis, hepatic cirrhosis, CNS damage, and intestinal obstruction.

Monitoring the patient
• Monitor patient for adverse effects.
• Monitor therapeutic response.

Information for the patient
• Instruct patient not to crush or chew extended-release forms.
• Inform parents that three or four tablets can cause serious iron poisoning in child.
• Warn patient to exercise, eat properly, and drink plenty of fluids to avoid constipation.

Geriatric patients
• Iron-induced constipation is common in elderly patients; stress proper diet.

Pediatric patients
• Iron extended-release capsules or tablets usually aren't recommended for children. Overdose may be fatal; treat immediately.

Breast-feeding patients
• Iron supplements often are recommended for breast-feeding women; no adverse effects have been documented.

Reactions may be *common*, uncommon, **life-threatening**, or COMMON AND LIFE-THREATENING.

fexofenadine hydrochloride
Allegra

Pharmacologic classification: H_1-receptor antagonist
Therapeutic classification: antihistaminic
Pregnancy risk category C

How supplied
Available by prescription only
Capsules: 60 mg

Indications, route, and dosage
Seasonal allergic rhinitis
Adults and children ages 12 and older: 60 mg P.O. b.i.d.
✦ *Dosage adjustment.* In patients with impaired renal function, 60 mg P.O. once daily.

Pharmacodynamics
Antihistaminic action: Principal effects are mediated through a selective inhibition of peripheral H_1 receptors.

Pharmacokinetics
• *Absorption:* Rapidly absorbed.
• *Distribution:* 60% to 70% bound to plasma protein.
• *Metabolism:* About 5% of drug metabolized.
• *Excretion:* Mainly excreted in feces; less so in urine. Mean elimination half-life is 14.4 hours.

Contraindications and precautions
Contraindicated in patients with hypersensitivity to drug or its components. Use cautiously in patients with impaired renal function.

Interactions
None reported.

Adverse reactions
CNS: fatigue, drowsiness.
GI: nausea, dyspepsia.
GU: dysmenorrhea.
Other: viral infection.

☑ Special considerations
• No information indicates that abuse or dependency occurs with fexofenadine use.
• Overdose of up to 800 mg didn't result in significant adverse reactions. If overdose occurs, treatment should be symptomatic or supportive.
• Drug isn't effectively removed by hemodialysis.

Monitoring the patient
• Monitor patient for adverse effects.
• Monitor therapeutic response.

Information for the patient
• Caution patient not to perform hazardous activities if drowsiness occurs with drug use.

• Instruct patient not to exceed prescribed dosage and to take drug only when needed.

Pediatric patients
• Safety and effectiveness in children under age 12 haven't been established.

Breast-feeding patients
• It's unknown if drug appears in breast milk. Use with caution in breast-feeding women.

filgrastim (granulocyte colony–stimulating factor, G-CSF)
Neupogen

Pharmacologic classification: biologic response modifier
Therapeutic classification: colony stimulating factor
Pregnancy risk category C

How supplied
Available by prescription only
Injection: 300 mcg/ml in 1-ml and 1.6-ml single-dose vials

Indications, route, and dosage
To decrease infection after cancer chemotherapy for nonmyeloid malignancies, chronic severe neutropenia, after bone marrow transplantation in cancer patients; to treat ◇ *agranulocytosis,* ◇ *pancytopenia with colchicine overdose,* ◇ *acute leukemia,* ◇ *myelodysplastic syndrome,* ◇ *hematologic toxicity with zidovudine antiviral therapy*
Adults: Initially, 5 mcg/kg S.C. or I.V. as a single daily dose; may increase dose incrementally by 5 mcg/kg for each course of chemotherapy according to duration and severity of absolute neutrophil count (ANC) nadir.
Don't administer earlier than 24 hours after or within 24 hours before chemotherapy.
Filgrastim should be given daily for up to 2 weeks until ANC nadir reaches $10,000/mm^3$ after the anticipated chemotherapy-induced ANC nadir. Duration of treatment depends on the myelosuppressive potential of the chemotherapy used. Stop if ANC nadir surpasses $10,000/mm^3$.
◇ *AIDS*
Adults: 0.3 to 3.6 mcg/kg/day S.C. or I.V.
◇ *Aplastic anemia*
Adults: 800 to 1,200 mcg/m^2/day S.C. or I.V.
◇ *Hairy cell leukemia, myelodysplasia*
Adults: 15 to 500 mcg/m^2/day S.C. or I.V.

Pharmacodynamics
Immunostimulant action: Naturally occurring cytokine glycoprotein that stimulates proliferation, differentiation, and functional activity of neutrophils, causing a rapid rise in WBC counts within 2 to ˚

days in patients with normal bone marrow function or 7 to 14 days in patients with bone marrow suppression. Blood counts return to pretreatment levels, usually within 1 week after therapy ends.

Pharmacokinetics
● *Absorption:* After S.C. bolus dose, blood levels suggest rapid absorption with peak levels in 2 to 8 hours.
● *Distribution:* No information available.
● *Metabolism:* No information available.
● *Excretion:* Elimination half-life is about 3½ hours.

Contraindications and precautions
Contraindicated in patients with hypersensitivity to proteins derived from *Escherichia coli* or to drug or its components.

Interactions
Drug-drug. *Chemotherapeutic drugs:* Cause rapidly dividing myeloid cells to be potentially sensitive to cytotoxic drugs. Don't use within 24 hours before or after a dose of one of these drugs.

Adverse reactions
CNS: headache, weakness, *fatigue.*
CV: *MI, arrhythmias,* chest pain, transient hypotension.
GI: *nausea, vomiting, diarrhea, mucositis,* stomatitis, constipation.
GU: increased serum creatinine.
Hematologic: *thrombocytopenia,* leukocytosis, transient increases in neutrophils.
Hepatic: elevated liver enzyme levels.
Metabolic: elevations in uric acid.
Musculoskeletal: *skeletal pain.*
Respiratory: dyspnea, cough.
Skin: *alopecia,* rash, cutaneous vasculitis, *hypersensitivity reactions.*
Other: *fever.*

☑ Special considerations
● Store drug in refrigerator; don't freeze. Avoid shaking. Before injection, allow to reach room temperature for a maximum of 24 hours. Discard after 24 hours. Use only one dose per vial; don't reenter vial.
● Obtain CBC and platelet counts before and twice weekly during therapy.
● Drug isn't compatible with normal saline solution.
● Adult respiratory distress syndrome (ARDS) may occur in patients with sepsis because of influx of neutrophils at inflammation site.
● MI and arrhythmias have occurred; closely monitor patients with preexisting cardiac conditions.
● Bone pain is most frequent adverse reaction and may be controlled with nonnarcotic analgesics if mild to moderate or may require narcotic analgesics if severe.
● Maximum tolerated dose hasn't been determined; no reports of overdose.

Monitoring the patient
● Monitor CBC with platelets before treatment and regularly during treatment.
● Monitor patients with preexisting cardiovascular disease for MI and arrhythmias.
● Monitor patients with history of peptic ulcer disease for the development of ARDS.

Information for the patient
● Review "Information for Patients" section of package insert with patient. Thorough instruction is essential if home use is prescribed.
● When drug can be safely and effectively self-administered, instruct patient in proper dosage and administration techniques.
● Manufacturer has hotline to answer questions about insurance reimbursement procedures. Hotline operates Monday through Friday 9 a.m. to 5 p.m. Eastern Standard Time: 1-800-272-9376.

Geriatric patients
● No age-related problems have been reported.

Pediatric patients
● Efficacy not established, but no evidence of greater toxicity in children than in adults.

Breast-feeding patients
● It's unknown if drug appears in breast milk. Assess risk-to-benefit ratio.

finasteride
Propecia, Proscar

Pharmacologic classification: steroid (synthetic 4-azasteroid) derivative
Therapeutic classification: androgen synthesis inhibitor
Pregnancy risk category X

How supplied
Available by prescription only
Tablets: 1 mg, 5 mg

Indications, route and dosage
Symptomatic benign prostatic hyperplasia (BPH), ◊ *adjuvant therapy after radical prostatectomy,* ◊ *first-stage prostate cancer,* ◊ *acne,* ◊ *hirsutism*
Adults: 5 mg P.O. daily, usually for 6 to 12 months.
◊ *Male pattern baldness (androgenetic alopecia)*
Adults: 1 mg P.O. daily, usually for 3 months or more. Continued use is recommended to sustain benefit. Withdrawal of treatment leads to reversal of effect within 12 months.

Pharmacodynamics
Androgen synthesis inhibition action: Competitively inhibits steroid 5μ-reductase, an enzyme responsible for formation of the potent androgen

5μ-dihydrotestosterone (DHT) from testosterone. Because DHT influences development of the prostate gland, decreasing levels of this hormone in men should relieve the symptoms associated with BPH. In men with male pattern baldness, the balding scalp contains miniaturized hair follicles and increased amounts of DHT. Drug decreases scalp and serum DHT levels in these men.

Pharmacokinetics
• *Absorption:* Average bioavailability 63%. Maximum plasma levels reached within 2 hours of administration.
• *Distribution:* About 90% bound to plasma proteins. Drug crosses blood-brain barrier.
• *Metabolism:* Extensively metabolized by liver; at least 2 metabolites identified. Metabolites responsible for less than 20% of drug's total activity.
• *Excretion:* 39% of oral dose excreted in urine as metabolites; 57% in feces. No unchanged drug found in urine.

Contraindications and precautions
Contraindicated in patients with hypersensitivity to drug. Although drug isn't used in women, manufacturer indicates pregnancy as a contraindication.

Interactions
Drug-drug. *Theophylline:* Small, insignificant increases in theophylline clearance and decreased half-life (10%). Monitor theophylline levels.

Adverse reactions
GU: impotence, decreased volume of ejaculate, decreased libido.

☑ Special considerations
• Because it isn't possible to identify prospectively which patients will respond to finasteride, a minimum of 6 months of therapy may be necessary.
• Long-term effects of drug on the complications of BPH, including acute urinary obstruction, or the incidence of surgery aren't known.
• Sustained increases in serum prostate-specific antigen (PSA) should be carefully evaluated. In patients receiving finasteride therapy, this could indicate noncompliance to therapy.
• Drug's effectiveness as adjuvant therapy after radical prostatectomy and as adjunctive treatment of prostate cancer, acne, and hirsutism not yet known.
• Finasteride will decrease levels of PSA even in prostate cancer. This doesn't indicate a beneficial effect.
• Experience with overdose is limited. Patients have received single doses of 400 mg and multiple doses of up to 80 mg daily for 3 months without adverse effects.

• Ensure that women of childbearing age aren't pregnant before therapy starts (drug is contraindicated in pregnancy).
• Counsel women of childbearing age regarding birth control.

Monitoring the patient
• Carefully monitor patients who have large residual urine volumes or severely diminished urine flows. Not all patients respond to drug, and these patients may not be candidates for finasteride therapy.
• Before starting therapy, closely monitor and evaluate patient for conditions that might mimic BPH, including hypotonic bladder, prostate cancer, infection, stricture, or other neurologic conditions.

Information for the patient
• Inform patient that Propecia treats male pattern hair loss in men only. It isn't indicated for use in women.
• Advise woman who is or may become pregnant not to handle crushed tablets because of risk of adverse effects on male fetus.
• Instruct man whose sexual partner is or may become pregnant to avoid exposing her to his semen or to stop drug.
• Explain to man that drug may decrease ejaculate volume but doesn't appear to impair normal sexual function. However, impotence and decreased libido have occurred in less than 4% of patients treated with drug.

Geriatric patients
• Although drug's elimination rate is decreased in elderly patients, dosage adjustments aren't necessary.

Pediatric patients
• Drug isn't indicated for use in children.

Breast-feeding patients
• It isn't known if drug appears in breast milk; however, drug isn't indicated for use in women.

---

flecainide acetate
Tambocor

Pharmacologic classification: benzamide derivative local anesthetic (amide)
Therapeutic classification: ventricular antiarrhythmic
Pregnancy risk category C

How supplied
Available by prescription only
Tablets: 50 mg, 100 mg, 150 mg

Indications, route, and dosage

Life-threatening ventricular tachycardia and PVCs

Adults: 100 mg P.O. q 12 hours; may increase in increments of 50 mg b.i.d. q 4 days until efficacy is achieved. Maximum dose is 400 mg daily.

Paroxysmal supraventricular tachycardia, paroxysmal atrial fibrillation or flutter in patients without structural heart disease

Adults: 50 mg P.O. q 12 hours; may increase in increments of 50 mg b.i.d. q 4 days until efficacy is achieved. Maximum dose is 300 mg/day.

✦ *Dosage adjustment.* Reduce dosage in patients with renal impairment (creatinine clearance below 35 ml/minute/1.73 m²) beginning at 100 mg/day (50 mg b.i.d.); increase dosage cautiously at intervals longer than 4 days. For patients with less severe renal failure, initial dose is 100 mg q 12 hours, increasing cautiously at intervals longer than 4 days.

Pharmacodynamics

Antiarrhythmic action: A class IC antiarrhythmic that suppresses SA node automaticity and prolongs conduction in the atria, AV node, ventricles, accessory pathways, and His-Purkinje system. Has the most pronounced effect on the His-Purkinje system, as shown by QRS complex widening; this leads to a prolonged QT interval. Has relatively little effect on action potential duration except in Purkinje's fibers, where it shortens it. A proarrhythmic (arrhythmogenic) effect may result from drug's potent effects on the conduction system. Effects on the sinus node are strongest in patients with sinus node disease (sick sinus syndrome). Also exerts a moderate negative inotropic effect.

Pharmacokinetics

• *Absorption:* Rapidly and almost completely absorbed from GI tract; bioavailability of commercially available tablets is 85% to 90%. Plasma levels usually peak within 2 to 3 hours.

• *Distribution:* Apparently well distributed throughout body. Only about 40% binds to plasma proteins. Trough serum levels ranging from 0.2 to 1 mcg/ml provide greatest therapeutic benefit. Trough serum levels higher than 0.7 mcg/ml have been associated with increased adverse effects.

• *Metabolism:* Metabolized in liver to inactive metabolites. About 30% of orally administered dose escapes metabolism; is excreted in urine unchanged.

• *Excretion:* Elimination half-life averages about 20 hours. Plasma half-life may be prolonged in patients with heart failure and renal disease.

Contraindications and precautions

Contraindicated in patients with hypersensitivity to drug and in those with cardiogenic shock or preexisting second- or third-degree AV block or right bundle branch block when associated with a left hemiblock (in the absence of an artificial pacemaker).

Use cautiously in patients with heart failure, cardiomyopathy, severe renal or hepatic disease, prolonged QT interval, sick sinus syndrome, or blood dyscrasia.

Proarrhythmic effects have occurred in patients with atrial fibrillation or flutter who are taking this drug; therefore drug isn't recommended for use in these patients.

Interactions

Drug-drug. *Acidifying and alkalizing drugs:* May change urinary pH, altering flecainide elimination; alkalization decreases renal flecainide excretion, and acidification increases it. Monitor patient closely if used together. When drugs that can markedly affect urine acidity (such as ammonium chloride) or alkalinity (such as high-dose antacids, carbonic anhydrase inhibitors, sodium bicarbonate) are given, watch for possible subtherapeutic or toxic levels and effects.

Amiodarone: May increase serum flecainide levels. Monitor serum flecainide levels.

Antiarrhythmics: May cause additive, synergistic, or antagonistic cardiac effects and additive adverse effects. Monitor patient closely.

Beta blockers (such as propranolol): May cause additive negative inotropic effects. Monitor patient closely.

Cimetidine: May decrease both renal and nonrenal clearance of flecainide. Monitor patient closely.

Digoxin: May cause increased serum digoxin levels. Avoid concomitant use.

Disopyramide: May cause an additive negative inotropic effect. Monitor patient closely.

Verapamil: May have an additive negative inotropic effect; may exacerbate AV nodal dysfunction. Monitor patient closely.

Drug-lifestyle. *Smoking:* May lower flecainide serum levels. Discourage use.

Adverse reactions

CNS: *dizziness, headache,* fatigue, tremor, anxiety, insomnia, depression, malaise, paresthesia, ataxia, vertigo, *light-headedness, syncope,* asthenia.

CV: **new or worsened arrhythmias,** chest pain, flushing, edema, **heart failure, cardiac arrest,** palpitations.

EENT: *blurred vision and other visual disturbances.*

GI: nausea, constipation, abdominal pain, dyspepsia, vomiting, diarrhea, anorexia.

Respiratory: *dyspnea.*

Skin: rash.

Other: fever.

Reactions may be *common*, uncommon, *life-threatening*, or COMMON AND LIFE-THREATENING.

☑ Special considerations
• Drug has been associated with excessive mortality or nonfatal cardiac arrest rate. Restrict use to patients for whom benefits outweigh risks.
• Drug is a strong negative inotrope and may cause or worsen heart failure, especially in patients with cardiomyopathy, preexisting heart failure, or low ejection fraction.
• Therapy should be initiated in the hospital with careful monitoring of patients with symptomatic heart failure, sinus node dysfunction, sustained ventricular tachycardia, or underlying structural heart disease and in patients changing from another antiarrhythmic in whom stopping current antiarrhythmic is likely to cause life-threatening arrhythmias.
• Loading doses may exacerbate arrhythmias and aren't recommended. Dosage adjustments should be made at intervals of at least 4 days because of drug's long half-life.
• Most patients can be adequately maintained on an every-12-hour dosage schedule, but some need drug every 8 hours.
• Twice-daily dosing improves patient compliance.
• Drug's full therapeutic effect may take 3 to 5 days. I.V. lidocaine may be administered while awaiting full effect.
• Drug may increase acute and chronic endocardial pacing thresholds and may suppress ventricular escape rhythms. Pacing threshold should be determined before drug is given, after 1 week of therapy, and regularly thereafter. Don't give to patients with preexisting poor thresholds or nonprogrammable artificial pacemakers unless pacing rescue is available.
• In patients with heart failure and myocardial dysfunction, initial dosage shouldn't exceed 100 mg every 12 hours; common initial dosage is 50 mg every 12 hours.
• Signs and symptoms of overdose include increased PR and QT intervals, increased QRS complex duration, decreased myocardial contractility, conduction disturbances, and hypotension.
• Treatment of overdose generally involves symptomatic and supportive measures along with ECG, blood pressure, and respiratory monitoring. Inotropic drugs, such as dopamine and dobutamine, may be used. Hemodynamic support, including use of an intra-aortic balloon pump and transvenous pacing, may be needed. Because of drug's long half-life, supportive measures may be needed for extended periods.
• Hemodialysis is ineffective in reducing serum drug levels.

Monitoring the patient
• Monitor serum potassium levels before initiating treatment and regularly during treatment. Hypokalemia or hyperkalemia may alter drug effects and should be corrected before drug therapy begins.
• Evaluate cardiac rhythm and QT intervals before treatment and regularly during treatment for the development of second- or third-degree AV block, development of right bundle-branch block in the presence of left hemiblock, atrial fibrillation, atrial flutter, and sick sinus syndrome.
• Watch for development or worsening of heart failure during treatment.
• Flecainide is a first class IC antiarrhythmic. Adverse effects increase when trough serum drug levels exceed 0.7 mcg/ml. Periodically monitor blood levels, especially in patients with renal failure or heart failure. Therapeutic levels range from 0.2 to 1.0 mcg/ml.
• Use in hepatic impairment hasn't been fully evaluated; however, because flecainide is metabolized extensively (probably in liver), use in patients with significant hepatic impairment only when benefits clearly outweigh risks. Dosage reduction may be necessary and patients should be monitored carefully for signs of toxicity. Also monitor serum levels.

Information for the patient
• Tell patient to report any syncope, orthostatic hypotension, chest pain, or shortness of breath.

Geriatric patients
• Elderly patients are more susceptible to adverse effects. Monitor patient carefully.

Pediatric patients
• Safety and efficacy haven't been established in children under age 18. Drug may be useful in management of paroxysmal reentrant supraventricular tachycardia.

Breast-feeding patients
• Drug appears in breast milk. Breast-feeding isn't recommended during therapy because of risk of adverse effects on infant.

floxuridine
FUDR

Pharmacologic classification: antimetabolite (cell cycle–phase specific, S phase)
Therapeutic classification: antineoplastic
Pregnancy risk category D

How supplied
Available by prescription only
Injection: 500-mg vials

Indications, route, and dosage
Dosage and indications may vary. Check current literature for recommended protocol.

Palliative management of GI adenocarcinoma metastatic to the liver; brain, head, neck, gallbladder, bile duct cancer
Adults: 0.1 to 0.6 mg/kg daily by intra-arterial infusion; or 0.4 to 0.6 mg/kg daily into hepatic artery.
◊ *Solid tumors*
Adults: 0.5 to 1 mg/kg daily by I.V. infusion for 6 to 15 days or until toxicity occurs; or 30 mg/kg daily by single injection for 5 days, then 15 mg/kg every other day for up to 11 days or until toxicity occurs.

Pharmacodynamics
Antineoplastic action: Exerts cytotoxic activity after conversion to its active form by competitively inhibiting the enzyme thymidylate synthetase; this halts DNA synthesis and leads to cell death.

Pharmacokinetics
• *Absorption:* Not administered orally.
• *Distribution:* Crosses blood-brain-barrier to limited extent.
• *Metabolism:* Metabolized to fluorouracil in liver after intra-arterial infusions and rapid I.V. injections.
• *Excretion:* About 60% of dose excreted through lungs as carbon dioxide; small amount excreted by kidneys as unchanged drug and metabolites.

Contraindications and precautions
Contraindicated in patients with poor nutritional state, bone marrow suppression, or serious infection. Use cautiously in patients following high-dose pelvic radiation therapy or using alkylating drugs and in those with impaired renal or hepatic function.

Interactions
Drug-lifestyle. *Sun exposure:* May increase skin reaction. Tell patient to take precautions in sun.

Adverse reactions
CNS: cerebellar ataxia, malaise, weakness, headache, lethargy, disorientation, confusion, euphoria.
CV: myocardial ischemia, angina, thrombophlebitis.
EENT: blurred vision, nystagmus, photophobia, epistaxis.
GI: *anorexia, stomatitis, nausea, vomiting, diarrhea, bleeding, enteritis,* GI ulceration.
Hematologic: *leukopenia, anemia, thrombocytopenia, agranulocytosis.*
Hepatic: elevated liver enzyme levels, increased bilirubin level, *drug-induced hepatotoxicity.*
Skin: *erythema,* dermatitis, pruritus, rash, alopecia, photosensitivity.
Other: *anaphylaxis,* fever.

☑ Special considerations
• To reconstitute, use 5 ml sterile water for injection to give a concentration of 100 mg/ml.

• Dilute to appropriate volume for infusion device with D_5W or normal saline solution.
• Administration by infusion pump maintains a continuous, uniform rate. Reconstituted drug solutions are stable for 14 days when refrigerated.
• Therapeutic effect may be delayed 1 to 6 weeks. Make sure patient is aware of time required for improvement.
• Signs and symptoms of overdose include myelosuppression, diarrhea, alopecia, dermatitis, and hyperpigmentation. Treatment is usually supportive and includes transfusion of blood components and antidiarrheals.

Monitoring the patient
• Monitor patient's intake and output, CBC, and renal and hepatic function.
• Monitor arterial perfused area. Check line for bleeding, blockage, displacement, or leakage. Drug is often administered via hepatic arterial infusion in treating hepatic metastases.
• Watch for severe skin and GI adverse reaction; stop drug if these occur.

Information for the patient
• Advise patient to report nausea, vomiting, stomach pain, signs of infection, or unusual bruising or bleeding.
• Inform patient that excellent mouth care can help prevent oral adverse reactions.

Breast-feeding patients
• It's unknown if drug appears in breast milk. However, because of risk of serious adverse reactions, mutagenicity, and carcinogenicity in infant, breast-feeding isn't recommended.

fluconazole
Diflucan

Pharmacologic classification: bistriazole derivative
Therapeutic classification: antifungal
Pregnancy risk category C

How supplied
Available by prescription only
Tablets: 50 mg, 100 mg, 150 mg, 200 mg
Injection: 200 mg/100 ml, 400 mg/200 ml
Suspension: 10 mg/ml, 40 mg/ml

Indications, route, and dosage
Oropharyngeal and esophageal candidiasis
Adults: 200 mg P.O. or I.V. on day 1; then 100 mg P.O. or I.V. once daily. As much as 400 mg daily has been used for esophageal disease. Treatment should continue for at least 2 weeks after resolution of symptoms.
Children: 6 mg/kg on day 1; then 3 mg/kg daily for at least 2 weeks.

Systemic candidiasis
Adults: Up to 400 mg P.O. or I.V. once daily. Treatment should be continued for at least 2 weeks after resolution of symptoms.

Cryptococcal meningitis
Adults: 400 mg I.V. or P.O. on day 1; then 200 mg once daily. Continue treatment for 10 to 12 weeks after CSF culture becomes negative. For suppression of relapse in patients with AIDS, give 200 mg once daily.

Vaginal candidiasis
Adults: 150 mg P.O. as single dose.

Urinary tract infection or peritonitis
Adults: 50 to 200 mg P.O. or I.V. daily.

Prophylaxis in patients undergoing bone marrow transplantation
Adults: 400 mg P.O. or I.V. daily for several days before transplantation and 7 days after neutrophil count rises above 1,000 cells/mm³.

◊ *Candidal infection, long-term suppression in patients with HIV infection*
Adults: 100 to 200 mg P.O. or I.V. daily.

◊ *Prophylaxis against mucocutaneous candidiasis, cryptococcosis, coccidioidomycosis, or histoplasmosis in patients with HIV infection*
Adults: 200 to 400 mg P.O. or I.V. daily.
Children and infants: 2 to 8 mg/kg P.O. daily.

✦ *Dosage adjustment.* Patients receiving hemodialysis should receive one full dose after each session.

Creatinine clearance (ml/min)	Percentage of usual adult dose
> 50	100
21 to 49	50
11 to 20	25

Pharmacodynamics
Antifungal action: Exerts fungistatic effects by inhibiting fungal cytochrome P-450 and interfering with sterols in the fungal cell. Spectrum of activity includes *Cryptococcus neoformans, Candida* (including systemic *C. albicans*), *Aspergillus flavus, A. fumigatus, Coccidioides immitis,* and *Histoplasma capsulatum.*

Pharmacokinetics
- *Absorption:* After oral administration, rapid and complete absorption. Plasma level peaks in 1 to 2 hours.
- *Distribution:* Well distributed to various sites, including CNS, saliva, sputum, blister fluid, urine, normal skin, nails, and blister skin. CNS levels approach 50% to 90% of that of serum. Drug is 12% protein-bound.
- *Metabolism:* Partially metabolized.

- *Elimination:* Primarily excreted via kidneys. Over 80% excreted unchanged in urine. Excretion rate diminishes as renal function decreases.

Contraindications and precautions
Contraindicated in patients with hypersensitivity to drug and other drugs in the same classification.

Interactions
Drug-drug. *Cimetidine:* May reduce fluconazole's serum levels. Monitor patient for desired effects.
Cyclosporine: May increase cyclosporine levels. Monitor cyclosporine levels.
Hydrochlorothiazide: Decreased clearance of fluconazole, raising drug serum levels. Monitor patient for side effects.
Isoniazid, phenytoin, rifampin, sulfonylureas, valproic acid: Elevated hepatic transaminase levels. Monitor liver function.
Phenytoin: May significantly increase serum phenytoin levels. Monitor serum phenytoin levels.
Rifampin: Lowered fluconazole levels. Monitor patient for desired effects.
Sulfonylureas (such as glipizide, glyburide, tolbutamide): Increased hypoglycemic effects. Monitor glucose levels.
Warfarin: Enhanced hypoprothrombinemic effects. Monitor INR.
Zidovudine: May increase activity of zidovudine. Monitor patient closely.
Drug-food. *Caffeine:* May increase plasma caffeine levels. (Ofloxacin or lomefloxacin are alternative drugs.) Discourage use.

Adverse reactions
CNS: headache.
GI: *nausea,* vomiting, abdominal pain, diarrhea.
Hepatic: Elevated liver enzyme levels.
Skin: rash.
Other: *anaphylaxis.*

☑ Special considerations
- Adjust dose in patients who have renal dysfunction.
- Fluconazole isn't compatible with other I.V. drugs.
- Bioavailability of oral drug is comparable to I.V. dosing. Administer drug via oral route whenever possible.
- Adverse reactions (including transaminase elevations) are more frequent and more severe in patients with severe underlying illness (including AIDS and malignancies).
- Overdose treatment is largely supportive.

Monitoring the patient
- Monitor serum phenytoin levels if patient is taking phenytoin.

● Monitor serum glucose if patient is taking oral antidiabetics.
● Monitor renal function before and during treatment.

Information for the patient
● Instruct patient to take drug as directed, even if he feels better.
● Instruct patient to report adverse effects immediately.

Breast-feeding patients
● Drug appears in breast milk at levels similar to those of plasma. Use in breast-feeding women isn't recommended.

---

flucytosine (5-FC)
Ancobon

Pharmacologic classification: fluorinated pyrimidine
Therapeutic classification: antifungal
Pregnancy risk category C

How supplied
Available by prescription only
Capsules: 250 mg, 500 mg

Indications, route, and dosage
Severe fungal infections caused by susceptible strains of Candida and Cryptococcus
Adults: 50 to 150 mg/kg/day P.O., administered in divided doses q 6 hours.
◊ *Chromomycosis*
Adults: 150 mg/kg P.O. daily.
✦ **Dosage adjustment.** In patients with renal failure who have a creatinine clearance of 50 ml/minute or less, reduce dosage by 20% to 80%. Or in patients with creatinine clearance of 20 to 40 ml/minute, increase dosage interval to q 12 hours; creatinine clearance of 10 to 20 ml/minute, increase dosage interval to q 24 hours; and for those with creatinine clearance below 10 ml/minute, increase dosage interval to q 24 to 48 hours. Serum levels should be monitored. Flucytosine is removed by hemodialysis and peritoneal dialysis.
    Dosage of 20 to 50 mg/kg P.O. immediately after hemodialysis q 2 to 3 days ensures therapeutic blood levels.

Pharmacodynamics
Antifungal action: Penetrates fungal cells and is then converted to fluorouracil, which interferes with pyrimidine metabolism; also may be converted to fluorodeoxyuredylic acid, which interferes with DNA synthesis. Because human cells lack the enzymes needed to convert drug to these toxic metabolites, flucytosine is selectively toxic to fungal, not host cells. Active against some strains of *Cryptococcus* and *Candida*.

Pharmacokinetics
● *Absorption:* About 75% to 90% of oral dose is absorbed. Serum levels peak at 2 to 6 hours. Food decreases absorption rate.
● *Distribution:* Distributed widely into liver, kidneys, spleen, heart, bronchial secretions, joints, peritoneal fluid, and aqueous humor. CSF levels vary from 60% to 100% of serum levels. 2% to 4% bound to plasma proteins.
● *Metabolism:* Only small amounts metabolized.
● *Excretion:* About 75% to 95% excreted unchanged in urine; less than 10% excreted unchanged in feces. Serum half-life is 2½ to 6 hours with normal renal function; as long as 1,160 hours with creatinine clearance below 2 ml/minute.

Contraindications and precautions
Contraindicated in patients with hypersensitivity to drug. Use cautiously in patients with impaired renal or hepatic function or bone marrow suppression.

Interactions
Drug-drug. *Amphotericin B:* May potentiate effects and toxicities. Avoid concomitant use.
Cytosine: May inactivate flucytosine. Monitor patient closely.

Adverse reactions
CNS: headache, vertigo, sedation, fatigue, weakness, confusion, hallucinations, psychosis, ataxia, hearing loss, paresthesia, parkinsonism, peripheral neuropathy.
CV: *cardiac arrest.*
GI: nausea, vomiting, diarrhea, abdominal pain, emesis, dry mouth, duodenal ulcer, **hemorrhage,** ulcerative colitis.
GU: azotemia, elevated creatinine and BUN levels, crystalluria, **renal failure.**
Hematologic: anemia, **leukopenia, bone marrow suppression, thrombocytopenia,** eosinophilia, **agranulocytosis, aplastic anemia.**
Hepatic: elevated liver enzyme levels, elevated serum alkaline phosphatase level, jaundice.
Metabolic: hypoglycemia, hypokalemia.
Respiratory: *respiratory arrest,* chest pain, dyspnea.
Skin: occasional rash, pruritus, urticaria, photosensitivity.

☑ Special considerations
● Give capsules over a 15-minute period to reduce nausea, vomiting, and GI distress.
● Prolonged serum levels in excess of 100 mcg/ml may be associated with toxicity; monitor serum levels, especially in patients with renal insufficiency.
● Flucytosine causes falsely elevated creatinine values on aminohydrolase enzymatic assay.
● Drug overdose may affect CV and pulmonary function. Treatment is largely supportive. Induced emesis or lavage may be useful within 4 hours

---

after ingestion. Activated charcoal and osmotic cathartics also may be helpful. Drug is readily removed by either hemodialysis or peritoneal dialysis.

Monitoring the patient
• Perform hematologic, renal, and hepatic function studies before therapy and frequently thereafter to evaluate dosage and watch for adverse effects.
• Monitor intake and output to ensure adequate renal function.

Information for the patient
• Teach patient signs and symptoms of adverse reactions and the importance of reporting them.
• Tell patient to call promptly if urine output decreases or bleeding or bruising occurs.
• Explain that adequate response may require several weeks or months of therapy. Advise patient to adhere to medical regimen and return as instructed for follow-up visits.

Pediatric patients
• Safety and effectiveness in children haven't been established.

Breast-feeding patients
• Safety in breast-feeding women hasn't been established.

fludarabine phosphate
Fludara

Pharmacologic classification: antimetabolite
Therapeutic classification: antineoplastic
Pregnancy risk category D

How supplied
Available by prescription only
Injection: 50 mg as lyophilized powder

Indications, route, and dosage
Treatment of B-cell chronic lymphocytic leukemia (CLL) in patients who haven't responded or responded inadequately to at least one standard alkylating drug regimen, ◇ **mycosis fungoides,** ◇ **hairy-cell leukemia,** ◇ **Hodgkin's and malignant lymphoma**
Adults: Usually, 25 mg/m² I.V. over 30 minutes (rapid I.V. injection or continuous I.V. infusion) for 5 consecutive days q 28 days. Therapy based on patient response and tolerance.
◇ **Chronic lymphocytic leukemia**
Adults: Usually, 18 to 30 mg/m² I.V. over 30 minutes (rapid I.V. injection or continuous I.V. infusion) for 5 consecutive days q 28 days. Therapy based on patient response and tolerance.

Pharmacodynamics
Antineoplastic action: Exact mechanism unknown. After rapid conversion of fludarabine to its active metabolite, the metabolite appears to inhibit DNA synthesis by inhibiting DNA polymerase alpha, ribonucleotide reductase, and DNA primase.

Pharmacokinetics
• *Absorption:* Administered I.V.
• *Distribution:* Widely distributed, with volume of distribution 96 to 98 L/m² at steady state.
• *Metabolism:* Rapidly dephosphorylated and then phosphorylated intracellularly to active metabolite.
• *Excretion:* 23% excreted in urine as unchanged active metabolite. Half-life is about 10 hours.

Contraindications and precautions
Contraindicated in patients with hypersensitivity to drug or its components. Use cautiously in patients with renal insufficiency.

Interactions
Drug-drug. *Myelosuppressives:* May cause additive toxicity when used with other myelosuppressives. Monitor patient closely.
Pentostatin: Increased risk of pulmonary toxicity. Monitor patient closely.

Adverse reactions
CNS: *fatigue, malaise, weakness, paresthesia,* peripheral neuropathy, headache, sleep disorder, depression, cerebellar syndrome, **CVA,** agitation, *confusion,* **coma.**
CV: *edema,* angina, transient ischemic attack, phlebitis, **arrhythmias, heart failure,** supraventricular tachycardia, deep venous thrombosis, **aneurysm, hemorrhage.**
EENT: *visual disturbances,* hearing loss, delayed blindness (with high doses), sinusitis, pharyngitis, epistaxis.
GI: *nausea, vomiting, diarrhea,* constipation, *anorexia,* stomatitis, *GI bleeding,* esophagitis, mucositis.
GU: *dysuria, urinary tract infection* or hesitancy, proteinuria, hematuria, **renal failure.**
Hematologic: **hemolytic anemia,** MYELOSUPPRESSION.
Hepatic: **liver failure,** cholelithiasis.
Metabolic: hypocalcemia, hyperkalemia, hyperglycemia, dehydration, hyperuricemia, hyperphosphatemia.
Musculoskeletal: *myalgia.*
Respiratory: *cough, pneumonia, dyspnea, upper respiratory tract infection,* allergic pneumonitis, hemoptysis, hypoxia, bronchitis.
Skin: alopecia, diaphoresis, *rash,* pruritus, seborrhea.
Other: *fever, chills, infection, pain,* tumor lysis syndrome, **anaphylaxis.**

☑ Special considerations
• Drug has been used as investigational treatment of malignant lymphoma, macroglobulinemic lymphoma, prolymphocytic leukemia or prolymphocytoid variant of CLL, mycosis fungoides, hairy cell leukemia, and Hodgkin's disease.
• Drug should be administered under the direct supervision of medical personnel experienced in antineoplastic therapy.
• Tumor lysis syndrome (hyperuricemia, hyperphosphatemia, hypocalcemia, metabolic acidosis, hyperkalemia, hematuria, urate crystalluria, and renal failure) has occurred in CLL patients with large tumors.
• Severe neurologic effects, including blindness, are seen when high doses are used to treat acute leukemia.
• Advanced age, renal insufficiency, and bone marrow impairment may predispose patient to severe toxicity; toxic effects are dose-dependent.
• Optimal duration of therapy hasn't been established; three additional cycles after achieving maximal response are recommended before stopping drug.
• To prepare, add 2 ml of sterile water for injection to solid cake of fludarabine. Dissolution should occur within 15 seconds and each ml will contain 25 mg of drug, 25 mg of mannitol, and sodium hydroxide. Use within 8 hours of reconstitution. Fludarabine has been further diluted in 100 ml or 125 ml of D_5W or normal saline solution.
• Follow institutional protocol and guidelines for proper handling and disposal of chemotherapeutic drugs.
• Irreversible CNS toxicity characterized by delayed blindness, coma, and death is associated with high doses. Severe thrombocytopenia and neutropenia secondary to bone marrow suppression also occur. There is no specific antidote; to treat, stop drug and provide supportive measures.

Monitoring the patient
• Monitor renal function before treatment starts.
• Careful hematologic monitoring, especially of neutrophil and platelet counts, is needed.
• Monitor patient for adverse neurologic effects (delayed blindness, coma).
• Watch for signs of infection.

Information for the patient
• Tell patient to avoid contact with infected persons and to report signs of infection or unusual bleeding immediately.

Geriatric patients
• Advanced age may increase toxicity potential.

Pediatric patients
• Safety and efficacy in children haven't been established.

Breast-feeding patients
• It's unknown if drug appears in breast milk. Determine risk-benefit ratio.

fludrocortisone acetate
Florinef

Pharmacologic classification: mineralocorticoid, glucocorticoid
Therapeutic classification: mineralocorticoid replacement therapy
Pregnancy risk category C

How supplied
Available by prescription only
Tablets: 0.1 mg

Indications, route, and dosage
Adrenal insufficiency (partial replacement), salt-losing adrenogenital syndrome
Adults: 0.1 to 0.2 mg P.O. daily.
Children: 0.05 to 0.1 mg P.O. daily.
Orthostatic hypotension in diabetic patients, orthostatic hypotension
Adults: 0.1 to 0.4 mg P.O. daily.
Orthostatic hypotension caused by levodopa therapy
Adults: 0.05 to 0.2 mg P.O. daily.

Pharmacodynamics
Adrenal hormone replacement: A synthetic glucocorticoid with potent mineralocorticoid activity that's used for partial replacement of corticosteroid hormones in adrenocortical insufficiency and in salt-losing forms of congenital adrenogenital syndrome. In treating adrenocortical insufficiency, an exogenous glucocorticoid must also be administered for adequate control. (Cortisone or hydrocortisone are usually the drugs of choice for replacement because they produce both mineralocorticoid and glucocorticoid activity.) Drug is administered on a variable schedule ranging from three times weekly to b.i.d., depending on individual requirements.

Pharmacokinetics
• *Absorption:* Absorbed readily from GI tract.
• *Distribution:* Removed rapidly from blood and distributed to muscle, liver, skin, intestines, and kidneys. Plasma half-life of about 30 minutes; extensively bound to plasma proteins (transcortin and albumin). Only unbound portion is active. Adrenocorticoids are distributed into breast milk and through placenta.
• *Metabolism:* Metabolized in liver to inactive glucuronide and sulfate metabolites.
• *Excretion:* Inactive metabolites and small amounts of unmetabolized drug excreted by kidneys. Insignificant quantities also excreted in feces. Biological half-life is 18 to 36 hours; plasma half-life is 3½ hours or more.

Reactions may be *common*, uncommon, *life-threatening*, or COMMON AND LIFE-THREATENING.

Contraindications and precautions
Contraindicated in patients with hypersensitivity to drug and in those with systemic fungal infections.

Use cautiously in patients with hypothyroidism, cirrhosis, ocular herpes simplex, emotional instability, psychotic tendencies, nonspecific ulcerative colitis, diverticulitis, fresh intestinal anastomoses, peptic ulcer, renal insufficiency, hypertension, osteoporosis, or myasthenia gravis.

Interactions
Drug-drug. *Amphotericin B, thiazide diuretics:* May enhance hypokalemia. Avoid concomitant use.
Barbiturates, phenytoin, rifampin: Possible decreased corticosteroid effects due to increased hepatic metabolism. Monitor patient for desired effects.
Cardiac glycosides: Hypokalemia may increase risk of toxicity in patients concurrently receiving these drugs. Monitor patient closely.
Drugs containing sodium: May increase blood pressure. Sodium intake may need to be adjusted.
Isoniazid, salicylates: May increase metabolism of these drugs. Avoid concomitant use.
Drug-food. *Foods containing sodium:* May increase blood pressure. Sodium intake may need to be adjusted.

Adverse reactions
CV: *sodium and water retention,* hypertension, cardiac hypertrophy, edema, **heart failure.**
Metabolic: increased serum sodium levels, hypokalemia.
Skin: bruising, diaphoresis, urticaria, allergic rash.

☑ Special considerations
Besides the recommendations relevant to all systemic adrenocorticoids, consider the following.
• Use only with other supplemental measures, such as glucocorticoids, control of electrolytes, and control of infection.
• Supplemental dosages may be required in times of physiologic stress due to serious illness, trauma, or surgery.
• Glucose tolerance tests should be performed only if necessary because addisonian patients tend to develop severe hypoglycemia within 3 hours of test.
• Acute toxicity occurs as an extension of therapeutic effect, such as disturbances in fluid and electrolyte balance, hypokalemia, edema, hypertension, and cardiac insufficiency. Provide symptomatic treatment and correct fluid and electrolyte imbalance.

Monitoring the patient
• Watch for significant patient weight gain, edema, hypertension, or severe headaches.
• Monitor therapeutic response.

Information for the patient
• Teach patient to recognize signs of electrolyte imbalance: muscle weakness, paresthesia, numbness, fatigue, anorexia, nausea, altered mental status, increased urination, altered heart rhythm, severe or continuing headaches, unusual weight gain, or swelling of feet.
• Tell patient to take missed doses as soon as possible, unless it's almost time for the next dose; don't double dose.

Pediatric patients
• Long-term use in children and adolescents may delay growth and maturation.

flumazenil
Romazicon

Pharmacologic classification: benzodiazepine antagonist
Therapeutic classification: antidote
Pregnancy risk category C

How supplied
Available by prescription only
Injection: 0.1 mg/ml in 5-ml and 10-ml multiple-dose vials

Indications, route, and dosage
Complete or partial reversal of the sedative effects of benzodiazepines after anesthesia or short diagnostic procedures (conscious sedation)
Adults: Initially, 0.2 mg I.V. over 15 seconds. If patient doesn't reach desired level of consciousness after 45 seconds, repeat dose. Repeat at 1-minute intervals until a cumulative dose of 1 mg has been given (initial dose plus four additional doses). Most patients respond after 0.6 to 1 mg of drug. If resedation occurs, dosage may be repeated after 20 minutes, but no more than 1 mg should be given at one time, and patient shouldn't receive more than 3 mg/hour.
Management of suspected benzodiazepine overdose
Adults: Initially, 0.2 mg I.V. over 30 seconds. If patient doesn't reach desired level of consciousness after 30 seconds, administer 0.3 mg over 30 seconds. If patient still doesn't respond adequately, give 0.5 mg over 30 seconds, then repeat 0.5-mg doses at 1-minute intervals until a cumulative dose of 3 mg has been given. Most patients with benzodiazepine overdose respond to cumulative doses between 1 and 3 mg; rarely, patients who respond partially after 3 mg may need additional doses. Don't give more than 5 mg over 5 minutes initially; sedation that persists after this dosage is unlikely to be caused by benzodiazepines. If resedation occurs, dosage may be repeated after 20 minutes, but no more than

1 mg should be given at one time, and patient shouldn't receive more than 3 mg/hour.

Pharmacodynamics
Antidote action: Competitively inhibits actions of benzodiazepines on the gamma-aminobutyric acid-benzodiazepine receptor complex.

Pharmacokinetics
• *Absorption:* Onset of action within 1 to 2 minutes after injection. 80% response within 3 minutes; peak effect at 6 to 10 minutes.
• *Distribution:* Redistributed rapidly (initial distribution half-life is 7 to 15 minutes). About 50% bound to plasma proteins.
• *Metabolism:* Rapidly extracted from blood and metabolized by liver. Metabolites identified are inactive. Ingestion of food during I.V. infusion enhances extraction of drug from plasma, probably by increasing hepatic blood flow.
• *Excretion:* About 90% to 95% appears in urine as metabolites; rest is excreted in feces. Plasma half-life is about 54 minutes.

Contraindications and precautions
Contraindicated in patients with hypersensitivity to drug or benzodiazepines; in patients who show evidence of serious tricyclic antidepressant overdose; and in those who received a benzodiazepine to treat a potentially life-threatening condition (such as status epilepticus).
   Use cautiously in alcohol-dependent or psychiatric patients, in those at high risk for developing seizures, and in those with head injuries, signs of seizures, or recent high intake of benzodiazepines (such as patients in the intensive care unit).

Interactions
Drug-drug. *Antidepressants, drugs that can cause arrhythmias or seizures:* May cause seizures or arrhythmias after flumazenil removes effects of benzodiazepine overdose. Don't use flumazenil in mixed overdose, especially in cases in which seizures (from any cause) are likely to occur. Monitor patient closely.

Adverse reactions
CNS: *dizziness, abnormal or blurred vision, headache, **seizures,** agitation, emotional lability, tremor, insomnia.
CV: ***arrhythmias,*** cutaneous vasodilation, palpitations.
GI: nausea, vomiting.
Respiratory: dyspnea, hyperventilation.
Skin: *diaphoresis,* pain at injection site.

☑ Special considerations
• Onset of action is usually evident within 1 to 2 minutes of injection, and effect peaks within 6 to 10 minutes. Because drug's duration of action is shorter than that of benzodiazepines, monitor pa-tient carefully and administer additional drug as needed. Duration and degree of effect depend on plasma levels of sedating benzodiazepine and dose of flumazenil.
• To minimize pain at injection site, give drug through free flowing I.V. solution running into large vein. Compatible solutions include D_5W, lactated Ringer's injection, and normal saline solution.
• Resedation may occur after reversal of benzodiazepine effect because drug has a shorter duration of action than that of benzodiazepines. Patients should be monitored for resedation according to duration of drug being reversed. Monitor closely after long-acting benzodiazepines (such as diazepam) or after high doses of shorter-acting benzodiazepines (such as 10 mg of midazolam). Usually, serious resedation is unlikely in patients who fail to show signs of resedation 2 hours after a 1-mg dose of flumazenil.
• Flumazenil can be administered by direct injection or diluted with a compatible solution. Discard unused drug that has been drawn into a syringe or diluted within 24 hours.
• Large doses of flumazenil were administered I.V. to volunteers in the absence of a benzodiazepine agonist. No serious adverse reactions, or altered laboratory tests were noted.
• In patients with benzodiazepine overdose, large doses of flumazenil may produce agitation or anxiety, hyperesthesia, increased muscle tone, or seizures. Treat seizures with barbiturates, phenytoin, or benzodiazepines.

Monitoring the patient
• Evaluate patient for history of seizures or alcohol-dependency. Patient is at greater risk for seizures with flumazenil administration.
• Monitor patient for resedation for up to 2 hours after reversal with flumazenil.

Information for the patient
• Because of resedation risk, advise patient to avoid alcohol, CNS depressants, OTC drugs, and hazardous activities such as driving a car within 24 hours of procedure.

Pediatric patients
• Drug use in children not recommended.

Breast-feeding patients
• It's unknown if drug appears in breast milk. Use cautiously in breast-feeding women.

Reactions may be *common*, uncommon, ***life-threatening***, or COMMON AND LIFE-THREATENING.

flunisolide
Nasal inhalant
Nasalide

Oral inhalant
AeroBid, AeroBid-M

Pharmacologic classification: glucocorticoid
Therapeutic classification: anti-inflammatory, antasthmatic
Pregnancy risk category C

How supplied
Available by prescription only
Nasal inhalant: 25 mcg/metered spray; 200 doses/bottle
Oral inhalant: 250 mcg/metered spray; at least 100 doses/inhaler

Indications, route, and dosage
Corticosteroid-dependent asthma
Adults: Two inhalations b.i.d. for total daily dose of 1 mg. Don't exceed 8 inhalations (2 mg)/day.
Children ages 6 and older: Two inhalations b.i.d. Don't exceed four inhalations daily.
Seasonal or perennial rhinitis
Adults: Two sprays (50 mcg) in each nostril b.i.d. (total dose 200 mcg/day). If needed, increase to two sprays in each nostril t.i.d. (total dose 300 mcg/day).
Children ages 6 to 14: One spray (25 mcg) in each nostril t.i.d. or two sprays (50 mcg) in each nostril b.i.d. (total dose 150 to 200 mcg/day).

Pharmacodynamics
Anti-inflammatory action: Stimulates synthesis of enzymes needed to decrease the inflammatory response. The anti-inflammatory and vasoconstrictor potency of topically applied flunisolide is several hundred times greater than that of hydrocortisone and about equal to that of an equal weight of triamcinolone; the metabolite, 6-beta-hydroxyflunisolide, has about three times the activity of hydrocortisone.
Antasthmatic action: The nasal inhalant form is used in the symptomatic treatment of seasonal or perennial rhinitis. In patients who require corticosteroids to control symptoms, the oral inhalant form is used to treat bronchial asthma.

Pharmacokinetics
• *Absorption:* About 50% of nasally inhaled dose absorbed systemically; plasma levels peak within 10 to 30 minutes. After oral inhalation, about 40% of dose absorbed from lungs and GI tract; only about 20% of orally inhaled dose reaches systemic circulation unmetabolized because of extensive metabolism in liver. Onset of action usually occurs in a few days but may take as long as 4 weeks.
• *Distribution:* Distribution after intranasal administration or oral inhalation hasn't been described. No evidence of tissue storage of flunisolide or metabolites.
• *Metabolism:* Drug that is swallowed undergoes rapid metabolism in liver or GI tract to several metabolites, one of which has glucocorticoid activity. Flunisolide and its 6-beta-hydroxy metabolite are eventually conjugated in liver, by glucuronic acid or surface sulfate, to inactive metabolites.
• *Excretion:* Unknown when given as inhalant; when given systemically, metabolites excreted in roughly equal portions in feces and urine. Biological half-life averages about 2 hours.

Contraindications and precautions
Contraindicated in patients with hypersensitivity to drug. Use of nasal inhalant is contraindicated in presence of untreated localized infection involving nasal mucosa; oral inhalant shouldn't be used in patients with status asthmaticus or respiratory infections.

Use nasal inhalant cautiously in patients with tuberculosis; untreated fungal, bacterial, or systemic viral or ocular herpes simplex infections; or septal ulcers, trauma, or surgery in the nasal region. Oral inhalant isn't recommended for patients with asthma controlled by bronchodilators or other noncorticosteroids alone or for patients with nonasthma bronchial diseases.

Interactions
None reported.

Adverse reactions
CNS: headache (with nasal inhalant); dizziness, irritability, nervousness (with oral inhalant).
CV: chest pain, edema (with oral inhalant).
EENT: nasopharyngeal fungal infection; *mild, transient nasal burning and stinging,* stinging, dryness, sneezing, epistaxis, watery eyes (with nasal inhalant).
GI: nausea, vomiting (with nasal inhalant); dry mouth, abdominal pain, decreased appetite, *nausea, vomiting, diarrhea, upset stomach (with oral inhalant).*
Respiratory: *upper respiratory tract infection* (with oral inhalant).
Skin: rash, pruritus (with oral inhalant).
Other: *cold symptoms, flu,* fever (with oral inhalant).

☑ Special considerations
• Recommendations for use of flunisolide and for care and teaching of patient during therapy are the same as those for all inhalant adrenocorticoids.

Monitoring the patient
• Evaluate patient for respiratory infection before therapy starts.
• Monitor patient for adverse effects.

Information for the patient
• Tell patient to avoid exposure to chickenpox or measles.
• To instill drug, instruct patient to shake the container before use; to blow nose to clear nasal passages; and to tilt head slightly forward and insert nozzle into nostril, pointing away from the septum. Tell him to hold the other nostril closed, inspire gently, and spray. The nosepiece should be cleaned with warm water if it becomes clogged.
• Explain that drug may take 2 to 3 weeks to have an effect.
• Advise patient to use drug as prescribed and not to exceed recommended dosage.
• Tell patient to stop drug and report if symptoms continue for 3 weeks, or if nasal irritation persists.

---

fluocinonide
Lidemol*, Lidex, Lidex-E, Lyderm*

Pharmacologic classification: topical adrenocorticoid
Therapeutic classification: anti-inflammatory
Pregnancy risk category C

How supplied
Available by prescription only
Cream, gel, ointment, solution: 0.05%

Indications, route, and dosage
Inflammation of corticosteroid-responsive dermatoses
Adults and children: Apply sparingly b.i.d. or t.i.d. Occlusive dressings may be used for severe or resistant dermatoses.

Pharmacodynamics
Anti-inflammatory action: Stimulates synthesis of enzymes needed to decrease inflammatory response. High-potency fluorinated glucocorticoid categorized as a group II topical corticosteroid.

Pharmacokinetics
• *Absorption:* Amount absorbed depends on amount applied and on nature and condition of skin at application site. Ranges from about 1% in areas of thick stratum corneum (such as palms, soles, elbows, and knees) to as high as 36% in areas of thin stratum corneum (face, eyelids, and genitals). Absorption increases in areas of skin damage, inflammation, or occlusion. Some systemic absorption of corticosteroids occurs, especially through oral mucosa.
• *Distribution:* After topical application, is distributed throughout local skin. Any drug absorbed into circulation is removed rapidly from blood and distributed into muscle, liver, skin, intestines, and kidneys.
• *Metabolism:* After topical administration, is metabolized primarily in skin. Small amount absorbed

into systemic circulation is metabolized primarily in liver to inactive compounds.
• *Excretion:* Inactive metabolites excreted by kidneys, primarily as glucuronides and sulfates, but also as unconjugated products. Small amounts of metabolites excreted in feces.

Contraindications and precautions
Contraindicated in patients with hypersensitivity to drug.

Interactions
None reported.

Adverse reactions
Metabolic: *hypothalamic-pituitary-adrenal axis suppression,* Cushing's syndrome, hyperglycemia, glycosuria.
Skin: burning, pruritus, irritation, dryness, erythema, folliculitis, hypertrichosis, hypopigmentation, acneiform eruptions, perioral dermatitis, allergic contact dermatitis; *maceration, secondary infection, atrophy, striae, miliaria* (with occlusive dressings).

☑ Special considerations
• Recommendations for use of fluocinonide, for care and teaching of patients during therapy, and for use in elderly patients, children, and breast-feeding women are the same as those for all topical adrenocorticoids.

Monitoring the patient
• Monitor patient for adverse effects.
• Watch for signs of systemic absorption.

Information for the patient
• Teach patient and family how to apply drug using gloves, sterile applicator, or with careful hand washing.
• Instruct patient not to leave occlusive dressings on for more than 12 hours each day, and not to use occlusive dressings on infected or exudative lesions.
• Tell patient to report skin irritation, ulceration, or infection.

---

fluorouracil (5-FU)
Adrucil, Efudex, Fluoroplex

Pharmacologic classification: antimetabolite (cell cycle–phase specific, S phase)
Therapeutic classification: antineoplastic
Pregnancy risk category D (injection), X (cream)

How supplied
Available by prescription only
Injection: 50 mg/ml in 10-ml, 20-ml, 50-ml, 100-ml vials

Reactions may be *common,* uncommon, **life-threatening**, or COMMON AND LIFE-THREATENING.

Cream: 1%, 5%
Topical solution: 1%, 2%, 5%

Indications, route, and dosage

Dosage and indications may vary. Check current literature for recommended protocol.

Palliative management of colon, rectal, breast, ◊ ovarian, ◊ cervical, gastric, ◊ bladder, ◊ liver, pancreatic cancers
Adults and children: 12 mg/kg I.V. for 4 days; then, if no toxicity occurs, give 6 mg/kg I.V. on days 6, 8, 10, and 12. Maintenance therapy is a repeated course q 30 days. Don't exceed 800 mg/day (400 mg/day in severely ill patients).

Actinic or solar keratoses
Adults: Sufficient cream or lotion to cover lesions b.i.d. for 2 to 4 weeks. Usually, 1% preparations are used on head, neck, and chest, 2% and 5% on hands.

Superficial basal cell carcinomas
Adults: 5% solution or cream in a sufficient amount to cover lesion b.i.d. for 3 to 6 weeks, up to 12 weeks.

Pharmacodynamics

Antineoplastic action: Exerts cytotoxic activity by acting as an antimetabolite, competing for the enzyme that is important in the synthesis of thymidine, an essential substrate for DNA synthesis. Therefore, DNA synthesis is inhibited. Also inhibits RNA synthesis to a lesser extent.

Pharmacokinetics

• *Absorption:* Given parenterally because absorbed poorly after oral administration.
• *Distribution:* Distributed widely into all areas of body water and tissues, including tumors, bone marrow, liver, and intestinal mucosa. Crosses blood-brain barrier to a significant extent.
• *Metabolism:* Small amount converted in tissues to active metabolite, with most of drug degraded in liver.
• *Excretion:* Metabolites primarily excreted through lungs as carbon dioxide. Small portion excreted in urine as unchanged drug.

Contraindications and precautions

Contraindicated in patients with hypersensitivity to drug and in those with bone marrow suppression (WBC counts of 5,000/mm³ or less or platelet counts of 100,000/mm³ or less) or potentially serious infections; in patients who are in a poor nutritional state; and in those who have had major surgery within the previous month.

Use cautiously in patients after high-dose pelvic radiation therapy or use of alkylating drugs. Also use with caution in patients with widespread neoplastic infiltration of bone marrow or impaired renal or hepatic function.

Interactions

Drug-drug. *Leucovorin calcium, prior treatment with alkylating drugs:* May enhance toxicity of fluorouracil. Monitor patient.
Drug-lifestyle. *Sun exposure:* May cause photosensitivity reactions. Tell patient to take precautions.

Adverse reactions

CNS: acute cerebellar syndrome, confusion, disorientation, euphoria, ataxia, headache, *weakness, malaise.*
CV: myocardial ischemia, angina.
EENT: nystagmus.
GI: *stomatitis, GI ulcer* (may precede leukopenia), *nausea, vomiting, diarrhea, anorexia,* GI bleeding.
Hematologic: *leukopenia, thrombocytopenia, agranulocytosis,* anemia; WBC count nadir 9 to 14 days after first dose; platelet count nadir in 7 to 14 days.
Metabolic: hypoalbuminemia because of drug-induced protein malabsorption.
Skin: *reversible alopecia; dermatitis; erythema; scaling; pruritus;* nail changes; pigmented palmar creases; erythematous, contact dermatitis; desquamative rash of hands and feet with long-term use ("hand-foot syndrome").
Other: *pain, burning,* soreness, suppuration, swelling (with topical use), thrombophlebitis, *anaphylaxis.*

☑ Special considerations

• Drug may be administered I.V. push over 1 to 2 minutes.
• Drug may be further diluted in D_5W or normal saline solution for infusions of up to 24 hours in duration.
• Use plastic I.V. containers for administering continuous infusions. Solution is more stable in plastic I.V. bags than in glass bottles.
• Don't use cloudy solution. If crystals form, redissolve by warming at a temperature of 140° F (60° C) with vigorous shaking. Allow solution to cool to body temperature before using.
• Use new vein site for each dose.
• Give antiemetic before administering to decrease nausea.
• Don't refrigerate fluorouracil.
• Drug can be diluted in 4 oz (120 ml) of water and administered orally; however, this isn't an FDA-approved method of administration, and absorption is erratic.
• General photosensitivity occurs for 2 to 3 months after dose.
• Apply topical drug while using plastic gloves. Wash hands immediately after handling. Avoid topical use with occlusive dressings.
• Apply topical solution with caution near eyes, nose, and mouth.
• Topical application to larger ulcerated areas may cause systemic toxicity.

• For superficial basal cell carcinoma confirmed by biopsy, use 5% strength. Apply 1% concentration on the face. Reserve higher concentrations for thicker-skinned areas or resistant lesions. Occlusion may be required.
• Don't continue to treat lesions resistant to fluorouracil; they should be biopsied.
• Signs and symptoms of overdose include myelosuppression, diarrhea, alopecia, dermatitis, hyperpigmentation, nausea, and vomiting. Treatment is usually supportive and includes transfusion of blood components, antiemetics, and antidiarrheals.

Monitoring the patient
• Monitor intake and output, CBC, and renal and hepatic function.
• Watch for extravasation; treat as a chemical phlebitis with warm compresses.
• Monitor patient for signs of serious infection.

Information for the patient
• Warn patient to avoid strong sunlight or ultraviolet light because it will intensify skin reaction. Encourage use of sunscreens.
• Tell patient to avoid exposure to people with infections. Advise patient to promptly report signs of infection or unusual bleeding.
• Reassure patient that hair should grow back after treatment ends.
• Tell patient to apply topical fluorouracil with gloves and wash hands thoroughly after application.
• Warn patient that treated area may be unsightly during therapy and for several weeks after therapy ends. Complete healing may not occur until 1 or 2 months after treatment ends.
• Advise woman of childbearing age to avoid becoming pregnant during therapy.

Breast-feeding patients
• It's unknown if drug appears in breast milk. Because of potential for serious adverse reactions, mutagenicity, and carcinogenicity in infant, breast-feeding isn't recommended.

---

fluoxetine
Prozac

Pharmacologic classification: selective serotonin reuptake inhibitor (SSRI)
Therapeutic classification: antidepressant
Pregnancy risk category C

How supplied
Available by prescription only
Capsules: 10 mg, 20 mg
Oral solution: 20 mg/5 ml

Indications, route, and dosage
Depression, ◇ panic disorder, ◇ bipolar disorder, ◇ alcohol dependence, ◇ cataplexy, ◇ myoclonus
Adults: 20 mg P.O. daily in the morning. Increase dosage, p.r.n., after several weeks to 40 mg daily with a dose in the morning and midday. Don't exceed 80 mg daily.
Obsessive-compulsive disorder
Adults: Initially, 20 mg P.O. daily. Gradually increase dosage, as needed and tolerated, to 60 to 80 mg daily.
◇ Obesity
Adults: 20 to 60 mg P.O. daily.
◇ Eating disorders
Adults: 60 to 80 mg P.O. daily.

Pharmacodynamics
Antidepressant action: Purportedly related to drug's inhibition of CNS neuronal uptake of serotonin. Blocks uptake of serotonin, but not of norepinephrine, into human platelets. Possibly a much more potent uptake inhibitor of serotonin than of norepinephrine.

Pharmacokinetics
• *Absorption:* Well absorbed after oral administration; absorption not altered by food.
• *Distribution:* Apparently highly protein-bound (about 95%).
• *Metabolism:* Metabolized primarily in liver to active metabolites.
• *Excretion:* Excreted by kidneys. Elimination half-life is 2 to 3 days. Norfluoxetine (primary active metabolite) elimination half-life of 7 to 9 days.

Contraindications and precautions
Contraindicated in patients with hypersensitivity to drug and in those taking MAO inhibitors within 14 days of starting therapy. Use cautiously in patients at high risk for suicide and in those with a history of seizures, diabetes mellitus, or renal, hepatic, or CV disease.

Interactions
Drug-drug. *Carbamazepine, flecainide, vinblastine:* May increase serum levels of these drugs. Monitor serum levels.
Cyproheptadine: May reverse or decrease pharmacologic effect. Monitor patient closely.
Insulin, oral antidiabetics: May alter blood glucose levels and possibly alter requirements for antidiabetics. Monitor serum glucose levels.
Lithium, tricyclic antidepressants: May cause increased adverse CNS effects. Monitor patient closely.
Phenytoin: May increase plasma phenytoin levels and risk of toxicity. Monitor phenytoin levels.
Tryptophan: May lead to increased adverse CNS effects (agitation, restlessness) and GI distress. Monitor patient closely.

~actions may be *common*, uncommon, **life-threatening**, or COMMON AND LIFE-THREATENING.

Warfarin, other highly protein-bound drugs: May increase plasma levels of fluoxetine or other highly protein-bound drugs. Monitor PT and INR.
Drug-lifestyle. *Alcohol:* May increase CNS depression. Discourage concomitant use.

Adverse reactions
CNS: *nervousness, anxiety, insomnia, headache, drowsiness, tremor, dizziness, asthenia,* fatigue.
CV: palpitations, hot flashes.
EENT: nasal congestion, pharyngitis, cough, sinusitis.
GI: *nausea, diarrhea, dry mouth, anorexia, dyspepsia,* constipation, abdominal pain, vomiting, flatulence, increased appetite.
GU: sexual dysfunction.
Musculoskeletal: muscle pain.
Respiratory: upper respiratory tract infection, respiratory distress.
Skin: *rash, pruritus,* diaphoresis.
Other: flulike syndrome, *weight loss,* fever.

☑ Special considerations
• Consider inherent risk of suicide until significant improvement of depressive state occurs. High-risk patients should have close supervision during initial drug therapy. To reduce risk of suicidal overdose, prescribe the smallest quantity of drug consistent with good management.
• Full antidepressant effect may be delayed until 4 weeks of treatment or longer.
• Treatment of acute depression usually requires at least several months of continuous drug therapy; optimal duration of therapy hasn't been established.
• Because of its long elimination half-life, changes in fluoxetine dosage won't be reflected in plasma for several weeks, affecting adjustment to final dose and withdrawal from treatment.
• Prescribe lower or less frequent dosages in patients with renal or hepatic impairment.
• Fluoxetine therapy may activate mania or hypomania.
• Symptoms of overdose include agitation, restlessness, hypomania, and other signs of CNS excitation, including seizures, and, in patients who took higher doses of fluoxetine, nausea and vomiting. Death has occurred. To treat, establish and maintain an airway; ensure adequate oxygenation and ventilation. Activated charcoal, which may be used with sorbitol, may be as effective as emesis or lavage.
• In overdose, monitor cardiac and vital signs, and provide the usual supportive measures. Fluoxetine-induced seizures that don't subside spontaneously may respond to diazepam. Forced diuresis, dialysis, hemoperfusion, and exchange transfusion are unlikely to be of benefit.

Monitoring the patient
• Monitor patient closely for risk of suicide before and during treatment.
• Monitor patient for adverse effects.

Information for the patient
• Inform patient that drug may cause dizziness or drowsiness. Patient should avoid hazardous tasks that require alertness until CNS response to drug is established.
• Caution patient to avoid ingestion of alcohol and to seek medical approval before taking other drugs.
• Tell patient to promptly report rash or hives, anxiety, nervousness, anorexia (especially in underweight patients), suspicion of pregnancy, or intent to become pregnant.

Geriatric patients
• Consider lower or less frequent dosages in elderly patients and others with concurrent disease or multiple drug therapy.

fluoxymesterone
Halotestin

Pharmacologic classification: androgen
Therapeutic classification: androgen replacement, antineoplastic
Controlled substance schedule III
Pregnancy risk category X

How supplied
Available by prescription only
Tablets: 2 mg, 5 mg, 10 mg

Indications, route, and dosage
Male hypogonadism
Adults: 5 to 20 mg P.O. daily in a single dose or in three or four divided doses.
Palliation of breast cancer in women
Adults: 10 to 40 mg P.O. daily in three or four divided doses.
Postpartum breast engorgement
Adults: 2.5 mg P.O. shortly after parturition; then 5 to 10 mg daily for 4 to 5 days in divided doses.
Vasomotor symptoms associated with menopause
Adults: 1 to 2 mg P.O. b.i.d. combined with ethinyl estradiol 0.02 or 0.04 mg P.O. b.i.d. for 21 days; then 7 days without drug. Repeat regimen when necessary.
Delayed puberty
Males: 2.5 to 20 mg daily. Most patients respond to dosages of 2.5 to 10 mg daily.

Pharmacodynamics
Androgenic action: Mimics action of the endogenous androgen testosterone by stimulating receptors in androgen-responsive organs and tissues. Exerts inhibitory, antiestrogenic effects

on hormone-responsive breast tumors and metastases.

Antianemic action: Enhances production of erythropoietic stimulating factors, thereby increasing production of RBCs.

Pharmacokinetics
- *Absorption:* No information available.
- *Distribution:* No information available.
- *Metabolism:* Eliminated primarily by hepatic metabolism.
- *Excretion:* No information available.

Contraindications and precautions
Contraindicated in patients with hypersensitivity to drug, in men with breast cancer or prostate cancer, in patients with cardiac, hepatic, or renal decompensation; during pregnancy; and in breast-feeding women.

Use cautiously in prepubertal boys and patients with benign prostatic hyperplasia or aspirin sensitivity.

Interactions
Drug-drug. *Anticoagulants:* Concomitant use may potentiate action. Monitor INR.
Hepatotoxic drugs: May increase risk of hepatotoxicity. Monitor patient closely.
Insulin, oral antidiabetics: Decreased blood glucose levels may need dosage adjustment. Monitor serum glucose levels.

Adverse reactions
CNS: headache, anxiety, depression, paresthesia, sleep apnea syndrome.
CV: edema.
GI: nausea.
GU: *hypoestrogenic effects in women (flushing; diaphoresis; vaginitis, including itching, dryness, and burning; vaginal bleeding; nervousness; emotional lability; menstrual irregularities); excessive hormonal effects in men* (prepubertal—*premature epiphyseal closure,* acne, *priapism, growth of body and facial hair,* phallic enlargement; postpubertal—*testicular atrophy, oligospermia,* decreased ejaculatory volume, impotence, gynecomastia, epididymitis).
Hematologic: polycythemia, elevated serum lipid levels, suppression of clotting factors, prolonged PT and INR.
Hepatic: reversible jaundice, *peliosis,* cholestatic hepatitis, elevated liver enzymes, *liver cell tumors.*
Metabolic: elevated serum sodium, potassium, calcium, phosphate, and cholesterol levels.
Skin: hypersensitivity skin manifestations.
Other: androgenic effects in women (acne, edema, *weight gain, hirsutism,* hoarseness, clitoral enlargement, deepening voice, *decreased breast size,* changes in libido, male-pattern baldness, *oily skin or hair).*

☑ Special considerations
Besides the recommendations relevant to all androgens, consider the following.
- Observe women carefully for signs of excessive virilization. If possible, stop drug at first sign of virilization because some adverse effects (deepening of voice, clitoral enlargement) aren't reversible.
- Patients with metastatic breast cancer should have regular determinations of serum calcium levels to identify potential for serious hypercalcemia.
- When drug is used in breast cancer, subjective effects may not appear for about 1 month; objective improvement not for 3 months.
- Halotestin contains tartrazine. Observe for signs of allergic reactions in patients sensitive to aspirin or tartrazine.
- Women with an intact uterus receiving drug with ethinyl estradiol must be monitored closely for endometrial carcinoma. Rule out malignancy if recurrent vaginal bleeding occurs.
- Fluoxymesterone may cause abnormal results of glucose tolerance test. Thyroid function test results (protein-bound iodine [131] uptake, thyroid-binding capacity) may decrease.

Monitoring the patient
- Monitor hepatic function before therapy starts and periodically during therapy.
- Monitor serum calcium level before therapy starts and periodically during therapy.
- Monitor serum blood glucose level if patient takes oral antidiabetics.
- Monitor serum coagulation studies if patient takes oral anticoagulants.
- In children, monitor X-rays frequently to evaluate closure of epiphyses.

Information for the patient
- Explain to patient taking drug for palliation of breast cancer that virilization usually occurs at dosage used. Tell patient to report androgenic effects immediately. Stopping drug will prevent further androgenic changes but probably won't reverse those already present.
- Tell woman to report menstrual irregularities and to stop therapy pending etiologic determination.
- Advise man to report overly frequent or persistent penile erections.
- Advise patient to report persistent GI distress, diarrhea, or onset of jaundice.

Geriatric patients
- Use with caution. Observe elderly men for prostatic hyperplasia. Development of symptomatic prostatic hyperplasia or prostatic cancer requires stopping drug.

Pediatric patients
- Use with extreme caution in children to avoid precocious puberty and premature closure of epi-

---

Reactions may be *common,* uncommon, *life-threatening,* or **COMMON AND LIFE-THREATENING.**

physes. X-ray examinations every 6 months are recommended to assess skeletal maturation.

Breast-feeding patients
• It's unknown if drug appears in breast milk. Because of potential adverse effects on infant, a decision should be made to stop either breast-feeding or drug, depending on patient's need for drug.

fluphenazine decanoate
Modecate*, Prolixin Decanoate

fluphenazine enanthate
Moditen Enanthate*, Prolixin Enanthate

fluphenazine hydrochloride
Permitil, Prolixin

Pharmacologic classification: phenothiazine (piperazine derivative)
Therapeutic classification: antipsychotic
Pregnancy risk category NR

How supplied
Available by prescription only
fluphenazine decanoate
Depot injection: 25 mg/ml
fluphenazine enanthate
Depot injection: 25 mg/ml
fluphenazine hydrochloride
Tablets: 1 mg, 2.5 mg, 5 mg, 10 mg
Oral concentrate: 5 mg/ml (Prolixin contains 14% alcohol and Permitil contains 1% alcohol)
Elixir: 2.5 mg/5 ml (with 14% alcohol)
I.M. injection: 2.5 mg/ml

Indications, route, and dosage
Psychotic disorders
Adults: Initially, 0.5 to 10 mg fluphenazine hydrochloride P.O. daily in divided doses q 6 to 8 hours; may increase cautiously to 20 mg. Maintenance dose is 1 to 5 mg P.O. daily. I.M. doses are one-third to one-half that of oral doses (starting dose is 1.25 mg I.M.).
✦ *Dosage adjustment.* Use lower doses for elderly patients (1 to 2.5 mg daily).

Pharmacodynamics
Antipsychotic action: Thought to exert antipsychotic effects by postsynaptic blockade of CNS dopamine receptors, thereby inhibiting dopamine-mediated effects. Has many other central and peripheral effects; produces both alpha and ganglionic blockade and counteracts histamine- and serotonin-mediated activity. Most prominent adverse reactions are extrapyramidal.

Pharmacokinetics
• *Absorption:* Rate and extent of absorption vary with route of administration; oral tablet absorption is erratic and variable. Oral and I.M. dosages have onset of action within 1 hour. Long-acting decanoate and enanthate salts act within 24 to 72 hours.
• *Distribution:* Distributed widely into body, including breast milk. CNS levels usually higher than those in plasma. 91% to 99% protein-bound. Effects of oral dose usually peak at 2 hours; steady-state serum levels achieved within 4 to 7 days.
• *Metabolism:* Metabolized extensively by liver, but no active metabolites formed; duration of action about 6 to 8 hours after oral administration; 1 to 6 weeks (average, 2 weeks) after I.M. depot administration.
• *Excretion:* Mostly excreted in urine via kidneys; some excreted in feces via biliary tract.

Contraindications and precautions
Contraindicated in patients with hypersensitivity to drug and in patients experiencing coma, CNS depression, bone marrow suppression or other blood dyscrasia, subcortical damage, or liver damage.

Use cautiously in elderly or debilitated patients and in those with pheochromocytoma, severe CV disease, peptic ulcer disease, exposure to extreme hot or cold (including antipyretic therapy), phosphorus insecticides, respiratory or seizure disorders, hypocalcemia, severe reaction to insulin or electroconvulsive therapy, mitral insufficiency, glaucoma, or prostatic hyperplasia. Use parenteral form cautiously in patients with asthma and in those allergic to sulfites.

Interactions
Drug-drug. *Antacids and antidiarrheals containing aluminum and magnesium; phenobarbital:* Possible pharmacokinetic alterations and subsequent decreased therapeutic response to fluphenazine. Enhanced renal excretion with phenobarbital; decreased absorption with antacids and antidiarrheals. Avoid concomitant use.
Antiarrhythmics, disopyramide, procainamide, quinidine: May result in additive effects, such as increased risk of arrhythmias and conduction defects. Avoid concomitant use.
Atropine, other anticholinergics (such as antidepressants, antihistamines, antiparkinsonians, MAO inhibitors, meperidine, phenothiazines): May result in oversedation, paralytic ileus, visual changes, and severe constipation. Avoid concomitant use.
Beta blockers: May inhibit fluphenazine metabolism, increasing plasma levels and toxicity. Monitor plasma levels closely.
Bromocriptine: May antagonize therapeutic effect on prolactin secretion. Avoid concomitant use.

Centrally acting antihypertensives (such as cloni-dine, guanabenz, guanadrel, guanethidine, meth-yldopa, reserpine): May inhibit blood pressure response to these drugs. Avoid concomitant use.
CNS depressants (such as analgesics; barbitu-rates; epidural, general, or spinal anesthetics; narcotics; parenteral magnesium sulfate; tran-quilizers): May result in additive effects. Avoid concomitant use.
Dopamine: Concomitant use may decrease vaso-constricting effects of high-dose regimen; may decrease effectiveness. Use cautiously togeth-er; monitor patient closely.
Levodopa: May increase toxicity (by dopamine blockade). Monitor patient closely.
Lithium: May result in severe neurologic toxicity with encephalitis-like syndrome, and decreased therapeutic response to fluphenazine. Monitor patient closely.
Metrizamide: Concomitant use may increase risk of seizures. Avoid concomitant use, but monitor closely if drug must be used.
Nitrates: May produce hypotension. Avoid con-comitant use.
Phenytoin, tricyclic antidepressants: May inhibit metabolism and increase toxicity of these drugs. Avoid concomitant use.
Propylthiouracil: Increased risk of agranulocyto-sis. Monitor patient closely.
Sympathomimetics (such as appetite suppres-sants, ephedrine, epinephrine, phenylephrine, phenylpropanolamine): May decrease their stim-ulatory and pressor effects. Avoid concomitant use.
Drug-food. *Caffeine:* May increase metabo-lism of fluphenazine. Discourage concomitant use.
Drug-lifestyle. *Alcohol:* May increase CNS de-pression. Discourage concomitant use.
Smoking: May increase drug metabolism. Dis-courage concomitant use.
Sun exposure: May increase risk of photosensi-tivity. Tell patient to take precautions.

Adverse reactions
CNS: *extrapyramidal reactions, tardive dyskine-sia, sedation, pseudoparkinsonism, EEG changes, drowsiness, **seizures,** dizziness.*
CV: *orthostatic hypotension,* tachycardia, ECG changes.
EENT: ocular changes, *blurred vision,* nasal con-gestion.
GI: *dry mouth, constipation.*
GU: *urine retention,* dark urine, menstrual irreg-ularities, gynecomastia, inhibited ejaculation.
Hematologic: *leukopenia, agranulocytosis,* eosinophilia, hemolytic anemia, **aplastic ane-mia, thrombocytopenia.**
Hepatic: cholestatic jaundice, abnormal liver func-tion test results.
Metabolic: elevated protein-bound iodine, weight gain, increased appetite.

Skin: *mild photosensitivity, **allergic reactions.***
After abrupt withdrawal of long-term ther-apy: gastritis, nausea, vomiting, dizziness, tremor, feeling of warmth or cold, diaphoresis, tachycar-dia, headache, insomnia.

☑ Special considerations
Besides the recommendations relevant to all phe-nothiazines, consider the following.
● Note that depot injection (25 mg/ml) and I.M. injection (2.5 mg/ml) aren't interchangeable.
● Depot injection isn't recommended for patients who aren't stabilized on a phenothiazine. This form has a prolonged elimination; its action couldn't be terminated if adverse reactions occur.
● Fluphenazine elevates test results for liver en-zymes and causes quinidine-like ECG effects.
● Fluphenazine causes false-positive test results for urinary porphyrins, urobilinogen, amylase, and 5-hydroxyindoleacetic acid because of darken-ing of urine by metabolites. Also causes false-positive urine pregnancy test results using hu-man chorionic gonadotropin.
● Overdose causes CNS depression character-ized by deep, unarousable sleep and possible coma. Other symptoms include hypotension or hypertension, extrapyramidal symptoms, dysto-nia, abnormal involuntary muscle movements, agitation, seizures, arrhythmias, ECG changes, hypothermia or hyperthermia, and autonomic nervous system dysfunction.
● Treatment of overdose is symptomatic and sup-portive, including maintaining vital signs, airway, stable body temperature, and fluid and electrolyte balance.
● In overdose, don't induce vomiting; drug inhibits cough reflex, and aspiration may occur. Use gas-tric lavage, then activated charcoal and saline cathartics; dialysis doesn't help. Regulate body temperature as needed. Treat hypotension with I.V. fluids; don't give epinephrine. Treat seizures with parenteral diazepam or barbiturates; ar-rhythmias with parenteral phenytoin (1 mg/kg with rate titrated to blood pressure); extrapyramidal reactions with benztropine 1 to 2 mg or parenteral diphenhydramine at 10 to 50 mg.

Monitoring the patient
● Monitor CBC and hepatic function before ther-apy starts and periodically throughout.
● Monitor patient for adverse effects.

Information for the patient
● Inform patient that drug may cause dizziness or drowsiness. Patient should avoid hazardous tasks that require alertness until CNS response to drug is established.
● Tell patient to avoid alcohol and to seek med-ical approval before taking other drugs.
● Instruct patient to promptly report rash or hives, anxiety, nervousness, anorexia (especially in un-

derweight patients), suspicion of pregnancy, or intent to become pregnant.

Pediatric patients
• Safety and efficacy in children under age 12 haven't been established.

Breast-feeding patients
• Drug appears in breast milk. Use with caution; potential benefits to mother should outweigh potential harm to infant.

flurandrenolide
Cordran, Cordran SP, Drenison*

Pharmacologic classification: topical adrenocorticoid
Therapeutic classification: anti-inflammatory
Pregnancy risk category C

How supplied
Available by prescription only
Cream: 0.025%, 0.05%
Lotion: 0.05%
Ointment: 0.025%, 0.05%
Tape: 4 mcg/cm²

Indications, route, and dosage
Inflammation of corticosteroid-responsive dermatoses
Adults and children: Apply cream, lotion, or ointment sparingly daily to q.i.d. Apply tape q 12 hours.
    Occlusive dressings may be used for severe or resistant dermatoses. The tape is usually applied as an occlusive dressing to clean, dry, affected areas.

Pharmacodynamics
Anti-inflammatory action: Stimulates synthesis of enzymes needed to decrease the inflammatory response. A group III (0.05%, 0.025%) fluorinated glucocorticoid.

Pharmacokinetics
• *Absorption:* Amount absorbed depends on strength of preparation, amount applied, and nature and condition of skin at application site. Ranges from about 1% in areas with thick stratum corneum (such as palms, soles, elbows, and knees) to as high as 36% in areas of thinnest stratum corneum (face, eyelids, and genitals). Absorption increases in areas of skin damage, inflammation, or occlusion. Some systemic absorption may occur, especially through oral mucosa.
• *Distribution:* After topical application, distributed throughout local skin. Any drug absorbed into circulation is removed rapidly from blood and

distributed into muscle, liver, skin, intestines, and kidneys.
• *Metabolism:* After topical administration, metabolized primarily in skin. Small amount absorbed into systemic circulation metabolized primarily in liver to inactive compounds.
• *Excretion:* Inactive metabolites excreted by kidneys, primarily as glucuronides and sulfates, but also as unconjugated products. Small amounts of metabolites also excreted in feces.

Contraindications and precautions
Contraindicated in patients with hypersensitivity to drug.

Interactions
None reported.

Adverse reactions
Metabolic: hyperglycemia, glucosuria, *hypothalamic-pituitary-adrenal axis suppression,* Cushing's syndrome.
Skin: burning, pruritus, irritation, dryness, erythema, folliculitis, hypertrichosis, hypopigmentation, acneiform eruptions, allergic contact dermatitis; *maceration, secondary infection, atrophy, striae, miliaria* (with occlusive dressings); purpura, stripping of epidermis, furunculosis (with tape).

☑ Special considerations
• Recommendations for use of flurandrenolide, for care and teaching of patients during therapy, and for use in elderly patients, children, and breast-feeding women are the same as those for all topical adrenocorticoids.

Monitoring the patient
• Monitor patient for adverse effects.
• Watch for signs of systemic absorption.

Information for the patient
• Teach patient and family how to apply drug.
• Instruct patient not to leave occlusive dressing in place for more than 12 hours each day.
• Tell patient to report signs of systemic absorption, skin irritation, hypersensitivity, or infection.

flurazepam hydrochloride
Apo-Flurazepam*, Dalmane, Novo-Flupam*

Pharmacologic classification: benzodiazepine
Therapeutic classification: sedative-hypnotic
Controlled substance schedule IV
Pregnancy risk category X

How supplied
Available by prescription only
Capsules: 15 mg, 30 mg

Indications, route, and dosage
Insomnia
Adults: 15 to 30 mg P.O. h.s.
✦ *Dosage adjustment.* In patients over age 65, 15 mg P.O. h.s.

Pharmacodynamics
Sedative action: Depresses the CNS at the limbic and subcortical levels of the brain. Produces a sedative effect by potentiating the effect of the neurotransmitter gamma-aminobutyric acid on its receptor in the ascending reticular activating system, which increases inhibition and blocks both cortical and limbic arousal.

Pharmacokinetics
Absorption: When administered orally, flurazepam is absorbed rapidly through the GI tract. Onset of action occurs within 20 minutes, with peak action in 1 to 2 hours. Duration of action is 7 to 10 hours.
Distribution: Distributed widely throughout the body. About 97% of administered dose is bound to plasma protein.
Metabolism: Metabolized in the liver to the active metabolite desalkylflurazepam.
Excretion: Desalkylflurazepam is excreted in urine; half-life is 50 to 100 hours.

Contraindications and precautions
Contraindicated in patients with hypersensitivity to drug and during pregnancy. Use cautiously in patients with impaired renal or hepatic function, chronic pulmonary insufficiency, mental depression, suicidal tendencies, or history of drug abuse.

Interactions
Drug-drug. *Antidepressants, antihistamines, barbiturates, general anesthetics, MAO inhibitors, narcotics, phenothiazines:* May potentiate CNS depressant effects. Avoid concomitant use.
Cimetidine, disulfiram, isoniazid, oral contraceptives, ritonavir: May decrease metabolism of benzodiazepines, leading to toxicity. Monitor patient closely.
Digoxin: Serum levels may increase, resulting in toxicity. Monitor digoxin levels.
Haloperidol: Decreased plasma levels of this drug. Avoid concomitant use.
Levodopa: Decreased therapeutic effects of levodopa. Avoid concomitant use.
Phenytoin: May increase phenytoin levels. Monitor phenytoin levels.
Rifampin: May enhance metabolism of benzodiazepines. Use cautiously together.
Theophylline: May act as antagonist with flurazepam. Use cautiously together.
Drug-lifestyle. *Alcohol:* May cause excessive CNS and respiratory depression. Discourage concomitant use.

Heavy smoking: Accelerated metabolism of flurazepam, lowering clinical effectiveness. Discourage concomitant use.

Adverse reactions
CNS: *daytime sedation, dizziness, drowsiness, disturbed coordination,* lethargy, confusion, *headache,* light-headedness, nervousness, hallucinations, staggering, ataxia, disorientation, changes in EEG patterns, *coma,* physical or psychological dependence.
GI: nausea, vomiting, heartburn, diarrhea, abdominal pain.
Hepatic: elevated liver enzyme levels.

☑ Special considerations
Besides the recommendations relevant to all benzodiazepines, consider the following.
● Drug has shown a carryover effect, being most effective after 3 or 4 nights of use because of long half-life. Don't increase dose more frequently than every 5 days.
● Drug is useful for patients who have trouble falling asleep and who awaken frequently at night and early in the morning.
● Although prolonged use isn't recommended, this drug has proven effective for up to 4 weeks of continuous use.
● Rapid withdrawal after prolonged use can cause withdrawal symptoms.
● Lower doses are effective in patients with renal or hepatic dysfunction.
● Signs and symptoms of overdose include somnolence, confusion, hypoactive reflexes, dyspnea, labored breathing, hypotension, bradycardia, slurred speech, unsteady gait or impaired coordination and, eventually, coma. Support blood pressure and respiration until drug effects subside; monitor vital signs. Mechanical ventilatory assistance via endotracheal (ET) tube may be required to maintain a patent airway and support adequate oxygenation. Use I.V. fluids to promote diuresis and vasopressors such as dopamine and phenylephrine to treat hypotension, as needed. Flumazenil, a specific benzodiazepine antagonist, may be useful as an adjunct to supportive therapy.
● If patient is conscious, induce emesis. Use gastric lavage if ingestion was recent, but only if ET tube is present to prevent aspiration. After emesis or lavage, administer activated charcoal with a cathartic as a single dose. Dialysis is of limited value. Don't use barbiturates if excitation occurs to avoid exacerbation of excitatory state or potentiation of CNS depressant effects.

Monitoring the patient
● If patient is of childbearing age, rule out pregnancy before treatment.
● Monitor hepatic function and AST, ALT, bilirubin, and alkaline phosphatase levels for changes.

Information for the patient
• Warn patient to avoid alcohol while taking drug.
• Advise woman not to take drug if pregnant. Tell her to call immediately if she suspects pregnancy.
• Emphasize potential for excessive CNS depression if drug is taken with alcohol, even if it's taken the evening before alcohol ingestion.
• Advise patient that rebound insomnia may occur after stopping drug.
• Warn patient not to stop drug abruptly after prolonged therapy.
• Advise patient not to exceed prescribed dosage.

Geriatric patients
• Elderly patients are more susceptible to CNS depressant effects of flurazepam. They may require assistance and supervision with walking and daily activities during start of therapy or after a dosage increase.
• Lower doses usually are effective in elderly patients because of decreased elimination.

Pediatric patients
• Closely observe neonate for withdrawal symptoms if mother took flurazepam during pregnancy. Use of flurazepam during labor may cause neonatal flaccidity.
• Drug isn't recommended for use in children under age 15.
• Neonates are more sensitive to flurazepam because of slower metabolism; possibility of toxicity is greatly increased.

Breast-feeding patients
• Drug appears in breast milk. A breast-fed infant may become sedated, have feeding difficulties, or lose weight. Avoid use in breast-feeding women.

---

flurbiprofen
Ansaid

Pharmacologic classification: NSAID, phenylalkanoic acid derivative
Therapeutic classification: antarthritic
Pregnancy risk category B

How supplied
Available by prescription only
Tablets: 50 mg, 100 mg

Indications, route, and dosage
Rheumatoid arthritis and osteoarthritis
Adults: 200 to 300 mg P.O. daily, divided b.i.d., t.i.d., or q.i.d.
✦ Dosage adjustment. Patients with end-stage renal disease may exhibit accumulation of flurbiprofen metabolites, but half-life of parent compound is unchanged. Monitor patient closely and adjust dosage accordingly.

Pharmacodynamics
Anti-inflammatory action: An NSAID that interferes with the synthesis of prostaglandins.

Pharmacokinetics
• *Absorption:* Well absorbed after oral administration, with levels peaking in about 1½ hours. Food alters rate but not extent of absorption.
• *Distribution:* More than 99% bound to plasma proteins.
• *Metabolism:* Metabolized primarily in liver. Major metabolite shows little anti-inflammatory activity.
• *Excretion:* Excreted primarily in urine. Average elimination half-life is 6 to 10 hours.

Contraindications and precautions
Contraindicated in patients with hypersensitivity to drug or history of aspirin- or NSAID-induced asthma, urticaria, or other allergic-type reactions. Use cautiously in elderly or debilitated patients and in those with history of peptic ulcer disease, herpes simplex keratitis, impaired renal or hepatic function, cardiac disease, or conditions associated with fluid retention.

Interactions
Drug-drug. *Aspirin:* May decrease flurbiprofen levels and increase GI toxicity. Monitor patient closely.
Beta blockers: Impaired antihypertensive effect. Monitor blood pressure.
Cyclosporine: Increased risk of nephrotoxicity. Avoid concomitant use.
Diuretics: Decreased diuretic effect. Monitor patient.
Lithium: Increased serum lithium levels. Monitor lithium levels.
Methotrexate: Increased risk of methotrexate toxicity. Monitor patient closely.
Oral anticoagulants: Increased PT and INR. Monitor patient closely.
Drug-lifestyle. *Alcohol:* May increase risk of adverse GI reactions. Discourage concomitant use.
Sun exposure: May potentiate photosensitivity reactions. Tell patient to take precautions.

Adverse reactions
CNS: *headache,* anxiety, insomnia, dizziness, increased reflexes, tremors, amnesia, asthenia, drowsiness, malaise, depression.
CV: *edema, heart failure,* hypertension, vasodilation.
EENT: rhinitis, tinnitus, visual changes, epistaxis.
GI: *dyspepsia, diarrhea, abdominal pain, nausea,* constipation, *bleeding,* flatulence, vomiting.
GU: *symptoms suggesting urinary tract infection,* hematuria, interstitial nephritis, *renal failure.*
Hematologic: *thrombocytopenia, neutropenia,* anemia, *aplastic anemia.*

Hepatic: *elevated liver enzyme levels, jaundice.*
Metabolic: weight changes.
Respiratory: asthma.
Skin: rash, photosensitivity, urticaria.
Other: *angioedema.*

☑ Special considerations
Besides the recommendations relevant to all NSAIDs, consider the following.
• Overdose has resulted in lethargy, coma, respiratory depression, epigastric pain and distress. Treatment should be supportive. Emptying stomach by emesis or lavage would be of little use if ingestion took place more than an hour before treatment, but is still recommended.

Monitoring the patient
• Closely monitor patient with impaired hepatic or renal function and elderly or debilitated patients; they may need lower doses. These patients may be at risk for renal toxicity. Periodically monitor renal function.
• Patients receiving long-term therapy should have periodic liver function studies, ophthalmologic and auditory examinations, and hematocrit determinations.

Information for the patient
• Teach patient signs and symptoms of GI bleeding; tell him to stop drug and call promptly if these occur.
• Tell patient to take drug with food, milk, or antacid to minimize GI upset.
• Advise patient to avoid hazardous activities that require alertness until the adverse CNS effects of drug are known.
• Tell patient to immediately report edema, substantial weight gain, black stools, rash, itching, or visual disturbances.

Pediatric patients
• Safe use in children hasn't been established.

Breast-feeding patients
• A breast-feeding woman taking 200 mg of flurbiprofen daily could deliver as much as 0.1 mg to infant daily. Breast-feeding isn't recommended while using drug.

flurbiprofen sodium
Ocufen Liquifilm

Pharmacologic classification: NSAID
Therapeutic classification: ophthalmic anti-inflammatory, antimiotic
Pregnancy risk category C

How supplied
Available by prescription only
Ophthalmic solution: 0.03%

Indications, route, and dosage
Inhibition of intraoperative miosis
Adults: Instill 1 drop into the eye undergoing surgery about q 30 minutes, beginning 2 hours before surgery. Give a total of 4 drops.

Pharmacodynamics
Anti-inflammatory action: Acts by inhibiting the cyclooxygenase enzyme essential in converting arachidonic acid to prostaglandin. When applied topically, it inhibits prostaglandin synthesis in the iris, ciliary body, and conjunctiva. Doesn't affect intraocular pressure or tonographic aqueous outflow resistance.
Antimiotic action: Inhibits or reduces miosis and possibly some manifestations of ocular inflammation induced by ocular trauma. When administered prophylactically, topical flurbiprofen inhibits intraoperative trauma-induced miosis. However, drug has little, if any, effect if administered after trauma-induced miosis is present. Doesn't inhibit or reduce light-induced miosis.

Pharmacokinetics
• *Absorption:* No information available on absorption after ophthalmic administration.
• *Distribution:* At least 99% bound to plasma proteins. Unknown if drug crosses placenta or is distributed into breast milk.
• *Metabolism:* After ophthalmic administration, absorbed systemically; metabolized primarily in liver where converted mainly to inactive glucuronide and sulfate compounds.
• *Excretion:* Inactive metabolites excreted by kidneys, primarily as glucuronides and sulfates. Biological half-life of orally administered flurbiprofen is 6 to 10 hours.

Contraindications and precautions
Contraindicated in patients with hypersensitivity to drug. Use cautiously in patients with history of herpes simplex keratitis, aspirin or NSAID allergy, bleeding tendencies, and those receiving drug that may prolong clotting times.

Interactions
Drug-drug. *Acetylcholine, carbachol:* May be rendered ineffective. Avoid use together.
Anticoagulants: May increase risk of bleeding if significant systemic absorption. Monitor patient closely.

Adverse reactions
EENT: transient burning and stinging on instillation, ocular irritation.

☑ Special considerations
• Store away from heat in a dark, tightly closed container; protect drug from freezing.

Monitoring the patient
• Monitor patient for adverse effects.

Information for the patient
• Teach patient not to touch eye dropper to eye.
• Remind patient to keep drug container closed tightly.
• Advise patient not to use more drug than amount prescribed or to use flurbiprofen for other eye problems unless prescribed.
• Instruct patient to discard drug when outdated or no longer needed.

Pediatric patients
• Safety and efficacy in children haven't been established.

flutamide
Eulexin

Pharmacologic classification: nonsteroidal antiandrogen
Therapeutic classification: antineoplastic
Pregnancy risk category D

How supplied
Available by prescription only
Capsules: 125 mg

Indications, route, and dosage
Treatment of metastatic prostatic carcinoma (stage D2) with luteinizing hormone–releasing hormone analogues such as leuprolide acetate
Adults: 250 mg P.O. q 8 hours.

Pharmacodynamics
Antitumor action: Inhibits androgen uptake or prevents binding of androgens in nucleus of cells within target tissues. Prostatic carcinoma is known to be androgen-sensitive.

Pharmacokinetics
• *Absorption:* Rapidly and completely absorbed after oral administration.
• *Distribution:* Drug concentrates in prostate. Drug and active metabolite about 95% protein-bound.
• *Metabolism:* Rapidly metabolized; at least six metabolites identified. More than 97% of drug metabolized within 1 hour of administration.
• *Excretion:* More than 95% excreted in urine.

Contraindications and precautions
Contraindicated in patients with hypersensitivity to drug.

Interactions
None reported.

Adverse reactions
CNS: *drowsiness, confusion, depression, anxiety, nervousness.*
CV: *peripheral edema, hypertension.*
GI: *diarrhea, nausea, vomiting.*
GU: *impotence, loss of libido.*
Hematologic: anemia, **leukopenia, thrombocytopenia,** hemolytic anemia.
Hepatic: elevated liver enzyme levels, ***hepatitis.***
Skin: rash, photosensitivity.
Other: *hot flashes,* gynecomastia.

☑ Special considerations
• Flutamide must be taken continuously with drug used for medical castration (such as leuprolide acetate) to produce full benefit of therapy. Leuprolide suppresses testosterone production, while flutamide inhibits testosterone action at cellular level. Together, they can impair androgen-responsive tumor growth.
• Elevation of plasma testosterone and estradiol levels has been reported.
• Dosage as high as 1,500 mg daily for 36 weeks has been used without serious adverse effects.

Monitoring the patient
• Monitor serum ALT, AST, bilirubin, and creatinine levels.
• Monitor patient for adverse effects.

Information for the patient
• Tell patient not to stop either leuprolide or flutamide without medical approval.
• Explain that some symptoms may worsen initially before they improve.

Pediatric patients
• Safe use in children hasn't been established.

Breast-feeding patients
• It's unknown if drug appears in breast milk. Avoid use in breast-feeding women.

fluticasone propionate
Cutivate, Flonase, Flovent

Pharmacologic classification: corticosteroid
Therapeutic classification: topical/inhalation anti-inflammatory
Pregnancy risk category C

How supplied
Available by prescription only
Cream: 0.05%
Ointment: 0.005%
Metered nasal spray: 50 mcg/actuation
Inhalation aerosol: 44 mcg/actuation, 110 mcg/actuation, 220 mcg/actuation
Inhalation powder: 50-mcg, 100-mcg, 250-mcg Rotadisk

Indications, route, and dosage
Relief of inflammation and pruritus of corticosteroid-responsive dermatoses
Adults: Apply sparingly to affected area b.i.d. and rub in gently and completely.
Allergic rhinitis
Adults: Two sprays in each nostril once daily or one spray b.i.d.
Management of nasal symptoms of seasonal and perennial allergic rhinitis in children
Adolescents and children ages 4 and older: Initially, one spray (50 mcg) in each nostril once daily. If patient doesn't respond or symptoms are severe, increase to two sprays in each nostril daily. Once adequate control is achieved, decrease dosage to one spray in each nostril daily. Maximum dose is two sprays in each nostril daily.
Maintenance treatment of asthma as prophylactic therapy
Adults and children ages 12 and older: 88 to 220 mcg inhalation aerosol b.i.d., adjusting to maximum 440 mcg inhalation aerosol b.i.d.
Adults and adolescents: 100 mcg inhalation powder b.i.d., adjusting to maximum 500 mcg inhalation powder b.i.d.
Children ages 4 to 11: 50 mcg inhalation powder b.i.d., adjusting to maximum 100 mcg inhalation powder b.i.d.
    See package insert for dosing considerations with oral corticosteroids.

Pharmacodynamics
Anti-inflammatory action: Stimulates synthesis of enzymes needed to decrease inflammation.

Pharmacokinetics
• *Absorption:* Amount of drug absorbed depends on amount applied, application site, vehicle used, use of occlusive dressing, and integrity of epidermal barrier. Some systemic absorption occurs.
• *Distribution:* Distributed throughout local skin.
• *Metabolism:* Metabolized primarily by skin. Absorbed drug extensively metabolized by liver.
• *Excretion:* Less than 5% excreted in urine as metabolites; rest excreted in feces as parent drug and metabolites.

Contraindications and precautions
Contraindicated in patients with hypersensitivity to drug or its components and in those with viral, fungal, herpetic, or tubercular skin lesions.
    Flovent inhalation aerosol and powder are contraindicated as the primary treatment in status asthmaticus or other acute episodes of asthma in which intensive measures are required.
    Use care when transferring patients from systemically active corticosteroids to Flovent inhalation aerosol or powder because deaths have occurred in asthmatic patients during and after transfer from systemic corticosteroids to less systemically available inhalation corticosteroids. During periods of stress or severe asthma attack, patients who have been withdrawn from systemic corticosteroids should be instructed to resume oral corticosteroids in large doses immediately and to call for further medical assistance.

Interactions
Drug-drug. *Ketoconazole:* May result in increased mean fluticasone levels. Use caution when fluticasone is administered with long-term ketoconazole and other known cytochrome P-450 3A4 inhibitors.

Adverse reactions
CNS: dizziness, giddiness.
GU: dysmenorrhea.
Metabolic: *hypothalamic-pituitary-adrenal axis suppression,* hyperglycemia, glycosuria, Cushing's syndrome.
Musculoskeletal: pain in joints, sprain or strain aches and pains, pain in limbs.
Respiratory: bronchitis, chest congestion.
Skin: stinging, burning, pruritus, irritation, dryness, erythema, folliculitis, skin atrophy, leukoderma, vesicles, numbness of fingers, rash, hypertrichosis, acneiform eruptions, hypopigmentation, perioral dermatitis, allergic contact dermatitis, secondary infection, striae, miliaria.
Other: fever.

☑ Special considerations
• Don't use for treatment of rosacea, perioral dermatitis, or acne.
• Mixing with other bases or vehicles may affect potency far beyond expectations.
• During withdrawal from oral corticosteroids, some patients may experience symptoms of systemically active corticosteroid withdrawal, such as joint or musculoskeletal pain, malaise, and depression, despite maintenance or improvement of respiratory function.
• Flovent inhalation aerosol and powder aren't indicated for relief of acute bronchospasm.

Monitoring the patient
• Because of possible systemic absorption of inhalation corticosteroids, patients treated with these drugs should be observed carefully for any evidence of systemic corticosteroid effects. Special care should be taken during periods of stress or postoperatively for adrenal insufficiency.
• With pediatric use, monitor growth velocity in children and teenagers (may see growth reduction).

Information for the patient
• Inform patient to apply topical form of drug sparingly and rub in lightly. Washing area before application may increase drug penetration.
• Instruct patient to report burning, irritation, or persistent or worsened condition.

Reactions may be *common*, uncommon, ***life-threatening***, or COMMON AND LIFE-THREATENING.

- Tell patient to avoid prolonged use, contact with eyes, or use around genital or rectal area, on face, and in skin creases.
- Inform patient to rinse mouth well after corticosteroid inhalation.
- Teach patient on inhalation corticosteroids to avoid exposure to chickenpox or measles; if exposed, he should call immediately.

Pediatric patients
- Safety and efficacy of topical form haven't been established in children. Safety and efficacy of nasal form haven't been established in children under age 12; use of drug isn't recommended in these patients.
- A reduction of growth velocity in children or teenagers may occur as a result of corticosteroid use for treatment or from inadequate control of chronic disease such as asthma. Benefits of asthma control from corticosteroid therapy must be weighed against possibility of growth suppression in these patients.

Breast-feeding patients
- It's unknown if topical or inhalation corticosteroids undergo sufficient absorption to produce systemic effects in infant; use with caution in breast-feeding women.

fluvastatin sodium
Lescol

Pharmacologic classification: hydroxy-methylglutaryl-coenzyme A (HMG-CoA) reductase inhibitor
Therapeutic classification: cholesterol-lowering antilipemic
Pregnancy risk category X

How supplied
Available by prescription only
Capsules: 20 mg, 40 mg

Indications, route, and dosage
Reduction of low-density lipoprotein and total cholesterol levels in patients with primary hypercholesterolemia (types IIa and IIb) when response to diet and other nonpharmacologic measures has been inadequate
Adults: Initially, 20 mg P.O. h.s. Increase dosage as necessary to a maximum of 40 mg daily.
✦ *Dosage adjustment.* With a persistent increase in ALT or AST levels of at least three times upper limit of normal, withdrawal of fluvastatin is recommended. Because fluvastatin is cleared hepatically, with less than 5% of the dose excreted in urine, dosage adjustments for mild to moderate renal impairment aren't necessary. Exercise caution with severe impairment.

Pharmacodynamics
Antilipemic action: A competitive inhibitor of HMG-CoA reductase, which is responsible for the conversion of HMG-CoA to mevalonate, a precursor of sterols, including cholesterol. This enzyme is an early (and rate-limiting) step in the synthetic pathway of cholesterol. Drug increases high-density lipoproteins and decreases low-density lipoproteins, very-low-density lipoproteins, and plasma triglycerides.

Pharmacokinetics
- *Absorption:* Absorbed rapidly; 98% absorbed after oral administration on empty stomach.
- *Distribution:* Over 98% of circulating drug is bound to plasma proteins.
- *Metabolism:* Completely metabolized in liver; has no active metabolites.
- *Excretion:* About 5% excreted in urine; 90% in feces.

Contraindications and precautions
Contraindicated in patients with hypersensitivity to drug; in those with active liver disease or conditions associated with unexplained persistent elevations of serum transaminase levels; in pregnant and breast-feeding women; and in women of childbearing age unless there is no risk of pregnancy.
    Use cautiously in patients with impaired renal function or history of hepatic disease or heavy alcohol consumption.

Interactions
Drug-drug. *Cholestyramine, colestipol:* May bind fluvastatin in GI tract and decrease absorption. Administer fluvastatin at bedtime, at least 2 hours after the resin, to avoid significant interaction from drug binding to resin.
Cimetidine, omeprazole, ranitidine: Decreased fluvastatin metabolism. Monitor patient closely.
Cyclosporine, erythromycin, gemfibrozil, niacin, other immunosuppressants: Increased risk of polymyositis and rhabdomyolysis when administered with fluvastatin. Avoid concomitant use.
Digoxin: May alter pharmacokinetics. Monitor serum digoxin levels carefully.
Rifampin: Enhanced fluvastatin metabolism and decreased plasma levels. Avoid concomitant use.
Warfarin: Increased anticoagulant effect with bleeding. Monitor patient.
Drug-lifestyle. *Alcohol:* May increase risk of hepatotoxicity. Discourage concomitant use.

Adverse reactions
CNS: headache, fatigue, dizziness, insomnia.
GI: dyspepsia, diarrhea, nausea, vomiting, abdominal pain, constipation, flatulence, tooth disorder.
Hepatic: increased liver enzyme levels, increased bilirubin levels.

Hematologic: *thrombocytopenia, leukopenia,* hemolytic anemia.
Metabolic: Thyroid function test abnormalities can occur.
Musculoskeletal: arthropathy, muscle pain.
Respiratory: sinusitis, *upper respiratory infection,* rhinitis, cough, pharyngitis, bronchitis.
Skin: *hypersensitivity reactions* (rash, pruritus).

☑ Special considerations
• Institute fluvastatin only after diet and other non-pharmacologic therapies have proven ineffective. Maintain patient on standard low-cholesterol diet during therapy.
• Drug may be taken without regard to meals; however, efficacy is enhanced if drug is taken in the evening.
• If accidental overdose occurs, treat symptomatically and institute supportive measures as needed.
• Dialyzability of fluvastatin and its metabolites is unknown.

Monitoring the patient
• Monitor CBC before treatment and periodically throughout.
• Liver function tests should be performed at the start of therapy, every 4 to 6 weeks during the first 3 months of therapy, every 6 to 12 weeks during the next 12 months, and at 6-month intervals thereafter.
• Monitor patient closely for signs of myositis.

Information for the patient
• Tell patient to take fluvastatin at bedtime to enhance effectiveness.
• Instruct patient on standard low-cholesterol diet and emphasize importance of dietary compliance as part of therapy. Also stress importance of weight control and exercise in controlling elevated serum lipid levels.
• Warn patient to restrict alcohol intake because of potentially serious adverse effects.
• Tell patient to report adverse reactions, particularly muscle aches and pains.

Pediatric patients
• Safety and effectiveness in patients under age 18 haven't been established. Use in children isn't recommended.

Breast-feeding patients
• Drug may appear in breast milk in a 2:1 ratio (milk:plasma). The potential for serious adverse reactions in breast-feeding infants indicates that breast-feeding women shouldn't take fluvastatin.

fluvoxamine maleate
Luvox

Pharmacologic classification: selective serotonin reuptake inhibitor (SSRI)
Therapeutic classification: anticompulsive
Pregnancy risk category C

How supplied
Available by prescription only
Tablets: 25 mg, 50 mg, 100 mg

Indications, route, and dosage
Obsessive-compulsive disorder
Adults: Initially, 50 mg P.O. daily h.s. Increase in 50-mg increments q 4 to 7 days until maximum benefit is achieved. Maximum daily dose is 300 mg. Total daily doses exceeding 100 mg should be given in two divided doses.
✦ *Dosage adjustment.* Because elderly patients and patients with hepatic impairment frequently have decreased clearance of fluvoxamine maleate, dosage adjustment may be appropriate.

Pharmacodynamics
Anticompulsive action: Exact mechanism unknown. A potent selective inhibitor of the neuronal uptake of serotonin, which is thought to improve obsessive-compulsive behavior.

Pharmacokinetics
• *Absorption:* Absolute bioavailability is 53%.
• *Distribution:* Mean apparent volume of distribution is about 25 L/kg. About 80% of drug is bound to plasma protein (mostly albumin).
• *Metabolism:* Extensively metabolized in liver mostly by oxidative demethylation and deamination.
• *Excretion:* Metabolites primarily excreted in urine.

Contraindications and precautions
Contraindicated in patients with hypersensitivity to drug or to other phenylpiperazine antidepressants and within 14 days of MAO inhibitor therapy. Use cautiously in patients with hepatic dysfunction, concomitant conditions that may affect hemodynamic responses or metabolism, or history of mania or seizures.

Interactions
Drug-drug. *Astemizole:* Decreased metabolism leading to increased levels of antihistamine and cardiotoxicity. Avoid use together.
Benzodiazepines, theophylline, warfarin: Concomitant use may cause reduced clearance. Use together cautiously.
Carbamazepine, clozapine, methadone, metoprolol, propranolol, tricyclic antidepressants: Concurrent use may cause elevated serum levels.

Reactions may be *common,* uncommon, **life-threatening**, or COMMON AND LIFE-THREATENING.

Use together with caution; monitor patient closely for adverse reactions. Dosage adjustments may be needed.

Diazepam: Reduced clearance of diazepam. The manufacturer doesn't recommend giving these drugs together.

Diltiazem: May cause bradycardia. Monitor patient's heart rate.

Lithium, tryptophan: May enhance fluvoxamine's effects. Use together cautiously.

MAO inhibitors: May cause severe excitation, hyperpyrexia, myoclonus, delirium, and coma. Avoid use together.

Drug-lifestyle. *Alcohol:* Enhanced CNS effects. Discourage alcoholic use.

Smoking: May decrease drug effectiveness. Discourage concomitant use.

Adverse reactions

CNS: headache, asthenia, somnolence, insomnia, nervousness, dizziness, tremor, anxiety, hypertonia, agitation, depression, CNS stimulation.
CV: palpitations, vasodilation.
EENT: amblyopia, taste perversion.
GI: *nausea, diarrhea, constipation, dyspepsia,* anorexia, *vomiting,* flatulence, tooth disorder, dysphagia, *dry mouth.*
GU: decreased libido, abnormal ejaculation, urinary frequency, impotence, anorgasmia, urine retention.
Respiratory: upper respiratory infection, dyspnea, yawning.
Skin: sweating.
Other: flulike syndrome, chills.

☑ Special considerations

• Allow at least 14 days after stopping fluvoxamine before patient begins an MAO inhibitor. Also, at least 14 days should be allowed before patient may start fluvoxamine after MAO inhibitor therapy ends.
• Record mood changes. Monitor patient for suicidal tendencies, and allow only a minimum supply of drug.
• Common signs and symptoms of overdose include drowsiness, vomiting, diarrhea, and dizziness; coma, tachycardia, bradycardia, hypotension, ECG abnormalities, liver function abnormalities, and seizures may also occur. Symptoms such as aspiration pneumonitis, respiratory difficulties, or hypokalemia may occur because of loss of consciousness or vomiting.
• Overdose treatment is supportive. Besides maintaining an open airway and monitoring vital signs and ECG, activated charcoal may be as effective as emesis or lavage. Because absorption with overdose may be delayed, measures to minimize absorption may be necessary for up to 24 hours postingestion. Dialysis isn't believed to be beneficial.

Monitoring the patient

• Evaluate patient closely for suicidal tendencies.
• Monitor hepatic function before treatment and periodically throughout.

Information for the patient

• Warn patient not to engage in hazardous activity until CNS effects are known.
• Advise patient to avoid alcoholic beverages while taking fluvoxamine.
• Alert patient that smoking may decrease effectiveness of drug.
• Instruct woman to call immediately if pregnancy is suspected or if she intends to become pregnant during therapy.
• Tell patient to report rash, hives, or related allergic reaction.
• Inform patient that several weeks of therapy may be required for full antidepressant effect. Once improvement is seen, advise patient not to stop drug until directed.
• Advise patient to call before taking OTC drugs because of possible drug interactions.

Geriatric patients

• Drug clearance is decreased by about 50% in elderly patients compared with younger patients. Administer drug cautiously to elderly patients and adjust dosage slowly during initiation of therapy.

Pediatric patients

• Safety and effectiveness in children under age 18 haven't been established.

Breast-feeding patients

• Drug appears in breast milk and shouldn't be given to breast-feeding women.

folic acid
Folvite

Pharmacologic classification: folic acid derivative
Therapeutic classification: vitamin supplement
Pregnancy risk category A

How supplied

Available by prescription only
Tablets: 1 mg
Injection: 10-ml vials (folic acid 5 mg/ml contains 1.5% benzyl alcohol and EDTA; Folvite 5 mg/ml contains 1.5% benzyl alcohol)
Available without a prescription
Tablets: 0.4 mg, 0.8 mg

Indications, route, and dosage

Megaloblastic or macrocytic anemia secondary to folic acid deficiency, hepatic di

ease, alcoholism, intestinal obstruction, excessive hemolysis
Pregnant and breast-feeding women: 0.8 mg P.O., S.C., or I.M. daily.
Adults and children ages 4 and older: 0.4 mg P.O., S.C., or I.M. daily for 4 to 5 days. After anemia secondary to folic acid deficiency is corrected, proper diet and RDA supplements are necessary to prevent recurrence.
Children under age 4: Up to 0.3 mg P.O., S.C., or I.M. daily.
Prevention of megaloblastic anemia of pregnancy and fetal damage
Adults: 1 mg P.O., S.C., or I.M. daily during pregnancy.
Nutritional supplement
Adults: Give 0.15 to 0.2 mg P.O., S.C., or I.M. daily for men; 0.15 to 0.18 mg P.O., S.C., or I.M. daily for women.
Children: 0.05 mg P.O. daily.
Tropical sprue
Adults: 3 to 15 mg P.O. daily.

Pharmacodynamics
Nutritional action: Exogenous folate is required to maintain normal erythropoiesis and to perform nucleoprotein synthesis. Folic acid stimulates production of RBCs, WBCs, and platelets in certain megaloblastic anemias.
　　Dietary folic acid is present in foods, primarily as reduced folate polyglutamate. This vitamin may be absorbed only after hydrolysis, reduction, and methylation occur in the GI tract. Conversion to active tetrahydrofolate may require vitamin B_{12}.
　　Oral synthetic form of folic acid is a monoglutamate and is absorbed completely after administration, even in malabsorption syndromes.

Pharmacokinetics
• *Absorption:* Absorbed rapidly from GI tract, mainly from proximal part of small intestine. Folate activity in blood peaks within 30 to 60 minutes after oral administration. Normal serum folate levels range from 0.005 to 0.015 mcg/ml. Usually, serum levels below 0.005 mcg/ml indicate folate deficiency; those below 0.002 mcg/ml usually result in megaloblastic anemia.
• *Distribution:* Active tetrahydrofolic acid and derivatives distributed into all body tissues; liver contains about half of total body folate stores. Folate actively concentrated in CSF; folic acid distributed into breast milk.
• *Metabolism:* Metabolized in liver to N-methyltetrahydrofolic acid, the main form of folate storage and transport.
• *Excretion:* A single 0.1-mg to 0.2-mg dose usually results in only a trace amount of drug in urine. After large doses, excessive folate excreted unchanged in urine. Small amounts of folic acid have been recovered in feces. About 0.05 mg/day of normal body folate stores is lost by a combination of urinary and fecal excretion and oxidative cleavage of molecule.

Contraindications and precautions
Contraindicated in patients with undiagnosed anemia because it may mask pernicious anemia, and in those with pernicious anemia and other megaloblastic anemias in which vitamin B_{12} is deficient.

Interactions
Drug-drug. *Aminosalicylic acid, chloramphenicol, methotrexate, oral contraceptives, pyrimethamine, sulfasalazine, triamterene, trimethoprim:* May act as antagonists to folic acid. Monitor patient for desired effects.
Anticonvulsants (such as phenobarbital, phenytoin): Increased anticonvulsant metabolism and decreased blood levels of anticonvulsants. Monitor patient closely.
Phenytoin, primidone: Decreased serum folate levels; symptoms of folic acid deficiency in long-term therapy. Monitor patient closely.
Pyrimethamine: May interfere with antimicrobial actions against toxoplasmosis. Monitor patient for desired effects.

Adverse reactions
CNS: general malaise.
Respiratory: *bronchospasm.*
Skin: allergic reactions (rash, pruritus, erythema).

☑ Special considerations
• RDA for folic acid is 25 to 200 mcg in children and 180 to 200 mcg in adults; 100 mcg/day is considered an adequate oral supplement. Pregnant women require 400 mcg daily. During the first 6 months of breast-feeding, women require 280 mcg daily; during the second 6 months, requirement decreases to 260 mcg daily.
• Preferred route of administration for folic acid is P.O. Manufacturer recommends deep I.M., S.C., or I.V. only when P.O. treatment isn't feasible or when malabsorption is suspected.
• Ensure that patients don't also have vitamin B_{12} deficiency; folic acid can improve hematologic measurements while allowing progression of neurologic damage. Don't use as sole treatment of pernicious anemia.
• Patients undergoing renal dialysis are at risk for folate deficiency.
• Protect folic acid injections from light.
• Folic acid therapy alters serum and erythrocyte folate levels; falsely low serum and erythrocyte folate levels may occur with the *Lactobacillus casei* assay in patients receiving anti-infectives such as tetracycline, which suppress growth of this organism.
• Folic acid is relatively nontoxic. Adverse GI and CNS effects have been reported rarely in patients receiving 15 mg of folic acid daily for 1 month.

Reactions may be *common*, uncommon, **life-threatening**, or COMMON AND LIFE-THREATENING.

Monitoring the patient
• Monitor CBC for effectiveness of therapy.
• Monitor patient for adverse effects.

Information for the patient
• Teach patient about dietary sources of folic acid, such as yeast, whole grains, leafy vegetables, beans, nuts, and fruit.
• Tell patient that folate is destroyed by over-cooking and canning.
• Stress importance of taking folic acid only under medical supervision.

Breast-feeding patients
• Folic acid appears in breast milk. Daily doses of 0.8 mg are sufficient to maintain normoblastic bone marrow after symptoms have subsided and blood components have returned to normal.

fomivirsen sodium
Vitravene

Pharmacologic classification: phospho-rothioate oligonucleotide
Therapeutic classification: antiviral
Pregnancy risk category C

How supplied
Available by prescription only
Intravitreal injection: preservative-free, single-use vials containing 0.25 ml, 6.6 mg/ml

Indications, route, and dosage
Local treatment of cytomegalovirus (CMV) retinitis in patients with AIDS, who are intolerant of or have a contraindication to other treatment or who were insufficiently responsive to previous treatment
Adults: Induction dose is 330 mcg (0.05 ml) by intravitreal injection every other week for two doses. Subsequent maintenance dose is 330 mcg (0.05 ml) by intravitreal injection once every 4 weeks after induction.

Pharmacodynamics
Antiviral action: Inhibits human CMV replication by binding to the target mRNA and subsequently inhibiting virus replication.

Pharmacokinetics
No information available.

Contraindications and precautions
Contraindicated in patients with hypersensitivity to drug or its components and in those who have been treated within 2 to 4 weeks with either I.V. or intravitreal cidofovir because of increased risk of exaggerated ocular inflammation.

Interactions
None reported.

Adverse reactions
CNS: asthenia, headache, abnormal thinking, depression, dizziness, neuropathy, pain.
CV: chest pain.
EENT: abnormal or blurred vision, anterior chamber inflammation, cataract, conjunctival hemorrhage, decreased visual acuity, desaturation of color vision, eye pain, floaters, increased intraocular pressure, *ocular inflammation, iritis,* photophobia, retinal detachment, retinal edema, retinal hemorrhage, retinal pigment changes, *uveitis, vitritis,* application site reaction, conjunctival hyperemia, conjunctivitis, corneal edema, decreased peripheral vision, eye irritation, hypotony, keratic precipitates, optic neuritis, photopsia, retinal vascular disease, visual field defect, vitreous hemorrhage, vitreous opacity, sinusitis.
GI: abdominal pain, anorexia, diarrhea, nausea, vomiting, oral candidiasis, *pancreatitis.*
GU: catheter infection, *kidney failure.*
Hematologic: anemia, lymphoma-like reaction, *neutropenia, thrombocytopenia.*
Hepatic: abnormal liver function, increased GTT level.
Metabolic: decreased weight, dehydration.
Musculoskeletal: back pain.
Respiratory: bronchitis, dyspnea, increased cough, pneumonia.
Skin: rash, sweating.
Other: allergic reactions, cachexia, fever, flulike syndrome, infection, *sepsis,* systemic CMV.

☑ Special considerations
• Drug is for ophthalmic use by intravitreal injection only.
• Drug provides localized therapy limited to treated eye and doesn't provide treatment for systemic CMV disease. Monitor patient for extraocular CMV disease or disease in the contralateral eye.
• Ocular inflammation (uveitis) is more common during induction dosing.

Monitoring the patient
• Monitor light perception and optic nerve head perfusion postinjection.
• Watch for increased intraocular pressure. This is usually transient and returns to normal without treatment or with temporary use of topical medications.

Information for the patient
• Inform patient that drug doesn't cure CMV retinitis and that some patients continue to experience progression of retinitis during and following treatment.
• Tell patient that drug treats only eye in which it has been injected and that CMV may also exist in body. Stress importance of follow-up visits to monitor progress and to check for additional infections.

- Instruct patient to have regular ophthalmologic follow-up examinations.
- Advise HIV-infected patient to continue taking antiretroviral therapy as indicated.

Geriatric patients
- Safety and efficacy in patients over age 65 haven't been established.

Pediatric patients
- Safety and efficacy in children haven't been established.

Breast-feeding patients
- It's unknown if drug appears in breast milk. Stop either drug or breast-feeding.

---

foscarnet sodium (phosphonoformic acid)
Foscavir

Pharmacologic classification: pyrophosphate analogue
Therapeutic classification: antiviral
Pregnancy risk category C

How supplied
Available by prescription only
Injection: 24 mg/ml in 250-ml and 500-ml vials

Indications, route, and dosage
Cytomegalovirus (CMV) retinitis in patients with AIDS
Adults: Initially, 60 mg/kg I.V. as an induction treatment in patients with normal renal function. Administer as an I.V. infusion over 1 hour q 8 hours for 2 or 3 weeks, depending on response. Follow with a maintenance infusion of 90 mg/kg daily administered over 2 hours; increase as needed and tolerated to 120 mg/kg daily if disease shows signs of progression.
Mucocutaneous acyclovir-resistant herpes simplex virus (HSV) infection
Adults: 40 mg/kg I.V. Administer as an I.V. infusion over 1 hour q 8 to 12 hours for 2 or 3 weeks, depending on response.
◊ **Varicella zoster infection**
Adults: 40 mg/kg I.V. q 8 hours for 10 to 21 days.
✦ **Dosage adjustment.** For adult patients with renal failure, calculate patient's weight-adjusted creatinine clearance (ml/minute/kg) from this equation:
For men:

$$\text{creatinine clearance} = \frac{(140 - \text{age})}{(\text{serum creatinine} \times 72)}$$

For women: Multiply the above value by 0.85.
Administer according to the tables on page 481.

Pharmacodynamics
Antiviral action: An organic analogue of pyrophosphate, a compound used in many enzymatic reactions, that inhibits all known herpes viruses in vitro by blocking the pyrophosphate binding site on DNA polymerases and reverse transcriptases.

Pharmacokinetics
- *Absorption:* No information available.
- *Distribution:* About 14% to 17% bound to plasma proteins. Drug is deposited in bone.
- *Metabolism:* No information available.
- *Excretion:* About 80% to 90% of drug appears in urine unchanged. Drug clearance dependent on renal function. Plasma half-life is about 3 hours.

Contraindications and precautions
Contraindicated in patients with hypersensitivity to drug. Use with extreme caution in patients with impaired renal function.

Interactions
Drug-drug. *Nephrotoxic drugs (such as aminoglycosides, amphotericin B):* May increase risk of nephrotoxicity. Avoid use together.
Pentamidine: May increase nephrotoxicity risk; severe hypocalcemia also reported. Avoid use together.
Zidovudine: May increase risk or severity of anemia. Monitor blood counts.

Adverse reactions
CNS: headache, **seizures,** fatigue, malaise, asthenia, paresthesia, dizziness, hypoesthesia, neuropathy, tremor, ataxia, generalized spasms, dementia, stupor, sensory disturbances, meningitis, aphasia, abnormal coordination, EEG abnormalities, depression, confusion, anxiety, insomnia, somnolence, nervousness, amnesia, agitation, aggressive reaction, hallucinations.
CV: *hypertension, palpitations, ECG abnormalities, sinus tachycardia,* cerebrovascular disorder, *first-degree AV block, hypotension, flushing,* edema.
EENT: visual disturbances, taste perversion, eye pain, conjunctivitis, sinusitis, pharyngitis, rhinitis.
GI: *nausea, diarrhea, vomiting, abdominal pain, anorexia,* constipation, dysphagia, rectal hemorrhage, dry mouth, dyspepsia, melena, flatulence, ulcerative stomatitis, **pancreatitis.**
GU: *abnormal renal function, decreased creatinine clearance and increased serum creatinine levels, albuminuria, dysuria, polyuria, urethral disorder, urine retention, urinary tract infections,* **acute renal failure,** candidiasis.
Hematologic: anemia, **granulocytopenia, leukopenia, bone marrow suppression, thrombocytopenia,** platelet abnormalities, thrombocytosis, WBC count abnormalities.
Hepatic: abnormal hepatic function, increased liver enzymes.

Reactions may be *common,* uncommon, *life-threatening,* or COMMON AND LIFE-THREATENING.

HSV INFECTION

Induction dose

Creatinine clearance (ml/min/kg)	Equivalent to 80 mg/kg/day (40 mg/kg q 12 hr)	Equivalent to 120 mg/kg/day (40 mg/kg q 8 hr)
> 1.4	40 q 12 hr	40 q 8 hr
> 1.0 – 1.4	30 q 12 hr	30 q 8 hr
> 0.8 – 1.0	20 q 12 hr	35 q 12 hr
> 0.6 – 0.8	35 q 24 hr	25 q 12 hr
> 0.5 – 0.6	25 q 24 hr	40 q 24 hr
≥ 0.4 – 0.5	20 q 24 hr	35 q 24 hr
< 0.4	Not recommended	Not recommended

CMV INFECTION

Induction dose

Creatinine clearance (ml/min/kg)	Equivalent to 180 mg/kg/day (60 mg/kg q 8 hr)	Equivalent to 180 mg/kg/day (90 mg/kg q 12 hr)
> 1.4	60 q 8 hr	90 q 12 hr
> 1.0 – 1.4	45 q 8 hr	70 q 12 hr
> 0.8 – 1.0	50 q 12 hr	50 q 12 hr
> 0.6 – 0.8	40 q 12 hr	80 q 24 hr
> 0.5 – 0.6	60 q 24 hr	60 q 24 hr
≥ 0.4 – 0.5	50 q 24 hr	50 q 24 hr
< 0.4	Not recommended	Not recommended

Maintenance dose

Creatinine clearance (ml/min/kg)	Equivalent to 90 mg/kg/day (Once daily)	Equivalent to 120 mg/kg/day (Once daily)
> 1.4	90 q 24 hr	120 q 24 hr
> 1.0 – 1.4	70 q 24 hr	90 q 24 hr
> 0.8 – 1.0	50 q 24 hr	65 q 24 hr
> 0.6 – 0.8	80 q 48 hr	105 q 48 hr
> 0.5 – 0.6	60 q 48 hr	80 q 48 hr
≥ 0.4 – 0.5	50 q 48 hr	65 q 48 hr
< 0.4	Not recommended	Not recommended

Metabolic: hypokalemia, hypomagnesemia, hypophosphatemia or hyperphosphatemia, hypocalcemia.

Musculoskeletal: leg cramps, back or chest pain, arthralgia, myalgia.

Respiratory: *cough, dyspnea,* pneumonitis, respiratory insufficiency, pulmonary infiltration, stridor, pneumothorax, **bronchospasm,** hemoptysis, flulike symptoms.

Skin: *rash, increased sweating,* pruritus, skin ulceration, erythematous rash, seborrhea, skin discoloration, facial edema.

Other: *fever,* lymphadenopathy, pain, infection, sepsis, rigors, inflammation and pain at infusion site, lymphoma-like disorder, sarcoma, bacterial or fungal infections, abscess.

☑ **Special considerations**
• Up to 33% of patients treated with drug experience anemia, which may be severe enough to require transfusions.
• Don't exceed recommended dosage, infusion rate, or frequency of administration. All doses must be individualized according to renal function.
• Use an infusion pump to administer foscarnet.
• Unlike ganciclovir, foscarnet doesn't need cellular activation by thymidine kinase or other kinases. Foscarnet may be active against certain CMV strains resistant to ganciclovir.

Monitoring the patient
• Monitor CBC and renal function before therapy and periodically throughout.
• Monitor patient for adverse effects.

Information for the patient
● Make sure that patient understands that adverse reactions to drug are common and that he should report for all laboratory studies and follow-up appointments to check progress.
● Advise patient to report perioral tingling, numbness in extremities, and paresthesia.

Geriatric patients
● It's unknown if age alters drug response. However, elderly patients are likely to have preexisting renal function impairment, which requires alterations in dosage.

Pediatric patients
● Safety and efficacy in children haven't been established. It's possible that up to 40% of dose is deposited in teeth and bones of growing children.

Breast-feeding patients
● It's unknown if drug appears in breast milk; however, drug may concentrate in breast milk when administered at high doses. Use with caution.

fosfomycin tromethamine
Monurol

Pharmacologic classification: phosphonic acid derivative
Therapeutic classification: antibiotic
Pregnancy risk category B

How supplied
Available by prescription only
Single-dose sachet: 3 g

Indications, route, and dosage
Uncomplicated urinary tract infections (acute cystitis) in women caused by susceptible strains of Escherichia coli *and* Enterococcus faecalis
Women over age 18: 1 sachet P.O. mixed with 3 to 4 oz (½ cup) of cold water just before ingestion.

Pharmacodynamics
Bactericidal action: Inhibits bacterial cell-wall synthesis. It's effective in the urinary tract because it reduces adherence of bacteria to uroepithelial cells.

Pharmacokinetics
● *Absorption:* Rapidly absorbed following oral administration and converted to free acid, fosfomycin. When drug is taken on empty stomach, levels peak within 2 hours; within 4 hours when taken with food.
● *Distribution:* Mean apparent steady-state volume of distribution is 136 L following oral administration. Not bound to plasma proteins; distributed to kidneys, bladder wall, prostate, and seminal vesicles. Crosses placenta.

● *Metabolism:* Not reported.
● *Excretion:* Excreted unchanged in both urine and feces.

Contraindications and precautions
Contraindicated in patients with hypersensitivity to drug. Use cautiously in patients with renal impairment.

Interactions
Drug-drug. *Metoclopramide:* Lowers serum level and urinary excretion of fosfomycin. Avoid concomitant use.
Other drugs that increase GI motility: May increase GI effects. Monitor patient.

Adverse reactions
CNS: asthenia, dizziness, *headache.*
EENT: pharyngitis, rhinitis.
GI: abdominal pain, *diarrhea,* dyspepsia, nausea.
GU: dysmenorrhea, vaginitis.
Musculoskeletal: back pain.
Skin: rash.

☑ Special considerations
● Using more than one single-dose sachet to treat a single episode of acute cystitis won't improve success and may cause adverse reactions.
● If overdose occurs, provide supportive treatment.

Monitoring the patient
● Obtain urine specimens for culture and sensitivity before and after therapy has been completed.
● Monitor therapeutic response.

Information for the patient
● Show patient how to properly take drug. Drug shouldn't be taken in its dry form. The entire contents of a single-dose sachet should be mixed with 3 to 4 oz (½ cup) cold water. Stir to dissolve, and drink immediately.
● Tell patient to call if symptoms don't improve in 2 to 3 days.
● Inform patient that drug may be taken without regard to food.

Geriatric patients
● There are no significant differences in drug effectiveness or safety in women age 65 or under compared with those over age 65.

Pediatric patients
● Safety and effectiveness in children age 12 and under haven't been established.

Breast-feeding patients
● It's unknown if drug appears in breast milk. Because many drugs appear in breast milk, a decision should be made to either stop breast-feeding or drug.

---

fosinopril sodium
Monopril

Pharmacologic classification: ACE inhibitor
Therapeutic classification: antihypertensive
Pregnancy risk category C (D in second and third trimesters)

How supplied
Available by prescription only
Tablets: 10 mg, 20 mg, 40 mg

Indications, route, and dosage
Hypertension
Adults: Initially, 10 mg P.O. daily; adjust dose based on blood pressure response at peak and trough levels. Usual dose 20 to 40 mg daily; maximum dose up to 80 mg daily. Dose may be divided.
Heart failure
Adults: Initially, 10 mg P.O. daily; maximum dose up to 40 mg daily. Dose may be divided.

Pharmacodynamics
Antihypertensive action: Believed to lower blood pressure primarily by suppressing the renin-angiotensin-aldosterone system, although it has also been effective in patients with low-renin hypertension.

Pharmacokinetics
• *Absorption:* Absorbed slowly through GI tract, primarily via proximal small intestine.
• *Distribution:* Over 95% protein-bound; levels peak in about 3 hours.
• *Metabolism:* Hydrolyzed primarily in liver and gut wall by esterases.
• *Excretion:* 50% of drug excreted in urine; rest in feces.

Contraindications and precautions
Contraindicated in patients with hypersensitivity to drug or other ACE inhibitors and in breast-feeding women. Use cautiously in patients with impaired renal or hepatic function.

Interactions
Drug-drug. *Antacids:* May impair absorption of fosinopril. Separate administration times by at least 2 hours.
Antihypertensives, diuretics: Excessive hypotension may be seen, especially if patient is volume-depleted. Avoid concomitant use. Effect may be minimized by stopping diuretic.
Lithium: May increase serum lithium levels; symptoms of lithium toxicity may occur. Increased risk of lithium toxicity if diuretic is also used. Monitor lithium levels frequently.

Potassium-sparing diuretics, potassium supplements: May result in hyperkalemia. Monitor potassium levels.
Drug-food. *Salt substitutes containing potassium:* Risk of hyperkalemia. Monitor potassium levels.

Adverse reactions
CNS: headache, dizziness, fatigue, syncope, paresthesia, sleep disturbance, *CVA.*
CV: chest pain, angina, *MI, hypertensive crisis*, rhythm disturbances, palpitations, hypotension, orthostatic hypotension.
EENT: tinnitus, sinusitis.
GI: nausea, vomiting, diarrhea, *pancreatitis*, dry mouth, abdominal distention, abdominal pain, constipation.
GU: sexual dysfunction, elevated BUN and serum creatinine levels, renal insufficiency.
Hematologic: decreases in hematocrit or hemoglobin may occur.
Hepatic: elevated liver function test results, *hepatitis.*
Metabolic: hyperkalemia, decreased libido.
Musculoskeletal: arthralgia, musculoskeletal pain, myalgia, gout.
Respiratory: *dry, persistent, tickling, nonproductive cough; bronchospasm.*
Skin: urticaria, rash, photosensitivity, pruritus.
Other: *angioedema.*

☑ Special considerations
• Diuretic therapy is usually stopped 2 to 3 days before start of ACE inhibitor therapy to reduce risk of hypotension. If fosinopril doesn't adequately control blood pressure, diuretic may be reinstituted with care. Monitor potassium levels.
• Risk of orthostatic hypotension is low.
• Blood pressure is lowered within 1 hour of a single dose of 10 to 40 mg, with peak reductions occurring 2 to 6 hours after dose. Antihypertensive effect lasts 24 hours.
• False low measurements of digoxin levels may result with the Digi-Tab radioimmunoassay kit for digoxin; other kits may be used.
• Overdose hasn't been reported; however, the most common sign of overdose is hypotension. Treat with infusion of normal saline. Hemodialysis and peritoneal dialysis aren't effective in removing drug.

Monitoring the patient
• Perform CBC with differential counts before therapy, then every 2 weeks for 3 months, and periodically thereafter.
• Monitor patient for adverse effects.

Information for the patient
• Tell patient to take dose 1 hour before or 2 hours after food or antacids.
• Tell patient to report light-headedness in the first few days of therapy and signs of infection such as fever or sore throat. Patient should also

stop drug immediately and call if the following occur: swelling of tongue, lips, face, mucous membranes, eyes, lips, or extremities; difficulty swallowing or breathing; or hoarseness.
• Advise patient to maintain same salt intake as before therapy; salt restriction can lead to precipitous drop in blood pressure with initial doses of drug. Large reductions in blood pressure may also occur with excessive perspiration and dehydration.
• Warn patient to avoid sudden position changes until effect of drug is known; however, orthostatic hypotension is infrequent.
• Instruct woman of childbearing age to call immediately if pregnancy is suspected.

Geriatric patients
• No age-related differences have been observed.

Pediatric patients
• Safety and efficacy in children haven't been established.

Breast-feeding patients
• Significant levels of drug appear in breast milk; avoid drug in breast-feeding women.

fosphenytoin sodium
Cerebyx

Pharmacologic classification: hydantoin derivative
Therapeutic classification: anticonvulsant
Pregnancy risk category D

How supplied
Available by prescription only
Injection: 2 ml (150 mg fosphenytoin sodium equivalent to 100 mg phenytoin sodium), 10 ml (750 mg fosphenytoin sodium equivalent to 500 mg phenytoin sodium)

Indications, route, and dosage
Status epilepticus
Adults: Give 15 to 20 mg phenytoin sodium equivalent (PE)/kg I.V. at 100 to 150 PE/minute as a loading dose, and then 4 to 6 mg PE/kg/day I.V. as a maintenance dose. (Phenytoin may be used instead of fosphenytoin as maintenance using the appropriate dose.)
Prevention and treatment of seizures during neurosurgery
Adults: Administer 10 to 20 mg PE/kg I.M. or I.V. at an I.V. infusion rate not exceeding 150 mg PE/minute as a loading dose. Maintenance dose is 4 to 6 mg PE/kg/day I.V.
Short-term substitution for oral phenytoin therapy
Adults: Same total daily dose as oral phenytoin sodium therapy given as a single daily dose I.M.

or I.V. at an I.V. infusion rate not exceeding 150 mg PE/minute. (Some patients may require more frequent dosing.)

Pharmacodynamics
Anticonvulsant action: Because fosphenytoin is a prodrug of phenytoin, its anticonvulsant action is that of phenytoin. Phenytoin stabilizes neuronal membranes and limits seizure activity by modulating voltage-dependent sodium channels of neurons, inhibiting calcium flux across neuronal membranes, modulating voltage-dependent calcium channels of neurons, and enhancing sodium-potassium adenosine triphosphatase activity of neurons and glial cells.

Pharmacokinetics
• *Absorption:* Plasma levels peak about 30 minutes after I.M. administration or at end of I.V. infusion.
• *Distribution:* About 95% to 99% bound to plasma proteins, primarily albumin. Volume of distribution increases with dose and rate and ranges from 4.3 to 10.8 L.
• *Metabolism:* Conversion half-life of fosphenytoin to phenytoin is about 15 minutes. Phosphatases believed to play major role in conversion.
• *Excretion:* No information available, although not excreted in urine.

Contraindications and precautions
Contraindicated in patients with hypersensitivity to drug or its components, phenytoin, or other hydantoins. Also contraindicated in patients with sinus bradycardia, SA block, second- and third-degree AV block, and Adams-Stokes syndrome because of the effect of parenteral phenytoin on ventricular automaticity.
    Use cautiously in patients with hypotension, severe myocardial insufficiency, impaired renal or hepatic function, hypoalbuminemia, porphyria, diabetes mellitus, and history of hypersensitivity to similarly structured drugs, such as barbiturates and succinimides.

Interactions
Drug-drug. *Carbamazepine, reserpine:* Decreased plasma phenytoin levels. Use cautiously together.
Coumarin, digitoxin, doxycycline, estrogens, furosemide, oral contraceptives, quinidine, rifampin, theophylline, vitamin D: Efficacy of these drugs may be decreased by phenytoin because of increased hepatic metabolism. Monitor patient closely; use drug cautiously.
Phenobarbital, sodium valproate, valproic acid: Possible increased or decreased plasma phenytoin levels. Effects of phenytoin on levels of these drugs is unpredictable. Monitor patient closely; use drug cautiously.
Phenytoin, other drugs that may increase plasma phenytoin levels (such as amiodarone, chlor-

amphenicol, chlordiazepoxide, cimetidine, di-azepam, dicumarol, disulfiram, estrogens, etho-suximide, fluoxetine, H_2 antagonists, halothane, isoniazid, methylphenidate, phenothiazines, phenylbutazone, salicylates, succinimides, sul-fonamides, tolbutamide, trazodone): Increased phenytoin effects. Use cautiously together.

Tricyclic antidepressants: May lower seizure threshold; may require adjustments in phenytoin dosage. Monitor patient closely.

Drug-lifestyle. Acute alcohol use: May increase plasma phenytoin level and its therapeutic ef-fects. Discourage concomitant use.

Chronic alcohol use: May decrease plasma phenytoin levels. Discourage concomitant use.

Adverse reactions

CNS: increased or decreased reflexes, speech disorders, dysarthria, asthenia, *intracranial hypertension, cerebral hemorrhage,* thinking abnor-malities, nervousness, hypesthesia, extrapyramidal syndrome, brain edema, headache, *nystagmus, dizziness, somnolence, ataxia,* stupor, incoordi-nation, paresthesia, agitation, tremor, vertigo.

CV: hypertension, *cardiac arrest,* palpitation, *si-nus bradycardia,* atrial flutter, *bundle-branch block,* cardiomegaly, orthostatic hypotension, *pulmonary embolus,* QT interval prolongation, thrombophlebitis, ventricular extrasystoles, *heart failure,* vasodilation, tachycardia, hypotension.

EENT: taste perversion, deafness, visual field defect, eye pain, conjunctivitis, photophobia, hy-peracusis, mydriasis, parosmia, ear pain, taste loss, tinnitus, diplopia, amblyopia, rhinitis, pharyn-gitis, sinusitis.

GI: constipation, dyspepsia, diarrhea, anorexia, GI hemorrhage, increased salivation, tenesmus, tongue edema, dysphagia, flatulence, gastritis, ileus, nausea, dry mouth, vomiting.

GU: urine retention, oliguria, dysuria, vaginitis, albuminuria, genital edema, *kidney failure,* polyuria, urethral pain, urinary incontinence, vagi-nal candidiasis.

Hematologic: *thrombocytopenia,* anemia, leukocytosis, hypochromic anemia, *leukopenia, agranulocytosis, granulocytopenia, pancy-topenia,* ecchymosis.

Hepatic: elevated liver enzyme levels.

Metabolic: diabetes insipidus, hypokalemia, hy-perglycemia, hypophosphatemia, alkalosis, aci-dosis, dehydration, hyperkalemia, ketosis, de-creased serum levels of T_4.

Musculoskeletal: myasthenia, myopathy, leg cramps, arthralgia, myalgia, pelvic pain, back pain.

Respiratory: cyanosis, pneumonia, hyperventi-lation, *apnea,* aspiration pneumonia, asthma, dyspnea, atelectasis, increased cough, increased sputum, epistaxis, hypoxia, pneumothorax, he-moptysis, bronchitis.

Skin: petechia, rash, maculopapular rash, ur-ticaria, sweating, skin discoloration, contact der-matitis, pustular rash, skin nodule, *pruritus.*

Other: lymphadenopathy.

☑ Special considerations

● Fosphenytoin should always be prescribed and dispensed in phenytoin sodium equivalent units (PE). Don't make adjustments in recommended doses when substituting fosphenytoin for pheny-toin and vice versa.

● Before I.V. infusion, dilute fosphenytoin in D_5W or normal saline solution for injection to a con-centration ranging from 1.5 to 25 mg PE/ml. Don't administer at a rate exceeding 150 mg PE/minute.

● Administer dose of I.V. fosphenytoin used to treat status epilepticus at a maximum rate of 150 mg PE/minute. Typical infusion of drug adminis-tered to a 110-lb patient takes 5 to 7 minutes; an identical molar dose of phenytoin can't be com-pleted in less than 15 to 20 minutes because of untoward CV effects that accompany direct I.V. administration of phenytoin at rates above 50 mg/minute. Don't use I.M. fosphenytoin because therapeutic phenytoin levels may not be reached as rapidly as with I.V. administration.

● If rapid phenytoin loading is a primary goal, I.V. administration of fosphenytoin is preferred be-cause the time to achieve therapeutic plasma phenytoin levels is greater following I.M. than that following I.V. administration.

● Patients receiving fosphenytoin at doses of 20 mg PE/kg at 150 mg PE/minute are expected to experience some sensory discomfort, with the groin being the most common location. Occur-rence and intensity of discomfort can be less-ened by slowing or temporarily stopping infusion.

● The phosphate load provided by fosphenytoin (0.0037 mmol phosphate/mg PE fosphenytoin) must be taken into consideration when treating patients who require phosphate restriction, such as those with severe renal impairment.

● Stop drug if rash appears. If rash is exfoliative, purpuric, or bullous or if lupus erythematosus, Stevens-Johnson syndrome, or toxic epidermal necrolysis is suspected, don't resume drug, and seek alternative therapy. If rash is mild (measles-like or scarlatiniform), therapy may be resumed after rash has completely disappeared. If rash re-curs on reinstitution of therapy, further fos-phenytoin or phenytoin administration is contra-indicated.

● Stop drug in patients with acute hepatotoxici-ty; don't readminister to these patients.

● I.M. drug administration generates systemic phenytoin levels that are similar enough to oral phenytoin sodium to allow essentially inter-changeable use.

● A dose of 15 to 20 mg PE/kg of fosphenytoin infused I.V. at 100 to 150 mg PE/minute yields plasma-free phenytoin levels over time that ap-proximate those achieved when an equivalent dose of phenytoin sodium (such as parenteral di-lantin) is administered at 50 mg/minute I.V.

• Following drug administration, it's recommended that phenytoin levels not be monitored until conversion to phenytoin is essentially complete; about 2 hours after the end of an I.V. infusion or 4 hours after I.M. administration.

• Interpretation of total phenytoin plasma levels should be made cautiously in patients with renal or hepatic disease or hypoalbuminemia because of an increased fraction in unbound phenytoin. Unbound phenytoin levels may be more useful in these patients. Also, these patients are at increased risk for both the frequency and severity of adverse reactions when fosphenytoin is administered I.V.

• Fosphenytoin may produce artificially low results in dexamethasone or metyrapone tests.

• Because fosphenytoin is a prodrug of phenytoin, overdose may be similar. Early signs of phenytoin overdose may include drowsiness, nausea, vomiting, nystagmus, ataxia, dysarthria, tremor, and slurred speech; hypotension, respiratory depression, and coma may follow. Death is caused by respiratory and circulatory depression. Estimated lethal dose of phenytoin in adults is 2 to 5 g.

• Formate and phosphate are metabolites of fosphenytoin and may contribute to signs of toxicity following overdose. Signs of formate toxicity are similar to those of methanol toxicity and are associated with severe anion-gap metabolic acidosis. Large amounts of phosphate, delivered rapidly, could potentially cause hypocalcemia with paresthesia, muscle spasms, and seizures. Ionized free calcium levels can be measured and, if low, used to guide treatment.

• Treat overdose with gastric lavage or emesis and follow by supportive treatment. Monitor vital signs and fluid and electrolyte balance. Forced diuresis is of little or no value. Hemodialysis or peritoneal dialysis may be helpful.

Monitoring the patient
• Evaluate patient's ECG before treatment (drug is contraindicated for sinus bradycardia, SA block, second- and third-degree AV block, and Adams-Stokes syndrome).

• Monitor renal and hepatic function before treatment and periodically throughout.

• Monitor patient's ECG, blood pressure, and respiration continuously throughout the period when maximal serum phenytoin levels occur, about 10 to 20 minutes after the end of fosphenytoin infusions. Severe CV complications are most commonly encountered in elderly or gravely ill patients. May require reducing rate of administration or stopping drug.

Information for the patient
• Warn patient that sensory disturbances may occur with I.V. drug administration.

• Tell patient to report adverse reactions immediately, especially rash.

Geriatric patients
• Elderly patients metabolize and excrete phenytoin slowly; fosphenytoin should be administered cautiously to older adults.

Pediatric patients
• Safety and effectiveness in children haven't been established.

Breast-feeding patients
• It's unknown if drug appears in breast milk; drug isn't recommended in breast-feeding women.

furosemide
Apo-Furosemide*, Lasix, Lasix Special*, Novosemide*, Uritol*

Pharmacologic classification: loop diuretic
Therapeutic classification: diuretic, antihypertensive
Pregnancy risk category C

How supplied
Available by prescription only
Tablets: 20 mg, 40 mg, 80 mg
Solution: 10 mg/ml, 40 mg/5 ml
Injection: 10 mg/ml

Indications, route, and dosage
Acute pulmonary edema
Adults: 40 mg I.V. injected slowly; then 80 mg I.V. within 1 hour, p.r.n.
Infants and children: 1 mg/kg I.M. or I.V. q 2 hours until response is achieved; maximum dose is 6 mg/kg.
Edema
Adults: 20 to 80 mg P.O. daily in morning, with second dose given in 6 to 8 hours, carefully adjusted up to 600 mg daily, p.r.n.; or 20 to 40 mg I.M. or I.V. Increase by 20 mg q 2 hours until desired response is achieved. I.V. dosage should be given slowly over 1 to 2 minutes.
Infants and children: 2 mg/kg/day P.O., increased by 1 to 2 mg/kg in 6 to 8 hours, p.r.n., carefully adjusted so as not to exceed 6 mg/kg/day.
Hypertension
Adults: 40 mg P.O. b.i.d. Adjust dosage according to response.
◊ Hypercalcemia
Adults: 80 to 100 mg I.V. q 1 to 2 hours; or 120 mg P.O. daily.
✦ *Dosage adjustment.* Reduced dosages may be indicated in elderly patients.

Pharmacodynamics
Diuretic action: Loop diuretics inhibit sodium and chloride reabsorption in the proximal part of the ascending loop of Henle, promoting excretion of sodium, water, chloride, and potassium.

Antihypertensive action: Drug's effect may be the result of renal and peripheral vasodilatation and a temporary increase in glomerular filtration rate and a decrease in peripheral vascular resistance.

Pharmacokinetics
• *Absorption:* About 60% absorbed from GI tract after oral administration. Food delays oral absorption but doesn't alter diuretic response. Diuresis begins in 30 to 60 minutes; diuresis peaks 1 to 2 hours after oral administration. Diuresis follows I.V. administration within 5 minutes and peaks in 20 to 60 minutes.
• *Distribution:* About 95% plasma protein–bound. Crosses placenta and appears in breast milk.
• *Metabolism:* Metabolized minimally by liver.
• *Excretion:* About 50% to 80% excreted in urine; plasma half-life is about 30 minutes. Duration of action is 6 to 8 hours after oral administration; about 2 hours after I.V. administration.

Contraindications and precautions
Contraindicated in patients with anuria or history of hypersensitivity to drug. Use cautiously in patients with hepatic cirrhosis and during pregnancy.

Interactions
Drug-drug. *Aminoglycoside antibiotics, cisplatin, ethacrynic acid:* Ototoxicity can be potentiated. Avoid concomitant use.
Amphotericin B, corticosteroids, corticotropin, metolazone: May increase risk of hypokalemia. Monitor potassium levels.
Antidiabetics: May decrease hypoglycemic effects. Monitor patient closely.
Antihypertensives: May increase risk of hypotension. Monitor blood pressure closely.
Cardiac glycosides, lithium, neuromuscular blockers: Furosemide-induced hypokalemia may increase risk of toxicity from these drugs. Monitor patient for arrhythmias.
NSAIDs: May inhibit diuretic response. Monitor intake and output.
Salicylates: May cause salicylate toxicity. Monitor patient closely; use drug cautiously.
Sucralfate: May reduce diuretic and antihypertensive effect. Monitor blood pressure and intake and output.
Drug-herb. *Aloe:* May increase drug effects. Use together cautiously.
Drug-lifestyle. *Sun exposure:* Potentiated photosensitivity reactions. Tell patient to take precautions.

Adverse reactions
CNS: vertigo, headache, dizziness, paresthesia, restlessness.
CV: volume depletion and dehydration, orthostatic hypotension.
EENT: transient deafness with too rapid I.V. injection, blurred vision.

GI: abdominal discomfort and pain, diarrhea, anorexia, nausea, vomiting, constipation, *pancreatitis.*
GU: nocturia, polyuria, frequent urination, altered renal function tests, oliguria.
Hematologic: *agranulocytosis, leukopenia, thrombocytopenia,* azotemia, anemia, *aplastic anemia.*
Hepatic: altered liver function test results.
Metabolic: hypokalemia; hypochloremic alkalosis; asymptomatic hyperuricemia; fluid and electrolyte imbalances, including dilutional hyponatremia, hypocalcemia, hypomagnesemia; hyperglycemia and impaired glucose tolerance.
Musculoskeletal: muscle spasm, weakness.
Skin: dermatitis, purpura.
Other: fever; transient pain (at I.M. injection site); thrombophlebitis (with I.V. administration).

☑ Special considerations
Besides the recommendations relevant to all loop diuretics, consider the following.
• Give I.V. furosemide slowly, over 1 to 2 minutes; for I.V. infusion, dilute furosemide in D_5W, normal saline solution, or lactated Ringer's solution, and use within 24 hours. If high-dose furosemide therapy is needed, administer as a controlled infusion not exceeding 4 mg/minute.
• Signs and symptoms of overdose include profound electrolyte and volume depletion, which may precipitate circulatory collapse. Treatment is chiefly supportive; replace fluids and electrolytes.

Monitoring the patient
• Monitor serum potassium and CBC before treatment and periodically throughout.
• Monitor patient for adverse effects.

Information for the patient
• Warn patient that photosensitivity reaction may occur. Explain that reaction is a photoallergy in which ultraviolet radiation alters drug structure, causing allergic reactions in some people.
• Tell patient that photosensitivity reactions occur 10 days to 2 weeks after first sun exposure.

Geriatric patients
• Elderly and debilitated patients need close observation; they are more susceptible to drug-induced diuresis. Excessive diuresis promotes rapid dehydration, leading to hypovolemia, hypokalemia, hyponatremia, and circulatory collapse.

Pediatric patients
• Use with caution in neonates. The common children's dosage can be used, but extend dosing intervals. Sorbitol content of oral preparations may cause diarrhea, especially at high doses.

Breast-feeding patients
• Drug appears in breast milk. Use caution when administering drug to breast-feeding women.

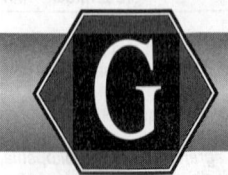

gabapentin
Neurontin

Pharmacologic classification: 1-amino-
methyl cyclohexoneacetic acid
Therapeutic classification: anticonvulsant
Pregnancy risk category C

How supplied
Available by prescription only
Capsules: 100 mg, 300 mg, 400 mg

Indications, route, and dosage
**Adjunctive treatment of partial seizures with
and without secondary generalization**
Adults: 300 mg P.O. on day 1, 300 mg P.O. b.i.d.
on day 2, and 300 mg P.O. t.i.d. on day 3. Increase
dosage as needed and tolerated to 1,800 mg daily, in three divided doses. Usual dosage is 300
to 600 mg P.O. t.i.d., although dosages up to 3,600
mg/day have been well tolerated.
✦ **Dosage adjustment.** In adult patients with renal failure, if creatinine clearance is above 60
ml/minute, give 400 mg P.O. t.i.d.; if creatinine
clearance is between 30 and 60 ml/minute, give
300 mg P.O. b.i.d.; if creatinine clearance is between 15 and 30 ml/minute, give 300 mg P.O.
daily; and if creatinine clearance is less than 15
ml/minute, give 300 mg P.O. every other day. Patients on hemodialysis should receive a loading
dose of 300 to 400 mg P.O.; then 200 to 300 mg
P.O. q 4 hours after hemodialysis.

Pharmacodynamics
Anticonvulsant action: Mechanism unknown. Although structurally related to gamma-aminobutyric
acid (GABA), drug doesn't interact with GABA
receptors, isn't converted metabolically into GABA
or a GABA agonist, and doesn't inhibit GABA uptake or degradation. Drug doesn't exhibit affinity
for other common receptor sites.

Pharmacokinetics
• *Absorption:* Bioavailability isn't dose proportional. For example, a 400-mg dose is about 25%
less bioavailable than a 100-mg dose. Differences
in bioavailability aren't large over recommended
dose range of 300 to 600 mg t.i.d.; bioavailability is about 60%. Food has no effect on rate or extent of absorption.

• *Distribution:* Circulates largely unbound (less
than 3%) to plasma protein. Crosses blood-brain
barrier with about 20% of corresponding plasma
levels found in CSF.
• *Metabolism:* Not appreciably metabolized.
• *Excretion:* Eliminated from systemic circulation
by renal excretion as unchanged drug. Elimination half-life is 5 to 7 hours. Drug can be removed
from plasma by hemodialysis.

Contraindications and precautions
Contraindicated in patients with hypersensitivity
to drug.

Interactions
Drug-drug. *Antacids:* Decreased absorption of
gabapentin. Separate administration times by at
least 2 hours.
Cimetidine: May decrease renal clearance of
gabapentin. Monitor patient closely.
Oral contraceptives: May alter pharmacokinetics
of oral contraceptives. Advise patient to use alternative method of birth control.

Adverse reactions
CNS: *fatigue, somnolence, dizziness, ataxia, nys-
tagmus, tremor,* nervousness, dysarthria, am-
nesia, depression, abnormal thinking, twitching,
incoordination.
CV: peripheral edema, vasodilation.
EENT: *diplopia, rhinitis,* pharyngitis, dry throat,
coughing, dental abnormalities, *amblyopia.*
GI: nausea, vomiting, dyspepsia, dry mouth, con-
stipation.
GU: impotence.
Hematologic: *leukopenia,* decreased WBC
count.
Metabolic: increased appetite, weight gain.
Musculoskeletal: back pain, myalgia, fractures.
Skin: pruritus, abrasion.

☑ Special considerations
• Discontinue drug therapy or substitute alternative drug gradually over at least 1 week to minimize risk of precipitating seizures. Don't suddenly withdraw other anticonvulsants in patients
starting gabapentin therapy.
• Don't use Ames N-Multistix SG dipstick to test
for urine protein; false-positive results can occur.
Use the more specific sulfosalicylic acid precipitation procedure to determine presence of urine
protein.

Reactions may be *common,* uncommon, *life-threatening,* or COMMON AND LIFE-THREATENING.

• Acute overdose of gabapentin may cause double vision, slurred speech, drowsiness, lethargy, and diarrhea. Supportive care is recommended.
• Drug can be removed by hemodialysis and may be indicated by patient's condition or in patients with significant renal impairment.

Monitoring the patient
• Routine monitoring of plasma drug levels isn't needed. Drug doesn't appear to alter plasma levels of other anticonvulsants.
• Monitor patient for adverse effects.

Information for the patient
• Warn patient to avoid driving or operating heavy machinery until CNS effects of drug are known.
• Instruct patient to take first dose at bedtime to minimize drowsiness, dizziness, fatigue, and ataxia.
• Inform patient that drug can be taken without regard to meals.

Pediatric patients
• Safety and effectiveness in children under age 12 haven't been established.

Breast-feeding patients
• It's unknown if drug appears in breast milk. Use in breast-feeding women only if benefits clearly outweigh risks.

ganciclovir (DHPG)
Cytovene, Vitrasert

Pharmacologic classification: synthetic nucleoside
Therapeutic classification: antiviral
Pregnancy risk category C

How supplied
Available by prescription only
Injection: 500-mg vial
Capsules: 250 mg
Implant: 4.5 mg

Indications, route, and dosage
Treatment of cytomegalovirus (CMV) retinitis
Adults: Initially, 5 mg/kg I.V. (given at a constant rate over 1 hour) q 12 hours for 14 to 21 days; then a maintenance dose of 5 mg/kg I.V. once daily for 7 days weekly; or 6 mg/kg I.V. once daily for 5 days weekly. These I.V. infusions should be given at a constant rate over 1 hour. Or a maintenance dose of 1,000 mg P.O. t.i.d. or 500 mg P.O. q 3 hours while awake (six times daily) may be used.
Prevention of CMV in transplant recipients
Adults: 5 mg/kg I.V. over 1 hour q 12 hours for 7 to 14 days; then a maintenance dose of 5 mg/kg once daily for 7 days weekly or 6 mg/kg once daily for 5 days weekly.

◇ *Other CMV infections*
Adults: 5 mg/kg I.V. over 1 hour q 12 hours for 14 to 21 days; or 2.5 mg/kg I.V. q 8 hours for 14 to 21 days.
✦ *Dosage adjustment.* Adjust dosage in patients with renal failure. A dosage reduction should also be considered for patients with neutropenia, anemia, or thrombocytopenia. For the treatment of CMV retinitis in patients with AIDS, the adult dosage should be one implant every 5 to 8 months.

Creatinine clearance (ml/min)	Dosage
I.V. induction dose	
≥ 70	5 mg/kg I.V. q 12 hr
50 to 69	2.5 mg/kg I.V. q 12 hr
25 to 49	2.5 mg/kg I.V. q 24 hr
10 to 24	1.25 mg/kg I.V. q 24 hr
< 10	1.25 mg/kg I.V. three times weekly following hemodialysis
P.O. dose	
≥ 70	1,000 mg P.O. t.i.d. or 500 mg q 3 hr, 6 times daily
50 to 69	1,500 mg P.O. daily or 500 mg P.O. t.i.d.
25 to 49	1,000 mg P.O. daily or 500 mg P.O. b.i.d.
10 to 24	500 mg P.O. daily
< 10	500 mg P.O. three times weekly following hemodialysis

Pharmacodynamics
Antiviral action: A synthetic nucleoside analogue of 2′-deoxyguanosine. Competitively inhibits viral DNA polymerase, and may be incorporated within viral DNA to cause early termination of DNA replication. Has shown activity against CMV, herpes simplex virus type 1 and type 2 (HSV-1 and HSV-2), varicella zoster virus, Epstein-Barr virus, and hepatitis B virus.

Pharmacokinetics
• *Absorption:* Administered I.V. because less than 7% is absorbed after oral administration.
• *Distribution:* Only 2% to 3% protein-bound. Prefers to concentrate within CMV-infected cells because of cellular kinases action that converts it to ganciclovir triphosphate.
• *Metabolism:* Over 90% excreted unchanged.
• *Excretion:* Elimination half-life is about 3 hours in patients with normal renal function; can be as long as 30 hours in patients with severe renal failure. Primarily excreted through kidneys by

glomerular filtration and some renal tubular secretion.

Contraindications and precautions
Contraindicated in patients with hypersensitivity to drug and in those with an absolute neutrophil count below 500/mm^3 or a platelet count below 25,000/mm^3. Use cautiously in patients with impaired renal function.

Interactions
Drug-drug. *Cytotoxic drugs:* Possible additive toxicity (bone marrow depression, stomatitis, alopecia). Monitor patient and CBC closely.
Didanosine: Administration with ganciclovir may result in mutual alteration of both drugs' pharmacokinetics. Avoid concomitant use.
Imipenem-cilastatin: Possible increased risk of seizures. Monitor patient closely.
Immunosuppressants (azathioprine, corticosteroids, cyclosporine): Enhanced immune and bone marrow suppression. Monitor patient.
Probenecid: May decrease renal clearance of ganciclovir. Avoid concomitant use.
Zidovudine: Possible increased risk of neutropenia in patients receiving zidovudine and ganciclovir. Monitor CBC.

Adverse reactions
CNS: altered dreams, confusion, ataxia, headache, *seizures, coma,* dizziness, somnolence, tremor, abnormal thinking, agitation, amnesia, anxiety, neuropathy, paresthesia, asthenia.
EENT: retinal detachment (in CMV retinitis patients).
GI: *nausea, vomiting, diarrhea, anorexia, abdominal pain,* flatulence, dyspepsia, dry mouth.
GU: increased serum creatinine levels.
Hematologic: granulocytopenia, *thrombocytopenia, leukopenia, anemia.*
Hepatic: abnormal liver function tests.
Respiratory: pneumonia.
Skin: rash; sweating; pruritus, inflammation, pain (at injection site).
Other: phlebitis, chills, sepsis, *fever,* infection.

☑ Special considerations
● Administer drug over 1 hour; don't administer as a rapid I.V. bolus. Don't give I.M. or S.C.
● Reconstitute with sterile water for injection. Don't reconstitute with bacteriostatic water for injection because this may lead to precipitate formation.
● Reconstituted solutions are stable for 12 hours. Don't refrigerate.
● Overdose may result in emesis, neutropenia, or GI disturbances. Treatment should be symptomatic and supportive. Hemodialysis may be useful. Hydrate patient to reduce plasma levels.

Monitoring the patient
● Monitor CBC to detect neutropenia, which may occur in as many as 40% of patients. Usually appears after about 10 days of therapy and may be associated with a higher dosage (15 mg/kg/day). Neutropenia is reversible, but may require interruption of therapy. Patients may resume drug therapy when blood counts return to normal.
● Monitor patient for retinitis through regular ophthalmic examinations.

Information for the patient
● Tell patient that maintenance infusions are necessary to prevent recurrence of disease.
● Instruct patient to have regular ophthalmic examinations to monitor retinitis.
● Advise patient to immediately report signs or symptoms of infection (fever, sore throat) or easy bruising or bleeding.
● Inform patient to take oral dose with food.

Geriatric patients
● Use cautiously in elderly patients with compromised renal function.

Pediatric patients
● Little data available on drug use in children under age 12. Use with extreme caution because of potential for carcinogenic and reproductive toxicity.

Breast-feeding patients
● It's unknown if drug appears in breast milk. Don't use drug in breast-feeding women. Instruct patient to stop breast-feeding until at least 72 hours after last treatment.

ganirelix acetate
Antagon

Pharmacologic classification: gonadotropin-releasing hormone (Gn-RH) antagonist
Therapeutic classification: fertility drug
Pregnancy risk category X

How supplied
Available by prescription only
Injection: 250 mcg/0.5 ml in prefilled syringes

Indications, route, and dosage
Inhibition of premature luteinizing hormone (LH) surges in women undergoing medically supervised, controlled ovarian hyperstimulation
Adults: 250 mcg S.C. once daily during early to midfollicular phase of menstrual cycle. Continue daily until enough follicles of sufficient size are confirmed by ultrasound; human chorionic go-

nadotropin will then be administered to induce final maturation of follicles.

Pharmacodynamics
LH suppression action: Gn-RH, secreted by the pituitary gland, stimulates synthesis and secretion of gonadotropins LH and follicle-stimulating hormone (FSH). In midcycle, a large increase in Gn-RH leads to a large surge in LH secretion, causing ovulation, a rise in progesterone levels, and a decrease in estradiol levels. Ganirelix blocks pituitary Gn-RH receptors and suppresses LH and, to a smaller degree, FSH secretions. By suppressing LH and FSH secretions in the early-to-mid menstrual cycle, ganirelix stops premature gonadotropin surges that could interfere with a trial of medically supervised, controlled ovarian hyperstimulation.

Pharmacokinetics
- *Absorption:* Rapidly absorbed after S.C. injection; average of 91.1% absorbed. Action peaks in 1 hour.
- *Distribution:* 81.9% bound to plasma proteins.
- *Metabolism:* Unmetabolized drug found in urine up to 24 hours after dose. Two metabolites detected in feces.
- *Excretion:* Primary excretion route is fecal; metabolites detected nearly 8 days after dose.

Contraindications and precautions
Contraindicated in patients with hypersensitivity to drug or its components or to Gn-RH or Gn-RH analogue. Also contraindicated in pregnant women. Use with caution in patients with potential hypersensitivity to Gn-RH and in those with latex allergies because the product packaging contains natural rubber latex.

Interactions
None reported.

Adverse reactions
CNS: headache.
GI: abdominal pain, nausea.
GU: vaginal bleeding, gynecologic abdominal pain, ovarian hyperstimulation syndrome.
Skin: injection site reaction.
Other: *fetal death.*

☑ Special considerations
- Before starting treatment, ensure that patient isn't pregnant.
- Use cautiously in patient who reports previous potential hypersensitivity to Gn-RH; monitor patient closely after first injection.
- Use cautiously in hypersensitive patients because natural rubber latex packaging of product may cause allergic reactions.
- Only health care providers experienced in fertility treatments should prescribe drug.

Monitoring the patient
- Monitor WBC count. Increased WBC count and decreased bilirubin levels and hematocrit have been observed in patients receiving ganirelix injections.
- Monitor patient for adverse effects.

Information for the patient
- Tell patient that correct use of ganirelix injection is extremely important to success of infertility treatments. Patient should be able to adhere to strict administration schedule.
- Teach patient proper technique for S.C. administration.
- Tell patient to use abdomen or upper thigh for injection and to vary injection site with each dose.
- Advise patient to store drug at room temperature, away from heat and light, and out of children's reach.
- Inform patient to discontinue drug and report suspected or known pregnancy.

Geriatric patients
- Drug hasn't been sufficiently studied in patients ages 65 and older.

Pediatric patients
- Drug hasn't been studied in children.

Breast-feeding patients
- Amount of drug appearing in breast milk is unknown; don't give drug to breast-feeding women.

gatifloxacin
Tequin

Pharmacologic classification: fluoroquinolone antibiotic
Therapeutic classification: antibiotic
Pregnancy risk category C

How supplied
Tablets: 200 mg, 400 mg
Injection: 200 mg/20-ml vial, 400 mg/40-ml vial; 200 mg in 100 ml D_5W, 400 mg in 200 ml D_5W

Indications, route, and dosage
Exacerbation of chronic bronchitis caused by Streptococcus pneumoniae, Haemophilus influenzae, H. parainfluenzae, Moraxella catarrhalis *or* Staphylococcus aureus; *complicated urinary tract infections caused by* Escherichia coli, Klebsiella pneumoniae, *or* Proteus mirabilis, *and acute pyelonephritis caused by* E. coli
Adults: 400 mg I.V. or P.O. daily for 7 to 10 days.
Acute sinusitis caused by S. pneumoniae *or* H. influenzae
Adults: 400 mg I.V. or P.O. daily for 10 days.
Community-acquired pneumonia caused by S. pneumoniae, H. influenzae, H. parainflu*

zae, M. catarrhalis, S. aureus, Mycoplasma pneumoniae, Chlamydia pneumoniae, or Legionella pneumophila
Adults: 400 mg I.V. or P.O. daily for 7 to 14 days.
✦ Dosage adjustment. For patients with creatinine clearance of less than 40 ml/min, those receiving hemodialysis, and those on continuous peritoneal dialysis, initial dose is 400 mg and subsequent doses are 200 mg daily. For patients on hemodialysis, administer after hemodialysis session is complete.
Uncomplicated urethral gonorrhea in men and cervical gonorrhea or acute uncomplicated rectal infections in women caused by Neisseria gonorrhoeae
Adults: 400 mg P.O. as single dose.
Uncomplicated urinary tract infection caused by E. coli, K. pneumoniae, or P. mirabilis
Adults: 400 mg I.V. or P.O. as single dose, or 200 mg I.V. or P.O. daily for 3 days.

Pharmacodynamics
Antibiotic action: Inhibits DNA gyrase and topoisomerase, preventing cell replication and division. Active against gram-positive and gram-negative organisms, including: *S. aureus, S. pneumoniae, E. coli, H. influenzae, H. parainfluenzae, K. pneumoniae, M. catarrhalis, N. gonorrhoeae, P. mirabilis, C. pneumoniae, L. pneumophila, M. pneumoniae.*

Pharmacokinetics
● *Absorption:* 96% absorbed after oral administration; levels peak in 1 to 2 hours.
● *Distribution:* 20% protein-bound; widely distributed into many tissues and fluids.
● *Metabolism:* Limited biotransformation.
● *Excretion:* More than 70% excreted unchanged by kidneys. Serum half-life is 7 to 14 hours.

Contraindications and precautions
Contraindicated in patients with a hypersensitivity to any fluoroquinolone. Don't use in patients with prolongation of the QTc interval or uncorrected hypokalemia.
Use cautiously in patients with clinically significant bradycardia, acute myocardial ischemia, known or suspected CNS disorders, or renal insufficiency.

Interactions
Drug-drug. *Antacids containing aluminum or magnesium; didanosine buffered solution tablets or buffered powder; products containing iron, magnesium, zinc:* Decreased absorption of gatifloxacin. Administer gatifloxacin 4 hours before these products.
Antidiabetics (glyburide, insulin): Possible symptomatic hypoglycemia or hyperglycemia. Monitor blood glucose level.

Antipsychotics, erythromycin, tricyclic antidepressants: Possible prolongation of QTc interval. Use cautiously.
Class IA (procainamide, quinidine) or class III (amiodarone, sotalol) antiarrhythmics: Potential for prolongation of QTc interval. Avoid concomitant use.
Digoxin: Levels may increase in some patients. Watch for signs of digoxin toxicity.
NSAIDs: May increase risks of CNS stimulation and convulsions. Use cautiously.
Probenecid: Increased gatifloxacin levels and prolonged half-life. Monitor patient closely.
Warfarin: Possible enhanced effects of warfarin. Monitor PT and INR.
Drug-lifestyle. *Sun exposure:* Photosensitivity reactions may occur. Patient should take precautions.

Adverse reactions
CNS: headache, dizziness, abnormal dreams, insomnia, paresthesia, tremor, vertigo.
CV: palpitations, chest pain, peripheral edema.
EENT: tinnitus, abnormal vision, pharyngitis, taste perversion.
GI: nausea, diarrhea, abdominal pain, constipation, dyspepsia, oral candidiasis, glossitis, stomatitis, mouth ulcer, vomiting
GU: dysuria, hematuria, vaginitis.
Musculoskeletal: arthralgia, myalgia, back pain.
Respiratory: dyspnea.
Skin: rash, sweating.
Other: redness at injection site, chills, fever, **anaphylaxis.**

☑ Special considerations
● For I.V. administration, dilute drug in single-use vials with D$_5$W or normal saline to a final concentration of 2 mg/ml before administration. Diluted solutions are stable for 14 days at room temperature or refrigerated. Frozen solutions are stable for up to 6 months except for 5% sodium bicarbonate solutions. Thaw at room temperature or in refrigerator. Don't mix with other drugs. Infuse over 60 minutes.
● Signs of overdose include decreased respiratory rate, vomiting, tremors, and convulsions. For oral gatifloxacin, empty stomach by induced vomiting or gastric lavage. Provide symptomatic and supportive treatment. Monitor ECG; maintain hydration.
● Drug isn't removed by hemodialysis or peritoneal dialysis.

Monitoring the patient
● Observe for rash; stop drug immediately if rash occurs.
● Monitor serum glucose level in diabetic patient.
● Monitor serum digoxin levels in patient taking digoxin.
● Monitor patient for seizures, increased intracranial pressure, psychosis, or CNS stimulation lead-

ing to tremors, light-headedness, confusion, restlessness, hallucinations, paranoia, depression, nightmares, and insomnia; stop drug immediately if these occur.
• Monitor renal function in patient with renal insufficiency.
• Monitor patient for signs of fainting or palpitations.
• Monitor patient for diarrhea (pseudomembranous colitis may occur).

Information for the patient
• Tell patient to take drug as prescribed and to finish drug even if symptoms disappear.
• Advise patient to take drug 4 hours before products containing aluminum, magnesium, zinc, or iron.
• Advise patient to use sunblock and protective clothing when exposed to excessive sunlight.
• Warn patient to avoid hazardous tasks until adverse CNS effects of drugs are known.
• Advise diabetic patient to monitor blood glucose levels and call if hypoglycemia occurs.
• Advise patient to report palpitations, fainting spells, skin rash, hives, difficulty swallowing or breathing, swelling of the lips, tongue, face, tightness in throat, hoarseness, or other symptoms of allergic reaction immediately.
• Advise patient to stop drug, refrain from exercise, and call if pain, inflammation, or rupture of tendon occurs.

Geriatric patients
• No dosage adjustment is necessary based on age.

Pediatric patients
• Safety and effectiveness haven't been established in children under age 18. Quinolones may cause arthropathy and osteochondrotoxicity in these patients.

Breast-feeding patients
• It's unknown if drug appears in breast milk. Administer cautiously to breast-feeding women.

---

gemcitabine hydrochloride
Gemzar

Pharmacologic classification: nucleoside analogue
Therapeutic classification: antitumor drug
Pregnancy risk category D

How supplied
Available by prescription only
Powder for injection: 200 mg/10-ml, 1 g/50-ml vials

Indications, route, and dosage
Locally advanced (nonresectable stage II or stage III) or metastatic pancreatic adenocar-

cinoma (stage IV) and in patients previously treated with fluorouracil
Adults: 1,000 mg/m² I.V. over 30 minutes once weekly for up to 7 weeks or until toxicity necessitates reducing or holding a dose. Monitor patient's CBC (including differential) and platelet count before each dose. Treatment course of 7 weeks; then 1 week rest. Subsequent dosage cycles consist of one infusion weekly for 3 out of 4 consecutive weeks.
✦ *Dosage adjustment.* Adjust dosage if bone marrow suppression is detected. Full dose should be given if absolute granulocyte count (AGC) is 1,000/mm³ or more and platelet count is 100,000/mm³ or more. If AGC is 500/mm³ to 999/mm³, or if platelet count is 50,000/mm³ to 99,000/mm³, give 75% of dose. Hold dose if AGC is below 500/mm³ or platelet count is below 50,000/mm³. Adjust dosage for subsequent cycles based on AGC and platelet count nadirs and degree of nonhematologic toxicity.

Pharmacodynamics
Cytotoxic action: Cell cycle–phase specific; inhibits DNA synthesis and blocks progression of cells through G1/S-phase boundary.

Pharmacokinetics
• *Absorption:* No information available.
• *Distribution:* Volume of distribution (V_d) increases with increased infusion time. After infusion lasting under 70 minutes, V_d was 50 L/m², suggesting that drug isn't extensively distributed. V_d rose to 370 L/m² for longer infusions, reflecting slow equilibration of gemcitabine with the tissue compartment. Plasma protein–binding is negligible. Longer infusion time results in longer drug half-life.
• *Metabolism:* Metabolized to inactive uracil metabolite.
• *Excretion:* Drug clearance decreases with increasing age; less clearance in women than men. Increased half-life with increased age and in women. In studies, 92% to 98% of drug recovered almost entirely in urine.

Contraindications and precautions
Contraindicated in patients with hypersensitivity to drug.

Interactions
None reported.

Adverse reactions
CNS: *paresthesia, somnolence.*
CV: *edema, peripheral edema.*
GI: *constipation, diarrhea, nausea, stomatitis, vomiting.*
GU: *elevated BUN* and creatinine, *hematuria, proteinuria.*
Hematologic: *anemia,* LEUKOPENIA, NEUTROPENIA, THROMBOCYTOPENIA, HEMORRHAGE.

Hepatic: *elevated liver enzyme levels.*
Respiratory: *bronchospasm, dyspnea.*
Skin: *alopecia, rash.*
Other: *fever, flulike symptoms,* INFECTION, *pain.*

☑ Special considerations
● Prolonged infusion time beyond 60 minutes and more frequently than weekly dosing increase drug toxicity.
● Follow institutional policy to reduce risks. Preparation and administration of parenteral form of drug is associated with mutagenic, teratogenic, and carcinogenic risks for personnel.
● Advanced age, female sex, and renal impairment may predispose patient to toxicity.
● No known antidote for drug overdose. If overdose is suspected, monitor appropriate blood counts and provide supportive therapy.

Monitoring the patient
● Perform renal and hepatic function tests before treatment and periodically thereafter.
● Monitor CBC, differential, and platelet count before giving each dose. Drug can suppress bone marrow function as evidenced by leukopenia, thrombocytopenia, and anemia.

Information for the patient
● Advise patient to watch for signs of infection (fever, sore throat, fatigue) and bleeding (easy bruising, nosebleeds, bleeding gums, melena). Also, tell patient to take temperature daily.
● Advise woman of childbearing age to avoid pregnancy and not to breast-feed during therapy.

Geriatric patients
● Drug clearance is affected by age. No evidence, however, that unusual dosage adjustments, other than those already recommended, are necessary. Grade 3 to 4 thrombocytopenia is more common in elderly patients.

Pediatric patients
● Safety and efficacy in children haven't been studied.

Breast-feeding patients
● It's unknown if drug appears in breast milk. Avoid drug in breast-feeding women.

gemfibrozil
Lopid

Pharmacologic classification: fibric acid derivative
Therapeutic classification: antilipemic
Pregnancy risk category C

How supplied
Available by prescription only
Tablets: 600 mg

Indications, route, and dosage
Types IV and V hyperlipidemia (hypertriglyceridemia) and severe hypercholesterolemia unresponsive to diet and other drugs; reducing risk of cardiac disease, only in type IIb patients without history of disease
Adults: 1,200 mg P.O. administered in two divided doses 30 minutes before morning and evening meals.

Pharmacodynamics
Antilipemic action: Decreases serum triglyceride levels and very-low-density lipoprotein (VLDL) cholesterol while increasing serum high-density lipoprotein cholesterol, inhibits lipolysis in adipose tissue, and reduces hepatic triglyceride synthesis. Closely related to clofibrate pharmacologically.

Pharmacokinetics
● *Absorption:* Well absorbed from GI tract; plasma levels peak 1 to 2 hours after oral dose. Plasma levels of VLDL decrease in 2 to 5 days; clinical effect peaks in 4 weeks. Further decreases in plasma VLDL levels occur over several months.
● *Distribution:* 95% protein-bound.
● *Metabolism:* Metabolized by liver.
● *Excretion:* Eliminated mostly in urine but some excreted in feces. After single dose, half-life is 1½ hours; after multiple doses, half-life decreases to about 1¼ hours.

Contraindications and precautions
Contraindicated in patients with hypersensitivity to drug and in those with hepatic or severe renal dysfunction (including primary biliary cirrhosis) or preexisting gallbladder disease.

Interactions
Drug-drug. *Lovastatin, pravastatin, simvastatin:* Possible myopathy with rhabdomyolysis. Avoid use together.
Oral anticoagulants: Increased risk of hemorrhage (gemfibrozil enhances anticoagulant effect). Adjust anticoagulant dose to maintain desired PT and INR; monitor frequently.

Adverse reactions
CNS: headache, fatigue, vertigo.
CV: atrial fibrillation.
GI: abdominal and epigastric pain, diarrhea, nausea, vomiting, *dyspepsia,* constipation, acute appendicitis.
Hematologic: anemia, *leukopenia,* eosinophilia, ***thrombocytopenia.***
Hepatic: bile duct obstruction, elevated liver enzyme levels.
Metabolic: hypokalemia.
Skin: rash, dermatitis, pruritus, eczema.

Reactions may be *common,* uncommon, *life-threatening,* or COMMON AND LIFE-THREATENING.

☑ Special considerations
- Because drug is pharmacologically related to clofibrate, adverse reactions associated with clofibrate may also occur with gemfibrozil. Clofibrate may increase risk of death from cancer, postcholecystectomy complications, and pancreatitis. These hazards haven't been studied in gemfibrozil but should be kept in mind.

Monitoring the patient
- Monitor coagulation studies if patient is taking anticoagulants.
- Monitor patient for adverse effects.

Information for the patient
- Stress importance of close medical supervision and tell patient to report adverse reactions promptly; encourage patient to comply with prescribed regimen, diet, and exercise.
- Warn patient not to exceed prescribed dose.
- Advise patient to take drug with food to minimize GI discomfort.

Pediatric patients
- Safety and efficacy in children under age 18 haven't been established.

Breast-feeding patients
- Safety in breast-feeding women hasn't been established.

gentamicin sulfate
Cidomycin*, Garamycin, Genoptic, Genoptic S.O.P., Gentacidin, Gentak, Jenamicin

Pharmacologic classification: aminoglycoside
Therapeutic classification: antibiotic
Pregnancy risk category NR

How supplied
Available by prescription only
Injection: 40 mg/ml (adult), 10 mg/ml (pediatric), 2 mg/ml (intrathecal)
Ophthalmic ointment: 3 mg/g
Ophthalmic solution: 3 mg/ml
Topical cream or ointment: 0.1%

Indications, route, and dosage
Serious infections caused by susceptible organisms
Adults with normal renal function: 3 mg/kg/day I.M. or I.V. infusion (in 50 to 100 ml of normal saline solution or D_5W infused over 30 minutes to 2 hours) daily in divided doses q 8 hours. May be given by direct I.V. push if needed. For life-threatening infections, patient may receive up to 5 mg/kg/day in three or four divided doses.
Children with normal renal function: 2 to 2.5 mg/kg I.M. or I.V. infusion q 8 hours.

Infants and neonates over age 1 week with normal renal function: 2.5 mg/kg I.M. or I.V. infusion q 8 hours.
Neonates under age 1 week: 2.5 mg/kg I.M. or I.V. infusion q 12 hours. For I.V. infusion, dilute in normal saline solution or D_5W and infuse over 30 minutes to 2 hours.
Meningitis
Adults: Systemic therapy as above; may also use 4 to 8 mg intrathecally daily.
Children: Systemic therapy as above; may also use 1 to 2 mg intrathecally daily.
Endocarditis prophylaxis for GI or GU procedure or surgery
Adults: 1.5 mg/kg I.M. or I.V. 30 to 60 minutes before procedure or surgery and q 8 hours after, for two doses. Given separately with aqueous penicillin G or ampicillin.
Children: 2 mg/kg I.M. or I.V. 30 to 60 minutes before procedure or surgery and q 8 hours after, for two doses. Given separately with aqueous penicillin G or ampicillin.
External ocular infections caused by susceptible organisms
Adults and children: Instill 1 to 2 drops in eye q 4 hours. In severe infections, may use up to 2 drops q hour. Apply ointment to lower conjunctival sac b.i.d. or t.i.d.
Primary and secondary bacterial infections; superficial burns; skin ulcers; and infected lacerations, abrasions, insect bites, or minor surgical wounds
Adults and children over age 1: Rub in small amount gently t.i.d. or q.i.d., with or without gauze dressing.
Pelvic inflammatory disease
Adults: Initially 2 mg/kg I.M. or I.V; then 1.5 mg/kg q 8 hours.
✦ *Dosage adjustment.* In patients with renal failure, initial dose is same as for those with normal renal function. Subsequent doses and frequency determined by renal function studies and blood levels; keep peak serum levels between 4 and 10 mcg/ml and trough serum levels between 1 and 2 mcg/ml. One method is to administer 1 mg/kg doses and adjust the dosing interval based on steady-state serum creatinine, using this formula:

$$\frac{\text{Creatinine}}{(\text{mg/100 ml})} \times 8 = \frac{\text{dosing interval}}{(\text{hours})}$$

Posthemodialysis to maintain therapeutic blood levels
Adults: 1 to 1.7 mg/kg I.M. or I.V. infusion after each dialysis.
Children: 2 to 2.5 mg/kg I.M. or I.V. infusion after each dialysis.

Pharmacodynamics
Antibiotic action: Bactericidal; binds directly to the 30S ribosomal subunit, thus inhibiting bac-

terial protein synthesis. Spectrum of activity includes many aerobic gram-negative organisms (including most strains of *Pseudomonas aeruginosa*) and some aerobic gram-positive organisms. May act against some bacterial strains resistant to other aminoglycosides; bacterial strains resistant to gentamicin may be susceptible to tobramycin, netilmicin, or amikacin.

Pharmacokinetics
● *Absorption:* Absorbed poorly after oral administration and is given parenterally; after I.M. administration, serum levels peak at 30 to 90 minutes.
● *Distribution:* Distributed widely after parenteral administration; poor intraocular penetration. Low CSF penetration even in patients with inflamed meninges. Intraventricular administration produces high levels throughout CNS. Minimal protein-binding. Drug crosses placenta.
● *Metabolism:* Not metabolized.
● *Excretion:* Excreted primarily in urine by glomerular filtration; small amounts may be excreted in bile and breast milk. Drug's elimination half-life in adults is 2 to 3 hours. In patients with severe renal damage, half-life may extend to 24 to 60 hours.

Contraindications and precautions
Contraindicated in patients with hypersensitivity to drug and in those who may exhibit cross-sensitivity with other aminoglycosides such as neomycin. Use systemic treatment cautiously in neonates, infants, elderly patients, and patients with renal or neuromuscular disorders.

Interactions
Drug-drug. *Acyclovir, amphotericin B, capreomycin, cephalosporins, cisplatin, methoxyflurane, polymyxin B, vancomycin, other aminoglycosides:* Potential for nephrotoxicity, ototoxicity, or neurotoxicity. Monitor patient closely.
Antiemetics, antivertigo drugs, dimenhydrinate: May mask gentamicin-induced ototoxicity. Monitor patient closely.
Bumetanide, ethacrynic acid, furosemide, mannitol, urea: Potential for ototoxicity. Monitor patient closely.
General anesthetics, neuromuscular blockers (such as succinylcholine, tubocurarine): May potentiate neuromuscular blockade. Monitor patient closely.
Indomethacin: May increase serum peak and trough levels of gentamicin. Monitor gentamicin levels.
Penicillin: Administration with gentamycin results in synergistic bactericidal effect against *Pseudomonas aeruginosa, Escherichia coli, Klebsiella, Citrobacter, Enterobacter, Serratia,* and *Proteus mirabilis;* however, the drugs are physically and chemically incompatible and are inactivated when mixed or given together. Avoid concomitant use.

Adverse reactions
CNS: headache, lethargy, encephalopathy, confusion, dizziness, *seizures,* numbness, peripheral neuropathy (with injected form).
CV: hypotension (with injected form).
EENT: *ototoxicity,* blurred vision (with injected form); burning, stinging, blurred vision (with ophthalmic ointment), transient irritation (with ophthalmic solution), conjunctival hyperemia (with ophthalmic form).
GI: vomiting, nausea (with injected form).
GU: *nephrotoxicity* (with injected form).
Hematologic: anemia, eosinophilia, *leukopenia, thrombocytopenia, granulocytopenia* (with injected form).
Musculoskeletal: muscle twitching, myasthenia gravis-like syndrome.
Respiratory: *apnea* (with injected form).
Skin: rash, urticaria, pruritus, tingling (with injected form); minor skin irritation, possible photosensitivity, allergic contact dermatitis (with topical administration).
Other: fever, pain at injection site (with injected form); *hypersensitivity reactions, anaphylaxis,* overgrowth of nonsusceptible organisms (with ophthalmic form and long-term use).

☑ Special considerations
Besides the recommendations relevant to all aminoglycosides, consider the following.
● For local application to skin infections, remove crusts by gently soaking with warm water and soap or wet compresses before applying ointment or cream; cover with protective gauze.
● Because drug is dialyzable, patients undergoing hemodialysis may need dosage adjustments.
● Systemic absorption from excessive use may cause systemic toxicities.
● Increased risk of toxicity is associated with prolonged peak serum level above 10 mcg/ml and trough serum level above 2 mcg/ml.
● Signs and symptoms of overdose include ototoxicity, nephrotoxicity, and neuromuscular toxicity. Drug can be removed by hemodialysis or peritoneal dialysis. Treatment with calcium salts or anticholinesterases reverses neuromuscular blockade.

Monitoring the patient
● Monitor renal function before initiating treatment and regularly throughout therapy.
● Monitor peak and trough gentamicin levels.

Information for the patient
● Teach patient proper topical application of drug; emphasize need to call promptly if lesions worsen or skin irritation occurs.

Reactions may be *common*, uncommon, *life-threatening*, OR COMMON AND LIFE-THREATENING.

glatiramer acetate
(formerly copolymer-1)
Copaxone

Pharmacologic classification: acetate salts of synthetic peptides containing four naturally occurring amino acids (L-alanine, L-glutamic acid, L-lysine, L-tyrosine)
Therapeutic classification: immune response modifier
Pregnancy risk category B

How supplied
Available by prescription only
Injection for S.C. use: sterile lyophilized material containing 20 mg glatiramer acetate and 40 mg mannitol, USP, in a single-use 2-ml vial (amber glass); 1-ml vials of sterile water for injection (in clear glass) are included for reconstitution

Indications, route, and dosage
To reduce frequency of relapses in patients with relapsing-remitting multiple sclerosis
Adults: 20 mg S.C. daily.

Pharmacodynamics
Immune response modifier action: Mechanism unknown. Thought to act by modifying immune processes responsible for the pathogenesis of multiple sclerosis.

Pharmacokinetics
Pharmacokinetics in patients with impaired renal function aren't known.
• *Absorption:* A substantial fraction of dose injected S.C. may be hydrolyzed locally. Some is presumed to enter lymphatic circulation and regional lymph nodes; some may enter systemic circulation.
• *Distribution:* No information available.
• *Metabolism:* No information available.
• *Excretion:* No information available.

Contraindications and precautions
Contraindicated in patients with hypersensitivity to drug or mannitol.

Interactions
None reported.

Adverse reactions
CNS: abnormal dreams, agitation, *anxiety, asthenia,* confusion, emotional lability, *hypertonia,* migraine, nervousness, speech disorder, stupor, tremor, vertigo.
CV: *chest pain,* hypertension, *palpitations, vasodilation,* syncope, tachycardia.
EENT: ear pain, eye disorder, laryngismus, nystagmus, *rhinitis.*

GI: anorexia, *diarrhea,* gastroenteritis, GI disorder, *nausea,* oral candidiasis, salivary gland enlargement, tooth caries, ulcerative stomatitis, vomiting.
GU: amenorrhea, bowel urgency, dysmenorrhea, hematuria, impotence, menorrhagia, suspicious Papanicolaou smear, *urinary urgency,* vaginal candidiasis, vaginal hemorrhage.
Hematologic: ecchymosis, *lymphadenopathy.*
Metabolic: edema, peripheral edema, weight gain.
Musculoskeletal: arthralgia, *back pain,* neck pain, foot drop.
Respiratory: bronchitis, *dyspnea,* hyperventilation.
Skin: eczema, erythema, herpes simplex and zoster, *pruritus, rash,* skin atrophy, skin nodule, *sweating,* urticaria, warts.
Other: bacterial infection, chills, cyst, facial edema, fever, *flulike syndrome, infection, injection site reaction* or hemorrhage, *pain.*

☑ Special considerations
• Administer drug by S.C. injection only.
• Store drug in refrigerator (36° to 46° F [2° to 8° C]); diluent can be kept at room temperature.
• Use immediately after reconstitution because drug doesn't contain preservatives. Discard unused drug.
• About 26% of patients experienced at least one episode of transient chest pain which usually began at least 1 month after treatment began; it wasn't accompanied by other symptoms and appeared not to be significant.

Monitoring the patient
• Monitor patient for immediate postinjection reactions. Such reactions have occurred in 10% of patients with multiple sclerosis; symptoms include flushing; chest pain, palpitations, anxiety, dyspnea, throat constriction, and urticaria. These reactions were transient, self-limited, and didn't require specific treatment. Onset may occur several months after therapy starts and patients may have more than one episode.
• Monitor patient for adverse effects.

Information for the patient
• Explain need for aseptic injection techniques and warn patient against reuse of needles and syringes.
• Instruct patient to call if pregnancy occurs, is suspected, or if pregnancy is being planned.
• Tell patient to call if she is breast-feeding.
• Advise patient not to change drug or dosing schedule or to stop drug without medical approval.
• Inform patient to call immediately if dizziness, hives, sweating, chest pain, difficulty breathing, or severe pain occurs following drug injection.

Geriatric patients
• Drug hasn't been studied specifically in elderly patients.

Pediatric patients
• Safety and efficacy haven't been established in children under age 18.

Breast-feeding patients
• It's unknown if drug appears in breast milk. Use with caution in breast-feeding women.

glimepiride
Amaryl

Pharmacologic classification: sulfonylurea
Therapeutic classification: antidiabetic
Pregnancy risk category C

How supplied
Available by prescription only
Tablets: 1 mg, 2 mg, 4 mg

Indications, route, and dosage
Adjunct to diet and exercise to lower blood glucose in patients with type 2 diabetes mellitus whose hyperglycemia can't be managed by diet and exercise alone
Adults: Initially, 1 to 2 mg P.O. once daily with first main meal of the day; usual maintenance dose is 1 to 4 mg P.O. once daily. Maximum recommended dose is 8 mg once daily. After dose of 2 mg is reached, increases in dosage should be made in increments not exceeding 2 mg at 1- to 2-week intervals based on patient's blood glucose response.
Adjunct to insulin therapy in patients with type 2 diabetes mellitus whose hyperglycemia can't be managed by diet and exercise with an oral hypoglycemic
Adults: 8 mg P.O. once daily with first main meal of the day in combination with low-dose insulin. Upward adjustments of insulin should be done weekly as needed and guided by patient's blood glucose response.
Adjunct to metformin therapy in patients with type 2 diabetes mellitus whose hyperglycemia can't be managed by diet, exercise, and glimepiride or metformin alone
Adults: 8 mg P.O once daily with first main meal of the day, with metformin if patient doesn't respond adequately to glimepiride monotherapy. Adjust dosages based on patient's blood glucose response to determine minimum effective dosage of each drug.
✦ *Dosage adjustment.* Patients with renal impairment require cautious dosing. Give 1 mg P.O. once daily with first main meal of the day, then appropriate dosage adjustment as necessary.

Pharmacodynamics
Antidiabetic action: Exact mechanism appears to depend on stimulating the release of insulin from functioning pancreatic beta cells. Also, drug therapy can lead to increased sensitivity of peripheral tissues to insulin.

Pharmacokinetics
• *Absorption:* Completely absorbed from GI tract. Significant absorption occurs within 1 hour after administration; drug levels peak at 2 to 3 hours.
• *Distribution:* Protein-binding is greater than 99.5%.
• *Metabolism:* Completely metabolized by oxidative biotransformation.
• *Excretion:* About 60% of metabolites excreted in urine; about 40% in feces.

Contraindications and precautions
Contraindicated in patients with hypersensitivity to drug and in those with diabetic ketoacidosis (with or without coma) because this condition should be treated with insulin. Use cautiously in debilitated or malnourished patients and in those with adrenal, pituitary, hepatic, or renal insufficiency because these patients are more susceptible to the hypoglycemic action of glucose-lowering drugs.

Interactions
Drug-drug. *Beta blockers:* May mask symptoms of hypoglycemia. Educate patient about possibility of hypoglycemia unawareness and alternative signs of hypoglycemia.
Corticosteroids, estrogens, isoniazid, nicotinic acid, oral contraceptives, phenothiazines, phenytoin, sympathomimetics, thiazides and other diuretics, thyroid products: Possible hyperglycemia. May require dosage adjustments. Monitor serum glucose levels.
Insulin: May increase potential for hypoglycemia. Monitor serum glucose.
NSAIDs, other highly protein-bound drugs (such as beta blockers, chloramphenicol, coumarins, MAO inhibitors, probenecid, salicylates, sulfonamides): May potentiate hypoglycemic action of sulfonylureas such as glimepiride. Monitor serum glucose levels.
Drug-lifestyle. *Alcohol:* May alter glycemic control; hypoglycemia may result. May also cause disulfiram-like reaction. Discourage concomitant use.

Adverse reactions
CNS: dizziness, asthenia, headache.
EENT: changes in accommodation, blurred vision.
GI: vomiting, abdominal pain, nausea, diarrhea.
Hematologic: *leukopenia,* hemolytic anemia, **agranulocytosis, thrombocytopenia, aplastic anemia, pancytopenia.**

Reactions may be *common*, uncommon, *life-threatening*, or COMMON AND LIFE-THREATENING.

Hepatic: cholestatic jaundice, elevated transaminase levels.
Metabolic: hypoglycemia.
Skin: allergic skin reactions (pruritus, erythema, urticaria, morbilliform or maculopapular eruptions).

☑ **Special considerations**
Besides the recommendations relevant to all sulfonylureas, consider the following.
• In elderly, debilitated, or malnourished patients or in patients with renal or hepatic insufficiency, the initial dosing, dose increments, and maintenance dosage should be conservative to avoid hypoglycemic reactions.
• During maintenance therapy, stop glimepiride if satisfactory lowering of blood glucose level is no longer achieved. Secondary failures to glimepiride monotherapy can be treated with glimepiride-insulin combination therapy.
• Oral hypoglycemic drugs have been associated with an increased risk of CV mortality compared with diet or diet and insulin therapy.
• Overdose of sulfonylureas can produce hypoglycemia. Mild hypoglycemic symptoms without loss of consciousness or neurologic findings should be treated aggressively with oral glucose and adjustments in drug dosage and meal patterns. Severe hypoglycemic reactions with coma, seizure, or other neurologic impairment occur infrequently but require immediate hospitalization. If hypoglycemic coma occurs or is suspected, give a rapid I.V. injection of concentrated (50%) glucose solution, then a continuous infusion of a more dilute (10%) glucose solution at a rate that will maintain blood glucose at a level above 100 mg/dl.
• Closely monitor patient for at least 24 to 48 hours because hypoglycemia may recur after apparent clinical recovery.

Monitoring the patient
• Monitor renal and hepatic function before initiating treatment.
• Monitor fasting blood glucose level periodically to determine therapeutic response. Monitor glycosylated hemoglobin, usually every 3 to 6 months, to more precisely assess long-term glycemic control.

Information for the patient
• Instruct patient to take drug with first meal of the day.
• Make sure patient understands that therapy relieves symptoms but doesn't cure disease.
• Stress importance of adhering to specific diet, weight reduction, exercise, and personal hygiene programs. Explain how and when to monitor blood glucose level.
• Teach patient how to recognize and manage the signs and symptoms of hyperglycemia and hypoglycemia.
• Advise patient to carry medical identification regarding diabetic status.

Geriatric patients
• Elderly patients may be more sensitive to effects of drug because of reduced metabolism and elimination.

Pediatric patients
• Safety and effectiveness in children haven't been established.

Breast-feeding patients
• It's unknown if drug appears in breast milk. Because of potential of hypoglycemia in breast-feeding infants, avoid use in breast-feeding women.

glipizide
Glucotrol, Glucotrol XL

Pharmacologic classification: sulfonylurea
Therapeutic classification: antidiabetic
Pregnancy risk category C

How supplied
Available by prescription only
Tablets: 5 mg, 10 mg
Tablets (extended-release): 5 mg, 10 mg

Indications, route, and dosage
Adjunct to diet to lower blood glucose levels in patients with non-insulin-dependent diabetes mellitus
Adults: Initially, 5 mg P.O. daily 30 minutes before breakfast; dose should be adjusted in increments of 2.5 to 5 mg. Usual maintenance dosage is 10 to 15 mg. Maximum recommended daily dose is 40 mg. Total daily doses above 15 mg should be divided except when using extended-release tablets.
✦ *Dosage adjustment.* Initial dosage in elderly patients or those with hepatic disease may be 2.5 mg.
Extended-release tablets
Adults: Initially, 5 mg P.O. daily. Titrate in 5-mg increments q 3 months based on level of glycemic control. Maximum daily dose is 20 mg.
To replace insulin therapy
Adults: If insulin dose is more than 20 units daily, patient may be started at usual dose of glipizide besides 50% of insulin dose. If insulin dose is below 20 units, insulin may be discontinued.

Pharmacodynamics
Antidiabetic action: Glipizide lowers blood glucose levels by stimulating insulin release from functioning beta cells in the pancreas. After prolonged administration, the drug's hypoglycemic effects appear to reflect extrapancreatic effects, possibly including reduction of basal hepatic glucose production and enhanced peripheral sensitivity to insulin. The latter may result from either

an increase in the number of insulin receptors or changes in events subsequent to insulin binding.

Pharmacokinetics

• *Absorption:* Absorbed rapidly and completely from GI tract. Onset of action occurs within 15 to 30 minutes, with maximum hypoglycemic effects within 2 to 3 hours.
• *Distribution:* Probably distributed within extracellular fluid; about 92% to 99% protein-bound.
• *Metabolism:* Metabolized almost completely by liver to inactive metabolites.
• *Excretion:* Drug and metabolites excreted primarily in urine; small amounts in feces. Renal clearance of unchanged drug increases with increasing urinary pH. Duration of action is 10 to 24 hours; half-life is 2 to 4 hours.

Contraindications and precautions

Contraindicated in patients with hypersensitivity to drug, diabetic ketoacidosis with or without coma, and during pregnancy or breast-feeding. Use cautiously in patients with impaired renal or hepatic function and in elderly, malnourished, or debilitated patients.

Interactions

Drug-drug. *Adrenocorticoids, amphetamines, baclofen, corticotropin, epinephrine, estrogens, ethacrynic acid, furosemide, glucocorticoids, oral contraceptives, phenytoin, thiazide diuretics, thyroid hormones, triamterene:* May increase glucose levels; may require dosage adjustments.
Anabolic steroids, chloramphenicol, clofibrate, guanethidine, insulin, MAO inhibitors, probenecid, salicylates, sulfonamides: May enhance hypoglycemic effect by displacing glipizide from its protein-binding sites. Monitor closely.
Anticoagulants: May increase plasma levels of both drugs; after continued therapy, may reduce plasma levels and effectiveness of anticoagulant. Monitor INR.
Beta blockers (such as ophthalmics): May mask symptoms of hypoglycemia, such as rising pulse rate and blood pressure; may prolong hypoglycemia by blocking gluconeogenesis. Educate patient for hypoglycemia unawareness and alternative signs of hypoglycemia.
Cimetidine: May potentiate hypoglycemic effects by preventing hepatic metabolism. Monitor patient closely.
Corticosteroids, glucagon, rifampin, thiazide diuretics: May decrease hypoglycemic response. Monitor glucose levels closely.
Hydantoins: May increase blood levels of hydantoins. Monitor hydantoin levels.
Drug-lifestyle. *Alcohol:* May alter glycemic control; hypoglycemia may result. May also cause disulfiram-like reaction with nausea, vomiting, abdominal cramps, and headaches. Discourage concomitant use.

Smoking: May increase corticosteroid release; patients who smoke may require higher dosages of glipizide. Discourage concomitant use.

Adverse reactions

CNS: dizziness, drowsiness, headache.
GI: nausea, constipation, diarrhea.
GU: altered BUN level.
Hematologic: *leukopenia,* hemolytic anemia, **agranulocytosis, thrombocytopenia, aplastic anemia.**
Hepatic: cholestatic jaundice, altered liver enzymes.
Metabolic: altered cholesterol, *hypoglycemia.*
Skin: rash, pruritus.

☑ Special considerations

Besides the recommendations relevant to all sulfonylureas, consider the following.
• To improve glucose control in patients who receive 15 mg/day or more, divided doses, usually given 30 minutes before morning and evening meals, are recommended.
• Some patients taking glipizide can be controlled effectively on a once-daily regimen; others show better response with divided dosing.
• Glipizide is a second-generation sulfonylurea oral hypoglycemic; appears to cause fewer adverse reactions than first-generation sulfonylureas.
• Drug has mild diuretic effect that may be useful in patients with heart failure or cirrhosis.
• When substituting glipizide for chlorpropamide, monitor patient carefully during the first week because of the prolonged retention of chlorpropamide.
• Patients who may be more sensitive to drug, such as elderly, debilitated, or malnourished patients, should begin therapy with lower dose (2.5 mg once daily).
• Use in pregnancy usually isn't recommended. If glipizide must be administered, manufacturer recommends that drug be stopped at least 1 month before expected delivery to prevent neonatal hypoglycemia.
• Oral antidiabetics have been associated with an increased risk of CV mortality as compared with diet or diet and insulin therapy.
• Signs and symptoms of overdose include low blood glucose levels, tingling of lips and tongue, hunger, nausea, decreased cerebral function (lethargy, yawning, confusion, agitation, and nervousness), increased sympathetic activity (tachycardia, sweating, and tremor), and ultimately seizures, stupor, and coma.
• Mild hypoglycemia (without loss of consciousness or neurologic findings) responds to treatment with oral glucose and dosage adjustments. If patient loses consciousness or experiences other neurologic changes, give a rapid injection of dextrose 50%, then continuous infusion of dextrose 10% at a rate to maintain blood glucose lev-

---

els more than 100 mg/dl. Monitor patient for 24 to 48 hours.

Monitoring the patient
• Monitor fasting serum glucose periodically to determine therapeutic response. Monitor glycosylated hemoglobin every 3 to 6 months to more precisely assess long-term glycemic control.
• Monitor patient for hypoglycemia when substituting glipizide for chlorpropamide during first week of therapy because chlorpropamide is retained longer in body.
• Monitor coagulation studies if patient is taking anticoagulants.

Information for the patient
• Emphasize importance of following prescribed diet, exercise, and medical regimen.
• Instruct patient to take drug at same time each day.
• Tell patient that, if a dose is missed, it should be taken immediately, unless it's almost time to take the next dose. Patient shouldn't take double doses.
• Advise patient to avoid alcohol when taking glipizide. Remind him that many foods and OTC products contain alcohol.
• Encourage patient to wear a medical identification bracelet or necklace.
• If glipizide causes GI upset, suggest that drug be taken with food.
• Teach patient how to monitor blood glucose, urine glucose, and ketone levels.
• Teach patient how to recognize and manage signs and symptoms of hyperglycemia and hypoglycemia.

Geriatric patients
• Elderly patients may be more sensitive to effects of drug.
• Hypoglycemia causes more neurologic symptoms in elderly patients.

Pediatric patients
• Glipizide is ineffective in type 1 diabetes. Safety and effectiveness in children haven't been established.

glucagon

Pharmacologic classification: antihypoglycemic
Therapeutic classification: antihypoglycemic, diagnostic
Pregnancy risk category B

How supplied
Available by prescription only
Powder for injection: 1 mg (1 unit)/vial, 10 mg (10 units)/vial

Indications, route, and dosage
Coma of insulin-shock therapy
Adults: 0.5 to 1 mg S.C., I.M., or I.V. 1 hour after coma develops; may repeat within 25 minutes, if needed. In deep coma, glucose 10% to 50% I.V. for faster response. When patient responds, give additional carbohydrate immediately.
Severe insulin-induced hypoglycemia during diabetic therapy
Adults: 0.5 to 1 mg S.C., I.M., or I.V.; may repeat q 20 minutes for two doses, if necessary.
Children: 0.025 mg/kg S.C., I.M., or I.V. 1 hour after coma develops; may repeat within 25 minutes, if needed. In deep coma, 10% to 50% glucose I.V. for faster response. When patient responds, give additional carbohydrate immediately.
Diagnostic aid for radiologic examination
Adults: 0.25 to 2 mg I.V. or I.M. before initiation of radiologic procedure.

Pharmacodynamics
Antihypoglycemic action: Increases plasma glucose levels and causes smooth-muscle relaxation and an inotropic myocardial effect because of the stimulation of adenylate cyclase to produce cAMP. cAMP initiates a series of reactions that leads to the degradation of glycogen to glucose. Hepatic stores of glycogen are necessary for glucagon to exert an antihypoglycemic effect.
Diagnostic action: Exact mechanism by which glucagon relaxes smooth muscles of the stomach, esophagus, duodenum, small bowel, and colon is unknown.

Pharmacokinetics
• *Absorption:* Destroyed in GI tract; must be given parenterally. After I.V. administration, hyperglycemic activity peaks within 30 minutes; relaxation of GI smooth muscle occurs within 1 minute. After I.M. administration, relaxation of GI smooth muscle occurs within 10 minutes. Administration to comatose hypoglycemic patients (with normal liver glycogen stores) usually produces a return to consciousness within 20 minutes.
• *Distribution:* Not fully understood.
• *Metabolism:* Degraded extensively by liver, in kidneys and plasma, and at its tissue receptor sites in plasma membranes.
• *Excretion:* Metabolic products excreted by kidneys. Half-life is about 3 to 10 minutes. Duration after I.M. administration is up to 32 minutes; after I.V. administration, up to 25 minutes.

Contraindications and precautions
Contraindicated in patients with hypersensitivity to drug and in those with pheochromocytoma. Use cautiously in patients with insulinoma.

Interactions
Drug-drug. *Anticoagulants:* Increased effects seen with glucagon. Monitor INR.

Epinephrine: Increased and prolonged hyperglycemic effect. Monitor patient closely.
Phenytoin: Appears to inhibit glucagon-induced insulin release. Use with caution as a diagnostic in patients with diabetes mellitus.

Adverse reactions
CV: hypotension.
GI: nausea, vomiting.
Metabolic: hypokalemia.
Respiratory: respiratory distress.
Other: *hypersensitivity reactions* (**bronchospasm,** rash, dizziness, light-headedness).

☑ Special considerations
● Glucagon should be used only under direct medical supervision.
● If patient experiences nausea and vomiting from glucagon administration and can't retain some form of sugar for 1 hour, consider administration of I.V. dextrose.
● For I.V. drip infusion, glucagon is compatible with dextrose solution but forms a precipitate in chloride solutions.
● Glucagon has a positive inotropic and chronotropic action on the heart and may be used to treat overdose of beta blockers.
● Glucagon may be used as a diagnostic aid in radiologic examination of stomach, duodenum, small intestine, and colon when a hypotonic state is desirable.
● Mixed solutions with diluent are stable for 48 hours when stored at 41° F (5° C). Use immediately after reconstitution with sterile water.
● Signs and symptoms of overdose include nausea, vomiting, and hypokalemia. Treat symptomatically.

Monitoring the patient
● Monitor level of consciousness and serum glucose levels until patient is stabilized.
● Monitor coagulation studies if patient is taking anticoagulants.

Information for the patient
● Teach patient how to mix and inject medication properly, using an appropriate-sized syringe and injecting at a 90-degree angle. Instructions for mixing injection: For 2 mg or less, must use manufacturer's diluent; for doses over 2 mg, use sterile water for injection rather than manufacturer's diluent.
● Instruct patient and family members how to administer glucagon and how to recognize hypoglycemia. Urge them to call immediately in emergencies.
● Tell patient to expect response usually within 20 minutes after injection and that injection may be repeated if no response occurs. Patient should seek medical assistance if second injection is needed.

Pediatric patients
● Drug shouldn't be used to treat newborn asphyxia or hypoglycemia in premature infants or in infants who have had intrauterine growth retardation.

Breast-feeding patients
● It's unknown if drug appears in breast milk. Because glucagon is destroyed in GI tract and because of its short-term use, it's unlikely to affect breast-feeding infant.

glyburide
DiaBeta, Glynase PresTab, Micronase

Pharmacologic classification: sulfonylurea
Therapeutic classification: antidiabetic
Pregnancy risk category C

How supplied
Available by prescription only
Tablets: 1.25 mg, 2.5 mg, 5 mg
Tablets (micronized): 1.5 mg, 3 mg, 6 mg

Indications, route, and dosage
Adjunct to diet to lower blood glucose levels in patients with type 2 diabetes mellitus
Adults: Initially, 2.5 to 5 mg P.O. daily with breakfast. Patients who are more sensitive to hypoglycemic drugs should be started at 1.25 mg daily. Usual maintenance dose is 1.25 to 20 mg daily, either as a single dose or in divided doses.
    For micronized tablets, initially give 1.5 to 3 mg P.O. with breakfast. Usual maintenance dose is 0.75 to 12 mg P.O. daily.
✦ Dosage adjustment. In elderly, debilitated, or malnourished patients or in those with renal or liver dysfunction, start therapy with 1.25 mg once daily.
To replace insulin therapy
Adults: If insulin dosage is more than 40 units/day, patient may be started on 5 mg of glyburide daily besides 50% of the insulin dose. Patients maintained on less than 20 units/day should receive 2.5 to 5 mg/day; those maintained on 20 to 40 units/day should receive 5 mg/day. In all patients, glyburide is substituted and insulin discontinued abruptly.
    For micronized tablets, if insulin dose is more than 40 units/day, give 3 mg P.O. with a 50% reduction in insulin. Patients maintained on 20 to 40 units/day should receive 3 mg P.O. as a single daily dose; those maintained on less than 20 units/day should receive 1.5 to 3 mg/day as a single dose.

Pharmacodynamics
Antidiabetic action: Lowers blood glucose levels by stimulating insulin release from functioning beta cells in the pancreas. After prolonged ad-

ministration, the drug's hypoglycemic effects appear to be related to extrapancreatic effects, possibly including reduction of basal hepatic glucose production and enhanced peripheral sensitivity to insulin. The latter may result either from an increase in the number of insulin receptors or from changes in events subsequent to insulin binding.

Pharmacokinetics
• *Absorption:* Almost completely absorbed from GI tract. Onset of action occurs within 2 hours; hypoglycemic effects peak within 3 to 4 hours. Micronized tablet results in significant absorption; 3-mg micronized tablet provides blood levels similar to 5-mg conventional tablet.
• *Distribution:* 99% protein-bound. Distribution not fully understood.
• *Metabolism:* Metabolized completely by liver to inactive metabolites.
• *Excretion:* Excreted as metabolites in urine and feces in equal proportions. Duration of action is 24 hours; half-life is 10 hours.

Contraindications and precautions
Contraindicated in patients with hypersensitivity to drug, in those with diabetic ketoacidosis with or without coma, and during pregnancy or breast-feeding. Use cautiously in patients with impaired renal or hepatic function and in elderly, malnourished, or debilitated patients.

Interactions
Drug-drug. *Adrenocorticoids, amphetamines, baclofen, corticotropin, diazoxide, epinephrine, ethacrynic acid, furosemide, glucagon, glucocorticoids, phenytoin, rifampin, thiazide diuretics, thyroid hormones, triamterene:* May cause hyperglycemia. Dosage adjustments may be needed; monitor blood glucose levels.
Anabolic steroids, chloramphenicol, clofibrate, guanethidine, insulin, MAO inhibitors, probenecid, salicylates, sulfonamides: May enhance hypoglycemic effect by displacing glyburide from its protein-binding sites. Monitor patient closely.
Anticoagulants: May increase plasma levels of both drugs; after continued therapy, may reduce plasma levels and anticoagulant effect. Monitor INR.
Beta blockers (such as ophthalmics): May increase risk of hypoglycemia, mask its symptoms (increased pulse rate and blood pressure), and prolong its effects by blocking gluconeogenesis. Educate patient to potential for hypoglycemia unawareness and to alternative signs of hypoglycemia.
Hydantoins: May increase blood levels of hydantoins. Monitor hydantoin levels.
Drug-lifestyle. *Alcohol:* May alter glycemic control, resulting in hypoglycemia. May also cause disulfiram-like reaction of nausea, vomiting, abdominal cramps, and headaches. Discourage concomitant use.

Smoking: May increase corticosteroid release; patients who smoke may require higher dosages of glipizide. Discourage concomitant use.

Adverse reactions
EENT: changes in accommodation or blurred vision.
GI: nausea, epigastric fullness, heartburn.
GU: altered BUN levels.
Hematologic: *leukopenia,* hemolytic anemia, *agranulocytosis, thrombocytopenia, aplastic anemia.*
Hepatic: cholestatic jaundice, *hepatitis,* abnormal liver function.
Metabolic: altered cholesterol level, *hypoglycemia.*
Musculoskeletal: arthralgia, myalgia.
Skin: rash, pruritus, other allergic reactions.
Other: *angioedema.*

☑ Special considerations
Besides the recommendations relevant to all sulfonylureas, consider the following.
• To improve control in patients receiving 10 mg/day or more, divided doses, usually given before the morning and evening meals, are recommended.
• Some patients taking glyburide may be controlled effectively on a once-daily regimen, whereas others show better response with divided dosing.
• Glyburide is a second-generation sulfonylurea oral antidiabetic; appears to cause fewer adverse reactions than first-generation drugs.
• Drug has mild diuretic effect that may be useful in patients who have chronic heart failure or cirrhosis.
• Oral antidiabetics have been associated with an increased risk of CV mortality compared with diet or diet and insulin therapy.
• Glyburide therapy alters cholesterol, alkaline phosphatase, and BUN levels.
• Signs and symptoms of overdose include low blood glucose levels, tingling of lips and tongue, hunger, nausea, decreased cerebral function (lethargy, yawning, confusion, agitation, and nervousness), increased sympathetic activity (tachycardia, sweating, and tremor) and ultimately seizures, stupor, and coma.
• Mild hypoglycemia, without loss of consciousness or neurologic findings, responds to treatment with oral glucose and dosage adjustments. The patient with severe hypoglycemia should be hospitalized immediately.
• If hypoglycemic coma is suspected, give rapid injection of dextrose 50%, then a continuous infusion of dextrose 10% at a rate to maintain blood glucose levels greater than 100 mg/dl. Monitor patient for 24 to 48 hours.

Monitoring the patient
• Monitor renal and hepatic function before initiating treatment.

• When substituting glyburide for chlorpropamide, monitor patient closely during first week because of the prolonged retention of chlorpropamide in body.
• Monitor serum glucose levels periodically to determine therapeutic response. Monitor glycosylated hemoglobin every 3 to 6 months to more precisely assess long-term glycemic control.

Information for the patient
• Emphasize importance of following prescribed diet, exercise, and medical regimen.
• Tell patient to take drug at same time each day. If a dose is missed, it should be taken immediately, unless it's almost time to take the next dose. Instruct patient not to take double doses.
• Advise patient to avoid alcohol while taking glyburide. Remind him that many foods and OTC drugs contain alcohol.
• Encourage patient to wear a medical identification bracelet or necklace.
• Suggest drug be taken with food if GI upset occurs.
• Teach patient how to monitor blood glucose, urine glucose and ketone levels.
• Teach patient how to recognize signs and symptoms of hyperglycemia and hypoglycemia and what to do if they occur.

Geriatric patients
• Elderly patients may be more sensitive to drug's effects because of reduced metabolism and elimination.
• Hypoglycemia causes more neurologic symptoms in elderly patients.

Pediatric patients
• Glyburide is ineffective in type 1 diabetes. Safety and effectiveness in children haven't been established.

glycerin (glycerol)
Fleet Babylax, Ophthalgan, Osmoglyn, Sani-Supp

Pharmacologic classification: trihydric alcohol, ophthalmic osmotic vehicle
Therapeutic classification: laxative (osmotic), ophthalmic osmotic, adjunct in treating glaucoma, lubricant
Pregnancy risk category C

How supplied
Available by prescription only
Ophthalmic solution: 7.5-ml containers
Oral solution: 50% (0.6 g/ml), 75% (0.94 g/ml)
Available without a prescription
Suppository: 1.5 g (for infants), 3 g (adults)
Rectal solution: 4 ml/applicator

Indications, route, and dosage
Constipation
Adults and children ages 6 and older: 3 g as a suppository or 5 to 15 ml as an enema.
Children under age 6: 1 to 1.5 g as a suppository or 2 to 5 ml as an enema.
Reduction of intraocular pressure
Adults: 1 to 2 g/kg P.O. 60 to 90 minutes preoperatively.

Drug is useful in acute angle-closure glaucoma; before iridectomy (with carbonic anhydrase inhibitors or topical miotics); in trauma or disease, such as congenital glaucoma and some secondary glaucoma forms; and before or after surgery, such as retinal detachment surgery, cataract extraction, or keratoplasty.
Reduction of corneal edema
Adults: 1 to 2 drops of ophthalmic solution topically before eye examination; 1 to 2 drops q 3 to 4 hours for corneal edema.

Drug is used to facilitate ophthalmoscopic and gonioscopic examination and to differentiate superficial edema and deep corneal edema.
To act as an osmotic diuretic
Adults: 1 to 2 g/kg P.O. 1 to 1½ hours before surgery.

Pharmacodynamics
Laxative action: Glycerin suppositories produce laxative action by causing rectal distention, thereby stimulating the urge to defecate; by causing local rectal irritation; and by triggering a hyperosmolar mechanism that draws water into the colon.
Antiglaucoma action: Orally administered glycerin helps reduce intraocular pressure by increasing plasma osmotic pressure, thereby drawing water into the blood from extravascular spaces. It also reduces intraocular fluid volume independently of routine flow mechanisms, decreasing intraocular pressure; it may cause tissue dehydration and decreased CSF pressure.

Topically applied glycerin produces a hygroscopic (moisture-retaining) effect that reduces edema and improves visualization in ophthalmoscopy or gonioscopy. Glycerin reduces fluid in the cornea via its osmotic action and clears corneal haze.

Pharmacokinetics
Rectal form
• *Absorption:* Absorbed poorly; after rectal administration, laxative effect occurs in 15 to 30 minutes.
• *Distribution:* Distributed locally.
• *Metabolism:* No information available.
• *Excretion:* Excreted in feces.
Oral form
• *Absorption:* Absorbed rapidly from GI tract, with serum levels peaking in 60 to 90 minutes with oral administration; intraocular pressure decreases in 10 to 30 minutes. Action peaks in 30 minutes to 2 hours, with effects persisting for 4 to 8 hours.

Reactions may be *common,* uncommon, *life-threatening,* or COMMON AND LIFE-THREATENING.

Intracranial pressure (ICP) decreases in 10 to 60 minutes; effect persists for 2 to 3 hours.
• *Distribution:* Distributed throughout blood but doesn't enter ocular fluid; drug may enter breast milk.
• *Metabolism:* About 80% metabolized in liver, 10% to 20% in kidneys.
• *Excretion:* Excreted in feces and urine.

Contraindications and precautions
Contraindicated in patients with hypersensitivity to drug. Rectal administration of drug is contraindicated in those with intestinal obstruction, undiagnosed abdominal pain, vomiting or other signs of appendicitis, fecal impaction, or acute surgical abdomen.
   Use oral form cautiously in elderly or dehydrated patients and in those with diabetes or cardiac, renal, or hepatic disease.

Interactions
Drug-drug. *Diuretics:* Possible additive effects. Avoid concomitant use.

Adverse reactions
CNS: mild headache, dizziness (with oral administration).
EENT: eye pain, irritation.
GI: cramping pain, thirst, nausea, vomiting, diarrhea (with oral administration); rectal discomfort, hyperemia of rectal mucosa (with rectal administration).
Metabolic: mild hyperglycemia, mild glycosuria.
   Note: Stop drug if hypersensitivity symptoms occur.

☑ Special considerations
• When administering glycerin orally, don't give hypotonic fluids to relieve thirst and headache from glycerin-induced dehydration; these will counteract drug's osmotic effects.
• Use topical tetracaine hydrochloride or proparacaine before ophthalmic instillation to prevent discomfort.
• Don't touch tip of dropper to eye, surrounding tissues, or tear-film; glycerin will absorb moisture.
• To prevent or relieve headache, have patient remain supine during and after oral administration.
• Monitor diabetic patients for possible alteration of serum and urine glucose levels; dosage adjustment may be necessary.
• Commercially available solutions may be poured over ice and sipped through a straw.
• Hyperosmolar laxatives are used most commonly to help laxative-dependent patients reestablish normal bowel habits.
• Other uses include reducing ICP in patients with CVA, meningitis, encephalitis, Reye's syndrome, or CNS trauma or tumors, reducing brain volume during neurosurgical procedures through oral or I.V. administration, or both.

• If excess glycerin is administered into eye, irrigate conjunctiva with sterile normal saline solution or water. Systemic effects aren't expected.

Monitoring the patient
• Monitor serum glucose level if patient is a diabetic.
• Monitor patient for adverse effects.

Information for the patient
• Instruct patient to call if severe headache is experienced from oral dose.
• Teach patient correct way to instill drops and warn him not to touch eye with dropper.
• Tell patient to lie down during and after administration of drug to prevent or relieve headache.

Geriatric patients
• Dehydrated elderly patients may experience seizures and disorientation.

Pediatric patients
• Safety and effectiveness of ophthalmic glycerin solutions in children haven't been established.

Breast-feeding patients
• Safety in breast-feeding women hasn't been established. Possible risks must be weighed against benefits.

glycopyrrolate
Robinul, Robinul Forte

Pharmacologic classification: anticholinergic
Therapeutic classification: antimuscarinic, GI antispasmodic
Pregnancy risk category B

How supplied
Available by prescription only
Tablets: 1 mg, 2 mg
Injection: 0.2 mg/ml in 1-ml, 2-ml, 5-ml, 20-ml vials

Indications, route, and dosage
Blockade of cholinergic effects of anticholinesterases used to reverse neuromuscular blockade
Adults and children: 0.2 mg I.V. for each 1 mg neostigmine or 5 mg of pyridostigmine. May be given I.V. without dilution or may be added to dextrose injection and given by infusion.
Preoperatively to diminish secretions and block cardiac vagal reflexes
Adults: 0.0044 mg/kg of body weight given I.M. 30 to 60 minutes before anesthesia.
Adjunctive therapy in peptic ulcers and other GI disorders
Adults: 1 to 2 mg P.O. t.i.d. or 0.1 mg I.M. t.i.d. or q.i.d. Dosage should be individualized.

Pharmacodynamics
Anticholinergic action: Inhibits acetylcholine's muscarinic actions on autonomic effectors innervated by postganglionic cholinergic nerves. That action blocks adverse muscarinic effects associated with anticholinesterases used to reverse curariform-induced neuromuscular blockade. Drug decreases secretions and GI motility by the same mechanism. Blocks cardiac vagal reflexes by blocking vagal inhibition of the SA node.

Pharmacokinetics
• *Absorption:* Poorly absorbed from GI tract (10% to 25%) after oral administration. Rapidly absorbed when given I.M.; serum levels peak in 30 to 45 minutes. Action begins in 1 minute after I.V.; 15 to 30 minutes after I.M. or S.C. administration.
• *Distribution:* Rapidly distributed. Because drug is a quaternary amine, doesn't cross blood-brain barrier or enter CNS.
• *Metabolism:* Exact metabolic fate unknown. Duration of effect up to 7 hours when given parenterally; up to 12 hours when given orally.
• *Excretion:* Small amount of drug eliminated in urine as unchanged drug and metabolites. Mostly excreted unchanged in feces or bile.

Contraindications and precautions
Contraindicated in patients with hypersensitivity to drug and in those with glaucoma, obstructive uropathy, obstructive disease of the GI tract, myasthenia gravis, paralytic ileus, intestinal atony, unstable CV status in acute hemorrhage, severe ulcerative colitis, or toxic megacolon.

Use cautiously in patients with autonomic neuropathy, hyperthyroidism, coronary artery disease, arrhythmias, heart failure, hypertension, hiatal hernia, hepatic or renal disease, or ulcerative colitis. Also use with caution in hot or humid conditions in which drug-induced heat stroke may occur.

Interactions
Drug-drug. *Antacids:* Concurrent administration decreases oral absorption of anticholinergics. Administer glycopyrrolate at least 1 hour before antacids.
Anticholinergics (such as ketoconazole, levodopa): Possible decreased GI absorption. Avoid concomitant administration.
Digoxin (slowly dissolving tablets): Increased digoxin levels. Monitor digoxin levels.
Drugs with anticholinergic effects (amantadine, antihistamines, antiparkinsonians, disopyramide, glutethimide, meperidine, phenothiazines, procainamide, quinidine, tricyclic antidepressants): May cause additive adverse effects. Monitor patient closely.
Oral potassium supplements (especially waxmatrix formulations): Possible increased risk of potassium-induced GI ulcerations. Use cautiously.

Adverse reactions
CNS: weakness, nervousness, insomnia, drowsiness, dizziness, headache, confusion or excitement (in elderly patients).
CV: palpitations, tachycardia.
EENT: *dilated pupils, blurred vision,* photophobia, increased intraocular pressure.
GI: *constipation, dry mouth,* nausea, loss of taste, abdominal distension, vomiting, epigastric distress.
GU: *urinary hesitancy, urine retention,* impotence.
Skin: urticaria, decreased sweating or anhidrosis, other dermal manifestations.
Other: fever, allergic reactions *(anaphylaxis)*.

☑ Special considerations
Besides the recommendations relevant to all anticholinergics, consider the following.
• Check all doses carefully. Even a slight overdose can lead to toxic effects.
• For immediate treatment of bradycardia, some clinicians prefer atropine over glycopyrrolate.
• Don't mix glycopyrrolate with I.V. solutions containing sodium chloride or bicarbonate.
• Drug may be administered with neostigmine or physostigmine in same syringe.
• Drug is incompatible in solution with thiopental, methohexital, secobarbital, pentobarbital, chloramphenicol, dimenhydrinate, and diazepam. Don't mix in the same syringe.
• Signs of overdose include such peripheral effects as dilated, nonreactive pupils; blurred vision; flushed, hot, dry skin; dryness of mucous membranes; dysphagia; decreased or absent bowel sounds; urine retention; hyperthermia; tachycardia; hypertension; and increased respiration.
• Treatment of overdose is primarily symptomatic and supportive, as needed. If patient is alert, induce emesis (or use gastric lavage), then use a saline cathartic and activated charcoal to prevent further drug absorption. In severe life-threatening cases, physostigmine may be administered to block glycopyrrolate's antimuscarinic effects. Give fluids, as needed, to treat shock. If urine retention occurs, catheterization may be necessary.

Monitoring the patient
• Monitor patient for adverse effects.
• Monitor therapeutic effect.

Information for the patient
• Instruct patient to take oral drug 30 to 60 minutes before meals.
• Warn patient to avoid activities that require alertness until drug's CNS effects are known.
• Advise patient to report signs of urinary hesitancy or retention.

Geriatric patients
• Administer glycopyrrolate cautiously to elderly patients. However, glycopyrrolate may be the preferred anticholinergic in elderly patients.

Pediatric patients
• Drug isn't recommended for children under age 12 for managing peptic ulcer.

Breast-feeding patients
• Drug may appear in breast milk and may decrease milk production; infant toxicity is possible. Avoid use in breast-feeding women.

gold sodium thiomalate
Aurolate

Pharmacologic classification: gold salt
Therapeutic classification: antarthritic
Pregnancy risk category C

How supplied
Available by prescription only
Injection: 50 mg/ml with benzyl alcohol

Indications, route, and dosage
Rheumatoid arthritis, ◊ psoriatic arthritis, ◊ Felty's syndrome
Adults: Initially, 10 mg I.M.; then 25 mg in second week and continue for a third dose the following week. Continue until 1 g (cumulative) has been given, unless toxicity occurs. If improvement occurs without toxicity before initial 1-g dose, a maintenance dose of 25 to 50 mg every other week for 2 to 20 weeks may be started. Then continue to every third then every fourth week indefinitely. Weekly injections may be restarted anytime, if needed. If patient doesn't respond after reaching initial 1-g dose, then stop therapy, or give 25 to 50 mg I.M. for an additional 10 weeks, or increase dose by 10 mg q 1 to 4 weeks (maximum dose per injection is 100 mg).
Children: Initiate therapy with 10-mg test dose; then give 1 mg/kg weekly. Continue dosage and administration as listed for adults. Maximum single dose for children under age 12 is 50 mg.
◊ Palindromic rheumatism
Adults: Initially, 10 to 15 mg I.M. weekly until dose of 1 g is reached.
◊ Pemphigus
Adults: Initially, 10 mg I.M.; then 25 mg I.M. for second week, then 50 mg I.M. weekly. When patient is off corticosteroid therapy, maintenance dose of 25 to 50 mg I.M. q 2 weeks may be administered.

Pharmacodynamics
Antarthritic action: Thought to be effective against rheumatoid arthritis by altering the immune system to reduce inflammation. Although exact mechanism unknown, these compounds have reduced serum levels of immunoglobulins and rheumatoid factors in patients with arthritis.

Pharmacokinetics
• *Absorption:* Rapid absorption; levels peak within 3 to 6 hours.
• *Distribution:* Higher tissue levels occur with parenteral gold salts, with a mean steady-state plasma level of 1 to 5 mcg/ml. Distributed widely throughout body in lymph nodes, bone marrow, kidneys, liver, spleen, and tissues. About 85% to 90% protein-bound.
• *Metabolism:* Not broken down into elemental form. Half-life with cumulative dosing is 14 to 40 days.
• *Excretion:* About 70% excreted in urine, 30% in feces.

Contraindications and precautions
Contraindicated in patients with hypersensitivity to drug; in those with history of severe toxicity from previous exposure to gold or heavy metals, hepatitis, or exfoliative dermatitis; and in patients with severe uncontrollable diabetes, renal disease, hepatic dysfunction, uncontrolled heart failure, systemic lupus erythematosus, colitis, or Sjögren's syndrome. Also contraindicated in patients with urticaria, eczema, hemorrhagic conditions, or severe hematologic disorders and in those who have recently received radiation therapy.
Use with extreme caution in patients with rash, marked hypertension, compromised cerebral or CV function, or history of renal or hepatic disease, drug allergies, or blood dyscrasias.

Interactions
Drug-drug. *Drugs known to cause blood dyscrasias:* May cause an additive risk of hematologic toxicity. Monitor patient closely.
Drug-lifestyle. *Sun, ultraviolet light exposure:* May cause photosensitivity reactions. Tell patient to take precautions.

Adverse reactions
CNS: confusion, hallucinations, **seizures.**
CV: **bradycardia,** hypotension.
EENT: corneal gold deposition, corneal ulcers.
GI: *metallic taste, stomatitis, diarrhea,* anorexia, abdominal cramps, nausea, vomiting, ulcerative enterocolitis.
GU: albuminuria, proteinuria, **nephrotic syndrome,** nephritis, acute tubular necrosis, hematuria, **acute renal failure.**
Hematologic: **thrombocytopenia** (with or without purpura), **aplastic anemia, agranulocytosis,** leukopenia, eosinophilia, anemia.
Hepatic: **hepatitis,** jaundice, elevated liver function test results.
Skin: diaphoresis, photosensitivity, *rash, dermatitis,* erythema, exfoliative dermatitis.
Other: **angioedema, anaphylaxis.**

☑ Special considerations
• Gold salts should be administered only under close medical supervision.

- Adverse reactions to gold are considered severe and potentially life-threatening.
- Most adverse reactions are readily reversible if drug is stopped immediately.
- Vasomotor adverse effects are more common with gold sodium thiomalate than with other gold salts.
- Administer all gold salts I.M., preferably intragluteally. Normal color of drug is pale yellow; don't use if it darkens.
- Observe patient for 30 minutes after administration because of possible anaphylactic reaction.
- When administering drug, advise patient to lie down and to remain recumbent for 10 to 20 minutes after injection.
- If adverse reactions are mild, some rheumatologists order resumption of gold therapy after 2 to 3 weeks' rest.
- Serum protein-bound iodine test, especially when done by the chloric acid digestion method, gives false readings during and for several weeks after gold therapy.
- When severe reactions to gold occur, corticosteroids, dimercaprol (a chelating drug), or penicillamine may be given to aid recovery. Prednisone 40 to 100 mg/day in divided doses is recommended to manage severe renal, hematologic, pulmonary, or enterocolitic reactions to gold. Dimercaprol may be used with corticosteroids to remove gold when corticosteroid treatment alone is ineffective.

Monitoring the patient
- Monitor renal and hepatic function before initiating treatment.
- Perform urinalysis for protein and sediment changes before each injection.
- Monitor patient's CBC and platelet count monthly or before every other injection.

Information for the patient
- Urge patient to have scheduled monthly platelet counts. Stop drug if platelet count falls below 100,000/mm³.
- Reassure patient that beneficial drug effect may be delayed for 3 months. However, if response is inadequate after 6 months, discontinue therapy.
- Explain that vasomotor adverse reactions (faintness, weakness, dizziness, flushing, nausea, vomiting, diaphoresis) may occur immediately after injection. Advise patient to lie down until symptoms subside.
- Advise patient to keep taking drug if mild diarrhea occurs but to call immediately if diarrhea persists or if blood appears in stools.
- Tell patient that stomatitis is often preceded by a metallic taste; this symptom must be reported immediately.
- Advise patient to report rash or other skin problems immediately.
- Encourage patient to take drug exactly as prescribed.

- Tell patient to continue taking concomitant drug therapy, such as NSAIDs, as prescribed.

Geriatric patients
- Administer usual adult dose. Use cautiously in patients with decreased renal function.

Pediatric patients
- Use in children under age 6 isn't recommended.

Breast-feeding patients
- Because drug appears in breast milk, it isn't recommended for use in breast-feeding women.

gonadorelin acetate
Lutrepulse

Pharmacologic classification: gonadotropin-releasing hormone (Gn-RH)
Therapeutic classification: fertility drug
Pregnancy risk category B

How supplied
Available by prescription only
Injection: 0.8 mg/10 ml, 3.2 mg/10 ml, in 10-ml vials
Supplied as a kit with I.V. supplies and portable infusion pump.

Indications, route, and dosage
To induce ovulation in women with primary hypothalamic amenorrhea
Adults: 5 mcg I.V. q 90 minutes (using a Lutrepulse pump, 0.8 mg solution at 50 microliters/pulse) for 21 days. If no response after three treatment intervals, dosage may be increased. Usual dose is 1 to 20 mcg.

Pharmacodynamics
Ovulation-stimulating action: Mimics action of Gn-RH, which results in synthesis and release of luteinizing hormone (LH) from the anterior pituitary. LH subsequently acts on the reproductive organs to regulate hormone synthesis.

Pharmacokinetics
- *Absorption:* Administered I.V. using a portable pump designed to administer drug in a pulsatile fashion to mimic endogenous hormone.
- *Distribution:* Low plasma volume of distribution (10 to 15 L) and high rate of clearance from plasma.
- *Metabolism:* Rapidly metabolized. Several biologically inactive peptide fragments identified.
- *Excretion:* Excreted primarily in urine. High initial clearance rate (half-life of 2 to 10 minutes) is followed by somewhat slower terminal half-life of 10 to 40 minutes.

Contraindications and precautions
Contraindicated in patients with hypersensitivity to drug, in women with conditions that could be complicated by pregnancy (such as prolactinoma), in those who are anovulatory from any cause other than a hypothalamic disorder, and in those with ovarian cysts.

Interactions
Drug-drug. *Ovarian-stimulating drugs:* Possible decreased risk of ovarian hyperstimulation. Avoid concomitant use.

Adverse reactions
GU: multiple pregnancy, ovarian hyperstimulation.
Skin: hematoma, local infection, inflammation, mild phlebitis.

☑ Special considerations
• Patients usually require pelvic ultrasound on days 7 and 14 after baseline scan, although interval between scans may be shortened.
• To mimic the action of naturally occurring hormone, gonadorelin requires a pulsatile administration with special portable infusion pump. The pulse period is set at 1 minute (drug is infused over 1 minute); pulse interval is set at 90 minutes.
• To give 2.5 mcg/pulse, reconstitute 0.8-mg vial with 8 ml of supplied diluent, and set pump to deliver 25 microliters/pulse. To give 5 mcg/pulse, use same dosage strength and dilution but set pump to deliver 50 microliters/pulse
• Some patients may require higher doses. To administer 10 mcg/pulse, reconstitute the 3.2-mg vial with 8 ml of supplied diluent, and set pump to deliver 25 microliters/pulse. To administer 20 mcg/pulse, use this dosage strength and dilution but set pump to deliver 50 microliters/pulse.
• No harmful effects are expected if pump malfunctions and delivers entire contents of highest concentration vial (3.2 mg). Bolus doses of up to 3,000 mcg haven't proven harmful; however, continuous exposure (nonpulsatile administration) to gonadorelin might temporarily reduce pituitary responsiveness.

Monitoring the patient
• Monitor patient for anaphylaxis initially.
• Monitor patient for adverse effects.

Information for the patient
• Because similar drugs have caused anaphylaxis, teach patient signs and symptoms of hypersensitivity reactions (hives, wheezing, difficulty breathing) and instruct her to report them immediately.
• Make sure patient understands that a multiple pregnancy is possible (about 12% possibility). Close monitoring of dosage and ultrasonography of ovaries are necessary to monitor drug response.

• Encourage patient to adhere to close monitoring schedule required by therapy. Regular pelvic examinations, midluteal phase serum progesterone determinations, and multiple ovarian ultrasound scans are necessary. Inspect I.V. site at each visit.
• Instruct patient about proper aseptic technique and I.V. site care. Provide written instructions. Catheter and I.V. site should be monitored and changed at appropriate intervals for type of catheter used.

Pediatric patients
• Safety and efficacy in children under age 18 haven't been established.

Breast-feeding patients
• It's unknown if drug appears in breast milk; however, there is no reason to administer drug to a breast-feeding woman.

goserelin acetate
Zoladex, Zoladex 3-Month

Pharmacologic classification: synthetic decapeptide
Therapeutic classification: luteinizing hormone–releasing hormone (LH–RH; Gn-RH) analogue
Pregnancy risk category X (10.8-mg implant); D (3.6-mg implant)

How supplied
Available by prescription only
Implant: 3.6 mg, 10.8 mg

Indications, route, and dosage
Palliative treatment of advanced carcinoma of the prostate, endometriosis, advanced breast carcinoma
Adults: 1 (3.6-mg) implant S.C. q 28 days into upper abdominal wall for 6 months. Treatment of endometriosis shouldn't exceed 6 months.
Palliative treatment of advanced carcinoma of the prostate
Men: 1 (10.8-mg) implant S.C. q 12 weeks into upper abdominal wall.

Pharmacodynamics
Hormonal action: Long-term administration of goserelin, an LH–RH, acts on the pituitary to decrease the release of follicle-stimulating hormone (FSH) and luteinizing hormone. In men, the result is dramatically lowered serum levels of testosterone.

Pharmacokinetics
• *Absorption:* Slowly absorbed from implant site. Drug levels peak in 12 to 15 days.
• *Distribution:* Implant results in measurable levels of drug in serum throughout dosing period.

• *Metabolism:* Rapid drug clearance following S.C. administration; combination of hepatic metabolism and urinary excretion.
• *Excretion:* Elimination half-life about 4.2 hours in patients with normal renal function. Substantial renal impairment prolongs half-life, but this doesn't appear to increase risk of adverse effects.

Contraindications and precautions
Contraindicated in patients with hypersensitivity to LH–RH, LH–RH agonist analogues, or to goserelin acetate. Also contraindicated during pregnancy or breast-feeding. The 10.8-mg implant is contraindicated in women.

Use cautiously in patients at risk for osteoporosis, in those with chronic alcohol or tobacco abuse, and in those taking anticonvulsants or corticosteroids.

Interactions
None reported.

Adverse reactions
CNS: lethargy, pain (worsened in the first 30 days), dizziness, *insomnia, asthenia,* anxiety, *depression, headache,* chills, *emotional lability.*
CV: edema, **heart failure, arrhythmias,** *peripheral edema, CVA,* hypertension, *MI,* peripheral vascular disorder, chest pain.
GI: nausea, vomiting, diarrhea, constipation, ulcer, anorexia, abdominal pain.
GU: *impotence, sexual dysfunction, lower urinary tract symptoms,* renal insufficiency, urinary obstruction, *vaginitis,* urinary tract infection, amenorrhea, increased serum testosterone levels during the first week of therapy.
Hematologic: anemia.
Metabolic: increased serum acid phosphatase initially (will decrease by week 4), hyperglycemia, weight increase.
Musculoskeletal: gout, back pain.
Respiratory: COPD, upper respiratory infection.
Skin: rash, *diaphoresis, acne, seborrhea,* hirsutism.
Other: *changes in libido, hot flashes, infection,* breast swelling and tenderness, *changes in breast size,* breast pain.

☑ Special considerations
• If patient is of childbearing age, rule out pregnancy before initiating treatment.
• Implant comes in preloaded syringe. If package is damaged, don't use syringe. Make sure drug is visible in translucent chamber of syringe.
• Drug should be given every 28 days for 3.6-mg implant and every 12 weeks for 10.8-mg implant, always under direct medical supervision. Local anesthesia may be used before injection.
• In the unlikely event of the need to surgically remove goserelin, it may be localized by ultrasound.

• Administer drug in upper abdominal wall using aseptic technique. After cleaning area with alcohol swab (and injecting a local anesthetic), stretch patient's skin with one hand while grasping barrel of syringe with other. Insert needle into S.C. fat, then change needle direction to parallel abdominal wall. Push needle in until hub touches patient's skin, then withdraw it about 1 cm (this creates a gap for the drug to be injected) before depressing plunger completely.
• After inserting needle, blood will be seen instantly in chamber if large vessel is penetrated (a new syringe and injection site will be needed). The Zoladex syringe doesn't permit aspiration.
• No information available on accidental or intentional overdose. Doses up to 1 mg/kg/day haven't produced non-endocrine-related symptoms.

Monitoring the patient
• Monitor patient for adverse effects.
• Monitor patient for therapeutic effect.

Information for the patient
• Advise patient to report every 28 days or 12 weeks, as appropriate, for a new implant. However, a delay of a few days is permissible.
• Tell patient to report chest pain, palpitations, light-headedness, or numbness of extremities.

Pediatric patients
• Safety and efficacy in children under age 18 haven't been established.

Breast-feeding patients
• It's unknown if drug appears in breast milk. Use with caution in breast-feeding women.

granisetron hydrochloride
Kytril

Pharmacologic classification: selective 5-hydroxytryptamine (5-HT$_3$) receptor antagonist
Therapeutic classification: antiemetic, antinauseant
Pregnancy risk category B

How supplied
Available by prescription only
Tablets: 1 mg
Injection: 1 mg/ml

Indications, route, and dosage
Prevention of nausea and vomiting associated with emetogenic cancer chemotherapy
Oral form
Adults: 1 mg P.O. b.i.d. Give first 1-mg tablet 1 hour before chemotherapy administration and second tablet 12 hours after first. Give only on days when chemotherapy is given. Continued treatment while not on chemotherapy isn't useful.

Reactions may be *common,* uncommon, *life-threatening,* or COMMON AND LIFE-THREATENING.

Intravenous form
Adults and children ages 2 to 16: 10 mcg/kg I.V. infused over 5 minutes. Begin infusion within 30 minutes before administration of chemotherapy.

Pharmacodynamics
Antiemetic action: Thought to bind to serotonin receptors of the 5-HT$_3$ type located peripherally on vagal nerve terminals and centrally in the chemoreceptor trigger zone of the area postrema. This binding blocks serotonin stimulation and subsequent vomiting after emetogenic stimuli such as cisplatin.

Pharmacokinetics
• *Absorption:* Not determined.
• *Distribution:* Distributed freely between plasma and RBCs. Plasma protein-binding is about 65%.
• *Metabolism:* Metabolized by liver, possibly mediated by cytochrome P-450 3A subfamily.
• *Excretion:* About 12% of drug eliminated unchanged in urine in 48 hours; rest excreted as metabolites, 48% in urine and 38% in feces.

Contraindications and precautions
Contraindicated in patients with hypersensitivity to drug.

Interactions
Drug-herb. *Horehound:* May enhance serotonergic effects. Avoid concomitant use.

Adverse reactions
CNS: *headache, asthenia,* somnolence, dizziness, anxiety.
CV: hypertension.
GI: diarrhea, *constipation,* abdominal pain, *nausea,* vomiting, decreased appetite.
Hematologic: *leukopenia,* anemia, **thrombocytopenia.**
Hepatic: elevated liver function test results.
Skin: alopecia.
Other: fever.

☑ Special considerations
• Dilute drug with normal saline injection or D$_5$W to a volume of 20 to 50 ml. Infuse I.V. over 5 minutes. Diluted solutions are stable for 24 hours at room temperature.
• Don't mix with other drugs; information about compatibility is limited.
• Although clearance is slower and half-life is prolonged in elderly patients and in patients with hepatic disease, dosage adjustments aren't necessary.
• No dosage adjustment is recommended in patients with renal impairment.
• No antidote for overdose exists. Provide symptomatic treatment. Overdose of up to 38.5 mg caused no adverse effects with the exception of a slight headache.

Monitoring the patient
• Monitor CBC.
• Monitor patient for adverse effects.

Information for the patient
• Tell patient to watch for signs of anaphylactoid reaction (local or generalized hives, chest tightness, wheezing, and dizziness or weakness) and to report them immediately.

Pediatric patients
• Safety and effectiveness in children under age 2 haven't been established. Safety and effectiveness in children haven't been established for oral form.

Breast-feeding patients
• It's unknown if drug appears in breast milk. Use with caution in breast-feeding women.

griseofulvin microsize
Fulvicin-U/F, Grifulvin V, Grisactin

griseofulvin ultramicrosize
Fulvicin P/G, Grisactin Ultra, Gris-PEG

Pharmacologic classification: penicillium antibiotic
Therapeutic classification: antifungal
Pregnancy risk category C

How supplied
Available by prescription only
Microsize
Capsules: 250 mg
Tablets: 250 mg, 500 mg
Oral suspension: 125 mg/5 ml
Ultramicrosize
Tablets: 125 mg, 165 mg, 250 mg, 330 mg
Tablets (film-coated): 125 mg, 250 mg

Indications, route, and dosage
Tinea corporis, tinea capitis, tinea barbae, tinea cruris infections
Adults: 330 mg ultramicrosize P.O. daily, or 500 mg microsize P.O. daily.
Children over age 2: 3.3 mg/lb ultramicrosize P.O. daily; or 125 to 250 mg microsize P.O. daily for children weighing 14 to 23 kg (30 to 50 lb), or 250 to 500 mg microsize P.O. daily for children weighing over 23 kg.
Tinea pedis, tinea unguium infections
Adults: 660 mg ultramicrosize P.O. daily or 1 g microsize P.O. daily.
Children over age 2: 3.3 mg/lb ultramicrosize P.O. daily; or 125 to 250 mg microsize P.O. daily for children weighing 14 to 23 kg, or 250 to 500 mg microsize P.O. daily for children weighing over 23 kg.

Pharmacodynamics
Antifungal action: Disrupts the fungal cell's mitotic spindle, interfering with cell division; it also may inhibit DNA replication. Drug is also deposited in keratin precursor cells, inhibiting fungal invasion. It's active against *Trichophyton, Microsporum,* and *Epidermophyton.*

Pharmacokinetics
• *Absorption:* Absorbed primarily in duodenum and varies among individuals. Ultramicrosize preparations absorbed almost completely; microsize absorption ranges from 25% to 70% and may be increased by giving with a high-fat meal. Levels peak at 4 to 8 hours.
• *Distribution:* Concentrated in skin, hair, nails, fat, liver, and skeletal muscle; tightly bound to new keratin.
• *Metabolism:* Oxidatively demethylated and conjugated with glucuronic acid to inactive metabolites in liver.
• *Excretion:* About 50% of drug and its metabolites excreted in urine and 33% in feces within 5 days. Less than 1% of dose appears unchanged in urine. Drug also excreted in perspiration. Elimination half-life is 9 to 24 hours.

Contraindications and precautions
Contraindicated in patients with hypersensitivity to drug and in those with porphyria or hepatocellular failure. Also contraindicated during pregnancy and in those who intend to become pregnant during therapy. Use cautiously in penicillin-sensitive patients.

Interactions
Drug-drug. *Barbiturates:* May impair absorption of griseofulvin. Increased dosage requirements may be needed.
Oral contraceptives: Possible decreased effectiveness. Avoid concomitant use.
Phenobarbital: Decreased griseofulvin blood levels due to decreased absorption or increased metabolism. Avoid using together or administer griseofulvin t.i.d.
Warfarin: Possible enzyme induction, decreasing anticoagulant effects. Avoid concomitant use.
Drug-food. *High-fat meals:* May increase absorption. Administer together.
Drug-lifestyle. *Alcohol:* Potentiates effects of alcohol, producing tachycardia, diaphoresis, and flushing. Discourage concomitant use.

Adverse reactions
CNS: headache (in early stages of treatment), transient decrease in hearing, fatigue with large doses, occasional mental confusion, impaired performance of routine activities, psychotic symptoms, dizziness, insomnia, paresthesia of the hands and feet after extended therapy.
EENT: oral thrush.

GI: nausea, vomiting, flatulence, diarrhea, epigastric distress, *bleeding.*
GU: proteinuria, menstrual irregularities.
Hematologic: *leukopenia, granulocytopenia* (requires discontinuation of drug), porphyria.
Hepatic: *hepatic toxicity.*
Skin: *rash, urticaria,* photosensitivity, angioneurotic edema.
Other: *hypersensitivity reactions,* lupus erythematosus.

☑ Special considerations
• Commercial formulation of drug has changed, decreasing dosage required for an equivalent therapeutic effect. Dosages equivalent to the original formulation (before 1971) for 1 g of griseofulvin are 250 mg ultramicrosize or 500 mg microsize. Dosages may vary slightly depending on manufacturer.
• Confirm identification of organism before therapy begins.
• Give drug with or after meals with high-fat content (if allowed), to minimize GI distress.
• Assess nutrition and monitor food intake; drug may alter taste sensation, suppressing appetite.
• Treatment of tinea pedis may need combined oral and topical therapy.
• Ultramicrosize griseofulvin is absorbed more rapidly and completely than microsize and is effective at ½ to ⅔ usual dose.
• Symptoms of overdose include headache, lethargy, confusion, vertigo, blurred vision, nausea, vomiting, and diarrhea. Treatment is supportive. After recent ingestion (within 4 hours), empty stomach by induced emesis or gastric lavage. Then use activated charcoal to decrease absorption; a cathartic may also be helpful.

Monitoring the patient
• Monitor hepatic and renal function before initiating treatment and periodically throughout.
• Check CBC regularly for possible adverse effects; monitor renal and liver function studies periodically.
• Monitor coagulation studies if patient is taking anticoagulants.

Information for the patient
• Encourage patient to maintain adequate nutritional intake; offer suggestions to improve taste of food.
• Stress importance of completing prescribed regimen to prevent relapse even though symptoms may abate quickly.
• Teach signs and symptoms of adverse effects and hypersensitivity, and tell patient to report them immediately.
• Advise patient to avoid exposure to intense indoor light and sunlight to reduce the risk of photosensitivity reactions.
• Explain that drug may potentiate alcohol effects; advise patient to avoid alcohol during therapy.

Reactions may be *common,* uncommon, **life-threatening,** or COMMON AND LIFE-THREATENING.

- Teach correct personal hygiene and skin care.

Pediatric patients
- Safety in children under age 2 hasn't been established.

Breast-feeding patients
- Safety in breast-feeding women hasn't been established.

---

guaifenesin
Anti-Tuss, Balminil Expectorant*, Breonesin, Fenesin, Gee-Gee, Genatuss, Glyate, Glycotuss, Glytuss, Guiatuss, Halotussin, Humibid L.A., Humibid Sprinkle, Hytuss, Hytuss 2X, Mytussin, Naldecon Senior EX, Organidin NR, Resyl*, Robitussin, Scot-Tussin, Uni-tussin

Pharmacologic classification: propanediol derivative
Therapeutic classification: expectorant
Pregnancy risk category C

How supplied
Available without a prescription
Tablets: 100 mg, 200 mg
Tablets (extended-release): 600 mg
Capsules: 200 mg
Capsules (extended-release): 300 mg
Syrup: 100 mg/5 ml, 200 mg/5 ml

Indications, route, and dosage
As expectorant
Adults and children ages 12 and older: 100 to 400 mg P.O. q 4 hours; maximum dose is 2.4 g/day.
Children ages 6 to 11: 100 to 200 mg P.O. q 4 hours; maximum dose is 1.2 g/day.
Children ages 2 to 5: 50 to 100 mg P.O. q 4 hours; maximum dose is 600 mg/day.
Children under age 2: Individualize dosage.
Extended-release
Adults and children over age 12: 600 to 1,200 mg P.O. q 12 hours, not to exceed 2,400 mg in 24 hours.
Children ages 6 to 12: 600 mg P.O. q 12 hours, not to exceed 1,200 mg in 24 hours.
Children ages 2 to 6: 300 mg P.O. q 12 hours, not to exceed 600 mg in 24 hours.

Pharmacodynamics
Expectorant action: Increases respiratory tract fluid by reducing adhesiveness and surface tension, decreasing viscosity of the secretions and thereby facilitating their removal.

Pharmacokinetics
No information available.

Contraindications and precautions
Contraindicated in patients with hypersensitivity to drug.

Interactions
None reported.

Adverse reactions
CNS: dizziness, headache.
GI: vomiting and nausea (with large doses).
Skin: rash.

☑ Special considerations
- Effectiveness of guaifenesin as an expectorant hasn't been clearly established.
- Drug should be taken with a glass of water to help loosen mucus in lungs.
- Drug may cause color interference with tests for 5-hydroxyindoleacetic acid and vanillylmandelic acid.

Monitoring the patient
- Monitor patient for adverse effects.
- Monitor therapeutic effect.

Information for the patient
- Tell patient to call if cough persists for more than 1 week, recurs, or is accompanied by fever, rash, or persistent headache.
- Advise patient to use sugarless throat lozenges to decrease throat irritation and associated cough.
- Recommend that patient use a humidifier to filter out dust, smoke, and air pollutants.
- Encourage patient to perform deep-breathing exercises.

Geriatric patients
- No specific recommendations available; however, most liquid preparations contain alcohol (3.5% to 10%).

Pediatric patients
- Individualize dosage for children under age 2.

Breast-feeding patients
- It's unknown if drug appears in breast milk. Safe use in breast-feeding women hasn't been established.

---

guanabenz acetate
Wytensin

Pharmacologic classification: centrally acting antiadrenergic
Therapeutic classification: antihypertensive
Pregnancy risk category C

How supplied
Available by prescription only
Tablets: 4 mg, 8 mg

Indications, route, and dosage
Hypertension (generally considered a step 2 drug)
Adults: Initially, 2 to 4 mg P.O. b.i.d. Dosage may be increased in increments of 4 to 8 mg/day q 1 to 2 weeks. Usual maintenance dose ranges from 8 to 16 mg daily. Maximum dose is 32 mg b.i.d.
Children ages 12 and older: Initially, 0.5 to 4 mg daily; maintenance dose ranges from 4 to 24 mg daily, administered in two divided doses.
◇ **Management of opiate withdrawal**
Adults: 4 mg P.O. b.i.d. to q.i.d.

Pharmacodynamics
Antihypertensive action: Lowers blood pressure by stimulating central alpha₂-adrenergic receptors, decreasing cerebral sympathetic outflow and thus decreasing peripheral vascular resistance. May also antagonize antidiuretic hormone (ADH) secretion and ADH activity in the kidney.

Pharmacokinetics
● *Absorption:* After oral administration, 70% to 80% is absorbed from GI tract; antihypertensive effect occurs within 60 minutes, peaking at 2 to 4 hours.
● *Distribution:* Appears to be distributed widely into body; about 90% protein-bound.
● *Metabolism:* Metabolized extensively in liver; several metabolites formed.
● *Excretion:* Drug and metabolites excreted primarily in urine; remaining drug excreted in feces. Duration of antihypertensive effect ranges from 6 to 12 hours.

Contraindications and precautions
Contraindicated in patients with hypersensitivity to drug. Use cautiously in elderly patients and in patients with impaired renal or hepatic function, severe coronary insufficiency, recent MI, or cerebrovascular disease.

Interactions
Drug-drug. *Barbiturates, benzodiazepines, phenothiazines, other sedatives:* Possible increased CNS depressant effects. Monitor patient.
Diuretics, other antihypertensives: May increase risk of excessive hypotension. Monitor blood pressure.
MAO inhibitors, tricyclic antidepressants: May inhibit antihypertensive effects of guanabenz. Monitor blood pressure.
Drug-lifestyle. *Alcohol:* May increase CNS depressant effects. Discourage concomitant use.

Adverse reactions
CNS: *drowsiness, sedation, dizziness, weakness,* headache.
CV: *rebound hypertension.*
GI: *dry mouth.*
Hepatic: elevations in liver enzyme levels.

Metabolic: slightly reduced serum cholesterol and total triglyceride levels.

☑ Special considerations
● To ensure overnight blood pressure control and minimize daytime drowsiness, give last dose at bedtime.
● Investigational uses include managing opiate withdrawal and adjunctive therapy in patients with chronic pain.
● Reduced dosages may be needed in patients with hepatic impairment.
● Signs and symptoms of overdose include bradycardia, CNS depression, respiratory depression, hypothermia, apnea, seizures, lethargy, agitation, irritability, diarrhea, and hypotension. Don't induce emesis; CNS depression occurs rapidly. After adequate respiration is assured, empty stomach by gastric lavage; then give activated charcoal and a saline cathartic to decrease absorption. Follow with symptomatic and supportive care.

Monitoring the patient
● Monitor blood pressure when discontinuing drug. Stopping drug abruptly will cause severe rebound hypertension; reduce dosage gradually over 2 to 4 days.
● Monitor patient for adverse effects.

Information for the patient
● Explain signs and symptoms of adverse effects and importance of reporting them.
● Warn patient to avoid hazardous activities that require mental alertness and to avoid alcohol and other CNS depressants.
● Suggest that patient take drug at bedtime until tolerance develops to sedation, drowsiness, and other CNS effects.
● Advise patient to avoid sudden position changes to minimize orthostatic hypotension, and to relieve dry mouth with ice chips or sugarless gum.
● Warn patient to seek medical approval before taking OTC cold preparations.
● Advise patient not to stop drug suddenly; severe rebound hypertension may occur.

Geriatric patients
● Elderly patients may be more sensitive to antihypertensive and sedative effects of guanabenz.

Pediatric patients
● Drug has been used to treat hypertension in a limited number of children over age 12; its safety and efficacy in younger children haven't been established.

Breast-feeding patients
● It's unknown if drug appears in breast milk; an alternative to breast-feeding is recommended during therapy.

guanadrel sulfate
Hylorel

Pharmacologic classification: adrenergic neuron blocker
Therapeutic classification: antihypertensive
Pregnancy risk category B

How supplied
Available by prescription only
Tablets: 10 mg, 25 mg

Indications, route, and dosage
Hypertension
Adults: Initially, 5 mg P.O. b.i.d.; adjust dosage until blood pressure is controlled. Most patients require 20 to 75 mg daily, usually given b.i.d. (400 mg daily is rarely used).
✦ *Dosage adjustment.* In patient with renal impairment, if creatinine clearance is 30 to 60 ml/minute, reduce dose to 5 mg q 24 hours; if creatinine clearance is below 30 ml/minute, increase dosing interval to q 48 hours.

Pharmacodynamics
Antihypertensive action: Reduces blood pressure by peripheral inhibition of norepinephrine release in adrenergic nerve endings, thus decreasing arteriolar vasoconstriction.

Pharmacokinetics
• *Absorption:* Absorbed rapidly and almost completely from GI tract. Antihypertensive effect usually occurs at ½ to 2 hours; effect peaks at 4 to 6 hours.
• *Distribution:* Distributed widely into body; about 20% protein-bound; doesn't enter CNS.
• *Metabolism:* About 40% to 50% metabolized by liver.
• *Excretion:* Drug and metabolites eliminated primarily in urine. Antihypertensive activity lasts for 4 to 14 hours. Plasma half-life is about 10 hours but varies considerably with each individual.

Contraindications and precautions
Contraindicated in patients with hypersensitivity to drug, known or suspected pheochromocytoma, or frank heart failure. Also contraindicated in patients receiving MAO inhibitors or within 1 week of discontinuing MAO inhibitor therapy.
 Use cautiously in patients with regional vascular disease, bronchial asthma, or peptic ulcer disease.

Interactions
Drug-drug. *Amphetamines, ephedrine, MAO inhibitors, methylphenidate, norepinephrine, phenothiazines, tricyclic antidepressants:* May antagonize antihypertensive effects of guanadrel.

Monitor blood pressure. Separate use of guanadrel and MAO inhibitors by 1 week.
Diuretics, other antihypertensive drugs: Increased antihypertensive effects of guanadrel. Monitor patient closely.
Metaraminol, norepinephrine: May potentiate pressor effects. Monitor patient for hypertension.
Drug-lifestyle. *Alcohol:* May increase risk of guanadrel-induced orthostatic hypotension. Discourage concomitant use.

Adverse reactions
CNS: *fatigue, drowsiness, faintness, headache,* confusion, paresthesia.
CV: *palpitations, chest pain, peripheral edema, orthostatic hypotension.*
EENT: *glossitis, visual disturbances.*
GI: *diarrhea,* dry mouth, *indigestion,* constipation, anorexia, nausea, vomiting, abdominal pain.
GU: impotence, *ejaculation disturbances, nocturia, urinary frequency.*
Metabolic: *weight gain.*
Musculoskeletal: *aching limbs, leg cramps.*
Respiratory: *shortness of breath, cough.*

☑ Special considerations
• Discontinue guanadrel 48 to 72 hours before surgery to minimize risk of vascular collapse during anesthesia.
• Signs and symptoms of overdose include hypotension, dizziness, blurred vision, and syncope. After acute ingestion, empty stomach by induced emesis or gastric lavage. Effect of activated charcoal in absorbing guanadrel hasn't been determined. Further treatment is usually symptomatic and supportive.

Monitoring the patient
• Monitor supine and standing blood pressure, especially during periods of dosage adjustment.
• Assess patient for signs and symptoms of edema.

Information for the patient
• Teach patient signs and symptoms of adverse effects and importance of reporting them; patient should also report excessive weight gain (more than 5 lb [2.25 kg] weekly).
• Explain that orthostatic hypotension can be minimized by rising slowly from a supine position and avoiding sudden position changes; it may be aggravated by fever, hot weather, hot showers, prolonged standing, exercise, and alcohol.
• Warn patient to avoid hazardous activities that require mental alertness and to take drug at bedtime until tolerance develops to sedation, drowsiness, and other CNS effects.
• Advise patient to use ice chips or sugarless hard candy or gum to relieve dry mouth.
• Warn patient to seek medical approval before taking OTC cold preparations.

Geriatric patients
• Elderly patients may be more sensitive to orthostatic hypotension.

Pediatric patients
• Safety and efficacy in children haven't been established; use drug only if potential benefit outweighs risk.

Breast-feeding patients
• It's unknown if drug appears in breast milk. An alternative to breast-feeding is recommended during therapy.

guanethidine monosulfate
Ismelin

Pharmacologic classification: adrenergic neuron blocker
Therapeutic classification: antihypertensive
Pregnancy risk category C

How supplied
Available by prescription only
Tablets: 10 mg, 25 mg

Indications, route, and dosage
Moderate to severe hypertension, ◊ signs and symptoms of thyrotoxicosis
Adults: Initially, 10 mg P.O. once daily; increase by 10 mg at weekly to monthly intervals, as needed. Usual dosage is 25 to 50 mg once daily; some patients may need up to 300 mg.

Pharmacodynamics
Antihypertensive action: Acts peripherally; decreases arteriolar vasoconstriction and reduces blood pressure by inhibiting norepinephrine release and depleting norepinephrine stores in adrenergic nerve endings.

Pharmacokinetics
• *Absorption:* Absorbed incompletely from GI tract. Maximal antihypertensive effects usually not evident for 1 to 3 weeks.
• *Distribution:* Distributed throughout body; not protein-bound but demonstrates extensive tissue binding.
• *Metabolism:* Partial hepatic metabolism to pharmacologically less active metabolites.
• *Excretion:* Drug and metabolites excreted primarily in urine; small amounts excreted in feces. Elimination half-life after long-term administration is biphasic.

Contraindications and precautions
Contraindicated in patients with hypersensitivity to drug and in those with pheochromocytoma and frank heart failure. Also contraindicated in those receiving MAO inhibitors. Use cautiously in patients with severe cardiac disease, recent MI, cerebrovascular disease, peptic ulcer, impaired renal function, or bronchial asthma and in those taking other antihypertensives.

Interactions
Drug-drug. *Amphetamines, ephedrine, MAO inhibitors, methylphenidate, norepinephrine, oral contraceptives, phenothiazines, tricyclic antidepressants:* May antagonize antihypertensive effect of guanethidine. Stop MAO inhibitor therapy 1 week before starting guanethidine. Monitor closely.
Cardiac glycosides: May result in additive bradycardia. Monitor ECG.
Diuretics, levodopa, other antihypertensives: Concomitant use may potentiate guanethidine's antihypertensive effect. Use together cautiously.
Metaraminol, norepinephrine, oral sympathomimetic nasal decongestants: Pressor effects may be potentiated. Avoid concomitant use.
Rauwolfia alkaloids (reserpine): May cause excessive orthostatic hypotension, bradycardia, and mental depression. Monitor closely.
Drug-lifestyle. *Alcohol:* May increase hypotensive effect of guanethidine. Discourage concomitant use.

Adverse reactions
CNS: *syncope, fatigue, headache, drowsiness, paresthesia, confusion.*
CV: *palpitations, chest pain, orthostatic hypotension, peripheral edema.*
EENT: *visual disturbances, glossitis.*
GI: *diarrhea, indigestion, constipation, anorexia, nausea, vomiting.*
GU: *nocturia, urination frequency, ejaculation disturbances, impotence.*
Metabolic: *weight gain.*
Musculoskeletal: *aching limbs, leg cramps.*
Respiratory: shortness of breath, cough.

☑ Special considerations
• Dosage requirements may be reduced in the presence of fever.
• If diarrhea develops, atropine or paregoric may be prescribed.
• Stop drug 2 to 3 weeks before elective surgery to reduce risk of CV collapse during anesthesia.
• When drug is replacing MAO inhibitors, wait at least 1 week before initiating guanethidine; if replacing ganglionic blocking drugs, withdraw them slowly to prevent a spiking blood pressure response during transfer period.
• Guanethidine has been used topically as a 5% ophthalmic solution to treat chronic open-angle glaucoma or endocrine ophthalmopathy.
• Signs and symptoms of overdose include hypotension, blurred vision, syncope, bradycardia, and severe diarrhea.
• After acute ingestion, empty stomach by induced emesis or gastric lavage and give acti-

vated charcoal to reduce absorption. Further treatment is usually symptomatic and supportive.

Monitoring the patient
• Monitor supine and standing blood pressure, especially during periods of dosage adjustment.
• Monitor patient for adverse effects.

Information for the patient
• Teach patient signs and symptoms of adverse effects and importance of reporting them; tell him to also report persistent diarrhea and excessive weight gain (5 lb [2.25 kg] weekly). Advise patient not to stop drug but to call for further instructions if adverse reactions occur.
• Warn patient to avoid hazardous activities that require mental alertness and to take drug at bedtime until tolerance develops to sedation, drowsiness, and other CNS effects.
• Advise patient to avoid sudden position changes, strenuous exercise, heat, and hot showers to minimize orthostatic hypotension and to relieve dry mouth with ice chips, hard candy, or gum.
• Tell patient not to double next scheduled dose if one is missed and to take next dose when scheduled.
• Advise patient to seek medical approval before taking OTC cold preparations.

Geriatric patients
• Elderly patients may be more sensitive to drug's antihypertensive effects.

Pediatric patients
• Safety and efficacy in children haven't been established.

Breast-feeding patients
• Small amounts of drug appear in breast milk; an alternative to breast-feeding is recommended during therapy.

---

guanfacine hydrochloride
Tenex

Pharmacologic classification: centrally acting antiadrenergic
Therapeutic classification: antihypertensive
Pregnancy risk category B

How supplied
Available by prescription only
Tablets: 1 mg, 2 mg

Indications, route, and dosage
Mild to moderate hypertension
Adults: Initially, 0.5 to 1 mg P.O. daily h.s. Average dose is 1 to 3 mg daily.

◊ *Heroin withdrawal*
Adults: 0.03 to 1.5 mg P.O. daily.
◊ *Migraine*
Adults: 1 mg P.O. daily for 12 weeks.

Pharmacodynamics
Antihypertensive action: Centrally acting alpha$_2$-adrenoreceptor agonist whose mechanism of action isn't clearly understood. Appears to stimulate central alpha$_2$-adrenergic receptors that decrease peripheral release of norepinephrine, thus decreasing peripheral vascular resistance and lowering blood pressure. Reduces heart rate by reducing sympathetic nerve impulses from the vasomotor center to the heart. Systolic and diastolic blood pressure are both decreased; cardiac output isn't altered.
  Elevated plasma renin activity and plasma catecholamine levels are lowered; however, there's no correlation with individual blood pressure. Single doses of guanfacine stimulate growth hormone secretion, but long-term use has no effect on growth hormone levels.

Pharmacokinetics
• *Absorption:* Absorbed well and completely after oral administration; about 80% bioavailable. Plasma levels peak in 1 to 4 hours.
• *Distribution:* About 70% protein-bound; high distribution to tissues suggested.
• *Metabolism:* Metabolized in liver.
• *Excretion:* About 50% of drug eliminated in urine unchanged, rest as conjugates of metabolites.

Contraindications and precautions
Contraindicated in patients with hypersensitivity to drug. Use cautiously in patients with renal or hepatic insufficiency, severe coronary insufficiency, recent MI, or cerebrovascular disease.

Interactions
Drug-drug. *Antihypertensives, diuretic combinations:* Antihypertensive effects may be potentiated; often used to therapeutic advantage. Avoid concomitant use.
CNS depressants (such as barbiturates, benzodiazepines, phenothiazines): May enhance depressant effects. Avoid concomitant use.
Estrogens, NSAIDs (especially indomethacin), sympathomimetics: May reduce antihypertensive effects of guanfacine. Indomethacin and other NSAIDs may inhibit renal prostaglandin synthesis or cause sodium and fluid retention, antagonizing antihypertensive activity of guanfacine. Blood pressure may increase via estrogen-induced fluid retention. Monitor patient carefully.
Tricyclic antidepressants: May inhibit antihypertensive effects. Avoid concurrent use.
Drug-lifestyle. *Alcohol:* May enhance CNS depressant effects. Discourage concomitant use.

Adverse reactions
CNS: *dizziness,* fatigue, headache, insomnia, *somnolence,* asthenia.
CV: *bradycardia.*
GI: *constipation,* diarrhea, nausea, *dry mouth.*
Metabolic: altered urinary catecholamine levels and urinary vanillylmandelic acid excretion (may be decreased during therapy but may increase on abrupt withdrawal); increased plasma growth hormone levels.
Skin: dermatitis, pruritus.

☑ Special considerations
• Give drug at bedtime to reduce daytime drowsiness.
• Withdrawal syndrome may occur if guanfacine is stopped abruptly or discontinued before surgery; therefore, anesthesiologist must be informed if drug was withdrawn more than 2 days before surgery or if drug hasn't been withdrawn.
• Dry mouth may contribute to development of dental caries, periodontal disease, oral candidiasis, and discomfort.
• Signs and symptoms of overdose include difficult breathing, extreme dizziness, faintness, slow heartbeat, severe or unusual tiredness or weakness. Treat symptomatically, with careful cardiac monitoring. Perform gastric lavage and infuse isoproterenol as appropriate.
• Guanfacine is dialyzed poorly.

Monitoring the patient
• Monitor blood pressure, especially standing and supine, at regular intervals.
• Monitor pulse rate.

Information for the patient
• Stress importance of diet and possible need for sodium restriction and weight reduction.
• Tell patient to take drug as directed even if feeling well and to take daily dose at bedtime to minimize daytime drowsiness.
• Advise patient that drug may cause drowsiness or dizziness. Urge patient to avoid use of alcohol and other CNS depressants, which may add to this effect. Tell patient to avoid driving or performing other tasks that require alertness until effects of drug are known.
• Inform patient to take a missed dose as soon as possible; if taking more than one dose per day when almost time for next dose, skip missed dose and return to regular schedule.
• If patient is to have surgery, including dental surgery, or emergency treatment, advise him to tell medical personnel that he is taking this drug.
• Advise chewing sugarless gum, candy, ice, or saliva substitute for treatment of dry mouth. If condition continues longer than 2 weeks, patient should call for further recommendations.
• Instruct patient not to take other drugs unless prescribed, particularly drugs for cough, cold, asthma, hay fever, or sinus conditions.

Geriatric patients
• Dizziness, drowsiness, hypotension, or faintness occur more frequently in elderly patients, who may be more sensitive to effects of guanfacine.

Breast-feeding patients
• It's unknown if drug appears in breast milk. Use cautiously in breast-feeding women.

Reactions may be *common,* uncommon, *life-threatening,* or COMMON AND LIFE-THREATENING.

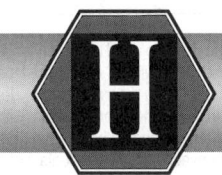

Haemophilus b vaccines

Haemophilus b conjugate vaccine, diphtheria CRM$_{197}$ protein conjugate (HbOC)
HibTITER

Haemophilus b conjugate vaccine, diphtheria toxoid conjugate (PRP-D)
ProHIBiT

Haemophilus b conjugate vaccine, meningococcal protein conjugate (PRP-OMP)
PedvaxHIB

Haemophilus b polysaccharide conjugate vaccine, tetanus toxoid
ActHIB, OmniHIB

Pharmacologic classification: vaccine
Therapeutic classification: bacterial vaccine
Pregnancy risk category C

How supplied
Available by prescription only
Conjugate vaccine, diphtheria CRM$_{197}$ protein conjugate
Injection: 10 mcg of purified *Haemophilus* b saccharide and about 25 mcg CRM$_{197}$ protein per 0.5 ml
Conjugate vaccine, diphtheria toxoid conjugate
Injection: 25 mcg of *Haemophilus influenzae* type B (Hib) capsular polysaccharide and 18 mcg of diphtheria toxoid protein per 0.5 ml
Conjugate vaccine, meningococcal protein conjugate
Powder for injection: 15 mcg *Haemophilus* b polysaccharide, 250 mcg *Neisseria meningitidis* OMPC per dose
Conjugate vaccine, tetanus toxoid
Powder for injection: 10 mcg *Haemophilus* b purified capsular polysaccharide, 24 mcg of tetanus toxoid, and 8.5% sucrose

Indications, route, and dosage
Routine immunization
Haemophilus b conjugate vaccine, diphtheria CRM$_{197}$ protein conjugate
Children ages 2 to 6 months: 0.5 ml I.M.; repeat in 2 months and again in 4 months (for total of three doses). A booster dose is required at age 15 months.
Previously unvaccinated children ages 7 to 11 months: 0.5 ml I.M.; repeat in 2 months (for total of two doses before age 15 months). A booster dose is required at age 15 months (but no sooner than 2 months after last vaccination).
Previously unvaccinated children ages 12 to 14 months: 0.5 ml I.M. A booster dose is required at age 15 months (but no sooner than 2 months after last vaccination).
Previously unvaccinated children ages 15 to 60 months: 0.5 ml I.M.
Haemophilus b conjugate vaccine, diphtheria toxoid conjugate
Children ages 15 to 60 months: 0.5 ml I.M.
Haemophilus b conjugate vaccine, meningococcal protein conjugate
Previously unvaccinated infants ages 2 to 10 months: 0.5 ml I.M. ideally at 2 months. Repeat 2 months later (or as soon as possible thereafter). A booster dose of 0.5 ml I.M. should be administered at 12 to 15 months (but no sooner than 2 months after last vaccination).
Previously unvaccinated children ages 11 to 14 months: 0.5 ml I.M.; repeat in 2 months.
Previously unvaccinated children ages 15 to 71 months: 0.5 ml I.M.
Haemophilus b polysaccharide conjugate vaccine, tetanus toxoid
Previously unvaccinated children ages 2 to 6 months: three 0.5-ml I.M. doses at 8-week intervals, then a booster dose at age 15 to 18 months.
Previously unvaccinated children ages 7 to 11 months: two 0.5-ml I.M. doses at 8-week intervals, then a booster dose at age 15 to 18 months.
Previously unvaccinated children ages 12 to 14 months: 0.5 ml I.M., then a booster dose at age 15 to 18 months. Administer no earlier than 2 months after previous dose.
Previously unvaccinated children ages 15 to 60 months: 0.5 ml I.M.

Pharmacodynamics

Prophylactic action: Vaccine promotes active immunity to *H. influenzae* type b.

Pharmacokinetics

• *Absorption:* After I.M. or S.C. administration, increases in *H. influenzae* type b capsular antibody levels in serum detectable in about 2 weeks; peak within 3 weeks.

• *Distribution:* Limited data indicate antibodies to *H. influenzae* type b detected in fetal blood and in breast milk after giving vaccine to pregnant and breast-feeding women.

• *Metabolism:* No information available.

• *Excretion:* Vaccine polysaccharide detected in urine for up to 11 days after administration to children.

Contraindications and precautions

Contraindicated in patients with hypersensitivity to any component of vaccine, including thimerosal, and in those with acute illness. Don't administer to patients less than 10 days before or during treatment with immunosuppressants or irradiation.

Interactions

Drug-drug. *Corticosteroids, immunosuppressants:* Concomitant use may impair immune response to vaccine. Avoid vaccination under these circumstances.

Immunoglobulin: Administration within 1 month may decrease antibody production. Avoid concomitant use.

Adverse reactions

CNS: irritability.
GI: diarrhea, vomiting.
Skin: *erythema, pain at injection site.*
Other: *anaphylaxis,* fever.

☑ Special considerations

• Obtain thorough history of patient's allergies and reactions to immunizations.

• Epinephrine solution 1:1,000 should be available to treat allergic reactions.

• Don't administer intradermally or I.V.

• Vaccine may be given simultaneously with diphtheria, tetanus, and pertussis (DTP) vaccine; measles, mumps, and rubella (MMR) vaccine; poliovirus vaccine, inactivated (IPV); meningococcal vaccine; or pneumococcal vaccine, but should be administered at different sites. Also may be given with oral poliovirus vaccine (OPV). Generally not recommended in pregnancy.

• Store vaccine in refrigerator and protect from light. Don't freeze.

• Children under age 24 months who develop invasive *H. influenzae* type b disease should be vaccinated because natural immunity may not develop.

• Vaccination shouldn't be used to prevent invasive disease associated with *H. influenzae* type b disease because of the time required to develop immunity. Instead, chemoprophylaxis (with drugs such as rifampin) should be used in both vaccinated and unvaccinated individuals since children with immunity may carry and transmit the organism. However, if every child in a household or day-care group has been fully vaccinated, chemoprophylaxis isn't needed.

• Note that a conjugate vaccine containing meningococcal proteins won't prevent meningococcal disease; one containing diphtheria proteins won't produce immunity against diphtheria; and one containing the tetanus toxoid conjugate won't produce immunity against tetanus toxoid. DTP vaccine should be administered according to recommended schedule.

Monitoring the patient

• Administer same vaccine throughout vaccination series; no data are available to support interchangeability of vaccines.

• Monitor for signs of anaphylaxis.

Information for the patient

• *H. influenzae* type b is a cause of meningitis in infants and preschool children. Explain to parents that this vaccine will protect children only against meningitis caused by this organism.

• Tell parents that child may experience swelling and inflammation at injection site and fever. Recommend acetaminophen liquid for fever.

• Tell parents to report worrisome or persistent adverse reactions promptly.

Pediatric patients

• These vaccines are indicated for use only in children between ages 2 months and 5 years.

• The U.S. Public Health Service's Advisory Committee on Immunization Practices currently recommends that beginning at age 2 months children receive one of the conjugate vaccines licensed for this age-group (*Haemophilus* b conjugate vaccine, diphtheria CRM_{197} protein conjugate [HibTITER] or *Haemophilus* b conjugate vaccine, meningococcal protein conjugate [PedvaxHIB], or *Haemophilus* b conjugate vaccine, tetanus toxoid conjugate). Check package insert to see if vaccine is licensed for use in specific age-groups.

haloperidol
Apo-Haloperidol*, Haldol,
Novo-Peridol*, Peridol*

haloperidol decanoate
Haldol Decanoate, Haldol Decanoate
100, Haldol LA*

haloperidol lactate
Haldol, Haldol Concentrate,
Haloperidol Intensol

Pharmacologic classification: butyro-
phenone
Therapeutic classification: antipsychotic
Pregnancy risk category C

How supplied
Available by prescription only
haloperidol
Tablets: 0.5 mg, 1 mg, 2 mg, 5 mg, 10 mg, 20 mg
Oral concentrate: 2 mg/ml
haloperidol decanoate
Injection: 50 mg/ml, 100 mg/ml
haloperidol lactate
Oral concentrate: 2 mg/ml
Injection: 5 mg/ml

Indications, route, and dosage
Psychotic disorders, ◊ alcohol dependence
Adults: Dosage varies for each patient and symptomatology. Initial dosage range is 0.5 to 5 mg
P.O. b.i.d. or t.i.d.; or 2 to 5 mg I.M. q 4 to 8 hours,
increased rapidly if needed for prompt control.
Maximum dose is 100 mg P.O. daily. Doses over
100 mg have been used for patients with severely
resistant conditions.
**Chronic psychotic patients who require pro-
longed therapy**
Adults: 100 mg I.M. of haloperidol decanoate q
4 weeks. Experience with doses over 450 mg
monthly is limited.
**Control of tics, vocal utterances in Tourette
syndrome**
Adults: 0.5 to 5 mg P.O. b.i.d. or t.i.d., increased
p.r.n.
Children ages 3 to 12: 0.05 to 0.075 mg/kg/day
given b.i.d. or t.i.d.

Pharmacodynamics
Antipsychotic action: Thought to exert antipsychotic effects by strong postsynaptic blockade of
CNS dopamine receptors, thereby inhibiting
dopamine-mediated effects; pharmacologic effects are most similar to those of piperazine antipsychotics. Mechanism of action in Tourette syndrome is unknown.

Has many other central and peripheral effects;
has weak peripheral anticholinergic and antiemetic effects, produces both alpha and ganglionic blockade, and counteracts histamine- and

serotonin-mediated activity. Most prominent adverse reactions are extrapyramidal.

Pharmacokinetics
• *Absorption:* Rate and extent of absorption vary
with route of administration. Oral tablet absorption yields 60% to 70% bioavailability; I.M. dose
is 70% absorbed within 30 minutes. After oral administration, plasma levels peak at 2 to 6 hours;
after I.M. administration, 30 to 45 minutes; after
long-acting I.M. (decanoate) administration, 6 to
7 days.
• *Distribution:* Distributed widely into body, with
high levels in adipose tissue. 90% to 92%
protein-bound.
• *Metabolism:* Metabolized extensively by liver;
possibly only one active metabolite less active
than parent drug.
• *Excretion:* About 40% excreted in urine within
5 days; about 15% excreted in feces via biliary
tract.

Contraindications and precautions
Contraindicated in patients with hypersensitivity
to drug and in those experiencing parkinsonism,
coma, or CNS depression.

Use cautiously in elderly or debilitated patients; in patients with history of seizures, EEG
abnormalities, CV disorders, allergies, narrow-
angle glaucoma, or urine retention; and in those
receiving anticoagulant, anticonvulsant, antiparkinsonian, or lithium drugs.

Interactions
Drug-drug. *Antacids containing aluminum and
magnesium, antidiarrheals, phenobarbital:* Pharmacokinetic alterations and subsequent decreased therapeutic response to haloperidol may
follow concomitant use. Monitor patient closely.
*Antiarrhythmics, disopyramide, procainamide,
quinidine:* Increased risk of arrhythmias and conduction defects. Use with extreme caution; monitor patient closely.
Anticholinergics, atropine: Oversedation, paralytic ileus, visual changes, severe constipation.
Avoid concomitant use.
*Appetite suppressants, sympathomimetics (such
as ephedrine, epinephrine, phenylephrine,
phenylpropanolamine):* May decrease stimulatory and pressor effects of these drugs. Monitor
patient closely.
Beta blockers: May inhibit haloperidol metabolism, increasing plasma levels and toxicity. Monitor haloperidol levels.
Bromocriptine: Haloperidol may antagonize therapeutic effect. Monitor patient closely.
*Centrally acting antihypertensive drugs (such as
clonidine, guanabenz, guanadrel, guanethidine,
methyldopa, reserpine):* Haloperidol may inhibit
blood pressure response to these drugs. Check
blood pressure frequently.

CNS depressants; epidural, general, or spinal anesthetics: Increased CNS depression. Avoid concomitant use.

Dopamine: May decrease vasoconstricting effects of high-dose dopamine. Monitor blood pressure.

Levodopa: May decrease effectiveness and increase toxicity of levodopa. Use together cautiously.

Lithium: May result in severe neurologic toxicity with encephalitis-like syndrome and decreased therapeutic response to haloperidol. Monitor patient.

Metrizamide: Increased risk of seizures. Use together with caution; monitor patient closely.

Nitrates: May cause hypotension. Monitor blood pressure closely.

Parenteral magnesium sulfate: Possible oversedation, respiratory depression, and hypotension. Avoid concomitant use.

Phenytoin: May inhibit metabolism and increase toxicity of phenytoin. Monitor phenytoin levels.

Propylthiouracil: Increased risk of agranulocytosis with concomitant use. Monitor patient closely.

Drug-herb. *Nutmeg:* May cause loss of symptom control with concomitant use or interfere with existing therapy for psychiatric illnesses. Discourage concomitant use.

Drug-lifestyle. *Alcohol:* Increased CNS depression. Discourage use.

Heavy smoking: Increased metabolism. Discourage concomitant use.

Adverse reactions

CNS: *severe extrapyramidal reactions, tardive dyskinesia,* sedation, drowsiness, lethargy, headache, insomnia, confusion, vertigo, **seizures.**

CV: tachycardia, hypotension, hypertension, ECG changes.

EENT: *blurred vision.*

GI: dry mouth, anorexia, constipation, diarrhea, nausea, vomiting, dyspepsia.

GU: urine retention, menstrual irregularities, gynecomastia, priapism.

Hematologic: *leukopenia,* leukocytosis.

Hepatic: altered liver function test results, jaundice.

Skin: rash, other skin reactions, diaphoresis.

Other: *neuroleptic malignant syndrome* (rare).

☑ Special considerations

• Drug has few CV adverse effects and may be preferred in patients with cardiac disease.

• Protect drug from light. Slight yellowing of injection or concentrate is common; doesn't affect potency. Discard markedly discolored solutions.

• Don't withdraw drug abruptly except when required because of severe adverse reaction.

• Dose of 2 mg is therapeutic equivalent of 100 mg chlorpromazine.

• When changing from tablets to decanoate injection, patient should initially receive 10 to 20 times the oral dose once monthly (maximum, 100 mg).

• Administer drug by deep I.M. injection. Don't administer decanoate form I.V.

• For overdose, use supportive measures according to symptoms. Gastric lavage may be used, then activated charcoal and saline cathartics; dialysis doesn't help.

• Coma and arrhythmias are signs of overdose.

Monitoring the patient

• Monitor ECG and vital signs frequently.

• Assess patient periodically for abnormal body movement. Abnormal involuntary muscle movements, agitation, and seizures are signs of overdose.

• Tardive dyskinesia may occur after prolonged use. It may not appear until months or years later and may disappear spontaneously or persist for life.

Information for the patient

• Warn patient against activities that require alertness and good psychomotor coordination until CNS response to drug is determined. Drowsiness and dizziness usually subside after a few weeks.

• Tell patient to report adverse effects, such as extrapyramidal reactions.

Geriatric patients

• Drug is especially useful for agitation associated with senile dementia.

• Elderly patients usually require lower initial doses and a more gradual dosage adjustment.

Pediatric patients

• Drug isn't recommended for children under age 3. Children are especially prone to extrapyramidal adverse reactions.

heparin sodium
Heparin Lock Flush, Hep-Lock, Hep-Lock U/P

Pharmacologic classification: anticoagulant
Therapeutic classification: anticoagulant
Pregnancy risk category C

How supplied
Available products are derived from bovine lung or porcine intestinal mucosa. All are injectable and available by prescription only.
heparin sodium
Vials: 1,000 units/ml, 5,000 units/ml, 10,000 units/ml, 20,000 units/ml, 40,000 units/ml
Unit-dose ampules: 1,000 units/ml, 5,000 units/ml, 10,000 units/ml

---

Disposable syringes: 1,000 units/ml, 2,500 units/ml, 5,000 units/ml, 7,500 units/ml, 10,000 units/ml, 20,000 units/ml
Carpuject: 5,000 units/ml
Premixed I.V. solutions: 1,000 units in 500 ml normal saline solution; 2,000 units in 1,000 ml normal saline solution; 12,500 units in 250 ml 0.45% saline solution; 25,000 units in 250 ml 0.45% saline solution; 25,000 units in 500 ml 0.45% saline solution; 10,000 units in 100 ml D_5W; 12,500 units in 250 ml D_5W; 25,000 units in 250 ml D_5W; 25,000 units in 500 ml D_5W

heparin sodium flush
Vials: 10 units/ml, 100 units/ml
Disposable syringes: 10 units/ml, 25 units/2.5 ml, 2,500 units/2.5 ml

Indications, route, and dosage

Deep vein thrombosis, pulmonary embolism
Adults: Initially, 5,000 to 10,000 units I.V. push, then adjust dose according to PTT results and give dose I.V. q 4 hours (usually 4,000 to 5,000 units); or 5,000 units I.V. bolus, then 20,000 to 40,000 units in 24 hours by I.V. infusion pump. Wait 4 to 6 hours after bolus dose, and adjust hourly rate based on PTT.
Children: Initially, 50 units/kg I.V. bolus. Maintenance dose is 50 to 100 units/kg I.V. drip q 4 hours. Constant infusion: 20,000 units/m² daily. Adjust dosage based on PTT.

Embolism prophylaxis, ◊ post MI, ◊ cerebral thrombosis in evolving stroke, ◊ left ventricular thrombi
Adults: 5,000 units S.C. q 8 to 12 hours.

Open-heart surgery
Adults: (total body perfusion) 150 to 400 units/kg continuous I.V. infusion.

DIC
Adults: 50 to 100 units/kg I.V. q 4 hours as a single injection or constant infusion. Stop if no improvement in 4 to 8 hours.
Children: 25 to 50 units/kg I.V. q 4 hours as a single injection or constant infusion. Stop if no improvement in 4 to 8 hours.

To maintain patency of I.V. indwelling catheters
Adults and children: 10 to 100 units as an I.V. flush (not intended for therapeutic use).

◊ Unstable angina
Adults: Keep PTT one and one-half to two times control during first week of anginal pain.

◊ Anticoagulation in blood transfusion and samples
Transfusions and samples: Mix 7,500 units and 100 ml of normal saline and add 6 to 8 ml of mixture to each 100 ml of whole blood or 70 to 150 units to each 10 to 20 ml of blood sample.

Note: Heparin dosing is highly individualized and depends on disease state, age, and renal and hepatic status.

Pharmacodynamics
Anticoagulant action: Accelerates formation of antithrombin III-thrombin complex; inactivates thrombin and prevents conversion of fibrinogen to fibrin.

Pharmacokinetics
• *Absorption:* Not absorbed from GI tract; must be given parenterally. After I.V. use, almost immediate onset of action; after S.C. injection, onset of action occurs in 20 to 60 minutes.
• *Distribution:* Extensively bound to lipoprotein, globulins, and fibrinogen; doesn't cross placenta.
• *Metabolism:* Not completely described; possibly removed by reticuloendothelial system, with some metabolism occurring in liver.
• *Excretion:* Little known; small fraction excreted in urine as unchanged drug. Not excreted into breast milk. Plasma half-life is 1 to 2 hours.

Contraindications and precautions
Contraindicated in patients with hypersensitivity to drug. Conditionally contraindicated in patients with active bleeding; blood dyscrasia; or bleeding tendencies, such as hemophilia, thrombocytopenia, or hepatic disease with hypoprothrombinemia; suspected intracranial hemorrhage; suppurative thrombophlebitis; inaccessible ulcerative lesions (especially of GI tract) and open ulcerative wounds; extensive denudation of skin; ascorbic acid deficiency and other conditions that cause increased capillary permeability; during or after brain, eye, or spinal cord surgery; during spinal tap or spinal anesthesia; during continuous tube drainage of stomach or small intestine; in subacute bacterial endocarditis; shock; advanced renal disease; threatened abortion; or severe hypertension. Although heparin use is clearly hazardous in these conditions, its risks and benefits must be evaluated.

Use cautiously in postpartum patients or women during menses; in patients with mild hepatic or renal disease, alcoholism, or history of asthma, allergies, or GI ulcer; and in those with occupations that have a high risk of accidents.

Interactions
Drug-drug. *Antihistamines, cardiac glycosides, nicotine, tetracyclines:* May partially counteract anticoagulant action of heparin. Monitor PT, PTT, and INR.
Oral anticoagulants, platelet inhibitors: Increased anticoagulant effect. Monitor PT, PTT, and INR.
Drug-herb. *Motherwort, red clover:* May increase risk of bleeding. Discourage concomitant use.

Adverse reactions
Hematologic: *hemorrhage* (with excessive dosage), *overly prolonged clotting time,* **thrombocytopenia.**

Other: irritation; mild pain; hematoma; ulceration; cutaneous or subcutaneous necrosis; *"white clot" syndrome; hypersensitivity reactions* (including chills, fever, pruritus, rhinitis, urticaria, *anaphylactoid reactions*).

☑ **Special considerations**
• Severe hemorrhage may require treatment with protamine sulfate. Usually, 1 mg protamine sulfate will neutralize 90 units of bovine heparin or 115 units of porcine heparin. For severe bleeding, transfusions may be needed.
• Obtain pretherapy baseline INR, PT, and PTT; measure PTT regularly. Anticoagulation is present when PTT values are one and one-half to two times control values; draw blood for PTT 4 to 6 hours after an I.V. bolus dose and 12 to 24 hours after an S.C. dose. Blood may be drawn at any time after 4 to 6 hours of constant I.V. infusion; if I.V. therapy is intermittent, draw blood 30 minutes before next scheduled dose to avoid falsely prolonged PTT. Never draw blood for PTT from the I.V. tubing of the heparin infusion or from vein of infusion; falsely prolonged PTT will result. Always draw blood from opposite arm.
• I.V. administration is preferred because S.C. and I.M. injections are irregularly absorbed. When possible, administer I.V. heparin by infusion pump for maximum safety.
• When using heparin flush solution, keep intermittent I.V. line patent by flushing it with saline solution before and after heparin; many drugs are incompatible with heparin and may form precipitates if they come in contact with heparin.
• For S.C. injection, use one needle to withdraw solution from vial and another to inject drug. Give low-dose S.C. injections sequentially between iliac crests in lower abdomen; give slowly and deep into subcutaneous fat. After inserting needle into skin, don't withdraw plunger to check for blood; to reduce risk of tissue injury and hematoma, leave needle in place for 10 seconds after S.C. injection. Alternate site every 12 hours: right for morning, left for evening. Don't massage after S.C. injection; watch for local bleeding, hematoma, or inflammation. Rotate site.
• Avoid excessive I.M. injection of other drugs to prevent or minimize hematomas. If possible, don't give any I.M. injections.
• Abrupt withdrawal may increase coagulability; heparin is usually followed by prophylactic oral anticoagulant therapy.

Monitoring the patient
• Check patient regularly for bleeding gums, bruises on arms or legs, petechiae, nosebleeds, melena, tarry stools, hematuria, or hematemesis. Monitor platelet counts regularly.
• Check I.V. infusions regularly, even when pumps are in good working order, to prevent overdose or underdose; don't piggyback other drugs into line while heparin infusion is running because many antibiotics and other drugs inactivate heparin. Never mix any drug with heparin in syringe when bolus therapy is used.

Information for the patient
• Teach injection technique and methods of record-keeping if patient or family will be giving drug.
• Encourage compliance with medication schedule, follow-up appointments, and need for routine monitoring of blood studies; teach patient and family signs of bleeding, and stress importance of calling immediately at first sign of excess bleeding.
• Caution patient not to take double doses if he misses one; tell him to call for instructions instead.
• Warn patient to seek medical approval before taking new medication, and to inform other medical personnel and dentist about heparin use.

Geriatric patients
• At least one manufacturer indicates that women over age 60 are at greatest risk for hemorrhage.

hepatitis A vaccine, inactivated
Havrix

Pharmacologic classification: vaccine
Therapeutic classification: viral vaccine
Pregnancy risk category C

How supplied
Available by prescription only
Injection: 360 Elisa units (EL.U.)/0.5 ml, 1,440 EL.U./1 ml

Indications, route, and dosage
Immunization against disease caused by hepatitis A virus
Adults: 1,440 EL.U./1 ml I.M. as a single dose. Give booster dose of 1,440 EL.U./1 ml I.M. anytime between 6 and 12 months after initial dosage to ensure highest antibody titers.
Children ages 2 to 18: Give two doses of 360 EL.U./0.5 ml I.M. 1 month apart and booster dose of 360 EL.U./0.5 ml I.M. anytime between 6 and 12 months after initial dosage to ensure highest antibody titers.

Pharmacodynamics
Immunostimulant action: Promotes active immunity to hepatitis A virus. Immunity isn't permanent or completely predictable.

Pharmacokinetics
No information available.

Contraindications and precautions
Contraindicated in patients with hypersensitivity to components of vaccine. Use cautiously in patients with thrombocytopenia or bleeding disorders and in those taking anticoagulants because bleeding may occur following I.M. injection in these individuals.

Interactions
Drug-drug. *Anticoagulants:* Increased risk of bleeding. Administer I.M. injections cautiously; monitor patient closely.

Adverse reactions
CNS: *malaise, fatigue,* headache, insomnia, photophobia, vertigo.
GI: *anorexia, nausea,* abdominal pain, diarrhea, dysgeusia, vomiting.
Hepatic: jaundice, *hepatitis.*
Musculoskeletal: arthralgia, myalgia.
Respiratory: pharyngitis, other upper respiratory tract infections.
Skin: pruritus, *rash,* urticaria, *induration, redness, swelling,* hematoma.
Other: *fever,* lymphadenopathy, hypertonic episode, elevation of CK, *anaphylaxis.*

☑ Special considerations
● As with any vaccine, administration of hepatitis A vaccine should be delayed, if possible, in patients with febrile illness.
● If vaccine is administered to immunosuppressed persons or those receiving immunosuppressive therapy, the expected immune response may not be obtained.
● Persons who should receive the vaccine include those traveling to or living in areas of high endemicity for hepatitis A (Africa, Asia [except Japan], the Mediterranean basin, Eastern Europe, the Middle East, Central and South America, Mexico, and parts of the Caribbean), military personnel, native people of Alaska and the Americas, persons engaging in high-risk sexual activity, and users of illicit injectable drugs. Also, certain institutional workers, employees of child daycare centers, laboratory workers who handle live hepatitis A virus, and handlers of primate animals may benefit from immunization.
● Shake vial or syringe well before withdrawal and use. With thorough agitation, vaccine is an opaque white suspension. Discard if it appears otherwise. No dilution or reconstitution necessary.
● Administer as I.M. injection into deltoid region in adults. Don't administer in gluteal region; such injections may result in suboptimal response. Never inject I.V., S.C., or intradermally.
● Hepatitis A vaccine won't prevent infection in persons with unrecognized hepatitis A infection at time of vaccination.

Monitoring the patient
● Although anaphylaxis is rare, keep epinephrine readily available to treat an anaphylactoid reaction.
● Observe for signs of hepatitis.

Information for the patient
● Inform patient that vaccine won't prevent hepatitis caused by other agents such as hepatitis B, hepatitis C, or hepatitis E virus; or other pathogens known to infect the liver.

Pediatric patients
● Vaccine is well tolerated, highly immunogenic, and effective in children ages 2 and older.

Breast-feeding patients
● It's unknown if vaccine appears in breast milk. Because many drugs appear in breast milk, administer cautiously in breast-feeding women.

hepatitis B immune globulin, human (HBIG)
H-BIG, HyperHep

Pharmacologic classification: immune serum
Therapeutic classification: hepatitis B prophylaxis
Pregnancy risk category C

How supplied
Available by prescription only
Injection: 1-ml, 4-ml, and 5-ml vials
Prefilled syringe: 0.5 ml

Indications, route, and dosage
Hepatitis B exposure
Adults and children: 0.06 ml/kg I.M. within 7 days after exposure. Repeat 28 days after exposure.
Neonates born to HBsAg-positive women: 0.5 ml I.M. within 12 hours of birth. Initiation of HB vaccination is also indicated.

The American College of Obstetricians and Gynecologists recommends use of HBIG in pregnancy for postexposure prophylaxis. Hepatitis B immune globulin should be given only if clearly needed.

Pharmacodynamics
Prophylactic action: HBIG provides passive immunity to hepatitis B.

Pharmacokinetics
● *Absorption:* Absorbed slowly after I.M. injection. Antibodies to hepatitis B surface antigen (HBsAg) appear in serum within 1 to 6 days, peak within 3 to 11 days, and persist for about 2 to 6 months.
● *Distribution:* Specific information not available; HBIG probably crosses placenta, as do other im-

munoglobulins. Data on distribution into breast milk not available.
- *Metabolism:* No information available.
- *Excretion:* Serum half-life for antibodies to HBsAg is reportedly 21 days.

Contraindications and precautions
Contraindicated in patients with history of thimerosal allergy or anaphylactic reactions to immune serum.

Interactions
Drug-drug. *Live virus vaccines:* May interfere with response to live virus vaccine. Defer immunization for 2 weeks before or 3 months after HBIG whenever possible.

Adverse reactions
Skin: urticaria, pain, tenderness at injection site.
Other: *anaphylaxis, angioedema.*

☑ Special considerations
- Obtain thorough history of patient's allergies and reactions to immunizations.
- Administer drug I.M. only. Severe, even fatal, reactions may occur if administered I.V.
- Gluteal or deltoid areas are preferred injection sites.
- HBIG may be given simultaneously, but at different sites, with hepatitis B vaccine.
- Store between 36° and 46° F (2° and 8° C). Don't freeze.
- Hospital staff should receive immunization if exposed to hepatitis B (for example, from a needlestick or direct contact).
- HBIG hasn't been associated with a higher risk of AIDS. The immune globulin is devoid of HIV. Immune globulin recipients don't develop antibodies to HIV.

Monitoring the patient
- Have epinephrine solution 1:1,000 available in case of allergic reactions.
- Observe for edema and signs of allergic reactions.

Information for the patient
- Explain that patient's chances of getting AIDS after receiving HBIG are very small.
- Inform patient that HBIG provides temporary protection against hepatitis B only.
- Tell patient to expect local pain, swelling, and tenderness at injection site after vaccination. Recommend acetaminophen to relieve minor discomfort.
- Encourage patient to promptly report headache, skin changes, or difficulty breathing.

Breast-feeding patients
- It's unknown if HBIG appears in breast milk. Use with caution in breast-feeding women.

hepatitis B vaccine, recombinant
Engerix-B, Recombivax HB, Recombivax HB Dialysis Formulation

Pharmacologic classification: vaccine
Therapeutic classification: viral vaccine
Pregnancy risk category C

How supplied
Available by prescription only
Injection: 2.5 mcg hepatitis B surface antigen (HBsAg)/0.5 ml (Recombivax HB pediatric formulation); 5 mcg HBsAg/0.5 ml (Recombivax HB adolescent/high-risk infant formulation); 10 mcg HBsAg/0.5 ml (Engerix-B, pediatric injection); 10 mcg HBsAg/ml (Recombivax HB); 20 mcg HBsAg/ml (Engerix-B); 40 mcg HBsAg/ml (Recombivax HB Dialysis Formulation)

Indications, route, and dosage
Immunization against infection from all known subtypes of hepatitis B; primary preexposure prophylaxis against hepatitis B; postexposure prophylaxis (when given with hepatitis B immune globulin)
Engerix-B
Adults ages 20 and older: Initially, give 20 mcg (1-ml adult formulation) I.M., then a second dose of 20 mcg I.M. 30 days later. Give a third dose of 20 mcg I.M. 6 months after the initial dose.
Neonates and children up to age 19: Initially, give 10 mcg (0.5-ml pediatric formulation) I.M., then a second dose of 10 mcg I.M. 30 days later. Give a third dose of 10 mcg I.M. 6 months after the initial dose.
Adults undergoing dialysis or receiving immunosuppressive therapy: Initially, give 40 mcg I.M. (divided into two 20-mcg doses and administered at different sites). Follow with a second dose of 40 mcg I.M. in 30 days, a third dose after 2 months, and a final dose of 40 mcg I.M. 6 months after the initial dose.
Note: Alternative dosing schedule in certain populations (neonates born to infected mothers, persons recently exposed to the virus, and travelers to high-risk areas) who may receive the initial vaccine dose (20 mcg for adults and children over age 10, and 10 mcg for neonates and children up to age 10 for this dosing schedule) then a second dose in 1 month and the third dose after 2 months. For prolonged maintenance of protective antibody titers, a booster dose is recommended 12 months after the initial dose.
Recombivax HB
Adults ages 20 and older: Initially, give 10 mcg (1-ml adult formulation) I.M., then a second dose of 10 mcg I.M. 30 days later. Give a third dose of 10 mcg I.M. 6 months after the initial dose.
Children ages 11 to 19: Initially, give 5 mcg (0.5-ml adolescent/high risk infant formulation) I.M.,

then a second dose of 5 mcg I.M. 30 days later. Give a third dose of 5 mcg I.M. 6 months after the initial dose.

Neonates born to HBsAg-negative mothers and children up to age 10: Initially, give 2.5 mcg (0.5-ml pediatric formulation), then a second dose of 2.5 mcg I.M. 30 days later. Give a third dose of 2.5 mcg I.M. 6 months after the initial dose.

Neonates born to HBsAg-positive mothers: Initially, give 5 mcg (0.5-ml adolescent/high-risk infant formulation) I.M. with 0.5 ml hepatitis B immune globulin. Follow with a second dose of 5 mcg I.M. 30 days later. Give a third dose of 5 mcg I.M. 6 months after the initial dose.

Adults undergoing dialysis or receiving immunosuppressive therapy: Initially, give 40 mcg I.M. (1-ml dialysis formulation). Follow with a second dose of 40 mcg I.M. in 30 days, and give a final dose of 40 mcg I.M. 6 months after the initial dose.

Pharmacodynamics
Prophylactic action: Promotes active immunity to hepatitis B.

Pharmacokinetics
• *Absorption:* After I.M. administration, antibody to HBsAg appears in serum within about 2 weeks, peaks after 6 months, and persists for at least 3 years.
• *Distribution:* No information available.
• *Metabolism:* No information available.
• *Excretion:* No information available.

Contraindications and precautions
Contraindicated in patients with hypersensitivity to yeast; recombinant vaccines are derived from yeast cultures. Use cautiously in patients with active infections or compromised cardiac and pulmonary status and in those to whom a febrile or systemic reaction could pose a risk.

Interactions
Drug-drug. *Corticosteroids, immunosuppressants:* May impair immune response to hepatitis B vaccine. Larger-than-usual doses of vaccine may be necessary to develop adequate circulating antibody levels.

Adverse reactions
CNS: headache, dizziness, insomnia, paresthesia, neuropathy, transient malaise.
EENT: pharyngitis.
GI: nausea, anorexia, diarrhea, vomiting.
Musculoskeletal: arthralgia, myalgia.
Skin: local inflammation, *soreness at injection site.*
Other: slight fever, flulike symptoms, ***anaphylaxis.***

☑ Special considerations
• Obtain thorough history of patient's allergies and reactions to immunizations.
• The Centers for Disease Control and Prevention reports that response to hepatitis B vaccine is significantly better when vaccine is injected into deltoid rather than gluteal muscle.
• Hepatitis B vaccine may be administered S.C. but only to persons who are at risk for hemorrhage from I.M. injection, such as hemophiliacs and patients with thrombocytopenia. Don't administer I.V.
• Hepatitis B vaccine may be given simultaneously, but at different sites, with hepatitis B immune globulin, influenza virus vaccine, *Haemophilus influenzae* type B conjugate vaccine, polyvalent pneumococcal vaccine, or DTP.
• Thoroughly agitate vial just before administration to restore a uniform suspension (slightly opaque and white).
• Store opened and unopened vial in refrigerator. Don't freeze.
• Although not necessary for most patients, serologic testing (to confirm immunity to hepatitis B after the three-dose regimen) is recommended for persons over age 50, those at high risk for needlestick injury (who might require postexposure prophylaxis), hemodialysis patients, immunocompromised patients, and those who inadvertently received one or more injections into gluteal muscle.

Monitoring the patient
• Have epinephrine solution 1:1,000 available in case of allergic reaction.
• Monitor for signs of allergic reactions.

Information for the patient
• Tell patient that there is no risk of contracting HIV infection or AIDS from hepatitis B vaccine because it's synthetically derived.
• Explain that hepatitis B vaccine provides protection against hepatitis B only, not against hepatitis A or hepatitis C.
• Tell patient to expect some discomfort at injection site and possible fever, headache, or upset stomach. Recommend acetaminophen to relieve such effects. Encourage patient to report distressing adverse reactions.

Pediatric patients
• Routine immunization is now recommended for all neonates, regardless of whether mother tests positive or negative for HBsAg. Vaccine is usually well tolerated and highly immunogenic in children and infants of all ages.

hetastarch (HES, hydroxyethyl starch)
Hespan

Pharmacologic classification: amylopectin derivative
Therapeutic classification: plasma volume expander
Pregnancy risk category C

How supplied
Available by prescription only
Injection: 500 ml (6 g/100 ml in normal saline solution)

Indications, route, and dosage
Plasma expander in shock and cardiopulmonary bypass surgery
Adults: 500 to 1,000 ml I.V. dependent on amount of blood lost and resultant hemoconcentration. Total dose usually shouldn't exceed 20 ml/kg, up to 1,500 ml/day. Up to 20 ml/kg (1.2 g/kg)/hour may be used in hemorrhagic shock; in burns or septic shock, rate should be reduced.
✦ **Dosage adjustment.** In patients with severe renal impairment (creatinine clearance less than 10 ml/minute), usual initial dose may be given, but subsequent doses should be reduced to 25% to 50% of usual dose.
Leukapheresis adjunct
Hetastarch is an adjunct in leukapheresis to improve harvesting and increase the yield of granulocytes.
Adults: Hetastarch 250 to 700 ml is infused at a constant fixed ratio, usually 1:8 to venous whole blood during continuous flow centrifugation (CFC) procedures. Up to 2 CFC procedures weekly, with total number of 7 to 10 procedures using hetastarch, have been found safe and effective. Safety of larger numbers of procedures is unknown.
Note: Hetastarch can be used as a priming fluid in pump oxygenators for perfusion during extracorporeal circulation or as a cryoprotective product for long-term storage of whole blood.

Pharmacodynamics
Plasma volume expanding action: Has an average molecular weight of 450,000 and exhibits colloidal properties similar to human albumin. After an I.V. infusion of hetastarch 6%, the plasma volume expands slightly in excess of the volume infused because of the colloidal osmotic effect. Maximum plasma volume expansion occurs in a few minutes and decreases over 24 to 36 hours. Hemodynamic status may improve for 24 hours or longer.
Leukapheresis adjunctive action: Enhances yield of granulocytes by centrifugal means.

Pharmacokinetics
• *Absorption:* After I.V. administration, plasma volume expands within a few minutes.
• *Distribution:* Distributed in blood plasma.
• *Metabolism:* Hetastarch molecules larger than 50,000 molecular weight are slowly, enzymatically degraded to molecules that can be excreted.
• *Excretion:* 40% of hetastarch molecules smaller than 50,000 molecular weight excreted in urine within 24 hours. Hetastarch molecules not hydroxyethylated are slowly degraded to glucose. About 90% of dose eliminated from body with average half-life of 17 days; remainder has half-life of 48 days.

Contraindications and precautions
Contraindicated in patients with severe bleeding disorders, severe heart failure, or renal failure with oliguria and anuria.

Interactions
None reported.

Adverse reactions
CNS: headache.
CV: peripheral edema of lower extremities.
EENT: periorbital edema.
GI: nausea, vomiting.
Musculoskeletal: muscle pain.
Respiratory: wheezing.
Skin: urticaria.
Other: mild fever, chills, *hypersensitivity reactions.*

☑ Special considerations
• To avoid circulatory overload, carefully monitor patients with impaired renal function and those at high risk for pulmonary edema or heart failure. Hetastarch 6% in normal saline contains 77 mEq sodium and chloride per 500 ml.
• When added to whole blood, hetastarch increases erythrocyte sedimentation rate.
• Don't administer as a substitute for blood or plasma.
• Discard partially used bottle; doesn't contain a preservative.
• Stop infusion if overdose occurs and treat supportively.

Monitoring the patient
• Monitor CBC, total leukocyte and platelet counts, leukocyte differential count, hemoglobin level, hematocrit, PT, PTT, and electrolyte, BUN, and creatinine levels.
• Assess vital signs and cardiopulmonary status to obtain baseline at start of infusion to prevent fluid overload.
• Monitor I.V. site for signs of infiltration and phlebitis.
• Observe patient for edema.

Reactions may be *common,* uncommon, *life-threatening,* or COMMON AND LIFE-THREATENING.

Information for the patient
• Explain use and administration of drug to patient and family.
• Instruct patient to report adverse reactions promptly.

Geriatric patients
• Use hetastarch with caution in elderly patients, who are more prone to fluid overload; a lower dosage may be sufficient to produce desired plasma volume expansion.

Pediatric patients
• Safety and efficacy in children haven't been established.

Breast-feeding patients
• Breast-feeding should be temporarily stopped in women receiving hetastarch.

homatropine hydrobromide
AK-Homatropine, I-Homatrine, Isopto Homatropine, Minims Homatropine*

Pharmacologic classification: anticholinergic
Therapeutic classification: cycloplegic, mydriatic
Pregnancy risk category C

How supplied
Available by prescription only
Ophthalmic solution: 2%, 5%

Indications, route, and dosage
Cycloplegic refraction
Adults: Instill 1 to 2 drops of 2% or 1 drop of 5% solution in eye; repeat in 5 to 10 minutes, p.r.n.
Children: Instill 1 drop of 2% solution in the eye; repeat at 10-minute intervals, p.r.n.
Uveitis
Adults: Instill 1 to 2 drops of 2% or 5% solution in eye up to q 3 or 4 hours.
Children: Instill 1 drop of 2% solution b.i.d. or t.i.d.

Pharmacodynamics
Cycloplegic and mydriatic actions: Anticholinergic action prevents the sphincter muscle of the iris and the muscle of the ciliary body from responding to cholinergic stimulation, resulting in unopposed adrenergic influence and producing pupillary dilation (mydriasis) and paralysis of accommodation (cycloplegia).

Pharmacokinetics
• *Absorption:* Peak effect reached in 40 to 60 minutes.
• *Distribution:* No information available.
• *Metabolism:* No information available.
• *Excretion:* Recovery from cycloplegic and mydriatic effects usually occurs within 1 to 3 days.

Contraindications and precautions
Contraindicated in patients with hypersensitivity to drug or other belladonna alkaloids such as atropine, and in those with glaucoma or those who have adhesions between the iris and lens. Use cautiously in the elderly and in those with increased ocular pressure.

Interactions
Drug-drug. *Carbachol, cholinesterase inhibitors, pilocarpine:* Homatropine may interfere with antiglaucoma effects of these drugs. Monitor patient.
Drug-lifestyle. *Sun exposure:* Photophobia may occur. Tell patient to take precautions.

Adverse reactions
CNS: confusion, somnolence, headache.
CV: tachycardia.
EENT: eye irritation, *blurred vision, photophobia,* increased intraocular pressure, transient stinging and burning, conjunctivitis, vascular congestion, edema.
GI: dry mouth.
Skin: dryness, rash.

☑ Special considerations
• Drug may produce symptoms of atropine sulfate poisoning, such as severe mouth dryness and tachycardia.
• Drug shouldn't be used internally. Treat accidental ingestion by emesis or activated charcoal.
• Patient may be photophobic and may benefit from wearing dark glasses to minimize discomfort.

Monitoring the patient
• Monitor patient for signs and symptoms of overdose such as flushed dry skin, dry mouth, blurred vision, ataxia, dysarthria, hallucinations, tachycardia, and decreased bowel sounds.
• Carefully monitor patients on antiglaucoma medications.

Information for the patient
• Teach patient how to instill drops and warn him not to touch the eye or surrounding area with dropper.
• Tell patient that vision will be temporarily blurred after instillation, and advise him to use caution when driving or operating machinery.
• Inform patient that drug may produce drowsiness.

Geriatric patients
• Use drug cautiously in these patients because of risk of undiagnosed glaucoma and increased sensitivity to drug's effects.

Pediatric patients
• Use drug cautiously in small children and infants. Increased risk of sensitivity in children with

Down syndrome, spastic paralysis, or brain damage. Feeding intolerance may result.

hyaluronidase
Wydase

Pharmacologic classification: protein enzyme
Therapeutic classification: adjunctive product
Pregnancy risk category C

How supplied
Available by prescription only
Injection (lyophilized powder): 150 USP units/vial, 1,500 USP units/vial
Injection (solution): 150 USP units/ml in 1-ml and 10-ml vials

Indications, route, and dosage
Adjunct to increase absorption and dispersion of other injected drugs
Adults and children: Add 150 USP units to solution containing other medication.
Adjunct to increase absorption rate of fluids given by hypodermoclysis
Adults and children: Inject 150 USP units into the rubber tubing close to the needle of the running clysis solution. Generally, 150 USP units will facilitate absorption of 1 L or more of solution, but dosage administration and type of solution should be individualized.
Adjunct in excretory urography
Adults and children: Administer 75 USP units S.C. over each scapula before administration of the contrast medium.

Pharmacodynamics
Diffusing action: Spreading or diffusing substance that modifies the permeability of connective tissue through the hydrolysis of hyaluronic acid. Drug enhances the diffusion of substances injected S.C. provided local interstitial pressure is adequate.

Pharmacokinetics
No information available.

Contraindications and precautions
Contraindicated in patients with hypersensitivity to drug.

Interactions
Drug-drug. *Local anesthetics:* May increase analgesia, hasten onset, and reduce local swelling; may also increase systemic absorption, increase toxicity, and shorten duration of action. Monitor patient closely.

Adverse reactions
None significant.

☑ Special considerations
● Give skin test for sensitivity before use with an intradermal injection using about 0.02 ml of hyaluronidase solution; a wheal with pseudopods appearing within 5 minutes after injection and lasting for 20 to 30 minutes along with urticaria indicates a positive reaction.
● Avoid contact with eyes; if contact occurs, flood with water immediately.
● Drug may be used to diffuse local anesthetics at injection site, especially in nerve block anesthesia. Has been used to enhance diffusion of drugs in management of I.V. extravasation.
● When considering administration of other drugs with hyaluronidase, consult appropriate references for compatibility.

Monitoring the patient
● Check for hypersensitivity reaction.
● Monitor patient for effect when used with local anesthetics.

Information for the patient
● Instruct patient to report unusual and significant adverse effects after injection.

Pediatric patients
● If administering drug for hypodermoclysis, take care to avoid overhydration. In children under age 3, clysis shouldn't exceed 200 ml; in premature neonates, clysis shouldn't exceed 25 ml/kg and the rate shouldn't exceed 2 ml/minute.

hydralazine hydrochloride
Apresoline

Pharmacologic classification: peripheral vasodilator
Therapeutic classification: antihypertensive
Pregnancy risk category C

How supplied
Available by prescription only
Tablets: 10 mg, 25 mg, 50 mg, 100 mg
Injection: 20 mg/ml

Indications, route, and dosage
Moderate to severe hypertension
Adults: Initially, 10 mg P.O. q.i.d. for 2 to 4 days, then increased to 25 mg q.i.d. for remainder of week. If necessary, increase dosage to 50 mg q.i.d. Maximum recommended dose is 200 mg daily, but some patients may require 300 to 400 mg daily.
For severe hypertension, 10 to 50 mg I.M. or 10 to 20 mg I.V. repeated, p.r.n. Switch to oral antihypertensives as soon as possible.
For hypertensive crisis associated with pregnancy, initially 5 mg I.V., then 5 to 10 mg I.V. q 20

Reactions may be *common*, uncommon, *life-threatening*, or COMMON AND LIFE-THREATENING.

to 30 minutes until adequate reduction in blood pressure is achieved (usual range, 5 to 20 mg).
Children: Initially, 0.75 mg/kg P.O. daily in four divided doses (25 mg/m² daily); may increase gradually to 7.5 mg/kg daily.

I.M. or I.V. drug dose is 0.4 to 1.2 mg/kg daily or 50 to 100 mg/m² daily in four to six divided doses. Initial parenteral dose shouldn't exceed 20 mg.

◊ *Management of severe heart failure*
Adults: Initially, 50 to 75 mg P.O., then adjusted according to patient response. Most patients respond to 200 to 600 mg daily, divided q 6 to 12 hours, but doses as high as 3 g daily have been used.

Pharmacodynamics
Antihypertensive action: Has direct vasodilating effect on vascular smooth muscle, thus lowering blood pressure. Drug's effect on resistance vessels (arterioles and arteries) is greater than that on capacitance vessels (venules and veins).

Pharmacokinetics
• *Absorption:* Absorbed rapidly from GI tract after oral administration; plasma levels peak in 1 hour; bioavailability is 30% to 50%. Antihypertensive effect occurs 20 to 30 minutes after oral dose, 5 to 20 minutes after I.V. administration, and 10 to 30 minutes after I.M. administration. Food enhances absorption.
• *Distribution:* Distributed widely throughout body; about 88% to 90% protein-bound.
• *Metabolism:* Metabolized extensively in GI mucosa and liver. Hydralazine is subject to polymorphic acetylation. Slow acetylators have higher plasma levels, generally requiring lower doses.
• *Excretion:* Mostly excreted in urine, primarily as metabolites; about 10% of oral dose excreted in feces. Antihypertensive effect persists 2 to 4 hours after oral dose, 2 to 6 hours after I.V. or I.M. administration.

Contraindications and precautions
Contraindicated in patients with hypersensitivity to drug, coronary artery disease, or mitral valvular rheumatic heart disease. Use cautiously in patients with suspected cardiac disease, CVA, or severe renal impairment and in those receiving other antihypertensives.

Interactions
Drug-drug. *Diazoxide, MAO inhibitors:* Profound hypotension may occur. Use together cautiously.
Diuretics, other antihypertensives: Hydralazine may potentiate effects of these drugs. Monitor blood pressure and intake and output closely.
Epinephrine: May decrease pressor response to epinephrine. Monitor patient closely.

Adverse reactions
CNS: peripheral neuritis, *headache,* dizziness.

CV: orthostatic hypotension, *tachycardia,* edema, angina, *palpitations.*
GI: *nausea, vomiting, diarrhea, anorexia,* constipation.
Hematologic: *neutropenia, leukopenia, agranulocytosis, agranulocytopenia, thrombocytopenia.*
Skin: rash.
Other: *lupus-like syndrome* (especially with high doses).

☑ Special considerations
• CBC, lupus erythematosus cell preparation, and antinuclear titer determinations should be performed before therapy and at regular intervals during long-term therapy.
• Risk of drug-induced systemic lupus erythematosus (SLE) syndrome is greatest in patients receiving more than 200 mg/day for prolonged periods.
• Headache and palpitations may occur 2 to 4 hours after first oral dose but should subside spontaneously.
• Orthostatic hypotension may occur.
• Food enhances oral absorption and helps minimize gastric irritation; adhere to consistent schedule.
• Some preparations contain tartrazine, which may precipitate allergic reactions, especially in aspirin-sensitive patients.
• Inject drug as soon as possible after draining through needle into syringe; drug changes color after contact with metal.
• Signs and symptoms of overdose are hypotension, tachycardia, headache, and skin flushing; arrhythmias and shock may occur. After acute ingestion, empty stomach by emesis or gastric lavage and give activated charcoal to reduce absorption.

Monitoring the patient
• With I.V. use, monitor blood pressure every 5 minutes until stable, then every 15 minutes; put patient in Trendelenburg's position if he is faint or dizzy. Too-rapid reduction in blood pressure can cause mental changes from cerebral ischemia.
• Sodium retention can occur with long-term use; monitor patient for signs of weight gain and edema.

Information for the patient
• Teach patient about disease and therapy and explain why drug should be taken exactly as prescribed, even when he feels well; advise him never to stop drug suddenly because severe rebound hypertension may occur.
• Explain adverse effects and advise patient to report unusual effects, especially symptoms of SLE (sore throat, fever, rash, and muscle and joint pain). Explain how to minimize impact of adverse effects.

- Tell patient to avoid operation of hazardous equipment until tolerance develops to sedation, drowsiness, and other CNS effects.
- Instruct patient to avoid sudden position changes to minimize orthostatic hypotension and to avoid alcohol.
- Advise patient to take drug with meals to enhance absorption and minimize gastric irritation.
- Reassure patient that headaches and palpitations occurring 2 to 4 hours after initial dose usually subside spontaneously; if not, he should report such effects.
- Instruct patient to weigh himself at least weekly. Advise him to report weight gain that exceeds 5 lb (2.3 kg) weekly.
- Warn patient to seek medical approval before taking OTC cold preparations.

Geriatric patients
- Elderly patients may be more sensitive to antihypertensive effects.

Pediatric patients
- Drug has had limited use in children. Safety and efficacy in children haven't been established; use only if potential benefit outweighs risk.

Breast-feeding patients
- It's unknown if drug appears in breast milk. An alternative to breast-feeding is recommended during therapy.

---

hydrochlorothiazide
Apo-Hydro*, Diuchlor H*, Esidrix, Hydro-chlor, Hydro-D, HydroDIURIL, Neo-Codema*, Novo-Hydrazide*, Oretic, Urozide*

Pharmacologic classification: thiazide diuretic
Therapeutic classification: diuretic, antihypertensive
Pregnancy risk category B

How supplied
Available by prescription only
Tablets: 25 mg, 50 mg, 100 mg
Solution: 50 mg/5 ml, 100 mg/ml

Indications, route, and dosage
Edema
Adults: Initially, 25 to 200 mg P.O. daily for several days or until dry weight is attained. Maintenance dose is 25 to 100 mg P.O. daily or intermittently. A few refractory patients may require up to 200 mg daily.
Children over age 6 months: 1 to 2 mg/kg P.O. daily divided b.i.d.
Children under age 6 months: Up to 3 mg/kg P.O. daily divided b.i.d.

Hypertension
Adults: 25 to 50 mg P.O. once daily or in divided doses. Increase or decrease daily dose based on blood pressure.

Pharmacodynamics
Diuretic action: Increases urinary excretion of sodium and water by inhibiting sodium reabsorption in the cortical diluting tubule of the nephron, thus relieving edema.
Antihypertensive action: Exact mechanism unknown. Action may result partially from direct arteriolar vasodilation and a decrease in total peripheral resistance.

Pharmacokinetics
- *Absorption:* Absorbed from GI tract; rate and extent of absorption vary with different formulations.
- *Distribution:* No information available.
- *Metabolism:* None.
- *Excretion:* Excreted unchanged in urine, usually within 24 hours; half-life is 5.6 to 14.8 hours.

Contraindications and precautions
Contraindicated in patients with hypersensitivity to other thiazides or other sulfonamide derivatives and in those with anuria. Use cautiously in patients with severely impaired renal or hepatic function or progressive hepatic disease.

Interactions
Drug-drug. *Amphetamines, quinidine:* May decrease urinary excretion of these drugs. Monitor patient.
Antihypertensives: Potentiated hypotensive effects of these drugs. Use cautiously for therapeutic advantage.
Cholestyramine, colestipol: May bind hydrochlorothiazide, preventing its absorption. Give drugs 1 hour apart.
Diazoxide: May potentiate hyperglycemic, hypotensive, and hyperuricemic effects of diazoxide. Use together cautiously.
Insulin, sulfonylureas: May decrease effectiveness and increase requirements in diabetic patients. Monitor serum glucose levels.
Lithium: Elevated serum lithium levels. May require reduction in lithium dosage by 50%.
Methenamine mandelate: Concomitant use may decrease therapeutic efficacy of drug. Monitor patient.
Drug-lifestyle. *Alcohol:* Increased orthostatic hypotension. Monitor patient closely.
Sun exposure: Possible photosensitivity reactions. Tell patient to take precautions.

Adverse reactions
CNS: dizziness, vertigo, headache, paresthesia, weakness, restlessness.

CV: volume depletion and dehydration, orthostatic hypotension, allergic myocarditis, vasculitis.
GI: anorexia, nausea, *pancreatitis,* epigastric distress, vomiting, abdominal pain, diarrhea, constipation.
GU: polyuria, frequent urination, *renal failure,* interstitial nephritis.
Hematologic: *aplastic anemia, agranulocytosis,* leukopenia, *thrombocytopenia,* hemolytic anemia.
Hepatic: jaundice.
Metabolic: hypokalemia; asymptomatic hyperuricemia; hyperglycemia and impaired glucose tolerance; fluid and electrolyte imbalances, including dilutional hyponatremia, hypochloremia, metabolic alkalosis, hypercalcemia.
Musculoskeletal: muscle cramps.
Respiratory: respiratory distress, pneumonitis.
Skin: dermatitis, photosensitivity, rash, purpura, alopecia.
Other: hypersensitivity reactions, gout, *anaphylactic reactions.*

☑ **Special considerations**
● Drug may cause glucose intolerance in some people. Monitor blood glucose level in patients with diabetes. May require dosage adjustment of insulin or oral antidiabetic.
● Hydrochlorothiazide may interfere with tests for parathyroid function and should be discontinued before such tests.
● Signs and symptoms of overdose are GI irritation and hypermotility, diuresis, and lethargy, which may progress to coma.

Monitoring the patient
● Monitor patient's vital signs, ECG, and fluid intake.
● Monitor patient's CBC and electrolyte status.

Information for the patient
● Instruct patient to take drug with food to avoid GI upset.
● Tell patient to take drug in morning or early afternoon to avoid nocturia.
● Advise patient to avoid sudden postural changes.

Geriatric patients
● Elderly and debilitated patients need close observation and may require reduced dosages. These patients are more sensitive to excess diuresis because of age-related changes in CV and renal function. Excess diuresis promotes orthostatic hypotension, dehydration, hypovolemia, hyponatremia, hypomagnesemia, and hypokalemia.

Breast-feeding patients
● Drug appears in breast milk; safety and effectiveness in breast-feeding women haven't been established.

hydrocortisone (systemic)
Cortef, Cortenema, Hycort*, Hydrocortone

hydrocortisone acetate
Cortifoam

hydrocortisone cypionate
Cortef

hydrocortisone sodium phosphate
Hydrocortone Phosphate

hydrocortisone sodium succinate
A-hydroCort, Solu-Cortef

Pharmacologic classification: glucocorticoid, mineralocorticoid
Therapeutic classification: adrenocorticoid replacement
Pregnancy risk category C

How supplied
Available by prescription only
hydrocortisone
Tablets: 5 mg, 10 mg, 20 mg
Injection: 25 mg/ml, 50 mg/ml suspension
Enema: 100 mg/60 ml
hydrocortisone acetate
Injection: 25 mg/ml, 50 mg/ml suspension
Enema: 10% aerosol foam (provides 90 mg/application)
hydrocortisone cypionate
Oral suspension: 10 mg/5 ml
hydrocortisone sodium phosphate
Injection: 50 mg/ml solution
hydrocortisone sodium succinate
Injection: 100 mg/vial, 250 mg/vial, 500 mg/vial, 1,000 mg/vial

Indications, route, and dosage
Severe inflammation, adrenal insufficiency
hydrocortisone
Adults: 5 to 30 mg P.O. b.i.d., t.i.d., or q.i.d. (as much as 80 mg P.O. q.i.d. may be given in acute situations).
Children: 2 to 8 mg/kg or 60 to 240 mg/m² P.O. daily.
hydrocortisone acetate
Adults: 10 to 75 mg into joints or soft tissue at 2- to 3-week intervals. Dose varies with size of joint. In many cases, local anesthetics are injected with dose.

hydrocortisone sodium phosphate
Adults: 15 to 240 mg S.C., I.M., or I.V. daily in divided doses q 12 hours.
hydrocortisone sodium succinate
Adults: Initially, 100 to 500 mg I.M. or I.V.; then 50 to 100 mg I.M. as indicated.
Shock (other than adrenal crisis)
hydrocortisone sodium phosphate
Children: 0.16 to 1 mg/kg I.M. daily or b.i.d.
hydrocortisone sodium succinate
Adults: 100 to 500 mg I.M. or I.V. q 2 to 6 hours.
Children: 0.16 to 1 mg/kg or 6 to 30 mg/m^2 I.M. or I.V. daily to b.i.d.
Life-threatening shock
hydrocortisone sodium succinate
Adults: 0.5 to 2 g I.V. initially, repeated at 2- to 6-hour intervals, p.r.n. High-dose therapy should be continued only until patient's condition has stabilized. Therapy shouldn't be continued beyond 48 to 72 hours.
Adjunctive treatment of ulcerative colitis and proctitis
hydrocortisone
Adults: one enema (100 mg) nightly for 21 days.
hydrocortisone acetate (rectal foam)
Adults: 90 mg (1 applicator) once or twice daily for 2 or 3 weeks; decrease frequency to every other day thereafter.

Pharmacodynamics

Adrenocorticoid replacement action: Hydrocortisone is an adrenocorticoid with both glucocorticoid and mineralocorticoid properties. It's a weak anti-inflammatory drug but a potent mineralocorticoid, having potency similar to that of cortisone and twice that of prednisone. Hydrocortisone (or cortisone) is usually drug of choice for replacement therapy in patients with adrenal insufficiency. It's usually not used for immunosuppressant activity because of the extremely large doses necessary and the unwanted mineralocorticoid effects.

Hydrocortisone and hydrocortisone cypionate may be administered orally. Hydrocortisone sodium phosphate may be administered by I.M., S.C., or I.V. injection or by I.V. infusion, usually at 12-hour intervals. Hydrocortisone sodium succinate may be administered by I.M. or I.V. injection or I.V. infusion every 2 to 10 hours, depending on the clinical situation. Hydrocortisone acetate is a suspension that may be administered by intra-articular, intrasynovial, intrabursal, intralesional, or soft tissue injection. It has a slow onset but a long duration of action. Injectable forms are usually used only when the oral forms can't be used.

Pharmacokinetics

- *Absorption:* Absorbed readily after oral administration. After oral and I.V. administration, effects peak in about 1 to 2 hours. Acetate suspension for injection has variable absorption over 24 to 48 hours, depending on whether injected into intra-articular space or muscle and blood supply to muscle.
- *Distribution:* Removed rapidly from blood and distributed to muscle, liver, skin, intestines, and kidneys. Bound extensively to plasma proteins (transcortin and albumin). Only the unbound portion is active. Adrenocorticoids are distributed into breast milk and through placenta.
- *Metabolism:* Metabolized in liver to inactive glucuronide and sulfate metabolites.
- *Excretion:* Inactive metabolites and small amounts of unmetabolized drug excreted by kidneys. Insignificant quantities of drug excreted in feces. Biological half-life is 8 to 12 hours.

Contraindications and precautions

Contraindicated in patients with hypersensitivity to drug or its components, in those with systemic fungal infections, and in premature infants (hydrocortisone sodium succinate).

Use hydrocortisone sodium phosphate or succinate cautiously in patients with a recent MI, GI ulcer, renal disease, hypertension, osteoporosis, diabetes mellitus, hypothyroidism, cirrhosis, diverticulitis, ulcerative colitis, recent intestinal anastomosis, thromboembolic disorders, seizures, myasthenia gravis, heart failure, tuberculosis, ocular herpes simplex, emotional instability, or psychotic tendencies.

Interactions

Drug-drug. *Amphotericin B, diuretics:* Hydrocortisone may enhance hypokalemia. Monitor patient and serum potassium levels closely.
Antacids, cholestyramine, colestipol: Decreased corticosteroid effect. Monitor patient closely.
Barbiturates, phenytoin, rifampin: May decrease corticosteroid effects. Increased doses may be necessary.
Cardiac glycosides: Increased risk of toxicity. Monitor patient and glycoside levels closely.
Estrogens: May reduce metabolism of corticosteroids. Monitor patient.
Isoniazid, salicylates: Increased metabolism of these drugs. Monitor patient closely.
NSAIDs: Increased risk of GI ulceration. Give together cautiously.
Oral anticoagulants: Decreased effects. Monitor PT and INR closely; alter dosage as necessary.
Skin-test antigens: Decreased response. Defer skin testing until after therapy.

Adverse reactions

Most adverse reactions to corticosteroids are dose- or duration-dependent.
CNS: *euphoria, insomnia,* psychotic behavior, pseudotumor cerebri, vertigo, headache, paresthesia, **seizures.**
CV: *heart failure,* hypertension, edema, **arrhythmias,** thrombophlebitis, **thromboembolism.**
EENT: cataracts, glaucoma.

Reactions may be *common*, uncommon, **life-threatening**, or COMMON AND LIFE-THREATENING.

GI: *peptic ulceration,* GI irritation, increased appetite, *pancreatitis,* nausea, vomiting.
GU: menstrual irregularities.
Metabolic: possible hypokalemia, hyperglycemia (requiring dosage adjustment in diabetics).
Musculoskeletal: muscle weakness, osteoporosis, growth suppression in children.
Skin: delayed wound healing, acne, various skin eruptions, easy bruising.
Other: hirsutism, susceptibility to infections, cushingoid state (moonface, buffalo hump, central obesity), carbohydrate intolerance, *acute adrenal insufficiency with increased stress (infection, surgery, trauma) or abrupt withdrawal (after long-term therapy),* suppression of the hypothalamic-pituitary-adrenal axis.

    After abrupt withdrawal: rebound inflammation, fatigue, weakness, arthralgia, fever, dizziness, lethargy, depression, fainting, orthostatic hypotension, dyspnea, anorexia, hypoglycemia. *After prolonged use, sudden withdrawal may be fatal.*

☑ Special considerations
• Recommendations for use of hydrocortisone and for care and teaching of patients during therapy are the same as those for all systemic adrenocorticoids.
• Determine if patient is sensitive to other corticosteroids.
• Give oral dose with food if possible.
• Give I.M. injection deeply into gluteal muscle. Rotate injection sites. Avoid S.C. injection.
• Hydrocortisone decreases ^{131}I uptake and protein-bound iodine levels in thyroid function tests.
• Don't confuse Solu-Cortef with Solu-Medrol.

Monitoring the patient
• Long-term use causes adverse physiologic effects, including suppression of the hypothalamic-pituitary-adrenal axis, cushingoid appearance, muscle weakness, and osteoporosis.
• Monitor patient's weight, blood pressure, and serum electrolyte levels.
• Watch for depression or signs of psychotic episodes.

Information for the patient
• Tell patient not to stop drug abruptly.
• Teach patient signs of early adrenal insufficiency.
• Advise patient to avoid exposure to people with infections.

Pediatric patients
• Long-term use in children and adolescents may delay growth and maturation.

hydrocortisone (topical)
Acticort 100, Aeroseb-HC, Ala-Cort, Ala-Scalp, Anusol-HC, Bactine, Barriere-HC*, CaldeCORT, Cetacort, Cortaid, Cortate*, Cort-Dome, Cortizone, Dermacort, DermiCort, Dermolate, Dermtex HC, Emo-Cort*, Hi-Cor, Hydro-Tex, Hytone, LactiCare-HC, Nutracort, Penecort, Rectocort*, S-T Cort, Synacort, Texacort, Unicort*

hydrocortisone acetate
Anusol-HC, CaldeCORT, Cortaid, Cort-Dome, Cortef, Corticaine, Corticreme*, Cortoderm*, Gynecort, Hyderm*, Lanacort, Novohydrocort*, Orabase-HCA, Pharma-Cort, Rhulicort

hydrocortisone buteprate
Pandel

hydrocortisone butyrate
Locoid

hydrocortisone valerate
Westcort

Pharmacologic classification: glucocorticoid
Therapeutic classification: anti-inflammatory
Pregnancy risk category C

How supplied
Available by prescription only (hydrocortisone 0.5% and 1% and hydrocortisone acetate 0.5% available without a prescription)
hydrocortisone
Cream: 0.5%, 1%, 2.5%
Ointment: 0.5%, 1%, 2.5%
Lotion: 0.25%, 0.5%, 1%, 2%, 2.5%
Gel: 0.5%, 1%
Solution: 0.5%, 1%, 2.5%
Aerosol: 0.5%, 1%
Pledgets (saturated with solution): 0.5%, 1%
hydrocortisone acetate
Cream: 0.5%, 1%
Ointment: 0.5%, 1%
Lotion: 0.5%
Suppositories: 25 mg
Rectal foam: 10%
Paste: 0.5%
Solution: 1%
hydrocortisone buteprate
Cream: 0.1%
hydrocortisone butyrate
Cream, ointment, solution: 0.1%
hydrocortisone valerate
Cream, ointment: 0.2%

Indications, route, and dosage

Inflammation of corticosteroid-responsive dermatoses, including those on face, groin, armpits, and under breasts; seborrheic dermatitis of scalp

Adults and children: Apply cream, lotion, ointment, foam, or aerosol sparingly once daily to q.i.d.

Aerosol
Shake can well. Direct spray onto affected area from a distance of 6 inches (15 cm). Apply for only 3 seconds (to avoid freezing tissues). Apply to dry scalp after shampooing; no need to massage or rub into scalp after spraying. Apply daily until acute phase is controlled; then reduce dosage to one to three times weekly, p.r.n., to maintain control.

Rectal administration
Shake can well. Apply once daily or b.i.d. for 2 to 3 weeks; then every other day, p.r.n.

Dental lesions
Adults and children: Apply paste b.i.d. or t.i.d. and h.s.

Pharmacodynamics

Anti-inflammatory action: Stimulates synthesis of enzymes needed to decrease the inflammatory response. Hydrocortisone, a corticosteroid secreted by the adrenal cortex, is about 1.25 times more potent an anti-inflammatory drug than equivalent doses of cortisone, but both have twice the mineralocorticoid activity of the other glucocorticoids.

Hydrocortisone 0.5%, 1%, and hydrocortisone acetate 0.5% are available without a prescription for the temporary relief of minor skin irritation, itching, and rashes caused by eczema, insect bites, soaps, and detergents.

Hydrocortisone is also administered rectally as a retention enema for the temporary treatment of acute ulcerative colitis. Hydrocortisone acetate suspension is also available as a rectal suppository or aerosol foam suspension for the temporary treatment of such inflammatory conditions of the rectum as hemorrhoids, cryptitis, proctitis, and pruritus ani.

Pharmacokinetics

• *Absorption:* Absorption depends on potency of preparation, amount applied, and nature and condition of skin at application site. Ranges from about 1% in areas with thick stratum corneum (such as palms, soles, elbows, and knees) to as high as 36% in areas where the stratum corneum is thinnest (face, eyelids, and genitals). Absorption increases in areas of skin damage, inflammation, or occlusion. Some systemic absorption occurs, especially through oral mucosa.
• *Distribution:* After topical application, is distributed throughout local skin layers. Any drug absorbed into circulation is removed rapidly from blood and distributed into muscle, liver, skin, intestines, and kidneys.
• *Metabolism:* After topical administration, is metabolized primarily in skin. Small amount absorbed into systemic circulation is metabolized primarily in liver to inactive compounds.
• *Excretion:* Inactive metabolites excreted by kidneys, primarily as glucuronides and sulfates, but also as unconjugated products. Small amounts of metabolites also excreted in feces.

Contraindications and precautions

Contraindicated in patients with hypersensitivity to drug.

Interactions

None reported.

Adverse reactions

CNS: *seizures, increased intracranial pressure.*
GU: glucosuria.
Metabolic: hyperglycemia.
Skin: burning, pruritus, irritation, dryness, erythema, folliculitis, hypertrichosis, hypopigmentation, acneiform eruptions, allergic contact dermatitis; *maceration, secondary infection, atrophy, striae, miliaria* (with occlusive dressings).
Other: *hypothalamic-pituitary-adrenal axis suppression,* Cushing's syndrome.

☑ Special considerations

• Recommendations for use of hydrocortisone, for care and teaching of patients during therapy, and for use in elderly patients, children, and breast-feeding women are the same as those for all topical adrenocorticoids.
• When using aerosol, cover patient's face and warn him not to inhale spray.

Monitoring the patient
• Check for skin infection, striae, and atrophy.
• Monitor patient for systemic effects.

Information for the patient
• Instruct patient to gently wash skin before applying. To prevent skin damage, rub drug in gently, leaving a thin coat. When treating hairy sites, part hair and apply directly to lesions.
• Tell patient to stop drug and report signs of systemic absorption, skin irritation or ulceration, hypersensitivity, infection, or no improvement.

Pediatric patients
• Avoid using plastic pants or tight fitting diapers on treated areas in young children. Children may absorb larger amounts of drug and be more prone to systemic toxicity.

Reactions may be *common*, uncommon, *life-threatening*, or **COMMON AND LIFE-THREATENING**.

hydromorphone hydrochloride
Dilaudid, Dilaudid-HP, Hydrostat IR

Pharmacologic classification: opioid
Therapeutic classification: analgesic, antitussive
Controlled substance schedule II
Pregnancy risk category C

How supplied
Available by prescription only
Tablets: 1 mg, 2 mg, 3 mg, 4 mg, 8 mg
Oral liquid: 5 mg/5 ml
Injection: 1 mg/ml, 2 mg/ml, 3 mg/ml, 4 mg/ml, 10 mg/ml
Suppository: 3 mg

Indications, route, and dosage
Moderate to severe pain
Adults: 2 to 10 mg P.O. q 3 to 6 hours, p.r.n., or around the clock; or 2 to 4 mg I.M., S.C., or I.V. q 4 to 6 hours, p.r.n., or around the clock (I.V. dose should be given over 3 to 5 minutes); or 3 mg rectal suppository q 6 to 8 hours, p.r.n., or around the clock. (Give 1 to 14 mg Dilaudid-HP S.C. or I.M. q 4 to 6 hours.)
Note: Drug should be given in the smallest effective dose to minimize development of tolerance and physical dependence. Dose must be individually adjusted based on patient's severity of pain, age, and size.
Cough
Adults: 1 mg P.O. q 3 to 4 hours, p.r.n.
Children ages 6 to 12: 0.5 mg P.O. q 3 to 4 hours, p.r.n.

Pharmacodynamics
Antitussive action: Acts directly on the cough center in the medulla, producing an antitussive effect.
Analgesic action: Has analgesic properties related to opiate receptor affinity, and is recommended for moderate-to-severe pain. No intrinsic limit to the analgesic effect of hydromorphone, unlike the other opioids.

Pharmacokinetics
• *Absorption:* Well absorbed after oral, rectal, or parenteral administration. Onset of action occurs in 15 to 30 minutes, with peak effect at ½ to 1 hour after dosing.
• *Distribution:* No information available.
• *Metabolism:* Metabolized primarily in liver, where it undergoes conjugation with glucuronic acid.
• *Excretion:* Excreted primarily in urine as glucuronide conjugate. Duration of action is 4 to 5 hours.

Contraindications and precautions
Contraindicated in patients with hypersensitivity to drug, in those with intracranial lesions associated with increased intracranial pressure, and whenever ventilator function is depressed, such as in status asthmaticus, COPD, cor pulmonale, emphysema, and kyphoscoliosis.
Use cautiously in elderly or debilitated patients and in those with hepatic or renal disease, Addison's disease, hypothyroidism, prostatic hyperplasia, or urethral strictures.

Interactions
Drug-drug. *Anticholinergics:* May cause paralytic ileus. Monitor patient.
Cimetidine, CNS depressants (antihistamines, barbiturates, benzodiazepines, general anesthetics, muscle relaxants, narcotic analgesics, phenothiazines, sedative-hypnotics, tricyclic antidepressants): Potentiated respiratory and CNS depression, sedation, and hypotensive effects of drug. Use together with extreme caution. Reduce hydromorphone dose and monitor patient's response.
Digitoxin, phenytoin, rifampin: Possible drug accumulation and enhanced effects. Monitor patient and drug levels.
Drug-lifestyle. *Alcohol:* May potentiate drug's CNS effects. Discourage concomitant use.

Adverse reactions
CNS: sedation, somnolence, clouded sensorium, dizziness, euphoria.
CV: *hypotension,* **bradycardia.**
EENT: blurred vision, diplopia, nystagmus.
GI: *nausea, vomiting, constipation,* ileus.
GU: *urine retention.*
Respiratory: **respiratory depression, bronchospasm.**
Other: induration (with repeated S.C. injections), physical dependence.

☑ Special considerations
Besides the recommendations relevant to all opioids, consider the following.
• Before administration, visually inspect all parenteral products for particulate matter and extreme yellow discoloration.
• Oral form is particularly convenient for patients with chronic pain because tablets are available in several strengths, enabling patient to adjust own dosage precisely.
• Dilaudid-HP, a highly concentrated form (10 mg/ml), may be administered in smaller volumes, preventing discomfort associated with large-volume injections.
• Common signs and symptoms of overdose are CNS depression, respiratory depression, and miosis (pinpoint pupils). Treatment is symptomatic and includes appropriate supportive measures. Manage airway and, when indicated, give a narcotic antagonist such as naloxone.

Monitoring the patient
• Monitor vital signs closely.

• With frequent use, observe patient carefully for signs of dependence.

Information for the patient
• Instruct patient to take or ask for drug before pain becomes intense.
• Tell patient to store suppositories in refrigerator.
• Encourage coughing or deep breathing to avoid atelectasis (postoperatively).
• Instruct patient to avoid hazardous activities that require mental alertness.
• Advise patient to avoid alcohol.

Geriatric patients
• Lower doses are usually indicated for elderly patients because they may be more sensitive to the therapeutic and adverse effects of drug.

Breast-feeding patients
• It's unknown if drug appears in breast milk; use with caution in breast-feeding women.

hydroxychloroquine sulfate
Plaquenil Sulfate

Pharmacologic classification: 4-aminoquinoline
Therapeutic classification: antimalarial, anti-inflammatory
Pregnancy risk category C

How supplied
Available by prescription only
Tablets: 200 mg (155 mg base)

Indications, route, and dosage
Suppressive prophylaxis of malarial attacks
Adults: 400 mg sulfate (310 mg base) P.O. weekly on exactly the same day each week. (Begin 2 weeks before entering and continue for 8 weeks after leaving the endemic area.)
Infants and children: 5 mg P.O., calculated as base per kg of body weight (shouldn't exceed the adult dose regardless of weight) on exactly the same day each week. Start 2 weeks before exposure. If unable, give 10-mg base/kg in two divided doses 6 hours apart.
Treatment of acute malaria attack
Adults: 800 mg (620 mg base) P.O.; then 400 mg (310 mg base) in 6 to 8 hours and 400 mg (310 mg base) on each of two consecutive days.
Infants and children: Initial dose, 10 mg base/kg (but not exceeding a single dose of 620 mg base) P.O. Second dose, 5 mg base/kg (but not exceeding a single dose of 310 mg base) 6 hours after first dose. Third dose, 5 mg base/kg 18 hours after second dose. Fourth dose, 5 mg base/kg 24 hours after third dose.

Lupus erythematosus (chronic discoid and systemic)
Adults: 400 mg P.O. daily or b.i.d., continued for several weeks or months, based on response. Prolonged maintenance dose is 200 to 400 mg P.O. daily.
◇ *Rheumatoid arthritis*
Adults: Initially, 400 to 600 mg P.O. daily. When good response occurs (usually in 4 to 12 weeks), reduce dose by half.

Pharmacodynamics
Antimalarial action: Binds to DNA, interfering with protein synthesis. Also inhibits DNA and RNA polymerases. Active against asexual erythrocytic forms of *Plasmodium malariae, P. ovale, P. vivax,* and many strains of *P. falciparum.*
Amebicidal action: Mechanism unknown.
Anti-inflammatory action: Mechanism unknown. May antagonize histamine and serotonin and inhibit prostaglandin effects by inhibiting conversion of arachidonic acid to prostaglandin F_2; may also inhibit chemotaxis of polymorphonuclear leukocytes, macrophages, and eosinophils.

Pharmacokinetics
• *Absorption:* Absorbed readily and almost completely, with plasma levels peaking at 1 to 2 hours.
• *Distribution:* Bound to plasma proteins. Concentrated in liver, spleen, kidneys, heart, and brain and is strongly bound in melanin-containing cells.
• *Metabolism:* Metabolized by liver to desethylchloroquine and desethylhydroxychloroquine.
• *Excretion:* Most of dose excreted unchanged in urine. Drug and its metabolites excreted slowly in urine; unabsorbed drug excreted in feces. Small amounts of drug may be present in urine for months after therapy ends. Drug appears in breast milk.

Contraindications and precautions
Contraindicated in patients with hypersensitivity to drug, in long-term therapy for children, and in patients with retinal or visual field changes or porphyria. Use cautiously in patients with severe GI, neurologic, or blood disorders.

Interactions
Drug-drug. *Cimetidine:* Decreased hepatic metabolism of hydroxychloroquine. Monitor patient for toxicity.
Digoxin: Increased serum digoxin levels. Monitor patient and digoxin levels closely.
Kaolin, magnesium trisilicate: Possible decreased absorption of hydroxychloroquine. Separate administration times.
Drug-lifestyle. *Sun exposure:* May cause drug-induced dermatoses. Tell patient to take precautions.

Reactions may be *common,* uncommon, **life-threatening,** or COMMON AND LIFE-THREATENING.

Adverse reactions
CNS: irritability, nightmares, ataxia, *seizures,* psychosis, vertigo, nystagmus, dizziness, hypoactive deep tendon reflexes, ataxia, lassitude, headache.
CV: inversion or depression of the T wave or widening of the QRS complex on ECG.
EENT: visual disturbances (blurred vision; difficulty in focusing; reversible corneal changes; typically irreversible, sometimes progressive or delayed retinal changes, such as narrowing of arterioles; macular lesions; pallor of optic disk; optic atrophy; visual field defects; patchy retinal pigmentation, commonly leading to blindness), ototoxicity (irreversible nerve deafness, tinnitus, labyrinthitis).
GI: anorexia, abdominal cramps, diarrhea, nausea, vomiting.
Hematologic: *agranulocytosis, leukopenia, thrombocytopenia, hemolysis (in patients with G6PD deficiency), aplastic anemia.*
Metabolic: weight loss.
Musculoskeletal: skeletal muscle weakness.
Skin: alopecia, bleaching of hair, pruritus, lichen planus eruptions, skin and mucosal pigmentary changes, pleomorphic skin eruptions.

☑ Special considerations
• Baseline and periodic ophthalmologic examinations are necessary in prolonged or high-dosage therapy.
• Give drug immediately before or after meals on same day each week to minimize gastric distress.
• Drug isn't effective for chloroquine-resistant strains of *P. falciparum.*
• Signs and symptoms of overdose (headache, drowsiness, visual changes, CV collapse, and seizures followed by respiratory and cardiac arrest) may appear within 30 minutes after ingestion. Treatment is symptomatic.

Monitoring the patient
• Monitor for blurred vision, increased sensitivity to light, hearing loss, pronounced GI disturbances, and muscle weakness.
• Monitor CBC and ECG.

Information for the patient
• To prevent drug-induced dermatoses, warn patient to avoid excessive sun exposure.

Pediatric patients
• Children are extremely susceptible to toxicity; monitor closely for adverse effects. Don't use drug for long-term therapy in children and don't exceed recommended dosage.

Breast-feeding patients
• Drug appears in breast milk. Safety hasn't been established. Use with caution in breast-feeding women.

hydroxyprogesterone caproate
Hy/Gestrone, Hylutin, Hyprogest, Prodrox

Pharmacologic classification: progestin
Therapeutic classification: progestin, antineoplastic
Pregnancy risk category X

How supplied
Available by prescription only
Injection: 125 mg/ml, 250 mg/ml

Indications, route, and dosage
Amenorrhea, uterine bleeding
Adults: 375 mg I.M. May be repeated at 4-week intervals, if needed. After 4 days of desquamation or if there is no bleeding within 21 days after administration, begin cyclic therapy with an estrogen.
Endometrial cancer
Adults: 1 g I.M. up to seven times weekly for 12 weeks or as indicated. Stop therapy if relapse occurs or if no objective response is seen after 12 weeks of therapy.

Pharmacodynamics
Progestational action: Suppresses ovulation, causes thickening of cervical mucous, and induces sloughing of the endometrium. Inhibits growth progression of progestin-sensitive uterine cancer tissue by an unknown mechanism.

Pharmacokinetics
• *Absorption:* Absorbed slowly after I.M. injection.
• *Distribution:* No information available.
• *Metabolism:* Primarily hepatic; not well characterized.
• *Excretion:* Primarily renal; not well characterized. Has a duration of action of 7 to 14 days when used as directed.

Contraindications and precautions
Contraindicated in patients with hypersensitivity to drug and in those with thromboembolic disorders, cerebral apoplexy, breast or genital organ cancer, undiagnosed abnormal vaginal bleeding, severe hepatic disease, or missed abortion. Also contraindicated during pregnancy.
    Use cautiously in patients with diabetes mellitus, seizures, migraine, cardiac or renal disease, asthma, mental depression, or impaired liver function.

Interactions
Drug-drug. *Bromocriptine:* May cause amenorrhea or galactorrhea, interfering with bromocriptine's action. Don't use concomitantly.

Adverse reactions
CNS: depression.
CV: thrombophlebitis, ***thromboembolism, CVA, pulmonary embolism,*** edema.
EENT: exophthalmos, diplopia.
GU: breakthrough bleeding, dysmenorrhea, amenorrhea, cervical erosion, abnormal secretions.
Hepatic: cholestatic jaundice.
Metabolic: changes in weight.
Skin: rash, acne, pruritus, melasma, irritation or pain at injection site.
Other: breast tenderness, enlargement, or secretion.

☑ Special considerations
Besides the recommendations relevant to all progestins, consider the following.
• Hydroxyprogesterone caproate is for I.M. administration only. Inject deep into large muscle mass, preferably gluteal muscle.
• Provide manufacturer's package insert to women receiving drug.

Monitoring the patient
• Monitor diabetic patients during therapy for signs of decreased glucose tolerance.
• Patients receiving drug should have a full physical examination, including a gynecologic examination and a Papanicolaou test, every 6 to 12 months.

Information for the patient
• Warn patient that edema and weight gain are likely.
• Remind patient that normal menstrual cycles may not resume for 2 to 3 months after therapy ends.
• Advise patient of potential risks to fetus if she becomes pregnant during therapy or is inadvertently exposed to drug during the first 4 months of pregnancy.

Breast-feeding patients
• Drug appears in breast milk; its use is contraindicated in breast-feeding women.

---

hydroxyurea
Hydrea, Droxia

Pharmacologic classification:
antimetabolite (cell cycle–phase specific, S phase)
Therapeutic classification: antineoplastic
Pregnancy risk category NR

How supplied
Available by prescription only
Capsules: 500 mg

Indications, route, and dosage
Dosage and indications may vary. Check current literature for recommended protocol.
Solid tumors
Adults: 80 mg/kg P.O. as a single dose q 3 days; or 20 to 30 mg/kg P.O. as a single daily dose.
Head and neck cancer
Adults: 80 mg/kg P.O. as a single dose q 3 days.
Resistant chronic myelocytic leukemia
Adults: 20 to 30 mg/kg P.O. as a single daily dose.
Sickle cell anemia
Adults: 15 mg/kg daily, administered as a single dose. Dose may be adjusted thereafter according to patient's blood cell counts.

Pharmacodynamics
Antineoplastic action: Exact mechanism unknown. Inhibits DNA synthesis without interfering with RNA or protein synthesis. May act as an antimetabolite, inhibiting the incorporation of thymidine into DNA, and may also damage DNA directly.

Pharmacokinetics
• *Absorption:* Well absorbed after oral administration, with serum levels peaking 2 hours after a dose. Higher serum levels achieved if drug is given as large, single dose rather than in divided doses.
• *Distribution:* Drug crosses blood-brain barrier.
• *Metabolism:* About 50% of oral dose degraded in liver.
• *Excretion:* Remaining 50% excreted in urine as unchanged drug. Metabolites excreted through lungs as carbon dioxide and in urine as urea.

Contraindications and precautions
Contraindicated in patients with hypersensitivity to drug and with marked bone marrow depression (leukopenia [less than 2,500 WBCs/mm^3], thrombocytopenia [less than 100,000 platelets/mm^3], or severe anemia).
  Use cautiously in patients with impaired renal function. Don't administer to pregnant women or women of childbearing age who may become pregnant unless potential benefit to patient outweighs possible risk to fetus.

Interactions
Drug-drug. *Fluorouracil:* May decrease activity of fluorouracil. Neurotoxicity may occur when these two drugs are administered together. Use together cautiously.

Adverse reactions
CNS: hallucinations, headache, dizziness, disorientation, ***seizures,*** malaise.
GI: *anorexia, nausea, vomiting, diarrhea,* stomatitis, constipation.
GU: increased BUN and serum creatinine levels.
Hematologic: *leukopenia, thrombocytopenia,* anemia, *megaloblastosis,* **bone marrow sup-**

---

pression, with rapid recovery (dose-limiting and dose-related).
Skin: rash, alopecia, erythema.
Other: fever, chills.

☑ Special considerations
● Dose modification may be needed following other chemotherapy or radiation therapy.
● Drug may exacerbate postirradiation erythema.
● Auditory and visual hallucinations and blood toxicity increase when renal function is decreased.
● Avoid all I.M. injections when platelet counts are below 100,000/mm³.
● Patient may need blood transfusions.
● Store capsules in tight container at room temperature. Avoid exposure to excessive heat.
● Signs and symptoms of overdose include ulceration of buccal and GI mucosa, facial erythema, maculopapular rash, disorientation, and hallucinations.

Monitoring the patient
● Monitor intake and output levels; keep patient hydrated.
● Obtain BUN, uric acid, and serum creatinine levels routinely.

Information for the patient
● Instruct patient to empty contents of capsule in water and drink immediately if capsule can't be swallowed.
● Emphasize importance of continuing therapy despite nausea and vomiting.
● Tell patient to call immediately if vomiting occurs shortly after taking a dose.
● Encourage daily intake of at least 2 L of fluid to increase urine output and facilitate excretion of uric acid.
● Tell patient to report unusual bruising or bleeding.
● Advise patient to avoid exposure to people with infections and to report signs and symptoms of infection immediately.

Geriatric patients
● Elderly patients may be more sensitive to drug's effects, requiring a lower dosage.

Pediatric patients
● Children may need a lower dosage.

Breast-feeding patients
● It's unknown if drug appears in breast milk. However, because of risk of serious adverse reactions, mutagenicity, and carcinogenicity in infant, breast-feeding isn't recommended.

hydroxyzine hydrochloride
Apo-Hydroxyzine*, Atarax, Hyzine-50, Multipax*, Novo-Hydroxyzin*, Vistazine-50

hydroxyzine pamoate
Vistaril

Pharmacologic classification: antihistamine (piperazine derivative)
Therapeutic classification: anxiolytic, sedative, antipruritic, antiemetic, antispasmodic
Pregnancy risk category C

How supplied
Available by prescription only
hydroxyzine hydrochloride
Capsules: 10 mg, 25 mg, 50 mg
Tablets: 10 mg, 25 mg, 50 mg, 100 mg
Syrup: 10 mg/5 ml
Injection: 25 mg/ml, 50 mg/ml
hydroxyzine pamoate
Capsules: 25 mg, 50 mg, 100 mg
Oral suspension: 25 mg/5 ml

Indications, route, and dosage
Anxiety, tension, hyperkinesia
Adults: 50 to 100 mg P.O. q.i.d.
Children over age 6: 50 to 100 mg P.O. daily in divided doses.
Children under age 6: 50 mg P.O. daily in divided doses.
Preoperative and postoperative adjunctive sedation; to control emesis; adjunct to asthma treatment
Adults: 25 to 100 mg I.M. q 4 to 6 hours.
Children: 1.1 mg/kg I.M. q 4 to 6 hours.

Pharmacodynamics
Anxiolytic and sedative actions: Produces sedative and antianxiety effects through suppression of activity at subcortical levels; analgesia occurs at high doses.
Antipruritic action: A direct competitor of histamine for binding at cellular receptor sites.
Other actions: Used as a preoperative and postoperative adjunct for its sedative, antihistaminic, and anticholinergic activity.

Pharmacokinetics
● *Absorption:* Absorbed rapidly and completely after oral administration. Serum levels peak within 2 to 4 hours. Sedation and other clinical effects usually noticed in 15 to 30 minutes.
● *Distribution:* Not well understood.
● *Metabolism:* Metabolized almost completely in liver.
● *Excretion:* Metabolites excreted primarily in urine; small amounts of drug and metabolites found in feces. Half-life of drug is 3 hours. Seda-

tive effects can last for 4 to 6 hours, antihistaminic effects for up to 4 days.

Contraindications and precautions
Contraindicated in patients with hypersensitivity to drug and during early pregnancy. Use cautiously with adjustments in dosage in elderly or debilitated patients.

Interactions
Drug-drug. *Anticholinergics:* Additive anticholinergic effects. Avoid concomitant use.
Barbiturates, opioids, tranquilizers, other CNS depressants: May add to or potentiate effects of these drugs. Reduce dosage of these drugs by 50%.
Epinephrine: May block epinephrine's vasopressor action. If a vasoconstrictor is needed, use norepinephrine or phenylephrine.
Drug-lifestyle. *Alcohol:* Increased effect of alcohol. Discourage concomitant use.

Adverse reactions
CNS: *drowsiness,* involuntary motor activity.
GI: *dry mouth.*
Other: marked discomfort at I.M. injection site, **hypersensitivity reactions** (wheezing, dyspnea, chest tightness).

☑ Special considerations
• Inject deep I.M. only; not for I.V., intra-arterial, or S.C. use. Aspirate injection carefully to prevent inadvertent intravascular administration.
• Drug causes falsely elevated urinary 17-hydroxycorticosteroid levels. May cause false-negative skin allergen tests by attenuating or inhibiting cutaneous response to histamine.
• Observe patients for excessive sedation, which could indicate overdose. Treatment is supportive.

Monitoring the patient
• Monitor vital signs closely.
• Monitor patient for CNS effects.

Information for the patient
• Tell patient to avoid tasks that require mental alertness or physical coordination until CNS effects of drug are known; advise against use of other CNS depressants with hydroxyzine unless prescribed. Patient should avoid alcohol ingestion.
• Instruct patient to seek medical approval before taking OTC cold or allergy preparations that contain antihistamine, which may potentiate effects of hydroxyzine.
• Advise patient to use sugarless gum or candy to help relieve dry mouth and to drink plenty of water to help with dry mouth or constipation.

Geriatric patients
• Elderly patients may experience greater CNS depression and anticholinergic effects. Lower doses are indicated.

Breast-feeding patients
• It's unknown if drug appears in breast milk. Safe use hasn't been established in breast-feeding women.

hyoscyamine
Cystospaz

hyoscyamine sulfate
Anaspaz, Cystospaz-M, Levsin, Levsin Drops, Levsinex Timecaps, Neoquess

Pharmacologic classification:
belladonna alkaloid
Therapeutic classification: anticholinergic
Pregnancy risk category C

How supplied
Available by prescription only
hyoscyamine
Tablets: 0.15 mg
hyoscyamine sulfate
Tablets: 0.125 mg
Capsules (extended-release): 0.375 mg
Oral solution: 0.125 mg/ml
Elixir: 0.125 mg/5 ml
Injection: 0.5 mg/ml

Indications, route, and dosage
GI tract disorders caused by spasm; adjunctive therapy for peptic ulcers
Adults: 0.125 to 0.25 mg P.O. or S.L. q.i.d. before meals and h.s.; 0.375 to 0.75 mg P.O. (extended-release form) q 12 hours; or 0.25 to 0.5 mg I.M., I.V., or S.C. q 4 hours b.i.d. to q.i.d. (Substitute oral medication when symptoms are controlled.)
Children ages 2 to 12: 0.033 mg at about 10 kg (22 lb); at about 20 kg (44 lb), 0.0625 mg; at about 40 kg (88 lb), 0.0938 mg; at about 50 kg (110 lb), 0.125 mg.
Children under age 2: 0.0125 mg at about 2.3 kg (5 lb); at about 3.4 kg (7.5 lb), 0.0167 mg; at about 5 kg (11 lb), 0.02 mg; at about 6.8 kg (15 lb), 0.025 mg; at about 10 kg (22 lb), 0.033 mg; at about 15 kg (33 lb), 0.05 mg.

Pharmacodynamics
Antispasmodic and antiulcer action: Competitively blocks acetylcholine at cholinergic neuroeffector sites, decreasing GI motility and inhibiting gastric acid secretion.

Pharmacokinetics
• *Absorption:* Well absorbed when taken orally. Onset of action usually occurs in 20 to 30 minutes with tablets, 5 to 20 minutes with elixir, 2 to 3 minutes with parenteral administration.
• *Distribution:* Well distributed throughout body; crosses blood-brain barrier. About 50% binds to plasma proteins.

Reactions may be *common,* uncommon, **life-threatening,** or COMMON AND LIFE-THREATENING.

- *Metabolism:* Metabolized in liver. Effect lasts up to 4 hours with standard oral and parenteral administration; up to 12 hours for extended-release preparation.
- *Excretion:* Drug and metabolites excreted in urine.

Contraindications and precautions
Contraindicated in patients with hypersensitivity to anticholinergics and in those with glaucoma, obstructive uropathy, obstructive disease of the GI tract, severe ulcerative colitis, myasthenia gravis, paralytic ileus, intestinal atony, unstable CV status in acute hemorrhage, or toxic mega-colon.

Use cautiously in patients with autonomic neuropathy, hyperthyroidism, coronary artery disease, arrhythmias, heart failure, hypertension, hiatal hernia with reflux esophagitis, hepatic or renal disease, or ulcerative colitis. Also use cautiously in hot or humid environments where drug-induced heat stroke can occur.

Interactions
Drug-drug. *Amantadine, phenothiazines:* May increase adverse anticholinergic effects such as confusion and hallucinations. Avoid concomitant use.
Antacids, antidiarrheals: May decrease hyoscyamine's absorption. Administer hyoscyamine 1 hour before these drugs.
Haloperidol, phenothiazines: May reduce antipsychotic effectiveness of these drugs. Monitor patient closely.
Drug-herb. *Jimsonweed:* May adversely effect CV function. Avoid concomitant use.

Adverse reactions
CNS: headache, insomnia, drowsiness, dizziness, nervousness, weakness; *confusion, excitement* (in elderly patients).
CV: *palpitations,* tachycardia.
EENT: *blurred vision,* mydriasis, increased intraocular pressure, cycloplegia, photophobia.
GI: *dry mouth,* dysphagia, *constipation,* heartburn, loss of taste, nausea, vomiting, *paralytic ileus.*
GU: *urinary hesitancy, urine retention,* impotence.
Skin: urticaria, decreased sweating or possible anhidrosis, other dermal manifestations.
Other: fever, allergic reactions.

☑ Special considerations
Besides the recommendations relevant to all anticholinergics, consider the following.
- Drug is usually administered P.O. but may be given I.V., I.M., S.C., or S.L. when therapeutic effect is needed or if oral administration isn't possible.
- Adjust dosage based on patient's response and tolerance.

- Signs and symptoms of overdose include curare-like symptoms, psychotic symptoms, and peripheral effects. Treatment is symptomatic and supportive.

Monitoring the patient
- Monitor patient for signs of overdose.
- Monitor elderly patients for CNS effects.

Information for the patient
- Advise patient to avoid driving or performing other hazardous activities if drowsiness, dizziness, or blurred vision occurs.
- Advise patient to avoid use of jimsonweed with hyoscyamine.
- Tell patient to drink fluids to avoid constipation.
- Instruct patient to report rash or other skin eruptions.

Geriatric patients
- Use drug cautiously in elderly patients; lower doses are indicated.

Breast-feeding patients
- Drug may appear in breast milk, possibly resulting in infant toxicity, and may decrease milk production. Avoid use in breast-feeding patients.

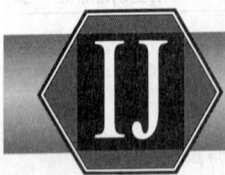

ibuprofen
Advil, Children's Advil, Medipren, Motrin, Motrin IB, Nuprin, PediaProfen, Rufen

Pharmacologic classification: NSAID
Therapeutic classification: nonnarcotic analgesic, antipyretic, anti-inflammatory
Pregnancy risk category B (D in third trimester)

How supplied
Available by prescription only
Tablets: 100 mg, 300 mg, 400 mg, 600 mg, 800 mg
Oral suspension: 100 mg/5 ml
Oral drops: 40 mg/ml
Available without a prescription
Tablets: 200 mg
Tablets (chewable): 50 mg, 100 mg
Oral suspension: 100 mg/5 ml
Liquid-filled capsules: 200 mg

Indications, route, and dosage
Arthritis, gout, and postextraction dental pain
Adults: 300 to 800 mg P.O. t.i.d. or q.i.d. Don't exceed 3,200 mg as total daily dose.
Primary dysmenorrhea
Adults: 400 mg P.O. q 4 to 6 hours.
Mild to moderate pain
Adults: 400 mg P.O. q 4 to 6 hours.
Children: 10 mg/kg P.O. q 6 to 8 hours; maximum dose, 40 mg/kg.
Juvenile arthritis
Children: 20 to 40 mg/kg/day P.O., divided into three or four doses. For mild disease, 20 mg/kg/day in divided doses.
Fever reduction
Adults: 200 to 400 mg P.O. q 4 to 6 hours, p.r.n. Don't exceed 1,200 mg/day or take for more than 3 days.
Children ages 6 months to 12 years: 5 mg/kg P.O. q 6 to 8 hours, p.r.n., if baseline temperature is 102.5° F (39.2° C) or below; 10 mg/kg P.O. q 6 to 8 hours, p.r.n., if baseline temperature is over 102.5° F. Recommended daily maximum dose, 40 mg/kg.

Pharmacodynamics
Analgesic, antipyretic, and anti-inflammatory actions: Mechanisms of action are unknown; ibuprofen is thought to inhibit prostaglandin synthesis.

Pharmacokinetics
● *Absorption:* 80% of oral dose absorbed from GI tract.
● *Distribution:* Highly protein-bound.
● *Metabolism:* Biotransformation in liver.
● *Excretion:* Excreted mainly in urine, with some biliary excretion. Plasma half-life ranges from 2 to 4 hours.

Contraindications and precautions
Contraindicated in patients with hypersensitivity to drug and in those who have syndrome of nasal polyps, angioedema, and bronchospastic reaction to aspirin or other NSAIDs.

Use cautiously in patients with impaired renal or hepatic function, GI disorders, peptic ulcer disease, cardiac decompensation, hypertension, or known coagulation defects. Because chewable tablets contain aspartame, use cautiously in patients with phenylketonuria.

Interactions
Drug-drug. *ACE inhibitors:* Ibuprofen may reduce blood pressure response to these drugs. Monitor blood pressure.
Acetaminophen, gold compounds, other anti-inflammatories: Possible increased nephrotoxicity. Avoid concomitant use.
Antacids: May decrease absorption of ibuprofen. Avoid concomitant use.
Anticoagulants, thrombolytics (coumarin derivatives, heparin, streptokinase, urokinase): May potentiate anticoagulant effects. Monitor PT and INR closely.
Antihypertensives, diuretics: May decrease effectiveness of these drugs. Monitor patient closely.
Anti-inflammatories, corticotropin, salicylates, corticosteroids: Increased GI adverse effects. Avoid concomitant use.
Aspirin: May decrease bioavailability of ibuprofen. Avoid concomitant use.
Aspirin, carbenicillin, cefamandole, cefoperazone, dextran, dipyridamole, mezlocillin, piperacillin, plicamycin, salicylates, sulfinpyrazone, ticarcillin, valproic acid, other anti-inflammatories: Possible bleeding problems if used with ibuprofen. Monitor patient closely.
Coumarin derivatives, nifedipine, phenytoin, verapamil: Increased toxicity risk. Monitor patient closely.
Insulin, oral antidiabetics: May potentiate hypoglycemic effects. Monitor serum glucose levels closely.

Reactions may be *common*, uncommon, ***life-threatening***, or COMMON AND LIFE-THREATENING.

Lithium, methotrexate: May decrease renal clearance of these drugs. Use together cautiously.
Drug-lifestyle. *Alcohol:* Increased risk of GI bleeding. Discourage use.
Sun exposure: May cause photosensitivity reactions. Tell patient to take precautions.

Adverse reactions
CNS: *headache, dizziness,* nervousness, aseptic meningitis.
CV: *peripheral edema,* fluid retention, edema.
EENT: *tinnitus.*
GI: *epigastric distress, nausea, occult blood loss, peptic ulceration,* diarrhea, constipation, dyspepsia, flatulence, heartburn, decreased appetite.
GU: *acute renal failure,* azotemia, cystitis, hematuria.
Hematologic: prolonged bleeding time, anemia, **neutropenia, pancytopenia, thrombocytopenia, aplastic anemia, leukopenia, agranulocytosis.**
Hepatic: elevated enzymes.
Respiratory: *bronchospasm.*
Skin: *rash,* urticaria, **Stevens-Johnson syndrome,** pruritus.

☑ Special considerations
Besides the recommendations relevant to all NSAIDs, consider the following.
• Maximum results in arthritis may require 1 to 2 weeks of continuous therapy with ibuprofen. Improvement may be seen, however, within 7 days.
• Administer drug on empty stomach, 1 hour before or 2 hours after meals for maximum absorption. However, it may be administered with meals to lessen GI upset.
• Establish safety measures, including raised side rails and supervised walking, to prevent possible injury from CNS effects.
• Signs and symptoms of overdose are dizziness, drowsiness, paresthesia, vomiting, nausea, abdominal pain, headache, sweating, nystagmus, apnea, and cyanosis. Empty stomach immediately by inducing emesis with ipecac syrup or by gastric lavage. Administer activated charcoal via nasogastric tube.

Monitoring the patient
• Monitor cardiopulmonary status closely; monitor vital signs, especially heart rate and blood pressure. Observe for possible fluid retention.
• Monitor auditory and ophthalmic functions periodically during therapy.

Information for the patient
• Instruct patient to seek medical approval before taking OTC products.
• Advise patient not to take ibuprofen for longer than 10 days for analgesic use and not to exceed maximum dose of six tablets (1.2 g) daily. Caution patient not to take drug if fever lasts longer than 3 days, unless prescribed.

• Tell patient to report adverse reactions; they are usually dose-related.
• Instruct patient in safety measures to prevent injury. Caution him to avoid hazardous activities that require mental alertness until CNS effects are known.
• Encourage patient to adhere to prescribed drug regimen and stress importance of medical follow-up.

Geriatric patients
• Patients over age 60 may be more susceptible to toxic effects of ibuprofen, especially adverse GI reactions. Use lowest possible effective dose.
• Effect of drug on renal prostaglandins may cause fluid retention and edema, a significant drawback for elderly patients, especially those with heart failure.

Pediatric patients
• Safety and efficacy in children under age 6 months haven't been established.

Breast-feeding patients
• Drug doesn't appear in breast milk in significant quantities. However, manufacturer recommends alternatives to breast-feeding during therapy.

ibutilide fumarate
Corvert

Pharmacologic classification: ibutilide derivative
Therapeutic classification: supraventricular antiarrhythmic
Pregnancy risk category C

How supplied
Available by prescription only
Injection: 0.1 mg/ml

Indications, route, and dosage
Rapid conversion of atrial fibrillation or atrial flutter of recent onset to sinus rhythm
Adults weighing 60 kg (132 lb) or more: 1 mg I.V. over 10 minutes.
Adults weighing below 60 kg: 0.01 mg/kg I.V. over 10 minutes.
  Note: Stop infusion if presenting arrhythmia is terminated or if sustained or nonsustained ventricular tachycardia or marked prolongation of QT or QTc interval occurs. If arrhythmia doesn't terminate within 10 minutes after infusion ends, a second 10-minute infusion of equal strength may be administered.

Pharmacodynamics
Antiarrhythmic action: An antiarrhythmic drug with predominantly class III properties that prolongs action potential duration in isolated cardiac my-

ocytes and increases both atrial and ventricular refractoriness.

Pharmacokinetics
- *Absorption:* Only given I.V.
- *Distribution:* Highly distributed and about 40% protein-bound.
- *Metabolism:* Not clearly defined.
- *Excretion:* Excreted mainly in urine with rest in feces; half-life of drug is about 6 hours.

Contraindications and precautions
Contraindicated in patients with hypersensitivity to drug or its components and in those with history of polymorphic ventricular tachycardia, such as torsades de pointes. Use cautiously in patients with hepatic or renal dysfunction.

Interactions
Drug-drug. *Class IA antiarrhythmics (disopyramide, procainamide, quinidine), other class III drugs (amiodarone, sotalol):* Increased potential for prolonged refractoriness. Avoid administering together; allow at least five half-lives before ibutilide dosing; allow 4 hours after ibutilide dosing.
Digoxin: Supraventricular arrhythmias may mask cardiotoxicity associated with excessive digoxin levels. Use together cautiously.
H_1-receptor antagonist antihistamines, phenothiazines, tetracyclic antidepressants, tricyclic antidepressants, other drugs that prolong QT interval: Increased risk of proarrhythmia. Monitor patient closely.

Adverse reactions
CNS: headache.
CV: ventricular extrasystoles, nonsustained ventricular tachycardia, hypotension, bundle-branch block, **sustained ventricular tachycardia**, AV block, hypertension, QT-interval prolongation, **bradycardia,** palpitation, tachycardia, **heart failure.**
GI: nausea.

☑ Special considerations
- Patients with atrial fibrillation of more than 2 to 3 days' duration must be given adequate anticoagulants, generally for at least 2 weeks.
- Proper equipment and facilities, including cardiac monitoring, intracardiac pacing facilities, cardioverter-defibrillator, and medication for treatment of sustained ventricular tachycardia, should be available during and after drug administration.
- Hypokalemia and hypomagnesemia should be corrected before therapy begins to reduce the potential for proarrhythmia.
- Administer drug undiluted or diluted in 50 ml diluent; may add to normal saline injection or D_5W injection before infusion. Contents of one 10-ml vial (0.1 mg/ml) also may be added to a 50-ml infusion bag to form an admixture of about 0.017 mg/ml ibutilide fumarate. Follow aseptic technique

strictly during admixture preparation. Drug is compatible with use of polyvinyl chloride plastic bags or polyolefin bags.
- Admixtures of product, with approved diluents, are chemically and physically stable for 24 hours at room temperature and for 48 hours at refrigerated temperatures.
- Inspect parenteral drug products for particulate matter and discoloration before use.
- Overdose could exaggerate expected prolongation of repolarization seen at usual doses.

Monitoring the patient
- Monitor patient's ECG continuously throughout drug administration and for at least 4 hours afterward or until QTc interval has returned to baseline because drug can induce or worsen ventricular arrhythmias in some patients. Longer monitoring is needed if arrhythmic activity is noted.
- In patients also receiving digoxin, monitor digoxin level closely.

Information for the patient
- Tell patient to report adverse reactions at once.
- Instruct patient to report discomfort at I.V. injection site.

Pediatric patients
- Safety and effectiveness in children under age 18 haven't been established.

Breast-feeding patients
- It's unknown if drug appears in breast milk; avoid use in breast-feeding women during therapy.

idarubicin
Idamycin

Pharmacologic classification: antibiotic antineoplastic
Therapeutic classification: antineoplastic
Pregnancy risk category D

How supplied
Available by prescription only
Injection: 5 mg, 10 mg, 20 mg (lyophilized powder) in single-dose vials with 50-, 100-, or 200-mg lactose

Indications, route, and dosage
Acute myelocytic leukemia in adults, including French-American-British classifications M1 through M7, with other approved antileukemic drugs
Adults: 12 mg/m^2 daily by slow I.V. injection (over 10 to 15 minutes) for 3 days. Administer with cytarabine 100 mg/m^2 daily by continuous infusion for 7 days, or give cytarabine as a 25-mg/m^2 bolus then 200 mg/m^2 daily by continuous I.V. infusion for 5 days. A second course may be administered if needed.

Reactions may be *common*, uncommon, **life-threatening**, or COMMON AND LIFE-THREATENING.

✦ *Dosage adjustment.* If patient experiences severe mucositis, delay administration until recovery is complete and reduce dosage by 25%. Also reduce dosage in patients with hepatic or renal impairment. Idarubicin shouldn't be given if bilirubin level is above 5 mg/dl.

Dosage and indications may vary. Check current literature for recommended protocol.

Pharmacodynamics
Antineoplastic action: Inhibits nucleic acid synthesis by intercalation and interacts with the enzyme topoisomerase II. It's highly lipophilic, which results in an increased rate of cellular uptake.

Pharmacokinetics
• *Absorption:* Peak cellular levels achieved within minutes of I.V. injection.
• *Distribution:* Highly lipophilic and 97% tissue-bound, with highest levels in nucleated blood and bone marrow cells. Its metabolite, idarubicinol, is detected in CSF; significance of this is under evaluation.
• *Metabolism:* Extensive extrahepatic metabolism indicated. Metabolite has cytotoxic activity.
• *Excretion:* Predominantly by biliary excretion as its metabolite and, to a lesser extent, by renal elimination. Mean terminal half-life is 22 hours (range, 4 to 46 hours) when used alone; 20 hours (range, 7 to 38 hours) when combined with cytarabine. Plasma levels of metabolite sustained for longer than 8 days.

Contraindications and precautions
No known contraindications. Use cautiously in patients with impaired renal or hepatic function and in those with bone marrow suppression induced by previous drug therapy or radiation therapy.

Interactions
Drug-drug. *Alkaline solutions, heparin:* Incompatible. Don't mix idarubicin with other drugs unless specific compatibility data are available.

Adverse reactions
CNS: *headache, changed mental status,* peripheral neuropathy, *seizures.*
CV: *heart failure,* atrial fibrillation, chest pain, *MI,* asymptomatic decline in left ventricular ejection fraction, *myocardial insufficiency, arrhythmias, hemorrhage, myocardial toxicity.*
GI: *nausea, vomiting, cramps, diarrhea, mucositis.*
GU: decreased renal function.
Hematologic: *myelosuppression.*
Hepatic: changes in hepatic function.
Skin: *alopecia, rash, urticaria, bullous erythrodermatous rash on palms and soles,* hives at injection site, erythema at previously irradiated sites, tissue necrosis at injection site (if extravasation occurs).

Other: INFECTION, *fever,* hyperuricemia, *hypersensitivity reactions.*

☑ Special considerations
• Control systemic infections before therapy.
• Administer drug over 10 to 15 minutes into a free-flowing I.V. infusion of saline solution or D₅W, which is running into a large vein.
• If extravasation or signs of extravasation occur, stop infusion immediately and restart in another vein. Treat with intermittent ice packs for 30 minutes four times daily for 4 days and evaluate affected extremity.
• Antiemetics may be used to prevent or treat nausea and vomiting.
• Reconstitute drug using 5, 10, or 20 ml saline solution for the 5-, 10-, or 20-mg vial, respectively, to give a final level of 1 mg/ml. Don't use bacteriostatic saline.
• Follow usual chemotherapy mixing precautions. Vial is under negative pressure.
• Reconstituted solutions are stable for 3 days (72 hours) at 59° to 86° F (15° to 30° C); 7 days if refrigerated. Discard unused solutions appropriately.
• If overdose occurs, supportive treatment, including platelet transfusions, antibiotics, and treatment of mucositis, may be needed.

Monitoring the patient
• Frequently monitor CBC and hepatic and renal function.
• Hyperuricemia may result from rapid lysis of leukemic cells; take appropriate preventive measures (including adequate hydration) before starting treatment.

Information for the patient
• Instruct patient to recognize signs and symptoms of extravasation and to report them if they occur.
• Tell patient to report signs and symptoms of infection, including persistent fever or sore throat.
• Tell patient to minimize dangerous behavior that can cause bleeding and to report bleeding or abnormal bruising.

Pediatric patients
• Safety and efficacy in children haven't been established.

Breast-feeding patients
• It's unknown if drug appears in breast milk. avoid risk of serious adverse reactions in in' stop breast-feeding before starting therar

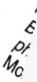

ifosfamide
Ifex

Pharmacologic classification: alkylating drug (cell cycle–phase nonspecific)
Therapeutic classification: antineoplastic
Pregnancy risk category D

How supplied
Injection: 1-g, 3-g vials

Indications, route, and dosage
Germ cell testicular cancer, ◇ **lung cancer,** ◇ **Hodgkin's and** ◇ **malignant lymphoma,** ◇ **breast cancer,** ◇ **acute and** ◇ **chronic lymphocytic leukemia,** ◇ **ovarian cancer,** ◇ **gastric cancer,** ◇ **pancreatic cancer,** ◇ **sarcomas**
Adults: 1.2 g/m²/day I.V. for 5 days. Regimen is usually repeated q 3 weeks.

Drug may be given by slow I.V. push, by intermittent infusion over at least 30 minutes, or by continuous infusion. Dosage and indications may vary. Check current literature for recommended protocol.

Pharmacodynamics
Antineoplastic action: Requires activation by hepatic microsomal enzymes to exert its cytotoxic activity. The active compound cross-links strands of DNA and also breaks the DNA chain.

Pharmacokinetics
- *Absorption:* Not administered orally.
- *Distribution:* Crosses blood-brain barrier along with its metabolites.
- *Metabolism:* About 50% metabolized in liver.
- *Excretion:* Drug and metabolites excreted primarily in urine. Terminal half-life reported to be about 7 hours at doses of 1.6 to 2.4 g/m²/day; about 15 hours at single dose of 3.8 to 5 g/m².

Contraindications and precautions
Contraindicated in patients with hypersensitivity to drug and in those with severe bone marrow suppression. Use cautiously in patients with renal or hepatic impairment, compromised bone marrow reserve as indicated by granulocytopenia, bone marrow metastases, prior radiation therapy, or therapy with cytotoxic drugs.

Interactions
Drug-drug. *Allopurinol:* May produce excessive ifosfamide effect. Monitor patient for signs of toxicity.
Anticoagulants, aspirin: Increased risk of bleeding. Avoid concomitant use.
Barbiturates, chloral hydrate, phenobarbital, phenytoin: May increase activity of ifosfamide. Monitor patient closely.

Adverse reactions
CNS: *somnolence, confusion, **coma, seizures,*** ataxia, hallucinations, depressive psychosis, dizziness, disorientation, cranial nerve dysfunction.
GI: *nausea, vomiting.*
GU: *hemorrhagic cystitis, hematuria, **nephrotoxicity.***
Hematologic: *leukopenia, thrombocytopenia, myelosuppression.*
Hepatic: elevated liver enzyme levels, liver dysfunction.
Skin: *alopecia.*
Other: *metabolic acidosis,* infection, phlebitis.

☑ Special considerations
- Follow all established procedures for safe handling, administration, and disposal of chemotherapeutic drugs.
- To reconstitute 1-g vial, use 20 ml of sterile water; for a 3-g vial, use 60 ml of sterile water for injection to give a level of 50 mg/ml. Normal saline solution also may be used for reconstitution.
- Push fluids (3 qt [3 L] daily) and administer with mesna (Mesnex) to prevent hemorrhagic cystitis. Avoid giving drug at bedtime because infrequent voiding during the night may increase the possibility of cystitis. Bladder irrigation with normal saline solution may decrease the possibility of cystitis.
- Dilutions not prepared with bacteriostatic water for injection (benzyl alcohol or parabens preserved) should be refrigerated and used within 6 hours.
- Drug can be further diluted with D₅W or normal saline solution for I.V. infusion. Solution is stable for 7 days at room temperature and 6 weeks at 41° F (5° C).
- Drug may be given by I.V. push injection in a minimum of 75 ml normal saline solution over 30 minutes.
- Infusing each dose over 2 hours or longer will decrease possibility of cystitis.
- Sterile phlebitis may occur at injection site; apply warm compresses.
- Treatment of overdose is usually supportive and includes transfusion of blood components, antiemetics, and bladder irrigation.

Monitoring the patient
- Assess patient for changes in mental status and cerebellar dysfunction. Dose may have to be decreased.
- Monitor CBC and renal and liver function tests.

Information for the patient
- Encourage patient to void every 2 hours during the day and twice during the night. Catheterization should be required for patient unable to void.
- Tell patient to ensure adequate fluid intake to prevent bladder toxicity and to facilitate excretion of uric acid.

• Warn patient to avoid exposure to people with infections. Tell him to report signs of infection or unusual bleeding immediately.
• Reassure patient that hair should grow back after treatment ends.
• Tell patient to call immediately if blood appears in urine.
• Advise both men and women to use contraception during therapy.

Pediatric patients
• Safety and effectiveness in children haven't been established.

Breast-feeding patients
• Drug appears in breast milk. Because of potential for serious adverse reactions, mutagenicity, and carcinogenicity in infant, breast-feeding isn't recommended.

imipenem and cilastatin sodium
Primaxin I.M., Primaxin I.V.

Pharmacologic classification: carbapenem (thienamycin class); beta-lactam antibiotic
Therapeutic classification: antibiotic
Pregnancy risk category C

How supplied
Available by prescription only
Powder (for I.M. injection): 500-mg, 750-mg vial
Injection: 250-mg, 500-mg vials, ADD-Vantage, and infusion bottles

Indications, route, and dosage
Mild to moderate lower respiratory tract, skin and skin-structure, gynecologic infections
Adults weighing at least 70 kg (154 lb): 500 to 750 mg I.M. q 12 hours.
Mild to moderate intra-abdominal infections
Adults weighing at least 70 kg: 750 mg I.M. q 12 hours.
Serious respiratory and urinary tract infections; intra-abdominal, gynecologic, bone, joint, or skin infections; bacterial septicemia; endocarditis
Adults weighing at least 70 kg: 250 mg to 1 g by I.V. infusion q 6 to 8 hours. Maximum daily dose is 50 mg/kg/day or 4 g/day, whichever is less.
◊ *Children:* 15 to 25 mg/kg q 6 hours.
✦ *Dosage adjustment.* In patients with renal failure and creatinine clearance of 6 to 20 ml/minute/1.73 m², 125 to 250 mg I.V. q 12 hours for most pathogens. There may be an increased risk of seizures when doses of 500 mg q 12 hours are administered to these patients. When creatinine clearance is 5 ml/minute/1.73 m² or less, drug shouldn't be given unless hemodialysis is instituted within 48 hours.

Note: In patients weighing less than 70 kg or in those with impaired renal function, dosages vary. Check current literature for recommended protocol.

Pharmacodynamics
Antibacterial action: A bactericidal drug, imipenem inhibits bacterial cell wall synthesis. Its spectrum of antimicrobial activity includes many gram-positive, gram-negative, and anaerobic bacteria, including *Staphylococcus* and *Streptococcus* species, *Escherichia coli, Klebsiella, Proteus, Enterobacter* species, *Pseudomonas aeruginosa,* and *Bacteroides* species, including *B. fragilis.* Resistant bacteria include methicillin-resistant staphylococci, *Clostridium difficile,* and other *Pseudomonas* species.
Cilastatin inhibits imipenem's enzymatic breakdown in the kidneys, making it effective in treating urinary tract infections.

Pharmacokinetics
• *Absorption:* Following I.M. administration, imipenem blood levels peak within 2 hours; cilastatin levels peak within 1 hour. After I.V. administration, levels of both drugs peak in about 20 minutes. Imipenem is about 75% and cilastatin about 95% bioavailable after I.M. administration compared with I.V. administration.
• *Distribution:* Both drugs distributed rapidly and widely. About 20% of imipenem is protein-bound; 40% of cilastatin.
• *Metabolism:* Imipenem metabolized by kidney dehydropeptidase I, resulting in low urine levels. Cilastatin inhibits this enzyme, reducing imipenem's metabolism.
• *Excretion:* About 70% of imipenem and cilastatin dose excreted unchanged by kidneys (when imipenem is combined with cilastatin) by tubular secretion and glomerular filtration. Imipenem is cleared by hemodialysis; a supplemental dose is required after this procedure. Half-life of drug is about 1 hour after I.V. administration. Prolonged absorption after I.M. administration results in longer half-life (2 to 3 hours).

Contraindications and precautions
Contraindicated in patients with hypersensitivity to drug. Imipenem and cilastatin sodium reconstituted with lidocaine hydrochloride for I.M. injection is contraindicated in patients with hypersensitivity to local anesthetics of the amide type and in patients with severe shock or heart block.
Use cautiously in patients with impaired renal function, seizure disorders, or allergy to penicillins or cephalosporins.

Interactions
Drug-drug. *Chloramphenicol:* May impede bactericidal effects of imipenem. Give chloramphenicol a few hours after imipenem and cilastatin.

Cyclosporine: Concomitant use may increase CNS effects of both drugs. Monitor patient closely.

Ganciclovir: Generalized seizures have occurred during combined imipenem and cilastatin and ganciclovir therapy. Avoid concomitant use.

Probenecid: May prevent tubular secretion of cilastatin (but not imipenem). Avoid concomitant use.

Adverse reactions
CNS: *seizures,* dizziness, somnolence.
CV: hypotension, thrombophlebitis.
GI: nausea, vomiting, diarrhea, *pseudomembranous colitis.*
Hematologic: *agranulocytosis,* thrombocytosis, *thrombocytopenia, leukopenia.*
Hepatic: transient increases in liver enzyme levels.
Skin: rash, urticaria, pruritus, pain at injection site.
Other: *hypersensitivity reactions (anaphylaxis),* fever.

☑ Special considerations
● Culture and sensitivity tests should be done before starting therapy.
● When reconstituting powder, shake until solution is clear. Solution may range from colorless to yellow; color variations within this range don't affect drug potency. After reconstitution, solution remains stable for 10 hours at room temperature and for 48 hours when refrigerated.
● Don't administer drug by direct I.V. bolus injection. Infuse 250- or 500-mg dose over 20 to 30 minutes; infuse 1-g dose over 40 to 60 minutes. If nausea occurs, slow infusion.
● Continue anticonvulsants in patients with known seizure disorders. Patients who exhibit CNS toxicity should receive phenytoin or benzodiazepines. Reduce dosage or stop drug if CNS toxicity continues.
● Drug has broadest antibacterial spectrum of any available antibiotic. It's most valuable for empiric treatment of unidentified infections and for mixed infections that would otherwise require a combination of antibiotics, possibly including an aminoglycoside.
● Prolonged use may result in overgrowth of non-susceptible organisms. In addition, use of imipenem and cilastatin as a sole course of therapy has resulted in resistance during therapy.
● Drug may be physically incompatible with aminoglycosides; avoid mixing.

Monitoring the patient
● Monitor vital signs frequently.
● Monitor patient for adverse reactions; stop drug if signs of overdose appear and treat symptomatically.

Information for the patient
● Tell patient to report discomfort at I.V. site.

● Tell patient to report adverse effects immediately.

Geriatric patients
● Administer cautiously to elderly patients because they may also have renal dysfunction.

Pediatric patients
● Safety and effectiveness in children under age 12 haven't been established; however, drug has been used in children ages 3 months to 13 years. Dosage range is 15 to 25 mg/kg every 6 hours.

Breast-feeding patients
● It's unknown if drug appears in breast milk. Use with caution in breast-feeding women.

imipramine hydrochloride
Apo-Imipramine*, Impril*, Novopramine*, Tofranil

imipramine pamoate
Tofranil-PM

Pharmacologic classification: dibenzazepine tricyclic antidepressant
Therapeutic classification: antidepressant
Pregnancy risk category B

How supplied
Available by prescription only
imipramine hydrochloride
Tablets: 10 mg, 25 mg, 50 mg
Injection: 25 mg/2 ml
imipramine pamoate
Capsules: 75 mg, 100 mg, 125 mg, 150 mg

Indications, route, and dosage
Depression
Adults: Initially, 75 to 100 mg P.O. or I.M. daily in divided doses, with 25- to 50-mg increments, up to 200 mg. Or start with lower doses (25 mg P.O.) and adjust slowly in 25-mg increments every other day. Maximum dose, 300 mg daily. Or entire dose may be given h.s. (I.M. route rarely used.) Maximum dose is 200 mg/day for outpatients, 300 mg/day for inpatients, 100 mg/day for elderly patients.
◇ **Childhood enuresis**
Children ages 6 and over: 25 to 75 mg P.O. daily, 1 hour before bedtime. Usual dose 1.5 mg/kg/day in three divided doses. Maximum dose, 5 mg/kg/day.

Pharmacodynamics
Antidepressant action: Thought to exert antidepressant effects by inhibiting reuptake of norepinephrine and serotonin in CNS nerve terminals (presynaptic neurons), which results in increased levels and enhanced activity of these neuro-

transmitters in the synaptic cleft. Also has anticholinergic activity and is used to treat nocturnal enuresis in children over age 6.

Pharmacokinetics
• *Absorption:* Absorbed rapidly from GI tract and muscle tissue after oral and I.M. administration.
• *Distribution:* Distributed widely into body, including CNS and breast milk. 90% protein-bound. Effect peaks in ½ to 2 hours; steady-state achieved within 2 to 5 days. Therapeutic plasma levels (parent drug and metabolite) thought to range from 150 to 300 ng/ml.
• *Metabolism:* Metabolized by liver to active metabolite desipramine. Significant first-pass effect may explain variability of serum levels in different patients taking same dosage.
• *Excretion:* Mostly excreted in urine.

Contraindications and precautions
Contraindicated in patients with hypersensitivity to drug, during acute recovery phase of MI, and in those receiving MAO inhibitors.

Use cautiously in patients at risk for suicide; in those with impaired renal or hepatic function, history of urine retention, angle-closure glaucoma, increased intraocular pressure, CV disease, hyperthyroidism, seizure disorders, or allergy to sulfites (injectable form only); and in patients receiving thyroid drugs.

Interactions
Drug-drug. *Antiarrhythmics, pimozide, thyroid drugs:* May increase risk of arrhythmias and conduction defects. Monitor ECG closely.
Anticholinergics, atropine: Possible oversedation, paralytic ileus, visual changes, and severe constipation. Use together cautiously.
Barbiturates, haloperidol, phenothiazines: Decreased therapeutic efficacy. Avoid concomitant use.
Beta blockers, cimetidine, methylphenidate, oral contraceptives, propoxyphene: Increased plasma levels. Monitor patient for toxicity.
Clonidine, guanabenz, guanadrel, guanethidine, methyldopa, reserpine: May decrease hypotensive effects of these drugs. Monitor patient and blood pressure closely.
CNS depressants: Additive CNS effects. Avoid concomitant use.
Disulfiram, ethchlorvynol: May cause delirium and tachycardia. Use with caution.
Metrizamide: Increased risk of seizures. Avoid concomitant use.
Sympathomimetics (ephedrine, epinephrine, phenylephrine, phenylpropanolamine): May increase blood pressure. Use with caution.
Warfarin: May prolong PT and cause bleeding. Monitor PT and INR closely.
Drug-lifestyle. *Alcohol:* Possible additive effects. Discourage use.

Heavy smoking: Induced imipramine metabolism and decreased therapeutic efficacy. Discourage use.
Sun exposure: Increased risk of photosensitivity reactions. Tell patient to take precautions.

Adverse reactions
CNS: *drowsiness, dizziness,* excitation, tremor, confusion, hallucinations, anxiety, ataxia, paresthesia, nervousness, EEG changes, *seizures,* extrapyramidal reactions.
CV: *orthostatic hypotension, tachycardia,* ECG changes, hypertension, **MI, stroke, arrhythmias, heart block, precipitation of heart failure.**
EENT: blurred vision, tinnitus, mydriasis.
GI: *dry mouth, constipation,* nausea, vomiting, anorexia, paralytic ileus, abdominal cramps.
GU: *urine retention,* gynecomastia (in men), testicular swelling, impotence.
Metabolic: increased or decreased blood glucose levels.
Skin: rash, urticaria, photosensitivity, pruritus.
Other: galactorrhea and breast enlargement (in women), altered libido, inappropriate antidiuretic hormone secretion syndrome, *diaphoresis,* **hypersensitivity reaction.**

After abrupt withdrawal of long-term therapy: nausea, headache, malaise (doesn't indicate addiction).

☑ Special considerations
Besides the recommendations relevant to all tricyclic antidepressants, consider the following.
• Drug may be used to treat nocturnal enuresis in children.
• Imipramine is associated with a high risk of orthostatic hypotension. Check sitting and standing blood pressures after initial dose.
• Don't withdraw drug abruptly, but taper gradually over time.
• Tolerance to drug's sedative effects usually develops over several weeks.
• Discontinue drug at least 48 hours before surgical procedures.
• Overdose is frequently life-threatening, particularly when combined with alcohol. Treatment is symptomatic and supportive, including maintaining airway, stable body temperature, and fluid or electrolyte balance.

Monitoring the patient
• Monitor closely for adverse effects.
• Monitor patient for CNS effects and exce~ anticholinergic activity.
• Monitor vital signs and ECG closely

Information for the patient
• Tell patient to take drug exac~
• Explain that full effects of dr~ apparent for up to 4 to 6 w~ apy.

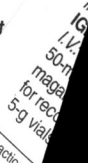

• Warn patient not to stop drug abruptly, not to share drug with others, and not to consume alcohol while taking drug.
• Advise patient to take drug with food or milk if it causes stomach upset.
• Suggest relieving dry mouth with sugarless chewing gum or hard candy. Encourage good dental prophylaxis because persistent dry mouth may lead to dental caries.
• Encourage patient to report unusual or troublesome effects immediately, including confusion, movement disorders, rapid heartbeat, dizziness, fainting, or difficulty urinating.

Geriatric patients
• Recommended dose is 30 to 40 mg P.O. daily, not to exceed 100 mg daily. Initiate therapy at low doses (10 mg) and adjust slowly. Elderly patients may be at greater risk for adverse cardiac reactions.

Pediatric patients
• Drug isn't recommended for treating depression in patients under age 12. Don't use pamoate salt for enuresis in children.

Breast-feeding patients
• Drug appears in breast milk in low levels. Potential benefit to mother should outweigh possible risks to infant.

immune globulin (gamma globulin, IG, immune serum globulin, ISG)

immune globulin for I.M. use (IGIM)

immune globulin for I.V. use (IGIV)

Gamimune N (5%, 10%), Gammagard S/D, Gammar-P IV, Iveegam, Polygam S/D, Sandoglobulin, Venoglobulin-I, Venoglobulin-S

Pharmacologic classification: immune serum
Therapeutic classification: stimulant for antibody production
Pregnancy risk category C

How supplied
Available by prescription only
IGIM
Injection: 2-ml, 10-ml vials
IV
Gamimune N—5% and 10% solution in 10-ml, [...]l, 100-ml, and 250-ml single-use vials; Gam[mag]rd S/D—2.5-g, 5-g, and 10-g single-use vials [for reco]nstitution; Gammar-P IV—1-g, 2.5-g, and [...] with diluent and 10-g vials with admin-

istration set and diluent; Iveegam—1-g, 2.5-g, and 5-g vials with diluent; Polygam S/D—2.5-g, 5-g, and 10-g single-use vials with diluent; Sandoglobulin—1-g, 3-g, 6-g, and 12-g vials or kits with diluent or bulk packs without diluent; Venoglobulin-I—2.5-g and 5-g vials with or without reconstitution kits with sterile water, 10-g vials with reconstitution kit and administration set, and 0.5-g vials with reconstitution kit; Venoglobulin-S—5% and 10% in 50-ml, 100-ml, and 200-ml vials.

Indications, route, and dosage
Agammaglobulinemia, hypogammaglobulinemia, immune deficiency (IGIV)
Adults and children: For Gamimune N only, 100 to 200 mg/kg or 2 to 4 ml/kg I.V. infusion monthly. Infusion rate is 0.01 to 0.02 ml/kg/minute for 30 minutes. Rate can then be increased to maximum of 0.08 ml/kg/minute for remainder of infusion.

For Gammagard S/D only, initially 200 to 400 mg/kg I.V., then 100 mg/kg monthly. Initiate infusion at 0.5 ml/kg/hour, gradually increasing to maximum of 4 ml/kg/hour.

For Gammar-P IV only, 200 to 400 mg/kg q 3 to 4 weeks. Infusion rate is 0.01 ml/kg/minute, increasing to 0.02 ml/kg/minute after 15 to 30 minutes, with gradual increase to 0.06 ml/kg/minute.

For Iveegam only, 200 mg/kg I.V. monthly. If response is inadequate, doses may be increased up to 800 mg/kg or the drug may be administered more frequently. Infuse at 1 to 2 ml/minute.

For Polygam S/D only, 100 mg/kg I.V. monthly. An initial dose of 200 to 400 mg/kg may be administered. Initiate infusion at 0.5 ml/kg/hour, gradually increasing to maximum of 4 ml/kg/hour.

For Sandoglobulin only, 200 mg/kg I.V. monthly. Start with 0.5 to 1 ml/minute of a 3% solution; increase up to 2.5 ml/minute gradually after 15 to 30 minutes.

For Venoglobulin-I only, 200 mg/kg I.V. monthly; may be increased to 300 to 400 mg/kg and may be repeated more frequently than once monthly. Infuse at 0.01 to 0.02 ml/kg/minute for 30 minutes, then increase to 0.04 ml/kg/minute or higher, if tolerated.

For Venoglobulin-S only, 200 mg/kg I.V. monthly. Increase dose to 300 to 400 mg/kg monthly or administer more frequently if adequate IgI levels aren't achieved. Initiate infusion at 0.01 to 0.02 ml/kg/minute for 30 minutes, then increase 5% solutions to 0.04 ml/kg/minute and 10% solutions to 0.05 ml/kg/minute, if tolerated.
Hepatitis A exposure (IGIM)
Adults and children: 0.02 to 0.04 ml/kg I.M. as soon as possible after exposure. Up to 0.1 ml/kg may be given after prolonged or intense exposure.
Measles exposure (IGIM)
Adults and children: 0.25 ml/kg within 6 days after exposure.

Postexposure prophylaxis of measles (IGIM)
Adults and children: 0.5 ml/kg I.M. within 6 days after exposure.

Chickenpox exposure (IGIM)
Adults and children: 0.6 to 1.2 ml/kg I.M. as soon as exposed.

Rubella exposure in first trimester of pregnancy (IGIM)
Women: 0.55 ml/kg I.M. as soon as exposed.

Idiopathic thrombocytopenic purpura (IGIV)
Adults and children: 400 mg/kg Sandoglobulin I.V. for 2 to 5 consecutive days; or 400 mg/kg Gamimune N 5% for 5 days or 1,000 mg/kg Gamimune N 10% for 1 to 2 days. Maintenance dose is 400 to 1,000 mg/kg I.V. of Gamimune N 10% as a single infusion to maintain a platelet count greater than 30,000/mm³.

Bone marrow transplantation (IGIV)
Adults over age 20: Gamimune N 10%, 500 mg/kg on day 7 and day 2 before transplantation; then weekly through 90 days posttransplant.

Pharmacodynamics
Immune action: Provides passive immunity by increasing antibody titer. Exact mechanism by which IGIV increases platelet counts in idiopathic thrombocytopenic purpura isn't known.

Pharmacokinetics
• *Absorption:* After slow I.M. absorption, serum levels peak within 2 days.
• *Distribution:* Distributed evenly between intravascular and extravascular spaces.
• *Metabolism:* No information available.
• *Excretion:* Serum half-life reportedly 21 to 24 days in immunocompetent patients.

Contraindications and precautions
Contraindicated in patients with hypersensitivity to drug.

Interactions
Drug-drug. *Live virus vaccines:* Immune globulin may interfere with immune response to vaccines. Don't administer live virus vaccines within 3 months after administration of immune globulin.

Adverse reactions
CNS: faintness, headache, malaise.
CV: chest pain, chest tightness.
GI: nausea, vomiting.
Musculoskeletal: hip pain, joint pain, muscle stiffness at injection site.
Respiratory: dyspnea, shortness of breath.
Skin: erythema, urticaria.
Other: fever, *anaphylaxis,* chills.

☑ Special considerations
• Obtain thorough history of allergies and reactions to immunizations.

• Epinephrine solution 1:1,000 should be available to treat allergic reactions.
• Excessively rapid I.V. infusion rate can precipitate anaphylactoid reaction.
• Inject I.M. formulation into different sites, preferably into buttocks. Don't inject more than 3 ml per injection site.
• Don't give for hepatitis A exposure if 2 weeks or more have elapsed since exposure or after onset of clinical illness.
• Immune globulin hasn't been associated with increased frequency of AIDS. It's devoid of HIV. Immune globulin recipients don't develop antibodies to HIV.
• Store Sandoglobulin and Gammagard S/D at room temperature not exceeding 77° F (25° C); Gamimune N and Iveegam at 36° to 46° F (2° to 8° C) but don't freeze; Gammar-P IV at room temperature below 86° F (30° C) but don't freeze; Venoglobulin-I at room temperature below 86° F.
• Immune globulin has been studied in the treatment of various conditions, including Kawasaki disease, asthma, allergic disorders, autoimmune neutropenia, myasthenia gravis, and platelet transfusion rejection. It's been used in prophylaxis of infections in immunocompromised patients.
• Gamimune N can be diluted with D_5W.
• Reconstitute Gammagard S/D with diluent (sterile water for injection) and transfer device provided by manufacturer. Administration set (provided) contains a 15-micron in-line filter that must be used during administration.
• Reconstitute Sandoglobulin with diluent supplied (normal saline).

Monitoring the patient
• Closely monitor blood pressure in patient receiving IGIV, especially if patient's first infusion of immune globulin.
• Monitor patient for local and systemic adverse reactions.

Information for the patient
• Explain to patient that chance of getting AIDS or hepatitis after receiving immune globulin is minute.
• Tell patient to expect local pain, swelling, and tenderness at injection site. Recommend acetaminophen for minor discomfort.
• Instruct patient to promptly report headach skin changes, or difficulty breathing.
• Although pregnancy isn't contraindicat' use, inform pregnant patient that it's unk' immune globulin can cause fetal harm

Breast-feeding patients
• It's unknown if immune globul' breast milk. Use with caution ir women.

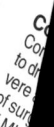

inamrinone lactate
Inocor

Pharmacologic classification: bipyridine derivative
Therapeutic classification: inotropic drug, vasodilator
Pregnancy risk category C

How supplied
Available by prescription only
Injection: 5 mg/ml

Indications, route, and dosage
Short-term management of heart failure
Adults: Initially, 0.75 mg/kg I.V. bolus over 2 to 3 minutes; then begin maintenance infusion of 5 to 10 mcg/kg/minute. Additional bolus of 0.75 mg/kg may be given 30 minutes after therapy starts. Maximum daily dose is 10 mg/kg.

Pharmacodynamics
Vasodilating action: Primary vasodilating effect seems to stem from a direct effect on peripheral vessels.

Inotropic action: The mechanism of action responsible for the apparent inotropic effect isn't fully understood; however, it may be associated with inhibition of phosphodiesterase activity, resulting in increased cellular levels of adenosine 3',5'-cyclic phosphate; this, in turn, may alter intracellular and extracellular calcium levels. The role of calcium homeostasis hasn't been determined. Effects include increased cardiac output mediated by reduced afterload and, possibly, inotropism.

Pharmacokinetics
• *Absorption:* With I.V. administration, onset of action occurs in 2 to 5 minutes, with peak effects in about 10 minutes. CV effects may persist for 1 to 2 hours.
• *Distribution:* Distribution volume is 1.2 L/kg. Distribution sites are unknown. Protein-binding ranges from 10% to 49%. Therapeutic steady-state serum levels range from 0.5 to 7 mcg/ml (ideal level: 3 mcg/ml).
• *Metabolism:* Metabolized in the liver to several metabolites of unknown activity.
• *Excretion:* In normal patients, excreted in the urine, with a terminal elimination half-life of about 4 hours. Half-life may be prolonged slightly in patients with heart failure.

Contraindications and precautions
Contraindicated in patients with hypersensitivity to drug or bisulfites. Don't use in patients with severe aortic or pulmonic valvular disease in place of surgical intervention or during an acute phase

Interactions
Drug-drug. *Disopyramide:* May cause severe hypotension. Avoid concurrent use.

Adverse reactions
CV: *arrhythmias,* hypotension.
GI: nausea, vomiting, anorexia, abdominal pain.
Hematologic: *thrombocytopenia* (based on dose and duration of therapy).
Hepatic: elevated liver enzymes.
Other: burning at injection site, *hypersensitivity reactions* (pericarditis, ascites, myositis vasculitis, pleuritis), fever, chest pain, decreased serum potassium levels.

☑ Special considerations
• Administer drug as supplied or dilute in normal or half-normal saline solution to concentration of 1 to 3 mg/ml. Don't dilute with solutions containing dextrose because a slow chemical reaction occurs over 24 hours. However, inamrinone can be injected into running dextrose infusions through Y-connector or directly into tubing. Use diluted solution within 24 hours.
• Don't administer furosemide in I.V. lines containing inamrinone because a chemical reaction occurs immediately.
• Watch for adverse GI effects (such as nausea, vomiting, and diarrhea); reduce dosage or discontinue drug if these occur.
• Drug is prescribed primarily for patients who haven't responded to therapy with cardiac glycosides, diuretics, and vasodilators.
• Effects of overdose include severe hypotension. Treatment may include administration of a potent vasopressor such as norepinephrine as well as other general supportive measures, including cautious fluid volume replacement.

Monitoring the patient
• Monitor blood pressure and heart rate throughout infusion. Infusion should be slowed or stopped if patient's blood pressure decreases or if arrhythmias (ventricular or supraventricular) occur. Dosage may need to be reduced.
• Monitor platelet counts. A count below 150,000/mm^3 usually necessitates dosage reduction. Thrombocytopenia usually occurs after prolonged treatment.
• Monitor electrolyte levels (especially potassium) because drug increases cardiac output, which may cause diuresis.
• Hemodynamic monitoring may be useful in guiding therapy.
• Monitor liver function tests to detect hepatic damage (rare).

Pediatric patients
• Safety and effectiveness in children under age 18 haven't been established.

Breast-feeding patients
● Drug may appear in breast milk. Safety in breast-feeding women hasn't been established.

indapamide
Lozol

Pharmacologic classification: thiazide-like diuretic
Therapeutic classification: diuretic, antihypertensive
Pregnancy risk category B

How supplied
Available by prescription only
Tablets: 1.25 mg, 2.5 mg

Indications, route, and dosage
Edema of heart failure
Adults: 2.5 mg P.O. as a single daily dose taken in the morning; increase dose to 5 mg daily after 1 week if response is poor.
Hypertension
Adults: 1.25 mg P.O. as a single daily dose taken in the morning; increase dose to 2.5 mg daily after 4 weeks if response is poor. Maximum daily dose, 5 mg.

Pharmacodynamics
Diuretic action: Increases urinary excretion of sodium and water by inhibiting sodium reabsorption in the cortical diluting tubule of the nephron, thus relieving edema.
Antihypertensive action: Exact mechanism unknown. This effect may result from direct arteriolar vasodilatation, via calcium channel blockade. Drug also reduces total body sodium.

Pharmacokinetics
● *Absorption:* After oral administration, absorbed completely from GI tract; serum levels peak at 2 to 2½ hours.
● *Distribution:* Distributed widely into body tissues because of its lipophilicity; drug is 71% to 79% plasma protein-bound.
● *Metabolism:* Significant hepatic metabolism.
● *Excretion:* About 60% excreted in urine within 48 hours; about 16% to 23% excreted in feces.

Contraindications and precautions
Contraindicated in patients with hypersensitivity to other sulfonamide-derived drugs and in those with anuria. Use cautiously in patients with severely impaired renal or hepatic function or progressive hepatic disease.

Interactions
Drug-drug. *Amphetamines, quinidine:* May decrease urinary excretion of these drugs. Monitor patient carefully.

Antihypertensives: Indapamide potentiates hypotensive effects of most other antihypertensives. May be used for therapeutic advantage.
Cholestyramine, colestipol: May bind indapamide, preventing its absorption. Give drugs 1 hour apart.
Diazoxide: Indapamide may potentiate hyperglycemic, hypotensive, and hyperuricemic effects. Use together cautiously.
Insulin, sulfonylureas: Increased hyperglycemic effect. Dose adjustment may be needed in diabetic patients.
Lithium: Elevated serum lithium levels. May necessitate reduction in lithium dosage by 50%.
Methenamine mandelate: Decreased therapeutic effectiveness. Monitor closely.

Adverse reactions
CNS: headache, nervousness, dizziness, lightheadedness, weakness, vertigo, restlessness, drowsiness, fatigue, anxiety, depression, numbness of extremities, irritability, agitation.
CV: volume depletion and dehydration, orthostatic hypotension, palpitations, PVCs, irregular heartbeat, vasculitis.
EENT: rhinorrhea.
GI: anorexia, nausea, epigastric distress, vomiting, abdominal pain, diarrhea, constipation.
GU: nocturia, polyuria, frequent urination, impotence.
Metabolic: asymptomatic hyperuricemia; fluid and electrolyte imbalances, including dilutional hyponatremia and hypochloremia, metabolic alkalosis, hypokalemia; gout; weight loss.
Musculoskeletal: muscle cramps and spasms.
Skin: rash, pruritus, flushing.

☑ Special considerations
● Recommendations for use of indapamide and for care and teaching of the patient during therapy are the same as those for all thiazide and thiazide-like diuretics.
● Indapamide therapy may interfere with tests for parathyroid function and should be discontinued before such tests.
● Signs of overdose are GI irritation and hypermotility, diuresis, and lethargy.

Monitoring the patient
● Monitor fluid intake and output, weight, blood pressure, and serum electrolyte levels.
● Watch for patient compliance in taking dru '

Information for the patient
● Instruct patient to take drug in the m prevent nocturia or with food if GI up
● Advise patient to avoid sudden po and to rise slowly to avoid orthc sion.
● Encourage high-potassiur

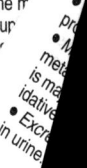

Geriatric patients
• Elderly and debilitated patients require close observation and may need reduced dosages. They are more sensitive to excess diuresis because of age-related changes in CV and renal function. Excess diuresis promotes orthostatic hypotension, dehydration, hypovolemia, hyponatremia, hypomagnesemia, and hypokalemia.

Pediatric patients
• Safety and effectiveness in children haven't been established.

Breast-feeding patients
• Drug appears in breast milk; drug's safety and effectiveness in breast-feeding women haven't been established.

indinavir sulfate
Crixivan

Pharmacologic classification: HIV protease inhibitor
Therapeutic classification: antiviral
Pregnancy risk category C

How supplied
Available by prescription only
Capsules: 200 mg, 400 mg

Indications, route, and dosage
Treatment of patients with HIV infection when antiretroviral therapy is warranted
Adults: 800 mg P.O. q 8 hours.
✦ *Dosage adjustment.* Reduce dosage to 600 mg P.O. q 8 hours in patients with mild to moderate hepatic insufficiency due to cirrhosis.

Pharmacodynamics
Antiviral action: Inhibits HIV protease, an enzyme required for the proteolytic cleavage of viral polyprotein precursors into individual functional proteins found in infectious HIV. By binding to the protease active site, indinavir prevents cleavage of the viral polyproteins, resulting in formation of immature noninfectious viral particles.

Pharmacokinetics
• *Absorption:* Rapidly absorbed in GI tract when taken on empty stomach. A meal high in calories, fat, and protein significantly interferes with drug absorption; lighter meals don't.
• *Distribution:* About 60% of drug is plasma protein-bound.
• *Metabolism:* Metabolized to at least seven metabolites. Cytochrome P-450 3A4 (CYP3A4) major enzyme responsible for formation of oxidized metabolites.
• *Excretion:* Less than 20% excreted unchanged

Contraindications and precautions
Contraindicated in patients with hypersensitivity to drug or its components. Use cautiously in patients with hepatic insufficiency due to cirrhosis.

Interactions
Drug-drug. *Didanosine:* Possible degradation of didanosine, formulated with buffers to increase pH. Administer at least 1 hour apart on an empty stomach.
INH: Increased INH levels. Don't administer together.
Ketoconazole: Increased plasma levels of indinavir. Consider a dosage reduction of indinavir when giving together.
Midazolam, triazolam: Possible inhibition of metabolism of these drugs; potential for serious or life-threatening events, such as arrhythmias or prolonged sedation. Don't administer together.
Quinidine, zidovudine: Increased indinavir levels. Separate administration times.
Rifabutin: Increased plasma levels. Reduce dosage of rifabutin if administered with indinavir.
Rifampin: Markedly reduced plasma levels of indinavir. Don't give together.
Drug-food. *Any food:* Substantially decreased absorption of oral indinavir. Don't give together.

Adverse reactions
CNS: malaise, headache, insomnia, dizziness, somnolence, asthenia, fatigue.
GI: abdominal pain, *nausea,* diarrhea, vomiting, acid regurgitation, anorexia, dry mouth, taste perversion.
GU: nephrolithiasis.
Hematologic: decreased hemoglobin level, platelet count, or neutrophil count.
Hepatic: elevations in ALT, AST, and serum amylase levels; *hyperbilirubinemia.*
Musculoskeletal: flank pain, back pain.

☑ Special considerations
• Dosage of indinavir is the same whether drug is used alone or with other antiretrovirals. However, antiretroviral activity of indinavir may be increased when used with approved reverse transcriptase inhibitors.
• Drug must be taken at 8-hour intervals.
• When giving with rifabutin, reduce dose of rifabutin by half. However, when giving with ketoconazole, decrease dosage of indinavir to 600 mg q 8 hours.

Monitoring the patient
• Monitor patient for adverse effects.
• Drug may cause nephrolithiasis. If signs and symptoms of nephrolithiasis occur, consider stopping drug for 1 to 3 days during acute phase. To prevent nephrolithiasis, patient should maintain adequate hydration.

...ay be *common,* uncommon, *life-threatening,* or COMMON AND LIFE-THREATENING.

Information for the patient
• Inform patient that indinavir doesn't cure HIV infection. He may continue to develop opportunistic infections and other complications associated with HIV disease. Drug also has not been shown to reduce risk of transmitting HIV to others through sexual contact or blood contamination.
• Caution patient not to adjust dosage or stop indinavir therapy without medical approval.
• Advise patient that if a dose of indinavir is missed, he should take the next dose at the regularly scheduled time and shouldn't double the dose.
• Instruct patient to take drug on an empty stomach with water 1 hour before or 2 hours after a meal. Or he may take it with other liquids (such as skim milk, juice, coffee, or tea) or with a light meal. Inform patient that a meal high in calories, fat, and protein reduces indinavir absorption.
• Tell patient to store capsules in original container and to keep desiccant in bottle; capsules are sensitive to moisture.
• Instruct patient to drink at least 1.5 qt (1.5 L) of fluid daily.

Pediatric patients
• Safety and effectiveness in children haven't been established.

Breast-feeding patients
• Drug may appear in breast milk. Because of potential for adverse effects in breast-feeding infants, and to prevent transmitting infection to infant, breast-feeding isn't recommended.

indomethacin, indomethacin sodium trihydrate
Apo-Indomethacin*, Indameth, Indocid*, Indocin, Indocin SR, Novomethacin*

Pharmacologic classification: NSAID
Therapeutic classification: nonnarcotic analgesic, antipyretic, anti-inflammatory
Pregnancy risk category NR

How supplied
Available by prescription only
Capsules: 25 mg, 50 mg
Capsules (sustained-release): 75 mg
Suspension: 25 mg/5 ml
Injection: 1-mg vials
Suppositories: 50 mg

Indications, route, and dosage
Moderate to severe arthritis, ankylosing spondylitis
Adults: 25 mg P.O. b.i.d. or t.i.d. with food or antacids; dose may be increased by 25 to 50 mg daily q 7 days up to 200 mg daily; or 50 mg P.R.

q.i.d. Or sustained-release capsules may be given: 75 mg to start, in the morning or h.s.; then, if necessary, 75 mg b.i.d.
Acute gouty arthritis
Adults: 50 mg t.i.d. Reduce dose as soon as possible; then stop drug. Don't use sustained-release capsules for this condition.
To close a hemodynamically significant patent ductus arteriosus in premature infants (I.V. form only)
Neonates under age 48 hours: 0.2 mg/kg I.V., then 2 doses of 0.1 mg/kg at 12- to 24-hour intervals.
Neonates ages 2 to 7 days: 0.2 mg/kg I.V., then 2 doses of 0.2 mg/kg at 12- to 24-hour intervals.
Neonates over age 7 days: 0.2 mg/kg I.V., then 2 doses of 0.25 mg/kg at 12- to 24-hour intervals.
Acute shoulder pain
Adults: 75 to 150 mg P.O. b.i.d. or t.i.d. with food or antacids; usual treatment is 7 to 14 days.
◊ **Dysmenorrhea**
Adults: 25 mg P.O. t.i.d. with food or antacids.
◊ **Bartter's syndrome**
Adults: 150 mg/day P.O. with food or antacids.
Children: 0.5 to 2 mg/kg in divided doses.

Pharmacodynamics
Analgesic, antipyretic, and anti-inflammatory actions: Exact mechanisms unknown; thought to produce analgesic, antipyretic, and anti-inflammatory effects by inhibiting prostaglandin synthesis and possibly by inhibiting phosphodiesterase.
Closure of patent ductus arteriosus: Mechanism unknown, but action is believed to be through inhibition of prostaglandin synthesis.

Pharmacokinetics
• Absorption: Absorbed rapidly and completely from GI tract.
• Distribution: Highly protein-bound.
• Metabolism: Metabolized in liver.
• Excretion: Excreted mainly in urine, with some biliary excretion.

Contraindications and precautions
Contraindicated in patients with hypersensitivity to drug and in those with history of aspirin- or NSAID-induced asthma, rhinitis, or urticaria; in pregnancy, or while breast-feeding. Also contraindicated in infants with untreated infection, tive bleeding, coagulation defects or thrombocytopenia, congenital heart disease in those whom patency of the ductus arteriosus essary for satisfactory pulmonary blood flow, necrotizing enterocolitis renal function. Suppositories are in patients with a history of proctal bleeding.
Use cautiously in elderly tients with history of GI d

or hepatic function, epilepsy, parkinsonism, CV disease, infection, mental illness, or depression.

Interactions

Drug-drug. *Acetaminophen, gold compounds, other anti-inflammatories:* Possible increased nephrotoxicity with coadministration. Don't use together.

Anticoagulants, thrombolytics: May potentiate anticoagulant effects. Monitor coagulation studies and patient for signs of bleeding.

Antihypertensives, diuretics: May decrease effectiveness of these drugs. Monitor patient's intake and output.

Anti-inflammatories, corticosteroids, corticotropin, salicylates: Increased GI adverse effects. Don't use together.

Aspirin, cefamandole, cefoperazone, dextran, dipyridamole, mezlocillin, parenteral carbenicillin, piperacillin, plicamycin, salicylates, sulfinpyrazone, ticarcillin, valproic acid, other anti-inflammatories: Decreased blood levels of indomethacin. Avoid concomitant use.

Coumarin derivatives, nifedipine, phenytoin, verapamil: Toxicity may occur with coadministration. Don't use together.

Diuretics, triamterene: Potential nephrotoxicity. Don't use together.

Insulin, oral antidiabetics: May potentiate hypoglycemic effects. Monitor serum glucose levels.

Lithium, methotrexate: May decrease renal clearance of these drugs. Monitor patient for toxicity.

Drug-herb. *Senna:* Blocked diarrheal effects. Avoid concomitant use.

Drug-lifestyle. *Alcohol:* Increased GI adverse effects. Discourage use.

Adverse reactions

P.O. and P.R. forms

CNS: headache, dizziness, depression, drowsiness, confusion, somnolence, fatigue, peripheral neuropathy, **seizures,** psychic disturbances, syncope, vertigo.

CV: hypertension, *edema,* **heart failure.**

EENT: blurred vision, corneal and retinal damage, hearing loss, tinnitus.

GI: nausea, anorexia, *diarrhea, peptic ulceration,* **GI bleeding,** constipation, dyspepsia, *pancreatitis.*

GU: hematuria, **acute renal failure,** proteinuria, interstitial nephritis.

Hematologic: *hemolytic anemia, aplastic anemia, agranulocytosis, leukopenia, thrombocytopenic purpura,* iron-deficiency anemia.

Metabolic: hyperkalemia.

Skin: pruritus, urticaria, *Stevens-Johnson syndrome.*

Other: hypersensitivity (rash, respiratory distress, **anaphylaxis, angioedema).**

proteinuria, interstitial nephritis, **renal fail-**

✓ Special considerations

Besides the recommendations relevant to all NSAIDs, consider the following.

● Don't mix oral suspension with liquids or antacids before administering.

● Patient should retain suppository in rectum for at least 1 hour after insertion to ensure maximum absorption.

● Reconstitute 1-mg vial of I.V. dose with 1 to 2 ml of sterile water for injection or normal saline injection. Prepare solution immediately before use to prevent deterioration. Don't use solution if discolored or contains a precipitate.

● Administer drug by direct I.V. injection over 5 to 10 seconds. Use a large vein to prevent extravasation.

● I.V. administration should be used only for premature neonates with patent ductus arteriosus. Don't administer a second or third I.V. dose if anuria or marked oliguria exists.

● If ductus arteriosus reopens, a second course of one to three doses may be given. If ineffective, surgery may be necessary.

● Signs and symptoms of overdose are dizziness, nausea, vomiting, intense headache, mental confusion, drowsiness, tinnitus, sweating, blurred vision, paresthesia, and seizures.

● To treat overdose, empty stomach immediately by inducing emesis with ipecac syrup or by gastric lavage. Administer activated charcoal via nasogastric tube.

Monitoring the patient

● Monitor I.V. site for complications.
● Monitor cardiopulmonary status for significant changes. Watch for signs and symptoms of fluid overload. Check weight and intake and output daily.
● Monitor renal function studies before start of therapy and frequently during therapy to prevent adverse effects.
● Severe headache may occur. If headache persists, decrease dose.
● Monitor carefully for bleeding and for reduced urine output.
● Observe patient for overdose.

Information for the patient

● Instruct patient in proper administration of dosage form prescribed, such as suppository, sustained-release capsule, or suspension.
● Advise patient to seek medical approval before taking OTC products.
● Caution patient to avoid hazardous activities that require alertness or concentration. Instruct him in safety measures to prevent injury.
● Tell patient to report signs and symptoms of adverse reactions. Encourage patient to adhere to prescribed drug regimen and recommended follow-up.

Geriatric patients
● Patients over age 60 may be more susceptible to toxic effects of indomethacin.
● The effect of drug on renal prostaglandins may cause fluid retention and edema, a significant drawback for elderly patients and those with heart failure.

Pediatric patients
● Safety of long-term drug use in children under age 14 hasn't been established.
● Use of I.V. indomethacin in premature infants for patent ductus arteriosus is considered an alternative to surgery.

Breast-feeding patients
● Drug appears in breast milk in levels similar to those in maternal plasma; avoid use in breast-feeding women.

---

infliximab
Remicade

Pharmacologic classification: mono-clonal antibody IgG1κ
Therapeutic classification: anti-inflammatory
Pregnancy risk category C

How supplied
Available by prescription only
Injection: 100 mg/20-ml vial

Indications, route, and dosage
Reduction of signs and symptoms in patients with moderately to severely active Crohn's disease with inadequate response to conventional therapy
Adults: 5 mg/kg single I.V. infusion over a period of not less than 2 hours.
Reduction in the number of draining enterocutaneous fistulas in patients with fistulizing Crohn's disease
Adults: 5 mg/kg I.V. infused over a period of not less than 2 hours. Additional doses of 5 mg/kg should be given at 2 and 6 weeks after initial infusion.

Pharmacodynamics
Anti-inflammatory action: Monoclonal antibody that binds to human tumor necrosis factor (TNF)-alpha to neutralize its activity and inhibit its binding with receptors reducing the infiltration of inflammatory cells and TNF-alpha production in inflamed areas of the intestine.

Pharmacokinetics
● *Absorption:* Administered I.V.; incomplete absorption.
● *Distribution:* No information available.
● *Metabolism:* No information available.

● *Excretion:* Terminal half-life is 9½ days.

Contraindications and precautions
Contraindicated in patients with hypersensitivity to murine proteins or other components of drug. Use with caution in elderly patients.

Interactions
None reported.

Adverse reactions
CNS: *headache, fatigue,* dizziness, malaise, insomnia.
CV: hypertension, hypotension, flushing, tachycardia, chest pain.
EENT: pharyngitis, rhinitis, sinusitis, conjunctivitis, toothache.
GI: *nausea, abdominal pain,* vomiting, constipation, dyspepsia, flatulence, intestinal obstruction, oral pain, ulcerative stomatitis.
GU: dysuria, increased micturition frequency.
Hematologic: anemia, hematoma, ecchymosis.
Hepatic: elevated liver enzyme levels.
Musculoskeletal: myalgia, arthralgia, arthritis, back pain.
Respiratory: *upper respiratory tract infections,* bronchitis, coughing, dyspnea, flu syndrome, respiratory tract allergic reaction.
Skin: rash, pruritus, candidiasis, acne, alopecia, eczema, erythema, erythematous rash, maculopapular rash, papular rash, dry skin, increased sweating, urticaria.
Other: *fever,* chills, pain, peripheral edema, hot flashes, abscess.

☑ Special considerations
● Drug may affect normal immune responses. Patient may develop autoimmune antibodies and lupus-like syndrome; drug therapy should be stopped. Symptoms can be expected to resolve.
● Some patients test positive for antinuclear antibody.
● Drug is incompatible with plasticized polyvinyl chloride equipment or devices; prepare only in glass infusion bottles or polypropylene or polyolefin infusion bags; administer through polyethylene-lined administration sets with an in-line, sterile, nonpyrogenic, low-protein-binding filter (pore size of 1.2 mm or less).
● Vials don't contain antibacterial preservatives; reconstituted dose should be used immediately. Reconstitute with 10 ml sterile water for injection using a syringe with a 21G or smaller nee~ Don't shake; gently swirl to dissolve powd~ lution should be colorless to light yel' opalescent; may develop a few trans' ticles. Don't use if other particles or is present.
● Dilute total volume of reconst~ ml with normal saline injecti~ tration range is 0.4 to 4 m~

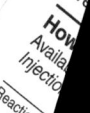

---

* Canada only

begin within 3 hours of preparation and must be administered over a period of not less than 2 hours.
● Don't infuse drug in same I.V. line with other drugs.

Monitoring the patient
● Watch for infusion-related reactions, such as fever, chills, pruritus, urticaria, dyspnea, hypotension, hypertension, and chest pain. If an infusion reaction occurs, stop drug and be prepared to give acetaminophen, antihistamines, corticosteroids, and epinephrine, as needed.
● Watch for development of lymphomas and infection. Patients with Crohn's disease of long duration and long-term exposure to immunosuppressive therapies are more prone to develop lymphomas and infections.

Information for the patient
● Tell patient about infusion-reaction symptoms and instruct him to report them if they occur.
● Inform patient of postinfusion side effects and instruct him to report them promptly.

Geriatric patients
● No information available regarding use in patients over age 65. Use with caution.

Pediatric patients
● Safety and efficacy in children haven't been established.

Breast-feeding patients
● It's unknown if drug appears in breast milk. Use cautiously; stop drug or breast-feeding, taking into account importance of drug to mother.

---

influenza virus vaccine, 2000–2001 trivalent types A & B (purified surface antigen)
Fluvirin

influenza virus vaccine, 2000–2001 trivalent types A & B (subvirion or purified subvirion)
Fluogen, FluShield, Fluzone

influenza virus vaccine, 2000–2001 trivalent types A & B (whole virion)
Fluzone

Pharmacologic classification: vaccine
Therapeutic classification: viral vaccine
Pregnancy risk category C

How supplied
Available by prescription only
Injection: 0.5-ml prefilled syringe; 5-ml vials

Indications, route, and dosage
Annual influenza prophylaxis in high-risk patients
Adults and children ages 13 and over: 0.5 ml I.M. (whole virus or split virus).
Children ages 9 to 12: 0.5 ml I.M. (split virus only).
Children ages 3 to 8: 0.5 ml I.M. (split virus only).
Infants and children ages 6 to 35 months: 0.25 ml I.M. (split virus only).
   Note: Second dose may be given in previously unvaccinated children under age 9 at least 1 month after first dose.
   Check package insert for annual changes and additional dosing recommendations.

Pharmacodynamics
Influenza prophylaxis: Promotes active immunity to influenza by inducing antibody production. Protection is provided only against those strains of virus from which the vaccine is prepared (or closely related strains).

Pharmacokinetics
● *Absorption:* Duration of immunity varies widely, but usually lasts about 1 year.
● *Distribution:* No information available.
● *Metabolism:* No information available.
● *Excretion:* No information available.

Contraindications and precautions
Contraindicated in patients with hypersensitivity to chicken eggs or any component of the vaccine such as thimerosal. Defer vaccination in patients with acute respiratory tract or other active infection and delay immunization in those with an active neurologic disorder.

Interactions
Drug-drug. *Aminopyrine, phenytoin:* Decreased serum levels of these drugs. Monitor serum levels.
Corticosteroids, immunosuppressants: May impair immune response to vaccine. Monitor patient closely.
Theophylline: Increased serum levels of theophylline. Monitor theophylline level.
Warfarin: Prolonged PT, GI bleeding, transient gross hematuria, and epistaxis. Monitor PT and INR; observe patient for signs of bleeding.

Adverse reactions
CNS: malaise.
Musculoskeletal: myalgia.
Skin: erythema, induration, *soreness at injection site.*
Other: *anaphylaxis,* fever.

☑ Special considerations
● Annual influenza prophylaxis is recommended for elderly patients and for adults and children with chronic CV, pulmonary, or renal disorders;

---

may be common, uncommon, life-threatening, or COMMON AND LIFE-THREATENING.

metabolic disease; severe anemia; or compromised immune function. Vaccine also is recommended for medical personnel who have extensive contact with high-risk patients, residents of nursing homes or other long-term care facilities, and teenagers or children (ages 6 months through 18 years) who are receiving long-term aspirin therapy and may be at risk for Reye's syndrome after influenza. Also, vaccine should be given to persons who wish to reduce their risk of acquiring influenza infection.

• Obtain thorough history of allergies, especially to eggs or chicken feathers, and of reactions to previous immunizations.

• Patients with a known or suspected hypersensitivity to egg protein should have a skin test to assess sensitivity to vaccine. Administer a scratch test with 0.05 to 0.1 ml of a 1:100 dilution in normal saline solution for injection. Patients with positive skin test reactions shouldn't receive vaccine.

• Have epinephrine solution 1:1,000 available to treat allergic reactions.

• Don't administer influenza vaccine to patients with active influenza infection. Such infection should be treated with amantadine.

• Preferred I.M. injection site is deltoid muscle in adults and older children and anterolateral thigh in infants and young children.

• To reduce frequency of adverse reactions, use only split-virus or purified surface antigen vaccine in children.

• Pneumococcal vaccine, DTP, or live attenuated measles virus vaccine may be given simultaneously but at a different injection site.

• Store vaccine between 36° and 46° F (2° and 8° C). Don't freeze.

Monitoring the patient
• Monitor patient for adverse reactions. Fever and malaise reactions occur most often in children and in others not exposed to other influenza viruses. Severe reactions in adults are rare.

• Observe patient for signs of allergy or anaphylaxis.

Information for the patient
• Tell patient that he may experience discomfort at injection site after immunization; he also may develop fever, malaise, and muscle aches 6 to 12 hours after vaccination that may persist for several days. Recommend acetaminophen to alleviate these effects.

• Encourage patient to report distressing adverse reactions promptly.

• Warn patient that many cases of Guillain-Barré syndrome were reported after vaccination for swine flu of 1976. This condition usually causes reversible paralysis and muscle weakness but can be fatal in some individuals. Influenza vaccines made after 1976 haven't been associated with as high a risk of Guillain-Barré syndrome, but condition still occurs, albeit rarely. Patients with history of Guillain-Barré syndrome have a greater risk for repeat episodes.

• Tell patient that he will need to be vaccinated annually.

Geriatric patients
• Annual vaccination is highly recommended for patients over age 65.

Pediatric patients
• Influenza vaccine is contraindicated in children under age 6 months.

Breast-feeding patients
• Breast-feeding isn't a contraindication for receiving vaccine.

---

insulin (regular)
Humulin-R, Novolin R, Novolin R PenFill, Regular Iletin I, Regular (Concentrated) Iletin II, Regular Insulin, Regular Purified Pork Insulin, Velosulin Human

insulin (lispro)
Humalog

isophane insulin suspension (NPH)
Humulin N, NPH Iletin*, NPH Iletin I, NPH Insulin*, NPH-N, Novolin N, Novolin N PenFill

insulin zinc suspension (lente)
Humulin L, Lente Iletin I, Lente Iletin II, Lente L, Novolin L

extended zinc insulin suspension (ultralente)
Humulin U Ultralente, Ultralente*

isophane insulin suspension and insulin injection (70% isophane insulin and 30% insulin injection)
Humulin 70/30, Novolin 70/30, Novolin 70/30 PenFill

isophane insulin suspension and ir injection (50% is

 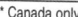

insulin and 50% insulin injection)
Humulin 50/50

Pharmacologic classification: pancreatic hormone
Therapeutic classification: antidiabetic
Pregnancy risk category NR

How supplied
Available by prescription only
insulin (lispro)
Injection (human): 100 units/ml
Cartridge (human): 1.5 ml
regular (concentrated) Iletin II insulin
Injection (pork): 500 units/ml
Available without a prescription
insulin (regular)
Injection (pork): 100 units/ml
Injection (human): 100 units/ml
isophane insulin suspension (NPH)
Injection (pork): 100 units/ml
Injection (human): 100 units/ml
insulin zinc suspension (lente)
Injection (pork): 100 units/ml
Injection (human): 100 units/ml
extended zinc insulin suspension (ultralente)
Injection (human): 100 units/ml

Indications, route, and dosage
Diabetic ketoacidosis (regular insulin)
Adults: Administer loading dose of 0.15 units/kg I.V., then 0.1 units/kg/hour as a continuous infusion. Rate of insulin infusion should be decreased when plasma glucose level reaches 300 mg/dl. Infusion of D_5W should be started separately from the insulin infusion when plasma glucose reaches 250 mg/dl. Thirty minutes before discontinuing insulin infusion, a dose of insulin should be administered S.C.; intermediate-acting insulin is recommended.

Alternative dosage schedule is 50 to 100 units I.V. and 50 to 100 units S.C. immediately; subsequent doses should be based on therapeutic response and glucose, acetone, or ketone levels monitored at 1- to 2-hour intervals, or 2.4 to 7.2 units I.V. loading dose, then 2.4 to 7.2 units/hour.
Children: 0.5 to 1 unit/kg in two divided doses, one given I.V. and the other S.C., then 0.5 to 1 unit/kg I.V. q 1 to 2 hours; or 0.1 unit/kg I.V. bolus, then 0.1 unit/kg/hour continuous I.V. infusion until serum glucose level decreases to 250 mg/dl; then start S.C. insulin.

Ketosis-prone and type 1 diabetes mellitus, diabetes mellitus inadequately controlled by diet and oral antidiabetics
Adults and children: Individualized dosage adjusted based on patient's blood and urine glucose levels.

Hyperkalemia
...to 10 units of regular insulin with 50 ml ...er 5 minutes. Or 25 units of regular in-

sulin given S.C. and an infusion of 1,000 ml dextrose 10% in water with 90 mEq sodium bicarbonate; infuse 330 ml over 30 minutes and the balance over 3 hours.
Provocative test for growth hormone secretion
Adults: Rapid I.V. injection of regular insulin 0.05 to 0.15 units/kg.

Pharmacodynamics
Antidiabetic action: Used as a replacement for the physiologic production of endogenous insulin in patients with type 1 diabetes mellitus and diabetes mellitus inadequately controlled by diet and oral hypoglycemic drugs. Insulin increases glucose transport across muscle and fat-cell membranes to reduce blood glucose levels. It also promotes conversion of glucose to its storage form, glycogen; triggers amino acid uptake and conversion to protein in muscle cells and inhibits protein degradation; stimulates triglyceride formation and inhibits release of free fatty acids from adipose tissue; and stimulates lipoprotein lipase activity, which converts circulating lipoproteins to fatty acids. Insulin is available in various forms and these differ mainly in onset, peak, and duration of action. Characteristics of the various insulin preparations are compared in chart on page 563.

Pharmacokinetics
• *Absorption:* Must be given parenterally because it's destroyed in GI tract. Preparations are formulated to differ in onset, peak, and duration after subcutaneous administration. Classified as rapid-acting (½ to 1-hour onset), intermediate-acting (1- to 2-hour onset), and long-acting (4- to 8-hour onset). Accompanying chart summarizes major pharmacokinetic differences.
• *Distribution:* Distributed widely throughout body.
• *Metabolism:* Some insulin is bound and inactivated by peripheral tissues, but the majority appears to be degraded in the liver and kidneys.
• *Excretion:* Insulin is filtered by the renal glomeruli and undergoes some tubular reabsorption. Plasma half-life is about 9 minutes after I.V. administration.

Contraindications and precautions
None known.

Interactions
Drug-drug. *Anabolic steroids, beta blockers, clofibrate, fenfluramine, MAO inhibitors, salicylates, tetracycline:* Prolonged hypoglycemic effect. Monitor blood glucose levels carefully.
Corticosteroids, dextrothyroxine sodium, epinephrine, thiazide diuretics: Diminished insulin response. Watch for hyperglycemia.

COMPARING INSULIN PREPARATIONS

The table below lists the various forms of insulin and their times of onset, peak, and duration. Individual responses can vary.

Preparation	Purified†	Onset (hr)	Peak (hr)	Duration (hr)
Rapid-acting insulins				
insulin injection (regular, crystalline zinc)				
Regular Insulin	No	½	2½ to 5	8 hr
Pork Regular Iletin II	Yes	½	2 to 4	6 to 8
Velosulin BR Human	Yes	½	1 to 3	8
Regular Purified Pork Insulin	Yes	½	2½ to 5	8
Humulin R	Not applicable	½	2 to 4	6 to 8
Novolin R/Novolin R PenFill	Not applicable	½	2½ to 5	8
insulin injection (lispro)				
Humalog	Yes	< ½	½ to 1½	< 6
Intermediate-acting Insulins				
isophane insulin suspension (NPH)				
NPH	No	1½	4 to 12	24
Pork NPH Iletin II	Yes	1 to 2	6 to 12	18 to 24
Humulin N	Not applicable	1 to 2	6 to 12	18 to 24
Novolin N/Novolin N PenFill	Not applicable	1½	4 to 12	24
insulin zinc suspension (lente)				
Lente Iletin II	Yes	1 to 3	6 to 12	18 to 24
Lente L	Yes	2½	7 to 15	22
Humulin L	Not applicable	1 to 3	6 to 12	18 to 24
Novolin L	Not applicable	2½	7 to 15	22
isophane (NPH) 70%, regular insulin 30%				
Humulin 70/30	Not applicable	½	4 to 8	24
Novolin 70/30/Novolin 70/30 PenFill	Not applicable	½	2 to 12	24
isophane (NPH) 50%, regular insulin 50%				
Humulin 50/50	Not applicable	½	4 to 8	24
Long-acting insulins				
extended insulin zinc suspension (ultralente)				
Ultralente	No	4	10 to 30	36
Humulin U Ultralente	Yes	4 to 6	8 to 20	24 to 28

† Contain < 10 ppm proinsulin.

Drug-herb. *Basil, bay, bee pollen, burdock, ginseng, glucomannan, horehound, marsh mallow, myrrh, sage:* May affect glycemic control. Monitor blood glucose levels carefully and avoid use together.
Garlic dust, ginseng: May decrease blood glucose levels. Monitor blood glucose levels.

Drug-lifestyle. *Alcohol:* Possible prolonged hypoglycemic effect. Discourage use and encourage careful monitoring of blood glucose levels. Discourage use.
Marijuana: Possible increased serum glucose levels. Discourage use.
Smoking: Decreases absorption of insulin administered S.C. Advise patient to avoid smoking within 30 minutes of insulin injection.

Adverse reactions

Skin: urticaria, pruritus, swelling, redness, stinging, warmth at injection site.

Other: *lipoatrophy, lipohypertrophy,* hypersensitivity reactions *(anaphylaxis,* rash), *hypoglycemia,* hyperglycemia (rebound, or Somogyi, effect).

☑ Special considerations

• Accuracy of measurement is very important, especially with regular insulin concentrated. Aids, such as magnifying sleeve, dose magnifier, or cornwall syringe, may help improve accuracy.
• With regular insulin concentrated, a secondary hypoglycemic reaction may occur 18 to 24 hours after injection. This may be caused by a repository effect of drug and the high concentration of insulin in the preparation (500 units/ml).
• Dosage is always expressed in USP units.
• Human insulin may benefit patients with type 2 diabetes mellitus who need intermittent or short-term therapy (such as for pregnancy, surgery, infection, or total parenteral nutrition therapy), patients with insulin resistance, or those who develop lipoatrophy.
• Lente and ultralente insulins may be mixed in any proportion.
• Regular insulin may be mixed with NPH or lente insulins in any proportion. However, in vitro binding will occur over time until an equilibrium is reached. These mixtures should be administered either immediately after preparation or after stability occurs (15 minutes for NPH regular, 24 hours for lente regular) in order to minimize variability in patient response. Switching from separate injections to a prepared mixture also may alter patient's response. When mixing two insulins, always draw regular insulin into syringe first.
• Lispro insulin may be mixed with Humulin N or Humulin U and should be given within 15 minutes before a meal to prevent a hypoglycemic reaction. The effects of mixing lispro insulin with pork insulin or insulin preparations produced by other manufacturers haven't been studied; a change in dosage may be needed.
• Store insulin in cool area. Refrigeration desirable but not essential, except with regular insulin concentrated.
• Don't use insulin that has changed color or becomes clumped or granular in appearance.
• Check expiration date on vial before using.
• Administration route is S.C. because it allows slower absorption and causes less pain than I.M. injections. Patients with type 1 diabetes mellitus and ketosis-prone, severely ill, and newly diagnosed diabetics with very high blood glucose levels may need hospitalization and I.V. treatment with regular fast-acting insulin. Ketosis-resistant diabetics may be treated as outpatients with intermediate-acting insulin after they have received instructions on how to alter dosage according to self-performed urine or blood glucose determinations. Some patients, primarily pregnant or brittle diabetics, may use a dextrometer to perform fingerstick blood glucose tests at home.
• Press but don't rub site after injection. Rotate injection sites. Record sites to avoid overuse of one area. However, unstable diabetics may achieve better control if injection site is rotated within same anatomic region.
• To mix insulin suspension, swirl vial gently or rotate between palms or between palm and thigh. Don't shake vigorously; this causes bubbling and air in syringe.
• In pregnant diabetic patients, insulin requirements increase, sometimes drastically, then decline immediately postpartum.
• Some patients may develop insulin resistance and need large insulin doses to control symptoms of diabetes. U-500 insulin is available for such patients as Purified Pork Iletin Regular Insulin, U-500. Although every pharmacy may not normally stock it, it's readily available. Patient should notify pharmacist several days before prescription refill is needed. Give hospital pharmacy sufficient notice before refill of inhouse prescription. Never store U-500 insulin in same area with other insulin preparations because of danger of severe overdose if given accidentally to other patients. U-500 insulin must be administered with a U-100 syringe because no syringes are made for this drug.
• Human insulin may help patients who are allergic to pork form. Humulin is synthesized by a genetically altered strain of *Escherichia coli.* Novolin brands are derived by enzymatic alteration of pork insulin.
• Treatment of overdose is directed toward treating hypoglycemia and is based on patient's symptoms. (If patient is responsive, give 10 to 15 g of a fast-acting oral carbohydrate. If patient's signs and symptoms persist after 15 minutes, give an additional 10 g carbohydrate. If patient is unresponsive, an I.V. bolus of dextrose 50% solution should immediately increase blood glucose.)

Monitoring the patient

• Monitor patient for insulin overdose, including signs and symptoms of hypoglycemia (tachycardia, palpitations, anxiety, hunger, nausea, diaphoresis, tremors, pallor, restlessness, headache, and speech and motor dysfunction).
• Monitor serum glucose levels.

Information for the patient

• Be sure patient knows that insulin therapy relieves symptoms but doesn't cure disease.
• Tell patient about nature of disease; importance of following therapeutic regimen, including specific diet, weight reduction, exercise, and personal hygiene; importance of avoiding infection; and timing of injection and eating.
• Instruct patient to strictly adhere to manufacturer's instructions regarding assembly, admin-

---

Reactions may be *common,* uncommon, **life-threatening,** or COMMON AND LIFE-THREATENING.

istration, and care of specialized delivery systems such as insulin pumps.
• Emphasize importance of regular meal times; don't skip meals.
• Teach patient that blood glucose monitoring is an essential guide to correct dosage and to therapeutic success.
• Emphasize importance of recognizing hypoglycemic symptoms because insulin-induced hypoglycemia is hazardous and may cause brain damage if prolonged.
• Advise patient to always wear a medical identification bracelet or pendant, to carry ample insulin supply and syringes on trips, to have carbohydrates (sugar or candy) on hand for emergency, and to note time-zone changes for dose schedule when traveling.
• Instruct patient not to change order of mixing insulins or change model or brand of syringe or needle. Be sure he knows that, when mixing two insulins, he should always draw regular insulin into syringe first.

interferon alfa-2a, recombinant
Roferon-A

interferon alfa-2b, recombinant
Intron A

Pharmacologic classification: biological response modifier
Therapeutic classification: antineoplastic
Pregnancy risk category C

How supplied
Available by prescription only
alfa-2a
Solution for injection: 3 million IU/vial, 9 million IU/vial, 9 million IU/multidose vial, 18 million IU/multidose vial, 36 million IU/multidose vial
Powder for injection with diluent: 18 million IU/multidose vial
alfa-2b
Powder for injection with diluent: 3 million IU/vial; 5 million IU/vial; 10 million IU/vial; 18 million IU/multidose vial; 25 million IU/vial; 50 million IU/vial
Solution for injection: 10 million IU/vial, 18 million IU/multidose vial, 25 million IU/vial

Indications, route, and dosage
Hairy cell leukemia
alfa-2a
Adults: For induction, 3 million IU S.C. or I.M. daily for 16 to 24 weeks. For maintenance, 3 million IU S.C. or I.M. three times weekly.
alfa-2b
Adults: For induction and maintenance, 2 million IU/m² I.M. or S.C. three times weekly.

Condylomata acuminata
alfa-2b
Adults: 1 million IU per lesion, intralesionally, three times weekly for 3 weeks.
Kaposi's sarcoma
alfa-2a
Adults: For induction, 36 million IU S.C. or I.M. daily for 10 to 12 weeks; for maintenance, 36 million IU three times weekly.
alfa-2b
Adults: 30 million IU/m² S.C. or I.M. three times weekly. Maintain dose unless disease progresses rapidly or intolerance occurs.
Chronic hepatitis C
Adults: 3 million IU (alfa-2b) S.C. or I.M. three times weekly. If response occurs, continue therapy for 6 months. If no response by 16 weeks, stop therapy.
Chronic hepatitis B
Adults: 30 to 35 million IU (alfa-2b) S.C. or I.M. weekly either as 5 million IU daily or 10 million IU three times weekly for 16 weeks.

Pharmacodynamics
Antineoplastic action: A sterile protein product produced by recombinant DNA techniques applied to genetically engineered *Escherichia coli* bacteria. The interferons are naturally occurring small protein molecules produced and secreted by cells in response to viral infections or synthetic and biological inducers. Their exact mechanism of action is unknown but appears to involve direct antiproliferative action against tumor cells or viral cells to inhibit replication and modulation of host immune response by enhancing the phagocytic activity of macrophages and augmenting specific cytotoxicity of lymphocytes for target cells. To date, three major classes of interferons have been identified: alfa, beta, and gamma.

Pharmacokinetics
• *Absorption:* More than 80% of dose absorbed after I.M. or S.C. injection.
• *Distribution:* Not applicable.
• *Metabolism:* Appears to be metabolized in liver and kidney.
• *Excretion:* Reabsorbed from glomerular filtrate with minor biliary elimination.

Contraindications and precautions
Contraindicated in patients with hypersensitivity to drug or to murine (mouse) immunoglobulin. Use cautiously in patients with CV or pulmonary disease, diabetes mellitus, coagulation disorders, or myelosuppression.

Interactions
Drug-drug. *Blood dyscrasia–causing drugs, bone marrow depressant therapy, radiation therapy:* Increased bone marrow depressant effects. Dosage reduction may be needed.

CNS depressants: Enhanced CNS effects. Avoid concomitant use.

Live virus vaccines: Increased adverse effects; decreased patient antibody response. Defer immunization if possible.

Methylxanthines: Interferon may substantially increase half-life. Monitor patient closely.

Drug-lifestyle. *Alcohol:* Increased risk of GI bleeding. Discourage concomitant use.

Adverse reactions

CNS: *dizziness, confusion,* paresthesia, numbness, lethargy, *depression, decreased mental status,* forgetfulness, ***coma,*** nervousness, insomnia, sedation, apathy, anxiety, irritability, fatigue, vertigo, gait disturbances, incoordination.
CV: hypotension, chest pain, ***arrhythmias,*** palpitations, syncope, ***heart failure,*** hypertension, edema, ***MI.***
EENT: *dryness or inflammation of the oropharynx,* rhinorrhea, sinusitis, conjunctivitis, earache, eye irritation.
GI: *anorexia, nausea, diarrhea, vomiting,* abdominal fullness, *abdominal pain,* flatulence, constipation, hypermotility, gastric distress, *weight loss, change in taste.*
GU: transient impotence.
Hematologic: *leukopenia, mild thrombocytopenia.*
Hepatic: *hepatitis.*
Respiratory: *cough, dyspnea.*
Skin: diaphoresis, *rash, dryness, pruritus, partial alopecia,* urticaria, flushing.
Other: *flulike syndrome (fever, fatigue, myalgia, headache, chills, arthralgia),* excessive salivation, cyanosis, night sweats, hot flashes.

☑ Special considerations

• When preparing antineoplastics for injection, take special precautions because of their potential for carcinogenicity and mutagenicity. Use of a biological containment cabinet is recommended. Don't shake vials.
• Use S.C. administration route in patients whose platelet count is below 50,000/mm³.
• Different brands of interferons may not be therapeutically interchangeable.
• Almost all patients experience flulike symptoms at start of therapy; however, they diminish with continued therapy.
• Make sure patient is well hydrated, especially during initial stages of treatment. Premedicate patient with acetaminophen to minimize flulike symptoms.
• Dosage reduction may be needed if headache persists. Hypotension may result from fluid depletion; may require supportive treatment.
• Administration of drug at bedtime minimizes inconvenience of fatigue.
• When using interferon alfa-2b for condylomata acuminata by intralesional injection, use only the 10 million-IU vial reconstituted with 1 ml of

diluent. Using other strengths or more diluent would produce a hypertonic solution. For administration, use a 25G to 30G needle and a tuberculin syringe. Up to five lesions may be treated simultaneously.
• The following indications aren't included in U.S. labeling, but drug may be used for these applications: chronic myelocytic leukemia; treatment of renal carcinoma or superficial bladder carcinoma; treatment of malignant lymphomas, especially nodular, poorly differentiated types; malignant melanoma; multiple myeloma; mycosis fungoides; papillomas; and laryngeal papillomatosis (interferon alfa-2b).

Monitoring the patient

• Monitor blood pressure, hematocrit, platelet count, total and differential leukocyte count, ECG, and BUN, ALT, AST, LD, alkaline phosphatase, serum bilirubin, creatinine, and uric acid levels.
• Watch for CNS adverse reactions, such as decreased mental status and dizziness. Periodic neuropsychiatric monitoring is recommended.
• Special precautions are needed for patients who develop thrombocytopenia: exercise extreme care in performing invasive procedures; inspect injection site and skin frequently for signs of bruising; limit frequency of I.M. injections; test urine, emesis fluid, stool, and secretions for occult blood.

Information for the patient

• Review patient instruction sheet if patient is to self-administer to ensure patient understanding of when and how to take drug. Stress importance of drinking extra fluids to prevent hypotension from fluid loss.
• Instruct patient in proper oral hygiene during treatment; drug's bone marrow depressant effects may increase risk of microbial infection, delayed healing, and gingival bleeding. Salivary flow may also decrease.
• Advise patient not to take a missed dose or to double next dose, but to call for further instructions.
• If patient is to self-administer drug, teach him to prepare injection, how to use disposable syringe, proper administration technique, and stability of drug.
• Inform patient to store drug in refrigerator; don't freeze.
• Caution patient against driving or performing tasks requiring alertness until response to drug is known.
• Advise patient to seek medical approval before taking OTC preparations for colds, coughs, allergies, and similar disorders; explain that interferons commonly cause flulike symptoms and patient may need to take acetaminophen before each dose.
• Emphasize need to follow instructions about taking and recording temperature, and how and when to take acetaminophen; not to have any im-

munization; and to avoid contact with persons who have taken oral polio vaccine. Because the body's resistance may be compromised, infection may occur.
• Tell patient drug may cause temporary loss of some hair. Normal hair growth should return when therapy ends.
• Inform patient to avoid aspirin and prolonged alcohol intake; may increase risk of GI bleeding.

Geriatric patients
• Neurotoxicity and cardiotoxicity are more common in elderly patients, especially those with underlying CNS or cardiac impairment.

Pediatric patients
• Safety and efficacy in children under age 18 haven't been established.

Breast-feeding patients
• Consider risk-to-benefit ratio. Drug usually isn't recommended in breast-feeding women because of potential for serious adverse effects in infants.

interferon beta-1a
Avonex

Pharmacologic classification: biological response modifier
Therapeutic classification: antiviral, immunoregulator
Pregnancy risk category C

How supplied
Available by prescription only
Lyophilized powder for injection: 33 mcg (6.6 million IU)

Indications, route, and dosage
To slow progression of physical disability and decrease the frequency of clinical exacerbations in relapsing multiple sclerosis
Adults: 30 mcg I.M. once weekly.

Pharmacodynamics
Antiviral and immunoregulator actions: Mechanisms by which interferon beta-1a exerts its actions in multiple sclerosis aren't clearly understood. However, it's known that the biological response-modifying properties of interferon beta-1a are mediated through its interactions with specific cell receptors found on the surface of human cells. The binding to these receptors induces the expression of a number of interferon-induced gene products that are believed to be the mediators of the biological actions of interferon beta-1a.

Pharmacokinetics
No information available.

Contraindications and precautions
Contraindicated in patients with history of hypersensitivity to natural or recombinant interferon beta, human albumin, or any other component of the formulation. Use cautiously in patients with depression, seizure disorders, or severe cardiac conditions.

Interactions
None reported.

Adverse reactions
CNS: malaise, *asthenia, headache, sleep difficulty, dizziness,* syncope, suicidal tendency, *seizures,* speech disorder, ataxia.
CV: chest pain, vasodilation.
EENT: otitis media, decreased hearing.
GI: *nausea, diarrhea, dyspepsia,* anorexia, abdominal pain.
GU: ovarian cyst, vaginitis.
Hematologic: anemia, elevated eosinophil levels, decreased hematocrit.
Hepatic: elevated AST levels.
Musculoskeletal: *muscle ache,* muscle spasm, arthralgia.
Respiratory: *upper respiratory tract infection,* sinusitis, dyspnea.
Skin: ecchymosis at injection site, injection site reaction, urticaria, alopecia, nevus, herpes zoster, herpes simplex.
Other: *flulike symptoms, pain, fever, chills, infection, hypersensitivity reaction.*

☑ Special considerations
• Safety and efficacy of interferon beta-1a in chronic progressive multiple sclerosis haven't been evaluated.
• Use of interferon beta-1a may cause depression and suicidal ideation. Not known whether these symptoms may be related to the underlying neurologic basis of multiple sclerosis, to interferon beta-1a treatment, or to a combination of both. Closely monitor patient for symptoms and consider stopping therapy if symptoms occur.
• To reconstitute drug, inject 1.1 ml of supplied diluent (sterile water for injection) into vial and gently swirl to dissolve drug. Don't shake.
• Use drug as soon as possible or within 6 hours after being reconstituted if stored at 36° to 46° F (2° to 8° C).
• Store drug vials in refrigerator. If refrigeration is unavailable, drug can be stored at 77° F (25° C) for up to 30 days. Don't expose drug to high temperatures or freezing.

Monitoring the patient
• Monitor patient with cardiac disease, such as angina, heart failure, or arrhythmia, for worsening of condition during initiation of therapy. Although drug doesn't cause any known direct-acting cardiac toxicity, it does cause flulike symp-

toms, which may be stressful to patients with severe cardiac conditions.
• The following laboratory tests are recommended before therapy starts and at periodic intervals thereafter: Complete and differential WBC counts, platelet counts, and blood chemistries, including liver function tests.

Information for the patient
• Teach patient or family member how to administer I.M. injections, including solution preparation, use of aseptic technique, rotation of injection sites, and equipment disposal. Periodically reevaluate patient's or family member's technique.
• Caution patient not to change dosage or administration schedule. If a dose is missed, tell him to take it as soon as he remembers, then resume regular schedule. Tell him that two injections shouldn't be administered within 2 days of each other.
• Inform patient that flulike symptoms are common following start of therapy. Recommend acetaminophen to relieve symptoms.
• Advise patient to report depression, suicidal ideation, or other adverse reactions.
• Tell patient to keep syringes and needles away from children. Also instruct patient not to reuse needles or syringes and to discard them in a syringe disposal unit.
• Advise woman of childbearing age not to become pregnant while taking interferon beta-1a because of the abortifacient potential of drug. If pregnancy does occur, instruct her to stop drug and call immediately.

Pediatric patients
• Safety and effectiveness in children under age 18 haven't been established.

Breast-feeding patients
• It's unknown if drug appears in breast milk. Because of potential for serious adverse reactions in breast-fed infants, stop either breast-feeding or therapy.

interferon beta-1b
Betaseron

Pharmacologic classification: biological response modifier
Therapeutic classification: antiviral, immunoregulator
Pregnancy risk category C

How supplied
Available by prescription only
Powder for injection, lyophilized: 9.6 million IU (0.3 mg)

Indications, route, and dosage
Reduction of the frequency of exacerbations in relapsing-remitting multiple sclerosis
Adults: 8 million IU (0.25 mg) S.C. every other day.

Pharmacodynamics
Antiviral and immunoregulator actions: Exact mechanisms by which interferon beta-1b exerts its actions in multiple sclerosis aren't known. However, it's known that the biological response-modifying properties of interferon beta-1b are mediated through its interactions with specific cell receptors found on the surface of human cells. The binding to these receptors induces the expression of a number of interferon-induced gene products that are believed to be the mediators of the biological actions of interferon beta-1b.

Pharmacokinetics
• *Absorption:* Serum levels undetectable after recommended dose; after higher doses, serum levels peak within 1 to 8 hours after S.C. administration.
• *Distribution:* No information available.
• *Metabolism:* No information available.
• *Excretion:* No information available on patients with multiple sclerosis; in healthy patients, elimination half-life ranged from 8 minutes to 4 hours.

Contraindications and precautions
Contraindicated in patients with hypersensitivity to interferon beta or human albumin. Use cautiously in women of childbearing age.

Interactions
Drug-lifestyle. *Sun exposure:* Potential photosensitivity reactions. Tell patient to take precautions.

Adverse reactions
CNS: *malaise,* depression, anxiety, emotional lability, depersonalization, **suicidal tendencies,** confusion, somnolence, *hypertonia, asthenia, migraine,* **seizures,** *headache, dizziness.*
CV: palpitations, hypertension, tachycardia, peripheral vascular disorder, **hemorrhage.**
EENT: laryngitis, *sinusitis, conjunctivitis,* abnormal vision.
GI: *diarrhea, constipation, abdominal pain, vomiting.*
GU: *menstrual disorders (bleeding or spotting, early or delayed menses, fewer days of menstrual flow, menorrhagia).*
Hematologic: *decreased WBC and absolute neutrophil counts.*
Hepatic: *elevated ALT and bilirubin levels.*
Respiratory: dyspnea.
Skin: *inflammation, pain, and necrosis at injection site, alopecia.*
Other: *flulike symptoms (fever, chills, myalgia, diaphoresis);* breast pain, *pelvic pain; lymph-*

Reactions may be *common,* uncommon, **life-threatening**, or COMMON AND LIFE-THREATENING.

adenopathy, generalized edema, *myasthenia, diaphoresis,* Cushing's syndrome, diabetes insipidus, diabetes mellitus, hypothyroidism, SIADH secretion.

☑ Special considerations
● Drug is being investigated for unlabeled uses in treatment of AIDS, AIDS-related Kaposi's sarcoma, metastatic renal-cell carcinoma, malignant melanoma, cutaneous T-cell lymphoma, and acute hepatitis C.
● Safety and efficacy in chronic progressive multiple sclerosis haven't been evaluated.
● Drug use may cause depression and suicidal ideation. Other mental disorders have been observed and include anxiety, emotional lability, depersonalization, and confusion. It's not known if these symptoms are related to the underlying neurologic basis of multiple sclerosis, to interferon beta-1b treatment, or to a combination of both. Closely monitor patient with these symptoms and consider stopping therapy.
● Having patient take drug at bedtime may minimize mild flulike symptoms that commonly occur.
● To reconstitute, inject 1.2 ml of supplied diluent (0.45% saline injection) into vial and gently swirl to dissolve drug. Don't shake. Reconstituted solution will contain 8 million IU (0.25 mg)/ml. Discard vial containing particulate material or discolored solution.
● Drug should be injected immediately after preparation.
● Refrigerate drug or reconstituted product (up to 3 hours) at 36° to 46° F (2° to 8° C). Don't freeze.

Monitoring the patient
● Perform the following laboratory tests before therapy starts and at periodic intervals thereafter: hemoglobin, complete and differential WBC counts, platelet counts, and blood chemistries, including liver function tests.
● Monitor patient for depression and suicidal behavior.

Information for the patient
● Teach patient how to self-administer S.C. injections, including solution preparation, use of aseptic technique, rotation of injection sites, and equipment disposal. Periodically reevaluate patient's technique.
● Instruct patient to rotate injection sites to minimize local reactions.
● Inform patient that flulike symptoms are common when therapy starts. Recommend taking drug at bedtime to help minimize symptoms.
● Caution patient not to change dosage or schedule of administration without medical consultation.
● Advise patient to report depression or suicidal ideation.
● Inform woman of childbearing age about drug's abortifacient potential.

Pediatric patients
● Safety and efficacy in children under age 18 haven't been established.

Breast-feeding patients
● It's unknown if drug appears in breast milk. Because of potential for serious adverse reactions in breast-fed infants, either stop breast-feeding or drug, taking into account importance of drug to mother.

ipecac syrup

Pharmacologic classification: alkaloid emetic
Therapeutic classification: emetic
Pregnancy risk category C

How supplied
Available with and without a prescription
Syrup: 70 mg powdered ipecac/ml

Indications, route, and dosage
To induce vomiting in poisoning
Adults: 15 to 30 ml P.O.; then 200 to 300 ml of water.
Children ages 1 and older: 15 ml P.O.; then 200 ml of water.
Children under age 1: 5 to 10 ml P.O.; then 100 to 200 ml of water.
    May repeat dose once after 20 minutes, if needed.

Pharmacodynamics
Emetic action: Directly irritates the GI mucosa and directly stimulates the chemoreceptor trigger zone through the effects of emetine and cephalin, its two alkaloids.

Pharmacokinetics
● *Absorption:* Absorbed in significant amounts mainly when it doesn't produce emesis. Onset of action usually occurs in 20 minutes.
● *Distribution:* No information available.
● *Metabolism:* No information available.
● *Excretion:* Emetine excreted in urine slowly, over a period lasting up to 60 days. Duration of effect is 20 to 25 minutes.

Contraindications and precautions
Contraindicated in semicomatose or unconscious patients and those with severe inebriation, seizures, shock, or loss of gag reflex. Don't give after ingestion of gasoline, kerosene, volatile oils, or caustic substances (lye).

Interactions
Drug-drug. *Activated charcoal:* May inactivate ipecac syrup. Don't give together; may give activated charcoal after vomiting.

Antiemetics: May decrease ipecac syrup's therapeutic effect. Don't give together.
Drug-food. *Carbonated beverages:* May cause abdominal distention. Avoid use together.
Milk (or milk products): May decrease ipecac syrup's therapeutic effect. Don't give together.
Vegetable oil: Delayed absorption. Don't use together.

Adverse reactions
CNS: depression, *drowsiness.*
CV: *arrhythmias, bradycardia,* hypotension; atrial fibrillation, *fatal myocarditis* (with excessive doses).
GI: diarrhea.

☑ Special considerations
• Administer ipecac syrup before giving activated charcoal, not after. Follow dose with 1 or 2 glasses of water. If vomiting doesn't occur after second dose, give activated charcoal to adsorb both ipecac syrup and ingested poison. Follow with gastric lavage.
• Inspect emesis for ingested substances, such as tablets or capsules.
• In over 90% of patients, ipecac syrup empties stomach completely within 30 minutes (average emptying time is 20 minutes).
• Don't confuse ipecac syrup with ipecac fluid extract, which is rarely used but 14 times more potent. Never store these two drugs together—the wrong drug could cause death.
• In antiemetic toxicity, ipecac syrup is usually effective if less than 1 hour has passed since ingestion of antiemetic.
• Little if any systemic toxicity occurs with doses of 30 ml or less.
• Drug may be abused by patients with eating disorders (such as bulimia or anorexia nervosa).
• Ipecac syrup may be used in small amounts as an expectorant in cough preparations; however, this use has doubtful therapeutic benefit.
• Signs and symptoms of overdose include diarrhea, persistent nausea or vomiting (longer than 30 minutes), stomach cramps or pain, arrhythmias, hypotension, myocarditis, difficulty breathing, and unusual fatigue or weakness. If overdose is suspected, stop drug and provide symptomatic and supportive care.

Monitoring the patient
• Monitor vital signs frequently.
• Monitor patient for response to drug.

Information for the patient
• Advise patient to seek medical attention immediately when poisoning is suspected.
• Caution patient to call poison information center before taking ipecac syrup.
• Advise patient to take syrup with 1 or 2 glasses of water.

• Warn parent not to let child sleep on his back after taking drug. Use a pillow to prop child on his side.

Pediatric patients
• Advise parents to keep ipecac syrup at home at all times but to keep it out of children's reach.

Breast-feeding patients
• Safety in breast-feeding infants hasn't been established; consider risk-to-benefit ratio.

ipratropium bromide
Atrovent

Pharmacologic classification: anticholinergic
Therapeutic classification: bronchodilator
Pregnancy risk category B

How supplied
Available by prescription only
Inhaler: Each metered dose supplies 18 mcg
Inhalation solution: 2.5 ml
Nasal spray: 0.03%, 0.06%

Indications, route, and dosage
Bronchospasm in chronic bronchitis and emphysema
Adults: Usually, 2 inhalations (36 mcg) q.i.d.; patient may take additional inhalations, p.r.n., but shouldn't exceed 12 inhalations in 24 hours or 500 mcg q 6 to 8 hours via oral nebulizer.
Rhinorrhea associated with allergic and nonallergic perennial rhinitis
0.03% nasal spray
Adults and children ages 12 and older: 2 sprays (42 mcg) per nostril b.i.d. or t.i.d.
Rhinorrhea associated with the common cold
0.06% nasal spray
Adults and children ages 12 and older: 2 sprays (84 mcg) per nostril t.i.d. or q.i.d.
Symptomatic relief of rhinorrhea associated with the common cold
Children ages 5 to 11: 2 sprays (84 mcg) per nostril three times daily.

Pharmacodynamics
Anticholinergic action: Appears to inhibit vagally mediated reflexes by antagonizing the action of acetylcholine. Anticholinergics prevent the increases in intracellular concentration of cyclic guanosine monophosphate (cyclic GMP) that result from interaction of acetylcholine with the muscarinic receptor on bronchial smooth muscle.
   The bronchodilation following inhalation is primarily a local, site-specific effect, not a systemic one.

Pharmacokinetics
- *Absorption:* Not readily absorbed into systemic circulation either from surface of lung or from GI tract as confirmed by blood levels and renal excretion studies. Much of inhaled dose is swallowed as shown by fecal excretion studies.
- *Distribution:* Not applicable.
- *Metabolism:* Metabolism is hepatic; elimination half-life is about 2 hours.
- *Excretion:* Mostly excreted unchanged in feces. Absorbed drug excreted in urine and bile.

Contraindications and precautions
Contraindicated in patients with hypersensitivity to drug or atropine or its derivatives and in those with a history of hypersensitivity to soya lecithin or related food products, such as soybeans and peanuts. Use cautiously in patients with angle-closure glaucoma, prostatic hyperplasia, and bladder-neck obstruction.

Interactions
Drug-drug. *Antimuscarinics:* May produce additive effects. Monitor patient closely.
Fluorocarbon propellant–containing oral inhalants (such as adrenocorticoids, cromolyn, glucocorticoids, sympathomimetics): Increased risk of fluorocarbon toxicity with too-closely timed administration of ipratropium and these drugs. A 5-minute interval between such drugs is recommended.
Drug-herb. *Jaborandi tree, pill-bearing spurge:* Decreased therapeutic effect of drug. Advise patient to use with caution; monitor effect closely.

Adverse reactions
CNS: dizziness, headache, nervousness.
CV: palpitations, chest pain.
EENT: cough, blurred vision, rhinitis, pharyngitis, sinusitis.
GI: nausea, GI distress, dry mouth.
Musculoskeletal: back pain.
Respiratory: *upper respiratory tract infection, bronchitis,* cough, dyspnea, **bronchospasm,** increased sputum.
Skin: rash.
Other: pain, flulike symptoms.

☑ Special considerations
- Because of delayed onset of bronchodilation, drug isn't recommended to treat acute respiratory distress.
- Store drug away from heat and direct sunlight; don't freeze.

Monitoring the patient
- Monitor vital signs and patient response to drug therapy.
- Monitor patient for adverse effects.

Information for the patient
- Tell patient to shake drug well before using.

- Initial nasal spray pump requires priming with 7 actuations of pump. If used regularly as recommended, no further priming is needed. If not used for over 24 hours, pump will require 2 actuations. If not used for over 7 days, pump will require 7 actuations to reprime.
- Tell patient that temporary blurred vision may result if aerosol is sprayed into eyes.
- Advise patient to allow 1 minute between inhalations.
- Instruct patient to take a missed dose as soon as possible—unless it's almost time for next scheduled dose, in which case he should skip the missed dose. Warn him to never double-dose.
- Suggest sugarless hard candy, gum, ice, or saliva substitute to relieve dry mouth. Tell patient to report dry mouth if it persists longer than 2 weeks.
- Instruct patient to call if he experiences no benefits within 30 minutes after use or if condition worsens.

Pediatric patients
- Safety and efficacy in children under age 12 haven't been established.

Breast-feeding patients
- It's unknown if drug appears in breast milk. Although lipid-insoluble quaternary bases appear in breast milk, ipratropium is unlikely to reach infant, especially when taken by aerosol. Use caution when administering to breast-feeding women.

---

irbesartan
Avapro

Pharmacologic classification: angiotensin II receptor antagonist
Therapeutic classification: antihypertensive
Pregnancy risk category C (D in second and third trimesters)

How supplied
Available by prescription only
Tablets: 75 mg, 150 mg, 300 mg

Indications, route, and dosage
Treatment of hypertension, alone or with other antihypertensives
Adults: Initially 150 mg P.O. once daily, increased to maximum of 300 mg once daily if needed, without regard to food.
✦ **Dosage adjustment.** In volume- and salt-depleted patients, give 75 mg P.O. initially.

Pharmacodynamics
Antihypertensive action: Blocks the vasoconstrictor and aldosterone-secreting effects of angiotensin II by selectively blocking the binding of angiotensin II to its receptor sites.

Pharmacokinetics
• *Absorption:* Absorbed rapidly and completely. Average absolute bioavailability is 60% to 80%; not affected by food. Plasma levels peak 1½ to 2 hours after ingestion.
• *Distribution:* Widely distributed; 90% bound to plasma proteins. May cross blood-brain barrier and placenta. Steady-state achieved within 3 days.
• *Metabolism:* Metabolized by conjugation and oxidation. Cytochrome P-450 2C9 is major enzyme responsible for formation of oxidative metabolites. Metabolites don't appear to add appreciably to pharmacologic activity.
• *Excretion:* Excreted in bile and urine. 20% excreted in urine; rest in feces. May also be excreted in breast milk. Elimination half-life is 11 to 15 hours.

Contraindications and precautions
Contraindicated in patients with hypersensitivity to drug or its components and in pregnant or breast-feeding women.
   Use cautiously in volume- or salt-depleted patients, in patients whose renal function may depend on the activity of the renin-angiotensin-aldosterone system (for example, patients with severe heart failure), and in those with unilateral or bilateral renal artery stenosis.

Interactions
None reported.

Adverse reactions
CNS: fatigue, anxiety, dizziness, headache.
CV: chest pain, edema, tachycardia.
EENT: pharyngitis, rhinitis, sinus abnormality.
GI: diarrhea, dyspepsia, abdominal pain, nausea, vomiting.
GU: urinary tract infection.
Musculoskeletal: musculoskeletal trauma or pain.
Respiratory: upper respiratory tract infection.
Skin: rash.

☑ Special considerations
• Pharmacokinetics of drug aren't altered in patients with renal impairment or in patients on hemodialysis. Irbesartan isn't removed by hemodialysis. Dosage adjustment isn't necessary in patients with mild to severe renal impairment unless patient with renal impairment is also volume depleted.
• Dosage adjustment isn't necessary in patients with hepatic insufficiency.
• Patients not adequately treated by maximum 300-mg once-daily dose are unlikely to derive additional benefit from higher dose or twice-daily dosing.

Monitoring the patient
• Monitor blood pressure regularly. A transient hypotensive response isn't a contraindication to

further treatment. Therapy can usually be continued once blood pressure has stabilized.
• Monitor patient for adverse drug reactions.

Information for the patient
• Tell patient drug may be taken once daily with or without food.
• Advise patient that if a dose is missed to take it as soon as possible, but not to take double doses.
• Warn patient about symptoms of hypotension and what to do if they occur.
• Caution patient not to stop drug without medical approval.
• Warn woman that drug is contraindicated during pregnancy because of potential danger to fetus. Advise her to call immediately if pregnancy occurs or if she plans to become pregnant.

Geriatric patients
• Dosage adjustment isn't necessary.

Pediatric patients
• Safety and effectiveness in children under age 18 haven't been established.

Breast-feeding patients
• Because of potential for serious adverse reactions in breast-fed infants, use an alternative to breast-feeding during therapy.

irinotecan hydrochloride
Camptosar

Pharmacologic classification: topoisomerase inhibitor
Therapeutic classification: antineoplastic
Pregnancy risk category D

How supplied
Available by prescription only
Injection: 100-mg vial

Indications, route, and dosage
Metastatic carcinoma of the colon or rectum in which the disease has recurred or progressed following fluorouracil (5-FU)-based therapy
Adults: Initially, 125 mg/m² I.V. infusion over 90 minutes. Recommended treatment regimen is 125 mg/m² I.V. administered once weekly for 4 weeks, then a 2-week rest period. Thereafter, additional courses of treatment may be repeated q 6 weeks (4 weeks on therapy, then 2 weeks off therapy). Subsequent doses may be adjusted to as high as 150 mg/m² or as low as 50 mg/m² in 25- to 50-mg/m² increments depending on patient's tolerance. Treatment with additional courses may continue indefinitely in patients who attain a response or in those whose disease remains stable provided intolerable toxicity doesn't occur.

Reactions may be *common,* uncommon, *life-threatening,* or COMMON AND LIFE-THREATENING.

Pharmacodynamics

Antineoplastic action: A derivative of camptothecin. Camptothecins interact specifically with the enzyme topoisomerase I, which relieves torsional strain in DNA by inducing reversible single-strand breaks. Irinotecan and its active metabolite bind to the topoisomerase I–DNA complex and prevent religation of these single-strand breaks.

Pharmacokinetics

- *Absorption:* Only administered I.V.
- *Distribution:* About 30% to 68% bound to plasma protein; active metabolite, SN-38, is about 95% protein-bound.
- *Metabolism:* Undergoes metabolic conversion in liver to its active metabolite SN-38.
- *Excretion:* Small amount of drug and SN-38 excreted in urine. Terminal half-life of irinotecan is 6 hours in patients who are ages 65 and older; 5½ hours in patients under age 65; mean terminal elimination half-life of SN-38 is about 10 hours.

Contraindications and precautions

Contraindicated in patients with hypersensitivity to drug. Use cautiously in elderly patients and in those who have previously received pelvic or abdominal irradiation because of increased risk of severe myelosuppression.

Interactions

Drug-drug. *Other antineoplastics:* Additive adverse effects such as myelosuppression and diarrhea. Monitor patient closely.
Pelvic or abdominal irradiation: Increased risk of severe myelosuppression. Avoid concurrent use.

Adverse reactions

CNS: *insomnia, dizziness, asthenia, headache.*
CV: *vasodilation, edema.*
EENT: *rhinitis.*
GI: DIARRHEA, *nausea, vomiting, anorexia, constipation, flatulence, stomatitis, dyspepsia, abdominal cramping and pain, abdominal enlargement.*
Hematologic: LEUKOPENIA, *anemia,* NEUTROPENIA.
Hepatic: *increased alkaline phosphatase and AST levels.*
Metabolic: *weight loss, dehydration.*
Musculoskeletal: *back pain.*
Respiratory: *dyspnea, increased coughing.*
Skin: *alopecia, sweating, rash.*
Other: *fever, pain, chills, minor infection.*

☑ Special considerations

- Premedicate patient with antiemetics on day of treatment starting at least 30 minutes before drug administration. Most patients receive 10 mg of dexamethasone with another antiemetic, for example a 5-HT$_3$ blocker such as ondansetron or granisetron. Patients should also receive an antiemetic regimen (prochlorperazine) for subsequent use as needed.

- Irinotecan is packaged in a backing/plastic blister to protect against inadvertent breakage and leakage. Inspect vial for damage and visible signs of leaks before removing backing/plastic blister. If damaged, incinerate unopened package. Store vial at room temperature of 59° to 86° F (15° to 30° C) and protect from light. Don't remove vial and backing/plastic blister from carton until time of use.

- Use caution in handling and preparing infusion solutions of irinotecan. Gloves should be worn. If drug solution comes in contact with skin, wash skin immediately and thoroughly with soap and water. If drug solution contacts mucous membranes, flush thoroughly with water.

- Drug must be diluted before infusion with D$_5$W injection (preferred) or normal saline injection to a final concentration range of 0.12 to 1.1 mg/ml.

- Drug solution is stable for up to 24 hours at room temperature of 77° F (25° C) and in ambient fluorescent lighting. Store solutions diluted in D$_5$W in refrigerator (35° to 46° F [2° to 8° C]) and protect from light; these are stable for 48 hours. However, because of possible microbial contamination during dilution, use admixture within 24 hours if refrigerated or within 6 hours if kept at room temperature. Refrigeration of admixtures using normal saline isn't recommended because of a low risk of visible particulates.

- Avoid freezing of drug and admixtures because drug may precipitate.

- Don't add other drugs to drug infusion.

- Routine administration of a colony-stimulating factor isn't necessary but may be helpful in patients experiencing significant neutropenia.

- Avoid drug extravasation. If extravasation occurs, flush site with sterile water and apply ice.

Monitoring the patient

- Withhold diuretic therapy during dosing with irinotecan and during periods of active vomiting or diarrhea because of potential risk of dehydration secondary to vomiting or diarrhea induced by irinotecan.

- Irinotecan can induce severe forms of diarrhea. Diarrhea occurring within 24 hours of drug administration may be preceded by complaints of diaphoresis and abdominal cramping; may be ameliorated by giving 0.25 to 1 mg of atropine I.V. unless contraindicated. Diarrhea occurring more than 24 hours after drug administration can be prolonged, may lead to dehydration and electrolyte imbalance, and can be life-threatening.

- Late diarrhea should be treated promptly with loperamide (4 mg at onset and then 2 mg every 2 hours until patient is diarrhea-free for at least 12 hours; during the night, patient may take 4 mg of loperamide every 4 hours). Premedication with loperamide isn't recommended. Monitor patient with severe diarrhea and give fluid and electrolyte

replacement if dehydration occurs. Interrupt drug therapy if severe diarrhea occurs.
• Therapy should be temporarily stopped if neutropenic fever occurs or if absolute neutrophil count drops below 500/mm³. Dose should be reduced if there is a significant decrease in total WBC count (less than 2,000/mm³), neutrophil count (below 1,000/mm³), hemoglobin (under 8 g/dl), or platelet count (under 100,000/mm³). Consult manufacturer for dosage guidelines in these situations.
• Careful monitoring of WBC count with differential, hemoglobin, and platelet count is recommended before each irinotecan dose.

Information for the patient
• Inform patient about risk of diarrhea and when and how to treat it if it occurs. Tell patient to have loperamide readily available; begin treatment for diarrhea that occurs more than 24 hours after drug administration at the first episode of poorly formed or loose stools or the earliest onset of bowel movements more frequent than normally expected for patient. Instruct patient to call if diarrhea occurs and to avoid drugs with laxative properties.
• Tell patient to call if vomiting occurs, fever or evidence of infection develops, or symptoms of dehydration (fainting, light-headedness, or dizziness) occur following drug administration.
• Warn patient that alopecia may occur.
• Advise woman of childbearing age to avoid pregnancy because drug may cause fetal harm.

Geriatric patients
• Use caution when administering drug to elderly patients, especially those with history of heart failure and hypotension.

Pediatric patients
• Safety and effectiveness in children haven't been established.

Breast-feeding patients
• It's unknown if drug appears in breast milk. Because of potential for serious adverse reactions in breast-fed infants, breast-feeding should be discontinued during therapy.

iron dextran
DexFerrum, InFeD, Infufer*

Pharmacologic classification: parenteral iron supplement
Therapeutic classification: hematinic
Pregnancy risk category C

How supplied
Available by prescription only
Injection: 50 mg elemental iron/ml in 2-ml, single-dose vials

Indications, route, and dosage
Iron-deficiency anemia
Adults and children: Dosage is highly individualized and is based on patient's weight and hemoglobin level. Drug is usually given I.M.; preservative-free solution can be given I.V. Check current literature for recommended protocol.

Pharmacodynamics
Hematinic action: A complex of ferric hydroxide and dextran in a colloidal solution. After I.M. injection, 10% to 50% remains in the muscle for several months; remainder enters bloodstream, increasing plasma iron level for up to 2 weeks. Iron is an essential component of hemoglobin.

Pharmacokinetics
• *Absorption:* I.M. doses absorbed in two stages: 60% after 3 days; up to 90% by 3 weeks. Remainder absorbed over several months or longer.
• *Distribution:* During first 3 days, local inflammation facilitates passage of drug into lymphatic system; drug then ingested by macrophages, which enter lymph and blood.
• *Metabolism:* After I.M. or I.V. administration, drug is cleared from plasma by reticuloendothelial cells of liver, spleen, and bone marrow.
• *Excretion:* In doses of 500 mg or less, half-life is 6 hours. Traces excreted in breast milk, urine, bile, and feces. Drug can't be removed by hemodialysis.

Contraindications and precautions
Contraindicated in patients with hypersensitivity to drug, in those with anemias except iron-deficiency anemia, and in those with acute infectious renal disease. Use cautiously in patients with impaired hepatic function, rheumatoid arthritis, or other inflammatory diseases.

Interactions
Drug-herb. *Oregano:* May reduce iron absorption. Separate administration time by at least 2 hours when giving with iron supplements or iron-containing foods.

Adverse reactions
CNS: headache, transitory paresthesia, dizziness, malaise.
CV: *hypotensive reaction, peripheral vascular flushing (with overly rapid I.V. administration).*
GI: nausea, anorexia.
Hematologic: false elevations of serum bilirubin level and false reductions in serum calcium level.
Musculoskeletal: arthralgia, myalgia.
Respiratory: *bronchospasm,* dyspnea.
Skin: rash, urticaria, purpura, *brown skin discoloration at I.M. injection site, phlebitis at I.V. injection site,* sterile abscess, necrosis, atrophy, fibrosis.

Reactions may be *common,* uncommon, **life-threatening**, or COMMON AND LIFE-THREATENING.

Other: *soreness, inflammation,* **anaphylaxis,** delayed sensitivity reactions, fever, chills.

☑ Special considerations
● Stop oral iron before giving iron dextran.
● Use 10-ml multidose vial only for I.M. injections because it contains phenol as a preservative; use only 2- or 5-ml ampule without preservative for I.V. administration.
● Administer test dose of 0.5 ml iron dextrose I.M. or I.V. Be alert for anaphylaxis on test dose; monitor vital signs for drug reaction. Keep epinephrine (0.5 ml of a 1:1,000 solution) readily available for such an emergency.
● Inject I.M. preparation deeply into upper outer quadrant of buttocks (never arm or other exposed area) using a 2- to 3-inch (5- to 8-cm), 19G or 20G needle. Use Z-track technique to avoid leakage into S.C. tissue and skin stains, and minimize staining by using a separate needle to withdraw drug from container.
● I.V. use is controversial; some facilities don't allow it.
● Give drug I.V. if patient has insufficient muscle mass for deep injection, impaired absorption from muscle because of stasis or edema, a risk of uncontrolled I.M. bleeding from trauma (as in hemophilia), or need for massive and prolonged parenteral therapy (as in chronic substantial blood loss). Don't administer more than 50 mg of iron/ minute (1 ml/minute) if using drug undiluted.
● After I.V. iron dextran administration, flush vein with 10 ml normal saline injection to minimize local irritation. Have patient rest for 15 to 30 minutes because orthostatic hypotension may occur.
● Iron dextran prevents meaningful measurement of serum iron level and total iron binding capacity for up to 3 weeks; I.M. injection may cause dense areas of activity on bone scans using technetium 99m diphosphonate for 1 to 6 days.
● Injected iron has much greater bioavailability than oral iron, but data on acute overdose are limited.

Monitoring the patient
● Monitor hemoglobin level, hematocrit, and reticulocyte count during therapy. An increase of about 1 g/dl weekly in hemoglobin is usual.
● Monitor patient for adverse effects.

Information for the patient
● Warn patient of possible skin staining with I.M. injections.
● Instruct patient to report adverse reactions promptly.

Pediatric patients
● Drug isn't recommended for use in children under age 4 months.

Breast-feeding patients
● Traces of unmetabolized iron dextran appear in breast milk; impact on infant is unknown.

isoniazid (INH)
Isotamine*, Nydrazid, PMS Isoniazid*

Pharmacologic classification: isonicotinic acid hydrazine
Therapeutic classification: antituberculotic
Pregnancy risk category C

How supplied
Available by prescription only
Tablets: 50 mg, 100 mg, 300 mg
Oral solution: 50 mg/5 ml
Injection: 100 mg/ml

Indications, route, and dosage
Primary treatment against actively growing tubercle bacilli
Adults: 5 mg/kg P.O. or I.M. daily in a single dose, up to 300 mg/day, continued for 9 months to 2 years.
Infants and children: 10 mg/kg P.O. or I.M. daily in a single dose, up to 300 mg/day, continued for 18 months to 2 years. Concomitant administration of at least one other effective antituberculotic is recommended.
Prophylaxis against tubercle bacilli of those closely exposed or with positive skin test
Adults: 300 mg P.O. daily single dose, continued for 6 months to 1 year.
Infants and children: 10 mg/kg P.O. daily single dose, up to 300 mg/day, continued for 6 months to 1 year.

Pharmacodynamics
Antitubercular action: Interferes with lipid and DNA synthesis, thus inhibiting bacterial cell wall synthesis. Its action is bacteriostatic or bactericidal, depending on organism susceptibility and drug concentration at infection site. Active against *Mycobacterium tuberculosis, M. bovis,* and some strains of *M. kansasii.*
Resistance by *M. tuberculosis* develops rapidly when INH is used to treat tuberculosis, and it's usually combined with another antituberculotic to prevent or delay resistance. During prophylaxis, however, resistance isn't a problem and isoniazid can be used alone.

Pharmacokinetics
● *Absorption:* Rapidly and completely absorbed from GI tract after oral administration; serum levels peak 1 to 2 hours after ingestion. Absorbed readily after I.M. injection.
● *Distribution:* Distributed widely into body tissues and fluids, including ascitic, synovial, pleural, and cerebrospinal fluids; lungs and other or-

gans; and sputum and saliva. Crosses placenta; enters breast milk in levels similar to plasma.
- *Metabolism:* Inactivated primarily in liver by genetically controlled acetylation. Rate of metabolism varies individually; fast acetylators metabolize drug five times as rapidly as others. About 50% of blacks and whites are slow acetylators of INH; over 80% of Chinese, Japanese, and Eskimos are fast acetylators.
- *Excretion:* About 75% excreted in urine as unchanged drug and metabolites in 24 hours; some drug excreted in saliva, sputum, feces, and breast milk. Plasma half-life in adults is 1 to 4 hours, depending on metabolic rate. Drug is removed by peritoneal dialysis or hemodialysis.

Contraindications and precautions
Contraindicated in patients with acute hepatic disease or drug-associated hepatic damage. Use cautiously in elderly patients and in patients with severe, non–INH-associated hepatic disease, seizure disorders (especially those taking phenytoin), severe renal impairment, or chronic alcoholism.

Interactions
Drug-drug. *Antacids containing aluminum, laxatives:* Decreased oral absorption of INH. Give isoniazid at least 1 hour before antacid or laxative.
Anticoagulants: May increase anticoagulant activity. Monitor PT and INR closely.
Benzodiazepines (such as diazepam), carbamazepine, phenytoin: INH-induced inhibition of metabolism and elevation of serum levels. Monitor patient closely.
Corticosteroids: May decrease INH efficacy. Monitor patient closely.
Cycloserine: Increased hazard of CNS toxicity, drowsiness, and dizziness. Avoid concomitant use.
Disulfiram: Possible coordination difficulties and psychotic episodes. Avoid concomitant use.
Rifampin: May accelerate INH metabolism to hepatotoxic metabolites. Monitor liver function tests.
Drug-food. *Foods containing tyramine (most cheeses, beer, broad bean pods, yeast, chicken liver):* Hypertensive crisis. Tell patient to avoid or eat in small quantities.
Drug-lifestyle. *Alcohol:* May increase risk of INH-induced hepatitis and seizures. Discourage use.

Adverse reactions
CNS: *peripheral neuropathy* (dose-related and especially in patients who are malnourished, alcoholic, diabetic, or slow acetylators), usually preceded by paresthesia of hands and feet, **seizures, toxic encephalopathy,** memory impairment, toxic psychosis.
EENT: optic neuritis, atrophy.
GI: nausea, vomiting, epigastric distress.
GU: gynecomastia.

Hematologic: *agranulocytosis,* hemolytic anemia, *aplastic anemia,* eosinophilia, **thrombocytopenia,** sideroblastic anemia.
Hepatic: *hepatitis* (occasionally severe and sometimes fatal, especially in elderly patients), jaundice, *elevated serum transaminase levels,* bilirubinemia, elevated liver function study results.
Metabolic: hyperglycemia, metabolic acidosis, pyridoxine deficiency, hypocalcemia, hypophosphatemia.
Skin: irritation at I.M. injection site.
Other: rheumatic and lupus-like syndromes, *hypersensitivity reactions* (fever, rash, lymphadenopathy, vasculitis).

☑ Special considerations
- At least 12 months of preventive therapy is recommended for persons with history of tuberculosis and for HIV-infected individuals.
- If compliance is a problem, twice-weekly supervised drug administration may be effective. Recommended twice-weekly dose for adults is 15 mg/kg P.O., not to exceed 900 mg.
- Oral doses should be taken on empty stomach for maximum absorption, or with food if gastric irritation occurs.
- Obtain specimens for culture and sensitivity testing before first dose, but therapy may begin before test results are complete; repeat periodically to detect drug resistance.
- INH alters results of urine glucose tests that use cupric sulfate method (Benedict's reagent, Diastix, or Chemstrip uG).
- Drug may hinder stabilization of serum glucose level in patients with diabetes mellitus.
- Improvement is usually evident after 2 to 3 weeks of therapy.
- Some recommend pyridoxine 50 mg P.O. daily to prevent peripheral neuropathy from large doses of INH. May also be useful in patients at risk for developing peripheral neuropathy (malnourished patients, diabetics, and alcohol abusers). Pyridoxine (50 to 200 mg daily) has been used to treat drug-induced neuropathy.
- To treat overdose, establish ventilation; control seizures with diazepam. Pyridoxine is administered to equal dose of INH. Initial dose is 1 to 4 g pyridoxine I.V., then 1 g every 30 minutes thereafter, until entire dose is given.
- Because drug is dialyzable, patients undergoing hemodialysis or peritoneal dialysis may need dosage adjustments.
- Hepatotoxicity appears to be age-related and may limit use for prophylaxis.

Monitoring the patient
- Monitor blood, renal, and hepatic function studies before and periodically during therapy to minimize toxicity; assess visual function periodically.
- Observe patient for adverse effects, especially hepatic dysfunction, CNS toxicity, and optic

---

Reactions may be *common,* uncommon, **life-threatening,** or COMMON AND LIFE-THREATENING.

neuritis. Establish safety measures in case orthostatic hypotension occurs.

Information for the patient
• Explain disease process and rationale for long-term therapy.
• Teach signs and symptoms of hypersensitivity and other adverse reactions, particularly visual disturbances, and emphasize need to report these; urge patient to report any unusual effects.
• Teach patient how and when to take drug; instruct patient to take INH on empty stomach, at least 1 hour before or 2 hours after meals. If GI irritation occurs, drug may be taken with food.
• Urge patient to comply with and complete prescribed regimen. Advise patient not to stop drug without medical approval; explain importance of follow-up appointments.
• Inform patient that drug therapy usually continues for 18 months to 2 years for treatment of active tuberculosis; 12 months for prophylaxis; 9 months if INH and rifampin therapy are combined.
• Emphasize importance of uninterrupted therapy to prevent relapse and spread of infection.

Geriatric patients
• Use with caution in elderly patients; risk of hepatic effects increases after age 35. Drug prophylaxis in patients with a positive purified protein derivative test may not be indicated in older patients because of risk of hepatotoxicity.

Pediatric patients
• Infants and children tolerate larger doses of drug.

Breast-feeding patients
• Drug appears in breast milk; use with caution in breast-feeding women and monitor infants for possible INH-induced toxicity.

isoproterenol
Isuprel

isoproterenol hydrochloride
Isuprel, Isuprel Mistometer

isoproterenol sulfate
Medihaler-Iso

Pharmacologic classification: adrenergic
Therapeutic classification: bronchodilator, cardiac stimulant
Pregnancy risk category C

How supplied
Available by prescription only
isoproterenol
Nebulizer inhaler: 0.25%, 0.5%, 1%
isoproterenol hydrochloride
Tablets (S.L.): 10 mg, 15 mg

Aerosol inhaler: 120 mcg/metered spray, 131 mcg/metered spray
Injection: 200 mcg/ml
isoproterenol sulfate
Aerosol inhaler: 80 mcg/metered spray

Indications, route, and dosage
Complete heart block after closure of ventricular septal defect
Adults: I.V. bolus, 0.02 to 0.06 mg (1 to 3 ml of a 1:50,000 dilution).
Children: I.V. bolus, 0.01 to 0.03 mg (0.5 to 1.5 ml of a 1:50,000 dilution).
To prevent heart block
Adults: 10 to 30 mg S.L. four to six times daily.
Maintenance therapy of AV block
Adults: Initially, 10 mg S.L.; then 5 to 50 mg, p.r.n. Or 5 mg (half of a 10-mg tablet) administered P.R.; then 5 to 15 mg, p.r.n.
Bronchospasm during mild acute asthma attacks
isoproterenol hydrochloride
Adults and children: Via aerosol inhalation, 1 inhalation initially, repeated, p.r.n., after 1 to 5 minutes, to maximum 6 inhalations daily. Maintenance dose is 1 to 2 inhalations four to six times daily at 3- to 4-hour intervals. Via hand-bulb nebulizer, 5 to 15 deep inhalations of a 0.5% solution; if needed, may be repeated in 5 to 10 minutes. May be repeated up to five times daily.
Or 3 to 7 deep inhalations of a 1% solution, repeated once in 5 to 10 minutes if needed. May be repeated up to five times daily.
isoproterenol sulfate
Adults and children: For acute dyspneic episodes, 1 inhalation initially; repeated if needed after 2 to 5 minutes. Maximum 6 inhalations daily. Maintenance dose is 1 to 2 inhalations up to six times daily.
Bronchospasm in COPD
isoproterenol hydrochloride
Adults and children: Via hand-bulb nebulizer: 5 to 15 deep inhalations of a 0.5% solution, or 3 to 7 deep inhalations of a 1% solution no more frequently than q 3 to 4 hours.
Bronchospasm during mild acute asthma attacks or in COPD
isoproterenol hydrochloride
Adults and children: Oral inhalation of 2 ml of 0.125% solution or 2.5 ml of 0.1% solution up to five times daily.
Acute asthma attacks unresponsive to inhalation therapy or control of bronchospasm during anesthesia
isoproterenol hydrochloride
Adults: 0.01 to 0.02 mg (0.5 to 1 ml of a 1:50,000 dilution) I.V. Repeat if needed.
Bronchodilation
isoproterenol hydrochloride
Adults: 10 to 20 mg S.L., not to exceed 60 mg daily.

Children: 5 to 10 mg S.L., not to exceed 30 mg daily.
Emergency treatment of arrhythmias
isoproterenol hydrochloride
Adults: Initially, 0.02 to 0.06 mg I.V. bolus. Subsequent doses 0.01 to 0.2 mg I.V. Or 5 mcg/minute titrated to patient's response. Range, 2 to 20 mcg/minute. Or 0.2 mg I.M. or S.C.; subsequent doses 0.02 to 1 mg I.M. or 0.15 to 0.2 mg S.C. In extreme cases, 0.02 mg (0.1 of 1:5,000) intracardiac injection.
Children: May give half of initial adult dose.
Immediate temporary control of atropine-resistant hemodynamically significant bradycardia
isoproterenol hydrochloride
Adults: 2 to 10 mcg/minute I.V. infusion, titrated to patient's response.
Children: 0.1 mcg/kg/minute, titrated to patient's response. Maximum rate 1 mcg/kg/minute.
Heart block, Stokes-Adams attacks, and shock
isoproterenol hydrochloride
Adults and children: 0.5 to 5 mcg/minute by continuous I.V. infusion to patient's response; or 0.02 to 0.06 mg I.V. boluses with 0.01 to 0.2 mg additional doses; or 0.2 mg I.M. or S.C. with 0.02 to 1 mg I.M. or 0.15 to 0.2 mg additional doses.

Pharmacodynamics
Bronchodilator action: Relaxes bronchial smooth muscle by direct action on beta$_2$-adrenergic receptors, relieving bronchospasm, increasing vital capacity, decreasing residual volume in lungs, and facilitating passage of pulmonary secretions. Also produces relaxation of GI and uterine smooth muscle via stimulation of beta$_2$ receptors. Peripheral vasodilation, cardiac stimulation, and relaxation of bronchial smooth muscle are the main therapeutic effects.
Cardiac stimulant action: Acts on beta$_1$-adrenergic receptors in the heart, producing a positive chronotropic and inotropic effect; it usually increases cardiac output. In patients with AV block, isoproterenol shortens conduction time and the refractory period of the AV node and increases the rate and strength of ventricular contraction.

Pharmacokinetics
• *Absorption:* After injection or oral inhalation, absorbed rapidly; after sublingual or rectal administration, absorption variable and often unreliable. Prompt onset of action after oral inhalation; lasts up to 1 hour. Effects persist for a few minutes after I.V. injection, up to 2 hours after S.C. or S.L. administration, and up to 4 hours after rectal administration of sublingual tablet.
• *Distribution:* Widely distributed throughout body.
• *Metabolism:* Metabolized by conjugation in GI tract and by enzymatic reduction in liver, lungs, and other tissues.

• *Excretion:* Primarily in urine as unchanged drug and its metabolites.

Contraindications and precautions
Contraindicated in patients with tachycardia caused by digitalis intoxication, preexisting arrhythmias (other than those that may respond to treatment with isoproterenol), and angina pectoris. Use cautiously in elderly patients and in patients with impaired renal function, CV disease, coronary insufficiency, diabetes, hyperthyroidism, or sensitivity to sympathomimetic amines.

Interactions
Drug-drug. *Beta blockers:* Antagonized cardiac-stimulating, bronchodilating, and vasodilating effects of isoproterenol. Monitor patient closely.
Cardiac glycosides, cyclopropane, halogenated hydrocarbon general anesthetics, potassium-depleting drugs, other drugs that affect cardiac rhythm: Arrhythmias may occur more readily. Use with caution; monitor ECG closely.
Epinephrine, other sympathomimetics: Additive CV reactions. Drugs may be used together if at least 4 hours elapse between administration of the two drugs.
Ergot alkaloids: May increase blood pressure. Monitor blood pressure.

Adverse reactions
CNS: *headache, mild tremor,* weakness, dizziness, *nervousness,* insomnia, **Stokes-Adams attacks.**
CV: palpitations, *tachycardia, anginal pain,* **arrhythmias, cardiac arrest,** *rapid rise and fall in blood pressure.*
GI: *nausea, vomiting, heartburn.*
Metabolic: hyperglycemia.
Respiratory: *bronchospasm,* bronchitis, sputum increase, pulmonary edema.
Skin: diaphoresis.
Other: swelling of parotid glands with prolonged use.

☑ Special considerations
Besides the recommendations relevant to all adrenergics, consider the following.
• Drug doesn't replace administration of blood, plasma, fluids, or electrolytes in patients with blood volume depletion.
• Severe paradoxical airway resistance may follow oral inhalations.
• Hypotension must be corrected before isoproterenol is administered.
• If three to five treatments within 6 to 12 hours provide minimal or no relief, reevaluate therapy.
• Prescribed I.V. infusion rate should include specific guidelines for regulating flow or terminating infusion in relation to heart rate, premature beats, ECG changes, precordial distress, blood pressure, and urine flow. Because of danger of precipitating arrhythmias, rate of infusion is usually

---

Reactions may be *common,* uncommon, *life-threatening,* or COMMON AND LIFE-THREATENING.

decreased or infusion may be temporarily stopped if heart rate exceeds 110 beats/minute.

• Constant-infusion pump prevents sudden infusion of excessive amounts of drug.

• S. L. doses shouldn't be given more frequently than every 3 to 4 hours nor more than t.i.d.

• S. L. tablet may be administered P.R.

• Monitor patient for rebound bronchospasm when drug's effects end.

• Isoproterenol has also been used to aid diagnosis of coronary artery disease and mitral regurgitation.

• Don't inject solutions intended for oral inhalation.

Monitoring the patient

• Continuously monitor ECG during I.V. administration.

• Carefully monitor response to therapy by frequent determinations of heart rate, ECG pattern, blood pressure, and central venous pressure as well as (for patients in shock) urine volume, blood pH, and partial pressure of carbon dioxide.

• Monitor vital signs closely. Sedatives (barbiturates) may be used to treat CNS stimulation. Use cardioselective beta blockers to treat tachycardia and arrhythmias. Use these drugs cautiously; they may induce asthmatic attack.

Information for the patient

• Remind patient to save applicator; refills may be available.

• Urge patient to call if no relief is gained or condition worsens.

• Advise patient to store oral forms away from heat and light (not in bathroom medicine cabinet where heat and moisture will cause deterioration). Keep drug out of reach of children.

Inhalation

• Give patient instructions on proper use of inhaler.

• Tell patient that saliva and sputum may appear red or pink after oral inhalation because isoproterenol turns red on exposure to air.

• Advise patient to rinse mouth with water after drug is absorbed completely and between doses.

Sublingual

• Tell patient to allow sublingual tablet to dissolve under tongue, without sucking, and not to swallow saliva (may cause epigastric pain) until drug has been absorbed completely.

• Warn patient that frequent use of sublingual tablets may damage teeth because of drug's acidity.

Geriatric patients

• Elderly patients may be more sensitive to therapeutic and adverse effects of drug.

Pediatric patients

• Use with caution in children.

Breast-feeding patients

• It's unknown if drug appears in breast milk; use cautiously in breast-feeding women.

isosorbide dinitrate

Apo-ISDN*, Coronex*, Dilatrate-SR, Isordil, Isordil Tembids, Isordil Titradose, Sorbitrate

Pharmacologic classification: nitrate
Therapeutic classification: antianginal, vasodilator
Pregnancy risk category C

How supplied

Available by prescription only
Tablets: 5 mg, 10 mg, 20 mg, 30 mg, 40 mg
Tablets (S.L.): 2.5 mg, 5 mg, 10 mg
Tablets (extended-release): 40 mg
Tablets (chewable): 5 mg, 10 mg
Capsules (extended-release): 40 mg

Indications, route, and dosage

Treatment or prophylaxis of acute anginal attacks; treatment of chronic ischemic heart disease (by preload reduction)
Adults: S.L. form—2.5 to 10 mg under tongue for prompt relief of angina pain, repeated q 2 to 3 hours during acute phase, or q 4 to 6 hours for prophylaxis.

Chewable form—2.5 to 10 mg, p.r.n., for acute attack or q 2 to 3 hours for prophylaxis, but only after initial test dose of 5 mg to determine risk of severe hypotension.

Oral form—10 to 20 mg P.O. t.i.d. or q.i.d. for prophylaxis only (use smallest effective dose).

Extended-release forms—20 to 40 mg P.O. q 8 to 12 hours.

◇ *Adjunctive treatment of heart failure*
Adults: 5 to 10 mg S.L. q 3 to 4 hours. Or give 20 to 40 mg P.O. (or chewable tablets) q 4 hours. Usually administered with vasodilators.

◇ *Diffuse esophageal spasm without gastroesophageal reflux*
Adults: 10 to 30 mg P.O. q 4 hours.

Pharmacodynamics

Antianginal action: Reduces myocardial oxygen demand through peripheral vasodilation, resulting in decreased venous filling pressure (preload) and, to a lesser extent, decreased arterial impedance (afterload). These combined effects result in decreased cardiac work and, consequently, reduced myocardial oxygen demands. Drug also redistributes coronary blood flow from epicardial to subendocardial regions.
Vasodilating action: Dilates peripheral vessels (primarily venous), helping to manage pulmonary edema and heart failure caused by decreased venous return to the heart (preload). Arterial vasodilatory effects also decrease arterial imped-

ance (afterload) and thus left ventricular work, benefiting the failing heart. These combined effects may help some patients with acute MI. (Use of isosorbide dinitrate in patients with heart failure and acute MI is currently unapproved.)

Pharmacokinetics

• *Absorption:* Oral form well absorbed from GI tract but undergoes first-pass metabolism, resulting in bioavailability of about 50% (depending on form used). With S.L. and chewable forms, onset of action is 3 minutes; with other oral forms, 30 minutes; with extended-release forms, 1 hour.

• *Distribution:* Limited information available on drug's plasma protein–binding and distribution. Like nitroglycerin, is distributed widely throughout body.

• *Metabolism:* Metabolized in liver to active metabolites.

• *Excretion:* Metabolites excreted in urine; elimination half-life is about 5 to 6 hours with oral administration; 2 hours with S.L. administration. About 80% to 100% of absorbed dose excreted in urine within 24 hours. Duration of effect is longer than that of S.L. preparations. With S.L. and chewable forms, duration of effect is 30 minutes to 2 hours; with other oral forms, 5 to 6 hours.

Contraindications and precautions

Contraindicated in patients with hypersensitivity or idiosyncrasy to nitrates, severe hypotension, shock, or acute MI with low left ventricular filling pressure. Use cautiously in patients with hypotension or blood volume depletion (such as from diuretic therapy).

Interactions

Drug-drug. *Antihypertensives, calcium channel blockers, phenothiazines, vasodilators:* May cause additive hypotensive effects. Monitor blood pressure closely.

Drug-lifestyle. *Alcohol:* May cause additive hypotensive effects. Discourage use.

Adverse reactions

CNS: *headache* (sometimes with throbbing), dizziness, weakness.
CV: *flushing, orthostatic hypotension, tachycardia, palpitations, ankle edema,* fainting.
GI: nausea, vomiting.
Skin: cutaneous vasodilation, rash.
Other: **hypersensitivity reactions,** sublingual burning.

☑ Special considerations

• Drug may cause headache, especially at first. Dose may need to be reduced temporarily, but tolerance usually develops to this effect. In the interim, patient may relieve headache with aspirin or acetaminophen.

• Additional dose may be given before anticipated stress or at bedtime if angina is nocturnal.

• Don't stop drug abruptly because this may cause coronary vasospasm.

• Store drug in cool place, in tightly closed container away from light.

• Maintenance of continuous 24-hour plasma levels may result in refractory tolerance. Dosing regimens should include dose-free intervals, which vary based on form of drug used.

• Drug may cause orthostatic hypotension. To minimize this, have patient change to upright position slowly, walk up and down stairs carefully, and lie down at first sign of dizziness.

• Isosorbide dinitrate may interfere with serum cholesterol determination tests using the Zlatkis-Zak color reaction, causing a falsely decreased value.

• Treatment of overdose includes gastric lavage, then activated charcoal to remove remaining gastric contents. An I.V. adrenergic agonist (such as phenylephrine) may be considered if further treatment is required.

Monitoring the patient

• Monitor blood pressure and intensity and duration of patient's response to drug.

• Blood gas measurements and methemoglobin levels should be monitored, as indicated, especially in suspected overdose of drug.

Information for the patient

• Instruct patient to take drug regularly, as prescribed, and to keep it easily accessible at all times. Drug is physiologically necessary but not addictive.

• Warn patient that headache may occur initially, but may respond to usual headache remedies or dosage reduction. Assure patient that headache usually subsides gradually with continued treatment.

• Tell patient to take oral tablets on empty stomach, either 30 minutes before or 1 to 2 hours after meals; to swallow oral tablets whole; and to chew chewable tablets thoroughly before swallowing.

• Advise patient to sit when taking S.L. tablets. He should lubricate tablet with saliva or place a few milliliters of fluid under tongue with tablet. If patient experiences tingling sensation with drug placed sublingually, he may try to hold tablet in buccal pouch. Dose may be repeated every 10 to 15 minutes for maximum of three doses. If no relief occurs, he should call or go to hospital emergency room.

• Warn patient to make positional changes gradually to avoid excessive dizziness.

• Advise patient to report blurred vision, dry mouth, or persistent headache.

• Caution patient not to stop long-term therapy abruptly.

Reactions may be *common*, uncommon, **life-threatening**, or COMMON AND LIFE-THREATENING.

isosorbide mononitrate **581**

Pediatric patients
● Methemoglobinemia may occur in infants receiving large doses of isosorbide dinitrate.

Breast-feeding patients
● It's unknown if drug appears in breast milk; use cautiously in breast-feeding women.

---

isosorbide mononitrate
Imdur, ISMO, Monoket

Pharmacologic classification: nitrate
Therapeutic classification: antianginal
Pregnancy risk category C

How supplied
Available by prescription only
Tablets: 10 mg, 20 mg
Tablets (extended-release): 30 mg, 60 mg, 120 mg

Indications, route, and dosage
Prevention of angina pectoris due to coronary artery disease (but not to abort acute anginal attacks)
Adults: 20 mg P.O. b.i.d., with doses 7 hours apart and first dose on awakening. For extended-release tablets, 30 to 60 mg P.O. once daily on arising; after several days, dose may be increased to 120 mg once daily; rarely, 240 mg may be required; extended-release tablets shouldn't be crushed or chewed.

Pharmacodynamics
Antianginal action: The major active metabolite of isosorbide dinitrate. Relaxes vascular smooth muscle and consequently dilates peripheral arteries and veins. Dilation of the veins promotes peripheral pooling of blood and decreases venous return to the heart, thereby reducing left ventricular end-diastolic pressure and pulmonary capillary wedge pressure (preload). Arteriolar relaxation reduces systemic vascular resistance, systolic arterial pressure, and mean arterial pressure (afterload). Dilation of the coronary arteries also occurs.

Pharmacokinetics
● *Absorption:* Absolute bioavailability is almost 100%. Serum levels peak 30 to 60 minutes after ingestion.
● *Distribution:* Volume of distribution is about 0.6 L/kg. Less than 4% bound to plasma proteins.
● *Metabolism:* Not subject to first-pass metabolism in liver.
● *Excretion:* Less than 1% eliminated in urine. Overall elimination half-life of drug is about 5 hours.

Contraindications and precautions
Contraindicated in patients with hypersensitivity or idiosyncrasy to nitrates and in those with se-

vere hypotension, shock, or acute MI with low left ventricular filling pressure. Use cautiously in patients with hypotension or blood volume depletion (such as from diuretic therapy).

Interactions
Drug-drug. *Calcium channel blockers, organic nitrates:* Marked symptomatic orthostatic hypotension when used in combination. Dosage adjustments of either class of drugs may be necessary.
Drug-lifestyle. *Alcohol:* Drug's vasodilating effects may be additive. Discourage use.

Adverse reactions
CNS: *headache* (sometimes with throbbing), dizziness, weakness.
CV: *flushing, orthostatic hypotension, tachycardia, palpitations, ankle edema,* fainting.
GI: nausea, vomiting.
Musculoskeletal: arthralgia.
Respiratory: bronchitis, pneumonia, upper respiratory tract infection.
Skin: cutaneous vasodilation, rash.
Other: *hypersensitivity reactions,* sublingual burning.

☑ Special considerations
● Drug-free interval sufficient to avoid tolerance to drug isn't completely defined. Recommended regimen involves two daily doses given 7 hours apart, with a gap of 17 hours between second dose of 1 day and first dose of next day. Considering the relatively long half-life of drug, this result is consistent with those obtained for other organic nitrates.
● The asymmetric twice-daily regimen successfully avoids significant rebound or withdrawal effects. In studies of other nitrates, the occurrence and magnitude of such phenomena appear to be highly dependent on the schedule of nitrate administration.
● Onset of action of oral drug isn't sufficiently rapid to be useful in aborting an acute anginal episode.
● Benefits of drug in patients with acute MI or heart failure haven't been established. Because drug's effects are difficult to terminate rapidly, its use isn't recommended in such patients. If it's used, however, careful clinical or hemodynamic monitoring must be performed to avoid hazards of hypotension and tachycardia.
● Methemoglobinemia has occurred in patients receiving other organic nitrates and probably could occur as an adverse reaction. Significant methemoglobinemia has occurred with moderate overdoses of organic nitrates. Suspect methemoglobinemia in patients who exhibit signs of impaired oxygen delivery despite adequate cardiac output and adequate partial pressure of arterial oxygen. Classically, methemoglobinemic blood is chocolate brown, without color change on ex-

posure to air. Treatment of choice for methemoglobinemia is methylene blue, 1 to 2 mg/kg I.V.
● Early symptoms of overdose include increased intracranial pressure; persistent, throbbing headache; confusion; moderate fever; vertigo; palpitations; visual disturbances; nausea and vomiting; syncope; air hunger; dyspnea. If drug is ingested, induce emesis or perform gastric lavage, then give activated charcoal.
● Drug is significantly removed from blood during hemodialysis.

Monitoring the patient
● Monitor vital signs and ECG closely.
● Monitor patient for adverse effects.

Information for the patient
● Tell patient to follow prescribed dosing schedule carefully (two doses taken 7 hours apart) to maintain antianginal effect and to prevent tolerance.
● Warn patient that daily headaches sometimes accompany treatment with nitrates, including isosorbide mononitrate, and are a marker of drug activity. Patient shouldn't alter treatment schedule because loss of headache may be associated with simultaneous loss of antianginal efficacy. Tell patient to treat headaches with aspirin or acetaminophen.
● Tell patient to rise slowly from recumbent or seated position to avoid light-headedness caused by sudden drop in blood pressure.

Pediatric patients
● Safety and effectiveness in children haven't been established.

Breast-feeding patients
● It's unknown if drug appears in breast milk; use with caution in breast-feeding women.

---

isotretinoin
Accutane

Pharmacologic classification: retinoic acid derivative
Therapeutic classification: antiacne, keratinization stabilizer
Pregnancy risk category X

How supplied
Available by prescription only
Capsules: 10 mg, 20 mg, 40 mg

Indications, route, and dosage
Severe recalcitrant nodular acne
Adults and adolescents: 0.5 to 2 mg/kg P.O. daily given in two divided doses and continued for 15 to 20 weeks.

◊ *Keratinization disorders resistant to conventional therapy,* ◊ *prevention of skin cancer*
Adults: Dosage varies with specific disease and severity of the disorder; doses up to 2 to 4 mg/kg P.O. daily have been used. Consult current literature for specific recommendations.

◊ *Squamous cell cancer of the head and neck*
Adults: 50 to 100 mg/m².

Pharmacodynamics
Antiacne action: Exact mechanism unknown. Decreases size and activity of sebaceous glands, which decreases secretion and probably explains the rapid clinical improvement. A reduction in *Propionibacterium acnes* in the hair follicles occurs as a secondary result of decreased nutrients.
Keratinizing action: Mechanism unknown. Has anti-inflammatory and keratinizing effects.

Pharmacokinetics
● *Absorption:* When administered orally, absorbed rapidly from GI tract. Levels peak in 3 hours, with peak levels of the metabolite 4-oxo-isotretinoin occurring in 6 to 20 hours. Therapeutic range for drug hasn't been established.
● *Distribution:* Distributed widely. Degree of placental transfer and of secretion in breast milk is unknown. Drug is 99.9% protein-bound, primarily to albumin.
● *Metabolism:* Metabolized in liver and possibly in gut wall. Major metabolite is 4-oxo-isotretinoin, with tretinoin and 4-oxo-tretinoin also found in blood and urine.
● *Excretion:* Not fully known; renal and biliary pathways used.

Contraindications and precautions
Contraindicated in women of childbearing age unless patient has had a negative serum pregnancy test within 2 weeks before beginning therapy, will begin drug therapy on day 2 or 3 of next menstrual period, and will comply with stringent contraceptive measures for 1 month before therapy, during therapy, and for at least 1 month after therapy. Severe fetal abnormalities may occur if used during pregnancy. Also contraindicated in patients hypersensitive to parabens, which are used as preservatives.

Interactions
Drug-drug. *Carbamazepine:* Decreased carbamazepine levels in plasma. Monitor carbamazepine levels.
Medicated "cover-ups," medicated cleansers and soaps, preparations containing alcohol, topical resorcinol peeling products (benzoyl peroxide): Cumulative drying effect. Monitor patient.
Tetracyclines: May increase potential for development of pseudotumor cerebri. Avoid concomitant use.

Vitamin A products: Possible additive toxic effect. Don't use together.

Drug-food. *Any food:* Enhanced drug absorption. Administer concurrently.

Drug-lifestyle. *Alcohol:* May increase plasma triglyceride levels. Discourage use.

Sun exposure: Increased photosensitivity reactions. Tell patient to take precautions.

Adverse reactions

CNS: headache, fatigue, *pseudotumor cerebri* (benign intracranial hypertension).

EENT: *conjunctivitis, drying of mucous membranes,* corneal deposits, dry eyes, visual disturbances, *epistaxis, dry nose.*

GI: nonspecific GI symptoms, gum bleeding and inflammation, *nausea, vomiting,* anorexia, *dry mouth, abdominal pain.*

Hematologic: anemia, elevated platelet count.

Hepatic: elevated AST, ALT, and alkaline phosphatase levels.

Metabolic: hyperglycemia.

Musculoskeletal: *musculoskeletal pain (skeletal hyperostosis).*

Skin: *cheilosis, rash, dry skin, facial skin desquamation,* peeling of palms and toes, skin infection, photosensitivity, *cheilitis, pruritus, fragility, petechiae, nail brittleness,* thinning of hair.

Other: *hypertriglyceridemia.*

☑ Special considerations

● Therapy usually lasts 15 to 20 weeks, then at least 8 weeks off drug before starting second course.

● Don't prescribe more than a 6-week supply at one time.

● Drug has been used in a limited number of patients to treat psoriasis (combined with psoralen and ultraviolet light); has also been used to treat cutaneous neoplasms.

Monitoring the patient

● Monitor baseline serum lipid levels and liver function tests before therapy begins and at regular intervals.

● Monitor blood glucose levels regularly and CK levels in patients who participate in vigorous physical activity.

● Monitor patient for visual problems.

Information for the patient

● Warn patient that isotretinoin is a potent teratogen and shouldn't be used by women who are pregnant or may become pregnant during therapy. Patient selection is important—informed consent must be obtained from patient or her legal guardian before therapy starts. The patient or responsible adult must fully understand consequences of fetal exposure to drug.

● Advise patient that reliable methods of contraception are essential for sexually active women taking isotretinoin.

● Inform patient that negative blood tests for pregnancy must be obtained before therapy.

● Instruct patient to schedule follow-up visits monthly during therapy. Pregnancy tests must be repeated monthly.

● Warn patient that acne may worsen during initial course of therapy and to call if irritation becomes severe.

● Warn patient not to donate blood or become pregnant while taking drug and for 30 days after therapy ends.

● Warn patient to be cautious when driving, particularly at night, because drug causes decreased night vision.

● Instruct patient not to crush capsules.

● Advise patient not to take vitamin supplements containing vitamin A while taking drug.

● Tell patient to avoid prolonged exposure to sunlight or sun lamps to prevent photosensitivity.

● Contact lenses may become uncomfortable during treatment; recommend use of artificial tears.

Breast-feeding patients

● It's unknown if drug appears in breast milk; breast-feeding isn't recommended during therapy.

isradipine
DynaCirc

Pharmacologic classification: calcium channel blocker

Therapeutic classification: antihypertensive

Pregnancy risk category C

How supplied

Available by prescription only

Capsules: 2.5 mg, 5 mg

Indications, route, and dosage

Management of hypertension

Adults: Individualize dosage. Initially, 2.5 mg P.O. b.i.d. alone or with thiazide diuretic. Maximal response may require 2 to 4 weeks; therefore, dose adjustments of 5 mg daily should be made at 2- to 4-week intervals up to maximum of 20 mg daily. Doses of 10 mg or more per day haven't been shown to be more effective but rather to lead to more adverse reactions. Same starting dose is used in elderly patients and in those with hepatic or renal impairment.

Pharmacodynamics

Antihypertensive action: A dihydropyridine calcium channel blocker that binds to calcium channels and inhibits calcium flux into cardiac and smooth muscle, which results in dilation of arterioles. This dilation reduces systemic resistance and lowers blood pressure while producing small increases in resting heart rate.

Pharmacokinetics
• *Absorption:* 90% to 95% of drug absorbed after oral administration; levels peak in 1½ hours.
• *Distribution:* 95% bound to plasma protein.
• *Metabolism:* Completely metabolized before elimination, with extensive first-pass metabolism.
• *Excretion:* 60% to 65% of drug excreted in urine; 25% to 30%, in feces.

Contraindications and precautions
Contraindicated in patients with hypersensitivity to drug. Use cautiously in patients with heart failure, especially if combined with a beta blocker.

Interactions
Drug-drug. *Fentanyl anesthesia:* Caused severe hypotension. Avoid concomitant use.

Adverse reactions
CNS: dizziness, *headache,* fatigue.
CV: edema, flushing, syncope, angina, tachycardia.
GI: nausea, diarrhea, abdominal discomfort, vomiting.
Respiratory: dyspnea.
Skin: rash.

☑ Special considerations
• Drug has no significant effect on heart rate and no adverse effects on cardiac contractility, conduction or digitalis clearance, or lipid or renal function.
• Administration with food significantly increases time to reach peak levels by about 1 hour. However, food has no effect on total bioavailability of drug.

Monitoring the patient
• Elevated liver function test results have been reported in some patients.
• Individualize dosage. Allow 2 to 4 weeks between dosage adjustments.

Information for the patient
• Instruct patient to report irregular heartbeat, shortness of breath, swelling of hands or feet, pronounced dizziness, constipation, nausea, or hypotension.

Geriatric patients
• No age-related problems have been reported.

Pediatric patients
• Safety and efficacy haven't been established in children under age 18.

Breast-feeding patients
• It's unknown if drug appears in breast milk. Consider potential risk of serious adverse reactions in infant.

itraconazole
Sporanox

Pharmacologic classification: synthetic triazole
Therapeutic classification: antifungal
Pregnancy risk category C

How supplied
Available by prescription only
Capsules: 100 mg

Indications, route, and dosage
Blastomycosis (pulmonary and extrapulmonary), histoplasmosis (including chronic cavitary pulmonary disease and disseminated nonmeningeal histoplasmosis)
Adults: 200 mg P.O. once daily. If condition doesn't improve or shows evidence of progressive fungal disease, increase dose in 100-mg increments to maximum of 400 mg daily. Give doses over 200 mg/day in two divided doses.
Aspergillosis (pulmonary and extrapulmonary) in patients who are intolerant of or refractory to amphotericin B therapy
Adults: 200 to 400 mg P.O. daily.
◇ *Superficial mycoses (dermatophytoses, pityriasis versicolor, sebopsoriasis, candidiasis [vaginal, oral, or chronic mucocutaneous], onychomycosis),* ◇ *systemic mycoses (candidiasis, cryptococcal infections [meningitis, disseminated],* ◇ *dimorphic infections [paracoccidioidomycosis, coccidioidomycosis]),* ◇ *subcutaneous mycoses (sporotrichosis, chromomycosis),* ◇ *cutaneous leishmaniasis,* ◇ *fungal keratitis,* ◇ *alternariatoxicosis, and* ◇ *zygomycosis*
Adults: 50 to 400 mg P.O. daily. Duration of therapy varies from 1 day to greater than 6 months, depending on the condition and mycologic response.
    Note: Stop drug if patient develops signs and symptoms consistent with liver disease that may be attributable to itraconazole.

Pharmacodynamics
Antifungal action: Synthetic triazole antifungal drug. In vitro, inhibits the cytochrome P-450–dependent synthesis of ergosterol, a vital component of fungal cell membranes.

Pharmacokinetics
• *Absorption:* Oral bioavailability maximal when taken with food; absolute oral bioavailability is 55%.

• *Distribution:* Plasma protein–binding is 99.8%; 99.5% for metabolite, hydroxyitraconazole.
• *Metabolism:* Extensively metabolized by liver into large number of metabolites, including hydroxyitraconazole, the major metabolite.
• *Excretion:* Fecal excretion of parent drug varies between 3% and 18% of dose. Renal excretion of parent drug is less than 0.03% of dose. About 40% of dose excreted as inactive metabolites in urine. Drug isn't removed by hemodialysis.

Contraindications and precautions
Contraindicated in patients with hypersensitivity to drug, in patients receiving terfenadine, and in breast-feeding patients because drug is excreted in breast milk.

Use cautiously in patients with hypochlorhydria or HIV infection and in those receiving drugs that are highly protein-bound.

Interactions
Drug-drug. *Cyclosporine:* Increased cyclosporine plasma levels. Reduce cyclosporine dosage by 50% when using itraconazole doses greater than 100 mg/day; monitor cyclosporine levels.
Digoxin: Increased digoxin levels. Monitor digoxin levels.
H_2 antagonists, isoniazid, phenytoin, rifampin: May reduce plasma itraconazole levels. Avoid concomitant use.
Nonsedating antihistamines: Itraconazole can increase plasma levels, resulting in rare instances of life-threatening arrhythmias and death. Avoid concurrent use.
Sulfonylureas: Possible hypoglycemia when used together. Monitor blood glucose level.
Warfarin: Enhanced anticoagulant effect. Monitor PT and INR.

Adverse reactions
CNS: malaise, fatigue, headache, dizziness, somnolence.
CV: edema, hypertension.
GI: *nausea,* vomiting, diarrhea, abdominal pain, anorexia.
GU: albuminuria, impotence.
Hepatic: impaired hepatic function.
Metabolic: hypokalemia.
Skin: rash, pruritus.
Other: fever, decreased libido.

☑ Special considerations
• In life-threatening situations, recommended loading dose is 200 mg three times daily (600 mg/day) for first 3 days. Continue treatment for minimum of 3 months and until clinical parameters and laboratory tests indicate that the active fungal infection has subsided. An inadequate period of treatment may lead to recurrence of active infection.
• Obtain specimens for fungal cultures and other relevant laboratory studies (wet mount, histopathology, serology) before therapy to isolate and identify causative organisms. Therapy may be instituted before results of cultures and other laboratory studies are known; once results become available, adjust anti-infective therapy accordingly.
• The clinical course of histoplasmosis in HIV-infected patients is more severe and usually requires maintenance therapy to prevent relapse. Because hypochlorhydia has occurred in HIV-infected patients, absorption of itraconazole may be decreased.

Monitoring the patient
• Monitor hepatic enzyme test values in patients with preexisting hepatic function abnormalities.
• Monitor therapeutic effect.

Information for the patient
• Instruct patient to take drug with food to enhance absorption.
• Tell patient to report signs and symptoms that may suggest liver dysfunction (jaundice, unusual fatigue, anorexia, nausea, vomiting, dark urine, pale stool) so that appropriate laboratory testing can be performed.

Pediatric patients
• Safety and effectiveness in children haven't been established.

Breast-feeding patients
• Because drug appears in breast milk, drug is contraindicated in breast-feeding women.

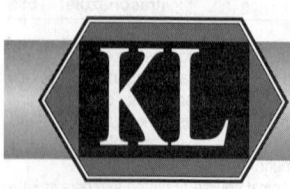

ketamine hydrochloride
Ketalar

Pharmacologic classification: dissociative anesthetic
Therapeutic classification: I.V. anesthetic
Pregnancy risk category NR

How supplied
Available by prescription only
Injection: 10 mg/ml, 50 mg/ml, 100 mg/ml

Indications, route, and dosage
Induction of general anesthesia, especially for short diagnostic or surgical procedures not requiring skeletal muscle relaxation; adjunct to other general anesthetics or low-potency drugs, such as nitrous oxide
Adults and children: 1 to 4.5 mg/kg I.V. administered over 60 seconds; or 6.5 to 13 mg/kg I.M. To maintain anesthesia, repeat in increments of half to full initial dose.

Pharmacodynamics
Anesthetic action: Induces a profound sense of dissociation from the environment by direct action on the cortex and limbic system.

Pharmacokinetics
• *Absorption:* Absorbed rapidly and well after I.M. injection. Induces surgical anesthesia in 30 seconds after I.V. administration; effect lasts 5 to 10 minutes. After I.M. injection, anesthesia begins in 3 to 4 minutes; lasts 12 to 25 minutes.
• *Distribution:* Rapidly enters CNS.
• *Metabolism:* Metabolized by liver to active metabolite with one-third potency of parent drug.
• *Excretion:* Excreted in urine.

Contraindications and precautions
Contraindicated in patients with schizophrenia or other acute psychosis because it may exacerbate the condition. Also contraindicated in those with CV disease in which a sudden rise in blood pressure would be harmful and in patients allergic to drug.

Interactions
Drug-drug. *Barbiturates, narcotics:* Possible prolonged recovery time if ketamine is used concomitantly. Use with caution. Don't give barbiturates in same syringe as ketamine.

Enflurane, halothane: Significant myocardial depression and hypotension. Avoid concomitant use.
Thyroid hormones: Possible hypertension and tachycardia. Monitor blood pressure and ECG closely.
Tubocurarine, other nondepolarizing muscle relaxants: May increase neuromuscular effects of these drugs if used together. Avoid concomitant use.

Adverse reactions
CNS: tonic-clonic movements, hallucinations, confusion, excitement, dreamlike states, irrational behavior, psychic abnormalities.
CV: *hypertension; tachycardia;* hypotension, **bradycardia** (if used with halothane); **arrhythmias.**
EENT: diplopia, nystagmus, laryngospasm.
GI: mild anorexia, nausea, vomiting, excessive salivation.
Respiratory: *respiratory depression* in high doses, *apnea* (if administered too rapidly).
Skin: transient erythema, measles-like rash.
 Note: Stop drug if hypersensitivity, laryngospasm, or severe hypotension or hypertension occurs.

☑ Special considerations
• Patients need physical support because of rapid induction; monitor vital signs perioperatively. Blood pressure begins to rise shortly after injection, peaks at 10% to 50% above preanesthetic levels, and returns to baseline within 15 minutes. Ketamine's effects on blood pressure make it particularly useful in hypovolemic patients as an induction drug that supports blood pressure.
• Keep verbal, tactile, and visual stimulation to a minimum during induction and recovery. Emergence reactions occur in 12% of patients, including dreams, visual imagery, hallucinations, and delirium and may occur for up to 24 hours postoperatively. They may be reduced by using lower dosage of ketamine with I.V. diazepam and can be treated with short-acting or ultrashort-acting barbiturates. Incidence is lower in patients under age 15 or over age 65 and when drug is given I.M.
• Dissociative and hallucinatory adverse effects have led to drug abuse.
• Barbiturates are incompatible in same syringe.
• For direct injection, dilute 100 mg/ml concentration with an equal volume of sterile water for

injection, normal saline, or D₅W. For continuous infusion, prepare a 1 mg/ml solution by adding 5 ml from the 100 mg/ml to 500 ml of D₅W or normal saline.

Monitoring the patient
• Monitor vital signs closely, especially respiratory status.
• Monitor cardiac rhythm during procedures.

Information for the patient
• Warn patient to avoid tasks requiring motor coordination and mental alertness for 24 hours after anesthesia.
• Instruct patient to report adverse effects immediately.

Geriatric patients
• Use drug with caution, especially in patients with suspected stroke, hypertension, or cardiac disease.

Pediatric patients
• Drug is safe and especially useful in managing minor surgical or diagnostic procedures and in repeated procedures that require large amounts of analgesia, such as changing of burn dressings.

---

ketoconazole
Nizoral

Pharmacologic classification: imidazole derivative
Therapeutic classification: antifungal
Pregnancy risk category C

How supplied
Available by prescription only
Tablets: 200 mg
Cream: 2%
Shampoo: 2%

Indications, route, and dosage
Severe fungal infections caused by susceptible organisms
Adults: Initially, 200 mg P.O. daily as a single dose. Dose may be increased to 400 mg once daily in patients who don't respond to lower dosage, or in patients with serious infections.
Children over age 2: 3.3 to 6.6 mg/kg P.O. daily as a single dose.
Topical treatment of tinea corporis, tinea cruris, tinea versicolor, and tinea pedis
Adults and children: Apply daily or b.i.d. for about 2 weeks; for tinea pedis apply for 6 weeks.
Seborrheic dermatitis
Adults and children: Apply b.i.d. for about 4 weeks.
◇ **Cushing's syndrome**
Adults: 800 to 1,200 mg/day P.O.

Dandruff
Adults: Apply for 1 minute, rinse, then reapply for 3 minutes. Shampoo twice weekly for 4 weeks with at least 3 days between shampoos.
◇ *Prostatic carcinoma*
Adults: 400 mg P.O. q 8 hours.

Pharmacodynamics
Antifungal action: Fungicidal and fungistatic, depending on levels. Inhibits demethylation of lanosterol, thereby altering membrane permeability and inhibiting purine transport. The in vitro spectrum of activity includes most pathogenic fungi. However, CSF levels following oral administration aren't predictable. Shouldn't be used to treat fungal meningitis, and specimens should be obtained for susceptibility testing before therapy. Currently available tests may not accurately reflect in vivo activity, so interpret results with caution.

Used orally to treat disseminated or pulmonary coccidiomycosis, paracoccidioidomycosis, or histoplasmosis; oral candidiasis; and candiduria (but low renal clearance may limit its usefulness).

Also useful in some dermatophytoses, including tinea capitis, tinea cruris, tinea pedis, tinea manus, and tinea unguium (onychomycosis) caused by *Epidermophyton, Microsporum,* or *Trichophyton.*

Pharmacokinetics
• *Absorption:* Converted to hydrochloride salt before absorption. Erratic absorption; decreased by raised gastric pH and may be increased in extent and consistency by food. Plasma levels peak at 1 to 4 hours.
• *Distribution:* Distributed into bile, saliva, cerumen, synovial fluid, and sebum; erratic and minimal CSF penetration. 84% to 99% bound to plasma proteins.
• *Metabolism:* Converted into several inactive metabolites in liver.
• *Excretion:* Over 50% excreted in feces within 4 days; drug and metabolites secreted in bile. About 13% excreted unchanged in urine. Probably excreted in breast milk. Half-life is biphasic; initially 2 hours, with a terminal half-life of 8 hours.

Contraindications and precautions
Contraindicated in patients with hypersensitivity to drug and in those taking astemizole because of the potential for serious CV adverse events. Use oral form cautiously in patients with hepatic disease. Because CSF levels of ketoconazole are unpredictable following oral administration, don't use drug alone to treat fungal meningitis.

Interactions
Drug-drug. *Antacids, antimuscarinics, cimetidine, famotidine, ranitidine:* Decreased absorption of drug. Wait at least 2 hours after ketoconazole dose before administering these drugs.

Corticosteroids: May result in increased plasma levels of corticosteroid. Monitor patient closely.
Cyclosporine: Increased serum levels of cyclosporine. Monitor serum levels of cyclosporine.
Oral sulfonylureas: May intensify effects of these drugs. Monitor patient closely.
Other hepatotoxic drugs: May enhance toxicity of these drugs. Monitor patient closely.
Phenytoin: May alter serum levels of both drugs. Monitor serum levels of both drugs.
Rifampin: May decrease ketoconazole to ineffective serum levels. Monitor patient for decreased antifungal effect.
Theophylline: May decrease theophylline plasma levels. Monitor serum levels and adjust dosage as needed.
Warfarin: Enhanced anticoagulant effects. Monitor INR, PT, and PTT; adjust dosage as needed.
Drug-herb. *Yew preparations:* Inhibited ketoconazole metabolism. Don't use concomitantly.

Adverse reactions
CNS: headache, nervousness, dizziness, somnolence, photophobia, *suicidal tendencies,* severe depression (with oral administration).
GI: *nausea, vomiting,* abdominal pain, diarrhea (with oral administration).
GU: gynecomastia with tenderness, impotence (with oral administration).
Hematologic: *thrombocytopenia,* hemolytic anemia, *leukopenia* (with oral administration).
Hepatic: elevated liver enzyme levels, *fatal hepatotoxicity* (with oral administration).
Skin: pruritus; severe irritation, stinging (with topical administration).
Other: fever, chills.

☑ Special considerations
• Identify organism, but don't delay therapy for results of laboratory tests.
• Give drug with citrus juice.
• Drug requires acidity for absorption and is ineffective in patients with achlorhydria.
• For overdose, induce emesis and use sodium bicarbonate lavage; then use activated charcoal and a cathartic.

Monitoring the patient
• Watch for signs of hepatotoxicity: persistent nausea, unusual fatigue, jaundice, dark urine, and pale stools.
• Monitor patient on long-term therapy for signs of adrenal crisis.

Information for the patient
• Teach achlorhydric patient how to take ketoconazole. He should dissolve each tablet in 4 ml of 0.2N (normal) hydrochloric acid solution or take with 200 ml of 0.1N hydrochloric acid, and administer through a glass or plastic straw to avoid damaging enamel on patient's teeth. Tell patient to drink a glass of water after each dose.

• Tell patient to avoid driving or performing other hazardous activities if dizziness or drowsiness occur; these often occur early in treatment but abate as treatment continues.
• Caution patient not to alter dose or dosage interval or to stop drug without medical approval. Explain that, to prevent recurrence, therapy must continue until active fungal infection is completely gone.
• Reassure patient that nausea will subside; to minimize reaction, patient may take drug with food or may divide dosage into two doses.
• Advise patient to avoid OTC preparations for GI distress (such as antacids). Some may alter gastric pH levels and interfere with drug action.
• Encourage patient to get specific medical approval before taking other drugs with ketoconazole.

Pediatric patients
• Safe use in children under age 2 hasn't been established. Use in children should be considered only when benefits outweigh risks.

Breast-feeding patients
• Drug may appear in breast milk. An alternative to breast-feeding is recommended.

ketoprofen
Actron, Orudis, Orudis KT, Oruvail

Pharmacologic classification: NSAID
Therapeutic classification: nonnarcotic analgesic, antipyretic, anti-inflammatory
Pregnancy risk category B

How supplied
Available by prescription only
Capsules: 25 mg, 50 mg, 75 mg
Capsules (extended-release): 100 mg, 150 mg, 200 mg
Available without a prescription
Tablets: 12.5 mg

Indications, route, and dosage
Rheumatoid arthritis and osteoarthritis
Adults: Usual dose is 75 mg t.i.d. or 50 mg q.i.d. P.O. Maximum dose is 300 mg/day or 200 mg (extended-release capsules) P.O. daily.
Mild to moderate pain; dysmenorrhea
Adults: 25 to 50 mg P.O. q 6 to 8 hours, p.r.n.
Temporary relief of mild aches and pain, fever (self-medication)
Adults: 12.5 mg q 4 to 6 hours. Don't exceed 75 mg in a 24-hour period.

Pharmacodynamics
Analgesic, antipyretic, and anti-inflammatory actions: Mechanisms unknown. Thought to inhibit prostaglandin synthesis.

Reactions may be *common,* uncommon, **life-threatening**, or COMMON AND LIFE-THREATENING.

Pharmacokinetics
• *Absorption:* Absorbed rapidly and completely from GI tract.
• *Distribution:* Highly protein-bound. Extent of body tissue fluid distribution not known, but therapeutic levels range from 0.4 to 6 mcg/ml.
• *Metabolism:* Metabolized in liver.
• *Excretion:* Excreted in urine as parent drug and metabolites.

Contraindications and precautions
Contraindicated in patients with hypersensitivity to drug and in those with history of aspirin- or NSAID-induced asthma, urticaria, or other allergic-type reactions. Use cautiously in patients with impaired renal or hepatic function, peptic ulcer disease, heart failure, hypertension, or fluid retention.

Interactions
Drug-drug. *Acetaminophen, diuretics, gold compounds, other anti-inflammatories:* Increased nephrotoxicity may occur with concomitant use. Monitor renal function.
Anticoagulants, thrombolytics: May potentiate anticoagulant effects. Monitor PT and INR closely.
Antihypertensives, diuretics: May decrease effectiveness of these drugs. Monitor patient closely.
Anti-inflammatories, corticotropin, salicylates, corticosteroids: Increased GI adverse effects. Avoid concomitant use.
Aspirin, cefamandole, cefoperazone, dextran, dipyridamole, mezlocillin, parenteral carbenicillin, piperacillin, plicamycin, salicylates, sulfinpyrazone, ticarcillin, valproic acid, other anti-inflammatories: Bleeding problems may occur if ketoprofen is used concomitantly. Avoid concomitant use.
Coumarin derivatives, lithium, methotrexate, nifedipine, phenytoin, verapamil: Toxicity may occur with concomitant use. Monitor patient closely.
Insulin, oral antidiabetics: May potentiate hypoglycemic effects. Monitor serum glucose levels closely.
Drug-lifestyle. *Alcohol:* May cause increased GI adverse effects. Discourage use.
Sun exposure: Increased risk of photosensitive reaction. Tell patient to take precautions.

Adverse reactions
CNS: *headache, dizziness, CNS excitation or depression.*
EENT: *tinnitus, visual disturbances.*
GI: *nausea, abdominal pain, diarrhea, constipation, flatulence, **peptic ulceration**, dyspepsia, anorexia, vomiting, stomatitis.*
GU: *nephrotoxicity,* elevated BUN level.
Hematologic: *prolonged bleeding time, **thrombocytopenia, agranulocytosis.***
Hepatic: elevated liver enzyme levels.

Respiratory: *dyspnea, **bronchospasm, laryngeal edema.***
Skin: rash, photosensitivity, ***exfoliative dermatitis.***
Other: peripheral edema.

☑ Special considerations
In addition to the recommendations relevant to all NSAIDs, consider the following.
• Administer tablets on empty stomach either 30 minutes before or 2 hours after meals to ensure adequate absorption. However, capsules may be taken with foods or antacids to minimize GI distress.
• Store suppositories in refrigerator.
• Signs and symptoms of overdose include nausea and drowsiness. To treat, induce emesis with ipecac syrup or empty stomach via gastric lavage; administer activated charcoal via nasogastric tube.
• Hemodialysis may be useful in removing ketoprofen and assisting in care of renal failure.

Monitoring the patient
• Monitor vital signs closely.
• Monitor CNS effects of drug. Institute safety measures, such as assisted walking, raised side rails, and gradual position changes, to prevent injury.
• Monitor laboratory test results for abnormalities.

Information for the patient
• Instruct patient in prescribed drug regimen and proper drug administration.
• Tell patient to seek medical approval before taking OTC products (especially aspirin and products containing aspirin).
• Caution patient to avoid activities that require alertness or concentration. Instruct him in safety measures to prevent injury.
• Instruct patient to report adverse reactions.

Geriatric patients
• Patients over age 60 may be more susceptible to toxic effects of ketoprofen. Use with caution.
• The effects of drug on renal prostaglandins may cause fluid retention and edema, a significant drawback for elderly patients and those with heart failure. The manufacturer recommends that initial dose be reduced by 33% to 50% in geriatric patients.

Pediatric patients
• Safe use in children under age 12 hasn't been established.

Breast-feeding patients
• Although most NSAIDs appear in breast milk, it's unknown if ketoprofen appears in breast milk. Avoid use in breast-feeding women.

ketorolac tromethamine
Toradol

Pharmacologic classification: NSAID
Therapeutic classification: analgesic
Pregnancy risk category C

How supplied
Available by prescription only
Tablets: 10 mg
Injection: 15 mg/ml (1-ml cartridge), 30 mg/ml (1-ml and 2-ml cartridges)

Indications, route, and dosage
Short-term management of pain
Adults under age 65: Dosage should be based on patient response; initially, 60 mg I.M. or 30 mg I.V. as a single dose, or multiple doses of 30 mg I.M. or I.V. q 6 hours. Maximum daily dose shouldn't exceed 120 mg.
✦ *Dosage adjustment.* In adults ages 65 and older, renally impaired patients, and those weighing less than 50 kg (110 lb), 30 mg I.M. or 15 mg I.V. initially as a single dose, or multiple doses of 15 mg I.M. or I.V. q 6 hours. Maximum daily dose shouldn't exceed 60 mg.
Short-term management of moderately severe, acute pain when switching from parenteral to oral administration
Adults under age 65: 20 mg P.O. as a single dose, then 10 mg P.O. q 4 to 6 hours, not to exceed 40 mg/day.
✦ *Dosage adjustment.* In adults ages 65 and older, renally impaired patients, and those weighing less than 50 kg, 10 mg P.O. as a single dose, then 10 mg P.O. q 4 to 6 hours, not to exceed 40 mg/day.

Pharmacodynamics
Analgesic action: An NSAID that acts by inhibiting the synthesis of prostaglandins.

Pharmacokinetics
• *Absorption:* Completely absorbed after I.M. administration. After oral administration, food delays absorption but doesn't decrease total amount absorbed.
• *Distribution:* Mean plasma levels peak about 30 minutes after a 50-mg dose and range from 2.2 to 3 mcg/ml. Over 99% protein-bound.
• *Metabolism:* Primarily hepatic; a para-hydroxy metabolite and conjugates identified; less than 50% of a dose metabolized. Liver impairment doesn't substantially alter drug clearance.
• *Excretion:* Primary excretion is in urine (over 90%); the rest in feces. Terminal plasma half-life is 3.8 to 6.3 hours (average 4½ hours) in young adults; substantially prolonged in patients with renal failure.

Contraindications and precautions
Contraindicated in patients with hypersensitivity to drug and in those with active peptic ulcer disease, recent GI bleeding or perforation, advanced renal impairment, risk of renal impairment due to volume depletion, suspected or confirmed cerebrovascular bleeding, hemorrhagic diathesis, incomplete hemostasis, or high risk of bleeding.

Also contraindicated in patients with history of peptic ulcer disease or GI bleeding, past allergic reactions to aspirin or other NSAIDs, and during labor and delivery or breast-feeding. In addition, drug is contraindicated as prophylactic analgesic before major surgery or intraoperatively when hemostasis is critical; in patients receiving aspirin, an NSAID, or probenecid; and in those requiring analgesics to be administered epidurally or intrathecally.

Use cautiously in patients with impaired renal or hepatic function.

Interactions
Drug-drug. *Diuretics:* Decreased efficacy of diuretic and enhanced nephrotoxicity. Monitor intake and output and renal function.
Lithium: Increased lithium levels. Monitor patient and serum lithium levels.
Methotrexate: Decreased methotrexate clearance and increased toxicity. Don't use together.
Salicylates, warfarin: Possible increased levels of free (unbound) salicylates or warfarin in blood. Monitor patient.

Adverse reactions
CNS: *drowsiness, sedation,* dizziness, *headache.*
CV: edema, hypertension, palpitations, ***arrhythmias.***
GI: *nausea, dyspepsia,* GI pain, diarrhea, ***peptic ulceration,*** vomiting, constipation, flatulence, stomatitis.
GU: *acute renal failure.*
Hematologic: decreased platelet adhesion, purpura, ***thrombocytopenia.***
Respiratory: ***bronchospasm.***
Skin: pain at injection site, pruritus, rash, diaphoresis.

☑ Special considerations
• Drug is intended for short-term pain management. Rate and severity of adverse reactions should be less than that observed in patients taking NSAIDs on a long-term basis.
• I.M. injections in patients with coagulopathies or those receiving anticoagulants may cause bleeding and hematoma at injection site.
• Combined duration of ketorolac I.M., I.V., or P.O. shouldn't exceed 5 days. Oral use is only for continuation of I.V. or I.M. therapy.

Reactions may be *common,* uncommon, ***life-threatening***, or COMMON AND LIFE-THREATENING.

Monitoring the patient
● Correct hypovolemia before starting ketorolac therapy.
● Watch for adverse effects, including GI irritation.

Information for the patient
● Warn patient that GI ulceration, bleeding, and perforation can occur at any time, with or without warning, in anyone taking NSAIDs on a long-term basis. Teach patient how to recognize signs and symptoms of GI bleeding.
● Instruct patient to avoid aspirin, products containing aspirin, and alcoholic beverages during therapy.

Geriatric patients
● Use lower initial doses (30 mg I.M.) in patients over age 65 or weighing less than 110 lb. Elderly patients have exhibited a longer terminal half-life of drug (average 7 hours in elderly patients compared with 4½ hours in healthy young adults).

Pediatric patients
● Safety and efficacy haven't been established. Drug isn't recommended for use in children.

Breast-feeding patients
● Drug appears in breast milk. Its use is contraindicated in breast-feeding women.

ketorolac tromethamine (ophthalmic)
Acular

Pharmacologic classification: NSAID
Therapeutic classification: ophthalmic anti-inflammatory
Pregnancy risk category C

How supplied
Available by prescription only
Ophthalmic solution: 0.5%

Indications, route, and dosage
Relief of ocular itching caused by seasonal allergic conjunctivitis
Adults: Instill 1 drop (0.25 mg) in conjunctival sac q.i.d. Efficacy hasn't been established beyond 1 week of continued use.
Postoperative ocular inflammation following cataract extraction
Adults: 1 drop q.i.d. beginning 24 hours after surgery and continuing for 2 weeks after surgery.

Pharmacodynamics
Anti-inflammatory action: Thought to be a result, in part, of its ability to inhibit prostaglandin biosynthesis. Drug reduces prostaglandin E_2 levels in aqueous humor with ocular administration. Has also demonstrated analgesic and antipyretic activity because of the same mechanism of action.

Pharmacokinetics
No information available.

Contraindications and precautions
Contraindicated in patients with hypersensitivity to drug or its components and in those wearing soft contact lenses. Use cautiously in patients with hypersensitivity to other NSAIDs or aspirin and in those with bleeding disorders.

Interactions
None reported.

Adverse reactions
EENT: *transient stinging and burning on instillation,* superficial keratitis, superficial ocular infections, ocular irritation.
Other: *hypersensitivity reactions.*

☑ Special considerations
● Ophthalmic solution has been safely administered with other ophthalmics, such as antibiotics, beta blockers, carbonic anhydrase inhibitors, cycloplegics, and mydriatics.
● Store drug at controlled room temperature and protect from light.
● If accidentally ingested, have patient drink fluids to dilute.

Monitoring the patient
● Monitor patient for sensitivity reactions.
● Monitor patient for signs of ocular infection.

Information for the patient
● Teach patient how to administer eyedrops and stress importance of not touching dropper to eye or surrounding area.
● Advise patient not to use more drops than prescribed or to use drug for other eye problems unless prescribed.
● Instruct patient to discard drug when outdated or no longer needed.

Pediatric patients
● Safety and efficacy in children haven't been established.

Breast-feeding patients
● Drug appears in breast milk. Use cautiously in breast-feeding women.

ketotifen fumarate
Zaditor

Pharmacologic classification: histamine
(H_1-receptor) antagonist and mast cell
stabilizer
Therapeutic classification: ophthalmic
antihistamine
Pregnancy risk category C

How supplied
Available by prescription only
Ophthalmic solution: 0.025%; supplied as 5-ml
solution in 7.5-ml bottles

Indications, route, and dosage
*Temporary prevention of itching of eye
caused by allergic conjunctivitis*
Adults and children ages 4 and older: Instill 1
drop in affected eye q 8 to 12 hours.

Pharmacodynamics
Antihistamine action: Selective, noncompetitive
histamine antagonist (H_1-receptor) and mast cell
stabilizer that inhibits release of mediators from
cells involved in hypersensitivity reactions, thus
providing temporary prevention of eye itching.

Pharmacokinetics
• *Absorption:* Effect is seen within minutes after
administration.
• *Distribution:* No information available.
• *Metabolism:* No information available.
• *Excretion:* No information available.

Contraindications and precautions
Contraindicated in persons with hypersensitivity
to drug or its component.

Interactions
None reported.

Adverse reactions
CNS: headaches.
EENT: conjunctival infection, rhinitis, ocular allergic reactions, burning or stinging of eyes, conjunctivitis, eye discharge, dry eyes, eye pain, eyelid disorder, itching of eyes, keratitis, lacrimation
disorder, mydriasis, photophobia, ocular rash,
pharyngitis.
Other: flulike syndrome.

☑ Special considerations
• Drug is for ophthalmic use only; not for injection or oral use.
• Drug isn't indicated for use with irritation related to contact lenses.
• Preservative in drug may be absorbed by soft
contact lenses. Contact lenses shouldn't be inserted until 10 minutes after drug is instilled.

Monitoring the patient
• Monitor patient for sensitivity reactions.
• Monitor patient for signs of infection.

Information for the patient
• Teach patient proper instillation technique. Tell
him to avoid contaminating dropper tip and solution and not to touch eyelids or surrounding areas with dropper tip of bottle.
• Tell patient not to wear contact lenses if eyes
are red. Warn patient not to use drug to treat irritation related to contact lenses.
• Instruct patient who wears soft contact lenses
and whose eyes aren't red to wait at least 10 minutes after instilling drug before inserting contact
lenses.
• Advise patient to report adverse reactions to
drug.
• Advise patient to keep bottle tightly closed when
not in use.

Pediatric patients
• Safety and effectiveness in children below age
3 haven't been established.

Breast-feeding patients
• It's unknown if topical ocular product appears
in breast milk. Use cautiously in breast-feeding
women.

labetalol hydrochloride
Normodyne, Trandate

Pharmacologic classification: alpha and
beta blocker
Therapeutic classification: antihypertensive
Pregnancy risk category C

How supplied
Available by prescription only
Tablets: 100 mg, 200 mg, 300 mg
Injection: 5 mg/ml in 20-, 40-, and 60-ml vials

Indications, route, and dosage
Hypertension
Adults: 100 mg P.O. b.i.d. with or without a diuretic. Dosage may be increased by 100 mg b.i.d.
q 2 or 4 days until optimum response is reached.
Usual maintenance dose is 200 to 400 mg b.i.d.;
maximum daily dose is 2,400 mg.
*Severe hypertension and hypertensive emer-
gencies; ◊ pheochromocytoma; ◊ clonidine
withdrawal hypertension*
Adults: Initially, 20-mg I.V. bolus slowly over 2
minutes; may repeat injections of 40 to 80 mg q
10 minutes to maximum dose of 300 mg.
   Or drug may be given as continuous I.V. infusion at an initial rate of 2 mg/minute until satisfactory response is obtained. Usual cumulative
dose is 50 to 200 mg.

◇ *Intraoperative hypertension*
Adults: Initially, 10 to 30 mg I.V. bolus slowly over 2 minutes; may repeat injections of 5 to 10 mg I.V., p.r.n.

Pharmacodynamics
Antihypertensive action: Inhibits catecholamine access to both beta- and postsynaptic alpha-adrenergic receptor sites. Drug also may have a vasodilating effect.

Pharmacokinetics
• *Absorption:* 90% to 100% oral absorption (however, drug undergoes extensive first-pass metabolism in liver; only about 25% of oral dose reaches systemic circulation unchanged). Antihypertensive effect occurs in 20 minutes to 2 hours, peaking in 1 to 4 hours. After direct I.V. administration, antihypertensive effect occurs in 2 to 5 minutes; maximal effect occurs in 5 to 15 minutes.
• *Distribution:* Distributed widely throughout body; about 50% protein-bound.
• *Metabolism:* Orally administered drug metabolized extensively in liver and possibly in GI mucosa.
• *Excretion:* About 5% excreted unchanged in urine; rest is excreted as metabolites in urine and feces (biliary elimination). Antihypertensive effect of oral dose lasts for about 8 to 24 hours; after I.V. administration, about 2 to 4 hours. Plasma half-life about 5½ hours after I.V. administration; 6 to 8 hours after oral administration.

Contraindications and precautions
Contraindicated in patients with hypersensitivity to drug and in those with bronchial asthma, overt cardiac failure, greater than first-degree heart block, cardiogenic shock, severe bradycardia, and other conditions associated with severe and prolonged hypotension.
    Use cautiously in patients with heart failure, hepatic failure, chronic bronchitis, emphysema, preexisting peripheral vascular disease, and pheochromocytoma.

Interactions
Drug-drug. *Beta-adrenergic agonists:* May blunt bronchodilator effect of these drugs in patients with bronchospasm. Greater than normal doses of these drugs may be required.
Cimetidine: May enhance labetalol's effect. Use with caution; adjust labetalol dosage as needed.
Diuretics, other antihypertensives: May potentiate antihypertensive effects of these drugs. Monitor patient and blood pressure.
Glutethimide: May decrease bioavailability of oral labetalol. May require adjustment of labetalol dosage.
Halothane: Synergistic antihypertensive effect; possible significant myocardial depression. Monitor blood pressure and ECG.

Nitroglycerin: Blunting of reflex tachycardia produced by nitroglycerin without preventing its hypotensive effect. If used concomitantly, additional antihypertensive effects may occur. Monitor patient closely.
Tricyclic antidepressants: May increase risk of labetalol-induced tremor. Monitor patient carefully.

Adverse reactions
CNS: vivid dreams, fatigue, headache, paresthesia, syncope, transient scalp tingling.
CV: *orthostatic hypotension, dizziness,* **ventricular arrhythmias.**
EENT: nasal stuffiness.
GI: nausea, vomiting, diarrhea.
GU: sexual dysfunction, urine retention.
Musculoskeletal: muscle spasm, toxic myopathy.
Respiratory: dyspnea, **bronchospasm.**
Skin: rash.

☑ Special considerations
Besides the recommendations relevant to all beta blockers, consider the following.
• Unlike other beta blockers, labetalol doesn't decrease resting heart rate or cardiac output.
• Dosage may need to be reduced in patients with hepatic insufficiency.
• Dizziness, the most troublesome adverse effect, tends to occur in early stages of treatment and in patients taking diuretics or receiving higher doses.
• Use specific radioenzyme or high performance liquid chromatography assay techniques to reduce risk of false-positive urine free and total catecholamine levels.
• Don't mix labetalol with 5% sodium bicarbonate injection because of incompatibility.
• When adjusting hospitalized patients from parenteral to oral labetalol, begin with 200 mg, then give 200 to 400 mg P.O. after 6 to 12 hours. Oral dosage may then be increased in usual increments at 1-day intervals, if needed, to achieve the desired blood pressure control. Daily dose may be given twice or three times daily.
• Signs and symptoms of overdose include severe hypotension, bradycardia, heart failure, and bronchospasm. For overdose, empty stomach by induced emesis or gastric lavage, and give activated charcoal to reduce absorption.

Monitoring the patient
• Monitor patient for adverse effects.
• Monitor vital signs and ECG.

Information for the patient
• Advise patient that transient scalp tingling may occur at start of therapy but usually subsides quickly.
• Warn patient to not abruptly stop drug; this may exacerbate angina and precipitate MI.

Geriatric patients
• Elderly patients may require lower maintenance doses of labetalol because of increased bio-availability or delayed metabolism; they also may experience enhanced adverse effects. Use drug with caution in elderly patients.

Pediatric patients
• Safety and efficacy in children haven't been established; use drug only if potential benefit outweighs risk.

Breast-feeding patients
• Small amounts of drug appear in breast milk; use cautiously in breast-feeding women.

---

lactulose
Cephulac, Cholac, Chronulac, Constilac, Constulose, Duphalac, Enulose

Pharmacologic classification: disaccharide
Therapeutic classification: laxative
Pregnancy risk category B

How supplied
Available by prescription only
Syrup: 10 g/15 ml
Rectal solution: 3.33 g/5 ml

Indications, route, and dosage
Constipation
Adults: 15 to 30 ml P.O. daily (may increase to 60 ml if needed).
To prevent and treat portal-systemic encephalopathy, including hepatic precoma and coma in patients with severe hepatic disease
Adults: Initially, 20 to 30 g (30 to 45 ml) P.O. t.i.d. or q.i.d., until two or three soft stools are produced daily. Usual dosage is 60 to 100 g daily in divided doses; can also be given by retention enema. For retention enema, mix 300 ml of lactulose with 700 ml of water or normal saline solution and retain for 60 minutes. May repeat q 4 to 6 hours.
Infants: Initially, 2.5 to 10 ml daily in divided doses. Adjust doses q 1 to 2 days to produce two to three loose stools daily.
Older children and adolescents: Initially, 40 to 90 ml daily in divided doses. Adjust doses q 1 to 2 days to produce two to three loose stools daily.
◊ *After barium meal examination*
Adults: 5 to 10 ml P.O. b.i.d. for 1 to 4 weeks.
◊ *To restore bowel movements after hemorrhoidectomy*
Adults: 15 ml P.O. twice during day before surgery and for 5 days postoperatively.

Pharmacodynamics
Laxative action: Because lactulose is indigestible, it passes through GI tract to the colon unchanged; there, it's digested by normally occurring bacteria. The weak acids produced in this manner increase the stool's fluid content and cause distention, thus promoting peristalsis and bowel evacuation.
   Lactulose also is used to reduce serum ammonia levels in patients with hepatic disease. Lactulose breakdown acidifies the colon; this, in turn, converts ammonia (NH_3) to ammonium ($NH4^+$), which isn't absorbed and is excreted in the stool. Furthermore, this "ion trapping" effect causes ammonia to diffuse from the blood into the colon, where it's excreted as well.

Pharmacokinetics
• *Absorption:* Absorbed minimally.
• *Distribution:* Distributed locally, primarily in colon.
• *Metabolism:* Metabolized by colonic bacteria (absorbed portion isn't metabolized).
• *Excretion:* Mostly excreted in feces; absorbed portion excreted in urine.

Contraindications and precautions
Contraindicated in patients on a low-galactose diet. Use cautiously in patients with diabetes mellitus.

Interactions
Drug-drug. *Neomycin, nonabsorbable antacids, other antibiotics:* May decrease lactulose effectiveness. Avoid concomitant use.

Adverse reactions
GI: *abdominal cramps, belching, gaseous distention, flatulence,* nausea, vomiting, *diarrhea* (with excessive dosage).

☑ Special considerations
• After giving drug via nasogastric tube, flush tube with water to clear it and ensure drug's passage to stomach.
• Dilute drug with water or fruit juice to minimize its sweet taste.
• For administration by retention enema, patient should retain drug for 30 to 60 minutes. If retained less than 30 minutes, dose should be repeated immediately. Begin oral therapy before discontinuing retention enemas.
• Don't administer drug with other laxatives because resulting loose stools may falsely indicate adequate dosage of lactulose.

Monitoring the patient
• Monitor frequency and consistency of stools.
• Monitor patient for adverse effects.

Information for the patient
• Advise patient to take drug with juice to improve taste.

Reactions may be *common*, uncommon, **life-threatening**, or COMMON AND LIFE-THREATENING.

• Instruct patient to report adverse effects immediately.

Geriatric patients
• Monitor patient's serum electrolyte levels; elderly patients are more sensitive to possible hypernatremia.

---

lamivudine (3TC)
Epivir, Epivir-HBV

Pharmacologic classification: synthetic nucleoside analogue
Therapeutic classification: antiviral
Pregnancy risk category C

How supplied
Available by prescription only
Epivir
Tablets: 150 mg
Oral solution: 10 mg/ml
Epivir-HBV
Tablets: 100 mg
Oral solution: 5 mg/ml

Indications, route, and dosage
Treatment of HIV infection, with zidovudine
Adults weighing 50 kg (110 lb) or more and children ages 12 and older: 150 mg P.O. b.i.d.
Adults weighing under 50 kg: 2 mg/kg P.O. b.i.d.
Children ages 3 months to 12 years: 4 mg/kg P.O. b.i.d. Maximum dose is 150 mg b.i.d.
✦ Dosage adjustment. For patients with renal failure, refer to chart below.

Creatinine clearance (ml/min)	Recommended dosage
≥ 50	150 mg b.i.d.
30 to 49	150 mg once daily
15 to 29	150 mg first dose; then 100 mg once daily
5 to 14	150 mg first dose; then 50 mg once daily
< 5	50 mg first; then 25 mg once daily

Chronic hepatitis B associated with evidence of hepatitis B viral replication and active liver inflammation
Adults: 100 mg P.O. once daily. Safety and effectiveness of treatment beyond 1 year haven't been established; optimum duration of treatment isn't known. Test patients for HIV before treatment and during therapy because formulation and dosage of lamivudine in Epivir-HBV aren't appropriate for those dually infected with hepatitis B virus (HBV) and HIV. If lamivudine is administered to patients with HBV and HIV, higher dosage indicated for HIV therapy should be used as part of an appropriate combination regimen.
✦ Dosage adjustment. In patients with renal impairment, if creatinine clearance is 30 to 49 ml/minute, 100 mg first dose; then 50 mg P.O. once daily. If clearance is 15 to 29 ml/minute, 100 mg first dose; then 25 mg P.O. once daily. If creatinine clearance is 5 to 14 ml/minute, 35 mg first dose; then 15 mg P.O. once daily. If less than 5 ml/minute, 35 mg first dose; then 10 mg P.O. once daily.

Pharmacodynamics
Antiviral action: Inhibits HIV reverse transcription via viral DNA chain termination. RNA- and DNA-dependent DNA polymerase activities are also inhibited.

Pharmacokinetics
• *Absorption:* Rapidly absorbed after oral administration in HIV-infected patients.
• *Distribution:* Believed to be distributed into extravascular spaces. Volume of distribution is independent of dose and doesn't correlate with body weight. Less than 36% is bound to plasma proteins.
• *Metabolism:* Minor route of elimination; only known metabolite is transsulfoxide metabolite.
• *Excretion:* Primarily eliminated unchanged in urine. Mean elimination half-life is 5 to 7 hours.

Contraindications and precautions
Contraindicated in patients with hypersensitivity to drug. Use with extreme caution, and only if there is no satisfactory alternative therapy, in children with history of pancreatitis or other significant risk factors for developing pancreatitis. Stop drug immediately if signs, symptoms, or laboratory abnormalities suggest pancreatitis.
    Use cautiously in patients with impaired renal function; dosage reduction in these patients is needed.

Interactions
Drug-drug. *Trimethoprim-sulfamethoxazole:* Increased blood levels of lamivudine. Monitor lamivudine levels.
Zidovudine: Increased serum zidovudine level. Monitor patient closely.

Adverse reactions
    Note: Adverse reactions are related to combination therapy of lamivudine and zidovudine.
CNS: *malaise, headache, fatigue, neuropathy, dizziness, insomnia and other sleep disorders,* depressive disorders.
EENT: *nasal symptoms, sore throat.*
GI: *nausea, diarrhea, vomiting, anorexia,* abdominal pain, abdominal cramps, dyspepsia, ***pancreatitis*** (in children ages 3 months to 12 years).
Hematologic: *neutropenia,* anemia, ***thrombocytopenia.***

Hepatic: elevated liver enzymes and bilirubin levels.
Musculoskeletal: *musculoskeletal pain,* myalgia, arthralgia.
Respiratory: *cough.*
Skin: rash.
Other: *fever, chills.*

☑ Special considerations
• When used to treat HIV infection, drug must be administered with zidovudine. Drug isn't intended for use as monotherapy.
• Safety and efficacy of treatment of HBV for periods over 1 year or in patients with decompensated liver disease or organ transplant haven't been established.
• Monotherapy with lamivudine in patients with HIV-HBV coinfection in HBV dosage is inadequate and may lead to rapid emergence of HIV resistance. Counseling and testing for HIV infection before and periodically during treatment are recommended. Use higher dosage with other appropriate antiretrovirals.
• An Antiretroviral Pregnancy Registry has been established to monitor maternal-fetal outcomes of pregnant women exposed to lamivudine. Pregnant patients can be registered by calling 1-800-258-4263.

Monitoring the patient
• Monitor patient for adverse effects.
• Monitor CBC, platelet count, and liver function studies throughout therapy because abnormalities may occur.

Information for the patient
• Inform patient that long-term effects of drug are unknown.
• Tell patient that tablets and oral solution are for oral ingestion only.
• Stress importance of taking drug exactly as prescribed.
• Instruct parents of children receiving drug about the signs and symptoms of pancreatitis and tell them to report such occurrences immediately.
• Inform patient receiving dosage below therapeutic levels for HIV treatment that HIV testing is recommended.

Pediatric patients
• No information available on use of lamivudine with zidovudine in children under age 12.

Breast-feeding patients
• To avoid transmitting HIV to infant, HIV-positive women shouldn't breast-feed.

lamivudine/zidovudine
Combivir

Pharmacologic classification: reverse transcriptase inhibitor
Therapeutic classification: antiretroviral
Pregnancy risk category C

How supplied
Available by prescription only
Tablets: each tablet contains 150 mg lamivudine and 300 mg zidovudine

Indications, route, and dosage
HIV infection
Adults and children over age 12 and weighing 50 kg (110 lb) or more: One tablet P.O. b.i.d.

Pharmacodynamics
Antiretroviral action: Lamivudine and zidovudine are phosphorylated intracellularly to active metabolites that inhibit reverse transcriptase via DNA chain termination. Both drugs are also weak inhibitors of mammalian DNA polymerase. Together, they have synergistic antiretroviral activity. Therapy with lamivudine and zidovudine aims to suppress or delay emergence of phenotypic and genotypic resistant strains that can occur with retroviral monotherapy because dual resistance requires many mutations.

Pharmacokinetics
• *Absorption:* Both drugs rapidly absorbed following oral administration; oral bioavailability of 86% and 64%, respectively.
• *Distribution:* Both drugs extensively distributed and exhibit low protein-binding.
• *Metabolism:* Only about 5% of lamivudine is metabolized; 74% of zidovudine metabolized in liver.
• *Excretion:* Lamivudine primarily eliminated unchanged in urine; zidovudine and its major metabolite primarily eliminated in urine. Elimination half-lives of lamivudine and zidovudine are 5 to 7 hours and $\frac{1}{2}$ to 3 hours, respectively. Because renal excretion is a principal route of elimination, dosage adjustments are necessary in patients with compromised renal function, making this fixed ratio combination unsuitable. Hemodialysis and peritoneal dialysis have negligible effect on removal of zidovudine, but removal of its metabolite, GZDV, is enhanced. Unknown effect of dialysis on lamivudine.

Contraindications and precautions
Contraindicated in patients with hypersensitivity to drug or its components, in those with body weight under 110 lb (50 kg) or creatinine clearance below 50 ml/minute, and in those experiencing dose-limiting adverse effects. Use com-

---

bination with caution in patients with bone marrow suppression or renal insufficiency.

Interactions
Drug-drug. *Atovaquone, fluconazole, methadone, probenecid, valproic acid:* Increased bioavailability of lamivudine. Monitor blood counts frequently.
Ganciclovir, interferon-alpha, other bone marrow suppressants or cytotoxic drugs: Increased hematologic toxicity of zidovudine. Monitor CBC.
Nelfinavir, ritonavir: Decreased bioavailability of zidovudine. Monitor patient for effect.
Nelfinavir, trimethoprim/sulfamethoxazole: Increased bioavailability of lamivudine. Check CBC frequently.

Adverse reactions
CNS: *headache,* malaise, *fatigue, insomnia, dizziness, neuropathy,* depression.
GI: *nausea, diarrhea, vomiting, anorexia,* abdominal pain, abdominal cramps, dyspepsia, *pancreatitis.*
EENT: *nasal signs and symptoms.*
Hematologic: *neutropenia,* anemia.
Musculoskeletal: *musculoskeletal pain,* myalgia, arthralgia, myopathy, myositis.
Respiratory: *cough.*
Skin: rash.
Other: *fever, chills.*

☑ Special considerations
• Don't use combination drug therapy in patients needing dosage adjustments, such as children and those with renal dysfunction.
• Lactic acidosis and severe hepatomegaly with steatosis have been reported in patients receiving lamivudine and zidovudine alone and in combination. Stop treatment if signs of lactic acidosis or hepatotoxicity develop. Hepatotoxic events may be more severe in patients with decompensated liver function due to hepatitis B. Myopathy and myositis associated with prolonged use of zidovudine may occur.
• Combination may be administered with or without food.

Monitoring the patient
• Watch for bone marrow toxicity with frequent blood counts, particularly in patients with advanced HIV infection.
• Monitor patients for signs of lactic acidosis and hepatotoxicity.
• Monitor patient's fine motor skills and peripheral sensation for evidence of peripheral neuropathies.

Information for the patient
• Advise patient that combination drug therapy isn't a cure for HIV infection, and that he may continue to experience illness, including opportunistic infections.

• Warn patient that transmission of HIV virus can still occur with drug therapy.
• Teach patient signs and symptoms of neutropenia and anemia, and instruct him to report such occurrences.
• Advise patient to seek medical approval before taking other drugs.
• Warn patient to report abdominal pain immediately.
• Stress importance of taking combination therapy exactly as prescribed to reduce development of resistance.

Geriatric patients
• Safety and effectiveness in patients over age 65 haven't been established.

Pediatric patients
• Don't use in patients under age 12; fixed-dose combination treatment can't be adjusted for this patient group.

Breast-feeding patients
• Although zidovudine appears in breast milk at levels similar to serum, no data are available for the presence of lamivudine and zidovudine. It's recommended that HIV-positive women not breast-feed because of risk of transmission of the virus.

lamotrigine
Lamictal

Pharmacologic classification: phenytriazine
Therapeutic classification: anticonvulsant
Pregnancy risk category C

How supplied
Available by prescription only
Tablets: 25 mg, 100 mg, 150 mg, 200 mg
Chewable tablets: 5 mg, 25 mg

Indications, route, and dosage
Adjunct therapy in treatment of partial seizures caused by epilepsy
Adults and children ages 16 and older: 50 mg P.O. daily for 2 weeks, then 100 mg daily in two divided doses for 2 weeks. Then, usual maintenance dose is 300 to 500 mg P.O. daily given in two divided doses. For patients also taking valproic acid, give 25 mg P.O. every other day for 2 weeks, then 25 mg P.O. daily for 2 weeks. Then, maximum dose is 150 mg P.O. daily in two divided doses.

Pharmacodynamics
Anticonvulsant action: Mechanism unknown. Possibly related to inhibition of release of glutamate and aspartate in the brain. This may occur by acting on voltage-sensitive sodium channels.

Pharmacokinetics
- *Absorption:* Rapidly and completely absorbed from GI tract with negligible first-pass metabolism. Absolute bioavailability is 98%.
- *Distribution:* About 55% bound to plasma proteins.
- *Metabolism:* Metabolized predominantly by glucuronic acid conjugation; major metabolite is an inactive 2-N-glucuronide conjugate.
- *Excretion:* Excreted primarily in urine; only small portion excreted in feces.

Contraindications and precautions
Contraindicated in patients with hypersensitivity to drug. Use cautiously in patients with impaired renal, hepatic, or cardiac function.

Interactions
Drug-drug. *Acetaminophen:* May reduce lamotrigine levels. Monitor lamotrigine levels.
Carbamazepine, phenobarbital, phenytoin, primidone: Decreased lamotrigine steady-state levels. Monitor patient closely.
Folate inhibitors (such as co-trimoxazole, methotrexate): Possible additive effects. Monitor patient closely.
Valproic acid: Decreased lamotrigine clearance, which increases drug's steady-state levels. Monitor patient closely for toxicity.
Drug-lifestyle. *Sun exposure:* Possible photosensitivity reactions. Tell patient to take precautions.

Adverse reactions
CNS: *dizziness, headache, ataxia, somnolence,* malaise, incoordination, insomnia, tremor, depression, anxiety, **seizures,** irritability, speech disorder, decreased memory, concentration disturbance, sleep disorder, emotional lability, vertigo, mind racing, **suicide attempts.**
CV: palpitations.
EENT: *diplopia, blurred vision,* vision abnormality, nystagmus, rhinitis, pharyngitis.
GI: *nausea, vomiting,* diarrhea, dyspepsia, abdominal pain, constipation, tooth disorder, anorexia, dry mouth.
GU: dysmenorrhea, vaginitis, amenorrhea.
Musculoskeletal: dysarthria, muscle spasm, neck pain.
Respiratory: cough, dyspnea.
Skin: **Stevens-Johnson syndrome,** *rash,* pruritus, hot flashes, alopecia, acne, epidermal neurolysis (rarely toxic), photosensitivity.
Other: flulike syndrome, fever, infection, chills.

☑ Special considerations
- Don't stop drug abruptly; risk of increasing seizure frequency. Instead, taper drug over at least 2 weeks.
- Stop drug immediately if drug-induced rash occurs.

- If lamotrigine is added to a multidrug regimen that includes valproate, reduce dose of lamotrigine. Use a lower maintenance dose in patients with severe renal impairment.

Monitoring the patient
- Evaluate patient for reduction in frequency and duration of seizures. Periodically evaluate adjunct anticonvulsant's serum levels.
- Monitor patient for adverse effects.

Information for the patient
- Inform patient that rash may occur, especially during first 6 weeks of therapy and in children. Combination therapy of valproic acid and lamotrigine is likely to precipitate a serious rash. Although rash may resolve with continued therapy, tell patient to report it immediately in case drug needs to be stopped.
- Warn patient not to perform hazardous activities until CNS effects are known.
- Advise patient to take protective measures against photosensitivity reactions until tolerance is known.

Geriatric patients
- Safety and effectiveness in patients over age 65 haven't been established.

Pediatric patients
- Recommended use for children ages 2 to 12 is very limited; carefully administer following detailed guidelines provided with drug. Risk of severe, potentially life-threatening rash in children is much higher than that reported in adults.

Breast-feeding patients
- Preliminary data indicate that lamotrigine appears in breast milk. Drug use in breast-feeding women isn't recommended.

lansoprazole
Prevacid

Pharmacologic classification: acid (proton) pump inhibitor
Therapeutic classification: antiulcerative
Pregnancy risk category B

How supplied
Available by prescription only
Capsules (delayed-release): 15 mg, 30 mg

Indications, route, and dosage
Short-term treatment of active duodenal ulcer
Adults: 15 mg P.O. daily before meals for 4 weeks.
Maintenance of healed duodenal ulcer
Adults: 15 mg P.O. once daily.

Reactions may be *common,* uncommon, **life-threatening,** or COMMON AND LIFE-THREATENING.

Short-term treatment of erosive esophagitis
Adults: 30 mg P.O. daily before meals for up to 8 weeks. If healing doesn't occur, an additional 8 weeks of therapy may be needed.
Maintenance of healing of erosive esophagitis
Adults: 15 mg P.O. once daily.
Long-term treatment of pathologic hypersecretory conditions, including Zollinger-Ellison syndrome
Adults: Initially 60 mg P.O. once daily. Increase dosage, p.r.n., to 180 mg/day. Daily doses exceeding 120 mg should be administered in divided doses.
Short-term treatment of gastric ulcer
Adults: 30 mg P.O. daily for up to 8 weeks.
Short-term treatment of symptomatic gastroesophageal reflux disease (GERD)
Adults: 15 mg P.O. daily for up to 8 weeks.
Helicobacter pylori *eradication to reduce risk of duodenal ulcer recurrence*
Adults: In patients receiving dual therapy, 30 mg P.O. lansoprazole with 1 g P.O. amoxicillin, each given q 8 hours for 14 days. In patients receiving triple therapy, 30 mg P.O. lansoprazole with 1 g P.O. amoxicillin and 500 mg P.O. clarithromycin, all given q 12 hours for 10 or 14 days.

Pharmacodynamics

Antiulcerative action: Inhibits activity of the acid (proton) pump and binds to hydrogen-potassium ATPase, located at the secretory surface of the gastric parietal cells, to block the formation of gastric acid.

Pharmacokinetics

• *Absorption:* Rapidly absorbed with absolute bioavailability of over 80%.
• *Distribution:* 97% bound to plasma proteins.
• *Metabolism:* Extensively metabolized in liver.
• *Excretion:* About two-thirds of dose excreted in feces; one-third in urine.

Contraindications and precautions

Contraindicated in patients with hypersensitivity to drug.

Interactions

Drug-drug. *Ampicillin esters, iron salts, ketoconazole:* May interfere with absorption of these drugs. Monitor patient closely.
Sucralfate: Delayed lansoprazole absorption. Give lansoprazole at least 30 minutes before sucralfate.
Theophylline: May cause mild increase in theophylline excretion. Use together cautiously. Dosage adjustment of theophylline may be necessary when lansoprazole is started or stopped.
Drug-herb. *Male fern:* Inactivated in alkaline stomach environment. Discourage concomitant use.

Adverse reactions

CNS: headache, asthenia, malaise, agitation, amnesia, anxiety, apathy, confusion, depression, dizziness or syncope, hallucinations, hemiplegia, aggravated hostility, decreased libido, nervousness, paresthesia, thinking abnormality.
CV: chest pain, edema, angina, ***CVA,*** hypertension or hypotension, ***MI, shock,*** palpitations, vasodilation, ***cardiospasm.***
EENT: amblyopia, deafness, epistaxis, eye pain, visual field deficits, otitis media, taste perversions, tinnitus.
GI: *diarrhea, nausea, abdominal pain,* halitosis, melena, anorexia, cholelithiasis, constipation, dry mouth, thirst, dyspepsia, dysphagia, eructation, esophageal stenosis, esophageal ulcer, esophagitis, fecal discoloration, flatulence, gastric nodules, fundic gland polyps, gastroenteritis, GI hemorrhage, hematemesis, increased appetite, increased salivation, rectal hemorrhage, stomatitis, tenesmus, ulcerative colitis.
GU: hematuria, impotence, kidney calculus, albuminuria, abnormal menses, breast tenderness, breast enlargement or gynecomastia.
Hematologic: anemia, hemolysis.
Hepatic: abnormal liver function test results.
Metabolic: diabetes mellitus, goiter, hyperglycemia, hypoglycemia, gout, weight gain or loss.
Musculoskeletal: arthritis, arthralgia, musculoskeletal pain, myalgia.
Respiratory: asthma, bronchitis, increased cough, dyspnea, hemoptysis, hiccups, pneumonia, upper respiratory tract inflammation.
Skin: acne, alopecia, pruritus, rash, urticaria.
Other: candidiasis, fever, flulike syndrome, infection, decreased libido.

☑ Special considerations

• Dosage adjustment may be required for patients with severe liver disease.
• For patients who have a nasogastric (NG) tube in place, capsules can be opened and intact granules mixed in 40 ml of apple juice and administered through tube into stomach. After administering granules, flush NG tube with additional apple juice to clear tube.
• A symptomatic response to lansoprazole therapy doesn't preclude presence of gastric malignancy.

Monitoring the patient

• Monitor patient's response to drug therapy.
• Monitor patient carefully for adverse effects.

Information for the patient

• Instruct patient to take drug before meals.
• Caution patient not to chew or crush capsules; capsules should be swallowed whole.
• Tell patient who has trouble swallowing capsules to open capsule, sprinkle contents over 1 tablespoon of applesauce, and swallow immediately.

Geriatric patients
● Although initial dosing regimen need not be altered for elderly patients, subsequent doses over 30 mg/day shouldn't be administered unless additional gastric acid suppression is needed.

Pediatric patients
● Safety and effectiveness in children haven't been established.

Breast-feeding patients
● It's unknown if drug appears in breast milk; either stop breast-feeding or discontinue drug.

---

latanoprost
Xalatan

Pharmacologic classification: prostaglandin analogue
Therapeutic classification: antiglaucoma drug; ocular antihypertensive
Pregnancy risk category C

How supplied
Available by prescription only
Ophthalmic solution: 0.005%

Indications, route, and dosage
Increased intraocular pressure (IOP) in patients with ocular hypertension or open-angle glaucoma who are intolerant of other IOP-lowering drugs or insufficiently responsive to other IOP-lowering drugs
Adults: Instill 1 drop in conjunctival sac of affected eye once daily in the evening.

Pharmacodynamics
Antiglaucoma and ocular antihypertensive actions: Exact mechanism unknown. May lower IOP by increasing the outflow of aqueous humor.

Pharmacokinetics
● *Absorption:* Absorbed through cornea. Levels in aqueous humor peak about 2 hours after topical administration.
● *Distribution:* Distribution volume is about 0.16 L/kg. Acid of latanoprost could be measured in aqueous humor during first 4 hours and in plasma only during first hour after local administration.
● *Metabolism:* Hydrolyzed by esterases in cornea to biologically active acid. Active acid of drug reaching systemic circulation is primarily metabolized by liver.
● *Excretion:* Metabolites mainly eliminated in urine.

Contraindications and precautions
Contraindicated in patients with hypersensitivity to drug, benzalkonium chloride, or other ingredi-

ents in the product. Use cautiously in patients with impaired renal or hepatic function.

Interactions
Drug-drug. *Eyedrops containing thimerosal:* Precipitation occurs when mixed with latanoprost. If used together, administer at least 5 minutes apart.

Adverse reactions
CV: chest pain; angina pectoris.
EENT: *blurred vision; burning; stinging;* itching; conjunctival hyperemia; foreign body sensation; increased pigmentation of iris; punctate epithelial keratopathy; dry eye; excessive tearing; photophobia; conjunctivitis; diplopia; eye pain or discharge; lid crusting, edema, erythema, discomfort, or pain.
Musculoskeletal: muscle, joint, or back pain.
Respiratory: upper respiratory tract infection.
Skin: rash; allergic skin reaction.
Other: cold, flu.

☑ Special considerations
● Latanoprost may gradually change eye color, increasing amount of brown pigment in iris. Color change occurs slowly and may not be noticeable for several months to years. The increased pigmentation may be permanent.
● Protect drug from light; refrigerate unopened bottle.

Monitoring the patient
● Monitor patient for adverse effects.
● Observe patient for response to drug therapy.

Information for the patient
● Patient who is receiving treatment in only one eye should be told about the potential for increased brown pigmentation in treated eye and thus heterochromia between the eyes.
● Teach patient to instill drops. Advise him to wash hands before and after instilling solution, and warn him not to touch dropper or tip to eye or surrounding tissue.
● Advise patient to apply light finger pressure on lacrimal sac for 1 minute after instillation to minimize systemic absorption of drug.
● Instruct patient to report ocular reactions, especially conjunctivitis and lid reactions.
● Tell patient using contact lenses to remove them before administration of the solution and not to reinsert them until 15 minutes after administration.
● Advise patient that, if more than one topical ophthalmic drug is being used, they should be administered at least 5 minutes apart.
● Stress importance of compliance with recommended therapy.

Pediatric patients
● Safety and effectiveness in children haven't been established.

Breast-feeding patients
● It's unknown if drug appears in breast milk. Use with caution in breast-feeding women.

leflunomide
Arava

Pharmacologic classification: pyrimidine synthesis inhibitor
Therapeutic classification: antirheumatic drug
Pregnancy risk category X

How supplied
Available by prescription only
Tablets: 10 mg, 20 mg, 100 mg

Indications, route, and dosage
Active rheumatoid arthritis to reduce signs and symptoms and to retard structural damage as evidenced by X-ray erosions and joint space narrowing
Adults: 100 mg P.O. q 24 hours for 3 days; then 20 mg (maximum daily dose) P.O. q 24 hours. Dose may be decreased to 10 mg daily if higher dose isn't well tolerated.

Pharmacodynamics
Immunomodulatory action: Inhibits dihydroorotate dehydrogenase, an enzyme involved in de novo pyrimidine synthesis, and has antiproliferative activity and anti-inflammatory effects.

Pharmacokinetics
● *Absorption:* Bioavailability is 80%; levels peak within 6 to 12 hours after loading dose. Without loading dose, plasma levels peak in about 2 months.
● *Distribution:* Over 99% bound to plasma proteins.
● *Metabolism:* Metabolized to active metabolite (M1), responsible for most of its activity.
● *Excretion:* Eliminated by renal and direct biliary excretion. About 43% excreted in urine; 48% in feces. Half-life of active metabolite is about 2 weeks.

Contraindications and precautions
Contraindicated in patients with hypersensitivity to drug or its components and in women who are or may become pregnant or who are breast-feeding. Drug isn't recommended for patients with hepatic insufficiency, hepatitis B or C, severe immunodeficiency, bone marrow dysplasia, or severe uncontrolled infections.

Vaccination with live vaccines isn't recommended. The long half-life of drug should be considered when contemplating administration of a live vaccine after stopping drug treatment.

Drug isn't recommended for use by men attempting to father a child.

Use cautiously in patients with renal insufficiency.

Interactions
Drug-drug. *Charcoal, cholestyramine:* Decreased plasma levels of leflunomide. Sometimes used for this effect in treating overdose.
Methotrexate, other hepatotoxic drugs: Increased risk of hepatotoxicity. Monitor liver enzyme levels.
NSAIDs (diclofenac, ibuprofen): Increased NSAID levels. Significance unknown.
Rifampin: Increased level of active leflunomide metabolite. Use together cautiously.
Tolbutamide: Increased levels of tolbutamide. Significance unknown.

Adverse reactions
CNS: asthenia, dizziness, headache, paresthesia, malaise, migraine, sleep disorder, vertigo, neuritis, anxiety, depression, insomnia, neuralgia.
CV: angina pectoris, *hypertension*, chest pain, palpitation, tachycardia, vasculitis, vasodilation, varicose vein, peripheral edema.
EENT: pharyngitis, rhinitis, sinusitis, epistaxis, mouth ulcer, oral candidiasis, enlarged salivary glands, stomatitis, tooth disorder, dry mouth, blurred vision, cataract, conjunctivitis, eye disorder, gingivitis, taste perversion.
GI: anorexia, *diarrhea*, dyspepsia, gastroenteritis, nausea, abdominal pain, vomiting, cholelithiasis, colitis, constipation, esophagitis, flatulence, gastritis, melena.
GU: urinary tract infection, albuminuria, cystitis, dysuria, hematuria, menstrual disorder, pelvic pain, vaginal candidiasis, prostate disorder, urinary frequency.
Hematologic: anemia, ecchymosis, hyperlipidemia.
Hepatic: elevated liver enzyme levels.
Metabolic: diabetes mellitus, hyperglycemia, hyperthyroidism, hypokalemia, weight loss.
Musculoskeletal: arthrosis, back pain, bursitis, muscle cramps, myalgia, bone necrosis, bone pain, arthralgia, leg cramps, joint disorder, neck pain, synovitis, tendon rupture, tenosynovitis.
Respiratory: bronchitis, increased cough, pneumonia, *respiratory tract infection,* asthma, dyspnea, lung disorder.
Skin: *alopecia,* eczema, pruritus, *rash,* dry skin, acne, contact dermatitis, fungal dermatitis, hair discoloration, hematoma, herpes simplex, herpes zoster, nail disorder, skin nodule, subcutaneous nodule, maculopapular rash, skin disorder, skin discoloration, skin ulcer, increased sweating.
Other: allergic reaction, fever, flu syndrome, injury or accident, pain, abscess, cyst, hernia, increased CK level.

☑ Special considerations
● Leflunomide can cause fetal harm when administered to pregnant women; women planning

to become pregnant should call immediately and stop drug.
• Men planning to father a child should stop therapy and follow recommended leflunomide removal protocol (8 g cholestyramine P.O. t.i.d. for 11 days).
• The risk of malignancy, particularly lymphoproliferative disorders, increases with use of some immunosuppressants, including leflunomide.
• Use of drug with antimalarials, intramuscular or oral gold, penicillamine, azathioprine, or methotrexate hasn't been adequately studied.

Monitoring the patient
• Monitor liver enzyme levels (ALT and AST) before starting therapy and then monthly until stable. Frequency can then be decreased based on clinical situation.
• Check blood pressure and heart rate and rhythm frequently.

Information for the patient
• Explain need for and frequency of required blood tests and monitoring.
• Instruct patient to use birth control during course of treatment and until drug is no longer active.
• Warn woman of childbearing potential to immediately call if signs or symptoms of pregnancy occur (such as late menses or breast tenderness).

Geriatric patients
• No significant differences noted compared to younger population.

Pediatric patients
• Safety in children and adolescents hasn't been established. Not recommended for children under age 18.

Breast-feeding patients
• Drug shouldn't be used by breast-feeding women.

letrozole
Femara

Pharmacologic classification: aromatase inhibitor
Therapeutic classification: hormone
Pregnancy risk category D

How supplied
Available by prescription only
Tablets: 2.5 mg

Indications, route, and dosage
Metastatic breast cancer in postmenopausal women with disease progression following antiestrogen therapy
Adults and elderly patients: 2.5 mg P.O. as a single daily dose, without regard to meals.

Pharmacodynamics
Hormone action: Inhibits conversion of androgens to estrogens by competitive inhibition of aromatase enzyme system. Decreased estrogens are likely to lead to decreased tumor mass or delayed progression of tumor growth in some women.

Pharmacokinetics
• *Absorption:* Rapidly and completely absorbed; food doesn't affect bioavailability. Steady-state plasma levels reached in 2 to 6 weeks after daily dosing.
• *Distribution:* Large volume of distribution (1.9 L/kg). Weakly protein-bound.
• *Metabolism:* Slowly metabolized to inactive form. In human liver microsomes, letrozole strongly inhibited cytochrome P-450 isozyme 2A6 and moderately inhibited isozyme 2C19.
• *Excretion:* Inactive glucuronide metabolite eliminated in urine.

Contraindications and precautions
Contraindicated in patients with hypersensitivity to drug or its components. Avoid use in pregnant women because drug may cause fetal harm. Use cautiously in patients with severe liver impairment.

Interactions
None reported.

Adverse reactions
CNS: headache, somnolence, dizziness, fatigue, asthenia.
CV: edema, hypertension, *thromboembolism,* chest pain.
GI: *nausea,* vomiting, constipation, diarrhea, abdominal pain, anorexia, dyspepsia.
Metabolic: weight gain.
Musculoskeletal: *bone pain, extremities and back pain,* arthralgias.
Respiratory: dyspnea, coughing.
Skin: hot flashes, rash, pruritus.
Other: hypercholesterolemia, viral infections.

☑ Special considerations
• No dosage adjustment is needed in patients with mild to moderate liver dysfunction or in renally impaired patients with creatinine clearance of 10 ml/minute or more.
• Patients treated with letrozole don't need glucocorticoid or mineralocorticoid replacement therapy. Letrozole significantly lowers serum estrone, estradiol, and estrone sulfate, but hasn't been shown to significantly affect adrenal corticosteroid synthesis, aldosterone synthesis, or synthesis of thyroid hormones.

Monitoring the patient
• Monitor renal function studies as indicated.
• Monitor patient for adverse effects.

Information for the patient
● Instruct patient to take drug exactly as prescribed.
● Tell patient that drug can be taken with or without food.
● Advise patient that drug treatment is long-term, and stress importance of follow-up appointments.
● Tell patient to call immediately if pregnancy is suspected or is being planned.

Breast-feeding patients
● It's unknown if drug appears in breast milk. Use with caution in breast-feeding women.

leucovorin calcium (citrovorum factor or folinic acid)
Wellcovorin

Pharmacologic classification: formyl derivative (active reduced form of folic acid)
Therapeutic classification: vitamin; antidote
Pregnancy risk category C

How supplied
Available by prescription only
Tablets: 5 mg, 15 mg, 25 mg
Injection: 1-ml ampule (3 mg/ml with 0.9% benzyl alcohol, 5 mg/ml with methyl and propyl parabens); 50-mg, 100-mg, and 350-mg vials for reconstitution (contain no preservatives)

Indications, route, and dosage
Overdose of folic acid antagonist
Adults and children: P.O., I.M., or I.V. dose equivalent to weight of antagonist given as soon as possible after overdose.
Leucovorin rescue after large methotrexate dose in treatment of cancer
Adults and children: Administer 24 hours after last dose of methotrexate according to protocol. Give 15 mg I.M., I.V., or P.O. q 6 hours until methotrexate serum level is less than 5×10^{-8} M.
Toxic effects of methotrexate used to treat severe psoriasis
Adults and children: 4 to 8 mg I.M. 2 hours after methotrexate dose.
Hematologic toxicity from pyrimethamine or trimethoprim therapy
Adults and children: 5 to 15 mg P.O. or I.M. daily.
Advanced colorectal cancer
Adults: 200 mg/m² by slow I.V. injection over 3 minutes, then 5-fluorouracil (5-FU) or 20 mg/m² by slow I.V. injection over 3 minutes, then 5-FU. Repeat treatment for 5 days. May repeat course at 4-week intervals for two courses and then at 4- to 5-week intervals provided the patient has recovered from toxic effects of previous treatment. Dosage of 5-FU should be individualized.

Megaloblastic anemia from congenital enzyme deficiency
Adults and children: 3 to 6 mg I.M. daily; then 1 mg P.O. daily for life.
Folate-deficient megaloblastic anemias
Adults and children: Up to 1 mg of leucovorin P.O. or I.M. daily. Duration of treatment depends on hematologic response.

Pharmacodynamics
Reversal of folic acid antagonism: Derivative of tetrahydrofolic acid, the reduced form of folic acid. Performs as a cofactor in 1-carbon transfer reactions in the biosynthesis of purines and pyrimidines of nucleic acids. Impairment of thymidylate synthesis in patients with folic acid deficiency may account for defective DNA synthesis, megaloblast formation, and megaloblastic and macrocytic anemias. A potent antidote for the hematopoietic and reticuloendothelial toxic effects of folic acid antagonists (trimethoprim, pyrimethamine, and methotrexate). "Leucovorin rescue" is used to prevent or decrease toxicity of massive methotrexate doses. Folinic acid rescues normal cells without reversing the oncolytic effect of methotrexate.

Pharmacokinetics
● *Absorption:* After oral administration, absorbed rapidly; serum folate levels peak less than 2 hours after a 15-mg dose. Increase in plasma and serum folate activity after oral administration is mainly from 5-methyltetrahydrofolate (major transport and storage form of folate in body).
● *Distribution:* Tetrahydrofolic acid and derivatives distributed throughout body; liver contains about half of total body folate stores.
● *Metabolism:* Metabolized in liver.
● *Excretion:* Drug excreted by kidneys as 10-formyl tetrahydrofolate and 5,10-methenyl tetrahydrofolate. Duration of action is 3 to 6 hours.

Contraindications and precautions
Contraindicated in patients with pernicious anemia and other megaloblastic anemias secondary to the lack of vitamin B_{12}.

Interactions
Drug-drug. *Fluorouracil:* Increased fluorouracil toxicity when used concomitantly. Use lower doses of fluorouracil.
Phenytoin: Decreased serum phenytoin levels; increased frequency of seizures. (This interaction has occurred solely in patients receiving folic acid.) Monitor patient closely; monitor phenytoin levels.
Phenytoin, primidone: Decreased serum folate levels; symptoms of folate deficiency. Monitor patient.

Adverse reactions
Skin: *hypersensitivity reactions* (urticaria, *anaphylactoid reactions*).

☑ Special considerations
● Maximum rate of leucovorin infusion shouldn't exceed 160 mg/minute because of calcium concentration of solution.
● When giving more than 25 mg, drug should be administered parenterally.
● Drug administration continues until plasma methotrexate levels are below 5×10^{-8} M.
● To prepare drug for parenteral use, add 5 ml of bacteriostatic water for injection to vial containing 50 mg of base drug.
● Don't use as sole treatment of pernicious anemia or vitamin B_{12} deficiency.
● After chemotherapy with folic acid antagonists, parenteral administration is preferable to oral dosing because vomiting may cause leucovorin loss.
● Leucovorin has no effect on other methotrexate toxicities.
● To treat overdose of folic acid antagonists, use drug within 1 hour; not effective after a 4-hour delay.
● Store at room temperature in a light-resistant container; protect from moisture.

Monitoring the patient
● Monitor patient for signs of drug allergy, such as rash, wheezing, pruritus, and urticaria.
● Monitor serum creatinine levels daily to detect possible renal function impairment.

Information for the patient
● Emphasize importance of taking leucovorin only under medical supervision.

Pediatric patients
● Drug may increase frequency of seizures in susceptible children.
● Don't use diluents containing benzyl alcohol when reconstituting drug for neonates.

Breast-feeding patients
● It's unknown if drug appears in breast milk; use with caution in breast-feeding women.

leuprolide acetate
Lupron, Lupron Depot, Lupron Depot-Ped, Lupron Depot-3 Month, Lupron Depot-4 month

Pharmacologic classification: gonadotropin-releasing hormone
Therapeutic classification: antineoplastic; luteinizing hormone–releasing hormone (LH-RH) analogue
Pregnancy risk category X

How supplied
Available by prescription only
Injection: 5 mg/ml in 2.8-ml multiple-dose vials
Suspension for depot injection: 3.75 mg, 7.5 mg, 11.25 mg, 15 mg, 22.5 mg, 30 mg

Indications, route, and dosage
Dosage and indications may vary. Check current literature for recommended protocol. The three different depot preparations aren't interchangeable.
Management of advanced prostate cancer
Adults: 7.5 mg I.M. (depot injection) once monthly or 1 mg S.C. daily; or 22.5 mg I.M. (depot injection) q 3 months or 30 mg I.M. q 4 months (depot injection).
Endometriosis
Adults: 3.75 mg I.M. (depot injection) once monthly for a maximum of 6 months.
◇ *Central precocious puberty (CPP)*
Children: Starting dose 0.3 mg/kg (minimum 7.5 mg), given as a single I.M. dose (depot injection) q 4 weeks. May adjust upward by 10 mcg/kg/day until total down-regulation is achieved. This becomes the maintenance dose.

Pharmacodynamics
Antineoplastic action: Synthetic analogue of LH-RH. Inhibits gonadotropin secretion and androgen or estrogen synthesis. Because of this effect, leuprolide may inhibit the growth of hormone-dependent tumors.
Hormonal action: Because leuprolide lowers levels of sex hormones, it reduces the size of endometrial implants, resulting in decreased dysmenorrhea and pelvic pain in women with endometriosis.

Pharmacokinetics
● *Absorption:* Drug is a polypeptide molecule destroyed in GI tract. After S.C. administration, drug is rapidly and, essentially, completely absorbed.
● *Distribution:* Distribution not determined; however, high levels may be distributed into kidney, liver, pineal, and pituitary tissue. About 7% to 15% of dose is bound to plasma proteins.
● *Metabolism:* Unclear, but drug may be metabolized in anterior pituitary and hypothalamus, similar to endogenous gonadotropin-releasing hormone.
● *Excretion:* Plasma elimination half-life reportedly 3 hours.

Contraindications and precautions
Contraindicated in patients with hypersensitivity to drug or other gonadotropin-releasing hormone analogues, during pregnancy or lactation, and in women with undiagnosed vaginal bleeding. Use cautiously in patients with hypersensitivity to benzyl alcohol.

Interactions
None reported.

Adverse reactions
CNS: *dizziness, depression, headache, pain,* insomnia, *asthenia.*

CV: *arrhythmias,* angina, *MI, peripheral edema, ECG changes,* hypertension, murmur.
GI: *nausea, vomiting,* anorexia, constipation.
GU: *impotence, vaginitis,* urinary frequency, hematuria, urinary tract infection, gynecomastia.
Hematologic: anemia.
Hepatic: elevated liver enzyme levels.
Metabolic: *weight gain or loss.*
Musculoskeletal: transient bone pain during first week of treatment, joint disorder, myalgia, neuromuscular disorder.
Respiratory: dyspnea, sinus congestion, pulmonary fibrosis.
Skin: skin reactions at injection site, dermatitis.
Other: *hot flashes, androgen-like effects.*

☑ **Special considerations**
• Use a 22G needle for monthly injection and a 23G needle for 3-month injection.
• When treating endometriosis, administer for a maximum of 6 months. Safety and efficacy of retreatment are unknown.
• Discard solution if particulate matter is visible or if solution is discolored.
• Refrigerate drug until used; don't freeze. Reconstituted suspension is stable for 24 hours.
• No unusual adverse effects were observed in patients who had received 20 mg daily for 2 years.
• Fetal harm may occur with use; drug is contraindicated in pregnant patients.

Monitoring the patient
• Erythema or induration may develop at injection site.
• When treating prostate cancer, leuprolide may aggravate signs and symptoms of disease during first 1 to 2 weeks of therapy. Temporary paresthesia and weakness may occur during first week of therapy.
• Measure serum testosterone and acid phosphatase levels before and during therapy.

Information for the patient
• Reassure patient that bone pain is transient and will disappear after about 1 week.
• Inform patient that a temporary reaction of burning, itching, and swelling at injection site may occur. Tell him to report persistent reactions.
• Advise patient to continue taking drug even if he experiences a sense of well-being.
• Instruct woman of childbearing age to use an effective nonhormonal method of contraception during therapy.

Pediatric patients
• Safety and efficacy in children for uses other than the treatment of central precocious puberty have not been established.

Breast-feeding patients
• Breast-feeding is not recommended due to potential risk to infant (unknown if drug appears in breast milk).

---

levalbuterol hydrochloride
Xopenex

Pharmacologic classification: beta$_2$ agonist
Therapeutic classification: bronchodilator
Pregnancy risk category C

How supplied
Available by prescription only
Solution for inhalation: 0.63 mg or 1.25 mg in 3-ml vials

Indications, route, and dosage
To prevent or treat bronchospasm in patients with reversible obstructive airway disease
Adults and adolescents ages 12 and older: 0.63 mg administered t.i.d. every 6 to 8 hours, by oral inhalation via a nebulizer. Patients with more severe asthma who don't respond adequately to a dosage of 0.63 mg may benefit from a dosage of 1.25 mg t.i.d.

Pharmacodynamics
Bronchodilator action: Activates beta$_2$ receptors on airway smooth muscle, which leads the smooth muscle in all airways—from the trachea to the terminal bronchioles—to relax, thereby relieving bronchospasm and reducing airway resistance. Also inhibits release of mediators from mast cells in the airway.

Pharmacokinetics
No information available.

Adverse reactions
CNS: dizziness, migraine, nervousness, tremor, anxiety, pain.
CV: tachycardia.
EENT: *rhinitis,* sinusitis, turbinate edema.
GI: dyspepsia.
Musculoskeletal: leg cramps.
Respiratory: increased cough, *viral infection.*
Other: flu syndrome, accidental injury.

Interactions
Drug-drug. *Beta blockers:* Possible reduced pulmonary effect of drug; possible severe bronchospasm. If use together is necessary, consider a cardioselective beta blocker but administer with extreme caution.
Digoxin: Decreased digoxin levels. Monitor serum digoxin levels.
Epinephrine, other short-acting sympathomimetic aerosol bronchodilators: Increased adrenergic adverse effects. Use with caution.

Loop or thiazide diuretics: Possible ECG changes and hypokalemia from concurrent administration. Use together cautiously.

MAO inhibitors, tricyclic antidepressants: Potentiated action of levalbuterol on vascular system. Use with extreme caution when administered concurrently or within 2 weeks of stopping these drugs.

Contraindications and precautions

Contraindicated in patients with hypersensitivity to levalbuterol or racemic albuterol.

Use cautiously in patients with cardiovascular disorders, especially coronary insufficiency, hypertension, and arrhythmias. Also use cautiously in patients with seizure disorders, hyperthyroidism, or diabetes mellitus and in patients who are unusually responsive to sympathomimetic amines.

☑ Special considerations

- Like other inhaled beta agonists, levalbuterol can produce paradoxical bronchospasm, which may be life-threatening. If this occurs, stop drug immediately and institute alternative therapy.
- Abuse of levalbuterol may result in cardiac arrest and death.
- Small, transient increases in blood glucose levels may occur after oral inhalation.
- Serum potassium levels may decrease slightly, but potassium supplementation is usually unnecessary.
- Keep unopened vials in foil pouch. Once foil pouch is opened, use vials within 2 weeks. If vials are removed from pouch but not used immediately, they should be protected from light and excessive heat and used within 1 week.
- Signs of overdose include seizures, angina, hypertension or hypotension, arrhythmias, nervousness, headache, tremor, dry mouth, palpitation, nausea, dizziness, fatigue, and sleeplessness.
- A cardioselective beta blocker may be used to treat overdose; monitor patient for bronchospasm.

Monitoring the patient

- Monitor vital signs frequently; watch for signs of overdose.
- Perform ECG and check electrolyte status in patients receiving diuretics concurrently.

Information for the patient

- Warn patient that he may experience paradoxical bronchospasm (difficulty breathing). Tell him to stop drug and call immediately if this occurs.
- Inform patient that common adverse effects include palpitations, rapid heart rate, headache, dizziness, tremor, and nervousness.
- Inform patient that effects of levalbuterol may last up to 8 hours.

- Warn patient not to increase dosage or frequency without calling.
- Advise patient to seek medical attention immediately if levalbuterol becomes less effective for treating signs and symptoms, signs and symptoms become worse, or he is using levalbuterol more frequently than usual.
- Caution patient to use other inhalants and antiasthma drugs only as directed while taking levalbuterol.
- Inform patient that once foil pouch is opened, vials should be used within 2 weeks. If opened pouch isn't used immediately, vials should be protected from light and excessive heat and used within 1 week.
- Tell patient to discard any vials containing discolored solution.
- Advise woman to call if she becomes pregnant or is breast-feeding.

Geriatric patients

- It's unknown if safety and efficacy are different in patients ages 65 and older. In general, patients in this age-group should be started at a dosage of 0.63 mg.

Pediatric patients

- Safety and efficacy in children under age 12 are unknown.

Breast-feeding patients

- Plasma levels of drug are very low after inhalation of therapeutic dosages. It's unknown if drug appears in breast milk. Use with caution in breast-feeding women.

levamisole hydrochloride
Ergamisol

Pharmacologic classification: immunomodulator
Therapeutic classification: antineoplastic
Pregnancy risk category C

How supplied

Available by prescription only
Tablets: 50 mg

Indications, route, and dosage

Adjuvant treatment with fluorouracil after surgical resection in patients with Dukes' stage C colon cancer

Adults: Initially, 50 mg P.O. q 8 hours for 3 days starting 7 to 30 days after surgery. Repeat q 14 days for 1 year. Administer with fluorouracil 450 mg/m² daily by rapid I.V. push for 5 days with a 3-day course of levamisole, starting 21 to 34 days after surgery.

If levamisole therapy begins 7 to 20 days after surgery, start fluorouracil with the second course of levamisole at 21 to 24 days. If levamisole

---

Reactions may be *common,* uncommon, ***life-threatening,*** or COMMON AND LIFE-THREATENING.

begins 21 to 30 days after surgery, start fluorouracil simultaneously with the first course of therapy.

Maintenance dose is 50 mg P.O. q 8 hours for 3 days q 2 weeks. Give with fluorouracil 450 mg/m² daily by rapid I.V. push weekly beginning 28 days after initiation of the 5-day course.

Note: If an acute neurologic syndrome occurs, consider stopping drug immediately.

Pharmacodynamics
Antineoplastic action: An immunomodulator. Mechanism of action with fluorouracil unknown. Its effects on the immune system are complete, but it appears to restore depressed immune function rather than stimulate response to abovenormal levels. It also can stimulate antibody formation; enhance T-cell responses by stimulating T-cell activation and proliferation; potentiate monocyte and macrophage formation, including phagocytosis and chemotaxis; increase neutrophil mobility adherence and chemotaxis; and inhibit alkaline phosphatase. Levamisole also has cholinergic activity.

Pharmacokinetics
• *Absorption:* Rapidly absorbed from GI tract; peak plasma levels occur in 1½ to 2 hours.
• *Distribution:* No information available.
• *Metabolism:* Extensively metabolized by liver.
• *Excretion:* 70% of metabolites excreted in urine over 3 days; 5%, in feces; less than 5% of unchanged drug excreted in urine; less than 2% in feces.

Contraindications and precautions
Contraindicated in patients with hypersensitivity to drug.

Interactions
Drug-drug. *Phenytoin:* Increased phenytoin levels. Monitor plasma phenytoin levels; decrease dosage as needed.
Warfarin: Possible excessive prolongation of PT and INR. Monitor PT and INR and adjust warfarin dosage as needed.
Drug-lifestyle. *Alcohol:* Disulfiram-like reaction if used together. Discourage use.

Adverse reactions
CNS: *dizziness, headache, paresthesia, somnolence, depression, nervousness, insomnia, anxiety, fatigue, fever.*
CV: chest pain, edema.
EENT: blurred vision, conjunctivitis, *stomatitis, dysgeusia, altered sense of smell.*
GI: *nausea, diarrhea, vomiting, anorexia, abdominal pain, constipation, flatulence, dyspepsia.*
Hematologic: **agranulocytosis, leukopenia, thrombocytopenia,** anemia.
Hepatic: hyperbilirubinemia.

Musculoskeletal: *arthralgia, myalgia.*
Skin: *alopecia,* dermatitis, **exfoliative dermatitis,** *pruritus, urticaria.*
Other: rigors, *infection.*

☑ Special considerations
• Fatalities have been reported after ingestion of 15 mg/kg by a 3-year-old child and of 32 mg/kg by an adult.
• Don't use drug in higher than recommended dosage or administer more frequently than indicated.
• Before drug therapy begins, patient should be ambulatory, maintain normal oral nutrition, have well-healed wounds, be fully recovered from any postsurgical complications, and not be hospitalized.
• In case of overdose, gastric lavage is recommended along with symptomatic and supportive measures.

Monitoring the patient
• Obtain CBC with differential, platelet counts, electrolyte levels, and liver function test results before therapy. CBC with differential and platelet counts should be performed weekly before each fluorouracil treatment; electrolyte and liver function tests every 3 months for 1 year. Modify doses as needed.
• If WBC count is 2,500 to 3,500/mm³, defer fluorouracil dose until count is over 3,500/mm³. If WBC count is below 2,500/mm³, defer fluorouracil dose until count is above 3,500/mm³; then reduce dose by 20%. If WBC count remains below 2,500/mm³ for more than 10 days even after deferring fluorouracil, stop drug. Defer both if platelet counts are below 100,000/mm³.
• If stomatitis or diarrhea develops during initial fluorouracil administration schedule, stop course before full five doses are given. If stomatitis or diarrhea occurs during weekly maintenance therapy, defer next dose of fluorouracil until it subsides. If adverse reactions are moderate to severe, reduce fluorouracil dose by 20% when treatment is resumed.

Information for the patient
• Advise patient to use a soft toothbrush and electric razor to avoid trauma and excessive bleeding.
• Tell patient to report unusual bruising or bleeding.
• Flulike syndrome frequently accompanies onset of agranulocytosis but may also occur in the absence of agranulocytosis. Instruct patient to report flulike symptoms immediately.
• Advise patient to avoid exposure to persons with infection.

Pediatric patients
• Safety and efficacy in children haven't been established.

Breast-feeding patients
● Although it's unknown if drug appears in breast milk, potential for serious adverse reactions in infants must be considered.

levetiracetam
Keppra

Pharmacologic classification: anticonvulsant
Therapeutic classification: anticonvulsant
Pregnancy risk category C

How supplied
Available by prescription only
Tablets: 250 mg, 500 mg, 750 mg

Indications, route, and dosage
Adjunctive therapy for partial seizures
Adults: Initially, 500 mg b.i.d. Dosage can be increased by 500 mg b.i.d., p.r.n., for seizure control at 2-week intervals to maximum dose of 1,500 mg b.i.d.
✦ *Dosage adjustment.* For patients with renal failure, if creatinine clearance is more than 80 ml/minute, give 500 to 1,500 mg q 12 hours; if 50 to 80 ml/minute, give 500 to 1,000 mg q 12 hours; if 30 to 50 ml/minute, give 250 to 750 mg q 12 hours; if less than 30 ml/minute, give 250 to 500 mg q 12 hours. For dialysis patients, give 500 to 1,000 mg q 24 hours. A 250- to 500-mg dose should be given after dialysis.

Pharmacodynamics
Anticonvulsant action: Mechanism unknown. Thought to inhibit kindling activity in hippocampus, thus preventing simultaneous neuronal firing that leads to seizure activity.

Pharmacokinetics
● *Absorption:* Rapidly absorbed in GI tract; serum levels peak in about 1 hour. Can be taken with food, but time to reach peak levels is delayed by about 1½ hours with slightly lower serum levels. Steady-state serum levels reached in about 2 days.
● *Distribution:* Minimal protein-binding.
● *Metabolism:* No active metabolites; isn't metabolized through cytochrome P-450 system.
● *Excretion:* Elimination half-life about 7 hours in patients with normal renal function. 66% of drug eliminated unchanged by glomerular filtration and tubular reabsorption.

Contraindications and precautions
Contraindicated in patients with hypersensitivity to drug. Use cautiously in immunocompromised patients and in those with poor renal function.

Interactions
Drug-drug. *Antihistamines, benzodiazepines, narcotics, tricyclic antidepressants, other drugs that cause drowsiness:* Possible severe sedation. Avoid concomitant use.
Drug-lifestyle. *Alcohol:* Possible severe sedation. Discourage use.

Adverse reactions
CNS: *asthenia, headache, somnolence,* dizziness, depression, vertigo, paresthesia, nervousness, hostility, emotional lability, ataxia, amnesia, anxiety.
EENT: diplopia.
GI: anorexia.
Respiratory: cough, pharyngitis, rhinitis, infection, sinusitis.
Musculoskeletal: pain.
Hematologic: *leukopenia, neutropenia.*

☑ Special considerations
● For patients with poor renal function, dosage reduction is based on creatinine clearance.
● Seizures can occur if drug is stopped abruptly. Tapering is recommended.
● Drug is approved only as an adjunctive drug for partial seizures.
● Drug can be taken with or without food.
● For overdose, emesis or gastric lavage may be helpful in early stages of treatment. Hemodialysis removes about 50% of drug if performed within 4 hours of overdose.

Monitoring the patient
● Baseline CBC with periodic follow-up may be advisable in immunocompromised patients because of reports of leukopenia and neutropenia.
● Monitor patients closely for such adverse reactions as dizziness, which may lead to falls.

Information for the patient
● Inform patient to call and not to stop drug suddenly if adverse reactions occur.
● Warn patient to use extra care when sitting or standing to avoid falling.
● Inform patient to take this drug in addition to other prescribed seizure drugs.

Geriatric patients
● Inform patient to use extra care when sitting up or standing to avoid falling.

Pediatric patients
● Drug is not recommended for children under age 16.

Breast-feeding patients
● It's unknown if drug appears in breast milk. Determine risks and benefits before administering to breast-feeding women.

Reactions may be *common,* uncommon, **life-threatening**, or COMMON AND LIFE-THREATENING.

levobunolol hydrochloride
AKBeta, Betagan

Pharmacologic classification: beta
blocker
Therapeutic classification: antiglaucoma
drug
Pregnancy risk category C

How supplied
Available by prescription only
Ophthalmic solution: 0.25%, 0.5%

Indications, route, and dosage
Chronic open-angle glaucoma and ocular hypertension
Adults: Instill 1 to 2 drops (0.5% solution) daily
or 1 to 2 drops (0.25% solution) b.i.d. in eye.

Pharmacodynamics
Antiglaucoma action: Exact mechanism unknown.
Reduces intraocular pressure and appears to reduce formation of aqueous humor.

Pharmacokinetics
• *Absorption:* Onset of activity usually occurs
within 60 minutes; peak effect in 2 to 6 hours.
• *Distribution:* No information available.
• *Metabolism:* No information available.
• *Excretion:* Duration of effect is 24 hours.

Contraindications and precautions
Contraindicated in patients with hypersensitivity
to drug and in those with bronchial asthma, history of bronchial asthma or severe COPD, sinus
bradycardia, second- or third-degree AV block,
cardiac failure, and cardiogenic shock. Use cautiously in patients with chronic bronchitis, emphysema, diabetes mellitus, hyperthyroidism, or
myasthenia gravis.

Interactions
Drug-drug. *Carbonic anhydrase inhibitors, epinephrine, pilocarpine:* Increased reductions in intraocular pressure. Use together cautiously.
Catecholamine-depleting drugs, reserpine: Enhanced hypotensive and bradycardiac effects of
these drugs. Monitor blood pressure and ECG.
Oral beta blockers: May increase systemic effect
of these drugs. Use together cautiously.
Drug-lifestyle. *Sun exposure:* Possible photophobia. Tell patient to take precautions.

Adverse reactions
CNS: headache, depression, insomnia.
CV: slight reduction in resting heart rate, ***bradycardia***, hypotension, **heart failure.**
EENT: *transient eye stinging and burning,* tearing, erythema, itching, keratitis, corneal punctate
staining, photophobia; decreased corneal sensitivity with long-term use.

GI: nausea.
Respiratory: *asthmatic attacks in patients
with history of asthma.*
Skin: urticaria.

☑ Special considerations
• Cardiac output is reduced in both healthy patients and those with heart disease. Drug may
decrease heart rate and blood pressure and produces beta blockade in bronchi and bronchioles.
No effect on pupil size or accommodation has
been noted.
• In some patients, a few weeks' treatment may
be required to stabilize pressure-lowering response; determine intraocular pressure after 4
weeks of treatment.
• Levobunolol is faster-acting than timolol.
• Signs and symptoms of overdose include bradycardia, hypotension, bronchospasm, heart block,
and cardiac failure. If accidental ingestion occurs,
emesis is most effective if started within 30 minutes.

Monitoring the patient
• Watch for signs and symptoms of overdose.
• In asthmatic patients, evaluate closely for
wheezing.

Information for the patient
• Warn patient not to touch dropper to eye or surrounding tissue.
• Show patient how to instill drug. Teach him to
press lacrimal sac lightly for 1 minute after drug
administration to decrease chance of systemic
absorption.
• Remind patient not to blink more than usual or
to close eyes tightly during treatment.
• Tell patient to call if reaction is severe, although
transient stinging and discomfort are common.

Geriatric patients
• Drug should be used with caution in elderly patients with cardiac or pulmonary disease, who
may experience exacerbation of symptoms, depending on extent of systemic absorption.

levodopa
Dopar, Larodopa

Pharmacologic classification: dopamine
precursor
Therapeutic classification: antiparkinsonian
Pregnancy risk category C

How supplied
Available by prescription only
Tablets: 100 mg, 250 mg, 500 mg
Capsules: 100 mg, 250 mg, 500 mg

Indications, route, and dosage

Parkinsonism
Levodopa is indicated in treating idiopathic, postencephalitic, arteriosclerotic parkinsonism and symptomatic parkinsonism that may follow injury to the nervous system by carbon monoxide intoxication and manganese intoxication.
Adults: Initially, 0.5 to 1 g P.O. daily, given b.i.d., t.i.d., or q.i.d. with food; increase by no more than 0.75 g daily q 3 to 7 days, as tolerated. The usual optimal dose is 3 to 6 g daily divided into three doses. Don't exceed 8 g daily, except for exceptional patients. A significant therapeutic response may not be obtained for 6 months. Larger dose requires close supervision.

Pharmacodynamics

Antiparkinsonian action: Exact mechanism unknown. A small percentage of each dose crossing the blood-brain barrier is decarboxylated. The dopamine then stimulates dopaminergic receptors in the basal ganglia to enhance the balance between cholinergic and dopaminergic activity, resulting in improved modulation of voluntary nerve impulses transmitted to the motor cortex.

Pharmacokinetics

• *Absorption:* Absorbed rapidly from small intestine by active amino acid transport system, with 30% to 50% reaching general circulation.
• *Distribution:* Distributed widely to most body tissues, but not to CNS; CNS receives less than 1% of dose because of extensive metabolism in periphery.
• *Metabolism:* 95% of levodopa is converted to dopamine by l-aromatic amino acid decarboxylase enzyme in lumen of stomach and intestines and on first pass through liver.
• *Excretion:* Excreted primarily in urine; 80% of dose excreted within 24 hours as dopamine metabolites. Half-life is 1 to 3 hours.

Contraindications and precautions

Contraindicated in patients with hypersensitivity to drug, in concurrent therapy with MAO inhibitors within 14 days, and in those with acute angle-closure glaucoma, melanoma, or undiagnosed skin lesions.

Use cautiously in patients with severe renal, CV, hepatic, or pulmonary disorders; peptic ulcer; psychiatric illness; MI with residual arrhythmias; bronchial asthma; emphysema; or endocrine disorders.

Interactions

Drug-drug. *Amantadine, benztropine, procyclidine, trihexyphenidyl:* Possible increased efficacy of levodopa. Monitor patient closely.
Anesthetics, hydrocarbon inhalation: Possible arrhythmias. Stop levodopa 6 to 8 hours before giving anesthetics such as halothane.

Antacids containing calcium, magnesium, or sodium bicarbonate: May increase absorption of levodopa. Give antacids 1 hour after levodopa.
Anticholinergics: Mild synergy and increased efficacy when used together. Gradual reduction in anticholinergic dosage is needed.
Anticonvulsants, benzodiazepines, haloperidol, papaverine, phenothiazines, rauwolfia alkaloids, thioxanthenes: Decreased therapeutic effects of levodopa. Avoid concomitant use.
Antihypertensives: Possible increased hypotensive effect. Monitor blood pressure carefully.
Bromocriptine: Additive effects. Reduce levodopa dosage as needed.
MAO inhibitors: Possible hypertensive crisis. Stop MAO inhibitors 2 to 4 weeks before starting levodopa.
Methyldopa: May alter antiparkinsonian effects of levodopa; possible additive toxic CNS effects. Avoid concomitant use.
Pyridoxine: Reversed antiparkinsonian effects of levodopa. Don't give together.
Sympathomimetics: Increased risk of arrhythmias. Dosage reduction of both drugs recommended.
Tricyclic antidepressants: Increased sympathetic activity, with sinus tachycardia and hypertension. Avoid concomitant use.
Drug-herb. *Jimsonweed:* May adversely affect CV function. Avoid use together.
Kava: Increased parkinsonian symptoms. Avoid use together.
Rauwolfia: May decrease effectiveness of levodopa. Avoid use together.
Drug-food. *Foods high in protein:* Decreased absorption of levodopa. Don't give together.
Drug-lifestyle. *Cocaine:* Increased risk of arrhythmias. Discourage use; monitor patient closely.

Adverse reactions

CNS: *aggressive behavior; choreiform, dystonic, and dyskinetic movements; involuntary grimacing, head movements, myoclonic body jerks,* **seizures,** *ataxia, tremor, muscle twitching;* bradykinetic episodes; psychiatric disturbances; mood changes, nervousness, anxiety, disturbing dreams, euphoria, malaise, fatigue; severe depression, **suicidal tendencies,** dementia, delirium, hallucinations (may require reduction or withdrawal of drug).
CV: *orthostatic hypotension,* cardiac irregularities, phlebitis.
EENT: blepharospasm, blurred vision, diplopia, mydriasis or miosis, activation of latent Horner's syndrome, oculogyric crises, excessive salivation.
GI: dry mouth, bitter taste, *nausea, vomiting, anorexia,* constipation, flatulence, diarrhea, abdominal pain.
GU: urinary frequency, urine retention, incontinence, darkened urine, priapism.

Reactions may be *common,* uncommon, **life-threatening,** or COMMON AND LIFE-THREATENING.

Hematologic: *hemolytic anemia, leukopenia, agranulocytosis.*
Hepatic: elevated liver enzyme levels, *hepatotoxicity.*
Metabolic: weight loss at start of therapy.
Respiratory: hyperventilation, hiccups.
Other: dark perspiration.

☑ Special considerations

• Drug should be given between meals and with low-protein snack to maximize drug absorption and minimize GI upset. Foods high in protein appear to interfere with transport of drug.
• Maximum effectiveness of drug may not occur for several weeks or months after therapy begins.
• Drug may interfere with some specific urine tests.
• Patients undergoing surgery should continue levodopa as long as oral intake is permitted, usually 6 to 24 hours before surgery. Drug should be resumed as soon as patient is able to take oral medication.
• If restarting therapy after a long period of interruption, adjust drug dosage gradually to previous level.
• Protect drug from heat, light, and moisture. If preparation darkens, it has lost potency and should be discarded.
• Although controversial, a medically supervised period of drug discontinuance (drug holiday) may reestablish the effectiveness of a lower dose regimen.
• Combination of levodopa and carbidopa usually reduces amount of levodopa needed, thus reducing adverse reactions.
• Levodopa has also been used to relieve pain of herpes zoster.
• Tablets and capsules may be crushed and mixed with applesauce or baby-food fruits for patients who have difficulty swallowing pills.
• Coombs' test occasionally becomes positive during extended use. Expect uric acid elevation with colorimetric method but not with uricase method.

Monitoring the patient

• Observe and monitor vital signs, especially while adjusting dose.
• Because of risk of precipitating a symptom complex resembling neuroleptic malignant syndrome, observe patient closely if levodopa dosage is reduced abruptly or stopped.
• Monitor patient for muscle twitching and blepharospasm (twitching of eyelids), and arrhythmias, which may be signs of drug overdose.
• Test patients on long-term therapy regularly for diabetes and acromegaly; monitor serum laboratory tests, including liver and kidney function studies, periodically for adverse effects. Leukopenia may require stopping therapy.
• Alkaline phosphatase, AST, ALT, lactic dehydrogenase, bilirubin, BUN, and protein-bound iodine levels show transient elevations in patients receiving levodopa; WBC, hemoglobin, and hematocrit levels show occasional reduction.

Information for the patient

• Warn patient and family not to increase drug dose without specific instruction. (They may be tempted to do this as parkinsonian symptoms progress.)
• Explain that therapeutic response may not occur for up to 6 months.
• Advise patient and family that multivitamin preparations, fortified cereals, and certain OTC products may contain pyridoxine (vitamin B_6), which can reverse the effects of levodopa.
• Warn patient of possible dizziness and orthostatic hypotension, especially at start of therapy. Tell patient to change position slowly and dangle legs before getting out of bed. Instruct patient in use of elastic stockings to control this adverse reaction if appropriate.
• Inform patient of signs and symptoms of adverse reactions and therapeutic effects and the need to report changes.
• Tell patient to take a missed dose as soon as possible; to skip dose if next scheduled dose is within 2 hours, but not to double doses.
• Advise patient not to take drug with food, but that eating something about 15 minutes after administration may help reduce GI upset.
• Warn patient of possible darkening of urine, sweat, and other body fluids.

Geriatric patients

• Smaller doses may be needed in this age-group because of reduced tolerance to drug's effects.
• Elderly patients, especially those with osteoporosis, should resume normal activity gradually because increased mobility may increase risk of fractures.
• Elderly patients are more likely to develop psychic adverse effects, such as anxiety, confusion, or nervousness; those with preexisting heart disease are more susceptible to levodopa's cardiac effects.

Pediatric patients

• Safe use of levodopa in children under age 12 hasn't been established.

Breast-feeding patients

• Drug may inhibit lactation and shouldn't be used by breast-feeding women.

levodopa-carbidopa
Sinemet, Sinemet CR

Pharmacologic classification: decarboxylase inhibitor dopamine precursor combination
Therapeutic classification: antiparkinsonian
Pregnancy risk category C

How supplied
Available by prescription only
Tablets: 10 mg carbidopa with 100 mg levodopa (Sinemet 10-100), 25 mg carbidopa with 100 mg levodopa (Sinemet 25-100), 25 mg carbidopa with 250 mg levodopa (Sinemet 25-250)
Tablets (sustained-release): 50 mg carbidopa with 200 mg levodopa (Sinemet CR 50-200), 25 mg carbidopa with 100 mg levodopa (Sinemet CR 25-100)

Indications, route, and dosage
Parkinsonism
Adults: Most patients respond to a 25 mg/100 mg combination (1 tablet t.i.d.). Dose may be increased q 1 or 2 days; or 1 tablet of 10 mg/100 mg t.i.d. or q.i.d. up to 2 tablets q.i.d.; or 1 sustained-release tablet b.i.d. at intervals at least 6 hours apart. Intervals may be adjusted based on patient response. Usual dose is 2 to 8 tablets daily in divided doses of 4 to 8 hours while awake.

Maintenance therapy must be carefully adjusted based on patient tolerance and desired therapeutic response.

Usual maintenance dose is 3 to 6 tablets of 25 mg carbidopa/250 mg levodopa daily in divided doses. Don't exceed 8 tablets of 25 mg carbidopa/250 mg levodopa daily. Optimum daily dose must be determined by careful adjustment for each patient.

Daily dose of carbidopa should be 70 mg or above to suppress the peripheral metabolism of levodopa but shouldn't exceed 200 mg.

Pharmacodynamics
Decarboxylase inhibiting action: Carbidopa inhibits the peripheral decarboxylation of levodopa, thus slowing its conversion to dopamine in extracerebral tissues. This results in an increased availability of levodopa for transport to the brain, where it undergoes decarboxylation to dopamine.

Pharmacokinetics
• *Absorption:* 40% to 70% of dose absorbed after oral administration. Plasma levodopa levels increase when carbidopa and levodopa are administered together because carbidopa inhibits peripheral metabolism of levodopa.
• *Distribution:* Carbidopa distributed widely in body tissues except the CNS; levodopa also distributed into breast milk.

• *Metabolism:* Carbidopa isn't metabolized extensively. It inhibits metabolism of levodopa in GI tract, thus increasing its absorption from GI tract and its level in plasma.
• *Excretion:* 30% of dose excreted unchanged in urine within 24 hours. When given with carbidopa, levodopa excreted unchanged in urine increases by about 6%. Half-life is 1 to 2 hours.

Contraindications and precautions
Contraindicated in patients with hypersensitivity to drug; in those with acute angle-closure glaucoma, melanoma, or undiagnosed skin lesions; and within 14 days of MAO inhibitor therapy.

Use cautiously in patients with severe CV, endocrine, pulmonary, renal, or hepatic disorders; peptic ulcer; psychiatric illness; MI with residual arrhythmias; bronchial asthma; emphysema; and well-controlled chronic open-angle glaucoma.

Interactions
Drug-drug. *Amantadine, benztropine, procyclidine, trihexyphenidyl:* May increase efficacy of levodopa. Monitor patient closely.
Anesthetics, hydrocarbon inhalation: Possible arrhythmias. Levodopa-carbidopa should be stopped 6 to 8 hours before administration of these drugs.
Antacids containing calcium, magnesium, or sodium bicarbonate: Possible increased absorption of levodopa. Administer antacids 1 hour after levodopa.
Anticonvulsants, benzodiazepines, droperidol, haloperidol, loxapine, metyrosine, papaverine, phenothiazines, rauwolfia alkaloids, thioxanthenes: May decrease therapeutic effects of levodopa. Monitor patient closely.
Antihypertensives: Possible increased hypotensive effect. Monitor blood pressure.
Bromocriptine: Possible additive effects. Reduce levodopa dosage.
MAO inhibitors: Possible hypertensive crisis. Stop MAO inhibitors for 2 to 4 weeks before starting levodopa-carbidopa.
Methyldopa: May alter antiparkinsonian effects of levodopa; possible additive toxic CNS effects. Avoid concomitant use.
Molindone: May inhibit antiparkinsonian effects of levodopa. Avoid concomitant use.
Sympathomimetics: Possible increased risk of arrhythmias. Reduced dosage of sympathomimetic is recommended; however, carbidopa with levodopa reduces tendency of sympathomimetics to cause dopamine-induced arrhythmias.

Adverse reactions
CNS: *choreiform, dystonic, dyskinetic movements; involuntary grimacing, head movements, myoclonic body jerks, ataxia,* tremor, muscle twitching; bradykinetic episodes; psychiatric disturbances, anxiety, disturbing dreams, euphoria, malaise, fatigue; severe depression, ***suicidal***

Reactions may be common, uncommon, **life-threatening**, or COMMON AND LIFE-THREATENING.

tendencies, dementia, delirium, hallucinations (may necessitate reduction or withdrawal of drug), confusion, insomnia, agitation.

CV: *orthostatic hypotension,* **cardiac irregularities,** phlebitis.

EENT: blepharospasm, blurred vision, diplopia, mydriasis or miosis, oculogyric crises, excessive salivation.

GI: *dry mouth,* bitter taste, *nausea, vomiting, anorexia,* constipation; flatulence; diarrhea; abdominal pain.

GU: urinary frequency, urine retention, urinary incontinence, darkened urine, priapism.

Hematologic: hemolytic anemia, thrombocytopenia, leukopenia, agranulocytosis.

Hepatic: *hepatotoxicity,* elevated levels of BUN, ALT, AST, alkaline phosphatase, serum bilirubin, LD, and serum protein-bound iodine.

Metabolic: weight loss at start of therapy.

Respiratory: hyperventilation, hiccups.

Other: dark perspiration, elevated serum gonadotropin levels.

☑ Special considerations
• Carefully monitor patient also receiving antihypertensives or hypoglycemics.
• Adjust dosage based on patient's response and tolerance to drug. Therapeutic and adverse reactions occur more rapidly with levodopa-carbidopa combination than with levodopa alone.
• If patient is being treated with levodopa, stop at least 8 hours before starting levodopa-carbidopa.
• Combination drug usually reduces amount of levodopa needed by 75%, thereby reducing adverse reactions.
• Pyridoxine (vitamin B$_6$) doesn't reverse beneficial effects of levodopa-carbidopa. Multivitamins can be taken without fear of losing control of symptoms.
• If therapy is interrupted temporarily, usual daily dose may be given as soon as patient resumes oral medications.
• Maximum effectiveness of drug may not occur for several weeks or months after therapy begins.
• Sustained-release tablets may be split, never crushed or chewed.
• Drug affects specific diagnostic urine tests.
• Muscle twitching and blepharospasm (twitching of eyelids), and arrhythmias may be signs of overdose. Treatment of overdose includes immediate gastric lavage and antiarrhythmics, if needed.

Monitoring the patient
• Observe and monitor vital signs, especially while dosage is being adjusted.
• Test patients on long-term therapy regularly for diabetes and acromegaly; periodically repeat laboratory tests, including liver and kidney function studies.

Information for the patient
• Instruct patient to report adverse reactions and therapeutic effects.
• Warn patient of possible dizziness or orthostatic hypotension, especially at start of therapy. Tell patient to change position slowly and dangle legs before getting out of bed. Elastic stockings may be helpful in some patients.
• Tell patient to take food shortly after taking drug to relieve gastric irritation.
• Inform patient that drug may cause urine or sweat to darken.
• Tell patient to take a missed dose as soon as possible, to skip a missed dose if next scheduled dose is within 2 hours, and never to double the dose.

Geriatric patients
• In elderly patients, smaller doses may be needed because of reduced tolerance to the effects of levodopa-carbidopa. Elderly patients, especially those with osteoporosis, should resume normal activity gradually because increased mobility may increase risk of fractures.
• Elderly patients are especially vulnerable to CNS adverse effects, such as anxiety, confusion, or nervousness; those with preexisting heart disease are more susceptible to cardiac effects.

Pediatric patients
• Safety in children under age 18 hasn't been established.

Breast-feeding patients
• Drug may inhibit lactation and shouldn't be used by breast-feeding women.

levofloxacin
Levaquin

Pharmacologic classification: fluorinated carboxyquinolone
Therapeutic classification: broad-spectrum antibacterial
Pregnancy risk category C

How supplied
Available by prescription only
Tablets: 250 mg, 500 mg
Single-use vials: 500 mg
Infusion (premixed): 250 mg in 50 ml D$_5$W, 500 mg in 100 ml D$_5$W

Indications, route, and dosage
Acute maxillary sinusitis caused by susceptible strains of Streptococcus pneumoniae, Moraxella catarrhalis, or Haemophilus influenzae
Adults: 500 mg P.O. or I.V. daily for 10 to 14 days.
Acute bacterial exacerbation of chronic bronchitis caused by Staphylococcus aureus, S.

pneumoniae, M. catarrhalis, H. influenzae, *or*
H. parainfluenzae
Adults: 500 mg P.O. or I.V. daily for 7 days.
Community-acquired pneumonia caused by
S. aureus, S. pneumoniae, M. catarrhalis, H.
influenzae, H. parainfluenzae, Klebsiella pneumoniae, Chlamydia pneumoniae, Legionella
pneumophila, *or* Mycoplasma pneumoniae
Adults: 500 mg P.O. or I.V. daily for 7 to 14 days.
*Uncomplicated skin and skin-structure in-
fections (mild to moderate) caused by* S. aureus *or* Streptococcus pyogenes
Adults: 500 mg P.O. or I.V. daily for 7 to 10 days.
✦ *Dosage adjustment.* If creatinine clearance
is 20 to 49 ml/minute, subsequent dosages are
half the initial dose. If creatinine clearance is 10
to 19 ml/minute, subsequent dosages are half
the initial dose and the interval is prolonged to q
48 hours.
*Complicated urinary tract infections (mild to
moderate) caused by* Enterococcus faecalis,
Enterobacter cloacae, Escherichia coli, K.
pneumoniae, Proteus mirabilis, *or* Pseudomonas aeruginosa
Adults: 250 mg P.O. or I.V. daily for 10 days.
*Acute pyelonephritis (mild to moderate)
caused by* E. coli
Adults: 250 mg P.O. or I.V. daily for 10 days.
✦ *Dosage adjustment.* If creatinine clearance
is 10 to 19 ml/minute, dosage interval is increased
to q 48 hours.

Pharmacodynamics

Antibacterial action: Inhibits bacterial DNA gyrase, an enzyme required for DNA replication,
transcription, repair, and recombination in susceptible bacteria.

Pharmacokinetics

• *Absorption:* Plasma level after I.V. administration is comparable to that of equivalent oral doses (on a mg/mg basis); oral and I.V. routes considered interchangeable. Plasma levels peak
within 1 to 2 hours after oral dosing. Steady-state
reached within 48 hours on a 500 mg/day regimen.
• *Distribution:* Mean volume of distribution ranges
from 89 to 112 L after single and multiple 500-
mg doses; widespread distribution into body tissues. Drug penetrates well into lung tissues; lung
tissue levels were generally two- to fivefold higher than plasma levels.
• *Metabolism:* Limited metabolism. Only identified metabolites are desmethyl and N-oxide
metabolites, which have little relevant pharmacologic activity.
• *Excretion:* Primarily excreted unchanged in
urine. Mean terminal half-life is about 6 to 8 hours.

Contraindications and precautions

Contraindicated in patients with hypersensitivity
to drug, its components, or quinolone antimicro-

bials. Safety during pregnancy hasn't been established.
Use cautiously in patients with history of seizure
disorders or other CNS diseases, such as cerebral arteriosclerosis, because quinolones can
cause CNS stimulation and increased intracranial pressure, which may lead to seizures (lowered seizure threshold), toxic psychoses, tremors,
restlessness, anxiety, light-headedness, confusion, hallucinations, paranoia, depression, nightmares, insomnia, and, rarely, suicidal thoughts or
acts. These reactions can occur after the first dose.

Interactions

Drug-drug. *Antacids containing aluminum or
magnesium, iron salts, products containing zinc,
sucralfate:* May interfere with GI absorption of levofloxacin. Administer at least 2 hours apart.
Antidiabetics: May alter blood glucose levels.
Monitor blood glucose levels closely.
NSAIDs: May increase CNS stimulation. Watch
for seizure activity.
Theophylline: Decreased clearance of theophylline. Monitor theophylline levels.
Warfarin: Possible increased oral anticoagulant
effect with some fluoroquinolones. Monitor PT
and INR.
Drug-lifestyle. *Sun exposure:* May cause photosensitivity. Tell patient to take precautions.

Adverse reactions

CNS: headache, insomnia, dizziness, enceph-
alopathy, paresthesia, *seizures,* abnormal EEG.
CV: chest pain, palpitations, vasodilation.
GI: nausea, diarrhea, constipation, vomiting, ab-
dominal pain, dyspepsia, flatulence, *pseudo-
membranous colitis.*
GU: vaginitis.
Hematologic: eosinophilia, hemolytic anemia.
Musculoskeletal: back pain, tendon rupture.
Respiratory: allergic pneumonitis.
Skin: rash, photosensitivity, pruritus, erythema
multiforme, **Stevens-Johnson syndrome.**
Other: pain, *hypersensitivity reactions,* injec-
tion site reaction, **anaphylaxis, multisystem or-
gan failure,** decreased glucose level and lymphocyte count.

☑ Special considerations

• If patient experiences symptoms of excessive
CNS stimulation (restlessness, tremor, confusion,
hallucinations), stop drug and institute seizure
precautions.
• Ruptures of tendons and tendonitis have occurred with quinolone therapy. Stop drug if pain,
inflammation, or tendon rupture occurs. These
ruptures can occur after therapy has been stopped.
• Because a rapid or bolus administration may result in hypotension, I.V. levofloxacin should be administered only by slow infusion over 60 minutes.
• If acute overdose occurs, empty stomach, maintain hydration, and observe.

Reactions may be *common*, uncommon, **life-threatening**, or COMMON AND LIFE-THREATENING.

Monitoring the patient
● Monitor vital signs closely.
● Watch for CNS changes.

Information for the patient
● Tell patient to take drug as prescribed, even if symptoms disappear.
● Advise patient to take drug with plenty of fluids and to avoid antacids, sucralfate, and products containing iron or zinc for at least 2 hours before and after each dose.
● Warn patient to avoid hazardous tasks until adverse CNS effects of drug are known.
● Tell patient to stop drug and call if rash or other signs of hypersensitivity develop.
● Tell patient to report pain or inflammation.
● Tell diabetic patient to monitor blood glucose levels and report if a hypoglycemic reaction occurs.

Geriatric patients
● Dosage adjustment based on age alone isn't necessary.

Pediatric patients
● Safety and effectiveness in children under age 18 haven't been established.

Breast-feeding patients
● Safety in breast-feeding women hasn't been established. Drug probably appears in breast milk. Because of potential for serious adverse reactions in breast-fed infants, a decision should be made to either stop drug or discontinue breast-feeding.

levonorgestrel implants
Norplant System

Pharmacologic classification: progestin
Therapeutic classification: contraceptive
Pregnancy risk category X

How supplied
Available by prescription only
Implants: 36 mg in each of 6 Silastic capsules; kits also include trocar, scalpel, forceps, syringe, two needles, package of skin closures, three packages of gauze sponges, stretch bandages, and surgical drape

Indications, route, and dosage
Long-term (up to 5 years), reversible prevention of pregnancy
Adults: Six Silastic capsules containing 36 mg each for a total of 216 mg are surgically implanted in superficial plane beneath skin of a woman's upper arm.

Pharmacodynamics
Contraceptive action: Synthetic, biologically active progestin, exhibiting no significant estrogenic activity. A continuous low dose of levonorgestrel is diffused through the wall of each capsule. Pregnancy is prevented by at least two mechanisms: inhibition of ovulation and thickening of cervical mucus.

Pharmacokinetics
● *Absorption:* Maximum or near maximum levels reached within 24 hours of implantation. Drug is 100% bioavailable. Plasma levels average 0.3 ng/ml over 5 years but are highly variable as a function of individual metabolism and body weight.
● *Distribution:* Bound by circulating protein sex hormone–binding globulin.
● *Metabolism:* Metabolized by liver.
● *Excretion:* Metabolites excreted in urine.

Contraindications and precautions
Contraindicated in patients with hypersensitivity to levonorgestrel or components of the Norplant System and in those with active thrombophlebitis or thromboembolic disorders, undiagnosed abnormal genital bleeding, acute liver disease, malignant or benign liver tumors, known or suspected breast cancer, known or suspected pregnancy, or history of idiopathic intracranial hypertension.
    Use cautiously in diabetic and prediabetic patients and in those with history of depression or hyperlipidemia.

Interactions
Drug-drug. *Carbamazepine, phenytoin:* Reduced efficacy of levonorgestrel; increased risk of pregnancy. Additional form of birth control may be needed.
Drug-food. *Caffeine:* May increase serum caffeine levels. Monitor patient for effects.
Drug-lifestyle. *Smoking:* Increased risk of adverse CV effects. Advise patient that, if smoking continues, alternative therapy may be needed.

Adverse reactions
CNS: headache, nervousness, dizziness, depression, tingling, numbness.
GI: nausea, *abdominal discomfort,* appetite change.
GU: *amenorrhea, many days of bleeding or prolonged bleeding, spotting, irregular onset of bleeding, frequent onset of bleeding, scanty bleeding, cervicitis, vaginitis, leukorrhea.*
Skin: dermatitis, acne, hirsutism, hypertrichosis, alopecia; infection, transient pain, itching (at implant site).
Other: adnexal enlargement, mastalgia, weight gain, *musculoskeletal pain, removal difficulty, breast discharge,* decreased thyroxine levels and increased T_3 uptake.

☑ Special considerations

- Total implanted dose is 216 mg. Implantation of all six capsules should be performed during the first 7 days of menstrual cycle. Insertion is subdermal in the midportion of inside of upper arm, 8 to 10 cm above elbow crease.
- Remove all previously implanted capsules before insertion of new set to prevent risk of overdose.
- Each capsule is 2.4 mm in diameter and 34 mm in length.
- Determine if patient has allergies to antiseptic or anesthetic to be used or contraindications to progestin-only contraception.
- During insertion, pay special attention to asepsis and correct placement of capsules; use careful technique to minimize tissue trauma.

Monitoring the patient

- Monitor patient's response to drug therapy.
- Watch for adverse effects.

Information for the patient

- Tell patient that altered bleeding patterns tend to become more regular after 9 to 12 months.
- Warn patient to report heavy bleeding.
- Advise patient to avoid bumping or wetting insertion site for at least 3 days after insertion.
- Explain that some tenderness in implant area may occur for 1 to 2 days.
- Tell patient that insertion usually takes 10 to 15 minutes and causes little or no discomfort because of the local anesthetic.
- Advise patient to disclose that she has levonorgestrel implants when laboratory studies are ordered.
- Advise patient to thoroughly review patient information booklet.

Breast-feeding patients

- Because drug appears in breast milk, its use during breast-feeding isn't recommended.

---

levothyroxine sodium (T₄ or L-thyroxine sodium)
Eltroxin, Levo-T, Levothroid, Levoxine, Levoxyl, Synthroid

Pharmacologic classification: thyroid hormone
Therapeutic classification: thyroid hormone replacement
Pregnancy risk category A

How supplied
Available by prescription only
Tablets: 25 mcg, 50 mcg, 75 mcg, 88 mcg, 100 mcg, 112 mcg, 125 mcg, 137 mcg, 150 mcg, 175 mcg, 200 mcg, 300 mcg
Injection: 200 mcg/vial, 500 mcg/vial

Indications, route, and dosage
Congenital hypothyroidism
Children under age 1: Initially, 25 to 50 mcg P.O. daily, increased to 50 mcg (in 4 to 6 weeks).
Myxedema coma
Adults: 300 to 500 mcg I.V. If no response occurs in 24 hours, give an additional 100 to 300 mcg I.V. in 48 hours. A maintenance dose of 50 to 200 mcg may be given until condition stabilizes and drug can be given orally.
Thyroid hormone replacement
Adults: For mild hypothyroidism—Initially, 50 mcg P.O. daily, increased by 25 to 50 mcg P.O. daily q 2 to 4 weeks until desired response is achieved; may be administered I.V. or I.M. when P.O. ingestion is precluded for long periods.

For severe hypothyroidism—12.5 to 25 mcg daily, increased by 25 to 50 mcg daily q 2 to 4 weeks until desired response is achieved.
Elderly: Start at 12.5 to 25 mcg daily and increase in 12.5- to 25-mcg increments q 2 to 8 weeks.
✦ *Dosage adjustment.* For patients with CV disease, start at 12.5 to 25 mcg daily and increase in 12.5- to 25-mcg increments q 2 to 8 weeks.
Children: Therapy may be initiated at the full therapeutic dose. Incremental doses aren't usually needed.
Children over age 12: Over 150 mcg or 2 to 3 mcg/kg/day.
Children ages 6 to 12: 100 to 150 mcg or 4 to 5 mcg/kg/day.
Children ages 1 to 5: 75 to 100 mcg or 5 to 6 mcg/kg/day.
Children ages 6 to 12 months: 50 to 75 mcg or 6 to 8 mcg/kg/day.
Children up to age 6 months: 25 to 50 mcg or 8 to 10 mcg/kg/day.

Pharmacodynamics
Thyroid hormone replacement: Affects protein and carbohydrate metabolism, promotes gluconeogenesis, increases the use and mobilization of glycogen stores, stimulates protein synthesis, and regulates cell growth and differentiation. Major effect of drug is to increase the metabolic rate of tissue.

Pharmacokinetics
- *Absorption:* Between 50% and 80% of drug absorbed from GI tract. Full effects don't occur for 1 to 3 weeks after oral therapy begins. After I.M. administration, poor and variable absorption. After an I.V. dose in patients with myxedema coma, increased responsiveness may occur within 6 to 8 hours, but maximum therapeutic effect may not occur for up to 24 hours.
- *Distribution:* Not fully described; however, is distributed into most body tissues and fluids. Highest levels found in liver and kidneys; 99% protein-bound.

- *Metabolism:* Metabolized in peripheral tissues, primarily in liver, kidneys, and intestines. About 85% of metabolized drug is deiodinated.
- *Excretion:* Fecal excretion eliminates 20% to 40% of drug; half-life is 6 to 7 days.

Contraindications and precautions

Contraindicated in patients with hypersensitivity to drug, acute MI and thyrotoxicosis uncomplicated by hypothyroidism, or uncorrected adrenal insufficiency. Use cautiously in elderly patients and in those with renal impairment, angina pectoris, hypertension, ischemia, or other CV disorders.

Interactions

Drug-drug. *Anticoagulants:* May alter anticoagulant effect. Increase in levothyroxine dosage may need a decrease in anticoagulant dosage. Monitor PT and INR.

Beta blockers: Decreased conversion of levothyroxine to liothyronine. Use with caution.

Cholestyramine: Delayed absorption of levothyroxine. Separate administration times by 4 to 5 hours.

Corticotropin: Concomitant use causes changes in thyroid status. Corticotropin dose may need adjustment.

Estrogens: Decreased free levothyroxines. Watch for decreased effectiveness of thyroid hormone.

Hepatic enzyme inducers (such as phenytoin): May increase hepatic degradation of levothyroxine. Increased dosage requirements of levothyroxine may be needed.

Insulin, oral antidiabetics: Altered serum glucose levels. Monitor serum glucose levels; dosage adjustments may be needed.

Somatrem: May accelerate epiphyseal maturation. Use with caution; monitor patient closely.

Sympathomimetics, tricyclic antidepressants: May increase effects of any or all of these drugs; possible coronary insufficiency or arrhythmias. Avoid concomitant use.

Theophylline: Decreased theophylline clearance in hypothyroid patients. Monitor serum theophylline levels.

Adverse reactions

CNS: *nervousness, insomnia, tremor,* headache.
CV: *tachycardia, palpitations,* **arrhythmias,** *angina pectoris,* **cardiac arrest.**
GI: diarrhea, vomiting.
GU: menstrual irregularities.
Metabolic: weight loss.
Skin: diaphoresis, allergic skin reactions.
Other: heat intolerance, fever.

☑ Special considerations

Besides the recommendations relevant to all thyroid hormones, consider the following.
- Administer as a single dose before breakfast.

- Patient with history of lactose intolerance may be sensitive to Levothroid, which contains lactose.
- Synthroid 100- and 300-mcg tablets contain tartrazine, a dye that causes allergic reactions in susceptible individuals.
- When switching from levothyroxine to liothyronine, stop levothyroxine when liothyronine treatment begins. After residual effects of levothyroxine have disappeared, liothyronine dosage can be increased in small increments. When switching from liothyronine to levothyroxine, levothyroxine therapy should begin several days before withdrawing liothyronine to avoid relapse.
- Patient taking levothyroxine who needs iodine[131] uptake studies must discontinue drug 4 weeks before test.
- Protect drug from moisture and light. Prepare I.V. immediately before injection. Don't mix with other I.V. solutions.
- Levothyroxine has predictable effects because of standard hormonal content; is the usual drug of choice for thyroid hormone replacement.
- Signs and symptoms of overdose are those of hyperthyroidism, such as weight loss, increased appetite, palpitations, nervousness, diarrhea, abdominal cramps, sweating, tachycardia, increased blood pressure, widened pulse pressure.
- If overdose occurs, use gastric lavage or induce emesis (then use activated charcoal up to 4 hours after ingestion).

Monitoring the patient

- Watch for aggravation of concurrent diseases, such as Addison's disease or diabetes mellitus, and for signs of overdose.
- Monitor vital signs and ECG.

Information for the patient

- Instruct patient to take drug at same time each day; encourage morning dosing to avoid insomnia.
- Tell patient to report headache, diarrhea, nervousness, excessive sweating, heat intolerance, chest pain, increased pulse rate, or palpitations.
- Encourage patient to use the same product consistently; all brands don't have equal bioavailability.
- Advise patient not to store drug in warm, humid areas, such as bathroom, to prevent deterioration of product.
- Tell patient that replacement therapy is to be taken essentially for life, except in cases of transient hypothyroidism.

Geriatric patients

- Elderly patients are more sensitive to effects of drug. In patients over age 60, initial dosage should be 25% lower than usual recommended dosage.

Pediatric patients
● Partial and temporary hair loss may occur during the first few months of therapy.

Breast-feeding patients
● Minimal amounts of drug appear in breast milk. Use with caution in breast-feeding women.

lidocaine (lignocaine)
Xylocaine

lidocaine hydrochloride
Anestacon, Dilocaine, L-Caine, Lidoderm Patch, Lidoject, LidoPen Auto-Injector, Nervocaine, Xylocaine, Xylocaine Viscous, Zilactin-L

Pharmacologic classification: amide derivative
Therapeutic classification: ventricular antiarrhythmic, local anesthetic
Pregnancy risk category B

How supplied
Available by prescription only
Injection: 5 mg/ml, 10 mg/ml, 15 mg/ml, 20 mg/ml, 40 mg/ml, 100 mg/ml, 200 mg/ml
Premixed solutions: 2 mg/ml, 4 mg/ml, 8 mg/ml in D$_5$W
Ointment: 5%
Topical solution: 2%, 4%
Jelly: 2%
Spray: 10%
Available without a prescription
Ointment: 2.5%
Liquid: 2.5%
Cream: 0.5%
Spray: 0.5%
Gel: 0.5%, 2.5%
Transdermal patch: 5%

Indications, route, and dosage
Ventricular arrhythmias from MI, cardiac manipulation, or cardiac glycosides
Adults: 50 to 100 mg (1 to 1.5 mg/kg) I.V. bolus at 25 to 50 mg/minute. Repeat bolus q 3 to 5 minutes until arrhythmias subside or adverse effects develop. Don't exceed 300-mg total bolus during a 1-hour period. Simultaneously, begin constant infusion of 1 to 4 mg/minute. If single bolus has been given, repeat smaller bolus (usually one-half initial bolus) 5 to 10 minutes after start of infusion to maintain therapeutic serum level. After 24 hours of continuous infusion, decrease rate by one-half.
Elderly: Give half the bolus amount and use slower infusion rate.
✦ *Dosage adjustment.* Give half the bolus amount to lightweight patients and to those with heart failure or hepatic disease. Use slower infu-

sion rate in those with heart failure or hepatic disease, or patients weighing under 50 kg (110 lb).
   For I.M. administration: 300 mg (4.3 mg/kg) in deltoid muscle has been used in early stages of acute MI.
Children: 0.5 to 1 mg/kg by I.V. bolus; then infusion of 20 to 50 mcg/kg/minute.
◇ **Status epilepticus**
Adults: 1 mg/kg I.V. bolus; then, if seizure continues, administer 0.5 mg/kg 2 minutes after first dose; infusion at 30 mcg/kg/minute may be used.
Local anesthesia of skin or mucous membranes, pain from dental extractions, stomatitis
Adults and children: Apply 2% to 5% solution or ointment or 15 ml of Xylocaine Viscous q 3 to 4 hours to oral or nasal mucosa.
Local anesthesia in procedures involving the urethra
Adults: Instill about 15 ml (male) or 3 to 5 ml (female) into urethra.
Pain, burning, or itching caused by burns, sunburn, or skin irritation
Adults and children: Apply liberally.
Relief of pain associated with postherpetic neuralgia
Adults: Apply one to three patches to intact skin, covering most painful area, once daily for up to 12 hours each day. Smaller areas of treatment are recommended in patients who are debilitated or have poor elimination. Excessive dosing by applying patch to larger areas or for longer than recommended wearing time could cause increased absorption of lidocaine and high lidocaine levels, leading to serious adverse effects.

Pharmacodynamics
Ventricular antiarrhythmic action: One of the oldest antiarrhythmics. As a class IB antiarrhythmic, the drug suppresses automaticity and shortens the effective refractory period and action potential duration of His-Purkinje fibers and suppresses spontaneous ventricular depolarization during diastole. Therapeutic levels of the drug don't significantly affect conductive atrial tissue and AV conduction.
   Unlike quinidine and procainamide, lidocaine doesn't significantly alter hemodynamics when given in usual doses. Drug seems to act preferentially on diseased or ischemic myocardial tissue; exerting its effects on the conduction system, it inhibits reentry mechanisms and halts ventricular arrhythmias.
Local anesthetic action: As a local anesthetic, lidocaine acts to block initiation and conduction of nerve impulses by decreasing the permeability of the nerve cell membrane to sodium ions.

Pharmacokinetics

● *Absorption:* Absorbed after oral administration; a significant first-pass effect occurs in liver and only about 35% of drug reaches systemic circulation. Oral doses high enough to achieve therapeutic blood levels result in unacceptable toxicity, probably from high levels of lidocaine.

● *Distribution:* Distributed widely throughout body; high affinity for adipose tissue. After I.V. bolus administration, early, rapid decline in plasma levels occurs; distribution into highly perfused tissues, such as kidneys, lungs, liver, and heart, then slower elimination phase where metabolism and redistribution into skeletal muscle and adipose tissue occur. First (early) distribution phase occurs rapidly, requiring constant infusion after an initial bolus dose. Distribution volume declines in patients with liver or hepatic disease, resulting in toxic levels with usual doses. About 60% to 80% of circulating drug is bound to plasma proteins. Usual therapeutic drug level is 1.5 to 5 mcg/ml. Although toxicity may occur within this range, levels greater than 5 mcg/ml are considered toxic and warrant dosage reduction.

● *Metabolism:* Metabolized in liver to two active metabolites. Less than 10% of a parenteral dose escapes metabolism and reaches kidneys unchanged. Metabolism affected by hepatic blood flow, which may decrease after MI and with heart failure. Liver disease also may limit metabolism.

● *Excretion:* Biphasic half-life; initial phase of 7 to 30 minutes, then terminal half-life of 1½ to 2 hours. Elimination half-life may be prolonged in patients with heart failure or liver disease. Continuous infusions longer than 24 hours may cause half-life increase.

Contraindications and precautions

Contraindicated in patients with hypersensitivity to amide-type local anesthetics and in those with Stokes-Adams syndrome, Wolff-Parkinson-White syndrome, and severe degrees of SA, AV, or intraventricular block in absence of artificial pacemaker. Also contraindicated in patients with inflammation or infection in puncture region, septicemia, severe hypertension, spinal deformities, and neurologic disorders.

Use cautiously in elderly patients; in those with renal or hepatic disease, complete or second-degree heart block, sinus bradycardia, or heart failure; and in those weighing less than 110 lb (50 kg).

Interactions

Drug-drug. *Beta blockers, cimetidine:* May cause lidocaine toxicity from reduced hepatic clearance. Monitor patient for toxicity.

Succinylcholine: May increase succinylcholine's neuromuscular effects. Monitor patient closely.

Other antiarrhythmics (such as phenytoin, procainamide, propranolol, quinidine): May cause additive or antagonist effects and additive toxicity. Monitor ECG and patient closely.

Drug-herb. *Pareira:* May add to or potentiate effects of neuromuscular blockade. Avoid use together.

Drug-lifestyle. *Smoking:* May increase metabolism of lidocaine. Discourage use; monitor patient closely.

Adverse reactions

CNS: anxiety, nervousness, lethargy, somnolence, paresthesia, muscle twitching; *confusion, tremor, stupor, restlessness, light-headedness,* hallucinations, *seizures* (with systemic form); apprehension, unconsciousness, confusion, tremors, stupor, restlessness, slurred speech, euphoria, depression, light-headedness, *seizures* (with topical use).

CV: *bradycardia, cardiac arrest;* hypotension, *new or worsened arrhythmias* (with systemic form); hypotension, myocardial depression, *arrhythmias* (with topical use), edema.

EENT: *tinnitus, blurred or double vision* (with systemic form); tinnitus, blurred or double vision (with topical use).

GI: nausea, vomiting (with topical use).

Respiratory: *respiratory depression and arrest.*

Skin: dermatologic reactions, sensitization, diaphoresis (with topical use), rash (with topical use).

Other: *anaphylaxis;* soreness at injection site, sensation of cold (with systemic form); *status asthmaticus.*

☑ Special considerations

● Monitor patient receiving I.V. lidocaine infusion and on cardiac monitor at all times. Use infusion pump or microdrip system and timer to monitor infusion precisely. Never exceed infusion rate of 4 mg/minute, if possible. A faster rate greatly increases risk of toxicity.

● Don't administer lidocaine with epinephrine (for local anesthesia) to treat arrhythmias. Use solutions with epinephrine cautiously in CV disorders and in body areas with limited blood supply (ears, nose, fingers, toes).

● Doses of up to 400 mg I.M. have been advocated in prehospital phase of acute MI.

● Patient receiving lidocaine I.M. will show a sevenfold increase in serum CK level. Such CK originates in skeletal muscle, not the heart. Test isoenzyme levels to confirm MI, if using I.M. route.

● Don't use solutions containing preservatives for spinal, epidural, or caudal block.

● With epidural use, inject a 2- to 5-ml test dose at least 5 minutes before giving total dose to check for intravascular or subarachnoid injection. Motor paralysis and extensive sensory anesthesia indicate subarachnoid injection.

● Discard partially used vials containing no preservatives.

• Drug has been used for investigational purposes to treat refractory status epilepticus.
• Therapeutic serum levels range from 2 to 5 mcg/ml.
• Effects of overdose include signs and symptoms of CNS toxicity, such as seizures or respiratory depression, and CV toxicity (as indicated by hypotension).
• Provide general supportive measures and stop drug. Maintain a patent airway and provide other respiratory support measures immediately.
• Diazepam or thiopental may be given to treat seizures.
• To treat significant hypotension, administer vasopressors (such as dopamine and norepinephrine).

Monitoring the patient
• Monitor vital signs and serum electrolyte, BUN, and creatinine levels.
• Monitor ECG constantly if administering drug I.V., especially in patients with liver disease, heart failure, hypoxia, respiratory depression, hypovolemia, or shock; these conditions may affect drug metabolism, excretion, or distribution volume, predisposing patient to drug toxicity.
• Watch for signs of excessive depression of cardiac conductivity (such as sinus node dysfunction, PR-interval prolongation, QRS-complex widening, and appearance or exacerbation of arrhythmias). If they occur, reduce dosage or stop drug.
• In many severely ill patients, seizures may be the first sign of toxicity. However, severe reactions are usually preceded by somnolence, confusion, and paresthesia. Regard all signs and symptoms of toxicity as serious, and promptly reduce dosage or stop therapy. Continued infusion could lead to seizures and coma. Give oxygen via nasal cannula, if not contraindicated. Keep oxygen and CPR equipment handy.

Information for the patient
• Instruct patient to alert nurse if discomfort occurs at I.V. site.
• Advise patient receiving I.M. injection that drug may cause soreness at injection site.
• Instruct patient to report adverse reactions promptly.

Geriatric patients
• Because of concurrent disease states and declining organ system function in elderly patients, use conservative lidocaine doses.

Pediatric patients
• Safety and effectiveness in children haven't been established. Use of an I.M. autoinjector device isn't recommended.

lindane
(gamma benzene hexachloride)
G-well, Kwell, Scabene

Pharmacologic classification: chlorinated hydrocarbon insecticide
Therapeutic classification: scabicide, pediculicide
Pregnancy risk category B

How supplied
Available by prescription only
Cream: 1%
Lotion: 1%
Shampoo: 1%

Indications, route, and dosage
Note: In no case should more than 2 oz be used by one person in one application.
Scabies
Adults and children: After bathing with soap and water, apply a thin layer of cream or lotion and gently massage it on all skin surfaces, moving from neck to toes. After 8 to 12 hours, remove drug by bathing and scrubbing well. Treatment may be repeated after 1 week if needed.
Pediculosis
Adults and children: Apply shampoo to dry, affected area and wait 4 minutes. Then add a small amount of water and lather for 4 to 5 minutes; rinse thoroughly. Comb hair to remove nits. Treatment may be repeated after 1 week if needed.

Pharmacodynamics
Scabicide and pediculicide actions: Toxic to the parasitic mite *Sarcoptes scabiei* and its eggs, and to lice (*Pediculus capitis, P. corporis,* and *Phthirus pubis*). Absorbed through organism's exoskeleton, causing death.

Pharmacokinetics
• *Absorption:* 10% of topical dose may be absorbed in 24 hours.
• *Distribution:* Stored in body fat.
• *Metabolism:* Occurs in liver.
• *Excretion:* Excreted in urine and feces.

Contraindications and precautions
Contraindicated in patients with hypersensitivity to drug, in those with raw or inflamed skin or seizure disorders, and in premature infants. Use cautiously in young patients (including infants); to be used not more than twice during pregnancy.

Interactions
Drug-lifestyle. *Oils, ointments:* May increase absorption of drug. If oil-based hair products are used, hair must be washed and dried before using lindane.

Adverse reactions
CNS: *dizziness, seizures.*
Skin: *irritation* (with repeated use).

☑ Special considerations
- Make sure patient's body is clean (scrubbed well) and dry before application.
- Avoid applying drug to acutely inflamed skin; raw, weeping surfaces; or open wounds, cuts, or sores.
- Place hospitalized patient in isolation with linen-handling precautions.
- Accidental ingestion may cause extreme CNS toxicity. To treat lindane ingestion, empty stomach by appropriate measures (emesis or lavage); then use saline catharsis (don't use oil laxative).

Monitoring the patient
- Monitor patient for adverse effects.
- Monitor patient for drug effect.

Information for the patient
- Explain correct use of drug.
- Warn patient that itching may continue for several weeks, even if treatment is effective, especially in scabies infestation.
- Tell patient that, if drug accidentally contacts eyes, flush with water and call for further instructions. Patient should avoid inhaling vapor.
- Explain that reapplication usually isn't necessary unless live mites are found; advise reapplication if drug is accidentally washed off, but caution against overuse.
- Tell patient he may use drug to clean combs and brushes, and to wash them thoroughly afterward; advise patient that all clothing and bed linen that may have been contaminated by him within the past 2 days should be machine washed in hot water and dried in hot dryer or dry-cleaned to avoid reinfestation or transmission of organism.
- Discourage repeated use of drug, which may irritate skin and cause systemic toxicity.
- Advise patient that family and close contacts, including sexual contacts, should be treated concurrently.

Pediatric patients
- Use cautiously, especially in infants and small children, who are much more susceptible to CNS toxicity. Discourage thumb sucking in children using lindane, to prevent drug ingestion. The Centers for Disease Control and Prevention recommends other scabicide therapies for children under age 10.

Breast-feeding patients
- Because low levels of drug appear in breast milk, an alternative to breast-feeding may be used for 4 days.

liothyronine sodium (T$_3$)
Cytomel, Triostat

Pharmacologic classification: thyroid hormone
Therapeutic classification: thyroid hormone replacement
Pregnancy risk category A

How supplied
Available by prescription only
Tablets: 5 mcg, 25 mcg, 50 mcg
Injection: 10 mcg/ml

Indications, route, and dosage
Congenital hypothyroidism
Children: 5 mcg P.O. daily, increased by 5 mcg q 3 to 4 days until desired response occurs.
Myxedema
Adults: Initially, 5 mcg daily, increased by 5 to 10 mcg q 1 to 2 weeks. Maintenance dose is 50 to 100 mcg daily.
Myxedema coma, precoma
Adults: Initially, 25 to 50 mcg I.V.; reassess after 4 to 12 hours, then switch to P.O. as soon as possible. Patients with known or suspected cardiac disease should receive 10 to 20 mcg I.V.
Nontoxic goiter
Adults: Initially, 5 mcg P.O. daily; may be increased by 5 to 10 mcg daily at intervals of 1 to 2 weeks until dosage of 25 mcg daily is reached. Then dosage may be increased by 12.5 to 25 mcg daily at intervals of 1 to 2 weeks until desired response is noted. Usual maintenance dose is 75 mcg daily.
Adults over age 65: Initially, 5 mcg P.O. daily, increased by 5-mcg increments q 1 to 2 weeks until dosage of 25 mcg is reached. Then dosage may be increased by 12.5 to 25 mcg daily q 1 to 2 weeks.
Children: Initially, 5 mcg P.O. daily, increased by 5-mcg increments at weekly intervals until desired response is achieved.
Thyroid hormone replacement
Adults: Initially, 25 mcg P.O. daily, increased by 12.5 to 25 mcg q 1 to 2 weeks until satisfactory response is achieved. Usual maintenance dose is 25 to 75 mcg daily.
Liothyronine suppression test to differentiate hyperthyroidism from euthyroidism
Adults: 75 to 100 mcg daily for 7 days.

Pharmacodynamics
Thyroid hormone replacement: Usually a second-line drug in the treatment of hypothyroidism, myxedema, and cretinism. This component of thyroid hormone affects protein and carbohydrate metabolism, promotes gluconeogenesis, increases the utilization and mobilization of glycogen stores, stimulates protein synthesis, and regulates cell growth and differentiation. The major

effect of liothyronine is to increase the metabolic rate of tissue. It may be most useful in syndromes of thyroid hormone resistance.

Pharmacokinetics
• *Absorption:* 95% absorbed from GI tract. Effect peaks within 24 to 72 hours.
• *Distribution:* Highly protein-bound; distribution not fully described.
• *Metabolism:* Not fully understood.
• *Excretion:* Half-life is 1 to 2 days.

Contraindications and precautions
Contraindicated in patients with hypersensitivity to drug and in those with acute MI uncomplicated by hypothyroidism, untreated thyrotoxicosis, or uncorrected adrenal insufficiency. Use cautiously in elderly patients and in those with angina pectoris, hypertension, ischemia, other CV disorders, renal insufficiency, diabetes, or myxedema.

Interactions
Drug-drug. *Adrenocorticoids, corticotropin:* Altered thyroid status. Changes in liothyronine dosages may also require dosage changes in adrenocorticoid or corticotropin.
Anticoagulants: May alter anticoagulant effects. Monitor PT and INR closely; adjust dosage as indicated.
Estrogens: Increased serum thyroxine-binding globulin levels. May increase liothyronine requirements.
Insulin, oral antidiabetics: May alter serum glucose levels. Dosage adjustment may be needed.
Sympathomimetics, tricyclic antidepressants: Increased effects of these drugs, causing coronary insufficiency or arrhythmias. Monitor patient closely.

Adverse reactions
CNS: *nervousness, insomnia, tremor,* headache.
CV: *tachycardia,* **arrhythmias,** angina pectoris, **cardiac decompensation and collapse.**
GI: diarrhea, vomiting.
GU: menstrual irregularities.
Metabolic: weight loss.
Musculoskeletal: accelerated bone maturation in infants and children.
Skin: diaphoresis, skin reactions.
Other: heat intolerance.

☑ Special considerations
Besides the recommendations relevant to all thyroid hormones, consider the following.
• Liothyronine may be preferred when rapid effect is desired or when GI absorption or peripheral conversion of levothyroxine to liothyronine is impaired.
• Oral absorption may be reduced in patients with heart failure.
• When switching from levothyroxine to liothyronine, stop levothyroxine and start liothyronine at low dosage, increasing in small increments after residual effects of levothyroxine have disappeared. When switching from liothyronine to levothyroxine, start levothyroxine several days before withdrawing liothyronine to avoid relapse.
• Stop drug 7 to 10 days before patient undergoes radioactive iodine uptake studies.
• Indications of overdose include signs and symptoms of hyperthyroidism, including weight loss, increased appetite, palpitations, diarrhea, nervousness, abdominal cramps, sweating, headache, tachycardia, and increased blood pressure.
• To treat overdose, use gastric lavage or induce emesis (then use activated charcoal up to 4 hours after ingestion).

Monitoring the patient
• Monitor patient for adverse effects.
• Monitor vital signs and ECG.

Information for the patient
• Tell patient to report headache, diarrhea, nervousness, excessive sweating, heat intolerance, chest pain, increased pulse rate, or palpitations.
• Advise patient not to store drug in warm, humid areas, such as the bathroom, to prevent deterioration of drug.
• Encourage patient to take drug at the same time each day, preferably in the morning, to avoid insomnia.

Geriatric patients
• Elderly patients are more sensitive to drug's effects. In patients over age 60, initial dosage should be 25% lower than usual recommended dosage.

Pediatric patients
• Partial hair loss may occur during first few months of therapy. Reassure child and parents that this is temporary.
• Infants and children may experience an accelerated rate of bone maturation.

Breast-feeding patients
• Minimal amounts of drug appear in breast milk. Use with caution in breast-feeding women.

liotrix
Thyrolar

Pharmacologic classification: thyroid hormone
Therapeutic classification: thyroid hormone replacement
Pregnancy risk category A

How supplied
Available by prescription only
Tablets: Thyrolar-1/4—levothyroxine sodium 12.5 mcg and liothyronine sodium 3.1 mcg

Thyrolar-1/2—levothyroxine sodium 25 mcg and liothyronine sodium 6.25 mcg
Thyrolar-1—levothyroxine sodium 50 mcg and liothyronine sodium 12.5 mcg
Thyrolar-2—levothyroxine sodium 100 mcg and liothyronine sodium 25 mcg
Thyrolar-3—levothyroxine sodium 150 mcg and liothyronine sodium 37.5 mcg

Indications, route, and dosage
Hypothyroidism
Dosages must be individualized to approximate deficit in patient's thyroid secretion.
Adults: Initially, 15 to 30 mg thyroid equivalent P.O. daily, increased by 15 to 30 mg thyroid equivalent q 1 to 2 weeks until desired response is achieved.
Children over age 12: 2 to 3 mcg/kg/day.
Children ages 6 to 12: 4 to 5 mcg/kg/day.
Children ages 1 to 5: 5 to 6 mcg/kg/day.
Children ages 6 to 12 months: 6 to 8 mcg/kg/day.
Children under age 6 months: 8 to 10 mcg/kg/day.

Pharmacodynamics
Thyroid stimulant and replacement: Affects protein and carbohydrate metabolism, promotes gluconeogenesis, increases the use and mobilization of glycogen stores, stimulates protein synthesis, and regulates cell growth and differentiation. The major effect of liotrix is to increase the metabolic rate of tissue. It's used to treat hypothyroidism (myxedema, cretinism, and thyroid hormone deficiency).

Liotrix is a synthetic preparation combining levothyroxine sodium and liothyronine sodium in a 4 to 1 ratio by weight. Such combination products were developed because circulating T_3 was assumed to result from direct release from the thyroid gland. About 80% of T_3 is now known to be derived from deiodination of T_4 in peripheral tissues, and patients receiving only T_4 have normal serum T_3 and T_4 levels. Therefore, there is no clinical advantage to combining thyroid drugs; actually, it could result in excessive T_3 levels.

Pharmacokinetics
- *Absorption:* 50% to 95% of drug absorbed from GI tract.
- *Distribution:* Not fully understood.
- *Metabolism:* Partially in peripheral tissues (liver, kidneys, and intestines).
- *Excretion:* Excreted partially in feces.

Contraindications and precautions
Contraindicated in patients with hypersensitivity to drug and in those with acute MI uncomplicated by hypothyroidism, untreated thyrotoxicosis, or uncorrected adrenal insufficiency.

Use cautiously in elderly patients and in those with impaired renal function, ischemia, angina pectoris, hypertension, other CV disorders, myxedema, and diabetes mellitus or insipidus.

Interactions
Drug-drug. *Adrenocorticoids, corticotropin:* Altered thyroid status. Changes in liotrix dosage may also require adrenocorticoid or corticotropin dosage changes.
Anticoagulants: Altered anticoagulant effect. Monitor PT and INR; may require a lower anticoagulant dose.
Beta blockers: Decreased conversion of T_4 to T_3. Monitor patient closely.
Cholestyramine: Delayed absorption of liotrix. Separate administration times by 4 to 5 hours.
Estrogens: Increased serum thyroxine-binding globulin levels. May require increasing liotrix dosage.
Hepatic enzyme inducers (such as phenytoin): Increased hepatic degradation of T_4, resulting in increased requirements of T_4. Monitor patient closely.
Insulin, oral antidiabetics: Altered serum glucose levels. Monitor serum glucose levels. Dosage adjustment may be needed.
Somatrem: Possible accelerated epiphyseal maturation. Monitor patient.
Sympathomimetics, tricyclic antidepressants: Possible coronary insufficiency or arrhythmias. Monitor ECG.

Adverse reactions
CNS: *nervousness, insomnia, tremor,* headache.
CV: *tachycardia,* **arrhythmias,** angina pectoris, **cardiac decompensation and collapse.**
GI: diarrhea, vomiting.
GU: menstrual irregularities.
Metabolic: weight loss.
Skin: diaphoresis, allergic skin reactions.
Other: heat intolerance, accelerated rate of bone maturation in infants and children.

☑ Special considerations
Besides the recommendations relevant to all thyroid hormones, consider the following.
- T_4 is drug of choice for hypothyroidism. Hepatic conversion of T_4 to T_3 is usually adequate. Excessive exogenous supplementation of T_3 is usually associated with toxicity.
- The two commercially prepared liotrix brands contain different amounts of each ingredient; don't switch brands without considering differences in potency.
- Liotrix therapy alters radioactive iodine (^{131}I) thyroid uptake, protein-bound iodine levels, and T_3 uptake.
- Evidence of overdose includes signs and symptoms of hyperthyroidism. Treatment requires reduction of GI absorption and efforts to counteract central and peripheral effects, primarily sympathetic activity. Thyroid therapy should be withdrawn gradually over 2 to 6 days, then resumed at a lower dosage.
- Protect drug from heat and moisture.

Monitoring the patient
● Monitor patient's pulse rate and blood pressure.
● Monitor ECG closely.

Information for the patient
● Tell patient to report headache, diarrhea, nervousness, excessive sweating, heat intolerance, chest pain, increased pulse rate, or palpitations.
● Advise patient not to store liotrix in warm and humid areas, such as the bathroom.
● Encourage patient to take a single daily dose in the morning to avoid insomnia.

Geriatric patients
● Elderly patients are more sensitive to drug's effects and may need a lower dosage.

Pediatric patients
● Partial hair loss may occur during first few months of therapy. Reassure child and parents that this is temporary.
● Infants and children may experience accelerated rate of bone maturation.

Breast-feeding patients
● Minimal amounts of drug appear in breast milk. Use with caution in breast-feeding women.

lisinopril
Prinivil, Zestril

Pharmacologic classification: ACE inhibitor
Therapeutic classification: antihypertensive
Pregnancy risk category C (D in second and third trimesters)

How supplied
Available by prescription only
Tablets: 2.5 mg, 5 mg, 10 mg, 20 mg, 40 mg

Indications, route, and dosage
Mild to severe hypertension
Adults: Initially, 10 mg P.O. daily. Most patients are well-controlled on 20 to 40 mg daily as a single dose. Doses up to 80 mg have been used.
Heart failure
Adults: Initially, 5 mg P.O. daily. Most patients are well-controlled on 5 to 20 mg daily as a single dose.
Acute MI
Adults: Initially, 5 mg P.O.; then give 5 mg after 24 hours, 10 mg after 48 hours, and 10 mg daily for 6 weeks.
   In patients with acute MI with low systolic blood pressure (below 120 mm Hg), give 2.5 mg P.O. when treatment is started or during the first 3 days after an infarct. If hypotension occurs, a daily maintenance dose of 5 mg may be given with temporary reductions to 2.5 mg if needed.

✦ *Dosage adjustment.* In adults with renal failure, initially, 5 mg/day P.O. if creatinine clearance is between 10 and 30 ml/minute, and 2.5 mg/day P.O. if it's less than 10 ml/minute. Dosage may be adjusted upward until blood pressure is controlled or to maximum of 40 mg daily. Dosage for patients with heart failure who have a creatinine clearance below 30 ml/minute is 2.5 mg/day P.O.

Pharmacodynamics
Antihypertensive action: Inhibits ACE, preventing the conversion of angiotensin I to angiotensin II, a potent vasoconstrictor. Reduced formation of angiotensin II decreases peripheral arterial resistance and aldosterone secretion, thereby reducing sodium and water retention and blood pressure.

Pharmacokinetics
● *Absorption:* Variable absorption after oral administration; average of about 25% of oral dose absorbed by test subjects. Serum levels peak in about 7 hours. Onset of antihypertensive activity occurs in about 1 hour; peaks in about 6 hours.
● *Distribution:* Distributed widely in tissues. Insignificant plasma protein-binding; minimal amounts enter brain. Preclinical studies indicate drug crosses placenta.
● *Metabolism:* Not metabolized.
● *Excretion:* Excreted unchanged in urine.

Contraindications and precautions
Contraindicated in patients with hypersensitivity to ACE inhibitors, in those with history of angioedema related to previous treatment with ACE inhibitor, and in women during the second and third trimester of pregnancy. Use cautiously in patients at risk for hyperkalemia and in those with impaired renal function.

Interactions
Drug-drug. *Diuretics:* Excessive hypotension. Monitor blood pressure.
Indomethacin: May attenuate hypotensive effect of lisinopril. Monitor blood pressure.
Lithium: May increase plasma lithium levels. Monitor serum lithium levels.
Potassium-sparing diuretics, potassium supplements: Possible hyperkalemia. Monitor serum potassium levels.
Drug-food. *Potassium-containing salt substitutes:* Possible hyperkalemia. Monitor serum potassium levels.

Adverse reactions
CNS: *dizziness, headache, fatigue, paresthesia.*
CV: hypotension, *orthostatic hypotension,* chest pain.
EENT: *nasal congestion.*
GI: *diarrhea,* nausea, dyspepsia.
GU: impotence.

Reactions may be *common,* uncommon, **life-threatening,** or COMMON AND LIFE-THREATENING.

Hematologic: *neutropenia, agranulocytopenia.*
Metabolic: hyperkalemia.
Respiratory: *dry, persistent, tickling, nonproductive cough;* dyspnea.
Skin: rash.
Other: *angioedema, anaphylaxis.*

☑ Special considerations
Besides the recommendations relevant to all ACE inhibitors, consider the following.
• Drug absorption is unaffected by food.
• Stop diuretics 2 to 3 days before lisinopril therapy to reduce risk of hypotension.
• If drug doesn't adequately control blood pressure, diuretics may be added.
• Lower dosage is necessary in patients with impaired renal function.
• Beneficial effects of lisinopril may require several weeks of therapy.
• The most likely sign of overdose is hypotension.

Monitoring the patient
• Monitor vital signs closely, especially blood pressure.
• Review WBC and differential counts before treatment, every 2 weeks for 3 months, and then periodically.

Information for the patient
• Tell patient to report light-headedness, especially in first few days of treatment, so dose can be adjusted; signs of infection such as sore throat or fever because drug may decrease WBC count; facial swelling or difficulty breathing because drug may cause angioedema; and loss of taste, which may require stopping drug.
• Advise patient to avoid sudden postural changes to minimize orthostatic hypotension.
• Warn patient to seek medical approval before taking OTC cold preparations.
• Instruct patient to avoid potassium-containing salt substitutes.
• Instruct patient to report any adverse events, including persistent dry cough.
• Warn patient of childbearing age to avoid pregnancy during therapy.

Geriatric patients
• Elderly patients may require lower doses because of impaired drug clearance. They also may be more sensitive to drug's hypotensive effects.

Pediatric patients
• Safety and efficacy in children haven't been established; use only if potential benefits outweigh risks.

Breast-feeding patients
• Drug may appear in breast milk; effect on infant is unknown. Use with caution in breast-feeding women.

lithium carbonate
Carbolith*, Duralith*, Eskalith, Eskalith CR, Lithane, Lithizine*, Lithobid, Lithonate, Lithotabs

lithium citrate
Cibalith-S

Pharmacologic classification: alkali metal
Therapeutic classification: antimanic, antipsychotic
Pregnancy risk category D

How supplied
Available by prescription only
lithium carbonate
Capsules: 150 mg, 300 mg, 600 mg
Tablets: 300 mg
Tablets (sustained-release): 300 mg, 450 mg
lithium citrate
Syrup (sugarless): 300 mg/5 ml (with 0.3% alcohol)

Indications, route, and dosage
Prevention or control of mania, prevention of depression in patients with bipolar illness
Adults: Acute and maintenance dose, 900 mg (sustained-release tablet) P.O. in morning and h.s., or 600 mg (tablet or capsule) in the morning, noon, and h.s.
◇ *Major depression,* ◇ *schizoaffective disorder,* ◇ *schizophrenic disorder,* ◇ *alcohol dependence*
Adults: 300 mg lithium carbonate P.O. t.i.d. or q.i.d.
◇ *Apparent mixed bipolar disorder in children*
Children: Initially, 15 to 60 mg/kg or 0.5 to 1.5 g/m² lithium carbonate P.O. daily in three divided doses. Don't exceed usual adult dosage. Adjust dosage based on patient response and serum lithium levels; usual dosage range is 150 to 300 mg daily in divided doses.
◇ *Chemotherapy-induced neutropenia in children and patients with AIDS receiving zidovudine*
Adults and children: 300 to 1,000 mg P.O. daily.

Pharmacodynamics
Antimanic action: Thought to exert antipsychotic and antimanic effects by competing with other cations for exchange at the sodium-potassium ion pump, thus altering cation exchange at the tissue level. Also inhibits adenyl cyclase, reducing intracellular levels of cAMP and, to a lesser extent, cyclic guanosine monophosphate.

Pharmacokinetics
• *Absorption:* Rate and extent of absorption vary with dosage form; absorption is complete within

6 hours of oral administration from conventional tablets and capsules.
• *Distribution:* Distributed widely into body, including breast milk; levels in thyroid gland, bone, and brain tissue exceed serum levels. Effects peak at 30 minutes to 3 hours; liquid peaks at 15 minutes to 1 hour. Steady-state serum level achieved in 12 hours; therapeutic effect begins in 5 to 10 days and is maximal within 3 weeks. Therapeutic and toxic serum levels and therapeutic effects show good correlation. Therapeutic range is 0.6 to 1.2 mEq/L; adverse reactions increase as level reaches 1.5 to 2 mEq/L—such levels may be necessary in acute mania. Toxicity usually occurs at levels above 2 mEq/L.
• *Metabolism:* Not metabolized.
• *Excretion:* Excreted 95% unchanged in urine; about 50% to 80% of dose excreted within 24 hours. Level of renal function determines elimination rate.

Contraindications and precautions
Contraindicated if therapy can't be closely monitored and during pregnancy. Use cautiously in elderly patients; in patients with thyroid disease, seizure disorders, renal or CV disease, severe dehydration or debilitation, or sodium depletion; and in those receiving neuroleptics, neuromuscular blockers, or diuretics.

Interactions
Drug-drug. *Antacids, drugs containing aminophylline, caffeine, calcium, sodium, theophylline:* Increased lithium excretion. Monitor serum lithium levels; monitor patient for lack of drug effectiveness.
Carbamazepine, mazindol, methyldopa, phenytoin, tetracyclines: Increased lithium toxicity. Monitor serum lithium levels.
Chlorpromazine: Decreased effects of chlorpromazine. Monitor patient.
Electroconvulsive therapy (ECT): Acute neurotoxicity with delirium in patients receiving concurrent therapy. Reduce or withdraw lithium dosage before ECT.
Fluoxetine: Increased serum lithium levels. Watch for toxicity.
Haloperidol: Possible severe encephalopathy. Use together cautiously.
Indomethacin, phenylbutazone, piroxicam, other NSAIDs: Decreased renal excretion of lithium. Monitor levels closely; may need 30% reduction in lithium dosage.
Neuromuscular blockers: May potentiate effects of these drugs. Monitor patient closely.
Sympathomimetics (such as norepinephrine): Lithium may interfere with pressor effects of these drugs. Monitor patient.
Thiazide diuretics: Decreased renal excretion; enhanced lithium toxicity. Monitor levels closely; diuretic dosage may need to be reduced by 30%.

Drug-herb. *Parsley:* May promote or produce serotonin syndrome. Advise patient to avoid use.
Psyllium seed: Inhibited GI absorption. Advise patient to avoid use.
Drug-food. *Caffeine:* Interferes with drug's effectiveness. Advise patient to avoid large amounts of caffeine.
Dietary sodium: Altered renal elimination of lithium. Monitor patient closely.

Adverse reactions
CNS: tremors, drowsiness, headache, confusion, restlessness, dizziness, psychomotor retardation, lethargy, *coma*, blackouts, *epileptiform seizures*, EEG changes, worsened organic mental syndrome, impaired speech, ataxia, muscle weakness, incoordination.
CV: *reversible ECG changes, arrhythmias*, hypotension, *bradycardia.*
EENT: tinnitus, blurred vision.
GI: dry mouth, metallic taste, nausea, vomiting, anorexia, diarrhea, *thirst*, abdominal pain, flatulence, indigestion.
GU: *polyuria*, glycosuria, *renal toxicity* with long-term use, decreased creatinine clearance, albuminuria.
Hematologic: *leukocytosis with WBC count of 14,000 to 18,000/mm³ (reversible)*, elevated neutrophil count.
Metabolic: goiter, transient hyperglycemia, hypothyroidism (lowered T_3, T_4, and protein-bound iodine, but elevated ^{131}I uptake), hyponatremia.
Skin: pruritus, rash, diminished or absent sensation, drying and thinning of hair, psoriasis, acne, alopecia.
Other: ankle and wrist edema.

☑ Special considerations
• Death has occurred in patients ingesting 10 to 60 g of lithium.
• Serum lithium levels above 3.4 mEq/L are potentially fatal.
• Determination of serum drug levels is crucial to safe use of drug. Don't use drug in patients who can't have regular serum drug level checks. Be sure patient or responsible family member can comply with instructions.
• When lithium blood levels are below 1.5 mEq/L, adverse reactions usually remain mild.
• Shake syrup formulation before administration.
• Administer drug with food or milk to reduce GI upset.
• Lithium has been used for investigational purposes to increase WBC count in patients undergoing cancer chemotherapy. Has also been used for investigational purposes to treat cluster headaches, aggression, organic brain syndrome, and tardive dyskinesia. Drug has been used to treat SIADH.
• Lithane tablets contain tartrazine, a dye that may precipitate an allergic reaction in certain individuals, particularly asthmatics sensitive to aspirin.

Reactions may be *common*, uncommon, *life-threatening*, or COMMON AND LIFE-THREATENING.

- Adjust fluid and salt ingestion to compensate if excessive loss occurs through protracted sweating or diarrhea. Patient should have fluid intake of 2,500 to 3,000 ml daily and a balanced diet with adequate salt intake.
- Arrange for outpatient follow-up of thyroid and renal functions every 6 to 12 months. Thyroid should be palpated to check for enlargement.
- Expect lag of 1 to 3 weeks before drug's beneficial effects are noticed. Other psychotropics (such as chlorpromazine) may be needed during interim period.
- Drug causes false-positive test results on thyroid function tests.
- Signs and symptoms of overdose (sedation, confusion, joint tremors) may progress to coma, movement abnormalities, tremors, seizures, and CV collapse. Vomiting and diarrhea occur within 1 hour of acute ingestion.

Monitoring the patient
- Monitor baseline ECG, thyroid and renal studies, and electrolyte levels. Monitor lithium blood levels 8 to 12 hours after first dose, usually before morning dose, two or three times weekly the first month, then weekly to monthly on maintenance therapy.
- Monitor fluid intake and output, especially when surgery is scheduled.
- Watch for signs of edema or sudden weight gain.
- Check urine for specific gravity level below 1.015, which may indicate diabetes insipidus.
- Drug may alter glucose tolerance in diabetic patients. Monitor blood glucose levels closely.
- Monitor serum levels and watch for signs of impending toxicity.
- Monitor drug dosing carefully when patient's initial manic symptoms begin to subside because the ability to tolerate high serum lithium levels decreases as symptoms resolve.
- EEG changes include diffuse slowing, widening of frequency spectrum, potentiation, and disorganization of background rhythm.

Information for the patient
- Explain that lithium has a narrow therapeutic margin of safety. A serum drug level that is even slightly high can be dangerous.
- Warn patient and family to watch for signs and symptoms of toxicity (diarrhea, vomiting, dehydration, drowsiness, muscle weakness, tremor, fever, and ataxia) and to expect transient nausea, polyuria, thirst, and discomfort during first few days. If toxic symptoms occur, tell patient to withhold one dose and call promptly.
- Warn patient to avoid activities that require alertness and good psychomotor coordination until CNS response to drug is determined.
- Advise patient to maintain adequate water intake and adequate (but not excessive) salt in diet.

- Explain importance of regular follow-up visits to measure serum lithium levels.
- Advise patient to call before initiating weight-loss program.
- Tell patient not to switch brands of lithium or take other prescription or OTC drugs without medical approval. Different brands may not provide equivalent effect.
- Warn patient against stopping drug abruptly.
- Tell patient to explain to close friend or family members signs and symptoms of lithium overdose in case emergency aid is needed.
- Instruct patient to carry medical identification and instruction card with toxicity and emergency information.

Geriatric patients
- Elderly patients are more susceptible to long-term overdose and toxic effects, especially dyskinesias. These patients usually respond to a lower dosage.

Pediatric patients
- Drug isn't recommended for use in children under age 12.

Breast-feeding patients
- Lithium level in breast milk is 33% to 50% that of maternal serum level. Avoid breast-feeding during therapy.

lomefloxacin hydrochloride
Maxaquin

Pharmacologic classification: fluoroquinolone
Therapeutic classification: broad-spectrum antibiotic
Pregnancy risk category C

How supplied
Available by prescription only
Tablets: 400 mg

Indications, route, and dosage
Acute bacterial exacerbations of chronic bronchitis caused by Haemophilus influenzae *or* Moraxella (Branhamella) catarrhalis
Adults: 400 mg P.O. daily for 10 days.
Uncomplicated urinary tract infections (cystitis) caused by Escherichia coli, Klebsiella pneumoniae, Proteus mirabilis, *or* Staphylococcus saprophyticus
Adults: 400 mg P.O. daily for 10 days.
Complicated urinary tract infections caused by E. coli, K. pneumoniae, P. mirabilis, *or* Pseudomonas aeruginosa; *possibly effective against infections caused by* Citrobacter diversus *or* Enterobacter cloacae
Adults: 400 mg P.O. daily for 14 days.

Prophylaxis of infections after transurethral surgical procedures
Adults: 400 mg P.O. 2 to 6 hours before surgery as a single dose.
✦ Dosage adjustment. In adults with renal failure and creatinine clearance of 10 to 40 ml/minute/1.73 m², give loading dose of 400 mg P.O. on first day, then 200 mg P.O. daily for duration of therapy. Periodic determination of blood drug levels is recommended. Hemodialysis removes negligible amounts of drug.

Pharmacodynamics
Antibiotic action: Bactericidal. Inhibits bacterial DNA gyrase, an enzyme necessary for bacterial replication.

Pharmacokinetics
● *Absorption:* Rapidly absorbed from GI tract; absolute bioavailability is 95% to 98%. Food reduces total amount absorbed and slows absorption rate.
● *Distribution:* Only 10% is bound to plasma proteins.
● *Metabolism:* About 10% is metabolized in liver.
● *Excretion:* Mostly excreted unchanged in urine; about 10% excreted as metabolites. Solubility in urine is pH dependent. About 10% of a dose appears unchanged in feces. Half-life is 8 hours; steady-state is reached after 2 days of once-daily therapy.

Contraindications and precautions
Contraindicated in patients with hypersensitivity to drug or other fluoroquinolones. Use cautiously in patients with known or suspected CNS disorders, such as seizures or cerebral arteriosclerosis.

Interactions
Drug-drug. *Antacids, sucralfate:* Bind with lomefloxacin in GI tract and impair its absorption. Administer no less than 4 hours before or 2 hours after a dose.
Cimetidine, other quinolones: Substantially increased plasma half-lives. Lomefloxacin hasn't been tested for these effects, however. Monitor patient for signs of toxicity.
NSAIDs: Possible increased CNS effects, including seizures. Observe patient for CNS effect.
Probenecid: Decreased excretion of lomefloxacin. Observe for signs of overdose.
Drug-lifestyle. *Sun exposure:* Photosensitivity reactions. Tell patient to take precautions.

Adverse reactions
CNS: *dizziness, headache,* abnormal dreams, fatigue, malaise, asthenia, agitation, anorexia, anxiety, confusion, depersonalization, depression, increased appetite, insomnia, nervousness, somnolence, **seizures, coma,** hyperkinesia, tremor, vertigo, paresthesia.

CV: flushing, hypotension, hypertension, edema, syncope, **arrhythmias,** tachycardia, **bradycardia,** extrasystoles, cyanosis, angina pectoris, **MI, cardiac failure, pulmonary embolism,** cerebrovascular disorder, cardiomyopathy, phlebitis.
EENT: epistaxis, abnormal vision, conjunctivitis, eye pain, earache, tinnitus, tongue discoloration, taste perversion.
GI: *diarrhea, nausea,* thirst, dry mouth, pseudomembranous colitis, abdominal pain, dyspepsia, vomiting, flatulence, constipation, inflammation, dysphagia, bleeding.
GU: dysuria, hematuria, anuria, leukorrhea, epididymitis, orchitis, vaginitis, vaginal moniliasis, intermenstrual bleeding, perineal pain.
Hematologic: thrombocythemia, ***thrombocytopenia,*** lymphadenopathy, increased fibrinolysis.
Hepatic: elevated liver enzyme levels.
Metabolic: hypoglycemia.
Musculoskeletal: leg cramps, arthralgia, myalgia.
Respiratory: dyspnea, **bronchospasm,** respiratory disorder or infection, increased sputum, stridor.
Skin: pruritus, skin disorder, skin exfoliation, eczema, increased diaphoresis, rash, urticaria, *photosensitivity.*
Other: *anaphylaxis,* chest or back pain, chills, allergic reaction, facial edema, flulike symptoms, decreased heat tolerance, gout.

☑ Special considerations
● Drug shouldn't be used for empiric treatment of acute exacerbations of chronic bronchitis when suspected pathogen is *Streptococcus pneumoniae;* organism demonstrates resistance to drug. Because blood drug levels don't readily exceed minimum inhibitory level against *Pseudomonas aeruginosa,* drug shouldn't be used to treat bacteremia caused by this organism. Drug has been used successfully to treat complicated urinary tract *Pseudomonas* infections.
● If overdose occurs, empty stomach by induced vomiting or gastric lavage, observe patient closely, and provide supportive care. Drug isn't significantly removed by hemodialysis or peritoneal dialysis.

Monitoring the patient
● Monitor patient's response to therapy.
● Evaluate patient for adverse effects; obtain ECG and CBC as needed.

Information for the patient
● Remind patient to take all of drug prescribed, even after he feels better.
● Advise patient to take drug on empty stomach.
● Tell patient to avoid hazardous tasks that require alertness, such as driving, until adverse CNS effects of drug are known.

Reactions may be *common,* uncommon, *life-threatening,* or COMMON AND LIFE-THREATENING.

• Caution patient to avoid mineral supplements or vitamins with iron or minerals within 2 hours before or after taking drug.
• Tell patient that sucralfate or antacids containing magnesium or aluminum shouldn't be taken within 4 hours before or 2 hours after taking drug.
• Instruct patient to drink plenty of fluids.

Pediatric patients
• Because studies have shown that quinolones can cause arthropathy, these drugs should be avoided in children.

Breast-feeding patients
• It's unknown if drug appears in breast milk. Because of risk of serious adverse effects on infant, stop either drug or breast-feeding.

lomustine (CCNU)
CeeNU

Pharmacologic classification: alkylating drug, nitrosourea (cell cycle–phase nonspecific)
Therapeutic classification: antineoplastic
Pregnancy risk category D

How supplied
Available by prescription only
Capsules: 10 mg, 40 mg, 100 mg

Indications, route, and dosage
Dosage and indications may vary. Check current literature for recommended protocol. Wait at least 6 weeks between repeat courses.
Brain, colon, lung, and renal cell cancer; Hodgkin's disease; lymphomas; melanomas; multiple myeloma
Adults and children: 100 to 130 mg/m² P.O. as single dose q 6 weeks.
✦ *Dosage adjustment.* Reduce dose according to bone marrow depression using the following guidelines: Repeat doses shouldn't be given until WBC count is more than 4,000/mm³ and platelet count is more than 100,000/mm³. Hematologic toxicity is delayed and cumulative; don't give repeat courses before 6 weeks.

Nadir after prior dose		Percentage of prior dose to be given
WBCs/mm³	Platelets/mm³	
> 4,000	100,000	100%
3,000 to 3,999	75,000 to 99,999	100%
2,000 to 2,999	25,000 to 74,999	70%
< 2,000	< 25,000	50%

Pharmacodynamics
Antineoplastic action: Exerts cytotoxic activity through alkylation, resulting in the inhibition of DNA and RNA synthesis. As with other nitrosourea compounds, lomustine is known to modify cellular proteins and alkylate proteins, resulting in an inhibition of protein synthesis. Cross-resistance exists between lomustine and carmustine.

Pharmacokinetics
• *Absorption:* Rapidly and well absorbed across GI tract after oral administration.
• *Distribution:* Distributed widely into body tissues. Because of its high lipid solubility, drug and metabolites cross blood-brain barrier to a significant extent.
• *Metabolism:* Metabolized rapidly and extensively in liver. Some metabolites have cytotoxic activity.
• *Excretion:* Metabolites excreted primarily in urine, with smaller amounts excreted in feces and through lungs. Biphasic plasma elimination; initial phase half-life of 6 hours and terminal phase of 1 to 2 days. Extended half-life of terminal phase thought to be caused by enterohepatic circulation and protein-binding.

Contraindications and precautions
Contraindicated in patients with hypersensitivity to drug. Use cautiously in patients with decreased platelet, WBC, or RBC counts and in those receiving other myelosuppressants.

Interactions
Drug-drug. *Anticoagulants, aspirin:* Increased risk of bleeding. Avoid concomitant use.
Myelosuppressants: Concomitant use can cause additive myelosuppression. Monitor patient.

Adverse reactions
CNS: disorientation, lethargy, ataxia.
GI: *nausea, vomiting,* stomatitis.
GU: *nephrotoxicity,* progressive azotemia, *renal failure.*
Hematologic: *anemia, leukopenia,* delayed up to 6 weeks, lasting 1 to 2 weeks; *thrombocytopenia,* delayed up to 4 weeks, lasting 1 to 2 weeks; *bone marrow suppression,* delayed up to 6 weeks.
Hepatic: *hepatotoxicity.*
Respiratory: *pulmonary fibrosis.*
Skin: alopecia.
Other: *secondary malignant disease.*

☑ Special considerations
• Give drug 2 to 4 hours after meals. Drug is more completely absorbed if taken when stomach is empty. To avoid nausea, give antiemetic before administering.
• Anorexia may persist for 2 to 3 days after a given dose.

• Avoid all I.M. injections when platelet count is below 100,000/mm³.
• Because drug crosses blood-brain barrier, it may be used to treat primary brain tumors.
• Signs and symptoms of overdose include myelosuppression, nausea, and vomiting. Treatment is usually supportive and includes antiemetics and transfusion of blood components.

Monitoring the patient
• Dose modification may be required in patients with decreased platelet, WBC, or RBC count.
• Monitor CBC weekly. Drug usually isn't administered more often than every 6 weeks; bone marrow toxicity is cumulative and delayed.
• Frequently assess renal and hepatic status.

Information for the patient
• Emphasize importance of continuing drug despite nausea and vomiting.
• Emphasize importance of taking exact dose.
• Tell patient to call immediately if vomiting occurs shortly after dose is taken.
• Advise patient to avoid exposure to people with infections.
• Caution patient to avoid alcoholic beverages for a short period after taking drug.
• Tell patient to promptly report sore throat, fever, or unusual bruising or bleeding.
• Advise patient to use effective contraceptive measures during therapy.

Breast-feeding patients
• Metabolites of lomustine appear in breast milk. Because of increased risk of serious adverse reactions, mutagenicity, and carcinogenicity in infant, breast-feeding should be discontinued during therapy.

---

loperamide hydrochloride
Imodium, Imodium A-D, Kaopectate II, Maalox Anti-Diarrheal, Pepto Diarrhea Control

Pharmacologic classification: piperidine derivative
Therapeutic classification: antidiarrheal
Pregnancy risk category B

How supplied
Available by prescription only
Capsules: 2 mg
Available without a prescription
Tablets: 2 mg
Solution: 1 mg/5 ml

Indications, route, and dosage
Acute, nonspecific diarrhea
Adults and children over age 12: Initially, 4 mg P.O., then 2 mg after each unformed stool. Maximum dose, 16 mg daily.

Children ages 9 to 11: 2 mg t.i.d. on first day.
Children ages 6 to 8: 2 mg b.i.d. on first day.
Children ages 2 to 5: 1 mg t.i.d. on first day.
Maintenance dose is one-third to one-half the initial dose.
Chronic diarrhea
Adults: Initially, 4 mg P.O., then 2 mg after each unformed stool until diarrhea subsides. Adjust dose to individual response.
Directions for patient self-medication
Adults: 4 teaspoons or 2 tablets after the first loose bowel movement, then 2 teaspoons or 1 tablet after each subsequent loose bowel movement. Don't exceed 8 teaspoons or 4 tablets daily.
Children ages 9 to 11 (27 to 43 kg [60 to 95 lb]): 2 teaspoons or 1 tablet after first loose bowel movement, then 1 teaspoon or ½ tablet after each subsequent loose bowel movement. Don't exceed 6 teaspoons or 3 tablets daily.
Children ages 6 to 8 (22 to 27 kg [48 to 59 lb]): 2 teaspoons or 1 tablet after first loose bowel movement, then 1 teaspoon or ½ tablet after each subsequent loose bowel movement. Don't exceed 4 teaspoons or 2 tablets daily.
Children ages 2 to 5 (11 to 21 kg [24 to 47 lb]): 1 teaspoon after first loose bowel movement, then 1 teaspoon after each subsequent loose bowel movement. Don't exceed 3 teaspoons daily.

Pharmacodynamics
Antidiarrheal action: Reduces intestinal motility by acting directly on intestinal mucosal nerve endings; tolerance to antiperistaltic effect doesn't develop. Also may inhibit fluid and electrolyte secretion by an unknown mechanism. Although chemically related to opiates, drug hasn't shown any physical dependence characteristics, and possesses no analgesic activity.

Pharmacokinetics
• *Absorption:* Absorbed poorly from GI tract.
• *Distribution:* Distribution not well characterized.
• *Metabolism:* Absorbed drug metabolized in liver.
• *Excretion:* Excreted primarily in feces; less than 2% excreted in urine.

Contraindications and precautions
Contraindicated in patients with hypersensitivity to drug, in children under age 2, and when constipation must be avoided. OTC use is contraindicated in patients with a temperature exceeding 101° F (38.3° C) or if blood is present in the stool. Use cautiously in patients with hepatic impairment.

Interactions
Drug-drug. *Opioid analgesics:* Possible severe constipation. Avoid concomitant use.

Adverse reactions
CNS: drowsiness, fatigue, dizziness.

Reactions may be *common*, uncommon, **life-threatening**, or COMMON AND LIFE-THREATENING.

GI: dry mouth; abdominal pain, distention, or discomfort; *constipation;* nausea; vomiting.
Skin: rash, *hypersensitivity reactions.*

☑ **Special considerations**
● After administration via nasogastric tube, flush tube to clear it and ensure drug's passage to stomach.
● Signs and symptoms of overdose include constipation, GI irritation, and CNS depression. Treat overdose with activated charcoal if ingestion was recent. If patient is vomiting, activated charcoal may be given in a slurry when patient can retain fluids. Or perform gastric lavage; then give activated charcoal slurry.
● Observe for CNS depression; treat respiratory depression with naloxone.

Monitoring the patient
● Monitor patient's response to drug therapy.
● Monitor intake and output.

Information for the patient
● Warn patient to take drug only as directed and not to exceed recommended dose.
● Caution patient to avoid driving and other tasks requiring alertness because drug may cause drowsiness and dizziness.
● Instruct patient to call if no improvement occurs in 48 hours or if fever develops.

Pediatric patients
● Drug is approved for use in children ages 2 and older; however, children may be more susceptible to adverse CNS effects.

Breast-feeding patients
● It's unknown if drug appears in breast milk. Use with caution in breast-feeding women.

loracarbef
Lorabid

Pharmacologic classification: synthetic beta-lactam antibiotic of carbacephem class
Therapeutic classification: antibiotic
Pregnancy risk category B

How supplied
Available by prescription only
Pulvules: 200 mg, 400 mg
Powder for oral suspension: 100 mg/5 ml, 200 mg/5 ml

Indications, route, and dosage
Secondary bacterial infections of acute bronchitis
Adults: 200 to 400 mg P.O. q 12 hours for 7 days.

Acute bacterial exacerbations of chronic bronchitis
Adults: 400 mg P.O. q 12 hours for 7 days.
Pneumonia
Adults: 400 mg P.O. q 12 hours for 14 days.
Pharyngitis, tonsillitis
Adults: 200 mg P.O. q 12 hours for 10 days.
Children ages 6 months to 12 years: 15 mg/kg P.O. daily in divided doses q 12 hours for 10 days.
Sinusitis
Adults: 400 mg P.O. q 12 hours for 10 days.
Acute otitis media
Children: 30 mg/kg (oral suspension) P.O. daily in divided doses q 12 hours for 10 days.
Uncomplicated skin and skin-structure infections
Adults: 200 mg P.O. q 12 hours for 7 days.
Impetigo
Children: 15 mg/kg P.O. daily in divided doses q 12 hours for 7 days.
Uncomplicated cystitis
Adults: 200 mg P.O. daily for 7 days.
Uncomplicated pyelonephritis
Adults: 400 mg P.O. q 12 hours for 14 days.
✦ **Dosage adjustment.** Adults and children with renal failure and creatinine clearance of 50 ml/minute or more don't require dose and interval changes. In patients with creatinine clearance of 10 to 49 ml/minute, give half usual dose at same interval or normal recommended dose at twice the usual dosage interval; in those with creatinine clearance below 10 ml/minute, give usual dose q 3 to 5 days. Hemodialysis patients should be given another dose after dialysis.

Pharmacodynamics
Antibiotic action: Exerts bactericidal action by binding to essential target proteins of the bacterial cell wall, leading to inhibition of cell-wall synthesis. Active against gram-positive aerobes, such as *Staphylococcus aureus, S. saprophyticus, Streptococcus pneumoniae,* and *S. pyogenes,* and gram-negative aerobes, such as *Escherichia coli, Haemophilus influenzae,* and *Moraxella (Branhamella) catarrhalis.*

Pharmacokinetics
● *Absorption:* After oral administration, about 90% absorbed from GI tract. When pulvules are taken with food, peak plasma levels are 50% to 60% of those achieved on empty stomach. (Effect of food on rate and extent of absorption of suspension form hasn't been studied to date.) Absorption of suspension form is greater than that of pulvule. Plasma levels of pulvule form peak in about 1¼ hours; those of suspension form peak in about ¾ hour.
● *Distribution:* About 25% of circulating drug bound to plasma proteins.
● *Metabolism:* Doesn't appear to be metabolized.

• *Excretion:* Eliminated primarily in urine. Elimination half-life in patients with normal renal function averages 1 hour.

Contraindications and precautions
Contraindicated in patients with hypersensitivity to drug or other cephalosporins and in patients with diarrhea caused by pseudomembranous colitis. Use cautiously in pregnant and breast-feeding women.

Interactions
Drug-drug. *Probenecid:* Decreased excretion of loracarbef, causing increased plasma levels. Monitor patient for toxicity.
Drug-food. *Any food:* Decreased absorption. Have patient take drug on empty stomach at least 1 hour before or 2 hours after a meal.

Adverse reactions
CNS: headache, somnolence, nervousness, insomnia, dizziness.
CV: vasodilation.
GI: diarrhea, nausea, vomiting, abdominal pain, anorexia, *pseudomembranous colitis.*
GU: vaginal candidiasis, transient increases in BUN and creatinine levels.
Hematologic: *transient thrombocytopenia, leukopenia,* eosinophilia, *neutropenia.*
Hepatic: transient elevations in AST, ALT, and alkaline phosphatase levels.
Skin: rash, urticaria, pruritus, *erythema multiforme.*
Other: *hypersensitivity reactions,* including *anaphylaxis.*

☑ Special considerations
• Consider increased rate of absorption if oral suspension is to be substituted for pulvule. Pulvules shouldn't be substituted for oral suspension when treating otitis media.
• Pseudomembranous colitis has been reported with nearly all antibacterial drugs and may range from mild to life-threatening. Therefore, diagnosis must be considered in patients who have diarrhea after drug administration.
• Obtain specimen for culture and sensitivity tests before giving first dose. Therapy may begin pending test results.
• Drug may cause overgrowth of nonsusceptible bacteria or fungi. Watch for signs and symptoms of superinfection.
• To reconstitute powder for oral suspension, add 30 ml of water in two portions to the 50-ml bottle or 60 ml of water in two portions to the 100-ml bottle; shake after each addition.
• After reconstitution, oral suspension is stable for 14 days at room temperature (59° to 86° F [15° to 30° C]).
• Drug can cause positive direct Coombs' test.

• Hemodialysis is effective in hastening elimination of loracarbef from plasma in patients with chronic renal failure.
• Toxic symptoms after overdose of beta-lactams (such as loracarbef) may include nausea, vomiting, epigastric distress, and diarrhea.

Monitoring the patient
• Monitor vital signs.
• Monitor patient's response to drug therapy.

Information for the patient
• Tell patient to take drug exactly as prescribed, even after he feels better.
• Inform patient that oral suspension can be stored at room temperature for 14 days. Instruct patient to discard unused portion after 14 days.

Pediatric patients
• Safety and effectiveness in infants under age 6 months haven't been established.

Breast-feeding patients
• It's unknown if drug appears in breast milk. Use with caution in breast-feeding women.

loratadine
Claritin

Pharmacologic classification: tricyclic antihistamine
Therapeutic classification: antihistamine
Pregnancy risk category B

How supplied
Available by prescription only
Tablets: 10 mg
Tablets (rapidly disintegrating): 10 mg
Syrup: 1 mg/ml

Indications, route, and dosage
Symptomatic treatment of seasonal allergic rhinitis; idiopathic chronic urticaria
Adults and children ages 6 and older: 10 mg P.O. daily.
✦ *Dosage adjustment.* In patients with liver failure or glomerular filtration rate below 30 ml/minute, adjust dose to 10 mg every other day.

Pharmacodynamics
Antihistaminic action: Long-acting tricyclic antihistamine with selective peripheral H_1-receptor antagonist activity.

Pharmacokinetics
• *Absorption:* Readily absorbed. Onset of action within 1 to 3 hours; reaches maximum at 8 to 12 hours; lasts more than 24 hours. Because peak plasma level may be delayed by 1 hour with a meal, give drug on empty stomach.

Reactions may be *common*, uncommon, *life-threatening*, or COMMON AND LIFE-THREATENING.

• *Distribution:* About 97% of drug bound to plasma protein. Doesn't readily cross blood-brain barrier.
• *Metabolism:* Extensively metabolized to active metabolite (descarboethoxyloratadine). Specific enzyme systems responsible for metabolism not identified.
• *Excretion:* About 80% of total dose equally distributed between urine and feces. Mean elimination half-life is 8.4 hours. Not eliminated by hemodialysis; not known if eliminated by peritoneal dialysis.

Contraindications and precautions
Contraindicated in patients with hypersensitivity to drug. Use cautiously in patients with hepatic impairment and in breast-feeding women.

Interactions
Drug-drug. *Cimetidine, macrolide antibiotics:* Increased loratadine plasma levels. Monitor patient closely.
Drugs known to inhibit hepatic metabolism: Definitive interactions unknown. Use together cautiously.
Drug-herb. *Licorice:* May prolong QT interval and be potentially additive. Advise patient to use together cautiously.
Drug-lifestyle. *Alcohol:* Increased CNS depression. Advise patient to use cautiously.
Sun exposure: Possible photosensitivity reactions. Tell patient to take precautions.

Adverse reactions
CNS: headache, somnolence, fatigue.
GI: dry mouth.

☑ Special considerations
• No information exists to indicate that drug abuse or dependency occurs.
• Somnolence, tachycardia, and headache have been reported with overdoses of 40 to 180 mg.
• If overdose occurs, institute symptomatic and supportive measures promptly and maintain for as long as needed. Induce emesis (ipecac syrup), except in patients with impaired consciousness; then administer activated charcoal.

Monitoring the patient
• Monitor vital signs.
• Monitor patient's response to drug therapy.

Information for the patient
• Instruct patient to take drug on empty stomach at least 2 hours after a meal and to avoid eating for at least 1 hour after taking drug.
• Tell patient to take drug only once daily. Tell him to call if symptoms persist or worsen.
• Warn patient to stop taking drug 4 days before allergy skin tests to preserve accuracy of tests.

Pediatric patients
• Safety and effectiveness in children under age 6 haven't been established.

Breast-feeding patients
• Drug appears in breast milk. Antihistamine therapy is contraindicated in breast-feeding women.

lorazepam
Apo-Lorazepam*, Ativan, Novo-Lorazem*

Pharmacologic classification: benzodiazepine
Therapeutic classification: anxiolytic, sedative-hypnotic
Controlled substance schedule IV
Pregnancy risk category D

How supplied
Available by prescription only
Tablets: 0.5 mg, 1 mg, 2 mg
Tablets (S.L.):* 1 mg, 2 mg
Injection: 2 mg/ml, 4 mg/ml

Indications, route, and dosage
Anxiety, tension, agitation, irritability, especially in anxiety neuroses or organic (especially GI or CV) disorders
Adults: 2 to 6 mg P.O. daily in divided doses; maximum dose 10 mg/day. Take largest dose h.s.
Insomnia
Adults: 2 to 4 mg P.O. h.s.
Preoperatively
Adults: 0.05 mg/kg I.M. 2 hours before surgery (maximum 4 mg). Or 0.044 mg/kg (maximum total dose 2 mg) I.V. 15 to 20 minutes before surgery; in adults below age 50, dosage may be increased to 0.05 mg/kg (maximum 4 mg) when increased lack of recall of preoperative events is desired.

Pharmacodynamics
Anxiolytic and sedative actions: Depresses the CNS at the limbic and subcortical levels of the brain. Produces an antianxiety effect by influencing the effect of the neurotransmitter gamma-aminobutyric acid on its receptor in the ascending reticular activating system, which increases inhibition and blocks both cortical and limbic arousal after stimulation of the reticular formation.

Pharmacokinetics
• *Absorption:* When administered orally, is well absorbed through GI tract. Levels peak in 2 hours.
• *Distribution:* Distributed widely throughout body. About 85% protein-bound.
• *Metabolism:* Metabolized in liver to inactive metabolites.
• *Excretion:* Metabolites excreted in urine as glucuronide conjugates.

Contraindications and precautions

Contraindicated in patients with hypersensitivity to drug or other benzodiazepines or its vehicle (used in parenteral dosage form) and in those with acute angle-closure glaucoma.

Use cautiously in patients with pulmonary, renal, or hepatic impairment and in elderly, acutely ill, or debilitated patients. Don't use in pregnant patients, especially during the first trimester.

Interactions

Drug-drug. *Antidepressants, antihistamines, barbiturates, general anesthetics, MAO inhibitors, narcotics, phenothiazines:* Lorazepam potentiates CNS depressant effects of these drugs. Avoid concomitant use.

Cimetidine, disulfiram: Diminished hepatic metabolism of lorazepam, which increases its plasma level. Monitor patient closely.

Scopolamine: Increased occurrence of hallucinations, irrational behavior, and increased sedation. Avoid concomitant use.

Drug-food. *Caffeine:* May interfere with drug's effectiveness. Tell patient to avoid products that contain large amounts of caffeine.

Drug-lifestyle. *Alcohol:* Lorazepam potentiates CNS depressant effects of alcohol. Discourage use.

Heavy smoking: Accelerates lorazepam's metabolism, thus lowering clinical effectiveness. Discourage use.

Adverse reactions

CNS: *drowsiness,* amnesia, insomnia, agitation, *sedation,* dizziness, weakness, unsteadiness, disorientation, depression, headache.

EENT: visual disturbances.

GI: abdominal discomfort, nausea, change in appetite.

Other: *acute withdrawal syndrome* (after sudden discontinuation in physically dependent persons).

☑ Special considerations

Besides the recommendations relevant to all benzodiazepines, consider the following.

● Arteriospasm may result from intra-arterial injection of lorazepam. Don't administer by this route.

● Lorazepam is one of the preferred benzodiazepines for patients with hepatic disease.

● Use lowest possible effective dose to avoid oversedation.

● Parenteral lorazepam appears to possess potent amnesic effects.

● For I.V. administration, dilute lorazepam with an equal volume of a compatible diluent, such as D_5W, sterile water for injection, or normal saline solution.

● Drug may be injected directly into vein or into tubing of a compatible I.V. infusion, such as normal saline solution or D_5W solution. The rate of lorazepam I.V. injection shouldn't exceed 2 mg/minute. Have emergency resuscitative equipment available when administering I.V.

● Administer diluted lorazepam solutions immediately.

● Don't use solution if discolored or precipitate is present.

● Administer I.M. dose of lorazepam undiluted, deep into a large muscle mass.

● Signs and symptoms of overdose include somnolence, confusion, coma, hypoactive reflexes, dyspnea, labored breathing, hypotension, bradycardia, slurred speech, and unsteady gait or impaired coordination. Treatment for overdose is symptomatic and supportive.

Monitoring the patient

● Periodically assess hepatic function to prevent cumulative effects and to ensure adequate drug metabolism.

● Monitor vital signs, especially respiratory status.

Information for the patient

● Caution patient not to make changes in drug regimen without specific instructions.

● Teach safety measures, such as gradual position changes and supervised walking, to protect patient from injury.

● Advise patient of possible retrograde amnesia after I.V. or I.M. use.

● Advise patient of potential for physical and psychological dependence with long-term use.

● Tell patient to discontinue drug slowly (over 8 to 12 weeks) after long-term therapy.

Geriatric patients

● Elderly patients are more sensitive to drug's CNS depressant effects. They may need supervision with walking and activities of daily living during initiation of therapy or after an increase in dose.

● Lower doses usually are effective in elderly patients because of decreased elimination.

● Parenteral administration of drug is more likely to cause apnea, hypotension, bradycardia, and cardiac arrest in elderly patients.

Pediatric patients

● Safe use of oral lorazepam in children under age 12 hasn't been established.

● Safe use of sublingual or parenteral lorazepam in children under age 18 hasn't been established.

● Closely observe neonate for withdrawal symptoms if mother took lorazepam for a prolonged period during pregnancy.

Breast-feeding patients

● Drug may appear in breast milk. Don't administer to breast-feeding women.

---

losartan potassium
Cozaar

Pharmacologic classification: angiotensin II receptor antagonist
Therapeutic classification: antihypertensive
Pregnancy risk category C (D in second and third trimesters)

How supplied
Available by prescription only
Tablets: 25 mg, 50 mg

Indications, route, and dosage
Hypertension
Adults: Initially, 25 to 50 mg P.O. daily. Maintenance dose is 25 to 100 mg P.O. once daily or b.i.d.

Pharmacodynamics
Antihypertensive action: Angiotensin II receptor antagonist that blocks the vasoconstrictor and aldosterone-secreting effects of angiotensin II by selectively blocking the binding of angiotensin II to its receptor sites found in many tissues, including vascular smooth muscle.

Pharmacokinetics
- *Absorption:* Well absorbed and undergoes substantial first-pass metabolism; systemic bioavailability is about 33%.
- *Distribution:* Drug and active metabolite highly bound to plasma proteins, primarily albumin.
- *Metabolism:* Cytochrome P-450 2C9 and 3A4 involved in biotransformation of drug to its metabolites.
- *Excretion:* Drug and metabolites primarily excreted in feces; small amount excreted in urine.

Contraindications and precautions
Contraindicated in patients with hypersensitivity to drug. Use cautiously in patients with impaired renal or hepatic function.

Interactions
Drug-drug. *Cimetidine:* Increased bioavailability without affecting pharmacokinetics of active metabolite. Monitor patient closely.
Phenobarbital: Decreased bioavailability of losartan and active metabolite. Monitor patient closely.

Adverse reactions
CNS: dizziness, insomnia.
EENT: nasal congestion, sinus disorder, sinusitis.
GI: diarrhea, dyspepsia.
Musculoskeletal: muscle cramps, myalgia, back or leg pain.

Respiratory: cough, upper respiratory tract infection.

☑ Special considerations
- Drugs such as losartan that act directly on the renin-angiotensin system can cause fetal and neonatal morbidity and death when administered to pregnant women; these problems haven't been detected when exposure has been limited to first trimester. If pregnancy is suspected, drug probably should be stopped.
- Use lowest dose (25 mg) initially in patients with impaired hepatic function and in those who are intravascularly volume-depleted (receiving diuretic therapy).
- Drug can be used alone or with other antihypertensives.
- If antihypertensive effect measured at trough (using once-daily dosing) is inadequate, a twice-daily regimen at the same total daily dose or an increased dose may give a more satisfactory response.
- The most likely signs of overdose are hypotension and tachycardia; bradycardia could occur from parasympathetic stimulation.

Monitoring the patient
- Monitor patient taking diuretics concurrently in treatment of hypertension for symptomatic hypotension.
- Regularly assess patient's renal function (serum creatinine and BUN levels).
- Patients with severe heart failure whose renal function depends on the angiotensin-aldosterone system have experienced acute renal failure during therapy with ACE inhibitors. Manufacturer of losartan states that drug would be expected to do the same. Closely monitor patient, especially during first few weeks of therapy.

Information for the patient
- Instruct patient not to stop drug abruptly.
- Tell patient to avoid sodium substitutes; these products may contain potassium, which can cause hyperkalemia in patients taking losartan.
- Inform woman of childbearing age about consequences of second- and third-trimester exposure to losartan; tell her to call immediately if pregnancy is suspected.

Pediatric patients
- Safety and effectiveness in children haven't been established.

Breast-feeding patients
- It's unknown if drug appears in breast milk. Because of potential for adverse effects on breast-fed infant, stop either drug or breast-feeding, taking into account importance of drug to mother.

lovastatin
Mevacor

Pharmacologic classification: lactone;
HMG-CoA reductase inhibitor
Therapeutic classification: cholesterol-lowering drug
Pregnancy risk category X

How supplied
Available by prescription only
Tablets: 10 mg, 20 mg, 40 mg

Indications, route, and dosage
Reduction of low-density lipoprotein and total cholesterol levels in patients with primary hypercholesterolemia (types IIa and IIb), atherosclerosis
Adults: Initially, 20 mg once daily with evening meal. For patients with severely elevated cholesterol levels (for example, over 300 mg/dl), initial dose should be 40 mg. Recommended range is 20 to 80 mg in single or divided doses.

Pharmacodynamics
Antilipemic action: Inactive lactone that is hydrolyzed to the beta-hydroxy acid, which specifically inhibits 3-hydroxy-3-methylglutaryl-coenzyme A reductase (HMG-CoA reductase). This enzyme is an early (and rate-limiting) step in the synthetic pathway of cholesterol. At therapeutic doses, the enzyme isn't blocked, and biologically necessary amounts of cholesterol can still be synthesized.

Pharmacokinetics
• *Absorption:* About 30% of oral dose absorbed. Administration with food improves plasma levels of total inhibitors by about 30%. Onset of action is about 3 days; maximal therapeutic effects in 4 to 6 weeks.
• *Distribution:* Less than 5% of oral dose reaches systemic circulation because of extensive first-pass hepatic extraction; liver is drug's principal site of action. Both parent compound and its principal metabolite are highly bound (more than 95%) to plasma proteins. Drug probably crosses placenta and blood-brain barrier.
• *Metabolism:* Coverted to active B hydroxy acid form in liver. Other metabolites include 6' hydroxy derivative and two unidentified compounds.
• *Excretion:* About 80% excreted primarily in feces; about 10% in urine.

Contraindications and precautions
Contraindicated in patients with hypersensitivity to drug, in those with active liver disease or conditions associated with unexplained persistent elevations of serum transaminase levels, in pregnant and breast-feeding patients, and in women of childbearing age unless there is no risk of pregnancy.

Use cautiously in patients who consume excessive amounts of alcohol or have history of liver disease.

Interactions
Drug-drug. *Cholestyramine, colestipol:* May enhance lipid-reducing effects but may decrease bioavailability of lovastatin. Separate administration times by at least 4 hours.
Cyclosporine, erythromycin, gemfibrozil, niacin: Increased risk of severe myopathy or rhabdomyolysis. Avoid concomitant use.
Isradipine: Increased clearance of lovastatin and its metabolites. Monitor patient.
Itraconazole: Increased HMG-CoA reductase inhibitor levels. Monitor patient closely.
Warfarin: Increased anticoagulant effect. Monitor PT and INR closely; adjust dosage, as indicated.
Drug-lifestyle. *Alcohol:* Increased risk of hepatotoxicity. Discourage use.
Sun exposure: Possible photosensitivity reaction. Tell patient to take precautions.

Adverse reactions
CNS: headache, dizziness, peripheral neuropathy, insomnia.
CV: chest pain.
EENT: blurred vision.
GI: constipation, diarrhea, dyspepsia, flatulence, abdominal pain or cramps, heartburn, nausea, vomiting.
Hepatic: elevated serum transaminase levels, abnormal liver test results.
Musculoskeletal: muscle cramps, myalgia, myositis, ***rhabdomyolysis.***
Skin: rash, pruritus, alopecia.
Other: photosensitivity.

☑ Special considerations
• Begin drug therapy only after diet and other nonpharmacologic therapies have proven ineffective. Patient should be following a standard cholesterol-lowering diet and should continue on this diet during therapy.
• Administer drug with evening meal; absorption is enhanced and cholesterol biosynthesis is greater in the evening.
• Therapeutic response occurs in about 2 weeks, with maximum effects in 4 to 6 weeks.
• Store tablets at room temperature in a light-resistant container.
• Don't exceed 20 mg/day if patient is receiving immunosuppressants.

Monitoring the patient
• Watch for signs of myositis; have patient report muscle aches and pains.
• Perform liver function tests frequently during start of therapy and then periodically.

Reactions may be *common,* uncommon, ***life-threatening,*** or COMMON AND LIFE-THREATENING.

Information for the patient
- Stress importance of lowering cholesterol.
- Advise patient to restrict alcohol intake.
- Instruct patient to take drug with evening meal.
- Tell patient to report adverse reactions, particularly muscle aches and pains, and to take precautions against exposure to sun and other ultraviolet light until tolerance is determined.

Pediatric patients
- Safety and efficacy in children haven't been established.

Breast-feeding patients
- An alternative to breast-feeding is recommended during therapy.

loxapine hydrochloride
Loxitane C, Loxitane IM

loxapine succinate
Loxapac*, Loxitane

Pharmacologic classification: dibenzoxazepine
Therapeutic classification: antipsychotic
Pregnancy risk category NR

How supplied
Available by prescription only
Capsules: 5 mg, 10 mg, 25 mg, 50 mg
Oral concentrate: 25 mg/ml
Injection: 50 mg/ml

Indications, route, and dosage
Psychotic disorders
Adults: 10 mg P.O. b.i.d. to q.i.d., rapidly increasing to 60 to 100 mg P.O. daily for most patients (dose varies from patient to patient) or 12.5 to 50 mg I.M. q 4 to 6 hours. Maximum daily dose, 250 mg. Don't administer drug I.V.

Pharmacodynamics
Antipsychotic action: The only tricyclic antipsychotic; structurally similar to amoxapine. Thought to exert antipsychotic effects by postsynaptic blockade of CNS dopamine receptors, thus inhibiting dopamine-mediated effects. Has many other central and peripheral effects; most prominent adverse reactions are extrapyramidal.

Pharmacokinetics
- *Absorption:* Absorbed rapidly and completely from GI tract. Levels of I.M. dose peak later than oral dose (5 hours versus 1 hour). First-pass metabolism results in lower systemic availability.
- *Distribution:* Distributed widely into body, including breast milk. Effect peaks at 1½ to 3 hours; steady-state serum level achieved within 3 to 4 days. 91% to 99% protein-bound.

- *Metabolism:* Metabolized extensively by liver, forming a few active metabolites; duration of action is 12 hours.
- *Excretion:* Mostly excreted as metabolites in urine; some excreted in feces via biliary tract. About 50% of drug excreted in urine and feces within 24 hours.

Contraindications and precautions
Contraindicated in patients with hypersensitivity to dibenzoxazepines and in patients experiencing coma, severe CNS depression, or drug-induced depressed states. Use cautiously in patients with seizure or CV disorders, glaucoma, or history of urine retention.

Interactions
Drug-drug. *Antacids containing aluminum and magnesium; antidiarrheals:* Decreased loxapine absorption; decreased therapeutic effects. Avoid concomitant use.
Antiarrhythmics, disopyramide, procainamide, quinidine: Increased risk of arrhythmias and conduction defects. Avoid concomitant use.
Appetite suppressants, sympathomimetics (ephedrine, epinephrine, phenylephrine, phenylpropanolamine): Decreased stimulatory and pressor effects. Loxapine may cause epinephrine reversal, an inhibition of epinephrine's vasopressor effect. Monitor patient.
Atropine, nitrates, other anticholinergics: Additive effects. Avoid concomitant use.
Beta blockers: May inhibit loxapine metabolism, increasing plasma levels and toxicity. Monitor patient closely.
Bromocriptine: May antagonize therapeutic effect of bromocriptine on prolactin secretion. Monitor patient.
Clonidine, guanabenz, guanadrel, guanethidine, methyldopa, reserpine: May inhibit blood pressure response to these drugs. Monitor blood pressure.
CNS depressants such as analgesics, anesthetics (epidural, general, spinal), barbiturates, narcotics, parenteral magnesium sulfate, tranquilizers: Additive effects. Avoid concomitant use.
Dopamine: Decreased vasoconstricting effects. Monitor patient for lack of effect.
Levodopa: Decreased effectiveness and increased toxicity of levodopa. Avoid concomitant use.
Lithium: Severe neurologic toxicity with an encephalitis-like syndrome and decreased therapeutic response to loxapine. Monitor serum lithium levels and patient closely.
Drug-lifestyle. *Alcohol:* Additive effects. Discourage use.

Adverse reactions
CNS: *extrapyramidal reactions, sedation, drowsiness, **seizures,** numbness, confusion, syncope,*

tardive dyskinesia, pseudoparkinsonism, EEG changes, dizziness, **neuroleptic malignant syndrome.**.
CV: *orthostatic hypotension,* **tachycardia,** ECG changes, hypertension.
EENT: *blurred vision,* nasal congestion.
GI: *dry mouth, constipation,* nausea, vomiting, paralytic ileus.
GU: *urine retention,* menstrual irregularities, gynecomastia.
Hematologic: *leukopenia,* **agranulocytosis, thrombocytopenia.**
Hepatic: jaundice.
Metabolic: weight gain.
Skin: *mild photosensitivity,* allergic reactions, rash, pruritus.

☑ **Special considerations**
● Assess patient periodically for abnormal body movement. Abnormal involuntary muscle movements may be a sign of overdose.
● Tardive dyskinesia may occur, usually after prolonged use. It may not appear until months or years after treatment and may disappear spontaneously or persist for life.
● Dose of 10 mg is therapeutic equivalent of 100 mg chlorpromazine.
● Photosensitivity warnings may apply with loxapine.
● Drug causes false-positive test results for urinary porphyrins, urobilinogen, amylase, and 5-hydroxyindoleacetic acid because of darkening of urine by metabolites.
● Overdose signs and symptoms include deep, unarousable sleep and coma. Treatment is symptomatic. Don't induce vomiting; drug inhibits cough reflex, and aspiration may occur.

Monitoring the patient
● Obtain baseline blood pressure measurements before starting therapy and monitor regularly.
● Monitor ECG closely for changes and signs of overdose such as arrhythmias.
● Periodic ophthalmic tests are recommended.
● Monitor patient for CNS effects.

Information for the patient
● Advise woman of childbearing age that drug causes false-positive urine pregnancy test results using human chorionic gonadotropin. Instruct her to call if planning pregnancy or if pregnancy is suspected.
● Warn against activities that require alertness and good psychomotor coordination until CNS response to drug is determined. Drowsiness and dizziness usually subside after first few weeks.
● Recommend sugarless gum or candy, mouthwash, ice chips, or artificial saliva to help alleviate dry mouth.
● Advise patient to dilute liquid concentrate with orange or grapefruit juice just before taking.

● Advise patient to get up slowly to avoid orthostatic hypotension.

Geriatric patients
● Elderly patients are highly sensitive to antimuscarinic, hypotensive, and sedative effects of drug and have a higher risk of developing extrapyramidal adverse reactions, such as parkinsonism and tardive dyskinesia. These patients develop higher plasma levels; they require lower initial dosage and more gradual dosage adjustment.

Pediatric patients
● Drug isn't recommended for children under age 16.

Lyme disease vaccine (recombinant OspA)
LYMErix

Pharmacologic classification: vaccine, bacterial-recombinant
Therapeutic classification: biological
Pregnancy risk category C

How supplied
Available by prescription only
Single-dose vials and prefilled syringes: 30 mcg/0.5 ml

Indications, route, and dosage
Active immunization against Lyme disease
Children and adults ages 15 to 70: 30 mcg I.M. in deltoid region; repeat dose at 1 and 12 months after first dose. Safety and efficacy of this vaccine are based on administration of second and third doses several weeks before the onset of *Borrelia burgdorferi* (a bacterial spirochete that causes Lyme disease) transmission season.

Pharmacodynamics
Lyme disease prophylaxis: Stimulates specific antibodies directed against *B. burgdorferi.* Contains lipoprotein OspA, an outer surface protein of *B. burgdorferi.*

Pharmacokinetics
No information available.

Contraindications and precautions
Contraindicated in patients with hypersensitivity to vaccine or its components. Don't give vaccine to patients with treatment-resistant Lyme arthritis (antibiotic refractory) or moderate or severe febrile illness. Lyme disease vaccine shouldn't be given to patients receiving anticoagulants unless potential benefit outweighs risk.
    Use cautiously in immunosuppressed patients or in those receiving immunosuppressive therapy because the expected immune response may

not occur. For patients receiving immunosuppressive therapy, consider deferring vaccination for 3 months after therapy.

Also use cautiously in persons who may have allergic reactions to packaging for the LYMErix syringe, which contains dry natural rubber. Note that the vial packaging doesn't contain rubber.

Interactions
None reported.

Adverse reactions
CNS: *headache, fatigue,* dizziness, depression, hypoesthesia, paresthesia.
EENT: pharyngitis, rhinitis, sinusitis.
GI: diarrhea, nausea.
Musculoskeletal: *arthralgia,* back pain, achiness, myalgia, arthritis, arthrosis, stiffness, tendinitis.
Respiratory: bronchitis, coughing, upper respiratory tract infection.
Skin: *rash, injection site pain, redness, soreness, swelling,* injection site reaction, contact dermatitis.
Other: chills or rigors, fever, viral infection, flulike symptoms.

☑ Special considerations
● Before immunization, review patient's history for possible vaccine sensitivity, allergies, previous vaccination-related adverse reactions, and occurrence of any adverse-event related signs or symptoms. Epinephrine injection (1:1000) and other appropriate drugs used for control of immediate allergic reactions must be immediately available.
● Shake well before withdrawal and use. Inspect visually for particulates or discoloration before administration. With thorough agitation, LYMErix is a turbid white suspension. Discard if it appears otherwise. Use vaccine as supplied, no dilution or reconstitution is necessary. Any vaccine remaining in a single-dose vial should be discarded.
● A separate sterile syringe and needle or a sterile disposable unit must be used for each patient to prevent transmission of infectious agents. Needles should be disposed of properly and shouldn't be recapped.
● Vaccine should be administered by I.M. injection in the deltoid region. Don't inject I.V., intradermally, or S.C.
● No data are available on immune response to vaccine when administered with other vaccines. When concomitant administration of other vaccines is needed, give with different syringes and at different injection sites.
● Store between 36° and 46° F (2° and 8° C). Don't freeze; discard if product has been frozen.
● LYMErix vaccination may result in a positive IgG enzyme-linked immunosorbent assay in the absence of infection.

Monitoring the patient
● Monitor patient's response to vaccine.
● Physicians are encouraged to register pregnant women who received the vaccine by calling 1-800-366-8900, ext. 5231.

Information for the patient
● Inform patient that this vaccine is specific for preventing, not treating, Lyme disease.
● Inform patient, parents, or guardians of the benefits and risks of immunization with vaccine and of the importance of completing the immunization series.
● Ask patient about signs and symptoms that may have occurred after a previous dose of same vaccine and advise him to report any adverse events.
● Instruct patient to disclose if he is taking anticoagulant drugs (warfarin, heparin) or other blood-thinning drugs such as aspirin.
● Advise patient to avoid tick contact (by wearing long-sleeved shirts, long pants, tucking pants into the socks, and treating clothing with tick repellents). Tell patient to carefully check himself for ticks when returning from endemic areas.
● Instruct patient on appropriate tick removal and to use fine-pointed tweezers to avoid squashing tick during removal from skin.

Geriatric patients
● Vaccine isn't indicated for patients who are over age 70.

Pediatric patients
● Safety and efficacy in children and adolescents under age 15 haven't been evaluated. Avoid giving to this age-group.

Breast-feeding patients
● It's unknown if vaccine appears in breast milk; use cautiously in breast-feeding women.

lymphocyte immune globulin (antithymocyte globulin [equine], ATG)
Atgam

Pharmacologic classification: immunoglobulin
Therapeutic classification: immunosuppressant
Pregnancy risk category C

How supplied
Available by prescription only
Injection: 50 mg of equine immunoglobulin G (IgG) per ml, in 5-ml ampules

Indications, route, and dosage
Prevention of acute renal allograft rejection
Adults and children: 15 mg/kg/day I.V. for 14 days; then same dosage every other day for next 14

days (to a total of 21 doses in 28 days). The first dose of ATG should be administered within 24 hours before or after transplantation.

Treatment of acute renal allograft rejection
Adults and children: 10 to 15 mg/kg/day for 14 days; if necessary, same dosage may be given every other day for another 14 days (to a total of 21 doses in 28 days). Therapy with ATG should begin at the first sign of acute rejection.

Aplastic anemia
Adults and children: 10 to 20 mg/kg I.V. daily for 8 to 14 days; then alternate day therapy for an additional 14 days (total of 21 doses in 28 days).

◊ *Skin allotransplantation*
Adults: 10 mg/kg 24 hours before allograft; then 10 to 15 mg/kg every other day. Maintenance dose is variable and can range from 5 to 40 mg/kg/day, based on response and clinical indicators of immunosuppressive activity. Therapy usually continues until allografts cover less than 20% of total body surface area; this frequently requires 40 to 60 days of treatment.

Bone marrow allotransplantation; ◊ *graft-versus-host disease after bone marrow trans-plantation*
Adults: 7 to 10 mg/kg I.V. every other day for six doses.

Pharmacodynamics

Immunosuppressive action: Exact mechanism unknown but may involve elimination of antigen-reactive T cells (T lymphocytes) in peripheral blood or alteration of T-cell function. The effects of antilymphocyte preparations, including ATG, on T cells are variable and complex. Whether the effects of ATG are mediated through a specific subset of T cells hasn't been determined.

Pharmacokinetics

• *Absorption:* Peak plasma levels of equine IgG after I.V. administration of ATG vary, depending on patient's ability to catabolize foreign IgG.
• *Distribution:* Distribution of ATG into body fluids and tissues not fully described. Because antilymphocyte serum reportedly is poorly distributed into lymphoid tissues (such as spleen, lymph nodes), it's likely that ATG is also poorly distributed into these tissues. No information available on transplacental distribution of ATG. Such distribution is likely because other immunoglobulins cross placenta. Virtually all transplacental passage of immunoglobulins occurs during last 4 weeks of pregnancy.
• *Metabolism:* No information available.
• *Excretion:* Plasma half-life averages about 6 days (range 1.5 to 13 days). About 1% of dose excreted in urine, principally as unchanged equine IgG. In one report, mean urinary level of equine IgG was about 4 mcg/ml after about 21 doses of ATG over 28 days.

Contraindications and precautions

Contraindicated in patients with hypersensitivity to drug. An intradermal skin test is recommended at least 1 hour before first dose. Marked local swelling or erythema larger than 10 mm indicates an increased potential for severe systemic reaction such as anaphylaxis. Severe reactions to skin test, such as hypotension, tachycardia, dyspnea, generalized rash, or anaphylaxis, usually preclude further administration of drug.

Use cautiously in patients receiving other immunosuppressants, such as corticosteroids or azathioprine.

Interactions

Drug-drug. *Other immunosuppressants (aza-thioprine, corticosteroids, graft irradiation):* May intensify immunosuppression; possible increased vulnerability to infection and risk of lymphoma or lymphoproliferative disorders. Drug may be used for this potential therapeutic advantage; however, monitor patient carefully.

Adverse reactions

CNS: malaise, *seizures, headache.*
CV: *hypotension,* chest pain, thrombophlebitis, tachycardia, edema, iliac vein obstruction, renal artery stenosis.
EENT: *laryngospasm.*
GI: *nausea, vomiting, diarrhea,* epigastric pain, abdominal distention, stomatitis.
Hematologic: LEUKOPENIA, THROMBOCYTOPENIA, *hemolysis, aplastic anemia.*
Hepatic: elevated liver enzyme level.
Metabolic: hyperglycemia.
Musculoskeletal: myalgia, arthralgia.
Respiratory: hiccups, *dyspnea, pulmonary edema.*
Skin: *rash, pruritus, urticaria.*
Other: *febrile reactions,* serum sickness, *ana-phylaxis, infections,* night sweats, lymphaden-opathy, *chills.*

☑ Special considerations

• Dilute drug concentrate for injection before I.V. infusion. Dilute required dose of ATG in normal saline or 0.45% saline injection (usually 250 to 1,000 ml); final level preferably shouldn't exceed 1 mg of equine IgG per ml. Infuse over at least 4 hours.
• Infusion in dextrose or highly acidic solutions isn't recommended.
• Invert I.V. infusion solution container into which ATG concentrate is added to prevent contact of undiluted ATG with air inside container. Refrigerate diluted solutions of ATG at 36° to 46° F (2° to 8° C) if administration is delayed. Reconstituted solutions shouldn't be used after 12 hours (including actual infusion time), even if stored at 36° to 46° F.
• Because of risk of severe systemic reaction (anaphylaxis), manufacturer recommends an in-

---

tradermal skin test before administration of initial dose of ATG. Procedure consists of intradermal injection of 0.1 ml of a 1:1,000 dilution of ATG concentrate for injection in normal saline injection (5 mcg of equine IgG). A control test using normal saline injection should be administered in the other arm to facilitate interpretation of the results. If a wheal or area of erythema exceeding 10 mm in diameter (with or without pseudopod formation) and itching or marked local swelling develops, infusion of ATG requires extreme caution; severe and potentially fatal systemic reactions can occur in patients with a positive skin test. A systemic reaction to the skin test such as generalized rash, tachycardia, dyspnea, hypotension, or anaphylaxis rules out further administration of ATG. The predictive value of the ATG skin test hasn't been clearly established, and an allergic reaction may occur despite a negative skin test.

• The manufacturer hasn't yet determined the total number of ATG doses (10 to 20 mg/kg per dose) that can be administered safely to a patient. Some renal allograft recipients have received up to 50 doses in 4 months; others, up to four 28-day courses of 21 doses each without an increased risk of adverse effects.

• Drug has been used to treat aplastic anemia, and as an adjunct in bone marrow and skin allotransplantation.

• Some clinicians elect to administer prophylactic platelet transfusion in patients receiving drug for aplastic anemia because of high risk of thrombocytopenia.

Monitoring the patient

• Anaphylaxis may occur at any time during drug therapy and may be indicated by hypotension, respiratory distress, or pain in chest, flank, or back.

• Observe patient receiving drug for signs of leukopenia, thrombocytopenia, and concurrent infection. To minimize risks of leukopenia and infection, some clinicians recommend that azathioprine and corticosteroid dosages be reduced by 50% when ATG is used with these drugs for the prevention or treatment of renal allograft rejection.

• Monitor patients for signs of infection during ATG therapy.

Information for the patient

• Warn patient to report adverse effects, especially signs of infection (fever, sore throat, fatigue).

• Tell patient to alert nurse immediately if discomfort develops at I.V. site.

• Advise woman to avoid becoming pregnant while on drug therapy.

Pediatric patients

• Safety and efficacy in children haven't been established. Drug has had limited use in children ages 3 months to 19 years.

Breast-feeding patients

• Although it's unknown if drug appears in breast milk, other immunoglobulins appear in breast milk. Breast-feeding women should consider an alternative to breast-feeding.

magaldrate (aluminum magnesium hydroxide sulfate)
Iosopan, Lowsium, Magaldrate, Riopan

Pharmacologic classification: aluminum-magnesium salt
Therapeutic classification: antacid
Pregnancy risk category C

How supplied
Available without a prescription
Suspension: 540 mg/5 ml

Indications, route, and dosage
Indigestion or hyperacidity associated with peptic ulcer, gastritis, peptic esophagitis, hiatal hernia
Adults: 5 to 10 ml (suspension) between meals and h.s. with water.

Pharmacodynamics
Antacid action: Neutralizes gastric acid, reducing the direct acid irritant effect. This increases gastric pH, which inactivates pepsin. Also enhances mucosal barrier integrity and improves gastroesophageal sphincter tone.

Pharmacokinetics
• *Absorption:* Aluminum may be absorbed systemically; magnesium also may be absorbed, posing a risk to patients with renal failure. Absorption is unrelated to mechanism of action.
• *Distribution:* Primarily local distribution.
• *Metabolism:* None.
• *Excretion:* Excreted in feces; some aluminum and magnesium may be excreted in breast milk. Duration of action is prolonged.

Contraindications and precautions
Contraindicated in patients with severe renal disease. Use cautiously in patients with mild renal impairment.

Interactions
Drug-drug. *Anticoagulants, antimuscarinics, chlordiazepoxide, coumadin chenodiol, diazepam, digoxin, isoniazid, phosphates, quinolones, tetracycline, vitamin A:* May decrease absorption and lessen effectiveness of these drugs. Separate administration times by 1 to 2 hours.

Enteric-coated drugs: May be released prematurely in stomach. Separate doses of magaldrate and all oral drugs by 1 to 2 hours.
Levodopa: Increased absorption; increased risk of toxicity. Avoid concomitant use.
Phenothiazines (especially chlorpromazine): May inhibit absorption of these drugs. Monitor patient closely.
Drug-herb. *Melatonin:* Additive inhibitory effects on NMDA receptor. Discourage concomitant use.

Adverse reactions
GI: mild constipation, diarrhea, decreased serum potassium levels.
Other: increased serum gastrin and urine pH levels.

☑ Special considerations
• Shake suspension well; give with small amounts of water or fruit juice.
• After administration through nasogastric tube, flush tube with water to clear it and ensure drug's passage to stomach.
• Magaldrate may antagonize pentagastrin's effect during gastric acid secretion tests.
• Suspension contains saccharin and sorbitol.
• Most formulations contain less than 0.5 mg of sodium per tablet (or 5 ml of liquid).

Monitoring the patient
• Monitor renal function and serum phosphate, potassium, and magnesium levels in patients with renal disease.
• Monitor patient for adverse effects.

Information for the patient
• Caution patient to take drug only as directed and 1 or 2 hours apart from other oral drugs.
• Remind patient to shake suspension well or to chew tablets thoroughly.
• Warn patient not to take more than 18 teaspoonful or 20 tablets in a 24-hour period.

Pediatric patients
• Use of drug as an antacid in children under age 6 needs a well-established diagnosis because children typically give vague descriptions of symptoms.

Breast-feeding patients
• Some aluminum and magnesium may appear in breast milk. However, no problems have been associated with use in breast-feeding women.

Reactions may be *common*, uncommon, *life-threatening*, or COMMON AND LIFE-THREATENING.

magnesium hydroxide (milk of magnesia)

Milk of Magnesia, Phillips' Milk of Magnesia, Concentrated Philips' Milk of Magnesia

Pharmacologic classification: magnesium salt
Therapeutic classification: antiulcerative, antacid, laxative
Pregnancy risk category NR

How supplied

Available without a prescription
Tablets: 300 mg, 600 mg
Tablets (chewable): 311 mg
Liquid: 400 mg/5 ml, 800 mg/5 ml
Suspension (concentrated): 10 ml (equivalent to 30 ml of milk of magnesia)
Suspension: 77.5 mg/g

Indications, route, and dosage

Constipation, bowel evacuation before surgery
Adults and children over age 6: 10 to 20 ml concentrated milk of magnesia P.O.; 15 to 60 ml milk of magnesia P.O.
Laxative
Adults: 30 to 60 ml P.O., usually h.s.
Children ages 6 to 12: 15 to 30 ml P.O.
Children ages 2 to 6: 5 to 15 ml P.O.
Antacid
Adults: 5 to 15 ml (liquid) P.O., p.r.n., up to q.i.d.; 2.5 to 7.5 ml (liquid concentrate) P.O., p.r.n., up to q.i.d.; 2 to 4 tablets P.O., p.r.n., up to q.i.d.
Children: 2.5 to 5 ml P.O., p.r.n.

Pharmacodynamics

Antiulcerative action: Neutralizes gastric acid, decreasing the direct acid irritant effect. This increases pH, which, in turn, leads to pepsin inactivation. Also enhances mucosal barrier integrity and improves gastric and esophageal sphincter tone.
Antacid action: Reacts rapidly with hydrochloric acid in the stomach to form magnesium chloride and water.
Laxative action: Produces laxative effect by increasing the osmotic gradient in the gut and drawing in water, causing distention that stimulates peristalsis and bowel evacuation.

Pharmacokinetics

● *Absorption:* About 15% to 30% of magnesium may be absorbed systemically (posing a potential risk to patients with renal failure).
● *Distribution:* None.
● *Metabolism:* None.
● *Excretion:* Unabsorbed drug excreted in feces; absorbed drug excreted rapidly in urine.

Contraindications and precautions

Contraindicated in patients with abdominal pain, nausea, vomiting, or other symptoms of appendicitis or acute surgical abdomen; in those with myocardial damage, heart block, fecal impaction, rectal fissures, intestinal obstruction or perforation, or renal disease; and in patients about to deliver.

Use cautiously in patients with rectal bleeding.

Interactions

Drug-drug. *Aluminum hydroxide, quinolones, tetracyclines:* When used together, magnesium hydroxide may decrease absorption of these drugs. Separate administration times.
Buffered or enteric-coated aspirin: Absorption increased by simultaneous administration. Separate administration times.
Enteric-coated drugs: May cause premature release of these drugs. Separate administration times.

Adverse reactions

GI: *abdominal cramping, nausea, diarrhea,* laxative dependence (with long-term or excessive use).
Metabolic: fluid and electrolyte disturbances (with daily use).

☑ Special considerations

● Give drug at least 1 hour apart from enteric-coated drugs; shake suspension well.
● After drug administration via nasogastric tube, flush tube with water to clear it.

Monitoring the patient

● Watch for signs and symptoms of hypermagnesemia, especially if patient has impaired renal function.
● Monitor patient for signs of overuse.

Information for the patient

● Caution patient to avoid overuse to prevent laxative dependence.
● Instruct patient to shake suspension well or to chew tablets well.

Pediatric patients

● Use as an antacid in children under age 6 needs a well-established diagnosis because children tend to give vague descriptions of symptoms.

Breast-feeding patients

● Some magnesium may appear in breast milk, but no problems have been reported with use in breast-feeding women.

magnesium salicylate
Extra Strength Doan's, Magan, Mobidin

Pharmacologic classification: salicylate
Therapeutic classification: nonnarcotic analgesic, anti-inflammatory, antipyretic
Pregnancy risk category C

How supplied
Available by prescription only
Tablets: 545 mg, 600 mg
Available without a prescription
Tablets: 325 mg, 500 mg

Indications, route, and dosage
Arthritis
Adults: 545 mg to 1.2 g t.i.d. or q.i.d.
Analgesia, antipyresis
Adults and children over age 11: 300 to 600 mg P.O. q 4 hours, p.r.n.
Analgesia (self-medicated)
Adults and children over age 11: 500 mg to 1 g P.O. initially, then 500 mg q 4 hours, p.r.n., not to exceed 3.5 g in 24 hours. Absorption of buffered or enteric-coated aspirin is increased by simultaneous administration. Use with caution in children; may receive the following doses q 4 hours, p.r.n., not to exceed five doses in 24 hours.
Children age 11: 450 mg P.O.
Children ages 9 to 10: 375 mg P.O.
Children ages 6 to 8: 300 mg P.O.
Children ages 4 to 5: 225 mg P.O.
Children ages 2 to 3: 150 mg P.O.
Children under age 2: Dose must be individualized.

Pharmacodynamics
Analgesic action: Produces analgesia by an ill-defined effect on the hypothalamus (central action) and by blocking generation of pain impulses (peripheral action). The peripheral action may involve inhibition of prostaglandin synthesis.
Anti-inflammatory action: Thought to exert anti-inflammatory effect by inhibiting prostaglandin synthesis; may also inhibit the synthesis or action of other mediators of inflammation.
Antipyretic action: Relieves fever by acting on the hypothalamic heat-regulating center to produce peripheral vasodilation. This increases peripheral blood supply and promotes sweating, which leads to loss of heat and to cooling by evaporation.

Pharmacokinetics
- *Absorption:* Magnesium salicylate is absorbed rapidly and completely from GI tract.
- *Distribution:* Highly protein-bound.
- *Metabolism:* Hydrolyzed in liver.
- *Excretion:* Metabolites excreted in urine.

Contraindications and precautions
Contraindicated in patients with hypersensitivity to drug, salicylates, or NSAIDs and in those with severe chronic renal insufficiency because of risk of magnesium toxicity. Also contraindicated in patients with bleeding disorders. Use cautiously in patients with hypoprothrombinemia or vitamin K deficiency.

Interactions
Drug-drug. *Ammonium chloride, other urine acidifiers:* Increased magnesium salicylate blood levels. Monitor patient for magnesium salicylate toxicity.
Antacids, other urine alkalizers: Decreased magnesium salicylate blood levels. Monitor patient for decreased salicylate effect.
Anticoagulants, thrombolytics: Potentiated platelet-inhibiting effects of magnesium salicylate. Monitor patient.
Corticosteroids: Enhanced magnesium salicylate elimination. Monitor patient for decreased salicylate effect.
Drugs that are highly protein-bound (such as phenytoin, sulfonylureas, warfarin): May cause displacement of either drug; possible adverse effects. Monitor patient.
Other GI-irritant drugs (antibiotics, corticosteroids, other NSAIDs): May potentiate adverse GI effects of magnesium salicylate. Use together with caution.
Drug-lifestyle. *Alcohol:* Increased risk of GI bleeding. Discourage use.

Adverse reactions
EENT: *tinnitus, hearing loss.*
GI: *nausea, vomiting, GI distress.*
Hepatic: abnormal liver function studies; increased serum levels of AST, ALT, alkaline phosphatase, and bilirubin; **hepatitis.**
Skin: *rash,* bruising.
Other: hypersensitivity reactions (**anaphylaxis,** asthma), **Reye's syndrome.**

☑ Special considerations
Besides the recommendations relevant to all salicylates, consider the following.
- Drug has been associated with a lower frequency of GI disturbances.
- Drug has a less profound effect on inhibiting platelet aggregation than other salicylates.
- High doses of drug may cause false-positive urine glucose test results using copper sulfate method; it may cause false-negative urine glucose test results using glucose enzymatic method.
- Signs and symptoms of overdose include metabolic acidosis with respiratory alkalosis. To treat, empty stomach immediately by inducing emesis with ipecac syrup if patient is conscious, or by gastric lavage. Administer activated charcoal via nasogastric tube.

Reactions may be *common*, uncommon, *life-threatening*, or COMMON AND LIFE-THREATENING.

Monitoring the patient
- Obtain hemoglobin and PT tests periodically.
- Monitor serum magnesium levels to prevent magnesium toxicity, especially in patients with renal insufficiency.
- Stop drug if dizziness, tinnitus, or hearing impairment occurs.

Information for the patient
- Instruct patient to follow prescribed regimen and to report problems.
- Advise patient not to take drug longer than 10 days without medical supervision.
- Caution patient to keep drug out of children's reach.

Geriatric patients
- Patients over age 60 may be more susceptible to the toxic effects of magnesium salicylate. Use with caution.
- The effects of salicylates on renal prostaglandins may cause fluid retention and edema, a significant drawback for elderly patients and those with heart failure.

Pediatric patients
- Safety of long-term magnesium salicylate use in children hasn't been established.
- Because of epidemiologic association with Reye's syndrome, the Centers for Disease Control and Prevention recommends that children with chickenpox or flulike symptoms not be given salicylates.
- Febrile, dehydrated children can develop toxicity rapidly.

Breast-feeding patients
- Salicylates appear in breast milk; avoid use of magnesium salicylate in breast-feeding women.

magnesium sulfate

Pharmacologic classification: mineral, electrolyte
Therapeutic classification: anticonvulsant
Pregnancy risk category A

How supplied
Available by prescription only
Injectable solutions: 4%, 8%, 10%, 12.5%, 50% in 2-ml, 5-ml, 8-ml, 10-ml, 20-ml, 30-ml, and 50-ml ampules, vials, and prefilled syringes

Indications, route, and dosage
Hypomagnesemic seizures
Adults: 1 to 2 g (as 10% solution) I.V. over 15 minutes, then 1 g I.M. q 4 to 6 hours, based on patient's response and magnesium blood levels.

Seizures secondary to hypomagnesemia in acute nephritis
Children: 0.2 ml/kg of 50% solution I.M. q 4 to 6 hours, p.r.n., or 100 mg/kg of 10% solution I.V. given slowly. Titrate dosage according to magnesium blood levels and seizure response.
Life-threatening arrhythmias
Adults: For patient with sustained ventricular tachycardia or torsades de pointes, give 1 to 6 g I.V. over several minutes, then 3 to 20 mg/minute I.V. infusion for 5 to 48 hours depending on patient response and serum magnesium levels. For patients with paroxysmal atrial tachycardia, give 3 to 4 g I.V. over 30 seconds.
Prevention or control of seizures in preeclampsia or eclampsia
Adults: Initially, 4 g I.V. in 250 ml D_5W and 4 to 5 g deep I.M. each buttock; then 4 g deep I.M. into alternate buttock q 4 hours, p.r.n. Or 4 g I.V. as a loading dose, then 1 to 2 g hourly as an I.V. infusion. Maximum daily dose 40 g.
Barium poisoning, ◊ asthma
Adults: 1 to 2 g I.V.
Mild hypomagnesemia
Adults: 1 g I.M. q 4 to 6 hours; or 5 g in 1 L of D_5W or dextrose 5% in normal saline solution I.V. over 3 hours.

Pharmacodynamics
Anticonvulsant action: Has CNS and respiratory depressant effects. Acts peripherally, causing vasodilation; moderate doses cause flushing and sweating, whereas high doses cause hypotension. Prevents or controls seizures by blocking neuromuscular transmission.
   Sometimes used in pregnant women to prevent or control preeclamptic or eclamptic seizures; also used in children with acute nephritis and to treat hypomagnesemic seizures in adults.

Pharmacokinetics
- *Absorption:* I.V. magnesium sulfate acts immediately; effects last about 30 minutes. After I.M. injection, acts within 60 minutes and lasts for 3 to 4 hours. Effective anticonvulsant serum levels are 2.5 to 7.5 mEq/L.
- *Distribution:* Distributed widely throughout body.
- *Metabolism:* None.
- *Excretion:* Excreted unchanged in urine; some excreted in breast milk.

Contraindications and precautions
Parenteral administration of drug contraindicated in patients with heart block or myocardial damage. Use cautiously in patients with impaired renal function and in women in labor. Don't give in toxemia of pregnancy during the 2 hours preceding delivery.

Interactions
Drug-drug. *Antidepressants, antipsychotics, anxiolytics, barbiturates, general anesthetics, hyp-*

notics, narcotics: May increase CNS depressant effects. Reduced dosages may be needed.
Cardiac glycosides: Concomitant use may exacerbate arrhythmias. Use together cautiously.
I.V. calcium: Changes in cardiac conduction in digitalized patients may lead to heart block if coadministered. Avoid concomitant use.
Succinylcholine, tubocurarine: Potentiated and prolonged neuromuscular blocking action of these drugs. Use with caution.
Drug-lifestyle. *Alcohol:* Increased CNS depressant effects. Discourage use.

Adverse reactions
CNS: drowsiness, *depressed reflexes,* flaccid paralysis.
CV: *hypotension, flushing,* **circulatory collapse,** depressed cardiac function.
Metabolic: hypocalcemia.
Respiratory: *respiratory paralysis.*
Skin: diaphoresis.
Other: hypothermia.

☑ Special considerations
● I.V. bolus must be injected slowly (to avoid respiratory or cardiac arrest).
● If available, administer by constant infusion pump; maximum infusion rate is 150 mg/minute. Rapid drip causes feeling of heat.
● Stop drug as soon as needed effect is achieved.
● Level of magnesium sulfate for I.V. administration shouldn't exceed 20% at a rate no greater than 150 mg/minute (1.5 ml of a 10% concentration or equivalent). For I.M. administration in adults, levels of 25% or 50% are generally used; in infants and children, levels shouldn't exceed 20%.
● To calculate grams of magnesium in a percentage of solution: $X\% = X$ g/100 ml (for example, 25% = 25 g/100 ml = 250 mg/ml).
● Signs and symptoms of overdose include a sharp drop in blood pressure and respiratory paralysis, ECG changes (increased PR and QT intervals and QRS complex), heart block, and asystole. Treatment requires artificial ventilation and I.V. calcium salt to reverse respiratory depression and heart block.

Monitoring the patient
● When giving repeated doses, test knee-jerk reflex before each dose; if absent, stop magnesium. Use of drug beyond this point risks respiratory center failure.
● Respiratory rate must be 16 breaths per minute or more before each dose. Keep I.V. calcium salts on hand.
● Monitor serum magnesium load and clinical status to avoid overdose.
● After use in toxemic women within 24 hours before delivery, watch newborn for signs of magnesium toxicity, including neuromuscular and respiratory depression.

Information for the patient
● Explain use and desired effects of drug to patient and family.
● Inform patient of possible adverse effects.

Pediatric patients
● Drug isn't indicated for use in children.

Breast-feeding patients
● Drug appears in breast milk; in patients with normal renal function, all magnesium sulfate is excreted within 24 hours of stopping drug. An alternative to breast-feeding is recommended during therapy.

mannitol
Osmitrol, Resectisol

Pharmacologic classification: osmotic diuretic
Therapeutic classification: diuretic, prevention and management of acute renal failure or oliguria, reduction of intracranial or intraocular pressure, treatment of drug intoxication
Pregnancy risk category C

How supplied
Available by prescription only
Injection: 5%, 10%, 15%, 20%, 25%
Urogenital solution: 5 g/100 ml distilled water

Indications, route, and dosage
Test dose for marked oliguria or suspected inadequate renal function
Adults and children over age 12: 200 mg/kg or 12.5 g as a 15% or 20% solution I.V. over 3 to 5 minutes. Response is adequate if 30 to 50 ml urine/hour is excreted over 2 to 3 hours.
◇ *Children under age 12:* 0.2 g/kg or 6 g/m² I.V. over 3 to 5 minutes.
Treatment of oliguria
Adults and children over age 12: 50 to 100 g as a 15% to 20% solution I.V. over 90 minutes to several hours.
Children under age 12: 2 g/kg or 60 g/m² I.V.
Prevention of oliguria or acute renal failure
Adults and children over age 12: 50 to 100 g, then a 5% to 10% solution I.V. Exact level is determined by fluid requirements.
Treatment of edema and ascites
Adults and children over age 12: 100 g as a 10% to 20% solution I.V. over 2 to 6 hours.
◇ *Children under age 12:* 2 g/kg or 60 g/m² I.V. as a 15% to 20% solution over 2 to 6 hours.
To reduce intraocular pressure or intracranial pressure
Adults and children over age 12: 1.5 to 2 g/kg as a 15% to 25% solution I.V. over 30 to 60 minutes administered 60 to 90 minutes before surgery.

◊ *Children under age 12:* 2 g/kg or 60 g/m² I.V. as a 15% to 20% solution over 30 to 60 minutes.

To promote diuresis in drug intoxication
Adults and children over age 12: 25 g loading dose; then an infusion maintaining 100 to 500 ml urine output/hour and positive fluid balance. For patients with barbiturate poisoning, give 0.5 g/kg; then a 5% to 10% solution.
◊ *Children under age 12:* 5% to 10% solution to maintain a 100 to 500 ml urine output/hour and positive fluid balance.

Urologic irrigation
Adults: 2.5% solution.

Pharmacodynamics
Diuretic action: Increases the osmotic pressure of glomerular filtrate, inhibiting tubular reabsorption of water and electrolytes, thus promoting diuresis and urinary elimination of certain drugs. This effect is useful for prevention and management of acute renal failure or oliguria and is also useful for reduction of intracranial or intraocular pressure because drug elevates plasma osmolality, enhancing flow of water into extracellular fluid.

Pharmacokinetics
● *Absorption:* Not absorbed from GI tract. I.V. mannitol lowers intracranial pressure in 15 minutes and intraocular pressure in 30 to 60 minutes; it produces diuresis in 1 to 3 hours.
● *Distribution:* Remains in the extracellular compartment. Doesn't cross blood-brain barrier.
● *Metabolism:* Minimally metabolized to glycogen in liver.
● *Excretion:* Drug is filtered by glomeruli; half-life in adults with normal renal function is about 100 minutes.

Contraindications and precautions
Contraindicated in patients with hypersensitivity to drug and in those with anuria, severe pulmonary congestion, frank pulmonary edema, severe heart failure, severe dehydration, metabolic edema, progressive renal disease or dysfunction, or active intracranial bleeding except during craniotomy. Use cautiously in pregnant patients.

Interactions
Drug-drug. *Cardiac glycosides:* May enhance possibility of digitalis toxicity. Monitor glycoside levels.
Lithium: May enhance renal excretion and lower serum lithium levels. Monitor lithium levels closely.
Other diuretics (such as carbonic anhydrase inhibitors): May increase effects of these drugs. Monitor patient closely.

Adverse reactions
CNS: *seizures,* dizziness, headache.

CV: edema, thrombophlebitis, hypotension, hypertension, *heart failure,* tachycardia, angina-like chest pain.
EENT: blurred vision, rhinitis, dry mouth.
GI: thirst, nausea, vomiting, *diarrhea.*
GU: urine retention.
Metabolic: fluid and electrolyte imbalance.
Skin: urticaria.
Other: dehydration, local pain, fever, chills.

☑ Special considerations
Besides the recommendations relevant to all osmotic diuretics, consider the following.
● For maximum pressure reduction during surgery, give drug 1 to 1½ hours preoperatively.
● Drug should be administered I.V. via an in-line filter with great care to avoid extravasation.
● Don't administer with whole blood; agglutination will occur.
● Mannitol solutions commonly crystallize at low temperatures; place crystallized solutions in a hot water bath, shake vigorously to dissolve crystals, and cool to body temperature before use. Don't use solutions with undissolved crystals.
● Drug therapy may interfere with tests for inorganic phosphorus level or blood ethylene glycol.
● If overdose is suspected, stop infusion and institute supportive measures. Hemodialysis removes mannitol and decreases serum osmolality.

Monitoring the patient
● Use with extreme caution in patients with compromised renal function; monitor vital signs (including CVP) hourly and input and output, weight, renal function, and fluid balance.
● Monitor serum and urinary sodium and potassium levels daily.

Information for the patient
● Tell patient he may feel thirsty or experience mouth dryness, and emphasize importance of drinking only the amount of fluids provided.
● With initial doses, warn patient to change position slowly, especially when rising from lying or sitting position, to prevent dizziness from orthostatic hypotension.
● Instruct patient to immediately report pain in chest, back, or legs; shortness of breath; or apnea.

Geriatric patients
● Elderly or debilitated patients require close observation and may need lower dosages. Excessive diuresis promotes rapid dehydration, leading to hypovolemia, hypokalemia, and hyponatremia.

Pediatric patients
● Dosage for children under age 12 hasn't been established.

Breast-feeding patients
• Safety of drug in breast-feeding women hasn't been established.

measles, mumps, and rubella virus vaccine, live
M-M-R II

Pharmacologic classification: vaccine
Therapeutic classification: viral vaccine
Pregnancy risk category C

How supplied
Available by prescription only
Injection: single-dose vial containing not less than 1,000 TCID$_{50}$ (tissue culture infective doses) of attenuated measles virus derived from Enders' attenuated Edmonston strain (grown in chick embryo culture); 20,000 TCID$_{50}$ of the Jeryl Lynn (B level) mumps strain (grown in chick embryo culture); and 1,000 TCID$_{50}$ of the Wistar RA 27/3 strain of rubella virus (propagated in human diploid cell culture)

Indications, route, and dosage
Measles, mumps, and rubella immunization
Adults (born after 1957) and children: 0.5 ml S.C. in outer aspect of the upper arm. Two doses are recommended for children. Give first dose, 0.5 ml S.C., when child is age 15 months or older, and give the second dose when child enters school or first grade (ages 4 to 6). Some local health officials may recommend giving the second dose at an older age.

Pharmacodynamics
Measles, mumps, and rubella prophylaxis: Promotes active immunity to measles (rubeola), mumps, and German measles (rubella) by inducing production of antibodies.

Pharmacokinetics
• *Absorption:* Antibodies usually evident 2 to 3 weeks after injection. Lifelong immunity expected.
• *Distribution:* No information available.
• *Metabolism:* No information available.
• *Excretion:* No information available.

Contraindications and precautions
Contraindicated in immunosuppressed patients; in those with cancer, blood dyscrasias, gamma globulin disorders, fever, active untreated tuberculosis, or anaphylactic or anaphylactoid reactions to neomycin or eggs; in those receiving corticosteroid or radiation therapy; and in pregnant women.

Interactions
Drug-drug. *Immune serum globulin, transfusions of blood or blood products:* May interfere with im-

mune response to vaccine. Whenever possible, vaccination should be deferred for 3 months in these situations.
Immunosuppressants: May interfere with response to vaccine. Monitor closely.
Tuberculin skin testing: Decreased response to tuberculin test. If a tuberculin skin test is necessary, administer either before or simultaneously with vaccine.

Adverse reactions
CNS: syncope, malaise, headache.
EENT: otitis media, conjunctivitis, sore throat.
GI: diarrhea, vomiting.
Respiratory: cough.
Skin: urticaria, rash.
Other: fever, regional lymphadenopathy, ***anaphylaxis***, vasculitis, erythema at injection site.

☑ Special considerations
• Obtain thorough history of allergies, especially to antibiotics, eggs, chicken, or chicken feathers, and of reactions to immunizations.
• Perform a skin test to assess vaccine sensitivity (against a control of normal saline solution in opposing extremity) in patients with history of anaphylactoid reactions to egg ingestion. Administer a prick (intracutaneous) or scratch test with a 1:10 dilution. Read results after 5 to 30 minutes. A positive reaction is a wheal with or without pseudopodia and surrounding erythema.
• Have epinephrine solution 1:1,000 available to treat allergic reactions.
• Most adults born before 1957 are believed to have been infected with naturally occurring disease, and vaccination isn't necessary; however, vaccination should be offered if they are considered susceptible.
• Don't administer I.V. Use a 25G, ⅝-inch needle and inject S.C., preferably into outer aspect of upper arm. Use a sterile syringe free of preservatives, antiseptics, and detergents for each injection because these substances may inactivate live virus vaccine.
• Solution may be used if red, pink, or yellow, but it must be clear.
• Use only the diluent supplied. Discard reconstituted solution after 8 hours.
• Vaccine shouldn't be given less than 1 month before or after immunization with other live virus vaccines—except for monovalent or trivalent live oral poliovirus vaccine, which may be administered simultaneously at separate sites using separate syringes.
• Vaccine may not offer any protection when given within a few days after exposure to natural measles, mumps, or rubella.
• Give passive immunization with immune serum globulin, if necessary, when immediate protection against measles is needed in patients who can't receive measles vaccine component. Don't

---

Reactions may be *common*, uncommon, ***life-threatening***, or COMMON AND LIFE-THREATENING.

administer any live virus vaccine component simultaneously with immune serum globulin.
- Revaccination is unnecessary if child received two doses of vaccine at least 1 month apart, beginning after the first birthday.
- Store vaccine at 36° to 46° F (2° to 8° C) and protect from light.

Monitoring the patient
- Monitor patient for sensitivity reaction to immunization.
- Monitor patient for adverse effects.

Information for the patient
- Tell patient to expect tingling sensations in extremities or joint aches and pains that may resemble arthritis, beginning several days to several weeks after vaccination. These symptoms usually resolve within 1 week. Other effects include pain and inflammation at injection site and a low-grade fever, a rash, or difficulty breathing. Recommend acetaminophen to alleviate adverse reactions such as fever.
- Tell patient to report distressing adverse reactions.
- Advise women of childbearing age not to become pregnant for 3 months after receiving vaccine.

Pediatric patients
- Children under age 15 months may not respond to one, two, or all three of vaccine components because retained maternal antibodies may interfere with immune response. However, vaccination at age 12 months is recommended if child lives in a high-risk area, because benefits outweigh risk of a slightly lower efficacy of vaccine.

Breast-feeding patients
- Not known if measles or mumps virus components appear in breast milk. Transfer of rubella virus or virus antigen into breast milk has occurred in about 68% of patients.
- Few adverse effects have been associated with breast-feeding after immunization with rubella-containing vaccines. The risk-benefit ratio suggests that breast-feeding women may be immunized with the rubella component, if necessary.

measles and rubella virus vaccine, live, attenuated
M-R-Vax II

Pharmacologic classification: vaccine
Therapeutic classification: viral vaccine
Pregnancy risk category C

How supplied
Available by prescription only
Injection: single-dose vial containing not less than 1,000 TCID$_{50}$ (tissue culture infective doses) each of attenuated measles virus derived from Enders' attenuated Edmonston strain (grown in chick embryo culture) and the Wistar RA 27/3 strain of rubella virus (propagated in human diploid cell culture)
Note: 10-dose and 50-dose vials are available to government agencies and institutions only.

Indications, route, and dosage
Measles and rubella immunization
Adults and children ages 15 months and over: 0.5 ml in outer aspect of upper arm. For adequate protection against measles, a two-dose schedule is recommended (at least 1 month between doses).

Pharmacodynamics
Measles and rubella prophylaxis: Promotes active immunity to measles (rubeola) and German measles (rubella) virus by inducing production of antibodies.

Pharmacokinetics
- *Absorption:* Antibodies usually detectable 2 to 3 weeks after injection. Lifelong immunity expected.
- *Distribution:* No information available.
- *Metabolism:* No information available.
- *Excretion:* No information available.

Contraindications and precautions
Contraindicated in immunosuppressed patients; in those with cancer, blood dyscrasias, gamma globulin disorders, fever, active untreated tuberculosis, or anaphylactic or anaphylactoid reactions to eggs or neomycin; in those receiving corticosteroid or radiation therapy; and in pregnant women.

Interactions
Drug-drug. *Immune serum globulin, transfusions of blood or blood products:* May interfere with immune response to vaccine. Defer vaccination for 3 months in these situations whenever possible.
Immunosuppressive drugs: May interfere with response to vaccine. Use cautiously.
Tuberculin skin testing: Vaccine may temporarily decrease response to tuberculin skin testing. If a tuberculin skin test is necessary, administer either before or simultaneously with measles and rubella vaccine.

Adverse reactions
CNS: syncope, malaise, headache.
EENT: sore throat.
GI: vomiting, diarrhea.
Respiratory: cough.
Skin: rash; erythema, burning, or stinging at injection site.
Other: fever, lymphadenopathy, vasculitis, *anaphylaxis.*

☑ Special considerations
- Obtain thorough history of allergies (especially to antibiotics, eggs, chicken, or chicken feathers) and of reactions to immunizations.
- Perform skin testing to assess vaccine sensitivity (against a control of normal saline solution in opposing extremity) in patients with history of anaphylactoid reactions to eggs. Administer a prick (intracutaneous) or scratch test with a 1:10 dilution. Read results after 5 to 30 minutes. A positive reaction is a wheal with or without pseudopodia and surrounding erythema.
- Have epinephrine solution 1:1,000 available to treat allergic reactions.
- Don't administer I.V. Use a 25G, ⅝-inch needle and inject S.C., preferably into outer aspect of upper arm.
- Use a sterile syringe free of preservatives, antiseptics, and detergents for each injection because these substances may inactivate live virus vaccine.
- Use only diluent supplied. Discard reconstituted solution after 8 hours.
- Store vaccine at 36° to 46° F (2° to 8° C), and protect from light. Solution may be used if red, pink, or yellow, but it must be clear.
- Vaccine shouldn't be given less than 1 month before or after immunization with other live virus vaccines, except for mumps virus vaccine and monovalent or trivalent live oral poliovirus vaccine, which may be administered simultaneously.
- Vaccine may not offer protection when given within a few days' exposure to natural measles or rubella.
- According to the Centers for Disease Control and Prevention recommendations, measles, mumps, and rubella (MMR) is the preferred vaccine.
- Give passive immunization with immune serum globulin when immediate protection against measles is required in patients who can't receive measles vaccine component. Don't administer either vaccine component simultaneously with immune serum globulin.
- Revaccination isn't necessary if primary vaccine is given at or after age 15 months.

Monitoring the patient
- Monitor patient for sensitivity reaction to immunization.
- Watch for signs of infection.

Information for the patient
- Tell patient to expect tingling sensations in extremities or joint aches and pains that may resemble arthritis, beginning several days to several weeks after vaccination. These symptoms usually resolve within 1 week. Other effects include pain and inflammation at the injection site and a low-grade fever, rash, or difficulty breathing. Recommend acetaminophen for relief of fever.

- Encourage patient to report distressing adverse reactions.
- Advise woman of childbearing age not to become pregnant for 3 months after receiving vaccine.

Pediatric patients
- Children under age 15 months may not respond to one or both of the vaccine components because retained maternal antibodies may interfere with immune response; revaccination is recommended after age 15 months.

Breast-feeding patients
- It's unknown if measles and rubella virus components appear in breast milk. Transfer of rubella virus or virus antigen into breast milk has occurred in about 68% of patients.
- Few adverse effects have been associated with breast-feeding after immunization with rubella-containing vaccines. The risk-benefit ratio suggests that breast-feeding women may be immunized with the rubella component, if necessary.

---

measles virus vaccine, live, attenuated
Attenuvax

Pharmacologic classification: vaccine
Therapeutic classification: viral vaccine
Pregnancy risk category C

How supplied
Available by prescription only
Injection: single-dose vial containing not less than 1,000 TCID$_{50}$ (tissue culture infective doses) per 0.5 ml of attenuated measles virus derived from Enders' attenuated Edmonston strain grown in chick embryo culture (10- and 50-dose vials available to government agencies and institutions only)

Indications, route, and dosage
Immunization
Adults and children ages 15 months and over: 0.5 ml (1,000 units) S.C. in outer aspect of upper arm. Administer two doses at least 1 month apart. For children, usual schedule is the first dose at age 15 months and a second dose at the entry of school (ages 4 to 6 years).

Pharmacodynamics
Measles prophylaxis: Promotes active immunity to measles virus by inducing production of antibodies.

Pharmacokinetics
- *Absorption:* Antibodies usually evident 2 to 3 weeks after injection. Immunity at least 13 to 16 years; probably lifelong in most immunized persons.

- *Distribution:* No information available.
- *Metabolism:* No information available.
- *Excretion:* No information available.

Contraindications and precautions
Contraindicated in immunosuppressed patients; in those with cancer, blood dyscrasias, gamma globulin disorders, fever, active untreated tuberculosis, or anaphylactic or anaphylactoid reactions to neomycin or eggs; in those receiving corticosteroid or radiation therapy; and in pregnant women.

Interactions
Drug-drug. *Immune serum globulin, transfusions of blood or blood products:* May interfere with immune response to vaccine. Defer vaccination for 3 months in these situations.
Immunosuppressants (such as interferon): May interfere with response to vaccine. Use together cautiously.
Meningococcal vaccine: Possible reduced seroconversion rate to meningococci. Defer vaccination if possible.
Tuberculin skin testing: Vaccine may decrease response to tuberculin skin testing. Should a tuberculin skin test be necessary, administer either before or simultaneously with measles vaccine.

Adverse reactions
CNS: *febrile seizures* (in susceptible children).
GI: anorexia.
Hematologic: *leukopenia.*
Skin: rash, erythema, swelling, tenderness (at injection site).
Other: fever, lymphadenopathy, *anaphylaxis.*

☑ Special considerations
- Obtain thorough history of allergies, especially to antibiotics, eggs, chicken, or chicken feathers, and of reactions to immunizations.
- Patients with a history of anaphylactoid reactions to eggs should first have a skin test to assess vaccine sensitivity (against a control of normal saline solution in other arm). Administer a prick (intracutaneous) or scratch test with a 1:10 dilution. Read results after 5 to 30 minutes. A positive reaction is a wheal with or without pseudopodia and surrounding erythema.
- Have epinephrine solution 1:1,000 available to treat allergic reactions.
- Don't administer I.V. Use a 25G, ⅝-inch needle and inject S.C., preferably into outer aspect of upper arm. Use a sterile syringe free of preservatives, antiseptics, and detergents for each injection because these substances may inactivate live virus vaccine.
- Use diluent supplied. Discard reconstituted solution after 8 hours.
- Measles vaccine shouldn't be given less than 1 month before or after immunization with other live virus vaccines—except for mumps virus vac-

cine, rubella virus vaccine, or monovalent or trivalent live oral poliovirus vaccine, which may be administered simultaneously.
- Vaccine may offer some protection when given within a few days after exposure to natural measles and substantial protection when given a few days before exposure.
- According to the Centers for Disease Control and Prevention recommendations, measles, mumps, and rubella (MMR) is the preferred vaccine.
- Give passive immunization with immune serum globulin if immediate protection against measles is required in patients who can't receive measles vaccine.
- Revaccination is unnecessary if primary vaccine is given at age 15 months or older.
- Store vaccine at 35° to 46° F (2° to 8° C), and protect from light. Solution may be used if red, pink, or yellow, but it must be clear.

Monitoring the patient
- Monitor patient for sensitivity reaction to vaccine.
- Watch for signs of infection.

Information for the patient
- Tell patient to expect pain and inflammation at the injection site, fever, rash, general malaise, or difficulty breathing. Recommend acetaminophen for relief of fever.
- Encourage patient to report distressing adverse reactions.
- Advise woman of childbearing age not to become pregnant for 3 months after receiving the vaccine.

Pediatric patients
- Children under age 15 months may not respond to the vaccine because retained maternal antibodies may interfere with the immune response; revaccination is recommended after age 15 months.

Breast-feeding patients
- It's unknown if vaccine appears in breast milk. Use with caution in breast-feeding women.

mebendazole
Vermox

Pharmacologic classification: benzimidazole
Therapeutic classification: anthelmintic
Pregnancy risk category C

How supplied
Available by prescription only
Tablets (chewable): 100 mg

Indications, route, and dosage

Pinworm infestations
Adults and children over age 2: 100 mg P.O. as a single dose. If infection persists 3 weeks later, repeat treatment.

Other roundworm, whipworm, and hookworm infestations
Adults and children over age 2: 100 mg P.O. b.i.d. for 3 days. If infection persists 3 weeks later, repeat treatment.

◇ *Trichinosis (second-line drug)*
Adults: 200 to 400 mg P.O. t.i.d. for 3 days; then 400 to 500 mg t.i.d. for 10 days.

◇ *Capillariasis*
Adults: 200 mg b.i.d. for 20 days.

◇ *Toxocariasis*
Adults: 100 to 200 mg b.i.d. for 5 days.

◇ *Dracunculiasis*
Adults: 400 to 800 mg daily for 6 days.

◇ *Mansonella perstans infestations*
Adults: 100 mg b.i.d. for 30 days.

◇ *Angiostrongylus cantonensis infestations*
Adults and children: 100 mg b.i.d. for 5 days.

Pharmacodynamics

Anthelmintic action: Inhibits uptake of glucose and other low-molecular weight nutrients in susceptible helminths, depleting the glycogen stores they need for survival and reproduction. Has a broad spectrum and may be useful in mixed infections. Considered a drug of choice in the treatment of ascariasis, capillariasis, enterobiasis, trichuriasis, and uncinariasis; has been used for investigational purposes to treat echinococciasis, onchocerciasis, and trichinosis.

Pharmacokinetics

● *Absorption:* About 5% to 10% of dose is absorbed; plasma levels peak at 2 to 4 hours. Absorption varies widely among patients.
● *Distribution:* Highly bound to plasma proteins; crosses placenta.
● *Metabolism:* Metabolized to inactive 2-amino-5(6)-benzimidazolyl phenylketone.
● *Excretion:* Most of dose excreted in feces; 2% to 10% excreted in urine in 48 hours as either unchanged drug or 2-amine metabolite. Half-life is 3 to 9 hours. Unknown if drug is excreted in breast milk.

Contraindications and precautions

Contraindicated in patients with hypersensitivity to drug.

Interactions

Drug-drug. *Anticonvulsants (such as carbamazepine, phenytoin):* May enhance metabolism of mebendazole and decrease its efficacy. Monitor patient closely.
Cimetidine: Inhibited mebendazole metabolism, possibly resulting in increased plasma levels of drug. Monitor drug levels.

Adverse reactions

GI: occasional, transient abdominal pain and diarrhea in massive infection and expulsion of worms.
Other: fever.

☑ Special considerations

● Tablets may be chewed, swallowed whole, or crushed and mixed with food.
● Laxatives, enemas, or dietary restrictions are unnecessary.
● Collect stool specimens in a clean, dry container and transfer to a properly labeled container to send to laboratory; ova may be destroyed by toilet bowl water, urine, and some drugs.
● Signs of overdose include GI effects and altered mental status. If overdose is suspected (for recent ingestion within 4 hours), empty stomach by induced emesis or gastric lavage. Follow with activated charcoal to decrease absorption.

Monitoring the patient
● Monitor patient's response to drug therapy.
● Monitor WBC as needed.

Information for the patient
● To prevent reinfection, teach patient and family members personal hygiene measures, such as washing perianal area and changing undergarments and bedclothes daily, washing hands and cleaning fingernails before meals and after defecation, and sanitary disposal of feces.
● Advise patient to bathe often, by showering, if possible.
● Advise patient to keep hands away from mouth, to keep fingernails short, and to wear shoes to avoid hookworm; explain that ova are easily transmitted directly and indirectly by hands, food, or contaminated articles. Washing clothes in household washing machine will destroy ova.
● Instruct patient to handle bedding carefully because shaking will send ova into the air, and to disinfect toilet facilities and vacuum or damp-mop floors daily to reduce number of ova.
● Encourage patient's family and contacts to be checked for infestation and treated, if necessary.

Pediatric patients
● Drug should be given to children under age 2 only when potential benefits justify risks.

Breast-feeding patients
● Safety in breast-feeding women hasn't been established.

mechlorethamine hydrochloride (nitrogen mustard)
Mustargen

Pharmacologic classification: alkylating drug (cell cycle–phase nonspecific)
Therapeutic classification: antineoplastic
Pregnancy risk category D

How supplied
Available by prescription only
Injection: 10-mg vials

Indications, route, and dosage
Dosage and indications may vary. Check current literature for recommended protocols.
Hodgkin's disease, bronchogenic carcinoma, chronic lymphocytic leukemia, chronic myelocytic leukemia, lymphosarcoma, polycythemia vera
Adults: 0.4 mg/kg I.V. per course of therapy as a single dose or 0.1 to 0.2 mg/kg on 2 to 4 successive days q 3 to 6 weeks. Give through running I.V. infusion. Dose reduced in prior radiation or chemotherapy to 0.2 to 0.4 mg/kg. Dose based on ideal or actual body weight, whichever is less.
Intracavitary doses for neoplastic effusions
Adults: 0.2 to 0.4 mg/kg.

Pharmacodynamics
Antineoplastic action: Exerts cytotoxic activity through the basic processes of alkylation. Causes cross-linking of DNA strands, single-strand breakage of DNA, abnormal base pairing, and interruption of other intracellular processes, resulting in cell death.

Pharmacokinetics
● *Absorption:* Well absorbed after oral administration; however, must be administered I.V. because drug is very irritating to tissue. After intracavitary administration, absorbed incompletely, probably from deactivation by body fluids in cavity.
● *Distribution:* Doesn't cross blood-brain barrier.
● *Metabolism:* Rapid chemical transformation and reacts quickly with various cellular components before being deactivated.
● *Excretion:* Metabolites excreted in urine. Less than 0.01% of an I.V. dose excreted unchanged in urine.

Contraindications and precautions
Contraindicated in patients with hypersensitivity to drug and in those with known infectious diseases. Use cautiously in patients with severe anemia or depressed neutrophil or platelet count and in those who have recently undergone chemotherapy or radiation therapy.

Interactions
Drug-drug. *Anticoagulants, aspirin:* Increased risk of bleeding. Avoid concomitant use.
Myelosuppressants: Possible additive myelosuppression. Monitor CBC and patient closely.

Adverse reactions
CNS: weakness, vertigo.
CV: *thrombophlebitis.*
EENT: tinnitus; deafness (with high doses).
GI: *nausea, vomiting, anorexia* (beginning within minutes, lasting 8 to 24 hours).
GU: menstrual irregularities, impaired spermatogenesis.
Hematologic: *thrombocytopenia,* lymphocytopenia, *agranulocytosis,* nadir of myelosuppression occurring by days 4 to 10 and lasting 10 to 21 days; mild anemia begins in 2 to 3 weeks.
Hepatic: jaundice.
Metabolic: hyperuricemia.
Skin: *alopecia,* rash, sloughing, severe irritation (if drug extravasates or touches skin).
Other: precipitation of herpes zoster, *anaphylaxis, secondary malignant disease,* amyloidosis.

☑ Special considerations
● To reconstitute powder, use 10 ml of sterile water for injection or normal saline solution to give a concentration of 1 mg/ml.
● When reconstituted, drug is a clear colorless solution. Don't use if solution is discolored or if droplets of water are visible within vial before reconstitution.
● Solution is very unstable. Prepare immediately before infusion and use within 15 minutes. Discard unused solution.
● Drug may be administered I.V. push over a few minutes into tubing of a freely flowing I.V. infusion.
● Dilution of drug into a large volume of I.V. solution isn't recommended; it may react with diluent and isn't stable for a prolonged period.
● Treatment of extravasation includes local injections of a 1/6 M sodium thiosulfate solution. Prepare solution by mixing 4 ml of sodium thiosulfate 10% with 6 ml of sterile water for injection. Also, apply ice packs for 6 to 12 hours to minimize local reactions.
● During intracavitary administration, patient should be turned from side to side every 15 minutes for 1 hour to distribute drug.
● To prevent hyperuricemia with resulting uric acid nephropathy, allopurinol may be given; keep patient well hydrated.
● Avoid all I.M. injections when platelet count is low.
● Avoid contact with skin or mucous membranes. Wear gloves when preparing solution and during administration to prevent accidental skin contact. If contact occurs, wash with copious amounts of water.

• Drug has been used topically to treat mycosis fungoides.

Monitoring the patient
• Monitor uric acid levels, CBC, and liver function tests.
• Monitor patient for signs of toxicity. Treatment is usually supportive and includes transfusion of blood components and antibiotic treatment of complicating infections.

Information for the patient
• Tell patient to avoid exposure to people with infections.
• Tell patient that adequate fluid intake is very important to facilitate excretion of uric acid.
• Reassure patient that hair should grow back after treatment has ended.
• Tell patient to promptly report signs or symptoms of bleeding or infection.
• Advise patient to use contraception while using drug.

Breast-feeding patients
• It's unknown if drug appears in breast milk. However, because of potential for serious adverse reactions, mutagenicity, and carcinogenicity in infant, breast-feeding isn't recommended.

meclizine hydrochloride
Antivert, Antivert/25, Antrizine, Bonine, Dizmiss, Meclizine, Meni-D

Pharmacologic classification: piperazine-derivative antihistamine
Therapeutic classification: antiemetic, antivertigo drug
Pregnancy risk category B

How supplied
Available with or without a prescription
Tablets: 12.5 mg, 25 mg, 50 mg
Tablets (chewable): 25 mg
Capsules: 25 mg, 30 mg

Indications, route, and dosage
Dizziness
Adults and children ages 12 and older: 25 to 100 mg P.O. daily in divided doses. Dosage varies with patient response.
Motion sickness
Adults and children ages 12 and older: 25 to 50 mg P.O. 1 hour before travel; may repeat dose daily for duration of journey.

Pharmacodynamics
Antiemetic action: Probably inhibits nausea and vomiting by centrally decreasing sensitivity of labyrinth apparatus that relays stimuli to the chemoreceptor trigger zone and stimulates the vomiting center in the brain.

Antivertigo action: Decreases labyrinth excitability and conduction in vestibular-cerebellar pathways.

Pharmacokinetics
• *Absorption:* Onset of action is about 60 minutes.
• *Distribution:* Well distributed throughout body; crosses placenta.
• *Metabolism:* Probably metabolized in liver.
• *Excretion:* Half-life is about 6 hours; action lasts for 8 to 24 hours. Excreted unchanged in feces; metabolites found in urine.

Contraindications and precautions
Contraindicated in patients with hypersensitivity to drug. Use cautiously in patients with asthma, glaucoma, or prostatic hyperplasia.

Interactions
Drug-drug. *CNS depressants:* Additive sedative and CNS depressant effects. Use together cautiously.
Ototoxic drugs (aminoglycosides, cisplatin, loop diuretics, salicylates, vancomycin): Meclizine may mask signs of ototoxicity. Don't use together.
Drug-lifestyle. *Alcohol:* Additive sedative and CNS depressant effects. Discourage use.

Adverse reactions
CNS: *drowsiness,* restlessness, excitation, nervousness, auditory and visual hallucinations.
CV: hypotension, palpitations, tachycardia.
EENT: blurred vision, diplopia, tinnitus, dry nose and throat.
GI: dry mouth, constipation, anorexia, nausea, vomiting, diarrhea.
GU: urine retention, urinary frequency.
Skin: urticaria, rash.

☑ Special considerations
Besides the recommendations relevant to all antihistamines, consider the following.
• Tablets may be placed in mouth and allowed to dissolve without water, or they may be chewed or swallowed whole.
• Abrupt withdrawal of drug after long-term use may cause paradoxical reactions or sudden reversal of improved state.
• Stop drug 4 days before diagnostic skin tests to avoid preventing, reducing, or masking test response.
• Signs and symptoms of moderate overdose may include hyperexcitability alternating with drowsiness. Seizures, hallucinations, and respiratory paralysis may occur in profound overdose. To treat overdose, use gastric lavage.

Monitoring the patient
• Monitor patient's response to drug therapy.
• Monitor patient for adverse effects.

Information for the patient
- Instruct patient to avoid activities that require mental alertness and physical coordination, such as driving and operating dangerous machinery.

Geriatric patients
- Elderly patients are usually more sensitive to adverse effects of antihistamines and are more likely than younger patients to experience dizziness, sedation, hyperexcitability, dry mouth, and urine retention.

Pediatric patients
- Safety and efficacy in children haven't been established. Don't use in children under age 12; infants and children under age 6 may experience paradoxical hyperexcitability.

Breast-feeding patients
- Safety in breast-feeding women hasn't been established.

medroxyprogesterone acetate
Amen, Curretab, Cycrin, Depo-Provera, Provera

Pharmacologic classification: progestin
Therapeutic classification: progestin, antineoplastic
Pregnancy risk category X

How supplied
Available by prescription only
Tablets: 2.5 mg, 5 mg, 10 mg
Injection: 150 mg/ml, 400 mg/ml

Indications, route, and dosage
Abnormal uterine bleeding from hormonal imbalance
Adults: 5 to 10 mg P.O. daily for 5 to 10 days beginning on day 16 or 21 of menstrual cycle. If patient has received estrogen, then 10 mg P.O. daily for 10 days beginning on day 16 of cycle.
Secondary amenorrhea
Adults: 5 to 10 mg P.O. daily for 5 to 10 days.
Endometrial or renal carcinoma
Adults: 400 to 1,000 mg I.M. weekly.
◇ **Paraphilia in men**
Adults: Initially, 200 mg I.M. b.i.d. or t.i.d. or 500 mg I.M. weekly. Adjust dosage based on response.
Contraception in women
Adults: 150 mg I.M. q 3 months; give first injection during first 5 days of menstrual cycle.

Pharmacodynamics
Progestational action: Parenteral medroxyprogesterone suppresses ovulation, causes thickening of cervical mucus, and induces endometrial sloughing.

Antineoplastic action: Mechanism unknown. May inhibit growth progression of progestin-sensitive endometrial or renal cancer tissue.

Pharmacokinetics
- *Absorption:* Slow absorption after I.M. administration.
- *Distribution:* Not well characterized.
- *Metabolism:* Primarily hepatic; not well characterized.
- *Excretion:* Primarily renal; not well characterized.

Contraindications and precautions
Contraindicated in patients with hypersensitivity to drug; in those with active thromboembolic disorders, past history of thromboembolic disorders or cerebral vascular disease or apoplexy, breast cancer, undiagnosed abnormal vaginal bleeding, missed abortion, or hepatic dysfunction; and during pregnancy. Tablets are also contraindicated in patients with liver dysfunction or known or suspected malignant disease of the genital organs.

Use cautiously in patients with diabetes mellitus, seizures, migraines, cardiac or renal disease, asthma, or mental depression.

Interactions
Drug-drug. *Aminoglutethimide:* May increase hepatic metabolism of medroxyprogesterone, possibly decreasing its therapeutic effect. Tell patient to use a nonhormonal contraceptive during therapy.
Bromocriptine: Progestins may cause amenorrhea or galactorrhea, interfering with action of bromocriptine. Concurrent use of these drugs isn't recommended.
Drug-food. *Caffeine:* May increase serum caffeine levels. Monitor patient for effects.
Drug-lifestyle. *Smoking:* Increased risk of adverse CV effects. If smoking continues, alternative therapy may be necessary.

Adverse reactions
CNS: depression.
CV: thrombophlebitis, **pulmonary embolism,** edema, **thromboembolism, CVA.**
EENT: exophthalmos, diplopia.
GU: breakthrough bleeding, dysmenorrhea, amenorrhea, cervical erosion, abnormal secretions.
Hepatic: cholestatic jaundice.
Metabolic: changes in weight.
Skin: rash, pain, induration, sterile abscesses, acne, pruritus, melasma, alopecia, hirsutism.
Other: breast tenderness, enlargement, or secretion.

☑ Special considerations
Besides the recommendations relevant to all progestins, consider the following.

• Parenteral form is for I.M. administration only. Inject deep into large muscle mass, preferably the gluteal muscle. Watch for development of sterile abscesses. Suspension must be shaken vigorously immediately before each use to ensure complete suspension of drug.
• Drug has been used to treat obstructive sleep apnea and to manage paraphilia.

Monitoring the patient
• When used for long-acting female contraception, rule out pregnancy before starting drug.
• Monitor patient for adverse effects, especially visual changes or migraines.

Information for the patient
• Caution patient to seek immediate treatment for chest pain, difficulty breathing, slurred speech, numbness or weakness of an extremity, or facial drooping.
• Tell patient that breakthrough bleeding may occur.
• Advise patient to report adverse effects.

Breast-feeding patients
• Drug appears in breast milk. In nursing mothers treated with drug, the milk composition, quality, and amount aren't adversely affected. Infants exposed to drug via breast milk have been studied for developmental and behavioral effects through puberty; no adverse effects have been noted.

---

megestrol acetate
Megace

Pharmacologic classification: progestin
Therapeutic classification: antineoplastic
Pregnancy risk category X

How supplied
Available by prescription only
Tablets: 20 mg, 40 mg
Suspension: 200 mg/5 ml

Indications, route, and dosage
Dosage and indications may vary. Check current literature for recommended protocol.
Palliative treatment of breast carcinoma
Adults: 40 mg (tablets) P.O. q.i.d.
Palliative treatment of endometrial carcinoma
Adults: 10 to 80 mg (tablets) P.O. q.i.d.
Anorexia, cachexia, or weight loss in patients with AIDS
Adults: 800 mg (suspension) P.O. daily; 100 to 400 mg for AIDS-related cachexia.

Pharmacodynamics
Antineoplastic action: Mechanism unknown. Inhibits growth and causes regression of progestin-sensitive breast and endometrial cancer tissue.

Treatment of anorexia, cachexia, or weight loss: Mechanism for weight gain is unknown. May stimulate appetite by interfering with production of mediators such as cachectin.

Pharmacokinetics
• *Absorption:* Well absorbed across GI tract after oral administration.
• *Distribution:* Appears to be stored in fatty tissue; highly bound to plasma proteins.
• *Metabolism:* Completely metabolized in liver.
• *Excretion:* Metabolites eliminated primarily through kidneys.

Contraindications and precautions
Contraindicated in patients with hypersensitivity to drug and during pregnancy (especially first 4 months). Use cautiously in patients with history of thrombophlebitis.

Interactions
Drug-drug. *Bromocriptine:* May cause amenorrhea or galactorrhea, interfering with action of bromocriptine. Concurrent use isn't recommended.

Adverse reactions
CV: thrombophlebitis, hypertension, edema, chest pain, *heart failure.*
EENT: pharyngitis.
GI: increased appetite, nausea, vomiting, diarrhea, flatulence.
GU: breakthrough menstrual bleeding, impotence.
Hepatic: hepatomegaly.
Metabolic: weight gain, hyperglycemia.
Respiratory: *pulmonary embolism,* dyspnea, pneumonia, cough.
Skin: alopecia, rash, pruritus, candidiasis.
Other: carpal tunnel syndrome, decreased libido.

☑ Special considerations
• Recommendations for administration of megestrol and for care and teaching of the patient during therapy are the same as those for all progestins.
• Blood glucose levels may increase in diabetic patients.
• Two months is usually an adequate trial when treating patients with cancer.

Monitoring the patient
• Monitor patient for adverse effects.
• Monitor blood pressure.

Information for the patient
• Advise patient of childbearing age to use effective form of birth control. Tell her to call immediately if she becomes pregnant or suspects she is pregnant.

Reactions may be *common,* uncommon, *life-threatening,* or COMMON AND LIFE-THREATENING.

• Inform patient of possible adverse reactions, and tell patient to seek care immediately for chest pain or shortness of breath.

Breast-feeding patients
• Use an alternative to breast-feeding during therapy because of possible infant toxicity.

---

melphalan
(phenylalanine mustard)
Alkeran

Pharmacologic classification: alkylating drug (cell cycle–phase nonspecific)
Therapeutic classification: antineoplastic
Pregnancy risk category D

How supplied
Available by prescription only
Tablets (scored): 2 mg
Powder for injection: 50 mg

Indications, route, and dosage
Dosage and indications may vary. Check current literature for recommended protocol.
Multiple myeloma
Adults: 6 mg P.O. daily for 2 to 3 weeks; then stop therapy for 4 weeks. When WBC and platelet counts begin to rise, start maintenance dose of 2 mg P.O. daily. Or give 0.15 mg/kg/day P.O. for 7 days administered at 2- to 6-week intervals or 0.25 mg/kg/day P.O. for 4 days at 4- to 6-week intervals; monitor patient's blood counts.
    For I.V. administration, give 16 mg/m² over 15 to 20 minutes once at 2-week intervals for four doses. Monitor patient's blood counts and reduce dose as necessary.
Epithelial ovarian cancer
Adults: 200 mcg/kg/day P.O. for 5 days, repeated q 4 to 6 weeks if blood counts return to normal.

Pharmacodynamics
Antineoplastic action: Exerts cytotoxic activity by forming cross-links of strands of DNA and RNA and inhibiting protein synthesis.

Pharmacokinetics
• *Absorption:* Incomplete and variable absorption from GI tract; absorption ranges from 25% to 89% after oral dose of 0.6 mg/kg.
• *Distribution:* Rapidly and widely distributed into total body water. Initially 50% to 60% bound to plasma proteins; eventually increases to 80% to 90%.
• *Metabolism:* Extensively deactivated by hydrolysis.
• *Excretion:* Biphasic; initial half-life of 8 minutes; terminal half-life of 2 hours. Drug and metabolites excreted primarily in urine; 10% of oral dose excreted as unchanged drug.

Contraindications and precautions
Contraindicated in patients with hypersensitivity to drug and in those whose disease is known to be resistant to drug. Patients hypersensitive to chlorambucil may have cross-sensitivity to melphalan.
    Use cautiously in patients with impaired renal function, severe leukopenia, thrombocytopenia, anemia, or chronic lymphocytic leukemia.

Interactions
Drug-drug. *Anticoagulants, aspirin:* Increased risk of bleeding. Avoid concomitant use.
Cimetidine: Inhibited GI absorption. Avoid use together.
Cisplatin, cyclosporine: Melphalan may increase cyclosporine-induced nephrotoxicity. Monitor renal function closely in patients receiving melphalan and cyclosporine together or melphalan and cisplatin together.
Interferon alpha: Decreased melphalan serum levels. Monitor closely.
Vaccines: Decreased effectiveness and risk of toxicity. Defer immunization for at least 3 months after last dose of melphalan.
Drug-food. *Any food:* Reduced bioavailability of oral melphalan. Give drug on empty stomach.

Adverse reactions
CV: hypotension, tachycardia, edema.
GI: nausea, vomiting, diarrhea, oral ulceration.
Hematologic: *thrombocytopenia, leukopenia, bone marrow suppression,* hemolytic anemia.
Hepatic: *hepatotoxicity.*
Respiratory: *pneumonitis, pulmonary fibrosis,* dyspnea, bronchospasm.
Skin: pruritus, alopecia, urticaria.
Other: *anaphylaxis, hypersensitivity,* secondary malignancy.

☑ Special considerations
• Oral dose may be taken all at one time.
• Stop therapy temporarily or reduce dosage if WBC count falls below 3,000/mm³ or platelet count falls below 100,000/mm³.
• Avoid I.M. injections when platelet count is below 100,000/mm³.
• Dosage reduction should be considered in patients with renal failure receiving I.V. melphalan. Increased bone marrow suppression was observed in patients with BUN levels of 30 mg/dl or more.
• Fever may enhance drug elimination.
• Signs and symptoms of overdose include myelosuppression, hypocalcemia, severe nausea, vomiting, ulceration of the mouth, decreased consciousness, seizures, muscular paralysis, and cholinomimetic effects.

Monitoring the patient
• Monitor hematologic studies, including CBC, to accurately adjust dosage and prevent toxicity.

• Monitor patient for adverse effects.

Information for the patient
• Instruct patient to continue taking drug despite nausea and vomiting.
• Tell patient to call immediately if vomiting occurs shortly after taking a dose.
• Explain that adequate fluid intake is important to facilitate excretion of uric acid.
• Instruct patient to avoid exposure to people with infections.
• Reassure patient that hair should grow back after treatment has ended.
• Tell patient to promptly report signs and symptoms of infection or bleeding.
• Advise woman of childbearing age to avoid becoming pregnant while receiving drug.

Breast-feeding patients
• It's unknown if drug appears in breast milk. However, because of risk of serious adverse reactions, mutagenicity, and carcinogenicity in infant, breast-feeding isn't recommended.

meningococcal polysaccharide vaccine
Menomune-A/C/Y/W-135

Pharmacologic classification: vaccine
Therapeutic classification: bacterial vaccine
Pregnancy risk category C

How supplied
Available by prescription only
Injection: a killed bacterial vaccine in single-dose, 10-dose, and 50-dose vials with vial of diluent

Indications, route, and dosage
Meningococcal meningitis prophylaxis
Adults and children over age 2: 0.5 ml S.C.

Pharmacodynamics
Meningitis prophylaxis: Promotes active immunity to meningitis caused by *Neisseria meningitidis.*

Pharmacokinetics
No information available.

Contraindications and precautions
Contraindicated in patients with hypersensitivity to thimerosal and in immunosuppressed and pregnant patients. Vaccination should be deferred in patients with acute illness.

Interactions
Drug-drug. *Immunosuppressants:* May reduce immune response to vaccine. Monitor patient.

Adverse reactions
CNS: headache, malaise.
Musculoskeletal: muscle cramps.
Skin: *pain, tenderness, erythema, and induration* at injection site.
Other: *anaphylaxis,* chills, fever.

☑ Special considerations
• Obtain thorough history of patient's allergies and reactions to immunizations.
• Don't give meningitis vaccine intradermally, I.M., or I.V.; safety and efficacy haven't been established.
• Have epinephrine solution 1:1,000 available to treat allergic reactions.
• Reconstitute vaccine with diluent provided. Shake until dissolved. Discard reconstituted solution after 5 days.
• Store vaccine between 36° and 46° F (2° and 8° C).
• Protective antibody levels may be achieved within 10 to 14 days after vaccination.

Monitoring the patient
• Monitor patient for sensitivity reaction to vaccine.
• Monitor patient for adverse effects.

Information for the patient
• Tell patient that pain and inflammation may occur at injection site. Recommend acetaminophen to alleviate adverse reactions such as fever.
• Encourage patient to report distressing adverse reactions.
• Explain that vaccine will provide immunity only to meningitis caused by one type of bacteria.
• Stress importance of avoiding pregnancy for 3 months after vaccination. Provide contraceptive information, if necessary.

Pediatric patients
• Vaccine isn't recommended for children under age 2.

Breast-feeding patients
• It's unknown if vaccine appears in breast milk. Use with caution in breast-feeding women.

menotropins
Humegon, Pergonal

Pharmacologic classification: gonadotropin
Therapeutic classification: ovulation stimulant, spermatogenesis stimulant
Pregnancy risk category X

How supplied
Available by prescription only
Injection: 75 IU of luteinizing hormone (LH) and 75 IU of follicle-stimulating hormone (FSH) ac-

tivity per ampule; 150 IU of LH and 150 IU of FSH activity per ampule

Indications, route, and dosage
Production of follicular maturation
Adults: 75 IU each of FSH and LH I.M. daily for 7 to 12 days, then 5,000 to 10,000 USP units human chorionic gonadotropin (HCG) I.M. 1 day after last dose of menotropins; repeat for two more menstrual cycles. Then, if ovulation or follicular development doesn't occur, increase to 150 IU each of FSH and LH I.M. daily for 7 to 12 days, then 5,000 to 10,000 USP units HCG I.M. 1 day after last dose of menotropins; repeat for two menstrual cycles.
Stimulation of spermatogenesis
Adults: After 4 to 6 months of treatment with HCG, 1 ampule (75 IU FSH/LH) I.M. three times weekly (given with 2,000 USP units HCG twice weekly) for at least 4 months. If no improvement occurs after 4 months, treatment may continue with 75 IU FSH/LH three times weekly or 150 IU FSH/LH three times weekly.

Pharmacodynamics
Ovulation stimulant action: Causes growth and maturation of the ovarian follicle in women who don't have primary ovarian failure by mimicking the action of endogenous LH and FSH. Additional treatment with HCG is usually needed to achieve ovulation.
Spermatogenesis stimulant action: Causes spermatogenesis when administered with HCG in men with primary or secondary pituitary hypofunction.

Pharmacokinetics
● *Absorption:* Must be administered parenterally for effectiveness.
● *Distribution:* No information available.
● *Metabolism:* Not fully known.
● *Excretion:* Excreted in urine.

Contraindications and precautions
Contraindicated in patients with hypersensitivity to drug; in women with primary ovarian failure, uncontrolled thyroid or adrenal dysfunction, pituitary tumor, abnormal uterine bleeding, uterine fibromas, or ovarian cysts or enlargement; in pregnant women; and in men with normal pituitary function, primary testicular failure, or infertility disorders other than hypogonadotropic hypogonadism.

Interactions
None reported.

Adverse reactions
CNS: headache, malaise, dizziness.
CV: *stroke,* tachycardia.
GI: nausea, vomiting, diarrhea, abdominal cramps, bloating.

GU: *ovarian enlargement with pain and abdominal distention, ovarian hyperstimulation syndrome* (sudden severe abdominal pain, distention, nausea, vomiting, weight gain, and dyspnea, then hypovolemia, hemoconcentration, electrolyte imbalance, pleural effusion, ascites, and hemoperitoneum), gynecomastia, ovarian cysts.
Musculoskeletal: musculoskeletal aches, joint pains.
Respiratory: *atelectasis, acute respiratory distress syndrome, pulmonary embolism, pulmonary infarction, arterial occlusion,* dyspnea, tachypnea.
Skin: rash.
Other: fever, multiple births, ectopic pregnancy, *hypersensitivity and anaphylactic reactions,* chills.

☑ Special considerations
● Drug is administered by I.M. route only.
● Reconstitute drug with 1 to 2 ml of sterile saline injection. Use immediately.
● Pregnancies that follow ovulation induced with menotropins show a relatively high frequency of multiple births.

Monitoring the patient
● Monitor patient for adverse effects from drug therapy.
● Patient should be examined at least every other day for signs of excessive ovarian stimulation during therapy and for 2 weeks after treatment ends.

Information for the patient
● Teach patient signs and tests that indicate time of ovulation, such as increase in basal body temperature and increase in appearance and volume of cervical mucus.
● Warn patient to immediately report symptoms of ovarian hyperstimulation syndrome, such as abdominal distention and pain, dyspnea, and vaginal bleeding.
● Warn patient that multiple births are possible. Ectopic pregnancy and congenital malformations have been reported in pregnancies following treatment.
● Encourage daily intercourse from day before HCG is given until ovulation occurs.

Breast-feeding patients
● Drug isn't indicated for use in breast-feeding women.

meperidine hydrochloride
(pethidine hydrochloride)
Demerol

Pharmacologic classification: opioid
Therapeutic classification: analgesic,
adjunct to anesthesia
Controlled substance schedule II
Pregnancy risk category C

How supplied
Available by prescription only
Tablets: 50 mg, 100 mg
Liquid: 50 mg/5 ml
Injection: 10 mg/ml, 25 mg/ml, 50 mg/ml, 75
mg/ml, 100 mg/ml

Indications, route, and dosage
Moderate to severe pain
Adults: 50 to 150 mg P.O., I.M., I.V., or S.C. q 3
to 4 hours.
Children: 1 to 1.8 mg/kg P.O., I.M., I.V., or S.C.
q 3 to 4 hours or 175 mg/m^2 daily in six divided
doses. Maximum single dose for children should
be no more than 100 mg.
Preoperatively
Adults: 50 to 100 mg I.M., I.V., or S.C. 30 to 90
minutes before surgery.
Children: 1 to 2 mg/kg I.M., I.V., or S.C. 30 to 90
minutes before surgery. Don't exceed adult dose.
Support of anesthesia
Adults: Repeated slow I.V. injections of fractional doses (10 mg/ml) or continuous I.V. infusion of
1 mg/ml. Dose should be titrated to meet patient's
needs.
Obstetric analgesia
Adults: 50 to 100 mg I.M. or S.C. when pain becomes regular; may repeat at 1- to 3-hour intervals.

Pharmacodynamics
Analgesic action: Narcotic agonist with actions
and potency similar to those of morphine, with
principal actions at the opiate receptors. Recommended for the relief of moderate to severe
pain.

Pharmacokinetics
• *Absorption:* Oral dose is only half as effective
as parenteral dose. Onset of analgesia occurs
within 10 to 45 minutes. Duration of action is 2 to
4 hours.
• *Distribution:* Distributed widely throughout body;
60% to 80% bound to plasma proteins.
• *Metabolism:* Primarily by hydrolysis in liver to
active metabolite, normeperidine.
• *Excretion:* About 30% of dose excreted in urine
as N-demethylated derivative; about 5% excreted unchanged. Excretion enhanced by acidifying urine. Half-life of parent compound is 3 to 5
hours; half-life of metabolite is 8 to 21 hours.

Contraindications and precautions
Contraindicated in patients with hypersensitivity
to drug and in those who have received MAO inhibitors within the past 14 days.
   Use cautiously in elderly or debilitated patients and in those with increased intracranial
pressure, head injury, asthma, other respiratory
conditions, supraventricular tachycardia, seizures,
acute abdominal conditions, renal or hepatic disease, hypothyroidism, Addison's disease, urethral stricture, or prostatic hyperplasia.

Interactions
Drug-drug. *Anticholinergics:* May cause paralytic ileus. Monitor closely.
Cimetidine, CNS depressants: Potentiated respiratory and CNS depression, sedation, and hypotensive effects of drug. Use together with extreme caution. Reduce meperidine dose.
General anesthetics: Possible severe CV depression. Use together with extreme caution. Reduce meperidine dose.
Isoniazid: Meperidine can potentiate adverse effects. Monitor patient closely.
MAO inhibitors: May precipitate unpredictable
and occasionally fatal reactions, even in patients
who may receive MAO inhibitors within 14 days
of receiving meperidine. Don't use together.
Narcotic antagonists: Patients physically dependent on drug may experience acute withdrawal
syndrome if given a narcotic antagonist. Monitor
patient closely.
Drug-herb. *Parsley:* May promote or produce
serotonin syndrome. Avoid concomitant use.
Drug-lifestyle. *Alcohol:* Potentiated respiratory
and CNS depression, sedation, and hypotensive
effects of drug. Discourage use.

Adverse reactions
CNS: *sedation, somnolence, clouded sensorium, euphoria, dizziness,* paradoxical excitement,
tremor, *seizures* (with large doses), headache,
hallucinations, syncope, *light-headedness.*
CV: *hypotension,* **bradycardia,** tachycardia, *cardiac arrest, shock.*
GI: *constipation,* ileus, dry mouth, *nausea, vomiting,* biliary tract spasms.
GU: urine retention.
Respiratory: *respiratory depression,* respiratory arrest.
Skin: pruritus, urticaria, *diaphoresis.*
Other: physical dependence, muscle twitching;
phlebitis (after I.V. delivery); pain at injection site;
local tissue irritation, induration (after S.C. injection), increased plasma amylase or lipase levels.

☑ Special considerations
Besides the recommendations relevant to all opioids, consider the following.
• Drug may be administered to some patients
who are allergic to morphine.

Reactions may be *common,* uncommon, **life-threatening,** or COMMON AND LIFE-THREATENING.

• Because drug toxicity commonly appears after several days of treatment, this drug isn't recommended for treatment of chronic pain.
• Meperidine may be given slowly through an I.V., preferably as a diluted solution. S.C. injection is very painful. During I.V. administration, tachycardia may occur, possibly as a result of drug's atropine-like effects.
• Oral dose is less than half as effective as parenteral dose. Give I.M. if possible. When changing from parenteral to oral route, dosage should be increased.
• Syrup has local anesthetic effect. Give with water.
• Alternating meperidine with a peripherally active nonopioid analgesic (aspirin, acetaminophen, NSAIDs) may improve pain control while allowing lower opioid dosages.
• Injectable meperidine is compatible with sodium chloride and D_5W solutions and their combinations, and with lactated Ringer's and sodium lactate solutions.
• The most common signs and symptoms of overdose are CNS depression, respiratory depression, skeletal muscle flaccidity, cold and clammy skin, mydriasis, bradycardia, and hypotension. If recent oral overdose (within 2 hours of ingestion), empty stomach immediately by inducing emesis (ipecac syrup) or using gastric lavage. Administer activated charcoal via nasogastric tube for further drug removal, and acidify urine to also remove drug.

Monitoring the patient
• Monitor patient for neurotoxic effects, especially in burn patients and those with poor renal function, sickle cell anemia, or cancer.
• Monitor vital signs closely, especially respiratory and CV status.

Information for the patient
• Instruct patient to ask for or take drug before pain becomes intense.
• Tell patient to take oral drug with food if GI upset occurs.
• Warn patient of CNS effects.

Geriatric patients
• Lower doses are usually indicated for elderly patients; they may be more sensitive to therapeutic and adverse effects of drug.

Pediatric patients
• Don't administer to infants under age 6 months.

Breast-feeding patients
• Drug appears in breast milk; use with caution in breast-feeding women.

mephenytoin
Mesantoin

Pharmacologic classification: hydantoin derivative
Therapeutic classification: anticonvulsant
Pregnancy risk category NR

How supplied
Available by prescription only
Tablets: 100 mg

Indications, route, and dosage
Generalized tonic-clonic or complex-partial seizures
Adults: 50 to 100 mg P.O. daily; may increase by 50 to 100 mg at weekly intervals, up to 200 mg P.O. q 8 hours. Doses up to 800 mg/day may be required.
Children: Initial dose is 50 to 100 mg P.O. daily. May increase slowly by 50 to 100 mg at weekly intervals up to 200 mg P.O. t.i.d., divided q 8 hours. Dosage must be adjusted individually. Usual maintenance dose is 100 to 400 mg/day (or 3 to 15 mg/kg/day or 100 to 450 mg/m²/day) administered in three equally divided doses.

Pharmacodynamics
Anticonvulsant action: Like other hydantoin derivatives, mephenytoin stabilizes the neuronal membranes and limits seizure activity by either increasing efflux or decreasing influx of sodium ions across cell membranes in the motor cortex during generation of nerve impulses. Like phenytoin, mephenytoin appears to have antiarrhythmic effects.
Mephenytoin is used for prophylaxis of tonic-clonic (grand mal), psychomotor, focal, and Jacksonian-type partial seizures in patients refractory to less toxic drugs. It's usually combined with phenytoin, phenobarbital, or primidone; phenytoin is preferred because it causes less sedation than barbiturates. Mephenytoin also is used with succinimides to control combined absence and tonic-clonic disorders; combined use with oxazolidinediones, paramethadione, or trimethadione isn't recommended because of the increased hazard of blood dyscrasias.

Pharmacokinetics
• *Absorption:* Absorbed from GI tract. Onset of action occurs in 30 minutes; lasts for 24 to 48 hours.
• *Distribution:* Distributed widely throughout body; good seizure control without toxicity occurs when serum levels of drug and major metabolite reach 25 to 40 mcg/ml.
• *Metabolism:* Metabolized by liver.
• *Excretion:* Drug and metabolites excreted in urine.

Contraindications and precautions
Contraindicated in patients with hydantoin hypersensitivity.

Interactions
Drug-drug. *Antihistamines, chloramphenicol, cimetidine, diazepam, diazoxide, disulfiram, isoniazid, oral anticoagulants, phenylbutazone, salicylates, sulfamethizole, valproate:* Mephenytoin's therapeutic effects and toxicity may be increased by concurrent use. Use together cautiously.
Folic acid: Mephenytoin's therapeutic effects may be decreased by concomitant use. Monitor patient closely.
Oral contraceptives: Possible decreased effects of oral contraceptives. Advise patient to use additional form of birth control.
Drug-lifestyle. *Alcohol:* May reduce drug's therapeutic effects. Avoid use together.

Adverse reactions
CNS: ataxia, *drowsiness,* fatigue, irritability, choreiform movements, depression, tremor, insomnia, dizziness (usually transient).
EENT: conjunctivitis, diplopia, nystagmus, gingival hyperplasia (with prolonged use).
GI: nausea and vomiting (with prolonged use).
Hematologic: *leukopenia, neutropenia, agranulocytosis, thrombocytopenia,* eosinophilia, leukocytosis.
Hepatic: elevated liver function test results.
Respiratory: *pulmonary fibrosis.*
Skin: rash, *exfoliative dermatitis, Stevens-Johnson syndrome, fatal dermatitides.*
Other: edema, lymphadenopathy, polyarthropathy.

☑ Special considerations
Besides the recommendations relevant to all hydantoin derivatives, consider the following.
● Decreased alertness and coordination are most pronounced at start of treatment. Patient may need help with walking and other activities for first few days.
● Drug shouldn't be stopped abruptly. Transition from mephenytoin to other anticonvulsant should progress over 6 weeks.
● Safe use of mephenytoin during pregnancy hasn't been established. Drug should be used during pregnancy only when clearly needed.
● Signs and symptoms of acute mephenytoin toxicity may include restlessness, dizziness, drowsiness, nausea, vomiting, nystagmus, ataxia, dysarthria, tremor, and slurred speech; hypotension, respiratory depression, and coma may follow. Treat overdose with gastric lavage or emesis and then give supportive treatment.

Monitoring the patient
● Carefully monitor vital signs and fluid and electrolyte balance.

● CBC and platelet counts should be performed before therapy, after 2 weeks of initial therapy, and after 2 weeks on maintenance dose; repeat tests every month for 1 year and, subsequently, at 3-month intervals.

Information for the patient
● Tell patient never to stop drug or change dosage except as prescribed and to avoid alcohol, which decreases effectiveness of drug and increases sedative effects.
● Explain that follow-up laboratory tests are essential for safe use.
● Instruct patient to report unusual changes immediately (cutaneous reaction, sore throat, glandular swelling, fever, mucous membrane swelling).

Pediatric patients
● Children usually need from 100 to 400 mg/day.

Breast-feeding patients
● Safe use in breast-feeding hasn't been established. Alternative to breast-feeding is recommended during therapy. Drug may appear in breast milk.

meprobamate
Apo-Meprobamate*, Equanil, Meprospan, Miltown, Neuramate

Pharmacologic classification: carbamate
Therapeutic classification: anxiolytic
Controlled substance schedule IV
Pregnancy risk category D

How supplied
Available by prescription only
Tablets: 200 mg, 400 mg, 600 mg
Capsules (sustained-release): 200 mg, 400 mg

Indications, route, and dosage
Anxiety, tension
Adults: 1.2 to 1.6 g P.O. daily in three or four equally divided doses. Maximum dose 2.4 g daily (sustained-release capsules, 400 to 800 mg b.i.d.).
Children ages 6 to 12: 100 to 200 mg P.O. b.i.d. or t.i.d. Not recommended for children under age 6 (sustained-release capsules, 200 mg b.i.d.).

Pharmacodynamics
Anxiolytic action: Cellular mechanism unknown. Causes nonselective CNS depression similar to that seen with barbiturates. Acts at several sites in the CNS, including the thalamus, hypothalamus, limbic system, and spinal cord, but not the medulla or reticular activating system.

Pharmacokinetics
● *Absorption:* Well absorbed after oral administration; serum levels peak in 1 to 3 hours. Sedation usually occurs within 1 hour.

• *Distribution:* Distributed throughout body; 20% is protein-bound. Excreted in breast milk at two to four times the serum level; drug crosses placenta.
• *Metabolism:* Metabolized rapidly in liver to inactive glucuronide conjugates. Half-life of drug is 6 to 17 hours.
• *Excretion:* Drug metabolites and 10% to 20% of single dose as unchanged drug are excreted in urine.

Contraindications and precautions
Contraindicated in patients with hypersensitivity to drug or related compounds (such as carisoprodol, mebutamate, tybamate, and carbromal) and in those with porphyria. Avoid drug during first trimester of pregnancy.

Use cautiously in elderly or debilitated patients and in those with impaired renal or hepatic function, seizure disorders, or suicidal tendencies.

Interactions
Drug-drug. *Antihistamines, barbiturates, narcotics, tranquilizers, other CNS depressants:* May add to or potentiate effects of these drugs. Avoid concomitant use.
Drug-lifestyle. *Alcohol:* May add to or potentiate effects of alcohol. Discourage use.

Adverse reactions
CNS: drowsiness, ataxia, dizziness, slurred speech, headache, syncope, vertigo, **seizures.**
CV: palpitations, tachycardia, hypotension, **arrhythmias.**
GI: nausea, vomiting, diarrhea.
Hematologic: aplastic anemia, thrombocytopenia, agranulocytosis.
Skin: pruritus, urticaria, erythematous maculopapular rash, **hypersensitivity reactions.**

After abrupt withdrawal of long-term therapy: severe generalized tonic-clonic seizures.

☑ Special considerations
• Serum levels above 100 mcg/ml may be fatal.
• Impose safety precautions, such as raised bed rails. Patient may need assistance when walking.
• Drug abuse and addiction may occur.
• Drug therapy may falsely elevate urinary 17-ketosteroids, 17-ketogenic steroids (as determined by the Zimmerman reaction), and 17-hydroxycorticosteroid levels (as determined by the Glenn-Nelson technique).
• Signs and symptoms of overdose include drowsiness, lethargy, ataxia, coma, hypotension, shock, and respiratory depression. Treatment is supportive and symptomatic.

Monitoring the patient
• Assess level of consciousness and vital signs frequently.
• Periodic evaluation of CBC is recommended during long-term therapy.

Information for the patient
• Advise patient not to increase dose or frequency and not to abruptly stop or decrease dose unless prescribed.
• Tell patient to avoid tasks that require mental alertness or physical coordination until drug's CNS effects are known.
• Recommend sugarless candy or gum or ice chips to relieve dry mouth.
• Advise patient to report sore throat, fever, or unusual bleeding or bruising.

Geriatric patients
• Elderly patients may have more pronounced CNS effects. Use lowest dose possible.

Pediatric patients
• Safety hasn't been established in children under age 6.

Breast-feeding patients
• Drug appears in breast milk at two to four times the serum level. Don't use in breast-feeding women.

mercaptopurine (6-MP)
Purinethol

Pharmacologic classification: antimetabolite (cell cycle–phase specific, S phase)
Therapeutic classification: antineoplastic
Pregnancy risk category D

How supplied
Available by prescription only
Tablets (scored): 50 mg

Indications, route, and dosage
Dosage and indications may vary. Check current literature for recommended protocols.
Acute lymphoblastic leukemia (in children), acute myeloblastic leukemia, chronic myelocytic leukemia
Adults: 2.5 mg/kg P.O. daily as a single dose, up to 5 mg/kg daily. Maintenance dose 1.5 to 2.5 mg/kg daily.
Children ages 5 and over: 2.5 mg/kg P.O. daily. Maintenance dose 1.5 to 2.5 mg/kg daily.
◇ **Regional enteritis (Crohn's disease) and ulcerative colitis**
Adults: Usual dose is 1.5 mg/kg/day, gradually increased to 2.5 mg/kg/day if tolerated.

Pharmacodynamics
Antineoplastic action: Converted intracellularly to its active form, which exerts its cytotoxic antimetabolic effects by competing for an enzyme required for purine synthesis. This results in inhibition of DNA and RNA synthesis. Cross-

resistance exists between mercaptopurine and thioguanine.

Pharmacokinetics
• *Absorption:* Incomplete and variable absorption after oral dose; about 50% of dose is absorbed. Serum levels peak 2 hours after a dose.
• *Distribution:* Distributed widely into total body water. Crosses blood-brain barrier, but CSF level is too low for treatment of meningeal leukemias.
• *Metabolism:* Extensively metabolized in liver. Appears to undergo extensive first-pass metabolism, contributing to its low bioavailability.
• *Excretion:* Drug and metabolites excreted in urine.

Contraindications and precautions
Contraindicated in patients whose disease has shown resistance to drug. Use cautiously after chemotherapy or radiation therapy in patients with depressed neutrophil or platelet counts and in those with impaired renal or hepatic function.

Interactions
Drug-drug. *Allopurinol:* Increased toxic effects of mercaptopurine, especially myelosuppression. Reduce dosage of drug to 25% to 30% when giving with allopurinol.
Hepatotoxic drugs: Increased potential for hepatotoxicity. Avoid concomitant use.
Trimethoprim-sulfamethoxazole: Possible enhanced marrow suppression. Monitor blood counts carefully.
Warfarin: Decreased anticoagulant activity. Monitor PT and INR.
Drug-lifestyle. *Alcohol:* Enhanced risk of hepatotoxicity. Discourage alcohol use.

Adverse reactions
GI: *nausea, vomiting, anorexia, painful oral ulcers, diarrhea, **pancreatitis**, GI ulceration.*
Hematologic: *leukopenia, thrombocytopenia,* anemia (all may persist several days after drug is stopped).
Hepatic: *jaundice, **hepatotoxicity.***
Skin: *rash, hyperpigmentation.*
Other: *hyperuricemia.*

☑ Special considerations
• Drug is sometimes called 6-mercaptopurine or 6-MP.
• Store tablets at room temperature and protect from light.
• Dose modifications may be required following chemotherapy or radiation therapy, in patients with depressed neutrophil or platelet count, and in patients with impaired hepatic or renal function.
• Hepatic dysfunction is reversible when drug is stopped. Watch for jaundice, clay-colored stools, and frothy dark urine. Drug should be stopped if hepatic tenderness occurs.

• Avoid all I.M. injections when platelet count is below 100,000/mm³.
• Advise woman of childbearing age not to become pregnant while receiving drug.

Monitoring the patient
• Monitor weekly blood counts; watch for precipitous fall.
• Monitor intake and output. Push fluids (3 qt [3 L]/day). Watch for nausea and vomiting.
• Monitor hepatic function and hematologic values weekly during therapy.
• Monitor serum uric acid levels. If allopurinol is necessary, use very cautiously.
• Observe for signs and symptoms of bleeding and infection.

Information for the patient
• Warn patient that improvement may take 2 to 4 weeks or longer.
• Tell patient to continue drug despite nausea and vomiting.
• Instruct patient to call immediately if vomiting occurs shortly after taking a dose.
• Warn patient to avoid alcoholic beverages while taking drug.
• Urge patient to ensure adequate fluid intake to increase urine output and facilitate excretion of uric acid.
• Advise patient to avoid exposure to people with infections. Tell patient to call immediately if signs and symptoms of unusual bleeding or infection occur.

Pediatric patients
• Adverse GI reactions are less common in children than in adults.

Breast-feeding patients
• It's unknown if drug appears in breast milk. However, because of potential for serious adverse reactions, mutagenicity, and carcinogenicity in infant, breast-feeding isn't recommended.

meropenem
Merrem I.V.

Pharmacologic classification: carbapenem derivative
Therapeutic classification: antibiotic
Pregnancy risk category B

How supplied
Available by prescription only
Powder for injection: 500 mg/15 ml, 500 mg/20 ml, 500 mg/100 ml, 1 g/15 ml, 1 g/30 ml, 1 g/100 ml

Indications, route, and dosage
Complicated appendicitis and peritonitis caused by viridans group streptococci, Es-

---

cherichia coli, Klebsiella pneumoniae, Pseudomonas aeruginosa, Bacteroides fragilis, B. thetaiotaomicron, *and* Peptostreptococcus sp.; *bacterial meningitis caused by* Streptococcus pneumoniae, Haemophilus influenzae, *and* Neisseria meningitidis
Note: Recommended concentration not to exceed 50 mg/ml.
Adults: Administer 1 g I.V. q 8 hours over 15 to 30 minutes as I.V. infusion or over about 3 to 5 minutes as I.V. bolus injection (5 to 20 ml). Dose shouldn't exceed 2 g every 8 hours.
Children ages 3 months and older: Give 20 mg/kg (intra-abdominal infection) or 40 mg/kg (bacterial meningitis) q 8 hours over 15 to 30 minutes as I.V. infusion or over about 3 to 5 minutes as I.V. bolus injection (5 to 20 ml).
Note: For children weighing over 50 kg (110 lb) give 1 g q 8 hours for treatment of intra-abdominal infections and 2 g q 8 hours for treatment of meningitis. Maximum dose is 2 g every 8 hours.
✦ *Dosage adjustment.* In adults with renal failure, give 1 g q 12 hours if creatinine clearance is 26 to 50 ml/minute, 500 mg q 12 hours if it's 10 to 25 ml/minute, and 500 mg q 24 hours if it's below 10 ml/minute. There is no clinical experience in children with renal impairment.

Pharmacodynamics
Antibiotic action: Inhibits cell-wall synthesis in bacteria. Readily penetrates the cell wall of most gram-positive and gram-negative bacteria to reach penicillin-binding protein targets.

Pharmacokinetics
- *Absorption:* Only given I.V.
- *Distribution:* Distributed into most body fluids and tissues, including CSF. Only about 2% bound to plasma protein.
- *Metabolism:* Possible minimal metabolism. One inactive metabolite identified.
- *Excretion:* Excreted unchanged primarily in urine. Elimination half-life in adults with normal renal function and children ages 2 and older is about 1 hour; 1½ hours in children ages 3 months to 2 years.

Contraindications and precautions
Contraindicated in patients with hypersensitivity to drug, its components, or other drugs in the same class and in those who have demonstrated anaphylactic reactions to beta-lactams. Use cautiously in patients with history of seizure disorders or impaired renal function.

Interactions
Drug-drug. *Probenecid:* Inhibited renal excretion of meropenem; significantly increased elimination half-life of meropenem and extent of systemic exposure. Avoid use together.

Adverse reactions
CNS: headache, syncope, insomnia, agitation, delirium, confusion, dizziness, *seizure,* nervousness, paresthesia, hallucinations, somnolence, anxiety, depression.
CV: *heart failure, cardiac arrest, MI, pulmonary embolism,* tachycardia, chest pain, hypertension, *bradycardia,* hypotension.
GI: diarrhea, nausea, vomiting, constipation, abdominal pain or enlargement, oral candidiasis, anorexia, flatulence.
GU: dysuria, *kidney failure,* increased creatinine clearance or BUN levels, presence of RBCs in urine.
Hematologic: anemia, increased or decreased platelet count, increased eosinophil count, prolonged or shortened PT and INR or partial thromboplastin time, positive direct or indirect Coombs' test, decreased hemoglobin or hematocrit, decreased WBC count.
Hepatic: *hepatic failure,* cholestatic jaundice, jaundice, ileus, increased levels of ALT, AST, alkaline phosphatase, LD, and bilirubin.
Musculoskeletal: back pain.
Respiratory: *apnea, hypoxia,* respiratory disorder, dyspnea.
Skin: rash, pruritus, urticaria, sweating.
Other: *hypersensitivity and anaphylactic reactions;* inflammation, pain, edema, phlebitis, or thrombophlebitis at injection site; bleeding events, pain, *sepsis, shock,* fever, peripheral edema.

☑ Special considerations
- Don't use to treat methicillin-resistant staphylococci.
- Obtain specimen for culture and sensitivity tests before giving first dose. Therapy may begin pending test results.
- For I.V. bolus administration, add 10 ml of sterile water for injection to 500 mg/20 ml vial size or 20 ml to 1 g/30 ml vial size. Shake to dissolve and let stand until clear.
- For I.V. infusion, infusion vials (500 mg/100 ml and 1 g/100 ml) may be directly reconstituted with a compatible infusion fluid. Or an injection vial may be reconstituted, then the resulting solution added to an I.V. container and further diluted with an appropriate infusion fluid. ADD-Vantage vials shouldn't be used.
- For ADD-Vantage vials, reconstitute only with half 0.45% saline injection, normal saline injection, or 5% dextrose injection in 50-, 100-, or 250-ml Abbott ADD-Vantage flexible diluent containers. Follow manufacturer guidelines closely when using ADD-Vantage vials.
- Don't mix with or physically add meropenem to solutions containing other drugs.
- Use freshly prepared solutions of meropenem immediately whenever possible. Stability of drug varies with type of drug used (injection vial, infusion vial, or ADD-Vantage container). Consult manufacturer's literature for details.

• Meropenem and its metabolite are readily dialyzable and effectively removed by hemodialysis.
• Serious and occasionally fatal hypersensitivity (anaphylactic) reactions have been reported in patients receiving therapy with beta-lactams. Before therapy is initiated, ascertain if previous hypersensitivity reactions to penicillins, cephalosporins, other beta-lactams, and other allergens have occurred.
• Stop drug immediately if allergic reaction occurs. Serious anaphylactic reactions require immediate emergency treatment with epinephrine, oxygen, I.V. corticosteroids, and airway management. Other therapy also may be needed as indicated by the patient's condition.
• Seizures and other CNS adverse reactions associated with meropenem therapy commonly occur in patients with CNS disorders, bacterial meningitis, and compromised renal function.
• If seizures occur during meropenem therapy, decrease dosage or stop drug.

Monitoring the patient
• Drug may cause overgrowth of nonsusceptible bacteria or fungi. Monitor patient for signs and symptoms of superinfection.
• Periodic assessment of organ system functions, including renal, hepatic, and hematopoietic, is recommended during prolonged therapy.
• Monitor vital signs closely.

Information for the patient
• Instruct patient to report adverse effects immediately.

Geriatric patients
• Use cautiously in elderly patients because of decreased renal function. Dosage adjustment is recommended in patients of advanced age whose creatinine clearance level is below 50 ml/minute.

Pediatric patients
• Safety and effectiveness haven't been established for children under age 3 months.

Breast-feeding patients
• It's unknown if drug appears in breast milk; use cautiously in breast-feeding women.

mesalamine
(5-aminosalicylic acid)
Asacol, Pentasa, Rowasa

Pharmacologic classification: salicylate
Therapeutic classification: anti-inflammatory
Pregnancy risk category B

How supplied
Available by prescription only
Capsules (controlled-release): 250 mg

Tablets (delayed-release): 400 mg
Suppositories: 500 mg
Rectal suspension: 4 g/60 ml, in units of 7 disposable bottles

Indications, route, and dosage
Active mild to moderate distal ulcerative colitis, proctosigmoiditis, proctitis
Adults: 800 mg (delayed-release tablets) P.O. t.i.d. for 6 weeks or 1 g (controlled-release capsules) q.i.d. for up to 8 weeks.

Or use 1 rectal suppository b.i.d. for 3 to 6 weeks. For maximum benefit, the suppository should be retained for 1 to 3 hours or longer. Usual dosage of mesalamine suspension enema in 60-ml units is one rectal instillation (4 g) once daily, preferably h.s., retained for about 8 hours.
   ◊ Lower doses of suspension enemas of 4 g q 2 to 3 nights or 1 g daily have been effective.

Pharmacodynamics
Anti-inflammatory action: Mechanism of action of mesalamine (and sulfasalazine) unknown, but appears to be topical rather than systemic. Mucosal production of arachidonic acid metabolites, both through cyclooxygenase pathways (such as prostaglandins) and through lipoxygenase pathways (such as leukotrienes and hydroxyeicosatetraenoic acids) is increased in patients with chronic inflammatory bowel disease; possibly, mesalamine may diminish inflammation by blocking cyclooxygenase and inhibiting prostaglandin production in the colon.

Sulfasalazine is split by bacterial action in the colon into sulfapyridine and mesalamine. The mesalamine component is considered therapeutically active in ulcerative colitis.

Pharmacokinetics
• *Absorption:* Poorly absorbed from colon when given rectally as a suppository or suspension enema. Extent of absorption depends on retention time, with considerable individual variation. Oral tablets coated with acrylic resin that delays drug release until tablet is beyond terminal ileum. About 72% of dose reaches colon; 28% is absorbed. Absorption not affected by food. Capsules formulated to release therapeutic levels throughout GI tract. About 20% to 30% absorbed.
• *Distribution:* Maximum plasma levels of oral mesalamine and N-acetyl 5-aminosalicylic acid are about twice as high as those seen with sulfasalazine therapy. At steady-state, about 10% to 30% of daily 4-g rectal dose recovered in cumulative 24-hour urine collections.
• *Metabolism:* Undergoes acetylation, but site is unknown. Most absorbed drug excreted in urine as N-acetyl-5-aminosalicylic acid metabolite. Elimination half-life of drug is $\frac{1}{2}$ to $1\frac{1}{2}$ hours; half-life of acetylated metabolite is 5 to 10 hours. Steady-state plasma levels show no accumulation of ei-

ther free or metabolized drug during repeated daily administrations.
• *Excretion:* After rectal administration, drug mostly excreted in feces as parent drug and metabolite. After oral administration, mostly excreted in urine as metabolite.

Contraindications and precautions
Contraindicated in patients with hypersensitivity to drug, its components (sulfite in rectal preparation), or salicylates. Use cautiously in patients with impaired renal function.

Interactions
Drug-drug. *Lactulose:* May impair release of delayed or extended-release preparations. Monitor patient closely.
Omeprazole: Increased absorption of mesalamine. Monitor patient closely.

Adverse reactions
CNS: headache, dizziness, fatigue, malaise, asthenia, chills, anxiety, depression, hyperesthesia, paresthesia, tremor.
CV: chest pain.
GI: abdominal pain, cramps, discomfort, flatulence, diarrhea, rectal pain, bloating, nausea, *pancolitis,* **pancreatitis,** vomiting, constipation, eructation.
GU: dysuria, hematuria, urinary urgency.
Musculoskeletal: arthralgia, myalgia, back pain.
Respiratory: wheezing.
Skin: itching, rash, urticaria, hair loss.
Other: fever, hypertonia.

☑ Special considerations
• Although drug's effects may be evident in 3 to 21 days, usual course of therapy is 3 to 6 weeks depending on symptoms and sigmoidoscopic findings. It's unknown if suspension enema will modify relapse rates after the 6-week, short-term treatment.

Monitoring the patient
• Monitor renal function studies periodically in patient on long-term therapy.
• Monitor patient for adverse effects.

Information for the patient
• Tell patient to swallow tablets whole and not to crush or chew them.
• Tell patient to retain suppository as long as possible (at least 1 to 3 hours) for maximum effectiveness.
• Instruct patient as follows in correct use of rectal suspension:
– Shake bottle well to make sure suspension is homogeneous.
– Remove protective sheath from applicator tip. Holding bottle at neck won't cause medication to be discharged.

– To administer, lie on left side (to facilitate migration into sigmoid colon) with lower leg extended and the upper right leg flexed forward for balance; or may use the knee-chest position.
– Gently insert applicator tip in rectum, pointing toward umbilicus.
– Steadily squeeze bottle to discharge preparation into colon.
• Patient instructions are included with every 7 units.

Pediatric patients
• Safety and efficacy for use in children haven't been established.

Breast-feeding patients
• It's unknown if drug or metabolites appear in breast milk. Avoid breast-feeding during therapy.

mesna
Mesnex

Pharmacologic classification: thiol derivative
Therapeutic classification: uroprotectant
Pregnancy risk category B

How supplied
Available by prescription only
Injection: 100 mg/ml in 2- and 10-ml ampules

Indications, route, and dosage
Prevention of ifosfamide-induced hemorrhagic cystitis
Adults: Calculate daily dose as 60% of the ifosfamide dose. Administer in three equally divided bolus doses: Give first dose at time of ifosfamide injection. Subsequent doses are given at 4 and 8 hours following ifosfamide.
Protocols that use 1.2 g/m^2 ifosfamide would employ 240 mg/m^2 mesna at 0, 4, and 8 hours after ifosfamide.
◊ *Prophylaxis in bone marrow recipients receiving cyclophosphamides*
Adults: 60% to 160% of the cyclophosphamide daily dose given in three to five divided doses or by continuous infusion.

Pharmacodynamics
Uroprotectant action: Mesna disulfide is reduced to mesna in the kidney and reacts with the urotoxic metabolites of ifosfamide to detoxify the drug and protect the urinary system.

Pharmacokinetics
• *Absorption:* Administered I.V.
• *Distribution:* Remains in vascular compartment; isn't distributed through tissues.
• *Metabolism:* Rapidly metabolized to mesna disulfide, its only metabolite.

• *Excretion:* In kidneys, 33% of dose eliminated in urine in 24 hours; half-life of mesna and mesna disulfide are 0.36 and 1.17 hours, respectively.

Contraindications and precautions
Contraindicated in patients with hypersensitivity to mesna or thiol-containing compounds.

Interactions
Drug-drug. *Cisplatin:* Drugs are physically incompatible. Don't mix with mesna.

Adverse reactions
CNS: headache, fatigue.
CV: hypotension.
GI: soft stools, nausea, vomiting, diarrhea, dysgeusia.
Musculoskeletal: limb pain.
Other: allergy.
   Note: Because mesna is used with ifosfamide and other chemotherapeutic drugs, it's difficult to determine adverse reactions attributable solely to mesna.

☑ Special considerations
• Mesnex multidose vials may be stored and used for up to 8 days.
• Discard unused mesna from open ampules. It will form an inactive oxidation product (dimesna) upon exposure to oxygen.
• Dilute appropriate dose in 5% dextrose injection, normal saline solution injection, or lactated Ringer's injection to a level of 20 mg/ml. Once diluted, solution is stable for 24 hours at room temperature.
• Mesna is physically incompatible with cisplatin. Don't add mesna to cisplatin infusions.
• Mesna may produce a false-positive test for urinary ketones. A red-violet color will return to violet with the addition of glacial acetic acid.

Monitoring the patient
• Monitor patient for hematuria.
• Monitor BUN and creatinine levels and intake and output.

Information for the patient
• Instruct patient to report hematuria or allergy immediately.

Pediatric patients
• Safety in children hasn't been established.

Breast-feeding patients
• It's unknown if drug appears in breast milk. Drug isn't recommended during breast-feeding.

mesoridazine besylate
Serentil

Pharmacologic classification: phenothiazine (piperidine derivative)
Therapeutic classification: antipsychotic
Pregnancy risk category NR

How supplied
Available by prescription only
Tablets: 10 mg, 25 mg, 50 mg, 100 mg
Oral concentrate: 25 mg/ml (0.6% alcohol)
Injection: 25 mg/ml

Indications, route, and dosage
Psychoneurotic manifestations (anxiety)
Adults and children over age 12: 10 mg P.O. t.i.d. up to maximum of 150 mg/day.
Schizophrenia
Adults and children over age 12: Initially, 50 mg P.O. t.i.d. to maximum of 400 mg/day; or 25 mg I.M. repeated in 30 to 60 minutes, p.r.n., not to exceed 200 mg I.M. daily.
Alcoholism
Adults and children over age 12: 25 mg P.O. b.i.d., up to maximum of 200 mg/day.
Behavioral problems associated with chronic brain syndrome
Adults and children over age 12: 25 mg P.O. t.i.d., up to maximum of 300 mg/day.

Pharmacodynamics
Antipsychotic action: A metabolite of thioridazine thought to exert antipsychotic effects by postsynaptic blockade of CNS dopamine receptors, thereby inhibiting dopamine-mediated effects.
   Has other central and peripheral effects; produces both alpha and ganglionic blockade and counteracts histamine- and serotonin-mediated activity. Most prominent adverse reactions are antimuscarinic and sedative; causes fewer extrapyramidal effects than other antipsychotics.

Pharmacokinetics
• *Absorption:* Seemingly well absorbed from GI tract following oral administration. I.M. dosage form absorbed rapidly.
• *Distribution:* Distributed widely into body, including breast milk. Effects peak at 2 to 4 hours; steady-state serum level achieved within 4 to 7 days. Drug is 91% to 99% protein-bound.
• *Metabolism:* Metabolized extensively by liver; no active metabolites formed. Duration of action 4 to 6 hours.
• *Excretion:* Mostly excreted as metabolites in urine; some excreted in feces via biliary tract.

Contraindications and precautions
Contraindicated in patients with hypersensitivity to drug and in those experiencing severe CNS depression or comatose states.

Reactions may be *common*, uncommon, **life-threatening**, or COMMON AND LIFE-THREATENING.

Interactions

Drug-drug. *Antacids containing aluminum and magnesium, antidiarrheals, phenobarbital:* Decreased therapeutic response to mesoridazine. Monitor patient; separate administration times.
Antiarrhythmics, disopyramide, procainamide, quinidine: Increased risk of arrhythmias and conduction defect. Use with extreme caution.
Anticholinergics (such as antidepressants, antihistamines, antiparkinsonians, MAO inhibitors, meperidine, phenothiazines), atropine: Possible oversedation, paralytic ileus, visual changes, and severe constipation. Monitor patient closely.
Appetite suppressants, sympathomimetics (ephedrine, epinephrine, phenylephrine, phenylpropanolamine): May decrease stimulatory and pressor effects. Monitor patient closely.
Beta blockers: Increased mesoridazine plasma levels and risk of toxicity. Monitor patient closely.
Bromocriptine: Mesoridazine may antagonize therapeutic effect. Monitor patient.
Centrally acting antihypertensives (clonidine, guanabenz, guanadrel, guanethidine, methyldopa, reserpine): May inhibit blood pressure response to these drugs. Monitor blood pressure.
CNS depressants: Additive effects likely. Use together cautiously.
High-dose dopamine: Decreased vasoconstricting effects. Monitor patient closely.
Levodopa: Decreased effectiveness and increased toxicity of levodopa by dopamine blockade. Avoid concomitant use.
Lithium: Severe neurologic toxicity with encephalitis-like syndrome; decreased therapeutic response to mesoridazine. Avoid concomitant use.
Metrizamide: Increased risk of seizures. Use together cautiously.
Nitrates: Increased risk of hypotension. Monitor blood pressure.
Phenothiazines: Possible epinephrine reversal and hypotension when epinephrine is used as a pressor drug. Avoid concomitant use.
Phenytoin: Possible inhibited metabolism and increased phenytoin toxicity. Avoid concomitant use.
Propylthiouracil: Increased risk of agranulocytosis. Monitor blood counts.
Drug-food. *Caffeine:* Increased metabolism of drug. Advise patient to limit caffeine use.
Drug-lifestyle. *Alcohol:* Additive CNS effects. Discourage use.
Smoking: Increased metabolism of drug. Discourage use.
Sun exposure: Increased risk of photosensitivity reactions. Tell patient to take precautions.

Adverse reactions

CNS: extrapyramidal reactions, *tardive dyskinesia, sedation, drowsiness, tremor, rigidity, weakness, EEG changes, dizziness.*
CV: *hypotension, tachycardia, ECG changes.*
EENT: *ocular changes, blurred vision, retinitis pigmentosa, nasal congestion.*
GI: *dry mouth, constipation, nausea, vomiting.*
GU: *urine retention, menstrual irregularities, gynecomastia, inhibited ejaculation.*
Hematologic: **leukopenia, agranulocytosis, aplastic anemia,** eosinophilia, **thrombocytopenia.**
Hepatic: jaundice, abnormal liver function test results.
Metabolic: weight gain.
Skin: *mild photosensitivity, allergic reactions, pain at I.M. injection site, sterile abscess, rash.*
Other: *neuroleptic malignant syndrome.*
  After abrupt withdrawal of long-term therapy: gastritis, nausea, vomiting, dizziness, tremor, feeling of warmth or cold, diaphoresis, tachycardia, headache, insomnia.

☑ Special considerations

• Recommendations for administration of mesoridazine, for care and teaching of the patient during therapy, and for use in elderly and breast-feeding patients are the same as those for all phenothiazines.
• I.M. dosage form is irritating.
• Drug elevates tests for protein-bound iodine. Drug causes false-positive test results for urinary porphyrins, urobilinogen, amylase, and 5-hydroxyindoleacetic acid because of darkening of urine by metabolites; it also causes false-positive urine pregnancy test results using human chorionic gonadotropin.
• Symptoms of overdose include drowsiness, confusion, disorientation, agitation, coma, and death. Dryness of mouth, edema of glottis, laryngeal spasms, nasal congestion, blurred vision, vomiting, hyperpyrexia, dilated pupils, muscle rigidity, hyperactive reflexes, areflexia, stupor, CNS depression, and cardiac abnormalities may also occur.
• Treatment of overdose is symptomatic and supportive, including maintaining vital signs, airway, stable body temperature, and fluid and electrolyte balance.
• Don't induce vomiting; drug inhibits cough reflex, and aspiration may occur. Use gastric lavage, then activated charcoal and saline cathartics; dialysis isn't useful.

Monitoring the patient

• Monitor vital signs carefully.
• Monitor patient for CNS effects.
• Monitor bilirubin tests weekly during first month, and perform periodic CBC and liver function tests.
• Opthalmic exams should be done periodically.

Information for the patient

• Advise patient to change position slowly.
• Warn patient to avoid activities that require alertness until CNS effects are known.

Pediatric patients

• Drug isn't recommended for children under age 12.

metaproterenol sulfate
Alupent

Pharmacologic classification: adrenergic
Therapeutic classification: broncho-
dilator
Pregnancy risk category C

How supplied
Available by prescription only
Tablets: 10 mg, 20 mg
Syrup: 10 mg/5 ml
Aerosol inhaler: 0.65 mg/metered spray
Nebulizer inhaler: 0.4%, 0.6%, 5% solution

Indications, route, and dosage
**Bronchial asthma and reversible broncho-
spasm**
Oral
*Adults and children over age 9 or weighing over
27 kg (60 lb):* 20 mg P.O. t.i.d. or q.i.d.
Children ages 6 to 9 or weighing below 27 kg:
10 mg P.O. t.i.d. or q.i.d.
Inhalation
Adults and children ages 12 and older: Administered by metered aerosol, 2 or 3 inhalations, with
at least 2 minutes between inhalations; no more
than 12 inhalations in 24 hours. Administered by
hand-bulb nebulizer, 10 inhalations of an undiluted 5% solution, or administered by intermittent positive pressure breathing (IPPB), 0.3 ml
(range, 0.2 to 0.3 ml of a 5% solution diluted in
about 2.5 ml of a normal saline solution or 2.5 ml
of a 0.4% or 0.6% solution for nebulization).

Pharmacodynamics
Bronchodilator action: Relaxes bronchial smooth
muscle and peripheral vasculature by stimulating beta$_2$-adrenergic receptors, thus decreasing
airway resistance via bronchodilation. It has lesser effect on beta$_1$ receptors and has little or no
effect on alpha-adrenergic receptors. In high doses, it may cause CNS and cardiac stimulation,
resulting in tachycardia, hypertension, or tremors.

Pharmacokinetics
• *Absorption:* Well absorbed from GI tract. Onset of action occurs within 1 minute after oral inhalation, 5 to 30 minutes after nebulization, and
15 to 30 minutes after oral administration; peak
effects seen in about 1 hour. Duration of action
after oral inhalation is 1 to 4 hours after single
dose, 1 to 2½ hours after multiple doses; after
nebulization, 2 to 6 hours after single dose, 4 to
6 hours after repeated doses; after oral administration, 1 to 4 hours.
• *Distribution:* Widely distributed throughout body.
• *Metabolism:* Extensively metabolized on first
pass through liver.
• *Excretion:* Excreted in urine, mainly as glucuronic acid conjugates.

Contraindications and precautions
Contraindicated in patients with hypersensitivity
to drug or its components, during anesthesia with
cyclopropane or halogenated hydrocarbon general anesthetics, and in those with tachycardia
and arrhythmias associated with tachycardia, peripheral or mesenteric vascular thrombosis, profound hypoxia, or hypercapnia.
    Use cautiously in patients with hypertension,
hyperthyroidism, heart disease, diabetes, or cirrhosis and in those receiving cardiac glycosides.

Interactions
Drug-drug. *Beta blockers (such as propranolol):*
Antagonized bronchodilating effects of metaproterenol. Monitor patient closely if used together.
*Cardiac glycosides, general anesthetics (such
as chloroform, cyclopropane, halothane, trichloroethylene), levodopa, theophylline derivatives, thyroid hormones:* Possible increased potential for
cardiac effects, including severe ventricular tachycardia, arrhythmias, and coronary insufficiency.
Avoid concomitant use.
MAO inhibitors, tricyclic antidepressants: May
potentiate CV actions. Avoid concomitant use.
Sympathomimetics: Possible additive effects and
toxicity. Use together cautiously.
*Xanthines, other CNS stimulating drugs, other
sympathomimetics:* Increased CNS stimulation.
Use with caution.

Adverse reactions
CNS: *nervousness, weakness, drowsiness,
tremor, vertigo, headache.*
CV: *tachycardia, hypertension, palpitations;* **car-
diac arrest** (with excessive use).
GI: *vomiting, nausea, heartburn, dry mouth.*
Respiratory: paradoxical bronchiolar constric-
tion with excessive use, cough, dry and irritated
throat.
Skin: rash, hypersensitivity reactions.

☑ Special considerations
Besides the recommendations relevant to all
adrenergics, consider the following.
• Adverse reactions are dose-related and characteristic of sympathomimetics and may persist
a long time because of metaproterenol's long duration of action.
• Excessive or prolonged use may lead to decreased effectiveness.
• Avoid simultaneous administration of adrenocorticoid inhalation aerosol. Allow at least 5 minutes to lapse between using the two aerosols.
• Drug may reduce sensitivity of spirometry in diagnosis of asthma.
• Aerosol treatments may be used with oral tablet
dosing.

Reactions may be *common*, uncommon, *life-threatening*, or COMMON AND LIFE-THREATENING.

Monitoring the patient
• Monitor patient for signs and symptoms of toxic effects (nausea and vomiting, tremors, and arrhythmias).
• Monitor vital signs closely. Support CV status.

Information for the patient
• Instruct patient to use only as directed and to take no more than two inhalations at one time with 1- to 2-minute intervals between. Remind patient to save applicator; refills may be available.
• Tell patient to take missed dose if remembered within 1 hour. If beyond 1 hour, patient should skip dose and resume regular schedule. Patient shouldn't double dose.
• Tell patient to store drug away from heat and light, and out of children's reach.
• Inform patient to call immediately if no relief occurs or condition worsens.
• Warn patient to avoid simultaneous use of adrenocorticoid aerosol and to allow at least 5 minutes to lapse between using the two aerosols.
• Tell patient that he may experience bad taste in mouth after using oral inhaler.
• Instruct patient to shake container, exhale through nose as completely as possible, then administer aerosol while inhaling deeply through mouth, and hold breath for 10 seconds before exhaling slowly. Patient should wait 1 to 2 minutes before repeating inhalations.
• Tell patient that drug may have shorter duration of action after prolonged use. Advise patient to report failure to respond to usual dose.
• Warn patient not to increase dose or frequency unless prescribed; serious adverse reactions are possible.

Geriatric patients
• Elderly patients may be more sensitive to the therapeutic and adverse effects of drug.

Pediatric patients
• Oral inhalation in children under age 12 isn't recommended; safety and efficacy haven't been established. Safety and efficacy of oral preparations in children under age 6 haven't been established.

---

metaraminol bitartrate
Aramine

Pharmacologic classification: adrenergic
Therapeutic classification: vasopressor
Pregnancy risk category C

How supplied
Available by prescription only
Injection: 10 mg/ml parenteral

Indications, route, and dosage
Prevention of hypotension
Adults: 2 to 10 mg I.M. or S.C.
Children: 0.1 mg/kg or 3 mg/m² S.C. or I.M.
Hypotension in severe shock
Adults: 0.5 to 5 mg direct I.V.; then I.V. infusion. If necessary, mix 15 to 100 mg (up to 500 mg has been used) in 500 ml normal saline solution or D₅W; titrate infusion based on blood pressure response.
Children: 0.01 mg/kg or 0.3 mg/m² direct I.V.; then I.V. infusion, if necessary, of 0.4 mg/kg or 12 mg/m² diluted and titrated to maintain desired blood pressure.
◊ *Priapism*
Adults: 1 to 2 mg injected into corpus cavernosum of penis.

Pharmacodynamics
Vasopressor action: Acts predominantly by direct stimulation of alpha-adrenergic receptors, which constrict both capacitance and resistance blood vessels, resulting in increased total peripheral resistance; increased systolic and diastolic blood pressure; decreased blood flow to vital organs, skin, and skeletal muscle; and constriction of renal blood vessels, which reduces renal blood flow. Also has direct stimulating effect on beta₁ receptors of the heart, producing a positive inotropic response, and an indirect effect, releasing norepinephrine from its storage sites, which, with repeated use, may result in tachyphylaxis.
    Also acts as a weak or false neurotransmitter by replacing norepinephrine in sympathetic nerve endings. Main effects are vasoconstriction and cardiac stimulation. Doesn't usually cause CNS stimulation but may cause contraction of pregnant uterus and uterine blood vessels because of alpha-adrenergic effects.

Pharmacokinetics
• *Absorption:* Onset of action after I.M. injection occurs within 10 minutes; after I.V. injection, within 1 to 2 minutes; after S.C. injection, within 5 to 20 minutes. Pressor effects may persist 20 to 90 minutes, depending on route of administration and patient variability.
• *Distribution:* Not completely known.
• *Metabolism:* In vitro tests suggest that metaraminol isn't metabolized. Effects appear to be terminated by uptake of drug into tissues and by urinary excretion.
• *Excretion:* Excreted in urine; may be accelerated by acidifying urine.

Contraindications and precautions
Contraindicated in patients with hypersensitivity to drug and in those receiving anesthesia with cyclopropane and halogenated hydrocarbon anesthetics.
    Use cautiously in patients with cardiac or thyroid disease, hypertension, peripheral vascular

disease, cirrhosis, history of malaria, or sulfite sensitivity; in those receiving cardiac glycosides; and during pregnancy.

Interactions
Drug-drug. *Alpha blockers:* Pressor effects may be decreased (but not completely blocked). Monitor patient.

Atropine: Blocked reflex bradycardia caused by metaraminol and enhanced pressor response. Use with caution.

Beta blockers: Mutual inhibition of therapeutic effects with increased potential for hypertension, and excessive bradycardia with possible heart block. Avoid concomitant use.

Cardiac glycosides, general anesthetics, levodopa, maprotiline, thyroid hormones, other sympathomimetics: Increased cardiac effects may result when used concomitantly. Monitor patient closely.

Diuretics used as antihypertensives, guanadrel, guanethidine, rauwolfia alkaloids: May decrease hypotensive effects of these drugs. Avoid concomitant use.

Doxapram, ergot alkaloids, mazindol, methylphenidate, trimethaphan: Increased pressor effects. Monitor patient closely.

MAO inhibitors: Prolonged and intensified cardiac stimulant and vasopressor effects of these drugs. Don't give metaraminol until 14 days after MAO inhibitors have been stopped.

Drug-lifestyle. *Cocaine:* Increased risk of adverse effects. Advise against illegal drug use. Monitor patient closely.

Adverse reactions
CNS: apprehension, dizziness, headache, tremor.
CV: hypertension; hypotension; palpitations; *arrhythmias,* including sinus or *ventricular tachycardia; cardiac arrest.*
GI: nausea.
Skin: flushing, diaphoresis.
Other: abscess, necrosis, sloughing upon extravasation.

☑ Special considerations
Besides the recommendations relevant to all adrenergics, consider the following.
● Correct blood volume depletion before administration. Metaraminol isn't a substitute for blood, plasma, fluids, or electrolyte replacement.
● Determine any allergies to sulfites before administering drug (vials contain sodium bisulfite).
● Drug must be diluted before I.V. use. Preferred solutions for dilution are normal saline solution or dextrose 5% injection. Select injection site carefully. I.V. route is preferred, using large veins. Avoid extravasation. Monitor infusion rate; use of infusion-controlling device preferred. Withdraw drug gradually; recurrent hypotension may follow abrupt withdrawal.

● When administering I.M. or S.C, allow at least 10 minutes to elapse before administering additional doses because maximum effect isn't immediately apparent.
● To treat extravasation, infiltrate site promptly with 10 to 15 ml normal saline solution containing 5 to 10 mg phentolamine, using fine needle.
● Cumulative effect possible after prolonged use. Excessive vasopressor response may persist after drug is withdrawn.
● Keep emergency drugs on hand to reverse effect of metaraminol (atropine for reflex bradycardia, phentolamine for extravasation, and propranolol for tachyarrhythmias).
● Don't mix in bag or syringe with other drugs.

Monitoring the patient
● Monitor blood pressure and ECG.
● Monitor diabetic patients; insulin adjustments may be needed.
● Monitor fluid and electrolyte status.

Information for the patient
● Inform patient that he will need frequent assessment of vital signs.
● Tell patient to report adverse reactions.

Geriatric patients
● Elderly patients may be more sensitive to drug's effects.

Pediatric patients
● Because safety hasn't been fully established, use cautiously in children.

Breast-feeding patients
● It's unknown if drug appears in breast milk; use cautiously in breast-feeding patients.

metformin hydrochloride
Glucophage

Pharmacologic classification: biguanide
Therapeutic classification: antidiabetic
Pregnancy risk category B

How supplied
Available by prescription only
Tablets: 500 mg, 850 mg

Indications, route, and dosage
Adjunct to diet and exercise to lower blood glucose in patients with type 2 diabetes mellitus
Adults: Initially, give 500 mg P.O. b.i.d. with morning and evening meals or 850 mg P.O. once daily with morning meal. When 500-mg dose is used, increase dose by 500 mg weekly to maximum dose of 2,500 mg daily, p.r.n. When 850-mg dose is used, increase dose 850 mg every other week to maximum daily dose of 2,550 mg, p.r.n.

Reactions may be *common*, uncommon, **life-threatening**, or COMMON AND LIFE-THREATENING.

Pharmacodynamics

Antidiabetic action: Decreases hepatic glucose production and intestinal absorption of glucose and improves insulin sensitivity (increases peripheral glucose uptake and utilization).

Pharmacokinetics

● *Absorption:* Absorbed from GI tract; absolute bioavailability about 50% to 60%. Food decreases extent of and slightly delays absorption.
● *Distribution:* Negligibly bound to plasma proteins. It partitions into erythrocytes, most likely as a function of time.
● *Metabolism:* Not metabolized.
● *Excretion:* 90% excreted in urine. Elimination half-life in plasma is about 6¼ hours and 17½ hours in blood.

Contraindications and precautions

Contraindicated in patients with hypersensitivity to drug and in those with renal disease or metabolic acidosis. Drug should be temporarily withheld in patients undergoing radiologic studies involving parenteral administration of iodinated contrast materials because use of such products may result in acute renal dysfunction. Stop drug if patient develops a hypoxic state. Avoid use in patients with hepatic disease.

Use cautiously in elderly, debilitated, or malnourished patients and in those with adrenal or pituitary insufficiency because of increased susceptibility to developing hypoglycemia.

Interactions

Drug-drug. *Calcium channel blockers, corticosteroids, estrogens, isoniazid, nicotinic acid, oral contraceptives, phenothiazines, phenytoin, sympathomimetics, thiazides, thyroid drugs, other diuretics:* Possible hyperglycemia. Monitor patient's glycemic control. Metformin dosage may need to be increased.
Cationic drugs (such as amiloride, cimetidine, digoxin, morphine, procainamide, quinidine, quinine, ranitidine, triamterene, trimethoprim, vancomycin): Increased metformin plasma levels. Monitor blood glucose level.
Nifedipine: Increased metformin plasma levels. Monitor patient closely. Metformin dosage may need to be decreased.
Radiologic contrast dye: Possible acute renal failure. Withhold metformin for 24 hours before procedure.
Drug-lifestyle. *Alcohol:* Potentiated effects of drug. Discourage use.

Adverse reactions

GI: unpleasant or metallic taste, diarrhea, nausea, vomiting, abdominal bloating, flatulence, anorexia.
Hematologic: *megaloblastic anemia.*
Skin: rash, dermatitis.
Other: *lactic acidosis.*

☑ Special considerations

● Assess patient's renal function before beginning therapy and annually thereafter. If renal impairment is detected, give another antidiabetic.
● Administer drug with meals; once-daily dose should be given with breakfast, twice-daily dose should be given with breakfast and dinner.
● When transferring patients from standard oral hypoglycemics other than chlorpropamide to metformin, no transition period is necessary. When transferring patients from chlorpropamide, exercise care during the first 2 weeks because of prolonged retention of chlorpropamide in the body, increasing risk of hypoglycemia during this time.
● Risk of drug-induced lactic acidosis is very low. Reported cases have occurred primarily in diabetic patients with significant renal insufficiency, multiple concomitant medical or surgical problems, and many concomitant drugs. Risk of lactic acidosis increases with advanced age and degree of renal impairment.
● Stop drug immediately if patient develops conditions associated with hypoxemia or dehydration because of risk of lactic acidosis associated with these conditions.
● Suspend therapy temporarily for surgical procedures (except minor procedures not associated with restricted intake of food and fluids); don't restart until patient's oral intake has resumed and renal function is normal.
● Hemodialysis may be useful for removing accumulated drug from patients in whom metformin overdose is suspected.

Monitoring the patient

● Monitor patient's blood glucose level regularly to evaluate effectiveness.
● If patient doesn't respond to 4 weeks of maximum dose of metformin, add an oral sulfonylurea while continuing metformin at the maximum dose. If patient still doesn't respond after several months of concomitant therapy at maximum doses, stop both drugs and initiate insulin therapy.
● Monitor patient closely during times of increased stress, such as infection, fever, surgery, or trauma. Insulin therapy may be required in these situations.
● Monitor patient's hematologic status for megaloblastic anemia. Patients with inadequate vitamin B_{12} or calcium intake or absorption appear to be predisposed to developing subnormal vitamin B_{12} levels. These patients should have serum vitamin B_{12} levels checked routinely at 2- to 3-year intervals.

Information for the patient

● Instruct patient to stop drug immediately and report unexplained hyperventilation, myalgia, malaise, unusual somnolence, or other nonspecific symptoms of early lactic acidosis.
● Instruct patient about nature of diabetes, importance of following therapeutic regimen, ad-

hering to specific diet, weight reduction, exercise and personal hygiene programs; and avoiding infection. Explain how and when to perform self-monitoring of blood glucose level, and teach recognition of hypoglycemia and hyperglycemia.
• Tell patient not to change drug dosage without medical approval. Encourage him to report abnormal blood glucose levels.
• Advise patient not to take other drugs, including OTC products, without medical approval.
• Instruct patient to carry medical identification regarding diabetic status.

Geriatric patients
• Because aging is associated with decreased renal function, administer cautiously to elderly patients.

Pediatric patients
• Safety and effectiveness in children haven't been established.

Breast-feeding patients
• It's unknown if drug appears in breast milk. Because of potential for serious adverse effects in nursing infants, drug shouldn't be administered to breast-feeding women.

methadone hydrochloride
Dolophine, Methadose

Pharmacologic classification: opioid
Therapeutic classification: analgesic, narcotic detoxification adjunct
Controlled substance schedule II
Pregnancy risk category C

How supplied
Available by prescription only
Tablets: 5 mg, 10 mg, 40 mg for oral solution (for narcotic abstinence syndrome)
Oral solution: 5 mg/5 ml, 10 mg/5 ml, 10 mg/ml (concentrate)
Injection: 10 mg/ml

Indications, route, and dosage
Severe pain
Adults: 2.5 to 10 mg P.O., I.M., or S.C. q 3 to 4 hours, p.r.n., or around-the-clock.
Narcotic abstinence syndrome
Adults: 15 to 20 mg P.O. daily (highly individualized).

　Maintenance dose is 20 to 120 mg P.O. daily. Adjust dose, p.r.n. Daily doses above 120 mg need special state and federal approval. If patient feels nauseated, give one-quarter of total P.O. dose in two injections, S.C. or I.M.

Pharmacodynamics
Analgesic action: Opiate agonist that has analgesic activity via an affinity for the opiate recep-

tors similar to that of morphine. Recommended for severe, chronic pain and is also used in detoxification and maintenance of patients with opiate abstinence syndrome.

Pharmacokinetics
• *Absorption:* Well absorbed from GI tract. Oral administration delays onset and prolongs duration of action as compared to parenteral administration. Onset of action occurs within 30 to 60 minutes; peak effect seen at ½ to 1 hour.
• *Distribution:* Highly bound to tissue protein, which may explain its cumulative effects and slow elimination.
• *Metabolism:* Primarily metabolized in liver by N-demethylation.
• *Excretion:* Duration of action is 4 to 6 hours. Half-life is prolonged (7 to 11 hours) in patients with hepatic dysfunction. Urinary excretion, the major route, is dose-dependent. Methadone metabolites also excreted in feces via bile.

Contraindications and precautions
Contraindicated in patients with hypersensitivity to drug. Use cautiously in elderly or debilitated patients and in those with severe renal or hepatic impairment, acute abdominal conditions, hypothyroidism, Addison's disease, prostatic hyperplasia, urethral stricture, head injury, increased intracranial pressure, asthma, or other respiratory disorders.

Interactions
Drug-drug. *Cimetidine, CNS depressants (antidepressants, antihistamines, barbiturates, benzodiazepines, general anesthetics, muscle relaxants, narcotic analgesics, phenothiazines, sedative-hypnotics):* Potentiated respiratory and CNS depression, sedation, and hypotensive effects of drug. Use together with extreme caution; monitor patient's response.
Opioid antagonists: Patients physically dependent on drug may experience acute withdrawal syndrome if given an opioid antagonist. Use with caution; monitor patient closely.
Rifampin: Reduced blood level of methadone. Use together cautiously.
Drug-lifestyle. *Alcohol:* Potentiated respiratory and CNS depression, sedation, and hypotensive effects of drug. Discourage use.

Adverse reactions
CNS: *sedation, somnolence, clouded sensorium, euphoria, dizziness, choreic movements, seizures* (with large doses), headache, insomnia, agitation, *light-headedness, syncope.*
CV: *hypotension,* **bradycardia, shock, cardiac arrest,** palpitations, edema.
EENT: visual disturbances.
GI: *nausea, vomiting, constipation, ileus, dry mouth, anorexia, biliary tract spasm,* increased plasma amylase level.

Reactions may be *common*, uncommon, *life-threatening*, or COMMON AND LIFE-THREATENING.

GU: *urine retention.*
Respiratory: *respiratory depression, respiratory arrest.*
Skin: *diaphoresis,* pruritus, urticaria.
Other: *decreased libido,* physical dependence; pain at injection site; tissue irritation, induration (after S.C. injection).

☑ Special considerations

Besides the recommendations relevant to all opioids, consider the following.

• Verify that patient is in a methadone maintenance program for management of narcotic addiction and, if so, at what dosage, and continue that program appropriately.

• Dispersible tablets may be dissolved in 4 oz (120 ml) of water or fruit juice; oral concentrate must be diluted to at least 3 oz (90 ml) with water before administration.

• Oral liquid form (not tablets) is legally required and is the only form available in drug maintenance programs.

• Regimented scheduling (around-the-clock) is beneficial in severe, chronic pain. When used for severe, chronic pain, tolerance may develop with long-term use, requiring a higher dose to achieve the same degree of analgesia.

• Patient treated for narcotic abstinence syndrome will usually need an additional analgesic if pain control is necessary.

• Physical and psychological tolerance or dependence may occur. Be aware of potential for abuse.

• The most common signs and symptoms of drug overdose are CNS depression, respiratory depression, and miosis (pinpoint pupils). To treat acute overdose, first establish adequate respiratory exchange; administer an opioid antagonist (naloxone) if indicated.

• If recent oral overdose (within 2 hours of ingestion), empty stomach immediately by inducing emesis (ipecac syrup) or using gastric lavage. Administer activated charcoal via nasogastric tube for further removal of drug.

Monitoring the patient

• Monitor laboratory values, vital signs, and neurologic status closely.

• Evaluate patient for compliance with therapy.

Information for the patient

• If appropriate, tell patient that constipation is often severe during maintenance with methadone. If not contraindicated, instruct him to increase fluid and fiber in diet. Instruct him to take a stool softener or other laxative.

• Caution patient to avoid activities that require full alertness, such as driving and operating machinery, because of potential for drowsiness.

Geriatric patients

• Lower doses are usually indicated for elderly patients because they may be more sensitive to the therapeutic and adverse effects of drug.

Pediatric patients

• Drug isn't recommended for use in children. Safe use as maintenance drug in adolescent addicts hasn't been established.

Breast-feeding patients

• Drug appears in breast milk. It may cause physical dependence in breast-feeding infants of women on methadone maintenance therapy. Women on methadone should not breast-feed.

methamphetamine hydrochloride
Desoxyn, Desoxyn Gradumet

Pharmacologic classification: amphetamine
Therapeutic classification: CNS stimulant, short-term adjunctive anorexigenic drug, sympathomimetic amine
Controlled substance schedule II
Pregnancy risk category C

How supplied

Available by prescription only
Tablets: 5 mg
Tablets (long-acting): 5 mg, 10 mg, 15 mg

Indications, route, and dosage

Attention deficit hyperactivity disorder
Children ages 6 and older: Initially, 5 mg P.O. once daily or b.i.d., with 5-mg increments weekly, p.r.n. Usual effective dose is 20 to 25 mg daily.
Short-term adjunct in exogenous obesity
Adults: 10 to 15 mg/day P.O. in morning. Don't use for more than a few weeks.

Pharmacodynamics

CNS stimulant action: Amphetamines are sympathomimetic amines with CNS stimulant activity; in hyperactive children, they have a paradoxical calming effect.
Anorexigenic action: Anorexigenic effects are thought to occur in the hypothalamus, where decreased smell and taste acuity decreases appetite; they may involve other systemic and metabolic effects. They may be tried for short-term control of refractory obesity, with caloric restriction and behavior modification.

The cerebral cortex and reticular activating system appear to be the primary sites of activity; amphetamines release nerve terminal stores of norepinephrine, promoting nerve impulse transmission. At high dosages, effects are mediated by dopamine.

Amphetamines are used to treat narcolepsy and as adjuncts to psychosocial measures in attention deficit disorder in children. The precise mechanisms of action in these conditions are unknown.

Pharmacokinetics
- *Absorption:* Rapidly absorbed from GI tract after oral administration; effects last 6 to 12 hours; prolonged absorption for sustained-release form.
- *Distribution:* Widely distributed throughout body. Crosses placenta and enters breast milk.
- *Metabolism:* Metabolized in liver to at least seven metabolites.
- *Excretion:* Excreted in urine.

Contraindications and precautions
Contraindicated in patients with moderate to severe hypertension, hyperthyroidism, symptomatic CV disease, advanced arteriosclerosis, glaucoma, hypersensitivity or idiosyncrasy to sympathomimetic amines, or history of drug abuse; within 14 days of MAO inhibitor therapy; and in agitated patients.

Use cautiously in elderly, debilitated, asthenic, or psychopathic patients and in those with history of suicidal or homicidal tendencies.

Interactions
Drug-drug. *Acetazolamide, antacids, sodium bicarbonate:* Enhanced reabsorption of methamphetamine and prolonged duration of action. Monitor patient for enhanced effects.
Antihypertensives: May antagonize effects of these drugs. Monitor blood pressure closely.
Ascorbic acid: Enhanced methamphetamine excretion; shortened duration of action. Monitor patient for decreased effects.
Barbiturates: Antagonize methamphetamine by CNS depression. Avoid concomitant use.
CNS stimulants: Additive effects. Avoid concomitant use.
General anesthesia: Increased risk of arrhythmias. Use with extreme caution; monitor ECG.
Haloperidol, phenothiazines: Decreased methamphetamine effects. Avoid concomitant use.
Insulin: Drug may alter insulin requirements. Monitor serum glucose levels.
MAO inhibitors: Severe hypertension or hypertensive crisis. Don't use together or within 14 days after stopping MAO inhibitor.
Drug-herb. *Melatonin:* Enhanced monoaminergic effects of methamphetamine; exacerbated insomnia. Avoid concomitant use.
Drug-food. *Caffeine:* Additive effects. Advise patient to avoid concomitant use.

Adverse reactions
CNS: *nervousness, insomnia, irritability,* talkativeness, dizziness, headache, hyperexcitability, tremor, euphoria.

CV: hypertension, *tachycardia, palpitations,* **arrhythmias.**
EENT: blurred vision, mydriasis.
GI: dry mouth, metallic taste, diarrhea, constipation, anorexia.
GU: impotence.
Skin: urticaria.
Other: altered libido.

☑ Special considerations
Besides the recommendations relevant to all amphetamines, consider the following.
- Drug isn't recommended for first-line treatment of obesity.
- Don't crush long-acting dosage forms.
- When treating behavioral disorders in children, consider periodically interrupting drug to evaluate effectiveness and need for continued therapy.
- Rapid withdrawal after prolonged use may lead to depression, somnolence, and increased appetite.
- Drug may elevate plasma corticosteroid levels and may interfere with urinary corticosteroid determinations.
- Symptoms of overdose include increasing restlessness, tremor, hyperreflexia, tachypnea, confusion, aggressiveness, hallucinations, and panic; fatigue and depression usually follow the excitement stage.
- To treat recent overdose (ingestion within 4 hours), use gastric lavage or emesis and sedate with barbiturate; monitor vital signs and fluid and electrolyte balance. Hemodialysis or peritoneal dialysis may be effective in severe cases.

Monitoring the patient
- Monitor patient's response to drug therapy.
- Monitor vital signs and encourage patient to report palpitations or irregular or rapid heartbeat.

Information for the patient
- Warn patient that potential for abuse is high. Discourage use to combat fatigue.
- Advise patient to take drug 1 hour before next meal, and to take last daily dose at least 6 hours before bedtime to prevent insomnia. Sustained-release (long-acting) forms should be taken at start of day.
- Warn patient not to increase dosage unless prescribed.
- Inform patient that drug may impair ability to engage in potentially hazardous activities, such as operating machinery or driving.

Geriatric patients
- Elderly or debilitated patients may be especially sensitive to methamphetamine's effects. Drug should be used with caution.

Pediatric patients
- Drug isn't recommended for weight reduction in children under age 12.

Reactions may be *common,* uncommon, **life-threatening,** or COMMON AND LIFE-THREATENING.

Breast-feeding patients
• Amphetamines appear in breast milk. An alternative to breast-feeding should be used.

---

methimazole
Tapazole

Pharmacologic classification: thyroid hormone antagonist
Therapeutic classification: antihyperthyroid drug
Pregnancy risk category D

How supplied
Available by prescription only
Tablets: 5 mg, 10 mg

Indications, route, and dosage
Hyperthyroidism, preparation for thyroidectomy, thyrotoxic crisis
Adults: 15 mg P.O. daily if mild; 30 to 40 mg P.O. daily if moderately severe; 60 mg P.O. daily if severe; all are given in three equally divided doses q 8 hours. Continue until patient is euthyroid; then start maintenance dose of 5 to 15 mg daily.
Children: 0.4 mg/kg/day divided q 8 hours. Continue until patient is euthyroid; then start maintenance dose of 0.2 mg/kg/day divided q 8 hours.

Pharmacodynamics
Antithyroid action: In treating hyperthyroidism, methimazole inhibits synthesis of thyroid hormone by interfering with the incorporation of iodide into tyrosyl. Methimazole also inhibits the formation of iodothyronine. As preparation for thyroidectomy, methimazole inhibits synthesis of the thyroid hormone and causes a euthyroid state, reducing surgical problems during thyroidectomy; as a result, the mortality for a single-stage thyroidectomy is low. Iodide reduces the vascularity of the gland, making it less friable. For treating thyrotoxic crisis (thyrotoxicosis), propylthiouracil (PTU) is preferred over methimazole because it inhibits peripheral deiodination of thyroxine to triiodothyronine.

Pharmacokinetics
• *Absorption:* Absorbed rapidly from GI tract (80% to 95% bioavailable). Plasma levels peak within 1 hour.
• *Distribution:* Readily crosses placenta; distributed into breast milk. Concentrated in thyroid. Isn't protein-bound.
• *Metabolism:* Hepatic metabolism.
• *Excretion:* About 80% of drug and metabolites excreted renally; 7% excreted unchanged. Half-life is between 5 and 13 hours.

Contraindications and precautions
Contraindicated in patients with hypersensitivity to drug and in breast-feeding patients. Use cautiously in pregnant women.

Interactions
Drug-drug. *Adrenocorticoids, corticotropin, PTU:* May alter response to drug therapy. Dosage adjustment of corticosteroid may be necessary when thyroid status changes.
Anticoagulants: Potentiated action of these drugs. Monitor PT, PTT, and INR closely.
Bone marrow depressants: Increased risk of agranulocytosis. Monitor blood count.
Cardiac glycosides: Increased serum levels. May need to decrease digitalis dose; monitor glycoside levels.
Hepatotoxic drugs: Increased risk of hepatotoxicity. Monitor liver function tests.
Iodinated glycerol, lithium, potassium iodide: May potentiate hypothyroid and goitrogenic effects. Dosage adjustment may be needed.

Adverse reactions
CNS: headache, drowsiness, vertigo, paresthesia, neuritis, neuropathies, CNS stimulation, depression.
GI: diarrhea, nausea, vomiting (may be dose-related), salivary gland enlargement, loss of taste, epigastric distress.
GU: nephritis.
Hematologic: *agranulocytosis, leukopenia, thrombocytopenia, aplastic anemia.*
Hepatic: jaundice, hepatic dysfunction, *hepatitis.*
Musculoskeletal: arthralgia, myalgia.
Skin: rash, urticaria, discoloration, pruritus, erythema nodosum, exfoliative dermatitis, lupus-like syndrome.
Other: fever, lymphadenopathy, hypothyroidism (mental depression; cold intolerance; hard, non-pitting edema; hypoprothrombinemia and bleeding).

☑ Special considerations
• Best response occurs if dosage is administered around-the-clock and given at the same time each day with respect to meals.
• Dosages of over 40 mg/day increase risk of agranulocytosis.
• A beta blocker, most often propranolol, is usually given to manage peripheral signs of hyperthyroidism, primarily tachycardia.
• Euthyroid state may take several months to develop.
• Signs and symptoms of overdose include nausea, vomiting, epigastric distress, fever, headache, arthralgia, pruritus, edema, and pancytopenia. If overdose occurs, induce emesis (if possible) or use gastric lavage.

Monitoring the patient
• Monitor patient for adverse effects; sulfonamide-type adverse reactions can occur.
• Check CBC, hepatic function, and coagulation studies periodically.

Information for the patient
• Tell patient to take drug at regular intervals around-the-clock and to take it at the same time each day in relation to meals.
• If GI upset occurs, advise patient to take drug with meals.
• Tell patient to call promptly if fever, sore throat, malaise, unusual bleeding, yellowing of eyes, nausea, or vomiting occurs.
• Advise patient not to store drug in bathroom; heat and humidity cause deterioration.
• Tell patient to inform other physicians and dentists of drug use.
• Teach patient how to recognize signs and symptoms of hyperthyroidism and hypothyroidism and what to do if they occur.

Breast-feeding patients
• Drug appears in breast milk; patient should stop breast-feeding before starting drug. If breast-feeding is necessary, PTU is the preferred anti-thyroid drug.

methocarbamol
Robaxin

Pharmacologic classification: carbamate derivative of guaifenesin
Therapeutic classification: skeletal muscle relaxant
Pregnancy risk category C

How supplied
Available by prescription only
Tablets: 500 mg, 750 mg
Injection: 100 mg/ml parenteral in 10-ml vial

Indications, route, and dosage
Adjunct in acute, painful musculoskeletal conditions
Adults: 1.5 g P.O. q.i.d. for 2 to 3 days. Maintenance dose 4 to 4.5 g P.O. daily in three to six divided doses. Or 1 g I.M. or I.V. Maximum dose 3 g daily I.M. or I.V. for 3 consecutive days.
Supportive therapy in tetanus management
Adults: 1 to 2 g I.V. push (300 mg/minute) and an additional 1 to 2 g may be added to I.V. solution. Total initial I.V. dose 3 g. Repeat I.V. infusion of 1 to 2 g q 6 hours until nasogastric tube can be inserted.
Children: 15 mg/kg or 500 mg/m² I.V. Don't inject faster than 180 mg/m²/minute. May be repeated q 6 hours if necessary to total dosage of 1.8 g/m² daily for 3 consecutive days.

Pharmacodynamics
Skeletal muscle relaxant action: Exact mechanism unknown. Doesn't relax skeletal muscle directly. Effects appear to be related to sedative action.

Pharmacokinetics
• *Absorption:* Rapidly and completely absorbed from GI tract. Onset of action within 30 minutes after single oral dose. Immediate onset of action after single I.V. dose.
• *Distribution:* Widely distributed throughout body.
• *Metabolism:* Extensively metabolized in liver via dealkylation and hydroxylation. Half-life is between 0.9 and 1.8 hours.
• *Excretion:* Rapidly and almost completely excreted in urine, mainly as its glucuronide and sulfate metabolites (40% to 50%), as unchanged drug (10% to 15%), and rest unidentified metabolites.

Contraindications and precautions
Contraindicated in patients with hypersensitivity to drug and in those with impaired renal function (injectable form) or seizure disorder (injectable form). Because safe use of methocarbamol in regard to fetal development hasn't been established, drug shouldn't be used in women who are or may become pregnant, especially during early pregnancy, unless benefits outweigh possible hazards.

Interactions
Drug-drug. *Anticholinesterases:* Patients with myasthenia gravis may experience severe weakness if given methocarbamol. Avoid concomitant use.
CNS depressants (such as anxiolytics, narcotics, psychotics, tricyclic antidepressants): May cause additive CNS depression. When used concomitantly, exercise care to avoid overdose.
Drug-lifestyle. *Alcohol:* Additive CNS depression. Discourage use.

Adverse reactions
CNS: drowsiness, dizziness, light-headedness, headache, syncope, mild muscular incoordination (with I.M. or I.V. use), **seizures** (with I.V. use only), vertigo.
CV: thrombophlebitis, flushing, hypotension, **bradycardia** (with I.M. or I.V. use).
EENT: blurred vision, conjunctivitis, nystagmus, diplopia.
GI: nausea, GI upset, metallic taste.
GU: hematuria (with I.V. use only), discoloration of urine.
Skin: urticaria, pruritus, rash.
Other: extravasation (with I.V. use only), fever, **anaphylactic reactions** (with I.M. or I.V. use).

☑ Special considerations
• Don't administer S.C. Give I.V. undiluted at a rate not exceeding 300 mg per minute. May also

---

Reactions may be *common*, uncommon, **life-threatening**, or COMMON AND LIFE-THREATENING.

be given by I.V. infusion after diluting in D_5W or normal saline solution.
● Patient should be supine during and for at least 10 to 15 minutes after I.V. injection.
● To give via nasogastric tube, crush tablets and suspend in water or normal saline solution.
● When used in tetanus, follow manufacturer's instructions.
● Extravasation of I.V. solution may cause thrombophlebitis and sloughing from hypertonic solution.
● Oral administration should replace parenteral use as soon as feasible.
● For I.M. administration, don't give more than 500 mg in each gluteal region.
● Patient's urine may turn black, blue, brown, or green if left standing.
● Methocarbamol therapy alters results of laboratory tests for urine 5-hydroxyindoleacetic acid using quantitative method of Udenfriend (false-positive) and for urine vanillylmandelic acid (false-positive when Gitlow screening test used; no problem when quantitative method of Sunderman used).
● Signs and symptoms of overdose include extreme drowsiness, nausea and vomiting, and arrhythmias. If ingestion is recent, empty stomach by emesis or gastric lavage; monitor urine output and vital signs.

Monitoring the patient
● Monitor patient for adverse effects; adverse reactions after oral administration are usually mild, transient, and subside with dosage reduction.
● In patients receiving CNS depressant drugs, observe carefully for increased depressant effects.

Information for the patient
● Tell patient urine may turn black, blue, green, or brown.
● Warn patient drug may cause drowsiness. Patient should avoid hazardous activities that require alertness until degree of CNS depression is known.
● Advise patient to make position changes slowly, particularly from recumbent to upright position, and to dangle legs before standing.
● Tell patient to store drug away from heat and light (not in bathroom medicine cabinet) and safely out children's reach.
● Tell patient to take missed dose if remembered within 1 hour. Beyond 1 hour, patient should skip that dose and resume regular schedule. Don't double dose.
● Inform athletes that skeletal muscle relaxants are banned in competition and tested for by the U.S. Olympic Committee and the National Collegiate Athletic Association.

Geriatric patients
● Lower doses are indicated because elderly patients are more sensitive to drug's effects.

Pediatric patients
● For children under age 12, use only as recommended for tetanus.

Breast-feeding patients
● Drug appears in breast milk in small amounts. Patient shouldn't breast-feed during treatment.

methohexital sodium
Brevital Sodium, Brietal Sodium*

Pharmacologic classification: barbiturate
Therapeutic classification: I.V. anesthetic
Controlled substance schedule IV
Pregnancy risk category B

How supplied
Available by prescription only
Injection: 500 mg, 2.5 g, 5 g powder for injection

Indications, route, and dosage
Induction of anesthesia; anesthesia for short procedures (such as electroconvulsive therapy [ECT])
Dosage is highly individualized.
Adults and children: For induction of anesthesia, administer a 1% solution at a rate of about 1 ml/5 seconds, possibly with inhalant anesthetics or skeletal muscle relaxants, or both. Induction dose may vary from 50 to 120 mg or more but averages about 70 mg; it usually provides anesthesia for 5 to 7 minutes. Maintenance of anesthesia may be achieved via intermittent injections of about 20 to 40 mg (2 to 4 ml of 1% solution), p.r.n., usually q 4 to 7 minutes; or by continuous I.V. infusion of a 0.2% solution (average rate of about 3 ml of a 0.2% solution per minute [1 drop/second]).

Pharmacodynamics
Anesthetic action: Produces anesthesia by direct depression of the polysynaptic midbrain reticular activating system; decreases presynaptic (via decreased neurotransmitter release) and postsynaptic excitation. These effects may be subsequent to increased gamma-aminobutyric acid (GABA), enhancement of GABA's effects, or a direct effect on GABA receptor sites.

Pharmacokinetics
● *Absorption:* Only given I.V.; is an ultrashort-acting barbiturate; levels in brain peak between 30 seconds and 2 minutes after administration.
● *Distribution:* Distributed throughout body; highest initial levels occur in vascular areas of brain, primarily gray matter.
● *Metabolism:* Metabolized extensively in liver.
● *Excretion:* Excretion of metabolites occurs via kidneys through glomerular filtration. Duration of action depends on tissue redistribution.

Contraindications and precautions

Contraindicated in patients with hypersensitivity to drug, in those with acute intermittent or variegate porphyria, and whenever general anesthesia is contraindicated.

Use cautiously in patients with circulatory, cardiac, renal, hepatic, endocrine, or pulmonary dysfunction; severe anemia; marked obesity or status asthmaticus (use extremely cautiously) because drug worsens these conditions. Also, use cautiously in patients with a full stomach because it blocks airway reflexes and may predispose the patient to aspiration.

Interactions

Drug-drug. *Antihistamines, benzodiazepines, hypnotics, narcotics, phenothiazines, sedatives:* May potentiate or add to CNS depressant effects of these drugs. Avoid concomitant use.

Ketamine (for anesthesia): Possible profound respiratory depression; ketamine potentiates methohexital. Avoid concomitant use.

Drug-lifestyle. *Alcohol:* Drug may potentiate or add to CNS depressant effects. Discourage use.

Adverse reactions

CNS: skeletal muscle hyperactivity, anxiety, restlessness, headache, emergence delirium, alteration of EEG patterns.

CV: thrombophlebitis, transient hypotension, tachycardia, *circulatory depression, peripheral vascular collapse.*

GI: abdominal pain, nausea, vomiting, excessive salivation.

Respiratory: *respiratory arrest, respiratory depression, apnea, laryngospasm, bronchospasm,* hiccups.

Skin: pain, swelling; ulceration, necrosis (on extravasation).

Other: pain at injection site, injury to adjacent nerves, *hypersensitivity reaction.*

Note: Stop drug if peripheral vascular collapse, respiratory arrest, or hypersensitivity reaction occurs.

☑ Special considerations

• Avoid extravasation or intra-arterial injection because of possible tissue necrosis and gangrene.

• Drug is physically incompatible with lactated Ringer's solution; with acidic solutions, such as atropine, metocurine, and succinylcholine; and with silicone. Avoid contact with rubber stoppers or parts of syringes that have been treated with silicone. The preferred diluent is sterile water, but D_5W or normal saline may be used. Don't use bacteriostatic diluents.

• Ensure maintenance of patent airway and adequate ventilation during induction and maintenance of anesthesia.

• Signs of overdose include respiratory depression, respiratory arrest, hypotension, and shock.

Treat supportively; use (as needed) mechanical ventilation and I.V. fluids or vasopressors (dopamine, phenylephrine) for hypotension.

Monitoring the patient

• Monitor vital signs closely and patient's response to drug.

• Monitor heart rate and rhythm during procedures.

Geriatric patients

• Lower doses may be indicated.

Pediatric patients

• Safety and efficacy in children haven't been established.

Breast-feeding patients

• Use cautiously in breast-feeding patients. It's unknown if drug appears in breast milk.

methotrexate, methotrexate sodium

Folex, Mexate, Mexate-AQ, Rheumatrex Dose Pack

Pharmacologic classification: antimetabolite (cell cycle–phase specific, S phase)
Therapeutic classification: antineoplastic
Pregnancy risk category X

How supplied

Available by prescription only
Tablets (scored): 2.5 mg
Injection: 20-mg, 25-mg, 50-mg, 100-mg, 250-mg, 1-g vials, lyophilized powder, preservative-free; 25-mg/ml vials, preservative-free solution; 2.5-mg/ml, 25-mg/ml vials, lyophilized powder, preserved

Indications, route, and dosage

Dosage and indications may vary. Check current literature for recommended protocols.

Trophoblastic tumors (choriocarcinoma, hydatidiform mole)

Adults: 15 to 30 mg P.O. or I.M. daily for 5 days. Repeat after 1 or more weeks, according to response or toxicity.

Acute lymphoblastic leukemia

Adults and children: 3.3 mg/m² P.O. daily for 4 to 6 weeks or until remission occurs; then 20 to 30 mg/m² P.O. or I.M. twice weekly or 2.5 mg/kg I.V. q 14 days. (Used with prednisone.)

Meningeal leukemia

Adults and children: 12 mg/m² intrathecally to a maximum dose of 15 mg q 2 to 5 days until CSF is normal. Use only vials of powder with no preservatives; dilute using normal saline solution injection without preservatives. Use only new vials of

---

drug and diluent. Use immediately after reconstitution.

Burkitt's lymphoma (stage I or II)
Adults: 10 to 25 mg P.O. daily for 4 to 8 days with 7- to 10-day rest intervals.

Lymphosarcoma (stage III; malignant lymphoma)
Adults: 0.625 to 2.5 mg/kg daily P.O., I.M., or I.V.

Mycosis fungoides (advanced)
Adults: 2.5 to 10 mg P.O. daily or 50 mg I.M. weekly; or 25 mg I.M. twice weekly.

Psoriasis (severe)
Adults: 10 to 25 mg P.O., I.M., or I.V. as single weekly dose.

Rheumatoid arthritis (severe, refractory)
Adults: 7.5 to 15 mg weekly P.O. in single or divided doses.

Adjunct treatment in osteosarcoma
Adults: Give 12 to 15 g/m^2 as a 4-hour I.V. infusion.

Pharmacodynamics
Antineoplastic action: Exerts its cytotoxic activity by tightly binding with dihydrofolic acid reductase, an enzyme crucial to purine metabolism, resulting in an inhibition of DNA, RNA, and protein synthesis.

Pharmacokinetics
• *Absorption:* Dose-related absorption across GI tract. Lower doses essentially completely absorbed; larger doses undergo incomplete and variable absorption. I.M. doses absorbed completely. Serum levels peak 30 minutes to 2 hours after I.M. dose; 1 to 4 hours after oral dose.
• *Distribution:* Distributed widely throughout body, with highest levels found in kidneys, gallbladder, spleen, liver, and skin. Crosses blood-brain barrier but doesn't achieve therapeutic levels in CSF. About 50% of drug is bound to plasma protein.
• *Metabolism:* Metabolized only slightly in liver.
• *Excretion:* Excreted primarily into urine as unchanged drug. Biphasic elimination; first phase half-life of 45 minutes and terminal phase half-life of 4 hours.

Contraindications and precautions
Contraindicated in patients with hypersensitivity to drug and during pregnancy or breast-feeding. Also contraindicated in patients with psoriasis or rheumatoid arthritis who also have alcoholism, alcoholic liver, chronic liver disease, immunodeficiency syndromes, or preexisting blood dyscrasias.

Use cautiously in very young or elderly or debilitated patients and in those with impaired renal or hepatic function, bone marrow suppression, aplasia, leukopenia, thrombocytopenia, anemia, folate deficiency, infection, peptic ulcer, or ulcerative colitis. Drug exits slowly from third space compartments, resulting in a prolonged terminal plasma half-life and risk of toxicity.

Interactions
Drug-drug. *Folic acid:* Decreased effectiveness of methotrexate. Avoid concomitant use, except for leucovorin rescue with high-dose methotrexate.
Immunizations: May not be effective when given during methotrexate therapy. Because of risk of disseminated infections, live virus vaccines generally aren't recommended during therapy.
NSAIDs, salicylates, sulfonamides, sulfonylureas: Increased therapeutic and toxic effects of methotrexate. Avoid concurrent use if possible.
Oral antibiotics (such as chloramphenicol, nonabsorbable broad-spectrum antibiotics, tetracycline): May decrease absorption of drug. Monitor patient.
Phenytoin: Serum levels may be decreased by chemotherapeutic regimens with methotrexate; increased risk of seizures. Monitor patient closely.
Probenecid, salicylates: Increased therapeutic and toxic effects of methotrexate. Combined use requires lower dosage of methotrexate.
Pyrimethamine: Drugs have similar pharmacologic action. Don't give concurrently.
Theophylline: Increased theophylline levels. Monitor levels closely.
Drug-food. *Any food:* Delayed absorption and reduced peak level of methotrexate. Don't give with food.
Drug-lifestyle. *Alcohol:* Increased hepatotoxicity. Discourage use.
Sun exposure: Increased photosensitivity reactions. Tell patient to take precautions.

Adverse reactions
CNS: *arachnoiditis* (within hours of intrathecal use), subacute *neurotoxicity* (may begin a few weeks later), *necrotizing demyelinating leukoencephalopathy* (may occur a few years later), malaise, fatigue, dizziness, headache, drowsiness, *seizures.*
EENT: pharyngitis, gingivitis, blurred vision.
GI: stomatitis, diarrhea, abdominal distress, anorexia, GI ulceration and bleeding, enteritis, *nausea, vomiting.*
GU: nephropathy, *tubular necrosis, renal failure,* hematuria, menstrual dysfunction, defective spermatogenesis, cystitis.
Hematologic: WBC and platelet count nadirs occurring on day 7; *anemia, leukopenia, thrombocytopenia* (all dose-related).
Hepatic: *acute toxicity* (elevated transaminase level), *chronic toxicity (*cirrhosis, *hepatic fibrosis).*
Musculoskeletal: arthralgia, myalgia.
Respiratory: *pulmonary fibrosis; pulmonary interstitial infiltrates,* pneumonitis; dry, nonproductive cough.
Skin: alopecia, *urticaria, pruritus, hyperpigmentation, erythematous rash, ecchymoses, pso-*

riatic lesions (aggravated by exposure to sun), rash, photosensitivity.
Other: osteoporosis (in children, with long-term use), fever, chills, reduced resistance to infection, septicemia, hyperuricemia, diabetes, ***sudden death.***

☑ Special considerations
● Methotrexate may be given undiluted by I.V. push injection.
● Drug can be diluted to a higher volume with normal saline solution for I.V. infusion.
● Use reconstituted solutions of preservative-free drug within 24 hours after mixing.
● For intrathecal administration, use preservative-free formulations only. Dilute with unpreserved normal saline.
● Avoid all I.M. injections in patients with thrombocytopenia.
● Leucovorin rescue is necessary with high-dose protocols (doses greater than 100 mg).
● The antidote for methotrexate's hematopoietic toxicity (diagnosed or anticipated) is calcium leucovorin, started as soon as possible and within 1 hour after administration of methotrexate.
● Dose modification may be needed in impaired hepatic or renal function, bone marrow depression, aplasia, leukopenia, thrombocytopenia, or anemia. Use cautiously in infection, peptic ulcer, ulcerative colitis, and in very young, old, or debilitated patients.
● GI adverse reactions may require stopping drug.
● Methotrexate may alter results of laboratory assay for folate by inhibiting organism used in assay, thus interfering with detection of folic acid deficiency.

Monitoring the patient
● Watch for rash, redness, or ulcerations in mouth or pulmonary adverse reactions; these may signal serious complications.
● Monitor uric acid levels.
● Monitor intake and output daily. Force fluids (2 to 3 qt [2 to 3 L] daily).
● Alkalinize urine by giving sodium bicarbonate tablets to prevent precipitation of drug, especially with high doses. Maintain urine pH at more than 6.5. Reduce dose if BUN level is 20 to 30 mg/dl or serum creatinine level is 1.2 to 2 mg/dl. Stop drug if BUN level is more than 30 mg/dl or serum creatinine level is more than 2 mg/dl.
● Watch for increases in AST, ALT, and alkaline phosphatase levels, which may signal hepatic dysfunction. Methotrexate shouldn't be used when the potential for "third spacing" exists.
● Watch for bleeding (especially GI) and infection.
● Monitor temperature daily, and watch for cough, dyspnea, and cyanosis.

Information for the patient
● Emphasize importance of continuing drug despite nausea and vomiting. Advise patient to call immediately if vomiting occurs shortly after taking a dose.
● Encourage patient to maintain adequate fluid intake to increase urine output, to prevent nephrotoxicity, and to facilitate excretion of uric acid.
● Instruct patient also taking leucovorin to take exactly as prescribed to avoid potentially serious adverse effects.
● Teach patient good mouth care to prevent superinfection of oral cavity.
● Advise patient that hair should grow back after treatment has ended.
● Recommend salicylate-free analgesics for pain relief or fever reduction.
● Tell patient to avoid exposure to people with infections and to report signs of infection immediately.
● Advise patient to report unusual bruising or bleeding promptly.
● Caution woman to avoid conception during and immediately after therapy because of possible abortion or congenital anomalies. Advise patient to call immediately if she becomes, or suspects she is, pregnant.

Breast-feeding patients
● Drug appears in breast milk. To avoid risk of serious adverse reactions, mutagenicity, and carcinogenicity in infant, stop breast-feeding during therapy.

methylcellulose
Citrucel

Pharmacologic classification: adsorbent
Therapeutic classification: bulk-forming laxative
Pregnancy risk category C

How supplied
Available without a prescription
Powder: 105 mg/g, 364 mg/g
Tablets: 500 mg

Indications, route, and dosage
Chronic constipation
Adults: Maximum dose is 6 g daily, divided into 0.45 to 3 g/dose.
Children ages 6 to 12: Maximum dose is 3 g daily, divided into 0.45 to 1.5 g/dose.

Pharmacodynamics
Laxative action: Adsorbs intestinal fluid and serves as a source of indigestible fiber, stimulating peristaltic activity.

Pharmacokinetics
• *Absorption:* Not absorbed. Action begins in 12 to 24 hours, but full effect may not occur for 2 to 3 days.
• *Distribution:* Distributed locally, in intestine.
• *Metabolism:* None.
• *Excretion:* Excreted in feces.

Contraindications and precautions
Contraindicated in patients with abdominal pain, nausea, vomiting, or other symptoms of appendicitis or acute surgical abdomen and in those with intestinal obstruction or ulceration, disabling adhesions, or difficulty swallowing.

Interactions
Drug-drug. *Oral drugs:* When used together, methylcellulose may absorb oral drugs. Separate administration time by at least 1 hour.

Adverse reactions
GI: *nausea, vomiting, diarrhea* (with excessive use); *esophageal, gastric, small intestinal, or colonic strictures* (when drug is chewed or taken in dry form); abdominal cramps, especially in severe constipation; laxative dependence (with long-term or excessive use).

☑ Special considerations
• Administer drug only with water or juice (at least 8 oz).
• Bulk laxatives most closely mimic natural bowel function and don't promote laxative dependence.
• Drug is especially useful in patients with postpartum constipation, chronic laxative abuse, irritable bowel syndrome, diverticular disease, or colostomies; in debilitated patients; and to empty colon before barium enema examinations.

Monitoring the patient
• Determine if patient has adequate fluid intake; monitor intake and output as needed.
• Watch for adverse reactions.

Information for the patient
• Instruct patient to take other oral drugs 1 hour before or after methylcellulose.
• Explain that drug's full effect may not occur for 2 to 3 days.

Breast-feeding patients
• Because drug isn't absorbed, use probably poses no risk to breast-feeding infants.

methyldopa
Aldomet, Apo-Methyldopa*, Dopamet*, Novomedopa*

Pharmacologic classification: centrally acting antiadrenergic
Therapeutic classification: antihypertensive
Pregnancy risk category B (oral); C (I.V.)

How supplied
Available by prescription only
Tablets: 125 mg, 250 mg, 500 mg
Oral suspension: 250 mg/5 ml
Injection (as methyldopate hydrochloride): 250 mg/5 ml in 5-ml vials

Indications, route, and dosage
Moderate to severe hypertension
Adults: Initially, 250 mg P.O. b.i.d. or t.i.d. in first 48 hours; then increased or decreased, p.r.n., q 2 days. Or 250 to 500 mg I.V. q 6 hours (maximum dose, 1 g q 6 hours). Adjust dosage if other antihypertensives are added to or deleted from therapy.
   Maintenance dose is 500 mg to 2 g P.O. daily in two to four divided doses. Maximum recommended daily dose is 3 g. I.V. infusion dose is 250 to 500 mg given over 30 to 60 minutes q 6 hours. Maximum I.V. dose is 1 g q 6 hours.
Children: Initially, 10 mg/kg P.O. daily or 300 mg/m^2 P.O. daily in two to four divided doses; or 20 to 40 mg/kg I.V. daily or 0.6 to 1.2 g/m^2 I.V. daily in four divided doses. Increase dosage at least q 2 days until desired response occurs. Maximum daily dose is 65 mg/kg, 2 g/m^2, or 3 g, whichever is least.

Pharmacodynamics
Antihypertensive action: Exact mechanism unknown. Thought to be caused by methyldopa's metabolite, alpha-methylnorepinephrine, which stimulates central inhibitory alpha-adrenergic receptors, decreasing total peripheral resistance; drug may act as a false neurotransmitter. May also reduce plasma renin activity.

Pharmacokinetics
• *Absorption:* Absorbed partially from GI tract. Absorption varies, but usually about 50% of oral dose absorbed. After oral administration, maximal decline in blood pressure occurs in 3 to 6 hours; full effect isn't evident for 2 to 3 days. No correlation exists between plasma level and antihypertensive effect. After I.V. administration, blood pressure usually begins to fall in 4 to 6 hours.
• *Distribution:* Distributed throughout body; bound weakly to plasma proteins.

• *Metabolism:* Metabolized extensively in liver and intestinal cells.
• *Excretion:* Drug and metabolites excreted in urine; unabsorbed drug excreted unchanged in feces. Elimination half-life is about 2 hours. Antihypertensive activity usually lasts up to 24 hours after oral administration; 10 to 16 hours after I.V. administration.

Contraindications and precautions
Contraindicated in patients with hypersensitivity to drug and in those with active hepatic disease (such as acute hepatitis) and active cirrhosis. Also contraindicated if previous methyldopa therapy has been associated with liver disorders. Use cautiously in patients with impaired hepatic function, in those receiving MAO inhibitors, and in breast-feeding women.

Interactions
Drug-drug. *Anesthetics:* Patients undergoing surgery may need reduced dosages of anesthetics. Use together cautiously.
Antihypertensives: May potentiate antihypertensive effects of these drugs. Monitor blood pressure.
Diuretics: Increased hypotensive effect of methyldopa. Monitor blood pressure.
Haloperidol: Possible dementia and sedation. Use together cautiously.
Lithium: Increased risk of lithium toxicity. Monitor lithium levels.
Oral iron therapy: Decreased hypotensive effects and increased serum levels of levodopa. Monitor levodopa levels and blood pressure.
Phenothiazines, tricyclic antidepressants: Reduced antihypertensive effects. Monitor blood pressure.
Phenoxybenzamine: Possible reversible urinary incontinence. Monitor patient.
Sympathomimetic amines: May potentiate pressor effects of these drugs. Use with caution.
Tolbutamide: Enhanced hypoglycemic effect of tolbutamide. Monitor serum glucose levels and patient closely.
Drug-herb. *Capsicum:* May reduce drug's antihypertensive effectiveness. Avoid use together.

Adverse reactions
CNS: *sedation, headache, weakness, dizziness,* decreased mental acuity, paresthesia, parkinsonism, involuntary choreoathetoid movements, psychic disturbances, depression, nightmares.
CV: *bradycardia,* orthostatic hypotension, aggravated angina, **myocarditis,** edema.
EENT: nasal congestion.
GI: nausea, vomiting, diarrhea, **pancreatitis,** *dry mouth,* constipation.
GU: gynecomastia, amenorrhea, impotence.
Hematologic: hemolytic anemia, thrombocytopenia, leukopenia, *bone marrow depression.*

Hepatic: *hepatic necrosis,* abnormal liver function tests, **hepatitis.**
Skin: rash.
Other: galactorrhea, drug-induced fever, decreased libido.

☑ Special considerations
• Patients with impaired renal function may require smaller maintenance doses of drug.
• Methyldopate hydrochloride is administered I.V.; I.M. or S.C. administration isn't recommended because of unpredictable absorption.
• Patients receiving drug may become hypertensive after dialysis because drug is dialyzable.
• Sedation and drowsiness usually disappear with continued therapy; bedtime dosage will minimize this effect. Orthostatic hypotension may indicate a need for dosage reduction. Some patients tolerate receiving the entire daily dose in the evening or h.s.
• Tolerance may develop after 2 to 3 weeks.
• Signs of hepatotoxicity may occur 2 to 4 weeks after therapy begins.
• Drug alters urine uric acid, serum creatinine, and AST levels; it may also cause falsely high levels of urine catecholamines, interfering with the diagnosis of pheochromocytoma. A positive direct antiglobulin (Coombs') test may also occur.

Monitoring the patient
• Monitor CNS status.
• At start of therapy (and periodically throughout), monitor hemoglobin level, hematocrit, and RBC count for hemolytic anemia; also monitor liver function tests.
• Take blood pressure in supine, sitting, and standing positions during dosage adjustment; take blood pressure at least every 30 minutes during I.V. infusion until patient is stable.
• Monitor intake and output and daily weights to detect sodium and water retention; voided urine exposed to air may darken because of methyldopa breakdown (or its metabolites).
• Watch for signs and symptoms of drug-induced depression.

Information for the patient
• Teach patient signs and symptoms of adverse effects, such as jerky movements, and stress reporting them; he should also report excessive weight gain (5 lb [2.25 kg] weekly), signs of infection, or fever.
• Teach patient to minimize adverse effects by taking drug at bedtime until tolerance develops to sedation, drowsiness, and other CNS effects; by avoiding sudden position changes to minimize orthostatic hypotension; and by using ice chips, hard candy, or gum to relieve dry mouth.
• Warn patient to avoid hazardous activities that require mental alertness until sedative effects subside.

Reactions may be *common,* uncommon, **life-threatening**, or COMMON AND LIFE-THREATENING.

• Instruct patient to call for instructions before taking OTC cold preparations.

Geriatric patients
• Dosage reductions may be needed in elderly patients because they are more sensitive to sedation and hypotension.

Pediatric patients
• Safety and efficacy in children haven't been established; use only if potential benefits outweigh risks.

Breast-feeding patients
• Drug appears in breast milk; the American Academy of Pediatrics considers methyldopa to be compatible with breast-feeding.

methylergonovine maleate
Methergine

Pharmacologic classification: ergot alkaloid
Therapeutic classification: oxytocic
Pregnancy risk category C

How supplied
Available by prescription only
Tablets: 0.2 mg
Injection: 0.2 mg/ml ampule

Indications, route, and dosage
Prevention and treatment of postpartum hemorrhage due to uterine atony or subinvolution
Adults: 0.2 mg I.M. or I.V. q 2 to 4 hours for maximum five doses. After initial I.M. or I.V. dose, may give 0.2 to 0.4 mg P.O. q 6 to 12 hours for maximum of 7 days. Decrease dose if severe cramping occurs.
◊ *Diagnosis of coronary artery spasm*
Adults: 0.1 to 0.4 mg I.V.

Pharmacodynamics
Oxytocic action: Stimulates contractions of uterine and vascular smooth muscle. The intense uterine contractions are followed by periods of relaxation. Produces vasoconstriction primarily of capacitance blood vessels, causing increased central venous pressure and elevated blood pressure. Increases the amplitude and frequency of uterine contractions and tone, thereby impeding uterine blood flow.

Pharmacokinetics
• *Absorption:* Rapid absorption, with 60% of oral dose appearing in bloodstream. Plasma levels peak in about 3 hours. Immediate onset of action I.V., 2 to 5 minutes for I.M., and 5 to 15 minutes for oral doses.
• *Distribution:* Rapidly distributed into tissues.

• *Metabolism:* Extensive first-pass metabolism precedes hepatic metabolism.
• *Excretion:* Excreted primarily in feces, with a small amount in urine.

Contraindications and precautions
Contraindicated in patients with toxemia, hypertension, or sensitivity to ergot preparations and in pregnant women. Use cautiously in patients with renal or hepatic disease, sepsis, or obliterative vascular disease and during the first stage of labor.

Interactions
Drug-drug. *Ergot alkaloids, sympathomimetic amines:* Enhanced vasoconstrictor potential of these drugs. Use together cautiously.
Local anesthetics: Use with vasoconstrictors (lidocaine with epinephrine) will enhance vasoconstriction. Use together cautiously.
Drug-lifestyle. *Smoking:* Enhanced vasoconstriction caused by drug. Discourage use.

Adverse reactions
CNS: dizziness, headache, *seizures, CVA* (with I.V. use), hallucinations.
CV: hypertension, transient chest pain, palpitations, hypotension, thrombophlebitis.
EENT: tinnitus, nasal congestion, foul taste.
GI: *nausea, vomiting, diarrhea.*
GU: hematuria.
Musculoskeletal: leg cramps.
Respiratory: dyspnea.
Skin: diaphoresis.

☑ Special considerations
• Contractions begin 5 to 15 minutes after P.O. administration, 2 to 5 minutes after I.M. injection, and immediately following I.V. injection; continue 3 hours or more after P.O. or I.M. administration, 45 minutes after I.V.
• Don't administer I.V. routinely because of the possibility of inducing sudden hypertension and CVA.
• Store tablets in tightly closed, light-resistant containers. Discard if discolored.
• Store I.V. solutions below 77° F (25° C). Administer only if solution is clear and colorless.
• If I.V. administration is considered essential as a life-saving measure, give slowly over no less than 60 seconds.
• Signs and symptoms of overdose include seizures and gangrene, with nausea, vomiting, diarrhea, dizziness, fluctuations in blood pressure, weak pulse, chest pain, tingling, and numbness and coldness in extremities. Treatment of oral overdose requires patient to drink tap water, milk, or vegetable oil to delay absorption; follow with gastric lavage or emesis, then activated charcoal and cathartics.

Monitoring the patient
• Monitor blood pressure, pulse rate, and uterine response; watch for sudden change in vital signs or frequent periods of uterine relaxation, and character and amount of vaginal bleeding.
• Monitor patient for adverse effects.

Information for the patient
• Advise patient to avoid smoking while taking drug.
• Advise patient of adverse reactions.

Breast-feeding patients
• Ergot alkaloids inhibit lactation. Drug appears in breast milk, and ergotism has been reported in breast-fed infants. Breast-feeding is not recommended.

---

methylphenidate hydrochloride
Concerta, Methylin, Methylin ER, Ritalin, Ritalin-SR

Pharmacologic classification: piperidine CNS stimulant
Therapeutic classification: CNS stimulant (analeptic)
Controlled substance schedule II
Pregnancy risk category NR; C (Concerta)

How supplied
Available by prescription only
Tablets: 5 mg, 10 mg, 20 mg
Tablets (sustained-release): 20 mg
Tablets (extended-relief): 10 mg, 18 mg, 20 mg, 36 mg

Indications, route, and dosage
Attention deficit hyperactivity disorder (ADHD; Ritalin, Methylin))
Children ages 6 and older: Initially, 5 mg P.O. daily before breakfast and lunch, increased in 5- to 10-mg increments weekly, p.r.n., until an optimum daily dose of 2 mg/kg is reached, not to exceed 60 mg/day.
Attention deficit hyperactivity disorder (Concerta)
Children ages 6 and older not currently on methylphenidate: Initially, 18 mg P.O. once daily in morning.
Children ages 6 and older currently on methylphenidate: If previous methylphenidate daily dose is 5 mg b.i.d. or t.i.d. or 20 mg sustained-release, give 18 mg P.O. q morning. If previous methylphenidate daily dose is 10 mg b.i.d. or t.i.d.or 40 mg sustained-release, give 36 mg P.O. q morning. If previous methylphenidate daily dose is 15 mg b.i.d. or t.i.d. or 60 mg sustained-release, give 54 mg P.O. q morning.

Adjust dosages in 18-mg increments weekly, p.r.n. Maximum dose is 54 mg/day.
Narcolepsy (Ritalin, Methylin)
Adults: 10 mg P.O. b.i.d. or t.i.d. 30 to 45 minutes before meals. Dosage varies with patient needs.
When using sustained-release tablets, calculate regular dose in q-8-hour intervals and administer as such.

Pharmacodynamics
Analeptic action: The cerebral cortex and reticular activating system appear to be the primary sites of activity; methylphenidate releases nerve terminal stores of norepinephrine, promoting nerve impulse transmission. At high doses, effects are mediated by dopamine.
Drug is used to treat narcolepsy and as an adjunctive to psychosocial measures in ADHD. Like amphetamines, it has a paradoxical calming effect in hyperactive children.

Pharmacokinetics
• *Absorption:* Absorbed rapidly and completely after oral administration; plasma levels peak at 1 to 2 hours. Duration of action usually 4 to 6 hours (with considerable individual variation); sustained-release tablets may act for up to 8 hours.
• *Distribution:* No information available.
• *Metabolism:* Metabolized by liver.
• *Excretion:* Excreted in urine.

Contraindications and precautions
Contraindicated in patients with hypersensitivity to drug and in those with glaucoma, motor tics, family history of or diagnosis of Tourette syndrome, or history of marked anxiety, tension, or agitation. Use cautiously in patients with history of seizures, drug abuse, hypertension, or EEG abnormalities.

Interactions
Drug-drug. *Anticonvulsants (phenobarbital, phenytoin, primidone), coumarin anticoagulants, phenylbutazone, tricyclic antidepressants:* May inhibit metabolism and increase serum levels of these drugs. Avoid concomitant use.
Bretylium, guanethidine: Decreased hypotensive effects of these drugs. Monitor blood pressure.
MAO inhibitors: May cause severe hypertension. Don't use together or within 14 days of such therapy.
Drug-food. *Caffeine:* May enhance methylphenidate's CNS stimulant effects and decrease drug's effectiveness in ADHD. Avoid use together.

Adverse reactions
CNS: *nervousness, insomnia, Tourette syndrome, dizziness, headache, akathisia, dyskinesia, **seizures,** drowsiness.*
CV: *palpitations, angina, tachycardia, changes in blood pressure and pulse rate, **arrhythmias.***
GI: nausea, abdominal pain, anorexia.

Reactions may be *common*, uncommon, **life-threatening**, or COMMON AND LIFE-THREATENING.

Hematologic: *thrombocytopenia, thrombocytopenic purpura, leukopenia,* anemia.
Metabolic: weight loss.
Skin: rash, urticaria, *exfoliative dermatitis, erythema multiforme.*

☑ Special considerations
● Methylphenidate is the drug of choice for ADHD. Therapy usually ends after puberty.
● Don't give Concerta to patients with preexisting severe GI narrowing.
● Monitor initiation of therapy closely; drug may precipitate Tourette syndrome.
● If paradoxical aggravation of symptoms occurs during therapy, reduce dosage or stop drug.
● Intermittent drug-free periods when stress is least evident (weekends, school holidays) may help prevent development of tolerance and permit decreased dosage when drug is resumed. Sustained-release form allows convenience of single, at-home dosing for school children.
● Drug has abuse potential; discourage use to combat fatigue. Some abusers dissolve tablets and inject drug.
● After high-dose and long-term use, abrupt withdrawal may unmask severe depression. Lower dosage gradually to prevent acute rebound depression.
● Drug impairs ability to perform tasks requiring mental alertness.
● Be sure patient obtains adequate rest; fatigue may result as drug wears off.
● Discourage methylphenidate use for analeptic effect; CNS stimulation superimposed on CNS depression may cause neuronal instability and seizures.
● Don't administer drug to women of childbearing age unless potential benefits outweigh possible risks.
● Symptoms of overdose may include euphoria, confusion, delirium, coma, toxic psychosis, agitation, headache, vomiting, dry mouth, mydriasis, self-injury, fever, diaphoresis, tremors, hyperreflexia, hyperpyrexia, muscle twitching, seizures, flushing, hypertension, tachycardia, palpitations, and arrhythmias. Treat symptomatically and supportively; use gastric lavage or emesis in patients with intact gag reflex.

Monitoring the patient
● Check vital signs regularly for increased blood pressure or other signs of excessive stimulation; avoid late-day or evening dosing, especially of long-acting dosage forms, to minimize insomnia.
● Monitor patient for seizures; drug may decrease seizure threshold in seizure disorders.
● Monitor CBC, differential, and platelet counts when patient is taking drug long-term.
● Monitor height and weight; drug has been associated with growth suppression.

Information for the patient
● Explain rationale for therapy and risks and benefits that may be anticipated.
● Tell patient to avoid drinks containing caffeine to prevent added CNS stimulation and not to alter dosage unless prescribed.
● Advise narcoleptic patient to take first dose on awakening; advise ADHD patient to take last dose several hours before bedtime to avoid insomnia.
● Tell patient not to chew or crush sustained-release dosage forms.
● Tell patient to swallow Concerta tablets whole with liquids, and not to chew, divide, or crush them.
● Warn patient not to use drug to mask fatigue, to obtain adequate rest, and to call if excessive CNS stimulation occurs.
● Advise patient to avoid hazardous activities that require mental alertness until degree of sedative effect is determined.

Pediatric patients
● Drug isn't recommended for ADHD in children under age 6. It's been associated with growth suppression; all patients should be monitored.

methylprednisolone (systemic)
Medrol

methylprednisolone acetate
depMedalone 40, depMedalone 80, Depoject-40, Depoject-80, Depo-Medrol, Depopred-40, Depopred-80, Duralone-40, Duralone-80, Medralone, Rep-Pred 40, Rep-Pred 80

methylprednisolone sodium succinate
A-MethaPred, Solu-Medrol

Pharmacologic classification: glucocorticoid
Therapeutic classification: anti-inflammatory, immunosuppressant
Pregnancy risk category C

How supplied
Available by prescription only
methylprednisolone
Tablets: 2 mg, 4 mg, 8 mg, 16 mg, 24 mg, 32 mg
methylprednisolone acetate
Injection: 20 mg/ml, 40 mg/ml, 80 mg/ml suspension
methylprednisolone sodium succinate
Injection: 40 mg, 125 mg, 500 mg, 1,000 mg, 2,000 mg/vial

Indications, route, and dosage
Multiple sclerosis
methylprednisolone
Adults: 200 mg P.O. daily for 1 week, then 80 mg every other day for 1 month.
Inflammation
methylprednisolone
Adults: 2 to 60 mg P.O. daily in four divided doses, depending on disease being treated.
Children: 0.117 to 1.66 mg/kg daily or 3.3 to 50 mg/m^2 P.O. daily in three to four divided doses.
methylprednisolone acetate
Adults: 10 to 80 mg I.M. daily; or 4 to 80 mg into joints and soft tissue, p.r.n., q 1 to 5 weeks; or 20 to 60 mg intralesionally.
methylprednisolone sodium succinate
Adults: 10 to 250 mg I.M. or I.V. q 4 hours.
Children: 0.03 to 0.2 mg/kg or 1 to 6.25 mg/m^2 I.M. or I.V. daily in divided doses.
Shock
methylprednisolone sodium succinate
Adults: 100 to 250 mg I.V. at 2- to 6-hour intervals.
◇ *Severe lupus nephritis*
Adults: 1 g I.V. over 1 hour for 3 days.
◇ *Treatment or minimization of motor and sensory defects caused by acute spinal cord injury*
Adults: Initially, 30 mg/kg I.V. over 15 minutes, then in 45 minutes by I.V. infusion of 5.4 mg/kg/hour for 23 hours.

Pharmacodynamics
Anti-inflammatory action: Methylprednisolone stimulates the synthesis of enzymes needed to decrease the inflammatory response. It suppresses the immune system by reducing activity and volume of the lymphatic system, thus producing lymphocytopenia (primarily of T lymphocytes), decreasing immunoglobulin and complement levels, decreasing passage of immune complexes through basement membranes, and possibly by depressing reactivity of tissue to antigen-antibody interactions.

Drug is an intermediate-acting glucocorticoid. It has essentially no mineralocorticoid activity but is a potent glucocorticoid, with five times the potency of an equal weight of hydrocortisone. It's used primarily as an anti-inflammatory and immunosuppressant.

Methylprednisolone may be administered orally. Methylprednisolone sodium succinate may be administered by I.M. or I.V. injection or by I.V. infusion, usually at 4- to 6-hour intervals. Methylprednisolone acetate suspension may be administered by intra-articular, intrasynovial, intrabursal, intralesional, or soft tissue injection. It has a slow onset but a long duration of action. Injectable forms usually are used only when the oral dosage forms can't be used.

Pharmacokinetics
● *Absorption:* Absorbed readily after oral administration. After oral and I.V. administration, effects peak in about 1 to 2 hours. Acetate suspension for injection has a variable absorption over 24 to 48 hours, depending on if injected into an intra-articular space or a muscle, and on blood supply to that muscle.
● *Distribution:* Distributed rapidly to muscle, liver, skin, intestines, and kidneys. Adrenocorticoids are distributed into breast milk and through placenta.
● *Metabolism:* Metabolized in liver to inactive glucuronide and sulfate metabolites.
● *Excretion:* Inactive metabolites and small amounts of unmetabolized drug excreted by kidneys. Insignificant quantities of drug excreted in feces. Biological half-life is 18 to 36 hours.

Contraindications and precautions
Contraindicated in patients allergic to any component of the formulation, in those with systemic fungal infections, and in premature infants (acetate and succinate).

Use cautiously in patients with renal disease, GI ulceration, hypertension, osteoporosis, diabetes mellitus, hypothyroidism, cirrhosis, diverticulitis, nonspecific ulcerative colitis, recent intestinal anastomoses, thromboembolic disorders, seizures, myasthenia gravis, heart failure, tuberculosis, emotional instability, ocular herpes simplex, and psychotic tendencies.

Interactions
Drug-drug. *Amphotericin B, diuretics:* Enhanced hypokalemia. Monitor serum potassium levels closely.
Antacids, cholestyramine, colestipol: Decreased corticosteroid effect; corticosteroid is adsorbed, decreasing amount absorbed. Monitor patient closely.
Anticholinesterase: Possible profound weakness. Monitor patient.
Barbiturates, phenytoin, rifampin: Decreased corticosteroid effects due to increased hepatic metabolism. Increase corticosteroid dose as ordered.
Cardiac glycosides: Increased risk of toxicity. Monitor glycoside levels.
Cyclosporine: Levels may increase. Monitor drug levels.
Estrogens: Reduced metabolism of corticosteroids. Monitor patient closely.
Insulin, oral antidiabetics: Cause hyperglycemia. Monitor serum glucose levels; may need dosage adjustment.
Isoniazid, salicylates: Glucocorticoids increase metabolism of these drugs. Monitor patient for lack of effect.
NSAIDs: May increase risk of GI ulceration. Give together cautiously.

Oral anticoagulants: Adrenocorticoids may decrease effects of these drugs. Monitor patient closely.

Skin test antigens: Decreased response. Defer test until after therapy.

Vaccines: Drug may decrease effectiveness. Avoid concomitant use.

Adverse reactions

Most adverse reactions to corticosteroids are dose-dependent or duration-dependent.

CNS: *euphoria, insomnia,* psychotic behavior, pseudotumor cerebri, vertigo, headache, paresthesia, *seizures.*

CV: *heart failure,* hypertension, edema, *arrhythmias,* thrombophlebitis, *thromboembolism, fatal arrest or circulatory collapse* (following rapid administration of large I.V. doses).

EENT: cataracts, glaucoma.

GI: *peptic ulceration,* GI irritation, increased appetite, *pancreatitis,* nausea, vomiting.

GU: menstrual irregularities, increased urine glucose and calcium levels.

Metabolic: hypokalemia, hyperglycemia, increased cholesterol levels, hypocalcemia, decreased thyroxine and triiodothyronine levels.

Musculoskeletal: muscle weakness.

Skin: delayed wound healing, acne, various skin eruptions.

Other: osteoporosis, hirsutism, susceptibility to infections, carbohydrate intolerance, growth suppression in children, cushingoid state (moonface, buffalo hump, central obesity), *acute adrenal insufficiency that may occur with increased stress (infection, surgery, or trauma) or abrupt withdrawal after long-term therapy.*

After abrupt withdrawal: rebound inflammation, fatigue, weakness, arthralgia, fever, dizziness, lethargy, depression, fainting, orthostatic hypotension, dyspnea, anorexia, hypoglycemia. *After prolonged use, sudden withdrawal may be fatal.*

☑ Special considerations

● Recommendations for use of methylprednisolone and for care and teaching of patients during therapy are the same as those for all systemic adrenocorticoids.

● Long-term use causes adverse physiologic effects, including suppression of the hypothalamus-pituitary-adrenal axis, cushingoid appearance, muscle weakness, and osteoporosis.

● Drug causes false-negative results in the nitroblue tetrazolium test for systemic bacterial infections; decreases ^{131}I uptake and protein-bound iodine levels in thyroid function tests.

Monitoring the patient

● Monitor patient's weight, blood pressure, serum electrolyte levels, and sleep patterns.

● Watch for signs of psychosis or depression.

● Watch for allergic reactions.

Information for the patient

● Tell patient not to stop drug abruptly or without medical consent.

● Instruct patient to take oral form with food or milk.

Geriatric patients

● In elderly patients, consider risk-benefit factors of corticosteroid use; lower doses are recommended. Monitor blood pressure and blood glucose and electrolyte levels at least every 6 months.

Pediatric patients

● Long-term use of adrenocorticoids in children and adolescents may delay growth and maturation.

methysergide maleate
Sansert

Pharmacologic classification: ergot alkaloid
Therapeutic classification: vasoconstrictor
Pregnancy risk category X

How supplied

Available by prescription only
Tablets: 2 mg

Indications, route, and dosage

Intervals of 3 to 4 weeks must separate each 6-month course of therapy.

Prevention of vascular headaches, including migraine and cluster headaches

Adults: 4 to 8 mg P.O. daily in divided doses with meals.

◊ *To control diarrhea in patients with carcinoid disease*

Adults: 2 mg P.O. t.i.d. Adjust dosage as needed and tolerated. Usual dosage range is 4 to 16 mg P.O. t.i.d.

Pharmacodynamics

Vasoconstrictor action: Competitively blocks serotonin peripherally and may act as a serotonin agonist in the CNS (brain stem). Drug's antiserotonin effects result in inhibition of peripheral vasoconstrictor and pressor effects of serotonin, inflammation induced by serotonin, and a reduction in the increased rate of platelet aggregation caused by serotonin.

Mechanism involved in prophylaxis of vascular headaches unknown. However, drug's effectiveness may result from humoral factors affecting the pain threshold and from its central serotonin-agonist effect.

Pharmacokinetics

● *Absorption:* Rapidly absorbed from GI tract.

• *Distribution:* Widely distributed in body tissues.
• *Metabolism:* Metabolized in liver to methyler-gonovine and glucuronide metabolites.
• *Excretion:* 56% of dose excreted in urine as un-changed drug and metabolites. Plasma elimina-tion half-life is 10 hours.

Contraindications and precautions
Contraindicated in patients with severe hyper-tension or arteriosclerosis, peripheral vascular insufficiency, renal or hepatic disease, coronary artery disease, phlebitis or cellulitis of lower limbs, collagen diseases, fibrotic processes, or valvu-lar heart disease; in debilitated patients; and dur-ing pregnancy.
  Use cautiously in patients with peptic ulcer or suspected coronary artery disease and in those with aspirin or tartrazine allergies.

Interactions
Drug-drug. *Beta blockers:* Possible peripheral ischemia, manifested by cold extremities with possible peripheral gangrene. Monitor patient closely.
Narcotic analgesics: Drug may reverse analgesic activity. Use with caution.
Drug-lifestyle. *Alcohol:* May worsen headaches. Discourage use.
Smoking: Increased adverse effects of drug. Dis-courage use.

Adverse reactions
CNS: insomnia, drowsiness, *euphoria, vertigo, ataxia,* light-headedness, hyperesthesia, weak-ness, hallucinations or feelings of dissociation, rapid speech, lethargy.
CV: *fibrotic thickening of cardiac valves and aor-ta, inferior vena cava, and common iliac branch-es (retroperitoneal fibrosis);* vasoconstriction, causing chest pain, abdominal pain, vascular in-sufficiency of lower limbs; cold, numb, painful ex-tremities with or without paresthesia and dimin-ished or absent pulses; flushing; orthostatic hypotension; tachycardia; peripheral edema; mur-murs; bruits.
GI: nausea, vomiting, diarrhea, constipation, heartburn.
Hematologic: *neutropenia,* eosinophilia.
Musculoskeletal: arthralgia, myalgia.
Respiratory: *pulmonary fibrosis* (causing dys-pnea, tightness and pain in chest, pleural friction rubs, and effusion).
Skin: hair loss, rash.

☑ Special considerations
Besides the recommendations relevant to all er-got alkaloids, consider the following.
• Adverse reactions occur in up to 50% of pa-tients.
• Drug may contain tartrazine, which can cause an allergic reaction.

• GI effects may be reduced by introducing drug gradually and by giving with food or milk.
• Don't use drug to treat acute episodes of mi-graine, vascular headache, or muscle contrac-tion headache.
• Dosage should be reduced gradually for 2 to 3 weeks before stopping drug.
• If drug is given for cluster headaches, it's usu-ally administered only during the cluster.
• Drug has also been used to control diarrhea in patients with carcinoid disease.
• Protective effect develops in 1 to 2 days and persists for 1 to 2 days after drug is stopped.
• Signs and symptoms of overdose include hy-peractivity, euphoria, dizziness, peripheral va-sospasm with diminished or absent pulses, coldness, mottling, and cyanosis of extremities. If patient is conscious and ingestion recent, in-duce emesis; if unconscious, insert cuffed en-dotracheal tube and perform gastric lavage. Ap-ply warmth (not direct heat) to ischemic extrem-ities if vasospasm occurs.

Monitoring the patient
• Monitor patient for adverse effects.
• Check WBC as indicated, vital signs, and ECG.

Information for the patient
• Tell patient to report immediately signs of numb-ness or tingling in hands or feet, red or violet blis-ters on hands and feet, flank or chest pain, short-ness of breath, leg cramps when walking, or oth-er signs or symptoms of impaired circulation.
• Tell patient to report illness or infection, which may increase sensitivity to drug effects.
• Advise patient to avoid prolonged exposure to very cold temperatures; cold may increase ad-verse effects of drug.
• Explain that, after stopping drug, patient's body may need time to adjust depending on amount of drug used and duration of time involved.
• Tell patient to take drug with food.
• Inform patient that drug may cause drowsiness and to use caution when driving or performing other tasks requiring alertness.
• Caution patient regarding caloric intake to avoid excessive weight gain.

Geriatric patients
• Use with caution in elderly patients.

Pediatric patients
• Drug isn't recommended for use in children be-cause of risk of fibrosis.

Breast-feeding patients
• Drug may appear in breast milk. Avoid breast-feeding during therapy.

Reactions may be *common*, uncommon, **life-threatening**, or COMMON AND LIFE-THREATENING.

metipranolol hydrochloride
OptiPranolol

Pharmacologic classification: beta blocker
Therapeutic classification: antiglaucoma drug
Pregnancy risk category C

How supplied
Available by prescription only
Ophthalmic solution: 0.3% in 5- or 10-ml dropper bottles with 0.004% benzalkonium chloride and ethylenediaminetetraacetic acid

Indications, route, and dosage
Ocular conditions in which lowering of intraocular pressure (IOP) would be beneficial (ocular hypertension, chronic open-angle glaucoma)
Adults: Instill 1 drop into affected eye(s) b.i.d. Larger dose or more frequent administration isn't known to be of benefit. If IOP isn't satisfactory, concomitant therapy to lower IOP may be instituted.

Pharmacodynamics
Antiglaucoma action: Exact mechanism unknown. Appears to be a reduction of aqueous humor production. A slight increase in outflow facility has been demonstrated with metipranolol. Like other noncardioselective beta blockers, metipranolol doesn't have significant local anesthetic (membrane-stabilizing) actions or intrinsic sympathomimetic activity. It does reduce elevated and normal IOP with or without glaucoma with little or no effect on pupil size or accommodation. In patients with IOP above 24 mm Hg, pressure is reduced an average of 20% to 26%.

Pharmacokinetics
• *Absorption:* Intended to act locally, but some systemic absorption may occur. Onset of action occurs in less than 30 minutes.
• *Distribution:* Local distribution.
• *Metabolism:* No information available.
• *Excretion:* No information available; maximum effect occurs in about 2 hours; duration of effect is 12 to 24 hours.

Contraindications and precautions
Contraindicated in patients with hypersensitivity to drug or its components and in those with bronchial asthma, history of bronchial asthma or severe COPD, sinus bradycardia, second- or third-degree AV block, cardiac failure, and cardiogenic shock.
    Use cautiously in patients with nonallergic bronchospasm, chronic bronchitis, emphysema, diabetes mellitus, hyperthyroidism, or cerebrovascular insufficiency.

Interactions
Drug-drug. *Antithyroid drugs, calcium channel blockers, catecholamine-depleting drugs, cimetidine, clonidine, digoxin, haloperidol, hydralazine, insulin, lidocaine, morphine, nondepolarizing neuromuscular blockers, NSAIDs, oral contraceptives, phenobarbital, phenothiazines, prazosin, rifampin, salicylates, sympathomimetics, theophylline, thyroid hormones:* May interfere with drug action. Use together cautiously.
Systemic beta blockers: Potential for additive effects. Use with caution.
Drug-lifestyle. *Smoking:* May interfere with drug's effect. Discourage use.

Adverse reactions
CNS: headache, anxiety, dizziness, depression, somnolence, nervousness, asthenia, brow ache.
CV: hypertension, *MI*, atrial fibrillation, angina, palpitations, *bradycardia.*
EENT: transient local eye discomfort, tearing, conjunctivitis, eyelid dermatitis, blurred vision, blepharitis, abnormal vision, photophobia, eye edema, rhinitis, epistaxis.
GI: nausea.
Musculoskeletal: myalgia.
Respiratory: dyspnea, bronchitis, cough.
Skin: rash.
Other: *hypersensitivity reactions.*

☑ Special considerations
• Pilocarpine and other miotics, dipivefrin, or systemic carbonic anhydrase inhibitors may be administered concomitantly if IOP isn't adequately controlled.
• Proper administration is essential for optimal therapeutic response; instruct patient in correct techniques.
• The normal eye can retain only about 10 mcl (microliters) of fluid; the average dropper delivers 25 to 50 mcl/drop. Thus, the value of more than 1 drop is questionable. If multiple-drop therapy is indicated, the best interval between drops is 5 minutes.
• If ocular overdose occurs, flush eye with copious amounts of water or normal saline solution.
• Systemic overdose, after accidental ingestion, may cause bradycardia, hypotension, bronchospasm, or acute cardiac failure. Stop therapy, institute supportive and symptomatic measures, and decrease further absorption (as with gastric lavage).

Monitoring the patient
• Monitor patient's response to drug therapy; watch for adverse effects.
• Monitor cardiac status carefully.

Information for the patient
• Tell patient to wash hands thoroughly before administration and then to follow these directions:
– Tilt head back or lie down and gaze upward.

– Gently grasp lower eyelid below eyelashes and pull eyelid away from eye to form a pouch.

– Place dropper directly over eye, avoiding contact of dropper with eye or any surface.

– Look up just before applying drop; look down for several seconds after applying drop. Slowly release eyelid.

– Close eyes gently for 1 to 2 minutes. Closing eyes tightly after instillation may expel drug from pouch.

– Apply gentle pressure to inside corner of eye at bridge of nose to retard drainage of solution from intended area.

● Tell patient to avoid rubbing eye and to minimize blinking.

● Tell patient not to rinse dropper after use.

● Advise patient to check expiration date on bottle before use and not to use eyedrops that have changed color.

● Tell patient who must use more than one drug to wait at least 5 minutes between instillations.

Pediatric patients
● Safety and efficacy in children haven't been established.

Breast-feeding patients
● It's unknown if drug appears in breast milk; systemic beta blockers appear in breast milk. Use with caution in breast-feeding women.

metoclopramide hydrochloride
Apo-Metoclop*, Clopra, Maxeran*, Maxolon, Octamide PFS, Reclomide, Reglan

Pharmacologic classification: para-aminobenzoic acid (PABA) derivative
Therapeutic classification: antiemetic, GI stimulant
Pregnancy risk category B

How supplied
Available by prescription only
Tablets: 5 mg, 10 mg
Syrup: 5 mg/5 ml
Injection: 5 mg/ml
Solution: 10 mg/ml

Indications, route, and dosage
Prevention or reduction of nausea and vomiting induced by highly emetogenic chemotherapy
Adults: 1 to 2 mg/kg I.V. q 2 hours for two doses, beginning 30 minutes before emetogenic chemotherapy drug administration, then q 3 hours for three doses.

Facilitation of small-bowel intubation and to aid in radiologic examinations
Adults: 10 mg I.V. as a single dose over 1 to 2 minutes.
Children ages 6 to 14: 2.5 to 5 mg I.V.
Children under age 6: 0.1 mg/kg I.V.
Delayed gastric emptying secondary to diabetic gastroparesis
Adults: 10 mg P.O. 30 minutes before meals and h.s. for 2 to 8 weeks, depending on response; or 10 mg I.V. over 2 minutes.
Gastroesophageal reflux
Adults: 10 to 15 mg P.O. q.i.d., p.r.n., taken 30 minutes before meals and h.s.
Postoperative nausea and vomiting
Adults: 10 to 20 mg I.M. near end of surgical procedure, repeated q 4 to 6 hours, p.r.n.
◇ *Lactation improvement*
Adults: 30 to 45 mg/day.
Vomiting
Adults: 10 mg P.O. taken 30 minutes before meals.

Pharmacodynamics
Antiemetic action: Inhibits dopamine receptors in the brain's chemoreceptor trigger zone to inhibit or reduce nausea and vomiting.
GI stimulant action: Relieves esophageal reflux by increasing lower esophageal sphincter tone and reduces gastric stasis by stimulating motility of the upper GI tract, thus reducing gastric emptying time.

Pharmacokinetics
● *Absorption:* After oral administration, absorbed rapidly and thoroughly from GI tract; action begins in 30 to 60 minutes. After I.M. administration, about 74% to 96% of drug is bioavailable; action begins in 10 to 15 minutes. After I.V. administration, onset of action occurs in 1 to 3 minutes.
● *Distribution:* Distributed to most body tissues and fluids, including brain. Crosses placenta; is distributed in breast milk.
● *Metabolism:* Not metabolized extensively; small amount metabolized in liver.
● *Excretion:* Mostly excreted in urine and feces. Hemodialysis and renal dialysis remove minimal amounts. Duration of effect is 1 to 2 hours.

Contraindications and precautions
Contraindicated in patients with hypersensitivity to drug, in those with pheochromocytoma or seizure disorders, and in those in whom stimulation of GI motility might be dangerous (for example, those with hemorrhage, obstruction, or perforation). Use cautiously in patients with history of depression, Parkinson's disease, and hypertension.

Interactions
Drug-drug. *Acetaminophen, aspirin, diazepam, ethanol, levodopa, lithium, tetracycline:* Increased

---

Reactions may be *common,* uncommon, ***life-threatening,*** or COMMON AND LIFE-THREATENING.

absorption of these drugs. Monitor patient carefully.

Anticholinergics, opiates: May antagonize metoclopramide's effect on GI motility. Use together cautiously.

Antihypertensives, CNS depressants: Increased CNS depression. Avoid concomitant use.

Butyrophenone antipsychotics, phenothiazine: May potentiate extrapyramidal reactions. Avoid concomitant use.

Cyclosporine: Increased absorption, possibly increasing its immunosuppressive and toxic effects. Monitor patient closely.

Digoxin: Decreased absorption of digoxin. Monitor patient and serum digoxin levels closely; dosage adjustment may be necessary.

MAO inhibitors: Metoclopramide releases catecholamines in patients with essential hypertension. Use with caution, if at all, in these patients.

Drug-lifestyle. *Alcohol:* Increased CNS depression. Discourage use.

Adverse reactions
CNS: *restlessness, anxiety, drowsiness, fatigue, lassitude, depression, akathisia, insomnia, confusion,* **suicidal ideation, seizures,** hallucinations, headache, dizziness, extrapyramidal symptoms, tardive dyskinesia, dystonic reactions.
CV: transient hypertension, hypotension, supraventricular tachycardia, **bradycardia.**
GI: nausea, bowel disturbances, diarrhea.
GU: urinary frequency, incontinence.
Hematologic: **neutropenia, agranulocytosis.**
Respiratory: **bronchospasm.**
Skin: rash, urticaria.
Other: fever, prolactin secretion, loss of libido, porphyria.

☑ Special considerations
• Don't use drug for more than 12 weeks.
• For I.V. push administration, use undiluted and inject over a 1- to 2-minute period. For I.V. infusion, dilute with 50 ml of D_2W, dextrose 5% in 0.45% saline injection, Ringer's injection, or lactated Ringer's injection, and infuse over at least 15 minutes.
• Administer by I.V. infusion 30 minutes before chemotherapy.
• Drug may be used to facilitate nasoduodenal tube placement.
• Drug isn't recommended for long-term use.
• Drug has been used for investigational purposes to treat anorexia nervosa, dizziness, migraine, intractable hiccups, and to promote postpartum lactation.
• Signs and symptoms of overdose (rare) include drowsiness, dystonia, seizures, and extrapyramidal effects. Diphenhydramine may be used to counteract extrapyramidal effects of high-dose metoclopramide.

Monitoring the patient
• Monitor vital signs and bowel sounds.
• Monitor patient's response to drug therapy.

Information for the patient
• Warn patient to avoid driving for 2 hours after each dose because drug may cause drowsiness.
• Advise patient to report twitching or involuntary movement.
• Instruct patient to take drug 30 minutes before each meal.

Geriatric patients
• Use drug with caution, especially if patient has impaired renal function; dosage may need to be decreased. Elderly patients are more likely to experience extrapyramidal symptoms and tardive dyskinesia.

Pediatric patients
• Children have an increased risk of adverse CNS effects.

Breast-feeding patients
• Because drug appears in breast milk, use with caution in breast-feeding women.

metolazone
Mykrox, Zaroxolyn

Pharmacologic classification: quinazoline derivative (thiazide-like) diuretic
Therapeutic classification: diuretic, antihypertensive
Pregnancy risk category B

How supplied
Available by prescription only
Tablets: 2.5 mg, 5 mg, 10 mg
Tablets (rapid-acting): 0.5 mg (Mykrox)

Indications, route, and dosage
Tablets
Edema (heart failure)
Adults: 5 to 10 mg P.O. daily.
Edema (renal disease)
Adults: 5 to 20 mg P.O. daily.
Hypertension
Adults: 2.5 to 5 mg P.O. daily; maintenance dose based on patient's blood pressure.
Rapid-acting tablets
Hypertension
Adults: 0.5 mg once daily; may be increased to maximum of 1 mg daily.

Pharmacodynamics
Diuretic action: Increases urinary excretion of sodium and water by inhibiting sodium reabsorption in the cortical diluting tubule of the nephron, thus relieving edema. May be more ef-

fective in edema associated with impaired renal function than thiazide or thiazide-like diuretics. *Antihypertensive action:* Exact mechanism unknown. May result from direct arteriolar vasodilatation. Also reduces total body sodium levels and total peripheral resistance.

Pharmacokinetics

• *Absorption:* About 65% is absorbed after oral administration to healthy subjects; in cardiac patients, absorption falls to 40%. Rate and extent of absorption vary among preparations. Blood levels peak in 2 to 4 hours with rapid-acting oral doses; 8 hours for other dose forms.
• *Distribution:* 50% to 70% erythrocyte-bound; about 33% protein-bound.
• *Metabolism:* Insignificant.
• *Excretion:* About 70% to 95% excreted unchanged in urine. Half-life is about 14 hours in healthy patients; may be prolonged in patients with decreased creatinine clearance.

Contraindications and precautions

Contraindicated in patients with anuria, hepatic coma or precoma, or hypersensitivity to thiazides or other sulfonamide-derived drugs. Use cautiously in patients with impaired renal or hepatic function.

Interactions

Drug-drug. *Amphetamines, quinidine:* Metolazone may decrease urinary excretion of some amines. Monitor patient closely.
Antihypertensives: Metolazone potentiates hypotensive effects. May be used to therapeutic advantage.
Cholestyramine, colestipol: May bind metolazone, preventing its absorption. Give drugs 1 hour apart.
Diazoxide: Metolazone may potentiate hyperglycemic, hypotensive, and hyperuricemic effects. Use together cautiously.
Digoxin: Metolazone may cause electrolyte disturbances and increase risk of toxicity. Monitor patient and blood levels.
Furosemide: Excessive volume and electrolyte depletion. Monitor patient closely; monitor serum electrolyte levels.
Insulin, sulfonylureas: Possible hyperglycemic effect. Monitor serum glucose levels; dosage requirements may increase.
Lithium: Elevated serum lithium levels. May necessitate 50% reduction in lithium dosage.
Methenamine compounds (such as methenamine mandelate): Decreased therapeutic efficacy. Monitor patient closely.
Drug-lifestyle. *Alcohol:* Increased orthostatic hypotension. Monitor patient and blood pressure closely; discourage use.
Sun exposure: Increased photosensitivity reactions. Tell patient to take precautions.

Adverse reactions

CNS: *dizziness, headache, fatigue, vertigo, paresthesia, weakness, restlessness, drowsiness, anxiety, depression, nervousness, blurred vision.*
CV: volume depletion and dehydration, orthostatic hypotension, palpitations, vasculitis.
GI: anorexia, nausea, ***pancreatitis***, epigastric distress, vomiting, abdominal pain, diarrhea, constipation, dry mouth.
GU: nocturia, polyuria, frequent urination, impotence.
Hematologic: *aplastic anemia, agranulocytosis,* leukopenia.
Hepatic: jaundice, hepatitis.
Metabolic: hyperglycemia and glucose tolerance impairment; fluid and electrolyte imbalances, including hypokalemia, dilutional hyponatremia and hypochloremia, metabolic alkalosis, hypercalcemia.
Musculoskeletal: muscle cramps.
Skin: dermatitis, photosensitivity, rash, purpura, pruritus, urticaria.

☑ Special considerations

Besides the recommendations relevant to all thiazide and thiazide-like diuretics, consider the following.
• Drug is effective in patients with decreased renal function.
• Metolazone is used as an adjunct in furosemide-resistant edema.
• Drug has been used with furosemide to induce diuresis in patients who didn't respond to either diuretic alone.
• Rapid-acting form (Mykrox) isn't interchangeable with other forms of metolazone. Dosage and uses vary.
• Drug may interfere with tests for parathyroid function; stop therapy before such tests.
• Signs and symptoms of overdose include orthostatic hypotension, dizziness, electrolyte abnormalities, GI irritation and hypermotility, diuresis, and lethargy, which may progress to coma. To treat, induce vomiting with ipecac in conscious patient; otherwise, use gastric lavage to avoid aspiration. Don't give cathartics; these promote additional loss of fluids and electrolytes.

Monitoring the patient

• Monitor vital signs closely.
• Monitor patient for adverse effects.

Information for the patient

• Tell patient to take drug in the morning to prevent nocturia.
• Advise patient to avoid sudden postural changes.

Geriatric patients

• Elderly and debilitated patients need close observation and may need reduced dosages. They are more sensitive to excess diuresis because of age-related changes in CV and renal function. Excess diuresis promotes orthostatic hypotension, dehydration, hypovolemia, hyponatremia, hypomagnesemia, and hypokalemia.

Pediatric patients
• Safety and effectiveness in children haven't been established.

Breast-feeding patients
• Drug may appear in breast milk; safety and effectiveness in breast-feeding women haven't been established.

metoprolol succinate
Toprol XL

metoprolol tartrate
Lopressor

Pharmacologic classification: beta blocker
Therapeutic classification: antihypertensive, adjunctive treatment of acute MI
Pregnancy risk category C

How supplied
Available by prescription only
metoprolol succinate
Tablets (extended-release): 50 mg, 100 mg, 200 mg
metoprolol tartrate
Tablets: 50 mg, 100 mg
Injection: 1 mg/ml in 5-ml ampules or prefilled syringes

Indications, route, and dosage
Mild to severe hypertension
Adults: Initially, 100 mg P.O. daily in single or divided doses; usual maintenance dose is 100 to 450 mg daily. Or 50 to 100 mg P.O. extended-release tablets daily (maximum dose 400 mg daily).
Early intervention in acute MI
Adults: Three 5-mg I.V. boluses q 2 minutes. Then, beginning 15 minutes after last dose, 50 mg P.O. q 6 hours for 48 hours. Maintenance dose 100 mg P.O. b.i.d. or 25 to 50 mg P.O. q 6 hours. (Late treatment 100 mg P.O. b.i.d.)
Angina
Adults: 100 mg in two divided doses. Maintenance dose 100 to 400 mg daily. Or 100 mg P.O. extended-release tablets daily (maximum dose 400 mg daily).

Pharmacodynamics
Antihypertensive action: Exact mechanism unknown. Metoprolol is classified as a cardioselective beta$_1$ antagonist. It may reduce blood pressure by blocking adrenergic receptors, thus decreasing cardiac output; by decreasing sympathetic outflow from the CNS; or by suppressing renin release.
Action after acute MI: Exact mechanism by which metoprolol decreases mortality after MI unknown. In patients with MI, metoprolol reduces heart rate, systolic blood pressure, and cardiac output. It also appears to decrease the occurrence of ventricular fibrillation in these patients.

Pharmacokinetics
• *Absorption:* Rapidly and almost completely absorbed from GI tract when given orally; food enhances absorption. Plasma levels peak in 90 minutes. After I.V. administration, maximum beta blockade occurs in 20 minutes. Maximum therapeutic effect occurs after 1 week of treatment.
• *Distribution:* Distributed widely throughout body; about 12% is protein-bound.
• *Metabolism:* Metabolized in liver.
• *Excretion:* About 95% of given dose is excreted in urine within 72 hours, largely as metabolites.

Contraindications and precautions
Contraindicated in patients with hypersensitivity to drug or other beta blockers. Also contraindicated in patients with sinus bradycardia, heart block greater than first-degree, cardiogenic shock, or overt cardiac failure when used to treat hypertension or angina. When used to treat MI, drug is contraindicated in patients with heart rate less than 45 beats/minute, second- or third-degree heart block, PR interval of 0.24 second or longer with first-degree heart block, systolic blood pressure less than 100 mm Hg, or moderate to severe cardiac failure.

Use cautiously in patients with impaired hepatic or respiratory function, diabetes, or heart failure.

Interactions
Drug-drug. *Cardiac glycosides:* Enhanced bradycardia. Use together cautiously. Monitor ECG.
Diuretics, other antihypertensives: May potentiate antihypertensive effects of these drugs. Monitor blood pressure.
Sympathomimetics: Antagonized beta-adrenergic effects. Use together cautiously.
Verapamil: Decreased bioavailability of metoprolol when given with antiarrhythmics. Use together cautiously.
Drug-food. *Any food:* Increased absorption. Give drug with food.

Adverse reactions
CNS: *fatigue, dizziness,* depression.
CV: *bradycardia,* hypotension, *heart failure, AV block.*
GI: nausea, diarrhea.
Respiratory: dyspnea, *bronchospasm.*
Skin: rash.

☑ Special considerations
Besides the recommendations relevant to all beta blockers, consider the following.
- Metoprolol may be administered daily as a single dose or in divided doses. If a dose is missed, patient should take only the next scheduled dose.
- Reduce dosage in patients with impaired hepatic function.
- Avoid late-evening doses to minimize insomnia.
- Signs and symptoms of overdose include severe hypotension, bradycardia, heart failure, and bronchospasm. After acute ingestion, empty stomach by induced emesis or gastric lavage, and give activated charcoal to reduce absorption.

Monitoring the patient
- Monitor vital signs and patient's response to drug therapy.
- Observe patient for signs of mental depression.

Information for the patient
- Tell patient to take drug exactly as prescribed and to take it with food.
- Tell patient not to stop drug suddenly, but to call if unpleasant reactions occur.

Geriatric patients
- Elderly patients may need lower maintenance doses because of delayed metabolism; they may also experience enhanced adverse effects. Use with caution.

Pediatric patients
- Safety and efficacy in children haven't been established. No dosage recommendation exists for children.

Breast-feeding patients
- Drug appears in breast milk. An alternative to breast-feeding is recommended during therapy.

metronidazole (systemic)
Apo-Metronidazole*, Flagyl, Flagyl ER, Metric-21, Novonidazol*, Protostat

metronidazole hydrochloride
Flagyl I.V., Flagyl I.V. RTU, Metro I.V.

Pharmacologic classification: nitroimidazole
Therapeutic classification: antibacterial, antiprotozoal, amebicide
Pregnancy risk category B

How supplied
Available by prescription only
Tablets: 250 mg, 500 mg
Tablets (film-coated): 250 mg, 500 mg
Capsules: 375 mg
Powder for injection: 500-mg single-dose vials
Injection: 500 mg/dl ready to use

Indications, route, and dosage
Amebic hepatic abscess
Adults: 500 to 750 mg P.O. t.i.d. for 5 to 10 days.
Children: 33 to 50 mg/kg P.O. daily (in three doses) for 10 days.
Intestinal amebiasis
Adults: 750 mg P.O. t.i.d. for 5 to 10 days. Centers for Disease Control and Prevention recommend addition of iodoquinol 650 mg P.O. t.i.d. for 20 days.
◊ *Children:* 35 to 50 mg/kg daily (in three doses) for 5 to 10 days. Follow this therapy with oral iodoquinol.
Trichomoniasis
Adults (both men and women): 375-mg capsule P.O. b.i.d. for 7 days, or 500-mg tablet P.O. b.i.d. for 7 days, or a single dose of 2 g P.O. or divided into two doses given on same day.
◊ *Children:* 15 mg/kg daily (in three doses) for 7 to 10 days.
Refractory trichomoniasis
Adults (women): 500 mg P.O. b.i.d. for 7 days.
Bacterial infections caused by anaerobic microorganisms
Adults: Loading dose is 15 mg/kg I.V. infused over 1 hour (about 1 g for a 70-kg [154-lb] adult). Maintenance dose is 7.5 mg/kg I.V. or P.O. q 6 hours (about 500 mg for a 70-kg adult). First maintenance dose should be administered 6 hours after the loading dose. Maximum dose shouldn't exceed 4 g daily.
Children: 7.5 mg/kg I.V. q 6 hours.
◊ *Giardiasis*
Adults: 250 mg P.O. t.i.d. for 5 days, or 2 g once daily for 3 days.
Children: 5 mg/kg P.O. t.i.d. for 5 days.
Prevention of postoperative infection in contaminated or potentially contaminated colorectal surgery
Adults: 15 mg/kg infused over 30 to 60 minutes and completed about 1 hour before surgery. Then 7.5 mg/kg infused over 30 to 60 minutes at 6 and 12 hours after initial dose.
◊ *Bacterial vaginosis*
Adults: 500 mg P.O. b.i.d. for 7 days, or 2 g P.O. as a single dose.
◊ *Pelvic inflammatory disease*
Adults: 500 mg P.O. b.i.d. for 14 days (given with 400 mg b.i.d. of ofloxacin).
◊ *Clostridium difficile*
Adults: 750 mg to 2 g P.O. daily, in three to four divided doses for 7 to 14 days.
◊ *Helicobacter pylori associated with peptic ulcer disease*
Adults: 250 to 500 mg P.O. t.i.d. (with other drugs).
Children: 15 to 20 mg/kg P.O. daily, divided in two doses for 4 weeks (with other drugs).

Pharmacodynamics
Bactericidal, amebicidal, and trichomonacidal actions: The nitro group of metronidazole is reduced inside the infecting organism; this reduc-

tion product disrupts DNA and inhibits nucleic acid synthesis. Drug is active in intestinal and extraintestinal sites. It's active against most anaerobic bacteria and protozoa, including *Bacteroides fragilis, B. melaninogenicus, Fusobacterium, Veillonella, Clostridium, Peptococcus, Peptostreptococcus, Entamoeba histolytica, Trichomonas vaginalis, Giardia lamblia*, and *Balantidium coli*.

Pharmacokinetics

• *Absorption:* About 80% of oral dose absorbed, with serum levels peaking at about 1 hour; food delays rate but not extent of absorption.
• *Distribution:* Distributed into most body tissues and fluids, including CSF, bone, bile, saliva, pleural and peritoneal fluids, vaginal secretions, seminal fluids, middle ear fluid, and hepatic and cerebral abscesses. CSF levels approach serum levels in patients with inflamed meninges; they reach about 50% of serum levels in patients with uninflamed meninges. Less than 20% is bound to plasma proteins. Readily crosses placenta.
• *Metabolism:* Metabolized to an active 2-hydroxymethyl metabolite and to other metabolites.
• *Excretion:* About 60% to 80% of dose excreted as parent compound or metabolites. About 20% of dose excreted unchanged in urine; about 6% to 15% excreted in feces. Drug's half-life is 6 to 8 hours in adults with normal renal function; its half-life may be prolonged in patients with impaired hepatic function.

Contraindications and precautions

Contraindicated in patients with hypersensitivity to drug or other nitroimidazole derivatives. Use cautiously in patients with history of blood dyscrasia or alcoholism, hepatic disease, retinal or visual field changes, or CNS disorders and in those receiving hepatotoxic drugs.

Interactions

Drug-drug. *Barbiturates, phenytoin:* Reduced antimicrobial effectiveness of metronidazole; increased metabolism. May require higher doses of metronidazole.
Cimetidine: Decreased metronidazole clearance; increased potential for adverse effects. Monitor patient.
Disulfiram: May precipitate psychosis and confusion. Avoid concomitant use.
Lithium: Increased lithium levels. Monitor serum lithium levels.
Oral anticoagulants: Increased anticoagulant effect. Monitor PT and INR.
Drug-lifestyle. *Alcohol:* May cause disulfiram-like reaction (nausea, vomiting, headache, abdominal cramps, and flushing) with drug. Discourage use during therapy and for 3 days after therapy ends.

Adverse reactions

CNS: vertigo, headache, ataxia, dizziness, syncope, incoordination, confusion, irritability, depression, weakness, insomnia, *seizures,* peripheral neuropathy.
CV: ECG change (flattened T wave), edema (with I.V. RTU preparation), thrombophlebitis (after I.V. infusion).
GI: abdominal cramping, stomatitis, metallic taste, epigastric distress, nausea, vomiting, anorexia, diarrhea, constipation, proctitis, dry mouth.
GU: darkened urine, polyuria, dysuria, cystitis, dyspareunia, dryness of vagina and vulva, vaginal candidiasis.
Hematologic: *transient leukopenia, neutropenia.*
Musculoskeletal: fleeting joint pain, sometimes resembling serum sickness.
Skin: flushing, rash.
Other: decreased libido; overgrowth of nonsusceptible organisms, especially *Candida* (glossitis, furry tongue); fever.

☑ Special considerations

• Confirm trichomoniasis by wet smear and amebiasis by culture before giving metronidazole.
• If indicated during pregnancy for trichomoniasis, the 7-day regimen is preferred over the single-dose regimen. Avoid treatment with metronidazole during the first trimester.
• I.V. form should be administered by slow infusion only; if used with a primary I.V. fluid system, stop the primary fluid during the infusion; don't give by I.V. push.
• When preparing powder for injection, follow manufacturer's instructions carefully; use solution prepared from powder within 24 hours. I.V. solutions must be prepared in three steps: reconstitution with 4.4 ml of normal saline solution injection (with or without bacteriostatic water); dilution with lactated Ringer's injection, D_5W, or normal saline solution; and neutralization with sodium bicarbonate, 5 mEq per 500 mg metronidazole.
• Drug may interfere with chemical analyses of aminotransferases and triglyceride, leading to falsely decreased values.
• Signs and symptoms of overdose include nausea, vomiting, ataxia, seizures, and peripheral neuropathy.

Monitoring the patient

• Monitor patient on I.V. drug for candidiasis.
• When treating amebiasis, monitor number and character of stools. Send fecal specimens to laboratory promptly; infestation is detectable only in warm specimens. Repeat fecal studies at 3-month intervals to ensure elimination of amebae.
• Monitor patient for adverse effects and toxicity.

Information for the patient
- Inform patient that drug may cause metallic taste and discolored (red-brown) urine.
- Tell patient to take tablets with meals to minimize GI distress; tablets may be crushed to facilitate swallowing.
- Counsel patient on need for medical follow-up after discharge.

Amebiasis patients:
- Explain that follow-up examinations of stool specimens are necessary for 3 months after treatment ends to ensure elimination of amebae.
- To help prevent reinfection, instruct patient and family members in proper hygiene; disposal of feces; hand washing after defecation and before handling, preparing, or eating food; risks of eating raw food; and the control of contamination by flies.
- Encourage other household members and suspected contacts to be tested and, if necessary, treated.

Trichomoniasis patients:
- Teach correct personal hygiene, including perineal care.
- Explain that asymptomatic sexual partners of patients being treated for trichomoniasis should be treated simultaneously to prevent reinfection; patient should refrain from intercourse during therapy, or condoms should be used.

Geriatric patients
- Monitoring of serum levels may be necessary to adjust dosage.

Pediatric patients
- Neonates may eliminate drug more slowly than older infants and children.

Breast-feeding patients
- Drug appears in breast milk. Avoid breast-feeding during therapy.

---

metronidazole (topical)
MetroGel, MetroGel-Vaginal, Metro-Cream, Noritate

Pharmacologic classification: nitro-imidazole
Therapeutic classification: antiprotozoal, antibacterial
Pregnancy risk category B

How supplied
Available by prescription only
Topical gel: 0.75%
Topical cream: 0.75%, 1%
Vaginal gel: 0.75%

Indications, route, and dosage
Topical treatment of acne rosacea, ◊ *pressure ulcer, inflammatory papules or pustules*
Adults: Apply a thin film b.i.d. to affected area in the morning and evening (once daily for Noritate). Significant results should be seen within 3 weeks and continue for first 9 weeks of therapy.
Topical treatment of bacterial vaginosis
Adults: One applicator b.i.d., vaginally, for 5 days.

Pharmacodynamics
Anti-inflammatory action: Exact mechanism unknown. Probably exerts an anti-inflammatory effect through antibacterial and antiprotozoal actions.

Pharmacokinetics
- *Absorption:* Under normal conditions, serum levels after topical administration are negligible; 20% to 25% is absorbed vaginally with serum levels peaking in 6 to 12 hours.
- *Distribution:* Less than 20% bound to plasma proteins.
- *Metabolism:* No information available.
- *Excretion:* Unknown after topical or intravaginal application.

Contraindications and precautions
Contraindicated in patients with hypersensitivity to drug or its components (such as parabens) and other nitroimidazole derivatives. Use cautiously in patients with history of blood dyscrasia. Use vaginal form cautiously in patients with history of CNS disease because of risk of seizures or peripheral neuropathy.

Interactions
Drug-drug. *Oral anticoagulants:* May potentiate anticoagulant effect. Monitor patient for potential adverse effects. Monitor PT and INR.
Drug-lifestyle. *Alcohol:* May cause disulfiram-like reaction. Discourage use.

Adverse reactions
CNS: dizziness, light-headedness, headache (with vaginal form).
EENT: lacrimation (if topical gel is applied around the eyes).
GI: decreased appetite, cramps, pain, nausea, diarrhea, constipation, metallic or bad taste in mouth (with vaginal form).
GU: *cervicitis, vaginitis,* urinary frequency (with vaginal form).
Skin: rash, *transient redness, dryness, mild burning, stinging* (with vaginal form).
Other: overgrowth of nonsusceptible organisms (with vaginal form).

☑ Special considerations
- Topical metronidazole therapy hasn't been associated with adverse reactions observed with parenteral or oral metronidazole therapy (including

---

Reactions may be *common*, uncommon, **life-threatening**, or COMMON AND LIFE-THREATENING.

disulfiram-like reaction following alcohol ingestion). However, some drug can be absorbed after topical use. Limited clinical experience hasn't shown any of these adverse effects.

Monitoring the patient
• Monitor patient for adverse effects.
• Monitor patient's response to drug therapy.

Information for the patient
• Advise patient to cleanse area thoroughly before applying drug. Patient may use cosmetics after applying drug.
• Instruct patient to avoid use of drug on eyelids; apply cautiously if drug must be used around eyes.
• If local reactions occur, advise patient to apply drug less frequently or to stop use and call for specific instructions.

Pediatric patients
• Safety in children hasn't been established.

Breast-feeding patients
• Drug appears in breast milk. Stop either drug or breast-feeding, after assessing importance of drug to mother.

mexiletine hydrochloride
Mexitil

Pharmacologic classification: lidocaine analogue, sodium channel antagonist
Therapeutic classification: ventricular antiarrhythmic
Pregnancy risk category C

How supplied
Available by prescription only
Capsules: 150 mg, 200 mg, 250 mg

Indications, route, and dosage
Life-threatening documented ventricular arrhythmias, including ventricular tachycardia
Adults: 200 mg P.O. q 8 hours. May increase or decrease dose in increments of 50 to 100 mg q 8 hours if satisfactory control isn't obtained. Or give a loading dose of 400 mg with maintenance dose of 200 mg P.O. q 8 hours. Some patients may respond well to 450 mg q 12 hours. Maximum daily dose shouldn't exceed 1,200 mg.
◊ **Diabetic neuropathy**
Adults: 150 mg daily for 3 days; then 300 mg daily for 3 days, followed by 10 mg/kg daily.

Pharmacodynamics
Antiarrhythmic action: Structurally similar to lidocaine and exerts similar electrophysiologic and hemodynamic effects. A class IB antiarrhythmic that suppresses automaticity and shortens the effective refractory period and action potential duration of His-Purkinje fibers and suppresses spontaneous ventricular depolarization during diastole. At therapeutic serum levels, doesn't affect conductive atrial tissue or AV conduction.

Unlike quinidine and procainamide, mexiletine doesn't significantly alter hemodynamics when given in usual doses. Its effects on the conduction system inhibit reentry mechanisms and halt ventricular arrhythmias. Drug doesn't have a significant negative inotropic effect.

Pharmacokinetics
• *Absorption:* About 90% absorbed from GI tract; serum levels peak in 2 to 3 hours. Absorption rate decreases with conditions that speed gastric emptying.
• *Distribution:* Widely distributed throughout body. About 50% to 60% of circulating drug is bound to plasma proteins. Usual therapeutic drug level is 0.5 to 2 mcg/ml. Although toxicity may occur within this range, levels above 2 mcg/ml are considered toxic and are associated with increased frequency of adverse CNS effects, warranting dosage reduction.
• *Metabolism:* Metabolized in liver to relatively inactive metabolites. Less than 10% of parenteral dose escapes metabolism and reaches kidneys unchanged. Metabolism affected by hepatic blood flow; may be reduced in patients who are recovering from MI and in those with heart failure. Liver disease also limits metabolism.
• *Excretion:* In healthy patients, drug's half-life is 10 to 12 hours. Elimination half-life may be prolonged in patients with heart failure or liver disease. Urinary excretion increases with urine acidification; slows with urine alkalinization.

Contraindications and precautions
Contraindicated in patients with cardiogenic shock or preexisting second- or third-degree AV block in the absence of an artificial pacemaker. Use cautiously in patients with hypotension, heart failure, first-degree heart block, ventricular pacemaker, preexisting sinus node dysfunction, or seizure disorders.

Interactions
Drug-drug. *Ammonium chloride:* Enhanced mexiletine excretion. Monitor patient closely.
Antacids containing aluminum-magnesium hydroxide, atropine, narcotics: Concomitant use may delay mexiletine absorption. Avoid administering drug within 1 hour of antacids containing aluminum-magnesium hydroxide. Monitor patient.
Cimetidine: May decrease mexiletine metabolism; increased serum levels. Monitor patient closely.
Drugs that alkalinize urine (such as carbonic anhydrase inhibitors, high-dose antacids, sodium bicarbonate): Decreased mexiletine excretion. Monitor patient closely.

Metoclopramide: Increased absorption. Monitor patient for toxicity.
Phenobarbital, phenytoin, rifampin: May induce hepatic metabolism of mexiletine; reduced serum drug levels. Monitor patient.
Theophylline: Increased serum theophylline levels. Monitor serum theophylline levels.

Adverse reactions
CNS: *tremor, dizziness, blurred vision, diplopia, confusion,* light-headedness, incoordination, changes in sleep habits, paresthesia, weakness, fatigue, speech difficulties, tinnitus, depression, *nervousness, headache.*
CV: *new or worsened arrhythmias,* palpitations, chest pain, nonspecific edema, angina.
GI: *nausea, vomiting, upper GI distress, heartburn, diarrhea, constipation, dry mouth, changes in appetite, abdominal pain.*
Skin: rash.

☑ Special considerations
• Dosage should be administered with meals, if possible.
• Because of proarrhythmic effects, drug generally isn't recommended for non-life-threatening arrhythmias.
• When changing from lidocaine to mexiletine, stop infusion when first mexiletine dose is given. Keep infusion line open, however, until arrhythmia appears to be satisfactorily controlled.
• Patients who aren't controlled by dosing every 8 hours may respond to dosing every 6 hours.
• Many patients who respond well to mexiletine (300 mg or less every 8 hours) can be maintained on an every-12-hour schedule. The same total daily dose is divided into twice-daily doses, which improves patient compliance.
• Liver function test results may be transiently altered during therapy.
• Signs and symptoms of overdose are primarily extensions of adverse CNS effects. Seizures are the most serious effect. In acute overdose, induce emesis or perform gastric lavage.

Monitoring the patient
• Monitor blood pressure and heart rate and rhythm for significant change.
• Tremor (usually a fine hand tremor) is common in patients taking higher doses of mexiletine.

Information for the patient
• Tell patient to take drug with food to reduce risk of nausea.
• Instruct patient to report unusual bleeding or bruising, signs of infection (such as fever, sore throat, stomatitis, or chills), or fatigue.

Geriatric patients
• Most elderly patients need reduced dosages because of reduced hepatic blood flow and de-

creased metabolism. Elderly patients also may be more susceptible to CNS adverse effects.

Breast-feeding patients
• Drug appears in breast milk. An alternative to breast-feeding should be used during therapy.

mezlocillin sodium
Mezlin

Pharmacologic classification: extended-spectrum penicillin, acyclaminopenicillin
Therapeutic classification: antibiotic
Pregnancy risk category B

How supplied
Available by prescription only
Injection: 1 g, 2 g, 3 g, 4 g
Infusion: 2 g, 3 g, 4 g
Pharmacy bulk package: 20 g

Indications, route, and dosage
Infections caused by susceptible organisms
Adults: 200 to 300 mg/kg I.V. daily given in four to six divided doses. Usual dosage is 3 g q 4 hours or 4 g q 6 hours. For serious infections, up to 24 g daily may be administered.
Children under age 12: 200 to 300 mg/kg per day I.M. or I.V. in divided doses q 4 to 6 hours.
✦ *Dosage adjustment.* In adult patients with renal failure, if creatinine clearance is 10 to 30 ml/minute, give 3 g q 6 to 8 hours for life-threatening or serious infection. For urinary tract infection (UTI), give 1.5 g q 6 to 8 hours. If creatinine clearance is below 10 ml/minute, give 2 g q 6 to 8 hours for life-threatening or serious infection. For UTI, give 1.5 g q 8 hours.
Patients on hemodialysis should be given 3 to 4 g after each dialysis session, then q 12 hours. Patients on peritoneal dialysis may receive 3 g q 12 hours.

Pharmacodynamics
Antibiotic action: Bactericidal. Adheres to bacterial penicillin-binding proteins, thereby inhibiting bacterial cell wall synthesis.
   Extended-spectrum penicillins are more resistant to inactivation by certain beta-lactamases, especially those produced by gram-negative organisms, but are still liable to inactivation by certain others.
   Drug's spectrum of activity includes many gram-negative aerobic and anaerobic bacilli, many gram-positive and gram-negative aerobic cocci, and some gram-positive aerobic and anaerobic bacilli, but a large number of these organisms are resistant to mezlocillin. Mezlocillin may be effective against some strains of carbenicillin-resistant and ticarcillin-resistant gram-negative bacilli. Mezlocillin shouldn't be used as sole therapy because of the rapid development of resis-

tance. Some clinicians feel that there is no evidence that it has any advantages over ticarcillin or carbenicillin, at least with respect to cure rates. Drug is less active against *Pseudomonas aeruginosa* than other members of this class, such as piperacillin.

Pharmacokinetics
• *Absorption:* After an I.M. dose, plasma levels peak at ¾ to 1½ hours.
• *Distribution:* Distributed widely. Penetrates minimally into CSF with uninflamed meninges, crosses placenta, and is 16% to 42% protein-bound.
• *Metabolism:* Partially metabolized; about 15% of dose metabolized to inactive metabolites.
• *Excretion:* Excreted primarily (39% to 72%) in urine by glomerular filtration and renal tubular secretion; up to 30% of dose is excreted in bile; some excreted in breast milk. Elimination half-life in adults is ¾ to 1½ hours; in extensive renal impairment, half-life extended to 2 to 14 hours. Drug removed by hemodialysis but not by peritoneal dialysis.

Contraindications and precautions
Contraindicated in patients with hypersensitivity to drug or other penicillins. Use cautiously in patients with bleeding tendencies, uremia, hypokalemia, or allergy to cephalosporins.

Interactions
Drug-drug. *Aminoglycoside antibiotics:* Drugs are physically and chemically incompatible; inactivated when mixed or given together. Give 1 hour apart, especially in patients with renal insufficiency.
Clavulanic acid: Synergistic bactericidal effect against certain beta-lactamase-producing bacteria. Don't use together.
Methotrexate: Delayed elimination and elevates serum levels of methotrexate. Avoid concomitant use.
Probenecid: Blocked tubular secretion of penicillins, raising their serum levels. Probenecid may be used for this effect.
Vecuronium bromide: Mezlocillin may prolong neuromuscular blockade. Use with caution.

Adverse reactions
CNS: neuromuscular irritability, *seizures.*
GI: nausea, diarrhea, vomiting, abnormal taste sensation, pseudomembranous colitis.
GU: interstitial nephritis.
Hematologic: *bleeding* (with high doses), *neutropenia, thrombocytopenia,* eosinophilia, *leukopenia, hemolytic anemia.*
Other: *hypersensitivity reactions (anaphylaxis),* edema, fever, chills, rash, pruritus, urticaria), overgrowth of nonsusceptible organisms, *hypokalemia, pain at injection site, vein irritation, phlebitis.*

☑ **Special considerations**
Besides the recommendations relevant to all penicillins, consider the following.
• Mezlocillin may be more suitable than carbenicillin or ticarcillin for patients on salt-free diets; mezlocillin contains only 1.85 mEq of sodium per gram.
• Drug is almost always used with another antibiotic, such as an aminoglycoside, in life-threatening infections.
• Inject I.M. dose slowly over 12 to 15 seconds to minimize pain. Don't exceed 2 g per site.
• If precipitate forms during refrigerated storage, warm to 98.6° F (37° C) in warm water bath and shake well. Solution should be clear.
• Because drug is partially dialyzable, dosage may need adjustment in patients undergoing hemodialysis.
• Drug alters tests for urinary or serum proteins; interferes with turbidimetric methods that use sulfosalicylic acid, trichloroacetic acid, acetic acid, or nitric acid; and causes positive Coombs' tests.
• Signs and symptoms of overdose include neuromuscular sensitivity or seizures; a 4- to 6-hour hemodialysis will remove 20% to 30% of drug.

Monitoring the patient
• Monitor serum potassium level and liver function studies.
• Monitor CBC and platelet counts regularly.
• Monitor patient with high serum levels for seizures.

Geriatric patients
• Half-life may be prolonged in elderly patients because of impaired renal function.

Breast-feeding patients
• Drug appears in breast milk; safe use in breast-feeding women hasn't been established. An alternative to breast-feeding is recommended during therapy.

miconazole nitrate
Femizol-M, Micatin, Monistat 3, Monistat 7, Monistat-Derm

Pharmacologic classification: imidazole derivative
Therapeutic classification: antifungal
Pregnancy risk category B

How supplied
Available by prescription only
Vaginal suppositories: 200 mg
Vaginal cream: 2%
Cream: 2%
Available without a prescription
Cream: 2%
Powder: 2%
Spray: 2%

Vaginal cream: 2%
Vaginal suppositories: 100 mg, 200 mg

Indications, route, and dosage
Cutaneous or mucocutaneous fungal infections caused by susceptible organisms
Topical use
Adults: Cover affected areas b.i.d. for 2 to 4 weeks.
Vaginal use
Adults: Insert 200-mg suppository h.s. for 3 days, or 100-mg suppository or 1 applicator of vaginal cream h.s. for 7 days.

Pharmacodynamics
Antifungal action: Fungistatic and fungicidal, depending on drug level, in *Coccidioides immitis, Candida albicans, Cryptococcus neoformans, Histoplasma capsulatum, Candida tropicalis, C. parapsilosis, Paracoccidioides brasiliensis, Sporothrix schenckii, Aspergillus flavus, Microsporum canis, Curvularia, Pseudallescheria boydii,* dermatophytes, and some gram-positive bacteria. Causes thickening of the fungal cell wall, altering membrane permeability; also may kill the cell by interference with peroxisomal enzymes, causing accumulation of peroxide within the cell wall. Attacks virtually all pathogenic fungi.

Pharmacokinetics
• *Absorption:* About 50% of an oral dose absorbed; however, no oral dosage form currently available. Small amount systemically absorbed after vaginal administration.
• *Distribution:* Penetrates well into inflamed joints, vitreous humor, and peritoneal cavity. Poor distribution into sputum and saliva; unpredictable CSF penetration. Over 90% is bound to plasma proteins.
• *Metabolism:* Metabolized in liver, predominantly to inactive metabolites.
• *Excretion:* Triphasic elimination; terminal half-life is about 24 hours. Between 10% and 14% of oral dose excreted in urine; 50% in feces. Up to 1% of vaginal dose excreted in urine; 14% to 22% of I.V. dose excreted in urine. Unknown if excreted in breast milk.

Contraindications and precautions
Topical form contraindicated in patients with hypersensitivity to drug. Use cautiously in patients with hepatic insufficiency.

Interactions
Drug-drug. *Amphotericin B:* May antagonize effects of amphotericin B. Monitor patient closely.
Phenytoin: Increased phenytoin levels. Monitor phenytoin levels.
Warfarin: Enhanced anticoagulant effect. Monitor PT and INR closely.

Adverse reactions
CNS: headache.

GU: vulvovaginal burning, pruritus, or irritation with vaginal cream; pelvic cramps.
Skin: irritation, burning, maceration, allergic contact dermatitis.

☑ Special considerations
• Clean affected area before applying cream. After application, massage area gently until cream disappears.
• Continue topical therapy for at least 1 month; improvement should begin in 1 to 2 weeks. If no improvement occurs by 4 weeks, reevaluate diagnosis.
• Don't use occlusive dressings.
• Insert vaginal applicator high into vagina.

Monitoring the patient
• Monitor patient for adverse effects and patient's response to therapy.
• In patients on phenytoin or warfarin, monitor drug levels closely due to enhanced phenytoin in serum and increased anticoagulant effects.

Information for the patient
• Teach patient symptoms of fungal infection, and explain treatment rationale.
• Encourage patient to adhere to prescribed regimen and follow-up visits and to report adverse effects.
• Teach patient correct procedure for intravaginal or topical applications.
• To prevent vaginal reinfection, teach correct perineal hygiene and recommend that patient abstain from sexual intercourse during therapy.

Pediatric patients
• Safe use in children under age 1 hasn't been established.

Breast-feeding patients
• Safety hasn't been established. It's unknown if drug appears in breast milk.

midazolam hydrochloride
Versed

Pharmacologic classification: benzodiazepine
Therapeutic classification: preoperative sedative, drug for conscious sedation, adjunct for induction of general anesthesia, amnesic drug
Controlled substance schedule IV
Pregnancy risk category D

How supplied
Available by prescription only
Injection: 1 mg/ml in 2-ml, 5-ml, and 10-ml vials; 5 mg/ml in 1-ml, 2-ml, 5-ml, and 10-ml vials; 5 mg/ml in 2-ml disposable syringe
Syrup: 2 mg/ml in 118-ml bottle

Indications, route, and dosage

Preoperative sedation (to induce sleepiness or drowsiness and relieve apprehension)
Adults under age 60: 0.07 to 0.08 mg/kg I.M. about 1 hour before surgery. May be administered with atropine or scopolamine and reduced doses of narcotics.

✦ *Dosage adjustment.* Reduce dosage in patients over age 60, those with COPD, those considered to be high-risk surgical patients, and in those who have received concomitant narcotics or other depressants.

Conscious sedation
Adults under age 60: Initially, 1 to 2.5 mg I.V. administered over at least 2 minutes; repeat in 2 minutes, if needed, in small increments of initial dose over at least 2 minutes to achieve desired effect. Total dose up to 5 mg may be used. Additional doses to maintain desired level of sedation may be given by slow titration in increments of 25% of dose used to reach the sedation endpoint.
Adults ages 60 and over: 1.5 mg or less over at least 2 minutes. If additional titration is needed, give at a rate not exceeding 1 mg over 2 minutes. Total doses exceeding 3.5 mg aren't usually necessary.

Induction of general anesthesia
Unpremedicated adults under age 55: 0.3 to 0.35 mg/kg I.V. over 20 to 30 seconds if patient hasn't received preanesthesia drugs, or 0.2 to 0.25 mg/kg I.V. over 20 to 30 seconds if patient has received preanesthesia drugs. Additional increments of 25% of the initial dose may be needed to complete induction.
Unpremedicated adults age 55 and over: Initially, 0.3 mg/kg. For debilitated patients, initial dose is 0.2 to 0.25 mg/kg. For premedicated patients, 0.15 mg/kg may be sufficient.

Continuous infusion for sedation of intubated and mechanically ventilated patients as a component of anesthesia or during treatment in the critical care setting
Adults: If a loading dose is necessary to rapidly initiate sedation, give 0.01 to 0.05 mg/kg slowly or infused over several minutes, with dose repeated at 10- to 15-minute intervals until adequate sedation is achieved. For maintenance of sedation, usual infusion rate is 0.02 to 0.10 mg/kg/hour (1 to 7 mg/hour). Infusion rate should be titrated to the desired amount of sedation. Drug can be titrated up or down by 25% to 50% of the initial infusion rate to achieve optimal sedation without oversedation.
Children: After a loading dose of 0.05 to 0.2 mg/kg over 2 to 3 minutes in intubated patients only, an infusion may be initiated at 0.06 to 0.12 mg/kg/hour (1 to 2 mcg/kg/minute). Dose may be titrated up or down by 25% of the initial or subsequent infusion rate to obtain optimal sedation.
Neonates: Use only on intubated neonates. No loading dose is used in neonates. Neonates less than 32 weeks receive infusion rates of 0.03 mg/kg/hour (0.5 mcg/kg/minute). In neonates older than 32 weeks, infusion rates are 0.06 mg/kg/hour (1 mcg/kg/minute). Infusion may be run more rapidly in the first few hours to obtain a therapeutic blood level. Rate of infusion should be frequently and carefully reassessed to administer the lowest possible amount of drug.

Sedation, anxiolysis and amnesia before diagnostic, therapeutic, or endoscopic procedures or before induction of anesthesia in children
Children (syrup only): Single dose 0.25 to 1 mg/kg P.O., with a maximum dose of 20 mg. Lower doses may provide adequate therapeutic effect for children ages 6 to 16 or cooperative patients.

Pharmacodynamics

Sedative and anesthetic actions: Exact mechanism unknown. As with other benzodiazepines, thought to facilitate the action of gamma-amino-butyric acid (GABA) to provide a short-acting CNS depressant action.
Amnesic action: Mechanism unknown.

Pharmacokinetics

• *Absorption:* After I.M. administration, 80% to 100%; serum levels peak in 45 minutes and are about one-half of those after I.V. administration. Sedation begins within 15 minutes after I.M. dose; within 2 to 5 minutes after I.V. injection. After I.V. administration, induction of anesthesia occurs in 1½ to 2½ minutes. Following oral doses of syrup in children ages 6 months to 2 years, serum levels peak in 10 to 15 minutes; in children ages 2 to 12 years, level peaks in 45 to 60 minutes. Absorption is slower, and peak levels lower, after oral doses of syrup in children ages 12 to 16 years.
• *Distribution:* Large volume of distribution; about 97% protein-bound. Crosses the placenta and enters fetal circulation.
• *Metabolism:* Metabolized in liver.
• *Excretion:* Metabolites excreted in urine. Half-life of drug is 1.2 to 12.3 hours. Duration of sedation usually 1 to 4 hours.

Contraindications and precautions

Contraindicated in patients with hypersensitivity to drug, in those with acute angle-closure glaucoma, and in those experiencing shock, coma, or acute alcohol intoxication. Use cautiously in patients with uncompensated acute illnesses and in elderly or debilitated patients.

Interactions

Drug-drug. *Antidepressants, antihistamines, barbiturates, narcotics, tranquilizers, other CNS and respiratory depressants:* May add to or potentiate effects of these drugs. Avoid concomitant use if possible; adjust dose of midazolam if used together.

Droperidol, fentanyl, narcotics: When used as preoperative drugs, potentiate hypnotic effect of midazolam. Avoid concomitant use.
Erythromycin: May decrease plasma clearance of midazolam. Use with caution.
Inhaled anesthetics: Midazolam may decrease needed dose of these drugs by depressing respiratory drive. Monitor patient closely.
Isoniazid: Decreased metabolism of midazolam. Use together with caution.
Drug-lifestyle. *Alcohol:* Midazolam may add to or potentiate effects. Discourage use.

Adverse reactions
CNS: headache, oversedation, drowsiness, amnesia.
CV: variations in blood pressure (hypotension) and pulse rate, *cardiac arrest.*
GI: *nausea,* vomiting.
Respiratory: *hiccups, decreased respiratory rate,* APNEA, *respiratory arrest.*
Other: *pain, tenderness (at injection site).*

☑ Special considerations
Besides the recommendations relevant to all benzodiazepines, consider the following.
• Individualize dosage; use smallest effective dose possible. Use with extreme caution and reduce dosage in elderly and debilitated patients.
• Medical personnel who administer midazolam should be familiar with airway management. Close monitoring of cardiopulmonary function is required. Continuously monitor patients who have received midazolam to detect potentially life-threatening respiratory depression.
• Solutions of D_5W, normal saline solution, and lactated Ringer's solution are compatible with drug.
• Before I.V. administration, ensure the immediate availability of oxygen and resuscitative equipment. Apnea and death have been reported with rapid I.V. administration. Avoid intra-arterial injection because the hazards of this route are unknown. Avoid extravasation. Administer I.V. dose slowly to prevent respiratory depression.
• There is a potential for adverse effects (hypotension, metabolic acidosis, kernicterus) related to neonate metabolism of benzyl alcohol. Consider the amount of benzyl alcohol when giving high doses of drugs (such as midazolam) containing the preservative.
• Administer I.M. dose deep into a large muscle mass to prevent tissue injury.
• Don't use solution that is discolored or contains a precipitate.
• Midazolam can be mixed in the same syringe with morphine, meperidine, atropine, and scopolamine.
• Syrup form must be given only to patients visually monitored by health care professionals.
• Signs and symptoms of overdose include confusion, stupor, coma, respiratory depression, and hypotension. Hypotension occurs more frequently in patients premedicated with narcotics.
• Laryngospasm and bronchospasm may occur rarely; countermeasures should be available.

Monitoring the patient
• Monitor vital signs closely.
• Cardiac monitoring of patient required during drug administration.
• Monitor neurologic status.

Information for the patient
• Advise patient to postpone tasks that require mental alertness or physical coordination until the drug's effects have worn off.
• Instruct patient, as needed, in safety measures, such as supervised walking and gradual position changes, to prevent injury.
• Advise patient to call for instructions before taking OTC drugs.

Geriatric patients
• Elderly or debilitated patients, especially those with COPD, are at significantly increased risk for respiratory depression and hypotension. Lower doses are indicated. Use with caution. Oral dosage forms aren't recommended for geriatric use.

Pediatric patients
• Safety and efficacy in children haven't been established for nonoral dosage forms.

Breast-feeding patients
• It's unknown if drug appears in breast milk; use with caution in breast-feeding women.

miglitol
Glyset

Pharmacologic classification: alpha-glucosidase inhibitor
Therapeutic classification: antidiabetic
Pregnancy risk category B

How supplied
Available by prescription only
Tablets: 25 mg, 50 mg, 100 mg

Indications, route, and dosage
Monotherapy adjunct to diet to improve glycemic control in patients with type 2 diabetes mellitus whose hyperglycemia can't be managed with diet alone, or with a sulfonylurea when diet plus either miglitol or sulfonylurea alone don't result in adequate glycemic control
Adults: 25 mg P.O. t.i.d. at the start (with the first bite) of each main meal; dose may be increased after 4 to 8 weeks to 50 mg P.O. t.i.d. Dosage may then be further increased after three months,

based on the glycosylated hemoglobin level, to a maximum of 100 mg P.O. t.i.d.

Pharmacodynamics
Antidiabetic action: Lowers blood glucose through reversible inhibition of the enzymes alpha-glucosidases in the brush border of small intestine. Alpha-glucosidases are responsible for the conversion of oligosaccharides and disaccharides to glucose. Inhibition of these enzymes results in delayed glucose absorption and a lowering of postprandial blood glucose. In contrast to sulfonylureas, miglitol doesn't affect insulin secretion.

Pharmacokinetics
● *Absorption:* Saturable absorption at high doses. A 25-mg dose is completely absorbed; 100-mg dose is only 50% to 70% absorbed; levels peak in 2 to 3 hours after oral dose.
● *Distribution:* Distributed primarily into extracellular fluid. Negligible protein-binding.
● *Metabolism:* Not metabolized.
● *Excretion:* Eliminated primarily by renal excretion. More than 95% recovered in urine as unchanged drug. Elimination half-life is about 2 hours.

Contraindications and precautions
Contraindicated in patients with hypersensitivity to drug or its components; in those with diabetic ketoacidosis, inflammatory bowel disease, colonic ulceration, or partial intestinal obstruction; and in patients predisposed to intestinal obstruction or those with chronic intestinal diseases associated with marked disorders of digestion or absorption, or with conditions that may deteriorate as a result of increased gas formation in the intestine.
   Drug isn't recommended in patients with significant renal dysfunction (serum creatinine greater than 2.0 mg/dL). Use cautiously in patients receiving insulin or oral sulfonylureas.

Interactions
Drug-drug. *Digoxin, propranolol, ranitidine:* Decreased bioavailability of these drugs. Monitor these drugs for loss of efficacy and adjust dose accordingly.
Insulin, oral sulfonylureas: Increased hypoglycemic potential. Use with caution. Monitor serum glucose levels closely.
Intestinal absorbents (such as charcoal), digestive enzyme preparations (such as amylase, pancreatin): Reduced effectiveness of miglitol. Avoid concomitant use.

Adverse reactions
GI: *abdominal pain, diarrhea, flatulence.*
Skin: rash.
Other: decreased serum iron levels.

☑ Special considerations
● Management of type 2 diabetes should also include diet control, exercise program, and regular testing of urine and blood glucose.
● Miglitol should be given with the first bite of each main meal.
● Treat mild to moderate hypoglycemia with a form of dextrose such as glucose tablets or gel. Severe hypoglycemia may require I.V. glucose or glucagon administration.

Monitoring the patient
● Monitor blood glucose regularly, especially during situations of increased stress, such as infection, fever, surgery, and trauma.
● Additionally, monitor glycosylated hemoglobin every 3 months to assess long-term glycemic control.

Information for the patient
● Instruct patient about the importance of adhering to dietary, weight reduction, and exercise instructions and to have blood glucose and glycosylated hemoglobin tested regularly.
● Inform patient that treatment relieves symptoms but doesn't cure diabetes.
● Teach patient to recognize signs and symptoms of hyperglycemia and hypoglycemia.
● Instruct patient to treat hypoglycemia with glucose tablets and to have a source of glucose readily available to treat symptoms of hypoglycemia when miglitol is taken with a sulfonylurea or insulin.
● Advise patient to seek medical advice promptly during periods of stress such as fever, trauma, infection, or surgery because drug requirements may change.
● Instruct patient to take miglitol three times a day with the first bite of each main meal.
● Show patient how and when to monitor blood glucose levels.
● Advise patient that adverse GI effects are most common during the first few weeks of therapy and should improve over time.
● Urge patient to carry medical identification at all times.

Geriatric patients
● No significant differences in the safety and effectiveness of miglitol have been observed between older and younger patients.

Pediatric patients
● Safety and effectiveness in children haven't been established.

Breast-feeding patients
● Although amount of drug that appears in breast milk is low, it's recommended that drug not be administered to breast-feeding women.

milrinone lactate
Primacor

Pharmacologic classification: bipyridine phosphodiesterase inhibitor
Therapeutic classification: inotropic vasodilator
Pregnancy risk category C

How supplied
Available by prescription only
Solution: 1 mg/ml in 10-ml and 20-ml vials
Cartridge: 5 ml
Injection, premixed: 200 mEq/ml in 5% dextrose

Indications, route, and dosage
Short-term I.V. therapy for heart failure
Adults: Initial loading dose of 50 mcg/kg I.V. over 10 minutes; then continuous infusion-maintenance dose of 0.375 to 0.75 mcg/kg/minute. Adjust infusion dose based on hemodynamic and clinical response.
✦ *Dosage adjustment.* For patients with renal impairment, refer to the table.

Creatinine clearance (ml/min/1.73 m²)	Infusion rate (mcg/kg/min)
5	0.20
10	0.23
20	0.28
30	0.33
40	0.38
50	0.43

Pharmacodynamics
Inotropic and vasodilator actions: Selective inhibitor of peak III cAMP phosphodiesterase isozyme in cardiac and vascular muscle. This inhibitory action is consistent with cAMP-mediated increases in intracellular ionized calcium and contractile force in cardiac muscle, as well as with cAMP-dependent contractile protein phosphorylation and relaxation in vascular muscle. In addition to increasing myocardial contractility, milrinone improves diastolic function, shown by improvements in left ventricular diastolic relaxation.

Pharmacokinetics
• *Absorption:* Not applicable.
• *Distribution:* About 70% bound to plasma protein.
• *Metabolism:* About 12% of dose metabolized to a glucuronide metabolite.
• *Excretion:* After I.V. administration, about 90% of drug excreted unchanged in urine within 8 hours.

Contraindications and precautions
Contraindicated in patients with hypersensitivity to drug, in those with severe aortic or pulmonic valvular disease in place of surgical correction, and during the acute phase of an MI. Use cautiously in patients with atrial fibrillation or flutter.

Interactions
Drug-drug. *Furosemide:* Forms precipitate when mixed with milrinone. Don't give in same I.V. line.

Adverse reactions
CNS: headache.
CV: VENTRICULAR ARRHYTHMIAS, *ventricular ectopic activity, nonsustained ventricular tachycardia,* SUSTAINED VENTRICULAR TACHYCARDIA, VENTRICULAR FIBRILLATION, hypotension, angina.

☑ Special considerations
• Drug isn't recommended for patients in acute phase of post-MI.
• Duration of therapy depends on patient response. Patients have been maintained on infusions of milrinone for up to 5 days.
• When furosemide is injected into an I.V. line containing milrinone, an immediate chemical interaction occurs, as evidenced by the formation of a precipitate. Furosemide shouldn't be administered in an I.V. line that contains milrinone.
• Hypotension may occur with milrinone overdose because of its vasodilator effect.

Monitoring the patient
• Monitor vital signs and ECG closely.
• If hypotension occurs, temporarily stop drug or reduce dosage until patient's condition stabilizes.
• Monitor renal function and fluid and electrolyte changes during therapy. Correct hypokalemia with potassium supplements before or during use of milrinone.

Information for the patient
• Instruct patient to report adverse effects immediately.
• Tell patient to alert nurse if discomfort occurs at I.V. site.

Pediatric patients
• Safety and efficacy in children haven't been established.

Breast-feeding patients
• It's unknown if drug appears in breast milk. Use with caution in breast-feeding women.

Reactions may be *common*, uncommon, **life-threatening**, or COMMON AND LIFE-THREATENING.

mineral oil
Agoral Plain, Fleet Enema Mineral Oil,
Kondremul*, Kondremul Plain,
Lansoÿl*, Nujol*, Petrogalar Plain

Pharmacologic classification: lubricant
oil
Therapeutic classification: laxative
Pregnancy risk category C

How supplied
Available without a prescription
Jelly: 180 ml
Emulsion: 2.5 ml/5 ml, 1.4 g/5 ml
Suspension: 1.4 ml/5 ml, 2.75 ml/5 ml, 4.75 ml/
5 ml
Rectal oil enema: 120 ml

Indications, route, and dosage
**Constipation, preparation for bowel studies
or surgery**
Adults and children ages 12 and older: 5 to 45
ml P.O. as a single dose or in divided doses, or
120-ml enema.
Children ages 6 to 11: 5 to 15 ml P.O. daily as a
single dose or in divided doses, or 30- to 60-ml
enema.
Children ages 2 to 6: 30- to 60-ml enema.

Pharmacodynamics
Laxative action: Acts mainly in the colon, lubricating the intestine and retarding colonic fluid absorption.

Pharmacokinetics
• *Absorption:* Normally absorbed minimally; with
emulsified drug form, significant absorption. Ac-
tion begins in 6 to 8 hours.
• *Distribution:* Distributed locally, primarily in colon.
• *Metabolism:* None.
• *Excretion:* Excreted in feces.

Contraindications and precautions
Contraindicated in patients with abdominal pain,
nausea, vomiting, or other symptoms of appendicitis or acute surgical abdomen, and in those
with fecal impaction or intestinal obstruction or
perforation. Also contraindicated in patients with
colostomy, ileostomy, ulcerative colitis, and diverticulitis.
　　Use cautiously in elderly or debilitated patients and in the young.

Interactions
Drug-drug. *Anticoagulants, cardiac glycosides,
fat-soluble vitamins (A, D, E, K), oral contraceptives, sulfonamides:* Mineral oil may impair absorption of these drugs, decreasing their therapeutic
effects. Monitor patient for vitamin deficiency.
Stool softeners (such as docusate): Increased
mineral oil absorption to potentially toxic levels.

Avoid use together; concurrent use may cause
lipid pneumonia.

Adverse reactions
GI: *nausea; vomiting; diarrhea* (with excessive
use); abdominal cramps, especially in severe constipation; decreased absorption of nutrients and
fat-soluble vitamins, resulting in deficiency; slowed
healing after hemorrhoidectomy.
Other: laxative dependence (with long-term or
excessive use), anal pruritus, anal irritation, hemorrhoids, perianal discomfort, *lipid pneumonia.*

☑ Special considerations
• Avoid administering drug to patients lying flat;
if drug is aspirated into the lungs, pneumonitis
may result.
• Don't give drug with food because this may delay gastric emptying, resulting in delayed drug
action and increased aspiration risk. Separate
administration times by at least 2 hours.
• To improve taste, give emulsion and suspension with fruit juice or carbonated beverages.
• Prescribe cleansing enema 30 minutes to 1
hour after retention enema.
• Reduce or divide dose or use emulsified drug
form to avoid leakage through anal sphincter.

Monitoring the patient
• Monitor patient's response to therapy.
• Monitor fluid balance.

Information for the patient
• Instruct patient not to take mineral oil with stool
softeners.
• Warn patient that mineral oil may leak through
anal sphincter, especially with repeated use or
with enema form. Undergarment protection may
be desired.

Geriatric patients
• Because of increased risk of aspiration, use
caution when administering drug to elderly patients.

Pediatric patients
• Mineral oil isn't recommended for children under age 6 because of risk of aspiration. Enema
form is contraindicated in children under age 2.

minocycline hydrochloride
Dynacin, Minocin

Pharmacologic classification: tetra-
cycline
Therapeutic classification: antibiotic
Pregnancy risk category NR

How supplied
Available by prescription only
Capsules: 50 mg, 100 mg

Tablets: 50 mg, 100 mg
Suspension: 50 mg/5 ml
Injection: 100 mg/vial

Indications, route, and dosage

Infections caused by sensitive organisms
Adults: Initially, 200 mg P.O. or I.V.; then 100 mg q 12 hours or 50 mg P.O. q 6 hours.
Children over age 8: Initially, 4 mg/kg P.O. or I.V.; then 4 mg/kg P.O. daily, divided q 12 hours. Give I.V. in 500- to 1,000-ml solution without calcium, over 6 hours.
Gonorrhea in patients sensitive to penicillin
Adults: Initially, 200 mg P.O., I.V., or I.M.; then 100 mg P.O. q 12 hours for 4 days.
Syphilis in patients sensitive to penicillin
Adults: Initially, 200 mg P.O., I.V., or I.M.; then 100 mg P.O. q 12 hours for 10 to 15 days.
Meningococcal carrier state
Adults: 100 mg P.O. q 12 hours for 5 days.
Uncomplicated urethral, endocervical, or rectal infection caused by Chlamydia trachomatis or Ureaplasma urealyticum
Adults: 100 mg P.O. q 12 hours for at least 7 days.
Uncomplicated gonococcal urethritis in men
Adults: 100 mg P.O. q 12 hours for 5 days.
Mycobacterium marinum
Adults: 100 mg P.O. q 12 hours for 6 to 8 weeks.
Cholera
Adults: Initially, 200 mg P.O.; then 100 mg P.O. q 12 hours for 72 hours.
Acne
Adults: 50 mg P.O. daily, b.i.d. or t.i.d.
◊ *Nocardiosis*
Adults: Usual dose for 12 to 18 months.
◊ *Sclerosis drug for pleural effusions*
Adults: 300 mg mixed in 40 to 50 ml normal saline solution, instilled through a thoracostomy tube.

Pharmacodynamics

Antibacterial action: Bacteriostatic. Binds reversibly to ribosomal units, thus inhibiting bacterial protein synthesis. Active against many gram-negative and gram-positive organisms, *Mycoplasma, Rickettsia, Chlamydia,* and spirochetes; may be more active against staphylococci than other tetracyclines.
   The potential vestibular toxicity and cost of minocycline limit its usefulness. It may be more active than other tetracyclines against *Nocardia asteroides;* it's also effective against *Mycobacterium marinum* infections. It has been used for meningococcal meningitis prophylaxis because of its activity against *Neisseria meningitidis.*

Pharmacokinetics

• *Absorption:* About 90% to 100% of drug absorbed after oral administration; serum levels peak at 2 to 3 hours.
• *Distribution:* Widely distributed into body tissues and fluids, including synovial, pleural, prostatic, and seminal fluids, bronchial secretions, saliva, and aqueous humor; poor CSF penetration. Crosses placenta; 55% to 88% protein-bound.
• *Metabolism:* Partially metabolized.
• *Excretion:* Excreted primarily unchanged in urine by glomerular filtration. Plasma half-life is 11 to 22 hours in adults with normal renal function. Some drug excreted in breast milk.

Contraindications and precautions

Contraindicated in patients with hypersensitivity to drug or other tetracyclines. Use cautiously in patients with impaired renal or hepatic function, in children under age 8, and during the last half of pregnancy.

Interactions

Drug-drug. *Antacids containing aluminum, calcium, magnesium; laxatives containing magnesium:* Decreased oral absorption of minocycline. Give antibiotic 1 hour before or 2 hours after these drugs.
Digoxin: Increased bioavailability. Monitor serum digoxin levels; adjust dosage as needed.
Oral anticoagulants: Enhanced anticoagulant effects. Monitor PT and INR; adjust dosage as necessary.
Oral contraceptives: May be less effective when administered with minocycline. Recommend use of nonhormonal birth control.
Oral iron products, sodium bicarbonate: Decreased absorption. Give drug 2 hours before or 3 hours after iron administration.
Penicillin: Tetracyclines may antagonize bactericidal effects. Administer penicillin 2 to 3 hours before minocycline.
Drug-food. *Any food, milk, other dairy products:* Decreased absorption of minocycline. Advise patient to take drug with full glass of water.
Drug-lifestyle. *Sun exposure:* Increased risk of photosensitivity reactions. Tell patient to take precautions.

Adverse reactions

CNS: headache, *intracranial hypertension (pseudotumor cerebri),* light-headedness, dizziness, vertigo.
CV: pericarditis, *thrombophlebitis.*
EENT: dysphagia, glossitis.
GI: *anorexia, epigastric distress, oral candidiasis, nausea, vomiting, diarrhea,* enterocolitis, inflammatory lesions in anogenital region.
GU: increased BUN level.
Hematologic: *neutropenia,* eosinophilia, *thrombocytopenia,* hemolytic anemia.
Hepatic: elevated liver enzyme levels.
Skin: *maculopapular and erythematous rashes, photosensitivity, increased pigmentation,* urticaria.
Other: hypersensitivity reactions (*anaphylaxis*); permanent discoloration of teeth, enamel defects, and bone growth retardation if used in children under age 8; superinfection.

Reactions may be *common*, uncommon, *life-threatening*, or COMMON AND LIFE-THREATENING.

☑ Special considerations
Besides the recommendations relevant to all tetracyclines, consider the following.
• Reconstitute 100 mg powder with 5 ml sterile water for injection, with further dilution of 500 to 1,000 ml for I.V. infusion.
• Reconstituted solution is stable for 24 hours at room temperature. However, final diluted solution should be used immediately.
• Drug causes false-negative results in urine glucose tests using glucose oxidase reagent (Diastix, Chemstrip uG, or glucose enzymatic test strip).
• Minocycline causes false elevations in fluorometric test results for urinary catecholamines.
• Signs and symptoms of overdose are usually limited to GI tract; give antacids or empty stomach by gastric lavage if recent ingestion (within 4 hours).

Monitoring the patient
• Monitor patient for adverse reactions and response to drug therapy.
• Watch for signs of superinfections.

Information for the patient
• Tell patient to take entire amount of drug, exactly as prescribed, even if feeling better.
• Warn patient of potential CNS effects, and to use caution until full effect is known.

Pediatric patients
• Drug isn't recommended for use in children under age 9.

Breast-feeding patients
• Avoid use in breast-feeding women; drug appears in breast milk.

---

minoxidil (systemic)
Loniten

Pharmacologic classification: peripheral vasodilator
Therapeutic classification: antihypertensive
Pregnancy risk category C

How supplied
Available by prescription only
Tablets: 2.5 mg, 10 mg

Indications, route, and dosage
Severe hypertension
Adults and children ages 12 and older: Initially, 5 mg P.O. as a single daily dose. Effective dosage range is usually 10 to 40 mg daily. Maximum dose is 100 mg/day.
Children under age 12: 0.2 mg/kg (maximum 5 mg) as a single daily dose. Effective dosage range is usually 0.25 to 1 mg/kg daily in one or two doses. Maximum dose is 50 mg/day.

Pharmacodynamics
Antihypertensive action: Produces its antihypertensive effect by a direct vasodilating effect on vascular smooth muscle; the effect on resistance vessels (arterioles and arteries) is greater than that on capacitance vessels (venules and veins).

Pharmacokinetics
• *Absorption:* Absorbed rapidly and almost completely from GI tract; antihypertensive effect occurs in 30 minutes; peaks at 2 to 3 hours.
• *Distribution:* Distributed widely into body tissues; not bound to plasma proteins.
• *Metabolism:* About 90% of dose metabolized.
• *Excretion:* Drug and metabolites excreted primarily in urine. Average plasma half-life is 4.2 hours; antihypertensive action lasts about 3 days.

Contraindications and precautions
Contraindicated in patients with hypersensitivity to drug and in those with pheochromocytoma. Use cautiously in patients with impaired renal function or after acute MI.

Interactions
Drug-drug. *Diuretics, guanethidine:* Possible profound orthostatic hypotension. Advise patient to stand slowly. Monitor blood pressure.

Adverse reactions
CV: *edema, tachycardia, pericardial effusion and tamponade,* **heart failure,** *ECG changes, rebound hypertension.*
GI: nausea, vomiting.
Metabolic: *weight gain.*
Skin: rash, **Stevens-Johnson syndrome.**
Other: *hypertrichosis (elongation, thickening, and enhanced pigmentation of fine body hair), breast tenderness.*

☑ Special considerations
• Drug is usually given with other antihypertensives, such as diuretics, beta blockers, or sympathetic nervous system suppressants.
• Patients with renal failure or on dialysis may need smaller maintenance doses of minoxidil. Because drug is removed by dialysis, it's recommended that, on the day of dialysis, the drug be administered immediately after dialysis if dialysis is at 9 a.m.; if dialysis is after 3 p.m., the daily dose is given at 7 a.m. (8 hours before dialysis).
• Signs and symptoms of overdose include hypotension, tachycardia, headache, and skin flushing. After acute ingestion, empty stomach by induced emesis or gastric lavage, and give activated charcoal to reduce absorption.

Monitoring the patient
• Monitor blood pressure and pulse after administration, and report significant changes; assess intake, output, and body weight for sodium and water retention.
• Monitor patient for heart failure, pericardial effusion, and cardiac tamponade; have phenylephrine, dopamine, and vasopressin on hand to treat hypotension.

Information for the patient
• Explain that drug is usually taken with other antihypertensives; emphasize importance of taking drug as prescribed.
• Caution patient to promptly report cardiac symptoms, such as increased heart rate (over 20 beats/minute over normal), rapid weight gain, shortness of breath, chest pain, severe indigestion, dizziness, light-headedness, or fainting.
• Tell patient to call for instructions before taking OTC cold preparations.
• Advise patient that hypertrichosis will disappear 1 to 6 months after drug ends.

Geriatric patients
• Elderly patients may be sensitive to drug's antihypertensive effects. Dosage adjustment may be necessary because of altered drug clearance.

Pediatric patients
• Because of limited experience in children, use with caution. Cautious dosage adjustment is necessary.

Breast-feeding patients
• Drug appears in breast milk. An alternative to breast-feeding is recommended during therapy.

---

minoxidil (topical)
Rogaine

Pharmacologic classification: direct-acting vasodilator
Therapeutic classification: hair-growth stimulant
Pregnancy risk category C

How supplied
Available without a prescription
Topical solution: 2%, 5% in 60-ml bottle

Indications, route, and dosage
Male pattern baldness (alopecia androgenetica), diffuse hair loss or thinning in women, ◊ adjunct to hair transplantation
Adults: Apply 1 ml to affected area b.i.d. for 4 months or longer.

Pharmacodynamics
Hair-growth stimulation: Exact mechanism unknown. May alter androgen metabolism in the scalp or may exert a local vasodilatation and enhance the microcirculation around the hair follicle. May also directly stimulate the hair follicle.

Pharmacokinetics
• *Absorption:* Poorly absorbed through intact skin. About 0.3% to 4.5% of topically applied dose reaches systemic circulation.
• *Distribution:* Serum levels generally negligible.
• *Metabolism:* Not fully described.
• *Excretion:* Eliminated primarily by kidneys. About 95% of topically applied dose eliminated after 4 days.

Contraindications and precautions
Contraindicated in patients with hypersensitivity to drug or its component and during pregnancy. Use cautiously in patients with renal, cardiac, or hepatic disease and in those over age 50.

Interactions
Drug-drug. *Petrolatum, topical corticosteroid, topical retinoids, other drugs that may enhance skin absorption:* Increased risk of systemic effects of minoxidil. Don't apply or mix minoxidil with other drugs.

Adverse reactions
CNS: headache, dizziness, light-headedness, faintness.
CV: edema, chest pain, hypertension, hypotension, palpitations, increased or decreased pulse rate.
EENT: sinusitis.
GI: diarrhea, nausea, vomiting.
GU: urinary tract infection, renal calculi, urethritis.
Metabolic: weight gain.
Musculoskeletal: back pain.
Respiratory: bronchitis, upper respiratory infection.
Skin: irritant dermatitis, allergic contact dermatitis, eczema, hypertrichosis, local erythema, pruritus, dry skin or scalp, flaking, alopecia, exacerbation of hair loss.
Other: tendinitis.

☑ Special considerations
• Rogaine is for topical use only; each milliliter contains 20 mg or 50 mg minoxidil and accidental ingestion could cause adverse systemic effects.
• Alcohol base will burn and irritate eyes and other sensitive surfaces (eyes, abraded skin, mucous membranes). If topical minoxidil contacts sensitive areas, flush copiously with cool water.
• Before starting treatment, check that patient has a normal, healthy scalp. Local abrasion or dermatitis may increase absorption and risk of adverse effects.
• Before treatment, patient should have a medical history obtained and physical performed and

should be advised of potential risks; a risk-benefit decision should be made. Patients with cardiac disease should realize that adverse effects may be especially serious. Alert patient to possibility of tachycardia and fluid retention, and monitor patient for increased heart rate, weight gain, or other systemic effects.
• If acute ingestion occurs, empty stomach by induced emesis or gastric lavage, and give activated charcoal to reduce absorption.

Monitoring the patient
• Monitor patient 1 month after starting topical drug therapy and at least every 6 months after; stop topical minoxidil if systemic effects occur.
• Monitor patient for adverse effects.

Information for the patient
• Tell patient to avoid inhaling spray.
• Teach patient to apply topical minoxidil as follows: Hair and scalp should be dry before application. Apply 1 ml to the total affected areas twice daily. Total daily dose shouldn't exceed 2 ml. If fingertips are used to apply drug, wash hands afterward.
• Encourage patient to carefully review patient information leaflet, which is included with each package and in the full product information.
• Inform patient that 4 months of use may be needed before results are seen.

Pediatric patients
• Safety and effectiveness haven't been established for children under age 18.

Breast-feeding patients
• It's unknown if drug appears in breast milk. Drug shouldn't be administered to breast-feeding women.

mirtazapine
Remeron

Pharmacologic classification: piperazinoazepine
Therapeutic classification: tetracyclic antidepressant
Pregnancy risk category C

How supplied
Available by prescription only
Tablets: 15 mg, 30 mg

Indications, route, and dosage
Depression
Adults: Initially, 15 mg P.O. h.s. Maintenance dose ranges from 15 to 45 mg daily. Dosage adjustments should be made at intervals no less than 1 to 2 weeks apart.

Pharmacodynamics
Antidepressant action: Mechanism unknown.

Pharmacokinetics
• Absorption: Rapidly and completely absorbed from GI tract. Absolute bioavailability of drug about 50%.
• Distribution: About 85% bound to plasma protein.
• Metabolism: Extensively metabolized in liver.
• Excretion: Predominantly eliminated in urine (75%); 15% excreted in feces. Half-life is between 20 and 40 hours.

Contraindications and precautions
Contraindicated in patients with hypersensitivity to drug. Administration with MAO inhibitors is contraindicated.
Use cautiously in patients with CV or cerebrovascular disease, seizure disorders, suicidal ideation, impaired hepatic and renal function, or history of mania or hypomania. Also, use cautiously in patients with conditions that predispose them to hypotension, such as dehydration, hypovolemia, or treatment with antihypertensives.

Interactions
Drug-drug. Diazepam, other CNS depressants: Additive CNS effects when administered with mirtazapine. Avoid use together.
MAO inhibitors: Potentially serious, sometimes fatal, reactions. Mirtazapine shouldn't be used with or within 14 days of starting or stopping MAO therapy.
Drug-lifestyle. Alcohol: Additive CNS effects when consumed with drug. Discourage use.

Adverse reactions
CNS: somnolence, dizziness, asthenia, abnormal dreams, abnormal thinking, tremor, confusion.
CV: edema.
GI: nausea, increased appetite, dry mouth, constipation.
GU: urinary frequency.
Metabolic: weight gain.
Musculoskeletal: back pain, myalgia.
Respiratory: dyspnea.
Other: flulike syndrome, peripheral edema.

☑ Special considerations
• Use with caution in patients with increased intraocular pressure or history of urine retention or narrow-angle glaucoma because of anticholinergic properties.
• Overdose may result in disorientation, drowsiness, impaired memory, and tachycardia. If overdose occurs, treatment should be the same as for any antidepressant overdose.

Monitoring the patient
• Monitor patient closely; it's unknown if drug causes physical or psychological dependence.
• Although risk of agranulocytosis is rare, stop drug and monitor patient closely if he develops a sore throat, fever, stomatitis, or other signs of infection with a low WBC count.

Information for the patient
• Caution patient not to perform hazardous activities if somnolence occurs with drug use.
• Instruct patient not to use alcohol or other CNS depressants while taking drug because of additive effect.
• Tell patient to report signs and symptoms of infection, such as fever, chills, sore throat, mucous membrane ulceration, or flulike symptoms.
• Stress importance of compliance with therapy.
• Instruct patient not to take any other drug without medical approval.
• Tell woman of childbearing age to report suspected pregnancy immediately.

Geriatric patients
• Administer drug cautiously to elderly patients because of decreased clearance in this age-group.

Pediatric patients
• Safety and effectiveness in children haven't been established.

Breast-feeding patients
• It's unknown if drug appears in breast milk; use cautiously in breast-feeding women.

misoprostol
Cytotec

Pharmacologic classification: prostaglandin E₁ analogue
Therapeutic classification: antiulcerative, gastric mucosal protectant
Pregnancy risk category X

How supplied
Available by prescription only
Tablets: 100 mcg, 200 mcg

Indications, route, and dosage
Prevention of gastric ulcer induced by NSAIDs
Adults: 200 mcg P.O. q.i.d with meals and h.s. Reduce dose to 100 mcg P.O. q.i.d. in patients who can't tolerate this dose.
◇ *Duodenal or gastric ulcer*
Adults: 100 to 200 mcg P.O. q.i.d. with meals and h.s.
◇ *Prevention of acute graft rejection in renal transplantation*
Adults: 200 mcg P.O. q.i.d. for 12 weeks.

Pharmacodynamics
Antiulcerative action: Enhances production of gastric mucous and bicarbonate and decreases basal, nocturnal, and stimulated gastric acid secretion.

Pharmacokinetics
• *Absorption:* Rapidly absorbed after oral administration.
• *Distribution:* Less than 90% bound to plasma proteins. Levels peak in about 12 minutes.
• *Metabolism:* Rapidly deesterified to misoprostol acid, the biologically active metabolite. Metabolite undergoes further oxidation in several body tissues.
• *Excretion:* About 15% of oral dose appears in feces; balance excreted in urine. Terminal half-life is 20 to 40 minutes.

Contraindications and precautions
Contraindicated in pregnant or breast-feeding patients and in those with known allergy to prostaglandins.

Interactions
Drug-drug. *Antacids:* Misoprostol levels decreased by coadministration. Effect not believed significant.
Aspirin: Decreased availability of aspirin. Effect not believed significant.
Drug-food. *Any food:* Reduced drug levels. Effect not believed significant.

Adverse reactions
CNS: headache.
GI: *diarrhea, abdominal pain, nausea, flatulence, dyspepsia, vomiting, constipation.*
GU: hypermenorrhea, dysmenorrhea, spotting, cramps, menstrual disorders.

☑ Special considerations
• Misoprostol shouldn't be prescribed for a woman of childbearing age unless she:
– needs NSAID therapy and is at high risk for developing gastric ulcers.
– is capable of complying with effective contraception.
– has received both oral and written warnings regarding hazards of misoprostol therapy, risk of possible contraception failure, and hazards drug would pose to other women of childbearing age who might take this drug by mistake.
– has had a negative serum pregnancy test within 2 weeks before beginning therapy, and she will begin therapy on the second or third day of her next normal menstrual period.
• Drug has been used for treatment and prophylaxis of reflux esophagitis, alcohol-induced gastritis, hemorrhagic gastritis, and fat malabsorption in cystic fibrosis.

- Misoprostol produces a modest decrease in basal pepsin secretion.
- Diarrhea is usually dose-related and develops within the first 2 weeks of therapy. Minimize by administering drug after meals and at bedtime, and by avoiding antacids containing magnesium.
- If overdose occurs, treatment should be supportive.

Monitoring the patient
- Monitor patient's response to drug therapy.
- Evaluate for adverse effects.

Information for the patient
- Explain importance of not giving drug to anyone else.
- Make sure woman understands that a miscarriage could result if drug is taken during pregnancy.

Pediatric patients
- Safety hasn't been established in children under age 18.

Breast-feeding patients
- Breast-feeding isn't recommended because of potential for drug-induced diarrhea in infant.

mitomycin
(mitomycin-C; MTC)
Mutamycin

Pharmacologic classification: antineoplastic antibiotic (cell cycle–phase nonspecific)
Therapeutic classification: antineoplastic
Pregnancy risk category NR

How supplied
Available by prescription only
Injection: 5-mg, 20-mg, 40-mg vials

Indications, route, and dosage
Dosage and indications may vary. Check current literature for recommended protocol. Not indicated as a single-drug primary therapy.
Stomach and pancreatic adenocarcinoma (with other chemotherapeutic drugs); ◊ *breast,* ◊ *colon,* ◊ *rectum,* ◊ *head,* ◊ *neck,* ◊ *lung,* ◊ *cervix, and* ◊ *bladder cancer*
Adults: 20 mg/m² as a single dose. Repeat cycle q 6 to 8 weeks, adjusting dosage, if needed, according to the following guidelines.
✦ *Dosage adjustment.* Stop drug if WBC count is below 4,000/mm³ or platelet count is below 100,000/mm³. No repeat dose should be given until blood counts go above these levels.

Nadir after prior dose		Percentage of prior dose to be given
WBCs/mm³	Platelets/mm³	
> 4,000	>100,000	100%
3,000 to 3,999	75,000 to 99,999	100%
2,000 to 2,999	25,000 to 74,999	70%
< 2,000	< 25,000	50%

Pharmacodynamics
Antineoplastic action: Exerts cytotoxic activity by a mechanism similar to that of the alkylating drugs. Converted to an active compound, which forms cross-links between strands of DNA, inhibiting DNA synthesis. Also inhibits RNA and protein synthesis to a lesser extent.

Pharmacokinetics
- *Absorption:* Because of its vesicant nature, drug must be administered I.V.
- *Distribution:* Distributed widely into body tissues; highest levels found in kidneys, then muscle, eyes, lungs, intestines, and stomach. Doesn't cross blood-brain barrier.
- *Metabolism:* Metabolized by hepatic microsomal enzymes; also deactivated in kidneys, spleen, brain, and heart.
- *Excretion:* Drug and metabolites excreted in urine; small portion eliminated in bile and feces.

Contraindications and precautions
Contraindicated in patients with hypersensitivity to drug and in those with thrombocytopenia, coagulation disorders, or an increase in bleeding tendency due to other causes. Contraindicated as primary therapy as a single drug to replace surgery or radiotherapy.

Interactions
Drug-drug. *Vinca alkaloids:* Acute shortness of breath and severe bronchospasm have occurred after drug use in patients who had previously or simultaneously received mitomycin. Monitor patient closely.

Adverse reactions
CNS: headache, neurologic abnormalities, confusion, drowsiness, fatigue.
EENT: blurred vision.
GI: *nausea, vomiting, anorexia, diarrhea.*
Hematologic: THROMBOCYTOPENIA, LEUKOPENIA (may be delayed up to 8 weeks and may be cumulative with successive doses), *microangiopathic hemolytic anemia, characterized by thrombocytopenia, renal failure, and hypertension.*

Respiratory: *interstitial pneumonitis,* pulmonary edema, dyspnea, nonproductive cough, adult respiratory distress syndrome.
Skin: *reversible alopecia;* desquamation, induration, pruritus, and pain at injection site.
Other: *septicemia,* cellulitis, ulceration, sloughing with extravasation, fever, pain.

☑ Special considerations
• To reconstitute 5-mg vial, use 10 ml of sterile water for injection; to reconstitute 20-mg vial, use 40 ml of sterile water for injection; to reconstitute a 40-mg vial, use 80 ml sterile water for injection, to give a concentration of 0.5 mg/ml. Allow to stand at room temperature until complete dissolution occurs.
• Drug may be administered by I.V. push injection slowly over 5 to 10 minutes into tubing of a free flowing I.V. infusion.
• Drug can be further diluted to 100 to 150 ml with normal saline solution or D₅W for I.V. infusion (over 30 to 60 minutes or longer).
• Reconstituted solution remains stable for 1 week at room temperature and for 2 weeks if refrigerated.
• Mitomycin has been used intra-arterially to treat certain tumors (for example, into hepatic artery for colon cancer). Has also been given as a continuous daily infusion.
• An unlabeled use of drug is to treat small bladder papillomas. It's instilled directly into bladder in a concentration of 20 mg/20 ml sterile water.
• Ulcers caused by extravasation develop late and dorsal to extravasation site. Apply cold compresses for at least 12 hours.
• Signs and symptoms of overdose include myelosuppression, nausea, vomiting, and alopecia. Treatment is supportive.

Monitoring the patient
• Observe patients for evidence of renal toxicity. Don't give to patients with a serum creatinine over 1.7 mg/dl.
• Continue CBC and blood studies at least 7 weeks after therapy is stopped. Monitor patient for signs of bleeding.

Information for the patient
• Tell patient to avoid exposure to people with infections.
• Warn patient not to receive immunizations during therapy and for several weeks afterward. Members of same household shouldn't receive immunizations during the same period.
• Reassure patient that hair should grow back after treatment ends.
• Tell patient to call promptly if he develops a sore throat or fever or notices unusual bruising or bleeding.

Breast-feeding patients
• It's unknown if drug appears in breast milk. To avoid risk of serious adverse reactions, mutagenicity, and carcinogenicity in infant, breast-feeding isn't recommended.

---

mitoxantrone hydrochloride
Novantrone

Pharmacologic classification: antibiotic antineoplastic
Therapeutic classification: antineoplastic
Pregnancy risk category D

How supplied
Available by prescription only
Injection: 2 mg mitoxantrone base/ml in 10-ml, 12.5-ml, 15-ml vials

Indications, route, and dosage
Initial treatment with other approved drugs for acute nonlymphocytic leukemia
Adults: For induction (in combination chemotherapy), 12 mg/m² daily by I.V. infusion on days 1 to 3, and 100 mg/m² of cytosine arabinoside by continuous I.V. infusion (over 24 hours) on days 1 to 7 for 7 days.
   Most complete remissions follow initial course of induction therapy. A second course may be given if antileukemic response is incomplete: give mitoxantrone for 2 days and cytosine for 5 days using the same daily dose. Second course of therapy should be withheld until toxicity clears if severe or life-threatening nonhematologic toxicity occurs.
Combined initial therapy for pain related to advanced hormone-refractory prostate cancer
Adults: 12 to 14 mg/m² I.V. infusion over 15 to 30 minutes q 21 days.

Pharmacodynamics
Antineoplastic action: Exact mechanism unknown. A DNA-reactive drug that has cytocidal effects on proliferating and nonproliferating cells, suggestive of lack of cell-phase specificity.

Pharmacokinetics
• *Absorption:* Only administered by I.V. infusion.
• *Distribution:* 78% plasma protein-bound.
• *Metabolism:* Metabolized by liver.
• *Excretion:* Excretion via renal and hepatobiliary systems; 6% to 11% of dose excreted in urine within 5 days: 65% unchanged drug; 35% two inactive metabolites. Within 5 days, 25% of dose excreted in feces.

Contraindications and precautions
Contraindicated in patients with hypersensitivity to drug. Use cautiously in patients with prior ex-

---

posure to anthracyclines or other cardiotoxic drugs.

Interactions
Drug-drug. *Heparin:* Physically incompatible. Don't mix.

Adverse reactions
CNS: *seizures,* headache.
CV: *heart failure, arrhythmias,* tachycardia.
EENT: conjunctivitis, temporary blue color to sclera.
GI: *bleeding, abdominal pain, diarrhea, nausea, mucositis, vomiting,* stomatitis.
GU: *renal failure.*
Hematologic: *myelosuppression.*
Hepatic: jaundice.
Respiratory: *dyspnea, cough.*
Skin: *alopecia, petechiae, ecchymoses.*
Other: hyperuricemia, *sepsis, fungal infections, fever.*

☑ Special considerations
• Safety of administration by routes other than I.V. hasn't been established. Don't use intrathecally.
• Hyperuricemia may result from rapid lysis of tumor cells. Monitor serum uric acid levels. Institute hypouricemic therapy before antileukemic therapy.
• To prepare, dilute solutions to at least 50 ml with either normal saline solution or D_5W. Inject slowly into tubing of a freely running I.V. solution of normal saline solution or D_5W over not less than 3 minutes. Discard unused infusion solutions appropriately. Don't mix for infusion with heparin; a precipitate may form. Specific compatibility data aren't available.
• If extravasation occurs, discontinue I.V. and restart in another vein. Mitoxantrone is a nonvesicant and the possibility of severe local reactions is minimal.
• Urine may appear blue-green for 24 hours after administration.

Monitoring the patient
• Close and frequent monitoring of hematologic and chemical laboratory parameters, including serial CBC and liver function tests, with frequent patient observation is recommended.
• Watch for bluish discoloration of sclera, which may be a sign of myelosuppression.
• Monitor AST and ALT levels. Transient elevations of AST and ALT levels have occurred 4 to 24 days after therapy.

Information for the patient
• Advise patient to call promptly if signs and symptoms of myelosuppression develop (fever, sore throat, easy bruising, or excessive bleeding).

• Advise patient to use contraception; tell patient to call if pregnancy is suspected.
• Tell patient to drink fluids to minimize uric acid nephropathy.
• Tell patient urine may appear blue-green for 24 hours after administration and sclera may appear bluish.

Pediatric patients
• Safety and efficacy in children haven't been established.

Breast-feeding patients
• It's unknown if drug appears in breast milk. Because of potential for serious adverse reactions in infants, breast-feeding should be stopped before therapy.

mivacurium chloride
Mivacron

Pharmacologic classification: nondepolarizing neuromuscular blocker
Therapeutic classification: skeletal muscle relaxant
Pregnancy risk category C

How supplied
Available by prescription only
Injection: 2 mg/ml in 5-ml and 10-ml vials
Infusion: 0.5 mg/ml in 50 ml D_5W

Indications, route, and dosage
Adjunct to general anesthesia, to facilitate endotracheal intubation, and to provide skeletal muscle relaxation during surgery or mechanical ventilation
Dosage is highly individualized. Note that all times of onset and duration of neuromuscular blockade are averages and considerable individual variation is normal.
Adults: Usually, 0.15 mg/kg I.V. push over 5 to 15 seconds provides adequate muscle relaxation within 2½ minutes for endotracheal intubation. Clinically sufficient neuromuscular blockade usually lasts about 15 to 20 minutes. Supplemental doses of 0.1 mg/kg I.V. q 15 minutes usually maintain muscle relaxation. Or maintain neuromuscular blockade with a continuous infusion of 4 mcg/kg/minute started simultaneously with initial dose, or 9 to 10 mcg/kg/minute started after evidence of spontaneous recovery of initial dose. When used with isoflurane or enflurane anesthesia, dosage is usually reduced about 35% to 40%.
✦ **Dosage adjustment.** Reduce infusion rate by 50% in end-stage renal and liver patients.
Children ages 2 to 12: 0.20 mg/kg I.V. push administered over 5 to 15 seconds.

Neuromuscular blockade is usually evident in less than 2 minutes. Although supplemental doses of 0.1 mg/kg I.V. q 15 minutes usually maintain muscle relaxation in adults, maintenance doses are usually needed more frequently in children. Or maintain neuromuscular blockade with a continuous infusion titrated to effect. Most children respond to 5 to 31 mcg/kg/minute (average 14 mcg/kg/minute).

Pharmacodynamics

Neuromuscular blocking action: Competes with acetylcholine for receptor sites at the motor endplate. Because this action may be antagonized by cholinesterase inhibitors, mivacurium is considered a competitive antagonist. Drug is a mixture of three stereoisomers, each possessing neuromuscular blocking activity: the cis-trans isomer (36% of the total) and the trans-trans isomer (57% of the total) are about 10 times as potent as the cis-cis isomer (only 6% of the total). The isomers don't interconvert in vivo.

Pharmacokinetics

• *Absorption:* Rapid absorption; may produce neuromuscular blockade in about 3.3 minutes with sufficient neuromuscular blockade lasting 15 to 20 minutes.
• *Distribution:* Small volume of distribution; indicates drug doesn't extensively distribute to tissues.
• *Metabolism:* Rapidly hydrolyzed by plasma pseudocholinesterase to inactive components.
• *Excretion:* Metabolites excreted in bile and urine. Of the highly active isomers, the cis-trans and trans-trans isomers each have an elimination half-life of under 2.3 minutes. The less active cis-cis isomer (only small portion of total drug) has an elimination half-life of 55 minutes.

Contraindications and precautions

Contraindicated in patients with hypersensitivity to drug. Use cautiously in patients with significant CV disease, metastatic cancer, severe electrolyte disturbances, or neuromuscular disease; in those who may be adversely affected by the release of histamine; and in those in whom neuromuscular blockade reversibility is difficult, such as patients with myasthenia gravis or myasthenic syndrome. Use with extreme caution in patients with reduced plasma cholinesterase activity; may cause prolonged neuromuscular blockade.

Interactions

Drug-drug. *Alkaline solutions (such as barbiturate solutions):* Physically incompatible; may form a precipitate. Don't administer through same I.V. line with any of these drugs.
Aminoglycosides (gentamicin, kanamycin, neomycin, streptomycin), bacitracin, colistimethate, colistin, magnesium salts, polymyxin B, tetracy-

clines: Increased muscle weakness. Use together cautiously.
Carbamazepine, phenytoin: Prolonged time to maximal block or shortened duration of blockade with neuromuscular blockers. Monitor patient closely.
Glucocorticosteroids, MAO inhibitors, oral contraceptives: Plasma cholinesterase activity may be diminished. Use together cautiously.
Inhalational anesthetics (such as enflurane, isoflurane), quinidine: Enhanced activity (or prolonged action) of nondepolarizing neuromuscular blockers. Monitor patient for excessive weakness.

Adverse reactions

CNS: dizziness.
CV: *flushing, tachycardia,* **bradycardia, arrhythmias,** *hypotension.*
Musculoskeletal: prolonged muscle weakness, muscle spasms.
Respiratory: **bronchospasm,** wheezing, **respiratory insufficiency or apnea.**
Skin: rash, urticaria, erythema.
Other: phlebitis.

☑ Special considerations

• When mivacurium is administered by I.V. push to adults receiving anesthetic combinations of nitrous oxide and opiates, neuromuscular blockade usually lasts 15 to 20 minutes; most patients recover 95% of muscle strength in 25 to 30 minutes.
• Duration of drug effect is increased about 150% in patients with end-stage renal disease and 300% in patients with hepatic dysfunction.
• Dosage should be adjusted to ideal body weight in obese patients (patients 30% or more above their ideal weight) because of reported prolonged neuromuscular blockade.
• A nerve stimulator and train-of-four monitoring are recommended to document antagonism of neuromuscular blockade and recovery of muscle strength. Before attempting pharmacologic reversal with neostigmine methylsulfate or edrophonium chloride, some evidence of spontaneous recovery should be evident.
• Experimental evidence suggests that acid-base and electrolyte balance may influence actions of and response to nondepolarizing neuromuscular blockers. Alkalosis may counteract paralysis; acidosis may enhance it.
• Note that mivacurium, like other neuromuscular blockers, doesn't have an effect on consciousness or pain threshold. To avoid patient distress, this drug shouldn't be administered until patient's consciousness is obtunded by general anesthetic.
• Drug is compatible with D_5W, normal saline solution injection, dextrose 5% in normal saline solution injection, lactated Ringer's injection, and dextrose 5% in lactated Ringer's injection. Dilut-

---

Reactions may be *common*, uncommon, **life-threatening**, or COMMON AND LIFE-THREATENING.

ed solutions are stable for 24 hours at room temperature.
● When diluted as directed, mivacurium is compatible with alfentanil, fentanyl, sufentanil, droperidol, and midazolam.
● Drug is available as premixed infusion in D_5W. After removing protective outer wrap, check container for minor leaks by squeezing bag before administering. Don't add other drugs to container, and don't use container in series connections.
● Overdose may result in prolonged neuromuscular blockade. Antagonists shouldn't be administered until there is some evidence of spontaneous recovery.

Monitoring the patient
● Monitor patient's response to drug.
● Monitor vital signs and ECG closely.

Information for the patient
● Reassure patient and family that he will be monitored at all times.

Pediatric patients
● Like other neuromuscular blockers, dosage requirements for children are higher on a mg/kg basis as compared with adults. Onset and recovery of neuromuscular blockade occur more rapidly in children.

Breast-feeding patients
● It's unknown if drug appears in breast milk. Use with caution in breast-feeding women.

modafinil
Provigil

Pharmacologic classification: non-amphetamine central nervous system stimulant
Therapeutic classification: analeptic
Controlled substance schedule IV
Pregnancy risk category C

How supplied
Available by prescription only
Tablets: 100 mg, 200 mg

Indications, route, and dosage
Improvement of wakefulness in patients with excessive daytime sleepiness associated with narcolepsy
Adults: 200 mg P.O. daily, given as a single dose in the morning.
✦ *Dosage adjustment.* In patients with severe hepatic impairment, 100 mg P.O. daily, given as a single dose in the morning.

Pharmacodynamics
CNS stimulant action: Exact mechanism by which modafinil promotes wakefulness unknown. Has

wake-promoting actions like sympathomimetics such as amphetamines, but is structurally distinct from amphetamines and doesn't appear to alter the release of either dopamine or norepinephrine to produce CNS stimulation.

Pharmacokinetics
● *Absorption:* Rapid absorption, with peak plasma levels at 2 to 4 hours.
● *Distribution:* Well distributed in body tissue. About 60% bound to plasma protein, primarily albumin.
● *Metabolism:* About 90% metabolized in liver, with subsequent renal elimination of metabolites.
● *Excretion:* Less than 10% renally excreted as unchanged drug.

Contraindications and precautions
Contraindicated in patients with hypersensitivity to drug. Don't use in patients with history of left ventricular hypertrophy or ischemic ECG changes, chest pain, arrhythmias, or other significant signs of mitral valve prolapse in association with CNS stimulant use.
Use with caution in patients with history of recent MI or unstable angina and in those with history of psychosis. Use cautiously, and in reduced dosages, in patients with severe hepatic impairment with or without cirrhosis. Also use cautiously in patients concurrently treated with monoamine oxidase inhibitors.

Interactions
Drug-drug. *Cyclosporine, theophylline:* Reduced serum levels of these drugs. Use together cautiously.
Diazepam, phenytoin, propranolol, other drugs metabolized by CYP2C19: Modafinil is a reversible inhibitor of cytochrome P-450 isoenzyme, CYP2C19, and may lead to increases in serum levels of these drugs. Use together cautiously. Adjust dosage as needed.
Itraconazole, ketoconazole, other inhibitors of CYP3A4; carbamazepine, phenobarbital, rifampin, other inducers of CYP3A4: Altered levels of modafinil. Monitor patient closely.
Methylphenidate: Delayed absorption of modafinil by about 1 hour when administered concurrently. Separate administration times of these drugs.
Phenytoin, warfarin: May cause concentration-dependent inhibition of CYP2C9 activity and may increase serum levels of these drugs. Monitor patient closely for signs of toxicity.
Steroidal contraceptives: Reduced serum levels of these drugs; reduced contraceptive effectiveness. Recommend alternative or concomitant method of contraception during modafinil therapy and for 1 month after therapy ends.
Tricyclic antidepressants (such as clomipramine, desipramine): Increased levels of tricyclics. Reduce dosage of these drugs as needed.

Drug-lifestyle. *Alcohol:* May interfere with drug action. Discourage concomitant use.

Adverse reactions
CNS: *headache,* nervousness, dizziness, syncope, depression, anxiety, cataplexy, insomnia, paresthesia, dyskinesia, hypertonia, confusion, amnesia, emotional lability, ataxia, tremor.
CV: hypotension, hypertension, vasodilation, *arrhythmias,* chest pain.
EENT: *rhinitis,* pharyngitis, epistaxis, amblyopia, abnormal vision, mouth ulcer, gingivitis, thirst.
GI: *nausea,* diarrhea, dry mouth, anorexia, vomiting.
GU: abnormal urine, urine retention, abnormal ejaculation, albuminuria.
Hematologic: eosinophilia.
Hepatic: abnormal liver function.
Metabolic: hyperglycemia.
Musculoskeletal: joint disorder, neck pain, rigid neck.
Respiratory: lung disorder, dyspnea, asthma.
Skin: herpes simplex, dry skin.
Other: chills, fever.

☑ Special considerations
• Safety and efficacy of dosage in patients with severe renal impairment haven't been determined.
• Although dosages of 400 mg daily as a single dose have been well tolerated, there is no consistent evidence that this dose confers additional benefit beyond the 200-mg dose.
• Although food has no effect on overall bioavailability, drug absorption may be delayed by about 1 hour if given with food.

Monitoring the patient
• Monitor patient for adverse effects and response to drug therapy.
• Monitor cardiac status.

Information for the patient
• Tell patient to call if he develops a rash, hives, or a related allergic reaction.
• Drug may impair judgment. Advise patient to use caution while driving or during other activities requiring alertness until effects of drug are known.
• Instruct patient to call before taking prescription or OTC drugs because of the potential for interactions.
• Advise woman to call if she becomes pregnant or intends to become pregnant during therapy.
• Caution patient regarding potential increased risk of pregnancy when using steroidal contraceptives (such as depot or implantable contraceptives) with modafinil tablets.

Geriatric patients
• Safety and effectiveness in patients over age 65 haven't been established. In elderly patients, a lower dosage may be considered because elim-

ination of drug and its metabolites may be reduced.

Pediatric patients
• Safety and effectiveness in children under age 16 haven't been established.

Breast-feeding patients
• It's unknown if drug appears in breast milk. Use cautiously in breast-feeding women.

---

moexipril hydrochloride
Univasc

Pharmacologic classification: ACE inhibitor
Therapeutic classification: antihypertensive
Pregnancy risk category C (D in second and third trimesters)

How supplied
Available by prescription only
Tablets: 7.5 mg, 15 mg

Indications, route, and dosage
Hypertension
Adults: Initially, 7.5 mg P.O. once daily before meals for patients not receiving diuretics. If control isn't adequate, dose can be increased or divided dosing may be attempted. Recommended dosage range is 7.5 to 30 mg daily, administered in one or two divided doses 1 hour before meals. For patients receiving diuretics, give 3.75 mg P.O. once daily before meals. Make subsequent dosage adjustments according to blood pressure response.

Pharmacodynamics
Antihypertensive action: Exact mechanism unknown. Thought to result primarily from suppression of the renin-angiotensin-aldosterone system. Moexipril's metabolite, moexiprilat, inhibits ACE and the production of angiotensin II (a potent vasoconstrictor and stimulator of aldosterone secretion). Other mechanisms may also be involved.

Pharmacokinetics
• *Absorption:* Incompletely absorbed from GI tract with bioavailability of about 13%. Food significantly decreases bioavailability.
• *Distribution:* Metabolite about 50% protein-bound.
• *Metabolism:* Metabolized extensively to active metabolite, moexiprilat.
• *Excretion:* Excreted primarily in feces; small amount excreted in urine. Half-life over 2 to 9 hours.

Contraindications and precautions
Contraindicated in patients with hypersensitivity to drug, in those with history of angioedema related to previous treatment with an ACE inhibitor, and during pregnancy. Use cautiously in patients with impaired renal function, heart failure, or renal artery stenosis and in breast-feeding women.

Interactions
Drug-drug. *Diuretics:* Increased risk of excessive hypotension. Stop diuretic or use lower dose of moexipril.
Lithium: Increased levels and lithium toxicity. Use together with caution; monitor serum lithium levels.
Potassium-sparing diuretics, potassium supplements: Increased risk of hyperkalemia. Monitor serum potassium.
Drug-food. *Sodium substitutes containing potassium:* Increased risk of hyperkalemia. Monitor serum potassium.

Adverse reactions
CNS: *dizziness,* headache, fatigue.
CV: peripheral edema, hypotension, orthostatic hypotension, chest pain, flushing.
EENT: pharyngitis, rhinitis, sinusitis.
GI: diarrhea, dyspepsia, nausea.
GU: urinary frequency.
Hematologic: *neutropenia.*
Metabolic: hyperkalemia.
Musculoskeletal: myalgia.
Respiratory: *dry, persistent, tickling, nonproductive cough;* upper respiratory tract infection.
Skin: rash.
Other: *anaphylactoid reactions, angioedema,* flu syndrome, pain.

☑ Special considerations
● If possible, stop diuretic therapy 2 to 3 days before starting moexipril to decrease potential for excessive hypotensive response. If drug doesn't adequately control blood pressure, reinstitute diuretic therapy with care.
● Because angioedema associated with tongue, glottis, or larynx may cause a fatal airway obstruction, have appropriate therapy, such as S.C. epinephrine 1:1,000 (0.3 to 0.5 ml) and equipment to ensure a patent airway readily available.
● In patients undergoing major surgery or anesthesia with drugs that produce hypotension, moexipril may block compensatory renin release. Hypotension can be treated with volume expansion.

Monitoring the patient
● Monitor vital signs closely, especially blood pressure.
● Other ACE inhibitors have been associated with agranulocytosis and neutropenia. Monitor CBC with differential counts before therapy, especially in patients who have collagen vascular disease with impaired renal function.

● Measure blood pressure at trough (just before a dose) to verify adequate blood pressure control. Drug is less effective in reducing trough blood pressures in blacks than in nonblacks.
● Assess renal function before treatment and periodically throughout therapy. Monitor serum potassium levels.

Information for the patient
● Instruct patient to take drug on empty stomach; meals, particularly those high in fat, can impair absorption.
● Inform patient that light-headedness can occur, especially during the first few days of therapy. Tell him to rise slowly to minimize this effect and to report symptoms. If fainting occurs, tell patient to stop drug and call immediately.
● Instruct patient to use caution in hot weather and during exercise. Inadequate fluid intake, vomiting, diarrhea, and excessive perspiration can lead to light-headedness and syncope.
● Advise patient to report signs of infection, such as fever and sore throat. Also tell patient to report easy bruising or bleeding; swelling of tongue, lips, face, eyes, mucous membranes, or extremities; difficulty swallowing or breathing; and hoarseness.
● Tell woman to report suspected pregnancy immediately. Drug will need to be stopped.

Pediatric patients
● Safety and effectiveness in children haven't been established.

Breast-feeding patients
● It's unknown if drug appears in breast milk; use with caution in breast-feeding women.

molindone hydrochloride
Moban

Pharmacologic classification: dihydro-indolone
Therapeutic classification: antipsychotic
Pregnancy risk category NR

How supplied
Available by prescription only
Tablets: 5 mg, 10 mg, 25 mg, 50 mg, 100 mg
Oral concentrate: 20 mg/ml

Indications, route, and dosage
Psychotic disorders
Adults: 50 to 75 mg P.O. daily, increased 100 mg daily in 3 to 4 days to a maximum of 225 mg daily. Maintenance dose for mild disease is 5 to 15 mg t.i.d. or q.i.d., for moderate disease 10 to 25 mg t.i.d. or q.i.d., and for severe disease 225 mg daily.

Pharmacodynamics

Antipsychotic action: Unrelated to all other antipsychotic drugs; thought to exert antipsychotic effects by postsynaptic blockade of CNS dopamine receptors, inhibiting dopamine-mediated effects.

Has many other central and peripheral effects; also produces alpha and ganglionic blockade. Most prominent adverse reactions are extrapyramidal.

Pharmacokinetics

- *Absorption:* Limited data; absorption appears rapid; effects peak within 1½ hours.
- *Distribution:* Distributed widely into body.
- *Metabolism:* Metabolized extensively; drug effects last for 24 to 36 hours.
- *Excretion:* Most of drug excreted as metabolites in urine; some excreted in feces via biliary tract. 90% of dose excreted within 24 hours.

Contraindications and precautions

Contraindicated in patients with hypersensitivity to drug and in those experiencing coma or severe CNS depression. Use cautiously in patients at risk for seizures or when high physical activity is harmful to patient.

Interactions

Drug-drug. *Antiarrhythmics, disopyramide, procainamide, quinidine:* Increased arrhythmias and conduction defects. Avoid concomitant use.

Appetite suppressants, ephedrine (often found in nasal sprays), epinephrine, phenylephrine, phenylpropanolamine: Decreased stimulatory and pressor effects. Because of its alpha-blocking potential, molindone may cause epinephrine reversal, a hypotensive response to epinephrine. Monitor patient closely.

Atropine, other anticholinergics (such as antidepressants, antihistamines, antiparkinsonians, MAO inhibitors, meperidine, phenothiazines): Oversedation, paralytic ileus, visual changes, and severe constipation. Monitor patient closely; use with caution.

Beta blockers: May inhibit molindone metabolism; increased plasma levels and toxicity. Monitor patient for toxicity.

Bromocriptine: Molindone may antagonize therapeutic effect. Monitor patient for drug effect.

Centrally acting antihypertensives (such as clonidine, guanabenz, guanadrel, guanethidine, methyldopa, reserpine): May inhibit blood pressure response to these drugs. Monitor blood pressure.

CNS depressants: Additive effects likely. Avoid concomitant use.

Dopamine: Decreased vasoconstricting effects of dopamine. Monitor blood pressure carefully.

Levodopa: Decreased effectiveness and increased toxicity of levodopa. Avoid concomitant use.

Metrizamide: Increased risk of seizures. Monitor patient closely.

Nitrates: Possible hypotension. Monitor patient and blood pressure closely.

Phenytoin, tetracyclines: Calcium sulfate in molindone tablets may inhibit absorption of phenytoin or tetracyclines. Don't give together.

Propylthiouracil: Increased risk of agranulocytosis and decreased therapeutic response to molindone. Avoid concomitant use.

Drug-lifestyle. *Alcohol:* Additive effects likely. Discourage use.

Sun exposure: Increased risk of photosensitivity reactions. Advise patient to take precautions.

Adverse reactions

CNS: *extrapyramidal reactions, tardive dyskinesia, sedation, drowsiness, depression, euphoria, pseudoparkinsonism, EEG changes, dizziness.*
CV: *orthostatic hypotension, tachycardia, ECG changes.*
EENT: *blurred vision.*
GI: *dry mouth, constipation, nausea.*
GU: *urine retention, menstrual irregularities, gynecomastia, inhibited ejaculation.*
Hematologic: **leukopenia,** leukocytosis.
Hepatic: jaundice, abnormal liver function test results.
Skin: *mild photosensitivity, allergic reactions.*

☑ Special considerations

- Drug may cause GI distress and should be administered with food or fluids.
- Dilute concentrate in 2 to 4 oz (60 to 120 ml) of liquid, preferably soup, water, juice, carbonated drinks, milk, or puddings.
- Drug may cause urine to turn pink to brown.
- Protect liquid form from light.
- Drug causes false-positive results in urine pregnancy tests using human chorionic gonadotropin; additive potential for causing seizures with metrizamide myelography.
- Signs and symptoms of overdose include CNS depression characterized by deep, unarousable sleep and possible coma, hypotension or hypertension, extrapyramidal symptoms, abnormal involuntary muscle movements, agitation, seizures, arrhythmias, ECG changes, hypothermia or hyperthermia, and autonomic nervous system dysfunction.
- If overdose occurs, don't induce vomiting; drug inhibits cough reflex, and aspiration may occur.

Monitoring the patient

- Monitor vital signs closely.
- Monitor CNS status.

Information for the patient

- Explain risks of dystonic reaction and tardive dyskinesia to patient, and advise him to report abnormal body movements.

Reactions may be common, uncommon, **life-threatening**, OR COMMON AND LIFE-THREATENING.

• Warn patient to avoid spilling liquid preparation on skin; rash and irritation may result.
• Advise patient to avoid temperature extremes (hot or cold baths, sunlamps, or tanning beds) because drug may cause thermoregulatory changes.
• Suggest sugarless gum or candy, ice chips, or artificial saliva to relieve dry mouth.
• Warn patient not to take drug with antacids or antidiarrheals; not to stop taking drug or take any other drug except as instructed; and to take drug exactly as prescribed, without doubling after missing a dose.
• Warn patient about sedative effect. Tell him to report difficult urination, sore throat, dizziness, or fainting.
• Advise patient to get up slowly from a recumbent or seated position to minimize effects of lightheadedness.
• Tell patient that drug may contain sodium metabisulfite, which can cause an allergic reaction in those with a sulfite allergy.

Geriatric patients
• Lower doses are recommended; 30% to 50% of usual dose may be effective. Elderly patients are at greater risk for tardive dyskinesia and other extrapyramidal effects.

Pediatric patients
• Drug isn't recommended for children under age 12.

---

montelukast sodium
Singulair

Pharmacologic classification: leukotriene receptor antagonist
Therapeutic classification: antasthmatic
Pregnancy risk category B

How supplied
Available by prescription only
Tablets: 10 mg
Tablets (chewable): 5 mg

Indications, route, and dosage
Prophylaxis and long-term treatment of asthma
Adults and adolescents: 10 mg P.O. once daily in evening.
Children ages 6 to 14: 5 mg (chewable tablet) P.O. once daily in the evening.

Pharmacodynamics
Antasthmatic action: Causes inhibition of airway cysteinyl leukotriene receptors. Binds with high affinity and selectivity to the $cysLT_1$ receptor and inhibits the physiologic action of the cysteinyl leukotriene LTD_4. This receptor inhibition reduces early- and late-phase bronchoconstriction due to antigen challenge.

Pharmacokinetics
• *Absorption:* Rapidly absorbed after oral administration; mean peak plasma levels achieved in 3 to 4 hours, and mean oral bioavailability is 64%. Food doesn't affect absorption. For chewable tablet, peak levels reached in 2 to 2½ hours, and mean oral bioavailability is 73%.
• *Distribution:* Minimally distributed to tissues; steady-state volume of distribution of 8 to 11 L. More than 99% bound to plasma proteins.
• *Metabolism:* Extensively metabolized; plasma levels of metabolites at therapeutic doses are undetectable. Metabolism involvement by cytochromes P-450 3A4 and 2C9.
• *Excretion:* About 86% of oral dose metabolized and excreted in feces; drug and metabolites excreted almost exclusively in bile. Half-life is 2.7 to 5.5 hours.

Contraindications and precautions
Contraindicated in patients with hypersensitivity to drug or its components. Also contraindicated in patients with acute asthmatic attacks or status asthmaticus. Although airway function is improved in patients with known aspirin hypersensitivity, these patients should avoid aspirin and NSAIDs.

Interactions
Drug-drug. *Drugs known to inhibit 3A4 and 2C9 enzymes:* Although plasma levels haven't been proven to be affected, use caution when montelukast is used with these drugs.
Phenobarbital, rifampin: Induce hepatic metabolism. Monitor patient closely.

Adverse reactions
CNS: *headache,* dizziness, fatigue, asthenia.
EENT: nasal congestion, dental pain.
GI: dyspepsia, infectious gastroenteritis, abdominal pain.
Respiratory: cough, influenza.
Skin: rash.
Other: fever, trauma.

☑ Special considerations
• Although dose of inhaled corticosteroids may be reduced gradually, montelukast shouldn't be abruptly substituted for inhaled or oral corticosteroids.
• Drug shouldn't be used as monotherapy for management of exercise-induced bronchospasm.
• No added benefit is achieved with doses above 10 mg daily.

Monitoring the patient
• Monitor vital signs and patient's response to drug therapy.
• Monitor patient for adverse effects.

Information for the patient
- Advise patient to take drug daily, even if asymptomatic, and to call if asthma isn't well controlled.
- Warn patient that drug isn't beneficial in acute asthma attacks, or in exercise-induced bronchospasm and advise him to keep appropriate rescue medications available.
- Advise patient with known aspirin sensitivity not to take aspirin and NSAIDs.
- Warn patient with phenylketonuria that chewable tablet contains phenylalanine, a component of aspartame.
- Advise patient to seek medical attention if short-acting bronchodilators are needed more often than usual or prescribed.

Geriatric patients
- No difference in safety and effectiveness of drug has been reported between elderly and younger patient populations.

Pediatric patients
- Safety and efficacy in children under age 6 haven't been established.

Breast-feeding patients
- It's unknown if drug appears in breast milk. Use cautiously in breast-feeding women.

---

moricizine hydrochloride
Ethmozine

Pharmacologic classification: sodium channel blocker
Therapeutic classification: anti-arrhythmic
Pregnancy risk category B

How supplied
Available by prescription only
Tablets: 200 mg, 250 mg, 300 mg

Indications, route, and dosage
Documented, life-threatening ventricular arrhythmias when benefit of treatment outweighs risks
Adults: Dosage must be individualized. Usual range is 600 to 900 mg daily, given q 8 hours in equally divided doses. Dosage may be adjusted within this range in increments of 150 mg daily at 3-day intervals until desired effect is obtained. Hospitalization is recommended for initiation of therapy because patient will be at high risk.

Pharmacodynamics
Antiarrhythmic action: Although moricizine is chemically related to the neuroleptic phenothiazines, it has no demonstrated dopaminergic activities. It does have potent local anesthetic activity and myocardial membrane stabilizing effects. A class I antiarrhythmic, it reduces the fast inward current carried by sodium ions. In patients with ventricular tachycardia, moricizine prolongs AV conduction but has no significant effect on ventricular repolarization. Intra-atrial conduction or atrial effective refractory periods aren't consistently affected and moricizine has minimal effect on sinus cycle length and sinus node recovery time. This may be significant in patients with sinus node dysfunction.

In patients with impaired left ventricular function, moricizine has minimal effects on measurements of cardiac performance: cardiac index, stroke volume, pulmonary artery wedge pressure, systemic or pulmonary vascular resistance, and ejection fraction either at rest or during exercise. A small but consistent increase in resting blood pressure and heart rate are seen. Moricizine has no effect on exercise tolerance in patients with ventricular arrhythmias, heart failure, or angina pectoris.

Moricizine has antiarrhythmic activity similar to that of disopyramide, propranolol, and quinidine. Arrhythmia "rebound" isn't noted after therapy ends.

Pharmacokinetics
- *Absorption:* Plasma levels usually peak within ½ to 2 hours. Giving within 30 minutes of mealtime delays absorption and lowers peak plasma levels, but has no effect on extent of absorption.
- *Distribution:* 95% plasma protein-bound.
- *Metabolism:* Significant first-pass metabolism; absolute bioavailability of about 38%. At least 26 metabolites identified; no single one representing at least 1% of administered dose. Induces its own metabolism.
- *Excretion:* 56% of drug excreted in feces; 39% in urine; some also recycled through enterohepatic circulation.

Contraindications and precautions
Contraindicated in patients with hypersensitivity to drug and in those with cardiogenic shock, pre-existing second- or third-degree AV block, or right bundle-branch block when associated with left hemiblock (bifascicular block) unless an artificial pacemaker is present. Discontinue drug or breast-feeding in breast-feeding women because drug is detected in breast milk.

Use cautiously in patients with impaired renal or hepatic function, sick sinus syndrome, coronary artery disease, or left ventricular function.

Interactions
Drug-drug. *Cimetidine:* Decreased moricizine clearance by 49%. Decrease dose of cimetidine (not more than 600 mg/day).
Digoxin, propranolol: Small additive increase in PR interval. Monitor patient and ECG closely.
Theophylline: Increased clearance and decreased plasma half-life with concomitant therapy. Moni-

---

tor plasma levels and patient's response when moricizine is added or discontinued.

Adverse reactions
CNS: *dizziness, headache, fatigue,* hyperesthesia, anxiety, asthenia, nervousness, paresthesia, sleep disorders.
CV: *proarrhythmic events (ventricular tachycardia, premature ventricular contractions, supraventricular arrhythmias),* ECG abnormalities (including *conduction defects, sinus pause, junctional rhythm,* or *AV block*), *heart failure,* palpitations, chest pain, *cardiac death,* hypotension, hypertension, vasodilation, cerebrovascular events, thrombophlebitis.
EENT: blurred vision.
GI: *nausea, vomiting, abdominal pain, dyspepsia, diarrhea, dry mouth.*
GU: urine retention, urinary frequency, dysuria.
Musculoskeletal: musculoskeletal pain.
Respiratory: dyspnea.
Skin: diaphoresis, rash.
Other: drug-induced fever.

☑ Special considerations
• When switching from another antiarrhythmic to moricizine, withdraw previous therapy one to two half-lives before starting moricizine.
• Initial dose for patients with renal or hepatic impairment is 600 mg daily or lower.
• Signs and symptoms of overdose include emesis, lethargy, coma, syncope, hypotension, conduction disturbances, exacerbation of heart failure, MI, sinus arrest, arrhythmias, and respiratory failure. Treatment is supportive.

Monitoring the patient
• Correct electrolyte imbalances before starting therapy; hypokalemia, hyperkalemia, or hypomagnesemia may alter drug's effects.
• Monitor vital signs.
• Monitor ECG before making dosage adjustments.

Information for the patient
• Instruct patient to take drug exactly as prescribed and to not abruptly stop drug.
• Tell patient to avoid activities that require alertness until CNS effects are known.

Pediatric patients
• Safety and efficacy in children haven't been established.

Breast-feeding patients
• Drug appears in breast milk. Because of potential for adverse reactions in breast-fed infant, a decision to stop either breast-feeding or therapy must be made.

morphine hydrochloride*
Morphitec*, M.O.S.*

morphine sulfate
Astramorph PF, Duramorph, Epimorph*, Infumorph, MS Contin, MSIR, MS/L, MS/S, OMS Concentrate, Oramorph SR, RMS Uniserts, Roxanol, Statex*

Pharmacologic classification: opioid
Therapeutic classification: narcotic analgesic
Controlled substance schedule II
Pregnancy risk category C

How supplied
Available by prescription only
morphine hydrochloride*
Tablets: 10 mg, 20 mg, 40 mg, 60 mg
Syrup: 1 mg/ml, 5 mg/ml, 10 mg/ml, 20 mg/ml, 50 mg/ml
Suppositories: 20 mg, 30 mg
morphine sulfate
Tablets: 15 mg, 30 mg
Tablets (extended-release): 15 mg, 30 mg, 60 mg, 100 mg, 200 mg
Tablets (soluble): 10 mg, 15 mg, 30 mg
Oral solution: 4 mg/ml, 10 mg/5 ml, 20 mg/5 ml, 20 mg/ml, 100 mg/5 ml
Injection (with preservative): 1 mg/ml, 2 mg/ml, 3 mg/ml, 4 mg/ml, 5 mg/ml, 8 mg/ml, 10 mg/ml, 15 mg/ml, 25 mg/ml, 50 mg/ml
Injection (without preservative): 500 mcg/ml, 1 mg/ml, 10 mg/ml, 25 mg/ml
Suppositories: 5 mg, 10 mg, 20 mg, 30 mg

Indications, route, and dosage
Severe pain
Adults: 10 mg q 4 hours S.C. or I.M., or 10 to 30 mg P.O., or 10 to 20 mg P.R. q 4 hours, p.r.n., or around the clock. May be injected slow I.V. (over 4 to 5 minutes) 2.5 to 15 mg diluted in 4 to 5 ml water for injection. May also administer controlled-release tablets 30 mg q 8 to 12 hours. As an epidural injection, 5 mg via an epidural catheter q 24 hours.
Children: 0.1 to 0.2 mg/kg S.C. q 4 hours. Maximum dose is 15 mg. In some situations, morphine may be administered by continuous I.V. infusion or by intraspinal and intrathecal injection.
Preoperative sedation and adjunct to anesthesia
Adults: 8 to 10 mg I.M., S.C., or I.V.
Control of pain associated with acute MI
Adults: 8 to 15 mg I.M., S.C., or I.V. Additional, smaller doses may be given in 3- to 4-hour intervals, p.r.n.

*Adjunctive treatment of acute pulmonary
edema*
Adults: 10 to 15 mg I.V. at a rate not exceeding
2 mg/minute.

Pharmacodynamics
Analgesic action: Drug is principal opium alkaloid, the standard for opiate agonist analgesic activity. Mechanism of action is thought to be via
the opiate receptors, altering patient's perception
of pain. Morphine is particularly useful in severe,
acute pain or severe, chronic pain. Morphine also
has a central depressant effect on respiration and
on the cough reflex center.

Pharmacokinetics
• *Absorption:* Variable absorption from GI tract.
Onset of analgesia within 15 to 60 minutes; anal-
gesia peaks ½ to 1 hour after dosing.
• *Distribution:* Distributed widely through body.
• *Metabolism:* Metabolized primarily in liver. One
metabolite, morphine 6-glucuromide, is active.
• *Excretion:* Duration of action is 3 to 7 hours.
Excreted in urine and bile. Morphine 6-glucuro-
mide may accumulate after continuous dosing in
patients with renal failure, leading to enhanced
and prolonged opiate activity.

Contraindications and precautions
Contraindicated in patients with hypersensitivity
to drug and in those with conditions that would
preclude administration of opioids by I.V. route
(acute bronchial asthma or upper airway obstruction).
   Use cautiously in elderly or debilitated patients and in those with head injury, increased intracranial pressure, seizures, pulmonary disease,
prostatic hyperplasia, hepatic or renal disease,
acute abdominal conditions, hypothyroidism, Addison's disease, or urethral strictures.

Interactions
Drug-drug. Anticholinergics: May cause paralytic ileus. Monitor patient.
*Cimetidine, CNS depressants (antihistamines,
barbiturates, benzodiazepines, general anesthetics, MAO inhibitors, muscle relaxants, narcotic analgesics, phenothiazines, sedative-
hypnotics, tricyclic antidepressants):* Potentiated
respiratory and CNS depression, sedation, and
hypotensive effects of drug. Use together with
extreme caution. Reduce morphine dose and
monitor patient's response.
General anesthetics: Possible severe CV depression. Use with extreme caution; monitor patient closely.
Narcotic antagonist: Patients who become physically dependent on this drug may experience
acute withdrawal syndrome if given a narcotic
antagonist. Monitor patient closely.

Drug-lifestyle. Alcohol: Potentiated respiratory
and CNS depressive, sedative, and hypotensive
effects of drug. Discourage use.

Adverse reactions
CNS: *sedation, somnolence, clouded sensorium, euphoria,* **seizures** *(with large doses), dizziness, nightmares (with long-acting oral forms),
light-headedness, hallucinations, nervousness,
depression, syncope.*
CV: *hypotension,* **bradycardia, shock, cardiac
arrest,** *tachycardia, hypertension.*
GI: *nausea, vomiting, constipation, ileus, dry
mouth, biliary tract spasms, anorexia,* increased
plasma amylase levels.
GU: *urine retention, decreased libido.*
Hematologic: *thrombocytopenia.*
Respiratory: *respiratory depression, apnea,
respiratory arrest.*
Skin: pruritus, skin flushing (with epidural administration); *diaphoresis; edema.*
Other: *physical dependence.*

☑ Special considerations
Besides the recommendations relevant to all opi-
oids, consider the following.
• Morphine is drug of choice in relieving pain of
MI; may cause transient decrease in blood pres-
sure.
• Regimented scheduling (around-the-clock) is
beneficial in severe, chronic pain.
• Oral solutions of various levels are available as
well as a new intensified oral solution.
• Note the disparity between oral and parenteral doses.
• Long-term therapy in patients with advanced
renal disease may lead to toxicity due to accumulation of the active metabolite.
• Some morphine injections contain sulfites, which
may cause allergic-type reactions.
• For S.L. administration, measure oral solution
with tuberculin syringe, and administer dose a
few drops at a time to allow maximal sublingual
absorption and to minimize swallowing.
• Refrigeration of rectal suppositories isn't necessary. Note that in some patients, rectal and oral
absorption may not be equivalent.
• Preservative-free preparations are available for
epidural and intrathecal administration. Use of
the epidural route is increasing.
• Epidural morphine has proven to be an excellent analgesic for patients with postoperative pain.
After epidural administration, monitor closely for
respiratory depression up to 24 hours after the
injection. Check respiratory rate and depth according to protocol (for example, every 15 minutes for 2 hours, then hourly for 18 hours). Some
clinicians advocate a dilute naloxone infusion (5
to 10 mcg/kg/hour) during the first 12 hours to
minimize respiratory depression without altering
pain relief.
• Morphine may worsen or mask gallbladder pain.

Reactions may be *common,* uncommon, *life-threatening,* or COMMON AND LIFE-THREATENING.

• Rapid I.V. administration may result in overdose because of the delay in maximum CNS effect (30 minutes).
• The most common signs and symptoms of morphine overdose are respiratory depression with or without CNS depression, and miosis (pinpoint pupils).

Monitoring the patient
• Monitor laboratory parameters, vital signs, and neurologic status closely.
• Observe patient carefully for respiratory depression.

Information for the patient
• Tell patient that oral liquid form of morphine may be mixed with a glass of fruit juice immediately before taken, if desired, to improve taste.
• Tell patient taking long-acting morphine tablets to swallow whole. Don't break, crush, or chew tablets before swallowing.

Geriatric patients
• Lower doses are usually indicated for elderly patients, who may be more sensitive to the therapeutic and adverse effects of drug.

Breast-feeding patients
• Drug appears in breast milk. A woman should wait 2 to 3 hours after last dose before breast-feeding to avoid sedating infant.

moxifloxacin hydrochloride
Avelox

Pharmacologic classification: fluoro-quinolone
Therapeutic classification: antibiotic
Pregnancy risk category C

How supplied
Available by prescription only
Tablets (film-coated): 400 mg

Indications, route, and dosage
Acute bacterial sinusitis caused by Strepto-coccus pneumoniae, Haemophilus influen-zae, *or* Moraxella catarrhalis
Adults: 400 mg P.O. once daily for 10 days.
Acute bacterial exacerbation of chronic bron-chitis caused by S. pneumoniae, H. influen-zae, H. parainfluenzae, Klebsiella pneumoni-ae, Staphylococcus aureus, *or* M. catarrhalis
Adults: 400 mg P.O. once daily for 5 days.
Mild to moderate community-acquired pneu-monia caused by S. pneumoniae, H. influen-zae, Mycoplasma pneumoniae, Chlamydia pneumoniae, *or* M. catarrhalis
Adults: 400 mg P.O. once daily for 10 days.

Pharmacodynamics
Antibactericidal action: Inhibits the activity of topo-isomerase I (DNA gyrase) and topoisomerase IV in susceptible bacteria. These enzymes are nec-essary for bacterial DNA replication, transcrip-tion, repair, and recombination.

Pharmacokinetics
• *Absorption:* Well absorbed after oral adminis-tration; absolute bioavailability of about 90%. Plas-ma levels peak within 1 to 3 hours; steady-state reached after 3 days on a 400-mg, once-daily dose.
• *Distribution:* Widely distributed; distribution vol-ume of 1.7 to 2.7 L/kg. Plasma protein–binding about 50%. Penetrates well into nasal and bronchial secretions, sinus mucosa, and saliva.
• *Metabolism:* Metabolized to inactive glucuronide and sulfate conjugates. About 14% of dose con-verted to glucuronide metabolite. Sulfate metabo-lite accounts for about 38% of dose.
• *Excretion:* About 45% excreted unchanged; about 20% in urine and 25% in feces. Sulfate metabolite eliminated primarily in feces; glu-curonide metabolite renally excreted. Mean elim-ination half-life about 12 hours.

Contraindications and precautions
Contraindicated in patients with hypersensitivity to drug or its components or fluoroquinolone an-timicrobials. Safety and efficacy haven't been doc-umented in children, adolescents under age 18, and pregnant or lactating women.
Use with caution in patients with prolonged QT interval and uncorrected hypokalemia. Use cautiously in patients with known or suspected CNS disorders or in the presence of other risk factors that may predispose patients to seizures or lower seizure threshold.

Interactions
Drug-drug. Antacids; didanosine; metal cations, such as aluminum, magnesium, iron, zinc; mul-tivitamins; sucralfate: Metal cations chelate with moxifloxacin, resulting in decreased absorption and lower serum levels. Administer drug at least 4 hours before or 8 hours after drugs containing metal cations.
Antipsychotics, erythromycin, tricyclic antide-pressants: May have additive effect when used with these drugs. Monitor patient and ECG close-ly; use with caution.
Class IA (such as procainamide, quinidine) or Class III (such as amiodarone, sotalol) antiar-rhythmics: Lack of clinical experience. Avoid con-current use.
NSAIDs: Increased risk of CNS stimulation and seizures. Don't use together.
Drug-lifestyle. Sun exposure: Although photo-sensitivity hasn't occurred with moxifloxacin, it has been reported with other fluoroquinolones. Tell patient to take precautions.

Adverse reactions
CNS: dizziness, headache.
CV: prolongation of QT interval.
EENT: taste perversion.
GI: abdominal pain; diarrhea; dyspepsia; nausea; vomiting; hyperlipidemia; increased amylase, gamma-glutamyltransferase, and lactate dehydrogenase levels.
Hematologic: thrombocythemia, ***thrombocytopenia,*** eosinophilia, ***leukopenia,*** increase or decrease in PT.
Hepatic: abnormal liver function test results.
Metabolic: hyperglycemia.

☑ Special considerations
• Drug may be administered without regard to meals. Administer at same time each day to provide consistent absorption. Provide liberal fluid intake.
• Advise patient to complete entire course of therapy.
• Administer moxifloxacin 4 hours before or 8 hours after antacids, sucralfate, and products containing iron or zinc.
• Store drug at controlled room temperature.
• NSAIDs may increase risk of CNS stimulation and seizures when used with fluoroquinolones such as moxifloxacin.
• Rupture of Achilles and other tendons has been associated with fluoroquinolones. If pain, inflammation, or rupture of a tendon occurs, stop drug.
• Drug hasn't been studied in patients with moderate to severe hepatotoxicity (Child Pugh Classes B and C) and isn't recommended in this setting.
• The most common adverse reactions are nausea, vomiting, stomach pain, diarrhea, dizziness, and headache.
• CNS reactions associated with fluoroquinolones include dizziness, confusion, tremors, hallucinations, depression, and, rarely, suicidal thoughts or acts. These reactions may occur after initial dose. Stop drug and institute appropriate therapy if any of these reactions occur.
• Serious hypersensitivity reactions, including anaphylaxis, have occurred in patients receiving fluoroquinolones. Stop drug and institute supportive measures as indicated.
• Pseudomembranous colitis may occur with moxifloxacin as with other antimicrobials. Consider this diagnosis if diarrhea develops after start of therapy.

Monitoring the patient
• Watch for hypersensitivity reactions, CNS toxicities including seizures, QT interval prolongation, pseudomembranous colitis, phototoxicity, and tendon rupture.
• Monitor response to drug therapy.

Information for the patient
• Tell patient to take drug once daily, at same time each day.
• Advise patient to finish entire course of therapy, even if condition has improved.
• Tell patient to drink plenty of fluids and to take drug 4 hours before or 8 hours after antacids, sucralfate, or products containing iron or zinc.
• Most common adverse reactions include nausea, vomiting, stomach pain, diarrhea, dizziness, and headache. Tell patient to avoid hazardous activities, such as driving an automobile or operating machinery, until effects of drug are known.
• Advise patient to call if he experiences allergic reaction, heart palpitations, fainting, persistent diarrhea, severe sunburn, injury to a muscle tendon, or seizures.

Geriatric patients
• Drug is safe and efficacious for use in elderly patients.

Pediatric patients
• Safety and efficacy haven't been established in children under age 18.

Breast-feeding patients
• Drug may appear in breast milk. Benefits of drug must be weighed against potential risks to breast-feeding infant.

mumps skin test antigen
MSTA

Pharmacologic classification: viral antigen
Therapeutic classification: skin test antigen
Pregnancy risk category C

How supplied
Available by prescription only
Injection: 40 complement-fixing units/ml suspension; 10 tests/1-ml vial

Indications, route, and dosage
Assessment of cell-mediated immunity
Adults and children: 0.1 ml intradermally into inner surface of forearm.

Pharmacodynamics
Antigenic action: Isn't indicated for the immunization, diagnosis, or treatment of mumps virus infection. The status of cell-mediated immunity can be determined from use of mumps with other antigens. In vitro tests (such as lymphocyte stimulation and assays for T and B cells) are necessary to diagnose a specific disorder.

Pharmacokinetics
• *Absorption:* After intradermal injection, examine test site in 48 to 72 hours.

• *Distribution:* Must be given intradermally; S.C. injection invalidates test.
• *Metabolism:* Not applicable.
• *Excretion:* Not applicable.

Contraindications and precautions
Contraindicated in persons sensitive to avian protein (chicken, eggs, or feathers) and in those hypersensitive to thimerosal. Use cautiously in elderly patients and in patients who are immunosuppressed.

Interactions
Drug-drug. *Cimetidine:* May augment or enhance delayed-sensitivity responses. Use cautiously.
Immunosuppressants, viral vaccines: Responses may be suppressed. Monitor patient closely.

Adverse reactions
CNS: headache, drowsiness.
GI: nausea, anorexia.
Other: tenderness, pruritus, and rash at injection site. Occasionally, a severe delayed-hypersensitivity reaction will produce vesiculation, local tissue necrosis, abscess, and scar formation, ***anaphylaxis,*** Arthus reaction, urticaria, ***angioedema,*** shortness of breath, excessive perspiration.

☑ Special considerations
• Obtain history of allergies and reactions to skin tests. In patients hypersensitive to feathers, eggs, or chicken, a severe reaction may follow administration of mumps skin test antigen.
• After injection, observe patient for 15 minutes for possible immediate-type systemic allergic reaction. Keep epinephrine 1:1,000 available.
• Accurate dosage (0.1 ml) and administration are essential with the use of mumps skin test antigen.
• Pseudopositive reactions may occur in patients with egg protein sensitivity.
• Examine injection site within 48 to 72 hours, interpreting as follows:
– *Positive reaction:* Induration of 5 mm or more, with or without erythema, indicates sensitivity.
– *Negative reaction:* Induration less than 5 mm means the individual hasn't been sensitized to mumps or is anergic.
• Reactivity to test may be depressed or suppressed for as long as 6 weeks in individuals who have received concurrent virus vaccines, in those who are receiving a corticosteroid or other immunosuppressants, in those who have had viral infections, and in malnourished patients.
• Mumps skin test antigen isn't used to assess exposure to mumps; it's used in assessing T-cell function for immunocompetence because most normal individuals will exhibit a positive reaction.
• Cold packs or topical corticosteroids may provide relief of pain, pruritus, and discomfort if a local reaction occurs.
• Store vial in refrigerator.

Monitoring the patient
• Watch for sensitivity or allergic reaction.
• Monitor patients on immunosuppressant drugs for response to therapy.

Information for the patient
• Tell patient to report unusual adverse effects.
• Explain that induration will disappear in a few days.

Geriatric patients
• Elderly patients who don't react to test are considered anergic.

Breast-feeding patients
• Although appearance of drug in breast milk is unlikely, benefit to breast-feeding patient should be weighed against possible risk to infant.

mumps virus vaccine, live
Mumpsvax

Pharmacologic classification: vaccine
Therapeutic classification: viral vaccine
Pregnancy risk category C

How supplied
Available by prescription only
Injection: Single-dose vial containing not less than 20,000 $TCID_{50}$ (tissue culture infective doses) of attenuated mumps virus derived from Jeryl Lynn mumps strain (grown in chick embryo culture) and vial of diluent

Indications, route, and dosage
Immunization
Adults and children over age 1: 1 vial (0.5 ml) S.C. in outer aspect of upper arm.

Pharmacodynamics
Mumps prophylaxis: Vaccine promotes active immunity to mumps.

Pharmacokinetics
• *Absorption:* Antibodies usually evident 2 to 3 weeks after injection. Duration of immunity at least 20 years and probably lifelong.
• *Distribution:* No information available.
• *Metabolism:* No information available.
• *Excretion:* No information available.

Contraindications and precautions
Contraindicated in immunosuppressed patients; in those with cancer, blood dyscrasias, gamma globulin disorders, fever, untreated active tuberculosis, or anaphylactic or anaphylactoid reactions to neomycin or eggs; in those receiving corticosteroid or radiation therapy; and in pregnant women.

Interactions
Drug-drug. *Immune serum globulin, transfusions of blood or blood products:* May interfere with immune response to vaccine. If possible, vaccination should be deferred for 3 months.
Immunosuppressants: May interfere with response to vaccine. Avoid concomitant use.
Tuberculin skin test: Decreased response to tuberculin skin testing. If tuberculin skin test is necessary, administer either before or simultaneously with mumps vaccine.

Adverse reactions
CNS: *malaise.*
GI: *diarrhea.*
Skin: *rash.*
Other: *anaphylaxis, slight fever, mild allergic reactions, mild lymphadenopathy, injection-site reaction.*

☑ Special considerations
● Mumps vaccine shouldn't be used in delayed hypersensitivity (anergy) skin testing.
● Obtain thorough history of allergies, especially to antibiotics, eggs, chicken, or chicken feathers, and of reactions to immunizations.
● Perform skin testing to assess vaccine sensitivity (against a control of normal saline solution in opposite arm) in patients with history of anaphylactoid reactions to egg ingestion. Administer an intradermal or scratch test with a 1:10 dilution. Read results after 5 to 30 minutes. A positive reaction is a wheal with or without pseudopodia and surrounding erythema. If sensitivity test is positive, consider desensitization.
● The FDA requires that the name of manufacturer, lot number, date of administration, and name, address, and title of person administering the vaccine be documented.
● Have epinephrine solution 1:1,000 available to treat allergic reactions.
● Don't administer vaccine I.V. Use a 25G, ⅝-inch needle and inject S.C., preferably into outer aspect of upper arm.
● Use only diluent supplied. Discard reconstituted solution after 8 hours.
● Store in refrigerator and protect from light. Solution may be used if red, pink, or yellow, but it must be clear.
● Don't give vaccine less than 1 month before or after immunization with other live virus vaccines—except for live, attenuated measles virus vaccine, live rubella virus vaccine, or monovalent or trivalent live oral poliovirus vaccine, which may be administered simultaneously.
● Vaccine doesn't offer protection when given after exposure to natural mumps.
● Revaccination isn't required if primary vaccine was given at age 1 or older.

Monitoring the patient
● Watch for hypersensitivity reactions.
● Monitor patient for adverse effects.

Information for the patient
● Tell patient that he may experience pain and inflammation at injection site and a low-grade fever, rash, or general malaise.
● Encourage patient to report adverse reactions.
● Recommend acetaminophen to alleviate adverse reactions such as fever.
● Tell woman of childbearing age to avoid pregnancy for 3 months after vaccination. Provide contraceptive information, if necessary.

Pediatric patients
● Vaccine isn't recommended for children under age 1 because retained maternal mumps antibodies may interfere with immune response.

Breast-feeding patients
● It's unknown if vaccine appears in breast milk. No problems have been reported. Use vaccine cautiously in breast-feeding women.

mupirocin
(pseudomonic acid A)
Bactroban, Bactroban Nasal

Pharmacologic classification: antibiotic
Therapeutic classification: topical antibacterial
Pregnancy risk category B

How supplied
Available by prescription only
Ointment: 2% (1-g single-use tubes, 15 g, 30 g)

Indications, route, and dosage
Topical treatment of impetigo caused by Staphylococcus aureus, *beta-hemolytic strep-tococcus,* and Streptococcus pyogenes
Adults and children: Apply a small amount to affected area t.i.d. The area treated may be covered with a gauze dressing if desired.
Eradication of nasal colonization of methi-cillin-resistant S. aureus
Adults: Apply one-half of a single-use tube to each nostril b.i.d. for 5 days.

Pharmacodynamics
Antibacterial action: Structurally unrelated to other drugs and is produced by fermentation of the organism *Pseudomonas fluorescens.* Inhibits bacterial protein synthesis by reversibly and specifically binding to bacterial isoleucyl transfer-RNA synthetase. Shows no cross-resistance with chloramphenicol, erythromycin, gentamicin, lincomycin, methicillin, neomycin, novobiocin, penicillin, streptomycin, or tetracycline.

Pharmacokinetics
- *Absorption:* Normal subjects showed no absorption after 24-hour application under occlusive dressings.
- *Distribution:* About 95% protein-bound. Expect substantial decrease in activity in presence of serum (as in exudative wounds).
- *Metabolism:* Slightly metabolized locally in skin to monic acid.
- *Excretion:* Eliminated locally by desquamation of skin.

Contraindications and precautions
Contraindicated in patients with hypersensitivity to drug. Use cautiously in patients with burns or impaired renal function.

Interactions
None reported.

Adverse reactions
CNS: headache (with nasal use).
EENT: rhinitis, pharyngitis, taste perversion, burning (with nasal use).
Respiratory: upper respiratory congestion, cough (with nasal use).
Skin: burning, pruritus, stinging, rash, pain, erythema (with topical administration).

☑ Special considerations
- Reevaluate patients not showing a clinical response within 3 to 5 days.
- If sensitivity or chemical irritation occurs, stop treatment and institute appropriate alternative therapy.
- When used on burns or to treat extensive open wounds, absorption of polyethylene glycol vehicle is possible and may result in serious renal toxicity.

Monitoring the patient
- Monitor patient for superinfection. Use of antibiotics (prolonged or repeated) may result in bacterial or fungal overgrowth of nonsusceptible organisms. Such overgrowth may lead to a secondary infection.
- Watch for sensitivity reactions.

Information for the patient
- Advise patient to wash and dry affected areas thoroughly and then to apply thin film, rubbing in gently.
- Tell patient to use single-use tube for nasal application one time only, then discard tube. He should apply one-half of ointment from tube into one nostril and remaining half into other nostril, morning and evening.
- Warn patient to avoid contact around eyes and mucous membranes.

Breast-feeding patients
- It's unknown if drug appears in breast milk. Use with caution in breast-feeding women.

muromonab-CD3
Orthoclone OKT3

Pharmacologic classification: monoclonal antibody
Therapeutic classification: immunosuppressant
Pregnancy risk category C

How supplied
Injection: 5 mg/5 ml in 5-ml ampules

Indications, route, and dosage
Acute allograft rejection in renal, cardiac, and hepatic transplant patients
Adults: 5 mg/day for 10 to 14 days. Begin treatment once acute renal rejection is diagnosed.
   Note: A reaction is common within ½ to 6 hours after the first dose, consisting of significant fever, chills, dyspnea, and malaise. Pulmonary edema may occur if patient isn't pretreated with a corticosteroid.

Pharmacodynamics
Immunosuppressive action: Reverses graft rejection, probably by interfering with T-cell function that promotes acute renal rejection. Interacts with and prevents the function of the T-cell antigen receptor complex in the cellular membrane, which influences antigen recognition and is essential for signal transduction. Reacts with most peripheral T cells in blood and in body tissues, and blocks all known T-cell functions.

Pharmacokinetics
- *Absorption:* Immediate after I.V. administration.
- *Distribution:* No information available.
- *Metabolism:* No information available.
- *Excretion:* No information available.

Contraindications and precautions
Contraindicated in patients with hypersensitivity to drug or to other products of murine (mouse) origin and in those with antimurine antibody titers of 1:1,000 or more; fluid overload, as evidenced by chest radiograph or a weight gain greater than 3% within week before treatment; or history of seizures or predisposition to seizures. Also contraindicated in pregnant and breast-feeding women.

Interactions
Drug-drug. *Live virus vaccines:* May potentiate replication and increase effects of virus vaccine. Defer immunization if possible. If given, monitor patient response.

Other immunosuppressants (azathioprine, cyclosporine): May potentiate immunosuppressive effects of these drugs. Monitor patient closely.

Adverse reactions
CNS: *tremor, headache,* **seizures, encephalopathy, cerebral edema, coma.**
CV: *chest pain, tachycardia, hypertension,* **cardiac arrest, heart failure.**
GI: *nausea, vomiting, diarrhea.*
Respiratory: **severe pulmonary edema, respiratory arrest,** *dyspnea, wheezing.*
Other: *fever, chills, tremors,* **infection, anaphylaxis,** increased serum creatinine, **cytokine release syndrome** (from flulike symptoms to shock), **aseptic meningitis, risk of neoplasia.**

☑ Special considerations
● To prepare solution, draw into a syringe through a low protein-binding 0.2 or 0.22 micrometer filter. Discard filter and attach needle for I.V. bolus injection.
● Because drug is a protein solution, it may develop a few fine translucent particles, which don't affect its potency.
● Administer as an I.V. bolus in less than 1 minute. Don't give by I.V. infusion or combined with other drug solutions.
● The manufacturer recommends that, if patient's temperature exceeds 100° F (37.8° C), lower it with antipyretics before giving drug.
● Immunosuppressive therapy increases susceptibility to infection and to lymphoproliferative disorders. Lymphomas may follow immunosuppressive therapy; their occurrence seems related to the intensity and duration of immunosuppression rather than specific drugs because most patients receive a combination of treatments.
● Reduce concomitant immunosuppressive therapy to daily dose of prednisone 0.5 mg/kg and azathioprine 25 mg. Reduce or stop cyclosporine. Maintenance immunosuppression can resume 3 days before stopping muromonab-CD3.
● Refrigerate drug at 36° to 46° F (2° to 8° C). Don't freeze or shake.

Monitoring the patient
● Chest radiograph taken within 24 hours before treatment must be clear of fluid; monitor WBC counts and differentials at intervals during treatment.
● Monitor drug's effect on circulating T cells using flow cytometry or by expressing the CD3 antigen by in vitro assay.

Information for the patient
● Inform patient of expected first-dose effects (fever, chills, dyspnea, chest pain, nausea, vomiting).

Pediatric patients
● Safety and efficacy in children haven't been established. Patients as young as age 2 have had no unexpected adverse effects.

Breast-feeding patients
● Safety in breast-feeding women hasn't been established. It's unknown if drug appears in breast milk.

mycophenolate mofetil
CellCept

mycophenolate mofetil hydrochloride
CellCept Intravenous

Pharmacologic classification: mycophenolic acid derivative
Therapeutic classification: immunosuppressant
Pregnancy risk category C

How supplied
Available by prescription only
Capsules: 250 mg
Tablets: 500 mg
Powder for injection: 500 mg

Indications, route, and dosage
Prophylaxis of organ rejection in patients receiving allogeneic renal transplants
Adults: 1 g P.O. or I.V. b.i.d. Use with corticosteroids and cyclosporine.
Prophylaxis of organ rejection in patients receiving cardiac transplants
Adults: 1.5 g P.O. or I.V. b.i.d. Use with corticosteroids and cyclosporine.

Pharmacodynamics
Immunosuppressive action: Inhibits proliferative responses of T- and B-lymphocytes, suppresses antibody formation by B-lymphocytes, and may inhibit recruitment of leukocytes into sites of inflammation and graft rejection.

Pharmacokinetics
● *Absorption:* Absorbed from GI tract. Absolute bioavailability of drug and active metabolite is 94%.
● *Distribution:* About 97% bound to plasma protein.
● *Metabolism:* Complete presystemic metabolism to mycophenolic acid.
● *Excretion:* Primarily excreted in urine; small amount excreted in feces. Half-life is about 17.9 hours.

Contraindications and precautions
Contraindicated in patients with hypersensitivity to drug or its components or mycophenolic acid.

Don't use during pregnancy unless the benefits outweigh the risks. Use cautiously in patients with GI disorders.

Interactions
Drug-drug. *Acyclovir, ganciclovir:* Increased risk of toxicity for both drugs. Monitor patient closely.
Antacids containing magnesium and aluminum hydroxides: Decreased absorption of mycophenolate mofetil. Separate administration times.
Cholestyramine: May interfere with enterohepatic recirculation; decreased mycophenolate bioavailability. Don't administer concurrently.
Oral contraceptives: Reduced efficacy. Advise patient to use alternative method of contraception.

Adverse reactions
CNS: *asthenia, tremor,* insomnia, dizziness, *headache.*
CV: *chest pain, hypertension, edema.*
EENT: pharyngitis.
GI: *diarrhea, constipation, nausea, dyspepsia, vomiting, oral candidiasis, abdominal pain,* **hemorrhage.**
GU: *urinary tract infection, hematuria,* kidney tubular necrosis.
Hematologic: *anemia,* LEUKOPENIA, THROMBOCYTOPENIA, hypochromic anemia, leukocytosis.
Metabolic: *hypercholesterolemia, hypophosphatemia, hypokalemia,* hyperkalemia, hyperglycemia.
Musculoskeletal: *back pain.*
Respiratory: *dyspnea, cough,* bronchitis, pneumonia.
Skin: *acne,* rash.
Other: *pain, fever,* **sepsis,** *possible immunosuppression-induced infection or lymphoma.*

☑ Special considerations
● Avoid doses exceeding 1 g b.i.d. in patients with severe chronic renal impairment (glomerular filtration rate below 25 ml/minute) outside the immediate posttransplant period.
● Because of potential teratogenic effects, don't open capsules and don't crush tablets. Also avoid inhalation or direct contact with skin or mucous membranes of powder contained in capsules. If such contact occurs, wash thoroughly with soap and water, rinse eyes with plain water.
● Immunosuppression-induced infection or lymphoma may occur.
● Don't administer I.V. solution by rapid or bolus method; must be given over 2 hours or more.
● Reconstitute with 5% dextrose injection to a solution of 6 mg/ml; drug is incompatible with other I.V. infusion solutions and must be administered through an exclusive site.

Monitoring the patient
● Monitor patient's CBC regularly. If neutropenia develops, interrupt therapy, reduce dosage, per-

form appropriate diagnostic tests, or give additional treatment.
● Evaluate patient for signs of infection.
● Monitor kidney function and electrolyte and cholesterol levels.

Information for the patient
● Warn patient not to open capsules or crush tablets; instruct him to swallow whole on empty stomach.
● Instruct patient of need for repeated appropriate laboratory tests during drug therapy.
● Give patient complete dosage instructions and inform him of increased risk of lymphoproliferative diseases and other malignancies.
● Explain that drug is used with other drug therapies. Stress importance of not interrupting or stopping these drugs without medical approval.
● Inform woman that a pregnancy test should be done within 1 week before therapy and that effective contraception must be used before, during, and for 6 weeks after therapy ends, even when there is history of infertility (unless due to hysterectomy). Also, two forms of contraception must be used simultaneously unless abstinence is chosen. If pregnancy occurs despite these measures, tell patient to call immediately.

Pediatric patients
● Safety and effectiveness in children haven't been established.

Breast-feeding patients
● It's unknown if drug appears in breast milk. Use in breast-feeding women isn't recommended.

nabumetone
Relafen

Pharmacologic classification: NSAID
Therapeutic classification: antarthritic
Pregnancy risk category C

How supplied
Available by prescription only
Tablets: 500 mg, 750 mg

Indications, route, and dosage
Acute and long-term treatment of rheumatoid arthritis or osteoarthritis
Adults: Initially, 1,000 mg P.O. daily as a single dose or in divided doses b.i.d. Adjust dosage based on patient response. Maximum recommended daily dose is 2,000 mg.

Pharmacodynamics
Anti-inflammatory action: Probably acts by inhibiting synthesis of prostaglandins. Also has analgesic and antipyretic action.

Pharmacokinetics
• *Absorption:* Well absorbed from GI tract. After absorption, about 35% is rapidly transformed to 6-methoxy-2-naphthylacetic acid (6MNA), principal active metabolite; balance transformed to unidentified metabolites. Food increases absorption rate and peak levels of 6MNA but doesn't change total drug absorbed. Levels peak in 2½ to 4 hours.
• *Distribution:* 6MNA more than 99% bound to plasma proteins.
• *Metabolism:* 6MNA metabolized to inactive metabolites in liver.
• *Excretion:* Metabolites excreted primarily in urine; about 9% in feces. Elimination half-life is about 24 hours; half-life increased in patients with renal failure.

Contraindications and precautions
Contraindicated in patients with hypersensitivity reactions; history of aspirin- or NSAID-induced asthma, urticaria, or other allergic-type reactions; and during third trimester of pregnancy.
Use cautiously in patients with impaired renal or hepatic function, heart failure, hypertension, conditions that predispose to fluid retention, or history of peptic ulcer disease.

Interactions
Drug-drug. *Drugs highly bound to plasma proteins (such as warfarin):* Increased risk of adverse reactions; nabumetone may displace drug. Use together with caution.

Adverse reactions
CNS: *dizziness, headache,* fatigue, insomnia, nervousness, somnolence.
CV: vasculitis, edema.
EENT: *tinnitus.*
GI: *diarrhea, dyspepsia, abdominal pain, constipation, flatulence, nausea,* dry mouth, gastritis, stomatitis, anorexia, vomiting, **bleeding,** ulceration.
Respiratory: dyspnea, pneumonitis.
Skin: *pruritus, rash,* increased diaphoresis.

☑ Special considerations
Besides the recommendations relevant to all NSAIDs, consider the following.
• Because NSAIDs impair the synthesis of renal prostaglandins, they can decrease renal blood flow and lead to reversible renal function impairment, especially in patients with preexisting renal failure, liver dysfunction, or heart failure; in elderly patients; and in those taking diuretics. Monitor these patients closely during therapy.

Monitoring the patient
• During long-term therapy, periodically monitor renal and liver function, CBC, and hematocrit.
• Monitor patient carefully for signs and symptoms of GI bleeding.

Information for the patient
• Tell patient to take drug with food, milk, or antacids to enhance drug absorption.
• Stress importance of follow-up examinations to detect adverse GI effects.
• Teach patient signs and symptoms of GI bleeding, and tell him to report them immediately.
• Advise patient to limit alcohol intake because of risk of additive GI toxicity.

Geriatric patients
• No differences in safety or efficacy have been noted in elderly patients.

Pediatric patients
• Safety and efficacy in children haven't been established.

Reactions may be *common*, uncommon, *life-threatening*, or COMMON AND LIFE-THREATENING.

Breast-feeding patients
● Because of risk of serious toxicity to infant, use in breast-feeding women isn't recommended.

nadolol
Corgard

Pharmacologic classification: beta blocker
Therapeutic classification: antihypertensive, antianginal
Pregnancy risk category C

How supplied
Available by prescription only
Tablets: 20 mg, 40 mg, 80 mg, 120 mg, 160 mg

Indications, route, and dosage
Hypertension
Adults: Initially, 20 to 40 mg P.O. once daily. Dosage may be increased in 40- to 80-mg increments daily at 2- to 14-day intervals until optimum response occurs. Usual maintenance dose is 40 or 80 mg once daily. Doses of up to 240 or 320 mg daily may be necessary.
Long-term prophylactic management of chronic stable angina pectoris
Adults: Initially, 40 mg P.O. once daily. Dosage may be increased in 40- to 80-mg increments daily at 3- to 7-day intervals until optimum response occurs. Usual maintenance dose is 40 or 80 mg once daily. Doses of up to 160 or 240 mg daily may be needed.
◊ Arrhythmias
Adults: 60 to 160 mg daily.
◊ Prophylaxis of vascular headache
Adults: 20 to 40 mg once daily; may gradually increase to 120 mg daily if necessary.
✦ *Dosage adjustment.* For renally impaired patients, refer to the table.

Creatinine clearance (ml/min/1.73 m²)	Dosing interval
> 50	q 24 hr
31 to 50	q 24 to 36 hr
10 to 30	q 24 to 48 hr
< 10	q 40 to 60 hr

Pharmacodynamics
Antihypertensive action: Mechanism unknown. May reduce blood pressure by blocking adrenergic receptors, thus decreasing cardiac output; by decreasing sympathetic outflow from the CNS; or by suppressing renin release.
Antianginal action: Decreases myocardial oxygen consumption, thus relieving angina, by blocking catecholamine-induced increases in heart rate, myocardial contraction, and blood pressure.

Pharmacokinetics
● *Absorption:* 30% to 40% of dose absorbed from GI tract; plasma levels peak in 2 to 4 hours. Absorption not affected by food.
● *Distribution:* Distributed throughout body; about 30% protein-bound.
● *Metabolism:* Not metabolized.
● *Excretion:* Most of a dose excreted unchanged in urine; remainder excreted in feces. Plasma half-life is about 20 hours. Antihypertensive and antianginal effects last for about 24 hours.

Contraindications and precautions
Contraindicated in patients with bronchial asthma, sinus bradycardia and greater than first-degree heart block, and cardiogenic shock. Use cautiously in patients with hyperthyroidism, heart failure, diabetes, chronic bronchitis, emphysema, or impaired renal or hepatic function and in those receiving general anesthesia before undergoing surgery.

Interactions
Drug-drug. *Antimuscarinics (such as atropine):* May antagonize nadolol-induced bradycardia. Use together cautiously.
Diuretics, other antihypertensives: Potentiate antihypertensive effects. Use together cautiously.
Epinephrine: Decreased pulse rate with first- and second-degree heart block and hypertension. Avoid using together.
Sympathomimetics (such as isoproterenol): May antagonize beta-adrenergic stimulating effects of these drugs. Monitor patient closely.
Tubocurarine and related drugs: Potentiated neuromuscular blocking effect. Use with caution.
Other antiarrhythmics: Additive or antagonistic cardiac effects and additive toxic effects. Use together cautiously.
Drug-lifestyle. *Cocaine:* May inhibit therapeutic effects of nadolol. Discourage concomitant use.

Adverse reactions
CNS: fatigue, dizziness.
CV: *bradycardia,* hypotension, *heart failure,* peripheral vascular disease, rhythm and conduction disturbances.
GI: nausea, vomiting, diarrhea, abdominal pain, constipation, anorexia.
Respiratory: *increased airway resistance.*
Skin: rash.
Other: fever.

☑ Special considerations
Besides the recommendations relevant to all beta blockers, consider the following.
● Dosage adjustments may be necessary in patients with renal impairment.
● Nadolol has been used as an antiarrhythmic and as a prophylactic for migraine headaches.
● If long-term therapy is used, gradually decrease dosage over 1 to 2 weeks before stopping drug.

Abrupt withdrawal can exacerbate angina and cause MI.
• Signs and symptoms of toxicity include severe hypotension, bradycardia, heart failure, and bronchospasm. After acute ingestion, empty stomach by induced emesis or gastric lavage, and give activated charcoal to reduce absorption. Magnesium sulfate may be given orally as a cathartic.

Monitoring the patient
• Monitor patient's renal function.
• Check blood pressure and ECG periodically.

Information for the patient
• Tell patient not to stop drug abruptly. Dosage should be tapered.

Geriatric patients
• Elderly patients may require lower maintenance doses because of increased bioavailability or delayed metabolism; they also may experience enhanced adverse effects.

Pediatric patients
• Safety and efficacy in children haven't been established; use only if potential benefit outweighs risk.

Breast-feeding patients
• Drug appears in breast milk; an alternative to breast-feeding is recommended during therapy.

nafcillin sodium
Nafcil, Nallpen, Unipen

Pharmacologic classification: penicillinase-resistant penicillin
Therapeutic classification: antibiotic
Pregnancy risk category B

How supplied
Available by prescription only
Capsules: 250 mg
Tablets: 500 mg
Injection: 500 mg, 1 g, 2 g
I.V. infusion piggyback: 1 g, 2 g

Indications, route, and dosage
Systemic infections caused by susceptible organisms (methicillin-sensitive Staphylococcus aureus)
Adults: 2 to 4 g P.O. daily, divided into doses given q 6 hours; 2 to 12 g I.M. or I.V. daily, divided into doses given q 4 to 6 hours.
Children over 1 month: 50 to 100 mg/kg P.O., I.M., or I.V. daily in equally divided doses q 6 hours. For more severe infections, 100 to 200 mg/kg I.V. or I.M. daily in equally divided doses q 4 to 6 hours.

Neonates: 30 to 40 mg/kg P.O. daily in three to four equally divided doses; or 20 mg/kg I.M. daily in two equally divided doses.
Neonates under 1 week, weighing less than 2 kg: 25 mg/kg I.V. q 12 hours or, if more than 2 kg, q 8 hours. If meningitis infection, 50 mg/kg q 12 hours if less than 2 kg, or q 8 hours if more than 2 kg.
Neonates over 1 week, weighing less than 2 kg: 25 mg/kg q 8 hours or, if more than 2 kg, q 6 hours. If meningitis infection, 50 mg/kg q 8 hours if less than 2 kg, or q 6 hours if more than 2 kg.

Pharmacodynamics
Antibiotic action: Bactericidal. Adheres to bacterial penicillin-binding proteins, thus inhibiting bacterial cell-wall synthesis.
   Resists the effects of penicillinases—enzymes that inactivate penicillin—and is thus active against many strains of penicillinase-producing bacteria; this activity is most important against penicillinase-producing staphylococci; some strains may remain resistant. Also active against a few gram-positive aerobic and anaerobic bacilli but has no significant effect on gram-negative bacilli.

Pharmacokinetics
• *Absorption:* Absorbed erratically and poorly from GI tract; serum levels peak at ½ to 2 hours after oral dose; 30 to 60 minutes after I.M. dose. Food decreases absorption.
• *Distribution:* Distributed widely; poor CSF penetration but enhanced by meningeal inflammation. Drug crosses placenta and is 70% to 90% protein-bound.
• *Metabolism:* Metabolized primarily in liver; undergoes enterohepatic circulation. Dosage adjustment isn't necessary for patients in renal failure.
• *Excretion:* Drug and metabolites excreted primarily in bile; about 25% to 30% excreted in urine unchanged. May also be excreted in breast milk. Elimination half-life in adults is ½ to 1½ hours.

Contraindications and precautions
Contraindicated in patients with hypersensitivity to drug or other penicillins. Use cautiously in patients with GI distress or sensitivity to cephalosporins.

Interactions
Drug-drug. *Aminoglycosides:* Synergistic bactericidal effects against *S. aureus.* However, drugs are physically and chemically incompatible. Don't mix or give together.
Cyclosporines: Subtherapeutic cyclosporine levels reported. When used concurrently in organ transplant patients, monitor cyclosporine levels.
Hepatotoxic drugs: Increased risk of hepatotoxicity. Monitor patient closely.

Drug-food. *Carbonated beverages, fruit juice:* Acid may inactivate drug. Don't give together. *Any food:* Decreased absorption. Drug should be taken on an empty stomach.

Adverse reactions
CV: thrombophlebitis.
GI: *nausea,* vomiting, diarrhea, **pseudomembranous colitis.**
Hematologic: transient leukopenia, **neutropenia, granulocytopenia, thrombocytopenia** with high doses.
Other: hypersensitivity reactions (chills, fever, rash, pruritus, urticaria, **anaphylaxis**), vein irritation.

☑ Special considerations
Besides the recommendations relevant to all penicillins, consider the following.
● Give drug with water only; acid in fruit juice or carbonated beverage may inactivate drug.
● Give dose on empty stomach; food decreases absorption.
● Nafcillin alters tests for urinary and serum proteins; turbidimetric urine and serum proteins are often falsely positive or elevated in tests using sulfosalicylic acid or trichloroacetic acid.
● Toxicity may cause neuromuscular irritability or seizures.
● Drug isn't appreciably removed by hemodialysis.

Monitoring the patient
● Renal, hepatic, and hematologic systems should be evaluated periodically during prolonged therapy.
● Monitor patient for adverse reactions, especially hypersensitivity reactions.

Information for the patient
● Tell patient to report severe diarrhea or allergic reactions promptly.

Geriatric patients
● Half-life may be prolonged in elderly patients because of impaired hepatic and renal function.

Pediatric patients
● Nafcillin reconstituted with bacteriostatic water for injection with benzyl alcohol shouldn't be used in neonates because of toxicity.

Breast-feeding patients
● Drug appears in breast milk; use with caution in breast-feeding women.

nalbuphine hydrochloride
Nubain

Pharmacologic classification: narcotic agonist-antagonist, opioid partial agonist
Therapeutic classification: analgesic, adjunct to anesthesia
Pregnancy risk category NR

How supplied
Available by prescription only
Injection: 10 mg/ml, 20 mg/ml

Indications, route, and dosage
Moderate to severe pain
Adults: 10 to 20 mg S.C., I.M., or I.V. q 3 to 6 hours, p.r.n., or around the clock. Maximum dose is 160 mg/day.
Supplement to anesthesia
Adults: 0.3 mg/kg to 3 mg/kg I.V. over 10 to 15 minutes; maintenance dose is 0.25 to 0.5 mg/kg I.V.

Pharmacodynamics
Analgesic action: Analgesia is believed to result from drug's action at opiate receptor sites in the CNS, relieving moderate to severe pain. The narcotic antagonist effect may result from competitive inhibition at opiate receptors. Like other opioids, nalbuphine causes respiratory depression, sedation, and miosis. In patients with coronary artery disease or MI, it appears to produce no substantial changes in heart rate, pulmonary artery or wedge pressure, left ventricular end-diastolic pressure, pulmonary vascular resistance, or cardiac index.

Pharmacokinetics
● *Absorption:* When administered orally, drug is about one-fifth as effective as an analgesic than when given I.M. because of first-pass metabolism in GI tract and liver. Onset of action within 15 minutes; peak effect seen at ½ to 1 hour.
● *Distribution:* Not appreciably bound to plasma proteins.
● *Metabolism:* Metabolized in liver; duration of action is 3 to 6 hours.
● *Excretion:* Excreted in urine and to some degree in bile.

Contraindications and precautions
Contraindicated in patients with hypersensitivity to drug. Use cautiously in patients with history of drug abuse, emotional instability, head injury, increased intracranial pressure, impaired ventilation, MI accompanied by nausea and vomiting, upcoming biliary surgery, and hepatic or renal disease.

Interactions

Drug-drug. *Barbiturate anesthetics (such as thiopental):* Nalbuphine may produce additive CNS and respiratory depressant effects; possible apnea. Monitor patient closely.

Cimetidine: May increase narcotic nalbuphine toxicity. If used together, be prepared to administer narcotic antagonist if toxicity occurs.

Digitoxin, phenytoin, rifampin: Drug accumulation and enhanced effects. Monitor patient for toxicity.

General anesthetics: Severe CV depression. Don't use together.

Narcotic antagonists: Acute withdrawal syndrome. Use with caution and monitor patient closely.

Other CNS depressants (antihistamines, barbiturates, benzodiazepines, muscle relaxants, narcotic analgesics, phenothiazines, sedative-hypnotics, tricyclic antidepressants): Potentiated effects of drug. May need to reduce nalbuphine dosage.

Drug-lifestyle. *Alcohol:* Potentiates drug's effects. Discourage concomitant use.

Adverse reactions

CNS: *headache, sedation, dizziness, vertigo,* nervousness, depression, restlessness, crying, euphoria, hostility, unusual dreams, confusion, hallucinations, speech difficulty, delusions.

CV: hypertension, hypotension, tachycardia, *bradycardia.*

EENT: blurred vision, *dry mouth.*

GI: cramps, dyspepsia, bitter taste, *nausea, vomiting,* constipation, biliary tract spasms.

GU: urinary urgency.

Respiratory: *respiratory depression,* dyspnea, asthma, *pulmonary edema.*

Skin: pruritus, burning, urticaria, *clamminess.*

☑ Special considerations

Besides the recommendations relevant to all opioid agonist-antagonists, consider the following.

● Nalbuphine may obscure signs and symptoms of an acute abdominal condition or worsen gallbladder pain.

● Before administration, visually inspect all parenteral products for particulate matter and discoloration.

● Parenteral administration of drug provides better analgesia than oral administration. I.V. doses should be given by slow I.V. injection, preferably in diluted solution. Rapid I.V. injection increases adverse effects.

● Drug causes respiratory depression, which at 10 mg is equal to respiratory depression produced by 10 mg of morphine.

● Drug acts as a narcotic antagonist; may precipitate abstinence syndrome in narcotic-dependent patients.

● Drug may interfere with enzymatic tests for detection of opioids.

● Toxicity may cause CNS depression, respiratory depression, and miosis (pinpoint pupils). Other acute toxic effects include hypotension, bradycardia, hypothermia, shock, apnea, cardiopulmonary arrest, circulatory collapse, pulmonary edema, and seizures.

● To treat acute overdose, first establish adequate respiratory exchange via a patent airway and ventilation as needed; administer a narcotic antagonist (naloxone) to reverse respiratory depression. Because the duration of action of nalbuphine is longer than that of naloxone, repeated naloxone dosing is necessary.

● Naloxone shouldn't be given in the absence of clinically significant respiratory or CV depression.

Monitoring the patient
● Drug may cause orthostatic hypotension in ambulatory patients.

● When drug is used during labor and delivery, observe neonate for signs of respiratory depression.

Information for the patient
● Instruct patient to avoid driving or operating machinery as drug may cause dizziness and fatigue.

Geriatric patients
● Lower doses are usually indicated for elderly patients, who may be more sensitive to the therapeutic and adverse effects of drug.

Pediatric patients
● Safety in children under age 18 hasn't been established.

Breast-feeding patients
● It's unknown if drug appears in breast milk; use with caution in breast-feeding women.

nalidixic acid
NegGram

Pharmacologic classification: quinolone antibiotic
Therapeutic classification: urinary tract anti-infective
Pregnancy risk category B

How supplied
Available by prescription only
Tablets: 250 mg, 500 mg, 1 g
Suspension: 250 mg/5 ml

Indications, route, and dosage
Acute and chronic urinary tract infections caused by susceptible gram-negative organisms
Adults: 1 g P.O. q.i.d. for 7 to 14 days; 2 g P.O. daily for long-term use. Up to 6 g daily have been used for severe urinary tract infection.

Children over age 3 months: 55 mg/kg P.O. daily divided q.i.d. for 7 to 14 days; 33 mg/kg P.O. daily divided q.i.d. for long-term use.

Pharmacodynamics
Antimicrobial action: Bactericidal. Inhibits microbial synthesis of DNA. Spectrum of action includes most gram-negative organisms except *Pseudomonas.* (About 2% to 14% of patients develop nalidixic acid-resistant organisms during therapy.)

Pharmacokinetics
• *Absorption:* Well absorbed from GI tract; levels peak in 1 to 2 hours.
• *Distribution:* Concentrates in renal tissue and seminal fluid; doesn't penetrate prostatic tissue; only minimal amounts appear in CSF and placenta. Drug is highly protein-bound.
• *Metabolism:* Metabolized to more active hydroxy-nalidixic acid and inactive conjugates in liver.
• *Excretion:* 13% of drug metabolites and 2% to 3% of unchanged drug excreted via kidneys. In patients with normal renal function, plasma half-life is 1 to 2½ hours. In anuric patients, half-life is prolonged up to 21 hours.

Contraindications and precautions
Contraindicated in patients with hypersensitivity to drug, in those with seizure disorders, and in infants under age 3 months. Use cautiously in patients with impaired renal or hepatic function, pulmonary disease, or severe cerebral arteriosclerosis and in prepubertal children.

Interactions
Drug-drug. *Antacids:* Decreased absorption of nalidixic acid. Don't give together.
Dicumarol, warfarin: Excessive anticoagulation. Monitor patient closely.
Other photosensitizing drugs: Possible additive effects. Inform patient about increased sensitivity to sun exposure and to use precautions.
Drug-lifestyle. *Sun exposure:* Photosensitivity reactions. Tell patient to take precautions.

Adverse reactions
CNS: drowsiness, weakness, headache, dizziness, vertigo, *seizures,* malaise, confusion, hallucinations, psychosis, *increased intracranial pressure and bulging fontanelles in infants and children.*
EENT: sensitivity to light, change in color perception, diplopia, blurred vision.
GI: *abdominal pain, nausea, vomiting,* diarrhea.
Hematologic: eosinophilia, *leukopenia, thrombocytopenia,* hemolytic anemia.
Musculoskeletal: arthralgia, joint stiffness.
Skin: pruritus, photosensitivity, urticaria, rash.
Other: *angioedema, anaphylactoid reaction.*

☑ Special considerations
• Drug is ineffective against *Pseudomonas* infection or infection found outside urinary tract.
• Resistant bacteria may emerge after first 48 hours of therapy (especially if inadequate doses are prescribed).
• Although CNS toxicity is rare, brief seizures, increased intracranial pressure, and toxic psychosis may occur in infants, children, and elderly patients.
• Drug can be used during second and third trimesters of pregnancy; however, safety hasn't been established for use in first trimester.
• False-positive reactions may occur in urine glucose tests using cupric sulfate reagents (such as Benedict's test, Fehling's solution, and Clinitest), from reaction between glucuronic acid (liberated by urinary metabolites of nalidixic acid) and cupric sulfate. Urine 17-ketosteroid and urine 17-ketogenic steroid levels may be falsely elevated because nalidixic acid interacts with *m*-dinitrobenzene, used to measure these urine metabolites. Urinary vanillylmandelic acid levels may also be falsely elevated.
• Toxicity may cause psychosis, seizures, increased intracranial pressure, metabolic acidosis, lethargy, nausea, and vomiting. However, because nalidixic acid is rapidly excreted, such reactions usually resolve in 2 to 3 hours.

Monitoring the patient
• Obtain culture and sensitivity tests before starting therapy and repeat as needed.
• Obtain CBC and renal and liver function studies periodically during long-term therapy.

Information for the patient
• Instruct patient to report visual disturbances; these usually disappear with dosage reduction.
• Warn patient that exposure to sunlight may cause photosensitivity. Inform him that photosensitivity reactions usually resolve within 2 to 8 weeks after therapy ends. Also warn him that bullae may continue after exposure to sunlight or mild skin trauma for up to 3 months after therapy ends.
• Advise patient to take drug with food or milk to avoid GI upset.
• Warn patient to use caution while driving because drug may cause drowsiness or blurred vision.

Pediatric patients
• Don't give drug to infants under age 3 months because safety hasn't been established; don't give to prepubertal children because drug can produce erosions to cartilage in weight-bearing joints.

Breast-feeding patients
• Low levels of drug appear in breast milk. In one case, hemolytic anemia occurred in infant of ure-

mic mother taking 1 g q.i.d. Lower drug excretion and elevated serum level resulted in higher level in milk. Use with caution in breast-feeding women.

naloxone hydrochloride
Narcan

Pharmacologic classification: narcotic (opioid) antagonist
Therapeutic classification: narcotic antagonist
Pregnancy risk category B

How supplied
Available by prescription only
Injection: 0.4 mg/ml, 1 mg/ml with preservatives, and 0.02 mg/ml, 0.4 mg/ml, 1 mg/ml parabens-free

Indications, route, and dosage
Known or suspected narcotic-induced respiratory depression, including that caused by natural and synthetic narcotics, methadone, nalbuphine, pentazocine, and propoxyphene
Adults: 0.4 to 2 mg I.V., S.C., or I.M., repeated q 2 to 3 minutes, p.r.n. If no response is observed after 10 mg have been administered, diagnosis of narcotic-induced toxicity should be questioned. *Children:* 0.01 mg/kg I.V.; give a subsequent dose of 0.1 mg/kg if needed. Dosage for continuous infusion is 0.024 to 0.16 mg/kg/hour. If I.V. route not available, dose may be given I.M. or S.C. in divided doses.
Postoperative narcotic depression
Adults: 0.1 to 0.2 mg I.V. q 2 to 3 minutes, p.r.n., until desired response is obtained.
Children: 0.005 to 0.01 mg/kg I.M., I.V., or S.C., repeated q 2 to 3 minutes, p.r.n., until desired degree of reversal is obtained.
Neonates (asphyxia neonatorum): 0.01 mg/kg I.V. into umbilical vein repeated q 2 to 3 minutes for three doses. Drug concentration for use in neonates and children is 0.02 mg/ml.
Naloxone challenge for diagnosing opiate dependence
Adults: 0.16 mg I.M. naloxone; if no signs of withdrawal after 20 to 30 minutes, give second dose of 0.24 mg I.V.

Pharmacodynamics
Narcotic (opioid) antagonist action: Essentially a pure antagonist. In patients who have received an opioid agonist or other analgesic with narcotic-like effects, naloxone antagonizes most of the opioid effects, especially respiratory depression, sedation, and hypotension. Because the duration of action of naloxone in most cases is shorter than that of the opioid, opiate effects may return as those of naloxone dissipate. Naloxone doesn't produce tolerance or physical or psychological dependence. The precise mechanism of action is unknown, but is thought to involve competitive antagonism of more than one opiate receptor in the CNS.

Pharmacokinetics
• *Absorption:* Rapidly inactivated after oral administration; given parenterally. Onset of action 1 to 2 minutes after I.V. administration; 2 to 5 minutes after I.M. or S.C. administration. Longer duration of action after I.M. use and higher doses when compared with I.V. use and lower doses.
• *Distribution:* Rapidly distributed into body tissues and fluids.
• *Metabolism:* Rapidly metabolized in liver, primarily by conjugation.
• *Excretion:* Excreted in urine. Duration of action about 45 minutes, depending on route and dose. Plasma half-life reported from 60 to 90 minutes in adults and 3 hours in neonates.

Contraindications and precautions
Contraindicated in patients with hypersensitivity to drug. Use cautiously in patients with cardiac irritability and opiate addiction. When given to a narcotic addict, naloxone may produce an acute abstinence syndrome. Use with caution, and monitor patient closely.

Interactions
Drug-drug. *Cardiotoxic drugs:* Potential serious CV effects. Avoid using together.

Adverse reactions
CNS: tremors, *seizures.*
CV: tachycardia, hypertension (with higher-than-recommended doses); hypotension; *ventricular fibrillation; cardiac arrest.*
GI: nausea, vomiting (with higher-than-recommended doses).
Respiratory: *pulmonary edema.*
Skin: diaphoresis.
Other: withdrawal symptoms (in narcotic-dependent patients with higher-than-recommended doses).

☑ Special considerations
Besides the recommendations relevant to all narcotic antagonists, consider the following.
• Before administration, visually inspect all parenteral products for particulate matter and discoloration.
• Take a careful drug history to rule out narcotic addiction and to avoid inducing withdrawal symptoms (apply same precautions to the baby of an addicted woman).
• Because naloxone's duration of activity is shorter than that of most narcotics, vigilance and repeated doses are usually necessary to manage acute narcotic overdose in a nonaddicted patient.

Reactions may be *common*, uncommon, **life-threatening**, or COMMON AND LIFE-THREATENING.

• Drug isn't effective in treating respiratory depression caused by nonopioid drugs.
• Drug can be diluted in dextrose 5% or normal saline solution. Use within 24 hours after mixing.
• Naloxone is the safest drug to use when cause of respiratory depression is uncertain.
• Drug may be given by continuous I.V. infusion, which is necessary in many cases to control adverse effects of epidurally administered morphine. Usual dose is 2 mg in 500 ml of D_5W or normal saline solution.

Monitoring the patient
• Monitor patient for cardiac function, oxygen saturation, and blood pressure.
• Don't neglect attention to the airway, breathing, and circulation. Maintain adequate respiratory and CV status at all times. Respiratory "overshoot" may occur; watch for respiratory rate higher than before respiratory depression. Respiratory rate increases in 1 to 2 minutes; effect lasts 1 to 4 hours.

Geriatric patients
• Lower doses are usually indicated for elderly patients because they may be more sensitive to the therapeutic and adverse effects of drug.

Breast-feeding patients
• It's unknown if drug appears in breast milk. Use with caution in breast-feeding women.

naltrexone hydrochloride
ReVia

Pharmacologic classification: narcotic (opioid) antagonist
Therapeutic classification: narcotic detoxification adjunct
Pregnancy risk category C

How supplied
Available by prescription only
Tablets: 50 mg

Indications, route, and dosage
Adjunct for maintenance of opioid-free state in detoxified individuals
Adults: Don't attempt treatment until naloxone challenge is negative (0.2 mg I.V., if no signs of withdrawal after 30 seconds, give additional 0.6 mg I.V.; Or administer 0.8 mg S.C. and observe for 20 minutes for signs of withdrawal). Don't attempt treatment until patient has remained opioid-free for 7 to 10 days, verified by analyzing urine. Initially, 25 mg P.O. If no withdrawal signs occur within 1 hour, administer an additional 25 mg. Once patient has been started on 50 mg q 24 hours, flexible maintenance schedule may be used. From 50 to 150 mg may be giv-

en daily, depending on schedule prescribed, but the average daily dose is 50 mg.
Alcoholism
Adults: 50 mg P.O. daily.

Pharmacodynamics
Opioid antagonist action: Essentially a pure opiate (narcotic) antagonist. Like naloxone, it has little or no agonist activity. Exact mechanism of action unknown, but it's thought to involve competitive antagonism of more than one opiate receptor in the CNS. When administered to patients who haven't recently received opiates, it exhibits little or no pharmacologic effect. At oral doses of 30 to 50 mg daily, it produces minimal analgesia, only slight drowsiness, and no respiratory depression. However, pharmacologic effects, including psychotomimetic effects, increased systolic or diastolic blood pressure, respiratory depression, and decreased oral temperature, which are suggestive of opiate agonist activity, have reportedly occurred in a few patients. In patients who have received single or repeated large doses of opiates, naltrexone attenuates or produces a complete but reversible block of the pharmacologic effects of the narcotic. Naltrexone doesn't produce physical or psychological dependence, and tolerance to its antagonist activity reportedly doesn't develop.

Pharmacokinetics
• *Absorption:* Well absorbed after oral administration, reaching peak plasma levels after 1 hour. Extensive first-pass hepatic metabolism; only 5% to 20% of oral dose reaches systemic circulation unchanged. Peak effect occurs within 1 hour.
• *Distribution:* About 21% to 28% protein-bound. Extent and duration of drug's antagonist activity appear directly related to plasma and tissue levels of drug. Widely distributed throughout body, but considerable individual variation exists.
• *Metabolism:* Oral naltrexone undergoes extensive first-pass hepatic metabolism. Major metabolite is pure antagonist and may contribute to efficacy. Drug and hepatic metabolites may undergo enterohepatic recirculation.
• *Excretion:* Excreted primarily by kidneys. Elimination half-life is about 4 hours; that of major active metabolite is about 13 hours.

Contraindications and precautions
Contraindicated in patients with hypersensitivity to drug, in those receiving opioid analgesics, in opioid-dependent patients, in patients in acute opioid withdrawal, in those with acute hepatitis or liver failure or positive urine screen for opioids.
Use cautiously in patients with mild hepatic disease or history of hepatic impairment.

Interactions
Drug-drug. *Opiates (or in nondetoxified patients physically dependent on opiates):* Potentially serious opiate withdrawal. Don't use together.
Opioid-containing drugs (antidiarrheals, cold and cough preparations, opioid analgesics): Attenuated opioid activity. Monitor patient carefully.
Thioridazine: Possible lethargy and somnolence. Monitor patient for this effect.
Other drugs that alter hepatic metabolism: Increased or decreased serum naltrexone levels. Monitor patient for effects.

Adverse reactions
CNS: *insomnia, anxiety, nervousness, headache,* depression, dizziness, fatigue, somnolence, *suicidal ideation.*
GI: *nausea, vomiting,* anorexia, *abdominal pain,* constipation, increased thirst.
GU: delayed ejaculation, decreased potency.
Hematologic: lymphocytosis.
Hepatic: *hepatotoxicity.*
Musculoskeletal: *muscle and joint pain.*
Skin: rash.
Other: chills.

☑ Special considerations
Besides the recommendations relevant to all narcotic (opioid) antagonists, consider the following.
● Administer a naloxone (Narcan) challenge test to the patient before naltrexone use. Naloxone (0.8 mg S.C. or I.V., incremental doses) is administered and the patient closely monitored for signs and symptoms of opiate withdrawal. If acute abstinence signs and symptoms are present, don't administer naltrexone.
● Before administering, take a careful drug history to rule out possible narcotic use. Don't attempt treatment until patient has been opiate-free for 7 to 10 days. Verify self-reporting of abstinence from narcotics by urinalysis for opioids. No withdrawal signs or symptoms should be reported by patient or be evident.
● In an emergency requiring analgesia that can only be achieved with opiates, patient who has been receiving naltrexone may need a higher than usual dose of narcotic, and the resulting respiratory depression may be deeper and more prolonged.
● Drug can cause hepatocellular injury if given at higher than recommended doses. Naltrexone can cause or exacerbate signs and symptoms of abstinence in anyone not completely opioid-free.

Monitoring the patient
● Perform liver function tests before naltrexone use to establish a baseline and to evaluate possible drug-induced hepatotoxicity.
● Monitor psychological status of patient.

Information for the patient
● Inform patient that opioids, such as cough and cold preparations, antidiarrheal products, and narcotic analgesics may not be effective; recommend nonnarcotic alternative if available.
● Warn patient not to take narcotics while taking naltrexone because serious injury, coma, or death may result.
● Explain that drug has no tolerance or dependence liability.
● Tell patient to report withdrawal signs and symptoms (tremors, vomiting, bone or muscle pains, sweating, abdominal cramps).
● Tell patient to carry a medical identification card that indicates he's taking naltrexone.

Geriatric patients
● Use in elderly patients isn't documented; consider reducing dosage in this age-group.

Pediatric patients
● Safe use in children under age 18 hasn't been established.

Breast-feeding patients
● It's unknown if drug appears in breast milk. Use with caution in breast-feeding women because of known hepatotoxicity.

nandrolone decanoate
Androlone-D 200, Deca-Durabolin, Hybolin Decanoate-50, Hybolin Decanoate-100, Neo-Durabolic

nandrolone phenpropionate
Durabolin, Hybolin Improved

Pharmacologic classification: anabolic steroid
Therapeutic classification: erythropoietic, anabolic (nandrolone decanoate); antineoplastic (nandrolone phenpropionate)
Controlled substance schedule III
Pregnancy risk category X

How supplied
Available by prescription only
decanoate
Injection: 50 mg/ml, 100 mg/ml, 200 mg/ml (in oil)
phenpropionate
Injection: 25 mg/ml, 50 mg/ml (in oil)

Indications, route, and dosage
Anemia associated with renal insufficiency
decanoate
Adults: 100 to 200 mg I.M. weekly in men; 50 to 100 mg weekly in women.
Children ages 2 to 13: 25 to 50 mg I.M. q 3 to 4 weeks.

Metastatic breast cancer
phenpropionate
Adults: 50 to 100 mg I.M. weekly.

Pharmacodynamics

Androgenic action: Exerts inhibitory effects on hormone-responsive breast tumors and metastases.

Erythropoietic action: Stimulates the kidneys' production of erythropoietin, leading to increases in red blood cell mass and volume.

Anabolic action: May reverse corticosteroid-induced catabolism and promote tissue development in severely debilitated patients.

Pharmacokinetics

● *Absorption:* Levels peak 1 to 6 days after I.M. administration.
● *Distribution:* Slowly released from I.M. depot after injection; hydrolyzed to free nandrolone by plasma esterase.
● *Metabolism:* Metabolized in liver.
● *Excretion:* Both unchanged drug and metabolites excreted in urine. Elimination half-life of drug is 6 to 8 days.

Contraindications and precautions

Contraindicated in patients with hypersensitivity to anabolic steroids, in men with breast cancer or prostate cancer, in patients with nephrosis, in those experiencing the nephrotic phase of nephritis, in women with breast cancer and hypercalcemia, during pregnancy, and who are breast-feeding.

Use cautiously in patients with renal, cardiac, or hepatic disease; diabetes; epilepsy; migraine; or other conditions that may be aggravated by fluid retention.

Interactions

Drug-drug. *Adrenocorticosteroids, adrenocorticotropic hormone:* Increased potential for fluid and electrolyte retention. Use together cautiously.
Insulin, oral antidiabetics: Decreased blood glucose levels. Adjust drug dosage.
Warfarin-type anticoagulants: Increased PT and INR. Monitor patient for this effect.

Adverse reactions

CNS: excitation, insomnia, habituation, depression.
CV: edema.
GI: nausea, vomiting, diarrhea.
GU: bladder irritability, *hypoestrogenic effects in women (flushing; diaphoresis; vaginitis, including itching, dryness, and burning; vaginal bleeding; nervousness; emotional lability; menstrual irregularities), excessive hormonal effects in men (prepubertal-premature epiphyseal closure, acne, priapism, growth of body and facial hair, phallic enlargement; postpubertal-testicular atrophy,*

oligospermia, decreased ejaculatory volume, impotence, gynecomastia, epididymitis).
Hematologic: elevated serum lipid levels, suppression of clotting factors.
Hepatic: reversible jaundice, peliosis hepatitis, elevated liver enzyme levels, *liver cell tumors.*
Metabolic: increased serum sodium, potassium, calcium and phosphate levels; abnormal results of fasting plasma glucose, glucose tolerance, and metyrapone tests; decreased thyroid function test results and 17-ketosteroid levels.
Skin: pain and induration at injection site.
Other: androgenic effects in women (acne, edema, *weight gain, hirsutism,* hoarseness, clitoral enlargement, *decreased breast size,* changes in libido, male-pattern baldness, *oily skin or hair*).

☑ Special considerations

● Nandrolone injections should be administered I.M. deeply into gluteal muscle.
● Adequate iron intake is necessary for maximum response when patient is receiving nandrolone decanoate injections.
● Therapy should be intermittent if possible.
● Duration is dependent on patient response and occurrence of adverse reactions.
● Surgically-induced anephric patients may be less responsive to effect on anemia.

Monitoring the patient

● Monitor hematologic studies, electrolytes, glucose and hepatic enzymes.
● Monitor patient for adverse effects.

Information for the patient

● Instruct diabetic patient to monitor glucose level closely because glucose tolerance may be altered.
● Tell woman to report menstrual irregularities, acne, deepening of voice, male-pattern baldness, or hirsutism.
● Tell patient to call if persistent GI upset, nausea, vomiting, changes in skin color, or ankle swelling occurs.

Geriatric patients

● Observe elderly men for the development of prostatic hypertrophy and prostatic carcinoma.

Pediatric patients

● Adverse effects of giving androgens to young children aren't fully understood, but the risk of serious disturbances (premature epiphyseal closure, masculinization of girls, or precocious development in boys) exists; weigh possible benefits against risks before starting therapy in young children.

Breast-feeding patients

● It's unknown if anabolic steroids appear in breast milk. Because of potential for serious adverse reactions in breast-fed infants, stop either breast-feeding or drug.

---

naphazoline hydrochloride
AK-Con, Albalon Liquifilm, Allerest, Clear Eyes, Comfort Eye Drops, Degest 2, Nafazair, Naphcon, Naphcon Forte, Privine, VasoClear, Vasocon

Pharmacologic classification: sympathomimetic
Therapeutic classification: decongestant, vasoconstrictor
Pregnancy risk category C

How supplied
Available by prescription only
Ophthalmic solution: 0.1%
Available without a prescription
Ophthalmic solution: 0.012%, 0.02%, 0.025% (generic), 0.03%
Nasal drops or sprays: 0.05% (solution)

Indications, route, and dosage
Ocular congestion, irritation, itching
Adults: Instill 1 to 3 drops (0.1% solution) or 1 to 2 drops (0.012% to 0.03% solution) in eye daily to q.i.d.
Nasal congestion
Adults and children over age 12: 1 or 2 drops or sprays (0.05% solution), p.r.n. Don't use drops more than q 3 hours or spray more often than q 4 to 6 hours.
Children ages 6 to 12: 1 to 2 drops or sprays (0.025% solution), p.r.n.

Pharmacodynamics
Decongestant action: Produces vasoconstriction by local and alpha-adrenergic action on blood vessels of the conjunctiva or nasal mucosa; therefore, it reduces blood flow and nasal congestion.

Pharmacokinetics
• *Absorption:* After intranasal application, local vasoconstriction occurs within 5 to 10 minutes; lasts for 5 to 6 hours with a gradual decline over next 6 hours.
• *Distribution:* No information available.
• *Metabolism:* No information available.
• *Excretion:* No information available.

Contraindications and precautions
Contraindicated in patients with hypersensitivity to drug and its components and in those with acute angle-closure glaucoma. Use of 0.1% solution is contraindicated in children. Use cautiously in patients with hyperthyroidism, cardiac disease, hypertension, or diabetes mellitus.

Interactions
Drug-drug. *MAO inhibitors:* Increased adrenergic response and hypertensive crisis. Avoid using together.
Maprotiline, tricyclic antidepressants: Increased pressor effects of naphazoline. Use together cautiously.

Adverse reactions
CNS: headache, dizziness, nervousness, weakness (with ophthalmic form), marked sedation (with nasal administration).
CV: hypertension, cardiac irregularities.
EENT: transient eye stinging, pupillary dilation, eye irritation, photophobia, blurred vision, increased intraocular pressure, keratitis, lacrimation (with ophthalmic form); rebound nasal congestion (with excessive or long-term use), sneezing, stinging, dryness of mucosa (with nasal administration).
GI: nausea (with ophthalmic form).
Skin: diaphoresis (with ophthalmic form).
Other: systemic effects in children after excessive or long-term use.

☑ Special considerations
• Naphazoline is the most widely used ocular decongestant.
• Don't shake container.
• Toxicity may cause CNS depression, sweating, decreased body temperature, bradycardia, shock-like hypotension, decreased respiration, CV collapse, and coma.
• Activated charcoal or gastric lavage may be used initially to treat accidental ingestion (administer early before sedation occurs). Treat seizures with I.V. diazepam.

Monitoring the patient
• Monitor patient for blurred vision, pain, or lid edema.
• Observe cardiac patient for irregular heart rhythm.

Information for the patient
• Teach patient how to instill ophthalmic or nasal medication; tell him not to share drug with others.
• Advise patient to report blurred vision, eye pain, or lid swelling that occurs when using ophthalmic product.
• Inform patient using ophthalmic solution that photophobia may follow pupil dilation; tell patient to report this effect promptly.
• Warn patient not to exceed recommended dosage; rebound nasal congestion and conjunctivitis also may occur with frequent or prolonged use.
• Tell patient to call if nasal congestion persists after 5 days of using nasal solution.

Reactions may be *common*, uncommon, *life-threatening*, or COMMON AND LIFE-THREATENING.

Geriatric patients
• Use drug with caution in elderly patients with severe cardiac disease or poorly controlled hypertension and in diabetics prone to diabetic ketoacidosis.

Pediatric patients
• Use in infants and children may result in CNS depression, leading to coma and marked reduction in body temperature. Although drug is available without a prescription, parents shouldn't use nasal solution containing 0.025% naphazoline hydrochloride in children under age 6 or 0.05% naphazoline hydrochloride in children under age 12.

naproxen
Naprosyn, EC-Naprosyn

naproxen sodium
Aleve, Anaprox, Naprelan

Pharmacologic classification: NSAID
Therapeutic classification: nonnarcotic analgesic, antipyretic, anti-inflammatory
Pregnancy risk category B

How supplied
Available by prescription only
naproxen
Tablets: 250 mg, 375 mg, 500 mg
Tablets (controlled-release): 375 mg, 500 mg
Tablets (delayed-release): 375 mg, 500 mg
Oral suspension: 125 mg/5 ml
naproxen sodium
Tablets (film-coated): 275 mg, 550 mg
   Note: 220 mg, 275 mg, 550 mg of naproxen sodium = 200 mg, 250 mg, or 500 mg of naproxen, respectively.
Available without a prescription
naproxen sodium
Tablets or capsules: 220 mg

Indications, route, and dosage
Mild to moderately severe musculoskeletal or soft tissue irritation
naproxen
Adults: 250 to 500 mg P.O. b.i.d. Or 250 mg in the morning and 500 mg in the evening; 375 to 500 mg P.O. b.i.d. (delayed release), or 750 to 1,000 mg P.O. daily (controlled release).
naproxen sodium
Adults: 275 to 550 mg P.O. b.i.d. Or 275 mg in the morning and 550 mg in the evening.
Mild to moderate pain, primary dysmenorrhea
naproxen
Adults: 500 mg P.O. to start, then 250 mg P.O. q 6 to 8 hours, p.r.n. Maximum daily dose shouldn't exceed 1.25 g. Or 1,000 mg P.O. daily (controlled-release).

naproxen sodium
Adults: 550 mg P.O. to start, then 275 mg P.O. q 6 to 8 hours, p.r.n. Maximum daily dose is 1.375 g naproxen sodium.
Self-medication: 220 mg q 8 to 12 hours. Maximum daily dose is 440 mg for adults ages 65 and older or 660 mg for adults below age 65. Don't take for more than 10 days.
Acute gout
naproxen
Adults: 750 mg initially, then 250 mg q 8 hours until episode subsides. Or 1,000 mg to 1,500 mg (controlled-release) P.O. daily on the first day, then 1,000 mg P.O. daily until attack subsides.
naproxen sodium
Adults: 825 mg initially, then 275 mg q 8 hours until attack has subsided.
Juvenile rheumatoid arthritis
naproxen
Children: 10 mg/kg/day in two divided doses.

Pharmacodynamics
Analgesic, antipyretic, and anti-inflammatory actions: Mechanisms unknown. Thought to inhibit prostaglandin synthesis.

Pharmacokinetics
• *Absorption:* Absorbed rapidly and completely from GI tract. Effect peaks at 2 to 4 hours.
• *Distribution:* Highly protein-bound. Crosses placenta; distributed into breast milk.
• *Metabolism:* Metabolized in liver.
• *Excretion:* Excreted in urine. Half-life is 10 to 20 hours.

Contraindications and precautions
Contraindicated in patients with hypersensitivity to drug or asthma, rhinitis, or nasal polyps. Use cautiously in elderly patients and in patients with history of peptic ulcer disease or renal, CV, GI, or hepatic disease.

Interactions
Drug-drug. *Acetaminophen, gold compounds, other anti-inflammatories:* Increased nephrotoxicity. Monitor renal function.
Anticoagulants, thrombolytics (coumadin derivatives, heparin, streptokinase, urokinase): Potentiated anticoagulant effects. Monitor PT and INR.
Antihypertensives, diuretics: Decreased clinical effectiveness of these drugs. Concomitant use may increase risk of nephrotoxicity. Avoid using together if possible.
Anti-inflammatories, corticotropin, salicylates, corticosteroids: Increased GI adverse reactions. Monitor if used together.
Aspirin: Decreased bioavailability of naproxen. Don't use together.
Aspirin, cefamandole, cefoperazone, dextran, dipyridamole, mezlocillin, parenteral carbenicillin, piperacillin, plicamycin, salicylates, sulfinpyra-

zone, ticarcillin, valproic acid, other anti-inflammatories: Increased bleeding problems. Monitor patient closely.

Coumadin derivatives, nifedipine, phenytoin, verapamil: Toxicity may occur. Monitor patient closely.

Insulin, oral antidiabetics: Potentiated hypoglycemic effects. Monitor patient closely.

Lithium, methotrexate: Decreased renal clearance of these drugs. Monitor patient for toxicity.

Protein-bound drugs: Naproxen may displace these drugs from binding sites. Monitor patient for clinical effect.

Drug-lifestyle. *Alcohol:* Increased GI adverse reactions. Discourage concomitant use.

Adverse reactions
CNS: *headache, drowsiness, dizziness,* vertigo.
CV: *edema,* palpitations.
EENT: visual disturbances, *tinnitus,* auditory disturbances.
GI: *epigastric distress, occult blood loss, nausea,* **peptic ulceration,** constipation, dyspepsia, heartburn, diarrhea, stomatitis, thirst.
GU: nephrotoxicity.
Hematologic: **thrombocytopenia,** eosinophilia, **agranulocytosis, neutropenia.**
Hepatic: elevated liver enzyme levels.
Respiratory: dyspnea.
Skin: *pruritus, rash,* urticaria, ecchymosis, diaphoresis, purpura.

☑ Special considerations
Besides the recommendations relevant to all NSAIDs, consider the following.
• Use lowest possible effective dose; 250 mg of naproxen is equivalent to 275 mg of naproxen sodium.
• Relief usually begins within 2 weeks after beginning therapy with naproxen.
• Institute safety measures to prevent injury resulting from possible CNS effects.
• Naproxen and its metabolites may interfere with urinary 5-hydroxyindoleacetic acid and 17-hydroxycorticosteroid determinations.
• Toxicity may cause drowsiness, heartburn, indigestion, nausea, and vomiting. Hemodialysis is ineffective in naproxen removal.

Monitoring the patient
• Monitor fluid balance. Watch for signs and symptoms of fluid retention, especially significant weight gain.
• Evaluate patient for signs of adverse GI effects.
• Evaluate hematologic and hepatic studies periodically.

Information for the patient
• Caution patient to avoid taking naproxen with OTC drugs.

• Teach patient signs and symptoms of possible adverse reactions and tell him to report them promptly.
• Instruct patient to check his weight every 2 to 3 days and to report any gain of 3 lb (1.4 kg) or more within 1 week.
• Instruct patient in safety measures; advise him to avoid activities that require alertness until CNS effects are known.
• Warn patient against combining naproxen (Naprosyn) with naproxen sodium (Anaprox); both drugs circulate in blood as naproxen anion.
• Teach patient not to break or crush controlled or delayed-released tablets.

Geriatric patients
• Patients over age 60 are more sensitive to adverse effects (especially GI toxicity) of drug.
• Naproxen's effect on renal prostaglandins may cause fluid retention and edema. This may be significant in elderly patients, especially those with heart failure.

Pediatric patients
• Safety in children under age 2 hasn't been established. Safety of naproxen sodium in children hasn't been established. No age-related problems have been reported.

Breast-feeding patients
• Naproxen and naproxen sodium appear in breast milk; avoid use in breast-feeding women.

---

naratriptan hydrochloride
Amerge

Pharmacologic classification: a selective 5-hydroxytryptamine$_1$ (5-HT$_1$) receptor subtype agonist
Therapeutic classification: antimigraine drug
Pregnancy risk category C

How supplied
Available by prescription only
Tablets: 1 mg, 2.5 mg

Indications, route, and dosage
Acute migraine attacks with or without aura
Adults: 1 or 2.5 mg P.O. as a single dose. Dose should be individualized, depending on the possible benefit of the 2.5-mg dose and the greater risk of adverse effects. If headache returns or if only partial response occurs, may repeat dose after 4 hours. Maximum dose is 5 mg within 24 hours.
✦ *Dosage adjustment.* In patients with mild to moderate renal or hepatic impairment, consider a lower initial dose; don't exceed maximum dose of 2.5 mg over a 24-hour period. Don't use in patients with severe renal or hepatic impairment.

Pharmacodynamics

Antimigraine action: Binds with high affinity to 5-HT_{1D} and 5-HT_{1B} receptors. One theory suggests that activation of 5-$HT_{1D/1B}$ receptors located on intracranial blood vessels leads to vasoconstriction, which is associated with the migraine relief. Another hypothesis suggests that activation of 5-$HT_{1D/1B}$ receptors on sensory nerve endings in the trigeminal system results in the inhibition of pro-inflammatory neuropeptide release.

Pharmacokinetics

• *Absorption:* Well absorbed, with about 70% oral bioavailability. Plasma levels peak in 2 to 4 hours.
• *Distribution:* Steady-state volume of drug's distribution is 170 L. Plasma protein binding 28% to 31%.
• *Metabolism:* In vitro, metabolized by many P-450 cytochrome isoenzymes to inactive metabolites.
• *Excretion:* Predominantly eliminated in urine; 50% of dose recovered unchanged and 30% as metabolites. Mean elimination half-life is 6 hours.

Contraindications and precautions

Contraindicated in patients with hypersensitivity to drug or its components and in those with history or signs and symptoms of ischemic cardiac, cerebrovascular (such as stroke or transient ischemic attack), or peripheral vascular syndromes (such as ischemic bowel disease). Also contraindicated in patients with significant underlying CV disease, including angina pectoris, MI, and silent myocardial ischemia. Don't give drug to patients with uncontrolled hypertension because of potential increase in blood pressure.

Contraindicated in patients with severe renal (creatinine clearance below 15 ml/minute) or hepatic (Child-Pugh grade C) impairment and in those with hemiplegic or basilar migraine.

Drug or other 5-HT_1 agonists are also contraindicated in patients with potential risk factors for coronary artery disease, such as hypertension, hypercholesterolemia, obesity, diabetes, strong family history of coronary artery disease, surgical or physiologic menopause (women), age over 40 (men), or smoking.

Interactions

Drug-drug. *Ergot-containing or ergot-type drugs, other 5-HT_1 agonists:* Prolonged vasospastic reactions. Use of these drugs within 24 hours of naratriptan is contraindicated.
Oral contraceptives: Slightly higher levels of naratriptan. Monitor patient for this effect.
Selective serotonin reuptake inhibitors (such as fluoxetine, fluvoxamine, paroxetine, sertraline): Possible weakness, hyperreflexia, and incoordination when given with 5-HT_1 agonists. Monitor patient closely if used together.
Drug-lifestyle. *Smoking:* Increased clearance of naratriptan by 30%. Discourage smoking.

Adverse reactions

CNS: paresthesia, dizziness, drowsiness, malaise, fatigue, vertigo.
CV: palpitations, increased blood pressure, tachyarrhythmias, *abnormal ECG changes (PR, QT interval prolongation; ST/T wave abnormalities; premature ventricular contractions; atrial flutter or fibrillation),* syncope.
EENT: ear, nose, and throat infections; photophobia.
GI: nausea, hyposalivation, vomiting.
Other: warm or cold temperature sensations; pressure, tightness, heaviness sensations.

☑ Special considerations

• Use drug only when a clear diagnosis of migraine has been established. It isn't intended for prophylactic therapy of migraines or for management of hemiplegic or basilar migraine.
• Administer first dose in a medically equipped facility for patients at risk for coronary artery disease but determined to have a satisfactory CV evaluation. Consider ECG monitoring.
• Safety and effectiveness haven't been established for cluster headaches.
• In case of overdose, blood pressure rises markedly ½ to 6 hours after drug ingestion. In some patients, it returns to normal in 8 hours; in others, antihypertensives are needed. Monitor patient for at least 24 hours after overdose or while symptoms persist.

Monitoring the patient

• Perform periodic cardiac reevaluation in patients who have or develop risk factors for coronary artery disease.
• Monitor patient for adverse effects.

Information for the patient

• Tell patient that drug is intended to relieve, not prevent, migraine headaches.
• Instruct patient not to use drug during pregnancy or if pregnancy is suspected.
• Teach patient to disclose risk factors for coronary artery disease.
• Instruct patient to take dose soon after headache starts. If there is no response to first tablet, tell patient to call before taking second tablet.
• Tell patient that, if more relief is needed after first tablet (such as when a partial response occurs or if the headache returns), he may take a second tablet but not sooner than 4 hours after first tablet. Inform him not to exceed two tablets within 24 hours.

Geriatric patients

• Don't use drug in elderly patients.

Pediatric patients

• Safety and effectiveness in children under age 18 haven't been established.

Breast-feeding patients
● Because it's unknown if drug appears in breast milk, use with caution in breast-feeding patients.

nedocromil sodium
Tilade

Pharmacologic classification: pyrano-quinoline
Therapeutic classification: anti-inflammatory respiratory inhalant
Pregnancy risk category B

How supplied
Available by prescription only
Inhalation aerosol: 1.75 mg per actuation in 16.2-g canister (U.S.); 2 mg per actuation in 16.2-g canister (Canada)

Indications, route, and dosage
Maintenance therapy in mild to moderate bronchial asthma
Adults and children age 6 and over: 2 inhalations q.i.d., preferably at regular intervals; may gradually decrease dosing interval to b.i.d.

Pharmacodynamics
Anti-inflammatory and antiallergic action: Inhibits activation and release of inflammatory mediators from various cell types in the lumen and mucosa of the bronchial tree. These mediators, which include the leukotrienes, histamine, and prostaglandins, are preformed or derived from arachidonic acid metabolism. A range of human cells associated with asthma may be involved. As a result, nedocromil exhibits specific anti-inflammatory properties when administered topically to the bronchial mucosa. It has demonstrated a significant inhibitory effect on allergen-induced early and late asthmatic reactions and on bronchial hyperresponsiveness. Nedocromil also may affect sensory nerves in the lung. The result is inhibition of bradykinin-induced bronchoconstriction.

Pharmacokinetics
● *Absorption:* 2% to 3% of amount swallowed after inhalation is absorbed. From 6% to 9% of drug deposited in lungs is completely absorbed. Onset of action within 30 minutes; peaks in 5 to 90 minutes and lasts 6 to 12 hours.
● *Distribution:* Distributed to plasma only. About 89% reversibly bound to plasma proteins when plasma levels range between 0.5 and 50 mcg/ml.
● *Metabolism:* Not metabolized.
● *Excretion:* Rapidly excreted unchanged in bile and urine. Half-life is about 1.5 to 3.3 hours.

Contraindications and precautions
Contraindicated in patients with hypersensitivity to drug or its components and in those experiencing an acute asthmatic attack or acute bronchospasm.

Interactions
None reported.

Adverse reactions
CV: chest pain.
CNS: headache, dysphagia, fatigue.
EENT: rhinitis, pharyngitis.
GI: nausea, vomiting, dyspepsia, abdominal pain, dry mouth, *unpleasant taste.*
Respiratory: upper respiratory tract infection, cough, increased sputum, bronchitis, dyspnea, **bronchospasm.**

☑ Special considerations
● Dosage may be reduced to two inhalations three times daily and then twice daily after several weeks, when patient's asthma is under control.
● In maintenance therapy, drug must be used regularly, even during symptom-free periods, to achieve benefit.
● When drug is added to an existing regimen of bronchodilators or given with inhaled or oral corticosteroids, a reduction in dosage of corticosteroid or bronchodilator may be achieved in some patients. However, reduction should be gradual and under close medical supervision to avoid exacerbating asthma.
● Don't exceed 16 mg within 24 hours.
● In some patients, bronchospasm may be prevented by a single dose of nedocromil before activities that precipitate asthma, such as exercise or exposure to cold air, pollutants, or allergens.

Monitoring the patient
● Monitor patient for reduced severity of symptoms or less need for accessory therapy; these are signs of improvement that usually occur in the first 2 weeks of therapy if patient responds to therapy.
● Evaluate patient's compliance with therapy.

Information for the patient
● Warn patient that drug has no direct bronchodilating action and can't replace bronchodilators during an acute asthmatic attack.
● Tell patient that drug is an adjunct to the regular bronchodilator regimen and may reduce the need for corticosteroids or bronchodilators.
● Emphasize that drug should be taken regularly for best results. Most patients report benefits after 1 week of use; some need longer treatment before improvement occurs.
● Teach patient how to use the inhaler. Instruct him to shake canister immediately before use and to invert it just before actuation. Prime inhaler with 3 actuations before first use or if unused for more than 7 days.
● Advise patient to clean inhaler at least twice weekly and to remove canister before rinsing in-

haler in hot running water. Allow inhaler to air dry overnight.

Pediatric patients
• Safety and efficacy haven't been established for children under age 6.

Breast-feeding patients
• It's unknown if drug appears in breast milk. Use cautiously in breast-feeding women.

nefazodone hydrochloride
Serzone

Pharmacologic classification: phenyl-piperazine
Therapeutic classification: antidepressant
Pregnancy risk category C

How supplied
Available by prescription only
Tablets: 100 mg, 150 mg, 200 mg, 250 mg

Indications, route, and dosage
Depression
Adults: Initially, 200 mg/day P.O. divided into two doses. Dose increased in 100- to 200-mg/day increments at intervals of no less than 1 week, p.r.n. Usual dosage range, 300 to 600 mg/day.

Pharmacodynamics
Antidepressive action: Exact mechanism unknown. Inhibits neuronal uptake of serotonin and norepinephrine. Also occupies central 5-HT$_2$ (serotonin) and alpha$_1$-adrenergic receptors.

Pharmacokinetics
• *Absorption:* Rapidly and completely absorbed; because of extensive metabolism, absolute bioavailability only about 20%.
• *Distribution:* Over 99% bound to plasma proteins.
• *Metabolism:* Extensively metabolized by n-dealkylation and aliphatic and aromatic hydroxylation.
• *Excretion:* Drug and metabolites excreted in urine. Half-life is 2 to 4 hours.

Contraindications and precautions
Contraindicated in patients with hypersensitivity to drug or other phenylpiperazine antidepressants. Don't use within 14 days of MAO inhibitor therapy.
    Use cautiously in patients with CV or cerebrovascular disease that could be exacerbated by hypotension (such as history of MI, angina, or CVA) and conditions that would predispose patients to hypotension (such as dehydration, hypovolemia, and antihypertensive treatment). Also use cautiously in patients with history of mania.

Interactions
Drug-drug. *Alprazolam, triazolam:* Potentiated effects of these drugs. Don't administer concurrently. However, if necessary, dosage of alprazolam and triazolam may need to be reduced greatly.
Buspirone: Increased buspirone levels, light-headedness, dizziness, asthenia. Monitor patient closely.
Carbamazepine: Increased carbamazepine levels. Monitor carbamazepine level.
CNS active drugs: May alter CNS activity. Use together cautiously.
Digoxin: Increased digoxin level. Use together cautiously and monitor digoxin levels.
HMG CoA reductase inhibitors: May increase risk of rhabdomyolysis and myositis. Use together cautiously.
MAO inhibitors: Possible severe excitation, hyperpyrexia, seizures, delirium, or coma. Avoid giving together. Don't use nefazodone within 14 days of MAO inhibitors.
Pimozide: QT interval prolongation and ventricular tachycardia. Don't use together.
Sibutramine, trazodone: May cause serotonin syndrome. Use together cautiously.
Other highly plasma protein-bound drugs: Increased incidence and severity of adverse reactions. Monitor patient closely.
Drug-herb. *St. John's wort:* Increased sedation. Discourage concomitant use.

Adverse reactions
CNS: *headache, somnolence, dizziness, asthenia,* insomnia, *light-headedness, confusion,* memory impairment, paresthesia, abnormal dreams, decreased concentration, ataxia, incoordination, taste perversion, psychomotor retardation, tremor, hypertonia.
CV: orthostatic hypotension, vasodilation, hypotension, peripheral edema.
EENT: *blurred vision, abnormal vision,* pharyngitis, tinnitus, visual field defect.
GI: *dry mouth, nausea, constipation,* dyspepsia, diarrhea, increased appetite, vomiting, thirst.
GU: urinary frequency, urinary tract infection, urine retention, vaginitis, breast pain.
Musculoskeletal: neck rigidity, arthralgia.
Respiratory: cough.
Skin: pruritus, rash.
Other: infection, flu syndrome, chills, fever.

☑ Special considerations
• Allow at least 1 week after stopping drug before giving patient an MAO inhibitor. Also, allow at least 14 days before patient is started on nefazodone after MAO inhibitor therapy has been stopped.
• Toxicity may cause nausea, vomiting, and somnolence. Provide symptomatic and supportive treatment in case of hypotension or excessive sedation.

Monitoring the patient
- Record mood changes. Monitor patient for suicidal tendencies and allow a minimum supply of drug.
- In patients on combined therapy, monitor patient for increased CNS effect.

Information for the patient
- Warn patient not to engage in hazardous activities until CNS effects are known.
- Tell man that if prolonged or inappropriate erections occur, he should stop drug immediately and call.
- Instruct woman to report if pregnancy is suspected or is being planned during therapy.
- Instruct patient not to drink alcoholic beverages during therapy.
- Tell patient to report rash, hives, or a related allergic reaction.
- Inform patient that several weeks of therapy may be required to obtain full antidepressant effect. Once improvement is seen, advise patient not to stop drug until directed.

Geriatric patients
- Because of increased systemic exposure to nefazodone, begin treatment at half usual dose, but increase dosage over same dosage range as in younger patients. Observe usual precautions in elderly patients who have ongoing medical illnesses or are receiving other drugs.

Pediatric patients
- Safety and effectiveness in children under age 18 haven't been established.

Breast-feeding patients
- It's unknown if drug appears in breast milk; use with caution in breast-feeding women.

---

nelfinavir mesylate
Viracept

Pharmacologic classification: HIV protease inhibitor
Therapeutic classification: antiviral
Pregnancy risk category B

How supplied
Available by prescription only
Tablets: 250 mg
Powder: 50 mg/g of powder

Indications, route, and dosage
HIV infection when antiretroviral therapy is warranted
Adults: 750 mg P.O. t.i.d with meal or light snack.
Children ages 2 to 13: 20 to 30 mg/kg/dose P.O. t.i.d with meal or light snack; don't exceed 750 mg t.i.d. Recommended pediatric doses given t.i.d. are shown in the following table.

Body weight (kg)	No. of level 1-g scoops	No. of level teaspoons	No. of tablets
7 to < 8.5	4	1	-
8.5 to < 10.5	5	1.25	-
10.5 to < 12	6	1.5	-
12 to < 14	7	1.75	-
14 to < 16	8	2	-
16 to < 18	9	2.25	-
18 to < 23	10	2.5	2
≥ 23	15	3.75	3

Pharmacodynamics
Antiviral action: An HIV protease inhibitor. Inhibition of the protease enzyme prevents cleavage of the viral polyprotein, resulting in the production of an immature, noninfectious virus.

Pharmacokinetics
- *Absorption:* Absolute bioavailability not determined. Food increases absorption. Levels peak 2 to 4 hours after giving drug with food.
- *Distribution:* Volume of drug's distribution is 2 to 7 L/kg. Over 98% of drug bound to plasma protein.
- *Metabolism:* Metabolized in liver by multiple cytochrome P-450 isoforms, including CYP3A.
- *Excretion:* Terminal half-life is 3½ to 5 hours. Primarily excreted in feces.

Contraindications and precautions
Contraindicated in patients with hypersensitivity to drug or its components. Use cautiously in patients with hepatic dysfunction or hemophilia types A and B.

Interactions
Drug-drug. *Amiodarone, ergot derivatives, midazolam, quinidine, triazolam:* Large increases in plasma levels of these drugs. Don't administer together.
Anti-HIV protease inhibitors (indinavir, ritonavir): May increase nelfinavir plasma levels. Reduce dosage of nelfinavir as needed.
Carbamazepine, phenobarbital, phenytoin: Reduced effectiveness of nelfinavir. Monitor patient for effect.
Drugs primarily metabolized by CYP3A (such as calcium channel blockers, dihydropyridine): Increased levels of other drug and decreased plasma level of nelfinavir. Use together cautiously.
Oral contraceptives (ethinyl estradiol, norethindrone): Decreased effectiveness. Advise patient to use alternative or additional contraceptive measures during nelfinavir therapy.
Reverse transcriptase inhibitors: Increased antiretroviral activity when used with approved re-

verse transcriptase inhibitors. Monitor patient for effect.

Rifabutin: Increased rifabutin plasma levels. Reduce dosage of rifabutin to one-half usual dose.

Rifampin: Decreased nelfinavir plasma levels. Don't use together.

Adverse reactions

CNS: anxiety, depression, dizziness, emotional lability, hyperkinesia, insomnia, malaise, migraine headache, paresthesia, *seizures,* sleep disorders, somnolence, *suicidal ideation.*

EENT: iritis, eye disorders, pharyngitis, rhinitis, sinusitis.

GI: abdominal pain, nausea, *diarrhea,* flatulence, anorexia, dyspepsia, epigastric pain, GI bleeding, *pancreatitis,* mouth ulceration, vomiting.

GU: sexual dysfunction, kidney calculus, urine abnormality.

Hematologic: anemia, *leukopenia, thrombocytopenia.*

Hepatic: *hepatitis.*

Metabolic: dehydration, diabetes mellitus, hyperlipidemia, hyperuricemia, hypoglycemia.

Musculoskeletal: back pain, arthralgia, arthritis, cramps, myalgia, myasthenia, myopathy.

Respiratory: dyspnea.

Skin: rash, dermatitis, folliculitis, fungal dermatitis, pruritus, sweating, urticaria.

Other: fever.

☑ Special considerations

● Decision to use drug is based on surrogate marker changes in patients who received drug with nucleoside analogues or alone for up to 24 weeks. Effect on opportunistic fungal infections is unknown.

● Drug dosage is same whether used alone or with other antiretrovirals.

● Administer oral powder in children unable to take tablets; may mix oral powder with water, milk, formula, soy formula, soy milk, or dietary supplements. Tell patient to drink entire contents.

● Don't reconstitute with water in its original container.

● Use reconstituted powder within 6 hours.

● Acidic foods or juice aren't recommended because of bitter taste.

● Dialysis isn't beneficial in case of overdose.

Monitoring the patient

● Monitor CBC with differential (especially neutrophils) and chemistry studies; few laboratory abnormalities have been reported.

● Increases in alkaline phosphatase, amylase, CK, LD, AST, ALT, and GGT levels may occur; monitor patient closely.

Information for the patient

● Advise patient to take drug with food.

● Inform patient that drug isn't a cure for HIV infection.

● Tell patient that long-term effects of drug are currently unknown and that there is evidence that drug reduces risk of HIV transmission to others. Use of a condom is still recommended.

● Advise patient to take drug daily as prescribed and not to alter dose or stop drug without medical approval.

● If patient misses a dose, tell him to take the dose as soon as possible and return to his normal schedule. If a dose is skipped, advise patient not to double dose.

● Tell patient that diarrhea is the most common adverse effect; can be controlled with loperamide if necessary.

● Instruct patient taking oral contraceptives to use alternative or additional contraceptive measures.

● Advise patient to report use of other prescribed or OTC drugs.

Pediatric patients

● Safety, efficacy, and pharmacokinetics haven't been established in children under age 2.

Breast-feeding patients

● It's unknown if drug appears in breast milk. Because safety hasn't been established, advise HIV-infected women not to breast-feed in order to avoid HIV transmission to infant.

---

neomycin sulfate

Mycifradin, Myciguent, Neo-Fradin, Neo-Tabs

Pharmacologic classification: aminoglycoside

Therapeutic classification: antibiotic

Pregnancy risk category D

How supplied

Available by prescription only

Tablets: 500 mg

Oral solution: 125 mg/5 ml

Otic: 5 mg/ml (with polymyxin B sulfate 10,000 units/ml and hydrocortisone 1%)

Available without a prescription

Cream: 0.5%

Ointment: 0.5%

Indications, route, and dosage

Infectious diarrhea caused by enteropathogenic Escherichia coli

Adults: 50 mg/kg P.O. daily in four divided doses for 2 to 3 days.

Children: 50 to 100 mg/kg P.O. daily divided q 4 to 6 hours for 2 to 3 days.

Suppression of intestinal bacteria preoperatively

Adults: 1 g P.O. q hour for four doses, then 1 g q 4 hours for rest of 24 hours. A saline cathartic should precede therapy.

Children: 40 to 100 mg/kg P.O. daily divided q 4 to 6 hours. First dose should be preceded by saline cathartic.

Adjunctive treatment in hepatic coma
Adults: 1 to 3 g P.O. q.i.d. for 5 to 6 days; 200 ml of 1% or 100 ml of 2% solution as enema retained for 20 to 60 minutes q 6 hours.
Children: 50 to 100 mg/kg P.O. daily in divided doses for 5 to 6 days.

External ear canal infection
Adults and children: 2 to 5 drops into ear canal t.i.d. or q.i.d.

Topical bacterial infections, burns, wounds, skin grafts, following surgical procedure, lesions, pruritus, trophic ulcerations, and edema
Adults and children: Rub in small amount gently b.i.d., t.i.d., or as directed.

✦ *Dosage adjustment.* Use reduced dosage in adults and children with renal failure. Specific recommendations aren't available.

Pharmacodynamics
Antibiotic action: Bactericidal. Binds directly to the 30S ribosomal subunit, thus inhibiting bacterial protein synthesis. Spectrum of action includes many aerobic gram-negative organisms and some aerobic gram-positive organisms. Drug is far less active against many gram-negative organisms than are amikacin, gentamicin, netilmicin, and tobramycin. Given orally or as retention enema, neomycin inhibits ammonia-forming bacteria in the GI tract, reducing ammonia and improving neurologic status of patients with hepatic encephalopathy. Rarely given systemically because of its high potential for ototoxicity and nephrotoxicity. The FDA recently revoked licensing of the parenteral preparation for this reason.

Pharmacokinetics
● *Absorption:* About 3% absorbed after oral administration, although oral administration is enhanced in patients with impaired GI motility or mucosal intestinal ulcerations. After oral administration, serum levels peak at 1 to 4 hours. Not absorbed through intact skin; may be absorbed from wounds, burns, or skin ulcers.
● *Distribution:* Crosses placenta. Oral administration restricts distribution to GI tract.
● *Metabolism:* Not metabolized.
● *Excretion:* Excreted primarily in urine by glomerular filtration. Elimination half-life in adults is 2 to 3 hours; in severe renal damage, half-life may extend to 24 hours. After oral administration, excreted primarily unchanged in feces.

Contraindications and precautions
Contraindicated in patients with hypersensitivity to drug. Oral form contraindicated in patients sensitive to other aminoglycosides and in those with intestinal obstruction.

Use oral form cautiously in elderly patients and in patients with impaired renal function, neuromuscular disorders, or ulcerative bowel lesions. Don't administer drug parenterally. Use topical form cautiously in patients with extensive dermatologic conditions.

Interactions
Drug-drug. *Oral anticoagulants:* Potentiated action of anticoagulants. Adjust dosage of anticoagulants as needed.

Adverse reactions
EENT: *ototoxicity* (with oral administration).
GI: nausea, vomiting, diarrhea, malabsorption syndrome, *Clostridium difficile–associated colitis* (with oral administration).
GU: *nephrotoxicity* (with oral administration).
Skin: *rash, contact dermatitis,* urticaria (with topical administration).
Other: *neuromuscular blockade* (with topical administration).

☑ Special considerations
Besides the recommendations relevant to all aminoglycosides, consider the following.
● Signs and symptoms of overdose include ototoxicity, nephrotoxicity, and neuromuscular toxicity. Remove drug by hemodialysis or peritoneal dialysis; treatment with calcium salts or anticholinesterase reverses neuromuscular blockade.

Preoperative bowel contamination
● Provide low-residue diet and cathartic immediately before administration of oral neomycin; follow-up enemas may be necessary to completely empty bowel.

Topical therapy
● Don't apply to more than 20% of body surface.
● Don't apply to any body surface of patient with decreased renal function without considering benefit-risk ratio.

Otic therapy
● Recapture persistent drainage.
● Drug best used with other antibiotics.
● Avoid touching ear with dropper.

Monitoring the patient
● Monitor renal function.
● In adjunctive treatment of hepatic coma, decrease patient's dietary protein, and assess neurologic status frequently during therapy.
● Monitor patient for hypersensitivity or contact dermatitis (otic therapy).

Information for the patient
● Instruct patient to report adverse reactions promptly.
● Encourage adequate fluid intake.

neostigmine bromide
neostigmine methylsulfate
Prostigmin

Pharmacologic classification: cholinesterase inhibitor
Therapeutic classification: muscle stimulant
Pregnancy risk category C

How supplied
Available by prescription only
Tablets: 15 mg
Injection: 0.25 mg/ml, 0.5 mg/ml, 1 mg/ml

Indications, route, and dosage
Antidote for nondepolarizing neuromuscular blockers
Adults: 0.5 to 2.5 mg slow I.V. Repeat, p.r.n.; maximum total dose is 5 mg. Give 0.6 to 1.2 mg atropine I.V. with or a few minutes before neostigmine.
Children: 0.025 to 0.08 mg/kg I.V. with 0.01 to 0.03 mg/kg of atropine.
Neonates and infants: 0.04 to 0.08 mg/kg I.V. with 0.02 mg/kg of atropine.
Postoperative abdominal distention and bladder atony
Adults: 0.5 to 1 mg I.M. or S.C. q 3 hours for five doses after bladder has emptied (treatment); 0.25 mg I.M. or S.C. q 4 to 6 hours for 2 to 3 days (prevention).
◇ *Diagnosis of myasthenia gravis*
Adults: 0.022 mg/kg I.M. If cholinergic reaction occurs, stop test and give atropine sulfate 0.4 to 0.6 mg I.V.
Children: 0.025 to 0.04 mg/kg I.M. preceded by 0.011 mg/kg S.C. of atropine sulfate.
Symptomatic control of myasthenia gravis
Adults: 0.5 mg S.C. or I.M. Oral dose can range from 15 to 375 mg/day (average 150 mg in 24 hours). Subsequent dosages must be individualized, based on response and tolerance of adverse effects. Therapy may be needed day and night.
Children: 7.5 to 15 mg P.O. t.i.d. or q.i.d.

Pharmacodynamics
Muscle stimulant action: Blocks acetylcholine's hydrolysis by cholinesterase, resulting in acetylcholine accumulation at cholinergic synapses. That leads to increased cholinergic receptor stimulation at the myoneural junction.

Pharmacokinetics
● *Absorption:* 1% to 2% absorbed from GI tract after oral administration. Action usually begins 45 to 75 hours after oral administration, 20 to 30 minutes after I.M. injection, and 4 to 8 minutes after I.V. dose.

● *Distribution:* About 15% to 25% binds to plasma proteins.
● *Metabolism:* Hydrolyzed by cholinesterases and metabolized by microsomal liver enzymes. Duration of effect varies considerably, depending on patient's physical and emotional status and on disease severity.
● *Excretion:* About 80% excreted in urine as unchanged drug and metabolites in first 24 hours after administration.

Contraindications and precautions
Contraindicated in patients with hypersensitivity to cholinergics or to bromide and in those with peritonitis or mechanical obstruction of the intestine or urinary tract. Use cautiously in patients with bronchial asthma, bradycardia, seizure disorders, recent coronary occlusion, vagotonia, hyperthyroidism, arrhythmias, or peptic ulcer.

Interactions
Drug-drug. *Aminoglycosides:* Increased neuromuscular blockade. Use together cautiously.
Atropine: Antagonized muscarinic effects of neostigmine. Used together for clinical effects.
Corticosteroids: Decreased cholinergic effects. Monitor patient closely.
General, local anesthetics: Decreased effects of neostigmine. Monitor patient for decreased effects.
Magnesium: May antagonize neostigmine's beneficial effects. Avoid using together.
Procainamide, quinidine: May reverse neostigmine's cholinergic effect on muscle. Monitor patient closely.
Succinylcholine: Prolonged respiratory depression. Monitor respiratory status of patient carefully.
Other cholinergics: May cause additive toxicity. Monitor patient closely.

Adverse reactions
CNS: dizziness, convulsions, headache, muscle weakness, loss of consciousness, drowsiness.
CV: *bradycardia,* hypotension, tachycardia, AV block, syncope, *cardiac arrest.*
EENT: blurred vision, lacrimation, miosis.
GI: *nausea, vomiting, diarrhea, abdominal cramps,* excessive salivation, flatulence, increased peristalsis.
GU: urinary frequency.
Musculoskeletal: *muscle cramps,* muscle fasciculations, arthralgia.
Respiratory: *bronchospasm,* dyspnea, respiratory depression, *respiratory arrest,* increased secretions.
Skin: rash, urticaria, diaphoresis, flushing.
Other: hypersensitivity reactions (*anaphylaxis*).

☑ Special considerations
Besides the recommendations relevant to all cholinesterase inhibitors, consider the following.

• If muscle weakness is severe, determine if this stems from drug toxicity or from exacerbation of myasthenia gravis. A test dose of edrophonium I.V. will aggravate drug-induced weakness but will temporarily relieve weakness resulting from disease.

• Hospitalized patients may be able to manage a bedside supply of tablets to take themselves.

• Give drug with food or milk to reduce chance for GI adverse effects.

• When administering drug to patient with myasthenia gravis, schedule largest dose before anticipated periods of fatigue. For example, if patient has dysphagia, schedule this dose 30 minutes before each meal.

• Stop all other cholinergics during neostigmine therapy because of risk of additive toxicity.

• When administering drug to prevent abdominal distention and GI distress, insertion of a rectal tube may be indicated to help passage of gas.

• Administering atropine with neostigmine can relieve or eliminate adverse reactions; these symptoms may indicate neostigmine overdose and will be masked by atropine.

• Patients may develop drug resistance.

• Signs and symptoms of overdose include headache, nausea, vomiting, diarrhea, blurred vision, miosis, excessive tearing, bronchospasm, increased bronchial secretions, hypotension, incoordination, excessive sweating, muscle weakness, cramps, fasciculations, paralysis, bradycardia or tachycardia, excessive salivation, and restlessness or agitation. Atropine may be given to block neostigmine's muscarinic effects but won't counter drug's paralytic effects on skeletal muscle. Avoid atropine overdose because it may lead to bronchial plug formation.

Monitoring the patient
• Monitor patient's vital signs.
• Watch for cardiac and respiratory depressant effects.

Information for the patient
• Instruct patient to observe and record changes in muscle strength.

Geriatric patients
• Elderly patients may be more sensitive to neostigmine's effects. Use with caution.

Pediatric patients
• Safety and effectiveness in children haven't been fully established.

Breast-feeding patients
• Drug may appear in breast milk; infant toxicity possible. Evaluate patient's status to see if breast-feeding or drug should be discontinued.

nevirapine
Viramune

Pharmacologic classification: non-nucleoside reverse transcriptase inhibitor
Therapeutic classification: antiviral
Pregnancy risk category C

How supplied
Available by prescription only
Tablets: 200 mg
Oral suspension: 50 mg/5 ml

Indications, route, and dosage
Adjunct treatment of patients with HIV-1 infection who have experienced clinical or immunologic deterioration
Adults: 200 mg P.O. daily for first 14 days, then 200 mg P.O. b.i.d. with nucleoside analogue antiretrovirals.
Adjunct treatment in children infected with HIV-1
Children ages 2 months to 8 years: 4 mg/kg P.O. once daily for first 14 days, then 7 mg/kg P.O. twice daily thereafter. Maximum daily dose shouldn't exceed 400 mg.
Children ages 8 and older: 4 mg/kg P.O. once daily for first 14 days, then 4 mg/kg P.O. twice daily thereafter. Maximum daily dose shouldn't exceed 400 mg.

Pharmacodynamics
Antiviral action: Binds directly to reverse transcriptase and blocks the RNA-dependent and DNA-dependent DNA polymerase activities by causing a disruption of the enzyme's catalytic site.

Pharmacokinetics
• *Absorption:* Readily absorbed.
• *Distribution:* Widely distributed, crosses placenta, and excreted in breast milk. About 60% bound to plasma proteins.
• *Metabolism:* Extensively metabolized in liver.
• *Excretion:* Drug metabolites primarily excreted in urine; small amount excreted in feces.

Contraindications and precautions
Contraindicated in patients with hypersensitivity to drug. Use cautiously in patients with impaired renal or hepatic function because drug's pharmacokinetics haven't been evaluated in these patient groups.

Interactions
Drug-drug. *Drugs extensively metabolized by P-450 CYP3A:* May lower plasma levels of these drugs. Dosage adjustment of these drugs may be needed.

Oral contraceptives, protease inhibitors: May decrease plasma levels of these drugs. Don't administer together.
Rifabutin, rifampin: Decreased nevirapine plasma levels. Monitor patient closely.

Adverse reactions
CNS: headache, peripheral neuropathy, paresthesia.
GI: nausea, diarrhea, abdominal pain, ulcerative stomatitis.
Hematologic: *decreased neutrophil count,* eosinophilia.
Hepatic: hepatitis, abnormal liver function test results, *hepatotoxicity.*
Musculoskeletal: myalgia.
Skin: *rash, Stevens-Johnson syndrome.*
Other: fever.

☑ Special considerations
• Use of a 200-mg dose as a lead-in period has been shown to decrease rash.
• Resistant virus emerges rapidly when drug is used as monotherapy. Always administer with at least one other antiretroviral.
• Stop drug if patient develops a severe rash or a rash accompanied by fever, blistering, oral lesions, conjunctivitis, swelling, muscle or joint aches, or general malaise. If rash occurs during initial 14 days, don't increase dose until resolved. Most rashes occur within first 6 weeks of therapy.
• Temporarily stop drug in patients experiencing moderate or severe liver function test abnormalities (excluding GGT) until returned to baseline. May restart drug at half previous dose level. If moderate or severe liver function test abnormalities recur, stop drug. Monitor liver function tests closely.
• If therapy is interrupted for over 7 days, restart therapy as if receiving drug for first time.
• If disease progresses during therapy, consider altering antiretroviral therapy.

Monitoring the patient
• Perform clinical chemistry tests, including liver function tests, before therapy and regularly throughout therapy.
• Monitor patient for adverse effects.

Information for the patient
• Inform patient that drug isn't a cure for HIV, and the illnesses associated with advanced HIV-1 infection may still occur. Also tell patient that drug doesn't reduce risk of transmission of HIV-1 to others through sexual contact or blood contamination.
• Instruct patient to report rash immediately. Therapy may need to be stopped temporarily.
• Stress importance of taking drug exactly as prescribed. If a dose is missed, tell patient to take next dose as soon as possible. However, if a dose is skipped, he shouldn't double the next dose.

• Tell patient not to use other drugs without medical approval.
• Advise woman of childbearing age to avoid oral contraceptives and other hormonal methods of birth control during therapy.

Pediatric patients
• The most frequently reported adverse effects in children were similar to those seen in adults, with the exception that granulocytopenia occurred more commonly in children. Nevirapine clearance adjusted for body weight reached maximum values by age 1 to 2 and then decreased with increasing age.

Breast-feeding patients
• Drug appears in breast milk. HIV-infected women shouldn't breast-feed.

niacin
(vitamin B₃, nicotinic acid)
Niacor, Niaspan, Nico-400, Nicobid, Nicolar, Nicotinex, Slo-Niacin

Pharmacologic classification: B-complex vitamin
Therapeutic classification: vitamin B₃, antilipemic, peripheral vasodilator
Pregnancy risk category A (C if greater than RDA)

How supplied
Available by prescription only
Capsules: 500 mg
Extended-release tablets: 500 mg, 750 mg, and 1,000 mg; and 21-day starter pack (7 each) 375 mg, 500 mg, and 750 mg.
Available without a prescription
Tablets: 25 mg, 50 mg, 100 mg, 125 mg, 250 mg, 400 mg, 500 mg
Tablets (timed-release): 250 mg, 500 mg, 750 mg
Capsules (timed-release): 125 mg, 250 mg, 300 mg, 400 mg, 500 mg, 750 mg
Elixir: 50 mg/5 ml

Indications, route, and dosage
Pellagra
Adults: 300 to 500 mg in divided doses P.O., depending on severity of niacin deficiency. Maximum recommended daily dose is 500 mg; should be divided into 10 doses, 50 mg each.
Children: Up to 300 mg P.O. daily, depending on severity of niacin deficiency.
    To prevent recurrence after symptoms subside, advise adequate nutrition and adequate supplements to meet RDA.
Peripheral vascular disease and circulatory disorders
Adults: 100 to 150 mg P.O. three to five times daily.

Adjunctive treatment of hyperlipidemias, especially those associated with hypercholesterolemia
Adults: 1.5 to 3 g daily in three divided doses with or after meals, increased at intervals to 6 g daily to maximum of 9 g daily.
Dietary supplement
Adults: 10 to 20 mg P.O. daily.

Pharmacodynamics
Vitamin replacement action: As a vitamin, niacin functions as a coenzyme essential to tissue respiration, lipid metabolism, and glycogenolysis. Niacin deficiency causes pellagra, which causes effects such as dermatitis, diarrhea, and dementia; administration of niacin cures pellagra. Niacin lowers cholesterol and triglyceride levels by an unknown mechanism.
Vasodilating action: Niacin acts directly on peripheral vessels, dilating cutaneous vessels and increasing blood flow, predominantly in the face, neck, and chest.
Antilipemic action: Mechanism unknown. Nicotinic acid inhibits lipolysis in adipose tissues, decreases hepatic esterification of triglyceride, and increases lipoprotein lipase activity. It reduces serum cholesterol and triglyceride levels.

Pharmacokinetics
• *Absorption:* Absorbed rapidly from GI tract. Plasma levels peak in 45 minutes. Cholesterol and triglyceride levels decrease after several days.
• *Distribution:* Niacin coenzymes distributed widely in body tissues; niacin distributed in breast milk.
• *Metabolism:* Metabolized by liver to active metabolites.
• *Excretion:* Excreted in urine.

Contraindications and precautions
Contraindicated in patients with hypersensitivity to drug and in those with hepatic dysfunction, active peptic ulcer, severe hypotension, or arterial hemorrhage. Use cautiously in patients with history of liver disease, peptic ulcer, allergy, gout, gallbladder disease, diabetes mellitus, or coronary artery disease.

Interactions
Drug-drug. *Aspirin:* Decreased metabolic clearance of nicotinic acid. Use together cautiously. *HMG CoA reductase inhibitors:* Possible myopathy or rhabdomyolysis. Monitor patient closely. *Sympathetic blockers:* Added vasodilation and hypotension. Use together cautiously.

Adverse reactions
Most reactions are dose-dependent.
CV: *excessive peripheral vasodilation,* hypotension, atrial fibrillation, **arrhythmias.**
EENT: *toxic amblyopia.*

GI: *nausea, vomiting, diarrhea,* possible activation of peptic ulceration, epigastric or substernal pain.
Hepatic: *hepatic dysfunction.*
Metabolic: hyperglycemia, hyperuricemia.
Skin: *flushing,* pruritus, dryness, tingling.

☑ Special considerations
• RDA of niacin in adult men is 19 mg; in adult women 15 mg; and in children 5 to 20 mg.
• Megadoses of niacin usually aren't recommended.
• Aspirin may reduce flushing response.
• Niacin therapy alters fluorometric test results for urine catecholamines and results for urine glucose tests using cupric sulfate (Benedict's reagent).

Monitoring the patient
• Monitor hepatic function and blood glucose levels during initial therapy.
• Evaluate patient for adverse reactions.

Information for the patient
• Explain disease process and rationale for therapy; stress that use of niacin to treat hyperlipidemia or to dilate peripheral vessels isn't simply taking a vitamin, but serious medicine. Emphasize importance of complying with therapy.
• Instruct patient not to substitute sustained-release (timed) tablets for intermediate-release tablets in equivalent doses. Severe hepatic toxicity, including necrosis, has occurred.
• Explain that cutaneous flushing and warmth commonly occur in first 2 hours; they will cease with continued therapy.
• Advise patient not to make sudden postural changes to minimize effects of orthostatic hypotension.
• Instruct patient to avoid hot liquids when initially taking drug to reduce flushing response.
• Advise patient to take drug with meals to minimize GI irritation.

Breast-feeding patients
• No problems have been reported in breast-feeding women taking normal daily doses as a dietary requirement. Drug appears in breast milk.

nicardipine hydrochloride
Cardene, Cardene SR

Pharmacologic classification: calcium channel blocker
Therapeutic classification: antianginal, antihypertensive
Pregnancy risk category C

How supplied
Available by prescription only
Capsules: 20 mg, 30 mg

Capsules (extended-release): 30 mg, 45 mg, 60 mg
Injection: 2.5 mg/ml in 10-ml ampules

Indications, route, and dosage
Hypertension; management of chronic stable angina
Adults: Initially, 20 mg P.O. t.i.d. Adjust dosage based on patient response. Usual dosage range is 20 to 40 mg t.i.d. Extended-release capsules (for hypertension only) can be initiated at 30 mg b.i.d. Usual dose is 30 to 60 mg b.i.d.
Short-term management of hypertension when oral therapy isn't feasible or possible
Adults: Initially, 5 mg/hour I.V. infusion; titrate infusion upward by 2.5 mg/hour q 15 minutes to a maximum of 15 mg/hour, p.r.n.
✦ Dosage adjustment. In patients with hepatic dysfunction, therapy should begin at 20 mg P.O. b.i.d.; carefully titrate subsequent dose based on patient response.

Pharmacodynamics
Antihypertensive and antianginal action: Inhibits the transmembrane flux of calcium ions into cardiac and smooth muscle cells. Appears to act specifically on vascular muscle, and may cause a smaller decrease in cardiac output than other calcium channel blockers because of vasodilatory effect.

Pharmacokinetics
• *Absorption:* Completely absorbed after oral administration. Plasma levels detectable within 20 minutes; peak in about 1 hour. Possible decreased absorption with food. Therapeutic serum levels 28 to 50 ng/ml.
• *Distribution:* More than 95% bound to plasma proteins.
• *Metabolism:* Substantial first-pass effect reduces absolute bioavailability to about 35%. Extensively metabolized in liver. Process is saturable; increasing dosage yields nonlinear increases in plasma levels.
• *Excretion:* Elimination half-life is about 8.6 hours after steady-state levels are reached.

Contraindications and precautions
Contraindicated in patients with hypersensitivity to drug and in those with advanced aortic stenosis. Use cautiously in patients with impaired renal or hepatic function, cardiac conduction disturbances, hypotension, or heart failure.

Interactions
Drug-drug. *Cimetidine:* Increased plasma levels of nicardipine. Monitor patient if used together.
Cyclosporine: Increased plasma levels of cyclosporine. Monitor patient carefully.
Digoxin: Increased serum digoxin levels. Monitor serum digoxin levels.

Fentanyl anesthesia: Severe hypotension. Monitor vital signs closely.

Adverse reactions
CNS: dizziness, light-headedness, headache, paresthesia, asthenia.
CV: *peripheral edema, palpitations,* angina, tachycardia.
GI: nausea, abdominal discomfort, dry mouth.
Skin: rash, *flushing.*

☑ Special considerations
Besides the recommendations relevant to all calcium channel blockers, consider the following.
• Allow at least 3 days between oral dosage changes to ensure achievement of steady-state plasma levels.
• When treating patients with chronic stable angina, S.L. nitroglycerin, prophylactic nitrate therapy, and beta blockers may be continued.
• Dilute solution in ampule before I.V. infusion. Recommended dilution is 0.1 mg/ml in dextrose or saline solution.
• Overdose may produce hypotension, bradycardia, drowsiness, confusion, and slurred speech. I.V. calcium gluconate may be useful to counteract drug effects.

Monitoring the patient
• When treating hypertension, measure blood pressure during times of plasma level trough (about 8 hours after dose or immediately before subsequent doses). Because of prominent effects that may occur during plasma level peaks, measure blood pressure 1 to 2 hours after dose.
• Monitor blood pressure during I.V. administration because nicardipine I.V. decreases peripheral resistance.

Information for the patient
• Tell patient to take oral form of drug exactly as prescribed.
• Advise patient to report chest pain immediately. Some patients may experience increased frequency, severity, or duration of chest pain at start of therapy or during dosage adjustments.

Pediatric patients
• Safety in children under age 18 hasn't been established.

Breast-feeding patients
• Drug may appear in breast milk. Breast-feeding isn't recommended.

nicotine
Habitrol, Nicoderm, Nicotrol,
Nicotrol NS, ProStep

Pharmacologic classification: nicotinic
cholinergic agonist
Therapeutic classification: smoking
cessation aid
Pregnancy risk category D

How supplied
Available with or without a prescription
Transdermal system: designed to release nico-
tine at a fixed rate
Habitrol: 21 mg/day, 14 mg/day, 7 mg/day
Nicoderm: 21 mg/day, 14 mg/day, 7 mg/day
Nicotrol: 15 mg/day, 10 mg/day, 5 mg/day
ProStep: 22 mg/day, 11 mg/day
Nasal spray: metered spray pump
Nicotrol NS: 10 mg/ml
Available by prescription only
Nicotrol inhaler: 10 mg cartridge, supplying 4 mg
of nicotine

Indications, route, and dosage
*Relief of nicotine withdrawal symptoms in
patients attempting smoking cessation*
Adults: One transdermal system applied to a non-
hairy part of upper trunk or upper outer arm.
Dosage varies slightly with product selected.
Habitrol, Nicoderm
Initially, apply one 21-mg/day system daily for 6
weeks. After 24 hours, the system should be removed and a new system applied to a different
site. Then, taper dosage to 14 mg/day for 2 to 4
weeks. Finally, taper dosage to 7 mg/day if necessary. Nicotine substitution and gradual withdrawal should take 8 to 12 weeks.
✦ *Dosage adjustment.* Patients who weigh under 45 kg (100 lb), have CV disease, or who
smoke less than half a pack of cigarettes daily
should start therapy with the 14-mg/day system.
Nicotrol
Adults: Initially, apply one 15-mg/day system daily for 12 weeks. The system should be applied
upon waking and removed h.s. Then, taper dose
to 10 mg/day for 2 weeks. Finally, taper dose to
5 mg/day for 2 weeks if necessary. Or dose may
be reduced in patients who have successfully abstained from smoking q 2 to 4 weeks until 5-
mg/day dose has been used for 2 weeks. Nicotine substitution and gradual withdrawal should
take 14 to 20 weeks.
Nicotrol NS
Adults: Initially, 1 or 2 doses/hour (1 dose = 2
sprays—one in each nostril). Encourage patient
to use at least the recommended minimum of
8 doses/day. Maximum recommended dose is
40 mg or 80 sprays/day. Duration of treatment
shouldn't exceed 3 months.

ProStep
Adults: Initially, apply one 22-mg/day system daily for 4 to 8 weeks. After 24 hours, system should
be removed and a new system applied to a different site. In patients weighing under 45 kg (100
lb), start therapy with the 11-mg/day system; those
who have successfully stopped smoking during
this period may stop drug. If therapy was initiated with the 22-mg/day system, treatment may
continue for an additional 2 to 4 weeks at lower
dose (11 mg/day). Nicotine substitution and gradual withdrawal should take 6 to 12 weeks.
Nicotrol inhaler
Adults: Initial dose is 6 to 16 cartridges daily. Best
effect is achieved with continuous puffing. Recommended treatment is up to 3 months and, if
needed, gradual reduction over the next 6 to 12
weeks.

Pharmacodynamics
Nicotinic cholinergic action: Nicotine transdermal
system and nasal spray provide nicotine, the chief
stimulant alkaloid found in tobacco products,
which stimulates nicotinic acetylcholine receptors in the CNS, neuromuscular junction, autonomic ganglia, and adrenal medulla.

Pharmacokinetics
• *Absorption:* Rapidly absorbed.
• *Distribution:* Plasma protein-binding below 5%.
• *Metabolism:* Metabolized by liver, kidney, and
lungs. Over 20 metabolites identified. Primary
metabolites are cotinine (15%) and trans-3-
hydroxycotinine (45%).
• *Excretion:* Excreted primarily in urine as metabolites; about 10% excreted unchanged. With high
urine flow rates or acidified urine, up to 30% excreted unchanged.

Contraindications and precautions
Contraindicated in patients with hypersensitivity
to nicotine or its components. Also contraindicated in nonsmokers and in patients with recent
MI, life-threatening arrhythmias, or severe or worsening angina pectoris.
   Use cautiously in patients with hyperthyroidism, pheochromocytoma, type 1 diabetes mellitus, or peptic ulcer disease.

Interactions
Drug-drug. *Acetaminophen, imipramine, oxazepam, pentazocine, propranolol, theophylline:*
Increased levels of these drugs with smoking cessation. Dosage reduction may be necessary.
Insulin: Smoking cessation may increase amount
of subcutaneous insulin absorbed. Insulin dosage
may be reduced.
Isoproterenol, phenylephrine: Cessation of smoking may decrease levels of circulating catecholamines. Higher doses of adrenergic agonists
may be required.

Reactions may be *common*, uncommon, **life-threatening**, or COMMON AND LIFE-THREATENING.

Labetalol, prazosin: Cessation of smoking may decrease levels of circulating catecholamines. Lower doses of adrenergic antagonists may be necessary.

Drug-herb. *Blue cohosh:* Increased effects of nicotine. Discourage concomitant use.

Drug-lifestyle. *Caffeine:* Increased levels with smoking cessation. Discourage use.

Adverse reactions

CNS: somnolence, dizziness, *headache, insomnia,* paresthesia, abnormal dreams, nervousness.
CV: hypertension.
EENT: pharyngitis, sinusitis.
GI: abdominal pain, constipation, dyspepsia, nausea, diarrhea, vomiting, dry mouth.
GU: dysmenorrhea.
Musculoskeletal: back pain, myalgia.
Respiratory: increased cough.
Skin: *local or systemic erythema, pruritus, burning at application site,* cutaneous hypersensitivity, rash, diaphoresis.

☑ Special considerations

● Discourage use of transdermal system for more than 3 months. Chronic nicotine consumption by any route can be dangerous and habit-forming.
● Patients who can't stop cigarette smoking during the initial 4 weeks of therapy probably won't benefit from continued use of drug. Patients who were unsuccessful may benefit from counseling to identify factors that led to unsuccessful attempt. Encourage patient to minimize or eliminate factors that contributed to treatment failure and to try again, possibly after some interval, before next attempt.
● Healthcare workers' exposure to nicotine within the transdermal systems should be minimal; however, avoid unnecessary contact with system. After contact, wash hands with water alone because soap can enhance absorption.
● Nicotrol NS isn't recommended in patients with chronic nasal disorders or severe reactive airway disease.
● Increased cough is common in patients using the inhaler.
● Toxicity may cause acute nicotine poisoning, including nausea, vomiting, diarrhea, weakness, respiratory failure, hypotension, and seizures. Barbiturates or benzodiazepines may be used to treat seizures, and atropine may attenuate excessive salivation or diarrhea. Administer fluids to treat hypotension; increase urine flow to enhance drug elimination.

Monitoring the patient

● Monitor patient for progress in smoking cessation.
● Evaluate patient for adverse effects.

Information for the patient

● Tell patient to stop patch use and to call immediately if a generalized rash or persistent or severe local skin reactions (pruritus, edema, or erythema) occur.
● Make sure patient understands that nicotine can evaporate from the transdermal system once it's removed from protective packaging. The patch shouldn't be altered in any way (folded or cut) before applied; apply quickly after removal of protective packaging. Tell patient not to store patch at temperatures above 86° F (30° C).
● Teach patient how to dispose of transdermal system. After removal, fold the patch in half, bringing adhesive sides together. If system comes in a protective pouch, dispose of the used patch in pouch that contained new system. Careful disposal is necessary to prevent accidental poisoning of children or pets.
● Be sure that patient reads and understands patient information dispensed with drug when prescription is filled.
● Inform patient to refrain from smoking while using system; he may experience adverse effects from increased nicotine levels.
● Explain that patient is likely to experience nasal irritation, which may become less bothersome with continued use of Nicotrol NS.

Pediatric patients

● Safety and efficacy in children haven't been established. The amount of nicotine contained in a patch could prove fatal to a child if ingested; even used patches contain a substantial amount of residual nicotine. Patients should take care to ensure that both used and unused transdermal systems and metered-spray bottles are kept out of the reach of children.

Breast-feeding patients

● Nicotine appears in breast milk and is readily absorbed after oral administration. Weigh infant's risk of exposure to nicotine against his risk of exposure from continued smoking by mother.

nicotine polacrilex (nicotine resin complex)
Nicorette

Pharmacologic classification: nicotinic agonist
Therapeutic classification: smoking cessation aid
Pregnancy risk category X

How supplied

Available with and without a prescription
Chewing gum: 2 mg, 4 mg nicotine resin complex per square

Indications, route, and dosage
Aid in managing nicotine dependence
Serves as a temporary aid to smoker seeking to give up smoking while participating in a behavior modification program under medical supervision. Generally, smoker with physical nicotine dependence is most likely to benefit from use of nicotine chewing gum.
Adults: Chew one piece of gum slowly and intermittently for 30 minutes whenever the urge to smoke occurs. Most patients need about 10 pieces of gum daily during first month. Patients using the 2-mg strength shouldn't exceed 30 pieces of gum daily; those using the 4-mg strength shouldn't exceed 20 pieces of gum daily.

Pharmacodynamics
Nicotine replacement action: An agonist at the nicotinic receptors in the peripheral nervous system and CNS and produces both behavioral stimulation and depression. Acts on the adrenal medulla to aid in overcoming physical dependence on nicotine during withdrawal from habitual smoking.
   CV effects are usually dose-dependent. Nonsmokers have experienced CNS-mediated symptoms of hiccuping, nausea, and vomiting, even with a small dose. A smoker chewing a 2-mg piece of gum every hour usually doesn't experience CV adverse effects.

Pharmacokinetics
• *Absorption:* Nicotine is bound to ion-exchange resin and is released only during chewing. Blood level depends upon vigor with which gum is chewed.
• *Distribution:* Distribution into tissues hasn't been fully characterized. Crosses placenta; appears in breast milk.
• *Metabolism:* Metabolized mainly by liver; less by kidneys and lungs. Main metabolites are cotinine and nicotine-19-N-oxide.
• *Excretion:* Both nicotine and metabolites excreted in urine, with about 10% to 20% excreted unchanged. Excretion of nicotine is increased in acid urine and by high urine output.

Contraindications and precautions
Contraindicated in nonsmokers; in patients with recent MI, life-threatening arrhythmias, severe or worsening angina pectoris, or active temporomandibular joint disease; and during pregnancy.
   Use cautiously in patients with hyperthyroidism, pheochromocytoma, type 1 diabetes mellitus, peptic ulcer disease, history of esophagitis, oral or pharyngeal inflammation, or dental conditions that might be exacerbated by chewing gum.

Interactions
Drug-drug. *Adrenergic agonists, adrenergic blockers:* Nicorette gum and smoking can in-

crease circulating levels of cortisol and catecholamines. Therapy with these drugs may need adjustments.
Imipramine, pentazocine, propoxyphene, theophylline: Smoking cessation may decrease metabolism of these drugs. Dosage adjustments may be needed.
Drug-herb. *Blue cohosh:* Increased effects of nicotine. Discourage concomitant use.
Drug-food. *Acidic beverages (coffee, carbonated soft drinks):* Lower saliva pH and decrease absorption of nicotine from gum. Avoid eating and drinking 15 minutes before and during chewing nicotine gum.
Drug-lifestyle. *Smoking:* Increased caffeine metabolism. Patient shouldn't smoke during therapy.

Adverse reactions
CNS: dizziness, light-headedness, irritability, insomnia, headache, paresthesia.
CV: atrial fibrillation.
EENT: throat soreness, jaw muscle ache (from chewing).
GI: nausea, vomiting, indigestion, eructation, anorexia, excessive salivation.
Other: hiccups, sweating.

☑ Special considerations
• Patients most likely to benefit from Nicorette gum are smokers with a high physical dependence. Typically, they smoke over 15 cigarettes daily; prefer brands of cigarettes with high nicotine levels; usually inhale smoke; smoke first cigarette within 30 minutes of arising; and find first morning cigarette the hardest to give up.
• The risk of overdose is minimized by early nausea and vomiting that result from excessive nicotine intake. Poisoning causes nausea, vomiting, salivation, abdominal pain, diarrhea, cold sweats, headache, dizziness, disturbed hearing and vision, mental confusion, and weakness.

Monitoring the patient
• Monitor patient for progress in smoking cessation.
• Monitor patient for adverse effects.

Information for the patient
• Instruct patient to chew gum slowly and intermittently for about 30 minutes to promote slow and even buccal absorption of nicotine. Fast chewing allows faster absorption and produces more adverse reactions. After about 15 chews, advise patient to hold the gum between cheek and gum for a few minutes.
• At initial visit, instruct patient to chew one piece of gum whenever urge to smoke occurs instead of having a cigarette. Most patients will require about 10 pieces of gum daily during first month of treatment.

- Tell patient who has successfully abstained to gradually withdraw gum use after 3 months; he shouldn't use gum for longer than 6 months.
- Inform patient that gum is sugar-free and usually doesn't stick to dentures.

Breast-feeding patients
- Nicotine appears in breast milk and is readily absorbed after oral administration. Weigh infant's risk of exposure to nicotine against his risk of exposure from continued smoking by mother.

nifedipine
Adalat, Adalat CC, Procardia, Procardia XL

Pharmacologic classification: calcium channel blocker
Therapeutic classification: antianginal
Pregnancy risk category C

How supplied
Available by prescription only
Capsules: 10 mg, 20 mg
Tablets (extended-release): 30 mg, 60 mg, 90 mg

Indications, route, and dosage
Management of Prinzmetal's or variant angina or chronic stable angina pectoris
Adults: Starting dose is 10 mg P.O. t.i.d. Usual effective dosage range is 10 to 20 mg t.i.d. Some patients may need up to 30 mg q.i.d. Maximum daily dose for capsules is 180 mg; for extended-release tablets, 120 mg.
Hypertension
Adults: Initially, 30 to 60 mg P.O. once daily (extended-release tablets). Adjust dosage at 7- to 14-day intervals based on patient tolerance and response. Maximum daily dose is 120 mg.

Pharmacodynamics
Antianginal action: Dilates systemic arteries, resulting in decreased total peripheral resistance and modestly decreased systemic blood pressure with a slightly increased heart rate, decreased afterload, and increased cardiac index. Reduced afterload and the subsequent decrease in myocardial oxygen consumption probably account for nifedipine's value in treating chronic stable angina. In Prinzmetal's angina, nifedipine inhibits coronary artery spasm, increasing myocardial oxygen delivery.

Pharmacokinetics
- *Absorption:* About 90% of dose absorbed rapidly from GI tract after oral administration; however, only about 65% to 70% of drug reaches systemic circulation because of significant first-pass effect in liver. Serum levels peak in 30 minutes to 2 hours; hypotensive effects may occur 5 minutes after S.L. administration. Therapeutic serum levels 25 to 100 ng/ml.
- *Distribution:* About 92% to 98% of circulating drug bound to plasma proteins.
- *Metabolism:* Metabolized in liver.
- *Excretion:* Excreted in urine and feces as inactive metabolites. Elimination half-life 2 to 5 hours. Duration of effect ranges from 4 to 12 hours.

Contraindications and precautions
Contraindicated in patients with hypersensitivity to drug. Use cautiously in elderly patients and in patients with heart failure or hypotension. Use extended-release form cautiously in patients with GI narrowing. Use cautiously in patients with unstable angina who aren't currently taking a beta blocker because a higher frequency of MI has been reported.

Interactions
Drug-drug. *Beta blockers:* Exacerbation of angina, heart failure, and hypotension. Monitor patient closely.
Cimetidine: Increased nifedipine drug levels. Use together cautiously.
Digoxin: Increased serum digoxin levels. Monitor serum digoxin levels.
Fentanyl: Excessive hypotension. Use together cautiously.
Hypotensive drugs: Excessive hypotension. Monitor patient's vital signs.
Phenytoin: Increased phenytoin levels. Monitor serum phenytoin levels.

Adverse reactions
CNS: *dizziness, light-headedness, flushing, headache, weakness, syncope, nervousness.*
CV: *peripheral edema, hypotension, palpitations, **heart failure, MI, pulmonary edema.***
EENT: nasal congestion.
GI: *nausea, diarrhea, constipation, abdominal discomfort.*
Hepatic: increased serum levels of alkaline phosphate, LD, AST, and ALT.
Musculoskeletal: muscle cramps.
Respiratory: dyspnea, cough.
Skin: rash, pruritus.
Other: hypokalemia, fever.

☑ Special considerations
- Initial doses or dosage increase may exacerbate angina briefly. Reassure patient that this symptom is temporary.
- Nifedipine isn't available in S.L. form. No advantage has been found in S.L. or intrabuccal use.
- Although rebound effect hasn't been observed when drug is stopped, reduce dose slowly.

Monitoring the patient
• Monitor blood pressure regularly, especially if patient is also taking beta blockers or antihypertensives.
• Monitor patient for antianginal drug effect.

Information for the patient
• Instruct patient to swallow capsules whole without breaking, crushing, or chewing them.
• Tell patient that he may experience annoying hypotensive effects during dosage adjustment and urge compliance with therapy.

Geriatric patients
• Use drug with caution in elderly patients because they may be more sensitive to drug's effects, and duration of effect may be prolonged.

nimodipine
Nimotop

Pharmacologic classification: calcium channel blocker
Therapeutic classification: cerebral vasodilator
Pregnancy risk category C

How supplied
Available by prescription only
Capsules: 30 mg

Indications, route, and dosage
Improvement of neurologic deficits after subarachnoid hemorrhage from ruptured congenital aneurysms
Adults: 60 mg P.O. q 4 hours for 21 days. Therapy should begin within 96 hours of subarachnoid hemorrhage.
✦ *Dosage adjustment.* In adults with hepatic impairment, 30 mg P.O. q 4 hours.
◇ *Migraine headache*
Adults: 120 mg P.O. daily in divided doses, 1 hour before or within 2 hours after meals.

Pharmacodynamics
Neuronal-sparing action: Inhibits calcium ion influx across cardiac and smooth muscle cells, thus decreasing myocardial contractility and oxygen demand, and dilates coronary arteries and arterioles. Although exact mechanism unknown, it's believed that dilation of the small cerebral resistance vessels with increased collateral circulation is possible.

Pharmacokinetics
• *Absorption:* Well absorbed after oral administration. However, because of extensive first-pass metabolism, bioavailability is only about 3% to 30%.
• *Distribution:* More than 95% protein-bound.

• *Metabolism:* Extensively metabolized in liver. Drug and metabolites undergo enterohepatic recycling.
• *Excretion:* Less than 1% excreted as parent drug. Elimination half-life is 1 to 9 hours.

Contraindications and precautions
No known contraindications. Use cautiously in patients with hepatic failure.

Interactions
Drug-drug. *Antihypertensives:* Enhanced hypotensive effect. Monitor patient's blood pressure.
Calcium channel blockers: May enhance CV effects of these drugs. Monitor patient closely.
Phenytoin: Increased phenytoin levels. Monitor serum phenytoin levels.
Drug-food. *Food:* Decreased absorption. Give drug 1 hour before or 2 hours after meals.

Adverse reactions
CNS: headache, psychic disturbances.
CV: decreased blood pressure, flushing, edema, tachycardia.
GI: nausea, diarrhea, abdominal discomfort.
Musculoskeletal: muscle cramps.
Respiratory: dyspnea.
Skin: dermatitis, rash.

☑ Special considerations
Besides the recommendations relevant to all calcium channel blockers, consider the following.
• Unlike other calcium channel blockers, nimodipine isn't used for angina pectoris or hypertension.
• Use lower doses in patients with hepatic failure. Initiate therapy at 30 mg P.O. every 4 hours, and closely monitor blood pressure and heart rate.
• If patient can't swallow capsules, puncture ends of liquid-filled capsule with an 18G needle and draw the contents into syringe. Instill dose into patient's nasogastric tube and rinse tube with 30 ml of normal saline solution.
• Toxicity may cause nausea, weakness, drowsiness, confusion, bradycardia, and decreased cardiac output. Calcium gluconate I.V. has been used to treat calcium channel blocker overdose.

Monitoring the patient
• Monitor blood pressure and heart rate in all patients, especially during initiation of therapy.
• Monitor patient for therapeutic effect.

Information for the patient
• Advise patient to rise from supine position slowly to avoid dizziness and hypotension, especially at start of therapy.
• Food decreases absorption. Advise patient to take drug 1 hour before or 2 hours after meals.

Pediatric patients
• Safety and efficacy in children haven't been established.

Breast-feeding patients
• Substantial amounts of drug may appear in breast milk. Avoid breast-feeding during therapy.

nisoldipine
Sular

Pharmacologic classification: calcium channel blocker
Therapeutic classification: antihypertensive
Pregnancy risk category C

How supplied
Available by prescription only
Tablets (extended-release): 10 mg, 20 mg, 30 mg, 40 mg

Indications, route, and dosage
Hypertension
Adults: Initially, 20 mg P.O. once daily, then increased by 10 mg/week or at longer intervals, p.r.n. Usual maintenance dose is 20 to 40 mg once daily. Don't exceed 60 mg daily.
✦ *Dosage adjustment.* In patients over age 65 or those with hepatic dysfunction, give starting dose of 10 mg P.O. once daily. Monitor blood pressure closely during any dosage adjustment.

Pharmacodynamics
Antihypertensive action: Prevents the entry of calcium ions into vascular smooth muscle cells, thereby causing dilation of the arterioles, which in turn decreases peripheral vascular resistance.

Pharmacokinetics
• *Absorption:* Relatively well absorbed from GI tract. High-fat foods significantly affect release of drug from coat-core formulation.
• *Distribution:* About 99% bound to plasma protein.
• *Metabolism:* Extensively metabolized; five major metabolites identified.
• *Excretion:* Excreted in urine; half-life ranges from 7 to 12 hours.

Contraindications and precautions
Contraindicated in patients with hypersensitivity to dihydropyridine calcium channel blockers. Use cautiously in patients receiving beta blockers or in those who have compromised ventricular or hepatic function and heart failure.

Interactions
Drug-drug. *Cimetidine:* Increased bioavailability of nisoldipine and increases peak level. Monitor patient closely.

Quinidine: Decreased bioavailability of nisoldipine. Monitor patient closely.
Drug-food. *Grapefruit juice, high-fat meal:* Decreased absorption. Don't give together.

Adverse reactions
CNS: *headache,* dizziness.
CV: vasodilation, palpitations, chest pain, *peripheral edema.*
EENT: pharyngitis, sinusitis.
GI: nausea.
Skin: rash.

☑ Special considerations
• Some patients, especially those with severe obstructive coronary artery disease, have developed increased frequency, duration, or severity of angina or even acute MI after initiation of calcium channel blocker therapy or at time of dosage increase.

Monitoring the patient
• Monitor blood pressure regularly, especially during initial administration and dosage adjustments.
• Evaluate patient for adverse drug effects.

Information for the patient
• Tell patient to take drug exactly as prescribed, even if he feels well.
• Instruct patient to swallow tablet whole; don't chew, divide, or crush tablets.
• Tell patient not to take drug with a high-fat meal or with grapefruit products.
• Advise patient to rise slowly from supine position to avoid dizziness and hypotension, especially at start of therapy.

Geriatric patients
• Elderly patients may have two- to threefold higher plasma levels than younger patients. Consider proper dosages carefully.

Pediatric patients
• Safety and effectiveness in children haven't been established.

Breast-feeding patients
• It's unknown if drug appears in breast milk. Not recommended for use in breast-feeding women.

nitrofurantoin macrocrystals
Macrobid, Macrodantin

nitrofurantoin
Furadantin

Pharmacologic classification: nitrofuran
Therapeutic classification: urinary tract anti-infective
Pregnancy risk category B

How supplied
Available by prescription only
macrocrystals
Capsules: 25 mg, 50 mg, 100 mg
Capsules (dual-release): 100 mg
nitrofurantoin
Suspension: 25 mg/5 ml

Indications, route, and dosage
Initial or recurrent urinary tract infections caused by susceptible organisms
Adults and children over age 12: 50 to 100 mg P.O. q.i.d. or 100 mg dual-release capsules q 12 hours.
Children ages 1 month to 12 years: 5 to 7 mg/kg/24 hours P.O. daily, divided q.i.d.
Long-term suppression therapy
Adults: 50 to 100 mg P.O. daily h.s. as a single dose.
Children: As low as 1 mg/kg/day in a single dose or two divided doses.

Pharmacodynamics
Antibacterial action: Exact mechanism unknown. Has bacteriostatic action in low levels and possible bactericidal action in high levels. May inhibit bacterial enzyme systems interfering with bacterial carbohydrate metabolism. Most active at an acidic pH.

Spectrum of activity includes many common gram-positive and gram-negative urinary pathogens, including *Escherichia coli, Staphylococcus aureus,* enterococci, and certain strains of *Klebsiella* and *Enterobacter.* Organisms that usually resist nitrofurantoin include *Acinetobacter, Proteus, Providencia, Pseudomonas,* and *Serratia.*

Pharmacokinetics
• *Absorption:* When administered orally, drug is well absorbed (mainly by small intestine) from GI tract. Food aids dissolution and speeds absorption. Slower dissolution and absorption of macrocrystal form; less GI distress.
• *Distribution:* Crosses into bile and placenta. 60% bound to plasma proteins. Plasma half-life about 20 minutes. Urine levels peak in about 30 minutes with microcrystals; somewhat later with macrocrystals.
• *Metabolism:* Metabolized partially in liver.

• *Excretion:* About 30% to 50% eliminated by glomerular filtration and tubular secretion into urine as unchanged drug within 24 hours. Some drug may be excreted in breast milk.

Contraindications and precautions
Contraindicated in pregnant patients at term (38 to 42 weeks' gestation), during labor and delivery, or when the onset of labor is imminent. Contraindicated in children age 1 month and less and in patients with moderate to severe renal impairment, anuria, oliguria, or creatinine clearance below 60 ml/minute.

Use cautiously in patients with impaired renal function, anemia, diabetes mellitus, electrolyte abnormalities, vitamin B deficiency, debilitating disease, or G6PD deficiency.

Interactions
Drug-drug. *Anticholinergics:* Enhanced bioavailability of nitrofurantoin. Monitor patient for effect.
Magnesium trisilicate antacids: May decrease nitrofurantoin absorption. Don't give together.
Probenecid, sulfinpyrazone: Increased serum and decrease urine nitrofurantoin levels. Watch for toxicity and decreased antibacterial effectiveness.
Quinolone derivatives (cinoxacin, ciprofloxacin, nalidixic acid, norfloxacin): May antagonize anti-infective effects. Monitor patient for effect.
Drug-food. *Any food:* Increased absorption. Give drug with food.

Adverse reactions
CNS: *peripheral neuropathy,* headache, dizziness, drowsiness, *ascending polyneuropathy* (with high doses or renal impairment).
GI: *anorexia, nausea, vomiting,* abdominal pain, diarrhea.
GU: overgrowth of nonsusceptible organisms in the urinary tract.
Hematologic: *hemolysis in patients with G6PD deficiency* (reversed after stopping drug), *agranulocytosis, thrombocytopenia.*
Hepatic: *hepatitis, hepatic necrosis,* elevated bilirubin and alkaline phosphatase.
Metabolic: decreased serum glucose.
Respiratory: *pulmonary sensitivity reactions* (cough, chest pain, fever, chills, dyspnea, pulmonary infiltration with consolidation or pleural effusion), *asthmatic attacks* in patients with history of asthma.
Skin: maculopapular, erythematous, or eczematous eruption; pruritus; urticaria; *exfoliative dermatitis; Stevens-Johnson syndrome;* transient alopecia.
Other: hypersensitivity reactions (*anaphylaxis*), drug fever.

Reactions may be *common,* uncommon, *life-threatening,* or COMMON AND LIFE-THREATENING.

☑ Special considerations
• Obtain culture and sensitivity tests before starting therapy, and repeat as needed.
• Oral suspension may be mixed with water, milk, fruit juice, and formulas.
• Continue treatment for at least 3 days after sterile urine specimens have been obtained.
• Long-term therapy may cause overgrowth of nonsusceptible organisms, especially *Pseudomonas*.
• Nitrofurantoin may cause false-positive results in urine glucose tests using cupric sulfate reagents (such as Benedict's test, Fehling's solution, or Clinitest) because it reacts with these reagents.
• Acute overdose may result in nausea and vomiting. Increase fluid intake to promote urinary excretion of drug. Nitrofurantoin is dialyzable.

Monitoring the patient
• Monitor CBC regularly.
• Monitor fluid intake and output and pulmonary status.

Information for the patient
• Instruct patient to take drug with food or milk to minimize GI distress. Have patient report any unpleasant side effects.
• Caution patient that drug may cause false-positive results in urine glucose tests using cupric sulfate reduction method (Clinitest) but not in glucose oxidase test (glucose enzymatic test strip, Diastix, or Chemstrip uG).
• Emphasize that bedtime dose is important because drug will remain in bladder longer.
• Warn patient that drug may turn urine brown or rust-yellow.

Pediatric patients
• Contraindicated in infants under age 1 month because their immature enzyme systems increase risk of hemolytic anemia.

Breast-feeding patients
• Drug appears in low levels in breast milk. Safety hasn't been established; however, no adverse reactions have been reported, except in infants with G6PD deficiency, who may develop hemolytic anemia.

---

nitrofurazone
Furacin

Pharmacologic classification: synthetic antibacterial nitrofuran derivative
Therapeutic classification: topical antibacterial
Pregnancy risk category C

How supplied
Available by prescription only
Topical solution: 0.2%

Ointment: 0.2% soluble dressing
Cream: 0.2%

Indications, route, and dosage
Adjunct for major burns (especially when resistance to other anti-infectives occurs), prevention of skin graft infection before or after surgery
Adults and children: Apply directly to lesion or to dressings used to cover affected area daily or as indicated, depending on severity of burn. Apply once daily or q few days, depending on dressing technique.

Pharmacodynamics
Antibacterial action: Exact mechanism unknown. However, it appears that drug inhibits bacterial enzymes involved in carbohydrate metabolism. Drug has a broad spectrum of activity.

Pharmacokinetics
• *Absorption:* Limited drug absorption with topical use.
• *Distribution:* None.
• *Metabolism:* None.
• *Excretion:* None.

Contraindications and precautions
Contraindicated in patients with hypersensitivity to drug. Use cautiously in patients with known or suspected renal impairment.

Interactions
None reported.

Adverse reactions
Skin: *erythema, pruritus,* burning, edema, severe reactions (vesiculation, denudation, ulceration), *allergic contact dermatitis.*

☑ Special considerations
• Avoid contact with eyes and mucous membranes.
• Use diluted solutions within 24 hours after preparation; discard diluted solution that becomes cloudy.

Monitoring the patient
• Monitor patient for overgrowth of nonsusceptible organisms, including fungi and *Pseudomonas.*

Information for the patient
• Teach patient proper application of drug and to apply directly on lesion or place on gauze.
• Tell patient to avoid exposing drug to direct sunlight, excessive heat, strong fluorescent lighting, and alkaline materials.

Breast-feeding patients
• Safety in breast-feeding women hasn't been established. It's unknown if drug appears in breast

milk; potential benefits to mother must be weighed against risks to infant.

nitroglycerin (glyceryl trinitrate)
Oral, extended-release
Niong, Nitro-Bid, Nitroglyn, Nitrong, Nitrong SR*

Sublingual
NitroQuick, Nitrostat

Translingual
Nitrolingual

Intravenous
Nitro-Bid IV, Tridil

Topical
Nitro-Bid, Nitrol

Transdermal
Deponit, Minitran, Nitro-Derm, Nitrodisc, Nitro-Dur, Transderm-Nitro

Transmucosal
Nitrogard

Pharmacologic classification: nitrate
Therapeutic classification: antianginal, vasodilator
Pregnancy risk category C

How supplied
Available by prescription only
Tablets (sustained-release): 2.6 mg, 6.5 mg, 9 mg
Tablets (S.L.): 0.3 mg, 0.4 mg, 0.6 mg
Tablets (buccal, controlled-release): 1 mg, 2 mg, 3 mg
Capsules (sustained-release): 2.5 mg, 6.5 mg, 9 mg, 13 mg
Aerosol (lingual): 0.4 mg/metered spray
I.V.: 0.5 mg/ml, 5 mg/ml
I.V. premixed solutions in dextrose: 100 mcg/ml, 200 mcg/ml, 400 mcg/ml
Topical: 2% ointment
Transdermal: 0.1-mg, 0.2-mg, 0.3-mg, 0.4-mg, 0.6 mg, 0.8 mg/hour systems

Indications, route, and dosage
Prophylaxis against chronic anginal attacks
Adults: One sustained-release capsule q 8 to 12 hours; or 2% ointment. Start with ½-inch ointment, increasing with ½-inch increments until headache occurs, then decreasing to previous dose. Range of dose with ointment is 2 to 5 inches. Usual dose is 1 to 2 inches. Or transdermal disc or pad may be applied to hairless site once daily. However, to prevent tolerance, topical forms shouldn't be worn overnight.

Relief of acute angina pectoris, prophylaxis to prevent or minimize anginal attacks when taken immediately before stressful events
Adults: One S.L. tablet dissolved under the tongue or in the buccal pouch immediately on indication of anginal attack. May repeat q 5 minutes for 15 to 30 minutes for a maximum of 3 doses. Or, using Nitrolingual spray, spray one or two doses into mouth, preferably onto or under the tongue. May repeat q 3 to 5 minutes to a maximum of three doses within a 15-minute period. Or, transmucosally, 1 to 3 mg q 3 to 5 hours during waking hours.

Control of hypertension associated with surgery, treatment of heart failure associated with MI, relief of angina pectoris in acute situations, production of controlled hypotension during surgery (by I.V. infusion)
Adults: Initial infusion rate is 5 mcg/minute. May be increased by 5 mcg/minute q 3 to 5 minutes until a response is noted. If a 20-mcg/minute rate doesn't produce desired response, dosage may be increased by as much as 20 mcg/minute q 3 to 5 minutes.
◇ *Hypertensive crisis*
Adults: Infuse at 5 to 100 mcg/minute.

Pharmacodynamics
Antianginal action: Relaxes vascular smooth muscle of both the venous and arterial beds, resulting in a net decrease in myocardial oxygen consumption. Also dilates coronary vessels, leading to redistribution of blood flow to ischemic tissue. Drug's systemic and coronary vascular effects (which may vary slightly with the various nitroglycerin forms) probably account for its value in treating angina.
Vasodilating action: Drug dilates peripheral vessels, making it useful (in I.V. form) in producing controlled hypotension during surgical procedures and in controlling blood pressure in perioperative hypertension. Because peripheral vasodilation decreases venous return to the heart (preload), nitroglycerin also helps to treat pulmonary edema and heart failure. Arterial vasodilation decreases arterial impedance (afterload), thereby decreasing left ventricular work and aiding the failing heart. These combined effects may prove valuable in treating some patients with acute MI.

Pharmacokinetics
• *Absorption:* Well absorbed from GI tract. However, because it undergoes first-pass metabolism in liver, is incompletely absorbed into systemic circulation. Onset of action for oral preparations is slow (except for sublingual tablets). After sublingual administration, absorption from the oral mucosa is relatively complete. Nitroglycerin also is well absorbed after topical administration as ointment or transdermal system. Onset of action for various preparations: I.V. 1 to 2 minutes;

S.L. 1 to 3 minutes; translingual spray 2 minutes; transmucosal tablet 3 minutes; ointment 20 to 60 minutes; oral (sustained-release) 40 minutes; transdermal 40 to 60 minutes.

• *Distribution:* Distributed widely throughout body. About 60% of circulating drug is bound to plasma proteins.

• *Metabolism:* Metabolized in liver and serum to 1,3 glyceryl dinitrate; 1,2 glyceryl dinitrate; and glyceryl mononitrate. Dinitrate metabolites have a slight vasodilatory effect.

• *Excretion:* Metabolites excreted in urine; elimination half-life about 1 to 4 minutes. Duration of effect for various preparations: I.V. 3 to 5 minutes; S.L. up to 30 minutes; translingual spray 30 to 60 minutes; transmucosal tablet 5 hours; ointment 3 to 6 hours; oral (sustained-release) 4 to 8 hours; transdermal 18 to 24 hours.

Contraindications and precautions

Contraindicated in patients with hypersensitivity to nitrates and in those with early MI (S.L. form), severe anemia, increased intracranial pressure, angle-closure glaucoma, orthostatic hypotension, and allergy to adhesives (transdermal form). I.V. form is contraindicated in patients with hypersensitivity to I.V. form, cardiac tamponade, restrictive cardiomyopathy, or constrictive pericarditis. Extended-release preparations shouldn't be used in patients with organic or functional GI hypermotility or malabsorption syndrome.

Use cautiously in patients with hypotension or volume depletion.

Interactions

Drug-drug. *Antihypertensives, phenothiazines:* Possible additive hypotensive effects. Monitor patient closely.

Ergot alkaloids: Increased bioavailability of ergot alkaloids; may precipitate angina. Avoid using together.

Sildenafil: Potentiated hypotensive effects of nitrates. Don't use together.

Drug-lifestyle. *Alcohol:* Additive hypotensive effects. Discourage concomitant use.

Adverse reactions

CNS: *headache, sometimes with throbbing; dizziness;* weakness.

CV: *orthostatic hypotension, tachycardia, flushing, palpitations,* fainting.

GI: nausea, vomiting, sublingual burning.

Skin: cutaneous vasodilation, contact dermatitis (patch), rash.

Other: *hypersensitivity reactions.*

☑ Special considerations

• Ask all male patients about the use of sildenafil (Viagra) before using nitrates.

• Use only S.L. and translingual forms to relieve acute angina attack.

• To apply ointment, spread in uniform thin layer to hairless part of skin except distal parts of arms or legs because absorption won't be maximal at these sites. Don't rub in. Cover with plastic film to aid absorption and to protect clothing. If using Tape-Surrounded Appli-Ruler (TSAR) system, keep TSAR on skin to protect patient's clothing and ensure that ointment remains in place. If serious adverse effects develop in patients using ointment or transdermal system, remove product at once or wipe ointment from skin. Avoid contact with ointment.

• Administration as I.V. infusion requires special nonabsorbent tubing supplied by manufacturer because regular plastic tubing may absorb up to 80% of drug. Infusion should be prepared in glass bottle or container.

• If drug causes headache (especially likely with initial doses), aspirin or acetaminophen may be indicated. Dose may need to be reduced temporarily.

• S.L. dose may be administered before anticipated stress or at bedtime if angina is nocturnal.

• Drug may cause orthostatic hypotension. To minimize this, patient should change to upright position slowly, go up and down stairs carefully, and lie down at the first sign of dizziness.

• When administering drug to patients during initial days after acute MI, monitor hemodynamic and clinical status carefully.

• Be sure to remove transdermal patch before defibrillation. Because of patch's aluminum backing, electric current may cause patch to explode.

• When ending transdermal nitroglycerin treatment for angina, gradually reduce dosage and frequency of application over 4 to 6 weeks.

• To prevent withdrawal symptoms, reduce dosage gradually after long-term use of oral or topical preparations.

• Nitroglycerin may interfere with serum cholesterol determination tests using the Zlatkis-Zak color reaction, resulting in falsely decreased values.

• Toxicity may cause hypotension, persistent throbbing headache, palpitations, visual disturbances, flushing of the skin, sweating (with skin later becoming cold and cyanotic), nausea and vomiting, colic, bloody diarrhea, orthostasis, initial hyperpnea, dyspnea, slow respiratory rate, bradycardia, heart block, increased intracranial pressure with confusion, fever, paralysis, tissue hypoxia (from methemoglobinemia) leading to cyanosis, and metabolic acidosis, coma, clonic seizures, and circulatory collapse. Death may result from circulatory collapse or asphyxia.

Monitoring the patient

• Monitor blood pressure and intensity and duration of patient's response to drug.

• Evaluate cardiac status regularly.

Information for the patient

- Instruct patient to take drug regularly, as pre-scribed, and to keep S.L. form accessible at all times. Drug is physiologically necessary but not addictive.
- Teach patient to take oral tablet on empty stomach, either 30 minutes before or 1 to 2 hours after meals, to swallow oral tablets whole, and to chew chewable tablets thoroughly before swallowing.
- Instruct patient to take S.L. tablet at first sign of angina attack. Tell him to wet tablet with saliva, place it under the tongue until completely absorbed, and sit down and rest. If no relief occurs after three tablets, he should call or go to hospital emergency room. If he complains of tingling sensation with drug placed sublingually, he may try holding tablet in buccal pouch.
- Advise patient to store S.L. tablets in original container or other container specifically approved for this use away from heat and light. Keep bottle tightly closed.
- Instruct patient to place transmucosal tablet under upper lip or in buccal pouch, to let it dissolve slowly over a 3- to 5-hour period; don't chew or swallow tablet. Advise him that dissolution rate may increase if he touches tablet with tongue or drinks hot liquids.
- If patient is receiving nitroglycerin lingual aerosol (Nitrolingual), show him how to use this device correctly. Remind him not to inhale spray but to release it onto or under the tongue. Also tell him not to swallow immediately after administering spray but to wait about 10 seconds before swallowing.
- Caution patient to use care when wearing transdermal patch near microwave oven because leaking radiation may heat patch's metallic backing and cause burns.
- Warn patient that headache may follow initial doses but that this symptom may respond to usual headache remedies or dosage reduction. (However, dose should be reduced only with medical approval.) Assure patient that headache usually subsides gradually with continued treatment.
- Instruct patient to avoid alcohol while taking drug because severe hypotension and CV collapse may occur.
- Warn patient that drug may cause dizziness or flushing and to move to an upright position slowly.
- Tell patient to report blurred vision, dry mouth, or persistent headache.

Pediatric patients

- Methemoglobinemia may occur in infants receiving large doses of nitroglycerin.

nitroprusside sodium

Nipride*, Nitropress

Pharmacologic classification: vaso-dilator
Therapeutic classification: antihyper-tensive
Pregnancy risk category C

How supplied

Available by prescription only
Injection: 50 mg/2-ml, 50 mg/5-ml vials

Indications, route, and dosage

Hypertensive emergencies

Adults and children: I.V. infusion titrated to blood pressure, with a range of 0.3 to 10 mcg/kg/minute. Maximum infusion rate is 10 mcg/kg/minute for 10 minutes.

Acute heart failure

Adults and children: I.V. infusion titrated to cardiac output and systemic blood pressure. Same dosage range as for hypertensive emergencies.

Pharmacodynamics

Antihypertensive action: Acts directly on vascular smooth muscle, causing peripheral vasodilation.

Pharmacokinetics

- *Absorption:* Administered by I.V. route; I.V. infusion reduces blood pressure almost immediately.
- *Distribution:* No information available.
- *Metabolism:* Metabolized rapidly in erythrocytes and tissues to a cyanide radical and then converted to thiocyanate in liver.
- *Excretion:* Excreted primarily as metabolites in urine. Blood pressure returns to pretreatment level 1 to 10 minutes after completion of infusion.

Contraindications and precautions

Contraindicated in patients with hypersensitivity to drug and in those with compensatory hypertension (such as in arteriovenous shunt or coarctation of the aorta), inadequate cerebral circulation, congenital optic atrophy, or tobacco-induced amblyopia.

Use cautiously in patients with renal or hepatic disease, increased intracranial pressure, hypothyroidism, hyponatremia, or low vitamin B_{12} levels.

Interactions

Drug-drug. *General anesthetics (enflurane, halothane), other antihypertensives:* Potentiated antihypertensive effects. Monitor patient closely. *Pressor drugs (epinephrine):* Increased blood pressure during nitroprusside therapy. Don't use together.

Reactions may be *common*, uncommon, **life-threatening**, or COMMON AND LIFE-THREATENING.

Sildenafil: Potentiated hypotensive effects of nitrates. Don't use together.

Adverse reactions

CNS: *headache, dizziness, loss of consciousness, apprehension, **increased intracranial pressure,** restlessness.*
CV: ***bradycardia,** hypotension, tachycardia, palpitations, ECG changes.*
GI: *nausea, abdominal pain, ileus.*
Metabolic: *acidosis, **thiocyanate toxicity, methemoglobinemia, cyanide toxicity,** hypothyroidism, increased serum creatinine.*
Musculoskeletal: *muscle twitching.*
Skin: pink color, flushing, rash, diaphoresis.
Other: *venous streaking, irritation at infusion site.*

☑ Special considerations

• Ask all male patients about the use of sildenafil (Viagra) before using nitrates.
• Prepare solution using D_5W solution; don't use bacteriostatic water for injection or sterile saline solution for reconstitution; because of light sensitivity, foil-wrap I.V. solution (but not tubing). Fresh solutions have faint brownish tint; discard after 24 hours.
• Infuse drug with infusion pump.
• Drug is best run piggyback through a peripheral line with no other drugs; don't adjust rate of main I.V. line while drug is running because even small boluses can cause severe hypotension.
• Drug also may be used to produce controlled hypotension during anesthesia to reduce bleeding from surgical procedure.
• Hypertensive patients are more sensitive to nitroprusside than normotensive patients. Also, patients taking other antihypertensives are extremely sensitive to nitroprusside. Nitroprusside has been used in patients with acute MI, refractory heart failure, and severe mitral regurgitation.
• Signs and symptoms of overdose include the adverse reactions listed above and increased tolerance to the drug's antihypertensive effects.
• Treat overdose by giving nitrites to induce methemoglobin formation. Stop drug and administer amyl nitrite inhalations for 15 to 30 seconds each minute until a 3% sodium nitrite solution can be prepared. Then administer the sodium nitrite solution by I.V. infusion at a rate not exceeding 2.5 to 5 ml/minute up to a total dose of 10 to 15 ml. Then give I.V. sodium thiosulfate infusion (12.5 g in 50 ml of D_5W solution) over 10 minutes. If necessary, repeat infusions of sodium nitrite and sodium thiosulfate at half the initial doses.

Monitoring the patient

• Check blood pressure at least every 5 minutes at start of infusion and every 15 minutes thereafter during infusion.

• Drug can cause cyanide toxicity. Check serum thiocyanate levels every 72 hours; levels above 100 mcg/ml are associated with cyanide toxicity, which can produce profound hypotension, metabolic acidosis, dyspnea, ataxia, and vomiting. If such symptoms occur, stop infusion and reevaluate therapy.

Information for the patient

• Warn patient to report CNS symptoms (such as headache or dizziness) promptly.

Geriatric patients

• Elderly patients may be more sensitive to drug's antihypertensive effects.

Breast-feeding patients

• It's unknown if drug appears in breast milk; use with caution in breast-feeding women.

nizatidine
Axid, Axid AR

Pharmacologic classification: H_2-receptor antagonist
Therapeutic classification: antiulcerative
Pregnancy risk category B

How supplied

Available by prescription only
Capsules: 150 mg, 300 mg
Available without a prescription
Capsules: 75 mg

Indications, route, and dosage

Treatment of active duodenal ulcer
Adults: 300 mg P.O. once daily h.s. Or may give 150 mg P.O. b.i.d.
Maintenance therapy for duodenal ulcer patients
Adults: 150 mg P.O. once daily h.s.
Gastroesophageal reflux disease
Adults: 150 mg P.O. b.i.d.
Heartburn (self-medication)
Adults: One 75-mg capsule P.O. ½ hour before meals; use up to b.i.d.
✦ ***Dosage adjustment.*** For adults with renal impairment, refer to the table.

Creatinine clearance (ml/min)	Active duodenal ulcer	Maintenance
20 to 50	150 mg/day	150 mg q other day
< 20	150 mg q other day	150 mg q 3 days

Pharmacodynamics
Antiulcerative action: Competitive, reversible inhibitor of H_2 receptors, particularly those in the gastric parietal cells.

Pharmacokinetics
• *Absorption:* More than 90% absorbed after oral administration. Absorption slightly enhanced by food; slightly impaired by antacids.
• *Distribution:* About 35% bound to plasma protein. Plasma levels peak in ½ to 3 hours.
• *Metabolism:* Probable hepatic metabolism. About 40% of excreted drug metabolized; remainder excreted unchanged.
• *Excretion:* More than 90% excreted in urine within 12 hours. Renal clearance is about 500 ml/minute, indicating excretion by active tubular secretion. Less than 6% of dose eliminated in feces. Elimination half-life is 1 to 2 hours. Moderate to severe renal impairment significantly prolongs half-life and decreases clearance. In anephric persons, half-life is 3½ to 11 hours; plasma clearance is 7 to 14 L/hour.

Contraindications and precautions
Contraindicated in patients with hypersensitivity to H_2 receptor antagonists. Use cautiously in patients with impaired renal function.

Interactions
Drug-drug. *High doses of aspirin (3,900 mg/day) with nizatidine (150 mg b.i.d.):* Increased serum salicylate levels. Avoid using together.
Drug-lifestyle. *Smoking:* May increase gastric acid secretion. Encourage patient not to smoke.

Adverse reactions
CNS: somnolence.
CV: *arrhythmias.*
Hematologic: eosinophilia.
Hepatic: hepatocellular injury, elevated liver function test results.
Metabolic: hyperuricemia.
Skin: *diaphoresis,* rash, urticaria.
Other: fever.

☑ Special considerations
• Because drug is excreted primarily by kidneys, reduce dosage in patients with moderate to severe renal insufficiency.
• Drug is partially metabolized in liver. In patients with normal renal function and uncomplicated hepatic dysfunction, the disposition of nizatidine is similar to that in patients with normal hepatic function.
• For patients on maintenance therapy, consider that effects of continuous drug therapy for over 1 year are unknown.
• False-positive tests for urobilinogen may occur during therapy.
• Toxicity may cause lacrimation, salivation, emesis, miosis, and diarrhea.

Monitoring the patient
• Monitor renal and hepatic functions.
• Monitor cardiac status regularly.

Information for the patient
• Advise patient not to smoke; this may increase gastric acid secretion and worsen disease.

Geriatric patients
• Safety and efficacy appear similar to those in younger patients. However, consider that elderly patients have reduced renal function.

Pediatric patients
• Safety and efficacy in children haven't been established.

Breast-feeding patients
• Drug may appear in breast milk. Use with caution in breast-feeding women.

norepinephrine bitartrate (levarterenol bitartrate)
Levophed

Pharmacologic classification: adrenergic (direct-acting)
Therapeutic classification: vasopressor
Pregnancy risk category C

How supplied
Available by prescription only
Injection: 1 mg/ml parenteral

Indications, route, and dosage
To maintain blood pressure in acute hypotensive states
Adults: Initially, 8 to 12 mcg/minute I.V. infusion, then titrated to maintain desired blood pressure; maintenance dose is 2 to 4 mcg/minute.
Children: Initially, 2 mcg/minute or 2 mcg/m²/minute I.V. infusion, then titrated to maintain desired blood pressure. For advanced cardiac life support, initial infusion rate is 0.1 mcg/kg/minute.
◊ *GI bleeding*
Adults: 8 mg in 250 ml normal saline solution given intraperitoneally, or 8 mg in 100 ml normal saline solution given via a nasogastric tube q hour for 6 to 8 hours, then q 2 hours for 4 to 6 hours.

Pharmacodynamics
Vasopressor action: Acts predominantly by direct stimulation of alpha-adrenergic receptors, constricting both capacitance and resistance blood vessels. That results in increased total peripheral resistance; increased systolic and diastolic blood pressure; decreased blood flow to vital organs, skin, and skeletal muscle; and constriction of renal blood vessels, which reduces

---

Reactions may be *common,* uncommon, **life-threatening,** or COMMON AND LIFE-THREATENING.

renal blood flow. Also has a direct stimulating effect on beta$_1$ receptors of the heart, producing a positive inotropic response. Main therapeutic effects are vasoconstriction and cardiac stimulation.

Pharmacokinetics
• *Absorption:* Pressor effect occurs rapidly after infusion, is of short duration, and stops within 1 to 2 minutes after infusion is stopped.
• *Distribution:* Localizes in sympathetic nerve tissues; crosses placenta but not blood-brain barrier.
• *Metabolism:* Metabolized in liver and other tissues to inactive compounds.
• *Excretion:* Excreted in urine primarily as sulfate and glucuronide conjugates; small amounts excreted unchanged in urine.

Contraindications and precautions
Contraindicated in patients with mesenteric or peripheral vascular thrombosis, profound hypoxia, hypercapnia, or hypotension resulting from blood volume deficit, and during cyclopropane and halothane anesthesia.
    Use cautiously in patients with sulfite allergies or in those receiving MAO inhibitors or triptyline- or imipramine-type antidepressants.

Interactions
Drug-drug. *Atropine:* Blocked reflex bradycardia caused by norepinephrine and enhanced pressor effects. This may have therapeutic advantage.
Beta blockers: Increased potential for hypertension. Use together cautiously.
Furosemide, other diuretics: Decreased arterial responsiveness. Use together cautiously.
General anesthetics: Increased arrhythmias. Monitor patient closely.
Guanethidine, MAO inhibitors, methyldopa, parenteral ergot alkaloids, some antihistamines, tricyclic antidepressants: Severe, prolonged hypertension. Use together cautiously.

Adverse reactions
CNS: anxiety, weakness, dizziness, tremor, restlessness, insomnia.
CV: *bradycardia, severe hypertension, arrhythmias.*
Respiratory: respiratory difficulties, *asthmatic episodes.*
Skin: irritation or necrosis with extravasation.
Other: *anaphylaxis.*

☑ Special considerations
Besides the recommendations relevant to all adrenergics, consider the following.
• Correct blood volume depletion before administration. Norepinephrine isn't a substitute for blood, plasma, fluid, or electrolyte replacement.

• Select injection site carefully. Administration by I.V. infusion requires an infusion pump or other device to control flow rate. If possible, infuse into antecubital vein of arm or femoral vein. Change injection sites for prolonged therapy. Drug must be diluted before use with 5% dextrose or with saline. (Dilution with saline alone not recommended.) Monitor infusion rate. Withdraw drug gradually; recurrent hypotension may follow abrupt withdrawal.
• Prepare infusion solution by adding 4 mg norepinephrine to 1 L of 5% dextrose. The resultant solution contains 4 mcg/ml.
• To treat extravasation, infiltrate site promptly with 10 to 15 ml saline solution containing 5 to 10 mg phentolamine, using a fine needle.
• Some clinicians add phentolamine (5 to 10 mg) to each liter of infusion solution to prevent sloughing should extravasation occur.
• In patients with previously normal blood pressure, adjust flow rate to maintain blood pressure at low normal (usually 80 to 100 mm Hg systolic); in hypertensive patients, maintain systolic no more than 40 mm Hg below preexisting pressure level.
• Protect solution from light. Discard solution that is discolored or contains a precipitate.
• Toxicity may cause severe hypertension, photophobia, retrosternal or pharyngeal pain, intense sweating, vomiting, cerebral hemorrhage, seizures, and arrhythmias. Treatment includes supportive and symptomatic measures. Use atropine for reflex bradycardia, phentolamine for extravasation, and propranolol for tachyarrhythmias.

Monitoring the patient
• Monitor intake and output. Norepinephrine reduces renal blood flow, which may cause decreased urine output initially.
• Monitor patient constantly during drug administration. Obtain baseline blood pressure and pulse before therapy, and repeat every 2 minutes until stabilization; repeat every 5 minutes during drug administration.
• In addition to vital signs, monitor patient's mental state, skin temperature of extremities, and skin color (especially earlobes, lips, and nail beds).

Information for the patient
• Inform patient of need for frequent monitoring of vital signs.
• Tell patient to report adverse reactions.

Geriatric patients
• Elderly patients are more sensitive to drug's effects. Decreased cardiac output may be harmful to elderly patients with poor cerebral or coronary circulation.

Pediatric patients
• Use with caution in children.

norethindrone
Micronor, Nor-Q.D.

norethindrone acetate
Aygestin, Norlutate*

Pharmacologic classification: progestin
Therapeutic classification: contraceptive
Pregnancy risk category X

How supplied
Available by prescription only
norethindrone
Tablets: 0.35 mg
norethindrone acetate
Tablets: 5 mg

Indications, route, and dosage
Amenorrhea, abnormal uterine bleeding, endometriosis
norethindrone acetate
Adults: 2.5 to 10 mg P.O. daily on days 5 to 10 of second half of menstrual cycle or on days 5 through 25 of menstrual cycle.
Endometriosis
norethindrone acetate
Adults: 5 mg P.O. daily for 14 days, then increase by 2.5 mg/day q 2 weeks up to 15 mg/day. Daily therapy may be continued consecutively for 6 to 9 months; if breakthrough bleeding occurs, therapy should be temporarily stopped.
Contraception
Adults: 0.35 mg norethindrone P.O. daily, beginning on day 1 of menstrual cycle and continuing uninterrupted thereafter.

Pharmacodynamics
Contraceptive action: Suppresses ovulation, causes thickening of cervical mucus, and induces sloughing of the endometrium.

Pharmacokinetics
• *Absorption:* Well absorbed after oral administration.
• *Distribution:* Distributed into bile and breast milk; is about 80% protein-bound.
• *Metabolism:* Primarily metabolized in liver; undergoes extensive first-pass metabolism.
• *Excretion:* Excreted primarily in feces. Elimination half-life is 5 to 14 hours.

Contraindications and precautions
Contraindicated in patients with hypersensitivity to drug and in those with thromboembolic disorders, cerebral apoplexy, or history of these conditions; breast cancer; undiagnosed abnormal vaginal bleeding; severe hepatic disease; or missed abortion; and during pregnancy.

Use cautiously in patients with diabetes mellitus, seizures, migraine, cardiac or renal disease, asthma, or mental depression.

Interactions
None reported.

Adverse reactions
CNS: depression.
CV: thrombophlebitis, *pulmonary embolism,* edema, *thromboembolism, CVA.*
EENT: exophthalmos, diplopia, retinal thrombosis.
GU: breakthrough bleeding, dysmenorrhea, amenorrhea, cervical erosion, abnormal secretions, breast tenderness, enlargement, or secretion.
Hepatic: cholestatic jaundice, increased serum alkaline phosphatase and amino acid levels.
Metabolic: changes in weight, decreased pregnanediol excretion, glucose tolerance.
Skin: melasma, rash, acne, pruritus.

☑ Special considerations
• Recommendations for administration of norethindrone, and for care and teaching of the patient during therapy, are the same as those for all progestins.
• Norethindrone acetate is twice as potent as norethindrone. Norethindrone acetate shouldn't be used for contraception.

Monitoring the patient
• Monitor patient for signs of edema.
• Monitor blood pressure.

Information for the patient
• Tell patient that FDA regulations require that, before receiving first dose, patient read package insert explaining possible adverse effects of progestin. Also give patient verbal explanation.
• Tell patient to report unusual symptoms immediately and to stop drug and call if visual disturbance or migraine occurs.
• Teach patient how to perform routine monthly breast self-examinations.
• Inform patient what to do if a dose is missed.

norfloxacin
Noroxin

Pharmacologic classification: fluoroquinolone
Therapeutic classification: broad-spectrum antibiotic
Pregnancy risk category C

How supplied
Available by prescription only
Tablets: 400 mg

Indications, route, and dosage

Complicated and uncomplicated urinary tract infections caused by various gram-negative and gram-positive bacteria

Adults: For complicated infection, 400 mg P.O. b.i.d. for 10 to 21 days; for uncomplicated infection, 400 mg P.O. b.i.d. for 3 to 10 days. Don't exceed 800 mg/day. Patients with creatinine clearance below 30 ml/minute should receive 400 mg/day for appropriate duration of therapy.

Uncomplicated gonorrhea

Adults: 800 mg P.O. as a single dose.

Prostatitis

Adults: 400 mg P.O. q 12 hours for 28 days.

◇ **Gastroenteritis**

Adults: 400 mg P.O. b.i.d. for 5 days.

◇ **Traveler's diarrhea**

Adults: 400 mg P.O. b.i.d. for up to 3 days.

Pharmacodynamics

Antibacterial action: Generally bactericidal. Inhibits DNA gyrase, blocking DNA synthesis. Spectrum of activity includes most aerobic gram-positive and gram-negative urinary pathogens, including *Pseudomonas aeruginosa.*

Pharmacokinetics

- *Absorption:* About 30% to 40% absorbed from GI tract; as dose increases, percentage of absorbed drug decreases. Food may reduce absorption.
- *Distribution:* Distributed into renal tissue, liver, gallbladder, prostatic fluid, testicles, seminal fluid, bile, and sputum. From 10% to 15% binds to plasma proteins.
- *Metabolism:* No information available.
- *Excretion:* Most of systemically absorbed drug is excreted by kidneys, with about 30% appearing in feces. In patients with normal renal function, plasma half-life is 3 to 4 hours; up to 8 hours in severe renal impairment.

Contraindications and precautions

Contraindicated in patients with hypersensitivity to fluoroquinolones. Use cautiously in patients with renal impairment or conditions predisposing them to seizure disorders, such as cerebral arteriosclerosis.

Interactions

Drug-drug. *Antacids:* Decreased absorption. Separate administration times by 2 hours.

Multivitamins containing divalent or trivalent cations: Interfered with absorption of norfloxacin. Separate administration times.

Nitrofurantoin: Decreased norfloxacin antibacterial activity. Avoid using together.

Probenecid: Increased serum norfloxacin levels. Monitor patient for toxicity.

Warfarin: Prolonged PT and INR. Monitor PT and INR.

Xanthine derivatives (aminophylline, theophylline): Increased theophylline levels. Monitor patient for toxicity.

Drug-food. *Any food:* Interfered with norfloxacin absorption. Give drug 1 hour before or 2 hours after meals.

Drug-lifestyle. *Sun exposure:* Possible photosensitivity reaction. Tell patient to take precautions.

Adverse reactions

CNS: fatigue, somnolence, headache, dizziness, **seizures,** depression, insomnia.

GI: nausea, constipation, flatulence, heartburn, dry mouth, abdominal pain, diarrhea, vomiting, anorexia.

GU: increased serum creatinine and BUN levels, crystalluria.

Hematologic: eosinophilia, **neutropenia,** decreased hematocrit.

Hepatic: transient elevations of AST, ALT, and alkaline phosphatase.

Musculoskeletal: back pain, tendinitis.

Skin: photosensitivity.

Other: hypersensitivity reactions (rash, **anaphylactoid reaction**), fever; hyperhidrosis.

☑ Special considerations

- Obtain culture and sensitivity tests before starting therapy, and repeat as needed throughout therapy.
- Make sure patient is well hydrated before and during therapy to avoid crystalluria.

Monitoring the patient

- Arrange for baseline and follow-up BUN and creatinine clearance level determinations, CBC, and liver function tests.
- Evaluate patient for signs and symptoms of resistant infection or reinfection.

Information for the patient

- Instruct patient to continue taking drug as directed, even if he feels better.
- Advise patient to take drug 1 hour before or 2 hours after meals and antacids.
- Warn patient that drug may cause dizziness that impairs his ability to perform tasks that require alertness and coordination.
- Instruct patient to avoid excessive exposure to sunlight.

Pediatric patients

- Contraindicated in children because of risk of arthropathy.

Breast-feeding patients

- Safety hasn't been established; alternative to breast-feeding is recommended during therapy. It's unknown if drug appears in breast milk.

norgestrel
Ovrette

Pharmacologic classification: progestin
Therapeutic classification: contraceptive
Pregnancy risk category X

How supplied
Available by prescription only
Tablets: 0.075 mg

Indications, route, and dosage
Contraception
Adults: 1 tablet P.O. daily, beginning on first day of menstruation.

Pharmacodynamics
Contraceptive action: Suppresses ovulation and causes thickening of cervical mucus.

Pharmacokinetics
• *Absorption:* Well absorbed after oral administration.
• *Distribution:* No information available.
• *Metabolism:* No information available.
• *Excretion:* No information available.

Contraindications and precautions
Contraindicated in patients with hypersensitivity to drug and in those with thromboembolic disorders, cerebral apoplexy, or history of these conditions; breast cancer; undiagnosed abnormal vaginal bleeding; severe hepatic disease; missed abortion; and during pregnancy.
   Use cautiously in patients with renal or cardiac disease, diabetes mellitus, migraine, seizures, asthma, or mental depression.

Interactions
None reported.

Adverse reactions
CNS: cerebral thrombosis or hemorrhage, migraine, depression.
CV: thrombophlebitis, *pulmonary embolism,* edema, *thromboembolism, CVA.*
EENT: exophthalmos, diplopia.
GU: *breakthrough bleeding, change in menstrual flow,* dysmenorrhea, spotting, amenorrhea, cervical erosion, breast tenderness, enlargement, or secretion.
Hepatic: cholestatic jaundice, increased serum alkaline phosphatase and amino acid levels.
Metabolic: changes in weight, decreased pregnanediol excretion, glucose tolerance.
Skin: melasma, rash, acne, pruritus.

☑ Special considerations
Besides the recommendations relevant to all progestins, consider the following.

• Failure rate of progestin-only contraceptive is about three times higher than that of combination contraceptives.
• Ovrette tablets contain tartrazine. Use cautiously in patients with tartrazine or aspirin sensitivity.
• Pregnanediol excretion may decrease; serum alkaline phosphatase and amino acid levels may increase. Glucose tolerance has been shown to decrease in a small percentage of patients receiving drug.

Monitoring the patient
• Monitor patient for adverse effects.
• Evaluate patient's compliance with therapy; suggest alternative contraception as indicated.

Information for the patient
• Tell patient to take drug at same time every day, even during menstruation. Norgestrel is also known as the "minipill."
• Advise patient of increased risk of serious CV adverse reactions associated with heavy smoking, especially while taking oral contraceptives.
• Tell patient that risk of pregnancy increases with each tablet missed. If one tablet is missed, she should take it as soon as she remembers and then take the next tablet at the regular time. If two tablets are missed, she should take one as soon as she remembers and then take the next regular dose at the usual time; she should use a nonhormonal method of contraception in addition to norgestrel until 14 tablets have been taken. If three or more tablets are missed, she should stop drug and use a nonhormonal method of contraception until after her period. Instruct patient to have a pregnancy test if her menstrual period doesn't occur within 45 days.
• Advise patient to report excessive bleeding or bleeding between menstrual cycles immediately.
• Instruct patient to use a second method of birth control for the first cycle on norgestrel, or for 3 weeks after starting the hormonal contraceptive, to ensure full protection.
• Advise patient who wishes to become pregnant to wait at least 3 months after stopping norgestrel to prevent birth defects.

Breast-feeding patients
• Drug appears in breast milk. If possible, advise breast-feeding patient not to use oral contraceptives until infant is completely weaned; drug may interfere with lactation by decreasing quantity and quality of breast milk. Recommend other means of contraception.

nortriptyline hydrochloride
Aventyl, Pamelor

Pharmacologic classification: tricyclic antidepressant
Therapeutic classification: antidepressant
Pregnancy risk category NR

How supplied
Available by prescription only
Capsules: 10 mg, 25 mg, 50 mg, 75 mg
Solution: 10 mg/5 ml (4% alcohol)

Indications, route, and dosage
Depression, ◇ panic disorder
Adults: 25 mg P.O. t.i.d. or q.i.d., gradually increasing to a maximum of 150 mg/day. Or entire dose may be given h.s.
Elderly or adolescents: 30 to 50 mg P.O. daily or in divided doses.

Pharmacodynamics
Antidepressant action: Thought to exert antidepressant effects by inhibiting reuptake of norepinephrine and serotonin in CNS nerve terminals (presynaptic neurons), which results in increased levels and enhanced activity of these neurotransmitters in the synaptic cleft. Inhibits reuptake of serotonin more actively than norepinephrine. Less likely than other tricyclic antidepressants to cause orthostatic hypotension.

Pharmacokinetics
• *Absorption:* Absorbed rapidly from GI tract after oral administration.
• *Distribution:* Distributed widely into body, including CNS and breast milk. 95% protein-bound. Plasma levels peak within 8 hours; steady-state serum levels achieved within 2 to 4 weeks. Therapeutic serum level ranges from 50 to 150 ng/ml.
• *Metabolism:* Metabolized by liver; significant first-pass effect may account for variability of serum levels in different patients taking same dosage.
• *Excretion:* Mostly excreted in urine; some in feces, via biliary tract.

Contraindications and precautions
Contraindicated in patients with hypersensitivity to drug, during acute recovery phase of MI, and within 14 days of MAO therapy. Use cautiously in patients with history of urine retention or seizures, glaucoma, suicidal tendencies, CV disease, or hyperthyroidism and in those receiving thyroid drugs.

Interactions
Drug-drug. *Antiarrhythmics (disopyramide, procainamide, quinidine), pimozide, thyroid drugs:* Increased arrhythmias and conduction defects. Use together with extreme caution; monitor ECG.
Atropine, other anticholinergics (such as antihistamines, antiparkinsonians, meperidine, phenothiazines): Additive effects. Watch for oversedation, paralytic ileus, visual changes, and severe constipation.
Barbiturates, haloperidol, phenothiazines: Decreased therapeutic efficacy. Monitor patient closely.
Beta blockers, cimetidine, methylphenidate, oral contraceptives, propoxyphene, quinolone antibiotics: Increased nortriptyline plasma levels. Monitor patient for toxicity.
Clonidine, guanabenz, guanadrel, guanethidine, methyldopa, reserpine: Decreased hypotensive effects of these drugs. Monitor blood pressure.
CNS depressants (such as analgesics, anesthetics, barbiturates, narcotics, tranquilizers): Additive effects. Monitor patient for increased sedation.
Disulfiram, ethchlorvynol: Delirium and tachycardia. Avoid using together.
MAO inhibitors: Hypertensive crises. Avoid concomitant use.
Metrizamide: Increased risk of seizures. Monitor patient closely.
Sympathomimetics (such as ephedrine, epinephrine, phenylephrine, phenylpropanolamine): Increased blood pressure. Use together cautiously.
Warfarin: Increased PT and INR. Monitor PT and INR.
Drug-lifestyle. *Alcohol:* Additive effects. Discourage use.
Heavy smoking: Decreased therapeutic efficacy. Discourage smoking.
Sun exposure: Increased risk of photosensitivity reaction. Tell patient to take precautions.

Adverse reactions
CNS: *drowsiness, dizziness, **seizures,** tremor,* weakness, confusion, headache, nervousness, EEG changes, extrapyramidal reactions, insomnia, nightmares, hallucinations, paresthesia, ataxia, agitation.
CV: *tachycardia,* hypertension, hypotension, ***MI, heart block, stroke;*** prolonged conduction time (elongation of QT and PR intervals, flattened T waves on ECG).
EENT: *blurred vision,* tinnitus, mydriasis.
GI: dry mouth, *constipation,* nausea, vomiting, anorexia, paralytic ileus.
GU: *urine retention.*
Hematologic: ***bone marrow depression, agranulocytosis,*** eosinophilia, **thrombocytopenia.**
Hepatic: elevated liver function test results.
Metabolic: increased serum glucose levels.
Skin: rash, urticaria, photosensitivity, *diaphoresis.*
Other: ***hypersensitivity reaction.***

After abrupt withdrawal of long-term therapy: nausea, headache, malaise (doesn't indicate addiction).

☑ Special considerations
Besides the recommendations relevant to all tricyclic antidepressants, consider the following.
• Drug may be administered at bedtime to reduce daytime sedation. Tolerance to sedative effects usually develops over the initial weeks of therapy.
• Withdraw drug gradually over a few weeks; however, discontinue at least 48 hours before surgical procedures.
• Drug is available in liquid form.
• In patients with bipolar disorders, drug may cause manic phase symptoms to emerge.
• Toxicity in the first 12 hours is characterized by excessive anticholinergic activity (agitation, irritation, confusion, hallucinations, hyperthermia, parkinsonian symptoms, seizures, urine retention, dry mucous membranes, pupillary dilation, constipation, and ileus). Then CNS depressant effects, including hypothermia, decreased or absent reflexes, sedation, hypotension, cyanosis, and cardiac irregularities, including tachycardia, conduction disturbances, and quinidine-like effects on the ECG.
• Severity of overdose is best indicated by prolonging QRS complex beyond 100 milliseconds, which usually indicates a serum level above 1,000 ng/ml. Metabolic acidosis may follow hypotension, hypoventilation, and seizures.
• In the case of overdose, dialysis is usually ineffective in removing drug. Consider giving cardiac glycosides or physostigmine if serious CV abnormalities or cardiac failure occurs. Treat seizures with parenteral diazepam or phenytoin, arrhythmias with parenteral phenytoin or lidocaine, and acidosis with sodium bicarbonate. Don't use quinidine, procainamide or disopyramide to treat arrhythmias because these drugs can further depress myocardial conduction and contractility. Don't give barbiturates, which may enhance CNS and respiratory depressant effects.

Monitoring the patient
• Monitor patient for mood changes, signs of psychosis, and suicidal tendencies.
• Monitor hematologic studies, serum glucose, and hepatic enzymes.

Information for the patient
• Explain that patient may not see full effects of drug for up to 4 weeks after start of therapy.
• Warn patient about sedative effects.
• Recommend taking full daily dose at bedtime to prevent daytime sedation.
• Instruct patient to avoid drinking alcoholic beverages, doubling doses after missing one, and stopping drug abruptly, unless instructed.

• Warn patient about possible dizziness. Tell patient to lie down for about 30 minutes after each dose at start of therapy and to avoid sudden orthostatic changes. Orthostatic hypotension is usually less severe than with amitriptyline.
• Urge patient to promptly report unusual reactions, such as confusion, movement disorders, fainting, rapid heartbeat, or difficulty urinating.
• Tell patient to store drug away from children.
• Suggest relieving dry mouth with sugarless gum or candy.
• Advise patient to avoid activities that require physical and mental alertness, such as driving or operating machinery

Geriatric patients
• Lower dosages may be indicated. Elderly patients are at greater risk for adverse cardiac effects. Nortriptyline is less likely to cause hypotension than other tricyclic antidepressants.

Pediatric patients
• Drug isn't recommended for children. Lower dosages may be indicated for adolescents.

Breast-feeding patients
• Low levels of drug appear in breast milk; potential benefit to mother should outweigh potential harm to infant.

nystatin
Mycostatin, Nilstat, Nystex

Pharmacologic classification: polyene macrolide
Therapeutic classification: antifungal
Pregnancy risk category B

How supplied
Available by prescription only
Tablets: 500,000 units
Suspension: 100,000 units/ml
Vaginal tablets: 100,000 units
Cream: 100,000 units/g
Ointment: 100,000 units/g
Powder: 100,000 units/g
Lozenges: 200,000 units

Indications, route, and dosage
GI infections
Adults: 500,000 to 1 million units as oral tablets, t.i.d.
Oral, vaginal, and intestinal infections caused by susceptible organisms
Adults: 500,000 to 1 million units of oral suspension t.i.d. for oral candidiasis. Or give 200,000 to 400,000 units (lozenges) four to five times daily; allow to dissolve in mouth.
Children and infants over age 3 months: 250,000 to 500,000 units of oral suspension q.i.d.

Newborn and premature infants: 100,000 units of oral suspension q.i.d.

Cutaneous or mucocutaneous candidal infections

Topical use: Apply to affected areas b.i.d. or t.i.d. until healing is complete.

Vaginal use: 100,000 units, as vaginal tablets, inserted high into vagina daily or b.i.d. for 14 days.

Pharmacodynamics

Antifungal action: Fungistatic and fungicidal. Binds to sterols in the fungal cell membrane, altering its permeability and allowing leakage of intracellular components. Acts against various yeasts and fungi, including *Candida albicans.*

Pharmacokinetics

• *Absorption:* Not absorbed from GI tract, nor through intact skin or mucous membranes.
• *Distribution:* No detectable amount available for tissue distribution.
• *Metabolism:* No detectable amount systemically available for metabolism.
• *Excretion:* Oral drug excreted almost entirely unchanged in feces.

Contraindications and precautions

Contraindicated in patients with hypersensitivity to drug.

Interactions

None reported.

Adverse reactions

GI: transient nausea, diarrhea (usually with large oral dosage), vomiting (with oral administration or vaginal tablets).
Skin: occasional contact dermatitis from preservatives in some forms (with topical administration or vaginal tablets).

☑ Special considerations

• Vaginal tablets may be used by pregnant women up to 6 weeks before term.
• Avoid hand contact with drug; hypersensitivity is rare but can occur.
• For treatment of oral candidiasis, patient should have clean mouth and should hold suspension in mouth for several minutes before swallowing; for infant thrush, drug should be swabbed on oral mucosa.
• May give immunosuppressed patient vaginal tablets (100,000 units) P.O. to provide prolonged drug contact with oral mucosa; or use clotrimazole troche.
• For candidiasis of feet, patient should dust powder on shoes and stockings as well as feet for maximal contact and effectiveness.
• Avoid occlusive dressings or ointment on moist covered body areas that favor yeast growth.
• To prevent maceration, use cream on intertriginous areas and powder on moist lesions.

• Clean affected skin gently before topical application; cool, moist compresses applied for 15 minutes between applications help soothe dry skin.
• Cleansing douches may be used by nonpregnant women if desired; they should use preparations that don't contain antibacterials, which may alter flora and promote reinfection.
• Protect drug from light, air, and heat.
• Drug is ineffective in systemic fungal infection.
• Drug overdose may result in nausea, vomiting, and diarrhea.

Monitoring the patient

• Monitor patient for therapeutic effect.

Information for the patient

• Teach patient signs and symptoms of candidal infection. Inform patient about predisposing factors, including use of antibiotics, oral contraceptives, and corticosteroids; diabetes; infected sexual partners; and tight-fitting pantyhose and undergarments.
• Teach good oral hygiene. Explain that overuse of mouthwash and poorly fitting dentures, especially in elderly patients, may alter flora and promote infection.
• Tell patient to continue using vaginal cream through menstruation; emphasize importance of washing applicator thoroughly after each use.
• Advise patient to change stockings and undergarments daily; teach good skin care.
• Teach patient how to administer each dosage form prescribed.
• Tell patient to continue drug for at least 48 hours after symptoms clear to prevent reinfection.

Breast-feeding patients

• It's unknown if drug appears in breast milk. Safety in breast-feeding patients hasn't been established.

octreotide acetate
Sandostatin

Pharmacologic classification: synthetic octapeptide
Therapeutic classification: somatotropic hormone
Pregnancy risk category B

How supplied
Available by prescription only
Injection: 0.05 mg/ml, 0.1 mg/ml, and 0.5 mg/ml in 1-ml ampules; 0.2 mg/ml and 1 mg/ml in 5-ml multidose vials

Indications, route, and dosage
Symptomatic treatment of flushing and diarrhea associated with carcinoid tumors
Adults: Initially, 100 to 600 mcg daily S.C. in two to four divided doses for first 2 weeks of therapy (usual daily dose is 300 mcg). Subsequent dosage based on individual response.
Symptomatic treatment of watery diarrhea associated with vasoactive intestinal peptide-secreting tumors (VIPomas)
Adults: Initially, 200 to 300 mcg daily S.C. in two to four divided doses for first 2 weeks of therapy. Subsequent dosage based on individual response, but usually won't exceed 450 mcg daily.
Acromegaly
Adults: Initially, 50 mcg t.i.d. S.C. Subsequent dosage based on individual response. Usual dosage is 100 mcg S.C. t.i.d., but some patients may require up to 500 mcg t.i.d. for maximum effectiveness.
◊ **Decrease output of rectal or pancreatic fistulas**
Adults: 50 to 200 mcg S.C. q 8 hours.
◊ **Variceal bleeding**
Adults: 25 to 50 mcg/hour via a continuous I.V. infusion.
◊ **Diarrheal states**
Adults: 100 to 500 mcg S.C. t.i.d.
◊ **Irritable bowel syndrome**
Adults: 100 mcg S.C. as a single dose to 125 mcg S.C. b.i.d.
◊ **Dumping syndrome**
Adults: 50 to 150 mcg S.C. daily.

Pharmacodynamics
Antidiarrheal action: Mimics the action of naturally occurring somatostatin and decreases the secretion of gastroenterohepatic peptides that may contribute to the adverse signs and symptoms seen in patients with metastatic carcinoid tumors and VIPomas. Unknown if drug affects the tumor directly.

Pharmacokinetics
• *Absorption:* Absorbed rapidly and completely after injection. Plasma levels peak in less than 30 minutes.
• *Distribution:* Distributed to plasma, where it binds to serum lipoprotein and albumin.
• *Metabolism:* Eliminated from plasma at a slower rate than naturally occurring hormone. Apparent half-life is about 1½ hours; effect lasts up to 12 hours.
• *Excretion:* About 35% of drug appears unchanged in urine.

Contraindications and precautions
Contraindicated in patients with hypersensitivity to drug or its components.

Interactions
Drug-drug. *Beta blockers, calcium channel blockers, electrolyte-controlling drugs, insulin, oral antidiabetics (sulfonylureas), oral diazoxide:* Altered absorption. May require dosage adjustments.
Cyclosporine: Decreased plasma levels of cyclosporine. Monitor cyclosporine level.

Adverse reactions
CNS: dizziness, light-headedness, fatigue, headache.
CV: *sinus bradycardia,* conduction abnormalities, *arrhythmias.*
EENT: blurred vision.
GI: *nausea, diarrhea, abdominal pain* or *discomfort, loose stools,* vomiting, fat malabsorption, gallstones or biliary sludge, flatulence, constipation.
GU: pollakiuria, urinary tract infection.
Metabolic: hyperglycemia, hypoglycemia, hypothyroidism, suppressed secretion of growth hormone and of gastroenterohepatic peptides gastrin, glucagon, insulin, motilin, pancreatic polypeptide, secretin, and VIP.
Musculoskeletal: backache, joint pain.
Skin: flushing, edema, wheals, erythema or pain at injection site, alopecia, pain or burning at the S.C. injection site.
Other: flulike symptoms.

Reactions may be *common,* uncommon, **life-threatening,** or COMMON AND LIFE-THREATENING.

☑ Special considerations

• Fluid and electrolyte balance may be altered after initiation of octreotide therapy.
• Half-life may be altered in patients with end-stage renal failure who are undergoing dialysis. Dosage adjustment may be necessary.
• Patients with acromegaly are more likely to experience GI side effects and bradycardia. Monitor patient closely.

Monitoring the patient

• Obtain baseline and periodic tests of thyroid function because drug's long-term effects on hypothalamic-pituitary function aren't known.
• Monitor laboratory values during therapy, such as urinary 5-hydroxyindoleacetic acid, plasma serotonin, plasma substance P for carcinoid tumors, and plasma VIP for VIPomas.
• Mild, transient hypoglycemia or hyperglycemia may occur during therapy. Observe patient for signs of glucose imbalance and monitor closely.
• Drug may alter fat absorption and aggravate fat malabsorption. Perform periodic assessment of 72-hour fecal fat and serum carotene.
• Drug may decrease vitamin B_{12} levels during long-term treatment. Monitor patient's vitamin B_{12} levels.

Information for the patient

• Because drug may cause gallstones, tell patient to report abdominal discomfort promptly.

Pediatric patients

• Doses of 1 to 10 mcg/kg appear to be well tolerated in children.

Breast-feeding patients

• It's unknown if drug appears in breast milk. Use cautiously in breast-feeding women.

ofloxacin
Floxin, Ocuflox

Pharmacologic classification: fluoro-quinolone
Therapeutic classification: antibiotic
Pregnancy risk category C

How supplied

Available by prescription only
Tablets: 200 mg, 300 mg, 400 mg
Injection: 200 mg in 50 ml D_5W; 400 mg in water for injection in 10- and 20-ml single-use vials; 400 mg in 100 ml D_5W.
Ophthalmic solution: 0.3%

Indications, route, and dosage

Conjunctivitis caused by known organism
Adults and children over age 1: Instill 1 to 2 drops in conjunctival sac q 2 to 4 hours, while awake, for first 2 days and then q.i.d. for up to 5 additional days.

Acute bacterial exacerbations of chronic bronchitis and pneumonia caused by susceptible organisms, mild to moderate skin and skin-structure infections, and community-acquired pneumonia
Adults: 400 mg P.O. or I.V. q 12 hours for 10 days.

Sexually transmitted diseases, such as acute uncomplicated urethral and cervical gonorrhea, nongonococcal urethritis and cervicitis, and mixed infections of urethra and cervix
Adults: For acute uncomplicated gonorrhea, 400 mg P.O. or I.V. once as a single dose; for cervicitis and urethritis, 300 mg P.O. or I.V. q 12 hours for 7 days.

Urinary tract infections
Adults: For cystitis caused by *Escherichia coli* or *Klebsiella pneumoniae,* 200 mg P.O. or I.V. q 12 hours for 3 days; for cystitis caused by other organisms, 200 mg P.O. or I.V. q 12 hours for 7 days.

Complicated urinary tract infections
Adults: 200 mg P.O. or I.V. q 12 hours for 10 days.

Prostatitis
Adults: 300 mg P.O. or I.V. q 12 hours for 6 weeks.

◊ **Adjunct in Brucella *infections***
Adults: 400 mg P.O. daily.

◊ **Peritonitis in patients receiving continuous ambulatory peritoneal dialysis**
Adults: 400 mg P.O. loading dose, then 300 mg P.O. daily for 7 to 10 days.

◊ **Typhoid fever**
Adults: 200 to 400 mg P.O. q 12 hours for 7 to 14 days.

◊ **Tuberculosis**
Adults: 300 mg P.O. daily.

◊ **Treatment of postoperative sternotomy or soft-tissue wounds caused by Mycobacterium fortuitum**
Adults: 300 to 600 mg P.O. daily for 3 to 6 months.

◊ **Leprosy**
Adults: 400 mg P.O. daily for 8 weeks.

◊ **Acute Q fever pneumonia**
Adults: 600 mg P.O. daily for up to 16 days.

◊ **Mediterranean spotted fever**
Adults: 200 mg P.O. q 12 hours for 7 days.

✦ **Dosage adjustment.** In patients with renal failure and creatinine clearance of 50 ml/minute or less, give initial dose as recommended; additional doses as follows: If creatinine clearance is 10 to 50 ml/minute, no dosage adjustment at 24-hour intervals; if below 10 ml/ minute, 50% of recommended dose q 24 hours.

Maximum daily dose in patients with hepatic function disorders is 400 mg.

Pharmacodynamics

Antibacterial action: Interferes with DNA gyrase, which is needed for synthesis of bacterial DNA.

Pharmacokinetics
• *Absorption:* Well absorbed after oral administration; maximum serum levels within 1 to 2 hours. Because oral bioavailability is about 98%, oral and I.V. dosage is the same.
• *Distribution:* Widely distributed to body tissues and fluids.
• *Metabolism:* Less than 10% of dose metabolized.
• *Excretion:* 70% to 80% excreted unchanged in urine; less than 5% in feces.

Contraindications and precautions
Contraindicated in patients with hypersensitivity to drug or other fluoroquinolones. Use oral and I.V. forms cautiously in patients with seizure disorders, CNS diseases (such as cerebral arteriosclerosis), hepatic disorders, or renal failure, and during pregnancy.

Interactions
Drug-drug. *Antacids:* Decreased serum ofloxacin levels. Separate administration times by 2 to 4 hours.
Antidiabetics: Hypoglycemia or hyperglycemia. Monitor serum glucose and adjust dosage as needed.
Theophylline: Increased serum theophylline levels. Monitor closely and adjust theophylline dosage as needed.
Warfarin: Prolonged PT and INR. Monitor PT and INR.
Drug-lifestyle. *Sun exposure:* Photosensitivity reactions. Tell patient to take precautions.

Adverse reactions
CNS: dizziness; headache, fatigue, lethargy, malaise, drowsiness, sleep disorders, nervousness, insomnia, visual disturbances, **seizures** (with oral or I.V. form).
CV: chest pain (with oral or I.V. form).
EENT: *transient ocular burning or discomfort,* stinging, redness, itching, photophobia, lacrimation, eye dryness (with ophthalmic form).
GI: *nausea,* **pseudomembranous colitis,** anorexia, abdominal pain or discomfort, diarrhea, vomiting, constipation, dry mouth, flatulence, dysgeusia (with oral or I.V. form).
GU: vaginitis, vaginal discharge, genital pruritus (with oral or I.V. form).
Hepatic: elevated liver enzymes.
Metabolic: increased blood glucose levels.
Musculoskeletal: trunk pain (with oral or I.V. form).
Skin: rash, pruritus, photosensitivity (with oral or I.V. form), phlebitis (with oral or I.V. form).
Other: hypersensitivity reactions (**anaphylactoid reaction**), fever.

☑ Special considerations
• Give I.V. ofloxacin by slow infusion only; don't give I.M., S.C., intrathecally, or by intraperitoneal injection. Administer over at least 60 minutes and avoid rapid or bolus injection. Compatible with most common I.V. solutions, including D_5W injection, normal saline injection, dextrose 5% in normal saline injection, dextrose 5% in 0.45% saline injection, dextrose 5% in lactated Ringer's solution, and 5% sodium bicarbonate injection.
• Drug isn't recommended for syphilis.

Monitoring the patient
• Perform periodic assessment of organ system functions during prolonged therapy.
• Evaluate patient for adverse reactions.

Information for the patient
• Advise patient to drink plenty of fluids.
• Advise patient to separate doses of antacids, vitamins, and ofloxacin by 2 hours.
• Tell patient that drug may be taken without regard to meals.
• Tell patient dizziness and light-headedness may occur. Advise caution when driving or operating hazardous machinery until effects of drug are known.
• Warn patient that hypersensitivity reactions may follow first dose; he should stop drug at first sign of rash or other allergic reaction and call immediately.
• Advise patient to avoid prolonged exposure to direct sunlight and to use a sunscreen when outdoors.

Pediatric patients
• Safety and efficacy in children under age 18 haven't been established. Similar drugs have caused arthropathy in some instances.

Breast-feeding patients
• Drug appears in breast milk in levels similar to those found in plasma. Because of the potential risk of serious adverse reactions, a decision must be made whether to discontinue breast-feeding or to discontinue the drug.

---

olanzapine
Zyprexa

Pharmacologic classification: thienobenzodiazepine derivative
Therapeutic classification: antipsychotic
Pregnancy risk category C

How supplied
Available by prescription only
Tablets: 2.5 mg, 5 mg, 7.5 mg, 10 mg

Indications, route, and dosage
Management of signs and symptoms of psychotic disorders
Adults: Initially, 5 to 10 mg P.O. once daily. Adjust dosage in 5-mg daily increments at intervals of

---

not less than 1 week. Most patients respond to 10 mg/day; don't exceed 20 mg/day.

Pharmacodynamics
Antipsychotic action: Unknown. Acts as an antagonist at dopamine (D_{1-4}) and serotonin ($5HT_{2A/2C}$) receptors; may also exhibit antagonist-binding at adrenergic, cholinergic, and histaminergic receptors.

Pharmacokinetics
• *Absorption:* Levels peak about 6 hours after oral dose. Food doesn't affect rate or extent of absorption. About 40% of dose eliminated by first-pass metabolism.
• *Distribution:* Distributed extensively throughout body; volume of distribution about 1,000 L. 93% protein-bound, primarily to albumin and alpha$_1$-acid glycoprotein.
• *Metabolism:* Metabolized by direct glucuronidation and cytochrome P-450-mediated oxidation.
• *Excretion:* About 57% of drug appears in urine; 30% in feces as metabolites. Only 7% of dose recovered unchanged in urine. Elimination half-life ranges from 21 to 54 hours.

Contraindications and precautions
Contraindicated in patients with hypersensitivity to drug. Use cautiously in patients with heart disease, cerebrovascular disease, conditions that predispose to hypotension (gradual dosage adjustment minimizes risk), history of seizures or conditions that might lower the seizure threshold, and hepatic impairment. Also use cautiously in elderly patients, in those with history of paralytic ileus, significant prostatic hypertrophy, or narrow-angle glaucoma, and in those at risk for aspiration pneumonia.

Interactions
Drug-drug. *Antihypertensives, diazepam:* Potentiated hypotensive effects. Monitor blood pressure closely.
Carbamazepine, omeprazole, rifampin: Increased clearance of olanzapine. Monitor patient for drug effect.
Dopamine agonists, levodopa: May cause antagonized effects of these drugs. Use together cautiously; monitor patient for drug effect.
Fluvoxamine: Inhibited olanzapine elimination. Watch for toxicity.
Drug-herb. *Nutmeg:* Loss of symptom control. Monitor patient closely.
Drug-lifestyle. *Alcohol:* Potentiated hypotensive effects. Monitor blood pressure closely; discourage alcohol use.

Adverse reactions
CNS: *somnolence, agitation, insomnia, headache, nervousness, hostility, parkinsonism, dizziness,* anxiety, personality disorder, *akathisia,* hypertonia, tremor, amnesia, articulation impairment, euphoria, stuttering, dystonic-dyskinetic events, tardive dyskinesia.
CV: orthostatic hypotension, tachycardia, chest pain, hypotension, edema.
EENT: amblyopia, blepharitis, corneal lesion, *rhinitis,* pharyngitis.
GI: constipation, dry mouth, abdominal pain, increased appetite, increased salivation, nausea, vomiting, thirst.
GU: premenstrual syndrome, hematuria, metrorrhagia, urinary incontinence, urinary tract infection.
Hematologic: increased eosinophil count.
Hepatic: increased ALT, AST, GGT levels.
Metabolic: weight gain or loss, increased serum prolactin and CK levels.
Musculoskeletal: joint pain, extremity pain, back pain, neck rigidity, twitching.
Respiratory: increased cough, dyspnea.
Skin: vesiculobullous rash.
Other: fever, intentional injury, flu syndrome, suicide attempt.

☑ Special considerations
• Initiate therapy with 5 mg in patients who are debilitated, predisposed to hypotension, or have an alteration in metabolism due to smoking status, sex, or age or who are pharmacologically sensitive to drug.
• Efficacy for long-term use (over 6 weeks) hasn't been established.
• Symptoms of overdose may include drowsiness and slurred speech, hypotension, circulatory collapse, obtundation, seizures, or dystonic reactions. Gastric lavage with activated charcoal and sorbitol may be effective. Drug isn't removed by dialysis. Avoid epinephrine, dopamine, or other sympathomimetics with beta-agonist activity.

Monitoring the patient
• Monitor patient for signs of neuroleptic malignant syndrome (hyperpyrexia, muscle rigidity, altered mental status, autonomic instability), a rare but frequently fatal adverse reaction that can occur with the administration of antipsychotics. Stop drug immediately; monitor and treat patient.
• Obtain baseline and periodic liver function tests.

Information for the patient
• Warn patient to avoid hazardous tasks until adverse CNS effects of drug are known.
• Caution patient against exposure to extreme heat; drug may impair body's ability to reduce core temperature.
• Instruct patient to avoid alcohol.
• Tell patient to rise slowly to avoid orthostatic hypotension.
• Advise patient to use ice chips or sugarless candy or gum to relieve dry mouth.

• Inform patient not to take prescription or OTC drugs without medical approval because of potential drug interactions.

Geriatric patients
• Drug may be initiated at lower dose because clearance may be decreased in elderly patients. Half-life is 1½ times greater in this population.

Pediatric patients
• Safety and efficacy in children under age 18 haven't been established.

Breast-feeding patients
• Drug appears in breast milk. Patient should use an alternative to breast-feeding during therapy.

olsalazine sodium
Dipentum

Pharmacologic classification: salicylate
Therapeutic classification: anti-inflammatory
Pregnancy risk category C

How supplied
Available by prescription only
Capsules: 250 mg

Indications, route, and dosage
Maintenance of remission of ulcerative colitis in patients intolerant of sulfasalazine
Adults: 1 g P.O. daily in two divided doses.

Pharmacodynamics
Anti-inflammatory action: Mechanism unknown but appears to be topical rather than systemic. Drug is converted to mesalamine (5-aminosalicylic acid; 5-ASA) in the colon. Presumably, mesalamine diminishes inflammation by blocking cyclooxygenase and inhibiting prostaglandin production in the colon.

Pharmacokinetics
• *Absorption:* After oral administration, about 2.4% of dose is absorbed; maximum levels in about 2 hours.
• *Distribution:* Once metabolized to 5-ASA, drug absorbed slowly from colon, resulting in very high local levels.
• *Metabolism:* 0.1% metabolized in liver; remainder will reach colon, where it's rapidly converted to 5-ASA by colonic bacteria.
• *Excretion:* Less than 1% of drug recovered in urine.

Contraindications and precautions
Contraindicated in patients with hypersensitivity to salicylates. Use cautiously in patients with existing renal disease.

Interactions
Drug-drug. *Warfarin:* Increased PT and INR. Monitor PT and INR.

Adverse reactions
CNS: headache, depression, vertigo, dizziness, fatigue.
GI: diarrhea, nausea, *abdominal pain,* dyspepsia, bloating, anorexia, stomatitis.
Musculoskeletal: arthralgia.
Skin: rash, itching.

☑ Special considerations
• Diarrhea was noted in 17% of patients, but it's difficult to distinguish from underlying condition.
• Toxicity may cause decreased motor activity and diarrhea can occur.

Monitoring the patient
• Monitor CBC with differential and liver function tests periodically.
• Monitor therapeutic effect.

Information for the patient
• Advise patient to take drug with food and in evenly divided doses.
• Inform patient to call if diarrhea develops.

Pediatric patients
• Safety and efficacy in children haven't been established.

Breast-feeding patients
• It's unknown if drug appears in breast milk. Use with caution in breast-feeding women.

omeprazole
Prilosec

Pharmacologic classification: substituted benzimidazole
Therapeutic classification: gastric acid suppressant
Pregnancy risk category C

How supplied
Available by prescription only
Capsules (delayed-release): 10 mg, 20 mg

Indications, route, and dosage
Active duodenal ulcer
Adults: 20 mg P.O. daily for 4 to 8 weeks.
Helicobacter pylori *eradication to reduce risk of duodenal ulcer recurrence*
Triple therapy (omeprazole/clarithromycin/amoxicillin)
Adults: 20 mg P.O. b.i.d., plus 500 mg clarithromycin P.O. b.i.d., plus 1,000 mg amoxicillin P.O. b.i.d. for 10 days. In patients with an ulcer present at the time of initiation of therapy, an additional 18 days of omeprazole 20 mg once daily

is recommended alone for ulcer healing and symptom relief.

Note: Refer to entries on clarithromycin and amoxicillin.

Dual therapy (omeprazole/clarithromycin)
Adults: 40 mg each morning, plus 500 mg clarithromycin t.i.d. for 14 days, then 14 days of omeprazole 20 mg daily.

Note: Refer to entry on clarithromycin.

Severe erosive esophagitis; symptomatic, poorly responsive gastroesophageal reflux disease (GERD)
Adults: 20 mg P.O. daily for 4 to 8 weeks. Patients with GERD should have failed initial therapy with an H_2 antagonist.

Pathologic hypersecretory conditions (such as Zollinger-Ellison syndrome)
Adults: Initial dosage is 60 mg P.O. daily; adjust dosage based on patient response. Administer daily doses exceeding 80 mg in divided doses. Doses up to 120 mg t.i.d. have been administered. Continue therapy as long as clinically indicated.

Gastric ulcer
Adults: 40 mg P.O. daily for 4 to 8 weeks.

Pharmacodynamics
Antisecretory action: Inhibits the activity of the acid (proton) pump, H^+/K^+ adenosine triphosphatase (ATPase), located at the secretory surface of the gastric parietal cell. This blocks the formation of gastric acid.

Pharmacokinetics
● *Absorption:* Drug is acid-labile; formulation contains enteric-coated granules that permit absorption after drug leaves stomach. Rapid absorption; levels peak in less than 3½ hours. Bioavailability about 40% because of instability in gastric acid and substantial first-pass effect. Bioavailability increases slightly with repeated dosing, possibly because of drug's effect on gastric acidity.
● *Distribution:* About 95% protein-bound.
● *Metabolism:* Primarily metabolized in liver.
● *Excretion:* Primarily excreted by kidneys. Plasma half-life is ½ to 1 hour, but drug effects may last for days.

Contraindications and precautions
Contraindicated in patients with hypersensitivity to drug or its components.

Interactions
Drug-drug. *Ampicillin esters, iron derivatives, itraconazole, ketoconazole:* Poor bioavailability. Avoid concomitant use.
Diazepam, phenytoin, propranolol, theophylline, warfarin: Impaired elimination of these drugs. Monitor patient for toxicity.
Drug-herb. *Male fern:* Inactivated in alkaline environments. Advise patient concerning this effect.

Pennyroyal: Drug may change rate of formation of toxic metabolites of pennyroyal. Discourage use.

Adverse reactions
CNS: headache, dizziness, asthenia.
GI: diarrhea, abdominal pain, nausea, vomiting, constipation, flatulence.
Metabolic: serum gastrin levels rise in most patients during first 2 weeks of therapy.
Musculoskeletal: back pain.
Respiratory: cough, upper respiratory infection.
Skin: rash.

☑ Special considerations
● Drug increases its own bioavailability with repeated administration. It's labile in gastric acid; less is lost to hydrolysis because drug raises gastric pH.
● Dosage adjustments aren't required for patients with impaired renal function; however, they are needed in those with hepatic impairment.
● Don't crush capsules.
● Toxicity may cause confusion, drowsiness, blurred vision, tachycardia, nausea, vomiting, diaphoresis, dry mouth, and headache.

Monitoring the patient
● Monitor hepatic function.
● Monitor therapeutic effect.

Information for the patient
● Explain importance of taking drug exactly as prescribed.
● Tell patient to take before meals; don't crush capsules.

Pediatric patients
● Safety in children hasn't been established.

Breast-feeding patients
● It's unknown if drug appears in breast milk. Avoid breast-feeding during therapy.

---

ondansetron hydrochloride
Zofran, Zofran ODT

Pharmacologic classification: serotonin (5-HT_3) receptor antagonist
Therapeutic classification: antiemetic
Pregnancy risk category B

How supplied
Available by prescription only
Tablets: 4 mg, 8 mg
Tablets (oral disintegrating): 4 mg, 8 mg
Oral solution: 4 mg/5 ml
Injection: 2 mg/ml in 20-ml multidose vials, 2-ml single-dose vials
Injection, premixed: 32 mg/50 ml in 5% dextrose single-dose vial

---

Indications, route, and dosage

Prevention of nausea and vomiting associated with initial and repeat courses of emetogenic cancer chemotherapy, including high-dose cisplatin
Adults and children ages 4 and older: Three I.V. doses of 0.15 mg/kg with first dose infused over 15 minutes beginning 30 minutes before start of chemotherapy, with subsequent doses of 0.15 mg/kg administered 4 and 8 hours after first dose. May also administer as a single dose of 32 mg, infused over 15 minutes, 30 minutes before start of chemotherapy.
Adults and children ages 12 and older: 8 mg P.O. b.i.d. starting 30 minutes before start of chemotherapy, with subsequent dose 8 hours after first dose, then 8 mg q 12 hours for 1 to 2 days after completion of chemotherapy.
Children ages 4 to 11: 4 mg P.O. t.i.d. dosed the same times as for adults.
Prevention of radiation-induced nausea and vomiting
Adults: 8 mg P.O. t.i.d.
Prevention of postoperative nausea and vomiting
Adults: 16 mg P.O. 1 hour before anesthesia or 4 mg I.V. immediately before anesthesia or shortly postoperatively.

Pharmacodynamics

Antiemetic action: Exact mechanism unknown; however, ondansetron isn't a dopamine-receptor antagonist. Because serotonin receptors of the 5-HT$_3$ type are present both peripherally on vagal nerve terminals and centrally in the chemoreceptor trigger zone, it isn't certain if ondansetron's antiemetic action is mediated centrally, peripherally, or in both sites.

Pharmacokinetics

• *Absorption:* Variable with oral administration. Level peaks within 2 hours; bioavailability of 50% to 60%.
• *Distribution:* 70% to 76% bound to plasma protein.
• *Metabolism:* Extensively metabolized by hydroxylation on the indole ring, then glucuronide or sulfate conjugation.
• *Excretion:* 5% of dose recovered in urine as parent compound. Half-life in adults is 3½ to 6 hours.

Contraindications and precautions

Contraindicated in patients with hypersensitivity to drug. Use cautiously in patients with hepatic failure.

Interactions

Drug-herb. *Horehound:* Enhanced serotonergic effects. Discourage use.

Adverse reactions

CNS: *headache, malaise, fatigue, dizziness, sedation.*
CV: chest pain.
GI: *diarrhea, constipation,* abdominal pain, xerostomia.
GU: urine retention, gynecologic disorders.
Hepatic: transient elevations in AST and ALT levels.
Musculoskeletal: *musculoskeletal pain.*
Respiratory: hypoxia.
Skin: rash, injection-site reaction.
Other: chills, fever.

☑ Special considerations

• Drug is stable at room temperature for 48 hours after dilution with normal saline, D$_5$W, 5% dextrose and normal saline, 5% dextrose and 0.45% saline, or 3% saline.

Monitoring the patient

• Monitor patient for adverse effects.
• Monitor therapeutic effect.

Information for the patient

• Explain to patient and his family the purpose of drug and its expected effects.

Geriatric patients

• No age-related problems have been reported.

Pediatric patients

• Little information is available for use in children age 3 and under.

Breast-feeding patients

• It's unknown if drug appears in breast milk; use cautiously in breast-feeding women.

---

opium tincture, deodorized (laudanum)

opium tincture, camphorated (paregoric)

Pharmacologic classification: opiate
Therapeutic classification: antidiarrheal
Controlled substance schedule II or III (depending on amount of opium contained in product)
Pregnancy risk category B (D for high doses or long-term use)

How supplied

Available by prescription only
opium tincture, deodorized
Alcoholic solution: Equivalent to morphine 10 mg/ml
opium tincture, camphorated
Alcoholic solution: Each 5 ml contains 2 mg morphine, 0.2 ml anise oil, 20 mg benzoic acid, 20

Reactions may be *common*, uncommon, ***life-threatening***, or COMMON AND LIFE-THREATENING.

mg camphor, 0.2 ml glycerin, and ethanol to make 5 ml

Indications, route, and dosage
Acute, nonspecific diarrhea
Don't confuse doses of opium tincture and camphorated opium tincture.
Adults: 0.6 ml opium tincture (range, 0.3 to 1 ml) P.O. q.i.d. (maximum dose is 6 ml daily); or 5 to 10 ml camphorated opium tincture daily, b.i.d., t.i.d., or q.i.d. until diarrhea subsides.
Children: 0.25 to 0.5 ml/kg camphorated opium tincture daily, b.i.d., t.i.d., or q.i.d. until diarrhea subsides.
Severe opiate withdrawal symptoms in neonates
Neonates: 1:25 dilution of opium tincture in water, administered as 0.2 ml P.O. q 3 hours. Adjust dosage to control withdrawal symptoms. Increase dosage by 0.05 ml q 3 hours until symptoms are controlled. Once symptoms are stabilized for 3 to 5 days, gradually decrease dosage over a 2- to 4-week period.

Pharmacodynamics
Antidiarrheal action: Opium, derived from the opium poppy, contains several ingredients. The most active ingredient, morphine, increases GI smooth-muscle tone, inhibits motility and propulsion, and diminishes secretions. By inhibiting peristalsis, the drug delays passage of intestinal contents, increasing water resorption and relieving diarrhea.

Pharmacokinetics
• *Absorption:* Morphine absorbed variably from gut.
• *Distribution:* Although opium alkaloids distributed widely in body, low doses used to treat diarrhea act primarily in GI tract. Camphor crosses placenta.
• *Metabolism:* Opium metabolized rapidly in liver.
• *Excretion:* Opium excreted in urine; opium alkaloids (especially morphine) enter breast milk. Drug effect lasts 4 to 5 hours.

Contraindications and precautions
Contraindicated in patients with acute diarrhea caused by poisoning until toxic material is removed from GI tract and in those with diarrhea caused by organisms that penetrate intestinal mucosa. Use cautiously in patients with asthma, prostatic hyperplasia, hepatic disease, or history of opium dependence.

Interactions
Drug-drug. *CNS depressants:* Additive effect. Use together cautiously.
Metoclopramide: Antagonized effects of metoclopramide. Monitor patient for this effect.

Adverse reactions
CNS: dizziness, light-headedness.
GI: nausea, vomiting.
Metabolic: increased serum amylase and lipase levels.
Other: physical dependence (after long-term use).

☑ Special considerations
• Mix drug with sufficient water to ensure passage to stomach.
• Opium tincture, deodorized (laudanum) is 25 times more potent than camphorated opium tincture (paregoric); don't confuse these drugs.
• Risk of physical dependence on drug increases with long-term use.
• Don't refrigerate drug.
• Opium tincture and camphorated opium tincture may prevent delivery of technetium 99m disofenin to small intestine during hepatobiliary imaging tests; delay test until 24 hours after last dose.
• Signs and symptoms of overdose include drowsiness, hypotension, seizures, and apnea. Use naloxone to treat respiratory depression.

Monitoring the patient
• Monitor vital signs and bowel function.
• Monitor patient for signs and symptoms of CNS or respiratory depression.

Information for the patient
• Warn patient that physical dependence may result from long-term use.
• Warn patient to use caution when driving or performing other tasks requiring alertness because drug may cause drowsiness, dizziness, and blurred vision.
• Because drug is indicated only for short-term use, instruct patient to report diarrhea that persists longer than 48 hours.
• Advise patient to take drug with food if it causes nausea, vomiting, or constipation.
• Instruct patient to call immediately if he has difficulty breathing or shortness of breath.
• Instruct patient to drink adequate fluids while diarrhea persists.

Pediatric patients
• Opium tincture has been used to treat withdrawal symptoms in infants whose mothers are narcotic addicts.

Breast-feeding patients
• Because opium alkaloids (especially morphine) appear in breast milk, drug's possible risks must be weighed against benefits.

oprelvekin
Neumega

Pharmacologic classification: recombinant human interleukin eleven
(rhIL-11)
Therapeutic classification: human
thrombopoietic growth factor
Pregnancy risk category C

How supplied
Available by prescription only
Injection: 5-mg, single-dose vial with diluent

Indications, route, and dosage
*Prevention of severe thrombocytopenia and
reduction of need for platelet transfusions after myelosuppressive chemotherapy in patients with nonmyeloid malignancies who are
at high risk for severe thrombocytopenia*
Adults: 50 mcg/kg S.C. once daily. Begin dosing
6 to 24 hours after completion of chemotherapy
and stop at least 2 days before starting the next
planned cycle of chemotherapy. Continue dosing until the postnadir platelet count is 50,000
cells/microliter more.

Pharmacodynamics
Thrombopoietic growth factor action: Thrombopoietic growth factor that directly stimulates
the proliferation of hematopoietic stem cells and
megakaryocyte progenitor cells. The primary
activity of oprelvekin is stimulation of megakaryocytopoiesis and thrombopoiesis. Platelets
produced in response to oprelvekin possess a
normal life-span and are functionally normal.
Bone-forming and bone-resorbing cells are potential targets for oprelvekin. In some instances,
platelet counts began to increase relative to baseline between 5 and 9 days after the start of
oprelvekin therapy. After treatment ceased,
platelet counts continued to increase for up to 7
days; platelet counts returned to baseline within 14 days.

Pharmacokinetics
• *Absorption:* When administered S.C., absolute
bioavailability is over 80%.
• *Distribution:* Plasma levels peak 3 to 5 hours
after S.C. dose.
• *Metabolism:* Mostly metabolized before excretion; routes of metabolism unknown.
• *Excretion:* Excreted primarily by kidneys; terminal half-life is about 7 hours.

Contraindications and precautions
Contraindicated in patients with hypersensitivity
to drug or its components. Use cautiously in patients with heart failure, in those at risk for the development of clinical heart failure, and in patients
with history of heart failure that is currently well
controlled. Also use cautiously in patients with
history of papilledema, atrial arrhythmias, or CNS
tumors. Use with caution in patients receiving
cardiac drugs, in those previously treated with
doxorubicin, and in elderly patients.

Interactions
None reported.

Adverse reactions
CNS: *asthenia, headache, insomnia, dizziness,*
paresthesia.
CV: *tachycardia, vasodilation, palpitations,* ATRIAL FLUTTER OR FIBRILLATION, *syncope, edema.*
EENT: blurred vision, *conjunctival injection,
pharyngitis, rhinitis,* eye hemorrhage.
GI: *oral candidiasis, nausea, vomiting, diarrhea,
mucositis.*
Hematologic: NEUTROPENIC FEVER, decrease in
hemoglobin, increased plasma fibrinogen.
Metabolic: dehydration; decreased serum albumin, other proteins (transferrin and gamma globulins), and calcium levels; increased Von Willebrand factor.
Respiratory: *dyspnea, cough,* PLEURAL EFFUSIONS.
Skin: *rash,* skin discoloration, exfoliative dermatitis, transient rash at injection site.
Other: *fever.*

☑ Special considerations
• Administer S.C. in abdomen, thigh, hip, or upper arm.
• Store drug and diluent in refrigerator until ready
for reconstitution.
• Reconstitute single-dose vial with 1 ml of supplied diluent. Avoid excessive or vigorous agitation. Discard unused drug.
• Use reconstituted drug within 3 hours.
• Some patients may develop antibodies to drug.
• If overdose occurs, stop drug and observe patient for cardiac signs of toxicity.

Monitoring the patient
• Closely monitor fluid and electrolyte status (especially potassium levels) in patients on long-term diuretic therapy. Severe hypokalemia resulting in death has occurred in patients concurrently receiving diuretics, ifosfamide, and
oprelvekin; use with caution.
• Obtain CBC before chemotherapy and at regular intervals during drug therapy. Drug isn't indicated following myeloablative chemotherapy.

Information for the patient
• Provide patient with information leaflet available from manufacturer. A copy can also be obtained from drug package insert.
• If patient is to self-administer, show him how to
prepare and administer drug.

- Advise patient to give each dose at about the same time each day.
- Tell patient to keep drug refrigerated before reconstitution and not to reconstitute until ready to use. Also inform patient that reconstituted drug is stable at room temperature or in refrigerator for up to 3 hours.
- Tell patient not to reuse vial that has been reconstituted and entered by a syringe, and to discard remaining solution after dose is administered.
- Instruct patient to call immediately if swelling, chest pain, irregular heart beat, blurred vision, difficulty breathing, or fatigue occurs.

Breast-feeding patients
- It's unknown if drug appears in breast milk. Depending on importance of drug to mother, stop either breast-feeding or drug.

orlistat
Xenical

Pharmacologic classification: lipase inhibitor
Therapeutic classification: antiobesity drug
Pregnancy risk category B

How supplied
Capsules: 120 mg

Indications, route, and dosage
Management of obesity, including weight loss and weight maintenance with a reduced-calorie diet; reduction of risk of weight regain after prior weight loss
Adults: 120 mg P.O. t.i.d. with each main meal containing fat (during or up to 1 hour after the meal).

Pharmacodynamics
Antiobesity action: As a reversible inhibitor of lipases, orlistat forms a bond with the active site of gastric and pancreatic lipases. These inactivated enzymes are thus unavailable to hydrolyze dietary fat, in the form of triglycerides, into absorbable free fatty acids and monoglycerides. Because the undigested triglycerides aren't absorbed, the resulting caloric deficit may have a positive effect on weight control. The recommended dosage of 120 mg t.i.d. inhibits dietary fat absorption by about 30%.

Pharmacokinetics
- *Absorption:* Minimal systemic exposure; only small amount of drug absorbed.
- *Distribution:* More than 99% of drug binds to plasma proteins; lipoproteins and albumin major binding proteins.

- *Metabolism:* Primarily metabolized within GI wall.
- *Excretion:* Majority of unabsorbed drug excreted in feces.

Contraindications and precautions
Contraindicated in patients with hypersensitivity to drug or its components and in those with chronic malabsorption syndrome or cholestasis. Also, exclude organic causes of obesity such as hypothyroidism before starting patient on orlistat therapy.

Use cautiously in patients with history of hyperoxaluria or calcium oxalate nephrolithiasis or a risk of anorexia nervosa or bulimia. Also use cautiously in patients receiving cyclosporine therapy because of the potential changes in cyclosporine absorption related to the variations in dietary intake.

Interactions
Drug-drug. *Fat-soluble vitamins (such as beta-carotene, vitamin E):* Decreased absorption of these vitamins. Separate administration times by 2 hours.
Pravastatin: Slightly increased pravastatin levels; additive lipid-lowering effects of drug. Monitor patient.
Warfarin: Possible change in coagulation parameters. Monitor INR.

Adverse reactions
CNS: *headache,* dizziness, fatigue, sleep disorder, anxiety, depression.
CV: pedal edema.
EENT: otitis, tooth and gingival disorders.
GI: *oily spotting, flatus with discharge, fecal urgency, fatty or oily stool, oily evacuation, increased defecation, abdominal pain,* fecal incontinence, nausea, infectious diarrhea, rectal pain, vomiting.
GU: menstrual irregularity, vaginitis, urinary tract infection.
Musculoskeletal: *back pain,* pain in lower extremities, arthritis, myalgia, joint disorder, tendinitis.
Respiratory: *influenza, upper respiratory tract infection,* lower respiratory tract infection.
Skin: rash, dry skin.

☑ Special considerations
- Drug is recommended for use in patients with initial body mass index (BMI) of 30 kg/m² or more, or 27 kg/m² or more and other risk factors (for example, hypertension, diabetes, or dyslipidemia).
- Patients should be advised to adhere to dietary guidelines. GI effects may increase when patients take orlistat with high-fat foods—specifically, when more than 30% of their total daily calories come from fat.

- Drug reduces absorption of some fat-soluble vitamins and beta-carotene. To ensure adequate nutrition, encourage patients to take a multivitamin supplement that contains fat-soluble vitamins during therapy.
- In diabetic patients, improved metabolic control may accompany weight loss; dosage of oral antidiabetic (such as sulfonylureas and metformin) or insulin may need to be reduced.
- It's unknown if orlistat is safe and effective to use in patients for more than 2 years.
- As with any weight-loss drug, the potential for misuse in certain patient populations, such as patients with anorexia nervosa or bulimia, exists.
- If an overdose occurs, stop drug and observe patient for 24 hours.

Monitoring the patient
- Monitor blood glucose level in diabetic patient.
- Monitor patient for adverse effects.

Information for the patient
- Advise patient to follow a nutritionally balanced, reduced-calorie diet that derives only 30% of calories from fat. The daily intake of fat, carbohydrate, and protein should be distributed over three main meals. If a meal is occasionally missed or contains no fat, tell the patient the dose of orlistat can be omitted.
- To ensure adequate nutrition, advise patient to take a daily multivitamin supplement that contains fat-soluble vitamins at least 2 hours before or after drug, such as at bedtime.
- Tell patient with diabetes that weight loss may improve glycemic control; dosage of his oral antidiabetic (such as sulfonylureas and metformin) or insulin may need to be reduced while he's taking drug.
- Tell woman to call if she is or plans to become pregnant or is breast-feeding.

Geriatric patients
- It's unknown if patients ages 65 and older respond differently to drug than younger patients.

Pediatric patients
- Safety and efficacy in children haven't been established.

Breast-feeding patients
- It's unknown if drug appears in breast milk. Don't give drug to breast-feeding women.

orphenadrine citrate
Banflex, Flexoject, Flexon, Myolin, Myotrol, Norflex

orphenadrine hydrochloride
Disipal*

Pharmacologic classification: diphenhydramine analogue
Therapeutic classification: skeletal muscle relaxant
Pregnancy risk category C

How supplied
Available by prescription only
Tablets: 100 mg
Tablets (extended-release): 100 mg
Injection: 30 mg/ml parenteral

Indications, route, and dosage
Adjunct in painful, acute musculoskeletal conditions
Adults: 100 mg P.O. b.i.d., or 60 mg I.V. or I.M. q 12 hours.
◊ **Leg cramps**
Adults: 100 mg P.O. h.s.

Pharmacodynamics
Skeletal muscle relaxant action: Doesn't relax skeletal muscle directly. Atropine-like central action on cerebral motor centers or on the medulla may be the mechanism by which it reduces skeletal muscle spasm. Reported analgesic effect may add to skeletal muscle relaxant properties.

Pharmacokinetics
- *Absorption:* Rapidly absorbed from GI tract; onset of action within 1 hour, peaks within 2 hours, lasts for 4 to 6 hours.
- *Distribution:* Widely distributed throughout body.
- *Metabolism:* Pathway unknown; drug almost completely metabolized to at least eight metabolites.
- *Excretion:* Excreted in urine, mainly as metabolites. Small amounts excreted unchanged. Half-life is about 14 hours.

Contraindications and precautions
Contraindicated in patients with hypersensitivity to drug and in those with glaucoma; prostatic hyperplasia; pyloric, duodenal, or bladder neck obstruction; myasthenia gravis; or peptic ulceration.

Use cautiously in elderly or debilitated patients and in those with tachycardia, cardiac disease, arrhythmias, or sulfite allergy.

Interactions
Drug-drug. *CNS depressants (antipsychotics, anxiolytics, tricyclic antidepressants), propoxy-*

---

phene: Additive CNS effects. Concurrent use requires reduction of both drugs.
MAO inhibitors: Increased CNS adverse effects. Monitor patient closely.
Other anticholinergics: Increased anticholinergic effects. Monitor patient closely.
Drug-lifestyle. *Alcohol:* Additive CNS effects. Discourage use.

Adverse reactions
CNS: weakness, *drowsiness,* light-headedness, confusion, agitation, tremor, headache, dizziness, hallucinations.
CV: palpitations, tachycardia, syncope.
EENT: dilated pupils, blurred vision, difficulty swallowing, increased intraocular pressure.
GI: constipation, *dry mouth,* nausea, vomiting, epigastric distress.
GU: urinary hesitancy, urine retention.
Hematologic: *aplastic anemia.*
Skin: urticaria, pruritus.
Other: *anaphylaxis.*

☑ Special considerations
● When giving drug I.V., inject slowly over 5 minutes. Keep patient supine during and 5 to 10 minutes after injection. Paradoxical initial bradycardia may occur when giving I.V.; usually disappears in 2 minutes.
● Some commercially available orphenadrine citrate injection formulations may contain sodium bisulfite, a sulfite that can cause allergic-type reactions, including anaphylaxis.
● Toxicity may cause dry mouth, blurred vision, urine retention, tachycardia, confusion, paralytic ileus, deep coma, seizures, shock, respiratory arrest, arrhythmias, and death.

Monitoring the patient
● Perform periodic blood, urine, and liver function tests during prolonged therapy.
● Monitor vital signs and intake and output, noting urine retention.

Information for the patient
● Recommend ice chips, sugarless gum, hard candy, or saliva substitutes to relieve dry mouth.
● Tell patient to avoid hazardous activities that require alertness or physical coordination until CNS depressant effects are known.
● Warn patient to avoid alcohol and to use cough and cold preparations cautiously because some contain alcohol.
● Tell patient to store drug away from heat and light (not in bathroom medicine cabinet) and safely out of reach of children.
● Instruct patient to take missed dose if remembered within 1 hour. If beyond 1 hour, patient should skip that dose and return to regular schedule. Patient shouldn't double doses.

Geriatric patients
● Elderly patients may be more sensitive to drug's effects. Advise cautious use

Pediatric patients
● Safety and efficacy in children under age 12 haven't been established.

oseltamivir phosphate
Tamiflu

Pharmacologic classification: neuraminidase inhibitor
Therapeutic classification: antiviral
Pregnancy risk category C

How supplied
Available by prescription only
Capsules: 75 mg

Indications, route, and dosage
Uncomplicated, acute illness due to influenza infection in patients who have been symptomatic for 2 days or less
Adults: 75 mg P.O. b.i.d. for 5 days.
✦ *Dosage adjustment.* For patients with creatinine clearance less than 30 ml/minute, reduce dosage to 75 mg P.O. once daily for 5 days.

Pharmacodynamics
Antiviral action: Oseltamivir carboxylate, the active form of oseltamivir, inhibits the enzyme neuraminidase within the influenza virus particles. This action is thought to inhibit viral replication, possibly by interfering with viral particle aggregation and release from the host cell.

Pharmacokinetics
● *Absorption:* Well absorbed after oral administration. More than 75% of dose reaches systemic circulation as oseltamivir carboxylate.
● *Distribution:* Serum protein-binding for oseltamivir is 42%; 3% for oseltamivir carboxylate.
● *Metabolism:* Oseltamivir extensively metabolized by hepatic esterases to active component, oseltamivir carboxylate.
● *Excretion:* Oseltamivir carboxylate almost entirely eliminated in urine via glomerular filtration and tubular secretion. Less than 20% of oral dose eliminated in feces.

Contraindications and precautions
Contraindicated in patients with hypersensitivity to drug or its components.

Interactions
None reported.

Adverse reactions
CNS: dizziness, insomnia, headache, vertigo, fatigue.

GI: abdominal pain, diarrhea, nausea, vomiting.
Respiratory: bronchitis, cough.

☑ Special considerations
● No evidence supporting drug use in treatment of viral infections other than influenza virus types A and B.
● Drug must be given within 2 days of onset of symptoms.
● Drug is used to treat flu symptoms, not to prevent influenza.
● Drug isn't a replacement for annual influenza vaccination. Patients for whom vaccine is indicated should continue to receive vaccine each fall.
● Safety and efficacy of repeated treatment courses haven't been established.
● Drug may be given with meals to decrease GI adverse effects.
● Store at controlled room temperature (59° to 86° F [15° to 30° C]).

Monitoring the patient
● Monitor patient for improvement of illness.
● Monitor patient for adverse effects.

Information for the patient
● Instruct patient to begin treatment as soon as possible after appearance of flu symptoms.
● Inform patient that drug may be taken with or without meals. If nausea or vomiting occurs, take with food or milk.
● Tell patient that if a dose is missed, it should be taken as soon as possible. He should skip missed dose, however, if next dose is due within 2 hours, and take the next dose on schedule.
● Advise patient to complete full 5 days of treatment, even if he feels better.
● Alert patient that drug isn't a replacement for annual influenza vaccination. Patients for whom vaccine is indicated should continue to receive vaccine each fall.

Geriatric patients
● Dosage reduction isn't needed for elderly patients unless creatinine clearance is less than 30 ml/minute.

Pediatric patients
● Safety and efficacy haven't been established in children under age 18.

Breast-feeding patients
● It's unknown if oseltamivir or oseltamivir carboxylate appears in breast milk. Use only if potential benefits to mother outweigh potential risks to infant.

---

oxacillin sodium
Bactocill

Pharmacologic classification: penicillinase-resistant penicillin
Therapeutic classification: antibiotic
Pregnancy risk category B

How supplied
Available by prescription only
Capsules: 250 mg, 500 mg
Oral solution: 250 mg/5 ml (after reconstitution)
Injection: 250 mg, 500 mg, 1 g, 2 g, 4 g
Pharmacy bulk package: 10 g
I.V. infusion: 1 g, 2 g, 4 g

Indications, route, and dosage
Systemic infections caused by Staphylococcus aureus
Adults and children weighing over 40 kg (88 lb): 2 to 6 g P.O. daily, divided into doses given q 4 to 6 hours; 1 to 12 g I.M. or I.V. daily, divided into doses given q 4 to 6 hours. Doses vary based on severity of infection.
Children over age 1 month weighing below 40 kg: 50 to 100 mg/kg P.O. daily, divided into doses given q 4 to 6 hours; 50 to 200 mg/kg I.M. or I.V. daily, divided into doses given q 4 to 6 hours. Doses vary based on severity of infection.
✦ *Dosage adjustment.* In adults with creatinine clearance below 10 ml/minute, 1 g I.M. or I.V. q 4 to 6 hours.

Pharmacodynamics
Antibiotic action: Bactericidal. Adheres to bacterial penicillin-binding proteins, thus inhibiting bacterial cell wall synthesis. Resists the effects of penicillinases—enzymes that inactivate penicillin—and is thus active against many strains of penicillinase-producing bacteria; this activity is most important against penicillinase-producing staphylococci; some strains may remain resistant. Also active against a few gram-positive aerobic and anaerobic bacilli but has no significant effect on gram-negative bacilli.

Pharmacokinetics
● *Absorption:* Absorbed rapidly but incompletely from GI tract; is stable in acid environment. Serum levels peak within ½ to 2 hours after oral dose; 30 minutes after I.M. dose. Food decreases absorption.
● *Distribution:* Distributed widely. Poor CSF penetration but enhanced by meningeal inflammation. Drug crosses placenta; is 89% to 94% protein-bound.
● *Metabolism:* Partially metabolized.
● *Excretion:* Drug and metabolites excreted primarily in urine by renal tubular secretion and glomerular filtration; also excreted in breast milk and small amounts in bile. Elimination half-life in

---

Reactions may be *common*, uncommon, **life-threatening**, or COMMON AND LIFE-THREATENING.

adults is ½ to 1 hour, extended to 2 hours in patients with severe renal impairment. Dosage adjustments not required in patients with creatinine clearance below 10 ml/minute.

Contraindications and precautions
Contraindicated in patients with hypersensitivity to drug or other penicillins. Use cautiously in patients with other drug allergies (especially to cephalosporins), in neonates, and in infants.

Interactions
Drug-drug. *Aminoglycosides:* Synergistic bactericidal effects against *S. aureus.* Monitor patient for this effect. Drugs are physically and chemically incompatible; inactivated when mixed or given together. Don't mix together in same I.V. solution.
Probenecid: Increased oxacillin serum levels. Probenecid may be used for this purpose.
Drug-food. *Any food:* Decreased absorption. Give drug on empty stomach.
Carbonated beverages, fruit juice: Interfered with absorption. Don't give together.

Adverse reactions
CNS: neuropathy, neuromuscular irritability, *seizures,* lethargy, hallucinations, anxiety, confusion, agitation, depression, dizziness, fatigue.
GI: oral lesions, nausea, vomiting, diarrhea, enterocolitis, pseudomembranous colitis.
GU: interstitial nephritis, nephropathy.
Hematologic: *thrombocytopenia,* eosinophilia, *hemolytic anemia, neutropenia,* anemia, *agranulocytosis.*
Hepatic: elevated liver enzymes.
Other: hypersensitivity reactions (fever, chills, rash, urticaria, *anaphylaxis,* overgrowth of nonsusceptible organisms, *thrombophlebitis*).

☑ Special considerations
Besides the recommendations relevant to all penicillins, consider the following.
• Give oral drug with water only; acid in fruit juice or carbonated beverage may inactivate drug.
• Give oral dose on empty stomach; food decreases absorption.
• Except in osteomyelitis, don't give I.M. or I.V. unless patient can't take oral dose.
• Drug alters tests for urinary and serum proteins; turbidimetric urine and serum proteins are often falsely positive or elevated in tests using sulfosalicylic acid or trichloroacetic acid. Oxacillin may falsely decrease serum aminoglycoside levels.
• Signs and symptoms of overdose include neuromuscular sensitivity or seizures. Drug isn't appreciably removed by peritoneal dialysis or hemodialysis.

Monitoring the patient
• Assess renal and hepatic functions; monitor patient for elevated AST and ALT levels.
• Monitor therapeutic effect.

Information for the patient
• Explain need to take oral preparations without food and to follow with water because acid content of fruit juice and carbonated beverages interferes with absorption.
• Tell patient to report allergic reactions or severe diarrhea promptly.
• Emphasize importance of completing full course of therapy.

Geriatric patients
• Drug's half-life may be prolonged in elderly patients because of impaired renal function.

Pediatric patients
• Drug elimination is reduced in neonates. Transient hematuria, azotemia, and albuminuria have occurred in some neonates receiving oxacillin; monitor renal function closely.

Breast-feeding patients
• Drug appears in breast milk; use with caution in breast-feeding women.

oxaprozin
Daypro

Pharmacologic classification: NSAID
Therapeutic classification: nonnarcotic analgesic, antipyretic, anti-inflammatory
Pregnancy risk category C

How supplied
Available by prescription only
Caplets: 600 mg

Indications, route, and dosage
Management of acute or chronic osteoarthritis or rheumatoid arthritis
Adults: Initially, 1,200 mg P.O. daily. Individualize to smallest effective dosage to minimize adverse reactions. Smaller patients or those with mild symptoms may require only 600 mg daily. Maximum daily dose is 1,800 mg or 26 mg/kg, whichever is lower, in divided doses.

Pharmacodynamics
Analgesic, antipyretic, anti-inflammatory actions: Exact mechanism unknown. Inhibits several steps along the arachidonic acid pathway of prostaglandin synthesis. One of the modes of action is presumed to be a result of the inhibition of cyclooxygenase activity and prostaglandin synthesis at inflammation site.

Pharmacokinetics
• *Absorption:* 95% oral bioavailability, with plasma levels peaking between 3 and 5 hours after dosing. Food may reduce rate but not extent of absorption.

• *Distribution:* About 99.9% bound to albumin in plasma.
• *Metabolism:* Primarily metabolized in liver by microsomal oxidation (65%) and glucuronic acid conjugation (35%).
• *Excretion:* Glucuronide metabolites excreted in urine (65%) and feces (35%). Elimination half-life in adults is 42 to 50 hours.

Contraindications and precautions
Contraindicated in patients with hypersensitivity to drug and in those with the syndrome of nasal polyps, angioedema, and bronchospastic reaction to aspirin or other NSAIDs. Use cautiously in patients with renal or hepatic dysfunction, history of peptic ulcer, hypertension, CV disease, or conditions predisposing to fluid retention.

Interactions
Drug-drug. *Aspirin:* Drug displaced salicylates from plasma protein–binding; increased risk of salicylate toxicity. Don't use together.
Beta blockers (such as metoprolol): Transient increase in blood pressure after 14 days of therapy. Perform routine blood pressure monitoring when starting oxaprozin therapy.
Oral anticoagulants: Increased risk of bleeding. Monitor PT and INR.
Drug-lifestyle. *Sun exposure.* Photosensitivity reactions. Tell patient to take precautions.

Adverse reactions
CNS: depression, sedation, somnolence, confusion, sleep disturbances.
EENT: tinnitus, blurred vision.
GI: *nausea, dyspepsia, diarrhea, constipation,* abdominal pain or distress, anorexia, flatulence, vomiting, **hemorrhage,** stomatitis, ulcer.
GU: dysuria, urinary frequency.
Hematologic: prolonged bleeding time.
Hepatic: elevated liver function test results (with long-term use).
Skin: *rash,* photosensitivity.

☑ Special considerations
• Serious GI toxicity, including peptic ulceration and bleeding, can occur in patients taking NSAIDs despite absence of GI symptoms. Patients at risk for developing peptic ulceration and bleeding are those with history of serious GI events, alcoholism, smoking, or other factors associated with peptic ulcer disease.
• Doses above 1,200 mg/day should be used for patients who weigh more than 110 lb (50 kg), who have normal renal and hepatic function, who are at low risk for peptic ulceration, and whose severity of disease justifies maximal therapy.
• Most patients tolerate once-daily dosing. Divided doses may be tried in patients unable to tolerate single doses.
• Signs and symptoms of toxicity may include lethargy, drowsiness, nausea, vomiting, and epi-

gastric pain and are generally reversible with supportive care. GI bleeding and coma have occurred after NSAID overdose.

Monitoring the patient
• Elevations of liver function tests can occur after prolonged use. These abnormal findings may persist, worsen, or resolve with continued therapy. Rarely, patients may progress to severe hepatic dysfunction. Periodically monitor liver function tests in patients receiving long-term therapy, and closely monitor patients with abnormal test results.
• Anemia may occur in patients receiving drug. Obtain hemoglobin level or hematocrit in patients receiving prolonged therapy at intervals appropriate for their condition.

Information for the patient
• Warn patient to call immediately if signs and symptoms of GI bleeding or visual or auditory adverse reactions occur.
• Tell patient to take drug with milk or meals if adverse GI reactions occur.
• Because photosensitivity reactions may occur, advise patient to use a sunblock, wear protective clothing, and avoid prolonged exposure to sunlight.

Geriatric patients
• Elderly patients may need a reduced dose because of low body weight or disorders associated with aging.
• Elderly patients are less likely than younger patients to tolerate adverse reactions associated with oxaprozin.

Pediatric patients
• Safety and effectiveness in children haven't been established.

Breast-feeding patients
• It's unknown if drug appears in breast milk. Use with caution in breast-feeding women.

oxazepam
Apo-Oxazepam*, Novoxapam*, Ox-pam*, Serax

Pharmacologic classification: benzodiazepine
Therapeutic classification: anxiolytic, sedative-hypnotic
Controlled substance schedule IV
Pregnancy risk category D

How supplied
Available by prescription only
Tablets: 15 mg
Capsules: 10 mg, 15 mg, 30 mg

Reactions may be *common,* uncommon, **life-threatening**, or COMMON AND LIFE-THREATENING.

Indications, route, and dosage
Alcohol withdrawal, severe anxiety
Adults: 15 to 30 mg P.O. t.i.d. or q.i.d.
Tension, mild to moderate anxiety
Adults: 10 to 15 mg P.O. t.i.d. or q.i.d.
Elderly: Give 10 mg P.O. t.i.d.; then increase to 15 mg t.i.d. or q.i.d., p.r.n.

Pharmacodynamics
Anxiolytic and sedative-hypnotic action: Depresses the CNS at the limbic and subcortical levels of the brain. Produces an antianxiety effect by enhancing the effect of the neurotransmitter gamma-aminobutyric acid on its receptor in the ascending reticular activating system, which increases inhibition and blocks both cortical and limbic arousal.

Pharmacokinetics
• *Absorption:* Well absorbed through GI tract when given orally. Onset of action at 1 to 2 hours; levels peak 3 hours after dosing.
• *Distribution:* Distributed widely throughout body. Drug is 85% to 95% protein-bound.
• *Metabolism:* Metabolized in liver to inactive metabolites.
• *Excretion:* Drug metabolites excreted in urine as glucuronide conjugates. Half-life of drug is 5.7 to 10.9 hours.

Contraindications and precautions
Contraindicated in patients with hypersensitivity to drug and in those with psychosis. Use cautiously in elderly or debilitated patients, in those with history of drug abuse, and in those in whom a decrease in blood pressure is associated with cardiac problems.

Interactions
Drug-drug. *Antacids:* Decreased rate of oxazepam absorption. Separate administration times.
Antidepressants, antihistamines, barbiturates, general anesthetics, MAO inhibitors, narcotics, phenothiazines: Potentiated CNS depressant effects of these drugs. Use together cautiously.
Cimetidine, disulfiram: Increased oxazepam plasma level. Monitor patient closely.
Levodopa: Inhibited therapeutic effects of levodopa. Monitor patient closely
Drug-lifestyle. *Alcohol:* Potentiated CNS depressant effects of alcohol. Discourage use.
Heavy smoking: Accelerated oxazepam metabolism, lowering clinical effectiveness. Discourage smoking.

Adverse reactions
CNS: *drowsiness, lethargy,* dizziness, vertigo, headache, syncope, tremor, slurred speech, changes in EEG patterns.
CV: edema.
GI: nausea.

GU: altered libido.
Hepatic: *hepatic dysfunction.*
Skin: rash.

☑ Special considerations
Besides the recommendations relevant to all benzodiazepines, consider the following.
• Oxazepam tablets contain tartrazine dye; check patient's history for allergy to this substance.
• Store drug in a cool, dry place away from light.
• Inform patient to reduce dose gradually (over 8 to 12 weeks) after long-term use.
• Toxicity may cause somnolence, confusion, coma, hypoactive reflexes, dyspnea, labored breathing, hypotension, bradycardia, slurred speech, and unsteady gait or impaired coordination.
• In case of overdose, flumazenil may be useful. Dialysis is of limited value.

Monitoring the patient
• Monitor hepatic and renal function studies to ensure normal function.
• Monitor patient for neurologic changes.

Information for the patient
• Advise patient not to change drug regimen without medical approval.
• Instruct patient in safety measures, such as gradual position changes and supervised walking, to prevent injury.
• Caution patient that sleepiness may not occur for up to 2 hours after taking drug.
• Advise patient of potential for physical and psychological dependence with long-term use.
• Tell patient not to stop drug suddenly if he's been taking it for prolonged periods.

Geriatric patients
• Elderly patients are more susceptible to CNS depressant effects of oxazepam. Some may need supervision with walking and activities of daily living during start of therapy or after an increase in dosage.
• Lower doses are usually effective in elderly patients because of decreased elimination.

Pediatric patients
• Safe use in children under age 12 hasn't been established. Closely observe neonate for withdrawal symptoms if mother took oxazepam for a prolonged period during pregnancy.

Breast-feeding patients
• Because drug appears in breast milk, the breast-fed infant of a mother who uses oxazepam may become sedated, have feeding difficulties, or lose weight. Avoid use in breast-feeding women.

oxybutynin chloride
Ditropan, Ditropan XL

Pharmacologic classification: synthetic tertiary amine
Therapeutic classification: antispasmodic
Pregnancy risk category B

How supplied
Available by prescription only
Tablets: 5 mg
Tablets (extended release): 5 mg, 10 mg, 15 mg
Syrup: 5 mg/5 ml

Indications, route, and dosage
Relief of symptoms of bladder instability associated with voiding in patients with uninhibited and reflex neurogenic bladder
Adults: 5 mg P.O. b.i.d. to t.i.d. to maximum of 5 mg q.i.d.
Children over age 5: 5 mg P.O. b.i.d. to maximum of 5 mg t.i.d.
Overactive bladder
Adults: 5 mg P.O. daily. Increase as needed in 5-mg increments at about 1-week intervals to a maximum dose of 30 mg/day.

Pharmacodynamics
Antispasmodic action: Reduces the urge to void, increases bladder capacity, and reduces the frequency of contractions to the detrusor muscle. Exerts a direct spasmolytic action and an antimuscarinic action on smooth muscle.

Pharmacokinetics
- *Absorption:* Absorbed rapidly, with peak levels in 3 to 6 hours. Action begins in 30 to 60 minutes; lasts for 6 to 10 hours.
- *Distribution:* No information available.
- *Metabolism:* Metabolized by liver.
- *Excretion:* Excreted principally in urine.

Contraindications and precautions
Contraindicated in patients with hypersensitivity to drug and in those with myasthenia gravis, GI obstruction, glaucoma, adynamic ileus, megacolon, severe colitis, ulcerative colitis when megacolon is present, or obstructive uropathy; in elderly or debilitated patients with intestinal atony; and in hemorrhaging patients with unstable CV status.
    Use cautiously in elderly patients and in patients with impaired renal or hepatic function, autonomic neuropathy, or reflux esophagitis.

Interactions
Drug-drug. *CNS depressants:* Additive sedative effects. Monitor patient for increased sedation.
Digoxin: Increased digoxin levels. Monitor serum digoxin level.

Haloperidol: Possible worsening of schizophrenia, decreased serum levels of haloperidol, and development of tardive dyskinesia. Avoid concomitant use.
Phenothiazine: Increased anticholinergic adverse effects. Monitor patient closely.

Adverse reactions
CNS: dizziness, insomnia, restlessness, hallucinations, asthenia.
CV: *palpitations, tachycardia,* vasodilation.
EENT: mydriasis, cycloplegia, decreased lacrimation, amblyopia.
GI: nausea, vomiting, *constipation, dry mouth,* decreased GI motility.
GU: *urinary hesitancy, urine retention,* suppressed lactation.
Skin: rash.
Other: decreased diaphoresis, fever.

☑ Special considerations
- Stop therapy periodically to determine if patient still needs drug.
- Toxicity may cause restlessness, excitement, psychotic behavior, flushing, hypotension, circulatory failure, and fever. In severe cases, paralysis, respiratory failure, and coma may occur. Physostigmine may be considered to reverse symptoms of anticholinergic intoxication.

Monitoring the patient
- Periodically prepare patient for cystometry to evaluate response to therapy.
- Monitor patient for adverse effects.

Information for the patient
- Instruct patient regarding drug and dosage schedule; tell him to take a missed dose as soon as possible but not to double a dose.
- Tell patient not to crush or chew extended-release tablets. They may be administered without regard to food.
- Warn patient about possibility of decreased mental alertness or visual changes.
- Remind patient to use drug cautiously when in warm climates to minimize risk of heatstroke that may occur because of decreased sweating.

Geriatric patients
- Elderly patients may be more sensitive to antimuscarinic effects. Use cautiously.

Pediatric patients
- Dosage guidelines haven't been established for children under age 5.

Breast-feeding patients
- It's unknown if drug appears in breast milk. Use with caution in breast-feeding women.

Reactions may be *common*, uncommon, **life-threatening**, or COMMON AND LIFE-THREATENING.

oxycodone hydrochloride
OxyContin, OxyFAST, OxyIR,
Percolone, Roxicodone, Supeudol*

Pharmacologic classification: opioid
Therapeutic classification: analgesic
Controlled substance schedule II
Pregnancy risk category C

How supplied
Available by prescription only
Tablets: 5 mg
Tablets (sustained-release): 10 mg, 20 mg, 40 mg, 80 mg
Oral solution: 5 mg/ml, 20 mg/ml

Indications, route, and dosage
Moderate to severe pain
Adults: 5 mg P.O. q 6 hours
Chronic pain
Adults: Initially, 10-mg sustained-release tablet q 12 hours; may increase dose q 1 to 2 days. Dosing frequency shouldn't be increased.

Pharmacodynamics
Analgesic action: Acts on opiate receptors, providing analgesia for moderate to moderately severe pain. Episodes of acute pain, rather than chronic pain, appear to be more responsive to treatment with oxycodone.

Pharmacokinetics
• *Absorption:* After oral administration, onset of analgesic effect within 15 to 30 minutes; peak effect reached within 1 hour.
• *Distribution:* Rapidly distributed.
• *Metabolism:* Metabolized in liver.
• *Excretion:* Excreted principally by kidneys. Duration of analgesia is 6 hours; for sustained-release tablets, 12 hours.

Contraindications and precautions
Contraindicated in patients with hypersensitivity to drug. Use cautiously in elderly or debilitated patients and in those with head injury, increased intracranial pressure, seizures, asthma, COPD, prostatic hyperplasia, severe hepatic or renal disease, acute abdominal conditions, urethral stricture, hypothyroidism, Addison's disease, or arrhythmias.

Interactions
Drug-drug. *Anticholinergics:* Paralytic ileus. Use together cautiously.
Anticoagulants: Oxycodone products containing aspirin may increase anticoagulant's effect. Monitor clotting times; use together cautiously.
Cimetidine: Increased respiratory and CNS depression, causing confusion, disorientation, apnea, or seizures. Avoid concomitant use.

Digitoxin, phenytoin, rifampin: Drug accumulation and enhanced effects may result from use with other drugs extensively metabolized in liver. Monitor patient for toxicity.
General anesthetics: Severe CV depression. Avoid concomitant use.
Opioid agonist-antagonist, single dose of an antagonist: Acute withdrawal syndrome in patients who become physically dependent on this drug. Avoid concomitant use.
Other CNS depressants (antihistamines, barbiturates, benzodiazepines, general anesthetics, muscle relaxants, narcotic analgesics, phenothiazines, sedative-hypnotics, tricyclic antidepressants): Potentiated drug's respiratory and CNS depression, sedation, and hypotensive effects. Monitor patient closely.
Drug-lifestyle. *Alcohol:* Potentiated drug's respiratory and CNS depression, sedation, and hypotensive effects. Discourage use.

Adverse reactions
CNS: *sedation, somnolence, clouded sensorium, euphoria, dizziness, light-headedness,* **seizures.**
CV: *hypotension,* **bradycardia.**
GI: *nausea, vomiting, constipation,* ileus, increased plasma amylase and lipase levels.
GU: *urine retention.*
Hepatic: increased liver enzyme levels.
Respiratory: *respiratory depression.*
Skin: *diaphoresis,* pruritus, rash.
Other: physical dependence.

☑ Special considerations
Besides the recommendations relevant to all opioids, consider the following.
• Single-drug oxycodone solution or tablets are ideal for patients who can't take aspirin or acetaminophen.
• Oxycodone has high abuse potential.
• Drug may obscure signs and symptoms of acute abdominal condition or worsen gallbladder pain.
• Consider prescribing stool softener for patients on long-term therapy.
• The 80-mg sustained-release tablets are for opioid-tolerant patients only.
• Severe toxicity may cause CNS depression, respiratory depression, and miosis (pinpoint pupils). Other acute toxic effects include hypotension, bradycardia, hypothermia, shock, apnea, cardiopulmonary arrest, circulatory collapse, pulmonary edema, and convulsions. Naloxone shouldn't be given unless patient has clinically significant respiratory or CV depression. Dialysis may be helpful if combination products containing aspirin or acetaminophen are involved.

Monitoring the patient
• Monitor circulatory and respiratory status. Withhold dose if respirations are shallow or if respiratory rate falls below 12 breaths/minute.

• Monitor patient for dependency and abuse of drug.
• Monitor patient's bowel and bladder patterns. Patient may need a laxative.

Information for the patient
• For full analgesic effect, teach patient to take drug before onset of intense pain.
• Warn patient about possibility of decreased alertness or visual changes.

Geriatric patients
• Lower doses are usually indicated for elderly patients, who may be more sensitive to therapeutic and adverse effects of drug.

Pediatric patients
• Dosage may be individualized for children; however, safety and effectiveness in children haven't been established.

Breast-feeding patients
• It's unknown if drug appears in breast milk; use with caution in breast-feeding women.

---

oxymetazoline hydrochloride
Afrin, Allerest 12 Hour Nasal, Chlorphed-LA, Dristan 12 Hr Spray, Duramist Plus, Duration, 4-Way Long Lasting Nasal, Genasal Decongestant Spray, Neo-Synephrine 12 Hour Spray, Nostrilla Long Acting Spray, NTZ, OcuClear, Sinarest 12 Hour Spray, Sinex, Visine L.R.

Pharmacologic classification: sympathomimetic
Therapeutic classification: decongestant, vasoconstrictor
Pregnancy risk category C

How supplied
Available without a prescription
Nasal solution: 0.025% (drops) for children
Nasal drops or spray: 0.05%
Ophthalmic solution: 0.025%

Indications, route, and dosage
Nasal congestion
Adults and children over age 6: Apply 2 to 3 drops or sprays of 0.05% solution in each nostril b.i.d. Use no more than 3 to 5 days.
Children ages 2 to 6: Apply 2 to 3 drops of 0.025% solution to nasal mucosa b.i.d. Use no more than 3 to 5 days. Dosage for younger children hasn't been established.
Relief of minor eye redness
Adults and children over age 6: Apply 1 to 2 drops in the conjunctival sac b.i.d. to q.i.d. (space at least 6 hours apart).

Pharmacodynamics
Decongestant action: Produces local vasoconstriction of arterioles through alpha receptors to reduce blood flow and nasal congestion.

Pharmacokinetics
• *Absorption:* After intranasal application, local vasoconstriction within 5 to 10 minutes; lasts for 5 to 6 hours with gradual decline over next 6 hours.
• *Distribution:* No information available.
• *Metabolism:* No information available.
• *Excretion:* No information available.

Contraindications and precautions
Contraindicated in patients with hypersensitivity to drug. Ophthalmic form contraindicated in patients with angle-closure glaucoma.
    Use cautiously in patients with hyperthyroidism, cardiac disease, or hypertension and in those receiving MAO inhibitors. Use nasal solution cautiously in patients with diabetes mellitus. Ophthalmic form should be used cautiously in those with eye disease, infection, or injury.

Interactions
Drug-drug. *Beta blockers:* Increased systemic adverse effects of beta blockers (ophthalmic form). Use together cautiously.
Local anesthetics: Increased absorption (ophthalmic form). Monitor patient for adverse effects.
Tricyclic antidepressants: Potentiated pressor effects of these drugs from significant systemic absorption of decongestant. Monitor patient closely.

Adverse reactions
CNS: headache, insomnia; drowsiness, dizziness, possible sedation (with nasal form); lightheadedness, nervousness, trembling (with ophthalmic form).
CV: palpitations; *CV collapse,* hypertension (with nasal form); tachycardia, **bradycardia,** irregular heartbeat (with ophthalmic form).
EENT: rebound nasal congestion or irritation with excessive or long-term use, dryness of nose and throat, increased nasal discharge, stinging, sneezing (with nasal form); *transient stinging upon instillation,* blurred vision, reactive hyperemia, keratitis, lacrimation, increased intraocular pressure (with ophthalmic form).
Other: systemic effects in children (with excessive or long-term use, with nasal form).

☑ Special considerations
• Toxicity may cause somnolence, sedation, sweating, CNS depression with hypertension, bradycardia, decreased cardiac output, rebound hypertension, CV collapse, depressed respirations, coma. If ingested, emesis isn't recommended unless given early because of rapid onset of sedation.

Reactions may be *common*, uncommon, *life-threatening*, or COMMON AND LIFE-THREATENING.

Monitoring the patient
● Watch carefully for adverse reactions in patients with CV disease, diabetes mellitus, or prostatic hypertrophy because systemic absorption can occur.
● Monitor therapeutic effect.

Information for the patient
● Emphasize that only one person should use dropper bottle or nasal spray.
● Advise patient not to exceed recommended dosage and to use drug only when needed.
● Tell patient to stop drug and call if symptoms persist after 3 days.
● Tell patient nasal mucosa may sting, burn, or become dry.
● Warn patient that excessive use may cause bradycardia, hypotension, dizziness, and weakness.
● Show patient how to apply. Have him bend head forward and sniff spray briskly or apply light pressure on lacrimal sac after instillation of eyedrop.

Geriatric patients
● Use drug with caution in elderly patients with cardiac disease, poorly controlled hypertension, or diabetes mellitus.

Pediatric patients
● Children may exhibit increased adverse effects from systemic absorption; 0.05% nasal solution is contraindicated in children under age 6; 0.025% nasal solution should be used in children under age 2 only under medical direction and supervision.

---

oxymorphone hydrochloride
Numorphan

Pharmacologic classification: opioid
Therapeutic classification: analgesic
Controlled substance schedule II
Pregnancy risk category C

How supplied
Available by prescription only
Injection: 1 mg/ml, 1.5 mg/ml
Suppository: 5 mg

Indications, route, and dosage
Moderate to severe pain
Adults: 1 to 1.5 mg I.M. or S.C. q 4 to 6 hours, p.r.n., or around the clock; 0.5 mg I.V. q 4 to 6 hours, p.r.n., or around the clock; or 1 suppository administered P.R. q 4 to 6 hours, p.r.n., or around the clock.
Note: Parenteral administration of drug is also indicated for preoperative medication, for support of anesthesia, for obstetric analgesia, and for relief of anxiety in dyspnea associated with acute left-sided heart failure and pulmonary edema.

Pharmacodynamics
Analgesic action: Effectively relieves moderate to severe pain via agonist activity at the opiate receptors. Has little or no antitussive effect.

Pharmacokinetics
● *Absorption:* Well absorbed after P.R., S.C., I.M., or I.V. administration. Onset of action within 5 to 10 minutes; peak analgesic effect at ½ to 1 hour.
● *Distribution:* Widely distributed.
● *Metabolism:* Primarily metabolized in liver.
● *Excretion:* Excreted primarily in urine as oxymorphone conjugates. Duration of action is 3 to 6 hours.

Contraindications and precautions
Contraindicated in patients with hypersensitivity to drug. Use cautiously in elderly or debilitated patients and in those with head injury, increased intracranial pressure, seizures, asthma, COPD, acute abdomen conditions, prostatic hyperplasia, severe renal or kidney disease, urethral stricture, respiratory depression, Addison's disease, arrhythmias, or hypothyroidism.

Interactions
Drug-drug. *Anticholinergics:* Paralytic ileus. Use together cautiously.
Cimetidine: Increased respiratory and CNS depression, causing confusion, disorientation, apnea, or seizures. Avoid concomitant use.
Digitoxin, phenytoin, rifampin: Drug accumulation and enhanced effects may result from use with other drugs extensively metabolized in liver. Monitor patient for toxicity.
General anesthetics: Severe CV depression. Avoid concomitant use.
Opioid agonist-antagonist, single dose of an antagonist: Acute withdrawal syndrome in patients who become physically dependent on this drug. Avoid concomitant use.
Other CNS depressants (antihistamines, barbiturates, benzodiazepines, general anesthetics, muscle relaxants, opiates, phenothiazines, sedative-hypnotics, tricyclic antidepressants): Potentiated respiratory and CNS depression, sedation, and hypotensive effects of drug. Monitor patient closely.
Drug-lifestyle. *Alcohol:* Potentiated drug's respiratory and CNS depression, sedation, and hypotensive effects. Discourage use.

Adverse reactions
CNS: *sedation, somnolence, clouded sensorium, euphoria,* dizziness, **seizures** (with large doses), *light-headedness, headache.*
CV: *hypotension,* **bradycardia.**
GI: *nausea, vomiting, constipation,* ileus, increased plasma amylase levels.

GU: *urine retention.*
Respiratory: *respiratory depression.*
Skin: pruritus.
Other: physical dependence.

☑ Special considerations
Besides the recommendations relevant to all opioids, consider the following.
• Refrigerate oxymorphone suppositories.
• Drug is well absorbed P.R. and is an alternative to opioids with more limited dosage forms.
• Drug may worsen gallbladder pain.
• Toxicity may cause CNS depression (extreme somnolence progressing to stupor and coma), respiratory depression, and miosis (pinpoint pupils). Other acute toxic effects include hypotension, bradycardia, hypothermia, shock, apnea, cardiopulmonary arrest, circulatory collapse, pulmonary edema, and seizures. Naloxone shouldn't be given unless patient has clinically significant respiratory or CV depression.

Monitoring the patient
• Monitor circulatory and respiratory status. Withhold dose if respirations are shallow or if respiratory rate falls below 12 breaths/minute.
• Watch for dependency and abuse of drug.
• Monitor patient's bowel and bladder patterns. Patient may need a laxative.

Geriatric patients
• Lower dosages are usually indicated for elderly patients, who may be more sensitive to therapeutic and adverse effects of drug.

Pediatric patients
• Don't use in children under age 12.

Breast-feeding patients
• It's unknown if drug appears in breast milk; use with caution in breast-feeding women.

oxytocin
Pitocin, Syntocinon

Pharmacologic classification: exogenous hormone
Therapeutic classification: oxytocic, lactation stimulant
Pregnancy risk category C

How supplied
Available by prescription only
Injection: 10-units/ml ampules, vials, and closed injection system

Indications, route, and dosage
Induction of labor
Adults: Initially, no more than 1 to 2 milliunits/minute I.V. infusion. Rate of infusion may be increased slowly. Decrease rate when labor is firmly established.
Augmentation of labor
Adults: Initially, 2 milliunits/minute I.V. infusion. Rate of infusion may be increased slowly to maximum of 20 milliunits/minute.
Reduction of postpartum bleeding after expulsion of placenta
Adults: 10 to 40 milliunits/minute I.V. infusion (or 10 units I.M.) after delivery of placenta.
To induce abortion
Adults: 10 units mixed in 500 ml D_5W or normal saline solution I.V. at 10 to 20 milliunits/minute.
◇ *Oxytocin challenge test to assess fetal distress in high-risk pregnancies greater than 31 weeks' gestation*
Adults: Prepare solution by adding 5 to 10 units oxytocin to 1 L of 5% dextrose injection (yielding a solution of 5 to 10 milliunits per ml). Infuse 0.5 milliunits/minute, gradually increasing at 15-minute intervals to maximum infusion of 20 milliunits/minute. Stop infusion when three moderate uterine contractions occur in a 10-minute interval. Response of fetal heart rate to test may be used to evaluate prognosis

Pharmacodynamics
Oxytocic action: Increases the sodium permeability of uterine myofibrils, indirectly stimulating the contraction of uterine smooth muscle. The threshold for response is lowered in the presence of high estrogen levels. Uterine response increases with the length of the pregnancy and increases further during active labor. Response mimics labor contractions.

Pharmacokinetics
• *Absorption:* Immediate onset after I.V. infusion; within 3 to 5 minutes of I.M. injection. Rapid but erratic absorption through nasal mucosa; acts within a few minutes. Destroyed in GI tract.
• *Distribution:* Distributed throughout extracellular fluid; small amounts may enter fetal circulation.
• *Metabolism:* Metabolized rapidly in kidneys and liver. In early pregnancy, a circulating enzyme, oxytocinase, can inactivate drug.
• *Excretion:* Only small amounts excreted in urine as oxytocin. Half-life is 3 to 5 minutes. Duration of action is 1 hour after I.V. infusion, 2 to 3 hours after I.M. injection, and 20 minutes after intranasal administration.

Contraindications and precautions
Contraindicated in patients with hypersensitivity to drug and in those with severe toxemia, hypertonic uterine patterns, total placenta previa, and vasoprevia. Also contraindicated when cephalopelvic disproportion is present or when delivery requires conversion, as in transverse lie; and in fetal distress when delivery isn't imminent, prematurity, and other obstetric emergencies.

Use cautiously during first and second stages of labor and in patients with history of cervical or uterine surgery (including cesarean section), grand multiparity, uterine sepsis, traumatic delivery, overdistended uterus, or invasive cervical cancer.

Interactions
Drug-drug. *Cyclopropane anesthesia:* May modify oxytocin's CV effects. Monitor patient closely.
Sympathomimetics: Increased pressor effects, possibly resulting in postpartum hypertension. Monitor vital signs carefully.
Thiopental: Delayed induction of thiopental anesthesia. Use together cautiously.

Adverse reactions
Maternal
CNS: *subarachnoid hemorrhage, seizures, or coma.*
CV: *hypertension,* increased heart rate, systemic venous return, and cardiac output, *arrhythmias, postpartum hemorrhage, water retention.*
GI: nausea, vomiting.
GU: tetanic uterine contractions, *abruptio placentae, impaired uterine blood flow,* pelvic hematoma, *increased uterine motility, uterine rupture.*
Hematologic: *afibrinogenemia.*
Other: hypersensitivity reactions (*anaphylaxis*).
Fetal
CV: *bradycardia, premature ventricular contractions, arrhythmias.*
Respiratory: *anoxia, asphyxia.*
Other: *brain damage, death, jaundice, low Apgar scores,* retinal hemorrhage.

☑ Special considerations
● Administer by I.V. infusion, not I.V. bolus injection. Use an infusion device.
● Drug may produce an antidiuretic effect; monitor fluid intake and output.
● Have magnesium sulfate (20% solution) available for relaxation of myometrium.
● Drug isn't recommended for routine I.M. use. However, 10 units may be administered I.M. after delivery of placenta to control postpartum uterine bleeding.
● Solution containing 10 milliunits/ml may be prepared by adding 10 units of oxytocin to 1 L of normal saline solution or D_5W. Solution containing 20 milliunits/ml may be prepared by adding 10 units of oxytocin to 500 ml of normal saline solution or D_5W.
● Toxicity may cause hyperstimulation of the uterus, causing tetanic contractions and possible uterine rupture, cervical laceration, abruptio placentae, impaired uterine blood flow, amniotic fluid embolism, and fetal trauma. Drug has very short half-life; therefore, therapy should be halted and supportive care initiated.

Monitoring the patient
● Monitor and record uterine contractions, heart rate, blood pressure, intrauterine pressure, fetal heart rate, and character of blood loss every 15 minutes.
● When administering oxytocin challenge test, monitor fetal heart rate and uterine contractions immediately before and during infusion. If fetal heart rate doesn't change during test, repeat in 1 week. If late deceleration in fetal heart rate is noted, consider terminating pregnancy.
● During long infusions, watch for signs of water intoxication.

Information for the patient
● Explain possible adverse effects of drug.

Breast-feeding patients
● Minimal amounts of drug appear in breast milk; evaluate benefits to mother versus risks to infant.

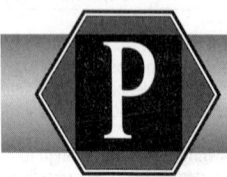

paclitaxel
Taxol

Pharmacologic classification: novel antimicrotubule
Therapeutic classification: antineoplastic
Pregnancy risk category D

How supplied
Available by prescription only
Injection: 30 mg/5 ml

Indications, route, and dosage
Metastatic ovarian cancer after failure of first-line or subsequent chemotherapy
Adults: 135 or 175 mg/m² I.V. over 3 hours q 3 weeks. Subsequent courses shouldn't be repeated until neutrophil count is at least 1,500 cells/mm³ and platelet count is at least 100,000 cells/mm³.
Breast carcinoma after failure of combination chemotherapy for metastatic disease or relapse within 6 months of adjuvant chemotherapy (prior therapy should have included an anthracycline unless clinically contraindicated)
Adults: 175 mg/m² I.V. over 3 hours q 3 weeks.
AIDS-related Kaposi's sarcoma
Adults: 135 mg/m² I.V. over 3 hours q 3 weeks, or 100 mg/m² I.V. over 3 hours q 2 weeks.

Pharmacodynamics
Antineoplastic action: Prevents depolymerization of cellular microtubules, thus inhibiting the normal reorganization of the microtubule network necessary for mitosis and other vital cellular functions.

Pharmacokinetics
• *Absorption:* No information available.
• *Distribution:* About 89% to 98% bound to serum proteins.
• *Metabolism:* Possibly metabolized in liver.
• *Excretion:* Not fully understood.

Contraindications and precautions
Contraindicated in patients with hypersensitivity to drug or polyoxyethylated castor oil, a vehicle used in drug solution, and in those with baseline neutrophil counts below 1,500/mm³. Use cautiously in patients who have received radiation therapy.

Interactions
Drug-drug. *Cisplatin:* Myelosuppression may be greater when cisplatin is given before rather than after paclitaxel. Consider this effect before therapy.
Cyclosporine, dexamethasone, diazepam, etoposide, ketoconazole, quinidine, teniposide, verapamil, vincristine: Inhibited paclitaxel metabolism. Use together cautiously.

Adverse reactions
CNS: *peripheral neuropathy.*
CV: ***bradycardia**, hypotension, abnormal ECG.*
GI: *nausea, vomiting, diarrhea, mucositis.*
Hematologic: NEUTROPENIA, LEUKOPENIA, THROMBOCYTOPENIA, anemia, *bleeding.*
Hepatic: *elevated liver enzyme levels.*
Musculoskeletal: *myalgia, arthralgia.*
Skin: *alopecia.*
Other: *hypersensitivity reactions (**anaphylaxis**), phlebitis, cellulitis at injection site, infections.*

☑ Special considerations
• Severe hypersensitivity reactions characterized by dyspnea, hypotension, angioedema, and generalized urticaria have occurred in 2% of patients receiving paclitaxel. To reduce risk or severity of these reactions, pretreat patients with corticosteroids (such as dexamethasone), antihistamines (such as diphenhydramine), and H₂-receptor antagonists (such as cimetidine or ranitidine).
• Don't rechallenge patients who experience severe hypersensitivity reactions to drug.
• In patients who experience severe neutropenia (neutrophil count below 500 cells/mm³ for 1 week or longer) or severe peripheral neuropathy during drug therapy, reduce dosage by 20% for subsequent courses. Risk and severity of neurotoxicity and hematologic toxicity increase with dose, especially above 190 mg/m².
• Use caution during drug preparation and administration; wear gloves. If solution contacts skin, wash skin immediately and thoroughly with soap and water. If drug contacts mucous membranes, flush membranes thoroughly with water. Mark all waste materials with CHEMOTHERAPY HAZARD labels.
• Concentrate must be diluted before infusion. Compatible solutions include normal saline injection, D₅W, dextrose 5% in normal saline injection, and 5% dextrose in lactated Ringer's

injection. Dilute to a final concentration of 0.3 to 1.2 mg/ml. Diluted solutions are stable for 27 hours at room temperature.
• Prepare and store infusion solutions in glass containers. Undiluted concentrate shouldn't contact polyvinyl chloride I.V. bags or tubing. Store diluted solution in glass or polypropylene bottles, or use polypropylene or polyolefin bags. Administer through polyethylene-lined administration sets, and use an in-line filter with a microporous membrane not exceeding 0.22 microns.
• Primary complications of overdose include bone marrow suppression, peripheral neurotoxicity, and mucositis.

Monitoring the patient
• Bone marrow toxicity is the most frequent and dose-limiting toxicity. Frequent blood count monitoring is necessary during therapy. Packed RBC or platelet transfusions may be necessary in severe cases. Institute bleeding precautions as appropriate.
• If patient develops significant conduction abnormalities during drug administration, provide appropriate therapy and monitor cardiac function continuously during subsequent drug therapy.
• Continuously monitor patient for 30 minutes after starting infusion. Continue close monitoring throughout infusion.

Information for the patient
• Advise woman of childbearing age to avoid becoming pregnant during therapy because of potential harm to fetus.
• Warn patient that alopecia occurs in almost all patients.
• Teach patient to recognize and immediately report signs and symptoms of peripheral neuropathy, such as tingling, burning, and numbness in extremities. Although mild symptoms are common, severe symptoms occur infrequently. Dosage reduction may be necessary.

Pediatric patients
• Safety and effectiveness in children haven't been established.

Breast-feeding patients
• It's unknown if drug appears in breast milk. Because of potential for serious adverse reactions in breast-fed infants, breast-feeding should be stopped during therapy.

palivizumab
Synagis

Pharmacologic classification: recombinant monoclonal antibody IgG1$_\kappa$
Therapeutic classification: respiratory syncytial virus (RSV) prophylaxis drug
Pregnancy risk category C

How supplied
Available by prescription only
Injection: 100 mg single-use vial

Indications, route, and dosage
Prevention of serious lower respiratory tract disease caused by RSV in children at high risk
Children: 15 mg/kg I.M. monthly throughout RSV season. Administer first dose before beginning of RSV season.

Pharmacodynamics
RSV prophylaxis drug action: Exhibits neutralizing and fusion-inhibitory activity against RSV, which inhibits RSV replication.

Pharmacokinetics
• *Absorption:* Not reported.
• *Distribution:* Not reported.
• *Metabolism:* Not reported.
• *Excretion:* Half-life is about 18 days.

Contraindications and precautions
Contraindicated in children with history of severe prior reaction to drug or its components. Use cautiously in patients with thrombocytopenia or any coagulation disorder.

Interactions
None reported.

Adverse reactions
CNS: nervousness.
EENT: *otitis media, rhinitis,* pharyngitis, sinusitis, conjunctivitis, oral candidiasis.
GI: diarrhea, vomiting, gastroenteritis.
Hematologic: anemia.
Hepatic: liver function abnormality (increased ALT, AST levels).
Respiratory: *upper respiratory tract infection,* cough, wheeze, bronchiolitis, *apnea,* pneumonia, bronchitis, asthma, croup, dyspnea.
Skin: *rash,* fungal dermatitis, eczema, seborrhea.
Other: pain, hernia, failure to thrive, injection site reaction, viral infection, flu syndrome.

☑ Special considerations
• Patient should receive monthly doses throughout RSV season, even if patient develops RSV

infection. In northern hemisphere, RSV season typically lasts from November to April.

• To reconstitute, slowly add 1 ml of sterile water for injection into a 100-mg vial. Gently swirl vial for 30 seconds to avoid foaming. Don't shake vial. Let reconstituted solution stand at room temperature for 20 minutes.

• Vial doesn't contain preservative; use within 6 hours of reconstitution.

• Administer drug in anterolateral aspect of thigh. Don't use gluteal muscle routinely as injection site because of risk of damage to sciatic nerve. Injection volumes over 1 ml should be given as a divided dose. Don't administer I.V.

• Anaphylactoid reactions after drug administration haven't been observed but can occur after administration of proteins. If anaphylaxis or severe allergic reaction occurs, give epinephrine (1:1,000) and provide supportive care as needed.

• Drug is intended for prophylaxis only. Not used for treatment of present RSV infection.

Monitoring the patient
• Monitor patient for adverse effects.
• Monitor hepatic enzymes.

Information for the patient
• Explain to parent or caregiver that drug is used to prevent RSV, not to treat it.
• Advise parent that monthly injections are recommended throughout RSV season (November to April in northern hemisphere).
• Advise parent to report adverse reactions immediately.

pamidronate disodium
Aredia

Pharmacologic classification: bisphosphonate, pyrophosphate analogue
Therapeutic classification: antihypercalcemic
Pregnancy risk category C

How supplied
Available by prescription only
Injection: 30 mg/vial, 60 mg/vial, 90 mg/vial

Indications, route, and dosage
Moderate to severe hypercalcemia associated with malignancy (with or without metastases)
Adults: Dosage depends on severity of hypercalcemia. Serum calcium levels should be corrected for serum albumin. Corrected serum calcium (CCa) is calculated using the following formula:

$$\frac{CCa}{(mg/dl)} = \frac{serum\ Ca}{(mg/dl)} + \frac{0.8\ (4 - serum\ albumin)}{(g/dl)}$$

Repeat doses shouldn't be given sooner than 7 days to allow for full response to initial dose.

✦ *Dosage adjustment.* Patients with moderate hypercalcemia (CCa levels of 12 to 13.5 mg/dl) may receive 60 to 90 mg by I.V. infusion over 24 hours. Patients with severe hypercalcemia (CCa levels over 13.5 mg/dl) may receive 90 mg as the initial dose.

Paget's disease
Adults: 30 mg I.V. daily over 4 hours for 3 consecutive days for total dose of 90 mg.

Osteolytic bone lesions of multiple myeloma
Adults: 90 mg I.V. over 4 hours once monthly.

Pharmacodynamics
Antihypercalcemic action: Inhibits resorption of bone. Adsorbs to hydroxyapatite crystals in bone and may directly block dissolution of calcium phosphate. Apparently doesn't inhibit bone formation or mineralization.

Pharmacokinetics
• *Absorption:* Rapid onset; duration of action up to 6 months in bone.
• *Distribution:* After I.V. administration, about 50% to 60% of dose rapidly absorbed by bone; drug also taken up by kidneys, liver, spleen, teeth, and tracheal cartilage.
• *Metabolism:* None.
• *Excretion:* Excreted by kidneys; average of 51% of dose excreted in urine within 72 hours of administration.

Contraindications and precautions
Contraindicated in patients with hypersensitivity to drug or other bisphosphonates, such as etidronate. Use with extreme caution in patients with impaired renal function.

Interactions
Drug-drug. *Solutions containing calcium:* Drug may form precipitate when mixed with solutions containing calcium. Don't mix together.

Adverse reactions
CNS: *seizures,* fatigue, headache, somnolence.
CV: atrial fibrillation, syncope, tachycardia, *hypertension.*
GI: *abdominal pain, anorexia, constipation, nausea, vomiting,* GI hemorrhage.
Hematologic: **leukopenia, thrombocytopenia,** anemia.
Metabolic: *hypophosphatemia, hypokalemia, hypomagnesemia, hypocalcemia.*
Musculoskeletal: *bone pain.*
Other: *fever, infusion-site reaction, generalized pain.*

☑ Special considerations
• Reconstitute vial with 10 ml sterile water for injection. Once drug is completely dissolved, add to 1,000 ml 0.45% or normal saline solution in-

jection or D$_5$W. Don't mix with infusion solutions that contain calcium, such as Ringer's injection or lactated Ringer's injection. Administer in single I.V. solution, in separate line from all other drugs. Visually inspect for precipitate before administering.
• Injection solution is stable for 24 hours when refrigerated. Give only by I.V. infusion. Nephropathy may occur when drug is given as a bolus.
• Consider retreatment if hypercalcemia recurs; wait a minimum of 7 days before retreatment to allow for full response to initial dose.

Monitoring the patient
• Because drug can cause electrolyte disturbances, careful monitoring of serum electrolytes (especially calcium, phosphate, and magnesium) is essential. Short-term administration of calcium may be necessary in patients with severe hypocalcemia. Also monitor hemoglobin and creatinine levels, CBC, differential, and hematocrit.
• Carefully monitor patients with preexisting anemia, leukopenia, or thrombocytopenia during first 2 weeks after therapy.
• Monitor patient's temperature. 27% of patients experience a slightly elevated temperature for 24 to 48 hours after therapy.

Information for the patient
• Explain use and administration of drug to patient and family.
• Instruct patient to report adverse reactions promptly.

Pediatric patients
• Safety and efficacy in children haven't been established.

Breast-feeding patients
• It's unknown if drug appears in breast milk. Use with caution in breast-feeding women.

pancreatin
Donnazyme, Hi-Vegi-Lip, 4X Pancreatin, 8X Pancreatin, Pancrezyme 4X

Pharmacologic classification: pancreatic enzyme
Therapeutic classification: digestant
Pregnancy risk category C

How supplied
Available without a prescription
Hi-Vegi-Lip
Tablets (enteric-coated): 2,400 mg pancreatin; 4,800 units lipase; 60,000 units protease; 60,000 units amylase

4X Pancreatin, Pancrezyme 4X
Tablets (enteric-coated): 2,400 mg pancreatin; 12,000 units lipase; 60,000 units protease; 60,000 units amylase
8X Pancreatin
Tablets (enteric-coated): 7,200 mg pancreatin; 22,500 units lipase; 180,000 units protease; 180,000 units amylase
Available by prescription only
Donnazyme
Tablets: 500 mg pancreatin; 1,000 units lipase; 12,500 units protease; 12,500 units amylase

Indications, route, and dosage
Exocrine pancreatic secretion insufficiency, digestive aid in cystic fibrosis, steatorrhea, and other disorders of fat metabolism secondary to insufficient pancreatic enzymes
Adults and children: 1 to 2 tablets P.O. with each meal.

Pharmacodynamics
Digestive action: The proteolytic, amylolytic, and lipolytic enzymes enhance the digestion of proteins, starches, and fats. Drug is sensitive to acids and is more active in neutral or slightly alkaline environments.

Pharmacokinetics
• *Absorption:* Not absorbed; acts locally in GI tract.
• *Distribution:* None.
• *Metabolism:* None.
• *Excretion:* Excreted in feces.

Contraindications and precautions
Contraindicated in patients with hypersensitivity to drug or pork protein or enzymes and in those with acute pancreatitis or acute exacerbations of chronic pancreatitis. Use cautiously in pregnant or breast-feeding women.

Interactions
Drug-drug. *Antacids containing calcium or magnesium:* Pancreatin activity may be reduced. Don't administer together.
Products containing iron: Decreased absorption of these drugs. Monitor patient for decreased effectiveness.

Adverse reactions
GI: nausea, diarrhea (with high doses).
Metabolic: increased serum uric acid.
Skin: perianal irritation, rash.
Other: *allergic reactions.*

☑ Special considerations
• For maximal effect, administer dose just before or during a meal.
• Tablets may not be crushed or chewed; follow with a glass of water to ensure complete swallowing.

- Diet should balance fat, protein, and starch intake properly to avoid indigestion. Dosage varies according to degree of maldigestion and malabsorption, amount of fat in diet, and enzyme activity of individual preparations.
- Adequate replacement decreases number of bowel movements and improves stool consistency.
- Use only after confirmed diagnosis of exocrine pancreatic insufficiency. Not effective in GI disorders unrelated to pancreatic enzyme deficiency.
- Enteric coating may reduce availability of enzyme in upper portion of jejunum and shouldn't be chewed. Swallow promptly to avoid mucosal irritation.
- Toxicity may include hyperuricuria, hyperuricemia, diarrhea, abdominal cramps, and transient intestinal upset.

Monitoring the patient
- Monitor dietary intake.
- Monitor therapeutic effect.

Information for the patient
- Explain use of drug, and advise storage away from heat and light.
- Be sure patient or family understands special dietary instructions for the particular disease. Tell him not to change brands without medical approval.

pancrelipase
Cotazym, Cotazym-S, Creon 5, Creon 10, Creon 20, Ilozyme, Ku-Zyme HP, Pancrease, Pancrease MT4, Pancrease MT10, Pancrease MT16, Pancrease MT20, Ultrase, Ultrase MT12, Ultrase MT18, Ultrase MT20, Viokase, Zymase

Pharmacologic classification: pancreatic enzyme
Therapeutic classification: digestant
Pregnancy risk category C

How supplied
Available by prescription only
Cotazym
Capsules: 8,000 units lipase; 30,000 units protease; 30,000 units amylase
Cotazym-S
Capsules: 5,000 units lipase; 20,000 units protease; 20,000 units amylase
Creon 5
Capsules (enteric-coated microspheres): 5,000 units lipase; 16,600 units protease; 18,750 units amylase
Creon 10
Capsules (delayed-release): 10,000 units lipase; 37,500 units protease; 33,200 units amylase

Creon 20
Capsules (delayed-release): 20,000 units lipase; 75,000 units protease; 66,400 units amylase
Ilozyme
Tablets: 11,000 units lipase; 30,000 units protease; 30,000 units amylase
Ku-Zyme HP
Capsules: 8,000 units lipase; 30,000 units protease; 30,000 units amylase
Pancrease
Capsules: 4,000 units lipase; 25,000 units protease; 20,000 units amylase
Pancrease MT4
Capsules (enteric-coated microtablets): 4,000 units lipase; 12,000 units protease; 12,000 units amylase
Pancrease MT10
Capsules (enteric-coated microtablets): 10,000 units lipase; 30,000 units protease; 30,000 units amylase
Pancrease MT16
Capsules (enteric-coated microtablets): 16,000 units lipase; 48,000 units protease; 48,000 units amylase
Pancrease MT20
Capsules (enteric-coated microtablets): 20,000 units lipase; 44,000 units protease; 56,000 units amylase
Ultrase
Capsules (enteric-coated microspheres): 4,500 units lipase; 25,000 units protease; 20,000 units amylase
Ultrase MT12
Capsules (enteric-coated microtablets): 12,000 units lipase; 39,000 units protease; 39,000 units amylase
Ultrase MT18
Enteric-coated minitablets: 18,000 units lipase; 58,500 units protease; 58,500 units amylase
Ultrase MT20
Capsules (enteric-coated microtablets): 20,000 units lipase; 65,000 units protease; 65,000 units amylase
Viokase
Powder: 16,800 units lipase; 70,000 units protease; 70,000 units amylase
Tablets: 8,000 units lipase; 30,000 units protease; 30,000 units amylase
Zymase
Capsules: 12,000 units lipase; 24,000 units protease; 24,000 units amylase

Indications, route, and dosage
Exocrine pancreatic secretion insufficiency, cystic fibrosis in adults and children, steatorrhea, other disorders of fat metabolism secondary to insufficient pancreatic enzymes
Adults: 4,000 to 20,000 units (or more) lipase with meals and snacks. Dose must be adjusted to patient's response.

Children ages 7 to 12: 4,000 to 12,000 units lipase with meals and snacks. Dose must be adjusted to patient's response.
Children ages 1 to 6: 4,000 to 8,000 units lipase with meals and 4,000 units with snacks. Dose must be adjusted to patient's response.
Children ages 6 to 12 months: 2,000 units lipase with meals and snacks. Dose must be adjusted to patient's response.
Patients with pancreatectomy or obstructive pancreatic duct
Adults: 8,000 to 16,000 units lipase at 2-hour intervals; may increase dose to 64,000 to 88,000 units in severe cases.

Pharmacodynamics
Digestive action: The proteolytic, amylolytic, and lipolytic enzymes enhance the digestion of proteins, starches, and fats. Drug is sensitive to acids and is more active in neutral or slightly alkaline environments.

Pharmacokinetics
● *Absorption:* Not absorbed; acts locally in GI tract.
● *Distribution:* None.
● *Metabolism:* None.
● *Excretion:* Excreted in feces.

Contraindications and precautions
Contraindicated in patients with severe hypersensitivity to pork and in those with acute pancreatitis or acute exacerbations of chronic pancreatic diseases. Use cautiously in pregnant or breast-feeding women.

Interactions
Drug-drug. *Antacids containing calcium or magnesium:* Pancrelipase activity may be reduced by these drugs. Don't give together.
Products containing iron: Decreased absorption of these drugs. Monitor patient for decreased effectiveness.

Adverse reactions
GI: *nausea,* cramping, diarrhea (high doses).
Metabolic: increased serum uric acid.
Other: *allergic reaction.*

☑ Special considerations
● For maximal effect, administer dose just before or during a meal. Patient should drink a glass of water or juice to ensure complete swallowing.
● Preparations may not be crushed or chewed.
● Use only after confirmed diagnosis of exocrine pancreatic insufficiency. Not effective in GI disorders unrelated to enzyme deficiency.
● For young children, mix powders (including content of capsules) with applesauce and give at mealtime. Avoid inhalation of powder. Older children may swallow capsules with food.

● Dosage varies with degree of maldigestion and malabsorption, amount of fat in diet, and enzyme activity of individual preparations.
● Adequate replacement decreases number of bowel movements and improves stool consistency.
● Enteric coating on some products may reduce availability of enzyme in upper portion of jejunum.
● Toxicity may cause hyperuricuria, hyperuricemia, diarrhea, and transient GI upset.

Monitoring the patient
● Monitor patient for effectiveness of therapy.
● Monitor patient for adverse effects.

Information for the patient
● Teach patient or family proper use of drug, and advise storage away from heat and light.
● Be sure patient or family understands special dietary instructions for the particular disease.
● Tell patient not to change brands without medical approval.

Pediatric patients
● Capsules may be opened to facilitate swallowing. Contents may be sprinkled on food, but a pH of 5.5 or greater is necessary to ensure stability. Dosage for children under age 6 months hasn't been established.

pancuronium bromide
Pavulon

Pharmacologic classification: nondepolarizing neuromuscular blocker
Therapeutic classification: skeletal muscle relaxant
Pregnancy risk category C

How supplied
Available by prescription only
Injection: 1 mg/ml, 2 mg/ml parenteral

Indications, route, and dosage
Adjunct to anesthesia to induce skeletal muscle relaxation, facilitate intubation and ventilation, and weaken muscle contractions in induced seizures
Dose depends on anesthetic used, individual needs, and response. Doses are representative and must be adjusted.
Adults and children over age 1 month: Initially, 0.04 to 0.1 mg/kg I.V.; then 0.01 mg/kg q 25 to 60 minutes if needed.

Pharmacodynamics
Skeletal muscle relaxant action: Prevents acetylcholine (ACh) from binding to the receptors on the motor end-plate, thus blocking depolarization. May increase heart rate through direct blocking effect on the ACh receptors of the heart; in-

crease is dose-related. Causes little or no histamine release and no ganglionic blockade.

Pharmacokinetics
- *Absorption:* After I.V. administration, onset of action within 30 to 45 seconds; peak effects seen in 2 to 3 minutes. Onset and duration are dose-related. After 0.06 mg/kg dose, effects begin to subside in 35 to 45 minutes. Repeated doses may increase magnitude and duration of action.
- *Distribution:* 87% bound to plasma proteins.
- *Metabolism:* No information available; small amounts may be metabolized by liver.
- *Excretion:* Mainly excreted unchanged in urine; some through biliary excretion.

Contraindications and precautions
Contraindicated in patients with hypersensitivity to bromides, in those with preexisting tachycardia, and in those for whom even a minor increase in heart rate is undesirable.

Use cautiously in elderly or debilitated patients and in those with impaired renal, pulmonary, or hepatic function; respiratory depression; myasthenia gravis; myasthenic syndrome of lung or bronchogenic cancer; dehydration; thyroid disorders; collagen diseases; porphyria; electrolyte disturbances; hyperthermia; or toxemic states. Also, use large doses cautiously in patients undergoing cesarean section.

Interactions
Drug-drug. *Aminoglycoside antibiotics, beta blockers, clindamycin, depolarizing neuromuscular blocking drugs, furosemide, general anesthetics, lincomycin, lithium, parenteral magnesium salts, polymyxin antibiotics, potassium-depleting drugs, quinidine, quinine, thiazide diuretics, other nondepolarizing neuromuscular blockers:* Potentiated pancuronium effects. Monitor patient closely.
Opioid analgesics: Increased respiratory depression. Monitor vital signs, especially respiratory rate.
Succinylcholine: Enhanced and prolonged neuromuscular blocking effects of pancuronium. Monitor patient closely.

Adverse reactions
CV: tachycardia, increased blood pressure.
Musculoskeletal: residual muscle weakness.
Respiratory: *prolonged, dose-related respiratory insufficiency or apnea.*
Skin: transient rashes.
Other: excessive salivation, *allergic or idiosyncratic hypersensitivity reactions.*

☑ Special considerations
- Administration requires direct medical supervision, with emergency respiratory support available.

- If using succinylcholine, allow its effects to subside before administering pancuronium.
- Store drug in refrigerator and not in plastic container or syringes. Plastic syringes may be used to administer dose.
- Don't mix in same syringe or give through same needle with barbiturates or other alkaline solutions.
- Reduce dosage when ether or other inhalation anesthetics that enhance neuromuscular blockade are used.
- Large doses may increase frequency and severity of tachycardia.
- Drug doesn't relieve pain or affect consciousness; be sure to assess need for analgesic or sedative.
- Toxicity may cause respiratory depression, apnea, and CV collapse. Use a peripheral nerve stimulator to monitor response and to evaluate neuromuscular blockade. Neostigmine, edrophonium, or pyridostigmine may be used to reverse effects.

Monitoring the patient
- Monitor baseline electrolyte levels, intake and output, and vital signs, especially heart rate and respiration.
- Monitor patient for cardiac function, oxygen saturation, and blood pressure.

Information for the patient
- Explain all events and procedures to patient because he can still hear.

Geriatric patients
- The usual adult dose must be individualized depending on response.

Pediatric patients
- Dosage for neonates under age 1 month must be carefully individualized. For infants over age 1 month and children, see adult dosage.

Breast-feeding patients
- It's unknown if drug appears in breast milk. Use with caution in breast-feeding women.

---

papaverine hydrochloride
Pavabid, Pavabid Plateau Caps

Pharmacologic classification: benzylisoquinoline derivative, opiate alkaloid
Therapeutic classification: peripheral vasodilator
Pregnancy risk category C

How supplied
Available by prescription only
Capsules (sustained-release): 150 mg
Injection: 30 mg/ml in 2- and 10-ml ampules

Indications, route, and dosage
Relief of cerebral and peripheral ischemia associated with arterial spasm and myocardial ischemia; treatment of coronary occlusion and certain cerebral angiospastic states
Adults: 75 to 300 mg P.O. three to five times daily or 150 to 300 mg sustained-release preparations q 8 to 12 hours; 30 to 120 mg I.M. or I.V. q 3 hours, as indicated. In treatment of extrasystoles, give two doses 10 minutes apart.
Children: 6 mg/kg I.M. or I.V. q.i.d.
◊ *Impotence*
Adults: 2.5 to 37.5 mg injected intracavernously.

Pharmacodynamics
Vasodilating action: Relaxes smooth muscle directly by inhibiting phosphodiesterase, thus increasing the level of cyclic adenosine monophosphate. There is considerable controversy regarding the clinical effectiveness of papaverine. Some clinicians find little objective evidence of any clinical value.

Pharmacokinetics
• *Absorption:* 54% of orally administered drug is bioavailable. Plasma levels peak 1 to 2 hours after oral dose; half-life varies from ½ to 24 hours, but levels can be maintained by giving drug at 6-hour intervals. Sustained-release forms sometimes absorbed poorly and erratically.
• *Distribution:* Tends to localize in adipose tissue and liver; remainder distributed throughout body. About 90% protein-bound.
• *Metabolism:* Metabolized by liver.
• *Excretion:* Excreted in urine as metabolites.

Contraindications and precautions
I.V. use is contraindicated in patients with Parkinson's disease or complete AV block. Use cautiously in patients with glaucoma or hepatic dysfunction.

Interactions
Drug-drug. *CNS depressants:* Papaverine's effects may be potentiated. Monitor patient closely.
Levodopa: Decreased antiparkinsonian effects; exacerbation of such symptoms as rigidity and tremors. Monitor patient for effect.
Morphine: Synergic response. Monitor patient closely.
Drug-lifestyle. *Heavy smoking:* May interfere with therapeutic effect of papaverine because nicotine constricts blood vessels. Discourage smoking.

Adverse reactions
CNS: *headache,* vertigo, drowsiness, sedation, malaise.
CV: *increased heart rate, increased blood pressure* (with parenteral use), depressed AV and intraventricular conduction, **arrhythmias.**

GI: constipation, *nausea,* anorexia, abdominal pain, diarrhea.
Hepatic: *hepatitis* (jaundice, eosinophilia, abnormal liver function tests), *cirrhosis.*
Respiratory: increased depth and rate of respiration.
Skin: *diaphoresis, flushing,* rash.

☑ Special considerations
• Papaverine is an opiate; however, it has strikingly different pharmacologic properties than other drugs in this group.
• Drug may be given orally, I.M., or, when immediate effect is needed, by slow I.V. injection. Inject I.V. slowly over 1 to 2 minutes; arrhythmias and fatal apnea may follow rapid injection.
• Papaverine injection is incompatible with lactated Ringer's injection; a precipitate will form.
• Signs of overdose include drowsiness, weakness, nystagmus, diplopia, incoordination, and lassitude, progressing to coma with cyanosis and respiratory depression. To slow drug absorption, give activated charcoal, water, or milk; then evacuate stomach contents by gastric lavage or emesis, then catharsis. Hemodialysis may be helpful.

Monitoring the patient
• Monitor vital signs and cardiac rhythm during and after I.V. administration.
• Monitor hepatic enzyme levels.

Information for the patient
• Advise patient to avoid sudden postural changes to minimize possible orthostatic hypotension.
• Instruct patient to report nausea, abdominal distress, anorexia, constipation, diarrhea, jaundice, rash, sweating, tiredness, or headache.

Geriatric patients
• Elderly patients are at greater risk for papaverine-induced hypothermia.

Pediatric patients
• Children's doses are administered parenterally.

Breast-feeding patients
• It's unknown if drug appears in breast milk. Safety in breast-feeding women hasn't been established.

paricalcitol
Zemplar

Pharmacologic classification: vitamin D
analogue
Therapeutic classification: hyperparathyroidism drug
Pregnancy risk category C

How supplied
Available by prescription only
Injection: 5 mcg/ml, 1-ml and 2-ml vials

Indications, route, and dosage
Prevention and treatment of secondary hy-
perparathyroidism associated with chronic
renal failure
Adults: 0.04 to 0.1 mcg/kg (2.8 to 7 mcg) I.V. bolus no more frequently than every other day during dialysis. Doses as high as 0.24 mcg/kg (16.8
mcg) have been safely administered. If satisfactory response isn't observed, dose may be increased by 2 to 4 mcg at 2- to 4-week intervals.

Pharmacodynamics
Antihyperparathyroid action: Synthetic vitamin D
analogue shown to reduce parathyroid hormone
(PTH) levels.

Pharmacokinetics
● *Absorption:* Administered I.V.
● *Distribution:* No information available.
● *Metabolism:* No information available.
● *Excretion:* Eliminated primarily by hepatobiliary
excretion; 74% in feces and 16% in urine. Half-
life is about 15 hours.

Contraindications and precautions
Contraindicated in patients with hypersensitivity
to drug or its components and in those with evidence of vitamin D toxicity or hypercalcemia. Use
cautiously in patients taking digitalis compounds.
Patients taking digoxin are at greater risk for digitalis toxicity during drug therapy secondary to
potential for hypercalcemia.

Interactions
None reported.

Adverse reactions
CNS: light-headedness, malaise.
CV: palpitation.
GI: dry mouth, GI bleeding, *nausea,* vomiting.
Hepatic: reduced serum total alkaline phos-
phatase level.
Respiratory: pneumonia.
Other: chills, edema, fever, flu syndrome, ***sep-***
sis.

☑ Special considerations
● In patients with chronic renal failure, appropriate types of phosphate-binding compounds may
be needed to control serum phosphorus levels,
but excessive use of compounds containing aluminum should be avoided.
● Drug is only administered as an I.V. bolus. Discard unused portion.
● Inspect drug for particulate matter and discoloration before use.
● Store drug at room temperature (59° to 86° F
[15° to 30° C]).
● As the PTH level is decreased, paricalcitol dose
may need to be decreased. Overdose may cause
hypercalcemia. Symptoms include weakness,
headache, nausea, vomiting, constipation, anorexia, pancreatitis, ectopic calcification, cardiac arrhythmias, and death. Treatment should include
correcting electrolyte abnormalities, assessing
cardiac abnormalities, and hemodialysis or peritoneal dialysis against a calcium-free dialysate.

Monitoring the patient
● Watch for ECG abnormalities.
● Monitor patient for symptoms of hypercalcemia.
● Monitor serum calcium and phosphorus levels
twice weekly when dose is being adjusted, and
then monitor monthly. PTH level should be measured every 3 months during therapy.

Information for the patient
● Stress importance of adhering to a dietary regimen of calcium supplementation and phosphorus restriction during therapy.
● Caution against use of phosphate or vitamin
D-related compounds during therapy.
● Explain need for frequent laboratory tests.
● Instruct patient with chronic renal failure to take
phosphate-binding compounds as prescribed but
to avoid excessive use of compounds containing
aluminum.
● Alert patient to early symptoms of hypercalcemia and vitamin D intoxication, such as weakness, headache, somnolence, nausea, vomiting,
dry mouth, constipation, muscle pain, bone pain,
and metallic taste.
● Instruct patient to promptly report adverse reactions.
● Remind patient taking digoxin to watch for signs
of digitalis toxicity.

Geriatric patients
● No significant difference in safety and efficacy
was reported in patients over age 65.

Pediatric patients
● Safety and efficacy in children haven't been established.

Reactions may be *common*, uncommon, ***life-threatening***, or COMMON AND LIFE-THREATENING.

Breast-feeding patients
● It's unknown if drug appears in breast milk. Use with caution in breast-feeding women.

---

paroxetine hydrochloride
Paxil

Pharmacologic classification: selective serotonin reuptake inhibitor (SSRI)
Therapeutic classification: anti-depressant
Pregnancy risk category C

How supplied
Available by prescription only
Tablets: 10 mg, 20 mg, 30 mg, 40 mg
Suspension: 10 mg/5ml

Indications, route, and dosage
Depression
Adults: Initially, 20 mg P.O. daily, preferably in the morning. Increase dosage by 10 mg/day at 1-week intervals, to maximum of 50 mg daily, if necessary.
Obsessive-compulsive disorder (OCD)
Adults: Initially, 20 mg P.O. daily, preferably in the morning. Increase dosage by 10 mg/day at 1-week intervals to target dose of 40 mg/day. Maximum dose is 60 mg/day.
Panic disorder
Adults: Initially, 10 mg P.O. daily, preferably in the morning. Increase dosage by 10 mg/day at 1-week intervals, to target dose of 40 mg/day. Maximum dose is 60 mg/day.
Social anxiety disorder
Adults: 20 mg P.O. daily.
✦ **Dosage adjustment.** For elderly or debilitated patients or patients with severe hepatic or renal disease, 10 mg P.O. daily, preferably in the morning. Increase dosage by 10 mg/day at 1-week intervals, p.r.n., to maximum of 40 mg daily.
◇ **Diabetic neuropathy**
Adults: 10 to 60 mg P.O. daily.
◇ **Headaches**
Adults: 10 to 50 mg P.O. daily.
◇ **Premature ejaculation**
Adults: 20 mg P.O. daily.

Pharmacodynamics
Antidepressant action: Exact mechanism unknown. Presumed to be linked to potentiation of serotonergic activity in the CNS, resulting from inhibition of neuronal reuptake of serotonin.

Pharmacokinetics
● *Absorption:* Completely absorbed after oral dosing.
● *Distribution:* Distributed throughout body, including CNS, with only 1% remaining in plasma. About 93% to 95% bound to plasma protein.

● *Metabolism:* About 36% metabolized in liver. Principal metabolites are polar and conjugated products of oxidation and methylation; readily cleared.
● *Excretion:* About 64% excreted in urine (2% as parent compound, 62% as metabolite).

Contraindications and precautions
Contraindicated in patients taking MAO inhibitors or within 14 days of discontinuing MAO inhibitors. Use cautiously in patients with history of seizures or mania; in those with severe, concurrent systemic illness; and in those at risk for volume depletion and those with hypersensitivity to SSRIs.

Interactions
Drug-drug. *Cimetidine:* Decreased hepatic metabolism of paroxetine; risk of toxicity. Dosage adjustments may be needed.
Digoxin: Decreased digoxin levels. Monitor patient closely.
MAO inhibitors: Increased risk of serious, sometimes fatal, adverse reactions. Avoid concomitant use and do not use paroxetine within 14 days of discontinuing MAO inhibitors.
Phenobarbital: Induced paroxetine metabolism; reduced plasma levels of drug. Adjust dosage as needed.
Phenytoin: Altered pharmacokinetics of phenytoin. Adjust dosage as needed.
Procyclidine: Increased procyclidine levels. Monitor patient for excessive anticholinergic effects.
Theophylline: Increased theophylline levels. Monitor patient closely.
Tryptophan: Increased adverse reactions, such as diaphoresis, headache, nausea, and dizziness. Avoid concomitant use.
Warfarin: Increased risk of bleeding. Monitor INR.
Drug-herb. *St. John's wort:* Sedative-hypnotic intoxication. Don't use together.
Drug-lifestyle. *Alcohol:* Increased risk of CNS adverse effects. Discourage use.

Adverse reactions
CNS: *somnolence, dizziness, insomnia, tremor, nervousness,* anxiety, paresthesia, confusion, *headache,* agitation, abnormal dreams.
CV: palpitations, vasodilation, orthostatic hypotension, chest pain.
EENT: lump or tightness in throat, dysgeusia, visual disturbances, double vision.
GI: *dry mouth, nausea, constipation, diarrhea,* flatulence, vomiting, dyspepsia, increased or decreased appetite, abdominal pain.
GU: ejaculatory disturbances, decreased libido, male genital disorders (including anorgasmia, erectile difficulties, delayed ejaculation or orgasm, impotence, and sexual dysfunction), urinary frequency, other urinary disorders, female genital disorders (including anorgasmia, difficulty with orgasm).

Musculoskeletal: myopathy, myalgia, myasthenia, *asthenia*.
Skin: *diaphoresis*, rash, pruritus.
Other: yawning.

☑ Special considerations

• At least 14 days should elapse between stopping an MAO inhibitor and starting drug therapy. Similarly, at least 14 days should elapse between stopping paroxetine and starting MAO inhibitor.
• Toxicity may cause nausea, vomiting, dizziness, sweating, facial flushing, drowsiness, sinus tachycardia, and dilated pupils. Perform gastric evacuation by emesis, lavage, or both. In most cases, 20 to 30 g of activated charcoal may then be used every 4 to 6 hours during the first 24 to 48 hours after ingestion.
• Special caution must be taken with a patient who currently receives or recently received paroxetine if the patient ingests an excessive quantity of a tricyclic antidepressant; accumulation of the parent tricyclic and its active metabolite may increase the possibility of clinically significant sequelae and extend the time needed for close medical observation.

Monitoring the patient

• Hyponatremia may occur with paroxetine use, especially in elderly patients, those taking diuretics, and those who are otherwise volume depleted. Monitor serum sodium levels.
• If signs of psychosis occur or increase, reduce dosage. Monitor patients for suicidal tendencies and allow them only a minimum supply of drug.

Information for the patient

• Caution patient not to operate hazardous machinery, including automobiles, until reasonably certain that drug doesn't affect ability to engage in such activity.
• Tell patient that he may notice improvement in 1 to 4 weeks but that he must continue with prescribed regimen to obtain continued benefits.
• Instruct patient to call before taking other drugs, including OTC preparations, while taking paroxetine.
• Tell patient to abstain from alcohol while taking drug.

Geriatric patients

• Use cautiously and in lower dosages in elderly patients.

Pediatric patients

• Safety and effectiveness in children haven't been established.

Breast-feeding patients

• Drug appears in breast milk. Use with caution in breast-feeding women.

pegaspargase
(PEG-L-asparaginase)
Oncaspar

Pharmacologic classification: modified version of the enzyme L-asparaginase
Therapeutic classification: antineoplastic
Pregnancy risk category C

How supplied

Available by prescription only
Injection: 750 IU/ml in single-use vial

Indications, route, and dosage

Acute lymphoblastic leukemia (ALL) in patients who need L-asparaginase but have developed hypersensitivity to the native forms of L-asparaginase
Adults and children with body surface area (BSA) of at least 0.6 m²: 2,500 IU/m² I.M. or I.V. q 14 days.
Children with BSA less than 0.6 m²: 82.5 IU/kg I.M. or I.V. q 14 days.
  Note: Moderate to life-threatening hypersensitivity reactions require stopping L-asparaginase treatment.

Pharmacodynamics

Antineoplastic action: Modified version of the enzyme L-asparaginase, which exerts its cytotoxic activity by inactivating the amino acid asparagine. Because leukemic cells can't synthesize their own asparagine, protein synthesis and eventually synthesis of DNA and RNA are inhibited.

Pharmacokinetics

No information available.

Contraindications and precautions

Contraindicated in patients with pancreatitis or a history of pancreatitis; in those who have had significant hemorrhagic events associated with prior L-asparaginase therapy; and in those with previous serious allergic reactions, such as generalized urticaria, bronchospasm, laryngeal edema, hypotension, or other unacceptable adverse reactions to pegaspargase.
  Use cautiously in patients with hepatic dysfunction and during pregnancy.

Interactions

Drug-drug. *Aspirin, dipyridamole, heparin, NSAIDs, warfarin:* Imbalances in coagulation factors; possible bleeding or thrombosis. Monitor patient for increased bleeding; monitor PT and INR.
Methotrexate: May interfere with action of drugs such as methotrexate that require cell replication for lethal effects. Watch for decreased effect.
Other protein-bound drugs: Increased toxicity of these drugs. Pegaspargase may also interfere

---

Reactions may be *common*, uncommon, **life-threatening**, or COMMON AND LIFE-THREATENING.

with enzymatic detoxification of other drugs, particularly in liver. Monitor patient closely.

Adverse reactions

CNS: *seizures,* headache, malaise, paresthesia, *status epilepticus,* somnolence, coma, mental status changes, dizziness, emotional lability, mood changes, parkinsonism, confusion, disorientation, fatigue.
CV: hypotension, tachycardia, chest pain, subacute bacterial endocarditis, hypertension, peripheral edema.
EENT: mouth tenderness, epistaxis.
GI: nausea, vomiting, abdominal pain, anorexia, diarrhea, constipation, indigestion, flatulence, GI pain, mucositis, *pancreatitis* (sometimes fulminant), increased serum amylase and lipase levels, severe colitis.
GU: increased BUN level, increased creatinine level, increased urinary frequency, hematuria, severe hemorrhagic cystitis, renal dysfunction, *renal failure.*
Hematologic: *thrombosis;* prolonged PT, prolonged partial thromboplastin time, decreased antithrombin III; *DIC;* decreased fibrinogen; hemolytic anemia; *leukopenia; pancytopenia; agranulocytosis; thrombocytopenia;* increased thromboplastin; easy bruising; ecchymoses; *hemorrhage.*
Hepatic: jaundice, abnormal liver function test results, bilirubinemia, increased ALT and AST levels, ascites, hypoalbuminemia, fatty changes in liver, *liver failure.*
Metabolic: hyperuricemia, hyponatremia, uric acid nephropathy, hypoproteinemia, proteinuria, weight loss, metabolic acidosis, increased blood ammonia level, hyperglycemia, hypoglycemia.
Musculoskeletal: arthralgia, myalgia, musculoskeletal pain, joint stiffness, cramps, pain in extremities.
Respiratory: cough, *severe bronchospasm,* upper respiratory tract infection.
Skin: itching, alopecia, fever blister, purpura, hand whiteness, fungal changes, nail whiteness and ridging, erythema simplex, petechial rash, injection pain or reaction, localized edema.
Other: hypersensitivity reactions, including *anaphylaxis,* rash, erythema, edema, pain, fever, chills, urticaria, dyspnea, or *bronchospasm;* night sweats; infection; *sepsis, septic shock.*

☑ Special considerations

● I.M. is preferred route because it has a lower risk of hepatotoxicity, coagulopathy, and GI and renal disorders than I.V. route.
● Drug shouldn't be administered if it has ever been frozen. Although there may not be an apparent change in drug's appearance, its activity is destroyed after freezing.
● Avoid excessive agitation; don't shake. Keep refrigerated at 36° to 46° F (2° to 8° C). Don't use if cloudy, if precipitate is present, or if stored at room temperature for more than 48 hours. Don't freeze. Discard unused portions. Use only one dose per vial; don't reenter vial. Don't save unused drug for later administration.
● When administering I.M., limit volume at a single injection site to 2 ml. If volume to be administered is greater than 2 ml, use multiple injection sites.
● When administered I.V., give over 1 to 2 hours in 100 ml of normal saline solution or 5% dextrose injection through an infusion that is already running.
● Pegaspargase should be the sole induction drug only when a combined regimen using other chemotherapeutic drugs is inappropriate because of toxicity or other specific patient-related factors or in patients refractory to other therapy.
● Because drug may be a contact irritant, handle and administer solution with care; wear gloves. Avoid inhalation of vapors and contact with skin or mucous membranes, especially eyes. In case of contact, wash with copious amounts of water for at least 15 minutes.

Monitoring the patient

● Hypersensitivity reactions to drug, including life-threatening anaphylaxis, may occur during therapy, especially in patients with known hypersensitivity to other forms of L-asparaginase. Observe patient for 1 hour and have available resuscitation equipment and other products necessary to treat anaphylaxis.
● A decrease in circulating lymphoblasts is common after initiating therapy. This may be accompanied by a marked rise in serum uric acid. As a guide to the effects of therapy, monitor patient's peripheral blood count and bone marrow. Obtain frequent serum amylase determinations to detect early evidence of pancreatitis. Monitor blood glucose level during therapy because hyperglycemia may occur. When using pegaspargase with hepatotoxic chemotherapy, monitor patient for liver dysfunction. Pegaspargase may affect some plasma proteins; therefore, monitoring of fibrinogen, PT, and partial thromboplastin time may be indicated.

Information for the patient

● Tell patient to report hypersensitivity reactions immediately.
● Instruct patient not to take other drugs, including OTC preparations, without medical approval; pegaspargase increases the risk of bleeding when given with certain drugs, such as aspirin, and may increase toxicity of other drugs.
● Instruct patient to report signs and symptoms of infection (fever, chills, malaise); drug may have immunosuppressive activity.

Pediatric patients

● Safety and efficacy in infants under age 1 haven't been established.

Breast-feeding patients
• It's unknown if drug appears in breast milk. Because of potential for serious adverse reactions in breast-fed infants, stop either breast-feeding or drug, taking into account importance of drug to mother.

---

pemoline
Cylert

Pharmacologic classification: oxazolidinedione derivative, CNS stimulant
Therapeutic classification: analeptic
Controlled substance schedule IV
Pregnancy risk category B

How supplied
Available by prescription only
Tablets: 18.75 mg, 37.5 mg, 75 mg
Tablets (chewable and containing povidone): 37.5 mg

Indications, route, and dosage
Attention deficit hyperactivity disorder (ADHD)
Children ages 6 and older: Initially, 37.5 mg P.O. given in the morning. Daily dosage can be raised by 18.75 mg weekly. Effective dose range is 56.25 to 75 mg daily; maximum is 112.5 mg daily.
Note: Because of its association with life-threatening hepatic failure, pemoline shouldn't be considered first-line therapy for ADHD.
◇ *Narcolepsy*
Adults: 50 to 200 mg daily, in divided doses after breakfast and lunch.

Pharmacodynamics
Analeptic action: Differs structurally from methylphenidate and amphetamines; however, like those drugs, pemoline has a paradoxical calming effect in children with ADHD.
Mechanism of action unknown. May be mediated through dopaminergic mechanisms. CNS stimulant effect has been studied in narcolepsy in adults, in fatigue, in depressed and schizophrenic states, and in elderly patients.

Pharmacokinetics
• *Absorption:* Well absorbed after oral administration. Peak therapeutic effects within 4 hours; last for about 8 hours.
• *Distribution:* No information available. Drug is 50% protein-bound.
• *Metabolism:* Metabolized by liver to active and inactive metabolites.
• *Excretion:* Drug and metabolites excreted in urine; 75% of oral dose excreted within 24 hours.

Contraindications and precautions
Contraindicated in patients with hypersensitivity or idiosyncrasy to drug and in those with hepat-

ic dysfunction. Use cautiously in patients with impaired renal function.

Interactions
Drug-drug. *Anticonvulsants:* Decreased seizure threshold. Monitor patient closely.
Drug-food. *Caffeine:* Decreased efficacy of pemoline in ADHD. Discourage use.

Adverse reactions
CNS: *insomnia,* dyskinetic movements, irritability, fatigue, mild depression, dizziness, headache, drowsiness, hallucinations, **seizures,** *Tourette syndrome,* abnormal oculomotor function.
GI: anorexia, abdominal pain, nausea.
Hematologic: **aplastic anemia.**
Hepatic: elevated liver enzyme levels, **hepatic failure.**
Skin: rash.

☑ Special considerations
• Give drug in a single morning dose for maximum daytime benefit and to minimize insomnia.
• Explain that therapeutic effects may not appear for 3 to 4 weeks and that intermittent drug-free periods when stress is least evident (weekends, school holidays) may help assess patient's condition, prevent development of tolerance, and permit decreased dosage when drug is resumed.
• Abrupt withdrawal after high-dose long-term use may unmask severe depression. Lower dosage gradually to prevent acute rebound depression.
• Drug impairs ability to perform tasks requiring mental alertness.
• Be sure patient obtains adequate rest; fatigue may result as drug wears off.
• Discourage pemoline use for analeptic effect because drug has abuse potential; CNS stimulation superimposed on CNS depression may cause neuronal instability and seizures.
• Carefully follow manufacturer's directions for reconstitution, storage, and administration of all preparations. Pemoline has been used to treat narcolepsy in adults (50 to 200 mg divided twice daily) as well as depression and schizophrenia, but these uses are controversial.
• Toxicity may cause irregular respiration, hyperreflexia, restlessness, tachycardia, hallucinations, excitement, and agitation.

Monitoring the patient
• Monitor initiation of therapy closely; drug may precipitate Tourette syndrome.
• Check vital signs regularly for increased blood pressure or other signs of excessive stimulation.
• Monitor blood and urine glucose levels in diabetic patients; drug may alter insulin requirements.
• Monitor CBC, differential, and platelet counts while patient is on long-term therapy.
• Determine baseline and periodically assess liver function tests. If abnormalities occur, stop drug.

Reactions may be *common,* uncommon, **life-threatening,** or COMMON AND LIFE-THREATENING.

- Monitor height and weight; drug has been associated with growth suppression.

Information for the patient
- Explain rationale for therapy and anticipated risks and benefits; teach signs and symptoms of adverse reactions and need to report these.
- Tell patient to avoid drinks containing caffeine to prevent added CNS stimulation, and not to alter dosage without medical approval.
- Warn patient not to use drug to mask fatigue, to be sure to obtain adequate rest, and to report excessive CNS stimulation.
- Advise diabetic patient to monitor blood glucose levels because drug may alter insulin needs.
- Advise patient to avoid tasks that require mental alertness until degree of sedative effect is determined.

Pediatric patients
- Drug isn't recommended for ADHD in children under age 6.

penbutolol sulfate
Levatol

Pharmacologic classification: beta blocker
Therapeutic classification: antihypertensive
Pregnancy risk category C

How supplied
Available by prescription only
Tablets: 20 mg

Indications, route, and dosage
Mild to moderate hypertension
Adults: 20 mg P.O. once daily. Usually given with other antihypertensives, such as thiazide diuretics. Doses as high as 40 to 80 mg daily and as low as 10 mg daily have been effective.

Pharmacodynamics
Antihypertensive action: Blocks both beta$_1$- and beta$_2$-adrenergic receptors. Antihypertensive effects may be related to peripheral antiadrenergic effects that lead to decreased cardiac output, a central effect that leads to decreased sympathetic tone, or decreased renin secretion by the kidneys.

Pharmacokinetics
- *Absorption:* Almost completely absorbed after oral administration. Plasma levels peak in 2 to 3 hours.
- *Distribution:* 80% to 98% bound to plasma proteins.
- *Metabolism:* Metabolized by liver. Several metabolites identified; some retain partial pharmacologic activity.

- *Excretion:* Average elimination half-life of parent drug is 5 hours; some metabolites persist for 20 hours or more. Most metabolites excreted in urine.

Contraindications and precautions
Contraindicated in patients with hypersensitivity to drug or other beta blockers and in those with sinus bradycardia, cardiogenic shock, overt cardiac failure, greater than first-degree heart block, bronchial asthma, bronchospastic disease, or chronic bronchitis.

Use cautiously in patients with heart failure controlled by drug therapy, diabetes, or history of bronchospastic disease.

Interactions
Drug-drug. *Clonidine:* Paradoxical hypertension when combined with beta blockers; enhanced rebound hypertension when clonidine is withdrawn. Use together cautiously.
Doxazosin, prazosin, terazosin: Enhanced first dose orthostatic hypotension with these drugs. Use together cautiously.
Insulin, oral antidiabetics: Altered hypoglycemic response. Monitor patient closely.
Lidocaine: Increased volume of distribution of lidocaine; may increase loading dose requirements in some patients. Adjust dosage as needed.
Oral calcium antagonists: Enhanced hypotensive effects of beta blockers; predispose patient to bradycardia and arrhythmias. Monitor patient closely.
Reserpine, other catecholamine-depleting drugs: Additive effects. Avoid using together.

Adverse reactions
CNS: *dizziness,* headache, fatigue, insomnia, asthenia.
CV: chest pain, **bradycardia, heart failure.**
GI: nausea, diarrhea, dyspepsia.
GU: impotence.
Metabolic: interference with glucose or insulin tolerance tests.
Respiratory: cough, dyspnea.
Skin: excessive diaphoresis.
Note: The potential for adverse effects associated with other beta blockers should be considered.

☑ Special considerations
Besides the recommendations relevant to all beta blockers, consider the following.
- Like other beta blockers, penbutolol may cause patients to exhibit hypersensitivity to catecholamines upon withdrawal.
- To discontinue drug, slowly taper dosage over a period of 1 to 2 weeks, especially in patients with ischemic heart disease. If symptoms of angina develop, immediately reinstitute therapy, at least temporarily, and take steps to control the patient's unstable angina.

• Toxicity may cause bradycardia, bronchospasm, heart failure, and severe hypotension.

Monitoring the patient
• Monitor blood pressure to determine effectiveness of therapy.
• Perform periodic ECG. Monitor patient for early signs of heart failure.

Information for the patient
• Advise patient not to stop drug abruptly because sudden withdrawal of other beta blockers has precipitated angina and MI.
• Tell patient to report adverse effects immediately, particularly slow heart rate, chest congestion, cough, wheezing, or shortness of breath from mild exertion.
• Teach about disease and therapy. Explain why it's important to continue taking drug, even when feeling well.
• Advise patient to report unpleasant adverse effects promptly.
• Inform patient to call before taking OTC products.

Geriatric patients
• Pharmacokinetic studies indicate no difference in plasma half-life in healthy elderly patients compared with patients on renal dialysis.

Pediatric patients
• Safety and effectiveness in children haven't been established.

Breast-feeding patients
• It's unknown if drug appears in breast milk. Use with caution in breast-feeding women.

---

penicillamine
Cuprimine, Depen

Pharmacologic classification: chelating drug
Therapeutic classification: heavy metal antagonist, antirheumatic
Pregnancy risk category NR

How supplied
Available by prescription only
Capsules: 125 mg, 250 mg
Tablets: 250 mg

Indications, route, and dosage
Wilson's disease
Adults: 250 mg P.O. q.i.d. ½ to 1 hour before meals and at least 2 hours after evening meal. Adjust dose to achieve urinary copper excretion of 0.5 to 1 mg daily. Doses over 2 g are seldom necessary.

Cystinuria
Adults: 250 mg P.O. daily in four divided doses; then gradually increase dosage. Usual dose is 2 g daily (range, 1 to 4 g daily). Adjust dose to achieve urinary cystine excretion of less than 100 mg daily when renal calculi are present, or 100 to 200 mg daily when no calculi are present.

Rheumatoid arthritis, ◊ Felty's syndrome
Adults: Initially, 125 to 250 mg P.O. daily, with increases of 125 to 250 mg daily at 1- to 3-month intervals if necessary. Maximum dose is 1.5 g daily.

◊ Adjunctive treatment of heavy metal poisoning
Adults: 500 to 1,500 mg P.O. daily for 1 to 2 months.

◊ Primary biliary cirrhosis
Adults: Initially, 250 mg P.O. daily, with increases of 250 mg q 2 weeks. Maximum dose is 1 g daily in divided doses.

Pharmacodynamics
Antirheumatic action: Mechanism unknown; depresses circulating IgM rheumatoid factor (but not total circulating immunoglobulin levels) and depresses T-cell but not B-cell activity. Also depolymerizes some macroglobulins (for example, rheumatoid factor).
Chelating action: Forms stable, soluble complexes with copper, iron, mercury, lead, and other heavy metals that are excreted in urine; particularly useful in chelating copper in patients with Wilson's disease. Also combines with cystine to form a complex more soluble than cystine alone, thereby reducing free cystine below the level of urinary stone formation.

Pharmacokinetics
• *Absorption:* Well absorbed after oral administration; peak serum levels at 3 hours.
• *Distribution:* Limited data available.
• *Metabolism:* Metabolized by liver to inactive compounds.
• *Excretion:* Only small amounts excreted unchanged; after 24 hours, about 50% of drug excreted in urine and about 50% in feces.

Contraindications and precautions
Contraindicated in patients with hypersensitivity to drug, history of penicillamine-related aplastic anemia or agranulocytosis, or significant renal or hepatic insufficiency; in pregnant women; and in patients receiving gold salts, immunosuppressants, antimalarials, or phenylbutazone because of the increased risk of serious hematologic effects.

Use cautiously in patients allergic to penicillin (cross reaction is rare); in those who receive a second course of therapy and who may have become sensitized and are more likely to have allergic reactions; and in patients who develop pro-

---

teinuria not associated with Goodpasture's syndrome.

Interactions

Drug-drug. *Antacids, iron salts:* Decreased absorption of penicillamine. Separate administration times.

Antimalarials, cytotoxic drugs, gold therapy, oxyphenbutazone, phenylbutazone: Serious hematologic and renal effects. Don't administer together.

Digoxin: Increased serum levels. Monitor serum digoxin level.

Adverse reactions

EENT: oral ulcerations, glossitis, cheilosis, tinnitus, optic neuritis.

GI: anorexia, nausea, vomiting, dyspepsia, alteration in sense of taste (salty and sweet), metallic taste, diarrhea, dysgeusia, *hypogeusia.*

GU: *proteinuria.*

Hematologic: eosinophilia, *leukopenia, thrombocytopenia, aplastic anemia, agranulocytosis,* thrombotic thrombocytopenia purpura, hemolytic anemia or iron deficiency anemia, lupus-like syndrome, *bone marrow suppression.*

Hepatic: cholestatic jaundice, *pancreatitis,* hepatic dysfunction.

Metabolic: thyroiditis.

Musculoskeletal: arthralgia, myasthenia gravis (with prolonged use).

Respiratory: pneumonitis, Goodpasture's syndrome.

Skin: *pruritus; erythematous rash;* intensely pruritic rash with scaly, macular lesions on trunk; pemphigoid reactions; urticaria; alopecia; *exfoliative dermatitis;* increased skin friability; purpuric or vesicular ecchymoses; wrinkling.

Other: lymphadenopathy, drug fever.

☑ Special considerations

• Stop drug if patient has signs of hypersensitivity or drug fever, usually with other allergic signs and symptoms (if Wilson's disease, may rechallenge); or if the following occur: rash developing 6 months or more after start of therapy; pemphigoid reaction; hematuria or proteinuria with hemoptysis or pulmonary infiltrates; gross or persistent microscopic hematuria or proteinuria greater than 2 g/day in patients with rheumatoid arthritis; platelet count below 100,000/mm³ or leukocyte count below 3,500/mm³, or if either shows three consecutive decreases (even within normal range).

• Patients with Wilson's disease or cystinuria may need daily pyridoxine (vitamin B₆) supplementation.

• Prescribe drug to be taken 1 hour before or 2 hours after meals or other drugs to facilitate absorption.

• For initial treatment of Wilson's disease, 10 to 40 mg of sulfurated potash should be administered with each meal during penicillamine therapy for 6 months to 1 year, then discontinued.

• Drug therapy may cause positive test results for antinuclear antibody with or without clinical systemic lupus erythematosus-like syndrome.

• Hemodialysis will remove penicillamine.

Monitoring the patient

• Perform urinalyses and CBC (including differential blood count) every 2 weeks for 6 months, then monthly. Perform kidney and liver functions studies, usually every 6 months. Watch for fever or allergic reactions (rash, joint pain, easy bruising). Check routinely for proteinuria, and handle patient carefully to avoid skin damage.

• About one-third of patients receiving drug experience an allergic reaction. Monitor patient for signs and symptoms of allergic reaction.

Information for the patient

• Provide health education for patients with Wilson's disease, rheumatoid arthritis, or cystinuria; explain disease process and rationale for therapy and explain that clinical results may not be evident for 3 months.

• Encourage patient compliance with therapy and follow-up visits.

• Stress importance of reporting immediately any fever, chills, sore throat, bruising, bleeding, or allergic reaction.

• Tell patient to take drug on an empty stomach 30 minutes to 1 hour before meals or 2 hours after ingesting food, antacids, mineral supplements, vitamins, or other drugs. Tell patient to drink large amounts of water, especially at night.

• Advise patient receiving drug for rheumatoid arthritis that an exacerbation of disease may occur during therapy. This usually can be controlled by concurrent use of NSAIDs.

• Advise patient taking drug for Wilson's disease to maintain a low-copper (less than 2 mg daily) diet by excluding foods with high copper content, such as chocolate, nuts, liver, and broccoli. Also, sulfurated potash may be administered with meals to minimize copper absorption.

Geriatric patients

• Lower doses may be indicated. Monitor renal and hepatic function closely. Toxicity may be more common in elderly patients.

Pediatric patients

• Check for possible iron deficiency resulting from long-term use. Safety and efficacy for juvenile rheumatoid arthritis haven't been established in children.

Breast-feeding patients

• It's unknown if drug appears in breast milk. Safety hasn't been established in breast-feeding women; an alternative to breast-feeding is recommended during therapy.

penicillin G benzathine
Bicillin L-A, Permapen

penicillin G benzathine and procaine
Bicillin C-R

penicillin G potassium
Pfizerpen

penicillin G procaine
Ayercillin*, Bicillin C-R, Wycillin

penicillin G sodium

Pharmacologic classification: natural penicillin
Therapeutic classification: antibiotic
Pregnancy risk category B

How supplied
Available by prescription only
penicillin G benzathine
Suspension: 250,000 units/5 ml*; 500,000 units/ml*
Injection: 300,000 units/ml; 600,000 units/ml; 1.2 million units/2 ml; 2.4 million units/4 ml
penicillin G benzathine and procaine
Injection: 300,000 units/ml; 600,000 units/ml
penicillin G potassium
Powder for injection: 1 million units, 5 million units, 10 million units, 20 million units
Injection (premixed, frozen): 1 million units/50 ml, 2 million units/50 ml, 3 million units/50 ml
penicillin G procaine
Injection: 600,000 units/ml
penicillin G sodium
Powder for injection: 1 million units*, 5 million units, 10 million units*

Indications, route, and dosage
Congenital syphilis
penicillin G benzathine
Children under age 2: 50,000 units/kg I.M. as a single injection.
Group A streptococcal upper respiratory infections, ◊ diphtheria, ◊ yaws, pinta, and bejel
penicillin G benzathine
Adults: 1.2 million units I.M. as a single injection.
Children who weigh 27 kg (60 lb) or more: 900,000 units I.M. in a single injection.
Children under 27 kg: 300,000 to 600,000 units I.M. in a single injection.
Prophylaxis of poststreptococcal rheumatic fever
penicillin G benzathine
Adults and children: 1.2 million units I.M. once monthly.

Syphilis of less than 1 year's duration
penicillin G benzathine
Adults: 2.4 million units I.M. in a single dose.
Syphilis of more than 1 year's duration
penicillin G benzathine
Adults: 2.4 million units I.M. weekly for 3 successive weeks.
Moderate to severe systemic infections
penicillin G potassium, sodium
Adults: 12 to 24 million units I.M. or I.V. daily, given in divided doses q 4 hours.
Children: 25,000 to 300,000 units/kg I.M. or I.V. daily, given in divided doses q 4 hours.
Moderate to severe systemic infections, pneumococcal pneumonia
penicillin G procaine
Adults: 600,000 to 1.2 million units I.M. daily as a single dose or q 6 to 12 hours.
Children: 300,000 units I.M. daily as a single dose.
Uncomplicated gonorrhea
penicillin G procaine
Adults and children over age 12: 1 g probenecid P.O; then, 30 minutes later, 4.8 million units of penicillin G procaine I.M., divided into two injection sites.
✦ *Dosage adjustment.* For patients with renal failure, refer to the table.

Creatinine clearance (ml/min)	Dosage (after full loading dose)
10 to 50	50% of usual dose q 4 to 5 hr; or, give usual dose q 8 to 12 hr
< 10	50% of usual dose q 8 to 12 hr; or, give usual dose q 12 to 18 hr

Pharmacodynamics
Antibiotic action: Bactericidal. Adheres to penicillin-binding proteins, thus inhibiting bacterial cell-wall synthesis. Spectrum of activity includes most non-penicillinase-producing strains of gram-positive and gram-negative aerobic cocci, spirochetes, and some gram-positive aerobic and anaerobic bacilli.

Pharmacokinetics
Penicillin G is available as four salts, each having the same bactericidal action, but designed to offer greater oral stability (potassium salt) or to prolong duration of action by slowing absorption after I.M. injection (benzathine and procaine salts).
• *Absorption:* Sodium and potassium salts of penicillin G absorbed rapidly after I.M. injection; peak serum levels within 15 to 30 minutes. Slower absorption of other salts. Serum levels of penicillin G procaine peak in 1 to 4 hours, with drug detectable in serum for 1 to 2 days; serum levels of penicillin G benzathine peak in 13 to 24 hours, with serum levels detectable for 1 to 4 weeks.

• *Distribution:* Penicillin G distributed widely into synovial, pleural, pericardial, ascitic fluids; bile, liver, skin, lungs, kidneys, muscle, intestines, tonsils, maxillary sinuses, saliva, and erythrocytes. Poor CSF penetration but enhanced in patients with inflamed meninges. Penicillin G crosses placenta; is 45% to 68% protein-bound.

• *Metabolism:* Between 16% and 30% of I.M. dose metabolized to inactive compounds.

• *Excretion:* Excreted primarily in urine by tubular secretion; 20% to 60% of dose recovered in 6 hours. Some drug excreted in breast milk. Elimination half-life in adults is about ½ to 1 hour. Severe renal impairment prolongs half-life; penicillin G is removed by hemodialysis and is only minimally removed by peritoneal dialysis.

Contraindications and precautions
Contraindicated in patients with hypersensitivity to drug or other penicillins. Use cautiously in patients with drug allergies (especially to cephalosporins or imipenem). Penicillin G potassium is contraindicated in patients with renal failure.

Interactions
Drug-drug. *Aminoglycosides:* Synergistic therapeutic effects, chiefly against enterococci; this combination is most effective in enterococcal bacterial endocarditis. However, drugs are physically and chemically incompatible; inactivated when mixed or given together. Administer separately.

Clavulanate: Enhanced effect of penicillin G against certain beta-lactamase-producing bacteria. Clavulanate may be used for this purpose.

Heparin, oral anticoagulants: Increased risk of bleeding. Monitor PTT, PT, and INR.

Methotrexate: Large doses of penicillin may interfere with renal tubular secretion of methotrexate; delayed elimination and elevated serum levels of methotrexate. Monitor patient for toxicity.

NSAIDs, sulfinpyrazone: Prolonged penicillin half-life. Monitor patient for clinical effectiveness.

Oral contraceptives: Decreased effectiveness. Suggest using alternative forms of contraception.

Potassium-sparing diuretics: Possible hyperkalemia when used with parenteral penicillin G potassium. Monitor serum potassium.

Probenecid: Blocked tubular secretion of penicillin, raising its serum levels. Probenecid may be used for this purpose.

Adverse reactions
CNS: neuropathy, *seizures* (with high doses), lethargy, hallucinations, anxiety, confusion, agitation, depression, dizziness, fatigue.

CV: thrombophlebitis (with penicillin G potassium only).

GI: nausea, vomiting, enterocolitis, pseudomembranous colitis.

GU: interstitial nephritis, nephropathy.

Hematologic: eosinophilia, hemolytic anemia, *thrombocytopenia, leukopenia,* anemia, *agranulocytosis.*

Metabolic: possible severe potassium poisoning with high doses (hyperreflexia, *seizures, coma*).

Other: hypersensitivity reactions (maculopapular and *exfoliative dermatitis,* chills, fever, edema, *anaphylaxis*); pain and sterile abscess at injection site; overgrowth of nonsusceptible organisms (with penicillin G potassium and procaine).

☑ Special considerations
Besides the recommendations relevant to all penicillins, consider the following.

• Have emergency equipment on hand to manage possible anaphylaxis.

• Because penicillins are dialyzable, patients undergoing hemodialysis may need dosage adjustments.

• Administer by deep I.M. injection in upper outer quadrant of buttock. In infants and small children, use midlateral aspect of thigh.

• Drug can be administered as a continuous infusion for meningitis.

• Penicillin G alters test results for urine and serum protein levels and interferes with turbidimetric methods using sulfosalicylic acid, trichloracetic acid, acetic acid, and nitric acid. It doesn't interfere with tests using bromophenol blue (Albustix, Albutest, Multistix), but alters urine glucose testing using cupric sulfate (Benedict's reagent); use Diastix, Chemstrip uG, or glucose enzymatic test strip instead. Penicillin G may cause falsely elevated results of urine specific gravity tests in patients with low urine output and dehydration, and falsely elevated Norymberski and Zimmermann test results for 17-ketogenic steroids; causes false-positive CSF protein test results (Folin-Ciocalteau method) and may cause positive Coombs' test results.

• Penicillin G may falsely decrease serum aminoglycoside levels. Adding beta-lactamase to sample inactivates penicillin, rendering assay more accurate. Or sample can be spun down and frozen immediately after collection.

• Signs and symptoms of overdose include neuromuscular irritability and seizures. Drug can be removed by hemodialysis.

Information for the patient
• Tell patient that drug must be injected deep into a large muscle mass.

• Instruct patient to report allergic symptoms and any adverse reactions.

Monitoring the patient
• Monitor closely for possible hypernatremia (with sodium) or hyperkalemia (with potassium).

• Patients with poor renal function are predisposed to high blood levels, which may cause seizures. Monitor renal function.

Geriatric patients
• Half-life is prolonged in elderly patients because of impaired renal function.

Breast-feeding patients
• Drug appears in breast milk; use in breast-feeding women may sensitize infant to penicillin.

penicillin V potassium
Betapen-VK, Ledercillin VK, Nadopen-V*, Pen Vee K, PVF K*, V-Cillin K, Veetids

Pharmacologic classification: natural penicillin
Therapeutic classification: antibiotic
Pregnancy risk category B

How supplied
Available by prescription only
Tablets: 250 mg, 500 mg
Tablets (film-coated): 250 mg, 500 mg
Solution: 125 mg/5 ml, 250 mg/5 ml (after reconstitution)

Indications, route, and dosage
Mild to moderate susceptible infections
Adults and children ages 12 and over: 125 to 500 mg (200,000 to 800,000 units) P.O. q 6 hours.
Children ages 1 month to 12 years: 15 to 62.5 mg/kg P.O. daily, divided into doses given q 6 to 8 hours.
Necrotizing ulcerative gingivitis
Adults: 250 to 500 mg P.O. q 6 to 8 hours.
◊ **Lyme disease**
Adults: 250 to 500 mg P.O. q.i.d. for 10 to 20 days.
◊ **Prophylaxis for pneumococcal infection**
Adults: 250 mg P.O. b.i.d.
Children over age 5: 125 mg P.O. b.i.d.

Pharmacodynamics
Antibiotic action: Bactericidal. Adheres to penicillin-binding proteins, thus inhibiting bacterial cell-wall synthesis. Spectrum of activity includes most non-penicillinase-producing strains of gram-positive and gram-negative aerobic cocci, spirochetes, and some gram-positive aerobic and anaerobic bacilli.

Pharmacokinetics
• *Absorption:* Penicillin V has greater acid stability and is absorbed more completely than penicillin G after oral administration. About 60% to 75% of oral dose of penicillin V absorbed. Serum levels peak at 60 minutes in fasting subjects; food has no significant effect.

• *Distribution:* Distributed widely into synovial, pleural, pericardial, ascitic fluids; bile, liver, skin, lungs, kidneys, muscle, intestines, tonsils, maxillary sinuses, saliva, and erythrocytes. Poor CSF penetration but is enhanced in patients with inflamed meninges. Penicillin V crosses placenta; is 75% to 89% protein-bound.
• *Metabolism:* Between 35% and 70% of dose metabolized to inactive compounds.
• *Excretion:* Excreted primarily in urine by tubular secretion; 26% to 65% of dose recovered in 6 hours. Some drug excreted in breast milk. Elimination half-life in adults is ½ hour; severe renal impairment prolongs half-life.

Contraindications and precautions
Contraindicated in patients with hypersensitivity to drug or other penicillins. Use cautiously in patients with drug allergies (especially to cephalosporins or imipenem).

Interactions
Drug-drug. *Aminoglycosides:* Synergistic therapeutic effects, chiefly against enterococci. However, drugs are physically and chemically incompatible; inactivated when given together. Don't administer together.
Anticoagulants, heparin: Increased risk of bleeding. Monitor PTT, PT, and INR.
Oral contraceptives containing estrogen: Decreased efficacy; possible breakthrough bleeding. Suggest alternative method of contraception.
Probenecid: Blocked tubular secretion of penicillin; higher serum levels of drug. Probenecid may be used for this purpose.
Sulfinpyrazone: Prolonged penicillin V half-life. Watch for clinical effectiveness.

Adverse reactions
CNS: neuropathy.
GI: *epigastric distress,* vomiting, diarrhea, *nausea,* black "hairy" tongue.
GU: nephropathy.
Hematologic: eosinophilia, hemolytic anemia, **leukopenia, thrombocytopenia.**
Other: hypersensitivity reactions (rash, urticaria, fever, laryngeal edema, **anaphylaxis**), overgrowth of nonsusceptible organisms.

☑ Special considerations
Besides the recommendations relevant to all penicillins, consider the following.
• Give oral dose 1 hour before or 2 hours after meals for maximum absorption.
• After reconstitution, oral solution is stable for 14 days if refrigerated.
• Penicillin V alters test results for urine and serum protein levels and interferes with turbidimetric methods using sulfosalicylic acid, trichloracetic acid, acetic acid, and nitric acid. Penicillin V doesn't interfere with tests using bromophe-

nol blue (Albustix, Albutest, Multistix) and may falsely decrease serum aminoglycoside levels.
● Signs and symptoms of overdose include neuromuscular sensitivity and seizures.

Information for the patient
● Tell patient to take drug on an empty stomach for maximum absorption.
● Instruct patient to swallow drug only with water because acid in fruit juices and carbonated beverages impairs absorption.

Monitoring the patient
● Monitor patient for overgrowth of nonsusceptible organisms.
● Monitor therapeutic effect.

Geriatric patients
● Half-life may be prolonged in elderly patients because of impaired renal function.

Breast-feeding patients
● Drug appears in breast milk; use in breast-feeding women may sensitize infant to penicillins.

pentamidine isethionate
NebuPent, Pentacarinat, Pentam 300

Pharmacologic classification: diamidine derivative
Therapeutic classification: antiprotozoal
Pregnancy risk category C

How supplied
Available by prescription only
Injection: 300-mg vials
Solution for inhalation: 300 mg

Indications, route, and dosage
Pneumonia caused by Pneumocystis carinii
Adults and children: 4 mg/kg I.V. or I.M. once a day for 14 to 21 days. As alternative dose in children, 150 mg/m² daily for 5 days; then 100 mg/m² for duration of therapy.
Prophylaxis against Pneumocystis carinii pneumonia (PCP) in persons at high risk for the disease
Adults: 300 mg by inhalation once q 4 weeks. Aerosol form of drug should be administered by the Respirgard II jet nebulizer.
◇ **Prophylaxis against Trypanosoma gambiense**
Adults: 4 mg/kg I.V. or I.M. usually q 3 to 6 months.
◇ **Leishmaniasis**
Adults: 2 to 4 mg/kg I.V. or I.M. daily or every other day up to 15 doses.

Pharmacodynamics
Antiprotozoal action: Mechanism unknown. May inhibit synthesis of RNA, DNA, proteins, or phospholipids. May also interfere with several metabolic processes, particularly certain energy-yielding reactions and reactions involving folic acid. Spectrum of activity includes *P. carinii* and *Trypanosoma* organisms.

Pharmacokinetics
● *Absorption:* Daily I.M. doses (4 mg/kg) produce surprisingly few plasma level fluctuations. Plasma levels usually increase slightly 1 hour after I.M. injection. Little information on pharmacokinetics with I.V. administration. Limited absorption after aerosol administration.
● *Distribution:* Extensively tissue-bound. Poor CNS penetration. Extent of plasma protein-binding unknown.
● *Metabolism:* No information available.
● *Excretion:* Mostly excreted unchanged in urine. Extensive tissue-binding may account for appearance in urine 6 to 8 weeks after therapy ends.

Contraindications and precautions
Contraindicated in patients with hypersensitivity to drug. Use cautiously in patients with hepatic or renal dysfunction, hypertension, hypotension, hypoglycemia, hypocalcemia, leukopenia, thrombocytopenia, or anemia.

Interactions
Drug-drug. *Aminoglycosides, amphotericin B, capreomycin, cisplatin, colistin, methoxyflurane, polymyxin B, vancomycin:* Additive nephrotoxic effects. Use together cautiously.

Adverse reactions
CNS: confusion, hallucinations, *fatigue, dizziness,* headache.
CV: *hypotension,* **ventricular tachycardia,** chest pain, edema.
EENT: metallic taste, pharyngitis, bad taste in mouth.
GI: nausea, decreased appetite, vomiting, diarrhea, abdominal pain, anorexia.
GU: *elevated serum creatinine,* **acute renal failure.**
Hematologic: *leukopenia, thrombocytopenia,* anemia.
Hepatic: elevated liver function test results.
Metabolic: hyperkalemia, hypocalcemia, *hypoglycemia,* hyperglycemia.
Musculoskeletal: myalgia.
Respiratory: *congestion, cough, bronchospasm, shortness of breath,* pneumothorax.
Skin: *rash,* **Stevens-Johnson syndrome.**
Other: *night sweats, chills, sterile abscess, pain or induration at injection site.*

☑ Special considerations
● Make sure patient is adequately hydrated before administering drug; dehydration may lead to hypotension and renal toxicity.
● I.V. infusion avoids risk of local reactions and is as safe as I.M. injection when given slowly, over

at least 60 minutes. To prepare drug for I.V. infusion, add 3 to 5 ml of sterile water for injection or D_5W to 300-mg vial to yield 100 mg/ml or 60 mg/ml, respectively. Withdraw desired dose and dilute further into 50 to 250 ml of D_5W; infuse over at least 60 minutes. Diluted solution remains stable for 48 hours.

• To prepare drug for I.M. injection, add 3 ml of sterile water for injection to 300-mg vial to yield 100 mg/ml. Withdraw desired dose and inject deep I.M.

• Keep emergency drugs and equipment (including emergency airway, vasopressors, and I.V. fluids) on hand.

• When inhalation solution is used for prophylaxis against PCP, high-risk individuals include persons infected with HIV with a history of PCP; patients who have never had an episode of PCP but whose CD4+ T cells are below 20% of total lymphocytes, or whose CD4+ T-cell count is below 200/mm².

• To administer by inhalation, dilute dose in 6 ml of sterile water and deliver at 6 L/minute from a 50-p.s.i. compressed air source until reservoir is dry. Alternative delivery systems (other than the Respirgard II) are under investigation but currently aren't recommended.

• Patients who develop wheezing or cough during pentamidine aerosol therapy may benefit by pretreatment (at least 5 minutes before pentamidine administration) with a bronchodilator.

Monitoring the patient

• To minimize risk of hypotension, patient should be supine during I.V. administration. Because sudden, severe hypotension may develop after I.M. injection or during I.V. infusion, closely monitor blood pressure during infusion and several times thereafter until patient is stable.

• Monitor daily blood glucose, BUN, and serum creatinine levels.

• Periodically monitor electrolyte levels, CBC, platelet count, and liver function tests.

• Observe patient for signs and symptoms of hypoglycemia.

Information for the patient

• Instruct patient to use aerosol device until chamber is empty, which may take up to 45 minutes.

• Warn patient that I.M. injection is painful.

• Instruct patient to complete full course of therapy, even if feeling better.

pentazocine hydrochloride
Talwin*, Talwin-Nx (with naloxone hydrochloride)

pentazocine lactate
Talwin

Pharmacologic classification: narcotic agonist-antagonist, opioid partial agonist
Therapeutic classification: analgesic, adjunct to anesthesia
Controlled substance schedule IV
Pregnancy risk category NR (C for Talwin-Nx)

How supplied
Available by prescription only
Tablets: 50 mg
Injection: 30 mg/ml

Indications, route, and dosage
Moderate to severe pain
Adults: 50 to 100 mg P.O. q 3 to 4 hours, p.r.n., or around the clock. Maximum oral dose is 600 mg daily. Or 30 mg I.M., I.V., or S.C. q 3 to 4 hours, p.r.n., or around the clock. Maximum parenteral dose is 360 mg daily. Doses above 30 mg I.V. or 60 mg I.M. or S.C. not recommended.

For patients in labor, give 30 mg I.M. or 20 mg I.V. in 2- to 3-hour intervals.

Pharmacodynamics
Analgesic action: Exact mechanism unknown. Believed to be a competitive antagonist at some receptors and an agonist at others, resulting in relief of moderate pain.

Can produce respiratory depression, sedation, miosis, and antitussive effects. Also may cause psychotomimetic and dysphoric effects. In patients with coronary artery disease, drug elevates mean aortic pressure, left ventricular end-diastolic pressure, and mean pulmonary artery pressure. In patients with acute MI, I.V. drug increases systemic and pulmonary arterial pressures and systemic vascular resistance.

Pharmacokinetics
• *Absorption:* Well absorbed after oral or parenteral administration. However, orally administered drug undergoes first-pass metabolism in liver; less than 20% of dose reaches systemic circulation unchanged. Increased bioavailability in patients with hepatic dysfunction; patients with cirrhosis absorb 60% to 70% of drug. Onset of analgesia in 15 to 30 minutes; peak effect at 15 to 60 minutes.

• *Distribution:* Widely distributed in body.

• *Metabolism:* Metabolized in liver, mainly by oxidation and secondarily by glucuronidation. Metabolism may be prolonged in patients with impaired hepatic function.

- *Excretion:* Duration of effect is 3 hours. Considerable variability among patients in its urinary excretion. Small amounts excreted in feces after oral or parenteral administration.

Contraindications and precautions

Contraindicated in patients with hypersensitivity to drug or its components and in children under age 12. Use cautiously in patients with impaired renal or hepatic function, acute MI, head injury, increased intracranial pressure, or respiratory depression.

Interactions

Drug-drug. *Barbiturates (such as thiopental):* If administered within a few hours of these drugs, pentazocine may produce additive CNS and respiratory depressant effects; possible apnea. Separate administration times if used together.
Cimetidine: Increased pentazocine toxicity; disorientation, respiratory depression, apnea, and seizures. Monitor patient; be prepared to administer naloxone if toxicity occurs.
General anesthetics: Concomitant use may cause severe CV depression. Avoid concomitant use.
Narcotic agonist-antagonist, single dose of an antagonist: Patients who become physically dependent on pentazocine may experience acute withdrawal syndrome. Use with caution; monitor patient closely.
Other CNS depressants (antihistamines, barbiturates, benzodiazepines, muscle relaxants, narcotic analgesics, phenothiazines, sedative-hypnotics, tricyclic antidepressants): Potentiated respiratory and CNS depression, sedation, and hypotensive effects. Reduced doses of pentazocine usually are needed.
Other drugs extensively metabolized in liver (digitoxin, phenytoin, rifampin): Drug accumulation and enhanced effects. Monitor patient for toxicity.
Drug-lifestyle. *Alcohol:* Potentiateed drug's respiratory and CNS depression, sedation, and hypotensive effects. Discourage use.

Adverse reactions

CNS: *sedation,* visual disturbances, hallucinations, drowsiness, *dizziness, light-headedness,* confusion, *euphoria,* headache, syncope, psychotomimetic effects.
CV: circulatory depression, **shock,** hypertension, hypotension.
EENT: dry mouth, blurred vision, nystagmus.
GI: *nausea, vomiting,* constipation, taste alteration.
GU: urine retention.
Hematologic: WBC depression.
Respiratory: *respiratory depression,* dyspnea, **apnea.**
Skin: induration, nodules, sloughing, and sclerosis of injection site; diaphoresis; pruritus.
Other: hypersensitivity reactions (**anaphylaxis**), physical and psychological dependence.

☑ Special considerations

Besides the recommendations relevant to all opioid (narcotic) agonist-antagonists, consider the following.
- Tablets aren't well absorbed.
- Don't mix in same syringe with soluble barbiturates.
- Pentazocine may obscure signs and symptoms of an acute abdominal condition or worsen gallbladder pain.
- Drug possesses narcotic antagonist properties. May precipitate abstinence syndrome in narcotic-dependent patients.
- Talwin-Nx, the available oral pentazocine, contains the narcotic antagonist naloxone, which prevents illicit I.V. use.
- Use S.C. route only when necessary. Severe tissue damage is possible at injection site.

Monitoring the patient
- Drug may cause orthostatic hypotension in ambulatory patients. Have patient sit down to relieve symptoms.
- Monitor blood pressure as needed.

Information for the patient
- Tell patient to report rash, confusion, disorientation, or other serious adverse effects.
- Warn patient that Talwin-Nx is for oral use only. Severe reactions may result if tablets are crushed, dissolved, and injected.
- Tell patient to avoid use of alcohol and other CNS depressants.

Geriatric patients
- Lower doses are usually indicated for elderly patients, who may be more sensitive to therapeutic and adverse effects of drug.

Pediatric patients
- Drug isn't recommended for children under age 12.

Breast-feeding patients
- It's unknown if drug appears in breast milk; use with caution in breast-feeding women.

---

pentobarbital sodium
Nembutal

Pharmacologic classification: barbiturate
Therapeutic classification: anticonvulsant, sedative-hypnotic
Controlled substance schedule II (suppositories, schedule III)
Pregnancy risk category D

How supplied

Available by prescription only
Elixir: 18.2 mg/5 ml
Capsules: 50 mg, 100 mg

Injection: 50 mg/ml, 1-ml and 2-ml disposable syringes; 2-ml, 20-ml, and 50-ml vials
Suppositories: 30 mg, 60 mg, 120 mg, 200 mg

Indications, route, and dosage
Sedation
Adults: 20 to 40 mg P.O. b.i.d., t.i.d., or q.i.d.
Children: 2 to 6 mg/kg P.O. daily in divided doses, to maximum of 100 mg/dose.
Insomnia
Adults: 100 mg P.O. h.s. or 150 to 200 mg deep I.M.; 120 to 200 mg P.R.
Children: 2 to 6 mg/kg I.M., up to maximum of 100 mg/dose. Or 30 mg P.R. (ages 2 months to 1 year), 30 to 60 mg P.R. (ages 1 to 4), 60 mg P.R. (ages 5 to 12), 60 to 120 mg P.R. (ages 12 to 14).
Preanesthetic
Adults: 150 to 200 mg I.M. or P.O. in two divided doses.
Anticonvulsant
Adults: Initially, 100 mg I.V.; after 1 minute additional doses may be given. Maximum dose is 500 mg.
Children: 50 mg initially; after 1 minute additional small doses may be given until desired effect is obtained.

Pharmacodynamics
Sedative-hypnotic action: Exact cellular site and mechanism of action unknown. Acts throughout the CNS as a nonselective depressant with a fast onset of action and short duration of action. Particularly sensitive to this drug is the reticular activating system, which controls CNS arousal. Pentobarbital decreases both presynaptic and postsynaptic membrane excitability by facilitating the action of gamma-aminobutyric acid (GABA).
Anticonvulsant action: Suppresses spread of seizure activity produced by epileptogenic foci in the cortex, thalamus, and limbic systems by enhancing the effect of GABA. Both presynaptic and postsynaptic excitability are decreased, and the seizure threshold is raised.

Pharmacokinetics
• *Absorption:* Absorbed rapidly after oral or rectal administration; onset of action in 10 to 15 minutes. Serum levels peak between 30 and 60 minutes after oral administration. After I.M. injection, onset of action is within 10 to 15 minutes. After I.V. administration, onset of action is immediate. Serum levels needed for sedation and hypnosis are 1 to 5 mcg/ml and 5 to 15 mcg/ml, respectively. After oral or rectal administration, duration of hypnosis is 1 to 4 hours.
• *Distribution:* Distributed widely throughout body. About 35% to 45% protein-bound. Accumulates in fat with long-term use.
• *Metabolism:* Metabolized in liver by penultimate oxidation.

• *Excretion:* 99% eliminated as glucuronide conjugates and other metabolites in urine. Terminal half-life ranges from 35 to 50 hours; duration of action 3 to 4 hours.

Contraindications and precautions
Contraindicated in patients with hypersensitivity to barbiturates and in those with porphyria or severe respiratory disease when dyspnea or obstruction is evident. Use cautiously in elderly or debilitated patients and in those with acute or chronic pain, mental depression, suicidal tendencies, history of drug abuse, or impaired hepatic function.

Interactions
Drug-drug. *Antidepressants, antihistamines, narcotics, sedative-hypnotics, tranquilizers:* Potentiated or added CNS and respiratory depressant effects. Monitor patient closely.
Corticosteroids, digitoxin, doxycycline, oral contraceptives (and other estrogens), theophylline (and other xanthines): Enhanced hepatic metabolism. Monitor patient for clinical effectiveness.
Disulfiram, MAO inhibitors, valproic acid: Decreased metabolism of pentobarbital. Monitor patient for toxicity.
Griseofulvin: Impaired effectiveness of this drug; decreased absorption from GI tract. Separate administration times.
Rifampin: Decreased pentobarbital levels; increases hepatic metabolism. Adjust dosage as needed.
Warfarin, other oral anticoagulants: Enhanced enzymatic degradation of these drugs. Increased doses of anticoagulants may be needed.
Drug-lifestyle. *Alcohol:* Potentiated or added CNS and respiratory depressant effects. Discourage use.

Adverse reactions
CNS: *drowsiness, lethargy, hangover,* paradoxical excitement in elderly patients, somnolence, syncope, hallucinations, change in EEG patterns.
CV: *bradycardia,* hypotension.
GI: nausea, vomiting.
Hematologic: exacerbation of porphyria.
Respiratory: *respiratory depression.*
Skin: rash, urticaria, STEVENS-JOHNSON SYNDROME.
Other: *angioedema,* physical and psychological dependence.

☑ Special considerations
Besides the recommendations relevant to all barbiturates, consider the following.
• Reserve I.V. injection for emergency treatment. Be prepared for emergency resuscitative measures.
• Avoid I.V. administration at a rate exceeding 50 mg/minute to prevent hypotension and respiratory depression.

- High-dose therapy for elevated intracranial pressure may require mechanically assisted ventilation.
- Administer I.M. dose deep into large muscle mass. Don't administer more than 5 ml into any one site.
- Discard solution that is discolored or contains precipitate.
- Administration of full loading doses over short periods of time to treat status epilepticus will require ventilatory support in adults.
- To assure accuracy of dosage, don't divide suppositories.
- Drug has no analgesic effect and may cause restlessness or delirium in patients with pain.
- Nembutal tablets contain tartrazine dye, which may cause allergic reactions in susceptible persons.
- To prevent rebound of rapid-eye-movement sleep after prolonged therapy, discontinue gradually over 5 to 6 days.
- Pentobarbital may cause a false-positive phentolamine test. Drug's physiologic effects may impair the absorption of cyanocobalamin Co 57; it may decrease serum bilirubin levels in neonates, epileptic patients, and patients with congenital nonhemolytic unconjugated hyperbilirubinemia.
- Toxicity may cause unsteady gait, slurred speech, sustained nystagmus, somnolence, confusion, respiratory depression, pulmonary edema, areflexia, and coma. Typical shock syndrome with tachycardia and hypotension may occur. Jaundice, hypothermia, then fever and oliguria also may occur. Serum levels greater than 10 mcg/ml may produce profound coma; levels greater than 30 mcg/ml may be fatal.
- Alkalinization of urine may be helpful in removing drug from body. Hemodialysis may be useful in severe overdose.

Monitoring the patient
- Monitor vital signs, especially respirations.
- Monitor patient for changes in neurologic status.

Information for the patient
- Advise pregnant patient of potential hazard to fetus or neonate when taking drug late in pregnancy. Withdrawal symptoms can occur.
- Tell patient not to take drug continuously for longer than 2 weeks.
- Emphasize the dangers of combining drug with alcohol. An excessive depressant effect is possible even if drug is taken the evening before ingestion of alcohol.

Geriatric patients
- Elderly patients usually need lower doses because of increased susceptibility to CNS depressant effects of pentobarbital. Confusion, disorientation, and excitability may occur in elderly patients. Use with caution.

Pediatric patients
- Barbiturates may cause paradoxical excitement in children. Use with caution.

Breast-feeding patients
- Drug appears in breast milk. Don't administer to breast-feeding women.

pentoxifylline
Trental

Pharmacologic classification: xanthine derivative
Therapeutic classification: hemorheologic
Pregnancy risk category C

How supplied
Available by prescription only
Tablets (extended-release): 400 mg

Indications, route, and dosage
Intermittent claudication from chronic occlusive vascular disease
Adults: 400 mg P.O. t.i.d. with meals.

Pharmacodynamics
Hemorheologic action: Improves capillary blood flow by increasing erythrocyte flexibility and reducing blood viscosity.

Pharmacokinetics
- *Absorption:* Absorbed almost completely from GI tract but undergoes first-pass hepatic metabolism. Absorption slowed by food. Levels peak in 2 to 4 hours; clinical effect requires 2 to 4 weeks of continued therapy.
- *Distribution:* No information available; bound to erythrocyte membrane.
- *Metabolism:* Metabolized extensively by erythrocytes and liver.
- *Excretion:* Metabolites excreted principally in urine; less than 4% of drug excreted in feces. Half-life of unchanged drug is about ½ to ¾ hour; half-life of metabolites is about 1 to 1½ hours.

Contraindications and precautions
Contraindicated in patients who are intolerant to pentoxifylline or methylxanthines (such as caffeine, theophylline, and theobromine) and in patients with recent cerebral or retinal hemorrhage. Use cautiously in elderly patients.

Interactions
Drug-drug. *Antihypertensives:* Increased hypotensive response. Monitor blood pressure.
Drugs that inhibit platelet aggregation, oral anticoagulants (such as warfarin): Bleeding abnormalities. Monitor PT and INR.
Theophylline: Increased theophylline levels. Monitor patient closely.

Adverse reactions
CNS: headache, dizziness.
CV: angina, chest pain.
GI: dyspepsia, nausea, vomiting, flatus, bloating.

☑ Special considerations
• If GI and CNS adverse effects occur, decrease dosage to twice daily. If adverse effects persist, stop drug.
• Drug is useful in patients who aren't good candidates for surgery.
• Don't crush or break timed-release tablets; make sure patient swallows whole.
• Signs and symptoms of overdose include flushing, hypotension, seizures, somnolence, loss of consciousness, fever, and agitation.

Monitoring the patient
• Monitor blood pressure regularly, especially in patients taking antihypertensives.
• Monitor INR, especially in patients taking anticoagulants such as warfarin.

Information for the patient
• Explain need for continuing therapy for at least 8 weeks; warn patient not to stop drug during this period without approval.
• Advise taking drug with meals to minimize GI distress.
• Tell patient to report GI or CNS adverse reactions; dosage reduction may be needed.

Geriatric patients
• Elderly patients may have increased bioavailability and decreased excretion of drug and, thus, are at higher risk for toxicity; adverse reactions may be more common in elderly patients.

Pediatric patients
• Safety and efficacy haven't been established for patients under age 18.

Breast-feeding patients
• Drug appears in breast milk. An alternative to breast-feeding is recommended during therapy.

pergolide mesylate
Permax

Pharmacologic classification: dopaminergic agonist
Therapeutic classification: antiparkinsonian
Pregnancy risk category B

How supplied
Available by prescription only
Tablets: 0.05 mg, 0.25 mg, 1 mg

Indications, route, and dosage
Adjunct to levodopa-carbidopa in the management of Parkinson's disease
Adults: Initially, 0.05 mg P.O. daily for first 2 days. Gradually increase dosage by 0.1 to 0.15 mg q third day over next 12 days of therapy. Subsequent dosage can be increased by 0.25 mg q third day until optimum response occurs. Mean therapeutic daily dose is 3 mg.
     Drug is usually administered in divided doses t.i.d. Gradual reductions in levodopa-carbidopa dosage may be made during dosage adjustment.

Pharmacodynamics
Antiparkinsonian action: Stimulates dopamine receptors at both D_1 and D_2 sites. Acts by directly stimulating postsynaptic receptors in the nigrostriatal system.

Pharmacokinetics
• *Absorption:* Well absorbed after oral administration. Half-life is about 24 hours.
• *Distribution:* About 90% bound to plasma proteins.
• *Metabolism:* Metabolized to at least 10 different compounds; some retain some pharmacologic activity.
• *Excretion:* Excreted primarily by kidneys.

Contraindications and precautions
Contraindicated in patients with hypersensitivity to drug or to ergot alkaloids. Use cautiously in patients prone to arrhythmias and underlying psychiatric disorders.

Interactions
Drug-drug. *Dopamine antagonists (such as butyrophenones, metoclopramide, phenothiazines, thioxanthenes):* Antagonized effects of pergolide. Use together cautiously.
Other drugs known to affect protein binding: Pergolide is extensively protein-bound. Use caution if pergolide is administered with these drugs.

Adverse reactions
CNS: headache, asthenia, *dyskinesia, dizziness, hallucinations, dystonia, confusion, somnolence,* insomnia, anxiety, depression, tremor, abnormal dreams, personality disorder, psychosis, abnormal gait, akathisia, extrapyramidal syndrome, incoordination, akinesia, hypertonia, neuralgia, speech disorder, twitching, paresthesia.
CV: *orthostatic hypotension,* vasodilation, palpitations, hypotension, syncope, hypertension, ***arrhythmias, MI.***
EENT: *rhinitis,* epistaxis, abnormal vision, diplopia, eye disorder.
GI: dry mouth, taste perversion, abdominal pain, *nausea, constipation,* diarrhea, dyspepsia, anorexia, vomiting.
GU: urinary frequency, urinary tract infection, hematuria.

Hematologic: anemia.
Metabolic: weight gain.
Musculoskeletal: chest, neck, and back pain; arthralgia; bursitis; myalgia.
Respiratory: dyspnea.
Skin: rash, diaphoresis.
Other: flulike syndrome; chills; infection; facial, peripheral, or generalized edema.

Note: The preceding adverse reactions, although not always attributable to drug, occurred in more than 1% of the study population.

☑ Special considerations

● Adverse effects (primarily hallucinations and confusion) have occurred in some patients taking pergolide.
● Toxicity may cause hypotension, vomiting, hallucinations, involuntary movements, palpitations, and arrhythmias.

Monitoring the patient

● Monitor blood pressure.
● Monitor patient for adverse effects.

Information for the patient

● Inform patient of potential for adverse effects. Warn patient to avoid activities that could expose him to injury secondary to orthostatic hypotension and syncope.
● Caution patient to rise slowly to avoid orthostatic hypotension, particularly at start of therapy.

Pediatric patients

● Safety in children hasn't been established.

Breast-feeding patients

● It's unknown if drug appears in breast milk. Safety in breast-feeding women hasn't been established.

---

perindopril erbumine
Aceon

Pharmacologic classification: angiotensin converting enzyme (ACE) inhibitor
Therapeutic classification: antihypertensive
Pregnancy risk category C (first trimester), D (second and third trimesters)

How supplied
Available by prescription only
Tablets: 2 mg, 4 mg, 8 mg

Indications, route, and dosage
Essential hypertension
Adults: Initially, 4 mg P.O. once daily. Increase dosage until blood pressure is controlled or to a maximum of 16 mg/day; usual maintenance dose is 4 to 8 mg once daily; may be given in two divided doses.
Elderly: Initially, 4 mg P.O. daily as one dose or in two divided doses. Dosage increases exceeding 8 mg/day should occur only under close medical supervision.

✦ *Dosage adjustment.* For renally impaired patients: initially, 2 mg P.O. daily with a maximum maintenance dose of 8 mg/day. Don't use in patients with creatinine clearance less than 30 ml/minute. For patients taking diuretics: initially, 2 to 4 mg P.O. daily as one dose or in two divided doses with close medical supervision for several hours and until blood pressure has stabilized. Adjust dosage based on patient's blood pressure response.

Pharmacodynamics
Antihypertensive action: A prodrug that is converted by the liver to the active metabolite perindoprilat. Perindoprilat is thought to lower blood pressure through inhibition of ACE activity, thereby preventing the conversion of angiotensin I to angiotensin II, a potent vasoconstrictor. Inhibition of ACE results in decreased vasoconstriction and decreased aldosterone, thus reducing sodium and water retention and lowering blood pressure.

Pharmacokinetics
● *Absorption:* Rapidly absorbed after oral administration; levels peak in about 1 hour. Absolute oral bioavailability around 75%. Plasma level of perindopril and perindoprilat increased about twofold in elderly patients.
● *Distribution:* Perindopril and perindoprilat about 60% and 10% to 20% bound to plasma proteins, respectively. Drug interaction resulting from effects on protein-binding aren't anticipated.
● *Metabolism:* Perindopril extensively metabolized by liver to perindoprilat.
● *Excretion:* About 4% to 12% of dose excreted in urine as unchanged drug. Reduced drug clearance in elderly patients and in those with heart failure or renal insufficiency.

Contraindications and precautions
Contraindicated in patients with hypersensitivity to perindopril or other ACE inhibitors and in those with history of angioedema secondary to ACE inhibitors. Also contraindicated in pregnant women.

Use cautiously in patients with history of angioedema unrelated to ACE inhibitor therapy. Also use cautiously in patients with impaired renal function, heart failure, ischemic heart disease, cerebrovascular disease or renal artery stenosis, and in patients with collagen vascular disease, such as systemic lupus erythematosus or scleroderma.

Interactions

Drug-drug. *Diuretics:* Additive hypotensive effect. Monitor patient closely.
Lithium: Increased serum lithium level; possible symptoms of lithium toxicity. Use of a diuretic may further increase risk of lithium toxicity. Use together cautiously; monitor serum lithium level.
Potassium-sparing diuretics (amiloride, spironolactone, triamterene), potassium supplements, other drugs capable of increasing serum potassium (cyclosporine, heparin, indomethacin): Additive hyperkalemic effect. Use together cautiously; monitor serum potassium level frequently.
Drug-food. *Salt substitutes containing potassium:* Increased risk of hyperkalemia. Use together cautiously.

Adverse reactions

CNS: dizziness, asthenia, sleep disorder, paresthesia, depression, somnolence, nervousness, *headache.*
CV: palpitation, edema, chest pain, abnormal ECG.
EENT: rhinitis, sinusitis, ear infection, pharyngitis, tinnitus.
GI: dyspepsia, diarrhea, abdominal pain, nausea, vomiting, flatulence.
GU: proteinuria, urinary tract infection, male sexual dysfunction, menstrual disorder.
Hepatic: increased ALT level.
Metabolic: increased triglyceride level.
Musculoskeletal: back pain, hypertonia, neck pain, joint pain, myalgia, arthritis, low or upper extremity pain.
Respiratory: *cough,* upper respiratory tract infection.
Skin: rash.
Other: viral infection, fever, injury, seasonal allergy.

☑ Special considerations

• Angioedema involving face, extremities, lips, tongue, glottis, and larynx reported in patients treated with perindopril. Stop drug and observe patient until swelling disappears. If swelling is confined to face and lips, it will probably resolve without treatment, but antihistamines may be useful in relieving symptoms. Angioedema associated with tongue, glottis, or larynx may be fatal because of airway obstruction. Appropriate therapy, such as subcutaneous epinephrine solution, should be promptly administered.
• Patients with history of angioedema unrelated to ACE inhibitor therapy may be at increased risk for angioedema while receiving an ACE inhibitor.
• Excessive hypotension can occur when drug is given with diuretics. If possible, diuretic therapy should be stopped 2 to 3 days before starting perindopril to decrease potential for excessive hypotensive response. If it isn't possible to stop diuretic, consider starting with a lower dose of perindopril or decreasing diuretic dose.

• Hypotension can occur when initiating therapy or adjusting doses in patients who have been volume- or salt-depleted as a result of prolonged diuretic therapy, dietary salt restriction, dialysis, diarrhea, or vomiting. Volume and salt depletion should be corrected before starting drug.
• ACE inhibitors have rarely been associated with a syndrome of cholestatic jaundice, fulminant hepatic necrosis, and death. Stop drug in patients who develop jaundice or marked elevations of hepatic enzyme levels during therapy.

Monitoring the patient

• Other ACE inhibitors have been associated with agranulocytosis and neutropenia. Monitor CBC with differential before therapy, especially in renally impaired patients with systemic lupus erythematosus or scleroderma.
• Monitor patients at risk for hypotension closely during start of therapy and for the first 2 weeks of treatment, and whenever perindopril dosage or concomitant diuretic is increased. If severe hypotension occurs, place patient in supine position and treat symptomatically.
• Monitor renal function before and periodically throughout therapy. Drug shouldn't be used in patients with creatinine clearance less than 30 ml/minute.
• Monitor serum potassium levels closely.

Information for the patient

• Inform patient that angioedema, including laryngeal edema, can occur during therapy, especially with first dose. Advise patient to stop taking drug and immediately report any signs or symptoms of angioedema (swelling of face, extremities, eyes, lips, or tongue; hoarseness; or difficulty in swallowing or breathing).
• Advise patient to report promptly any sign of infection (such as sore throat, fever) or jaundice (yellowing of eyes or skin).
• Advise patient to avoid salt substitutes containing potassium unless instructed otherwise.
• Caution patient that light-headedness may occur, especially during first few days of therapy. Advise patient to report light-headedness and, if fainting occurs, to stop drug and call promptly.
• Caution patient that inadequate fluid intake or excessive perspiration, diarrhea, or vomiting can lead to an excessive drop in blood pressure.
• Advise woman of childbearing age of consequences of second and third trimester exposure to drug. Advise her to call immediately if pregnancy is suspected.

Geriatric patients

• Plasma levels of both perindopril and perindoprilat in patients over age 70 are about twice those observed in younger patients. With the exception of dizziness and possibly rash, adverse effects don't appear to increase in elderly patients. Doses above 8 mg/day should be administered with caution and under close medical supervision.

Pediatric patients
• Safety and effectiveness of drug in children haven't been established.

Breast-feeding patients
• It's unknown if drug appears in breast milk. Because many drugs appear in breast milk, use with caution in breast-feeding women.

permethrin
Acticin, Elimite, Nix

Pharmacologic classification: synthetic pyrethroid
Therapeutic classification: scabicide, pediculicide
Pregnancy risk category B

How supplied
Available by prescription only
Acticin, Elimite
Cream: 5%
Available without a prescription
Nix
Liquid: 60 ml (1%)

Indications, route, and dosage
Pediculosis
Adults and children: Apply sufficient volume to saturate the hair and scalp. Allow to remain on hair for 10 minutes before rinsing.
Scabies
Adults and children: Thoroughly massage into skin from head to soles of feet. Treat infants on hairline, neck, scalp, temple, and forehead. Remove cream by washing after 8 to 14 hours. One application is curative.

Pharmacodynamics
Scabicide action: Acts on the parasites' nerve cell membranes to disrupt the sodium channel current, thereby paralyzing the parasites.

Pharmacokinetics
• *Absorption:* Not entirely investigated; probably less than 2% of amount applied.
• *Distribution:* No information available.
• *Metabolism:* Rapidly metabolized by ester hydrolysis to inactive metabolites.
• *Excretion:* Metabolites excreted in urine. Residue on hair detectable for up to 10 days.

Contraindications and precautions
Contraindicated in patients with hypersensitivity to pyrethrins or chrysanthemums.

Interactions
None reported.

Adverse reactions
Skin: pruritus, *burning, stinging,* edema, tingling, numbness or scalp discomfort, mild erythema, scalp rash.

☑ Special considerations
• A single treatment is usually effective. Although combing of nits isn't needed for effectiveness, drug package supplies a fine-tooth comb.
• A second application may be needed if lice are seen 7 days after initial application.
• Permethrin has been shown to be at least as effective as lindane (Kwell) in treating head lice.

Monitoring the patient
• Monitor patient for clinical effectiveness of treatment.

Information for the patient
• Tell patient or caregiver to wash hair with shampoo, rinse it thoroughly, and then towel dry.
• Tell patient or caregiver to apply sufficient amount to saturate hair and scalp.
• Instruct patient to report itching, redness, or swelling of scalp.
• Advise patient that drug is for external use only and to avoid contact with mucous membranes.

Pediatric patients
• Safety and efficacy in children under age 2 haven't been established.

Breast-feeding patients
• It's unknown if drug appears in breast milk. Either discontinue breast-feeding temporarily or stop drug.

perphenazine
Apo-Perphenazine*, Trilafon

Pharmacologic classification: phenothiazine (piperazine derivative)
Therapeutic classification: antipsychotic, antiemetic
Pregnancy risk category NR

How supplied
Available by prescription only
Tablets: 2 mg, 4 mg, 8 mg, 16 mg
Oral concentrate: 16 mg/5 ml
Injection: 5 mg/ml

Indications, route, and dosage
Psychosis
Adults: Initially, 8 to 16 mg P.O. b.i.d., t.i.d., or q.i.d., increasing to 64 mg daily. Or administer 5 to 10 mg I.M.; change to P.O. as soon as possible.
Mental disturbances, acute alcoholism, nausea, vomiting, hiccups
Adults: 5 to 10 mg I.M., p.r.n. Maximum dose is 15 mg daily in ambulatory patients; 30 mg daily

in hospitalized patients; or 8 to 16 mg P.O. daily in divided doses.

Perphenazine may be given slowly by I.V. drip at a rate of 1 mg/2 minutes with continuous blood pressure monitoring (rarely used). A maximum of 5 mg I.V. diluted to 0.5 mg/ml with normal saline solution may be given for severe hiccups or vomiting. Extended-release preparation may be given 8 to 16 mg P.O. b.i.d. for outpatients; 8 to 32 mg P.O. b.i.d. for inpatients.

Pharmacodynamics

Antipsychotic action: Thought to exert antipsychotic effects by postsynaptic blockade of CNS dopamine receptors, thus inhibiting dopamine-mediated effects; antiemetic effects are attributed to dopamine receptor blockade in the medullary chemoreceptor trigger zone. Has many other central and peripheral effects: produces both alpha and ganglionic blockade and counteracts histamine- and serotonin-mediated activity. Most serious adverse reactions are extrapyramidal.

Pharmacokinetics

• *Absorption:* Rate and extent of absorption vary with administration route. Oral tablet absorption erratic and variable, with onset of action ranging from ½ to 1 hour; oral concentrate absorption much more predictable. I.M. drug absorbed rapidly.
• *Distribution:* Distributed widely into body, including breast milk. 91% to 99% protein-bound. After oral tablet administration, peak effect at 2 to 4 hours; steady-state serum levels achieved within 4 to 7 days.
• *Metabolism:* Metabolized extensively by liver; no active metabolites formed.
• *Excretion:* Mostly excreted in urine via kidneys; some in feces via biliary tract.

Contraindications and precautions

Contraindicated in patients with hypersensitivity to drug; in patients experiencing coma; in those with CNS depression, blood dyscrasia, bone marrow depression, liver damage, or subcortical damage; and in those receiving large doses of CNS depressants.

Use cautiously in elderly or debilitated patients; in those with alcohol withdrawal, psychic depression, suicidal tendencies, adverse reaction to other phenothiazines, impaired renal function, or respiratory disorders; and in patients receiving other CNS depressants or anticholinergics.

Interactions

Drug-drug. *Antacids containing aluminum and magnesium, antidiarrheals:* Inhibited absorption. Separate administration times by at least 2 hours. *Antiarrhythmics, disopyramide, procainamide, quinidine:* Increased risk of arrhythmias and conduction defects. Monitor patient closely.

Appetite suppressants, sympathomimetics (such as ephedrine [commonly found in nasal sprays], epinephrine, phenylephrine, phenylpropanolamine): Decreased stimulatory and pressor effects. Monitor patient closely.
Atropine, other anticholinergics (such as antidepressants, antihistamines, antiparkinsonians, MAO inhibitors, meperidine, phenothiazines): Oversedation, paralytic ileus, visual changes, and severe constipation. Monitor patient closely.
Beta blockers: Inhibited perphenazine metabolism; increased plasma levels. Watch for toxicity.
Bromocriptine: Antagonized prolactin secretion. Monitor patient closely.
Centrally acting antihypertensives (such as clonidine, guanabenz, guanadrel, guanethidine, methyldopa, reserpine): Inhibited blood pressure response. Monitor blood pressure.
CNS depressants (such as analgesics; barbiturates; epidural, general, spinal anesthetics; narcotics; tranquilizers), parenteral magnesium sulfate: Oversedation, respiratory depression, and hypotension. Monitor patient closely.
Epinephrine: Phenothiazines can cause epinephrine reversal and hypotensive response when epinephrine is used for pressor effects. Avoid concomitant use.
High-dose dopamine: Decreased vasoconstricting effects. Monitor patient closely.
Levodopa: Decreased effectiveness; increased risk of levodopa toxicity. Use together cautiously.
Lithium: Severe neurologic toxicity with encephalitis-like syndrome; decreased therapeutic response to perphenazine. Avoid using together.
Metrizamide: Increased risk of seizures. Monitor patient closely.
Nitrates: Hypotension. Monitor blood pressure.
Phenobarbital: Enhanced renal excretion of perphenazine. Adjust dosage as needed.
Phenytoin: Inhibited metabolism and increased risk of phenytoin toxicity. Monitor patient closely.
Propylthiouracil: Increased risk of agranulocytosis. Monitor hematologic studies.
Drug-food. *Caffeine:* Decreased therapeutic response to perphenazine. Discourage use.
Drug-lifestyle. *Alcohol:* Additive effects. Discourage use.
Heavy smoking: Decreased therapeutic response to perphenazine. Discourage smoking.
Sun exposure: Possible photosensitivity reactions. Tell patient to take precautions.

Adverse reactions

CNS: *extrapyramidal reactions, tardive dyskinesia,* sedation, pseudoparkinsonism, EEG changes, dizziness, adverse behavioral effects, **seizures,** drowsiness.
CV: *orthostatic hypotension,* tachycardia, ECG changes, **cardiac arrest.**
EENT: ocular changes, *blurred vision,* nasal congestion.

GI: *dry mouth, constipation,* nausea, vomiting, diarrhea, ileus.

GU: *urine retention,* dark urine, menstrual irregularities, gynecomastia, inhibited ejaculation.

Hematologic: *leukopenia,* galactorrhea, *agranulocytosis,* eosinophilia, *hemolytic anemia, thrombocytopenia.*

Hepatic: jaundice, abnormal liver function test results.

Metabolic: hyperglycemia, hypoglycemia, weight gain.

Skin: *mild photosensitivity, allergic reactions,* pain at I.M. injection site, sterile abscess.

Other: SIADH, *neuroleptic malignant syndrome.*

After abrupt withdrawal of long-term therapy: gastritis, nausea, vomiting, dizziness, tremor, feeling of warmth or cold, diaphoresis, tachycardia, headache, insomnia.

☑ Special considerations

Besides the recommendations relevant to all phenothiazines, consider the following.

- Oral formulations may cause stomach upset; administer with food or fluid.
- Dilute the concentrate in 2 to 4 oz (60 to 120 ml) of liquid (water, caffeine-free carbonated drinks, fruit juice, tomato juice, milk, or puddings). Dilute every 5 ml of concentrate with 60 ml of suitable fluid. Shake oral concentrate before administration.
- Liquid formulation may cause rash upon contact with skin.
- I.M. injection may cause skin necrosis; avoid extravasation.
- Administer I.M. injection deep into upper outer quadrant of buttocks. Massaging injection site may prevent formation of abscesses.
- Don't administer drug for injection if it's excessively discolored or contains precipitate.
- Perphenazine causes false-positive test results for urinary porphyrins, urobilinogen, amylase, and 5-hydroxyindoleacetic acid because of darkening of urine by metabolites; also causes false-positive urine pregnancy test results using human chorionic gonadotropin.
- CNS depression is characterized by deep, unarousable sleep and possible coma, hypotension or hypertension, extrapyramidal symptoms, dystonia, abnormal involuntary muscle movements, agitation, seizures, arrhythmias, ECG changes, hypothermia or hyperthermia, and autonomic nervous system dysfunction.
- In case of overdose, treat hypotension with I.V. fluids. Don't give epinephrine. Treat seizures with parenteral diazepam or barbiturates; arrhythmias with parenteral phenytoin (1 mg/kg with rate titrated to blood pressure); and extrapyramidal reactions with benztropine at 1 to 2 mg or parenteral diphenhydramine at 10 to 50 mg.

Monitoring the patient

- Monitor blood pressure before and after parenteral administration.
- Monitor serum glucose level, CBC, and liver function tests.

Information for the patient

- Explain risks of dystonic reactions and tardive dyskinesia, and tell patient to report abnormal body movements.
- Instruct patient to avoid sun exposure and to wear sunscreen when going outdoors to prevent photosensitivity reactions and to avoid using sun lamps and tanning beds, which may cause burning of the skin or skin discoloration.
- Tell patient to avoid spilling liquid; contact with skin may cause rash and irritation.
- Warn patient not to take extremely hot or cold baths and to avoid exposure to temperature extremes; drug may cause thermoregulatory changes.
- Advise patient to take drug exactly as prescribed and not to double missed doses.
- Inform patient that interactions with many other drugs are possible. Advise patient to seek medical approval before taking OTC products.
- Instruct patient not to stop taking drug suddenly; any adverse reactions may be alleviated by a dosage reduction. Patient should promptly report difficulty urinating, sore throat, dizziness, or fainting.
- Tell patient to avoid hazardous activities that require alertness until drug's effect is known. Reassure patient that sedative effects of drug should become tolerable within a few weeks.
- Tell patient not to drink alcohol or take other drugs that may cause excessive sedation.
- Explain which fluids are appropriate for diluting the concentrate (not apple juice or drinks containing caffeine); explain dropper technique of measuring dose.
- Recommend sugarless hard candy or chewing gum, ice chips, or artificial saliva to relieve dry mouth.
- Tell patient not to crush or chew sustained-release form.

Geriatric patients

- Use lower doses in elderly patients. Dose must be adjusted to effects; 30% to 50% of the usual dose may be effective. Elderly patients are at greater risk for adverse effects, especially tardive dyskinesia and other extrapyramidal effects.

Pediatric patients

- Drug isn't recommended for children under age 12.

Breast-feeding patients

- Drug appears widely in breast milk; use with caution. Potential benefits to mother should outweigh potential harm to infant.

---

phenazopyridine hydrochloride
Azo-Standard, Baridium, Geridium, Phenazo*, Prodium, Pyridiate, Pyridium, Urogesic

Pharmacologic classification: azo dye
Therapeutic classification: urinary analgesic
Pregnancy risk category B

How supplied
Available by prescription only
Tablets: 100 mg, 200 mg
Available without prescription
Tablets: 95 mg

Indications, route, and dosage
Pain with urinary tract irritation or infection
Adults: 200 mg P.O. t.i.d. Give drug after meals.

Pharmacodynamics
Analgesic action: Mechanism unknown. Has a local anesthetic effect on urinary tract mucosa.

Pharmacokinetics
• *Absorption:* No information available.
• *Distribution:* Traces thought to enter CSF and cross placenta.
• *Metabolism:* Metabolized in liver.
• *Excretion:* Excreted by kidneys; 65% excreted unchanged in urine. Totally excreted on average in 20.4 hours.

Contraindications and precautions
Contraindicated in patients with hypersensitivity to drug and in those with glomerulonephritis, severe hepatitis, uremia, pyelonephritis during pregnancy, or renal insufficiency.

Interactions
None reported.

Adverse reactions
CNS: headache.
GI: nausea, GI disturbances.
Hematologic: hemolytic anemia.
Skin: rash, pruritus.
Other: *anaphylactoid reactions,* methemoglobinemia.

☑ Special considerations
• Drug colors urine red or orange; may stain fabrics.
• Use only as an analgesic.
• May be used with an antibiotic to treat urinary tract infections.
• Discontinue drug in 2 days with concurrent antibiotic use.
• Drug may alter results of Diastix, Chemstrip uG, glucose enzymatic test strip, Acetest, and Ketostix. Clinitest should be used to obtain accurate urine glucose test results. Drug may also interfere with Ehrlich's test for urine urobilinogen; phenolsulfonphthalein excretion tests of kidney function; sulfobromophthalein excretion tests of liver function; and urine tests for protein, corticosteroids, or bilirubin.
• Toxicity may cause methemoglobinemia (most obvious as cyanosis), along with renal and hepatic impairment and failure.
• To treat overdose, empty stomach immediately by inducing emesis with ipecac syrup or by gastric lavage. Administer methylene blue, 1 to 2 mg/kg I.V., or 100 to 200 mg ascorbic acid P.O. to reverse methemoglobinemia.

Monitoring the patient
• Monitor patient for decrease in pain associated with urinary tract infection.
• Watch for continued symptoms of urinary tract infection.
• Repeat urinalysis as indicated.

Information for the patient
• Instruct patient in measures to prevent urinary tract infection.
• Advise patient of possible adverse reactions; caution that drug colors urine red or orange and may stain clothing.
• Tell patient that stains on clothing may be removed with a 0.25% solution of sodium dithionite or hydrosulfite.
• Advise patient to take missed dose as soon as possible but not to double doses.
• Instruct patient to report symptoms that worsen or don't resolve.

Geriatric patients
• Use with caution in elderly patients because of possible decreased renal function.
• Administer with food or fluids to reduce GI upset.
• Evaluate response to therapy; assess urinary function, such as output, complaints of burning, pain, and frequency.
• Monitor vital signs, especially temperature.
• Encourage patient to force fluids (if not contraindicated). Monitor intake and output.

Breast-feeding patients
• It's unknown if drug appears in breast milk. Safe use in breast-feeding women hasn't been established.

Reactions may be *common*, uncommon, *life-threatening*, or COMMON AND LIFE-THREATENING.

phenelzine sulfate
Nardil

Pharmacologic classification: MAO inhibitor
Therapeutic classification: antidepressant
Pregnancy risk category C

How supplied
Available by prescription only
Tablets: 15 mg

Indications, route, and dosage
Severe depression
Adults: 15 mg P.O. t.i.d. Increase rapidly to 60 mg/day; maximum daily dose is 90 mg. Onset of maximum therapeutic effect is 2 to 6 weeks. Some clinicians reduce dosage after response occurs; maintenance dose may be as low as 15 mg daily or every other day.

Pharmacodynamics
Antidepressant action: Depression is thought to result from low CNS levels of neurotransmitters, including norepinephrine and serotonin. Phenelzine inhibits MAO, an enzyme that normally inactivates amine-containing substances, thus increasing the level and activity of these substances.

Pharmacokinetics
• *Absorption:* Absorbed rapidly and completely from GI tract.
• *Distribution:* No information available.
• *Metabolism:* Metabolized in liver.
• *Excretion:* Excreted primarily in urine within 24 hours; some drug excreted in feces via biliary tract. Relatively short half-life, but enzyme inhibition is prolonged and unrelated to half-life.

Contraindications and precautions
Contraindicated in patients with hypersensitivity to drug and in those with heart failure, pheochromocytoma, hypertension, liver disease, or CV disease. Also contraindicated during therapy with other MAO inhibitors (isocarboxazid, tranylcypromine); within 14 days of such therapy or within 14 days of elective surgery requiring general anesthesia; with cocaine use; or with local anesthesia containing sympathomimetic vasoconstrictors. Contraindicated within 2 weeks of selective serotonin reuptake inhibitor antidepressant use. Contraindicated by some manufacturers in patients over age 60 because of possibility of existing cerebrosclerosis with damaged vessels.

Use cautiously in patients at risk for diabetes, suicide, or seizure disorders and in those receiving thiazide diuretics or spinal anesthetics.

Interactions
Drug-drug. *Amphetamines, ephedrine, phenylephrine, phenylpropanolamine, other related drugs:* Enhanced pressor effects. Avoid concomitant use.
Barbiturates, dextromethorphan, narcotics, tricyclic antidepressants, other sedatives: Increased adverse reactions. Use cautiously and reduce dosage of phenelzine.
Disulfiram: Possible tachycardia, flushing, or palpitations. Monitor patient closely.
General, spinal anesthetics: Severe hypotension and excessive CNS depression. Avoid concomitant use.
Local anesthetics (lidocaine, procaine): Decreased effectiveness of these drugs; poor nerve block. Stop phenelzine for at least 1 week before giving these drugs.
OTC cold, hay fever, weight-reduction products: Serious CV toxicity. Avoid concomitant use.
Serotonergic drugs (fluoxetine, fluvoxamine, paroxetine, sertraline), tricyclic antidepressants: Serious adverse effects. At least a 2-week waiting period between drug use is recommended.
Drug-herb. *Cacao:* Potentiated vasopressor effects. Discourage use.
Ginseng: Possible adverse reactions, including headache, tremors, mania. Discourage use.
Drug-food. *Foods high in caffeine, tryptophan, tyramine:* May precipitate hypertensive crisis. Discourage use.
Drug-lifestyle. *Alcohol:* Increased adverse reactions. Use cautiously; reduce drug dosage.

Adverse reactions
CNS: *dizziness,* vertigo, headache, hyperreflexia, tremor, muscle twitching, *insomnia,* drowsiness, weakness, fatigue.
CV: orthostatic hypotension, edema.
GI: dry mouth, *anorexia,* nausea, constipation.
GU: elevated urinary catecholamine levels, sexual disturbances.
Hematologic: elevated WBC count.
Hepatic: elevated liver function test results.
Metabolic: weight gain.
Skin: diaphoresis.

☑ Special considerations
• Exercise precautions for use of MAO inhibitors, given alone or with other drugs, for 14 days after stopping drug.
• Consider inherent risk of suicide until significant improvement of depressive state occurs. High-risk patients should have close supervision during initial therapy. To reduce risk of suicidal overdose, prescribe smallest quantity of tablets consistent with good management.
• At start of therapy, patient should lie down for 1 hour after taking phenelzine; to prevent dizziness from orthostatic blood pressure changes, sudden changes to standing position should be avoided.

• Unlike therapy with other MAO inhibitors, therapy with phenelzine and tricyclic antidepressants is generally well tolerated.
• Signs and symptoms of toxicity become apparent slowly (within 24 to 48 hours) and may last for up to 2 weeks. Agitation, flushing, tachycardia, hypotension, hypertension, palpitations, increased motor activity, twitching, increased deep tendon reflexes, seizures, hyperpyrexia, cardiorespiratory arrest, and coma may occur. Doses of 375 mg to 1.5 g have been ingested with fatal and nonfatal results. Give 5 to 10 mg phentolamine I.V. push for hypertensive crisis; treat seizures, agitation, or tremors with I.V. diazepam; tachycardia with beta blockers; and fever with cooling blankets. Monitor vital signs and fluid and electrolyte balance. Use of sympathomimetics (such as norepinephrine or phenylephrine) is contraindicated in hypotension caused by MAO inhibitors.

Monitoring the patient
• Monitor blood pressure closely at start of therapy.
• Monitor patient for adverse effects.

Information for the patient
• Warn patient not to take alcohol, other CNS depressants, or OTC products (such as cold, hay fever, or diet preparations) without medical approval.
• Explain that many foods and beverages (such as wine, beer, cheeses, preserved fruits, meats, and vegetables) may interact with drug. A list of foods to avoid can usually be obtained from the dietary department or pharmacy at most hospitals.
• Tell patient to avoid hazardous activities that require alertness until drug's full CNS effects are known. Suggest taking drug at bedtime to minimize daytime sedation.
• Instruct patient to take drug exactly as prescribed and not to double dose if a dose is missed.
• Tell patient not to stop drug abruptly and to report any problems; dosage reduction can relieve most adverse reactions.

Geriatric patients
• Drug isn't recommended for patients over age 60.

Pediatric patients
• Drug isn't recommended for children under age 16.

phenobarbital
Barbita, Solfoton

phenobarbital sodium
Luminal

Pharmacologic classification: barbiturate
Therapeutic classification: anticonvulsant, sedative-hypnotic
Controlled substance schedule IV
Pregnancy risk category D

How supplied
Available by prescription only
Tablets: 15 mg, 16 mg, 30 mg, 60 mg, 100 mg
Capsules: 16 mg
Elixir: 15 mg/5 ml; 20 mg/5 ml
Injection: 30 mg/ml, 60 mg/ml, 65 mg/ml, 130 mg/ml

Indications, route, and dosage
All forms of epilepsy except absence seizures, febrile seizures in children
Adults: 60 to 100 mg P.O. daily, divided t.i.d. or given as single dose h.s. Or give 200 to 300 mg I.M. or I.V. and repeat q 6 hours, p.r.n.
Children: 1 to 6 mg/kg P.O. daily, usually divided q 12 hours. It can, however, be administered once daily. Or give 4 to 6 mg/kg I.V. or I.M. daily and monitor patient's blood levels.
Status epilepticus
Adults and children: 10 to 20 mg/kg I.V. over 10 to 15 minutes (don't exceed 60 mg/min). Repeat if necessary.
Sedation
Adults: 30 to 120 mg P.O., I.M., or I.V. daily in two or three divided doses. Maximum dose is 400 mg/24 hours.
Children: 8 to 32 mg P.O. daily.
Insomnia
Adults: 100 to 200 mg P.O. or 100 to 320 mg I.M.
Preoperative sedation
Adults: 100 to 200 mg I.M. 60 to 90 minutes before surgery.
Children: 1 to 3 mg/kg I.V. or I.M. 60 to 90 minutes before surgery.

Pharmacodynamics
Anticonvulsant action: Exact cellular site and mechanism of action unknown. Suppresses spread of seizure activity produced by epileptogenic foci in the cortex, thalamus, and limbic systems by enhancing the effect of GABA. Both presynaptic and postsynaptic excitability are decreased; also raises the seizure threshold.
Sedative-hypnotic action: Acts throughout the CNS as a nonselective depressant with a slow onset of action and a long duration of action. Particularly sensitive to this drug is the reticular activating system, which controls CNS arousal. Phenobarbital decreases both presynaptic and post-

synaptic membrane excitability by facilitating the action of GABA.

Pharmacokinetics

• *Absorption:* Well absorbed after oral administration, with 70% to 90% reaching bloodstream. 100% absorption after I.M. administration. After oral administration, serum levels peak in 1 to 2 hours; levels in CNS peak at 1 to 3 hours. Onset of action occurs 20 to 60 minutes or longer after oral dosing; onset after I.V. administration is about 5 minutes. Serum level of 10 mcg/ml needed to produce sedation; 40 mcg/ml usually produces sleep. Levels of 20 to 40 mcg/ml considered therapeutic for anticonvulsant therapy.

• *Distribution:* Distributed widely throughout body. About 25% to 30% protein-bound.

• *Metabolism:* Metabolized by hepatic microsomal enzyme system.

• *Excretion:* 25% to 50% of dose eliminated unchanged in urine; remainder excreted as metabolites of glucuronic acid. Drug's half-life is 5 to 7 days.

Contraindications and precautions

Contraindicated in patients with barbiturate hypersensitivity or history of manifest or latent porphyria, hepatic dysfunction, respiratory disease with dyspnea or obstruction, or nephritis.

Use cautiously in elderly or debilitated patients and in those with acute or chronic pain, depression, suicidal tendencies, history of drug abuse, blood pressure alterations, CV disease, shock, or uremia.

Interactions

Drug-drug. *Antidepressants, antihistamines, narcotics, phenothiazines, tranquilizers, other sedative-hypnotics:* Potentiated CNS and respiratory depressant effects. Monitor patient closely.
Corticosteroids, digitoxin, doxycycline, oral contraceptives (and other estrogens), theophylline (and other xanthines): Enhanced hepatic metabolism of these drugs. Monitor patient for clinical effectiveness; adjust dosage as needed.
Disulfiram, MAO inhibitors, valproic acid: Decreased metabolism of phenobarbital and increased toxicity. Monitor serum levels.
Griseofulvin: Decreased absorption from GI tract. Separate administration times by at least 2 hours.
Rifampin: Decreased phenobarbital levels due to increased hepatic metabolism. Monitor serum levels; adjust dosage as needed.
Warfarin, other oral anticoagulants: Enhanced enzymatic degradation of these drugs. Increased dosages of anticoagulant may be needed.
Drug-lifestyle. *Alcohol:* Potentiated CNS and respiratory depressant effects. Discourage use.

Adverse reactions

CNS: *drowsiness, lethargy, hangover,* paradoxical excitement in elderly patients, somnolence, change in EEG patterns.
CV: *bradycardia,* hypotension.
GI: nausea, vomiting.
Hematologic: exacerbation of porphyria.
Respiratory: *respiratory depression, apnea.*
Skin: rash, *erythema multiforme, Stevens-Johnson syndrome,* urticaria, pain, swelling, thrombophlebitis, necrosis, nerve injury at injection site.
Other: *angioedema,* physical and psychological dependence.

☑ Special considerations

Besides the recommendations relevant to all barbiturates, consider the following.

• Oral solution may be mixed with water or juice to improve taste.

• Don't crush or break extended-release form; this will impair drug action.

• Reconstitute powder for injection with 2.5 to 5 ml sterile water for injection. Roll vial in hands; don't shake.

• Use a larger vein for I.V. administration to prevent extravasation.

• Avoid I.V. administration at a rate exceeding 60 mg/minute to prevent hypotension and respiratory depression. It may take up to 30 minutes after I.V. administration to achieve maximum effect.

• Administer parenteral dose within 30 minutes of reconstitution because drug hydrolyzes in solution and on exposure to air.

• Keep emergency resuscitation equipment on hand when administering phenobarbital I.V.

• Administer I.M. dose deep into large muscle mass to prevent tissue injury.

• Don't use injectable solution if it contains a precipitate.

• Administration of full loading doses over short periods of time to treat status epilepticus will require ventilatory support in adults.

• Full therapeutic effects aren't seen for 2 to 3 weeks, except when loading dose is used.

• Drug may cause a false-positive phentolamine test. The physiologic effects of drug may impair absorption of cyanocobalamin Co 57; it may decrease serum bilirubin levels in neonates, epileptics, and in patients with congenital nonhemolytic unconjugated hyperbilirubinemia. Barbiturates may increase sulfobromophthalein retention.

• Toxicity may cause unsteady gait, slurred speech, sustained nystagmus, somnolence, confusion, respiratory depression, pulmonary edema, areflexia, and coma. Typical shock syndrome with tachycardia and hypotension along with jaundice, oliguria, and chills then fever may occur.

• Alkalinization of urine may be helpful in removing drug from body; hemodialysis may be useful in severe overdose. Oral activated charcoal may enhance drug elimination regardless of its route of administration.

Monitoring the patient
• Monitor vital signs when giving via I.V. route.
• Monitor phenobarbital levels as needed.

Information for the patient
• Advise patient of potential for physical and psychological dependence with prolonged use.
• Warn patient to avoid alcohol and other CNS depressants while taking drug. An excessive depressant effect is possible even if drug is taken the evening before alcohol ingestion.
• Caution patient not to stop taking drug suddenly because this could cause a withdrawal reaction.
• Advise patient to avoid driving and other hazardous activities that require alertness until adverse CNS effects of drug are known.

Geriatric patients
• Elderly patients are more sensitive to drug's effects and usually need lower doses. Confusion, disorientation, and excitability may occur in elderly patients.

Pediatric patients
• Paradoxical hyperexcitability may occur in children. Use with caution. Use of phenobarbital extended-release capsules isn't recommended in children under age 12.

Breast-feeding patients
• Drug appears in breast milk; avoid use in breast-feeding women.

phentermine hydrochloride
Adipex-P, Fastin, Ionamin, Obe-Nix, Phentride, Teramine

Pharmacologic classification: amphetamine congener
Therapeutic classification: short-term adjunctive anorexigenic, indirect-acting sympathomimetic amine
Controlled substance schedule IV
Pregnancy risk category X

How supplied
Available by prescription only
Capsules and tablets: 8 mg, 15 mg, 18.75 mg, 30 mg, 37.5 mg
Capsules (resin complex, sustained-release): 15 mg, 30 mg, 37.5 mg

Indications, route, and dosage
Short-term adjunct in exogenous obesity
Adults: 8 mg P.O. t.i.d. ½ hour before meals; or 15 to 37.5 mg daily before breakfast; or 15 to 30 mg daily before breakfast (resin complex).

Pharmacodynamics
Anorexigenic action: Indirect-acting sympathomimetic amine; causes fewer and less severe adverse reactions from CNS stimulation than do amphetamines, and potential for addiction is lower. Anorexigenic effects are thought to follow direct stimulation of the hypothalamus; they may involve other CNS and metabolic effects.

Pharmacokinetics
• *Absorption:* Absorbed readily after oral administration; therapeutic effects last 4 to 6 hours.
• *Distribution:* Distributed widely throughout body.
• *Metabolism:* No information available.
• *Excretion:* Excreted in urine.

Contraindications and precautions
Contraindicated in patients with hypersensitivity or idiosyncrasy to sympathomimetic amines and in those with hyperthyroidism, moderate to severe hypertension, advanced arteriosclerosis, symptomatic CV disease, or glaucoma. Also contraindicated within 14 days of MAO inhibitor therapy and in agitated patients. Use cautiously in patients with mild hypertension.

Interactions
Drug-drug. *Acetazolamide, antacids, sodium bicarbonate:* Increased renal reabsorption of phentermine and prolonged duration of action. Monitor patient closely.
General anesthetics: Arrhythmias. Monitor patient closely.
Guanethidine, other antihypertensives: Decreased hypotensive effects. Monitor blood pressure.
Haloperidol, phenothiazines: Decreased phentermine effects. Monitor patient for clinical effect.
Insulin: Altered insulin requirements in diabetic patient. Monitor blood glucose levels.
MAO inhibitors (drugs with MAO-inhibiting effects): Concomitant use or use within 14 days may cause hypertensive crisis. Avoid concomitant use.
Drug-food. *Caffeine:* Additive CNS stimulation. Discourage excessive use.

Adverse reactions
CNS: overstimulation, headache, euphoria, dysphoria, dizziness, *insomnia.*
CV: *palpitations, tachycardia,* increased blood pressure.
GI: dry mouth, dysgeusia, constipation, diarrhea, other GI disturbances.
GU: impotence, dysuria, polyuria, urinary frequency, altered libido.
Skin: urticaria.

☑ Special considerations
Besides the recommendations relevant to all amphetamines, consider the following.
• Intermittent courses of treatment (6 weeks on, then 4 weeks off) are equally as effective as continuous use.

Reactions may be *common,* uncommon, *life-threatening,* or COMMON AND LIFE-THREATENING.

• Greatest weight loss occurs in first weeks of therapy and diminishes in succeeding weeks. When such tolerance to drug effect develops, drug should be discontinued instead of increasing dosage.

• Don't crush sustained-release forms.

• Give morning dose 2 hours after breakfast.

• Toxicity may cause restlessness, tremor, hyperreflexia, fever, tachypnea, dizziness, confusion, aggressive behavior, hallucinations, blood pressure changes, arrhythmias, nausea, vomiting, diarrhea, and cramps. Fatigue and depression usually follow CNS stimulation; then possible seizures, coma, and death. Chlorpromazine may antagonize CNS stimulation. Acidification of urine may hasten excretion.

Monitoring the patient

• Monitor patient's weight loss.

• Monitor patient for adverse effects.

Information for the patient

• Advise patient to take morning dose 2 hours after breakfast, not to crush or chew sustained-release products, and to avoid drinks containing caffeine.

• Tell patient to take last daily dose at least 6 hours before bedtime to prevent insomnia.

• Warn patient not to take drug more frequently than prescribed.

• Advise patient that drug may produce dizziness, fatigue, or drowsiness.

• Tell patient to call if palpitations occur.

• Tell diabetic patients to closely monitor blood glucose level. Adjustment in eating habits, body weight, and activity and change in dosage of antidiabetic may be needed.

Pediatric patients

• Drug isn't recommended for children under age 12.

---

phentolamine mesylate
Regitine

Pharmacologic classification: alpha-adrenergic blocker
Therapeutic classification: antihypertensive for pheochromocytoma; cutaneous vasodilator
Pregnancy risk category C

How supplied
Available by prescription only
Injection: 5 mg/ml in 1-ml vials

Indications, route, and dosage
Aid for diagnosis of pheochromocytoma
Adults: 5 mg I.V. or I.M.
Children: 1 mg I.V., or 3 mg I.M

Control or prevention of paroxysmal hypertension immediately before or during pheochromocytomectomy
Adults: 5 mg I.M. or I.V. 1 to 2 hours preoperatively, repeated as necessary; 5 mg I.V. during surgery if indicated.
Children: 1 mg I.M. or I.V. 1 to 2 hours preoperatively, repeated as necessary; 1 mg I.V. during surgery if indicated.
Prevention or treatment of dermal necrosis and sloughing of extravasation after I.V. administration of norepinephrine or ◇ dopamine
Adults and children: Inject 5 to 10 mg in 10 ml of normal saline solution into affected area, or add 10 mg to each liter of I.V. fluids containing norepinephrine.
◇ Adjunctive treatment of left-sided heart failure secondary to acute MI
Adults: 170 to 400 mcg/minute by I.V. infusion.
◇ Treatment adjunct for men with impotence (neurogenic or vascular)
Adults: 0.5 to 1 mg by intracavernosal injection. Usually administered with 30 mg papaverine injection.
◇ Hypertensive crisis from sympathomimetic amines
Adults: 5 to 15 mg I.V.

Pharmacodynamics
Antihypertensive action: Competitively antagonizes endogenous and exogenous amines at presynaptic and postsynaptic alpha-adrenergic receptors, decreasing both preload and afterload.
Cutaneous vasodilation action: Blocks epinephrine- and norepinephrine-induced vasoconstriction.

Pharmacokinetics
• *Absorption:* Immediate effect after I.V. administration.
• *Distribution:* No information available.
• *Metabolism:* No information available.
• *Excretion:* About 10% of dose excreted unchanged in urine; excretion of remainder unknown. Short duration of action; plasma half-life is 19 minutes after I.V. administration.

Contraindications and precautions
Contraindicated in patients with hypersensitivity to drug and in those with angina, coronary artery disease, or MI or history of MI. Use cautiously in patients with peptic ulcer or gastritis.

Interactions
Drug-drug. *Ephedrine, epinephrine:* Antagonized vasoconstrictor and hypertensive effects of these drugs. Avoid using together.

Adverse reactions
CNS: *dizziness, weakness, flushing, **cerebrovascular occlusion,** cerebrovascular spasm.*

CV: *hypotension,* **shock, arrhythmias,** tachycardia, **MI.**
EENT: *nasal congestion.*
GI: *diarrhea, nausea, vomiting.*

☑ **Special considerations**
Besides the recommendations relevant to all alpha-adrenergic blockers, consider the following.
• Usual doses of phentolamine have little effect on blood pressure of normal individuals or patients with essential hypertension.
• Before test for pheochromocytoma, have patient rest in supine position until blood pressure is stabilized. When drug is administered I.V., inject dose rapidly after effects of venipuncture on blood pressure have passed. A marked decrease in blood pressure will be seen immediately, with maximum effect seen within 2 minutes.
• When possible, sedatives, analgesics, and all other drugs should be withdrawn at least 24 hours (preferably 48 to 72 hours) before phentolamine test; antihypertensives should be withdrawn and test shouldn't be performed until blood pressure returns to pretreatment levels; rauwolfia drugs should be withdrawn at least 4 weeks before test.
• Drug has been used to treat hypertension resulting from clonidine withdrawal and to treat reaction to sympathetic amines or other drugs or foods in patients taking MAO inhibitors.
• Drug has been used in patients with MI associated with left-sided heart failure in an attempt to reduce infarct size and decrease left ventricular ejection impedance. Drug has also been used to treat supraventricular premature contractions.
• Toxicity may cause hypotension, dizziness, fainting, tachycardia, vomiting, lethargy, and shock. Use norepinephrine if necessary to increase blood pressure. Don't use epinephrine; it stimulates both alpha and beta receptors and will cause vasodilation and further drop in blood pressure.

Monitoring the patient
• When testing for pheochromocytoma, record blood pressure immediately after injection, at 30-second intervals for first 3 minutes, and at 1-minute intervals for next 7 minutes. When drug is given I.M., maximum effect occurs within 20 minutes. Record blood pressure every 5 minutes for 30 to 45 minutes after injection.
• Watch for test response. A positive test response occurs when patient's blood pressure decreases at least 35 mm Hg systolic and 25 mm Hg diastolic; a negative test response occurs when patient's blood pressure remains unchanged, is elevated, or decreases less than 35 mm Hg systolic and 25 mm Hg diastolic.

Information for the patient
• Teach patient about phentolamine test, if indicated.
• Tell patient to report adverse effects at once.

• Tell patient not to take sedatives or narcotics for at least 24 hours before test.

Geriatric patients
• Administer cautiously because elderly patients may be more sensitive to adverse effects.

Pediatric patients
• Administer cautiously.

Breast-feeding patients
• It's unknown if drug appears in breast milk; because of possible adverse reactions in infant, stop either breast-feeding or drug based on importance of drug to mother.

phenylephrine hydrochloride
Nasal products
Alconefrin 12, Alconefrin 25, Neo-Synephrine, Nostril, Rhinall, Sinex

Parenteral
Neo-Synephrine

Ophthalmic
AK-Dilate, AK-Nefrin, Isopto Frin, Mydfrin, Neo-Synephrine, Prefrin Liquifilm

Pharmacologic classification: adrenergic
Therapeutic classification: vasoconstrictor
Pregnancy risk category C

How supplied
Available by prescription only
Injection: 10 mg/ml parenteral
Ophthalmic solution: 0.12%, 2.5%, 10%
Available without a prescription
Nasal solution: 0.125%, 0.16%, 0.25%, 0.5%, 1%
Nasal spray: 0.25%, 0.5%, 1%

Indications, route, and dosage
Hypotensive emergencies during spinal anesthesia
Adults: Initially, 0.1 to 0.2 mg I.V.; subsequent doses should also be low (0.1 mg).
Prevention of hypotension during spinal or inhalation anesthesia
Adults: 2 to 3 mg S.C. or I.M. 3 to 4 minutes before anesthesia.
Mild to moderate hypotension
Adults: 1 to 10 mg S.C. or I.M. (initial dose shouldn't exceed 5 mg). Additional doses may be given in 1 to 2 hours if needed. Or 0.1 to 0.5 mg slow I.V. injection (initial dose shouldn't exceed 0.5 mg). Additional doses may be given q 10 to 15 minutes.
Children: 0.1 mg/kg or 3 mg/m² I.M. or S.C.

Reactions may be common, uncommon, **life-threatening,** or COMMON AND LIFE-THREATENING.

Paroxysmal supraventricular tachycardia
Adults: Initially, 0.5 mg rapid I.V.; subsequent doses may be increased in increments of 0.1 to 0.2 mg. Maximum dose shouldn't exceed 1 mg.

Prolongation of spinal anesthesia
Adults: 2 to 5 mg added to anesthetic solution.

Adjunct in the treatment of severe hypotension or shock
Adults: 0.1 to 0.18 mg/minute I.V. infusion. After blood pressure stabilizes, maintain at 0.04 to 0.06 mg/minute, adjusted to patient response.

Vasoconstrictor for regional anesthesia
Adults: 1 mg phenylephrine added to 20 ml local anesthetic.

Mydriasis (without cycloplegia)
Adults: Instill 1 or 2 drops 2.5% or 10% solution in eye before procedure. May be repeated in 10 to 60 minutes if needed.

Posterior synechia (adhesion of iris)
Adults: Instill 1 drop of 10% solution in eye 3 or more times daily with atropine sulfate.

Diagnosis of Horner's or Raeder's syndrome
Adults: Instill a 1% or 10% solution in both eyes.

Initial treatment of postoperative malignant glaucoma
Adults: Instill 1 drop of a 10% solution with 1 drop of a 1% to 4% atropine sulfate solution 3 or more times daily.

Nasal, ◊ sinus, or eustachian tube congestion
Adults and children over age 12: Apply 2 to 3 drops or 1 to 2 sprays of 0.25% to 1% solution instilled in each nostril; or a small quantity of 0.5% nasal jelly applied into each nostril. Apply jelly or spray to nasal mucosa.
Children ages 6 to 12: Apply 2 to 3 drops or 1 to 2 sprays in each nostril.
Children under age 6: Apply 2 to 3 drops or sprays of 0.125% or 0.16% solution in each nostril.
Drops, spray, or jelly can be given q 4 hours, p.r.n.

Conjunctival congestion
Adults: 1 to 2 drops of 0.08% to 0.25% solution applied to conjunctiva q 3 to 4 hours, p.r.n.

Pharmacodynamics
Vasopressor action: Acts predominantly by direct stimulation of alpha-adrenergic receptors, which constrict resistance and capacitance blood vessels, resulting in increased total peripheral resistance; increased systolic and diastolic blood pressure; decreased blood flow to vital organs, skin, and skeletal muscle; and constriction of renal blood vessels, reducing renal blood flow. Main therapeutic effect is vasoconstriction.

Also may act indirectly by releasing norepinephrine from its storage sites. Doesn't stimulate beta receptors except in large doses (activates beta$_1$ receptors). Tachyphylaxis (tolerance) may follow repeated injections.

Other alpha-adrenergic effects include action on the dilator muscle of the pupil (producing contraction) and local decongestant action in the arterioles of the conjunctiva (producing constriction).

Acts directly on alpha-adrenergic receptors in the arterioles of conjunctiva nasal mucosa, producing constriction. Vasoconstricting action on skin, mucous membranes, and viscera slows the vascular absorption rate of local anesthetics, which prolongs their action, localizes anesthesia, and decreases the risk of toxicity.

May cause contraction of pregnant uterus and constriction of uterine blood vessels.

Pharmacokinetics
• *Absorption:* Pressor effects almost immediately after I.V. injection; last 15 to 20 minutes. After I.M. injection, onset is within 10 to 15 minutes; lasts ½ to 2 hours. After S.C. injection, onset is within 10 to 15 minutes; lasts 50 to 60 minutes. Nasal or conjunctival decongestant effects last 30 minutes to 4 hours. Peak effects for mydriasis 15 to 60 minutes for 2.5% solution; 10 to 90 minutes for 10% solution. Mydriasis recovery time is 3 hours for 2.5% solution; 3 to 7 hours for 10% solution.
• *Distribution:* No information available.
• *Metabolism:* Metabolized in liver and intestine by MAO.
• *Excretion:* No information available.

Contraindications and precautions
All forms are contraindicated in patients with hypersensitivity to drug. Injected form is also contraindicated in those with severe hypertension or ventricular tachycardia. Ophthalmic form is also contraindicated in patients with angle-closure glaucoma and in those who wear soft contact lenses.

Use all forms cautiously in elderly patients and in patients with hyperthyroidism or cardiac disease. Use nasal and ophthalmic forms cautiously in patients with type 1 diabetes mellitus, hypertension, or advanced arteriosclerotic changes and in children who have low body weight. Use injectable form cautiously in patients with severe atherosclerosis, bradycardia, partial heart block, myocardial disease, or allergy to sulfites.

Interactions
Drug-drug. *Alpha blockers, antihypertensives, diuretics used as antihypertensives, guanadrel, guanethidine, nitrates, rauwolfia alkaloids:* Decreased pressor response (hypotension). Monitor patient closely.
Cardiac glycosides, epinephrine, general anesthetics (cyclopropane, halothane), guanadrel, guanethidine, levodopa, MAO inhibitors, tricyclic antidepressants, other sympathomimetics: Increased risk of arrhythmias, including tachycardia. Monitor patient closely; don't use with MAO inhibitors.

Cycloplegic antimuscarinics (such as atropine): Increased mydriatic response to phenylephrine. Use together cautiously.

Doxapram, ergot alkaloids, MAO inhibitors, mazindol, methyldopa, oxytocics: Potentiated pressor effects. Monitor patient closely; don't use with MAO inhibitors.

Levodopa: Decreased mydriatic response to phenylephrine. Use together cautiously.

Nitrates: Reduced antianginal effects. Evaluate response to therapy.

Thyroid hormones: Increased effects of either drug. Monitor patient closely.

Adverse reactions

CNS: *headache;* excitability (with injected form); brow ache (with ophthalmic form); tremor, dizziness, nervousness (with nasal form).

CV: **bradycardia, arrhythmias,** hypertension (with injected form); *hypertension* (with 10% solution), tachycardia, palpitations, **PVCs, MI** (with ophthalmic form); *palpitations, tachycardia,* **PVCs,** hypertension, pallor (with nasal form).

EENT: transient eye burning or stinging on instillation, blurred vision, increased intraocular pressure, keratitis, lacrimation, reactive hyperemia of eye, allergic conjunctivitis, rebound miosis (with ophthalmic form); transient burning or stinging, dryness of nasal mucosa, rebound nasal congestion with continued use (with nasal form).

GI: nausea (with nasal form).

Respiratory: *asthmatic episodes.*

Skin: pallor, dermatitis (with ophthalmic form), tissue sloughing with extravasation (with injected form), diaphoresis (with ophthalmic form).

Other: tachyphylaxis (may occur with continued use), **anaphylaxis, decreased organ perfusion** (with prolonged use), trembling.

☑ Special considerations

Besides the recommendations relevant to all adrenergics, consider the following.

• Give I.V. through large veins, and monitor flow rate. To treat extravasation ischemia, infiltrate site promptly and liberally with 10 to 15 ml of saline solution containing 5 to 10 mg of phentolamine through fine needle. Topical nitroglycerin has also been used.

• Hypovolemic states should be corrected before administration of drug; phenylephrine shouldn't be used in place of fluid, blood, plasma, and electrolyte replacement.

• Drug is chemically incompatible with butacaine, sulfate, alkalies, ferric salts, and oxidizing drugs and metals.

• Toxicity may cause exaggeration of common adverse reactions, palpitations, paresthesia, vomiting, arrhythmias, and hypertension. Use atropine sulfate to block reflex bradycardia; phentolamine to treat excessive hypertension; and propranolol to treat cardiac arrhythmias, or levodopa to reduce excessive mydriatic effect of ophthalmic preparation as necessary.

Ophthalmic

• Apply digital pressure to lacrimal sac during and for 1 to 2 minutes after instillation to prevent systemic absorption.

• Prolonged exposure to air or strong light may cause oxidation and discoloration. Don't use if solution is brown or contains precipitate.

• To prevent contamination, don't touch applicator tip to any surface. Instruct patient in proper technique.

• Drug may cause false-normal tonometry readings.

Nasal

• Prolonged or long-term use may result in rebound congestion and chronic swelling of nasal mucosa.

• To reduce risk of rebound congestion, use weakest effective dose.

• After use, rinse tip of spray bottle or dropper with hot water and dry with clean tissue. Wipe tip of nasal jelly container with clean, damp tissues.

Monitoring the patient

• During I.V. administration, monitor pulse, blood pressure, and CVP every 2 to 5 minutes. Control flow rate and dosage to prevent excessive increases. I.V. overdoses can induce ventricular arrhythmias.

• Monitor patient for adverse effects.

Information for the patient

• Tell patient to store away from heat, light, and humidity (not in bathroom medicine cabinet) and out of children's reach.

• Warn patient to use only as directed. If using OTC product, patient should follow directions on label and not use more often or in larger doses than prescribed or recommended.

• Caution patient not to exceed recommended dosage regardless of formulation; patient shouldn't double, decrease, or omit doses nor change dosage intervals unless so instructed.

• Tell patient to call if drug provides no relief in 2 days after using ophthalmic solution or 3 days after using nasal solution.

• Explain that systemic absorption from nasal and conjunctival membranes can occur. Patient should report systemic reactions, such as dizziness and chest pain, and stop drug.

Ophthalmic

• Instruct patient not to use if solution is brown or contains a precipitate.

• Tell patient to wash hands before applying and to use finger to apply pressure to lacrimal sac during and for 1 to 2 minutes after instillation to decrease systemic absorption.

• Warn patient to avoid touching tip to any surface to prevent contamination.

• Inform patient that after applying drops, pupils will become unusually large. Patient should use

---

Reactions may be *common,* uncommon, *life-threatening,* or COMMON AND LIFE-THREATENING.

sunglasses to protect eyes from sunlight and other bright lights, and call if effects persist 12 hours or more.

Nasal

• After use, tell patient to rinse tip of spray bottle or dropper with hot water and dry with clean tissue or wipe tip of nasal jelly container with clean, damp tissues.

• Instruct patient to blow nose gently (with both nostrils open) to clear nasal passages before using drug.

• Teach patient appropriate method:

– Drops: Tilt head back while sitting or standing up, or lie on bed and hang head over side. Stay in position a few minutes to permit drug to spread through nose.

– Spray: With head upright, squeeze bottle quickly and firmly to produce 1 or 2 sprays into each nostril; wait 3 to 5 minutes, blow nose and repeat dose.

– Jelly: Place in each nostril and sniff well back into nose.

• Tell patient that increased fluid intake helps keep secretions liquid.

• Warn patient to avoid using OTC drugs with phenylephrine to prevent possible hazardous interactions.

Geriatric patients

• Effects may be exaggerated in elderly patients. In patients over age 50, phenylephrine (ophthalmic solution) appears to alter the response of the dilator muscle of the pupil so that rebound miosis may occur the day after drug is administered.

Pediatric patients

• Infants and children may be more susceptible than adults to drug's effects. Because of risk of precipitating severe hypertension, only ophthalmic solutions containing 0.5% or less should be used in infants under age 1. The 10% ophthalmic solution is contraindicated in infants. Most manufacturers recommend that the 0.5% nasal solution not be used in children under age 12 except under medical supervision, and the 0.25% nasal solution shouldn't be used in children under age 6 except under medical supervision.

Breast-feeding patients

• It's unknown if drug appears in breast milk; use with caution in breast-feeding women.

phenytoin, phenytoin sodium, phenytoin sodium (extended)
Dilantin, Dilantin Infatab, Dilantin Kapseals, Dilantin-125

phenytoin sodium (prompt)

Pharmacologic classification: hydantoin derivative
Therapeutic classification: anticonvulsant
Pregnancy risk category D

How supplied
Available by prescription only
phenytoin
Tablets (chewable): 50 mg
Oral suspension: 30 mg/5 ml*, 125 mg/5 ml
phenytoin sodium
Injection: 50 mg/ml
phenytoin sodium (extended)
Capsules: 30 mg, 100 mg
phenytoin sodium (prompt)
Capsules: 100 mg

Indications, route, and dosage

Generalized tonic-clonic seizures, status epilepticus, nonepileptic seizures (post–head trauma, Reye's syndrome)
Adults: Loading dose is 10 to 15 mg/kg I.V. slowly, not to exceed 50 mg/minute; oral loading dose is 1 g divided into three doses (400 mg, 300 mg, 300 mg) given at 2-hour intervals. Once controlled, maintenance dose is 300 mg P.O. daily (extended only); initially use a dose divided t.i.d. (extended or prompt).
Children: Loading dose is 15 to 20 mg/kg I.V. at 50 mg/minute, or P.O. divided q 8 to 12 hours; then start maintenance dose of 4 to 8 mg/kg P.O. or I.V. daily, divided q 12 hours.
Neuritic pain (migraine, trigeminal neuralgia, and Bell's palsy)
Adults: 200 to 600 mg P.O. daily in divided doses.
Skeletal muscle relaxant
Adults: 200 to 600 mg P.O. daily, p.r.n.
◊ *Ventricular arrhythmias unresponsive to lidocaine or procainamide, and arrhythmias induced by cardiac glycosides*
Adults: 50 to 100 mg q 10 to 15 minutes, p.r.n., not to exceed 15 mg/kg. Infusion rate should never exceed 50 mg/minute (slow I.V. push).
Alternative method: 100 mg I.V. q 15 minutes until adverse effects develop, arrhythmias are controlled, or 1 g has been given. Also may administer entire loading dose of 1 g I.V. slowly at 25 mg/minute. Can be diluted in normal saline solution. I.M. route isn't recommended because of pain and erratic absorption.

Prophylactic control of seizures during neurosurgery

Adults: 100 to 200 mg I.V. at intervals of about 4 hours during perioperative and postoperative periods.

Pharmacodynamics

Anticonvulsant action: Like other hydantoin derivatives, phenytoin stabilizes neuronal membranes and limits seizure activity by either increasing efflux or decreasing influx of sodium ions across cell membranes in the motor cortex during generation of nerve impulses. Phenytoin exerts its antiarrhythmic effects by normalizing sodium influx to Purkinje's fibers in patients with cardiac glycoside–induced arrhythmias. It's indicated for generalized tonic-clonic (grand mal) and partial seizures.

Other actions: Inhibits excessive collagenase activity in patients with epidermolysis bullosa.

Pharmacokinetics

- *Absorption:* Absorbed slowly from small intestine; absorption is formulation-dependent and bioavailability may differ among products. For extended-release capsules, serum levels peak at 4 to 12 hours; for prompt-release products, levels peak at 1½ to 3 hours. I.M. doses absorbed erratically; about 50% to 75% of I.M. dose absorbed in 24 hours.
- *Distribution:* Widely distributed throughout body; therapeutic plasma levels 10 to 20 mcg/ml; 5 to 10 mcg/ml in some patients. Lateral nystagmus may occur at levels above 20 mcg/ml; ataxia usually at levels above 30 mcg/ml; significantly decreased mental capacity at 40 mcg/ml. About 90% protein-bound; less so in uremic patients.
- *Metabolism:* Metabolized by liver to inactive metabolites.
- *Excretion:* Excreted in urine; exhibits dose-dependent (zero-order) elimination kinetics. Above a certain dosage level, small increases in dosage disproportionately increase serum levels.

Contraindications and precautions

Contraindicated in patients with hydantoin hypersensitivity, sinus bradycardia, SA block, second- or third-degree AV block, or Adams-Stokes syndrome.

Use cautiously in elderly or debilitated patients; in those with hepatic dysfunction, hypotension, myocardial insufficiency, diabetes, or respiratory depression; and in those receiving hydantoin derivatives.

Interactions

Drug-drug. Phenytoin interacts with many drugs. Diminished therapeutic effects and toxic reactions commonly are the result of recent changes in drug therapy.

Allopurinol, amiodarone, benzodiazepines, chloramphenicol, chlorpheniramine, cimetidine, diazepam, disulfiram, fluconazole, ibuprofen, imipramine, isoniazid, metronidazole, miconazole, omeprazole, phenacemide, phenylbutazone, salicylates, succinimides, trimethoprim, valproic acid: Increased therapeutic effects of phenytoin. Monitor patient.

Amiodarone, APAP, carbamazepine, corticosteroids, cyclosporine, dicumarol, digitoxin, disopyramide, dopamine, doxycycline, estrogens, furosemide, haloperidol, levodopa, mebendazole, meperidine, methadone, metyrapone, oral contraceptives, phenothiazines, quinidine, sulfonylureas: Decreased effects of these drugs via increased hepatic metabolism. Adjust dosages as needed.

Antacids, antineoplastics, barbiturates, calcium, calcium gluconate, carbamazepine, charcoal, diazoxide, folic acid, loxapine, nitrofurantoin, pyridoxine, rifampin, sucralfate, theophylline: Decreased therapeutic effects of phenytoin. Monitor patient.

Antipsychotic drugs: Lowered seizure threshold. Use together cautiously.

Drug-lifestyle. *Alcohol:* Decreased therapeutic effects. Discourage use.

Adverse reactions

CNS: *ataxia, slurred speech,* dizziness, insomnia, nervousness, twitching, headache, *mental confusion, decreased coordination.*

CV: periarteritis nodosa, hypotension.

EENT: *nystagmus, diplopia,* blurred vision, gingival hyperplasia (especially in children).

GI: nausea, vomiting, constipation.

Hematologic: *thrombocytopenia, leukopenia, agranulocytosis, pancytopenia,* macrocythemia, megaloblastic anemia.

Hepatic: *toxic hepatitis.*

Metabolic: hyperglycemia, decreased protein-bound iodine.

Musculoskeletal: osteomalacia.

Skin: scarlatiniform or morbilliform rash; bullous, *exfoliative,* or purpuric dermatitis; *Stevens-Johnson syndrome;* lupus erythematosus; *hirsutism; toxic epidermal necrolysis;* photosensitivity; pain, necrosis, and inflammation at injection site; discoloration of skin (purple glove syndrome) if given by I.V. push in back of hand.

Other: lymphadenopathy, hypertrichosis.

☑ Special considerations

Besides the recommendations relevant to all hydantoin derivatives, consider the following.

- Only extended-release capsules are approved for once-daily dosing; all other forms are given in divided doses every 8 to 12 hours.
- Oral or nasogastric feeding may interfere with absorption of oral suspension; separate dosing and feeding times as much as possible, but by

no less than 1 hour. During continuous tube feeding, tube should be flushed before and after dose.
• If suspension is used, shake well.
• I.M. administration should be avoided; it's painful and drug absorption is erratic.
• Mix I.V. doses in normal saline solution and use within 30 minutes; mixtures with D_5W will precipitate. Don't refrigerate solution; don't mix with other drugs. In-line filter is recommended.
• If using I.V. bolus, use slow (50 mg/minute) I.V. push or constant infusion; too-rapid I.V. injection may cause hypotension and circulatory collapse. Don't use I.V. push in veins on back of hand; larger veins are needed to prevent discoloration associated with purple glove syndrome.
• Abrupt withdrawal may precipitate status epilepticus.
• Phenytoin commonly is abbreviated as DPH (diphenylhydantoin), an older drug name.
• Drug may interfere with the 1-mg dexamethasone suppression test.
• Early toxicity may cause drowsiness, nausea, vomiting, nystagmus, ataxia, dysarthria, tremor, and slurred speech; then hypotension, arrhythmias, respiratory depression, and coma. Death is caused by respiratory and circulatory depression. Estimated lethal dose in adults is 2 to 5 g.

Monitoring the patient
• Monitoring of serum levels is essential because of dose-dependent excretion.
• When giving I.V., continuous monitoring of ECG, blood pressure, and respiratory status is essential.

Information for the patient
• Tell patient to use same brand of phenytoin consistently. Changing brands may change therapeutic effect.
• Instruct patient to take drug with food or milk to minimize GI distress.
• Warn patient not to stop drug, except with medical supervision; to avoid hazardous activities that require alertness until CNS effect is determined; and to avoid alcoholic beverages, which can decrease effectiveness of drug and increase adverse reactions.
• Encourage patient to wear a medical identification bracelet or necklace.
• Stress good oral hygiene to minimize overgrowth and sensitivity of gums.

Geriatric patients
• Elderly patients metabolize and excrete drug slowly; they may require lower dosages.

Pediatric patients
• Special pediatric-strength suspension (30 mg/5 ml) is available in Canada only. Take extreme care to use correct strength. Don't confuse with adult strength (125 mg/5 ml).

Breast-feeding patients
• Drug appears in breast milk; an alternative to breast-feeding is recommended during therapy.

---

physostigmine salicylate
Antilirium

physostigmine sulfate
Eserine

Pharmacologic classification: cholinesterase inhibitor
Therapeutic classification: antimuscarinic antidote, antiglaucoma drug
Pregnancy risk category C

How supplied
Available by prescription only
Injection: 1 mg/ml
Ophthalmic ointment: 0.25%

Indications, route, and dosage
Tricyclic antidepressant and anticholinergic poisoning
Adults: 0.5 to 2 mg I.M. or I.V. given slowly (not to exceed 1 mg/minute I.V.). Dosage individualized and repeated, p.r.n., q 10 minutes.
Children: Reserve for life-threatening situations only. Initial pediatric I.V. or I.M. dose of physostigmine salicylate is 0.02 mg/kg. Dose may be repeated at 5- to 10-minute intervals to maximum of 2 mg if no adverse cholinergic signs are present.
Postanesthesia care
Adults: 0.5 to 1 mg I.M. or I.V. given slowly (not to exceed 1 mg/minute I.V.). Dosage individualized and repeated, p.r.n., q 10 to 30 minutes.
Open-angle glaucoma
Adults: Apply ointment to lower fornix up to t.i.d.

Pharmacodynamics
Antimuscarinic action: Competitively blocks acetylcholine hydrolysis by cholinesterase, resulting in acetylcholine accumulation at cholinergic synapses; that antagonizes the muscarinic effects of overdose with antidepressants and anticholinergics. With ophthalmic use, miosis and ciliary muscle contraction increase aqueous humor outflow and decrease intraocular pressure.

Pharmacokinetics
• *Absorption:* Well absorbed from GI tract, mucous membranes, and subcutaneous tissues when given I.M. or I.V.; effects peak within 5 minutes. After ophthalmic use, may be absorbed orally after passage through nasolacrimal duct.
• *Distribution:* Distributed widely; crosses blood-brain barrier.
• *Metabolism:* Cholinesterase hydrolyzes drug relatively quickly. Duration of effect is 1 to 2 hours

---

after I.V. administration, 12 to 48 hours after ophthalmic use.
• *Excretion:* Only small amount excreted in urine. Exact mode of excretion unknown.

Contraindications and precautions
Injected form contraindicated in patients with mechanical obstruction of the intestine or urogenital tract, asthma, gangrene, diabetes, CV disease, or vagotonia and in those receiving choline esters or depolarizing neuromuscular blockers.

Ophthalmic form is contraindicated in patients with intolerance to physostigmine and in those with active uveitis or corneal injury. Use injectable form cautiously during pregnancy.

Interactions
Drug-drug. *Succinylcholine:* Prolonged respiratory depression due to inhibition of succinylcholine hydrolysis by plasma esterases. Monitor patient closely.
Systemic cholinergic drugs: Additive toxicity. Monitor patient for toxicity.
Drug-herb. *Jaborandi tree, pill-bearing spurge:* Additive effects when used together. Use with caution to avoid toxicity.

Adverse reactions
CNS: weakness; headache (with ophthalmic form); *seizures, restlessness, excitability* (with injected form).
CV: slow or irregular heartbeat (with ophthalmic form); *bradycardia,* hypotension (with injected form).
EENT: blurred vision, eye pain, burning, redness, stinging, eye irritation, twitching of eyelids, watering of eyes (with ophthalmic form); miosis (with injected form).
GI: nausea, vomiting, diarrhea; epigastric pain, *excessive salivation* (with injected form).
GU: loss of bladder control (with ophthalmic form); urinary urgency (with injected form).
Respiratory: *bronchospasm,* bronchial constriction, shortness of breath, dyspnea (with injected form).
Skin: diaphoresis.

☑ Special considerations
Besides the recommendations relevant to all cholinesterase inhibitors, consider the following.
• Toxicity may cause headache, nausea, vomiting, diarrhea, blurred vision, miosis, myopia, excessive tearing, bronchospasm, increased bronchial secretions, hypotension, incoordination, excessive sweating, muscle weakness, bradycardia, excessive salivation, restlessness or agitation, and confusion.
Injectable
• Observe solution for discoloration. Don't use if darkened.

• Atropine sulfate injection should always be available as an antagonist and antidote for most of physostigmine's effects.
• The commercially available formulation of physostigmine salicylate injection contains sodium bisulfite, a sulfite that can cause allergic-type reactions, including anaphylaxis and life-threatening or less severe asthmatic episodes in susceptible individuals.
Ophthalmic
• After applying ointment, have patient close eyelids and roll eyes.

Monitoring the patient
• Monitor patient's vital signs during administration.
• Monitor patient for adverse effects.

Information for the patient
• Teach patient how to administer ophthalmic ointment.
• Instruct patient not to close his eyes tightly or blink unnecessarily after instilling ointment.
• Warn patient that he may experience blurred vision and difficulty seeing after initial instillation.
• Instruct patient to report abdominal cramps, diarrhea, or excessive salivation.
• Remind patient to wait 10 minutes after instillation before using another eye preparation.

Geriatric patients
• Use caution when administering to elderly patients because they may be more sensitive to drug's effects.

Breast-feeding patients
• It's unknown if drug appears in breast milk. Safety and efficacy in breast-feeding women haven't been established.

pilocarpine hydrochloride (ophthalmic)
Adsorbocarpine, Akarpine, Isopto Carpine, Minims Pilocarpine*, Miocarpine*, Ocusert Pilo, Pilocar, Pilopine HS

pilocarpine nitrate
Pilagan

Pharmacologic classification: cholinergic agonist
Therapeutic classification: miotic
Pregnancy risk category C

How supplied
Available by prescription only
pilocarpine hydrochloride
Solution: 0.25%, 0.5%, 1%, 2%, 3%, 4%, 5%, 6%, 8%, 10%
Gel: 4%

Releasing-system insert: 20 mcg/hour, 40 mcg/hour
pilocarpine nitrate
Solution: 1%, 2%, 4%

Indications, route, and dosage

Chronic open-angle glaucoma; before or instead of emergency surgery in acute narrow-angle glaucoma
Adults and children: Instill 1 or 2 drops of a 1% to 4% solution in the lower conjunctival sac q 4 to 12 hours (dosage should be based on periodic tonometric readings) or apply ½-inch ribbon of 4% gel (Pilopine HS) h.s.

Or apply one Ocusert Pilo System (20 or 40 mcg/hour) q 7 days.
Emergency treatment of acute narrow-angle glaucoma
Adults and children: 1 drop of 2% solution q 5 minutes for three to six doses; then 1 drop q 1 to 3 hours until pressure is controlled.
To counteract mydriatic effects of sympathomimetics
Adults: 1 drop of 1% solution in affected eye.

Pharmacodynamics

Miotic action: Stimulates cholinergic receptors of the sphincter muscles of the iris, resulting in miosis. Also produces ciliary muscle contraction, resulting in accommodation with deepening of the anterior chamber, and vasodilation of conjunctival vessels of the outflow tract.

Pharmacokinetics

• *Absorption:* Drops act within 10 to 30 minutes; peak effect at 2 to 4 hours. With Ocusert Pilo System, 0.3 to 7 mg of drug are released during initial 6-hour period; during remainder of 1-week insertion period, release rate is within 20% of rated value. Effect seen in 1½ to 2 hours; maintained for the 1-week life of insertion.
• *Distribution:* No information available.
• *Metabolism:* No information available.
• *Excretion:* Duration of effect of drops is 4 to 6 hours.

Contraindications and precautions

Contraindicated in patients with hypersensitivity to drug or when cholinergic effects such as constriction are undesirable (for example, in acute iritis, some forms of secondary glaucoma, pupillary block glaucoma, acute inflammatory disease of the anterior chamber).

Use cautiously in patients with acute cardiac failure, bronchial asthma, peptic ulcer, hyperthyroidism, GI spasm, urinary obstruction, and Parkinson's disease.

Interactions

Drug-drug. *Demecarium, echothiophate, isoflurophate:* Decreased pharmacologic effects of pilocarpine. Monitor patient closely.

Epinephrine derivatives, timolol: Enhanced reductions in intraocular pressure. Monitor patient closely.

Adverse reactions

CV: hypertension, tachycardia.
EENT: periorbital or supraorbital headache, *myopia,* ciliary spasm, *blurred vision,* conjunctival irritation, transient stinging and burning, keratitis, lens opacity, retinal detachment, lacrimation, changes in visual field, *brow pain.*
GI: nausea, vomiting, diarrhea, salivation.
Respiratory: *bronchoconstriction, pulmonary edema.*
Skin: diaphoresis.
Other: *hypersensitivity reactions.*

☑ Special considerations

• Drug may be used alone or with mannitol, urea, glycerol, or acetazolamide. May be used to counteract effects of mydriatic and cycloplegic products after surgery or ophthalmoscopic examination and may be used alternately with atropine to break adhesions.
• Toxicity may cause flushing, vomiting, bradycardia, bronchospasm, increased bronchial secretion, sweating, tearing, involuntary urination, hypotension, and tremors. Vomiting is usually spontaneous with accidental ingestion; if not, induce emesis and then use activated charcoal or cathartic. Treat dermal exposure by washing areas twice with water. Use epinephrine to treat CV responses. Atropine sulfate is antidote of choice. Flush eye with water or sodium chloride to treat local overdose. Doses up to 20 mg are generally considered nontoxic.

Monitoring the patient
• Monitor tonometric readings.
• Monitor patient for adverse effects.

Information for the patient
• Warn patient that vision will be temporarily blurred, that miotic pupil may make surroundings appear dim and reduce peripheral field of vision, and that transient brow ache and myopia are common at first; assure patient that adverse effects subside 10 to 14 days after therapy begins.
• Instruct patient to check for presence of pilocarpine ocular system at bedtime and upon arising.
• Tell patient that if systems in both eyes are lost, they should be replaced as soon as possible. If one system is lost, it may be replaced with a fresh system or the system remaining in other eye may be removed and both systems replaced with fresh systems so that both systems will subsequently be replaced on same schedule.
• Instruct patient that if Ocusert System falls out of eye during sleep, he should wash hands, then

rinse Ocusert in cool tap water and reposition it in eye. Don't use insert if deformed.
• Inform patient that systems should be replaced every 7 days.
• Provide patient with a copy of manufacturer's instructions for pilocarpine ocular system.
• Tell patient to use caution in night driving and other activities in poor illumination because miotic pupil diminishes side vision and illumination.
• Stress importance of complying with prescribed medical regimen.
• Reassure patient that adverse effects will subside.
• Teach patient correct way to instill drops and to apply light finger pressure on lacrimal sac for 1 minute after administration to minimize systemic absorption.
• Instruct patient to apply gel at bedtime because it will cause blurred vision.

---

pilocarpine hydrochloride (oral)
Salagen

Pharmacologic classification: cholinergic agonist
Therapeutic classification: antixerostomia
Pregnancy risk category C

How supplied
Available by prescription only
Tablets: 5 mg

Indications, route, and dosage
Treatment of symptoms of xerostomia from salivary gland hypofunction caused by radiotherapy for cancer of the head and neck
Adults: 5 mg P.O. t.i.d. Dosage may be increased to 10 mg P.O. t.i.d., p.r.n.

Pharmacodynamics
Antixerostomia action: Increases secretion of the salivary glands, which eliminates dryness.

Pharmacokinetics
• *Absorption:* Absorbed in GI tract. High-fat meal may decrease absorption rate.
• *Distribution:* No information available.
• *Metabolism:* Inactivation thought to occur at neuronal synapses and probably in plasma.
• *Excretion:* Drug and minimally active or inactive degradation products excreted in urine.

Contraindications and precautions
Contraindicated in patients with hypersensitivity to pilocarpine, in those with uncontrolled asthma, and when miosis is undesirable, such as in acute iritis and narrow-angle glaucoma.
    Use cautiously in patients with CV disease, controlled asthma, chronic bronchitis, COPD,

cholelithiasis, biliary tract disease, nephrolithiasis, and cognitive or psychiatric disturbances.

Interactions
Drug-drug. *Beta-adrenergic antagonists:* Increased risk of conduction disturbances. Use together cautiously.
Drugs with anticholinergic effects: Antagonized anticholinergic effects of oral pilocarpine. Use together cautiously.
Drugs with parasympathomimetic effects: Additive pharmacologic effects. Monitor patient closely.

Adverse reactions
CNS: *dizziness, headache,* tremor.
CV: hypertension, tachycardia, edema.
EENT: *rhinitis,* lacrimation, amblyopia, pharyngitis, voice alteration, conjunctivitis, epistaxis, sinusitis, abnormal vision.
GI: *nausea,* dyspepsia, diarrhea, abdominal pain, vomiting, dysphagia, taste perversion.
GU: *urinary frequency.*
Musculoskeletal: *asthenia,* myalgia.
Skin: *flushing,* rash, pruritus.
Other: *sweating,* chills.

☑ Special considerations
• Patient should undergo careful examination of fundus before therapy begins; retinal detachment has been reported with pilocarpine use in patients with preexisting retinal disease.
• Taking 100 mg of oral pilocarpine is considered potentially fatal. Treat with atropine titration (0.5 mg to 1 mg S.C. or I.V.) and supportive measures to maintain respiration and circulation. Epinephrine (0.3 mg to 1 mg S.C. or I.M.) may also be useful during severe CV depression or bronchoconstriction.

Monitoring the patient
• Monitor patient for signs and symptoms of pilocarpine toxicity characterized by exaggeration of its parasympathomimetic effects, including headache, visual disturbance, lacrimation, sweating, respiratory distress, GI spasm, nausea, vomiting, diarrhea, AV block, tachycardia, bradycardia, hypotension, hypertension, shock, mental confusion, cardiac arrhythmia, and tremors.

Information for the patient
• Warn patient that drug may cause visual disturbances (especially at night) that could impair the ability to drive safely.
• Tell patient to drink plenty of fluids to prevent dehydration if drug causes excessive sweating. If adequate fluid intake can't be maintained, tell patient to call.

Pediatric patients
• Safety and effectiveness in children haven't been established.

Reactions may be *common,* uncommon, **life-threatening**, or COMMON AND LIFE-THREATENING.

Breast-feeding patients
● It's unknown if drug appears in breast milk. Because of potential for serious adverse reactions in breast-feeding infants, stop either breast-feeding or drug, taking into account importance of drug to mother.

pimozide
Orap

Pharmacologic classification: diphenyl-butylpiperidine
Therapeutic classification: antipsychotic
Pregnancy risk category C

How supplied
Available by prescription only
Tablets: 2 mg

Indications, route, and dosage
Suppression of severe motor and phonic tics in patients with Tourette syndrome
Adults and children over age 12: Initially, 1 to 2 mg/day in divided doses. Then, increase dosage, p.r.n., every other day.
Maintenance dose: From 7 to 16 mg/day. Maximum dose is 20 mg/day.
Children under age 12: 0.05 mg/kg h.s.; increase at 3-day intervals to maximum of 0.2 mg/kg. Maximum dose is 10 mg/day.

Pharmacodynamics
Antipsychotic action: Mechanism unknown. Thought to exert effects by postsynaptic or presynaptic blockade of CNS dopamine receptors, thus inhibiting dopamine-mediated effects. Also has anticholinergic, antiemetic, and anxiolytic effects and produces mild alpha blockade.

Pharmacokinetics
● *Absorption:* Absorbed slowly and incompletely from GI tract; bioavailability about 50%. Peak plasma levels from 4 to 12 hours (usually in 6 to 8 hours).
● *Distribution:* Distributed widely into body.
● *Metabolism:* Metabolized by liver; a significant first-pass effect exists.
● *Excretion:* About 40% of dose excreted in urine as parent drug and metabolites in 3 to 4 days; about 15% excreted in feces via biliary tract within 3 to 6 days.

Contraindications and precautions
Contraindicated in patients with hypersensitivity to drug, in treatment of simple tics or tics other than those associated with Tourette syndrome, with drug therapy known to cause motor and phonic tics, and in congenital long QT interval syndrome or history of arrhythmias. Also contraindicated in patients with severe toxic CNS depression and in those experiencing coma.
   Use cautiously in patients with impaired renal or hepatic function, glaucoma, prostatic hyperplasia, seizure disorders, or EEG abnormalities.

Interactions
Drug-drug. *Amphetamines, methylphenidate, pemoline:* Tourette-like tic; exacerbation of existing tics. Monitor patient closely.
Anticonvulsants (carbamazepine, phenobarbital, phenytoin): Seizures. An anticonvulsant dosage increase may be needed.
Antidepressants, disopyramide, phenothiazines, procainamide, quinidine, other antiarrhythmics, other antipsychotics: Further depress cardiac conduction and prolong QT interval, resulting in serious arrhythmias. Monitor patient closely if concomitant use is necessary.
CNS depressants (such as analgesics; anxiolytics; barbiturates; epidural, general, spinal anesthetics; narcotics; parenteral magnesium sulfate; tranquilizers): Oversedation and respiratory depression due to additive CNS depressant effects. Avoid concomitant use.
Drug-lifestyle. *Alcohol:* Oversedation and respiratory depression due to additive CNS depressant effects. Discourage use.

Adverse reactions
CNS: *parkinsonian-like symptoms,* drowsiness, headache, insomnia, **neuroleptic malignant syndrome,** other extrapyramidal signs and symptoms (dystonia, akathisia, hyperreflexia, opisthotonos, oculogyric crisis), *tardive dyskinesia, sedation, adverse behavioral effects.*
CV: *ECG changes (prolonged QT interval),* hypotension, hypertension, tachycardia.
EENT: visual disturbances.
GI: *dry mouth, constipation.*
GU: impotence, urinary frequency.
Musculoskeletal: muscle rigidity.
Skin: rash, diaphoresis.

☑ Special considerations
● Elderly patients may be at greater risk for adverse CV effects.
● Extrapyramidal reactions develop in about 10% to 15% of patients at normal doses. Reactions are especially likely to occur during early days of therapy.
● If excessive restlessness and agitation occur, therapy with a beta blocker, such as propranolol or metoprolol, may be helpful.
● Signs of overdose include severe extrapyramidal reactions, hypotension, respiratory depression, coma, and ECG abnormalities, including QT interval prolongation, inversion or flattening of T waves, and new appearance of U waves. Treat with gastric lavage to remove unabsorbed

drug. Maintain blood pressure with I.V. fluids, plasma expanders, or norepinephrine. Don't use epinephrine. Treat extrapyramidal symptoms with parenteral diphenhydramine. Monitor patient for adverse effects for at least 4 days because of drug's prolonged half-life (55 hours).

Monitoring the patient
• Obtain baseline ECG before therapy and then periodically to monitor CV effects.
• Maintain patient's serum potassium level within normal range; decreased potassium levels increase risk of arrhythmias. Monitor potassium level in patients with diarrhea and in those who are taking diuretics.
• Assess patient periodically for abnormal body movement.

Information for the patient
• Inform patient of risks and signs and symptoms of dystonic reactions and tardive dyskinesia.
• Advise patient to take drug exactly as prescribed, not to double missed doses, not to share drug with others, and not to stop taking it suddenly.
• Explain that drug's therapeutic effect may not be seen for several weeks.
• Urge patient to report unusual effects immediately.
• Tell patient not to take drug with alcohol, sleeping medications, or other drugs that may cause drowsiness without medical approval.
• Recommend use of sugarless hard candy or chewing gum, ice chips, or artificial saliva to relieve dry mouth.
• To prevent dizziness at start of therapy, tell patient to lie down for 30 minutes after taking each dose and to avoid sudden changes in posture, especially when rising to upright position.
• To minimize daytime sedation, suggest taking entire daily dose at bedtime.
• Warn patient to avoid hazardous activities that require alertness until drug's effects are known.

Geriatric patients
• Elderly patients are more likely to develop cardiac toxicity and tardive dyskinesia even at normal doses.

Pediatric patients
• Use and efficacy in children under age 12 are limited. Dosage should be kept at lowest possible level. Use of drug in children for any disorder other than Tourette syndrome isn't recommended.

pindolol
Visken

Pharmacologic classification: beta blocker
Therapeutic classification: antihypertensive
Pregnancy risk category B

How supplied
Available by prescription only
Tablets: 5 mg, 10 mg

Indications, route, and dosage
Hypertension
Adults: Initially, 5 mg P.O. b.i.d. increased by 10 mg/day q 3 to 4 weeks up to maximum of 60 mg/day. Usual dosage is 10 to 30 mg daily, given in two or three divided doses. In some patients, once-daily dosing may be possible.
◇ *Angina*
Adults: 15 to 40 mg daily P.O. in three or four divided doses.

Pharmacodynamics
Antihypertensive action: Exact mechanism unknown. Doesn't consistently affect cardiac output or renin release, and other mechanisms such as decreased peripheral resistance probably contribute to hypotensive effect. Because pindolol has some intrinsic sympathomimetic activity—that is, beta-agonist sympathomimetic activity—it may be useful in patients who develop bradycardia with other beta blockers. It's a nonselective beta blocker, inhibiting both $beta_1$ and $beta_2$ receptors.

Pharmacokinetics
• *Absorption:* After oral administration, absorbed rapidly from GI tract; peak plasma levels in 1 to 2 hours. Effect on heart rate usually occurs in 3 hours. Food doesn't reduce bioavailability but may increase rate of GI absorption.
• *Distribution:* Distributed widely throughout body; 40% to 60% protein-bound.
• *Metabolism:* About 60% to 65% of dose metabolized by liver.
• *Excretion:* In adults with normal renal function, 35% to 50% of dose excreted unchanged in urine; half-life about 3 to 4 hours. Antihypertensive effect usually lasts 24 hours.

Contraindications and precautions
Contraindicated in patients with hypersensitivity to drug and in those with bronchial asthma, severe bradycardia, heart block greater than first degree, cardiogenic shock, or overt cardiac failure.

Use cautiously in patients with heart failure, nonallergic bronchospastic disease, diabetes, hyperthyroidism, or impaired renal or hepatic function.

Interactions

Drug-drug. *Other antihypertensives:* Potentiated antihypertensive effects. Monitor blood pressure.

Adverse reactions

CNS: *insomnia, fatigue, dizziness, nervousness,* vivid dreams, weakness, paresthesia.
CV: *edema,* **bradycardia, heart failure,** chest pain.
GI: *nausea,* abdominal discomfort.
Hepatic: elevated serum transaminase, alkaline phosphatase, LD, and uric acid levels.
Musculoskeletal: *muscle pain, joint pain.*
Respiratory: *increased airway resistance,* dyspnea.
Skin: rash, pruritus.

☑ Special considerations

Besides the recommendations relevant to all beta blockers, consider the following.
• Maximum therapeutic response may not be seen for 2 weeks or more.
• Toxicity may cause severe hypotension, bradycardia, heart failure, and bronchospasm.

Monitoring the patient

• Monitor patient for clinical effects.
• Monitor hepatic studies.

Information for the patient

• Tell patient to take drug exactly as prescribed.
• Tell patient to report adverse reactions immediately.

Geriatric patients

• Elderly patients may need lower maintenance drug doses because of increased bioavailability or delayed metabolism; they also may experience enhanced adverse effects. Half-life of drug may be increased in elderly patients.

Pediatric patients

• Safety and efficacy in children haven't been established; use only if potential benefit outweighs risk.

Breast-feeding patients

• Drug appears in breast milk; an alternative to breast-feeding is recommended during therapy.

pioglitazone hydrochloride
Actos

Pharmacologic classification: thiazolidinedione
Therapeutic classification: antidiabetic
Pregnancy risk category C

How supplied

Available by prescription only
Tablets: 15 mg, 30 mg, 45 mg

Indications, route, and dosage

Monotherapy adjunct to diet and exercise to improve glycemic control in patients with type 2 diabetes mellitus; combination therapy with a sulfonylurea, metformin, or insulin when diet and exercise plus single drug doesn't result in adequate glycemic control
Adults: Initially, 15 or 30 mg P.O. once daily. For patients who respond inadequately to initial dose, dose may be increased in increments; maximum dose is 45 mg/day. If used in combination therapy, maximum dose shouldn't exceed 30 mg/day.

Pharmacodynamics

Antidiabetic action: Lowers blood glucose levels by decreasing insulin resistance in the periphery and in the liver, resulting in increased insulin-dependent glucose disposal and decreased glucose output by the liver. Potent and highly selective agonist for receptors found in insulin-sensitive tissues, such as adipose tissue, skeletal muscle, and liver. Activation of these receptors modulates the transcription of a number of insulin-responsive genes involved in control of glucose and lipid metabolism.

Pharmacokinetics

• *Absorption:* When taken on empty stomach, rapidly absorbed and measurable in serum within 30 minutes; levels peak within 2 hours. Food delays time to peak serum levels slightly (to 3 to 4 hours), but doesn't affect overall extent of absorption.
• *Distribution:* Drug and metabolites more than 98% protein-bound, primarily to serum albumin.
• *Metabolism:* Extensively metabolized by liver. Three pharmacologically active metabolites: M-II, M-III, and M-IV.
• *Excretion:* About 15% to 30% of dose recovered in urine, primarily as metabolites and their conjugates. Majority of oral dose excreted into bile and eliminated in feces. Half-life ranges from 3 to 7 hours.

Contraindications and precautions

Contraindicated in patients with hypersensitivity to drug or its components. Drug shouldn't be used in patients with type 1 diabetes mellitus or for the treatment of diabetic ketoacidosis, in patients with clinical evidence of active liver disease or serum ALT level greater than two and one-half times upper limit of normal, or in those who experienced jaundice while taking troglitazone. Don't use in patients with New York Heart Association Class III or IV heart failure. Use cautiously in patients with edema or heart failure.

Interactions
Drug-drug. *Ketoconazole:* May inhibit metabolism of pioglitazone. Monitor patient's blood glucose levels more frequently.
Oral contraceptives: Decreased effectiveness of contraceptives. Advise patient to consider additional birth control measures.

Adverse reactions
CNS: headache.
CV: *edema* (with insulin).
EENT: sinusitis, pharyngitis, tooth disorder.
Hematologic: anemia.
Metabolic: *hypoglycemia* (with combination therapy), aggravated diabetes mellitus, weight gain, decreased triglyceride levels, increased high-density lipoprotein cholesterol.
Musculoskeletal: myalgia.
Respiratory: *upper respiratory tract infection.*

☑ Special considerations
• Because ovulation may resume in premenopausal, anovulatory women with insulin resistance, contraceptive measures may need to be considered.
• Drug should be used in pregnancy only if benefit justifies risk to fetus. Insulin is the preferred antidiabetic for use during pregnancy.
• Management of type 2 diabetes should include diet control. Because caloric restrictions, weight loss, and exercise help improve insulin sensitivity and help make drug therapy effective, these measures are essential for proper diabetes management.

Monitoring the patient
• Liver enzyme levels should be measured at start of therapy, every 2 months for first year, and then periodically. Liver function tests also should be performed in patients who develop signs and symptoms of liver dysfunction, such as nausea, vomiting, abdominal pain, fatigue, anorexia, or dark urine. Stop drug if patient develops jaundice or if results of liver functions tests show ALT elevations greater than three times upper limit of normal.
• Patients with heart failure should be observed for increased edema during therapy.
• While patient is receiving drug, hemoglobin levels and hematocrit may decrease, usually during the first 4 to 12 weeks of therapy. Monitor patient.

• Watch for hypoglycemia in patients receiving drug with insulin and adjust dosage of these products as needed.
• Besides having blood glucose levels checked regularly, patients should also have glycosylated hemoglobin checked periodically to evaluate therapeutic response to drug.

Information for the patient
• Instruct patient to adhere to dietary instructions and to have blood glucose levels and glycosylated hemoglobin tested regularly.
• Teach patient taking pioglitazone with insulin or oral antidiabetics the signs and symptoms of hypoglycemia.
• Advise patient to call during periods of stress, such as fever, trauma, infection, or surgery, because drug requirements may change.
• Notify patient that blood tests for liver function will be performed before therapy, every 2 months for the first year, and then periodically.
• Tell patient to report unexplained nausea, vomiting, abdominal pain, fatigue, anorexia, or dark urine immediately because these may indicate potential liver problems.
• Inform patient that drug can be taken with or without meals.
• Tell patient that, if a dose is missed, he shouldn't double dose the next day.
• Advise anovulatory, premenopausal women with insulin resistance that drug may cause resumption of ovulation and contraceptive measures may need to be considered.

Geriatric patients
• No significant differences in drug safety and effectiveness have been observed between patients ages 65 and older and younger patients.

Pediatric patients
• Safety and effectiveness in children haven't been evaluated.

Breast-feeding patients
• It's unknown if drug appears in breast milk. Because many drugs appear in breast milk, pioglitazone shouldn't be administered to breast-feeding women.

pipecuronium bromide
Arduan

Pharmacologic classification: non-depolarizing neuromuscular blocker
Therapeutic classification: skeletal muscle relaxant
Pregnancy risk category C

How supplied
Available by prescription only
Injection: 10 mg/vial

Indications, route, and dosage

To provide skeletal muscle relaxation during surgery as an adjunct to general anesthesia

Adults and children: Dosage is highly individualized. The following doses may serve as a guide, assuming that patient isn't obese and has normal renal function. Initially, doses of 70 to 85 mcg/kg I.V. are used to provide conditions considered ideal for endotracheal intubation and will maintain paralysis for 1 to 2 hours. If succinylcholine is used for endotracheal intubation, initial doses of pipecuronium 50 mcg/kg will provide good relaxation for 45 minutes or more. Maintenance doses of 10 to 15 mcg/kg provide relaxation for about 50 minutes.

✦ *Dosage adjustment.* For patients with renal impairment, refer to the table.

Creatinine clearance (ml/min)	Dose (mcg/kg)
100	85
80	70
60	55
40	50

Pharmacodynamics

Muscle relaxant action: Like other nondepolarizing muscle relaxants, pipecuronium competes with acetylcholine for receptor sites at the motor end plate. Because this action may be antagonized by cholinesterase inhibitors, it's considered a competitive antagonist.

Pharmacokinetics

• *Absorption:* No information available regarding use by any route other than I.V. Maximum onset of action within 5 minutes.
• *Distribution:* Volume of distribution (V_D) about 0.25 L/kg; increases in patients with renal failure. Other conditions associated with increased V_D (edema, old age, CV disease) may delay onset.
• *Metabolism:* Only about 20% to 40% of dose metabolized, probably in liver. One metabolite (3-desacetyl pipecuronium) has about 50% of neuromuscular blocking activity of parent drug.
• *Excretion:* Primarily excreted by kidneys. Half-life estimated at 1.7 hours; may increase to 4 hours or more in patients with severe renal disease.

Contraindications and precautions

Contraindicated in patients with hypersensitivity to drug. Use cautiously in patients with renal failure.

Interactions

Drug-drug. *Aminoglycosides (gentamicin, kanamycin, neomycin, streptomycin), bacitracin, co-*

listimethate sodium, colistin, polymyxin B, tetracyclines: Use of pipecuronium with parenteral or intraperitoneal administration of certain antibiotics in high doses has been associated with muscle weakness; weakness may worsen in presence of a nondepolarizing neuromuscular blocker. Observe patient closely.

Magnesium salts: Enhanced and prolonged neuromuscular blockade. Monitor patient for enhanced drug effects.

Quinidine: Prolonged action of nondepolarizing neuromuscular blocking drugs. Monitor patient closely.

Succinylcholine: Pipecuronium may be administered after succinylcholine when the latter is used to facilitate intubation. Don't use pipecuronium before succinylcholine. Use with other nondepolarizing neuromuscular blockers isn't recommended.

Volatile inhalational anesthetics: Intensified or prolonged action of nondepolarizing neuromuscular blocking drugs. Monitor patient for drug effect.

Adverse reactions

CV: hypotension, *bradycardia,* hypertension, myocardial ischemia, *CVA,* thrombosis, atrial fibrillation, *ventricular extrasystole.*
GU: anuria.
Metabolic: increased creatinine levels.
Musculoskeletal: prolonged muscle weakness.
Respiratory: dyspnea, respiratory depression, *respiratory insufficiency or apnea.*
Skin: rash, urticaria.

☑ Special considerations

• Because of its prolonged duration of action, drug is recommended only for procedures that take 90 minutes or longer.
• Adjust dosage to ideal body weight in obese patients.
• Store powder at room temperature or in refrigerator (36° to 86° F [2° to 30° C]).
• Reconstitute with 10 ml solution before use to yield a solution of 1 mg/ml. Large volumes of diluent or addition of drug to a hanging I.V. solution isn't recommended.
• When reconstituted with sterile water for injection or other compatible I.V. solutions, such as normal saline injection, D_5W, lactated Ringer's injection, and dextrose 5% in saline, drug is stable for 24 hours if refrigerated.
• If reconstituted with solution other than bacteriostatic water for injection, discard unused portions of drug.
• When reconstituted with bacteriostatic water for injection, drug is stable for 5 days at room temperature or in refrigerator. Note that bacteriostatic water contains benzyl alcohol and isn't intended for use in neonates.
• Experimental evidence suggests that acid-base balance may influence drug's actions. Alkalosis

may counteract paralysis; acidosis may enhance it. Electrolyte disturbances may also influence response.
• Edrophonium 0.5 mg/kg isn't as effective as neostigmine 0.04 mg/kg in reversing pipecuronium's effects. No information is available on the effects of higher doses of edrophonium and pyridostigmine.
• In case of overdose, antagonists such as neostigmine shouldn't be used until there is some evidence of spontaneous recovery of neuromuscular function. A nerve stimulator is recommended to document antagonism of neuromuscular blockade.

Monitoring the patient
• Monitor patient's vital signs and cardiac rhythm carefully during administration and through recovery period.
• Monitor oxygen saturation; have emergency equipment ready in case of severe respiratory depression.

Information for the patient
• Explain drug's purpose.
• Reassure patient and family that patient will be monitored at all times.

Pediatric patients
• Drug isn't recommended for use in children under age 3 months. Limited evidence suggests that children (ages 1 to 14) under balanced anesthesia or halothane anesthesia may be less sensitive than adults to effects of drug.

Breast-feeding patients
• It's unknown if drug appears in breast milk. Use with caution in breast-feeding women.

piperacillin sodium
Pipracil

Pharmacologic classification: extended-spectrum penicillin, acylaminopenicillin
Therapeutic classification: antibiotic
Pregnancy risk category B

How supplied
Available by prescription only
Injection: 2 g, 3 g, 4 g
Infusion: 2 g, 3 g, 4 g
Bulk vial: 40 g

Indications, route, and dosage
Infections caused by susceptible organisms
Adults and children over age 12: Serious infection: 12 to 18 g/day I.V. in divided doses q 4 to 6 hours. Uncomplicated urinary tract infection (UTI) and community-acquired pneumonia: 6 to 8 g/day I.V. in divided doses q 6 to 12 hours. Complicat-

ed UTI: 8 to 16 g/day I.V. in divided doses q 6 to 8 hours. Uncomplicated gonorrhea: 2 g I.M. as a single dose. Maximum daily dose is 24 g.
◊ *Children 1 month to 12 years:* 50 mg/kg I.V. over 30 minutes q 4 hours.
Prophylaxis of surgical infections
Adults: Intra-abdominal surgery: 2 g I.V. before surgery, 2 g during surgery, and 2 g q 6 hours after surgery for no more than 24 hours. Vaginal hysterectomy: 2 g I.V. before surgery, 2 g 6 hours after first dose then 2 g 12 hours after second dose. Cesarean section: 2 g I.V. after cord is clamped; then 2 g q 4 hours for two doses. Abdominal hysterectomy: 2 g I.V. before surgery, 2 g in postanesthesia care unit, and 2 g after 6 hours.
✦ *Dosage adjustment.* For adults with renal impairment, refer to the table.

Creatinine clearance (ml/min)	Urinary tract infection		Serious systemic infection
	Uncomplicated	Complicated	
20 to 40	*	3 g q 8 hr	4 g q 8 hr
< 20	3 g q 12 hr	3 g q 12 hr	4 g q 12 hr

*No dosage adjustment necessary

Pharmacodynamics
Antibiotic action: Bactericidal. Adheres to bacterial penicillin-binding proteins, thus inhibiting bacterial cell-wall synthesis.
  Extended-spectrum penicillins are more resistant to inactivation by certain beta-lactamases, especially those produced by gram-negative organisms, but are still liable to inactivation by certain others. Because of the potential for rapid development of bacterial resistance, drug shouldn't be used as a sole drug in the treatment of an infection.
  Piperacillin's spectrum of activity includes many gram-negative aerobic and anaerobic bacilli, many gram-positive and gram-negative aerobic cocci, and some gram-positive aerobic and anaerobic bacilli. Piperacillin may be effective against some strains of carbenicillin-resistant and ticarcillin-resistant gram-negative bacilli. Piperacillin is more active against *Pseudomonas aeruginosa* than are other extended-spectrum penicillins.

Pharmacokinetics
• *Absorption:* Plasma levels peak 30 to 50 minutes after I.M. dose.
• *Distribution:* Distributed widely after parenteral administration; penetrates minimally into uninflamed meninges and slightly into bone and

sputum. 16% to 22% protein-bound; crosses placenta.

• *Metabolism:* None significant.

• *Excretion:* 42% to 90% excreted in urine by renal tubular secretion and glomerular filtration; also excreted in bile and breast milk. Elimination half-life in adults is about ½ to 1½ hours; in extensive renal impairment, half-life extended to about 2 to 6 hours; in combined hepatorenal dysfunction, half-life may extend from 11 to 32 hours. Drug is removed by hemodialysis but not by peritoneal dialysis.

Contraindications and precautions
Contraindicated in patients with hypersensitivity to drug or other penicillins. Use cautiously in patients with other drug allergies (especially to cephalosporins), bleeding tendencies, uremia, or hypokalemia.

Interactions
Drug-drug. *Aminoglycoside antibiotics:* Synergistic bactericidal effects against *Pseudomonas aeruginosa, Escherichia coli, Klebsiella, Citrobacter, Enterobacter, Serratia,* and *Proteus mirabilis.* However, drugs are physically and chemically incompatible; inactivated when mixed or given together. Don't give together.

Clavulanic acid, sulbactam, tazobactam: Synergistic bactericidal effects against certain beta-lactamase-producing bacteria. May be used together for this effect.

Methotrexate: Large doses of penicillins may interfere with renal tubular secretion of methotrexate; delayed elimination and elevated serum levels of methotrexate. Monitor patient for toxicity.

Oral contraceptives: Decreased efficacy. Suggest other means of contraception.

Probenecid: Blocked tubular secretion of piperacillin, raising serum levels of drug. Probenecid may be used for this purpose.

Vecuronium: Prolonged neuromuscular blockade. Monitor patient closely.

Adverse reactions
CNS: *seizures,* headache, dizziness, fatigue.
GI: nausea, diarrhea, vomiting, pseudomembranous colitis.
GU: interstitial nephritis.
Hematologic: *bleeding* (with high doses), *neutropenia,* eosinophilia, *leukopenia, thrombocytopenia.*
Hepatic: elevations in liver function studies.
Metabolic: *hypokalemia,* hypernatremia.
Musculoskeletal: prolonged muscle relaxation.
Other: hypersensitivity reactions (edema, fever, chills, rash, pruritus, urticaria, *anaphylaxis*), overgrowth of nonsusceptible organisms, pain at injection site, vein irritation, phlebitis.

☑ Special considerations
Besides the recommendations relevant to all penicillins, consider the following.

• Piperacillin is almost always used with another antibiotic such as an aminoglycoside in life-threatening situations.

• Drug may be more suitable than carbenicillin or ticarcillin for patients on salt-free diets; piperacillin contains only 1.85 mEq of sodium per gram.

• Drug may be administered by direct I.V. injection, given slowly over at least 5 minutes; chest discomfort occurs if injection is given too rapidly.

• Patients with cystic fibrosis are most susceptible to fever or rash from piperacillin.

• Use reduced dosage in patients with creatinine clearance below 40 ml/minute.

• Because drug is dializable, patients undergoing hemodialysis may need dosage adjustments.

• Drug may falsely decrease serum aminoglycoside levels; drug may cause positive Coombs' tests.

• Signs and symptoms of overdose include neuromuscular hypersensitivity and seizures resulting from CNS irritation by high drug levels. A 4- to 6-hour hemodialysis will remove 10% to 50% of drug.

Monitoring the patient
• Monitor serum electrolytes, especially potassium.

• Monitor neurologic status. High serum levels of this drug may cause seizures.

• Monitor CBC, differential, and platelets. Drug may cause thrombocytopenia. Observe patient carefully for signs of occult bleeding.

Information for the patient
• Tell patient to report adverse reactions promptly.

• Advise patient to limit salt intake during therapy because drug contains 1.85 mEq of sodium/g.

Geriatric patients
• Half-life may be prolonged in elderly patients because of impaired renal function.

Pediatric patients
• Safe use in children under age 12 hasn't been established.

Breast-feeding patients
• Drug appears in breast milk; use with caution in breast-feeding women.

piperacillin sodium and tazobactam sodium
Zosyn

Pharmacologic classification: extended-spectrum penicillin/beta-lactamase inhibitor
Therapeutic classification: antibiotic
Pregnancy risk category B

How supplied
Available by prescription only
Powder for injection (equivalent to piperacillin/tazobactam in a ratio of 8 to 1): 2.25 g, 3.375 g, 4.5 g

Indications, route, and dosage
Moderate to severe infections caused by piperacillin-resistant, piperacillin/tazobactam-susceptible, beta-lactamase-producing strains of microorganisms in the following conditions: appendicitis (complicated by rupture or abscess) and peritonitis caused by Es-cherichia coli, Bacteroides fragilis, B. ovatus, B. thetaiotaomicron, B. vulgatus; *skin and skin-structure infections caused by* Staphylococcus aureus; *postpartum endometritis or pelvic inflammatory disease caused by* E. coli; *moderately severe community-acquired pneumonia caused by* Haemophilus influenzae
Adults: 3.375 g (3 g piperacillin/0.375 g tazobactam) q 6 hours as a 30-minute I.V. infusion.
+ Dosage adjustment. For adult or child over 12 years with creatinine clearance 20 to 40 ml/minute, 2.25 g (2 g piperacillin/0.25 g tazobactam) q 6 hours and if less than 20 ml/minute, same dose q 8 hours. In hemodialysis patients, give same dose q 8 hours with a supplemental dose of 0.75 g (0.67 g piperacillin/0.08 g tazobactam) after each dialysis period.
Note: Stop therapy if hypersensitivity reactions or signs and symptoms of bleeding occur.

Pharmacodynamics
Antibiotic action: Piperacillin is an extended-spectrum penicillin that inhibits cell-wall synthesis during microorganism multiplication; tazobactam increases piperacillin effectiveness by inactivating beta-lactamases, which destroy penicillins.

Pharmacokinetics
• *Absorption:* No information available.
• *Distribution:* Both piperacillin and tazobactam are about 30% bound to plasma proteins.
• *Metabolism:* Piperacillin metabolized to minor microbiologically active desethyl metabolite; tazobactam metabolized to single metabolite that lacks pharmacologic and antibacterial activities.
• *Excretion:* Both piperacillin and tazobactam eliminated via kidneys by glomerular filtration and tubular secretion. Piperacillin excreted rapidly as unchanged drug (68% of dose); tazobactam excreted as unchanged drug (80%) in urine. Piperacillin, tazobactam, and desethyl piperacillin also secreted into bile.

Contraindications and precautions
Contraindicated in patients with hypersensitivity to drug or other penicillins. Use cautiously in patients with drug allergies (especially to cephalosporins), bleeding tendencies, uremia, or hypokalemia.

Interactions
Drug-drug. *Aminoglycosides:* Substantial inactivation of aminoglycoside. Don't mix in same I.V. container.
Heparin, oral anticoagulants, other drugs affecting blood coagulation system or thrombocyte function: Prolonged effectiveness. Monitor coagulation parameters more frequently.
Probenecid: Increased blood levels of piperacillin/tazobactam. Probenecid may be used for this purpose.
Vecuronium: Prolonged neuromuscular blockade of vecuronium. Monitor patient closely.

Adverse reactions
CNS: *headache, insomnia,* agitation, dizziness, anxiety.
CV: hypertension, tachycardia, chest pain, edema.
EENT: rhinitis.
GI: *diarrhea, nausea, constipation,* vomiting, dyspepsia, stool changes, abdominal pain.
GU: interstitial nephritis.
Hematologic: *leukopenia,* anemia, eosinophilia, *thrombocytopenia.*
Respiratory: dyspnea.
Skin: rash (including maculopapular, bullous, urticarial, and eczematoid), pruritus.
Other: fever; pain; candidiasis; inflammation, phlebitis at I.V. site; *anaphylaxis.*

☑ Special considerations
• Pseudomembranous colitis has been reported with nearly all antibacterial drugs, including piperacillin/tazobactam, and may range in severity from mild to life-threatening. Therefore, consider this diagnosis in patients with diarrhea after piperacillin/tazobactam administration.
• Bacterial and fungal superinfection may occur and warrants appropriate measures.
• Use piperacillin/tazobactam with an aminoglycoside to treat infections caused by *Pseudomonas aeruginosa.*
• Piperacillin/tazobactam contains 2.35 mEq (54 mg) of sodium per g of piperacillin in combination product. Consider this when treating patients requiring restricted sodium intake.

• As with other semisynthetic penicillins, piperacillin has been associated with increased risk of fever and rash in patients with cystic fibrosis.
• Reconstitute piperacillin/tazobactam with 5 ml of diluent per 1 g of piperacillin. Appropriate diluents include sterile or bacteriostatic water for injection, normal saline injection, bacteriostatic normal saline injection, D_5W, dextrose 5% in normal saline solution injection, or dextran 6% in normal saline injection. Don't use lactated Ringer's injection. Shake until dissolved. Further dilution can be made to a final desired volume.
• Infuse over at least 30 minutes. Stop primary infusion during administration if possible. Don't mix with other drugs.
• Use single-dose vials immediately after reconstitution. Discard unused drug after 24 hours if held at room temperature; 48 hours if refrigerated. Once diluted, drug is stable in I.V. bags for 24 hours at room temperature or 1 week if refrigerated.
• Change I.V. site every 48 hours.
• As with other penicillins, piperacillin/tazobactam may result in false-positive reaction for urine glucose using a copper-reduction method such as Clinitest. Glucose tests based on enzymatic glucose oxidase reactions (such as Diastix or glucose enzymatic test strip) are recommended.

Monitoring the patient
• Obtain specimen for culture and sensitivity tests before giving first dose. Therapy may begin pending results.
• Perform periodic electrolyte determinations in patients with low potassium reserves; hypokalemia can occur when patient with potentially low potassium reserves receives cytotoxic therapy or diuretics.

Information for the patient
• Tell patient to report adverse reactions immediately.

Pediatric patients
• Safety and effectiveness in children under age 12 haven't been established.

Breast-feeding patients
• Low levels of piperacillin appear in breast milk (no information on tazobactam levels). Use piperacillin/tazobactam with caution in breast-feeding women.

pirbuterol acetate
Maxair

Pharmacologic classification: beta-adrenergic agonist
Therapeutic classification: bronchodilator
Pregnancy risk category C

How supplied
Available by prescription only
Inhaler: 0.2 mg per inhalation

Indications, route, and dosage
Prevention and reversal of bronchospasm; asthma
Adults and children ages 12 and over: 1 or 2 inhalations (0.2 to 0.4 mg) repeated q 4 to 6 hours. Not to exceed 12 inhalations daily.

Pharmacodynamics
Bronchodilating action: Stimulates $beta_2$-adrenergic receptors and increases the activity of intracellular adenylate cyclase, an enzyme that catalyzes the conversion of adenosine triphosphate to cyclic adenosine monophosphate (cAMP). Elevated cellular cAMP is associated with bronchodilation and inhibition of the cellular release of mediators of immediate hypersensitivity.

Pharmacokinetics
• *Absorption:* Serum levels achieved after inhalation of usual dose.
• *Distribution:* Drug acts locally.
• *Metabolism:* Metabolized in liver.
• *Excretion:* About 50% of inhaled dose recovered in urine as parent drug and metabolites.

Contraindications and precautions
Contraindicated in patients with hypersensitivity to drug. Use cautiously in patients with CV disorders, hyperthyroidism, diabetes, or seizure disorders and in those who are sensitive to sympathomimetic amines.

Interactions
Drug-drug. *MAO inhibitors, tricyclic antidepressants:* Enhanced vascular effects of beta-adrenergic agonists. Use together cautiously.
Propranolol, other beta blockers: Decreased bronchodilating effects of beta agonists. Avoid using together.

Adverse reactions
CNS: tremor, nervousness, dizziness, insomnia, headache, vertigo.
CV: tachycardia, palpitations, chest tightness.
EENT: dry or irritated throat, dry mouth, cough.
GI: nausea, vomiting, diarrhea.

☑ Special considerations
Besides the recommendations relevant to all adrenergics, consider the following.
• Don't administer to patients who are receiving other beta-adrenergic bronchodilators.
• Anginal pain, hypertension, and tachycardia may result from overdose. Sedatives or barbiturates may be necessary to counteract any adverse CNS effects; cautious use of beta blockers may be useful to counteract cardiac effects.

Monitoring the patient
• Monitor patients for worsening symptoms of asthma.
• Watch for increased inhaler use.

Information for the patient
• Warn patient not to exceed recommended maximum dose of 12 inhalations daily. He should call if a previously effective dosage doesn't control symptoms because this may signify a worsening of disease.
• Tell patient to call promptly if he experiences increased bronchospasm after using drug.
• Teach patient how to use metered dose inhaler correctly. Have him shake container, exhale through the nose, administer aerosol while inhaling deeply on mouthpiece of inhaler, hold breath for a few seconds, then exhale slowly. Tell him to allow at least 2 minutes between inhalations, and to wait at least 5 minutes before using his corticosteroid inhalant (if he's also taking inhalational corticosteroids).

Pediatric patients
• Use in children under age 12 isn't recommended.

Breast-feeding patients
• It's unknown if drug appears in breast milk. Use with caution in breast-feeding women.

---

piroxicam
Apo-Piroxicam*, Feldene, Novo-Pirocam*

Pharmacologic classification: NSAID
Therapeutic classification: nonnarcotic analgesic, antipyretic, anti-inflammatory
Pregnancy risk category B (D in third trimester or near delivery)

How supplied
Available by prescription only
Capsules: 10 mg, 20 mg

Indications, route, and dosage
Osteoarthritis, rheumatoid arthritis
Adults: 20 mg P.O. once daily. If desired, the dose may be divided.

◊ *Juvenile rheumatoid arthritis*
Children weighing 15 to 30 kg (33 to 67 lb): 5 mg P.O.
Children weighing 31 to 45 kg (68 to 100 lb): 10 mg P.O.
Children weighing 46 to 55 kg (101 to 121 lb): 15 mg P.O.

Pharmacodynamics
Analgesic, antipyretic, and anti-inflammatory actions: Exact mechanisms unknown. Thought to inhibit prostaglandin synthesis.

Pharmacokinetics
• *Absorption:* Absorbed rapidly from GI tract. Peak effect seen 3 to 5 hours after dosing. Food delays absorption.
• *Distribution:* Highly protein-bound.
• *Metabolism:* Metabolized in liver.
• *Excretion:* Excreted in urine. Long half-life (about 50 hours) allows for once-daily dosing.

Contraindications and precautions
Contraindicated in patients with hypersensitivity to drug, in those with bronchospasm or angioedema precipitated by aspirin or NSAIDs, during pregnancy, or while breast-feeding.
    Use cautiously in elderly patients and in patients with GI disorders, hypertension, conditions predisposing to fluid retention, or history of renal, peptic ulcer, or cardiac disease.

Interactions
Drug-drug. *Acetaminophen, gold compounds, other anti-inflammatories:* Increased nephrotoxicity. Monitor patient for toxicity.
Anticoagulants, thrombolytics (coumarin derivatives, heparin, other highly protein-bound drugs): May potentiate anticoagulant effects. Monitor PTT, PT, and INR.
Antihypertensives, diuretics: Decreased effectiveness of these drugs; using piroxicam with diuretics may increase risk of nephrotoxicity. Monitor patient.
Anti-inflammatories, corticotropin, salicylates, corticosteroids: GI adverse effects, including ulceration and hemorrhage. Use together cautiously.
Aspirin: Decreased bioavailability of piroxicam. Don't administer together.
Coumarin derivatives, nifedipine, phenytoin, verapamil: Piroxicam may displace highly protein-bound drugs. Monitor patient for toxicity.
Drugs that inhibit platelet aggregation (such as aspirin, cefamandole, cefoperazone, dextran, dipyridamole, mezlocillin, piperacillin, plicamycin, salicylates, sulfinpyrazone, ticarcillin, valproic acid, other anti-inflammatories): Possible bleeding problems. Monitor patient.
Insulin, oral antidiabetics: Potentiated hypoglycemic effects. Monitor serum glucose level.
Lithium, methotrexate: Decreased renal clearance of these drugs. Monitor plasma levels.

Reactions may be *common*, uncommon, **life-threatening**, or COMMON AND LIFE-THREATENING.

Drug-lifestyle. *Alcohol:* Increased GI adverse effects, including ulceration and hemorrhage. Avoid alcohol use.
Sun exposure: Photosensitivity reaction. Tell patient to take precautions.

Adverse reactions
CNS: headache, drowsiness, dizziness, somnolence, vertigo.
CV: peripheral edema.
EENT: auditory disturbances.
GI: *epigastric distress, nausea, occult blood loss,* **peptic ulceration, severe GI bleeding,** diarrhea, constipation, abdominal pain, dyspepsia, flatulence, anorexia, stomatitis.
GU: *nephrotoxicity,* elevated BUN level.
Hematologic: prolonged bleeding time, anemia, *leukopenia, aplastic anemia, agranulocytosis,* eosinophilia, **thrombocytopenia.**
Hepatic: elevated liver enzyme levels.
Skin: pruritus, rash, urticaria, *photosensitivity.*

☑ Special considerations
Besides the recommendations relevant to all NSAIDs, consider the following.
• Drug is usually administered as a single dose.
• Adverse skin reactions are more common with piroxicam than with other NSAIDs; photosensitivity reactions are the most common.
• Drug hasn't been proven safe for fetus.

Monitoring the patient
• Effectiveness isn't usually seen for at least 2 weeks after therapy begins. Evaluate response to drug as evidenced by reduced symptoms.
• Monitor renal and hepatic function and CBC periodically during therapy.

Information for the patient
• Advise patient to call before taking OTC products.
• Caution patient to avoid hazardous activities requiring alertness until CNS effects are known. Instruct patient in safety measures to prevent injury.
• Instruct patient in signs and symptoms of adverse effects. Tell patient to report them immediately.
• Encourage patient to comply with recommended medical follow-up.
• Tell patient to avoid aspirin and alcohol during therapy.

Geriatric patients
• Patients over age 60 are more sensitive to drug's adverse effects. Use with caution.
• Because of its effect on renal prostaglandins, drug may cause fluid retention and edema. This may be significant in elderly patients and in those with heart failure.

Pediatric patients
• Safe use of long-term piroxicam in children hasn't been established.

Breast-feeding patients
• Drug may inhibit lactation. Drug appears in breast milk at 1% of maternal serum levels; avoid use in breast-feeding women.

plasma protein fraction
Plasmanate, Plasma-Plex, Plasmatein, Protenate

Pharmacologic classification: blood derivative
Therapeutic classification: plasma volume expander
Pregnancy risk category C

How supplied
Available by prescription only
Injection: 5% solution in 50-ml, 250-ml, 500-ml vials

Indications, route, and dosage
Shock
Adults: Varies with patient's condition and response, but usually 250 to 500 ml (12.5 to 25 g protein) I.V., not to exceed 10 ml/minute.
Children: 22 to 33 ml/kg I.V. infused at rate of 5 to 10 ml/minute.
Small children and infants: 15 ml/2.2 kg (1 lb) I.V. infused at rate of 5 to 10 ml/minute (Plasma-Plex).
Hypoproteinemia
Adults: 1,000 to 1,500 ml I.V. daily. Maximum infusion rate is 8 ml/minute (500 ml infused in 30 to 45 minutes).

Pharmacodynamics
Plasma-expanding action: Supplies colloid to the blood and expands plasma volume. Causes fluid to shift from interstitial spaces into the circulation and slightly increases the plasma protein level. Comprised mostly of albumin, but may contain up to 17% alpha and beta globulins and not more than 1% gamma globulin.

Pharmacokinetics
The pharmacokinetics of plasma protein fraction (PPF) are similar to its chief constituent, albumin (about 83% to 90%).
• *Absorption:* Albumin isn't adequately absorbed from GI tract.
• *Distribution:* Albumin accounts for about 50% of plasma proteins. Distributed into intravascular space and extravascular sites, including skin, muscle, and lungs. In patients with reduced circulating blood volumes, hemodilution secondary to albumin administration lasts for many hours; in patients with normal blood volume, excess flu-

id and protein are lost from intravascular space within a few hours.
• *Metabolism:* Albumin synthesized in liver, but liver isn't involved in clearance of albumin from plasma in healthy individuals.
• *Excretion:* Little is known about albumin excretion in healthy individuals. Administration of albumin decreases hepatic albumin synthesis and increases albumin clearance if plasma oncotic pressure is high. In certain pathologic states, liver, kidneys, or intestines may provide elimination mechanisms.

Contraindications and precautions
Contraindicated in patients with severe anemia or heart failure and in those undergoing cardiac bypass. Use cautiously in patients with impaired renal or hepatic function, low cardiac reserve, or restricted salt intake.

Interactions
None reported.

Adverse reactions
CNS: headache.
CV: hypotension (after rapid infusion or intra-arterial administration), ***vascular overload*** (after rapid infusion), tachycardia.
GI: nausea, vomiting, hypersalivation.
Metabolic: increased plasma protein levels.
Musculoskeletal: back pain.
Respiratory: dyspnea, ***pulmonary edema.***
Skin: rash.
Other: flushing, chills, fever.

☑ Special considerations
• Don't use solution if cloudy, contains sediment, or has been frozen. Store at room temperature; freezing may break bottle and allow bacterial contamination.
• Use opened solution promptly, discarding unused portion after 4 hours; solution contains no preservatives and becomes unstable.
• One unit is usually considered to be 250 ml of the 5% concentration.
• Avoid rapid I.V. infusion. Rate is individualized according to patient's age, condition, and diagnosis. Maximum dose is 250 g/48 hours; don't give faster than 10 ml/minute. Decrease infusion rate to 5 to 8 ml/minute as plasma volume approaches normal.
• PPF is also used in treatment of burns; dosage depends on extent and severity of burn.
• No cross-matching is needed. PPF shouldn't be administered with same administration set of solutions containing protein hydrolysates, amino acid solutions, or alcohol.
• If patient is dehydrated, give additional fluids either P.O. or I.V.
• Each liter contains 130 to 160 mEq of sodium before dilution with any additional I.V. fluids; a 250-ml container of the 5% concentration contains about 33 to 40 mEq sodium.

Monitoring the patient
• Monitor blood pressure frequently; slow or stop infusion if hypotension suddenly occurs. Vital signs should return to normal gradually.
• Observe patient for signs of vascular overload (heart failure, pulmonary edema, widening pulse pressure indicating increased cardiac output) and signs of hemorrhage or shock (after surgery or trauma); be alert for bleeding sites not evident at lower blood pressure.
• Monitor intake and output (watch especially for decreased output), hemoglobin and serum protein and electrolyte levels, and hematocrit to help determine ongoing dosage.

Information for the patient
• Explain use and administration of drug to patient and family.
• Tell patient to report adverse reactions immediately.

plicamycin
Mithracin

Pharmacologic classification: antibiotic antineoplastic (cell cycle–phase nonspecific)
Therapeutic classification: antineoplastic, hypocalcemic
Pregnancy risk category X

How supplied
Available by prescription only
Injection: 2,500-mcg vials

Indications, route, and dosage
Dosage and indications may vary. Check current literature for recommended protocol.
Hypercalcemia
Adults: 25 mcg/kg I.V. daily over 4 to 6 hours for 3 to 4 days. Repeat at intervals of 1 week, p.r.n.
Testicular cancer
Adults: 25 to 30 mcg/kg I.V. daily over 4 to 6 hours for up to 10 days (based on ideal body weight or actual weight, whichever is less).
◇ **Paget's disease**
Adults: 15 mcg/kg I.V. daily over 4 to 6 hours for up to 10 days.

Pharmacodynamics
Antineoplastic action: Exerts cytotoxic activity by intercalating between DNA base pairs and also binding to the outside of the DNA molecule. The result is inhibition of DNA-dependent RNA synthesis.
Hypocalcemic action: Exact mechanism unknown. May block the hypercalcemic effect of vitamin D or may inhibit the effect of parathyroid hormone

upon osteoclasts, preventing osteolysis. Both mechanisms reduce serum calcium levels.

Pharmacokinetics
- *Absorption:* Not administered orally.
- *Distribution:* Distributed mainly into Kupffer's cells of liver, into renal tubular cells, and along formed bone surfaces. Crosses blood-brain barrier; achieves appreciable levels in CSF.
- *Metabolism:* Poorly understood.
- *Excretion:* Eliminated primarily through kidneys.

Contraindications and precautions
Contraindicated in patients with thrombocytopenia, bone marrow suppression, or coagulation and bleeding disorders and in women who are or who may become pregnant. Use cautiously in patients with impaired renal or hepatic function.

Interactions
None reported.

Adverse reactions
CNS: drowsiness, weakness, lethargy, headache, malaise.
GI: *nausea, vomiting,* anorexia, diarrhea, stomatitis.
GU: increased BUN and serum creatinine levels.
Hematologic: *leukopenia, thrombocytopenia, bleeding syndrome* (from epistaxis to generalized hemorrhage).
Hepatic: *elevated liver enzyme levels, hepatotoxicity.*
Metabolic: *decreased serum calcium,* potassium, and phosphorus levels.
Skin: facial flushing, rash.
Other: *death,* fever, cellulitis with extravasation, phlebitis.

☑ Special considerations
- To reconstitute drug, use 4.9 ml of sterile water to give a concentration of 500 mcg/ml. Reconstitute drug immediately before administration, and discard unused solution.
- Drug may be further diluted with normal saline solution or D_5W to a volume of 1,000 ml and administered as an I.V. infusion over 4 to 6 hours.
- To reduce nausea, give antiemetics before administering drug.
- Although drug may be administered by I.V. push injection, this method is discouraged because of the higher risk and greater severity of GI toxicity. Nausea and vomiting are greatly diminished as infusion rate is decreased.
- Infusions of plicamycin in 1,000 ml D_5W are stable for up to 24 hours.
- If I.V. infiltrates, infusion should be stopped immediately and ice packs applied before restarting an I.V. in other arm.

- Therapeutic effect in hypercalcemia may not be seen for 24 to 48 hours; may last 3 to 15 days.
- Avoid drug contact with skin or mucous membranes.
- Store lyophilized powder in refrigerator.
- Toxicity may cause myelosuppression, electrolyte imbalance, and coagulation disorders. Treatment includes transfusion of blood components. Patient's renal and hepatic status should be closely monitored.

Monitoring the patient
- Monitor LD, AST, ALT, alkaline phosphatase, BUN, creatinine, potassium, calcium, and phosphorus levels.
- Monitor platelet count and PT before and during therapy.
- Check serum calcium levels. Monitor patient for tetany, carpopedal spasm, Chvostek's sign, and muscle cramps because a sharp drop in calcium levels is possible.
- Watch for signs of bleeding. Facial flushing may be an early indicator.

Information for the patient
- Tell patient to use salicylate-free drugs for pain relief or fever reduction.
- Instruct patient to avoid exposure to people with infections and to call immediately if signs of infection or unusual bleeding occur.
- Inform patient that he and household members shouldn't receive immunizations during therapy and for several weeks after therapy.
- Advise patient to use contraceptive measures during therapy.

Breast-feeding patients
- It's unknown if drug appears in breast milk. Because of potential for serious adverse reactions, mutagenicity, and carcinogenicity in infant, breast-feeding isn't recommended.

pneumococcal vaccine, polyvalent
Pneumovax 23, Pnu-Imune 23

Pharmacologic classification: vaccine
Therapeutic classification: bacterial vaccine
Pregnancy risk category C

How supplied
Available by prescription only
Injection: 25 mcg each of 23 polysaccharide isolates of *Streptococcus pneumoniae* per 0.5-ml dose, in 1-ml and 5-ml vials and disposable syringes.

Indications, route, and dosage
Pneumococcal immunization
Adults and children over age 2: 0.5 ml I.M. or S.C. as a one-time dose.

Pharmacodynamics
Pneumonia prophylaxis: Promotes active immunity against the 23 most prevalent pneumococcal types.

Pharmacokinetics
• *Absorption:* Protective antibodies produced within 3 weeks after injection. Duration of vaccine-induced immunity at least 5 years in adults.
• *Distribution:* No information available.
• *Metabolism:* No information available.
• *Excretion:* No information available.

Contraindications and precautions
Contraindicated in patients with hypersensitivity to drug or its components (phenol). Also contraindicated in patients with Hodgkin's disease who have received extensive chemotherapy or nodal irradiation.

Interactions
Drug-drug. *Corticosteroids, other immunosuppressants:* Impaired immune response to vaccine; vaccination should be avoided.

Adverse reactions
CNS: headache.
GI: nausea, vomiting.
Musculoskeletal: myalgia, arthralgia.
Skin: rash.
Other: adenitis, *anaphylaxis,* serum sickness, *slight fever, soreness at injection site,* severe local reaction associated with revaccination within 3 years.

☑ Special considerations
• Obtain thorough history of allergies and reactions to immunizations.
• Persons with asplenia who received the 14-valent vaccine should be revaccinated with the 23-valent vaccine.
• Have epinephrine solution 1:1,000 available to treat allergic reactions.
• Use deltoid or midlateral thigh. Don't inject I.V. Avoid intradermal administration because this may cause severe local reactions.
• Polyvalent pneumococcal vaccine also may be administered to children to prevent pneumococcal otitis media.
• Candidates for pneumococcal vaccine include persons ages 65 and older; adults and children ages 2 and older with chronic illness, asplenia, or splenic dysfunction; and those with sickle-cell anemia and HIV infection.
• Vaccine also is recommended for patients awaiting organ transplants, those receiving radiation

therapy or cancer chemotherapy, persons in nursing homes and orphanages, and bedridden individuals.
• If different sites and separate syringes are used, pneumococcal vaccine may be administered simultaneously with influenza, DTP, poliovirus, or *Haemophilus* b polysaccharide vaccines.
• Store vaccine at 36° to 46° F (2° to 8° C). Reconstitution or dilution is unnecessary.

Monitoring the patient
• Monitor patient for adverse effects.

Information for the patient
• Tell patient to expect redness, soreness, swelling, and pain at injection site after vaccination. Patient may also develop fever, joint or muscle aches and pains, rash, itching, general weakness, or difficulty breathing.
• Encourage patient to report distressing adverse reactions promptly.
• Advise patient to use acetaminophen to relieve adverse reactions promptly.

Pediatric patients
• Children under age 2 don't respond satisfactorily to pneumococcal vaccine. Safety and efficacy of vaccine haven't been established.

Breast-feeding patients
• It's unknown if vaccine appears in breast milk. Use with caution in breast-feeding women.

---

poliovirus vaccine, inactivated (IPV)
IPOL

poliovirus vaccine, live, oral, trivalent (Sabin vaccine, TOPV)
Orimune

Pharmacologic classification: vaccine
Therapeutic classification: viral vaccine
Pregnancy risk category C

How supplied
Available by prescription only
poliovirus vaccine, inactivated (IPV)
Injectable suspension: 40 D antigen units of type 1 (Mahoney), 8 D antigen units of type 2 (MEF-1), and 32 D antigen units of type 3 (Saukett) per 0.5 ml
poliovirus vaccine, live, oral, trivalent
Oral vaccine: mixture of three viruses (types 1, 2, and 3), grown in monkey kidney tissue culture, in 0.5-ml single-dose Dispettes

---

Indications, route, and dosage

Poliovirus immunization (IPV)

Infants and children (primary series): 0.5 ml S.C. or I.M. at 2 months, 4 months, 6 to 18 months, and at 4 to 6 years. Minimum interval between doses is 4 weeks. Or use sequential IPV/oral poliovirus vaccine (OPV) regimen: IPV given at 2 and 4 months of age, then OPV at 12 to 18 months and 4 to 6 years.

Adults: Three doses: Two doses 0.5 ml S.C. or I.M., 4 to 8 weeks apart, and third dose given 6 to 12 months after second dose.

Poliovirus immunization (primary series)

Infants and children ages 6 weeks and older: 0.5 ml P.O. at ages 2 months, 4 months, and 6 to 18 months. All children entering elementary school (ages 4 to 6) who have completed the primary series should receive a single follow-up dose of TOPV. Booster vaccination beyond elementary school isn't routinely recommended.

Adults ages 18 and over: TOPV shouldn't be given to persons ages 18 and over who haven't received at least one prior dose of TOPV. Inactivated polio vaccine (IPV) should be used if polio vaccination is indicated.

If less than 4 weeks are available before protection is needed, a single dose of TOPV or IPV may be given.

Persons traveling to countries with endemic or epidemic polio who previously completed a primary series should receive a single follow-up dose of TOPV.

Pharmacodynamics

Polio prophylaxis: TOPV and IPV promote immunity to poliomyelitis by inducing humoral and secretory antibodies and antibodies in the lymphatic tissue of the GI tract.

Pharmacokinetics

- *Absorption:* Antibody response to vaccine occurs within 7 to 10 days after ingestion; peaks around 21 days. Duration of immunity thought to be lifelong.
- *Distribution:* No information available.
- *Metabolism:* No information available.
- *Excretion:* No information available.

Contraindications and precautions

Oral vaccine is contraindicated in immunosuppressed patients, in those with cancer or immunoglobulin abnormalities, and in those receiving radiation, antimetabolite, alkylating drug, or corticosteroid therapy. These patients should receive IPV. Injectable vaccine is contraindicated in patients hypersensitive to neomycin, streptomycin, or polymyxin B.

Use cautiously in siblings of children with known immunodeficiency syndrome.

Interactions

Drug-drug. *Corticosteroids, other immunosuppressants:* Impaired immune response to vaccine. Defer vaccination with TOPV until immunosuppressant is stopped; or inactivated poliovirus vaccine may be used.

Immune serum globulin, transfusions of blood or blood products: Interference with immune response to vaccine. Defer vaccination for 3 months in these situations.

Adverse reactions

CNS: sleepiness.
GI: decreased appetite.
Skin: erythema.
Other: crying, *fever,* **hypersensitivity reactions, poliomyelitis,** induration, *pain at injection site.*

☑ Special considerations

- IPV regimen is currently recommended for routine primary immunization in healthy infants.
- OPV is no longer recommended for routine immunization but is recommended for outbreak control.
- Obtain thorough history of allergies, especially to antibiotics, and of reactions to immunizations.
- Vaccine isn't effective in modifying or preventing existing or incubating poliomyelitis.
- Adults and immunocompromised persons who haven't been vaccinated should receive IPV (Salk) in three doses, given 1 month apart, before other household contacts are immunized with TOPV.
- TOPV isn't for parenteral use. Dose may be administered directly or mixed with distilled water, chlorine-free tap water, simple syrup USP, or milk. It also may be placed on bread, cake, or a sugar cube.
- Keep TOPV frozen until used. It may be refrigerated up to 30 days once thawed, if unopened. Opened vials may be refrigerated up to 7 days. IPV should be refrigerated; don't freeze.
- Color change from pink to yellow has no effect on efficacy of TOPV as long as vaccine remains clear. Yellow color results from storage at low temperatures.
- Vaccine may temporarily decrease response to tuberculin skin testing. If a tuberculin test is necessary, administer either before, simultaneously with, or at least 8 weeks after TOPV.

Monitoring the patient

- Check parents' immunization history when they bring in child for vaccine; this is an excellent time for parents to receive booster immunizations.
- Monitor patient for adverse effects.

Information for the patient

- Inform patient that risk of vaccine-associated paralysis is extremely small for vaccines, susceptible family members, and other close con-

tacts (about 1 case per 2.6 million patients receiving the vaccines).
● Encourage patient to report distressing adverse reactions promptly.

Pediatric patients
● Poliovirus vaccine shouldn't be administered to neonates under age 6 weeks.

Breast-feeding patients
● It's unknown if drug appears in breast milk. Breast-feeding doesn't interfere with successful immunization; no interruption in feeding schedule is necessary.

polyethylene glycol-electrolyte solution (PEG-ES)
Colovage, CoLyte, GoLYTELY, NuLytely, OCL

Pharmacologic classification: polyethylene glycol 3350 nonabsorbable solution
Therapeutic classification: laxative and bowel evacuant
Pregnancy risk category C

How supplied
Available by prescription only
Powder for oral solution: polyethylene glycol (PEG) 3350 (6 g), anhydrous sodium sulfate (568 mg), sodium chloride (146 mg), potassium chloride (74.5 mg/100 ml) (Colovage); PEG 3350 (120 g), sodium sulfate (3.36 g), sodium chloride (2.92 g), potassium chloride (1.49 g/2 L) (CoLyte); PEG 3350 (236 g), sodium sulfate (22.74 g), sodium bicarbonate (6.74 g), sodium chloride (5.86 g), potassium chloride (2.97 g/4.8 L) (GoLYTELY); PEG 3350 (420 g), sodium bicarbonate (5.72 g), sodium chloride (11.2 g), potassium chloride (1.48 g/4 L) (NuLytely); PEG 3350 (6 g), sodium sulfate decahydrate (1.29 g), sodium chloride (146 mg), potassium chloride (75 mg), polysorbate-80 (30 mg/100 ml) (OCL)

Indications, route, and dosage
Bowel preparation before GI examination
Adults: 240 ml P.O. q 10 minutes until 4 L are consumed or rectal effluent is clear. Typically, administer 4 hours before examination, allowing 3 hours for drinking and 1 hour for bowel evacuation.
Note: If a patient experiences severe bloating, distention, or abdominal pain, slow or temporarily stop administration until symptoms abate.

Pharmacodynamics
Laxative and bowel evacuant action: Acts as an osmotic product. With sodium sulfate as the major sodium source, active sodium absorption is

markedly reduced. Diarrhea results, which rapidly cleans the bowel, usually within 4 hours.

Pharmacokinetics
● *Absorption:* Nonabsorbable solution. Onset of action within 30 to 60 minutes.
● *Distribution:* Not applicable; not absorbed.
● *Metabolism:* Not applicable; not absorbed.
● *Excretion:* Excreted via GI tract.

Contraindications and precautions
Contraindicated in patients with GI obstruction or perforation, gastric retention, toxic colitis, ileus, or megacolon.

Interactions
Drug-drug. *Oral drugs:* Drug given within 1 hour before start of therapy may be flushed from GI tract and not absorbed. Avoid oral drug within this time frame.

Adverse reactions
EENT: rhinorrhea.
GI: *nausea, bloating, cramps, vomiting, abdominal fullness,* anal irritation.
Skin: urticaria, dermatitis.
Other: *anaphylaxis.*

☑ Special considerations
● Drug may be given via nasogastric tube (at 20 to 30 ml/minute, or 1.2 to 1.8 L/hour) to patients unwilling or unable to drink preparation. First bowel movement should occur within 1 hour.
● Tap water may be used to reconstitute solution. Shake container vigorously several times to ensure powder is completely dissolved. After reconstitution to 4 L with water, the solution contains PEG 3350 17.6 mmol/L, sodium 125 mmol/L, sulfate 40 mmol/L (CoLyte 80 mmol/L), chloride 35 mmol/L, bicarbonate 20 mmol/L, and potassium 10 mmol/L (1 mmol/L = 1 mEq/L).
● Store reconstituted solution in refrigerator (chilling before administration improves palatability); use within 48 hours.
● Don't add flavorings or additional ingredients to solution before use.
● No major shifts in fluid or electrolyte balance have been reported.
● Patient preparation for barium enema may be less satisfactory with this solution because it may interfere with barium coating of colonic mucosa using the double-contrast technique.

Monitoring the patient
● Monitor patient for adverse GI reactions.

Information for the patient
● Instruct patient to fast about 3 to 4 hours before ingesting solution.
● Tell patient not to take solid foods less than 2 hours before solution is administered. Also inform him that no foods except clear liquids are

---

Reactions may be *common*, uncommon, *life-threatening*, or COMMON AND LIFE-THREATENING.

permitted after administration of solution until examination is completed.

---

polysaccharide-iron complex
Hytinic, Niferex, Niferex-150, Nu-Iron, Nu-Iron 150

Pharmacologic classification: oral iron supplement
Therapeutic classification: hematinic
Pregnancy risk category NR

How supplied
Available without a prescription
Tablets (film-coated): 50 mg
Capsules: 150 mg
Solution: 100 mg/5 ml

Indications, route, and dosage
Uncomplicated iron-deficiency anemia
Adults and children ages 12 and older: 150 to 300 mg P.O. daily as capsules or tablets or 1 to 2 teaspoonfuls of elixir P.O. daily.
Children ages 6 to 12: 150 mg to 300 mg P.O. daily as tablets or 1 teaspoonful of elixir P.O. daily.
Children ages 2 to 6: ½ teaspoonful of elixir P.O. daily.

Pharmacodynamics
Hematinic action: Provides elemental iron, an essential component in the formation of hemoglobin.

Pharmacokinetics
• *Absorption:* Although iron is absorbed from entire length of GI tract, duodenum and proximal jejunum are primary absorption sites. Up to 10% of iron absorbed by healthy individuals; patients with iron-deficiency anemia may absorb up to 60%. Enteric coating and some extended-release formulas have decreased absorption; designed to release iron past points in GI tract of highest absorption. Food may decrease absorption by 33% to 50%.
• *Distribution:* Iron is transported through GI mucosal cells directly into blood; immediately bound to a carrier protein, transferrin, and transported to bone marrow for incorporation into hemoglobin. Iron is highly protein-bound.
• *Metabolism:* Iron is liberated by hemoglobin destruction but is conserved and reused by body.
• *Excretion:* Healthy individuals lose only small amounts of iron each day. Men and postmenopausal women lose about 1 mg/day; premenopausal women about 1.5 mg/day. Loss usually occurs in nails, hair, feces, and urine; trace amounts lost in bile and sweat.

Contraindications and precautions
Contraindicated in patients with hypersensitivity to drug or its components and in those with hemochromatosis and hemosiderosis.

Interactions
Drug-drug. *Antacids, cholestyramine resin, cimetidine, tetracycline, vitamin E:* Decreased iron absorption. Separate administration times by 2 to 4 hours.
Chloramphenicol: Delayed response to iron therapy. Monitor patient closely.
Fluoroquinolones, levodopa, methyldopa, penicillamine: Decreased absorption of these drugs, possibly resulting in decreased serum levels or efficacy. Monitor patient.
Vitamin C: Increased iron absorption. Give together.
Drug-food. *Coffee, dairy products, eggs, tea, whole-grain breads and cereals:* Decreased iron absorption. Separate use by 2 to 4 hours.
Foods high in vitamin C: Increased iron absorption. Give with these foods.

Adverse reactions
GI: nausea, constipation, black stools, epigastric pain. (Associated with iron therapy; however, few, if any, occur with polysaccharide-iron complex. Iron-containing liquids may cause temporary staining of teeth.)

☑ Special considerations
• Administer iron with juice (preferably orange juice) or water, but not with milk or antacids.
• Polysaccharide-iron complex is nontoxic and there are relatively few, if any, GI adverse effects associated with other iron preparations.
• Oral iron may turn stools black. This unabsorbed iron is harmless; however, it could mask melena.
• Polysaccharide-iron complex may blacken feces and may interfere with test for occult blood in stool; guaiac and orthotoluidine tests may yield false-positive results. Benzidine test usually isn't affected. Iron overload may decrease uptake of technetium 99m and interfere with skeletal imaging.
• The lethal dose of iron is between 200 and 250 mg/kg. Symptoms may follow ingestion of 20 to 60 mg/kg. Signs and symptoms of acute overdose may occur as follows. Between ½ and 8 hours after ingestion, patient may experience lethargy, nausea and vomiting, green then tarry stools, weak and rapid pulse, hypotension, dehydration, acidosis, and coma. If death isn't immediate, symptoms may clear for about 24 hours. At 12 to 48 hours, symptoms may return, accompanied by diffuse vascular congestion, pulmonary edema, shock, seizures, anuria, hyperthermia, then possibly death.
• Follow emesis with lavage, using 1% sodium bicarbonate solution to convert iron to less irritating, poorly absorbed form. (Phosphate solu-

tions have been used, but carry risk of other adverse effects.) Perform radiographic evaluation of abdomen to determine continued presence of excess iron; if serum iron levels exceed 350 mg/dl, deferoxamine may be used for systemic chelation. Survivors are likely to sustain organ damage, including pyloric or antral stenosis, hepatic cirrhosis, CNS damage, and intestinal obstruction.

Monitoring the patient

• Monitor hemoglobin level and hematocrit and reticulocyte counts during therapy.

Information for the patient

• Inform parents that as few as three or four tablets can cause serious iron poisoning in children.
• If patient misses a dose, tell him to take it as soon as he remembers but not to double dose.
• Advise patient to avoid certain foods that may impair oral iron absorption, including yogurt, cheese, eggs, milk, whole-grain breads and cereals, tea, and coffee.
• Teach patient dietary measures to follow for preventing constipation.

Geriatric patients

• Because iron-induced constipation is common in elderly patients, stress proper diet to minimize this adverse effect. Elderly patients may need higher doses of iron because reduced gastric secretions and achlorhydria may lower capacity for iron absorption.

Pediatric patients

• Iron overdose may be fatal in children; treat patient immediately.

Breast-feeding patients

• Iron supplements are often recommended for breast-feeding women; no adverse effects documented.

---

potassium iodide (KI, SSKI)
Pima, Thyro-Block

Pharmacologic classification: electrolyte
Therapeutic classification: antihyperthyroid drug, expectorant
Pregnancy risk category D

How supplied
Available by prescription only
Tablets: 130 mg
Syrup: 325 mg/5 ml
Saturated solution (SSKI): 1 g/ml
Strong iodine solution (Lugol's solution): iodine 50 mg/ml and potassium iodide 100 mg/ml

Indications, route, and dosage
Expectorant
Adults: 300 to 600 mg t.i.d. or q.i.d.
Children: 60 to 250 mg q.i.d.
Preoperative thyroidectomy
Adults and children: 50 to 250 mg (or 1 to 5 drops) SSKI t.i.d.; or 0.1 to 0.3 ml (or 3 to 5 drops) Lugol's solution t.i.d.; give drug for 10 to 14 days before surgery.
Nuclear radiation protection
Adults and children: 0.13 ml P.O. of SSKI (130 mg) immediately before or after initial exposure will block 90% of radioactive iodine. Same dosage given 3 to 4 hours after exposure will provide 50% block. Drug should be administered for up to 10 days under medical supervision.
Infants under age 1: Half the adult dosage.
◇ *To replenish iodine*
Adults: 5 to 10 mg/day.
Children: 1 mg/day.
Management of thyrotoxic crisis
Adults: 500 mg P.O. q 4 hours (about 10 drops of a potassium iodide solution containing 1 g/ml). Or 1 ml of strong iodine solution P.O. t.i.d.
◇ *Graves' disease in neonates*
Neonates: 1 drop P.O. of strong iodine solution q 8 hours.
◇ *Cutaneous sporotrichosis*
Adults: 65 to 325 mg P.O. t.i.d.

Pharmacodynamics
Expectorant action: Exact mechanism unknown. Thought to reduce viscosity of mucus by increasing respiratory tract secretions.
Antihyperthyroid action: Acts directly on the thyroid gland to inhibit synthesis and release of thyroid hormone.

Pharmacokinetics
• *Absorption:* Absorption similar to iodinated amino acids.
• *Distribution:* Distributed extracellularly.
• *Metabolism:* No information available.
• *Excretion:* Excreted by kidneys.

Contraindications and precautions
Contraindicated in patients with tuberculosis, acute bronchitis, iodide hypersensitivity, or hyperkalemia. Some formulations contain sulfites, which may precipitate allergic reactions in hypersensitive individuals.
    Use cautiously in patients with hypocomplementemic vasculitis, goiter, or autoimmune thyroid disease.

Interactions
Drug-drug. *Drugs containing potassium, potassium-sparing diuretics:* Possible hyperkalemia and subsequent arrhythmia or cardiac arrest. Avoid concomitant use.

Reactions may be *common*, uncommon, **life-threatening**, or COMMON AND LIFE-THREATENING.

Lithium: Potentiated hypothyroid and goitrogenic effects of potassium iodide. Use together cautiously.

Adverse reactions

EENT: inflammation of salivary glands, periorbital edema.
GI: nausea, vomiting, stomach pain, diarrhea, burning mouth and throat, sore teeth and gums, *metallic taste.*
Metabolic: altered thyroid function tests.
Skin: acneiform rash.
Other: fever, *hypersensitivity reactions.*

☑ Special considerations

• Dilute with 6 oz (180 ml) of water, fruit juice, or broth to reduce GI distress and disguise strong, salty metallic taste; advise patient to use a straw to avoid tooth discoloration.
• Store in light-resistant container because exposure to light liberates traces of free iodine; if crystals develop in solution, dissolve them by placing container in warm water and carefully agitating it.
• Drug may cause flare-up of adolescent acne or other rash.
• Sudden withdrawal may precipitate thyroid storm.
• Maintain fluid intake when using drug as an expectorant; adequate hydration encourages optimal expectorant action.
• Acute overdose is rare; angioedema, laryngeal edema, and cutaneous hemorrhages may occur. Treat hyperkalemia immediately; salt and fluid intake help eliminate iodide. Iodism (chronic iodine poisoning) may follow prolonged use; symptoms include metallic taste, sore mouth, swollen eyelids, sneezing, skin eruptions, nausea, vomiting, epigastric pain, and diarrhea.

Monitoring the patient

• Monitor serum potassium levels before and during therapy; patient taking any diuretic, especially potassium-sparing diuretics, is at risk for hyperkalemia.
• Monitor patient for adverse effects.

Information for the patient

• Enteric-coated tablets are seldom used because of reports of small-bowel lesions with possible obstruction, perforation, and hemorrhage; when prescribed, give tablet with small amount of water, and tell patient to swallow tablet whole (don't crush or chew) and follow with 8 oz (240 ml) of water or juice.
• Advise patient to drink all of solution prepared and to use a straw to avoid discoloring teeth.
• Review signs and symptoms of iodism with patient, and instruct patient to report such symptoms, especially abdominal pain, distention, nausea, vomiting, or GI bleeding.

• Caution patient not to use OTC drugs without approval; many preparations contain iodides and could potentiate drug. For the same reason, patient should report ingestion of iodized salt and shellfish.

Geriatric patients

• Serum potassium determinations may be needed in elderly patients with renal dysfunction.

Pediatric patients

• Strong iodine solution is used for treating Graves' disease in neonates (1 drop every 8 hours).

Breast-feeding patients

• Drug appears in breast milk. Avoid use breast-feeding women; it may cause rash and thyroid suppression in infant.

---

potassium salts (oral)

potassium acetate

potassium bicarbonate
K+ Care ET, K-Electrolyte, K-Ide, Klor-Con/EF, K-Lyte, K-Vescent

potassium chloride
Apo-K*, Cena-K, Gen-K, K-8, K-10*, Kalium Durules*, Kaochlor S-F, Kaon-Cl, Kaon-Cl-10, Kato, Kay Ciel, K+ Care, KCL*, K-Dur, K-Ide, K-Lease, K-Long*, K-Lor, Klor-Con, Klorvess, Klotrix, K-Lyte/Cl Powder, K-Med 900*, K-Norm, K-Sol, K-Tab, Micro-K Extencaps, Micro-K 10 Extencaps, Potasalan, Rum-K, Slow-K, Ten-K

potassium gluconate
Glu-K, Kaon

Pharmacologic classification: potassium supplement
Therapeutic classification: therapeutic drug for electrolyte balance
Pregnancy risk category C

How supplied
Available by prescription only
Tablets (effervescent): 20 mEq, 25 mEq, 50 mEq
Liquid: 15 mEq/15 ml, 20 mEq/15 ml, 30 mEq/15 ml, 40 mEq/15 ml
potassium acetate
Vials: 2 mEq/ml, 4 mEq/ml in 20-ml vials
potassium chloride
Tablets (sustained-release): 6.7 mEq, 8 mEq, 10 mEq, 20 mEq
Powder: 15 mEq/package, 20 mEq/package, and 25 mEq/package

---

potassium gluconate
Liquid: 20 mEq/15 ml
Tablets: 2 mEq

Indications, route, and dosage
Hypokalemia
Adults and children: 40- to 100-mEq tablets divided into two to four doses daily. Use I.V. potassium chloride when oral replacement isn't feasible or when hypokalemia is life-threatening. Dosage up to 20 mEq/hour in concentration of 60 mEq/L or less. Further dose based on serum potassium determinations. Don't exceed total daily dose of 150 mEq (3 mEq/kg in children).

Further doses are based on serum potassium levels and blood pH. I.V. potassium replacement should be carried out only with ECG monitoring and frequent serum potassium determinations.

Prevention of hypokalemia
Adults and children: Initially, 20 mEq of potassium supplement P.O. daily, in divided doses. Adjust dosage, p.r.n., based on serum potassium levels.

Potassium replacement
Adults and children: Potassium chloride should be diluted in a suitable I.V. solution (not more than 40 mEq/L) and administered at rate not exceeding 20 mEq/hour. Don't exceed total dosage of 400 mEq/day (3 mEq/kg/day or 40 mEq/m^2/day for children). I.V. potassium replacement should be carried out only with ECG monitoring and frequent serum potassium determinations.

Pharmacodynamics
Potassium replacement action: Potassium, the main cation in body tissue, is necessary for physiologic processes such as maintaining intracellular tonicity, maintaining a balance with sodium across cell membranes, transmitting nerve impulses, maintaining cellular metabolism, contracting cardiac and skeletal muscle, maintaining acid-base balance, and maintaining normal renal function.

Pharmacokinetics
• *Absorption:* Well absorbed from GI tract. Should be taken with meals and sipped slowly over a 5- to 10-minute period to decrease irritation. Potassium bicarbonate doesn't correct hypochloremic alkalosis.
• *Distribution:* Normal serum levels of potassium range from 3.8 to 5 mEq/L. Plasma potassium levels up to 7.7 mEq/L may be normal in neonates. Up to 60 mEq/L of potassium may be found in gastric secretions and diarrhea fluid.
• *Metabolism:* None significant.
• *Excretion:* Excreted largely by kidneys. Small amounts may be excreted via skin and intestinal tract, but intestinal potassium usually is reabsorbed. A healthy patient on a potassium-free diet will excrete 40 to 50 mEq of potassium daily.

Contraindications and precautions
Contraindicated in patients with severe renal impairment with oliguria, anuria, or azotemia; in those with untreated Addison's disease; and in those with acute dehydration, heat cramps, hyperkalemia, hyperkalemic form of familial periodic paralysis, or conditions associated with extensive tissue breakdown.

Use cautiously in patients with cardiac or renal disease.

Interactions
Drug-drug. *ACE inhibitors (captopril), potassium-sparing diuretics:* Severe hyperkalemia. Use with caution.
Anticholinergics that slow GI motility: Increased chance of GI irritation and ulceration. Use together cautiously.
Digoxin: Potential for arrhythmias. Potassium isn't recommended in digitalized patients with severe or complete heart block.
Products containing potassium: Hyperkalemia within 1 to 2 days. Monitor patient closely.
Drug-food. *Salt substitutes containing potassium salts:* Severe hyperkalemia. Avoid concurrent use.

Adverse reactions
Signs of hyperkalemia
CNS: paresthesia of the extremities, listlessness, mental confusion, weakness or heaviness of legs, flaccid paralysis.
CV: hypotension, *arrhythmias, cardiac arrest, heart block,* ECG changes.
GI: nausea, vomiting, abdominal pain, diarrhea.
Metabolic: hyperkalemia.
Respiratory: *respiratory paralysis.*
Other: pain and redness at infusion site, fever.

☑ Special considerations
• In patients receiving cardiac glycosides, removing potassium too rapidly may result in digitalis toxicity.
• Don't give potassium during immediate postoperative period until urine flow is established.
• Give parenteral potassium by slow infusion only, never by I.V. push or I.M. Dilute I.V. potassium preparations with large volume of parenteral solutions.
• Give oral potassium supplements with extreme caution because its many forms deliver varying amounts of potassium. Patient may tolerate one product better than another.
• Potassium gluconate doesn't correct hypokalemic hypochloremic alkalosis.
• Enteric-coated tablets aren't recommended because of potential for GI bleeding and small-bowel ulcerations.
• Tablets in wax matrix sometimes lodge in esophagus and cause ulceration in cardiac patients who have esophageal compression due to enlarged left atrium. In such patients and in those

---

with esophageal or GI stasis or obstruction, use liquid form.

• Drug is often used orally with diuretics that cause potassium excretion. Potassium chloride is most useful because diuretics waste chloride ions. Hypokalemic alkalosis is treated best with potassium chloride.

• Don't crush sustained-released potassium products.

• Toxicity is evidenced by increased serum potassium level and characteristic ECG changes, including tall peaked T waves, depression of ST segment, disappearance of P wave, prolonged QT interval, and widening and slurring of the QRS complex. Late signs of toxicity include weakness, paralysis of voluntary muscles, respiratory distress, and dysphagia. These may precede severe or fatal cardiac toxicity. Hyperkalemia produces symptoms paradoxically similar to those of hypokalemia.

• In patients with a potassium level greater than 6.5 mEq/L, supportive therapy may include the following interventions (with continuous ECG monitoring): Infuse 40 to 160 mEq sodium bicarbonate I.V. over a 5-minute interval; repeat in 10 to 15 minutes if ECG abnormalities persist. Infuse 300 to 500 ml of dextrose 10% to 25% over 1 hour. Insulin (5 to 10 units per 20 g of dextrose) should be added to the infusion or, ideally, administered as a separate injection.

• Patients with absent P waves or broad QRS complex who aren't receiving cardiotonic glycosides should immediately be given 0.5 g to 1 g of calcium gluconate or another calcium salt I.V. over a 2-minute period (with continuous ECG monitoring) to antagonize cardiotoxic effect of potassium. May be repeated in 1 to 2 minutes if ECG abnormalities persist.

• To remove potassium from body, use sodium polystyrene sulfonate resin, hemodialysis, or peritoneal dialysis. Administer potassium-free I.V. fluids when hyperkalemia is associated with water loss.

Monitoring the patient
• Monitor serum potassium, BUN, and serum creatinine levels before starting therapy.

• Monitor ECG, pH, serum potassium levels, and other electrolytes during therapy.

Information for the patient
• Tell patient potassium is available only with a prescription because the wrong amount may cause severe reactions.

• Suggest diluting liquid potassium product in at least 4 to 8 oz (120 to 240 ml) of water; to take it after meals; and to sip liquid potassium slowly to minimize GI irritation.

• Tell patient to dissolve powder, soluble tablets, or granules completely in at least 4 oz (120 ml) of water or juice, and to allow fizzing to finish before drinking.

• Instruct patient not to crush or chew sustained-release capsules; contents of capsule can be opened and sprinkled onto applesauce or other soft food.

• Tell patient to stop taking drug and report immediately if the following reactions occur: confusion; irregular heartbeat; numbness of feet, fingers, or lips; shortness of breath; anxiety; excessive tiredness or weakness of legs; unexplained diarrhea; nausea and vomiting; stomach pain; or bloody or black stools. Such reactions are rare.

• Tell patient that expelling a whole tablet (sustained-release tablet) in stool is normal. The body eliminates the shell after absorbing the potassium.

• Warn patient to avoid salt substitutes except when prescribed.

Pediatric patients
• Use cautiously in children.

Breast-feeding patients
• Potassium supplements appear in breast milk. Safety in breast-feeding women hasn't been established; use potassium only when benefits to mother outweigh risks to infant.

---

pralidoxime chloride (2-PAM chloride, 2-pyridine aldoxime methochloride)
Protopam Chloride

Pharmacologic classification: quaternary ammonium oxime
Therapeutic classification: antidote
Pregnancy risk category C

How supplied
Available by prescription only
Injection: 1 g/20 ml vial (without diluent or syringe); 1 g/20 ml vial with diluent, syringe, needle, alcohol swab (emergency kit); 600 mg/2 ml auto-injector, parenteral

Indications, route, and dosage
Organophosphate pesticide poisoning
Adults: 1 to 2 g I.V. in 100 ml of normal saline over 15 to 30 minutes. May repeat in 1 hour if muscle weakness continues. For subconjunctival injection, give 0.1 to 0.2 ml of a 5% solution.
Children: 20 to 40 mg/kg I.V. in 100 ml of normal saline over 15 to 30 minutes. May repeat in 1 hour if muscle weakness continues.

Drug is most effective when administered within 24 hours of exposure. It should be administered with atropine.
Anticholinesterase overdose
Adults: 1 to 2 g I.V.; then increments of 250 mg q 5 minutes.

Pharmacodynamics

Antidote action: Reactivates cholinesterase that has been inactivated by phosphorylation due to exposure to an organophosphate pesticide or related compound. One of the few drugs that correct a biochemical lesion, pralidoxime acts by removing the phosphoryl group from the active site of the inhibited enzyme, freezing and reactivating acetylcholinesterase. It also directly reacts with and detoxifies the organophosphorus molecule and may also react with cholinesterase to protect it from inhibition.

Cholinesterase reactivation occurs primarily at the neuromuscular junction where pralidoxime exerts its most critical effect—reversal of respiratory paralysis or paralysis of other skeletal muscles. Reactivation also occurs at autonomic effector sites and, to a lesser degree, within the CNS. Pralidoxime is effective against nicotinic signs and symptoms but it doesn't substantially influence muscarinic effects. Therefore, it's used in conjunction with atropine, which ameliorates muscarinic symptoms and directly blocks the effects of accumulation of excess acetylcholine at various sites, including the respiratory center.

Pharmacokinetics

• *Absorption:* After I.V. administration, plasma levels peak in 5 to 15 minutes; after I.M., in 10 to 20 minutes.
• *Distribution:* Distributed throughout extracellular water; not appreciably bound to plasma protein. Doesn't readily pass into CNS. Distribution into breast milk is unknown. Therapeutic levels achieved in eye after subconjunctival injection.
• *Metabolism:* Exact mechanism unknown; likely hepatic metabolism.
• *Excretion:* Excreted rapidly in urine as unchanged drug and metabolite; 80% to 90% of I.V. or I.M. dose excreted unchanged within 12 hours.

Contraindications and precautions

Contraindicated in patients with hypersensitivity to drug or its components. Use cautiously in patients with myasthenia gravis.

Interactions

Drug-drug. *Barbiturates:* Potentiated by anticholinesterase. Use with caution.
CNS depressants, drugs that lower seizure threshold (aminophylline, morphine, phenothiazines, reserpine, succinylcholine, theophylline, other respiratory depressants), skeletal muscle relaxants: Possible potentiation or decreased effect of these drugs. Avoid in patients with anticholinesterase poisoning.

Adverse reactions

CNS: dizziness, headache, drowsiness.
CV: tachycardia, hypertension.
EENT: blurred vision, diplopia, impaired accommodation.

GI: nausea.
Hepatic: transient AST and ALT elevations, transient elevation in CK levels, transient elevation of liver enzyme levels.
Musculoskeletal: muscle weakness.
Respiratory: hyperventilation.
Other: mild to moderate pain at injection site.

☑ Special considerations

• Reconstitute drug with 20 ml of sterile water for injection to provide a solution containing 50 mg/ml. For I.V. infusion, dilute calculated dose to a volume of 100 ml with normal saline injection. Use within a few hours.
• Drug usually is administered by I.V. infusion over 15 to 30 minutes. Rapid administration has produced tachycardia, laryngospasm, muscle rigidity, and transient neuromuscular blockade. Hypertension may also occur, related to dose and rate of infusion; it may be treated by stopping infusion or slowing rate of infusion. Phentolamine 5 mg I.V. quickly reverses pralidoxime-induced hypertension.
• In patients with pulmonary edema, or when I.V. infusion isn't practical, or a more rapid effect is needed, drug may be given by slow I.V. injection over at least 5 minutes. It may also be given I.M. or S.C.
• Institute treatment of organophosphate poisoning without waiting for laboratory test results. Begin pralidoxime and atropine therapy simultaneously. Give 2 to 6 mg of atropine I.V. (I.M. if patient is cyanotic) every 5 to 60 minutes in adults until muscarinic effects (dyspnea, cough, salivation, bronchospasm) subside. Repeat dosage if signs reappear. Maintain some degree of atropinism for at least 48 hours.
• Use reduced dosage in renally impaired patients.
• Treatment is most effective when started within first 24 hours, preferably within a few hours after poisoning. Even severe poisoning may be reversed if drug is given within 48 hours. Monitor effect of therapy by ECG because of possible heart block due to the anticholinesterase. Continued absorption of the anticholinesterase from the lower bowel constitutes new toxic exposure that may require additional doses of pralidoxime every 3 to 8 hours, or over several days.
• After dermal exposure, patient's clothing should be removed and hair and skin should be washed with sodium bicarbonate, soap, water, or alcohol as soon as possible. While cleaning patient, caregiver should wear gloves and protective clothing to avoid contamination. Patient may need a second washing.
• Drug isn't effective in treating toxic exposure to phosphorus, inorganic phosphates, or organophosphates that don't have anticholinesterase activity.
• Give I.V. sodium thiopental or diazepam if seizures interfere with respiration.

Reactions may be *common*, uncommon, **life-threatening**, or COMMON AND LIFE-THREATENING.

• Subconjunctival injection is currently an unapproved method of administration but has been used to reverse adverse ocular effects resulting from systemic overdose or splashing of an organophosphate into eye.
• Toxicity may cause dizziness, headache, blurred vision, diplopia, impaired accommodation, nausea, and tachycardia. However, these effects may also result from organophosphate toxicity or the use of atropine.

Monitoring the patient
• Assess vital signs and insert I.V. line. Drug administration requires close medical supervision and close observation of patient for at least 24 hours.
• Draw blood for RBC and cholinesterase levels before giving pralidoxime.
• Closely monitor blood pressure during infusion.

Information for the patient
• Warn patient that mild to moderate pain may occur 20 to 40 minutes after I.M. injection.

Pediatric patients
• Safety hasn't been established.

Breast-feeding patients
• It's unknown if drug appears in breast milk. Use caution when administering drug to breast-feeding women.

pramipexole hydrochloride
Mirapex

Pharmacologic classification: nonergot dopamine agonist
Therapeutic classification: antiparkinsonian
Pregnancy risk category C

How supplied
Available by prescription only
Tablets: 0.125 mg, 0.25 mg, 0.5 mg, 1 mg, 1.5 mg

Indications, route, and dosage
Idiopathic Parkinson's disease
Adults: Initially, 0.375 mg P.O. daily given in three divided doses; don't increase more than q 5 to 7 days. Increase dose by 0.75 mg in divided doses weekly until maximum dose of 1.5 mg t.i.d. is reached after 7 weeks of therapy. Maintenance dose ranges from 1.5 to 4.5 mg daily administered in three divided doses.
✦ *Dosage adjustment.* For patients with impaired renal function and creatinine clearance of 35 to 59 ml/minute, initial dose is 0.125 mg P.O. b.i.d. and maintenance maximum dose is 1.5 mg b.i.d. For patients with creatinine clearance of 15 to 34

ml/minute, initial dose is 0.125 mg P.O. daily and maintenance maximum dose is 1.5 mg daily.

Pharmacodynamics
Antiparkinsonian action: Thought to stimulate dopamine (D_2 and D_3) receptors in striatum; pramipexole influences striatal neuronal firing rates via activation of dopamine receptors in the striatum and the substantia nigra, the site of neurons that send projections to the striatum.

Pharmacokinetics
• *Absorption:* Rapidly absorbed; levels peak in about 2 hours. Absolute bioavailability over 90%, suggesting it's well absorbed and undergoes little presystemic metabolism. Food doesn't affect extent of absorption, but increases time of maximum plasma level by about 1 hour.
• *Distribution:* Extensively distributed; volume of distribution of about 500 L. About 15% bound to plasma proteins; also distributed into RBCs. Terminal half-life 8 to 12 hours; steady-state reached within 2 days of dosing.
• *Metabolism:* 90% of dose excreted unchanged in urine.
• *Excretion:* Excreted mainly in urine. Nonrenal routes may contribute a small extent to elimination; no metabolites identified in plasma or urine. Drug secreted by renal tubules, probably by organic transport system.

Contraindications and precautions
Contraindicated in patients with hypersensitivity to drug or its components. Use with caution in those who have renal impairment, such as elderly patients, because dosing may need to be adjusted.

Interactions
Drug-drug. *Cimetidine, diltiazem, quinidine, quinine, ranitidine, triamterene, verapamil:* Decreased clearance of pramipexole. Adjust pramipexole dose if used together.
Dopamine antagonists (butyrophenones, metoclopramide, phenothiazines, thiothixenes): Diminished effectiveness of pramipexole. Monitor patient closely.
Levodopa: Increased levodopa maximum plasma levels. Adjust levodopa dosage as needed.

Adverse reactions
CNS: *dizziness,* somnolence, malaise, *insomnia,* hallucinations, *confusion,* amnesia, hypoesthesia, dystonia, akathisia, thought abnormalities, myoclonus, *asthenia, dyskinesia, extrapyramidal syndrome, dream abnormalities,* gait abnormalities, hypertonia, paranoid reaction, delusions, sleep disorders.
CV: chest pain, peripheral edema, *orthostatic hypotension,* general edema.
EENT: accommodation abnormalities, diplopia, dry mouth, rhinitis, vision abnormalities.

GI: anorexia, *constipation,* dysphagia, nausea.
GU: decreased libido, impotence, urinary frequency, urinary tract infection, urinary incontinence.
Musculoskeletal: arthritis, twitching, bursitis, myasthenia.
Respiratory: dyspnea, pneumonia.
Skin: skin disorders.
Other: fever, unevaluable reaction, *accidental injury.*

☑ Special considerations
● If drug needs to be discontinued, do so over a 1-week period.
● Neuroleptic malignant syndrome (elevated temperature, muscular rigidity, altered consciousness, and autonomic instability) without obvious cause has occurred with rapid dose reduction or withdrawal of or changes in antiparkinsonian therapy.
● Adjust dosage gradually. Increase dosage to achieve maximum therapeutic effect, balanced against the main adverse effects of dyskinesia, hallucinations, somnolence, and dry mouth.

Monitoring the patient
● Drug may cause orthostatic hypotension, especially during dose escalation; monitor patient carefully.
● Monitor patient for adverse effects.

Information for the patient
● Tell patient to take drug only as prescribed.
● Instruct patient not to rise rapidly after sitting or lying down because of risk of orthostatic hypotension.
● Caution patient not to drive or operate complex machinery until response to drug is known.
● Tell patient to use caution before taking drug with other CNS depressants.
● Advise patient to take drug with food if nausea develops.
● Caution patient to not stop drug abruptly.

Geriatric patients
● Drug clearance decreases with age because half-life and clearance are about 40% longer and 30% lower, respectively, in patients ages 65 and older.

Pediatric patients
● Safety and efficacy in children haven't been established.

Breast-feeding patients
● It's unknown if drug appears in breast milk. Use with caution in breast-feeding women.

pravastatin sodium
Pravachol

Pharmacologic classification: HMG-CoA reductase inhibitor
Therapeutic classification: antilipemic
Pregnancy risk category X

How supplied
Available by prescription only
Tablets: 10 mg, 20 mg, 40 mg

Indications, route, and dosage
Reduction of low-density lipoprotein and total cholesterol levels in patients with primary hypercholesterolemia (types IIa and IIb), primary prevention of coronary events
Adults: Initially, 10 to 20 mg P.O. daily h.s. Adjust dosage q 4 weeks based on patient tolerance and response; maximum daily dose is 40 mg. Most elderly patients respond to a daily dose of 20 mg or less.

Pharmacodynamics
Antilipemic action: Inhibits the enzyme 3-hydroxy-3-methylglutaryl-coenzyme A (HMG-CoA) reductase. This hepatic enzyme is an early (and rate limiting) step in the synthetic pathway of cholesterol.

Pharmacokinetics
● *Absorption:* Rapidly absorbed; plasma levels peak in 1 to 1½ hours. Average oral absorption is 34%; absolute bioavailability of 17%. Food reduces bioavailability, but same drug effects if drug is taken with or 1 hour before meals.
● *Distribution:* Plasma levels proportional to dose, but don't necessarily correlate perfectly with lipid-lowering effects. About 50% bound to plasma proteins. Undergoes extensive first-pass extraction, possibly because of active transport system into hepatocytes.
● *Metabolism:* Metabolized by liver. At least six metabolites identified; some active.
● *Excretion:* Excreted by liver and kidneys.

Contraindications and precautions
Contraindicated in patients with hypersensitivity to drug; in those with active liver disease or conditions that cause unexplained, persistent elevations of serum transaminase levels; in pregnant and breast-feeding women; and in women of childbearing age unless there is no risk of pregnancy.
    Use cautiously in patients who consume large quantities of alcohol or have history of liver disease.

Interactions
Drug-drug. *Cholestyramine, colestipol:* Decreased plasma levels of pravastatin. Administer

---

Reactions may be *common,* uncommon, **life-threatening,** or COMMON AND LIFE-THREATENING.

pravastatin 1 hour before or 4 hours after these drugs.
Cimetidine, ketoconazole, spironolactone: Increased risk of endocrine dysfunction. No intervention appears necessary; take complete drug history in patients who develop endocrine dysfunction.
Erythromycin, fibric acid derivatives (clofibrate, gemfibrozil), high doses of niacin (1 g or more nicotinic acid daily), immunosuppressants (such as cyclosporine): Increased risk of rhabdomyolysis. Monitor patient closely if drugs must be given together.
Gemfibrozil: Decreased protein-binding and urinary clearance of pravastatin. Avoid concomitant use.
Hepatotoxic drugs: Increased risk of hepatotoxicity. Use together cautiously.
Drug-lifestyle. *Chronic alcohol abuse:* Increased risk of hepatotoxicity. Monitor patient closely.
Sun exposure: Photosensitivity reaction. Tell patient to take precautions.

Adverse reactions
CNS: headache, dizziness, fatigue.
CV: chest pain.
EENT: rhinitis.
GI: vomiting, diarrhea, heartburn, abdominal pain, constipation, flatulence, nausea.
GU: *renal failure* secondary to myoglobinuria, urinary abnormality.
Hepatic: increased AST, ALT, CK, alkaline phosphatase, and bilirubin levels.
Metabolic: abnormal thyroid function test.
Musculoskeletal: myositis, myopathy, *localized muscle pain,* myalgia, **rhabdomyolysis.**
Respiratory: cough.
Skin: rash.
Other: flulike symptoms, photosensitivity, influenza, common cold.

☑ Special considerations
● Stop drug temporarily in patients with an acute condition that suggests a developing myopathy or in patients with risk factors that may predispose them to development of renal failure secondary to rhabdomyolysis (including severe acute infection; severe endocrine, metabolic, or electrolyte disorders; hypotension; major surgery; or uncontrolled seizures).
● Initiate drug therapy only after diet and other nonpharmacologic therapies have proved ineffective. Patients should continue a cholesterol-lowering diet during therapy.
● Give drug in evening, preferably at bedtime. Drug may be given without regard to meals.
● Dosage adjustments should be made about every 4 weeks. May reduce dosage if cholesterol levels fall below target range.

Monitoring the patient
● Watch for signs of myositis. Rarely, myopathy and marked elevations of CK level, possibly leading to rhabdomyolysis and renal failure secondary to myoglobinuria, have occurred.
● Monitor therapeutic effect.

Information for the patient
● Teach patient appropriate dietary management (restricting total fat and cholesterol intake), weight control, and exercise. Explain importance of these interventions in controlling serum lipids.
● Because of drug's possible impact on liver function, advise patient to restrict alcohol intake.
● Tell patient to call if he experiences adverse reactions, particularly muscle aches and pains.
● Inform patient to take drug at bedtime.

Geriatric patients
● Maximum effectiveness is usually evident with daily doses of 20 mg or less.

Pediatric patients
● Safety and efficacy in children under age 18 haven't been established.

Breast-feeding patients
● Drug appears in breast milk. Women shouldn't breast-feed while taking drug.

prazosin hydrochloride
Minipress

Pharmacologic classification: alpha-adrenergic blocker
Therapeutic classification: antihypertensive
Pregnancy risk category C

How supplied
Available by prescription only
Capsules: 1 mg, 2 mg, 5 mg

Indications, route, and dosage
Hypertension
Adults: Initially, 1 mg P.O. b.i.d. or t.i.d.; gradually increased to maximum of 20 mg daily. Usual maintenance dose is 6 to 15 mg daily in divided doses. If other antihypertensives or diuretics are added to prazosin therapy, reduce dose of prazosin to 1 or 2 mg t.i.d. and then gradually increase as necessary.
◇ *Benign prostatic hyperplasia*
Adults: Initially, 2 mg P.O. b.i.d. Dose may range from 1 to 9 mg/day.

Pharmacodynamics
Antihypertensive action: Selectively and competitively inhibits alpha-adrenergic receptors, causing arterial and venous dilation, reducing peripheral vascular resistance and blood pressure.

Hypertrophic action: Alpha blockade in nonvascular smooth muscle causes relaxation, notably in prostatic tissue, thereby reducing urinary symptoms in men with benign prostatic hyperplasia.

Pharmacokinetics

- *Absorption:* Variable absorption from GI tract. Antihypertensive effect begins in about 2 hours; peaks in 2 to 4 hours. Full antihypertensive effect may not occur for 4 to 6 weeks.
- *Distribution:* Distributed throughout body; about 97% protein-bound.
- *Metabolism:* Metabolized extensively in liver.
- *Excretion:* Over 90% of dose excreted in feces via bile; remainder excreted in urine. Plasma half-life is 2 to 4 hours. Antihypertensive effect lasts less than 24 hours.

Contraindications and precautions

No known contraindications. Use cautiously in patients receiving antihypertensives and in those with chronic renal failure.

Interactions

Drug-drug. *Diuretics, other antihypertensives:* Increased hypotensive effects. Monitor blood pressure regularly.
Other highly protein-bound drugs: Prazosin is highly bound to plasma proteins and may interact with these drugs. Monitor patient closely.
Drug-herb. *Butcher's broom:* Reduced effects of drug. Discourage use.

Adverse reactions

CNS: *dizziness,* headache, drowsiness, nervousness, paresthesia, weakness, *first-dose syncope,* depression.
CV: edema, orthostatic hypotension, *palpitations.*
EENT: blurred vision, tinnitus, conjunctivitis, nasal congestion, epistaxis.
GI: vomiting, diarrhea, abdominal cramps, constipation, *nausea.*
GU: increased BUN levels, priapism, impotence, urinary frequency, incontinence.
Hematologic: transient fall in leukocyte count.
Hepatic: liver function test abnormalities.
Metabolic: increased serum uric acid levels.
Musculoskeletal: arthralgia, myalgia.
Respiratory: dyspnea.
Skin: pruritus.
Other: fever.

☑ Special considerations

Besides the recommendations relevant to all alpha blockers, consider the following.
- First-dose syncope (light-headedness, dizziness, and syncope) may occur within ½ to 1 hour after initial dose; it may be severe, with loss of consciousness, if initial dose exceeds 2 mg. Effect is transient and may be diminished by giving drug at bedtime, by limiting initial dose of prazosin to 1 mg, by subsequently increasing dosage

gradually, and by introducing other antihypertensives into patient's regimen cautiously; it's more common during febrile illness and more severe if patient has hyponatremia. Always increase dosage gradually and have patient sit or lie down if he experiences dizziness.
- Prazosin's effect is most pronounced on diastolic blood pressure.
- Drug has been used to treat vasospasm associated with Raynaud's syndrome. It also has been used with diuretics and cardiac glycosides to treat severe heart failure, to manage the signs and symptoms of pheochromocytoma preoperatively, and to treat ergotamine-induced peripheral ischemia.
- Drug alters results of screening tests for pheochromocytoma and causes increases in levels of the urinary metabolite of norepinephrine and vanillylmandelic acid.
- Toxicity may cause hypotension and drowsiness. Prazosin isn't dialyzable.

Monitoring the patient
- Monitor blood pressure, especially at start of therapy and with changes in dosing.
- Monitor patient for adverse effects.

Information for the patient
- Teach patient about his disease and therapy, and explain that he must take drug exactly as prescribed, even when feeling well; advise him never to stop drug suddenly because severe rebound hypertension may occur, and to promptly report malaise or unusual adverse effects.
- Tell patient to avoid hazardous activities that require mental alertness until tolerance develops to sedation, drowsiness, and other CNS effects; to avoid sudden position changes to minimize orthostatic hypotension; and to use ice chips, candy, or gum to relieve dry mouth.
- Warn patient to seek medical approval before taking OTC cold preparations.

Geriatric patients
- Elderly patients may be more sensitive to hypotensive effects and may need lower doses because of altered drug metabolism.

Pediatric patients
- Safety and efficacy in children haven't been established; use only when potential benefit outweighs risk.

Breast-feeding patients
- Small amounts of drug appear in breast milk; an alternative to breast-feeding is recommended during therapy.

Reactions may be *common,* uncommon, **life-threatening**, OR COMMON AND LIFE-THREATENING.

prednisolone (systemic)
Delta-Cortef, Prelone

prednisolone acetate
Cotolone, Key-Pred-25, Predalone-50, Predcor-50

prednisolone sodium phosphate
Hydeltrasol, Key-Pred SP, Pediapred

prednisolone tebutate
Nor-Pred T.B.A., Predate TBA, Predcor-TBA, Prednisol TBA

Pharmacologic classification: glucocorticoid, mineralocorticoid
Therapeutic classification: anti-inflammatory, immunosuppressant
Pregnancy risk category C

How supplied
Available by prescription only
prednisolone
Tablets: 5 mg
Syrup: 5 mg/ml, 15 mg/5 ml
prednisolone acetate
Injection: 25 mg/ml, 50 mg/ml suspension
prednisolone sodium phosphate
Oral liquid: 6.7 mg (5 mg base)/5 ml
Injection: 20 mg/ml solution
prednisolone tebutate
Injection: 20 mg/ml suspension

Indications, route, and dosage
Severe inflammation, modification of body's immune response to disease
Adults: 2.5 to 15 mg P.O. b.i.d., t.i.d., or q.i.d.
Children: 0.14 to 2 mg/kg or 4 to 60 mg/m² daily in divided doses.
prednisolone acetate
Adults: 2 to 30 mg I.M. q 12 hours.
prednisolone sodium phosphate
Adults: 2 to 30 mg I.M. or I.V. q 12 hours, or into joints, lesions, and soft tissue, p.r.n.
prednisolone tebutate
Adults: 4 to 40 mg into joints and lesions, p.r.n.

Pharmacodynamics
Anti-inflammatory action: Prednisolone stimulates the synthesis of enzymes needed to decrease the inflammatory response. It suppresses the immune system by reducing activity and volume of the lymphatic system, thus producing lymphocytopenia (primarily of T-lymphocytes), decreasing immunoglobulin and complement levels, decreasing passage of immune complexes through basement membranes, and possibly by depressing reactivity of tissue to antigen-antibody interactions.

The mineralocorticoids regulate electrolyte homeostasis by acting renally at the distal tubules to enhance the reabsorption of sodium ions (and thus water) from the tubular fluid into the plasma and enhance the excretion of both potassium and hydrogen ions.
Prednisolone is an adrenocorticoid with both glucocorticoid and mineralocorticoid properties. It's a weak mineralocorticoid with only half the potency of hydrocortisone but is a more potent glucocorticoid, having four times the potency of equal weight of hydrocortisone. It's used primarily as an anti-inflammatory drug and an immunosuppressant. It's not used for mineralocorticoid replacement therapy because of the availability of more specific and potent drugs.
Prednisolone may be administered orally. Prednisolone sodium phosphate is highly soluble, has a rapid onset and a short duration of action, and may be given I.M. or I.V. Prednisolone acetate and tebutate are suspensions that may be administered by intra-articular, intrasynovial, intrabursal, intralesional, or soft-tissue injection. They have a slow onset but a long duration of action.

Pharmacokinetics
● *Absorption:* Absorbed readily after oral administration. After oral and I.V. administration, effects peak in about 1 to 2 hours. Acetate and tebutate suspensions for injection have a variable absorption rate over 24 to 48 hours, depending on if injected into intra-articular space or muscle, and on blood supply to that muscle. Slow systemic absorption after intra-articular injection.
● *Distribution:* Removed rapidly from blood and distributed to muscle, liver, skin, intestines, and kidneys. Extensively bound to plasma proteins (transcortin and albumin); only unbound portion is active. Adrenocorticoids distributed into breast milk and through placenta.
● *Metabolism:* Metabolized in liver to inactive glucuronide and sulfate metabolites.
● *Excretion:* Inactive metabolites, and small amounts of unmetabolized drug, excreted in urine. Insignificant drug quantities excreted in feces. Biological half-life 18 to 36 hours.

Contraindications and precautions
Contraindicated in patients with hypersensitivity to drug or its components and in those with and systemic fungal infections.
Use cautiously in patients with a recent MI, GI ulcer, renal disease, hypertension, osteoporosis, diabetes mellitus, hypothyroidism, cirrhosis, diverticulitis, nonspecific ulcerative colitis, recent intestinal anastomoses, thromboembolic disorders, seizures, myasthenia gravis, heart failure, tuberculosis, ocular herpes simplex, emotional instability, or psychotic tendencies.

Interactions
Drug-drug. *Amphotericin B, diuretics:* Enhanced hypokalemia. Monitor serum potassium level.
Antacids, cholestyramine, colestipol: Decreased prednisolone absorption. Separate administration times.
Barbiturates, phenytoin, rifampin: Decreased corticosteroid effects because of increased hepatic metabolism. Monitor patient.
Cardiac glycosides: Possible hypokalemia may increase risk of toxicity in patients receiving these drugs. Monitor serum potassium level.
Estrogens: Reduced metabolism of prednisolone via increased level of transcortin; half-life of corticosteroid prolonged because of increased protein-binding. Adjust dosage as needed.
Insulin, oral antidiabetics: Hyperglycemia. Adjust dosages of these drugs as needed.
Isoniazid, salicylates: Increased metabolism of these drugs. Monitor patient closely.
Oral anticoagulants: Decreased effects. Monitor PT and INR.
Ulcerogenic drugs (such as NSAIDs): Increased risk of GI ulceration. Use together cautiously.

Adverse reactions
Most adverse reactions to corticosteroids are dose- or duration-dependent.
CNS: *euphoria, insomnia,* psychotic behavior, pseudotumor cerebri, vertigo, headache, paresthesia, *seizures.*
CV: *heart failure, thromboembolism,* hypertension, edema, *arrhythmias,* thrombophlebitis.
EENT: cataracts, glaucoma.
GI: *peptic ulceration,* GI irritation, increased appetite, *pancreatitis,* nausea, vomiting.
GU: menstrual irregularities.
Metabolic: hypokalemia, hyperglycemia, carbohydrate intolerance.
Musculoskeletal: muscle weakness, osteoporosis, growth suppression in children.
Skin: delayed wound healing, acne, various skin eruptions, hirsutism.
Other: susceptibility to infections; *acute adrenal insufficiency (with increased stress from infection, surgery, or trauma);* cushingoid state (moonface, buffalo hump, central obesity).
After abrupt withdrawal: rebound inflammation, fatigue, weakness, arthralgia, fever, dizziness, lethargy, depression, fainting, orthostatic hypotension, dyspnea, anorexia, hypoglycemia. *After prolonged use, sudden withdrawal may cause acute adrenal insufficiency and death.*

☑ Special considerations
● Recommendations for use of prednisolone are the same as those for all systemic adrenocorticoids.
● Prednisolone suppresses reactions to skin tests; causes false-negative results in the nitroblue tetrazolium test for systemic bacterial infections.

Monitoring the patient
● Monitor patient's weight, blood pressure, and serum electrolyte levels.
● Monitor serum glucose level in diabetic patients.

Information for the patient
● Recommendations for care and teaching of patients are the same as those for all systemic adrenocorticoids.
● Tell patient to report fluid retention when it occurs.
● Instruct patient to not become immunized during drug therapy.
● Advise patient to be aware of signs of infection; some of these signs may be masked during drug use.

Pediatric patients
● Prolonged use of adrenocorticoids or corticotropin may suppress growth and maturation in children and adolescents.

---

prednisolone acetate (ophthalmic)
Econopred, Pred Forte, Pred Mild

prednisolone sodium phosphate
AK-Pred, Inflamase Forte, Inflamase Mild, I-Pred, Ocu-Pred

Pharmacologic classification: corticosteroid
Therapeutic classification: ophthalmic anti-inflammatory
Pregnancy risk category C

How supplied
Available by prescription only
prednisolone acetate
Suspension: 0.12%, 0.125%, 1%
prednisolone sodium phosphate
Solution: 0.125%, 1%

Indications, route, and dosage
Inflammation of palpebral and bulbar conjunctiva, cornea, and anterior segment of globe; corneal injury; graft rejection
Adults and children: Instill 1 or 2 drops in eye. In severe conditions, may be used hourly, tapering to discontinuation as inflammation subsides. In mild conditions, may be used four to six times daily.

Pharmacodynamics
Anti-inflammatory action: Corticosteroids stimulate the synthesis of enzymes needed to decrease the inflammatory response. Prednisolone, a synthetic corticosteroid, has about four times the anti-inflammatory potency of an equal weight of hydrocortisone. Prednisolone acetate is poorly

soluble and therefore has a slower onset of action, but a longer duration of action, when applied in a liquid suspension. The sodium phosphate salt is highly soluble and has a rapid onset but short duration of action.

Pharmacokinetics
● *Absorption:* After ophthalmic use, absorbed through aqueous humor. Systemic absorption rarely occurs.
● *Distribution:* After ophthalmic use, distributed throughout local tissue layers. Any drug absorbed into circulation is rapidly removed from blood and distributed into muscle, liver, skin, intestines, and kidneys.
● *Metabolism:* After ophthalmic use, corticosteroids primarily metabolized locally. Small amount absorbed into systemic circulation is metabolized primarily in liver to inactive compounds.
● *Excretion:* Inactive metabolites excreted by kidneys, primarily as glucuronides and sulfates, but also as unconjugated products. Small amounts of metabolites excreted in feces.

Contraindications and precautions
Contraindicated in patients with acute, untreated, purulent ocular infections; acute superficial herpes simplex (dendritic keratitis); vaccinia, varicella, or other viral or fungal eye diseases; or ocular tuberculosis. Use cautiously in patients with corneal abrasions that may be contaminated (especially with herpes).

Interactions
None reported.

Adverse reactions
EENT: increased intraocular pressure; thinning of cornea, interference with corneal wound healing, increased susceptibility to viral or fungal corneal infection, corneal ulceration; with excessive or long-term use: discharge, discomfort, foreign body sensation, glaucoma exacerbation, cataracts, visual acuity and visual field defects, optic nerve damage.
Other: systemic effects and adrenal suppression with excessive or long-term use.

☑ Special considerations
● Shake suspension and check dosage before administering. Store in tightly covered container.

Monitoring the patient
● Monitor tonometric readings in patients on long-term therapy.
● Monitor therapeutic effect.

Information for the patient
● Teach patient how to apply eyedrops.
● Tell patient not to share drug, washcloths, or towels with family members.

● Tell patient to call if improvement doesn't occur within several days or if pain, itching, or swelling of eye occurs.

prednisone
Apo-Prednisone*, Deltasone, Meticorten, Orasone, Prednicen-M, Sterapred, Winpred*

Pharmacologic classification: adrenocorticoid
Therapeutic classification: immunosuppressant, anti-inflammatory
Pregnancy risk category C

How supplied
Available by prescription only
Tablets: 1 mg, 2.5 mg, 5 mg, 10 mg, 20 mg, 50 mg
Oral solution: 5 mg/ml, 5 mg/5 ml
Syrup: 5 mg/5 ml

Indications, route, and dosage
Severe inflammation, modification of body's immune response to disease
Adults: 5 to 60 mg P.O. daily in single dose or divided doses. Maximum daily dose is 250 mg. Maintenance dose given once daily or every other day. Dosage must be individualized.
Children: 0.14 to 2 mg/kg or 4 to 60 mg/m² P.O. daily in divided doses; or may use the following dosage schedule:
Children ages 11 to 18: 20 mg P.O. q.i.d.
Children ages 5 to 10: 15 mg P.O. q.i.d.
Children ages 18 months to 4 years: 7.5 to 10 mg P.O. q.i.d.
◊ *Adjunct to anti-infective therapy in treatment of moderate to severe* **Pneumocystis carinii** *pneumonia*
Adults or children over age 13 with AIDS: 40 mg P.O. b.i.d. for 5 days; then 40 mg. P.O. once daily for 5 days; then 20 mg P.O. once daily for 11 days (or until completion of the concurrent anti-infective regimen).

Pharmacodynamics
Immunosuppressant action: Stimulates the synthesis of enzymes needed to decrease the inflammatory response. Suppresses the immune system by reducing activity and volume of the lymphatic system, thus producing lymphocytopenia (primarily of T-lymphocytes), decreasing immunoglobulin and complement levels, decreasing passage of immune complexes through basement membranes, and possibly by depressing reactivity of tissue to antigen-antibody interactions.
Anti-inflammatory action: One of the intermediate-acting glucocorticoids, with greater glucocorticoid activity than cortisone and hydrocortisone but less anti-inflammatory activity than betamethasone, dexamethasone, and parametha-

sone. About four to five times more potent as an anti-inflammatory than hydrocortisone, but has only half the mineralocorticoid activity of an equal weight of hydrocortisone. The oral glucocorticoid of choice for anti-inflammatory or immunosuppressive effects.

Pharmacokinetics
• *Absorption:* Absorbed readily after oral administration; effects peak in about 1 to 2 hours.
• *Distribution:* Distributed rapidly to muscle, liver, skin, intestines, and kidneys. Extensively bound to plasma proteins (transcortin and albumin); only unbound portion is active. Distributed into breast milk and through placenta.
• *Metabolism:* Metabolized in liver to active metabolite prednisolone, which is then metabolized to inactive glucuronide and sulfate metabolites.
• *Excretion:* Inactive metabolites and small amounts of unmetabolized drug excreted by kidneys. Insignificant drug quantities also excreted in feces. Biological half-life of prednisone is 18 to 36 hours.

Contraindications and precautions
Contraindicated in patients with hypersensitivity to drug and in those with systemic fungal infections.
    Use cautiously in patients with GI ulcer, renal disease, hypertension, osteoporosis, diabetes mellitus, hypothyroidism, cirrhosis, diverticulitis, nonspecific ulcerative colitis, recent intestinal anastomoses, thromboembolic disorders, seizures, myasthenia gravis, heart failure, tuberculosis, ocular herpes simplex, emotional instability, and psychotic tendencies.

Interactions
Drug-drug. *Amphotericin B, diuretics:* Enhanced hypokalemia. Monitor serum potassium level.
Antacids, cholestyramine, colestipol: Decreased prednisone absorption. Separate administration times.
Barbiturates, phenytoin, rifampin: Decreased corticosteroid effects because of increased hepatic metabolism. Monitor patient.
Cardiac glycosides: Possible hypokalemia may increase risk of toxicity in patients receiving these drugs. Monitor serum potassium level.
Estrogens: Reduced metabolism of prednisone via increased level of transcortin; half-life of corticosteroid prolonged because of increased protein binding. Adjust dosage as needed.
Insulin, oral antidiabetics: Hyperglycemia. Adjust dosages of these drugs as needed.
Isoniazid, salicylates: Increased metabolism of these drugs. Monitor patient closely.
Oral anticoagulants: Decreased effects. Monitor PT and INR.

Ulcerogenic drugs (such as NSAIDs): Increased risk of GI ulceration. Use together cautiously.

Adverse reactions
Most adverse reactions to corticosteroids are dose- or duration-dependent.
CNS: *euphoria, insomnia,* psychotic behavior, pseudotumor cerebri, vertigo, headache, paresthesia, **seizures.**
CV: hypertension, edema, **arrhythmias,** thrombophlebitis, **thromboembolism, heart failure.**
EENT: cataracts, glaucoma.
GI: *peptic ulceration,* GI irritation, increased appetite, **pancreatitis,** nausea, vomiting.
GU: menstrual irregularities.
Metabolic: hypokalemia, hyperglycemia, carbohydrate intolerance.
Musculoskeletal: muscle weakness, osteoporosis, growth suppression in children.
Skin: delayed wound healing, acne, various skin eruptions, hirsutism.
Other: susceptibility to infections; *acute adrenal insufficiency (with increased stress from infection, surgery, or trauma);* cushingoid state (moonface, buffalo hump, central obesity).
    After abrupt withdrawal: rebound inflammation, fatigue, weakness, arthralgia, fever, dizziness, lethargy, depression, fainting, orthostatic hypotension, dyspnea, anorexia, hypoglycemia. *After prolonged use, sudden withdrawal may cause acute adrenal insufficiency and death.*

☑ Special considerations
• Recommendations for use of prednisone are the same as those for all systemic adrenocorticoids.
• For patients who can't swallow tablets, liquid forms are available. The oral concentrate (5 mg/ml) may be diluted in juice or another flavored diluent or mixed in semisolid food (such as applesauce) before administration.
• Prednisone suppresses reactions to skin tests; causes false-negative results in the nitroblue tetrazolium test for systemic bacterial infections.

Monitoring the patient
• Monitor patient's weight, blood pressure, and serum electrolyte levels.
• Monitor serum glucose in diabetic patients.

Information for the patient
• Recommendations for care and teaching of patients are the same as those for all systemic adrenocorticoids.
• Tell patient to report fluid retention when it occurs.
• Instruct patient to not become immunized during drug therapy.
• Advise patient to be aware of signs of infection; some of these signs may be masked during drug use.

Pediatric patients
● Prolonged use of prednisone in children or adolescents may delay growth and maturation.

---

primaquine phosphate

Pharmacologic classification: 8-amino-quinoline
Therapeutic classification: antimalarial
Pregnancy risk category C

How supplied
Available by prescription only
Tablets: 26.3 mg (15-mg base)

Indications, route, and dosage
Radical cure of relapsing vivax malaria, eliminating symptoms and infection completely, and prevention of relapse
Adults: 15 mg (base) P.O. daily for 14 days (26.3-mg tablet equals 15 mg of base), or 79 mg (45-mg base) once weekly for 8 weeks.
Children: 0.3 mg (base)/kg/day for 14 days, or 0.9 mg (base)/kg/day once weekly for 8 weeks.
◊ **Pneumocystis carinii** *pneumonia*
Adults: 15 to 30 mg (base) P.O. daily.

Pharmacodynamics
Antimalarial action: Disrupts the parasitic mitochondria, thereby interrupting metabolic processes requiring energy. Spectrum of activity includes preerythrocytic and exoerythrocytic forms of *Plasmodium falciparum, P. malariae, P. ovale,* and *P. vivax.* Nifurtimox (Lampit), an investigational drug available from the Centers for Disease Control and Prevention, is preferred for intracellular parasites.

Pharmacokinetics
● *Absorption:* Well absorbed from GI tract; levels peak in 2 to 6 hours.
● *Distribution:* Distributed widely into liver, lungs, heart, brain, skeletal muscle, and other tissues.
● *Metabolism:* Carboxylated rapidly in liver.
● *Excretion:* Only small amount of drug excreted unchanged in urine. Plasma half-life is 4 to 10 hours.

Contraindications and precautions
Contraindicated in patients with systemic diseases in which granulocytopenia may develop (such as lupus erythematosus or rheumatoid arthritis) and in those taking bone marrow suppressants and potentially hemolytic drugs.

Use cautiously in patients with previous idiosyncratic reaction (manifested by hemolytic anemia, methemoglobinemia, or leukopenia) and in those with family or personal history of favism, erythrocytic G6PD deficiency, or nicotinamide adenine dinucleotide (NADH) methemoglobin reductase deficiency.

Interactions
Drug-drug. *Aluminum salts, magnesium:* Decreased GI absorption. Separate administration times.
Quinacrine: Potentiated toxic effects of primaquine. Use together cautiously.

Adverse reactions
GI: nausea, vomiting, epigastric distress, abdominal cramps.
Hematologic: *leukopenia, hemolytic anemia in G6PD deficiency,* methemoglobinemia in NADH methemoglobin reductase deficiency.

☑ Special considerations
● Primaquine is often used with a fast-acting antimalarial such as chloroquine.
● Light-skinned patients taking more than 30 mg daily, dark-skinned patients taking more than 15 mg daily, and patients with severe anemia or suspected sensitivity should have frequent blood studies and urine examinations. A sudden fall in hemoglobin levels or erythrocyte or leukocyte counts, or a marked darkening of urine suggests impending hemolytic reaction.
● Toxicity may cause abdominal distress, vomiting, CNS and CV disturbances, cyanosis, methemoglobinemia, leukocytosis, leukopenia, and anemia.

Monitoring the patient
● Before starting therapy, screen patients for possible G6PD deficiency.
● Perform periodic blood studies and urinalyses to monitor patient for impending hemolytic reactions.

Information for the patient
● Teach patient signs and symptoms of adverse reactions and to report them if they occur.
● Advise patient to check urine color at each voiding and to report if urine darkens, becomes tinged with red, or decreases in volume.
● Tell patient to take drug with meals to minimize gastric irritation. Don't take with antacids, which may decrease absorption.
● Advise patient to complete entire course of therapy.

Breast-feeding patients
● It's unknown if drug appears in breast milk. Safety in breast-feeding women hasn't been established.

primidone
Mysoline

Pharmacologic classification: barbiturate analogue
Therapeutic classification: anticonvulsant
Pregnancy risk category NR

How supplied
Available by prescription only
Tablets: 50 mg, 250 mg
Suspension: 250 mg/5 ml

Indications, route, and dosage
Generalized tonic-clonic seizures, focal seizures, complex-partial (psychomotor) seizures
Adults and children ages 8 and over: 100 to 125 mg P.O. h.s. on days 1 to 3; 100 to 125 mg P.O. b.i.d. on days 4 to 6; 100 to 125 mg P.O. t.i.d. on days 7 to 9; and maintenance dose of 250 mg P.O. t.i.d. on day 10. May need up to 2 g/day.
Children under age 8: 50 mg P.O. h.s. on days 1 to 3; 50 mg P.O. b.i.d. on days 4 to 6; 100 mg P.O. t.i.d. on days 7 to 9; and maintenance dose of 125 to 250 mg P.O. t.i.d. on day 10.
Benign familial tremor (essential tremor)
Adults: 750 mg P.O. daily.

Pharmacodynamics
Anticonvulsant action: Mechanism unknown. Acts as a nonspecific CNS depressant used alone or with other anticonvulsants to control refractory tonic-clonic seizures and to treat psychomotor or focal seizures. Some activity may be from phenobarbital, an active metabolite.

Pharmacokinetics
• *Absorption:* Drug absorbed readily from GI tract; serum levels peak at about 3 hours. Phenobarbital appears in plasma after several days of continuous therapy; most laboratory assays detect both phenobarbital and primidone. Therapeutic levels 5 to 12 mcg/ml for primidone; 10 to 30 mcg/ml for phenobarbital.
• *Distribution:* Primidone distributed widely throughout body.
• *Metabolism:* Primidone metabolized slowly by liver to phenylethylmalonamide (PEMA) and phenobarbital; PEMA is major metabolite.
• *Excretion:* Primidone excreted in urine; substantial amounts excreted in breast milk.

Contraindications and precautions
Contraindicated in patients with phenobarbital hypersensitivity or porphyria.

Interactions
Drug-drug. *Acetazolamide, succinimides:* Decreased levels of primidone. Monitor patient closely.
Carbamazepine, phenytoin: Possible decreased effects of primidone; increased conversion to phenobarbital. Monitor serum levels to prevent toxicity.
CNS depressants (such as narcotic analgesics): Excessive depression in patients taking primidone. Avoid using together.
Oral contraceptives: Barbiturates may render oral contraceptives ineffective. Advise patient to consider a different birth control method.
Drug-lifestyle. *Alcohol:* Excessive depression in patients taking primidone. Discourage use.

Adverse reactions
CNS: *drowsiness, ataxia,* emotional disturbances, vertigo, hyperirritability, fatigue, paranoia.
EENT: *diplopia,* nystagmus.
GI: anorexia, nausea, vomiting.
GU: impotence, polyuria.
Hematologic: megaloblastic anemia, **thrombocytopenia.**
Hepatic: abnormalities in liver function test results.
Skin: morbilliform rash.

☑ Special considerations
Besides the recommendations relevant to all barbiturates, consider the following.
• Abrupt withdrawal of drug may cause status epilepticus; dosage should be reduced gradually.
• Barbiturates impair ability to perform tasks requiring mental alertness such as driving.
• Signs and symptoms of toxicity resemble those of barbiturate intoxication, including CNS and respiratory depression, areflexia, oliguria, tachycardia, hypotension, hypothermia, and coma. Shock may occur. Alkalinization of urine and forced diuresis may hasten excretion. Hemodialysis may be necessary.

Monitoring the patient
• Perform a CBC and liver function tests every 6 months.
• Monitor patient for adverse effects.

Information for the patient
• Explain rationale for therapy and potential risks and benefits.
• Teach patient signs and symptoms of adverse reactions.
• Tell patient to avoid alcohol and other sedatives to prevent added CNS depression.
• Instruct patient not to stop drug or to alter dosage without medical approval.
• Advise patient to avoid hazardous tasks that require mental alertness until degree of sedative effect is determined. Tell patient that dizziness

---

Reactions may be *common*, uncommon, **life-threatening**, or COMMON AND LIFE-THREATENING.

and incoordination are common at first but will disappear.
● Recommend that patient wear a medical identification bracelet or necklace identifying him as having a seizure disorder and listing drug.
● Tell patient to shake oral suspension well before use.

Geriatric patients
● Reduce dosage in elderly patients; many have decreased renal function.

Pediatric patients
● Drug may cause hyperexcitability in children under age 6.

Breast-feeding patients
● Considerable amounts of drug appear in breast milk. Use an alternative to breast-feeding during therapy.

probenecid
Benemid

Pharmacologic classification: sulfonamide derivative
Therapeutic classification: uricosuric
Pregnancy risk category NR

How supplied
Available by prescription only
Tablets: 500 mg

Indications, route, and dosage
Adjunct to penicillin therapy
Adults and children over age 14 or weighing over 50 kg (110 lb): 500 mg P.O. q.i.d.
Children age 2 to 14 or weighing under 50 kg: Initially, 25 mg/kg or 700 mg/m² daily; then 40 mg/kg or 1.2 g/m² divided q.i.d.
Single-dose penicillin treatment of gonorrhea
Adults: 1 g P.O. given together with penicillin treatment, or 1 g P.O. 30 minutes before I.M. dose of penicillin.
Hyperuricemia associated with gout
Adults: 250 mg P.O. b.i.d. for first week, then 500 mg b.i.d., to maximum of 2 to 3 g daily.
◊ **To diagnose parkinsonian syndrome or mental depression**
Adults: 500 mg P.O. q 12 hours for five doses.

Pharmacodynamics
Uricosuric action: Competitively inhibits the active reabsorption of uric acid at the proximal convoluted tubule, thereby increasing urinary excretion of uric acid.
Adjunctive action in antibiotic therapy: Competitively inhibits secretion of weak organic acids, such as penicillins, cephalosporins, and other beta-lactam antibiotics, thereby increasing serum levels of these drugs.

Pharmacokinetics
● *Absorption:* Completely absorbed after oral administration; serum levels peak in 2 to 4 hours.
● *Distribution:* Distributed throughout body; about 75% protein-bound. CSF levels about 2% of serum levels.
● *Metabolism:* Metabolized in liver to active metabolites, with some uricosuric effect.
● *Excretion:* Drug and metabolites excreted in urine; drug (but not metabolites) actively reabsorbed.

Contraindications and precautions
Contraindicated in patients with hypersensitivity to drug, in those with uric acid kidney stones or blood dyscrasias; in acute gout attack; and in children under age 2. Use cautiously in patients with impaired renal function or peptic ulcer.

Interactions
Drug-drug. *Aminosalicylic acid, dapsone, methotrexate, nitrofurantoin:* Increased serum levels; increased risk of toxicity of these drugs. Monitor patient for toxicity.
Bumetanide, ethacrynic acid, furosemide: Impaired natriuretic effects of these drugs. Adjust dosages as needed.
Cephalosporins, ketamine (possibly), penicillins, sulfonamides, thiopental (possibly), other beta-lactam antibiotics: Significant increased or prolonged effects of these drugs. Monitor patient closely.
Chlorpropamide, other oral sulfonylureas: Enhanced hypoglycemic effects. Adjust dosages as needed.
Diuretics, pyrazinamide: Decrease uric acid levels of probenecid. Increased doses of probenecid may be needed.
Indomethacin, naproxen: Decreased excretion of these drugs. Use lower dosages.
Salicylates: Inhibited uricosuric effect of probenecid only in doses that achieve levels of 50 mcg/ml or more; occasional use of low-dose aspirin doesn't interfere.
Weak organic acids: Inhibited urinary excretion of these drugs. Monitor patient.
Zidovudine: Increased bioavailability of zidovudine; cutaneous eruptions accompanied by systemic symptoms (including malaise, myalgia, or fever) possible. Monitor patient for toxicity.
Drug-lifestyle. *Alcohol:* Decreased uric acid levels of probenecid. Increased doses of probenecid may be needed with alcohol use.

Adverse reactions
CNS: *headache,* dizziness.
GI: anorexia, nausea, vomiting, sore gums.
GU: urinary frequency, renal colic, nephrotic syndrome.
Hematologic: *hemolytic anemia, aplastic anemia,* anemia.
Hepatic: *hepatic necrosis.*

Skin: dermatitis, pruritus.
Other: flushing, fever, exacerbation of gout, hypersensitivity reactions (including *anaphylaxis*).

☑ Special considerations
● When used for hyperuricemia associated with gout, probenecid has no analgesic or anti-inflammatory actions and no effect on acute attacks; start therapy after attack subsides. Because drug may increase frequency of acute attacks during first 6 to 12 months of therapy, prophylactic doses of colchicine or an NSAID should be given during first 3 to 6 months of probenecid therapy.
● Give with food, milk, or prescribed antacids to lessen GI upset.
● Maintain adequate hydration with high fluid intake to prevent formation of uric acid stones. Also maintain alkalinization of urine.
● Drug has been used in the diagnosis of parkinsonian syndrome and mental depression.
● Probenecid causes false-positive test results for urinary glucose with tests using cupric sulfate reagent (Benedict's reagent, Clinitest, and Fehling's test); perform tests with glucose oxidase reagent (Diastix, Chemstrip uG, or glucose enzymatic test strip) instead.
● Toxicity may cause nausea, copious vomiting, stupor, coma, and tonic-clonic seizures.

Monitoring the patient
● Monitor BUN and serum creatinine levels closely; drug is ineffective in severe renal insufficiency.
● Monitor uric acid levels and adjust dosage to lowest dose that maintains normal uric acid levels.

Information for the patient
● Instruct patient not to stop drug without medical approval.
● Warn patient not to use drug for pain or inflammation and not to increase dose during gouty attack.
● Tell patient to drink 8 to 10 glasses of fluid daily and to take drug with food to minimize GI upset.
● Warn patient to avoid aspirin and other salicylates, which may antagonize probenecid's uricosuric effect.
● Caution diabetic patients to use glucose enzymatic test strip, Diastix, or Chemstrip uG for urine glucose testing.

Geriatric patients
● Lower dosages are indicated in elderly patients.

Pediatric patients
● Drug is contraindicated in infants under age 2.

Breast-feeding patients
● It's unknown if drug appears in breast milk. An alternative to breast-feeding is recommended during therapy.

procainamide hydrochloride
Procanbid, Pronestyl, Pronestyl-SR

Pharmacologic classification: procaine derivative
Therapeutic classification: ventricular antiarrhythmic, supraventricular antiarrhythmic
Pregnancy risk category C

How supplied
Available by prescription only
Tablets: 250 mg, 375 mg, 500 mg
Tablets (extended-release): 500 mg, 1 g
Tablets (sustained-release): 250 mg, 500 mg, 750 mg
Capsules: 250 mg, 375 mg, 500 mg
Injection: 100 mg/ml, 500 mg/ml

Indications, route, and dosage
Symptomatic PVCs; life-threatening ventricular tachycardia; ◇ atrial fibrillation and flutter unresponsive to quinidine; ◇ paroxysmal atrial tachycardia
Adults: 50 to 100 mg q 5 minutes by slow I.V. push, no faster than 25 to 50 mg/minute, until arrhythmias disappear, adverse effects develop, or 500 mg has been given. When arrhythmias disappear, give continuous infusion of 1 to 6 mg/minute. Usual effective loading dose is 500 to 600 mg. If arrhythmias recur, repeat bolus as above and increase infusion rate. For I.M. administration, give 50 mg/kg divided q 3 to 6 hours; during surgery, 100 to 500 mg I.M. For oral therapy, initiate dosage at 50 mg/kg P.O. in divided doses q 3 hours until therapeutic levels are reached. Once patient is stable, may substitute sustained-release form q 6 hours or extended-release form at dose of 50 mg/kg in two divided doses q 12 hours.
◇ *Loading dose to prevent atrial fibrillation or paroxysmal atrial tachycardia*
Adults: 1 to 1.25 g P.O. If arrhythmias persist after 1 hour, give additional 750 mg. If no change occurs, give 500 mg to 1 g q 2 hours until arrhythmias disappear or adverse effects occur.
Loading dose to prevent ventricular tachycardia
Adults: 1 g P.O. Maintenance dose is 50 mg/kg/day given at 3-hour intervals; average is 250 to 500 mg q 4 hours but 1 to 1.5 g q 4 to 6 hours may be needed.
◇ *Malignant hyperthermia*
Adults: 200 to 900 mg I.V.; then an infusion.

Pharmacodynamics
Antiarrhythmic action: A class IA antiarrhythmic that depresses phase 0 of the action potential. Considered a myocardial depressant because it decreases myocardial excitability and conduction velocity and may depress myocardial con-

tractility. Also possesses anticholinergic activity, which may modify direct myocardial effects. In therapeutic doses, drug reduces conduction velocity in the atria, ventricles, and His-Purkinje system. Its effectiveness in controlling atrial tachyarrhythmias stems from its ability to prolong the effective refractory period (ERP) and increase the action potential duration in the atria, ventricles, and His-Purkinje system. Because ERP prolongation exceeds action potential duration, tissue remains refractory even after returning to resting membrane potential (membrane-stabilizing effect).

Procainamide shortens the effective refractory period of the AV node. Drug's anticholinergic action also may increase AV node conductivity. Suppression of automaticity in the His-Purkinje system and ectopic pacemakers accounts for drug's effectiveness in treating ventricular premature beats. At therapeutic doses, procainamide prolongs the PR and QT intervals. (This effect may be used as an index of drug effectiveness and toxicity.) The QRS complex usually isn't prolonged beyond normal range; the QT interval isn't prolonged to the extent achieved with quinidine.

Procainamide exerts a peripheral vasodilatory effect; with I.V. administration, it may cause hypotension, which limits the administration rate and amount of drug deliverable.

Pharmacokinetics

• *Absorption:* Rate and extent of absorption from intestines vary; usually, 75% to 95% of oral dose absorbed. With tablets and capsules, plasma levels peak in about 1 hour. Extended-release tablets formulated to provide sustained and relatively constant rate of release and absorption throughout small intestine. After drug's release, extended wax matrix isn't absorbed and may appear in feces after 15 minutes to 1 hour. With I.M. injection, onset of action in about 10 to 30 minutes; peak levels in about 1 hour.

• *Distribution:* Distributed widely in most body tissues, including CSF, liver, spleen, kidneys, lungs, muscles, brain, and heart. Only about 15% binds to plasma proteins. Usual therapeutic range of serum procainamide levels is 4 to 8 mcg/ml. Some experts suggest that a range of 10 to 30 mcg/ml for the sum of procainamide and N-acetyl procainamide (NAPA) serum levels is therapeutic.

• *Metabolism:* Drug is acetylated in liver to form NAPA. Acetylation rate determined genetically and affects NAPA formation. (NAPA also exerts antiarrhythmic activity.)

• *Excretion:* Procainamide and NAPA metabolite excreted in urine. Procainamide's half-life is about 2½ to 4¾ hours; NAPA's half-life is about 6 hours. In patients with heart failure or renal dysfunction, half-life increases; in such patients, dosage reduction required to avoid toxicity.

Contraindications and precautions

Contraindicated in patients with hypersensitivity to procaine and related drugs; in those with complete, second-, or third-degree heart block in the absence of an artificial pacemaker; and in patients with myasthenia gravis or systemic lupus erythematosus. Also contraindicated in patients with atypical ventricular tachycardia (torsades de pointes) because procainamide may aggravate this condition.

Use cautiously in patients with ventricular tachycardia during coronary occlusion, heart failure or other conduction disturbances (bundle-branch heart block, sinus bradycardia, cardiac glycoside intoxication), impaired renal or hepatic function, preexisting blood dyscrasia, or bone marrow suppression.

Interactions

Drug-drug. *Anticholinergics (atropine, diphenhydramine, tricyclic antidepressants):* Additive anticholinergic effects. Monitor patient closely.

Antihypertensives: Additive hypotensive effects (most common with I.V. procainamide). Monitor blood pressure.

Cholinergics (neostigmine, pyridostigmine, which are used to treat myasthenia gravis): May negate effects of these drugs. Increase dosage.

Cimetidine: Impaired renal clearance of procainamide and NAPA, with elevated serum drug levels. Adjust dose if used together.

Neuromuscular blockers (such as decamethonium bromide, gallium triethiodide, metocurine iodide, pancuronium bromide, succinylcholine chloride, tubocurarine chloride): Potentiated effects of neuromuscular blockers. Monitor patient closely.

Other antiarrhythmics: Additive or antagonistic cardiac effects; possible additive toxic effects. Monitor patient for toxicity.

Drug-herb. *Jimsonweed:* Possible adverse effect on cardiovascular system function. Discourage use.

Licorice: Possible prolonged QT interval; potentially additive. Use together cautiously.

Adverse reactions

CNS: hallucinations, confusion, *seizures,* depression, dizziness.

CV: *hypotension,* **ventricular asystole, bradycardia, AV block, ventricular fibrillation** (after parenteral use).

GI: nausea, vomiting, anorexia, diarrhea, bitter taste.

Hematologic: **thrombocytopenia, neutropenia** (especially with sustained-release forms), **agranulocytosis, hemolytic anemia.**

Hepatic: increased liver function tests.

Skin: *maculopapular rash, urticaria, pruritus, flushing, angioneurotic edema.*

Other: *fever, lupuslike syndrome* (especially after prolonged administration), positive antinuclear antibody (ANA) titers, positive direct antiglobulin (Coombs') tests.

☑ Special considerations
• In treating atrial fibrillation and flutter, ventricular rate may accelerate because of vagolytic effects on the AV node; to prevent this effect, a cardiac glycoside may be administered before procainamide therapy begins.
• Infusion pump or microdrip system and timer should be used to monitor infusion precisely.
• For initial oral therapy, use conventional capsules and tablets; use extended-release tablets only for maintenance therapy.
• I.V. drug form is more likely to cause adverse cardiac effects, possibly resulting in severe hypotension.
• Procainamide will invalidate bentiromide test results; discontinue at least 3 days before bentiromide test. Procainamide may alter edrophonium test results.
• Toxicity may cause severe hypotension, widening QRS complex, junctional tachycardia, intraventricular conduction delay, ventricular fibrillation, oliguria, confusion and lethargy, and nausea and vomiting. Phenylephrine or norepinephrine may be used to treat hypotension after adequate hydration has been ensured. Hemodialysis may be effective in removing procainamide and NAPA. A 1/6 M solution of sodium lactate may reduce procainamide's cardiotoxic effect.

Monitoring the patient
• Monitor patient receiving infusions at all times.
• Monitor blood pressure and ECG continuously during I.V. administration. Watch for prolonged QT interval and QRS complex (50% or greater widening), heart block, or increased arrhythmias. When these ECG signs appear, stop drug and monitor patient closely.
• Monitor therapeutic serum levels of procainamide: 3 to 10 mcg/ml (most patients are controlled at 4 to 8 mcg/ml; may exhibit toxicity at levels greater than 16 mcg/ml). Monitor NAPA levels as well; some clinicians feel that procainamide and NAPA levels should be 10 to 30 mcg/ml.
• Baseline and periodic determinations of ANA titers, lupus erythematosus cell preparations, and CBCs may be indicated because procainamide therapy (usually long-term) has been associated with a syndrome resembling systemic lupus erythematosus.
• In prolonged use of oral form, perform ECGs occasionally to determine continued need for drug.

Information for the patient
• Stress importance of taking drug exactly as prescribed.

• Instruct patient to report fever, rash, muscle pain, diarrhea, bleeding, bruises, or pleuritic chest pain.
• Tell patient not to crush or break sustained-release tablets.
• Reassure patient who is taking extended-release form that a wax-matrix "ghost" from tablet may be passed in stools. Drug is completely absorbed before this occurs.

Geriatric patients
• Elderly patients may need reduced dosage. Because of highly variable metabolism, monitoring of serum levels is recommended.

Pediatric patients
• Manufacturer hasn't established dosage guidelines for children. For treating arrhythmias, the suggested dosage is 40 to 60 mg/kg of standard tablets or capsules, P.O. daily, given in four to six divided doses; or 3 to 6 mg/kg I.V. over 5 minutes, then a drip of 0.02 to 0.08 mg/kg/minute.

Breast-feeding patients
• Procainamide and NAPA appear in breast milk. An alternative to breast-feeding is recommended for breast-feeding women.

procarbazine hydrochloride
Matulane, Natulan*

Pharmacologic classification: antibiotic antineoplastic (cell cycle–phase specific, S phase)
Therapeutic classification: antineoplastic
Pregnancy risk category D

How supplied
Available by prescription only
Capsules: 50 mg

Indications, route, and dosage
Dosage and indications may vary. Check current literature for recommended protocol.
Hodgkin's disease, lymphomas, brain and lung cancer
Adults: 2 to 4 mg/kg/day P.O. in single or divided doses for the first week; then 4 to 6 mg/kg/day until response or toxicity occurs. Maintenance dose is 1 to 2 mg/kg/day.
Children: 50 mg/m² daily P.O. for first week; then 100 mg/m² daily until response or toxicity occurs. Maintenance dose is 50 mg/m² P.O. daily after bone marrow recovery.

Pharmacodynamics
Antineoplastic action: Exact mechanism unknown. Appears to have several sites of action, resulting in inhibition of DNA, RNA, and protein synthesis. Has also been reported to damage DNA direct-

---

Reactions may be *common*, uncommon, **life-threatening**, or COMMON AND LIFE-THREATENING.

ly and to inhibit the mitotic S phase of cell division.

Pharmacokinetics

• *Absorption:* Rapidly and completely absorbed after oral administration.
• *Distribution:* Distributed widely into body tissues; highest levels found in liver, kidneys, intestinal wall, and skin. Crosses blood-brain barrier.
• *Metabolism:* Extensively metabolized in liver. Some metabolites have cytotoxic activity.
• *Excretion:* Drug and metabolites excreted primarily in urine.

Contraindications and precautions

Contraindicated in patients hypersensitive to drug and in those with inadequate bone marrow reserve as shown by bone marrow aspiration. Use cautiously in patients with impaired renal or hepatic function.

Interactions

Drug-drug. *CNS depressants:* Enhanced CNS depression through additive mechanism. Monitor patient.
Digoxin: Possible decreased serum digoxin levels. Monitor serum digoxin levels.
Levodopa: Flushing and significant rise in blood pressure. Use together cautiously.
MAO inhibitors, selective serotonin reuptake inhibitors, sympathomimetics, tricyclic antidepressants: Inhibition of MAO by procarbazine; hypertensive crisis, tremors, excitation, and cardiac palpitations. Don't use together.
Meperidine: Severe hypotension and death. Don't use together.
Drug-food. *Foods containing tyramine:* Inhibition of MAO by procarbazine; hypertensive crisis, tremors, excitation, and cardiac palpitations. Don't give together.
Drug-lifestyle. *Alcohol:* Disulfiram-like reaction. Discourage use.
Sun exposure: Photosensitivity reactions. Tell patient to take precautions.

Adverse reactions

CNS: nervousness, depression, headache, dizziness, *coma, seizures,* insomnia, nightmares, paresthesia, neuropathy, *hallucinations,* confusion.
CV: hypotension, tachycardia, syncope.
EENT: retinal hemorrhage, nystagmus, photophobia.
GI: *nausea, vomiting,* anorexia, stomatitis, dry mouth, dysphagia, diarrhea, constipation.
GU: hematuria, urinary frequency, nocturia, gynecomastia.
Hematologic: *bleeding tendency, thrombocytopenia, leukopenia, anemia,* hemolytic anemia.
Respiratory: *pleural effusion,* pneumonitis, cough.

Skin: dermatitis, pruritus, rash, reversible alopecia.
Other: *allergic reactions.*

☑ Special considerations

• Nausea and vomiting may be decreased if drug is taken at bedtime and in divided doses.
• Procarbazine inhibits MAO. Use procarbazine cautiously with MAO inhibitors, tricyclic antidepressants and selective serotonin reuptake inhibitors, other drugs that interact with MAO inhibitors, or tyramine-rich foods.
• Use cautiously in patients with inadequate bone marrow reserve, leukopenia, thrombocytopenia, anemia, and impaired hepatic or renal function.
• Store capsules in dry environment.
• Toxicity may cause myalgia, arthralgia, fever, weakness, dermatitis, alopecia, paresthesia, hallucinations, tremors, seizures, coma, myelosuppression, nausea, and vomiting.

Monitoring the patient

• Watch for signs of bleeding and monitor patient for other adverse effects..

Information for the patient

• Emphasize importance of continuing drug despite nausea and vomiting.
• Advise patient to call immediately if vomiting occurs shortly after taking dose.
• Warn patient that drowsiness may occur, so patient should avoid hazardous activities that require alertness until drug's effect is established.
• Warn patient not to drink alcoholic beverages or eat foods containing tyramine while taking drug.
• Instruct patient to stop drug and call immediately if disulfiram-like reaction occurs (chest pains, rapid or irregular heartbeat, severe headache, stiff neck).
• Tell patient to avoid exposure to people with infections.
• Warn patient to avoid prolonged sun exposure because photosensitivity occurs during therapy.
• Tell patient to call if a sore throat or fever or unusual bruising or bleeding occurs.

Pediatric patients

• Severe reactions, such as tremors, seizures, and coma, have occurred in children receiving drug.

Breast-feeding patients

• It's unknown if drug appears in breast milk. Because of potential for serious adverse reactions, mutagenicity, and carcinogenicity in infant, breast-feeding isn't recommended.

prochlorperazine
Compazine, Stemetil*

prochlorperazine edisylate
Compazine

prochlorperazine maleate
Compazine, Compazine Spansule, Stemetil*

Pharmacologic classification: phenothiazine (piperazine derivative)
Therapeutic classification: antipsychotic, antiemetic, anxiolytic
Pregnancy risk category C

How supplied
Available by prescription only
prochlorperazine maleate
Tablets: 5 mg, 10 mg, 25 mg
prochlorperazine edisylate
Spansules (sustained-release): 10 mg, 15 mg, 30 mg
Syrup: 1 mg/ml
Injection: 5 mg/ml
Suppositories: 2.5 mg, 5 mg, 25 mg

Indications, route, and dosage
Preoperative nausea control
Adults: 5 to 10 mg I.M. 1 to 2 hours before induction of anesthesia, repeated once in 30 minutes if necessary; or 5 to 10 mg I.V. 15 to 30 minutes before induction of anesthesia, repeated once if necessary; or 20 mg/L D₅W and normal saline solution by I.V. infusion, added to infusion 15 to 30 minutes before induction. Maximum parenteral dose is 40 mg daily.
Severe nausea, vomiting
Adults: 5 to 10 mg P.O. t.i.d. or q.i.d.; or 15 mg of sustained-release form P.O. on arising; or 10 mg of sustained-release form P.O. q 12 hours; or 25 mg P.R. b.i.d.; or 5 to 10 mg I.M. injected deeply into upper outer quadrant of gluteal region. Repeat q 3 to 4 hours, p.r.n. May be given I.V. Maximum parenteral dose is 40 mg daily.
Children weighing 18 to 39 kg (39 to 86 lb): 2.5 mg P.O. or P.R. t.i.d.; or 5 mg P.O. or P.R. b.i.d.; or 0.132 mg/kg deep I.M. injection. (Control usually obtained with one dose.) Maximum dose is 15 mg daily.
Children weighing 14 to 17 kg (31 to 38 lb): 2.5 mg P.O. or P.R. b.i.d. or t.i.d.; or 0.132 mg/kg deep I.M. injection. (Control usually obtained with one dose.) Maximum dose is 10 mg daily.
Children weighing 9 to 14 kg (20 to 30 lb): 2.5 mg P.O. or P.R. daily or b.i.d.; or 0.132 mg/kg deep I.M. injection. (Control usually obtained with one dose.) Maximum dose is 7.5 mg daily.
Anxiety
Adults: 5 mg P.O. t.i.d. or q.i.d.

Psychotic disorders
Adults: 5 to 10 mg P.O. or 10 to 20 mg I.M. t.i.d. or q.i.d.; up to 150 mg daily P.O. for hospitalized patients.

Pharmacodynamics
Antipsychotic action: Thought to exert antipsychotic effects by postsynaptic blockade of CNS dopamine receptors, thus inhibiting dopamine-mediated effects.
Antiemetic action: Effects attributed to dopamine receptor blockade in the medullary chemoreceptor trigger zone.
  Has many other central and peripheral effects: Produces alpha and ganglionic blockade and counteracts histamine- and serotonin-mediated activity. Most prevalent adverse reactions are extrapyramidal. Used primarily as an antiemetic; ineffective against motion sickness.

Pharmacokinetics
• *Absorption:* Rate and extent of absorption vary with administration route. Oral tablet absorption is erratic and variable; onset of action ranging from ½ to 1 hour. Oral concentrate absorption more predictable. I.M. drug absorbed rapidly.
• *Distribution:* Distributed widely into body, including breast milk. 91% to 99% protein-bound. Peak effect at 2 to 4 hours; steady-state serum levels within 4 to 7 days.
• *Metabolism:* Metabolized extensively by liver; no active metabolites formed. Duration of action about 3 to 4 hours; 10 to 12 hours for extended-release form.
• *Excretion:* Mostly excreted in urine via kidneys; some excreted in feces via biliary tract.

Contraindications and precautions
Contraindicated in patients with hypersensitivity to phenothiazines and in those with CNS depression including coma; during pediatric surgery; when using spinal or epidural anesthetic, adrenergic blockers, or ethanol; and in infants under age 2.
  Use cautiously in patients with impaired CV function, glaucoma, or seizure disorders; in those who have been exposed to extreme heat; and in children with acute illness.

Interactions
Drug-drug. *Antacids containing aluminum and magnesium; antidiarrheals:* Inhibited absorption. Separate administration times by at least 2 hours.
Antiarrhythmics, disopyramide, procainamide, quinidine: Increased risk of arrhythmias and conduction defects. Avoid using together.
Appetite suppressants, sympathomimetics (such as ephedrine [commonly found in nasal sprays], epinephrine, phenylephrine, phenylpropanolamine): Decreased stimulatory and pressor effects; possible epinephrine reversal (hypotensive

response to epinephrine). Use together cautiously; don't use with epinephrine.

Atropine, other anticholinergics (such as antidepressants, antihistamines, antiparkinsonians, MAO inhibitors, meperidine, phenothiazines): Oversedation, paralytic ileus, visual changes, and severe constipation. Avoid concomitant use.

Beta blockers: Inhibited prochlorperazine metabolism, increasing plasma levels and toxicity. Adjust dosage as needed.

Bromocriptine: Antagonized prolactin secretion. Monitor patient closely.

Centrally acting antihypertensives (such as clonidine, guanabenz, guanadrel, guanethidine, methyldopa, reserpine): Inhibited blood pressure response. Monitor blood pressure.

CNS depressants (such as anesthetics [epidural, general, spinal], barbiturates, narcotics, parenteral magnesium sulfate, tranquilizers): Oversedation, respiratory depression, and hypotension. Monitor patient closely.

High-dose dopamine: Decreased vasoconstricting effects. Monitor patient closely.

Levodopa: Decreased effectiveness and increased toxicity of levodopa. Monitor patient for drug effect.

Lithium: Severe neurologic toxicity with encephalitis-like syndrome; decreased therapeutic response to prochlorperazine. Avoid concomitant use.

Metrizamide: Increased risk of seizures. Use together cautiously.

Nitrates: Hypotension. Monitor blood pressure.

Phenobarbital: Enhanced renal excretion of perphenazine. Adjust dosage as needed.

Phenytoin: Inhibited metabolism and increased toxicity of phenytoin. Monitor patient closely.

Propylthiouracil: Increased risk of agranulocytosis. Monitor hematologic studies.

Drug-food. *Caffeine:* Decreased therapeutic response to prochlorperazine. Discourage use.

Drug-lifestyle. *Alcohol:* Additive effects. Discourage use.

Heavy smoking: Increased prochlorperazine metabolism. Discourage smoking.

Sun exposure: Photosensitivity reactions. Tell patient to take precautions.

Adverse reactions

CNS: *extrapyramidal reactions,* sedation, pseudoparkinsonism, EEG changes, dizziness.
CV: *orthostatic hypotension,* tachycardia, ECG changes.
EENT: *ocular changes, blurred vision.*
GI: *dry mouth, constipation,* ileus, increased appetite.
GU: *urine retention,* dark urine, menstrual irregularities, inhibited ejaculation, hyperprolactinemia, gynecomastia.
Hematologic: *transient leukopenia, agranulocytosis, thrombocytopenia, hemolytic anemia.*

Hepatic: *cholestatic jaundice.*
Metabolic: weight gain, hyperglycemia or hypoglycemia.
Skin: mild photosensitivity, *allergic reactions, exfoliative dermatitis.*

☑ Special considerations

Besides the recommendations relevant to all phenothiazines, consider the following.
● Liquid and injectable formulations may cause a rash after contact with skin.
● Drug may cause a pink to brown discoloration of urine.
● Drug is associated with a high risk of extrapyramidal effects and, in institutionalized psychiatric patients, photosensitivity reactions; patient should avoid exposure to sunlight or heat lamps.
● Oral formulations may cause stomach upset. Administer with food or fluid.
● Don't give sustained-release form to children.
● Solution for injection may be slightly discolored. Don't use if excessively discolored or if a precipitate is evident. Contact pharmacist.
● Dilute concentrate in 60 to 120 ml (2 to 4 oz) of water. Store suppository form in a cool place.
● Give I.V. dose slowly (5 mg/minute). I.M. injection may cause skin necrosis; take care to prevent extravasation. Don't mix with other drugs in syringe. Don't administer S.C.
● Administer I.M. injection deep into upper outer quadrant of buttock. Massaging area after administration may prevent formation of abscesses.
● Drug is ineffective in treating motion sickness.
● Protect liquid formulation from light.
● Prochlorperazine causes false-positive test results for urinary porphyrins, urobilinogen, amylase, and 5-hydroxyindoleacetic acid because of darkening of urine by metabolites; also causes false-positive urine pregnancy results in tests using human chorionic gonadotropin as the indicator.
● Toxicity may cause CNS depression characterized by deep, unarousable sleep and possible coma, hypotension or hypertension, extrapyramidal symptoms, dystonia, abnormal involuntary muscle movements, agitation, seizures, arrhythmias, ECG changes, hypothermia or hyperthermia, and autonomic nervous system dysfunction.
● To treat overdose, don't induce vomiting. Drug inhibits cough reflex, and aspiration may occur. Use gastric lavage, then activated charcoal and saline cathartics; dialysis doesn't help. Regulate body temperature as needed. Treat hypotension with I.V. fluids. Don't give epinephrine. Treat seizures with parenteral diazepam or barbiturates; arrhythmias with parenteral phenytoin (1 mg/kg with rate titrated to blood pressure); and extrapyramidal reactions with benztropine or parenteral diphenhydramine 2 mg/kg/minute.

Monitoring the patient
• Monitor patient's blood pressure before and after parenteral administration.
• Monitor therapeutic effect.

Information for the patient
• Explain risks of dystonic reactions and tardive dyskinesia. Tell patient to promptly report abnormal body movements.
• Tell patient to avoid sun exposure and to wear sunscreen when going outdoors to prevent photosensitivity reactions. (Note that heat lamps and tanning beds also may cause skin burning or skin discoloration.)
• Tell patient to avoid spilling liquid form. Contact with skin may cause rash and irritation.
• Warn patient to avoid extremely hot or cold baths and exposure to temperature extremes, sunlamps, or tanning beds; drug may cause thermoregulatory changes.
• Advise patient to take drug exactly as prescribed, not to double doses after missing one, and not to share drug with others.
• Warn patient to avoid alcohol or taking other drugs that may cause excessive sedation.
• Tell patient to dilute concentrate in water; explain dropper technique of measuring dose; teach correct use of suppository.
• Tell patient that hard candy, chewing gum, or ice chips can alleviate dry mouth.
• Urge patient to store drug safely away from children.
• Inform patient that interactions are possible with many drugs. Warn him to seek medical approval before taking OTC products.
• Warn patient not to stop taking drug suddenly and to promptly report difficulty urinating, sore throat, dizziness, or fainting. Reassure patient that most reactions can be relieved by reducing dosage.
• Caution patient to avoid hazardous activities that require alertness until drug's effect is known. Reassure patient that sedative effects subside and become tolerable in several weeks.

Geriatric patients
• Elderly patients tend to require lower dosages, adjusted to individual effects. These patients are at greater risk for adverse reactions, especially tardive dyskinesia, other extrapyramidal effects, and hypotension.

Pediatric patients
• Drug isn't recommended for patients under age 2 or weighing less than 20 lb (9 kg).

Breast-feeding patients
• Drug may appear in breast milk; use with caution. Potential benefits to mother should outweigh potential harm to infant.

progesterone
Crinone

Pharmacologic classification: progestin
Therapeutic classification: progestin, contraceptive
Pregnancy risk category X

How supplied
Available by prescription only
Gel: 4% (45 mg), 8% (90 mg)
Injection: 50 mg/ml (in oil)

Indications, route, and dosage
Amenorrhea
Adults: 5 to 10 mg I.M. daily for 6 to 8 days. Or, for secondary amenorrhea, one application of 4% gel vaginally every other day up to a total of six doses. If no response, may use Crinone 8% every other day up to a total of six doses.
Dysfunctional uterine bleeding
Adults: 5 to 10 mg I.M. daily for 6 days. Or a single 50 to 100 mg I.M. dose.
Corpus luteum insufficiency
Adults: 12.5 mg I.M. initiated within several days of ovulation and continuing for 2 weeks. May continue for up to 11th week of gestation. Or, for infertility, one application of 8% gel vaginally, daily or b.i.d. If pregnancy occurs, treatment may be continued until placental autonomy is achieved up to 10 to 12 weeks.

Pharmacodynamics
Contraceptive action: Suppresses ovulation, thickens cervical mucus, and induces endometrial sloughing.

Pharmacokinetics
• *Absorption:* Must be administered parenterally; inactivated by liver after oral administration.
• *Distribution:* Little information available.
• *Metabolism:* Progesterone reduced to pregnanediol in liver, then conjugated with glucuronic acid. Short plasma half-life of progesterone (several minutes).
• *Excretion:* Glucuronide-conjugated pregnanediol excreted in urine.

Contraindications and precautions
Contraindicated in patients with hypersensitivity to drug and in those with thromboembolic disorders or cerebral apoplexy (or history of these conditions), breast cancer, undiagnosed abnormal vaginal bleeding, severe hepatic disease, or missed abortion.
    Use cautiously in patients with diabetes mellitus, seizures, migraines, cardiac or renal disease, asthma, or mental depression.

Interactions
Drug-drug. *Bromocriptine:* Progesterone may cause amenorrhea or galactorrhea, interfering with bromocriptine's action. Don't use concurrently.

Adverse reactions
CNS: depression, somnolence, headache.
CV: thrombophlebitis, ***thromboembolism, CVA, pulmonary embolism,*** edema.
GI: nausea, constipation, diarrhea, vomiting.
GU: breakthrough bleeding, dysmenorrhea, amenorrhea, cervical erosion, abnormal secretions, nocturia, breast tenderness, enlargement, or secretion; decreased pregnanediol excretion.
Hepatic: cholestatic jaundice.
Metabolic: increased serum alkaline phosphatase and amino acid levels.
Skin: melasma, rash, acne, pruritus, pain at injection site.

☑ Special considerations
Besides the recommendations relevant to all progestins, consider the following.
• Parenteral form is for I.M. administration only. Inject deep into large muscle mass, preferably gluteal muscle.
• Large doses of progesterone may cause a moderate catabolic effect and a transient increase in sodium and chloride excretion.

Monitoring the patient
• Check parenteral injection sites for irritation.
• Monitor patient for adverse effects.

Information for the patient
• Advise patient that withdrawal bleeding usually occurs 2 to 3 days after stopping drug.
• Instruct patient to call promptly if she suspects pregnancy during therapy.
• For patient using Crinone gel, advise her not to use gel concurrently with other local intravaginal therapy. If other local intravaginal therapy is used concurrently, there should be at least a 6-hour period before or after gel administration.

Breast-feeding patients
• Because drug appears in breast milk, its use is contraindicated in breast-feeding women.

promethazine hydrochloride
Anergan 25, Anergan 50, Histantil*, Phencen-50, Phenergan, Phenergan Fortis, Phenergan Plain, Phenoject-50, V-Gan-25, V-Gan-50

Pharmacologic classification: phenothiazine derivative
Therapeutic classification: antiemetic antivertigo drug, antihistamine (H_1-receptor antagonist), preoperative, postoperative, or obstetric sedative and adjunct to analgesics
Pregnancy risk category NR

How supplied
Available by prescription only
Tablets: 12.5 mg, 25 mg, 50 mg
Syrup: 6.25 mg/5 ml, 25 mg/5 ml
Suppositories: 12.5 mg, 25 mg, 50 mg
Injection: 25 mg/ml, 50 mg/ml

Indications, route, and dosage
Motion sickness
Adults: 25 mg P.O. b.i.d.
Children: 12.5 to 25 mg P.O., I.M., or P.R. b.i.d.
Nausea
Adults: 12.5 to 25 mg P.O., I.M., or P.R. q 4 to 6 hours, p.r.n.
Children: 0.25 to 0.5 mg/kg I.M. or P.R. q 4 to 6 hours, p.r.n.
Rhinitis, allergy symptoms
Adults: 12.5 to 25 mg P.O. before meals and h.s., or 25 mg P.O. h.s.
Children: 6.25 to 12.5 mg P.O. t.i.d., or 25 mg P.O. or P.R. h.s.
Sedation
Adults: 25 to 50 mg P.O. or I.M. h.s. or p.r.n.
Children: 12.5 to 25 mg P.O., I.M., or P.R. h.s.
Routine preoperative or postoperative sedation or as an adjunct to analgesics
Adults: 25 to 50 mg I.M., I.V., or P.O.
Children: 12.5 to 25 mg I.M., I.V., or P.O.
Obstetric sedation
25 to 50 mg I.M. or I.V. in early stages of labor, and 25 to 75 mg after labor is established; repeat q 2 to 4 hours, p.r.n. Maximum daily dose is 100 mg.

Pharmacodynamics
Antiemetic and antivertigo actions: The central antimuscarinic actions of antihistamines probably are responsible for their antivertigo and antiemetic effects; promethazine also is believed to inhibit the medullary chemoreceptor trigger zone.
Antihistamine action: Competes with histamine for the H_1-receptor, thereby suppressing allergic rhinitis and urticaria; drug doesn't prevent the release of histamine.

Sedative action: Mechanism unknown; probably causes sedation by reducing stimuli to the brainstem reticular system.

Pharmacokinetics

- *Absorption:* Well absorbed from GI tract. Onset begins 20 minutes after P.O., P.R., or I.M. administration; within 3 to 5 minutes after I.V. administration. Effects usually last 4 to 6 hours but may last for 12 hours.
- *Distribution:* Distributed widely throughout body; crosses placenta.
- *Metabolism:* Metabolized in liver.
- *Excretion:* Metabolites excreted in urine and feces.

Contraindications and precautions

Contraindicated in patients with hypersensitivity to drug; in those with intestinal obstruction, prostatic hyperplasia, bladder neck obstruction, seizure disorders, coma, CNS depression, or stenosing peptic ulcerations; in newborns, premature neonates, and breast-feeding patients; and in acutely ill or dehydrated children.

Use cautiously in patients with asthma or cardiac, pulmonary, or hepatic disease.

Interactions

Drug-drug. *Epinephrine:* Partial adrenergic blockade; further hypotension. Monitor blood pressure.
Levodopa: Possible block of levodopa's antiparkinsonian action. Monitor patient.
MAO inhibitors: Interference with detoxification of antihistamines and phenothiazines; prolonged and intensified sedative and anticholinergic effects. Avoid concomitant use.
Other antihistamines or CNS depressants (such as anxiolytics, barbiturates, sleeping aids, tranquilizers): Additive CNS depression. Use together cautiously.
Drug-lifestyle. *Alcohol:* Additive CNS depression. Discourage use.
Sun exposure: Photosensitivity reactions. Tell patient to take precautions.

Adverse reactions

CNS: *sedation,* confusion, sleepiness, dizziness, disorientation, extrapyramidal symptoms, *drowsiness.*
CV: hypotension, hypertension.
EENT: blurred vision.
GI: nausea, vomiting, *dry mouth.*
GU: urine retention.
Hematologic: *leukopenia, agranulocytosis, thrombocytopenia.*
Metabolic: hyperglycemia.
Skin: photosensitivity, rash.

☑ Special considerations

Besides the recommendations relevant to all phenothiazines, consider the following.

- Pronounced sedative effects may limit use in some ambulatory patients.
- The 50 mg/ml concentration is for I.M. use only; inject deep into large muscle mass. Don't administer drug S.C.; this may cause chemical irritation and necrosis. Drug may be administered I.V., in concentrations not to exceed 25 mg/ml and at a rate not to exceed 25 mg/minute. When using I.V. drip, wrap in aluminum foil to protect drug from light.
- Promethazine and meperidine (Demerol) may be mixed in same syringe.
- Stop drug 4 days before diagnostic skin tests to avoid preventing, reducing, or masking test response. Promethazine may cause either false-positive or false-negative pregnancy test results. It also may interfere with blood grouping in the ABO system.
- Toxicity may cause CNS depression (sedation, reduced mental alertness, apnea, and CV collapse) or CNS stimulation (insomnia, hallucinations, tremors, or seizures). Atropine-like signs and symptoms, such as dry mouth, flushed skin, fixed and dilated pupils, and GI symptoms, are common, especially in children. Urinary acidification promotes excretion of drug.

Monitoring the patient

- Monitor patient for adverse effects.

Information for the patient

- Warn patient about possible photosensitivity and ways to avoid it.
- When treating motion sickness, tell patient to take first dose 30 to 60 minutes before travel; on succeeding days, he should take dose upon arising and with evening meal.

Geriatric patients

- Elderly patients are usually more sensitive to adverse effects of antihistamines and are especially likely to experience a greater degree of dizziness, sedation, hyperexcitability, dry mouth, and urine retention than younger patients. Symptoms usually respond to a decrease in dosage.

Pediatric patients

- Use cautiously in children with respiratory dysfunction. Safety and efficacy in children younger than age 2 haven't been established; don't give drug to infants under age 3 months.

Breast-feeding patients

- Antihistamines such as promethazine shouldn't be used during breast-feeding. Many of these drugs appear in breast milk, exposing infants to risks of unusual excitability, especially premature infants and other neonates, who may experience seizures.

Reactions may be *common,* uncommon, **life-threatening,** or COMMON AND LIFE-THREATENING.

propafenone hydrochloride
Rythmol

Pharmacologic classification: sodium
channel antagonist
Therapeutic classification: antiarrhythmic
Pregnancy risk category C

How supplied
Available by prescription only
Tablets: 150 mg, 225 mg, 300 mg

Indications, route, and dosage
**Suppression of documented life-threatening
ventricular arrhythmias**
Adults: Initially, 150 mg P.O. q 8 hours. Dose may
be increased to 225 mg q 8 hours after 3 or 4
days; if necessary, increase dose to 300 mg q 8
hours. Maximum daily dose is 900 mg.
♦ Dosage adjustment. Reduce dosage in patients with hepatic failure to 20% to 30% of usual dosage.

Pharmacodynamics
Antiarrhythmic action: Reduces the inward sodium current in myocardial cells and Purkinje fibers;
also has weak beta-adrenergic blocking effects.
Slows the upstroke velocity of the action potential (phase 0 depolarization) and slows conduction in the AV node, His-Purkinje system, and intraventricular conduction system and prolongs
the refractory period in the AV node.

Pharmacokinetics
• *Absorption:* Well absorbed from GI tract; absorption not affected by food. Significant first-pass
effect; limited bioavailability. Increases with dosage.
Absolute bioavailability is 3.4% with 150-mg tablet;
10.6% with 300-mg tablet. Plasma levels peak
about 3½ hours after administration.
• *Distribution:* Rapidly distributed into lung, liver,
and heart tissue. The degree of protein binding
is concentration dependent. Drug crosses the
placenta and appears in breast milk. Distribution
of drug and its metabolites hasn't been fully described.
• *Metabolism:* Metabolized in liver, with a significant first-pass effect. Two active metabolites identified: 5-hydroxypropafenone and N-depropyl-
propafenone. 10% of all patients and patients receiving quinidine metabolize drug more slowly.
Little (if any) 5-hydroxypropafenone present in
plasma.
• *Excretion:* Elimination half-life 2 to 10 hours in
normal metabolizers (about 90% of patients); can
be as long as 10 to 32 hours in slow metabolizers.

Contraindications and precautions
Contraindicated in patients with hypersensitivity
to drug and in those with severe or uncontrolled
heart failure; cardiogenic shock; SA, AV, or intraventricular disorders of impulse conduction in
the absence of a pacemaker; bradycardia; marked
hypotension; bronchospastic disorders; or electrolyte imbalance.
  Use cautiously in patients with renal or hepatic failure or heart failure, and in those receiving other cardiac depressant drugs.

Interactions
Drug-drug. *Beta blockers (such as metoprolol,
propranolol):* Increased plasma levels of these
drugs. Use together cautiously.
Cimetidine: Increased plasma levels of propafenone. Monitor patient closely.
Digoxin: Dose-related increase in plasma digoxin levels, ranging from 35% at 450 mg/day to 85%
at 900 mg/day. Monitor plasma digoxin levels
closely; adjust dosage of digoxin as necessary.
Local anesthetics: Increased risk of CNS toxicity. Use together cautiously.
Quinidine: Competitively inhibits one of the metabolic pathways for propafenone, increasing its
half-life. Don't give together.
Warfarin: Increased INR. Monitor PT and INR.

Adverse reactions
CNS: anxiety, ataxia, *dizziness,* drowsiness, fatigue, headache, insomnia, syncope, tremor.
CV: atrial fibrillation, bradycardia, bundle-branch
block, angina, chest pain, edema, first-degree
AV block, hypotension, increased QRS complex
duration, intraventricular conduction delay, palpitations, **heart failure, proarrhythmic events
(ventricular tachycardia, PVCs, ventricular
fibrillation).**
EENT: blurred vision.
GI: abdominal pain or cramps, constipation, diarrhea, dyspepsia, anorexia, flatulence, *nausea,
vomiting,* dry mouth, unusual taste.
Musculoskeletal: joint pain.
Respiratory: dyspnea.
Skin: diaphoresis, rash.

☑ Special considerations
• Propafenone pharmacokinetics are complex;
studies have shown that a threefold increase in
daily dose (from 300 to 900 mg/day) may produce a tenfold increase in plasma levels. Dosage
must be individualized for each patient.
• Toxicity symptoms usually develop within 3
hours of ingestion. Hypotension, somnolence,
bradycardia, conduction disturbances, ventricular arrhythmias, and seizures have been reported. Rhythm and blood pressure may be controlled
with dopamine and isoproterenol; seizures may
respond to I.V. diazepam.

Monitoring the patient
• Monitor patient with impaired hepatic function carefully.
• Watch for toxicity, especially if there has been a recent dosage change.

Information for the patient
• Instruct patient to report signs and symptoms of infection, such as sore throat, chills, and fever.

Geriatric patients
• In elderly patients and patients with substantial heart disease, increase dosage more gradually during initial phase of treatment.

Breast-feeding patients
• It's unknown if drug appears in breast milk. Because of potential for serious toxicity in infant, consider an alternative to breast-feeding during therapy.

propantheline bromide
Pro-Banthine, Propanthel*

Pharmacologic classification: anticholinergic
Therapeutic classification: antimuscarinic, GI antispasmodic
Pregnancy risk category C

How supplied
Available by prescription only
Tablets: 7.5 mg, 15 mg

Indications, route, and dosage
Adjunctive treatment of peptic ulcer, irritable bowel syndrome, and other GI disorders; to reduce duodenal motility during diagnostic radiologic procedures
Adults: 15 mg P.O. t.i.d. before meals, and 30 mg h.s. up to 60 mg q.i.d.
Elderly patients: 7.5 mg P.O. t.i.d. before meals.
Children: Antispasmodic dose 2 to 3 mg/kg/day P.O. divided q 4 to 6 hours and h.s. Antisecretory dose 1.5 mg/kg/day P.O. divided q 6 to 8 hours.

Pharmacodynamics
Anticholinergic action: Competitively blocks acetylcholine's actions at cholinergic neuroeffector sites, decreasing GI motility and inhibiting gastric acid secretion.

Pharmacokinetics
• *Absorption:* Only about 10% to 25% of drug absorbed (absorption varies among patients).
• *Distribution:* Doesn't cross blood-brain barrier; little else known about distribution.
• *Metabolism:* Appears to undergo considerable metabolism in upper small intestine and liver.
• *Excretion:* Absorbed drug excreted in urine as metabolites and unchanged drug.

Contraindications and precautions
Contraindicated in patients with hypersensitivity to anticholinergics and in those with angle-closure glaucoma, obstructive uropathy, obstructive disease of the GI tract, severe ulcerative colitis, myasthenia gravis, paralytic ileus, intestinal atony, unstable CV status in acute hemorrhage, or toxic megacolon.
   Use cautiously in patients with impaired renal or hepatic function, autonomic neuropathy, hyperthyroidism, coronary artery disease, arrhythmias, heart failure, hypertension, hiatal hernia associated with gastric reflux, or ulcerative colitis and in those living in a hot or humid environment.

Interactions
Drug-drug. *Antacids:* Decreased oral absorption of anticholinergics. Administer propantheline at least 1 hour before antacids.
Atenolol: Increased absorption; enhanced atenolol effects. Use together cautiously.
Digoxin: Slowly dissolving tablets may yield higher serum digoxin levels when administered with anticholinergics. Monitor serum digoxin levels.
Drugs with anticholinergic effects: Additive toxicity. Use together cautiously.
Ketoconazole, levodopa: Decreased GI absorption. Monitor patient.
Oral potassium supplements (especially wax-matrix formulations): Increased potassium-induced GI ulcerations. Monitor patient closely.

Adverse reactions
CNS: headache, insomnia, drowsiness, dizziness, *confusion or excitement in elderly patients,* nervousness, weakness.
CV: *palpitations,* tachycardia.
EENT: *blurred vision,* mydriasis, increased intraocular pressure, cycloplegia, drying of salivary secretions.
GI: *dry mouth,* constipation, loss of taste, nausea, vomiting, paralytic ileus, bloated feeling.
GU: *urinary hesitancy, urine retention,* impotence.
Skin: urticaria, decreased sweating or possible anhidrosis, other dermal signs and symptoms.
Other: allergic reactions (*anaphylaxis*).

☑ Special considerations
Besides the recommendations relevant to all anticholinergics, consider the following.
• Drug may be used with histamine$_2$ receptor to treat Zollinger-Ellison syndrome as an unlabeled use.
• Adjust drug until therapeutic effect is obtained or adverse effects become intolerable.
• Toxicity may cause curare-like symptoms such as respiratory paralysis and such peripheral effects as headache; dilated, nonreactive pupils; blurred vision; flushed, hot, dry skin; dryness of mucous membranes; dysphagia; decreased or absent bowel sounds; urine retention; hyper-

thermia; tachycardia; hypertension; and increased respirations. In severe cases, physostigmine may be administered to block propantheline's antimuscarinic effects.

Monitoring the patient
• Monitor patient for adverse effects.

Information for the patient
• Instruct patient to swallow tablets whole rather than chewing or crushing them.

Geriatric patients
• Administer drug cautiously to elderly patients. Lower dosages are recommended.

Breast-feeding patients
• Drug may appear in breast milk, possibly resulting in infant toxicity. Don't use in breast-feeding women. Drug may decrease milk production.

---

propofol
Diprivan

Pharmacologic classification: phenol derivative
Therapeutic classification: anesthetic
Pregnancy risk category B

How supplied
Available by prescription only
Injection: 10 mg/ml in 20-ml ampules and 50-ml and 100-ml infusion vials

Indications, route, and dosage
Induction and maintenance of sedation in mechanically ventilated intensive care unit patients
Adults: Initially, 5 mcg/kg/minute I.V. for 5 minutes (0.3 mg/kg/hour). Subsequent increments of 5 to 10 mcg/kg/minute (0.3 to 0.6 mg/kg/hour) over 5 to 10 minutes until desired level of sedation is achieved. Maintenance rates of 5 to 50 mcg/kg/minute (0.3 to 3 mg/kg/hour) or higher may be needed. Minimum amount necessary should be used. Lower dosages are needed for patients over age 55.
Induction of anesthesia
Adults: Individualize doses based on patient's condition and age. Most patients classified as American Society of Anesthesiologists (ASA) Physical Status category (PS) I or II under age 55 need 2 to 2.5 mg/kg I.V. Drug is usually administered in a 40-mg bolus q 10 seconds until desired response is obtained.
Children ages 3 and over: 2.5 to 3.5 mg/kg I.V. over 20 to 30 seconds.
Elderly, debilitated, or hypovolemic patients or patients in ASA PS III or IV: Half of the usual induction dose (20-mg bolus q 10 seconds).

Maintenance of anesthesia
Adults: May give as a variable rate infusion, titrated to clinical effect. Most patients may be maintained with 0.1 to 0.2 mg/kg/minute (6 to 12 mg/kg/hour).
Elderly, debilitated, or hypovolemic patients or patients in ASA PS III or IV: Half the usual maintenance dose (0.05 to 0.1 mg/kg/minute or 3 to 6 mg/kg/hour).
Children ages 3 and over: 125 to 300 mcg/kg/minute I.V.

Pharmacodynamics
Anesthetic action: Produces a dose-dependent CNS depression similar to benzodiazepines and barbiturates. However, it can be used to maintain anesthesia through careful titration of infusion rate.

Pharmacokinetics
• *Absorption:* Must be administered I.V.
• *Distribution:* Terminal half-life of 1 to 3 days.
• *Metabolism:* Metabolized within liver and tissues; metabolites not fully characterized.
• *Excretion:* Excreted through kidneys. However, termination of drug action is probably caused by redistribution out of CNS as well as metabolism.

Contraindications and precautions
Contraindicated in patients with hypersensitivity to propofol or components of the emulsion, including soybean oil, egg lecithin, and glycerol. Because drug is administered as an emulsion, administer with caution to patients with a disorder of lipid metabolism (such as pancreatitis, primary hyperlipoproteinemia, and diabetic hyperlipidemia). Use cautiously if patient is receiving lipids as part of a total parenteral nutrition infusion; I.V. lipid dose may need to be reduced. Use cautiously in elderly or debilitated patients and in those with circulatory disorders.
Don't use drug in obstetric anesthesia because safety of fetus hasn't been established. Also avoid in patients with increased intracranial pressure or impaired cerebral circulation because the reduction in systemic arterial pressure caused by drug may substantially reduce cerebral perfusion pressure.
Don't use drug in children under age 3 and in those in intensive care units or under monitored anesthesia care sedation.
Drug should be administered under direct medical supervision by persons familiar with airway management and the administration of I.V. anesthetics.

Interactions
Drug-drug. *Inhalational anesthetics (enflurane, halothane, isoflurane), supplemental anesthetics (nitrous oxide, opiates):* Enhanced anesthetic and CV actions of propofol expected. Use together cautiously.

Opiate analgesics or sedatives: Intensified reduction of systolic, diastolic, mean arterial pressure, and cardiac output. Decrease induction dose requirements as needed.

Adverse reactions
CNS: headache, dizziness, twitching, clonic-myoclonic movement.
CV: *hypotension,* **bradycardia,** hypertension.
GI: nausea, vomiting, abdominal cramping.
GU: discolored urine.
Metabolic: hyperlipidemia.
Respiratory: *apnea,* cough, hiccups.
Skin: flushing.
Other: fever, *injection site burning or stinging, pain,* tingling or numbness, coldness.

☑ Special considerations
● Although the hemodynamic effects of drug can vary, its major effect in patients maintaining spontaneous ventilation is arterial hypotension (arterial pressure can decrease as much as 30%) with little or no change in heart rate and cardiac output. However, significant depression of cardiac output may occur in patients undergoing assisted or controlled positive pressure ventilation.
● Drug has no vagolytic activity. Premedication with anticholinergics, such as glycopyrrolate or atropine, may help manage potential increases in vagal tone caused by other drugs or surgical manipulations.
● Don't mix propofol with other drugs or blood products. If it's to be diluted before infusion, use only D_5W and don't dilute to a concentration of less than 2 mg/ml. After dilution, drug appears to be more stable in glass containers than plastic.
● When administered into a running I.V. catheter, emulsion is compatible with D_5W, lactated Ringer's injection, lactated Ringer's and 5% dextrose injection, 5% dextrose and 0.45% saline injection, and 5% dextrose and 0.2% saline injection.
● Store emulsion above 40° F (4° C) and below 72° F (22° C). Refrigeration isn't recommended.
● If used for sedation of mechanically ventilated patients, wake patient every 24 hours.
● Use strict aseptic technique when administering drug; discard unused drug after 12 hours.

Monitoring the patient
● Monitor patient for signs and symptoms of significant hypotension or bradycardia. Treatment may include increased rate of fluid administration, pressor drugs, elevation of lower extremities, or atropine.
● Watch for apnea during induction; may persist for longer than 60 seconds. Ventilatory support may be needed.

Geriatric patients
● Drug's pharmacokinetics aren't influenced by chronic hepatic cirrhosis, chronic renal failure, or gender.

Pediatric patients
● Safety in children hasn't been established.

Breast-feeding patients
● Drug appears in breast milk; don't use in breast-feeding women.

---

propoxyphene hydrochloride
Darvon

propoxyphene napsylate
Darvocet-N 50, Darvocet-N 100,
Darvon-N

Pharmacologic classification: opioid
Therapeutic classification: analgesic
Controlled substance schedule IV
Pregnancy risk category NR

How supplied
Available by prescription only
propoxyphene hydrochloride
Capsules: 65 mg
propoxyphene napsylate
Tablets: 100 mg
Suspension: 50 mg/5 ml
propoxyphene napsylate and acetaminophen
Tablets: 50 mg propoxyphene napsylate, 325 mg acetaminophen; 100 mg propoxyphene napsylate, 650 mg acetaminophen

Indications, route, and dosage
Mild to moderate pain
Adults: 65 mg (hydrochloride) P.O. q 4 hours, p.r.n., or 100 mg (napsylate) P.O. q 4 hours, p.r.n.

Pharmacodynamics
Analgesic action: Exerts analgesic effect via opiate agonist activity and alters patient's response to painful stimuli, particularly mild to moderate pain.

Pharmacokinetics
● *Absorption:* After oral administration, absorbed primarily in upper small intestine. Equimolar doses of the hydrochloride and napsylate salts provide similar plasma levels. Onset of analgesia in 20 to 60 minutes; analgesic effects peak in 2 to 2½ hours.
● *Distribution:* Enters CSF. Assumed to cross placental barrier; however, placental fluid and fetal blood levels not determined.
● *Metabolism:* Degraded mainly in liver; about one-quarter of dose metabolized to norpropoxyphene, an active metabolite.
● *Excretion:* Excreted in urine. Duration of effect 4 to 6 hours.

Contraindications and precautions
Contraindicated in patients with hypersensitivity to drug. Use cautiously in patients with impaired

---

Reactions may be *common*, uncommon, **life-threatening**, or COMMON AND LIFE-THREATENING.

renal or hepatic function, emotional instability, or history of drug or alcohol abuse.

Interactions

Drug-drug. *Antidepressants such as doxepin:* Propoxyphene may inhibit metabolism of these drugs. Lower dosage of antidepressant as needed.

Carbamazepine: Increased carbamazepine's effects. Monitor serum carbamazepine levels.

Cimetidine: Enhanced respiratory and CNS depression; confusion, disorientation, apnea, or seizures. Avoid concomitant use.

Drugs highly metabolized in liver (digitoxin, phenytoin, rifampin): Possible accumulation of either drug. Withdrawal symptoms may result if used together. Avoid using together.

General anesthetics: Possible severe CV depression. Use with caution and monitor patient closely.

Opiate antagonist: Patients who become physically dependent on propoxyphene may experience acute withdrawal syndrome when given a single dose. Use with caution and monitor closely.

Other CNS depressants (antidepressants, antihistamines, barbiturates, benzodiazepines, general anesthetics, muscle relaxants, narcotic analgesics, phenothiazines, sedative-hypnotics): Potentiation of adverse effects (respiratory depression, sedation, hypotension). Reduced doses of propoxyphene are usually needed.

Drug-lifestyle. *Alcohol:* Potentiated CNS depressant effects of propoxyphene. Discourage use.

Adverse reactions

CNS: *dizziness, sedation,* headache, euphoria, light-headedness, weakness, hallucinations.
GI: *nausea, vomiting,* constipation, abdominal pain.
Hepatic: abnormal liver function tests.
Respiratory: *respiratory depression.*
Other: psychological and physical dependence.

☑ Special considerations

Besides the recommendations relevant to all opioids, consider the following.

• Propoxyphene may obscure signs and symptoms of an acute abdominal condition or worsen gallbladder pain.

• Don't prescribe for drug maintenance purposes in narcotic addiction.

• Drug can be considered a mild narcotic analgesic, but pain relief is equivalent to that of aspirin.

• Drug may cause false decrease in test for urinary corticosteroid excretion.

• Toxicity may cause CNS depression, respiratory depression, and miosis (pinpoint pupils); hypotension, bradycardia, hypothermia, shock, apnea, cardiopulmonary arrest, circulatory collapse, pulmonary edema, and seizures may also occur.

• Drug is known to cause ECG changes (prolonged QRS complex) and nephrogenic diabetes insipidus in acute toxic doses. Death from acute overdose is most likely to occur within first hour. Signs and symptoms of overdose with propoxyphene combination products may include salicylism from aspirin or acetaminophen toxicity.

• Administer a narcotic antagonist (naloxone) to reverse respiratory depression. Don't give naloxone in the absence of clinically significant respiratory or CV depression. Dialysis may be helpful in the treatment of overdose with propoxyphene combination products containing aspirin or acetaminophen.

Monitoring the patient

• Monitor patient for effectiveness of treatment.
• Watch for signs of dependence.

Information for the patient

• Warn patient not to exceed recommended dosage.

• Tell patient to avoid use of alcohol because it will cause additive CNS depressant effects.

• Warn patient of additive depressant effect that can occur if drug is prescribed for medical conditions requiring use of sedatives, tranquilizers, muscle relaxants, antidepressants, or other CNS-depressant drugs.

• Tell patient to take drug with food if GI upset occurs.

Geriatric patients

• Lower doses are usually indicated for elderly patients because they may be more sensitive to therapeutic and adverse effects of drug.

Breast-feeding patients

• Drug appears in breast milk; use with caution in breast-feeding women.

propranolol hydrochloride
Inderal, Inderal LA

Pharmacologic classification: beta blocker
Therapeutic classification: antihypertensive, antianginal, antiarrhythmic, adjunctive therapy of migraine, adjunctive therapy of MI
Pregnancy risk category C

How supplied

Available by prescription only
Tablets: 10 mg, 20 mg, 40 mg, 60 mg, 80 mg, 90 mg
Capsules (extended-release): 60 mg, 80 mg, 120 mg, 160 mg
Injection: 1 mg/ml

Solution: 4 mg/ml, 8 mg/ml, 20 mg/5 ml, 40 mg/5 ml, 80 mg/ml (concentrated)

Indications, route, and dosage

Hypertension
Adults: Initially, 80 mg P.O. daily in two to four divided doses or sustained-release form once daily. Increase at 3- to 7-day intervals to maximum daily dose of 640 mg. Usual maintenance dose is 160 to 480 mg daily.
◊ *Children:* 1 mg/kg P.O. daily (maximum daily dose is 16 mg/kg).

Management of angina pectoris
Adults: 10 to 20 mg t.i.d. or q.i.d., or one 80-mg sustained-release capsule daily. Dosage may be increased at 7- to 10-day intervals. Average optimum dose is 160 to 240 mg daily.

Supraventricular, ventricular, and atrial arrhythmias; tachyarrhythmias caused by excessive catecholamine action during anesthesia, hyperthyroidism, and pheochromocytoma
Adults: 1 to 3 mg I.V. diluted in 50 ml D$_5$W or normal saline solution infused slowly, not to exceed 1 mg/minute. After 3 mg have been infused, another dose may be given in 2 minutes; subsequent doses no sooner than q 4 hours. Usual maintenance dose is 10 to 30 mg P.O. t.i.d. or q.i.d.

Prevention of frequent, severe, uncontrollable, or disabling migraine or vascular headache
Adults: Initially, 80 mg daily in divided doses or one sustained-release capsule once daily. Usual maintenance dose is 160 to 240 mg daily, divided t.i.d. or q.i.d.

To reduce mortality after MI
Adults: 180 to 240 mg P.O. daily in divided doses. Usually administered in three to four doses daily, beginning 5 to 21 days after infarct.

Hypertrophic subaortic stenosis
Adults: 10 to 20 mg P.O. t.i.d. or q.i.d. before meals and h.s.

Preoperative pheochromocytoma
Adults: 60 mg P.O. daily.

◊ **Adjunctive treatment of anxiety**
Adults: 10 to 80 mg P.O. 1 hour before anxiety-provoking activity.

◊ **Essential, familial, or senile movement tremors**
Adults: 40 mg P.O. b.i.d., as tolerated and needed.

Pharmacodynamics

Antihypertensive action: Exact mechanism unknown. May reduce blood pressure by blocking adrenergic receptors (thus decreasing cardiac output), by decreasing sympathetic outflow from the CNS, and by suppressing renin release.
Antianginal action: Decreases myocardial oxygen consumption by blocking catecholamine access to beta-adrenergic receptors, thus relieving angina.
Antiarrhythmic action: Decreases heart rate and prevents exercise-induced increases in heart rate. Also decreases myocardial contractility, cardiac output, and SA and AV nodal conduction velocity.
Migraine prophylactic action: Thought to result from inhibition of vasodilation.
MI prophylactic action: Exact mechanism unknown.

Pharmacokinetics

● *Absorption:* Absorbed almost completely from GI tract; food enhances absorption. Plasma levels peak 60 to 90 minutes after giving regular-release tablets. After I.V. administration, peak levels in about 1 minute, with virtually immediate onset of action.
● *Distribution:* Distributed widely throughout body; more than 90% protein-bound.
● *Metabolism:* Almost total hepatic metabolism; oral dosage form undergoes extensive first-pass metabolism.
● *Excretion:* About 96% to 99% of given dose excreted in urine as metabolites; remainder excreted in feces as unchanged drug and metabolites. Biological half-life about 4 hours.

Contraindications and precautions

Contraindicated in patients with bronchial asthma, sinus bradycardia and heart block greater than first-degree, cardiogenic shock, and heart failure (unless failure is secondary to a tachyarrhythmia that can be treated with propranolol).

Use cautiously in elderly patients; in patients with impaired renal or hepatic function, nonallergic bronchospastic diseases, diabetes mellitus, or thyrotoxicosis; and in those receiving other antihypertensives.

Interactions

Drug-drug. *Aluminum hydroxide antacid:* Decreased GI absorption. Separate administration times.
Antidiabetics, insulin: Altered dosage requirements in previously stable diabetic patients. Monitor serum glucose level.
Atropine, tricyclic antidepressants, other drugs with anticholinergic effects: Possible antagonized propranolol-induced bradycardia. Monitor patient closely.
Calcium channel blockers (especially I.V. verapamil): Depressed myocardial contractility or AV conduction. Rarely, concurrent I.V. use of a beta blocker and verapamil has resulted in serious adverse reactions, especially in patients with severe cardiomyopathy, heart failure, or recent MI. Use together cautiously.
Cimetidine: Decreased clearance of propranolol via inhibition of hepatic metabolism. Watch for enhanced beta-blocking effects.

Reactions may be *common*, uncommon, **life-threatening**, or COMMON AND LIFE-THREATENING.

Epinephrine: Severe vasoconstriction. Monitor blood pressure and observe patient carefully.
NSAIDs: Possible antagonized hypotensive effects. Monitor patient closely.
Phenytoin, rifampin: Accelerated clearance of propranolol. Adjust dosage as needed.
Sympathomimetics (such as isoproterenol, MAO inhibitors): Antagonized beta-adrenergic stimulating effects. Monitor patient closely.
Tubocurarine and related compounds: High doses of propranolol may potentiate neuromuscular blocking effect. Monitor patient closely.
Other antihypertensives (especially catecholamine-depleting drugs such as reserpine): Potentiated antihypertensive effects. Monitor blood pressure.
Drug-herb. *Betel palm:* Reduced temperature-elevating effects and enhanced CNS effects. Don't use together.
Drug-lifestyle. *Alcohol:* Slowed rate of absorption. Discourage use.

Adverse reactions
CNS: *fatigue, lethargy,* vivid dreams, hallucinations, mental depression, light-headedness, insomnia.
CV: *bradycardia,* hypotension, *heart failure,* intermittent claudication, **intensification of AV block.**
GI: nausea, vomiting, diarrhea, abdominal cramping.
GU: increased BUN levels.
Hematologic: *agranulocytosis.*
Hepatic: elevated serum transaminase, alkaline phosphatase, and LD levels.
Respiratory: *bronchospasm.*
Skin: rash.
Other: fever.

☑ Special considerations
Besides the recommendations relevant to all beta blockers, consider the following.
- Propranolol also has been used to treat aggression and rage, stage fright, recurrent GI bleeding in cirrhotic patients, and menopausal symptoms.
- Never administer propranolol as an adjunct in treatment of pheochromocytoma unless patient has been pretreated with alpha blockers.
- Toxicity may cause severe hypotension, bradycardia, heart failure, and bronchospasm. Treat bradycardia with atropine (0.25 to 1 mg); if no response, administer isoproterenol cautiously. Treat cardiac failure with cardiac glycosides and diuretics and hypotension with glucagon or vasopressors; epinephrine is preferred. Treat bronchospasm with isoproterenol and aminophylline.

Monitoring the patient
- Monitor serum glucose level; drug may mask signs of hypoglycemia.
- Monitor patient for adverse effects.

Information for the patient
- Warn patient not to stop drug abruptly.
- Instruct patient on proper use, dosage, and potential adverse effects of drug.
- Tell patient to call before taking OTC drugs that may interact with propranolol, such as nasal decongestants or cold preparations.

Geriatric patients
- Elderly patients may need lower maintenance doses because of increased bioavailability or delayed metabolism; they also may experience enhanced adverse effects.

Pediatric patients
- Safety and efficacy in children haven't been established; use only if potential benefit outweighs risk.

Breast-feeding patients
- Drug appears in breast milk; an alternative to breast-feeding is recommended during therapy.

propylthiouracil (PTU)
Propyl-Thyracil*

Pharmacologic classification: thyroid hormone antagonist
Therapeutic classification: antihyperthyroid drug
Pregnancy risk category D

How supplied
Available by prescription only
Tablets: 50 mg

Indications, route, and dosage
Hyperthyroidism
Adults: 300 to 450 mg P.O. daily in divided doses. Continue until patient is euthyroid; then start maintenance dose of 100 mg daily to t.i.d.
Neonates and children: 5 to 7 mg/kg P.O. daily in divided doses q 8 hours. Or give according to age.
Children age 6 to 10: 50 to 150 mg P.O. daily in divided doses q 8 hours.
Children over age 10: 100 mg P.O. t.i.d. Continue until patient is euthyroid; then start maintenance dose of 25 mg t.i.d. to 100 mg b.i.d.

Pharmacodynamics
Antithyroid action: When used to treat hyperthyroidism, PTU inhibits synthesis of thyroid hormone by interfering with the incorporation of iodine into thyroglobulin; it also inhibits the formation of iodothyronine. Besides blocking hormone synthesis, it also inhibits the peripheral deiodination of thyroxine to triiodothyronine (liothyronine). Clinical effects become evident only when the preformed hormone is depleted and circulating hormone levels decline.

As preparation for thyroidectomy, PTU inhibits synthesis of the thyroid hormone and causes a euthyroid state, reducing surgical problems during thyroidectomy; as a result, the mortality for a single-stage thyroidectomy is low. Iodide reduces the vascularity of the gland and makes it less friable.

When used in treating thyrotoxic crisis, PTU inhibits peripheral deiodination of thyroxine to triiodothyronine. Theoretically, it's preferred over methimazole in thyroid storm because of its peripheral action.

Pharmacokinetics
• *Absorption:* About 80% absorbed rapidly and readily from GI tract. Levels peak in 1 to 1½ hours.
• *Distribution:* Appears to be concentrated in thyroid gland. Readily crosses placenta; distributed into breast milk. 75% to 80% protein-bound.
• *Metabolism:* Metabolized rapidly in liver.
• *Excretion:* About 35% of dose excreted in urine. Half-life is 1 to 2 hours in patients with normal renal function; 8½ hours in anuric patients.

Contraindications and precautions
Contraindicated in patients with hypersensitivity to drug and in breast-feeding patients. Use cautiously in pregnant patients.

Interactions
Drug-drug. *Adrenocorticoids, corticotropin:* Altered effects. May require dosage adjustment of the steroid when thyroid status changes.
Bone marrow depressants: Increased risk of agranulocytosis. Monitor hematologic studies.
Hepatotoxic drugs: Increased risk of hepatotoxicity. Monitor patient for toxicity.
Iodinated glycerol, lithium, potassium iodide: Potentiated hypothyroid effects. Monitor patient carefully.
Oral anticoagulants: Potentiated by anti–vitamin K activity attributed to PTU. Monitor PT and INR.

Adverse reactions
CNS: headache, drowsiness, vertigo, paresthesia, neuritis, neuropathies, CNS stimulation, depression.
CV: vasculitis.
EENT: visual disturbances.
GI: diarrhea, *nausea, vomiting* (may be dose-related), epigastric distress, salivary gland enlargement, loss of taste.
GU: nephritis.
Hematologic: *agranulocytosis, thrombocytopenia, aplastic anemia, leukopenia,* altered INR.
Hepatic: altered AST, ALT, and LD levels, jaundice, *hepatotoxicity.*
Metabolic: altered selenomethionine levels and liothyronine uptake, dose-related hypothyroidism (mental depression; hypoprothrombinemia and

bleeding; cold intolerance; hard, nonpitting edema).
Musculoskeletal: arthralgia, myalgia.
Skin: rash, urticaria, skin discoloration, pruritus, erythema nodosum, exfoliative dermatitis, lupuslike syndrome.
Other: fever, lymphadenopathy.

☑ Special considerations
• Best response occurs when drug is administered around the clock and given at the same time each day in respect to meals.
• A beta blocker, usually propranolol, commonly is given to manage peripheral signs of hyperthyroidism, which are primarily cardiac-related (tachycardia).
• Stop drug if patient develops severe rash or enlarged cervical lymph nodes.
• Toxicity may cause nausea, vomiting, epigastric distress, fever, headache, arthralgia, pruritus, edema, and pancytopenia.
• Treatment of toxicity includes withdrawal of drug in the presence of agranulocytosis, pancytopenia, hepatitis, fever, or exfoliative dermatitis. For depression of bone marrow, treatment may require antibiotics and transfusions of fresh whole blood. For hepatitis, treatment includes rest, adequate diet, and symptomatic support, including analgesics, gastric lavage, I.V. fluids, and mild sedation.

Monitoring the patient
• Watch for signs and symptoms of hypothyroidism (mental depression; cold intolerance; hard, nonpitting edema; hair loss).
• Monitor therapeutic effect.

Information for the patient
• Warn patient to avoid using self-prescribed cough medicines; many contain iodine.
• Suggest taking drug with meals to reduce GI adverse effects.
• Instruct patient to store drug in a light-resistant container and not to store in the bathroom; heat and humidity may cause drug to deteriorate.
• Tell patient to promptly report fever, sore throat, malaise, unusual bleeding, yellowing of eyes, nausea, or vomiting.
• Advise patient to have medical review of thyroid status before undergoing surgery (including dental surgery).
• Teach patient how to recognize signs of hyperthyroidism and hypothyroidism and what to do if they occur.

Breast-feeding patients
• Drug appears in breast milk. Avoid breast-feeding during treatment. However, if breast-feeding is necessary, PTU is the preferred antithyroid drug.

---

protamine sulfate

Pharmacologic classification: antidote
Therapeutic classification: heparin antagonist
Pregnancy risk category C

How supplied
Available by prescription only
Injection: 10 mg/ml in 5-ml ampule, 25-ml ampule, 5-ml vial, 10-ml vial, 25-ml vial

Indications, route, and dosage
Heparin overdose
Adults and children: Dosage based on venous blood coagulation studies, usually 1 mg for each 90 units of heparin derived from lung tissue or 1 mg for each 115 units of heparin derived from intestinal mucosa. Give by slow I.V. injection over 1 to 3 minutes. Maximum dose is 50 mg in any 10-minute period.

Pharmacodynamics
Heparin antagonism: Has weak anticoagulant activity; however, when given in the presence of heparin, forms a salt that neutralizes anticoagulant effects of both drugs.

Pharmacokinetics
• *Absorption:* Heparin-neutralizing effect within 30 to 60 seconds.
• *Distribution:* No information available.
• *Metabolism:* Fate of heparin-protamine complex unknown; appears to be partially degraded, with release of some heparin.
• *Excretion:* Binding action lasts about 2 hours.

Contraindications and precautions
Contraindicated in patients with hypersensitivity to drug. Use cautiously after cardiac surgery.

Interactions
None reported.

Adverse reactions
CV: fall in blood pressure, ***bradycardia, circulatory collapse.***
GI: nausea, vomiting.
Hematologic: shortens heparin-prolonged PTT.
Respiratory: dyspnea, ***pulmonary edema, acute pulmonary hypertension.***
Other: transitory flushing, feeling of warmth, ***anaphylaxis, anaphylactoid reactions,*** lassitude.

☑ Special considerations
• Check for possible fish allergy.
• Dosage is based on blood coagulation studies as well as on route of administration of heparin and time elapsed since heparin was administered.
• Don't mix protamine with any other drug.

• Reconstitute powder by adding 5 ml sterile water to 50-mg vial (25 ml to 250-mg vial); discard unused solution.
• Slow I.V. administration (over 1 to 3 minutes) decreases adverse effects; have antishock equipment available.
• Overdose may cause bleeding secondary to interaction with platelets and proteins including fibrinogen. Replace blood loss with blood transfusions or fresh frozen plasma. If hypotension occurs, consider treating with fluids, epinephrine, dobutamine, or dopamine.

Monitoring the patient
• Watch for sudden fall in blood pressure. Monitor patient continually, and check vital signs frequently.
• Monitor therapeutic effect.

Information for the patient
• Advise patient that he may experience transitory flushing or feel warm after I.V. administration.

pseudoephedrine hydrochloride

pseudoephedrine sulfate
Cenafed, Decofed, Efidac/24, Genaphed, Novafed, PediaCare Infants' Decongestant Drops, Pseudogest, Sudafed, Triaminic AM

Pharmacologic classification: adrenergic
Therapeutic classification: decongestant
Pregnancy risk category B

How supplied
Available without a prescription
Oral solution: 7.5 mg/0.8 ml, 15 mg/5 ml, 30 mg/5 ml
Tablets: 30 mg, 60 mg
Tablets (extended-release): 120 mg, 240 mg
Capsules: 60 mg
Capsules (extended-release): 120 mg

Indications, route, and dosage
Nasal and eustachian tube decongestant
Adults and children ages 12 and over: 60 mg P.O. q 4 to 6 hours. Maximum dose is 240 mg daily, or 120 mg extended-release tablet q 12 hours.
Children ages 6 to 11: Administer 30 mg P.O. q 4 to 6 hours. Maximum dose is 120 mg daily.
Children ages 2 to 5: 15 mg P.O. q 4 to 6 hours. Maximum dose is 60 mg/day, or 4 mg/kg or 125 mg/m^2 P.O. divided q.i.d.

Pharmacodynamics
Decongestant action: Directly stimulates alpha-adrenergic receptors of respiratory mucosa to produce vasoconstriction; shrinkage of swollen

nasal mucous membranes; reduction of tissue hyperemia, edema, and nasal congestion; an increase in airway (nasal) patency and drainage of sinus excretions; and opening of obstructed eustachian ostia. Relaxation of bronchial smooth muscle may result from direct stimulation of beta-adrenergic receptors. Mild CNS stimulation may also occur.

Pharmacokinetics

- *Absorption:* Nasal decongestion within 30 minutes; lasts 4 to 6 hours after oral dose of 60-mg tablet or oral solution. Effects last 8 hours after 60-mg dose; up to 12 hours after 120-mg dose of extended-release form.
- *Distribution:* Widely distributed throughout body.
- *Metabolism:* Incompletely metabolized in liver by n-demethylation to inactive compounds.
- *Excretion:* 55% to 75% of dose excreted unchanged in urine; remainder excreted as unchanged drug and metabolites.

Contraindications and precautions

Contraindicated in patients with severe hypertension or severe coronary artery disease; in those receiving MAO inhibitors; and in breast-feeding women. Extended-release preparations are contraindicated in children under age 12.

Use cautiously in elderly patients and in patients with hypertension, cardiac disease, diabetes, glaucoma, hyperthyroidism, or prostatic hyperplasia.

Interactions

Drug-drug. *Beta blockers:* Increased pressor effects of pseudoephedrine. Monitor patient.
MAO inhibitors: Potentiated pressor effects of pseudoephedrine. Use together cautiously.
Methyldopa, reserpine: Reduced antihypertensive effects. Monitor blood pressure.
Tricyclic antidepressants: Antagonized effects of pseudoephedrine. Monitor patient.
Other sympathomimetics: Additive effects. Monitor patient for toxicity.

Adverse reactions

CNS: anxiety, transient stimulation, tremor, dizziness, headache, insomnia, *nervousness.*
CV: **arrhythmias,** *palpitations,* tachycardia.
GI: anorexia, nausea, vomiting, dry mouth.
GU: difficulty urinating.
Respiratory: respiratory difficulties.
Skin: pallor.

☑ Special considerations

Besides the recommendations relevant to all adrenergics, consider the following.

- Administer last daily dose several hours before bedtime to minimize insomnia.
- If symptoms persist longer than 5 days or fever is present, reevaluate therapy.

- Toxicity may cause exaggeration of common adverse reactions, particularly seizures, arrhythmias, and nausea and vomiting.
- Treatment of toxicity may include an emetic and gastric lavage within 4 hours of ingestion. Charcoal is effective only if administered within 1 hour, unless extended-release form was used. Forced diuresis will increase elimination. Don't force diuresis in severe overdose. I.V. propranolol may control cardiac toxicity; I.V. diazepam may be helpful to manage delirium or seizures; dilute potassium chloride solutions (I.V.) may be given for hypokalemia.

Monitoring the patient

- Observe patient for complaints of headache or dizziness.
- Monitor blood pressure.

Information for the patient

- If patient finds swallowing capsules difficult, suggest opening capsules and mixing contents with applesauce, jelly, honey, or syrup. Mixture must be swallowed without chewing.
- Tell patient that dry mouth may occur and suggest using ice chips, sugarless gum, or hard candy for relief.
- Instruct patient to take missed dose if remembered within 1 hour. If beyond 1 hour, patient should skip missed dose and resume regular schedule; he shouldn't double dose.
- Tell patient to store drug away from heat and light (not in bathroom medicine cabinet) and safely out of reach of children.
- Caution patient that many OTC preparations may contain sympathomimetics, which can cause additive, hazardous reactions.
- Advise patient to take last dose at least 2 to 3 hours before bedtime to avoid insomnia.

Geriatric patients

- Elderly patients may be sensitive to effects of drug; lower dose may be needed. Overdose may cause hallucinations, CNS depression, seizures, and death in patients over age 60. Use extended-release preparations with caution in elderly patients.

Pediatric patients

- Don't use extended-release form in children under age 12.

Breast-feeding patients

- Drug appears in breast milk. Avoid use in breast-feeding women; infant may be susceptible to drug effects.

Reactions may be *common,* uncommon, **life-threatening,** or COMMON AND LIFE-THREATENING.

psyllium
Cillium, Fiberall, Hydrocil Instant,
Konsyl, Konsyl-D, Metamucil, Naturacil,
Reguloid, Serutan, Syllact, V-Lax

Pharmacologic classification: adsorbent
Therapeutic classification: bulk laxative
Pregnancy risk category C

How supplied
Available without a prescription
Powder: 3.3 g/teaspoon, 3.4 g/teaspoon, 3.5 g/
teaspoon, 4.94 g/teaspoon
Powder (effervescent): 3.4 g/packet, 3.7 g/
packet
Granules: 2.5 g/teaspoon, 4.03 g/teaspoon
Chewable pieces: 1.7 g/piece, 3.4 g/piece
Wafers: 1.7 g/wafer, 3.4 g/wafer

Indications, route, and dosage
**Constipation, bowel management, irritable
bowel syndrome**
Adults: 1 to 2 rounded teaspoons P.O. in full glass
of liquid daily, b.i.d., or t.i.d., then second glass
of liquid; or 1 packet P.O. dissolved in water daily; or 2 wafers b.i.d. or t.i.d.
Children over age 6: 1 level teaspoon P.O. in ½
glass of liquid h.s.

Pharmacodynamics
Laxative action: Adsorbs water in the gut; also
serves as a source of indigestible fiber, increasing stool bulk and moisture, thus stimulating peristaltic activity and bowel evacuation.

Pharmacokinetics
• *Absorption:* None; onset of action varies from
12 hours to 3 days.
• *Distribution:* Distributed locally in gut.
• *Metabolism:* Not metabolized.
• *Excretion:* Excreted in feces.

Contraindications and precautions
Contraindicated in patients with hypersensitivity
to drug; in those with abdominal pain, nausea,
vomiting, or other symptoms of appendicitis; and
in those with intestinal obstruction or ulceration,
disabling adhesions, or difficulty swallowing.

Interactions
Drug-drug. *Anticoagulants, cardiac glycosides,
salicylates:* Psyllium may adsorb oral drugs. Separate administration times by at least 2 hours.

Adverse reactions
GI: nausea, vomiting, diarrhea (with excessive
use); esophageal, gastric, small intestinal, and
rectal obstruction when drug is taken in dry form;
abdominal cramps, especially in severe constipation.

☑ Special considerations
• Before administering drug, add at least 8 oz
(240 ml) of water or juice and stir for a few seconds (improves drug's taste). Have patient drink
mixture immediately to prevent it from congealing; then have him drink another glass of fluid.
• Drug may reduce appetite if administered before meals.
• Psyllium and other bulk laxatives most closely
mimic natural bowel function and don't cause laxative dependence; they are especially useful for
patients with postpartum constipation or diverticular disease, for debilitated patients, for irritable bowel syndrome, and for chronic laxative
users.
• Give diabetic patients a sugar-free and sodium-
free psyllium product.

Monitoring the patient
• Monitor patient for adverse GI effects.
• Monitor therapeutic effect.

Information for the patient
• Warn patient not to swallow drug in dry form;
he should mix it with at least 8 oz (240 ml) of fluid, stir briefly, drink immediately (to prevent mixture from congealing), and then drink another 8
oz of fluid.
• Explain that drug may reduce appetite if taken
before meals; recommend taking drug 2 hours
after meals and any other oral drug.
• Advise diabetic patient and patient with restricted sodium or sugar intake to avoid psyllium
products containing salt or sugar. Advise patient
who must restrict phenylalanine intake to avoid
psyllium products containing aspartame.

Breast-feeding patients
• Because drug isn't absorbed, it's presumably
safe for use in breast-feeding women.

pyrantel pamoate
Antiminth, Combantrin*, Pin-X,
Reese's Pinworm

Pharmacologic classification: pyrimidine
derivative
Therapeutic classification: anthelmintic
Pregnancy risk category C

How supplied
Available by prescription only
Tablets: 62.5 mg
Oral suspension: 50 mg/ml

Indications, route, and dosage
Roundworm and pinworm infections
Adults and children over age 2: Single dose of
11 mg/kg P.O. Maximum dose is 1 g. For pinworm
infection, dose should be repeated in 2 weeks.

Pharmacodynamics

Anthelmintic action: Causes the release of acetylcholine and inhibits cholinesterases, paralyzing the worms. Active against *Ancylostoma duodenale, Ascaris lumbricoides, Enterobius vermicularis, Necator americanus,* and *Trichostrongylus orientalis.*

Pharmacokinetics

• *Absorption:* Absorbed poorly; peak levels in 1 to 3 hours.
• *Distribution:* Little information available.
• *Metabolism:* Small amount of absorbed drug metabolized partially in liver.
• *Excretion:* Over 50% of oral dose excreted unchanged in feces; about 7% excreted in urine as unchanged drug or known metabolites.

Contraindications and precautions

Contraindicated in patients with hypersensitivity to drug and during pregnancy. Use cautiously in patients with hepatic dysfunction or severe malnutrition or anemia.

Interactions

Drug-drug. *Piperazine:* Antagonized effects of piperazine. Avoid using together.

Adverse reactions

CNS: headache, dizziness, drowsiness, insomnia.
GI: anorexia, nausea, vomiting, gastralgia, abdominal cramps, diarrhea, tenesmus.
Hepatic: transient elevation of AST level.
Skin: rash.
Other: fever, weakness.

☑ Special considerations

• Shake suspension well before measuring to ensure accurate dosage.
• Drug may be given with milk, fruit juice, or food.
• Laxatives, enemas, or dietary restrictions are unnecessary.
• Protect drug from light.
• Treat all family members.

Monitoring the patient

• Monitor patient for adverse effects.
• Monitor therapeutic effect.

Information for the patient

• Tell patient to wash perianal area daily and to change undergarments and bedclothes daily.
• To help prevent reinfection, instruct patient and family members in personal hygiene, including sanitary disposal of feces and hand washing and nail cleaning after defecation and before handling, preparing, or eating food.
• Explain routes of transmission and tell patient to encourage other household members and suspected contacts to be tested and, if necessary, treated.

Pediatric patients

• Safety and efficacy in children under age 2 haven't been established.

Breast-feeding patients

• It's unknown if drug appears in breast milk. Safety in breast-feeding women hasn't been established.

pyrazinamide
PMS-Pyrazinamide*, Tebrazid*

Pharmacologic classification: synthetic pyrazine analogue of nicotinamide
Therapeutic classification: antituberculotic
Pregnancy risk category C

How supplied

Available by prescription only
Tablets: 500 mg

Indications, route, and dosage

Adjunctive treatment of tuberculosis (when primary and secondary antituberculotics can't be used or have failed)
Adults: 15 to 30 mg/kg P.O. daily, in one or more doses. Maximum dose is 3 g daily. Or a twice-weekly dose of 50 to 70 mg/kg (based on lean body weight) has been developed to promote patient compliance. Lower dosage is recommended in patients with decreased renal function.

Pharmacodynamics

Antibiotic action: Mechanism unknown. May be bactericidal or bacteriostatic depending on organism susceptibility and drug level at infection site. Active only against *Mycobacterium tuberculosis.* Considered adjunctive in tuberculosis therapy and is given with other drugs to prevent or delay development of resistance to pyrazinamide by *M. tuberculosis.*

Pharmacokinetics

• *Absorption:* Well absorbed after oral administration; serum levels peak 2 hours after oral dose.
• *Distribution:* Distributed widely into body tissues and fluids, including lungs, liver, and CSF; 50% protein-bound. Not known if drug crosses placenta.
• *Metabolism:* Hydrolyzed in liver; some hydrolysis occurs in stomach.
• *Excretion:* Excreted almost completely in urine by glomerular filtration. Not known if excreted in breast milk. Elimination half-life in adults is 9 to 10 hours; prolonged half-life in renal and hepatic impairment.

Contraindications and precautions

Contraindicated in patients with hypersensitivity to drug and in those with severe hepatic disease

---

or acute gout. Use cautiously in patients with diabetes mellitus, renal failure, or gout.

Interactions
Drug-lifestyle. *Sun exposure:* Possible photosensitivity reactions. Tell patient to take precautions.

Adverse reactions
CNS: malaise.
GI: anorexia, nausea, vomiting.
GU: dysuria, interstitial nephritis.
Hematologic: sideroblastic anemia, ***thrombocytopenia.***
Hepatic: *increased liver enzyme levels,* **hepatitis.**
Metabolic: temporarily decreased 17-ketosteroid levels; increased protein-bound iodine and urate levels, hyperuricemia and gout.
Musculoskeletal: *arthralgia, myalgia.*
Skin: rash, urticaria, pruritus, photosensitivity.
Other: fever, porphyria.

☑ Special considerations
● In patients with diabetes mellitus, pyrazinamide therapy may hinder stabilization of serum glucose levels.
● In many cases, drug elevates serum uric acid levels. Although usually asymptomatic, a uricosuric drug, such as probenecid or allopurinol, may be necessary.
● Patients with concomitant HIV infection may need a longer course of treatment.
● Pyrazinamide may interfere with urine ketone determinations.

Monitoring the patient
● Monitor liver function, especially enzyme and bilirubin levels, and renal function, especially serum uric acid levels, before therapy and thereafter at 2- to 4-week intervals.
● Observe patient for signs of liver damage or decreased renal function.

Information for the patient
● Explain disease process and rationale for long-term therapy.
● Teach patient signs and symptoms of hypersensitivity and other adverse reactions, and emphasize need to report them; urge patient to report unusual reactions, especially signs of gout.
● Be sure patient understands how and when to take drugs; urge patient to complete entire prescribed regimen, to comply with instructions for around-the-clock dosage, and to keep follow-up appointments.

Geriatric patients
● Because elderly patients commonly have diminished renal function, which decreases drug excretion, drug should be used with caution.

Pediatric patients
● Drug isn't recommended for use in children.

Breast-feeding patients
● Drug appears in breast milk. Safety in breast-feeding women hasn't been established. An alternative to breast-feeding is recommended during therapy.

pyridostigmine bromide
Mestinon, Regonol

Pharmacologic classification: cholinesterase inhibitor
Therapeutic classification: muscle stimulant
Pregnancy risk category NR

How supplied
Available by prescription only
Tablets: 60 mg
Tablets (sustained-release): 180 mg
Syrup: 60 mg/5 ml
Injection: 5 mg/ml in 2-ml ampule or 5-ml vial

Indications, route, and dosage
Reversal of the effects of nondepolarizing drugs, curariform antagonist (postoperatively)
Adults: 10 to 20 mg I.V. preceded by atropine sulfate 0.6 to 1.2 mg I.V.
Myasthenia gravis
Adults: 60 to 180 mg P.O. b.i.d. or q.i.d. Usual dose is 600 mg daily, but higher doses may be needed (up to 1,500 mg daily). Give one-thirtieth of oral dose I.M. or I.V. Adjust dosage based on patient response and tolerance of adverse effects. Sustained-release and rapid-release forms are often used together depending on patient's symptoms.
Children: 7 mg/kg/24 hours P.O. divided into five or six doses.
Neonates of myasthenic mothers: 0.05 to 0.15 mg/kg I.M.

Pharmacodynamics
Muscle stimulant action: Blocks acetylcholine's hydrolysis by cholinesterase, resulting in acetylcholine accumulation at cholinergic synapses, increasing stimulation of cholinergic receptors at the myoneural junction.

Pharmacokinetics
● *Absorption:* Poorly absorbed from GI tract. Onset of action usually occurs 30 to 45 minutes after oral administration; 2 to 5 minutes after I.V.; 15 minutes after I.M.
● *Distribution:* Little information available; however, may cross placenta, especially when given in large doses.
● *Metabolism:* Exact metabolic fate unknown. Duration of effect usually 3 to 6 hours after oral dose

and 2 to 3 hours after I.V. dose, depending on patient's physical and emotional status and disease severity. Drug hydrolyzed by cholinesterase.
• *Excretion:* Drug and metabolites excreted in urine.

Contraindications and precautions
Contraindicated in patients with hypersensitivity to anticholinesterases and in those with mechanical obstruction of the intestine or urinary tract. Use cautiously in patients with bronchial asthma, bradycardia, or arrhythmias.

Interactions
Drug-drug. *Aminoglycoside antibiotics:* Mild but definite nondepolarizing blocking action of these drugs may accentuate neuromuscular block. Monitor patient for pyridostigmine effectiveness.
Corticosteroids: Decreased cholinergic effect of drug; when corticosteroids are stopped, this effect may increase, possibly affecting muscle strength. Monitor patient.
Ganglionic blockers: Decreased blood pressure; effect usually preceded by abdominal symptoms. Monitor patient and blood pressure closely.
Magnesium: Antagonized beneficial effects of pyridostigmine. Monitor patient for pyridostigmine effectiveness.
Procainamide, quinidine: Reversal of pyridostigmine's cholinergic effect on muscle. Monitor patient for pyridostigmine effectiveness.
Succinylcholine: Prolonged respiratory depression from plasma esterase inhibition, delaying succinylcholine hydrolysis. Monitor patient closely.

Adverse reactions
CNS: headache (with high doses), weakness.
CV: *bradycardia,* hypotension, thrombophlebitis.
EENT: miosis.
GI: abdominal cramps, nausea, vomiting, diarrhea, excessive salivation, increased peristalsis.
Musculoskeletal: muscle cramps, muscle fasciculations.
Respiratory: *bronchospasm, bronchoconstriction,* increased bronchial secretions.
Skin: rash, diaphoresis.

☑ Special considerations
Besides the recommendations relevant to all anticholinesterases, consider the following.
• If muscle weakness is severe, determine if this effect stems from drug toxicity or exacerbation of myasthenia gravis. A test dose of edrophonium I.V. will aggravate drug-induced weakness but will temporarily relieve weakness that results from the disease.
• Avoid giving large doses to patients with decreased GI motility because toxicity may result once motility has been restored.
• Give drug with food or milk to reduce risk of muscarinic adverse effects.

• Atropine sulfate should always be readily available as an antagonist for the muscarinic effects of pyridostigmine.
• Stop all other cholinergics during drug therapy to avoid additive toxicity.
• Toxicity may cause nausea, vomiting, diarrhea, blurred vision, miosis, excessive tearing, bronchospasm, increased bronchial secretions, hypotension, incoordination, excessive sweating, muscle weakness, cramps, fasciculations, paralysis, bradycardia or tachycardia, excessive salivation, and restlessness or agitation. Atropine may be given to block muscarinic effects; however, it won't counter skeletal muscle paralysis. Avoid atropine overdose because it may lead to bronchial plug formation.

Monitoring the patient
• Monitor therapeutic effect.
• Watch for resistance to drug.

Information for the patient
• When drug is used in patient with myasthenia gravis, stress importance of taking drug exactly as ordered, on time, and in evenly spaced doses.
• If patient is taking sustained-release tablets, explain how these work and instruct him to take them at the same time each day; swallow tablets whole rather than crushing them.
• Teach patient how to evaluate muscle strength; instruct him to observe changes in muscle strength and to report muscle cramps, rash, or fatigue.

Breast-feeding patients
• It's unknown if drug appears in breast milk. Because of potential for serious adverse reactions in breast-fed infant, stop either breast-feeding or drug, taking into account importance of drug to mother.

---

pyridoxine hydrochloride (vitamin B₆)
Aminoxin, Nestrex

Pharmacologic classification: water-soluble vitamin
Therapeutic classification: nutritional supplement
Pregnancy risk category A (C if greater than RDA)

How supplied
Available by prescription only
Injection: 10-ml vial (100 mg/ml), 30-ml vial (100 mg/ml), 10-ml vial (100 mg/ml, with 1.5% benzyl alcohol), 30-ml vial (100 mg/ml, with 1.5% benzyl alcohol), 10-ml vial (100 mg/ml, with 0.5% chlorobutanol), 1-ml vial (100 mg/ml)

Available without a prescription
Tablets: 10 mg, 25 mg, 50 mg, 100 mg, 200 mg, 250 mg, 500 mg, 500 mg timed-release

Indications, route, and dosage
RDA
Neonates and infants to age 6 months: 0.3 mg daily.
Infants ages 6 months to 1 year: 0.6 mg daily.
Children ages 1 to 3: 1 mg daily.
Children ages 4 to 6: 1.1 mg daily.
Children ages 7 to 10: 1.4 mg daily.
Females ages 11 to 14: 1.4 mg daily.
Females ages 15 to 18: 1.5 mg daily.
Females ages 19 and older: 1.6 mg daily.
Women during pregnancy: 2.2 mg daily.
Breast-feeding women: 2.1 mg daily.
Males ages 11 to 14: 1.7 mg daily.
Males ages 15 and over: 2 mg daily.

Dietary vitamin B_6 deficiency
Adults: 2.5 to 10 mg P.O., I.M., or I.V. daily for 3 weeks; then 2 to 5 mg daily as a supplement to a proper diet.
Children: 10 to 100 mg I.M. or I.V. to correct deficiency; then an adequate diet with supplementary RDA doses to prevent recurrence.

Seizures related to vitamin B_6 deficiency or dependency
Adults and children: 100 mg I.M. or I.V. in single dose.

Vitamin B_6–responsive anemias or dependency syndrome (inborn errors of metabolism)
Adults: 200 to 600 mg P.O. daily for 1 to 2 months; then 30 to 50 mg P.O. daily.
Children: 100 mg I.M. or I.V.; then 2 to 10 mg I.M. or 10 to 100 mg P.O. daily.

◊ **Premenstrual syndrome**
Adults: 40 to 500 mg P.O., I.M., or I.V. daily.

◊ **Hyperoxaluria type I**
Adults: 25 to 300 mg P.O., I.M., or I.V. daily.

Seizures secondary to isoniazid overdose
Adults and children: A dose of pyridoxine hydrochloride equal to the amount of isoniazid ingested is usually given; generally, 1 to 4 g I.V. initially and then 1 g I.M. every 30 minutes until the entire dose has been given.

Prevention of isoniazid- or penicillamine-induced anemia
Adults: 10 to 50 mg P.O. daily.

Pharmacodynamics
Metabolic action: Natural vitamin B_6 contained in plant and animal foodstuffs is converted to physiologically active forms of vitamin B_6, pyridoxal phosphate, and pyridoxamine phosphate. Exogenous forms of the vitamin are metabolized. Vitamin B_6 acts as a coenzyme in protein, carbohydrate, and fat metabolism and participates in the decarboxylation of amino acids in protein metabolism. Vitamin B_6 also helps convert tryptophan to niacin as well as facilitate the deamination, transamination, and transulfuration of amino acids. Finally, vitamin B_6 is responsible for the breakdown of glycogen to glucose-1-phosphate in carbohydrate metabolism. The total adult body store consists of 16 to 27 mg of pyridoxine. The need for pyridoxine increases with the amount of protein in the diet.

Pharmacokinetics
• *Absorption:* After oral administration, drug and its substituents absorbed readily from GI tract. GI absorption may be diminished in patients with malabsorption syndromes or after gastric resection. Normal serum levels are 30 to 80 ng/ml.
• *Distribution:* Stored mainly in liver. Total body store about 16 to 27 mg. Pyridoxal and pyridoxal phosphate most common forms found in blood; highly protein-bound. Pyridoxal crosses placenta; fetal plasma levels five times greater than maternal plasma levels. After maternal intake of 2.5 to 5 mg/day of pyridoxine, level of vitamin in breast milk is about 240 ng/ml.
• *Metabolism:* Degraded to 4-pyridoxic acid in liver.
• *Excretion:* In erythrocytes, pyridoxine is converted to pyridoxal phosphate; pyridoxamine is converted to pyridoxamine phosphate. Phosphorylated form of pyridoxine is transaminated to pyridoxal and pyridoxamine, which is phosphorylated rapidly. Conversion of pyridoxine phosphate to pyridoxal phosphate requires riboflavin. Biological half-life is 15 to 20 days.

Contraindications and precautions
Contraindicated in patients with hypersensitivity to pyridoxine.

Interactions
Drug-drug. *Cycloserine, hydralazine, isoniazid, oral contraceptives, penicillamine:* Increased pyridoxine requirements. Adjust dosages as necessary.
Levodopa: Reversed therapeutic effects. Monitor patient closely.
Phenobarbital, phenytoin: Possible 50% decrease in serum levels of these anticonvulsants. Use together cautiously.

Adverse reactions
CNS: paresthesia, unsteady gait, numbness, somnolence.

☑ Special considerations
• Prepare a dietary history. A single vitamin deficiency is unusual; lack of one vitamin often indicates a deficiency of others.
• A dosage of 25 mg/kg/day is well tolerated. Adults consuming 200 mg/day for 33 days and on a normal dietary intake develop vitamin B_6 dependency.
• Don't mix with sodium bicarbonate in the same syringe.

- Patients receiving levodopa shouldn't take pyridoxine in doses above 5 mg/day.
- Store in a tight, light-resistant container.
- Don't use injection solution if it contains precipitate. Slight darkening is acceptable.
- Pyridoxine is sometimes useful for treating nausea and vomiting during pregnancy.
- Pyridoxine therapy alters determinations for urobilinogen in the spot test using Ehrlich's reagent, resulting in a false-positive reaction.
- Toxicity may cause ataxia and severe sensory neuropathy after long-term consumption of high daily doses of pyridoxine (2 to 6 g). These neurologic deficits usually resolve after pyridoxine is discontinued.

Monitoring the patient
- Monitor protein intake; excessive protein intake increases pyridoxine requirements.

Information for the patient
- Teach patient about dietary sources of vitamin B_6, such as yeast, wheat germ, liver, whole grain cereals, bananas, and legumes.

Pediatric patients
- Safety and efficacy in children haven't been established.
- The use of large doses of pyridoxine during pregnancy has been implicated in pyridoxine-dependency seizures in neonates.

Breast-feeding patients
- Drug appears in breast milk. Use caution when administering to breast-feeding women. Pyridoxine may inhibit lactation by suppression of prolactin.

---

pyrimethamine
Daraprim

Pharmacologic classification: aminopyrimidine derivative (folic acid antagonist)
Therapeutic classification: antimalarial
Pregnancy risk category C

How supplied
Available by prescription only
Tablets: 25 mg of pyrimethamine

Indications, route, and dosage
Malaria prophylaxis and transmission control
Adults and children over age 10: 25 mg P.O. weekly.
Children ages 4 to 10: 12.5 mg P.O. weekly.
Children under age 4: 6.25 mg P.O. weekly.
    Dosage should be continued for all age-groups for at least 10 weeks after leaving endemic areas.

Acute attacks of malaria
Not recommended alone in nonimmune persons; use with faster-acting antimalarials, such as chloroquine, for 2 days to initiate transmission control and suppressive cure. For chloroquine-resistant strain, administer with sulfonamides and possibly quinine.
Adults and children over age 15: 50 mg P.O. daily for 2 days.
Toxoplasmosis
Adults: 50 to 75 mg P.O. daily for 3 to 4 weeks, with sulfadiazine 2 to 8 g P.O. daily in three or four divided doses.
◇ *Children:* 1 mg/kg/day P.O. (maximum daily dose is 25 mg) in divided doses q 12 hours for 3 days; then 1 mg/kg/day P.O. for 4 weeks. Administer with sulfadoxine 100 to 200 mg P.O. daily in divided doses.
◇ **Isosporiasis**
Adults: 50 to 75 mg P.O. daily.

Pharmacodynamics
Antimalarial action: Inhibits the reduction of dihydrofolate to tetrahydrofolate, thereby blocking folic acid metabolism needed for survival of susceptible organisms. This mechanism is distinct from sulfonamide-induced folic acid antagonism. Drug is active against the asexual erythrocytic forms of susceptible plasmodia and against *Toxoplasma gondii*.

Pharmacokinetics
- *Absorption:* Well absorbed from intestinal tract; serum levels peak within 2 hours.
- *Distribution:* Distributed to kidneys, liver, spleen, and lungs; about 80% bound to plasma proteins.
- *Metabolism:* Metabolized to several unidentified compounds.
- *Excretion:* Excreted in urine and breast milk; elimination half-life 2 to 6 days. Half-life not changed in end-stage renal disease.

Contraindications and precautions
Contraindicated in patients with hypersensitivity to drug and in those with megaloblastic anemia due to folic acid deficiency. Use cautiously in patients with impaired renal or hepatic function, severe allergy or bronchial asthma, G6PD deficiency, or seizure disorders and in those who have been treated with chloroquine.

Interactions
Drug-drug. *Co-trimoxazole, other sulfonamides:* Additive adverse effects. Pyrimethamine and sulfadoxine combination shouldn't be given with these drugs.
Folic acid, para-aminobenzoic acid: Reduced antitoxoplasmic effects of pyrimethamine. May need dosage adjustment.
Lorazepam: Mild hepatotoxicity. Monitor liver function.

Reactions may be *common*, uncommon, **life-threatening**, or COMMON AND LIFE-THREATENING.

Sulfonamides: Pyrimethamine and sulfonamides act synergistically against some organisms; each inhibits folic acid synthesis at a different level. Monitor patient if used together.

Adverse reactions
GI: anorexia, vomiting, atrophic glossitis.
Hematologic: *aplastic anemia,* megaloblastic anemia, *leukopenia, thrombocytopenia, pancytopenia.*
    Note: Adverse drug reactions related to sulfadiazine are similar to those of sulfonamides.

☑ Special considerations
● No longer considered a first-line antimalarial. Other antimalarials (mefloquine, chloroquine, sulfadoxine) are generally preferred.
● Give drug with meals to minimize GI distress.
● Because severe reactions may occur, pyrimethamine with sulfadoxine should be given only to patient traveling to areas where chloroquine-resistant malaria is prevalent and only if traveler will be in such areas longer than 3 weeks.
● Toxicity may cause anorexia, vomiting, and CNS stimulation, including seizures. Megaloblastic anemia, thrombocytopenia, leukopenia, glossitis, and crystalluria may also occur. Treatment of overdose consists of gastric lavage, then a cathartic; barbiturates may help to control seizures. Leucovorin (folinic acid) in a dosage of 5 to 15 mg/day P.O., I.M., or I.V. for 3 days or longer is used to restore decreased platelet or leukocyte counts.

Monitoring the patient
● Monitor CBC, including platelet counts, twice weekly.
● Monitor patient for signs of folate deficiency or bleeding when platelet count is low; if abnormalities appear, decrease dosage or stop drug. Leucovorin (folinic acid) may be prescribed to raise blood counts while reducing dosage or after drug is stopped.

Information for the patient
● Teach patient how to recognize signs and symptoms of adverse blood reactions and tell him to report them immediately. Teach emergency measures to control overt bleeding.
● Teach patient signs and symptoms of folate deficiency.
● Counsel patient about need to report adverse effects and to keep follow-up medical appointments.
● Tell patient to keep drug out of reach of children.

Pediatric patients
● Use with caution in children.

Breast-feeding patients
● Pyrimethamine is contraindicated in breast-feeding women because of the risk of serious adverse reactions in breast-fed infants.

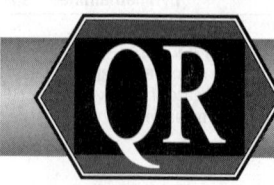

quetiapine fumarate
Seroquel

Pharmacologic classification: dibenzo-thiazepine derivative
Therapeutic classification: antipsychotic
Pregnancy risk category C

How supplied
Available by prescription only
Tablets: 25 mg, 100 mg, 200 mg

Indications, route, and dosage
Management of signs and symptoms of psychotic disorders
Adults: Initially, 25 mg P.O. b.i.d., with increases in increments of 25 to 50 mg b.i.d. or t.i.d. on days 2 and 3, as tolerated to a target dose range of 300 to 400 mg daily by day 4, divided into two or three doses. Further dosage adjustments, if indicated, should generally occur at intervals of not less than 2 days. Dosages can be increased or decreased by 25 to 50 mg b.i.d. Antipsychotic efficacy is generally in range of 150 to 750 mg/day. Safety of doses above 800 mg/day hasn't been evaluated.

✦ **Dosage adjustment.** In elderly or debilitated patients or those who have hepatic impairment or a predisposition to hypotensive reactions, consider lower doses, slower adjustment, and careful monitoring during initial dosing period. No specific dosing recommendations are given.

Pharmacodynamics
Antipsychotic action: Exact mechanism unknown. A dibenzothiazepine derivative thought to exert antipsychotic activity through antagonism of dopamine type 2 (D_2) and serotonin type 2 ($5\text{-}HT_2$) receptors. Antagonism at serotonin $5\text{-}HT_{1A}$, D_1, H_1, and alpha$_1$- and alpha$_2$-adrenergic receptors may explain other effects.

Pharmacokinetics
• *Absorption:* Rapidly absorbed after oral administration. Plasma levels peak in about 1½ hours. Food affects absorption; maximum level increases 25% and bioavailability increases 15%.
• *Distribution:* Apparent volume of distribution is 6 to 14 L/kg. 83% plasma protein-bound. Steady-state levels reached within 2 days.
• *Metabolism:* Extensively metabolized by liver via sulfoxidation and oxidation. Cytochrome P-450 3A4 is major isoenzyme involved.
• *Excretion:* Less than 1% of dose excreted as unchanged drug. About 73% recovered in urine; 20% in feces. Mean terminal half-life about 6 hours.

Contraindications and precautions
Contraindicated in patients with hypersensitivity to drug or its components. Use cautiously in patients with known CV or cerebrovascular disease or conditions that would predispose patient to hypotension; history of seizures or with conditions that potentially lower the seizure threshold; and in those at risk for aspiration pneumonia because of associated esophageal dysmotility and aspiration. Also use with caution in patients with conditions that may contribute to an elevation in core body temperature.

Interactions
Drug-drug. *Antihypertensives:* Potentiated hypotensive effect of both drugs. Monitor blood pressure.
Centrally acting drugs: Increased CNS depression. Use cautiously.
Cimetidine: Decreased mean oral clearance of quetiapine. Adjust quetiapine dosage as needed.
Cytochrome P-450 3A inhibitors (erythromycin, fluconazole, itraconazole, ketoconazole): Decreased quetiapine clearance. Use cautiously.
Dopamine agonists, levodopa: Possible antagonized effect of these drugs. Monitor patient closely.
Lorazepam: Reduced mean oral clearance when administered with quetiapine. Monitor patient.
Phenytoin: Fivefold increase in mean oral clearance of quetiapine. Adjust quetiapine dosage as needed.
Thioridazine: 65% increase in oral clearance of quetiapine. Adjust quetiapine dosage as needed.
Drug-lifestyle. *Alcohol:* Potentiated cognitive and motor effects. Discourage use.

Adverse reactions
CNS: *dizziness, headache, somnolence,* hypertonia, asthenia, dysarthria.
CV: orthostatic hypotension, tachycardia, palpitations, peripheral edema.
EENT: pharyngitis, rhinitis, ear pain.
GI: dry mouth, dyspepsia, abdominal pain, constipation, anorexia.

Hematologic: *leukopenia.*
Metabolic: *weight gain.*
Musculoskeletal: back pain.
Respiratory: increased cough, dyspnea.
Skin: rash, diaphoresis.
Other: fever, flulike syndrome.

☑ Special considerations
• A decrease in total and free T_4 may occur; usually isn't clinically significant. Although rare, some patients experience increased thyroid-stimulating hormone and need thyroid replacement.
• Increases in cholesterol and triglycerides have been observed.
• Asymptomatic, transient, and reversible increases in serum transaminases (primarily ALT) have been reported. These elevations usually occur within the first 3 weeks of therapy and promptly return to pretreatment levels with continued use.
• Neuroleptic malignant syndrome, a potentially fatal syndrome, has been reported with use of antipsychotics. Signs and symptoms include hyperpyrexia, muscle rigidity, altered mental status, and evidence of autonomic instability. Carefully monitor at-risk patients.
• Use smallest effective dose for shortest duration to minimize risk of tardive dyskinesia.
• Toxicity may cause drowsiness, sedation, tachycardia, hypotension. Hypokalemia and first-degree heart block may also occur. Avoid use of disopyramide, procainamide, quinidine, and bretylium if antiarrhythmic therapy is indicated. Administer I.V. fluids or sympathomimetics (not epinephrine or dopamine) to treat hypotension and circulatory collapse. For severe extrapyramidal symptoms, administer anticholinergic drugs.

Monitoring the patient
• Examine the lens before therapy begins or shortly thereafter, and at 6-month intervals during long-term treatment for possible cataract formation.
• Monitor thyroid function, serum cholesterol and triglyceride levels, and hepatic function.
• Closely supervise schizophrenic patient during drug therapy because of inherent risk of suicide attempt.

Information for the patient
• Advise patient of risk of orthostatic hypotension, especially during the 3- to 5-day period of initial dosage adjustment and when dose is increased or treatment reinitiated.
• Tell patient to avoid becoming overheated or dehydrated.
• During initial dosage adjustment period or dosage increases, warn patient to avoid activities that require mental alertness, such as driving or operating hazardous machinery until CNS effects of drug are known.
• Advise patient to avoid alcohol while taking drug.

• Remind patient to have an initial eye examination at beginning of therapy and every 6 months during treatment to watch for cataract formation.
• Tell patient to call before taking other prescription or OTC drugs.
• Instruct woman to call if pregnancy is being planned or is suspected. Advise her not to breast-feed during therapy.

Geriatric patients
• There appears to be no difference in tolerability in patients ages 65 and older. However, the presence of factors that may decrease pharmacokinetic clearance, increase pharmacodynamic response to drug, or cause poorer tolerance or orthostasis should indicate use of a lower starting dose, slower adjustment, and careful monitoring during initial dosing period.

Pediatric patients
• Safety and effectiveness in children haven't been established.

Breast-feeding patients
• It's unknown if drug appears in breast milk; breast-feeding isn't recommended during therapy.

quinapril hydrochloride
Accupril

Pharmacologic classification: ACE inhibitor
Therapeutic classification: antihypertensive
Pregnancy risk category C (D second and third trimesters)

How supplied
Available by prescription only
Tablets: 5 mg, 10 mg, 20 mg, 40 mg

Indications, route, and dosage
Hypertension
Adults: Initially, 10 mg P.O. daily. Adjust dosage based on response at intervals of about 2 weeks. Most patients are controlled at 20, 40, or 80 mg daily, as a single dose or in two divided doses.
Hypertension in patients receiving diuretics, management of heart failure
Adults: Initially, 5 mg P.O. b.i.d. when added to diuretic and cardiac glycoside therapy. Adjust dosage weekly based on response. Usual dosage is 20 to 40 mg daily in two equally divided doses.
✦ *Dosage adjustment.* In adults with renal impairment, initial dose is 10 mg P.O. daily if creatinine clearance exceeds 60 ml/minute; 5 mg if it's 30 to 60 ml/minute; and 2.5 mg if it's 10 to 30 ml/minute. No dose recommendations are available for creatinine clearance below 10 ml/minute.

Pharmacodynamics

Antihypertensive action: Quinapril and its active metabolite, quinaprilat, inhibit ACE, preventing conversion of angiotensin I to angiotensin II, a potent vasoconstrictor. Reduced formation of angiotensin II decreases peripheral arterial resistance, decreases aldosterone secretion, reduces sodium and water retention, and lowers blood pressure. Quinapril also has antihypertensive activity in patients with low-renin hypertension.

Pharmacokinetics

● *Absorption:* At least 60% of drug absorbed; plasma levels peak within 1 hour. Rate and extent of absorption decrease 25% to 30% when administered during high-fat meal.
● *Distribution:* About 97% of drug and active metabolite bound to plasma proteins.
● *Metabolism:* About 38% of oral dose deesterified in liver to quinaprilat.
● *Excretion:* Primarily excreted in urine; terminal elimination half-life about 25 hours.

Contraindications and precautions

Contraindicated in patients with hypersensitivity to ACE inhibitors or history of angioedema related to treatment with an ACE inhibitor. Use cautiously in patients with impaired renal function.

Interactions

Drug-drug. *Diuretics, other antihypertensives:* Increased risk of excessive hypotension. Discontinue diuretic or lower dosage of quinapril as needed.
Lithium: Increased serum lithium levels. Monitor patient for lithium toxicity.
Potassium-sparing diuretics, potassium supplements: Increased risk of hyperkalemia. Don't use together.
Tetracycline: Significantly impaired absorption of tetracycline. Avoid concomitant use.
Drug-food. *Salt substitutes containing potassium:* Hyperkalemia. Don't use together.

Adverse reactions

CNS: somnolence, vertigo, nervousness, headache, dizziness, fatigue, depression.
CV: palpitations, tachycardia, angina, hypertensive crisis, orthostatic hypotension, chest pain, *rhythm disturbances.*
GI: dry mouth, abdominal pain, constipation, vomiting, nausea, hemorrhage.
Hematologic: *thrombocytopenia, agranulocytosis.*
Hepatic: elevated liver enzyme levels.
Metabolic: hyperkalemia.
Respiratory: *dry, persistent, tickling, nonproductive cough.*
Skin: pruritus, *exfoliative dermatitis, photosensitivity,* diaphoresis.
Other: *angioedema.*

☑ Special considerations

● Because administration with diuretics is associated with risk of excessive hypotension, diuretic therapy should end 2 to 3 days before start of quinapril, if possible. If quinapril alone doesn't adequately control blood pressure, a diuretic may be carefully added to regimen.
● Like other ACE inhibitors, drug may cause a dry, persistent, tickling cough; reversible when therapy ends.

Monitoring the patient

● Blood pressure measurements should be taken when drug levels are at their peak (2 to 6 hours after dosing) and at their trough (just before a dose) to verify adequate blood pressure control.
● Assess renal and hepatic function before and periodically throughout therapy. Also monitor CBC and serum potassium levels.

Information for the patient

● Tell patient that drug should be taken on an empty stomach because meals, particularly high-fat meals, can impair absorption.
● Tell patient to immediately report signs or symptoms of angioedema (swelling of face, eyes, lips, tongue, or difficulty breathing). If these occur, patient should stop drug and seek immediate medical attention.
● Warn patient that light-headedness may occur, especially during first few days of therapy. Tell him to arise slowly to minimize this effect and to report persistent or severe symptoms. If syncope (fainting) occurs, patient should stop drug and call immediately.
● Inadequate fluid intake, vomiting, diarrhea, and excessive perspiration can lead to light-headedness and syncope. Patient should take care in hot weather and during periods of exercise to avoid dehydration and overheating.
● Tell patient not to use sodium substitutes; they contain potassium and can cause hyperkalemia.
● Tell patient to immediately report signs or symptoms of infection (sore throat, fever) or easy bruising or bleeding. Other ACE inhibitors have been associated with development of agranulocytosis and neutropenia.

Geriatric patients

● Elderly patients have demonstrated higher peak plasma levels and slower elimination of drug; these changes were related to decreased renal function that often occurs in elderly patients. No overall differences in safety or efficacy have been seen in elderly patients.

Pediatric patients

● Safety and efficacy in children haven't been established.

Reactions may be *common,* uncommon, *life-threatening,* or COMMON AND LIFE-THREATENING.

Breast-feeding patients
● It's unknown if drug appears in breast milk. Use with caution in breast-feeding women.

quinidine gluconate
Quinaglute Dura-Tabs, Quinalan

quinidine polygalacturonate
Cardioquin

quinidine sulfate
Apo-Quinidine*, Quinidex Extentabs, Quinora

Pharmacologic classification: cinchona alkaloid
Therapeutic classification: ventricular antiarrhythmic, supraventricular antiarrhythmic, atrial antitachyarrhythmic
Pregnancy risk category C

How supplied
Available by prescription only
Tablets: 325 mg* (gluconate); 275 mg (polygalacturonate); 200 mg, 300 mg (sulfate);
Tablets (extended-release): 300 mg (sulfate); 324 mg (gluconate)
Injection: 80 mg/ml (gluconate); 190 mg/ml (sulfate)*

Indications, route, and dosage
Atrial flutter or fibrillation
Adults: 200 mg (sulfate or equivalent base) P.O. q 2 to 3 hours for five to eight doses with subsequent daily increases until sinus rhythm is restored or toxic effects develop. Administer quinidine only after digitalization to avoid increasing AV conduction. Maximum dose is 3 to 4 g daily.
Maintenance dose is 200 to 400 mg P.O. t.i.d. or q.i.d., or 600 mg P.O. q 8 to 12 hours daily (extended-release).
Paroxysmal supraventricular tachycardia
Adults: 400 to 600 mg (sulfate) P.O. q 2 to 3 hours until toxic effects develop or arrhythmia subsides.
Premature atrial contractions, PVCs, paroxysmal AV junctional rhythm or atrial or ventricular tachycardia, maintenance of cardioversion
Adults: Give test dose of 50 to 200 mg P.O. of sulfate (or 200 mg gluconate I.M.); then monitor vital signs before beginning therapy: 200 to 400 mg P.O. sulfate or equivalent base q 4 to 6 hours; or, initially, 600 mg of gluconate I.M., then up to 400 mg q 2 hours, p.r.n.; or 800 mg I.V. gluconate diluted in 40 ml of D₅W, infused at 16 mg (1 ml)/minute. Or give 300 to 600 mg of sulfate (extended-release), or 324 to 648 mg of gluconate (extended-release), q 8 to 12 hours.
Children: Give test dose of 2 mg/kg, then 30 mg/kg/day P.O. or 900 mg/m²/day P.O. in five divided doses.

◊ *Malaria (when quinine dihydrochloride is unavailable)*
Adults: Administer quinidine gluconate by continuous I.V. infusion. Initial loading dose of 10 mg/kg diluted in 250 ml of normal saline injection and infused over 1 to 2 hours, then a continuous maintenance infusion of 0.02 mg/kg/minute (20 mcg/kg/minute) for 72 hours or until parasitemia is reduced to less than 1% or oral therapy can be started; or 10 mg/kg quinidine sulfate P.O. q 8 hours for 5 to 7 days. Contact the Centers for Disease Control and Prevention (CDC) Malaria Branch for protocol instructions and recommendations.

Pharmacodynamics
Antiarrhythmic action: A class IA antiarrhythmic that depresses phase O of the action potential. Considered a myocardial depressant because it decreases myocardial excitability and conduction velocity and may depress myocardial contractility. Also exerts anticholinergic activity, which may modify direct myocardial effects. In therapeutic doses, reduces conduction velocity in the atria, ventricles, and His-Purkinje system. Helps control atrial tachyarrhythmias by prolonging the effective refractory period (ERP) and increasing the action potential duration in the atria, ventricles, and His-Purkinje system. Because ERP prolongation exceeds action potential duration, tissue remains refractory even after returning to resting membrane potential (membrane-stabilizing effect).
Shortens the effective refractory period of the AV node. Because quinidine's anticholinergic action may increase AV node conductivity, a cardiac glycoside should be administered for atrial tachyarrhythmias before quinidine therapy begins to prevent ventricular tachyarrhythmias. Quinidine also suppresses automaticity in the His-Purkinje system and ectopic pacemakers, making it useful in treating PVCs. At therapeutic doses, quinidine prolongs the QRS complex duration and QT interval; these ECG effects may be used as an index of drug effectiveness and toxicity.

Pharmacokinetics
● *Absorption:* Although all quinidine salts are well absorbed from GI tract, individual serum drug levels vary greatly. Onset of action of quinidine sulfate from 1 to 3 hours. For extended-release forms, onset of action may be slightly slower but duration of effect longer; drug delivery system allows longer-than-usual dosing intervals. Plasma levels peak in 3 to 4 hours for quinidine gluconate; 6 hours for quinidine polygalacturonate.
● *Distribution:* Well distributed in all tissues except brain; concentrates in heart, liver, kidneys, and skeletal muscle. Distribution volume decreases in patients with heart failure, possibly re-

quiring reduction in maintenance dose. About 80% bound to plasma proteins; the unbound (active) fraction may increase in patients with hypoalbuminemia from various causes, including hepatic insufficiency. Usual therapeutic serum levels depend on assay method and range as follows:
– Specific assay (enzyme multiplied immunoassay technique, high-performance liquid chromatography, fluorescence polarization): 2 to 5 mcg/ml.
– Nonspecific assay (fluorometric): 4 to 8 mcg/ml.
• *Metabolism:* About 60% to 80% of drug metabolized in liver to two metabolites that may have some pharmacologic activity.
• *Excretion:* About 10% to 30% of dose excreted in urine within 24 hours as unchanged drug. Urine acidification increases quinidine excretion; alkalinization decreases excretion. Most of dose eliminated in urine as metabolites; elimination half-life ranges from 5 to 12 hours (usual half-life is about 6½ hours). Duration of effect ranges from 6 to 8 hours.

Contraindications and precautions
Contraindicated in patients with idiosyncrasy or hypersensitivity to quinidine or related cinchona derivatives and in those with intraventricular conduction defects, cardiac glycoside toxicity when AV conduction is grossly impaired, abnormal rhythms due to escape mechanisms, and history of drug-induced torsades de pointes or QT syndrome.

Use cautiously in patients with impaired renal or hepatic function, asthma, muscle weakness, or infection accompanied by a fever because hypersensitivity reactions may be masked.

Interactions
Drug-drug. *Antacids, sodium bicarbonate, thiazide diuretics:* Decreased quinidine elimination when urine pH increased. Monitor levels and adjust dosage as needed.
Antiarrhythmics (such as amiodarone, lidocaine, phenytoin, procainamide, propranolol): Additive or antagonistic cardiac effects and additive toxic effects. Monitor patient closely.
Anticholinergics: Additive anticholinergic effects. Monitor patient closely.
Anticonvulsants (such as phenobarbital, phenytoin): Increased rate of quinidine metabolism. Adjust dosage as needed.
Cholinergics: Quinidine antagonizes cholinergics' vagal excitation effect on atria and AV node. Use other drugs to terminate paroxysmal supraventricular tachycardia.
Coumarin: Potentiated anticoagulant effect. Monitor PT and INR.
Digitoxin, digoxin: Increased (possibly toxic) serum digoxin levels. Monitor serum digoxin levels and reduce dosage as needed.
Hypotensive drugs: Additive hypotensive effects. Monitor blood pressure.

Neostigmine, pyridostigmine: Decreased effects of these drugs when used to treat myasthenia gravis. Monitor patient.
Neuromuscular blockers (such as metocurine iodide, pancuronium bromide, succinylcholine chloride, tubocurarine chloride): Potentiated anticholinergic effects. Use of quinidine should be avoided immediately after use of these drugs; if quinidine must be used, respiratory support may be needed.
Nifedipine: Decreases quinidine levels. Adjust dosage as needed.
Phenothiazines, reserpine: Possible additive cardiac depressant effects. Monitor patient.
Rifampin: Increased quinidine metabolism; decreased serum quinidine levels. Adjust dosage as needed.
Verapamil: Significant hypotension in some patients with hypertrophic cardiomyopathy. Monitor vital signs.
Drug-herb. *Jimsonweed:* May adversely affect cardiovascular system function. Avoid using together.
Licorice: Possible prolonged QT interval; potentially additive. Use cautiously together.

Adverse reactions
CNS: *vertigo, headache, light-headedness,* confusion, ataxia, depression, dementia.
CV: *PVCs; **ventricular tachycardia; atypical ventricular tachycardia (torsades de pointes);** hypotension; **complete AV block,** tachycardia; ECG changes (particularly widening of QRS complex, widened QT and PR intervals).*
EENT: *tinnitus,* excessive salivation, blurred vision, diplopia, photophobia.
GI: *diarrhea, nausea, vomiting,* anorexia, abdominal pain.
Hematologic: *hemolytic anemia, thrombocytopenia, agranulocytosis.*
Hepatic: *hepatotoxicity.*
Respiratory: acute asthmatic attack, *respiratory arrest.*
Skin: rash, petechial hemorrhage of buccal mucosa, pruritus, urticaria, lupus erythematosus, photosensitivity.
Other: *angioedema,* fever, cinchonism.

☑ Special considerations
• When drug is used to treat atrial tachyarrhythmias, ventricular rate may be accelerated from drug's anticholinergic effects on AV node. This can be prevented by previous treatment with a cardiac glycoside.
• Because conversion of chronic atrial fibrillation may be associated with embolism, anticoagulant should be administered for several weeks before quinidine therapy begins.
• I.V. route should be used for acute arrhythmias only; it's generally avoided because of potential for severe hypotension.

• Don't use discolored (brownish) quinidine solution.
• For maintenance, give only by oral or I.M. route. Dosage requirements vary. Some patients may need drug q 4 hours, others q 6 hours. Adjust dose by both clinical response and blood levels.
• When changing administration route, alter dosage to compensate for variations in quinidine base content.
• Decrease dosage in patients with heart failure and hepatic disease.
• Lidocaine may be effective in treating quinidine-induced arrhythmias because it increases AV conduction.
• Quinidine may cause hemolysis in patients with G6PD deficiency.
• Small amounts of quinidine are removed by hemodialysis; drug isn't removed by peritoneal dialysis.
• Amount of quinidine in the different salt forms varies as follows:
– Gluconate: 62% quinidine (324 mg of gluconate, 202 mg sulfate).
– Polygalacturonate: 60% quinidine (275 mg polygalacturonate, 166 mg sulfate).
– Sulfate: 83% quinidine. The sulfate form is considered the standard dosage preparation.
• Quinidine gluconate is reported to be as or more active in vitro against *Plasmodium falciparum* than quinine dihydrochloride. Because the latter drug is only available through the CDC, quinidine gluconate may be useful in the treatment of severe malaria when delay of therapy may be life-threatening. The current CDC protocol involves follow-up treatment with either tetracycline or sulfadoxine and pyrimethamine.
• Toxicity may cause severe hypotension, ventricular arrhythmias (including torsades de pointes), and seizures. QRS complexes and QT and PR intervals may be prolonged, and ataxia, anuria, respiratory distress, irritability, and hallucinations may develop. Urine acidification may be used to help increase quinidine elimination. Metaraminol or norepinephrine may be used to reverse hypotension (after adequate hydration has been ensured).
• CNS depressants should be avoided because CNS depression may occur, possibly with seizures. Cardiac pacing may be necessary.
• Isoproterenol or ventricular pacing possibly may be used to treat torsades de pointes tachycardia.
• I.V. infusion of 1/6 M sodium lactate solution reduces quinidine's cardiotoxic effect. Hemodialysis, although rarely warranted, also may be effective.

Monitoring the patient
• Check apical pulse rate, blood pressure, and ECG tracing before starting therapy.
• Monitor ECG, especially when large doses of drug are being administered. Quinidine-induced

cardiotoxicity is evidenced by conduction defects (50% widening of the QRS complex), ventricular tachycardia or flutter, frequent PVCs, and complete AV block. When these ECG signs appear, stop drug and monitor patient closely.
• Monitor liver function tests during first 4 to 8 weeks of therapy.
• Drug may increase toxicity of cardiac glycoside derivatives. Use cautiously in patients receiving cardiac glycosides. Monitor digoxin levels and expect to reduce dosage of cardiac glycoside derivatives; many clinicians recommend that digoxin dosage be reduced by 50% when quinidine therapy is initiated.
• GI adverse effects, especially diarrhea, are signs of toxicity. Check quinidine blood levels; suspect toxicity when they exceed 8 mcg/ml. GI symptoms may be minimized by giving drug with meals.

Information for the patient
• Instruct patient to report rash, fever, unusual bleeding, bruising, ringing in ears, or visual disturbance.

Geriatric patients
• Dosage reduction may be needed in elderly patients. Because of highly variable metabolism, monitor serum levels.

Breast-feeding patients
• Drug appears in breast milk. An alternative to breast-feeding is recommended during therapy.

quinine sulfate

Pharmacologic classification: cinchona alkaloid
Therapeutic classification: antimalarial
Pregnancy risk category D

How supplied
Available by prescription only
Tablets: 260 mg, 325 mg
Capsules: 260 mg, 325 mg

Indications, route, and dosage
Malaria (chloroquine-resistant)
Adults: 650 mg P.O. q 8 hours for 10 days, with 25 mg pyrimethamine q 12 hours for 3 days and with 500 mg sulfadiazine q.i.d. for 5 days.
Children: 25 mg/kg/day divided into three doses for 10 days.
Babesia microti *infections*
Adults: 650 mg P.O. q 6 to 8 hours for 7 days.
Children: 25 mg/kg/day divided into three doses for 7 days.
◊ *Nocturnal recumbency leg muscle cramps*
Adults: 200 to 300 mg P.O. h.s. Stop if leg cramps don't occur after several days to determine if continued therapy is necessary.

Pharmacodynamics

Antimalarial action: Intercalates into DNA, disrupting the parasite's replication and transcription; also depresses its oxygen uptake and carbohydrate metabolism. Active against the asexual erythrocytic forms of *Plasmodium falciparum, P. malariae, P. ovale,* and *P. vivax* and is used for chloroquine-resistant malaria.

Skeletal muscle relaxant action: Increases the refractory period, decreases excitability of the motor end plate, and affects calcium distribution within muscle fibers.

Pharmacokinetics

• *Absorption:* Almost completely absorbed; serum levels peak in 1 to 3 hours.
• *Distribution:* Distributed widely into liver, lungs, kidneys, and spleen; CSF levels reach 2% to 5% of serum levels. About 70% bound to plasma proteins; readily crosses placenta.
• *Metabolism:* Metabolized in liver.
• *Excretion:* Less than 5% of single dose excreted unchanged in urine; small amounts of metabolites appear in feces, gastric juice, bile, saliva, and breast milk. Half-life is 7 to 21 hours in healthy or convalescing persons; longer in patients with malaria. Urine acidification hastens elimination.

Contraindications and precautions

Contraindicated in patients with hypersensitivity to drug, during pregnancy, and in those with G6PD deficiency, optic neuritis, tinnitus, or history of blackwater fever or thrombocytopenic purpura associated with previous quinine ingestion.

Use cautiously in patients with arrhythmias and in those taking sodium bicarbonate.

Interactions

Drug-drug. *Acetazolamide, sodium bicarbonate:* Increased level of quinine via decreased urinary excretion. Adjust quinine dosage as needed.

Antacids containing aluminum: Delayed or decreased absorption of quinine. Separate administration times.

Digitoxin, digoxin: Increased plasma levels. Monitor serum digoxin levels.

Mefloquine: Additive cardiac effects. Don't use together.

Neuromuscular blockers: Potentiated effects of these drugs. Monitor patient closely.

Warfarin: Quinine depresses synthesis of vitamin K–dependent clotting factors. Monitor PT and INR.

Adverse reactions

CNS: severe headache, apprehension, excitement, confusion, delirium, syncope, hypothermia, vertigo, *seizures* (with toxic doses).
CV: hypotension, *CV collapse* (with overdose or rapid I.V. administration), conduction disturbances.
EENT: altered color perception, photophobia, blurred vision, night blindness, amblyopia, scotoma, diplopia, mydriasis, optic atrophy, tinnitus, impaired hearing.
GI: epigastric distress, diarrhea, nausea, vomiting.
GU: renal tubular damage, anuria.
Hematologic: hemolytic anemia, *thrombocytopenia, agranulocytosis,* hypoprothrombinemia, thrombosis at infusion site.
Metabolic: hypoglycemia.
Respiratory: asthma, dyspnea.
Skin: rash, pruritus.
Other: flushing, fever, facial edema.

☑ Special considerations

• Administer quinine after meals to minimize gastric distress; don't crush tablets because drug irritates gastric mucosa.
• Stop drug if signs of idiosyncrasy or toxicity occur.
• Quinine is no longer used for acute malarial attack by *P. vivax* or for suppression of malaria from resistant organisms.
• Drug causes false elevations of urinary catecholamines and may interfere with 17-hydroxycorticosteroid and 17-ketogenic steroid tests.
• Toxicity may cause tinnitus, vertigo, headache, fever, rash, CV effects, GI distress (including vomiting), blindness, apprehension, confusion, and seizures. Urinary acidification may increase elimination of quinine but will also augment renal obstruction. Hemodialysis or hemoperfusion may be helpful. Vasodilator therapy or stellate blockage may relieve visual disturbances.

Monitoring the patient

• Serum levels of 10 mcg/ml or more may confirm toxicity as the cause of tinnitus or hearing loss.
• Monitor CBC and coagulation studies as needed.

Information for the patient

• Teach patient about adverse reactions, especially tinnitus and hearing impairment, and the need to report these immediately.
• Tell patient to avoid concurrent use of antacids containing aluminum because these may alter drug absorption.
• Instruct patient to keep drug out of reach of children.

Geriatric patients

• Use with caution in patients with conduction disturbances.

Breast-feeding patients

• Drug appears in breast milk. Before drug is given to breast-feeding mother, evaluate infant for possible G6PD deficiency.

---

quinupristin/dalfopristin
Synercid

Pharmacologic classification: streptogramin
Therapeutic classification: antibiotic
Pregnancy risk category B

How supplied
Available by prescription only
Injection: 500 mg/10 ml (150 mg quinupristin and 350 mg dalfopristin)

Indications, route, and dosage
Serious or life-threatening infections associated with vancomycin-resistant Enterococcus faecium (VREF) bacteremia
Adults and adolescents ages 16 and older: 7.5 mg/kg I.V. infusion over 1 hour every 8 hours. Treatment duration should be determined by site and severity of infection.
Complicated skin and skin-structure infections due to Staphylococcus aureus (methicillin susceptible) or Streptococcus pyogenes
Adults and adolescents ages 16 and older: 7.5 mg/kg I.V. infusion over 1 hour every 12 hours for at least 7 days.

Pharmacodynamics
Antibiotic action: The two antibiotics, quinupristin and dalfopristin, work synergistically to inhibit or destroy susceptible bacteria through combined inhibition on protein synthesis in bacterial cells. Dalfopristin inhibits the early phase of protein synthesis in the bacterial ribosome while quinupristin inhibits the late phase of protein synthesis. Without the ability to manufacture new proteins, the bacterial cells are inactivated or die.

Pharmacokinetics
• *Absorption:* Quinupristin and dalfopristin have different pharmacokinetic profiles. After multiple infusion doses of 7.5 mg/kg every 8 hours, levels of quinupristin and metabolites peak at 3.2 mcg/ml; dalfopristin levels peak at 8 mcg/ml.
• *Distribution:* Moderate protein-binding.
• *Metabolism:* Quinupristin and dalfopristin converted to several active major metabolites by nonenzymatic reactions.
• *Excretion:* About 75% of both drugs and their metabolites excreted in feces. About 15% of quinupristin and 19% of dalfopristin excreted in urine. Elimination half-life of quinupristin and dalfopristin is about 0.85 and 0.70 hours, respectively.

Contraindications and precautions
Contraindicated in patients with hypersensitivity to drug or other streptogramin antibiotics.

Interactions
Drug-drug: *Cyclosporine:* Reduced metabolism; levels may increase. Monitor cyclosporine levels.
Drugs metabolized by cytochrome P-450 3A4 (such as carbamazepine, delavirdine, diazepam, diltiazem, disopyramide, docetaxel, indinavir, lidocaine, lovastatin, methylprednisolone, midazolam, nevirapine, nifedipine, paclitaxel, ritonavir, tacrolimus, verapamil, vinblastine): Increased plasma levels of these drugs; possible increased therapeutic effects and adverse reactions. Use together cautiously.
Drugs metabolized by cytochrome P-450 3A4 that may prolong QT_c interval (such as quinidine): Decreased metabolism of these drugs resulting in prolongation of QT_c interval. Avoid concomitant use.

Adverse reactions
CNS: headache.
CV: thrombophlebitis.
GI: nausea, diarrhea, vomiting.
Hepatic: *elevated total and conjugated bilirubin level,* altered liver function studies.
Musculoskeletal: arthralgia, myalgia.
Skin: rash, pruritus.
Other: *inflammation, pain, edema at infusion site; infusion site reaction,* pain.

☑ Special considerations
• Quinupristin/dalfopristin isn't active against *Enterococcus faecalis.* Appropriate blood cultures are needed to avoid misidentifying *E. faecalis* as *E. faecium.*
• Reconstitute powder for injection by adding 5 ml of either sterile water for injection or D_5W and gently swirling vial by manual rotation to ensure dissolution; avoid shaking to limit foaming. Reconstituted solutions must be further diluted within 30 minutes.
• Quinupristin/dalfopristin is incompatible with saline and heparin solutions. Don't dilute drug with solutions containing saline or infuse into lines that contain saline or heparin. Flush line with D_5W before and after each dose.
• The appropriate dose, according to patient's weight, of reconstituted solution should be added to 250 ml of D_5W to make a final concentration of no more than 2 mg/ml. This diluted solution is stable for 5 hours at room temperature or 54 hours if refrigerated.
• Administer all doses by I.V. infusion over 1 hour. An infusion pump or device may be used to control rate of infusion.
• Fluid-restricted patients with a central venous catheter may receive dose in 100 ml of D_5W. This concentration isn't recommended for peripheral venous administration.
• If moderate to severe peripheral venous irritation occurs, consider increasing infusion volume to 500 or 750 ml, changing injection site, or infusing by a central venous catheter.

• Because mild to life-threatening pseudomembranous colitis has been reported with use of quinupristin/dalfopristin, consider this diagnosis in patients who develop diarrhea during or after therapy.
• Adverse reactions, such as arthralgia and myalgia, may be reduced by decreasing dosage interval to every 12 hours.
• Drug isn't removed by peritoneal dialysis or hemodialysis.

Monitoring the patient
• Because overgrowth of nonsusceptible organisms may occur, monitor patient closely for signs and symptoms of superinfection.
• Monitor liver function tests during therapy.

Information for the patient
• Advise patient to immediately report irritation at I.V. site, pain in joints or muscles, and diarrhea.
• Tell patient about importance of reporting persistent or worsening signs and symptoms of infection, such as pain and erythema.

Geriatric patients
• No dosage adjustment is needed in elderly patients.

Pediatric patients
• Safety and efficacy of drug in patients under age 16 haven't been established. However, under emergency conditions, patients have been given 7.5 mg every 8 or 12 hours.

Breast-feeding patients
• It's unknown if drug appears in breast milk. Use with caution in breast-feeding women.

---

rabeprazole sodium
Aciphex

Pharmacologic classification: proton pump inhibitor
Therapeutic classification: antiulcerative
Pregnancy risk category B

How supplied
Available by prescription only
Tablets (delayed-release): 20 mg

Indications, route, and dosage
Healing of erosive or ulcerative gastroesophageal reflux disease (GERD)
Adults: 20 mg P.O. daily for 4 to 8 weeks. Additional 8-week course may be considered, if necessary.
Maintenance of healing of erosive or ulcerative GERD
Adults: 20 mg P.O. daily.
Healing of duodenal ulcers
Adults: 20 mg P.O. daily after morning meal for up to 4 weeks.

Treatment of pathological hypersecretory conditions, including Zollinger-Ellison syndrome
Adults: 60 mg P.O. daily; may be increased, p.r.n., to 100 mg P.O. daily or 60 mg P.O. twice daily.

Pharmacodynamics
Antiulcerative action: Blocks activity of the acid (proton) pump by inhibiting gastric hydrogen-potassium adenosine triphosphatase at the secretory surface of the gastric parietal cell, thereby blocking gastric acid secretion.

Pharmacokinetics
• *Absorption:* Acid labile; enteric coating allows drug to pass through stomach relatively intact. Plasma levels peak over a period of 2 to 5 hours.
• *Distribution:* 96.3% plasma protein-bound.
• *Metabolism:* Extensively metabolized by liver to inactive compounds.
• *Excretion:* 90% eliminated in urine as metabolites. Remaining 10% of metabolites eliminated in feces. Plasma half-life is 1 to 2 hours.

Contraindications and precautions
Contraindicated in patients with hypersensitivity to rabeprazole, other benzimidazoles (lansoprazole, omeprazole), or components in these formulations. Use cautiously in patients with severe hepatic impairment.

Interactions
Drug-drug. *Cyclosporine:* Inhibited cyclosporine metabolism. Use together cautiously.
Digoxin, ketoconazole, other gastric pH-dependent drugs: Decreased or increased drug absorption at increased pH values. Monitor patient closely when used concomitantly.

Adverse reactions
CNS: headache, dizziness, malaise, asthenia, migraine, syncope, insomnia, anxiety, depression, nervousness, somnolence, neuralgia, vertigo, *seizures,* abnormal dreams, neuropathy, paresthesia, tremor.
CV: substernal chest pain, hypertension, *myocardial infarction,* electrocardiogram abnormalities, angina, bundle-branch block, palpitations, *sinus bradycardia,* tachycardia, edema.
EENT: epistaxis, cataracts, amblyopia, glaucoma, dry eyes, abnormal vision, tinnitus, otitis media.
GI: diarrhea, nausea, abdominal pain, vomiting, dyspepsia, flatulence, constipation, dry mouth, eructation, gastroenteritis, rectal hemorrhage, melena, anorexia, cholelithiasis, mouth ulceration, stomatitis, dysphagia, gingivitis, cholecystitis, increased appetite, abnormal stools, colitis, esophagitis, glossitis, *pancreatitis,* proctitis.
GU: cystitis, urinary frequency, dysmenorrhea, dysuria, renal calculi, metrorrhagia, polyuria, decreased libido.
Hematologic: anemia.

Reactions may be *common*, uncommon, *life-threatening*, or COMMON AND LIFE-THREATENING.

Metabolic: hyperthyroidism, hypothyroidism, weight gain, weight loss, dehydration.
Musculoskeletal: neck rigidity, myalgia, arthritis, leg cramps, bone pain, arthrosis, bursitis, hypertonia.
Respiratory: bronchitis, dyspnea, asthma, laryngitis, hiccups, hyperventilation.
Skin: rash, pruritus, sweating, urticaria, alopecia, photosensitivity reaction.
Other: infection, fever, *allergic reaction,* chills, lymphadenopathy, ecchymosis, gout.

☑ Special considerations
● Consider additional courses of therapy when duodenal ulcer or GERD isn't healed after first course of therapy.
● Symptomatic response to therapy doesn't preclude presence of gastric malignancy.

Monitoring the patient
● Monitor patient for improvement of symptoms.
● Perform periodic evaluations of ECG.

Information for the patient
● Explain importance of taking drug exactly as prescribed.
● Advise patient that delayed-release tablets should be swallowed whole; don't crush, chew, or split.
● Advise patient that drug may be taken without regard to meals.

Geriatric patients
● No differences in safety and effectiveness have been observed in elderly patients.

Pediatric patients
● Safety and efficacy in children haven't been established.

Breast-feeding patients
● It's unknown if drug appears in breast milk. Taking into account importance of drug to mother, stop either drug or breast-feeding.

rabies immune globulin, human (RIG)
Hyperab, Imogam Rabies Immune Globulin

Pharmacologic classification: immune serum
Therapeutic classification: rabies prophylaxis
Pregnancy risk category C

How supplied
Available by prescription only
Injection: 150 IU/ml in 2-ml and 10-ml vials

Indications, route, and dosage
Rabies exposure
Adults and children: 20 IU/kg at time of first dose of rabies vaccine. Use half dose to infiltrate wound area. Give remainder I.M. (gluteal area preferred). Don't give rabies vaccine and RIG in same syringe or at same site.

Pharmacodynamics
Postexposure rabies prophylaxis: Provides passive immunity to rabies.

Pharmacokinetics
● *Absorption:* After slow I.M. absorption, rabies antibody appears in serum within 24 hours; peaks within 2 to 13 days.
● *Distribution:* Probably crosses placenta and distributed into breast milk.
● *Metabolism:* No information available.
● *Excretion:* Serum half-life for rabies antibody titer is about 24 days.

Contraindications and precautions
Don't give repeated doses once vaccine treatment has been started. Use cautiously in patients with immunoglobulin A deficiency or history of prior systemic allergic reactions after administration of human immunoglobulin preparations and in those with known hypersensitivity to thimerosal.

Interactions
Drug-drug. *Corticosteroids, immunosuppressants:* May interfere with immune response to RIG. Whenever possible, avoid using these drugs during postexposure immunization period.
Live virus vaccine (such as measles, mumps, rubella): May interfere with immune response to these vaccines. Don't administer live virus vaccines within 3 months after administration of RIG.

Adverse reactions
GU: *nephrotic syndrome.*
Skin: *rash,* pain, redness, induration at injection site.
Other: slight fever, *anaphylaxis, angioedema.*

☑ Special considerations
● Obtain a thorough history of the animal bite, allergies, and reactions to immunizations.
● Have epinephrine solution 1:1,000 available to treat allergic reactions.
● Repeated doses of RIG shouldn't be given after rabies vaccine is started.
● Don't administer more than 5 ml I.M. at one injection site; divide I.M. doses over 5 ml and administer them at different sites.
● Don't confuse drug with rabies vaccine, which is a suspension of attenuated or killed microorganisms used to confer active immunity. These two drugs are commonly given together prophy-

lactically after exposure to known or suspected rabid animals.

• Because rabies can be fatal if untreated, use of RIG during pregnancy appears justified. No fetal risk from RIG use has been reported to date.

• Ask patient when he received his last tetanus immunization; a booster may be indicated.

• Patients previously immunized with a tissue culture-derived rabies vaccine and those who have confirmed adequate rabies antibody titers should receive only the vaccine.

• RIG hasn't been associated with an increased frequency of AIDS. The immune globulin is devoid of HIV. Immune globulin recipients don't develop antibodies to HIV.

• Store between 36° and 46° F (2° to 8° C). Don't freeze.

Monitoring the patient
• Monitor patient for adverse effects.
• Check renal function studies as needed.

Information for the patient
• Explain that the body needs about 1 week to develop immunity to rabies after receiving vaccine. Therefore, patients receive RIG to provide antibodies in their blood for immediate protection against rabies.

• Reactions to antirabies serum may occur up to 12 days after product is given. Tell patient to report skin changes, difficulty breathing, or headache.

• Tell patient that local pain, swelling, and tenderness at injection site may occur. Recommend acetaminophen to alleviate these minor effects.

Breast-feeding patients
• RIG probably appears in breast milk. Safety in breast-feeding women hasn't been established. An alternative to breast-feeding is recommended.

---

rabies vaccine, adsorbed

Pharmacologic classification: vaccine
Therapeutic classification: viral vaccine
Pregnancy risk category C

How supplied
Available by prescription only
Injection: 1 ml single-dose vial

Indications, route, and dosage
Preexposure prophylaxis rabies immunization for persons in high-risk groups
Adults and children: 1 ml I.M. at 0, 7, and 21 or 28 days for a total of three injections. Patients at increased risk for rabies should be checked q 6 months and given a booster vaccination, 1 ml I.M., p.r.n., to maintain adequate serum titer.

Postexposure rabies prophylaxis
Adults and children not previously vaccinated against rabies: 20 IU/kg of human rabies immune globulin (HRIG) I.M. and five 1-ml injections of rabies vaccine, adsorbed, I.M. given one each on days 0, 3, 7, 14, and 28.
Adults and children previously vaccinated against rabies: Two 1-ml injections of rabies vaccine, adsorbed, I.M. given one each on days 0 and 3. HRIG shouldn't be given.

Pharmacodynamics
Vaccine action: Promotes active immunity to rabies.

Pharmacokinetics
• *Absorption:* Antibodies detected consistently in serum samples about 2 weeks after last injection in series. People at high risk should be retested for rabies antibody titer every 6 months.
• *Distribution:* No information available.
• *Metabolism:* No information available.
• *Excretion:* No information available.

Contraindications and precautions
Contraindicated in patients who have experienced life-threatening allergic reactions to previous injections of vaccine or its components, including thimerosal. Use cautiously in patients with history of non-life-threatening allergic reactions to previous injections of vaccine or hypersensitivity to monkey proteins.

Interactions
Drug-drug. *Antimalarials, corticosteroids, immunosuppressants:* Decreased response to rabies vaccine. Don't use together.
Rabies immune globulin (RIG): May delay antibody response to vaccine. Don't give more than recommended dose of RIG.

Adverse reactions
CNS: *headache, dizziness, fatigue.*
GI: *abdominal pain, nausea.*
Musculoskeletal: aching of injected muscle, *myalgia.*
Skin: erythema, swelling, itching, mild inflammatory reaction (at injection site).
Other: *anaphylaxis, slight fever,* serum sickness-like reactions; transient pain.

☑ Special considerations
• Keep epinephrine 1:1,000 readily available.
• Administer I.M. into deltoid region in adults and older children; midanterolateral aspect of thigh is acceptable for younger children. Vaccine shouldn't be used by intradermal route. Don't inject vaccine close to a peripheral nerve or in adipose and subcutaneous tissue.
• Vaccine is normally a light pink color because of presence of phenol red in suspension.

• Preexposure immunization should be delayed in patients with acute intercurrent illness.

Monitoring the patient
• Monitor patient for adverse effects.
• If patient experiences a serious adverse reaction to vaccine, report this promptly to Michigan Department of Public Health (517) 335-8165 during working hours or (517) 335-9030 at other times.

Information for the patient
• Tell patient that headache, stomach upset, fever, or pain, swelling, and itching at injection site may occur.
• Recommend acetaminophen to alleviate headache, fever, and muscle aches.

Pediatric patients
• Use caution when administering vaccine to children because of limited experience with this age-group.

rabies vaccine, human diploid cell (HDCV)
Imovax Rabies I.D. Vaccine (inactivated whole virus), Imovax Rabies Vaccine

Pharmacologic classification: vaccine
Therapeutic classification: viral vaccine
Pregnancy risk category C

How supplied
Available by prescription only
I.M. injection: 2.5 IU of rabies antigen/ml, in single-dose vial with diluent
I.D. injection: 0.25 IU rabies antigen per dose

Indications, route, and dosage
Preexposure prophylaxis immunization for persons in high-risk groups
Adults and children: Three 0.1-ml injections intradermally or three 1-ml injections I.M. Give first dose on day 0 (first day vaccination), second dose on day 7, and third dose on either day 21 or 28.
Booster: Persons exposed to rabies virus at their workplace should have antibody titers checked q 6 months. Those persons with continued risk of exposure should have antibody titers checked q 2 years. When the titers are inadequate, administer a booster dose.
Primary postexposure dosage
Five 1-ml doses I.M. on each of days 3, 7, 14, and 28 (in conjunction with rabies immune globulin [RIG] on day 0). A sixth dose may be given on day 90. For patients who previously received the full HDCV vaccination regimen or who have demonstrated rabies antibody, give two 1-ml doses I.M. Give first dose on day 0 and the second 3 days later. RIG shouldn't be given.

Pharmacodynamics
Rabies prophylaxis: Promotes active immunity to rabies.

Pharmacokinetics
• *Absorption:* After I.D. injection, rabies antibodies appear in serum within 7 to 10 days; peak at 30 to 60 days. Vaccine-induced immunity persists for about 1 year.
• *Distribution:* No information available.
• *Metabolism:* No information available.
• *Excretion:* No information available.

Contraindications and precautions
No contraindications reported for persons after exposure. An acute febrile illness contraindicates use of vaccine for persons previously exposed. Use cautiously in patients with history of hypersensitivity.

Interactions
Drug-drug. *Corticosteroids, immunosuppressants:* May interfere with development of active immunity to rabies vaccine. Avoid using together.

Adverse reactions
CNS: headache, dizziness, *fatigue.*
GI: abdominal pain, diarrhea, *nausea.*
Musculoskeletal: muscle aches.
Skin: pain, erythema, swelling, *itching at injection site.*
Other: **anaphylaxis,** fever, *serum sickness.*

☑ Special considerations
• I.D. form is for preexposure use only.
• Obtain a thorough history of allergies, especially to antibiotics, and of reactions to immunizations.
• Epinephrine solution 1:1,000 should be available to treat allergic reactions.
• I.M. injections should be made in deltoid or upper outer quadrant of gluteus muscle in adults and children. In infants and small children, use midlateral aspect of thigh.
• Reconstitute with diluent provided. Gently shake vial until vaccine is completely dissolved.
• Store vaccine at 36° to 46° F (2° to 8° C). Don't freeze.

Monitoring the patient
• Monitor patient for adverse effects.

Information for the patient
• Tell patient that pain, swelling, and itching at injection site as well as headache, stomach upset, or fever may occur after vaccination.
• Recommend acetaminophen to alleviate headache, fever, and muscle aches.

Breast-feeding patients
• It's unknown if HDCV appears in breast milk or if transmission to breast-feeding infant presents

risk. Breast-feeding women should choose an alternative to breast-feeding.

raloxifene hydrochloride
Evista

Pharmacologic classification: selective estrogen receptor modulator
Therapeutic classification: antiosteoporotic
Pregnancy risk category X

How supplied
Available by prescription only
Tablets: 60 mg

Indications, route, and dosage
Prevention of osteoporosis in postmenopausal women
Adults: One 60-mg tablet P.O. once daily.

Pharmacodynamics
Antiosteoporotic action: Decreases bone turnover and reduces bone resorption. These effects are manifested as reductions in serum and urine levels of bone turnover markers and increases in bone mineral density. Raloxifene's biologic actions are mediated through binding to estrogen receptors resulting in differential expression of multiple estrogen-regulated genes in different tissues.

Pharmacokinetics
• *Absorption:* Rapidly absorbed. Peak levels depend upon systemic interconversion and enterohepatic cycling of drug and metabolites. After oral administration, about 60% absorbed. Because of extensive presystemic glucuronide conjugation, absolute bioavailability is 2%.
• *Distribution:* Apparent volume of distribution is 2,348 L/kg; doesn't depend on dose given. Highly bound to plasma proteins, both albumin and alpha-1 acid glycoprotein; doesn't appear to interact with binding of warfarin, phenytoin, or tamoxifen to plasma proteins.
• *Metabolism:* Extensive first-pass metabolism to glucuronide conjugates.
• *Excretion:* Primarily excreted in feces; less than 6% of dose eliminated as glucuronide conjugates in urine. Less than 0.2% of dose excreted unchanged in urine.

Contraindications and precautions
Contraindicated in patients with hypersensitivity to drug or constituents of tablet. Also contraindicated in pregnant women or those planning pregnancy and in women with past history of or currently active venous thromboembolic events, including pulmonary embolism, retinal vein thrombosis, and deep vein thrombosis. Use with hormone replacement therapy or systemic estrogen hasn't been evaluated and isn't recommended.

Use with caution in patients with severe hepatic impairment.

Interactions
Drug-drug. *Ampicillin:* Decreased absorption of raloxifene. Monitor patient closely.
Cholestyramine: Significantly reduced absorption of raloxifene. Don't use concomitantly.
Warfarin: Decreased PT. Monitor PT and INR.
Other highly protein-bound drugs (clofibrate, diazepam, diazoxide, ibuprofen, indomethacin, naproxen): May interfere with binding sites. Use together cautiously.

Adverse reactions
CNS: depression, insomnia.
CV: *hot flashes,* chest pain, migraine, peripheral edema.
EENT: *sinusitis,* pharyngitis, laryngitis.
GI: nausea, dyspepsia, vomiting, flatulence, GI disorder, gastroenteritis, abdominal pain.
GU: vaginitis, urinary tract infection, cystitis, leukorrhea, endometrial disorder, vaginal bleeding, breast pain.
Metabolic: weight gain; increased apolipoprotein A1 and reduced serum total cholesterol, low-density lipoprotein cholesterol, fibrinogen, apolipoprotein B, and lipoprotein; increased hormone-binding globulin levels.
Musculoskeletal: *arthralgia,* myalgia, arthritis, leg cramps.
Respiratory: increased cough, pneumonia.
Skin: rash, sweating.
Other: *infection, flu syndrome,* fever.

☑ Special considerations
• Stop drug at least 72 hours before prolonged immobilization.
• No association between breast enlargement, breast pain, or an increased risk of breast cancer has been shown. Evaluate breast abnormalities that occur during treatment.
• A decrease in total and low-density lipoprotein cholesterol by 6% and 11%, respectively, has been reported. No effect on high-density lipoprotein or triglycerides has been shown.
• There are no data to support drug use in premenopausal women; avoid use in this population.
• Safety and efficacy in men haven't been evaluated.
• Effect on bone mineral density beyond 2 years of treatment isn't known. Safety and efficacy haven't been established beyond 2 years.

Monitoring the patient
• Monitor patient for blood clots. The greatest risk of thromboembolic events (deep vein thrombosis, pulmonary embolism, retinal vein thrombosis) occurs during first 4 months of treatment.
• Endometrial proliferation hasn't been associated with drug use. Evaluate unexplained uterine bleeding.

Information for the patient
• Tell patient to avoid long periods of restricted movement (such as during traveling) because of an increased risk of venous thromboembolic events (such as deep vein thrombosis and pulmonary embolism).
• Inform patient that hot flashes or flushing may occur and don't disappear with drug use.
• Tell patient to take supplemental calcium and vitamin D if dietary intake is inadequate.
• Encourage patient to perform weight-bearing exercises. Also advise her to stop alcohol consumption and smoking.
• Tell patient that drug may be taken without regard to food.

Geriatric patients
• No age-related differences have been observed in patients ages 42 to 84.

Pediatric patients
• Drug hasn't been evaluated in children; don't use in this age-group.

Breast-feeding patients
• It's unknown if drug appears in breast milk. Don't use in breast-feeding women.

ramipril
Altace

Pharmacologic classification: ACE inhibitor
Therapeutic classification: antihypertensive
Pregnancy risk category C (D in second and third trimesters)

How supplied
Available by prescription only
Capsules: 1.25 mg, 2.5 mg, 5 mg, 10 mg

Indications, route, and dosage
Hypertension either alone or with thiazide diuretics
Adults: Initially, 2.5 mg P.O. daily in patients not receiving concomitant diuretic therapy. Adjust dosage based on blood pressure response. Usual maintenance dose is 2.5 to 20 mg daily as a single dose or in two equal doses.
In patients receiving diuretic therapy, symptomatic hypotension may occur. To minimize this, discontinue diuretic, if possible, 2 to 3 days before starting ramipril. When this isn't possible, initial dose of ramipril should be 1.25 mg.
✦ *Dosage adjustment.* In renally impaired patients with creatinine clearance below 40 ml/minute (serum creatinine above 2.5 mg/dl), recommended initial dose is 1.25 mg daily, adjusted upward to maximum dose of 5 mg based on blood pressure response.

Heart failure post MI
Adults: Initially, 2.5 mg P.O. b.i.d. Adjust to target dose of 5 mg P.O. b.i.d.

Pharmacodynamics
Antihypertensive action: Ramipril and its active metabolite, ramiprilat, inhibit ACE, preventing conversion of angiotensin I to angiotensin II, a potent vasoconstrictor. Reduced formation of angiotensin II decreases peripheral arterial resistance and, in turn, decreases aldosterone secretion, reduces sodium and water retention, and lowers blood pressure. Ramipril also has antihypertensive activity in patients with low-renin hypertension.

Pharmacokinetics
• *Absorption:* 50% to 60% of drug absorbed after oral administration; levels peak within 1 hour. Plasma levels peak in 2 to 4 hours.
• *Distribution:* 73% serum protein-bound; ramiprilat, 56%.
• *Metabolism:* Ramipril almost completely metabolized to ramiprilat, which has six times more ACE inhibitory effects than parent drug.
• *Excretion:* 60% of drug excreted in urine; 40% in feces. Less than 2% of dose excreted in urine as unchanged drug.

Contraindications and precautions
Contraindicated in patients with hypersensitivity to ACE inhibitors and in those with history of angioedema related to treatment with an ACE inhibitor. Use cautiously in patients with impaired renal function.

Interactions
Drug-drug. *Diuretics:* Excessive hypotension. Stop diuretic or lower dosage of ramipril, as needed.
Indomethacin: Decreased hypotensive effects. Monitor blood pressure.
Lithium: Increased serum lithium levels. Monitor patient for lithium toxicity.
Potassium-sparing diuretics, potassium supplements: Hyperkalemia. Monitor serum potassium level.
Drug-food. *Salt substitutes containing potassium:* Possible hyperkalemia. Don't use together.
Drug-lifestyle. *Sun exposure:* Photosensitivity reaction. Tell patient to take precautions.

Adverse reactions
CNS: asthenia, dizziness, fatigue, headache, malaise, light-headedness, anxiety, amnesia, **seizures,** depression, insomnia, nervousness, neuralgia, neuropathy, paresthesia, somnolence, tremor, vertigo.
CV: orthostatic hypotension, syncope, angina, **arrhythmias, MI,** chest pain, palpitations, edema.
EENT: epistaxis, tinnitus.

GI: nausea, vomiting, abdominal pain, anorexia, constipation, diarrhea, dyspepsia, dry mouth, gastroenteritis.
GU: impotence, increased BUN and creatinine levels.
Hematologic: decreased hemoglobin levels and hematocrit, hemolytic anemia, *pancytopenia, neutropenia, thrombocytopenia.*
Hepatic: elevations of liver enzyme, serum bilirubin, and uric acid levels; *hepatitis.*
Metabolic: hyperkalemia, weight gain, increased blood glucose.
Musculoskeletal: arthralgia, arthritis, myalgia.
Respiratory: *dry, persistent, tickling, nonproductive cough;* dyspnea.
Skin: *hypersensitivity reactions,* rash, dermatitis, pruritus, photosensitivity, increased diaphoresis.
Other: *angioedema.*

☑ **Special considerations**
• Diuretic therapy should be discontinued 2 to 3 days before starting ramipril therapy, if possible, to decrease potential for excessive hypotensive response.
• Like other ACE inhibitors, ramipril may cause a dry, persistent, tickling, nonproductive cough, which is reversible when drug is stopped.

Monitoring the patient
• Assess renal and hepatic function before and periodically throughout therapy.
• Monitor serum potassium levels.

Information for the patient
• Tell patient to immediately report signs or symptoms of angioedema (swelling of face, eyes, lips or tongue or difficulty breathing). Tell him to stop taking drug and seek medical attention if these occur.
• Warn patient that light-headedness can occur, especially during first few days of therapy. Tell him to change positions slowly to reduce hypotensive effect and to report these symptoms. If syncope (fainting) occurs, instruct patient to stop drug and call immediately.
• Warn patient that inadequate fluid intake, vomiting, diarrhea, or excessive perspiration can lead to light-headedness and syncope. Advise caution in excessive heat and during exercise.
• Tell patient to avoid using sodium substitutes containing potassium unless instructed.
• Tell patient to immediately report signs of infection, such as sore throat or fever.

Geriatric patients
• No age-related differences in safety or efficacy have been observed.

Pediatric patients
• Safety and efficacy in children haven't been established.

Breast-feeding patients
• Drug may appear in breast milk. Don't give drug to breast-feeding women.

ranitidine
Zantac, Zantac 75, Zantac EFFERdose, Zantac GELdose

Pharmacologic classification: H_2-receptor antagonist
Therapeutic classification: antiulcerative
Pregnancy risk category B

How supplied
Available by prescription only
Tablets: 150 mg, 300 mg
Tablets (effervescent): 150 mg
Capsules: 150 mg, 300 mg
Granules (effervescent): 150 mg
Injection: 25 mg/ml
Injection (premixed): 50 mg/50 ml, 50 mg/100 ml
Syrup: 15 mg/ml
Available without a prescription
Tablets: 75 mg

Indications, route, and dosage
Duodenal and gastric ulcer (short-term treatment); pathologic hypersecretory conditions such as Zollinger-Ellison syndrome
Adults: 150 mg P.O. b.i.d. or 300 mg h.s. Doses up to 6 g/day may be given to patients with Zollinger-Ellison syndrome. May give drug parenterally: 50 mg I.V. or I.M. q 6 to 8 hours.
Maintenance therapy in duodenal ulcer
Adults: 150 mg P.O. h.s.
Prophylaxis of stress ulcer
Adults: Continuous I.V. infusion of 150 mg in 250 ml compatible solution delivered at a rate of 6.25 mg/hour using an infusion pump.
Gastroesophageal reflux disease
Adults: 150 mg P.O. b.i.d.
Erosive esophagitis
Adults: 150 mg or 10 ml (2 teaspoonfuls equivalent to 150 mg of ranitidine) P.O. q.i.d.
Self-medication for relief of occasional heartburn, acid indigestion, and sour stomach
Adults and adolescents ages 12 and older: 75 mg once or twice daily; maximum dose is 150 mg in 24 hours.

Pharmacodynamics
Antiulcerative action: Competitively inhibits histamine's action at H_2-receptors in gastric parietal cells. This reduces basal and nocturnal gastric acid secretion as well as that caused by histamine, food, amino acids, insulin, and pentagastrin.

Pharmacokinetics
• *Absorption:* About 50% to 60% of oral dose absorbed; food doesn't significantly affect absorp-

tion. After I.M. injection, absorbed rapidly from parenteral sites.
• *Distribution:* Distributed to many body tissues; appears in CSF and breast milk. Drug is about 10% to 19% protein-bound.
• *Metabolism:* Metabolized in liver.
• *Excretion:* Excreted in urine and feces. Half-life is 2 to 3 hours.

Contraindications and precautions
Contraindicated in patients with hypersensitivity to drug and in those with history of acute porphyria. Use cautiously in patients with impaired renal or hepatic function.

Interactions
Drug-drug. *Antacids:* Decreased ranitidine absorption. Separate administration times by at least 1 hour.
Diazepam: Decreased absorption of diazepam. Monitor patient.
Glipizide: Increased hypoglycemic effect. Dosage adjustment of glipizide may be needed.
Procainamide, warfarin: Decreased renal clearance of these drugs. Monitor serum levels and adjust dosages as needed.

Adverse reactions
CNS: malaise, vertigo.
EENT: blurred vision.
GU: increased serum creatinine level.
Hematologic: *reversible leukopenia, pancytopenia, granulocytopenia, thrombocytopenia.*
Hepatic: elevated liver enzyme levels, jaundice.
Other: burning, itching at injection site; *anaphylaxis;* angioneurotic edema.

☑ Special considerations
• When administering I.V. push, dilute to a total volume of 20 ml and inject over 5 minutes. No dilution necessary when administering I.M. Drug also may be administered by intermittent I.V. infusion. Dilute 50 mg ranitidine in 100 ml of D_5W and infuse over 15 to 20 minutes.
• Dosage adjustment may be needed in patients with impaired renal function.
• Dialysis removes ranitidine; administer drug after treatment.
• Drug may cause false-positive results in urine protein tests using Multistix.

Monitoring the patient
• Monitor patients with impaired renal function.
• Check CBC periodically.

Information for the patient
• Instruct patient to take drug as directed, even after pain subsides, to ensure proper healing.
• If patient is taking a single daily dose, advise him to take it at bedtime.

• Instruct patient not to take OTC preparations continuously for longer than 2 weeks without medical approval.
• Tell patient to swallow oral form whole with water; don't chew.

Geriatric patients
• Elderly patients may experience more adverse reactions because of reduced renal clearance. Debilitated patients may experience reversible confusion, agitation, depression, and hallucinations.

Breast-feeding patients
• Drug appears in breast milk; use with caution in breast-feeding women.

ranitidine bismuth citrate
Tritec

Pharmacologic classification: H_2-receptor antagonist, antimicrobial
Therapeutic classification: antiulcerative
Pregnancy risk category C

How supplied
Available by prescription only
Tablets: 400 mg

Indications, route, and dosage
With clarithromycin for treatment of active duodenal ulcer associated with Helicobacter **pylori** *infection*
Adults: 400 mg P.O. b.i.d for 28 days with clarithromycin 500 mg P.O. t.i.d for first 14 days.

Pharmacodynamics
Antiulcerative activity: Reduces gastric acid secretion by competitively inhibiting histamine at the H_2 receptor of the gastric parietal cells. Bismuth is a topical drug that disrupts the integrity of bacterial cell walls, prevents adhesion of *H. pylori* to gastric epithelium, decreases the development of resistance, and inhibits *H. pylori* urease, phospholipase, and proteolytic activity.

Pharmacokinetics
• *Absorption:* Drug dissociates to ranitidine and bismuth after ingestion. Mean peak plasma levels of ranitidine within ½ to 5 hours. Variable oral bioavailability of bismuth, with mean peak plasma levels 15 to 60 minutes after a 400-mg dose.
• *Distribution:* Volume of distribution of ranitidine is 1.7 L/kg. Ranitidine and bismuth are 15% and 98% protein-bound, respectively.
• *Metabolism:* Metabolized by liver. Not known if bismuth undergoes biotransformation.
• *Excretion:* Ranitidine primarily eliminated by kidneys. Elimination half-life of ranitidine is about 3 hours. Bismuth excreted primarily in feces. Bismuth also undergoes minor excretion in bile and

urine. Terminal elimination half-life of bismuth is 11 to 28 days.

Contraindications and precautions
Contraindicated in patients with hypersensitivity to drug or its components.

Interactions
Drug-drug. *Diazepam:* Decreased diazepam absorption. Stagger administration times.
Glipizide: Increased hypoglycemic effect. Dosage adjustment of glipizide may be needed.
High-dose antacids (170 mEq): Decreased plasma levels of ranitidine and bismuth. Separate administration times.
Procainamide, warfarin: Decreased renal clearance of these drugs. Monitor serum levels and adjust dosages as needed.

Adverse reactions
CNS: headache.
GI: constipation, diarrhea.

☑ Special considerations
● Drug shouldn't be prescribed alone for treatment of active duodenal ulcers.
● If drug therapy in combination with clarithromycin isn't successful, patient is considered to have clarithromycin-resistant *H. pylori* and shouldn't be retreated with another regimen containing clarithromycin.
● Ranitidine bismuth citrate with clarithromycin shouldn't be used in patients with history of acute porphyria. This combination isn't recommended in patients with creatinine clearance below 25 ml/minute.
● Dialysis removes ranitidine; administer drug after treatment.
● Drug may cause false-positive results in urine protein tests using Multistix; test with sulfosalicylic acid if needed.

Monitoring the patient
● Monitor patient for improvement of clinical condition.
● Monitor patient for adverse effects.

Information for the patient
● Inform patient that drug may be administered without regard to food.
● Instruct patient to take drug as directed, even after pain has subsided.
● Tell patient that it's important to take clarithromycin with drug for specified length of time.
● Inform patient that a temporary and harmless darkening of tongue or stool may occur with drug use.

Geriatric patients
● Serum drug levels may be increased in elderly patients.

Pediatric patients
● Safety and efficacy in children haven't been established.

Breast-feeding patients
● Drug appears in breast milk; use with caution in breast-feeding women.

rapacuronium bromide
Raplon

Pharmacologic classification: nondepolarizing neuromuscular blocker
Therapeutic classification: skeletal muscle relaxant
Pregnancy risk category C

How supplied
Available by prescription only
Injection: 20 mg/ml

Indications, route, and dosage
Adjunct to general anesthesia to facilitate tracheal intubation and to provide skeletal muscle relaxation during short surgical procedures
Dosage is highly individualized. The following dosages should serve as a guide only.
Adults: Initially, 1.5 mg/kg I.V. provides conditions considered ideal for tracheal intubation within 60 to 90 seconds and maintains paralysis for about 15 minutes. After intubating dose, up to three maintenance doses of 0.5 mg/kg I.V. may be administered as needed. Repeat dosing is based on clinical duration of previous dose and shouldn't be administered until recovery of neuromuscular function is evident.
Adult women undergoing cesarean section with thiopental induction: 2.5 mg/kg I.V. is recommended intubating dose.
Children ages 13 to 17: Individualize dose considering physical maturity, height, and weight and using the other recommendations as a guide.
Children ages 1 month to 12 years: 2 mg/kg I.V. bolus will produce acceptable intubating conditions within 60 to 90 seconds; muscle paralysis should last about 15 minutes.

Pharmacodynamics
Skeletal muscle relaxant action: Competes with acetylcholine for cholinergic receptors at the motor end plate, thus blocking depolarization. Action can be reversed by neostigmine, an acetylcholinesterase inhibitor.

Pharmacokinetics
● *Absorption:* Onset within 60 to 90 seconds of administration; peak effect in about 90 seconds. Duration of action about 15 minutes for recommended adult dose of 1.5 mg/kg.
● *Distribution:* About 50% to 88% protein-bound.

- *Metabolism:* Undergoes hydrolysis to the 3-hydroxy metabolite, the major and active metabolite.
- *Excretion:* About 28% of drug excreted in urine and 28% in feces (total of 56%).

Contraindications and precautions
Contraindicated in patients with hypersensitivity to drug. Repeat dosing in children or adults who have been given intubating doses greater than 1.5 mg/kg isn't recommended.

Use cautiously in patients with myasthenia gravis, myasthenic syndrome, renal or hepatic dysfunction, acid-base abnormalities, electrolyte disturbances, burns, disuse atrophy, cachexia, and carcinomatosis. Also use cautiously in debilitated patients and in patients with neuromuscular disease.

Interactions
Drug-drug. *Anticonvulsants (carbamazepine, phenytoin):* Reduced duration of action of rapacuronium, resulting in higher infusion rates and development of resistance. Monitor patient.
Certain antibiotics (aminoglycosides, bacitracin, polymyxin, tetracyclines, vancomycin), inhalation anesthetics (desflurane, enflurane, halothane, isoflurane, sevoflurane), lithium, local anesthetics, magnesium salts, procainamide, quinidine: Enhanced neuromuscular blocking action of rapacuronium. Use together cautiously; consider lower doses of rapacuronium.

Adverse reactions
CV: hypotension, tachycardia, ***bradycardia.***
GI: vomiting, nausea.
Respiratory: *bronchospasm.*
Skin: rash.

☑ Special considerations
- Adequate anesthesia or sedating drugs must accompany administration of rapacuronium because drug has no effect on consciousness or pain.
- Don't administer additional doses until there is a definite response to nerve stimulation.
- In morbidly obese patients (body mass index greater than 40 kg/m²), base initial dose on ideal body weight. In all other patients, base dose on actual body weight.
- Reconstitute drug with sterile water for injection or other compatible I.V. solutions, such as normal saline, 5% dextrose in water, 5% dextrose in saline, lactated Ringer's, or bacteriostatic water for injection.
- Drug is physically incompatible with cefuroxime, danaparoid sodium, diazepam, nitroglycerin, and thiopental.
- Only those experienced in use of neuromuscular blockers and techniques of airway management should prescribe this drug. Don't administer unless an antagonist and equipment for

artificial respiration, oxygen therapy, and intubation are within reach.
- Drug shouldn't be administered by infusion, particularly during long surgical procedures or in intensive care unit setting.
- Use within 24 hours of reconstitution. Prepared solutions may be stored at room temperature or refrigerated (36° to 77° F [2° to 25° C]). Don't use if particulates are present.
- Profound neuromuscular blockade can be reversed by neostigmine.

Monitoring the patient
- Assess baseline electrolyte levels (electrolyte imbalance can potentiate neuromuscular blocking effects).
- Monitor vital signs, especially respirations and heart rate.
- Use a peripheral nerve stimulator to measure neuromuscular function during administration in order to monitor drug effect, determine need for additional doses, and confirm recovery from neuromuscular block.
- In patients with end-stage renal disease, monitor closely for return of neuromuscular function because condition increases clearance time of drug.

Information for the patient
- Explain all events and procedures to patient.
- Reassure patient and family that he will be monitored at all times.

Geriatric patients
- No dosage adjustment is recommended for elderly patients.

Pediatric patients
- Safety and efficacy in infants less than age 1 month haven't been established.

Breast-feeding patients
- It's unknown if drug appears in breast milk. Use with caution in breast-feeding women.

repaglinide
Prandin

Pharmacologic classification: meglitinide
Therapeutic classification: antidiabetic
Pregnancy risk category C

How supplied
Available by prescription only
Tablets: 0.5 mg, 1 mg, 2 mg

Indications, route, and dosage
Adjunct to diet and exercise in lowering blood glucose in patients with type 2 diabetes mel-

litus whose hyperglycemia can't be controlled by diet and exercise alone
Adults: For patients not previously treated or whose HbA$_{1c}$ is below 8%, starting dose is 0.5 mg P.O. with each meal given 15 minutes before meal; however, time may vary from immediately before to as long as 30 minutes before meal. For patients previously treated with glucose-lowering drugs and whose HbA$_{1c}$ is 8% or more, initial dose is 1 to 2 mg P.O. with each meal. Recommended dosage range is 0.5 to 4 mg with meals b.i.d., t.i.d., or q.i.d. Maximum daily dose is 16 mg.

Dosage should be determined by blood glucose response. May double dosage up to 4 mg with each meal until satisfactory blood glucose response is achieved. At least 1 week should elapse between dosage adjustments to assess response to each dose.

Metformin may be added if repaglinide monotherapy is inadequate.

Pharmacodynamics
Antidiabetic action: Stimulates release of insulin from the beta cells in the pancreas. Closes ATP-dependent potassium channels in the beta cell membrane, which causes opening of the calcium channels. The increased calcium influx induces insulin secretion; the overall effect is to lower the blood glucose level.

Pharmacokinetics
• *Absorption:* Rapidly and completely absorbed with oral administration; plasma levels peak within 1 hour.
• *Distribution:* Mean volume of distribution after I.V. administration is 31 L; protein-binding to albumin exceeds 98%.
• *Metabolism:* Completely metabolized by oxidative biotransformation and conjugation with glucuronic acid. P-450 isoenzyme system (specifically CYP 3A4) also involved in N-dealkylation of repaglinide. All metabolites are inactive; don't contribute to blood glucose–lowering effect.
• *Excretion:* About 90% of dose occurs in feces as metabolites. About 8% of dose recovered in urine as metabolites, less than 0.1% as parent drug. Half-life about 1 hour.

Contraindications and precautions
Contraindicated in patients with hypersensitivity to drug or its inactive ingredients and in those with type 1 diabetes mellitus or ketoacidosis. Use cautiously in patients with hepatic insufficiency in whom reduced metabolism could cause elevated blood levels of repaglinide and hypoglycemia.

Interactions
Drug-drug. *Beta blockers, chloramphenicol, coumarins, MAO inhibitors, NSAIDs, probenecid, salicylates, sulfonamides, other highly protein-bound drugs:* Potentiated hypoglycemic action of repaglinide. Monitor serum glucose level and adjust repaglinide dosage as needed.
Calcium channel blockers, corticosteroids, estrogens, isoniazid, nicotinic acid, oral contraceptives, phenothiazines, phenytoin, sympathomimetics, thiazides, thyroid products, other diuretics: Hyperglycemia resulting in loss of glycemic control. Monitor serum glucose level and adjust repaglinide dosage as needed.
Erythromycin, ketoconazole, miconazole, other similar inhibitors of P-450 cytochrome system 3A4: Inhibited repaglinide metabolism. Monitor patient closely.
Inducers of P-450 cytochrome system 3A4 (such as barbiturates, carbamazepine, rifampin, troglitazone): Increased metabolism of repaglinide. Monitor patient closely.

Adverse reactions
CNS: *headache.*
CV: chest pain, angina.
EENT: tooth disorder, rhinitis.
GI: nausea, diarrhea, constipation, vomiting, dyspepsia.
GU: urinary tract infection.
Metabolic: HYPOGLYCEMIA.
Musculoskeletal: arthralgia, back pain.
Respiratory: bronchitis, sinusitis, *upper respiratory tract infection.*

☑ Special considerations
• Administration of other oral antidiabetics has been reported to be associated with increased CV mortality compared with diet treatment alone. Although not specifically evaluated for repaglinide, this warning may also apply.
• Loss of glycemic control can occur during stress, such as fever, trauma, infection, or surgery. If this occurs, stop drug and administer insulin.
• Hypoglycemia may be difficult to recognize in elderly patients and in patients taking beta blockers.
• Use caution when increasing drug dosage in patients with impaired renal function or renal failure requiring dialysis.
• In case of overdose, monitor patient closely for minimum of 24 to 48 hours because hypoglycemia may reoccur after apparent clinical recovery.

Monitoring the patient
• Monitor patient's blood glucose periodically to determine minimum effective dose.
• Monitor long-term efficacy by measuring HbA$_{1c}$ levels every 3 months.

Information for the patient
• Instruct patient on importance of diet and exercise with drug therapy.
• Discuss symptoms of hypoglycemia with patient and family.
• Tell patient to take drug before meals, usually 15 minutes before start of meal; however, time

can vary from immediately preceding meal to up to 30 minutes before meal.
• Tell patient that, if a meal is skipped or an extra meal added, he should skip the dose or add an extra dose of drug for that meal.

Geriatric patients
• No increase in the frequency or severity of hypoglycemia in older patients has been found.

Pediatric patients
• Safety and efficacy in children haven't been established.

Breast-feeding patients
• It's unknown if drug appears in breast milk. Because the potential for hypoglycemia in a breast-fed infant exists, stop either drug or breast-feeding.

reteplase, recombinant
Retavase

Pharmacologic classification: tissue-plasminogen activator
Therapeutic classification: thrombolytic enzyme
Pregnancy risk category C

How supplied
Available by prescription only
Injection: 10.8 units (18.8 mg)/vial (supplied in kit with components for reconstitution and administration of two single-use vials)

Indications, route, and dosage
Management of acute MI
Adults: Double-bolus injection of 10 + 10 units. Give each bolus I.V. over 2 minutes. If no complications occur after first bolus, such as serious bleeding or anaphylactoid reactions, give second bolus 30 minutes after start of first bolus. Initiate treatment soon after onset of symptoms of acute MI. There is no experience of repeat courses with reteplase.

Pharmacodynamics
Thrombolytic action: Catalyzes the cleavage of plasminogen to generate plasmin, which leads to fibrinolysis.

Pharmacokinetics
• *Absorption:* Given I.V.
• *Distribution:* Cleared from plasma at a rate of 250 to 450 ml/minute.
• *Metabolism:* Metabolized primarily by liver and kidneys.
• *Excretion:* Drug's plasma half-life is 13 to 16 minutes.

Contraindications and precautions
Contraindicated in patients with active internal bleeding, known bleeding diathesis, history of CVA, recent intracranial or intraspinal surgery or trauma, severe uncontrolled hypertension, intracranial neoplasm, arteriovenous malformation, or aneurysm.

Use cautiously in patients undergoing obstetric delivery, organ biopsy, trauma, or within 10 days of major surgery; in patients with previous puncture of noncompressible vessels, cerebrovascular disease, recent GI or GU bleeding, hypertension (systolic pressure 180 mm Hg or more or diastolic pressure 110 mm Hg or more), likelihood of left-sided heart thrombus, subacute bacterial endocarditis, acute pericarditis; hemostatic defects, diabetic hemorrhagic retinopathy, septic thrombophlebitis, other conditions in which bleeding would be difficult to manage; in patients who are pregnant; and in patients ages 75 and older.

Interactions
Drug-drug. *Heparin, oral anticoagulants, platelet inhibitors (abciximab, aspirin, dipyridamole), vitamin K antagonists:* Increased risk of bleeding. Use together cautiously.

Adverse reactions
CNS: *intracranial hemorrhage.*
CV: *arrhythmias, cholesterol embolization.*
GI: *hemorrhage.*
GU: hematuria.
Hematologic: *anemia, bleeding tendency.*
Other: *bleeding at puncture site, hemorrhage.*

☑ Special considerations
• Drug is administered I.V. as a double-bolus injection. If bleeding or anaphylactoid reactions occur after first bolus, second bolus may be withheld.
• Reconstitute drug according to manufacturer's instructions using items provided in kit.
• Don't administer drug with other I.V. drugs through same I.V. line. Heparin and reteplase are incompatible in solution.
• Potency is expressed in terms of units specific for reteplase and not comparable to other thrombolytic drugs.
• Avoid use of noncompressible pressure sites during therapy. If an arterial puncture is needed, an upper extremity vessel should be used. Apply pressure for at least 30 minutes; then apply a pressure dressing. Check site frequently.
• Drug may alter coagulation studies; it remains active in vitro and can lead to degradation of fibrinogen in sample. Collect blood samples in the presence of PPACK (chloromethylketone) at 2- micromolar levels.

Monitoring the patient
• Carefully monitor ECG during treatment. Coronary thrombolysis may result in arrhythmias as-

sociated with reperfusion. Be prepared to treat bradycardia or ventricular irritability.
• Monitor patient for bleeding. Avoid I.M. injections, invasive procedures, and nonessential handling of patient. Bleeding is most common adverse reaction and may occur internally or at external puncture sites. If local measures don't control serious bleeding, stop concurrent anticoagulation therapy. Withhold second bolus of reteplase.

Information for the patient
• Explain to patient and family use and administration of drug.
• Tell patient to report adverse reactions such as signs and symptoms of bleeding or allergic reaction immediately.
• Advise patient about proper dental care to avoid excessive gum trauma.

Geriatric patients
• Use cautiously in elderly patients. Risk of intracranial hemorrhage increases with age.

Pediatric patients
• Safety and efficacy in children haven't been established.

Breast-feeding patients
• It's unknown if drug appears in breast milk. Use with caution in breast-feeding women.

Rh₀(D) immune globulin, human
Gamulin Rh, HypRho-D, RhoGAM

Rh₀(D) immune globulin, microdose
HypRho-D Mini-Dose, MICRhoGAM, Mini-Gamulin Rh

Pharmacologic classification: immune serum
Therapeutic classification: anti-Rh₀(D)-positive prophylaxis
Pregnancy risk category C

How supplied
Available by prescription only
Injection: 300 mcg of Rh₀(D) immune globulin/vial (standard dose); 50 mcg of Rh₀(D) immune globulin/vial (microdose)

Indications, route, and dosage
Rh-positive exposure (full-term pregnancy or termination of pregnancy beyond 13 weeks' gestation), threatened abortion
Women: Administer 1 vial I.M. for each 15 ml of estimated fetal packed RBC volume entering patient's blood, as determined by a modified Kleihauer-Betke technique to determine fetal

packed RBC volume. Usual (standard) dose after delivery of full-term infant is 1 vial; it must be given within 72 hours after delivery or miscarriage.
If Rh₀(D) immune globulin is indicated before delivery, administer 1 vial (standard dose) at about 28 weeks' gestation and give a second vial within 72 hours of delivery.
Transfusion accidents
Premenopausal women: Consult blood bank or transfusion unit at once. The number of vials (standard dose) to administer is calculated via the following formula:

$$\text{Number of vials} = \frac{\text{volume of whole blood transfused}}{15} \times \text{donor unit hematocrit}$$

Dose must be given within 72 hours.
Termination of pregnancy (spontaneous or induced abortion or ectopic pregnancy) up to and including 12 weeks' gestation
Women: 1 vial of microdose immune globulin I.M.; ideally, given within 3 hours but may give up to 72 hours after abortion or miscarriage.
Amniocentesis or abdominal trauma during pregnancy
Women: Dosage varies, based on extent of estimated fetomaternal hemorrhage.

Pharmacodynamics
Rh reaction prophylaxis: Suppresses the active antibody response and formation of anti-Rh₀(D) in Rh₀(D)-negative or Dᵘ-negative individuals exposed to Rh-positive blood. Provides passive immunity to women exposed to Rh-positive fetal blood during pregnancy. Prevents formation of maternal antibodies (active immunity), which prevents hemolytic disease of the Rh-positive newborn in another pregnancy.

Pharmacokinetics
No information available.

Contraindications and precautions
Contraindicated in Rh₀(D)-positive or D-positive patients and those previously immunized to Rh₀(D) blood factor. Also contraindicated in patients with anaphylactic or severe systemic reaction to human globulin. Use with extreme caution in patients with immunoglobulin A deficiency because of increased risk of an anaphylactic reaction.

Interactions
Drug-drug. *Live virus vaccines (measles, mumps, rubella):* Rh₀(D) immune globulin may interfere with immune response to these vaccines. Don't administer live virus vaccines within 3 months after administration of Rh₀(D) immune globulin. If postpartum women receive both Rh₀(D) immune globulin and rubella virus vaccine within a 3-month

---

Reactions may be *common*, uncommon, **life-threatening**, or COMMON AND LIFE-THREATENING.

period, serologic tests should be performed 6 to 8 weeks after vaccination to confirm seroconversion.

Adverse reactions
Other: discomfort at injection site, slight fever.

☑ Special considerations
• Obtain thorough history of allergies and reactions to immunizations.
• Have epinephrine solution 1:1,000 available to treat allergic reactions.
• For best results, $Rh_o(D)$ immune globulin must be administered within 72 hours of Rh-incompatible delivery, spontaneous or induced abortion, or transfusion.
• The microdose formulation is recommended for use after every spontaneous or induced abortion up to and including 12 weeks' gestation unless mother is $Rh_o(D)$-positive or D^u-positive, she has Rh antibodies, or father or fetus is Rh-negative.
• Administer I.M. in anterolateral aspect of upper thigh and deltoid muscle. Don't give I.V.
• $Rh_o(D)$ immune globulin hasn't been associated with an increased frequency of AIDS. The immune globulin is devoid of HIV. Immune globulin recipients don't develop antibodies to HIV.
• Store product between 36° and 46° F (2° and 8° C). Don't freeze.

Monitoring the patient
• Immediately after delivery, send a sample of infant's cord blood to laboratory for typing and cross matching and direct antiglobulin test. Infant must be $Rh_o(D)$-positive or D^u-positive. Confirm that mother is $Rh_o(D)$-negative and D^u-negative.

Information for the patient
• Inform patient that she is receiving this product because her blood has been exposed to the Rh-positive factor. Tell postpartum patient that her body will naturally develop antibodies to destroy this factor, which could threaten future Rh-positive pregnancies.
• Tell patient there is no known risk of HIV infection after receiving product.
• Tell patient local pain, swelling, and tenderness at injection site may occur after vaccination. Recommend acetaminophen to ease minor discomfort.
• Tell patient to report headache, skin changes, or difficulty breathing.

Breast-feeding patients
• Immune globulins appear in breast milk. Safety in breast-feeding women hasn't been established.

ribavirin
Virazole

Pharmacologic classification: synthetic nucleoside
Therapeutic classification: antiviral
Pregnancy risk category X

How supplied
Available by prescription only
Powder to be reconstituted for inhalation: 6 g in 100-ml glass vial

Indications, route, and dosage
Hospitalized infants and young children infected by respiratory syncytial virus (RSV)
Infants and young children: Solution in concentration of 20 mg/ml delivered via the Viratek Small Particle Aerosol Generator (SPAG-2) results in a mist with a concentration of 190 mcg/L. Treatment is carried out for 12 to 18 hours/day for at least 3, and no more than 7, days with a flow rate of 12.5 L of mist per minute.
   For ventilated patients, use same dose with a pressure- or volume-cycled ventilator in conjunction with SPAG-2. Patient should be suctioned q 1 to 2 hours and pulmonary pressures checked q 2 to 4 hours.

Pharmacodynamics
Antiviral action: Probably involves inhibition of RNA and DNA synthesis, inhibition of RNA polymerase, and interference with completion of viral polypeptide coat.

Pharmacokinetics
• *Absorption:* Some drug absorbed systemically.
• *Distribution:* Concentrates in bronchial secretions; plasma levels are subtherapeutic for plaque inhibition.
• *Metabolism:* Metabolized to 1,2,4-triazole-3-carboxamide (deribosylated ribavirin).
• *Excretion:* Mostly excreted renally. First phase of drug's plasma half-life is 9½ hours; second phase has extended half-life of 40 hours (from slow drug release from RBC binding sites).

Contraindications and precautions
Contraindicated in patients with hypersensitivity to drug and in women who are or may become pregnant during treatment.

Interactions
None reported.

Adverse reactions
CV: *cardiac arrest,* hypotension.
EENT: conjunctivitis, erythema of eyelids.
Hematologic: anemia, reticulocytosis.

Respiratory: worsening respiratory state, *apnea,* bacterial pneumonia, pneumothorax, *bronchospasm.*
Skin: rash.

☑ Special considerations
● Ribavirin aerosol is indicated only for lower respiratory tract infection caused by RSV. (Although treatment may begin before test results are available, RSV infection must eventually be confirmed.)
● Administer ribavirin aerosol only by SPAG-2. Don't use other aerosol-generating devices.
● To prepare drug, reconstitute solution with USP sterile water for injection or inhalation, then transfer aseptically to sterile 500-ml Erlenmeyer flask. Dilute further with sterile water to 300 ml to yield final level of 20 mg/ml. Solution remains stable for 24 hours at room temperature.
● Don't use bacteriostatic water (or any other water containing antimicrobial product) to reconstitute drug.
● Discard unused solution in SPAG-2 unit before adding newly reconstituted solution. Solution should be changed at least every 24 hours.
● Drug is most useful for infants with most severe RSV form—typically premature infants and those with underlying disorders such as cardiopulmonary disease. (Most other infants and children with RSV infection don't need treatment because disease is self-limiting.)
● Drug therapy must be accompanied by appropriate respiratory and fluid therapy.

Monitoring the patient
● Monitor ventilator-dependent patients carefully because drug may precipitate in ventilatory apparatus. Change heated wire connective tubing and bacteria filters in series in expiratory limb of the system frequently (such as every 4 hours).
● Monitor cardiac rhythm, blood pressure and oxygen saturation, and respirations carefully.

Information for the patient
● Explain use of drug and administration to children and their parents.
● Tell children and parents to report worsening symptoms.

---

riboflavin (vitamin B₂)
Pharmacologic classification: water-soluble vitamin
Therapeutic classification: vitamin B complex vitamin
Pregnancy risk category A (C if more than RDA)

How supplied
Available without a prescription, as appropriate
Tablets: 25 mg, 50 mg, 100 mg

Indications, route, and dosage
Riboflavin deficiency or adjunct to thiamine treatment for polyneuritis or cheilosis secondary to pellagra
Adults and adolescents over age 12: 5 to 30 mg P.O. daily, depending on severity.
Children under age 12: 3 to 10 mg P.O. daily, depending on severity.
Microcytic anemia associated with splenomegaly and glutathione reductase deficiency
Adults: 10 mg P.O. daily for 10 days.
Dietary supplementation
Adults: 1 to 4 mg P.O. daily. For maintenance, increase nutritional intake and supplement with vitamin B complex.

Pharmacodynamics
Metabolic action: Riboflavin, a coenzyme, functions in the forms of flavin adenine dinucleotide (FAD) and flavin mononucleotide (FMN) and plays a vital metabolic role in numerous tissue respiration systems. FAD and FMN act as hydrogen-carrier molecules for several flavoproteins involved in intermediary metabolism. Riboflavin is also directly involved in maintaining erythrocyte integrity.

Pharmacokinetics
● *Absorption:* Absorbed readily from GI tract, but limited extent of absorption. Absorption occurs at a specialized segment of mucosa; absorption limited by duration of drug's contact with this area. Before being absorbed, riboflavin-5-phosphate is rapidly dephosphorylated in GI lumen. GI absorption increases when drug is given with food; decreases when hepatitis, cirrhosis, biliary obstruction, or probenecid is present.
● *Distribution:* FAD and FMN distributed widely to body tissues. Free riboflavin present in retina. Riboflavin stored in limited amounts in liver, spleen, kidneys, and heart, mainly in the form of FAD. FAD and FMN are about 60% protein-bound in blood. Drug crosses placenta; breast milk contains about 400 ng/ml.
● *Metabolism:* Metabolized in liver.
● *Excretion:* After single oral dose, biological half-life is about 66 to 84 minutes in healthy individuals. Metabolized to FMN in erythrocytes, GI mucosal cells, and liver; FMN is converted to FAD in liver. About 9% of drug excreted unchanged in urine after normal ingestion. Excretion involves renal tubular secretion and glomerular filtration. Amount renally excreted unchanged is directly proportional to dose. Drug removal by hemodialysis is slower than by natural renal excretion.

Contraindications and precautions
None known.

Interactions
Drug-drug. *Oral contraceptives:* Altered absorption. Riboflavin dose may need to be increased.
Propantheline bromide: Delayed absorption rate of riboflavin but increased total amount absorbed. Monitor patient.
Drug-lifestyle. *Alcohol:* Impaired intestinal absorption of riboflavin. Discourage use.

Adverse reactions
GU: bright yellow urine (with high doses).

☑ Special considerations
• RDA of riboflavin is 0.4 to 1.8 mg/day in children, 1.2 to 1.7 mg/day in adults, and 1.6 to 1.8 mg/day in pregnant and breast-feeding women.
• Give oral preparation of riboflavin with food to increase absorption.
• Riboflavin therapy alters urinalysis based on spectrophotometry or color reactions. Large doses of drug result in bright yellow urine. Riboflavin produces fluorescent substances in urine and plasma, which can falsely elevate fluorometric determinations of catecholamines and urobilinogen.
• Riboflavin deficiency causes a clinical syndrome with the following symptoms: cheilosis, angular stomatitis, glossitis, keratitis, scrotal skin changes, ocular changes, and seborrheic dermatitis. In severe deficiency, normochromic, normocytic anemia, and neuropathy may occur. Clinical signs may become evident after 3 to 8 months of inadequate riboflavin intake. Administration of riboflavin reverses signs of deficiency. Riboflavin deficiency rarely occurs alone and is commonly associated with deficiency of other B vitamins and protein.
• Obtain dietary history because other vitamin deficiencies may coexist.

Monitoring the patient
• Monitor patient for signs and symptoms of riboflavin deficiency.
• Monitor CBC, as indicated.

Information for the patient
• Inform patient that riboflavin may cause a yellow discoloration of the urine.
• Teach patient about good dietary sources of riboflavin, such as whole grain cereals and green vegetables. Liver, kidney, heart, eggs, and dairy products are also dietary sources but may not be appropriate based on patient's serum cholesterol and triglyceride levels.
• Tell patient to store riboflavin in a tight, light-resistant container.

Breast-feeding patients
• Drug crosses placenta; during pregnancy and lactation, riboflavin requirements are increased. Increased food intake during this time usually provides adequate amounts of vitamin. The National Research Council recommends daily intake of 1.8 mg/day during first 6 months of breast-feeding.

---

rifabutin
Mycobutin

Pharmacologic classification: semisynthetic ansamycin
Therapeutic classification: antibiotic
Pregnancy risk category B

How supplied
Available by prescription only
Capsules: 150 mg

Indications, route, and dosage
Prevention of disseminated Mycobacterium avium complex (MAC) disease in patients with advanced HIV infection
Adults: 300 mg P.O. daily as a single dose or divided b.i.d. with food.

Pharmacodynamics
Antibiotic action: Inhibits DNA-dependent RNA polymerase in susceptible strains of *Escherichia coli* and *Bacillus subtilis,* but not in mammalian cells. Unknown whether rifabutin inhibits this enzyme in *M. avium* or in *M. intracellulare,* which compose MAC.

Pharmacokinetics
• *Absorption:* Readily absorbed from GI tract. Plasma levels peak 2 to 4 hours after oral dose.
• *Distribution:* High lipophilicity; drug has high propensity for distribution and intracellular tissue uptake. About 85% of drug bound in concentration-independent manner to plasma proteins.
• *Metabolism:* Metabolized in liver to five identified metabolites. The 25-0-desacetyl metabolite has activity equal to parent drug and contributes up to 10% of total antimicrobial activity.
• *Excretion:* Less than 10% excreted in urine as unchanged drug. About 53% of oral dose excreted in urine, primarily as metabolites. About 30% excreted in feces.

Contraindications and precautions
Contraindicated in patients with hypersensitivity to drug or other rifamycin derivatives (such as rifampin) and in patients with active tuberculosis because single-drug therapy with rifabutin increases the risk of inducing bacterial resistance to both rifabutin and rifampin.

Use cautiously in patients with preexisting neutropenia and thrombocytopenia.

◇ Unlabeled clinical use

Interactions
Drug-drug. *Oral contraceptives:* Decreased contraceptive efficacy. Instruct patient to use non-hormonal forms of birth control.
Zidovudine: Decreased zidovudine serum levels; doesn't affect zidovudine's inhibition of HIV. Monitor patient.

Adverse reactions
CNS: headache, insomnia.
GI: dyspepsia, eructation, flatulence, diarrhea, nausea, vomiting, abdominal pain, altered taste.
GU: *discolored urine* (brown-orange).
Hematologic: NEUTROPENIA, LEUKOPENIA, *thrombocytopenia,* eosinophilia.
Musculoskeletal: myalgia.
Skin: *rash.*
Other: fever.

☑ Special considerations
• Evaluate patient who develops complaints consistent with active tuberculosis during rifabutin prophylaxis immediately so that active disease may be given an effective combination regimen of antituberculosis medications. Administration of single-drug rifabutin to patients with active tuberculosis likely leads to development of tuberculosis that is resistant to rifabutin and rifampin.
• High-fat meals slow rate but not extent of drug absorption.

Monitoring the patient
• Because rifabutin may be associated with neutropenia, and more rarely thrombocytopenia, consider obtaining hematologic studies periodically in patients receiving rifabutin prophylaxis.
• Monitor patient for adverse effects.

Information for the patient
• Inform woman using oral contraceptives that drug may decrease their effectiveness. Recommend that she use a nonhormonal form of birth control during therapy.
• Tell patient with swallowing difficulty to mix drug with soft foods such as applesauce.
• Advise patient with nausea, vomiting, or other GI upset to take drug with food, in two divided doses.
• Warn patient that urine and other body fluids may become discolored (brown-orange). Clothes and soft contact lenses may become permanently discolored.

Pediatric patients
• Although safety and effectiveness in children haven't been fully established, drug may be helpful in children at maximum daily dose of 5 mg/kg.

Breast-feeding patients
• It's unknown if drug appears in breast milk. Because of potential for serious adverse effects in breast-fed infants, stop either drug or breast-feeding, depending on importance of drug to mother.

---

rifampin
Rifadin, Rimactane

Pharmacologic classification: semisynthetic rifamycin B derivative (macrocyclic antibiotic)
Therapeutic classification: antituberculotic
Pregnancy risk category C

How supplied
Available by prescription only
Capsules: 150 mg, 300 mg
Injection: 600 mg/vial

Indications, route, and dosage
Primary treatment in pulmonary tuberculosis
Adults: 600 mg P.O. or I.V. daily as a single dose (give P.O. dose 1 hour before or 2 hours after meals).
Children: 10 to 20 mg/kg P.O. or I.V. daily as a single dose (give P.O. dose 1 hour before or 2 hours after meals). Maximum daily dose is 600 mg. Concurrent administration of other effective antituberculotics is recommended. Treatment usually lasts 6 to 9 months.
Asymptomatic meningococcal carriers
Adults: 600 mg P.O. b.i.d. for 2 days.
Infants and children over age 1 month: 10 mg/kg P.O. b.i.d. for 2 days.
Neonates under age 1 month: 5 mg/kg P.O. b.i.d. for 2 days.
✦ Dosage adjustment. Reduce dosage in patients with hepatic dysfunction.
Prophylaxis of Haemophilus influenzae type B
Adults and children: 20 mg/kg (up to 600 mg) once daily for 4 consecutive days.
◇ *Leprosy*
Adults: 600 mg P.O. once monthly, usually used with other drugs.

Pharmacodynamics
Antibiotic action: Impairs RNA synthesis by inhibiting DNA-dependent RNA polymerase. May be bacteriostatic or bactericidal, depending on organism susceptibility and drug level at infection site.
Acts against *Mycobacterium bovis, M. kansasii, M. marinum,* and *M. tuberculosis,* some strains of *M. avium, M. avium-intracellulare,* and *M. fortuitum,* and many gram-positive and some gram-negative bacteria. Resistance to rifampin by *M. tuberculosis* can develop rapidly; rifampin is usually given with other antituberculotics to prevent or delay resistance.

Reactions may be *common,* uncommon, *life-threatening,* or COMMON AND LIFE-THREATENING.

Pharmacokinetics

• *Absorption:* Absorbed completely from GI tract after oral administration; serum levels peak 1 to 4 hours after ingestion. Food delays absorption.

• *Distribution:* Distributed widely into body tissues and fluids, including CSF, tears, saliva, liver, prostate, lungs, bone, and ascitic, pleural, and seminal fluids. Drug crosses placenta; 84% to 91% protein-bound.

• *Metabolism:* Metabolized extensively in liver by deacetylation; undergoes interohepatic circulation.

• *Excretion:* Undergoes enterohepatic circulation; drug and metabolite excreted primarily in bile; drug, but not metabolite, is reabsorbed. From 6% to 30% of rifampin and metabolite appear unchanged in urine in 24 hours; about 60% excreted in feces. Some drug excreted in breast milk. Plasma half-life in adults is 1½ to 5 hours; serum levels rise in obstructive jaundice. Dosage adjustment not necessary for patients with renal failure. Drug isn't removed by either hemodialysis or peritoneal dialysis.

Contraindications and precautions

Contraindicated in patients with hypersensitivity to drug. Use cautiously in patients with hepatic disease.

Interactions

Drug-drug. *Anticoagulants, barbiturates, beta blockers, cardiac glycoside derivatives, chloramphenicol, clofibrate, corticosteroids, cyclosporine, dapsone, disopyramide, estrogens, methadone, oral contraceptives, oral sulfonylureas, phenytoin, quinidine, tocainide, verapamil:* Reduced effectiveness of these drugs. Monitor patient and adjust dosages as needed.

Isoniazid: Accelerated metabolic conversion of isoniazid to hepatotoxic metabolites; increased hazard of isoniazid hepatotoxicity. Monitor patient for toxicity if used together.

Para-aminosalicylate: Decreased oral absorption of rifampin, lowering serum levels. Administer drugs 8 to 12 hours apart.

Drug-lifestyle. *Alcohol:* Increased risk of hepatotoxicity. Discourage use.

Adverse reactions

CNS: headache, fatigue, drowsiness, behavioral changes, dizziness, ataxia, mental confusion, generalized numbness.

EENT: visual disturbances, exudative conjunctivitis.

GI: epigastric distress, anorexia, nausea, vomiting, abdominal pain, diarrhea, flatulence, sore mouth and tongue, pseudomembranous colitis, *pancreatitis.*

GU: hemoglobinuria, hematuria, menstrual disturbances, *acute renal failure.*

Hematologic: eosinophilia, *thrombocytopenia, transient leukopenia,* hemolytic anemia.

Hepatic: *hepatotoxicity,* transient abnormalities in liver function tests.

Metabolic: hyperuricemia.

Musculoskeletal: osteomalacia.

Respiratory: shortness of breath, wheezing.

Skin: pruritus, urticaria, rash.

Other: flulike syndrome, discoloration of body fluids, *shock,* porphyria exacerbation.

☑ Special considerations

• Give drug 1 hour before or 2 hours after meals for maximum absorption; capsule contents may be mixed with food or fluid to enhance swallowing.

• Reconstituted solution is stable for 24 hours at room temperature. Infusion solutions of 100 to 500 ml should be used within 4 hours.

• Rifampin alters standard serum folate and vitamin B_{12} assays. Drug may cause temporary retention of sulfobromophthalein in liver excretion test; may also interfere with contrast material in gallbladder studies and urinalysis based on spectrophotometry.

• Signs and symptoms of overdose include lethargy, nausea, vomiting and, if massive overdose, hepatotoxicity (hepatomegaly, jaundice, elevated liver function studies and bilirubin levels, and loss of consciousness). Red-orange discoloration of skin, urine, sweat, saliva, tears, and feces may occur. Treat by gastric lavage, then activated charcoal; if necessary, force diuresis. Perform bile drainage if hepatic dysfunction lasts beyond 24 to 48 hours.

Monitoring the patient

• Obtain specimens for culture and sensitivity testing before giving first dose, but don't delay therapy; repeat periodically to detect drug resistance.

• Observe patient for adverse reactions and monitor hematologic, renal and liver function studies, and serum electrolytes to minimize toxicity. Watch for signs and symptoms of hepatic impairment (anorexia, fatigue, malaise, jaundice, dark urine, liver tenderness).

• Increased liver enzyme activity inactivates certain drugs (especially warfarin, corticosteroids, and oral hypoglycemics), requiring dosage adjustments.

Information for the patient

• Explain disease process and rationale for long-term therapy.

• Teach signs and symptoms of hypersensitivity and other adverse reactions, and emphasize need to call if these occur; urge patient to report any unusual reactions.

• Tell patient to take drug on empty stomach, at least 1 hour before or 2 hours after a meal. If GI irritation occurs, patient may need to take drug with food.

- Urge patient to comply with prescribed regimen, not to miss doses, and not to stop drug without approval. Explain importance of follow-up appointments.
- Encourage patient to promptly report any flu-like signs or symptoms, weakness, sore throat, loss of appetite, unusual bruising, rash, itching, tea-colored urine, clay-colored stools, or yellow discoloration of eyes or skin.
- Explain that drug turns all body fluids red-orange color; advise patient of possible permanent stains on clothes and soft contact lenses.
- Advise woman using oral contraceptives to substitute other methods; rifampin inactivates such drugs and may alter menstrual patterns.

Geriatric patients
- Usual dose in elderly and debilitated patients is 10 mg/kg once daily. Monitor renal function closely because elderly patients may be more susceptible to toxic effects.

Pediatric patients
- Safety in children under age 5 hasn't been established.

Breast-feeding patients
- Drug may appear in breast milk. Use with caution in breast-feeding women.

rifapentine
Priftin

Pharmacologic classification: cyclopentyl rifamycin
Therapeutic classification: antituberculotic
Pregnancy risk category C

How supplied
Tablets (film-coated): 150 mg

Indications, route, and dosage
Pulmonary tuberculosis, with at least one other antituberculotic to which the isolate is susceptible
Adults: During the intensive phase of short-course therapy, 600 mg P.O. twice weekly for 2 months, with an interval between doses of not less than 3 days (72 hours).
   During the continuation phase of short-course therapy, 600 mg P.O. once weekly for 4 months with isoniazid or another drug to which the isolate is susceptible.

Pharmacodynamics
Antituberculotic action: Inhibits DNA-dependent RNA polymerase in susceptible strains of *Mycobacterium tuberculosis.* Has bactericidal activity against the organism both intra- and extra-

cellularly. Rifapentine and rifampin share similar antimicrobial action.

Pharmacokinetics
- *Absorption:* Relative bioavailablity after oral absorption is 70%. Maximum levels achieved 5 to 6 hours after oral dose.
- *Distribution:* Bound primarily to albumin.
- *Metabolism:* No information available.
- *Excretion:* Appears to be excreted through urine and feces.

Contraindications
Contraindicated in patients with history of hypersensitivity to a rifamycin (rifapentine, rifampin, or rifabutin).

Interactions
Drug-drug. *Antiarrhythmics (disopyramide, mexiletine, quinidine, tocainide), antibiotics (chloramphenicol, clarithromycin, dapsone, doxycycline, fluoroquinolones), anticonvulsants (phenytoin), antifungals (fluconazole, itraconazole, ketoconazole), barbiturates, benzodiazepines (diazepam), beta blockers, calcium channel blockers (diltiazem, nifedipine, verapamil), cardiac glycosides, clofibrate, corticosteroids, haloperidol, HIV protease inhibitors (indinavir, nelfinavir, ritonavir, saquinavir), immunosuppressants (cyclosporine, tacrolimus), levothyroxine, narcotic analgesics (methadone), oral anticoagulants (warfarin), oral hypoglycemics (sulfonylureas), oral or other systemic hormonal contraceptives, progestins, quinine, reverse transcriptase inhibitors (delavirdine, zidovudine), sildenafil, theophylline, tricyclic antidepressants (amitriptyline, nortriptyline):* Decreased activity of these drugs via induced metabolism of the hepatic cytochrome P-450 enzyme system. Monitor patient and adjust drug dosages as needed.

Adverse reactions
CNS: headache, dizziness.
CV: hypertension.
GI: anorexia, nausea, vomiting, dyspepsia, diarrhea.
GU: pyuria, proteinuria, hematuria, urinary casts.
Hematologic: *neutropenia,* lymphopenia, anemia, *leukopenia,* thrombocytosis.
Hepatic: elevated AST and ALT levels.
Metabolic: *hyperuricemia.*
Musculoskeletal: arthralgia, pain.
Respiratory: hemoptysis.
Skin: rash, pruritus, acne, maculopapular rash.

☑ Special considerations
- Coadministration of pyridoxine (vitamin B_6) is recommended in malnourished patients, in those predisposed to neuropathy (alcoholics, diabetics), and in adolescents.
- Drug must be given with appropriate daily companion drugs. Compliance with all medication

---

regimens, especially of daily companion drugs on the days when rifapentine isn't given, is crucial for early sputum conversion and protection from relapse of tuberculosis.

• Administration of drug during last 2 weeks of pregnancy may lead to postnatal hemorrhage in mother or infant. Monitor clotting parameters closely if drug is given.

• Drug can turn body tissues and fluids red-orange. This can lead to permanent staining of contact lenses.

• In case of overdose, neither hemodialysis nor forced diuresis is suggested.

Monitoring the patient
• Use drug cautiously and with frequent monitoring in patients with liver disease.
• Rifamycin antibiotics have been associated with hepatotoxicity. Monitor liver function test results before beginning therapy.
• Drug therapy may affect liver function test results, CBC, and platelet counts; monitor patient carefully.
• Monitor patient for persistent or severe diarrhea.

Information for the patient
• Stress importance of strict compliance with drug and daily companion drugs as well as necessary follow-up visits and laboratory tests.
• Advise patient to use nonhormonal methods of birth control.
• Tell patient to take drug with food if nausea, vomiting, or GI upset occurs.
• Instruct patient to call if the following occur: fever, loss of appetite, malaise, nausea, vomiting, darkened urine, yellowish discoloration of skin and eyes, pain or swelling of joints, and excessive loose stools or diarrhea.
• Instruct patient to protect pills from excessive heat.
• Tell patient that drug can turn body fluids red-orange. If patient wears contact lenses, these can become permanently stained.

Pediatric patients
• Safety and efficacy in children under age 12 haven't been established.

Breast-feeding patients
• Drug may appear in breast milk and isn't recommended for breast-feeding women.

riluzole
Rilutek

Pharmacologic classification: benzothiazole
Therapeutic classification: neuroprotector
Pregnancy risk category C

How supplied
Available by prescription only
Tablets: 50 mg

Indications, route, and dosage
Amyotrophic lateral sclerosis (ALS)
Adults: 50 mg P.O. q 12 hours on an empty stomach.

Pharmacodynamics
Neuroprotector action: Mechanism unknown.

Pharmacokinetics
• *Absorption:* About 90% absorbed from GI tract (with average absolute oral bioavailability of about 60%. A high-fat meal decreases absorption.
• *Distribution:* 96% protein-bound.
• *Metabolism:* Extensively metabolized in liver to six major and several minor metabolites, not all identified.
• *Excretion:* Excreted primarily in urine; small amount in feces. Half-life is 12 hours with repeated doses.

Contraindications and precautions
Contraindicated in patients with history of severe hypersensitivity reactions to drug or components in tablets. Use cautiously in patients with hepatic or renal dysfunction and in elderly patients. Also use cautiously in women and Japanese patients who may possess a lower metabolic capacity to eliminate drug.

Interactions
Drug-drug. *Hepatotoxic drugs (such as allopurinol, methyldopa, sulfasalazine):* Increased risk of hepatotoxicity. Monitor hepatic function.
Inducers of CYP 1A2 (omeprazole, rifampin): Increased riluzole elimination. Observe patient for drug effect.
Potential inhibitors of CYP 1A2 (amitriptyline, caffeine, phenacetin, quinolones, theophylline): Decreased riluzole elimination. Monitor patient closely.
Drug-food. *Any food:* Decreased bioavailability. Administer 1 hour before or 2 hours after meals.
Charbroiled foods: Increased riluzole elimination. Avoid concomitant use.
Drug-lifestyle. *Alcohol:* Increased risk of hepatotoxicity. Discourage excessive use.
Smoking: Increased riluzole elimination. Discourage smoking.

Adverse reactions
CNS: headache, aggravation reaction, hyperto-nia, malaise, depression, dizziness, insomnia, somnolence, vertigo, circumoral paresthesia.
CV: hypertension, tachycardia, palpitation, or-thostatic hypotension, peripheral edema.
EENT: rhinitis, sinusitis.
GI: abdominal pain, *nausea*, vomiting, dyspep-sia, anorexia, diarrhea, flatulence, stomatitis, tooth disorder, oral candidiasis, dry mouth.
GU: urinary tract infection, dysuria.
Metabolic: weight loss.
Musculoskeletal: *asthenia*, back pain, arthral-gia.
Respiratory: *decreased lung function*, increased cough.
Skin: pruritus, eczema, alopecia, exfoliative der-matitis.
Other: phlebitis.

☑ Special considerations
● Give drug at least 1 hour before or 2 hours af-ter a meal to avoid a food-related decrease in bioavailability.

Monitoring the patient
● Baseline elevations in liver function studies (es-pecially elevated bilirubin) should preclude use of riluzole. Perform liver function studies period-ically during therapy. In many patients, drug may cause serum aminotransferase elevations; stop drug if levels exceed 10 times upper limit of nor-mal or if jaundice develops.
● Monitor therapeutic effect.

Information for the patient
● Tell patient or caregiver that drug must be tak-en regularly and at the same time each day. If a dose is missed, tell patient to take the next tablet as originally planned.
● Instruct patient to report febrile illness because the patient's WBC count should be checked.
● Warn patient to avoid hazardous activities un-til CNS effects of drug are known.
● Advise patient to avoid excessive alcohol in-take while taking drug.
● Tell patient to store drug at room temperature and protect it from bright light.
● Stress importance of keeping drug out of reach of children.

Geriatric patients
● Age-related decreased renal and hepatic func-tion may cause a decrease in clearance of rilu-zole; administer drug cautiously to this age-group.

Pediatric patients
● Safety and effectiveness in children haven't been established.

Breast-feeding patients
● It's unknown if drug appears in breast milk. Be-cause of potential for serious adverse reactions in infants, use of drug in breast-feeding women isn't recommended.

rimantadine hydrochloride
Flumadine

Pharmacologic classification: adaman-tine
Therapeutic classification: antiviral
Pregnancy risk category C

How supplied
Available by prescription only
Tablets: 100 mg
Syrup: 50 mg/5 ml

Indications, route, and dosage
Prophylaxis against influenza A virus
Adults and children ages 10 and older: 100 mg P.O. b.i.d.
✦ *Dosage adjustment.* For patients with severe hepatic dysfunction or renal failure (creatinine clearance 10 ml/minute or less) and for elderly nursing home patients, a dosage reduction to 100 mg P.O. daily is recommended.
Children under age 10: 5 mg/kg P.O. once daily. Maximum dose is 150 mg.
Treatment of illness caused by various strains of influenza A virus
Adults: 100 mg P.O. b.i.d. for 7 days from initial onset of symptoms.
✦ *Dosage adjustment.* For patients with severe hepatic dysfunction or renal failure (creatinine clearance 10 ml/minute or less) and for elderly nursing home patients, a dose reduction to 100 mg P.O. daily is recommended.
Note: If seizures develop, stop drug.

Pharmacodynamics
Antiviral action: Exact mechanism unknown. Ap-pears to exert its inhibitory effect early in the vi-ral replicative cycle, possibly inhibiting the un-coating of the virus. A virus protein specified by the virion M^2 gene may play an important role in the susceptibility of influenza A virus to inhibition by rimantadine.

Pharmacokinetics
● *Absorption:* Tablet and syrup formulations equal-ly absorbed after oral administration. Levels peak in about 6 hours in an otherwise healthy adult.
● *Distribution:* Plasma protein-binding is about 40%.
● *Metabolism:* Extensively metabolized in liver.
● *Excretion:* Less than 25% excreted in urine as unchanged drug. Elimination half-life about 25.4 to 32 hours. Hemodialysis doesn't contribute to drug clearance.

Reactions may be *common*, uncommon, **life-threatening**, or COMMON AND LIFE-THREATENING.

Contraindications and precautions

Contraindicated in patients with hypersensitivity to drug or to amantadine. Use cautiously during pregnancy and in patients with impaired renal or hepatic function or seizure disorders (especially epilepsy).

Interactions

Drug-drug. *Acetaminophen, aspirin:* Reduced levels of amantadine. Monitor effectiveness of rimantadine.

Cimetidine: Decreased total rimantadine clearance by about 16%. Monitor patient for adverse effects associated with rimantadine use.

Adverse reactions

CNS: insomnia, headache, dizziness, nervousness, fatigue, asthenia.
GI: nausea, vomiting, anorexia, dry mouth, abdominal pain.

☑ Special considerations

● For illnesses associated with various strains of influenza A, treatment should begin as soon as possible (preferably within 48 hours after onset of signs and symptoms) to reduce duration of fever and systematic symptoms.
● An increased frequency of seizures has been observed in some patients with history of seizures who weren't taking anticonvulsant medication during rimantadine therapy. If seizures develop, stop drug.
● Influenza A–resistant strains can emerge during therapy. Patients taking drug may still be able to spread the disease.
● In case of overdose, administration of I.V. physostigmine (1 to 2 mg in adults and 0.5 mg in children; repeated as needed but not to exceed 2 mg/hour) has been reported anecdotally to benefit patients with CNS effects from overdose of amantadine (a related drug).

Monitoring the patient

● Because of risk of accumulation of drug metabolites during multiple dosing, monitor patient with any degree of renal insufficiency for adverse effects, and adjust dosage as necessary.

Information for the patient

● Tell patient to take drug several hours before bedtime to prevent insomnia.
● Inform patient that taking drug doesn't prevent him from spreading the disease; he should limit contact with others until fully recovered.
● Warn patient that drug may cause adverse CNS effects; he shouldn't drive or perform activities that require mental alertness until these effects are known.
● Tell patient with history of epilepsy to stop taking drug and call if seizure activity occurs.

Geriatric patients

● Adverse reactions associated with drug occur more frequently in elderly patients than in the general population. Monitor these patients closely.

Pediatric patients

● Drug is recommended for prophylaxis of influenza A. Safety and effectiveness of drug in treating symptomatic influenza infection in children haven't been established. Prophylaxis studies with rimantadine haven't been performed in children under age 1.

Breast-feeding patients

● It's unknown if drug appears in human breast milk. Don't give drug to breast-feeding women because of potential adverse effects in infant.

Ringer's injection

Pharmacologic classification: electrolyte solution
Therapeutic classification: electrolyte and fluid replenishment
Pregnancy risk category C

How supplied

Available by prescription only
Injection: 250 ml, 500 ml, 1,000 ml

Indications, route, and dosage

Fluid and electrolyte replacement

Adults and children: Dose highly individualized according to patient's size and clinical condition.

Pharmacodynamics

Fluid and electrolyte replacement: Replaces fluid and supplies important electrolytes: sodium 147 mEq/L, potassium 4 mEq/L, calcium 4.5 mEq/L, and chloride 155.5 mEq/L. However, clinically, the addition of potassium and calcium only slightly increases the therapeutic value of an isotonic sodium chloride solution. Neither potassium nor calcium is present in sufficient level in Ringer's injection to correct a deficit of these ions adequately. Large volumes of Ringer's injection usually cause minimal distortion of cation composition of the extracellular fluid. The solution may alter the acid-base balance.

Pharmacokinetics

● *Absorption:* Given by direct I.V. infusion.
● *Distribution:* Widely distributed.
● *Metabolism:* None significant.
● *Excretion:* Excreted primarily in urine.

Contraindications and precautions

Contraindicated in patients with renal failure, except as emergency volume expander. Use cautiously in patients with heart failure, circulatory insufficiency, renal dysfunction, hypoproteinemia, or pulmonary edema.

Interactions
Drug-drug. *Several drugs as well as packed RBCs:* Incompatible with Ringer's solution. Consult specialized references for further information.

Adverse reactions
CV: fluid overload.

☑ Special considerations
● Ringer's injection is a colorless, odorless solution with a salty taste and a pH between 5.0 and 7.5.

Monitoring the patient
● Monitor patient for acid-base imbalance when large volume of solution is infused.
● Monitor weight in cardiac and renal patients.

Information for the patient
● Explain need for I.V. therapy.
● Tell patient to report adverse reactions immediately.

Ringer's injection, lactated

Pharmacologic classification: electrolyte-carbohydrate solution
Therapeutic classification: electrolyte and fluid replenishment
Pregnancy risk category C

How supplied
Available by prescription only
Injection: 150 ml, 250 ml, 500 ml, 1,000 ml

Indications, route, and dosage
Fluid and electrolyte replacement
Adults and children: Dose highly individualized. Solution approximates the contents of the blood more closely than Ringer's injection does; however, additional electrolytes may have to be added to meet the patient's needs. Specific formulations of I.V. solutions are generally preferred to this premixed formulation.

Pharmacodynamics
Fluid and electrolyte replacement: Replaces fluid and supplies important electrolytes: sodium 130 mEq/L, potassium 4 mEq/L, calcium 3 mEq/L, chloride 109.7 mEq/L, and lactate 28 mEq/L. However, clinically, the addition of potassium and calcium only slightly increases the therapeutic value of an isotonic sodium chloride solution. Neither potassium nor calcium is present in sufficient level in lactated Ringer's injection to correct a deficit of these ions. Large volumes of lactated Ringer's injection usually cause minimal distor-

tion of cation composition of the extracellular fluid. The solution may alter the acid-base balance.

Lactated Ringer's injection may be used for its alkalinizing effect because the lactate is ultimately metabolized to bicarbonate. In persons with normal cellular oxidative activity, the alkalinizing effect will be fully realized in 1 to 2 hours.

Pharmacokinetics
● *Absorption:* Given by direct I.V. infusion.
● *Distribution:* Distributed widely.
● *Metabolism:* None significant for electrolytes; lactate is oxidized to bicarbonate.
● *Excretion:* Excreted primarily in urine.

Contraindications and precautions
Contraindicated in patients with renal failure, except as emergency volume expander. Use cautiously in patients with heart failure, circulatory insufficiency, renal dysfunction, hypoproteinemia, or pulmonary edema.

Interactions
Drug-drug. *Several drugs as well as packed RBCs:* Incompatible with lactated Ringer's injection. Consult specialized references for further information.

Adverse reactions
CV: fluid overload.

☑ Special considerations
● Solution is colorless and odorless with a salty taste and a pH between 6 and 7.5. The absence of bicarbonate from the solution stabilizes the calcium, which may precipitate as calcium bicarbonate. It contains no antibacterial product.

Monitoring the patient
● Monitor patient for acid-base imbalance when large volume of solution is infused.
● Monitor weight in patients at risk for excessive fluid retention.

Information for the patient
● Explain need for I.V. therapy.
● Tell patient to report adverse reactions immediately.

---

risperidone
Risperdal

Pharmacologic classification: benzisoxazole derivative
Therapeutic classification: antipsychotic
Pregnancy risk category C

How supplied
Available by prescription only
Tablets: 0.25 mg, 0.5 mg, 1 mg, 2 mg, 3 mg, 4 mg
Oral solution: 1 mg/ml

Indications, route, and dosage
Psychosis
Adults: Initially, 1 mg P.O. b.i.d. Increase in increments of 1 mg b.i.d. on days 2 and 3 of treatment to a target dose of 3 mg b.i.d. Wait at least 1 week before adjusting dosage further. Doses above 6 mg/day were not found to be more effective than lower doses and were associated with more extrapyramidal effects.

✦ Dosage adjustment. Elderly or debilitated patients, hypotensive patients, or patients with severe renal or hepatic impairment should initially receive 0.5 mg P.O. b.i.d. Increase dosage in increments of 0.5 mg b.i.d. on second and third day of treatment to target dose of 1.5 mg P.O. b.i.d. Wait at least 1 week before increasing dosage further.

Pharmacodynamics
Antipsychotic action: Exact mechanism unknown. Antipsychotic activity may be mediated through a combination of dopamine type 2 (D_2) and serotonin type 2 ($5-HT_2$) antagonism. Antagonism at receptors other than D_2 and $5-HT_2$ may explain other effects of drug.

Pharmacokinetics
• Absorption: Well absorbed after oral administration. Absolute oral bioavailability is 70%. Food doesn't affect rate or extent of absorption.
• Distribution: Plasma protein-binding about 90% for drug; 77% for its major active metabolite, 9-hydroxyrisperidone.
• Metabolism: Extensively metabolized in liver to 9-hydroxyrisperidone; is the predominant circulating species. Appears about equi-effective with risperidone with respect to receptor binding activity. (About 6% to 8% of whites and a low percentage of Asians show little or no receptor binding activity and are poor metabolizers.)
• Excretion: Metabolite excreted by kidneys. Clearance of drug and metabolite reduced in renally impaired patients.

Contraindications and precautions
Contraindicated in patients with hypersensitivity to drug and in breast-feeding patients. Use cautiously in patients with prolonged QT interval, CV disease, cerebrovascular disease, dehydration, hypovolemia, history of seizures, or exposure to extreme heat or conditions that could affect metabolism or hemodynamic responses.

Interactions
Drug-drug. Antihypertensives: Increased hypotension. Monitor vital signs closely.
Carbamazepine: Increased clearance of risperidone. Monitor patient closely.
Clozapine: Decreased clearance of risperidone. Monitor patient for toxicity.
Dopamine agonists, levodopa: Antagonized effects of these drugs. Monitor patient closely.

Other CNS depressants: Additive CNS depression when administered together. Use together with caution.
Drug-lifestyle. Alcohol: Additive CNS depression when administered together. Discourage use.
Sun exposure: Photosensitivity reactions. Tell patient to take precautions.

Adverse reactions
CNS: somnolence, extrapyramidal symptoms, headache, insomnia, agitation, anxiety, tardive dyskinesia, aggressiveness.
CV: tachycardia, chest pain, orthostatic hypotension, prolonged QT interval.
EENT: rhinitis, sinusitis, pharyngitis, abnormal vision.
GI: constipation, nausea, vomiting, dyspepsia.
Metabolic: increased serum prolactin levels.
Musculoskeletal: arthralgia, back pain.
Respiratory: coughing, upper respiratory tract infection.
Skin: rash, dry skin, photosensitivity.
Other: fever.

☑ Special considerations
• Risperidone and 9-hydroxyrisperidone appear to lengthen the QT interval in some patients, although there is no average increase in treated patients, even at 12 to 16 mg/day (well above recommended dose). Other drugs that prolong the QT interval have been associated with torsades de pointes, a life-threatening arrhythmia. Bradycardia, electrolyte imbalance, use with other drugs that prolong the QT interval, or congenital prolongation of the QT interval can increase risk for occurrence of this arrhythmia.
• If antiarrhythmic therapy is administered, disopyramide, procainamide, and quinidine carry a theoretical hazard of QT interval–prolonging effects that might be additive to those of risperidone. Similarly, it's reasonable to expect that the alpha-blocking properties of bretylium might be additive to those of risperidone, resulting in problematic hypotension.
• An antiemetic effect may occur, masking signs and symptoms of overdose or of such conditions as intestinal obstruction, Reye's syndrome, and brain tumor.
• Tardive dyskinesia may occur after prolonged therapy. It may not appear until months or years later and may disappear spontaneously or persist for life despite stopping drug.
• Neuroleptic malignant syndrome is rare but in many cases fatal. It isn't necessarily related to length of drug use or type of neuroleptic. Monitor patient closely for symptoms, including hyperpyrexia, muscle rigidity, altered mental status, irregular pulse, alteration in blood pressure, and diaphoresis.

• When restarting drug for patients who have been off drug, follow initial 3-day dose initiation schedule.
• When switching patient from another antipsychotic to risperidone, immediately stop other antipsychotic on initiation of risperidone when medically appropriate.
• Toxicity may cause drowsiness and sedation, tachycardia and hypotension, and extrapyramidal symptoms. Hyponatremia, hypokalemia, prolonged QT interval, widened QRS complex, and seizures also have been reported.

Monitoring the patient
• Monitor blood pressure.
• Perform periodic ECG to monitor patient for adverse cardiac reactions.

Information for the patient
• Advise patient to rise slowly from a recumbent or seated position to minimize light-headedness.
• Warn patient not to drive or operate hazardous machinery until drug's effects are known.
• Tell woman to call if pregnancy is being planned or is suspected.
• Tell patient to call before taking new drugs, including OTC drugs, because of potential for interactions.
• Advise patient to avoid alcohol during therapy.

Geriatric patients
• A lower starting dose is recommended for elderly patients because they have decreased pharmacokinetic clearance; a greater incidence of hepatic, renal, or cardiac dysfunction; and a greater tendency toward orthostatic hypotension.

Pediatric patients
• Safety and efficacy in children haven't been established.

Breast-feeding patients
• It's unknown if drug appears in breast milk. Patient should discontinue breast-feeding while receiving drug.

---

ritodrine hydrochloride
Yutopar

Pharmacologic classification: beta-receptor agonist
Therapeutic classification: adjunct in suppression of preterm labor
Pregnancy risk category B

How supplied
Available by prescription only
Injection (ampule): 10 mg/ml, 15 mg/ml
Injection (premixed): 0.3 mg/ml

Indications, route, and dosage
Management of preterm labor
Adults: Initially, 0.05 mg/minute I.V. infusion; increase q 10 minutes, p.r.n., or until maternal heart rate is 130 beats/minute, in 0.05-mg increments to effective dose (usually 0.15 to 0.35 mg/minute). Continue for at least 12 hours after uterine contractions cease. Dose shouldn't exceed 0.35 mg/minute.

Pharmacodynamics
Tocolytic action: Beta-receptor agonist that exerts a preferential effect on beta$_2$-adrenergic receptors (such as uterine smooth muscle). Stimulation of the beta$_2$-receptors inhibits contractility of the uterine smooth muscle. Drug also may act to affect directly the interaction between actin and myosin in muscle to decrease the intensity and frequency of contractions.

Pharmacokinetics
• *Absorption:* 100% absorbed by I.V. route.
• *Distribution:* Peak serum levels are 32 to 50 ng/ml after an I.V. infusion of 60 minutes. I.V. dose has a distribution half-life of 6 to 9 minutes.
• *Metabolism:* Metabolized in liver, primarily to inactive sulfate and glucuronide conjugates.
• *Excretion:* About 70% to 90% of I.V. dose excreted in urine in 10 to 12 hours as unchanged drug and its conjugates. Drug can be removed by dialysis.

Contraindications and precautions
Contraindicated in patients with hypersensitivity to drug and in those with preexisting maternal medical conditions, such as hypovolemia, pheochromocytoma, or uncontrolled hypertension, that would seriously be affected by the known pharmacologic properties of drug. Also contraindicated in pregnant women before the 20th week of pregnancy and in women with antepartum hemorrhage, eclampsia, intrauterine fetal death, chorioamnionitis, maternal cardiac disease, pulmonary hypertension, maternal hyperthyroidism, or uncontrolled maternal diabetes mellitus.

Use cautiously in patients with sulfite allergies.

Interactions
Drug-drug. *Atropine:* Worsened hypertension. Avoid concomitant use.
Beta blockers (propranolol): Inhibited action of ritodrine. Avoid concurrent use.
Corticosteroids: Additive diabetogenic effects, pulmonary edema, and possibly death in mother. Stop drugs if pulmonary edema occurs. Monitor patient closely during concurrent use.
Diazoxide, magnesium sulfate, meperidine: Potentiated CV effects. Use together with caution.
Sympathomimetic amines: Additive effect (especially CV). Use together with caution.

Reactions may be *common*, uncommon, **life-threatening**, or COMMON AND LIFE-THREATENING.

Adverse reactions
CNS: nervousness, anxiety, *headache,* emotional upset, malaise.
CV: *palpitation; dose-related alterations in blood pressure, tachycardia,* **pulmonary edema.**
GI: *nausea, vomiting.*
Hematologic: *leukopenia, agranulocytosis.*
Metabolic: *hyperglycemia,* hypokalemia.
Skin: rash, *erythema.*
Other: *anaphylactic shock.*

☑ Special considerations
• Prepare I.V. solution by diluting 150 mg ritodrine in 500 ml of D₅W to produce a solution containing 300 mcg (0.3 mg) of ritodrine per milliliter. Use of saline diluents (normal saline solution, Ringer's solution, and Hartmann's solution) should be reserved for cases in which dextrose solution is medically undesirable because of increased probability of pulmonary edema.
• Stop drug if pulmonary edema occurs.
• Don't use drug I.V. if solution is discolored or contains a precipitate. Don't use more than 48 hours after preparation.
• Control infusion rate by use of a microdrip chamber I.V. infusion set or an infusion control device.
• Place patient in left lateral recumbent position to reduce risk of hypotension.
• Drug may uncover a previously unknown cardiac pathologic condition. Sinus bradycardia may follow drug withdrawal.
• Maternal tachycardia or decreased diastolic blood pressure usually reverses with a dosage reduction but requires stopping drug in 1% of patients.
• Overdose produces signs and symptoms similar to those of excessive beta-adrenergic stimulation (maternal and fetal tachycardia, palpitations, cardiac arrhythmia, hypotension, nervousness, tremor, nausea, and vomiting).
• Treat overdose by stopping infusion and administering appropriate beta blocker (such as propranolol) as an antidote.

Monitoring the patient
• Because CV responses are common, closely monitor maternal pulse rate and blood pressure and fetal heart rate. A maternal tachycardia of over 140 beats/minute or persistent respiratory rate of over 20 breaths/minute may be signs of impending pulmonary edema.
• Monitor blood glucose levels during ritodrine infusions, especially in mothers predisposed to diabetes mellitus.
• Monitor amount of I.V. fluid administered to prevent circulatory overload.

Information for the patient
• Advise patient to keep scheduled follow-up appointments and to report adverse reactions immediately.

• Teach patient how to time contractions and when to contact physician.
• Tell patient to immediately report leakage of fluid, vaginal bleeding, or severe abdominal pain.

ritonavir
Norvir

Pharmacologic classification: HIV protease inhibitor
Therapeutic classification: antiviral
Pregnancy risk category B

How supplied
Available by prescription only
Capsules: 100 mg
Oral solution: 80 mg/ml

Indications, route, and dosage
HIV infection when antiretroviral therapy is warranted
Adults: 600 mg P.O. b.i.d. with meals. If nausea occurs, increased dosage may provide some relief: 300 mg b.i.d. for 1 day, 400 mg b.i.d. for 2 days, 500 mg b.i.d. for 1 day; then 600 mg b.i.d. thereafter.

Pharmacodynamics
Antiviral action: HIV protease inhibitor. HIV protease is an enzyme required for the proteolytic cleavage of the viral polyprotein precursors into the individual functional proteins found in infectious HIV. Drug binds to the protease active site and inhibits the activity of the enzyme. This inhibition prevents cleavage of the viral polyproteins, resulting in the formation of immature noninfectious viral particles.

Pharmacokinetics
• *Absorption:* Absorbed better when taken with food; absolute bioavailability not determined.
• *Distribution:* 98% to 99% bound to plasma proteins.
• *Metabolism:* Metabolized in liver; P-450 3A (CYP3A) is major isoform in metabolism.
• *Excretion:* Primarily excreted in feces; small amount found in urine. Half-life is 3 to 5 hours.

Contraindications and precautions
Contraindicated in patients with hypersensitivity to drug or its components. Use cautiously in patients with hepatic insufficiency.

Interactions
Drug-drug. *Alprazolam, clorazepate, diazepam, estazolam, flurazepam, midazolam, triazolam, zolpidem:* Extreme sedation and respiratory depression. Don't use together.
Amiodarone, bepridil, bupropion, clozapine, encainide, flecainide, meperidine, piroxicam, propafenone, propoxyphene, quinidine, rifabutin:

Large increases in plasma levels of these drugs; increased risk of arrhythmias, hematologic abnormalities, seizures, or other potentially serious adverse effects. Don't use together.

Clarithromycin (in patients with impaired renal function): Reduced creatinine clearance. Patients need a 50% reduction in clarithromycin if creatinine clearance is 30 to 60 ml/minute and a 75% reduction if below 30 ml/minute.

Desipramine: Increased desipramine levels. Adjust dosage as needed.

Disulfiram, metronidazole: Disulfiram-like reactions; ritonavir formulations contain alcohol. Monitor patient.

Drugs that increase CYP3A activity (such as carbamazepine, dexamethasone, phenytoin, rifabutin, rifampin, phenobarbital): Increased clearance of ritonavir. Monitor patient closely.

Glucuronosyltransferases: Decreased therapeutic effects. Use of these drugs with ritonavir should be accompanied by therapeutic drug level monitoring and increased monitoring of therapeutic and adverse effects. Adjust dosages as needed. A dosage reduction greater than 50% may be needed for those drugs extensively metabolized by CYP3A.

Oral contraceptives: Decreased effectiveness. Patient may need dosage increase in use of contraceptive or alternative contraceptive measures.

Theophylline: Decreased theophylline serum levels. Increase dosage of theophylline may be needed.

Drug-lifestyle. *Smoking:* Decreased level of ritonavir. Discourage smoking.

Adverse reactions

CNS: *asthenia,* headache, malaise, circumoral paresthesia, dizziness, insomnia, paresthesia, peripheral paresthesia, somnolence, thinking abnormality, migraine headache, syncope, abnormal dreams, abnormal gait, agitation, amnesia, anxiety, aphasia, ataxia, confusion, depression, emotional lability, euphoria, *generalized tonic-clonic seizure,* hallucinations, hyperesthesia, incoordination, nervousness, neuralgia, neuropathy, paralysis, peripheral neuropathy, peripheral sensory neuropathy, personality disorder, tremor, vertigo.

CV: vasodilation, *hemorrhage,* hypertension, palpitation, peripheral vascular disorder, orthostatic hypotension, tachycardia, chest pain, peripheral edema, edema.

EENT: abnormal electrooculogram, abnormal electroretinogram, abnormal vision, amblyopia, blurred vision, blepharitis, diplopia, ear pain, epistaxis, eye pain, hearing impairment, increased cerumen, iritis, parosmia, pharyngitis, photophobia, rhinitis, taste loss, *taste perversion,* tinnitus, uveitis, visual field defect, local throat irritation.

GI: abdominal pain, anorexia, constipation, *diarrhea, nausea, vomiting,* dyspepsia, flatulence, enlarged abdomen, abnormal stools, bloody diarrhea, cheilitis, cholangitis, colitis, dry mouth, dysphagia, eructation, esophagitis, gastritis, gastroenteritis, GI disorder, *GI hemorrhage,* gingivitis, ileitis, mouth ulcer, oral moniliasis, *pancreatitis,* periodontal abscess, rectal disorder, tenesmus, thirst.

GU: decreased libido, kidney pain, dysuria, hematuria, impotence, kidney calculus, *kidney failure,* nocturia, penis disorder, polyuria, pyelonephritis, urethritis, urine retention, urinary frequency.

Hematologic: anemia, ecchymosis, *leukopenia,* lymphadenopathy, lymphocytosis, *thrombocytopenia.*

Hepatic: *hepatitis,* hepatomegaly, liver damage, liver function test abnormality.

Metabolic: altered hormonal levels, diabetes mellitus, avitaminosis, glycosuria, gout, hypercholestererua, increased CK level, hyperlipidemia, cachexia, hypothermia, dehydration.

Musculoskeletal: arthralgia, arthrosis, joint disorder, muscle cramps, muscle weakness, myalgia, myositis, twitching, back pain, neck pain, neck rigidity, unspecified, substernal chest pain.

Respiratory: asthma, dyspnea, hiccups, hypoventilation, increased cough, interstitial pneumonia, lung disorder.

Skin: rash, sweating, photosensitivity reaction, acne, contact dermatitis, dry skin, eczema, folliculitis, maculopapular rash, molluscum contagiosum, pruritus, psoriasis, seborrhea, urticaria, vesiculobullous rash.

Other: fever, *allergic reaction,* chills, facial edema, facial pain, flu syndrome.

☑ Special considerations

● Drug may be administered alone or with nucleoside analogues.

● GI tolerance may be improved in patients initiating combination regimens with ritonavir and nucleosides by initiating ritonavir alone and subsequently adding nucleosides before completing 2 weeks of ritonavir monotherapy.

Monitoring the patient

● Periodically monitor liver function tests.
● Monitor CBC and serum amylase and lipase levels.

Information for the patient

● Inform patient that drug isn't a cure for HIV infection. He may continue to develop opportunistic infections and other complications associated with HIV infection. Drug hasn't been shown to reduce risk of transmitting HIV to others through sexual contact or blood contamination.

● Caution patient not to adjust dosage or stop drug without medical approval.

● Tell patient that he may improve taste of oral solution by mixing with chocolate milk, Ensure, or Advera within 1 hour of dosing.

Reactions may be *common,* uncommon, **life-threatening,** or COMMON AND LIFE-THREATENING.

- Instruct patient to take drug with meals to improve absorption.
- Tell patient to take a missed dose as soon as possible. However, if a dose is skipped, he shouldn't double the next dose.
- Advise patient to report use of other drugs, including OTC preparations, because of possible drug interactions.

Pediatric patients
- Safety and effectiveness in children under age 12 haven't been established.

Breast-feeding patients
- It's unknown if drug appears in breast milk. However, to prevent transmission of infection, HIV-positive women shouldn't breast-feed.

rituximab
Rituxan

Pharmacologic classification: monoclonal antibody
Therapeutic classification: antineoplastic
Pregnancy risk factor C

How supplied
Available by prescription only
Injection: 10 mg/ml; 10 ml, 50 ml single-use vials

Indications, route, and dosage
Relapsed or refractory low-grade or follicular, CD20 positive, B-cell malignant lymphoma
Adults: 375 mg/m² I.V. infusion once weekly for four doses (days 1, 8, 15, 22). Initial infusion should be started at 50 mg/hour. If hypersensitivity or infusion-related events don't occur, increase rate to 50 mg/hour q 30 minutes to maximum of 400 mg/hour. Administer subsequent infusions at initial rate of 100 mg/hour and increase by increments of 100 mg/hour at 30-minute intervals, to maximum of 400 mg/hour as tolerated.

Pharmacodynamics
Antineoplastic action: A murine/human monoclonal antibody directed against CD20 antigen found on the surface of normal and malignant B-lymphocytes. CD20 regulates early steps in cell cycle initiation and differentiation processes. Binding to this antigen mediates the lysis of the B cells.

Pharmacokinetics
No information available.

Contraindications and precautions
Contraindicated in patients with type I hypersensitivity or anaphylactic reactions to murine proteins or to any component of drug.

Interactions
None reported.

Adverse reactions
CNS: dizziness, *asthenia, headache,* fatigue, paresthesia, malaise, agitation, insomnia, hypoesthesia, hypertonia, nervousness, anxiety.
CV: *hypotension, arrhythmias,* hypertension, peripheral edema, chest pain, tachycardia, orthostatic hypotension, *bradycardia.*
EENT: sore throat, rhinitis, sinusitis, lacrimation disorder, conjunctivitis.
GI: *nausea,* vomiting, abdominal pain or enlargement, diarrhea, dyspepsia, anorexia, increased lactate dehydrogenase, taste perversion.
Hematologic: LEUKOPENIA, *thrombocytopenia, neutropenia,* anemia.
Metabolic: hyperglycemia, hypocalcemia.
Musculoskeletal: arthralgia, back pain, myalgia.
Respiratory: *bronchospasm,* dyspnea, cough increase, bronchitis.
Skin: *pruritus, rash,* urticaria, flushing.
Other: ANGIOEDEMA, *fever, chills, rigor,* pain, pain at injection site, tumor pain.

☑ Special considerations
- Drug must be given as I.V. infusion; don't give as an I.V. push or bolus. Drug may be diluted to a final concentration of 1 to 4 mg/ml in normal saline solution or D₅W.
- Consider medicating patient with acetaminophen and diphenhydramine before each infusion because hypersensitivity reactions may occur.
- Stop infusion if serious or life-threatening cardiac arrhythmias occur.
- Human anti-murine antibody (HAMA) and human antichimeric antibody (HACA) have been detected in less than 1% of patients. If HAMA or HACA titers appear, patient may develop allergic or hypersensitivity reactions to drug or other murine or chimeric monoclonal antibody preparations.
- Immunization safety or efficacy during drug therapy hasn't been studied.
- Because transient hypotension may occur during infusion, consider withholding antihypertensives 12 hours before infusion.

Monitoring the patient
- Monitor patient closely for signs and symptoms of hypersensitivity reaction.
- Hypotension, bronchospasm, and angioedema have occurred as part of an infusion-related symptom complex. Have such drugs as epinephrine, diphenhydramine, and corticosteroids available to immediately treat such a reaction. Monitor patient's blood pressure closely during infusion. If an infusion-related symptom complex occurs, stop infusion and restart at a 50% rate reduction when symptoms resolve. Recommended symptom treatment includes aceta-

minophen, diphenhydramine; bronchodilators or
I.V. saline may be indicated. In most cases, patients have been able to proceed with a full course
of therapy.
• Patients with preexisting cardiac conditions, including arrhythmias and angina, could have recurrences during drug therapy and should be
monitored throughout infusion period.
• Perform cardiac monitoring during and after
subsequent drug infusions in patients who develop clinically significant infusion-related symptoms.
• Obtain CBCs at regular intervals and more frequently in patients who develop cytopenias.

Information for the patient
• Tell patient to report unusual symptoms during
and after infusion.
• Advise patient to disclose history of cardiac
problems.
• Instruct patient not to receive any vaccinations
(especially live viral vaccines) during therapy unless approved.
• Inform patient that frequent CBCs may be necessary.

Pediatric patients
• Safety and effectiveness in children haven't
been established.

Breast-feeding patients
• It's unknown if drug appears in breast milk. Because other antibodies can appear, advise patient to stop breast-feeding until circulation levels of drug are undetectable.

---

rizatriptan benzoate
Maxalt, Maxalt-MLT

Pharmacologic classification: selective
5-hydroxytryptamine (5-HT$_{1b/1d}$) receptor agonist
Therapeutic classification: antimigraine
drug
Pregnancy risk category C

How supplied
Tablets: 5 mg, 10 mg
Tablets (orally disintegrating): 5 mg, 10 mg

Indications, route, and dosage
*Acute migraine headaches with or without
aura*
Adults: Initially, 5 or 10 mg P.O. If first dose is ineffective, another dose can be given at least 2
hours after first dose. Maximum dose is 30 mg
within a 24-hour period. For patients receiving
propranolol, 5 mg P.O. up to maximum of three
doses (15 mg) in 24 hours.

Pharmacodynamics
Antimigraine action: Believed to exert effect by
acting as an agonist at serotonin receptors on
the extracerebral intracranial blood vessels, which
results in vasoconstriction of the affected vessels, inhibition of neuropeptide release, and reduction of pain transmission in the trigeminal
pathways.

Pharmacokinetics
• *Absorption:* Bioavailablity after oral administration is 45%. Plasma levels peak in 1 to 1½
hours.
• *Distribution:* Minimally plasma-bound.
• *Metabolism:* Primary metabolism via oxidative
deamination by monoamine oxidase, A to the indole acetic acid metabolite.
• *Excretion:* 82% excreted in urine; 12% in feces.

Contraindications and precautions
Contraindicated in patients with hypersensitivity
to drug or its components and in those with ischemic heart disease (angina pectoris, history
of MI, or documented silent ischemia) or symptoms or findings consistent with ischemic heart
disease, coronary artery vasospasm (Prinzmetal's variant angina), or other significant underlying CV disease. Also contraindicated in patients
with uncontrolled hypertension or within 24 hours
of treatment with another 5-HT agonist or an ergotamine-containing or ergot-type drug such as
dihydroergotamine or methysergide.
    Use cautiously in patients with hepatic or renal impairment and in those with risk factors for
coronary artery disease (hypertension, hypercholesterolemia, smoking, obesity, diabetes,
strong family history of coronary artery disease,
women with surgical or physiologic menopause,
or men over 40), unless a cardiac evaluation provides evidence that patient is free from cardiac
disease.
    Don't use within 2 weeks of discontinuation
of MAO inhibitor.

Interactions
Drug-drug. *Drugs containing ergot, ergot-type
drugs (dihydroergotamine, methysergide), other 5-HT$_1$ agonists:* Prolonged vasospastic reactions. Don't use within 24 hours of rizatriptan.
*MAO inhibitors (moclobemide), nonselective MAO
inhibitors (types A and B, such as isocarboxazid,
pargyline, phenelzine, tranylcypromine):* Increased
plasma levels of rizatriptan. Avoid concurrent use;
allow at least 14 days between ending an MAO
inhibitor and starting rizatriptan.
Propranolol: Increased rizatriptan levels. Reduce
rizatriptan dose to 5 mg.
Selective serotonin reuptake inhibitors (fluoxetine, fluvoxamine, paroxetine, sertraline): Possible weakness, hyperreflexia, and incoordination.
Monitor patient.

Adverse reactions
CNS: dizziness, headache, somnolence, paresthesia, asthenia, fatigue, hypoesthesia, decreased mental acuity, euphoria, tremor.
CV: chest pain, pressure or heaviness, palpitations.
EENT: neck, throat and jaw pain, pressure, or heaviness.
GI: dry mouth, nausea, diarrhea, vomiting.
Respiratory: dyspnea.
Skin: flushing.
Other: pain, hot flashes,warm or cold sensations.

☑ Special considerations
• Drug should be used only after a definite diagnosis of migraine is established.
• Don't use for prophylactic therapy of migraines or in patients with hemiplegic or basilar migraine or cluster headaches.
• Safety of treating, on average, more than four headaches in a 30-day period hasn't been established.
• Orally disintegrating tablets contain phenylalanine.

Monitoring the patient
• Patients with risk factors that have a satisfactory cardiac evaluation should be closely monitored after first dose.
• Assess CV status in patients who develop risk factors for coronary artery disease during treatment.

Information for the patient
• Inform patient that drug doesn't prevent migraine headaches.
• For Maxalt-MLT, tell patient to remove blister pack from pouch, then remove drug from blister pack immediately before use. Tablet shouldn't be popped out of blister pack, but pack should be carefully peeled away with dry hands, and tablet placed on tongue and allowed to dissolve. Tablet is then swallowed with saliva. No water is necessary or recommended. Tell patient that orally dissolving tablet doesn't provide more rapid headache relief.
• Advise patient that if headache returns after initial dose, a second dose may be taken with medical approval at least 2 hours after first dose. Patient shouldn't take more than 30 mg in a 24-hour period.
• Inform patient that drug may cause somnolence and dizziness and warn him to avoid hazardous activities until effects are known.
• Tell patient that food may delay drug's onset of action.
• Advise patient to call if pregnancy occurs or is suspected.

Pediatric patients
• Safety and effectiveness in children under age 18 haven't been established.

Breast-feeding patients
• It's unknown if drug appears in breast milk. Instruct patient not to breast-feed because effects on infant are unknown.

rocuronium bromide
Zemuron

Pharmacologic classification: non-depolarizing neuromuscular blocker
Therapeutic classification: skeletal muscle relaxant
Pregnancy risk category B

How supplied
Available by prescription only
Injection: 10 mg/ml

Indications, route, and dosage
Adjunct to general anesthesia, facilitation of endotracheal intubation, or skeletal muscle relaxation during surgery or mechanical ventilation
Adults and children ages 3 months and older: Initially, 0.6 to 1.2 mg/kg I.V. bolus. In most patients, tracheal intubation may be performed within 2 minutes; muscle paralysis should last about 31 minutes. Maintenance dose of 0.1 mg/kg should provide an additional 12 minutes of muscle relaxation (0.15 mg/kg will add 17 minutes; 0.2 mg/kg will add 24 minutes). Or maintenance dose by continuous I.V. infusion of 4 to 16 mcg/kg/minute.
Note: Dosage depends on anesthetic used, individual needs, and response. Dosages are representative and must be adjusted.

Pharmacodynamics
Skeletal muscle relaxation action: Acts by competing for cholinergic receptors at the motor end plate. This action is antagonized by acetylcholinesterase inhibitors, such as neostigmine and edrophonium.

Pharmacokinetics
• *Absorption:* Given I.V.
• *Distribution:* Rapid distribution half-life is 1 to 2 minutes; slower distribution half-life is 14 to 18 minutes. Drug is about 30% bound to plasma proteins.
• *Metabolism:* No information available, but hepatic clearance could be significant. The rocuronium analogue 17-desacetyl-rocuronium, a metabolite, has rarely been observed in plasma or urine.
• *Excretion:* About 33% of dose recovered in urine within 24 hours.

Contraindications and precautions
Contraindicated in patients with hypersensitivity to bromides. Use cautiously in patients with hepatic disease, severe obesity, bronchogenic carcinoma, electrolyte disturbances, neuromuscular disease, or altered circulation time caused by age and CV or edematous states.

Interactions
Drug-drug. *Aminoglycosides, bacitracin, colistimethate sodium, colistin, polymyxins, quinidine, tetracyclines, vancomycin:* Enhanced neuromuscular blocking action of rocuronium. Use cautiously during surgical procedure and in postoperative period.
Anticonvulsants (carbamazepine, phenytoin): Diminished magnitude of neuromuscular block or shortened clinical duration. Monitor patient closely.
Enflurane, isoflurane: Prolonged duration of action of initial and maintenance doses of rocuronium; decrease average infusion requirement of rocuronium by 40% compared with opioid, nitrous oxide, or oxygen anesthesia. Adjust dosage as needed.

Adverse reactions
CV: tachycardia, abnormal ECG, transient hypotension and hypertension.
GI: nausea, vomiting.
Respiratory: asthma, hiccups.
Skin: rash, edema, pruritus.

☑ Special considerations
• Drug should be used only by those experienced in airway management.
• Keep airway clear. Have emergency respiratory support equipment (endotracheal equipment, ventilator, oxygen, atropine, edrophonium, epinephrine, and neostigmine) available.
• Neuromuscular blockers don't obtund consciousness or alter pain threshold. Patients should receive sedatives or general anesthetics before neuromuscular blockers are administered.
• Drug is well tolerated in patients with renal failure.
• In obese patients, initial dose should be based on patient's actual body weight.
• A peripheral nerve stimulator should be used to measure neuromuscular function during drug administration to monitor drug effect, determine need for additional doses, and confirm recovery from neuromuscular block. Once spontaneous recovery starts, drug-induced neuromuscular blockade may be reversed with an anticholinesterase.
• Drug, which has an acid pH, shouldn't be mixed with alkaline solutions (such as barbiturate solutions) in same syringe or administered simultaneously during I.V. infusion through same needle.

• Store reconstituted solution in refrigerator. Discard after 24 hours.

Monitoring the patient
• Monitor patients with liver disease because they may need larger doses of drug to achieve adequate muscle relaxation. These patients may also experience prolonged effects from drug.
• Monitor vital signs, especially respirations, until patient is fully recovered from drug effects.

Information for the patient
• Explain all events and procedures to patient because he can still hear.

Pediatric patients
• Use in children under age 3 months hasn't been studied.

rofecoxib
Vioxx

Pharmacologic classification: cyclooxygenase-2 (COX-2) inhibitor
Therapeutic classification: nonnarcotic analgesic, anti-inflammatory
Pregnancy risk category C

How supplied
Available by prescription only
Tablets: 12.5 mg, 25 mg
Oral suspension: 12.5 mg/5 ml, 25 mg/5 ml

Indications, route, and dosage
Relief of signs and symptoms of osteoarthritis
Adults: Initially, 12.5 mg P.O. once daily, increased as needed to a maximum of 25 mg P.O. once daily.
Management of acute pain, treatment of primary dysmenorrhea
Adults: 50 mg P.O. once daily as needed for up to 5 days.

Pharmacodynamics
Analgesic and anti-inflammatory actions: Exact mechanism unknown. Anti-inflammatory and analgesic effects along with antipyretic activity may come from drug's ability to inhibit prostaglandin synthesis, which it does by inhibiting the COX-2 isoenzyme. At therapeutic serum levels, rofecoxib doesn't inhibit the cyclooxygenase-1 (COX-1) isoenzyme.

Pharmacokinetics
• *Absorption:* Well absorbed, with a mean bioavailability of 93%. Median time for peak serum levels is 2 to 3 hours; range is 2 to 9 hours.
• *Distribution:* About 87% of drug binds to proteins.
• *Metabolism:* Metabolized in liver to inactive metabolites.

• *Excretion:* Eliminated predominantly through hepatic metabolism. Less than 1% eliminated from kidneys as unchanged drug. Half-life is about 17 hours.

Contraindications and precautions

Contraindicated in patients with hypersensitivity to drug or its components and in those who have experienced asthma, urticaria, or allergic-type reactions after taking aspirin or other NSAIDs. Drug should be avoided in patients with advanced kidney disease or moderate or severe hepatic insufficiency and in pregnant women because it may cause the ductus arteriosus to close prematurely.

Use cautiously in patients with preexisting asthma, renal disease, liver dysfunction, or abnormal liver function tests. Also use cautiously in patients with a history of ulcer disease or GI bleeding. Use cautiously in patients being treated with oral corticosteroids or anticoagulants, in patients with a history of smoking or alcoholism, and in geriatric or debilitated patients because of increased risk of GI bleeding.

Use cautiously in patients with considerable dehydration. Rehydration is recommended before therapy begins. Use cautiously, and initiate therapy at the lowest recommended dosage, in patients with fluid retention, hypertension, or heart failure.

Interactions

Drug-drug. *ACE inhibitors:* Decreased antihypertensive effects of these drugs. Monitor patient closely.
Aspirin: Increased rate of GI ulceration and other complications. Don't use together, if possible. If used together, monitor patient closely for GI bleeding.
Furosemide, thiazide diuretics: Potentially reduced efficacy of these drugs. Monitor patient closely.
Lithium: Increased plasma lithium levels; decreased lithium clearance. Monitor patient closely for toxic reaction to lithium.
Methotrexate: Increased plasma methotrexate levels. Monitor patient closely for toxic reaction to methotrexate.
Rifampin: Decreased rofecoxib levels by about 50%. Initiate therapy with a higher dosage of rofecoxib.
Warfarin: Increased effects of warfarin. Monitor INR more frequently in first few days after therapy with rofecoxib begins or is changed.
Drug-lifestyle. *Chronic alcohol use, smoking:* Increased risk of GI bleeding. Monitor patient closely for such bleeding.

Adverse reactions

CNS: headache, asthenia, fatigue, dizziness.
CV: hypertension, lower-extremity edema.
EENT: sinusitis.

GI: diarrhea, dyspepsia, epigastric discomfort, heartburn, nausea, abdominal pain.
GU: urinary tract infection.
Musculoskeletal: back pain.
Respiratory: bronchitis, upper respiratory tract infection.
Other: flulike syndrome.

☑ Special considerations

• Patient may be allergic to rofecoxib if he has an allergy to aspirin or other NSAIDs.
• NSAIDs may cause serious GI toxicity. Signs and symptoms include bleeding, ulceration, and perforation of stomach and small and large intestines. Such toxicity can occur any time, with or without warning. To minimize risk of adverse GI event, the lowest effective dosage of rofecoxib should be used for the shortest possible duration.
• Rehydrate patients who are dehydrated before starting drug.
• Fluid retention and edema have occurred in patients taking drug. Use the lowest recommended dosage cautiously in patients with fluid retention, hypertension, or heart failure.
• Hemodialysis doesn't remove drug; it's unknown if peritoneal dialysis removes it.

Monitoring the patient

• Rofecoxib may be hepatotoxic. Monitor patient for signs and symptoms of liver toxicity. Drug should be stopped if signs and symptoms of liver disease develop.
• Patients undergoing long-term treatment should have hemoglobin level and hematocrit checked if they experience signs or symptoms of anemia or blood loss.
• Monitor patient closely for GI bleeding.

Information for the patient

• Warn patient that he may experience GI bleeding. Signs and symptoms include bloody vomitus, blood in urine and stool, and black, tarry stools. Advise patient to call if he experiences any of these signs or symptoms.
• Advise patient to report rash, unexplained weight gain, or edema.
• Tell patient that drug may be taken without regard to food, though taking with food may decrease GI upset.
• Tell patient that the most common minor adverse effects are dyspepsia, epigastric discomfort, heartburn, and nausea. Taking drug with food may help minimize these effects.
• Tell patient to avoid aspirin and products containing aspirin unless instructed otherwise.
• Inform patient to avoid OTC anti-inflammatories such as ibuprofen unless instructed otherwise.
• Tell patient that all NSAIDs, including rofecoxib, may adversely affect the liver. Signs and symptoms of liver toxicity include nausea, fatigue, lethar-

gy, itching, jaundice, right upper quadrant tenderness, and flulike symptoms. Advise patient to stop therapy and call immediately if he experiences any of these signs or symptoms.
● Instruct woman to call if she becomes pregnant or is planning pregnancy while taking drug.

Geriatric patients
● No substantial differences in safety and effectiveness exist between elderly and younger patients. Although dosage doesn't need to be adjusted in elderly patients, rofecoxib should be initiated at the lowest recommended dosage.

Pediatric patients
● Safety and effectiveness in children younger than age 18 haven't been evaluated.

Breast-feeding patients
● It's unknown if drug appears in breast milk. However, because breast-fed infants are at risk for serious adverse reactions, women taking this drug shouldn't breast-feed.

---

ropinirole hydrochloride
Requip

Pharmacologic classification: nonergoline dopamine agonist
Therapeutic classification: antiparkinsonian
Pregnancy risk category C

How supplied
Available by prescription only
Tablets: 0.25 mg, 0.5 mg, 1 mg, 2 mg, 5 mg

Indications, route and dosage
Signs and symptoms of idiopathic Parkinson's disease
Adults: Initially, 0.25 mg P.O. t.i.d. Based on patient response, dosage should then be adjusted at weekly intervals: 0.5 mg t.i.d. after week 1, 0.75 mg t.i.d. after week 2, and 1 mg t.i.d. after week 3. After week 4, dose may be increased by 1.5 mg/day on a weekly basis up to a dose of 9 mg/day; then increased weekly by up to 3 mg/day to maximum dose of 24 mg/day.

Pharmacodynamics
Antiparkinsonian action: Exact mechanism unknown. A nonergoline dopamine agonist thought to stimulate postsynaptic dopamine D_2 receptors within the caudate-putamen in the brain.

Pharmacokinetics
● *Absorption:* Rapidly absorbed, reaching peak level in 1 to 2 hours. Absolute bioavailability is 55%.

● *Distribution:* Widely distributed throughout body; apparent volume of distribution of 7.5 L/kg. Up to 40% bound to plasma proteins.
● *Metabolism:* Extensively metabolized by cytochrome P-450 CYP 1A2 isoenzyme to inactive metabolites.
● *Excretion:* Less than 10% of dose excreted unchanged in urine. Elimination half-life is 6 hours.

Contraindications and precautions
Contraindicated in patients with hypersensitivity to drug or its components. Use cautiously in patients with severe renal or hepatic impairment.

Interactions
Drug-drug. *Ciprofloxacin:* Increased ropinirole levels when coadministered. Adjust dosage as needed.
CNS depressants (antidepressants, antipsychotics, benzodiazepines): Increased CNS effects. Use cautiously.
Dopamine antagonists (butyrophenones, metoclopramide, phenothiazines, thioxanthenes): Decreased effectiveness of ropinirole when administered together. Avoid concomitant use.
Estrogens: Reduced clearance of ropinirole. Adjust ropinirole dosage if estrogens are started or stopped during ropinirole treatment.
Inhibitors or substrates of cytochrome P-450 CYP 1A2 (ciprofloxacin, fluvoxamine, mexiletine, norfloxacin): Altered clearance. Dosage adjustment of ropinirole may be needed.
Drug-lifestyle. *Alcohol:* Increased CNS effects. Advise patient to use cautiously.
Smoking: Increased clearance of ropinirole. Monitor patient closely.

Adverse reactions
Early Parkinson's disease (without levodopa)
CNS: asthenia, hallucinations, *dizziness,* aggravated Parkinson's disease, *somnolence, fatigue,* headache, confusion, hyperkinesia, hypoesthesia, vertigo, amnesia, impaired concentration, malaise.
CV: orthostatic hypotension, orthostatic symptoms, hypertension, *syncope,* edema, chest pain, extrasystoles, **atrial fibrillation,** palpitation, tachycardia.
EENT: pharyngitis, dry mouth, abnormal vision, eye abnormality, xerophthalmia, rhinitis, sinusitis.
GI: *nausea, vomiting, dyspepsia,* flatulence, abdominal pain, anorexia.
GU: urinary tract infection, impotence.
Respiratory: bronchitis, dyspnea.
Skin: flushing, increased sweating.
Other: *viral infection,* pain, yawning, peripheral ischemia.
Advanced Parkinson's disease (with levodopa)
CNS: *dizziness,* aggravated parkinsonism, *somnolence, headache,* insomnia, *hallucinations,* ab-

normal dreaming, confusion, tremor, *dyskinesia,* anxiety, nervousness, amnesia, hypokinesia, paresthesia, paresis.
CV: hypotension, syncope.
EENT: diplopia, dry mouth.
GI: *nausea,* abdominal pain, vomiting, constipation, diarrhea, dysphagia, flatulence, increased saliva.
GU: urinary tract infection, pyuria, urinary incontinence.
Hematologic: anemia.
Metabolic: weight decrease.
Musculoskeletal: arthralgia, arthritis.
Respiratory: upper respiratory infection, dyspnea.
Skin: increased sweating.
Other: injury, *falls,* viral infection, increased drug level, pain.

☑ **Special considerations**
• Dosage adjustment isn't needed in patients with mild to moderate renal impairment.
• Adjust drug with caution in patients with severe renal or hepatic impairment.
• Drug may cause increased alkaline phosphatase and BUN levels.
• Although not reported with ropinirole, a symptom complex resembling neuroleptic malignant syndrome (elevated temperature, muscular rigidity, altered consciousness, and autonomic instability) has been reported with rapid dose reduction or withdrawal of antiparkinsonians. If this complex occurs, stop drug gradually over 7 days and reduce frequency of administration to twice daily for 4 days and then once daily over remaining 3 days.
• Other adverse events reported with dopaminergic therapy may occur with ropinirole; these include withdrawal emergent hyperpyrexia and confusion, and fibrotic complications.
• Ropinirole can potentiate the dopaminergic adverse effects of levodopa and may cause or exacerbate existing dyskinesia. If this occurs, levodopa dosage may need to be decreased.
• Symptoms of overdose include mild or facial dyskinesia, agitation, increased dyskinesia, grogginess, sedation, orthostatic hypotension, chest pain, confusion, vomiting, and nausea.

Monitoring the patient
• Monitor renal and hepatic function.
• Symptomatic hypotension may occur due to dopamine agonists' impairment of systemic regulation of blood pressure. Monitor patient carefully for orthostatic hypotension, especially during dosage escalation.
• Syncope, with or without bradycardia, has been reported. Monitor patient carefully, especially after 4 weeks of initiation of therapy and with dosage increases.

Information for the patient
• Inform patient to take drug with food to reduce nausea.
• Advise patient that hallucinations may occur.
• Instruct patient to rise slowly after sitting or lying down because of risk of orthostatic hypotension, which may occur during initial therapy or after a dosage increase.
• Advise patient to use caution when driving or operating machinery until CNS effects of drug are known.
• Advise patient to avoid alcohol and other CNS depressants.
• Tell woman to call if pregnancy is suspected or is being planned; also disclose if she is breast-feeding.

Geriatric patients
• Dosage adjustments aren't necessary.
• Elderly patients are at greater risk for hallucinations than younger patients with Parkinson's disease.

Pediatric patients
• Safety and effectiveness in children haven't been established.

Breast-feeding patients
• Drug inhibits prolactin secretion and could potentially inhibit lactation. It's unknown if drug appears in breast milk. Stop either drug or breast-feeding, taking into account importance of drug to mother.

ropivacaine hydrochloride
Naropin

Pharmacologic classification: aminoamide
Therapeutic classification: local anesthetic
Pregnancy risk category B

How supplied
Available by prescription only
E-Z off single-dose vials: 7.5 mg/ml, 10 mg/ml in 10-ml vials
Single-dose vials: 2 mg/ml, 7.5 mg/ml, 10 mg/ml in 20-ml vials; 5 mg/ml in 30-ml vials
Single-dose ampules: 2 mg/ml, 7.5 mg/ml, 10 mg/ml in 20-ml ampules; 5 mg/ml in 30-ml ampules
Infusion bottles: 2 mg/ml in 100-ml and 200-ml bottles
Sterile-pak single-dose vials: 2 mg/ml, 7.5 mg/ml, 10 mg/ml in 20-ml vials; 5 mg/ml in 30-ml vials

Indications, route, and dosage
Surgical anesthesia
Adults: Lumbar epidural administration in surgery: 75 to 200 mg doses (duration, 2 to 6 hours). Lum-

bar epidural administration for cesarean section: 100 to 150 mg (duration, 2 to 4 hours). Thoracic epidural administration: 25 to 75 mg to establish block for postoperative pain relief. Major nerve block (for example, brachial plexus block): 175 to 250 mg (duration, 5 to 8 hours). Field block (such as minor nerve blocks and infiltration): 5 to 200 mg (duration, 2 to 6 hours).

Labor pain management
Adults: Lumbar epidural administration: initially, 20 to 40 mg (duration, 0.5 to 1.5 hours); then 12 to 28 mg/hour as continuous infusion or 20 to 30 mg/hour as incremental injections.

Postoperative pain management
Adults: Lumbar epidural administration: 12 to 20 mg/hour as continuous infusion. Thoracic epidural administration: 8 to 16 mg/hour as continuous infusion. For infiltration (minor nerve block): 2 to 200 mg (duration, 2 to 6 hours).

Pharmacodynamics
Anesthetic action: Blocks the generation and conduction of nerve impulses, presumably by increasing the threshold for electrical excitation in the nerve by slowing the propagation of the nerve impulse and by reducing the rate of the action potential. Generally, progression of anesthesia is related to the diameter, myelination, and conduction velocity of affected nerve fibers. Clinically, the order of loss of nerve function is as follows: pain, temperature, touch, proprioception, and skeletal muscle tone.

Pharmacokinetics
• *Absorption:* Depends on total dose and level of drug, route of administration, patient's hemodynamic or circulatory condition, and vascularity of administration site. From the epidural space, drug shows complete and biphasic absorption; mean half-lives of two phases are 14 minutes and 4.2 hours, respectively. Slow absorption is a rate-limiting factor in elimination of drug. Terminal half-life is longer after epidural than after I.V. administration.
• *Distribution:* After intravascular infusion, drug has steady-state volume of distribution of 34 to 48 L. Drug is 94% protein-bound, mainly to alpha$_1$ acid glycoprotein. An increase in total plasma levels during continuous epidural infusion has been observed, secondary to a postoperative increase in alpha$_1$ acid glycoprotein.
• *Metabolism:* Extensively metabolized in liver, via cytochrome P4501A to 3-hydroxy ropivacaine. About 37% of dose excreted in urine as free drug and as conjugated metabolites. Urinary excretion of metabolites accounts for only 3% of dose.
• *Excretion:* Primarily excreted by kidneys; 86% of dose appears in urine after I.V. administration, only 1% of which relates to unchanged drug.

Contraindications and precautions
Contraindicated in patients with hypersensitivity to drug or local anesthetics of amide type.

Use with caution in debilitated, elderly, and acutely ill patients because accumulation may result. Also use cautiously in patients with hypotension, hypovolemia, impaired CV function, or heart block and in those with hepatic disease, especially with repeat doses of drug.

Interactions
Drug-drug. *Amide-type anesthetics:* Additive effects if given with ropivacaine. Use with caution.
Fluvoxamine, imipramine, theophylline, verapamil: Possible competitive inhibition of ropivacaine. Use with caution.

Adverse reactions
CNS: anxiety, dizziness, headache, hypoesthesia, pain, paresthesia.
CV: *bradycardia,* chest pain, *hypotension,* hypertension, tachycardia; FETAL BRADYCARDIA, *fetal tachycardia.*
GI: *nausea,* neonatal vomiting, vomiting.
GU: oliguria, urine retention.
Hematologic: anemia.
Hepatic: neonatal jaundice.
Musculoskeletal: back pain.
Respiratory: *neonatal tachypnea, respiratory distress.*
Skin: pruritus.
Other: FETAL DISTRESS, fever, neonatal fever, postoperative complications, rigors.

☑ Special considerations
• Don't inject drug rapidly. Have emergency equipment and personnel immediately available.
• Drug should be used only by personnel familiar with drug.
• Increase dosages in incremental steps.
• Don't use in emergency situations in which a rapid onset of surgical anesthesia is necessary. Drug shouldn't be used for production of obstetric paracervical block anesthesia, retrobulbar block, or spinal anesthesia (subarachnoid block) because of insufficient data to support use. I.V. regional anesthesia (bier block) shouldn't be performed because of lack of clinical experience and risk of obtaining toxic blood levels of ropivacaine.
• To reduce risk of potentially serious adverse reactions, attempts should be made to optimize patients who may be at risk, such as those with complete heart block or hepatic or renal impairment.
• Use an adequate test dose (3 to 5 ml of short-acting local anesthetic solution containing epinephrine) before induction of complete block.
• In case of unintentional subarachnoid injection of drug, establish a patent airway and administer 100% oxygen. This may prevent seizures if

---

they haven't already occurred. Administer medication to control seizures as appropriate.
• Don't use drug in ophthalmic surgery.

Monitoring the patient
• Monitor patient for adverse effects.
• Watch for toxicity. Early signs and symptoms of CNS toxicity include restlessness, anxiety, incoherent speech, light-headedness, numbness and tingling of mouth and lips, metallic taste, tinnitus, dizziness, blurred vision, tremors, twitching, depression, and drowsiness.

Information for the patient
• Tell patient that he may experience a temporary loss of sensation and motor activity in anesthetized body part after proper administration of lumbar epidural anesthesia. Also explain adverse reactions that may occur.

Pediatric patients
• Don't use drug in children under age 12.

Breast-feeding patients
• It's unknown if drug appears in breast milk; use with caution in breast-feeding women.

rosiglitazone maleate
Avandia

Pharmacologic classification: thiazolidinedione
Therapeutic classification: antidiabetic
Pregnancy risk category C

How supplied
Available by prescription only
Tablets: 2 mg, 4 mg, 8 mg

Indications, route, and dosage
Monotherapy adjunct to diet and exercise to improve glycemic control in patients with type 2 diabetes mellitus or with metformin when diet, exercise, and rosiglitazone alone or diet, exercise, and metformin alone don't provide adequate glycemic control in patients with type 2 diabetes mellitus
Adults: Initially, 4 mg P.O. daily in the morning or in divided doses b.i.d. in the morning and evening. Dosage may be increased to 8 mg P.O. daily or in divided doses b.i.d. if fasting plasma glucose level doesn't improve after 12 weeks of treatment.

Pharmacodynamics
Antidiabetic action: Lowers blood glucose levels by improving insulin sensitivity. Highly selective and potent agonist for the receptors, which are found in key target areas for insulin action, such as adipose tissue, skeletal muscle, and liver.

Pharmacokinetics
• *Absorption:* Plasma levels peak about 1 hour after dosing. Absolute bioavailability is 99%.
• *Distribution:* About 99.8% binds to plasma proteins, primarily albumin.
• *Metabolism:* Extensively metabolized; no unchanged drug excreted in urine. Primarily metabolized through N-demethylation and hydroxylation.
• *Excretion:* After oral administration, about 64% and 23% of dose is eliminated in urine and feces, respectively. The elimination half-life is 3 to 4 hours.

Contraindications and precautions
Contraindicated in patients with hypersensitivity to drug or its components and in patients with New York Heart Association Class III and IV cardiac status unless the expected benefits outweigh the potential risks. Don't use in patients with active liver disease, increased baseline liver enzyme levels (ALT level is greater than 2½ times the upper limit of normal), type 1 diabetes mellitus, or diabetic ketoacidosis or in patients who experienced jaundice while taking troglitazone.

Because metformin is contraindicated in patients with renal impairment, therapy with metformin and rosiglitazone is also contraindicated in patients with renal impairment. Rosiglitazone can be used as monotherapy in patients with renal impairment. Use cautiously in patients with edema or heart failure.

Interactions
None reported.

Adverse reactions
CNS: headache, fatigue.
CV: edema.
EENT: sinusitis.
GI: diarrhea.
Hematologic: anemia.
Metabolic: hyperglycemia.
Musculoskeletal: back pain.
Respiratory: upper respiratory tract infection.
Other: injury.

☑ Special considerations
• Management of type 2 diabetes mellitus should include diet control. Because caloric restriction, weight loss, and exercise help improve insulin sensitivity and help make drug therapy effective, these measures are essential to proper diabetes treatment.
• Because ovulation may resume in premenopausal, anovulatory women with insulin resistance, contraceptive measures may need to be considered.
• Hemoglobin level and hematocrit may decrease while patient is receiving drug, usually during first 4 to 8 weeks of therapy. Increases in total cholesterol, low-density lipoprotein, and high-density

lipoprotein levels and decreases in free fatty acid levels may also occur.
• For patients whose blood glucose levels are inadequately controlled with metformin, rosiglitazone should be added to—not substituted for—metformin.

Monitoring the patient
• Liver enzyme levels should be checked before therapy starts, every 2 months for the first 12 months of treatment, and then periodically afterward. If ALT levels are elevated during treatment, recheck levels as soon as possible. Stop drug if levels remain elevated.
• In addition to regular blood glucose level checks, patients should also have glycosylated hemoglobin level checked periodically to monitor therapeutic response to drug.

Information for the patient
• Advise patient that drug can be taken with or without food.
• Inform patient that blood will be tested to check liver function before therapy starts, every 2 months for the first 12 months, and then periodically thereafter.
• Tell patient to immediately report unexplained signs and symptoms (such as nausea, vomiting, abdominal pain, fatigue, anorexia, or dark urine) because these may indicate potential liver problems.
• Inform premenopausal, anovulatory women with insulin resistance that ovulation may resume and contraceptive measures may need to be considered.
• Advise patient that management of diabetes should include diet control. Because caloric restriction, weight loss, and exercise help improve insulin sensitivity and help make drug therapy effective, these measures are essential to proper diabetes treatment.

Geriatric patients
• No substantial differences in safety and effectiveness exist between patients older than 65 and younger patients. No dosage adjustments are needed for elderly patients.

Pediatric patients
• Safety and effectiveness in children haven't been established.

Breast-feeding patients
• It's unknown if drug appears in breast milk. Because many drugs appear in breast milk, drug shouldn't be used in breast-feeding women.

rubella and mumps virus vaccine, live
Biavax II

Pharmacologic classification: vaccine
Therapeutic classification: viral vaccine
Pregnancy risk category C

How supplied
Available by prescription only
Injection: single-dose vial containing not less than 1,000 $TCID_{50}$ (tissue culture infective doses) of the Wistar RA 27/3 rubella virus (propagated in human diploid cell culture) and not less than 20,000 $TCID_{50}$ of the Jeryl Lynn mumps strain (grown in chick embryo cell culture)

Indications, route, and dosage
Rubella (German measles) and mumps immunization
Adults and children over age 1: 1 vial (0.5 ml) S.C. in outer aspect of upper arm.

Pharmacodynamics
Live rubella and mumps prophylaxis: Promotes active immunity to rubella and mumps by inducing production of antibodies.

Pharmacokinetics
• *Absorption:* Antibodies usually detectable within 2 to 6 weeks; lifelong duration of vaccine-induced immunity expected.
• *Distribution:* No information available.
• *Metabolism:* No information available.
• *Excretion:* No information available.

Contraindications and precautions
Contraindicated in pregnant or immunosuppressed patients; in those with cancer, blood dyscrasia, gamma globulin disorders, fever, active untreated tuberculosis, or history of anaphylaxis or anaphylactoid reactions to neomycin or eggs; and in those receiving corticosteroids (except those receiving corticosteroids as replacement therapy) or radiation therapy.

Interactions
Drug-drug. *Immune serum globulin, transfusions of blood and blood products:* Impaired immune response to vaccine. Defer vaccination for 3 months in these situations.
Immunosuppressants: May interfere with response to vaccine. Monitor patient closely.

Adverse reactions
CNS: polyneuritis.
GI: diarrhea.
Hematologic: thrombocytopenic purpura.
Musculoskeletal: arthritis, arthralgia.
Skin: rash, urticaria.

Reactions may be *common*, uncommon, *life-threatening*, or COMMON AND LIFE-THREATENING.

Other: fever, *anaphylaxis,* lymphadenopathy; pain, erythema, induration (at injection site).

☑ Special considerations
● Obtain thorough history of allergies (especially to antibiotics, eggs, chicken, or chicken feathers) and of reactions to immunizations.
● Have epinephrine solution 1:1,000 available to treat allergic reactions.
● Perform skin testing first to assess vaccine sensitivity (against a control of normal saline solution in the opposite arm) in patients with history of anaphylactoid reactions to egg ingestion. Administer I.D. or scratch test with a 1:10 dilution. Read results after 5 to 30 minutes. Positive reaction is a wheal with or without pseudopodia and surrounding erythema.
● Women who have rubella antibody titers of 1:8 or greater (by hemagglutination inhibition) need not be vaccinated with the rubella vaccine component.
● Rubella and mumps vaccine shouldn't be given less than 1 month before or after immunization with other live virus vaccines—except for monovalent or trivalent live poliovirus vaccine or live, attenuated measles virus vaccine, which may be administered simultaneously.
● Use only the diluent supplied. Discard reconstituted vaccine after 8 hours.
● Inject S.C. (not I.M.) into outer aspect of upper arm.
● Revaccination or booster isn't needed if patient was previously vaccinated at age 1 or older; however, there is no conclusive evidence of increased risk of adverse reactions for persons who are already immune when vaccinated.
● Vaccine won't offer protection when given after exposure to natural rubella or mumps, but there is no evidence that it would be harmful.
● Although rubella vaccine should be deferred in patients with febrile illness, it may be administered to susceptible children with mild illness such as upper respiratory infection.
● According to CDC recommendations, measles, mumps, and rubella is the preferred vaccine.
● Women who aren't immune to rubella are at risk for congenital rubella injury to fetus if exposed during pregnancy.
● Rubella and mumps vaccine temporarily may decrease response to tuberculin skin testing. Should a tuberculin skin test be necessary, administer either before or simultaneously with rubella and mumps vaccine.
● Store vaccine at 36° to 46° F (2° to 8° C) and protect from light. Solution may be used if red, pink, or yellow, but it must be clear.

Monitoring the patient
● Monitor patient for adverse effects.

Information for the patient
● Tell patient that tingling sensations in extremities, or joint aches and pains that may resemble arthritis, may occur beginning several days to several weeks after vaccination. These symptoms usually resolve within 1 week. Pain and inflammation at injection site and low-grade fever, rash, or breathing difficulties also may occur. Encourage patient to report distressing adverse reactions.
● Recommend acetaminophen to relieve fever or other minor discomfort.
● Tell women of childbearing age to avoid pregnancy for 3 months after immunization. Provide contraceptive information if necessary.

Pediatric patients
● Live rubella and mumps virus vaccine isn't recommended for children under age 1 because retained maternal antibodies may interfere with immune response.

Breast-feeding patients
● Some reports have shown transfer of rubella virus or virus antigen into breast milk in about 68% of patients. Few adverse effects have been associated with breast-feeding after immunization with vaccines containing rubella. Use caution when administering vaccine to breast-feeding women.

rubella virus vaccine, live
Meruvax II

Pharmacologic classification: vaccine
Therapeutic classification: viral vaccine
Pregnancy risk category C

How supplied
Available by prescription only
Injection: single-dose vial containing not less than 1,000 $TCID_{50}$ (tissue culture infective doses) of the Wistar RA 27/3 strain of rubella virus propagated in human diploid cell culture

Indications, route, and dosage
Rubella (German measles) immunization
Adults and children over age 1: 1 vial (0.5 ml) S.C.

Pharmacodynamics
Rubella prophylaxis: Vaccine promotes active immunity to rubella by inducing production of antibodies.

Pharmacokinetics
● *Absorption:* Antibodies usually detectable 2 to 6 weeks after injection; lifelong duration of vaccine-induced immunity expected.
● *Distribution:* No information available.
● *Metabolism:* No information available.
● *Excretion:* No information available.

Contraindications and precautions

Contraindicated in pregnant or immunosuppressed patients; in those with cancer, blood dyscrasia, gamma globulin disorders, fever, active untreated tuberculosis, or history of hypersensitivity to neomycin; and in patients receiving corticosteroid (except those receiving corticosteroids as replacement therapy) or radiation therapy.

Interactions

Drug-drug. *Immune serum globulin, transfusions of blood and blood products:* Impaired immune response to the vaccine. If possible, defer vaccination for 3 months in these situations.

Adverse reactions

CNS: polyneuritis, malaise, headache.
EENT: sore throat.
Hematologic: thrombocytopenic purpura.
Musculoskeletal: arthralgia, arthritis.
Skin: rash; urticaria; pain, erythema, induration at injection site.
Other: fever, ***anaphylaxis,*** lymphadenopathy.

☑ Special considerations

• Obtain thorough history of allergies, especially to antibiotics, and of reactions to immunizations.
• Women who have rubella antibody titers of 1:8 or greater (by hemagglutination inhibition) need not be vaccinated with rubella virus vaccine.
• Have epinephrine solution 1:1,000 available to treat allergic reactions.
• Don't give rubella vaccine less than 1 month before or after immunization with other live virus vaccines—except for monovalent or trivalent live poliovirus vaccine; live, attenuated measles virus vaccine; or live mumps virus vaccine, which may be administered simultaneously.
• Don't inject I.M. Inject S.C. into outer aspect of upper arm.
• Use only diluent supplied. Discard 8 hours after reconstituting.
• Store vaccine at 36° to 46° F (2° to 8° C), and protect from light. Solution may be used if red, pink, or yellow, but it must be clear.
• Vaccine won't offer protection when given after exposure to natural rubella, although there is no evidence that it would be harmful.
• Revaccination or booster dose is needed if patient was previously vaccinated under age 1. The Advisory Committee on Immunization Practices and the American Academy of Pediatrics currently recommends that a second dose be routinely given at age 4 to 6. It may be given at any other time provided at least 1 month has elapsed since the first dose. There is no conclusive evidence of increased risk of adverse reactions for persons who are already immune when revaccinated.

• Although rubella vaccine administration should be deferred in patients with febrile illness, it may be administered to susceptible children with mild illnesses such as upper respiratory tract infection.
• Women who aren't immune to rubella are at risk for congenital rubella injury to fetus if exposed during pregnancy.
• Rubella vaccine may temporarily decrease response to tuberculin skin testing. If a tuberculin test is necessary, administer either before, simultaneously with, or at least 8 weeks after rubella vaccine.

Monitoring the patient

• Monitor patient for adverse effects.

Information for the patient

• Tell patient that tingling sensations in extremities, or joint aches and pains that resemble arthritis, may occur several days to several weeks after vaccination. The symptoms usually resolve within 1 week. Pain and inflammation at injection site and low-grade fever, rash, or breathing difficulties may also occur. Encourage patient to report distressing symptoms.
• Recommend acetaminophen to relieve fever or other minor discomfort after vaccination.
• Tell woman of childbearing age to avoid pregnancy for 3 months after rubella immunization. Provide contraceptive information, if necessary.

Pediatric patients

• Live, attenuated rubella virus vaccine isn't recommended for children under age 1 because retained maternal antibodies may impair immune response.

Breast-feeding patients

• Reports have shown transfer of rubella virus or virus antigen into breast milk in about 68% of patients. Few adverse effects have been associated with breast-feeding after immunization with vaccines containing rubella. Risk-benefit ratio suggests that breast-feeding women may be immunized if necessary.

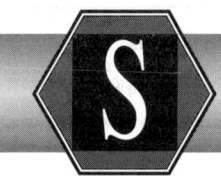

salmeterol xinafoate
Serevent

Pharmacologic classification: selective beta$_2$-adrenergic agonist
Therapeutic classification: bronchodilator
Pregnancy risk category C

How supplied
Available by prescription only
Inhalation aerosol: 25 mcg per activation in 6.5-g canister (60 activations), 25 mcg per activation in 13-g canister (120 activations)
Inhalation powder: 0.046 mg base/inhalation; 50 mcg blister packs

Indications, route, and dosage
Long-term maintenance treatment of asthma; prevention of bronchospasm in patients with nocturnal asthma or reversible obstructive airway disease who need regular treatment with short-acting beta agonists
Adults and children over age 12: Two inhalations b.i.d. in the morning and evening. One powder inhalation q 12 hours.
Prevention of exercise-induced bronchospasm
Adults and children over age 12: Two inhalations at least 30 to 60 minutes before exercise. One powder inhalation 30 minutes before exercise.
Note: Paradoxical bronchospasms (which can be life-threatening) have been reported after use of salmeterol. If they occur, stop salmeterol immediately and institute alternative therapy.
◊ **COPD or emphysema**
Adults and children over age 12: Two oral inhalations twice daily in the morning and evening.

Pharmacodynamics
Bronchodilator action: Selectively stimulates beta$_2$-adrenergic receptors, resulting in bronchodilation. Also blocks the release of histamine from mast cells lining the respiratory tract, which produces vasodilation and increases ciliary motility.

Pharmacokinetics
• *Absorption:* Because of low therapeutic dose, systemic levels of drug are low or undetectable after inhalation of recommended doses.
• *Distribution:* 94% to 99% bound to plasma proteins.

• *Metabolism:* Extensively metabolized by hydroxylation.
• *Excretion:* Excreted primarily in feces.

Contraindications and precautions
Contraindicated in patients with hypersensitivity to drug or its components. Use cautiously in patients with coronary insufficiency, arrhythmias, hypertension, other CV disorders, thyrotoxicosis, or seizure disorders and in those unusually responsive to sympathomimetics.

Interactions
Drug-drug. *Beta-adrenergic agonists, theophylline, other methylxanthines:* Possible adverse cardiac effects with excessive use of salmeterol. Monitor patient closely.
MAO inhibitors, tricyclic antidepressants: Risk of severe adverse CV effects. Avoid use of salmeterol within 14 days of MAO therapy.

Adverse reactions
CNS: *headache,* sinus headache, tremor, nervousness, giddiness.
CV: tachycardia, palpitations, ***ventricular arrhythmias.***
EENT: *nasopharyngitis,* nasal cavity or sinus disorder.
GI: nausea, vomiting, diarrhea, heartburn.
Musculoskeletal: joint and back pain, myalgia.
Respiratory: cough, lower respiratory infection, *upper respiratory infection,* **bronchospasm.**
Other: hypersensitivity reactions (rash, urticaria).

☑ Special considerations
• Don't use drug in patients whose asthma can be managed by occasional use of a short-acting, inhaled beta$_2$-agonist such as albuterol.
• Salmeterol inhalation shouldn't be used more than twice daily (morning and evening) at the recommended dose. Provide patient with a short-acting inhaled beta$_2$-agonist for treatment of symptoms that occur despite regular twice-daily use of salmeterol.
• Patients who are taking a short-acting inhaled beta$_2$-agonist daily should be advised to use it only as needed if they develop asthma symptoms while taking salmeterol.
• Salmeterol isn't a substitute for oral or inhaled corticosteroids.
• Patients receiving drug twice daily shouldn't use additional doses for prevention of exercise-induced bronchospasm.

• Signs and symptoms of overdose may include exaggerated effects associated with beta-adrenoceptor agonists (tachycardia, arrhythmias, tremor, headache, and muscle cramps). Significant prolongation of QT interval possible, producing ventricular arrhythmias. Cardiac arrest and death may be associated with salmeterol abuse. Other signs of overdose may include hypokalemia and hyperglycemia.

• In case of overdose, stop salmeterol and all beta-adrenergic-stimulant drugs. Provide supportive therapy. Use a beta blocker cautiously; bronchospasm is possible with use of such drugs. Cardiac monitoring is recommended. Dialysis isn't appropriate.

Monitoring the patient
• Monitor respiratory status, cardiac status, and therapeutic effects.
• Monitor patient for adverse effects.

Information for the patient
• Advise patient on proper use of salmeterol inhalation device; review illustrated instructions in package insert.
• Remind patient to shake container well before using.
• Remind patient to take drug at 12-hour intervals for optimum effect and to take it even when feeling better.
• Inform patient that drug isn't meant to relieve acute asthmatic symptoms. Instead, acute symptoms should be treated with an inhaled, short-acting bronchodilator that has been prescribed for symptomatic relief.
• Tell patient to call if the short-acting agonist no longer provides sufficient relief or if more than four inhalations are being used daily. This may be a sign that asthma symptoms are worsening.
• Advise patient already receiving short-acting beta$_2$-agonist to stop the regular daily-dosing regimen for drug and to use the short-acting drug only if asthma symptoms are experienced while taking salmeterol.
• Tell patient taking an inhaled corticosteroid to continue to use it regularly. Warn patient not to take other drugs without medical approval.
• If drug is being used to prevent exercise-induced bronchospasm, tell patient to take it 30 to 60 minutes before exercise.

Geriatric patients
• As with other beta$_2$-agonists, use with extreme caution in elderly patients who have CV disease that could be adversely affected by this class of drugs.

Pediatric patients
• Safety and effectiveness in children under age 12 haven't been established.

Breast-feeding patients
• It's unknown if drug appears in breast milk. Use with caution in breast-feeding women.

saquinavir
Fortovase

saquinavir mesylate
Invirase

Pharmacologic classification: HIV-1 and HIV-2 proteinase inhibitor
Therapeutic classification: antiviral
Pregnancy risk category B

How supplied
Available by prescription only
saquinavir
Capsules (soft gelatin): 200 mg
saquinavir mesylate
Capsules (hard gelatin): 200 mg

Indications, route, and dosage
Adjunct treatment of advanced HIV infection in selected patients
Adults: 600 mg (Invirase, three 200-mg capsules) P.O. t.i.d. taken within 2 hours after a full meal and with a nucleoside analogue such as zalcitabine at a dosage of 0.75 mg P.O. t.i.d. or 200 mg zidovudine P.O. t.i.d. Or 1,200 mg (Fortovase, six 200-mg capsules) t.i.d. within 2 hours after a full meal with a nucleoside analogue.
✦ *Dosage adjustment.* For toxicities that may occur with saquinavir or saquinavir mesylate, interrupt drug therapy. In therapy with nucleoside analogues, dosage adjustments of the nucleoside analogue should be based on the known toxicity profile of specific drug.

Pharmacodynamics
Antiviral action: Inhibits the activity of HIV protease and prevents the cleavage of HIV polyproteins, which are essential for the maturation of HIV.

Pharmacokinetics
• *Absorption:* Poorly absorbed from GI tract. Higher saquinavir levels achieved with Fortovase compared with Invirase. (Fortovase has a relative bioavailability of 331% of Invirase.)
• *Distribution:* About 98% bound to plasma proteins.
• *Metabolism:* Rapidly metabolized.
• *Excretion:* Excreted mainly in feces.

Contraindications and precautions
Contraindicated in patients with hypersensitivity to drug or components contained in the capsule. Safety of drug hasn't been established in pregnant women.

Interactions
Drug-drug. *Clarithromycin, ketoconazole:* Increased steady-state level of saquinavir. Use together cautiously.
Rifabutin, rifampin: Reduced steady state level of saquinavir. Use together cautiously.
Drug-food. *Any food:* Increased drug absorption. Give drug with food.

Adverse reactions
CNS: paresthesia, headache, asthenia.
EENT: pharyngitis, rhinitis, epistaxis.
GI: diarrhea, ulcerated buccal mucosa, abdominal pain, nausea.
Musculoskeletal: musculoskeletal pain.
Respiratory: bronchitis, dyspnea, hemoptysis, upper respiratory tract disorder, cough.
Skin: rash.

☑ Special considerations
• If a serious or severe toxicity occurs during treatment, stop drug until the cause is identified or the toxicity resolves. Dose modification isn't needed when drug is resumed.
• Invirase will be phased out and replaced by Fortovase. Note dosing differences.

Monitoring the patient
• Evaluate CBC, platelets, electrolytes, uric acid, liver enzymes, and bilirubin before therapy and then at appropriate intervals during therapy.
• Monitor patient for adverse effects.

Information for the patient
• Inform patient that drug should be taken within 2 hours after a full meal.
• Tell patient to report adverse reactions.
• Inform patient that drug is usually given with other AIDS-related antivirals.
• Tell patient to use Fortovase within 3 months when stored at room temperature or refer to expiration date on label if capsules are refrigerated.

Pediatric patients
• Safety and effectiveness in children under age 16 haven't been established.

Breast-feeding patients
• Drug's safety hasn't been established in breast-feeding women; it's unknown if drug appears in breast milk. To avoid transmitting virus to infant, women with HIV infection shouldn't breast-feed.

sargramostim (granulocyte macrophage-colony stimulating factor, GM-CSF)
Leukine

Pharmacologic classification: biological response modifier
Therapeutic classification: colony stimulating factor
Pregnancy risk category C

How supplied
Available by prescription only
Injection (preservative-free): 250 mcg, 500 mcg (as lyophilized powder) in single-dose vials
Liquid: 500 mcg/ml vials

Indications, route, and dosage
Acceleration of hematopoietic reconstitution after autologous bone marrow transplantation in patients with malignant lymphoma, acute lymphoblastic leukemia, or Hodgkin's disease
Adults: 250 mcg/m^2 daily for 21 consecutive days given as a 2-hour I.V. infusion, beginning 2 to 4 hours after the bone marrow transplant. Don't administer within 24 hours of last dose of chemotherapy or within 12 hours after last dose of radiotherapy because of potential sensitivity of rapidly dividing progenitor cells to cytotoxic chemotherapeutic or radiologic therapies.
✦ *Dosage adjustment.* Reduce dosage by half or temporarily stop therapy if severe adverse reactions occur. Therapy may be resumed when reaction abates. If blast cells appear or increase to 10% or more of the WBC count or if progression of the underlying disease occurs, stop therapy. If absolute neutrophil count is more than 20,000 cells/mm^3 or if WBC counts are more than 50,000 cells/mm^3, therapy should be temporarily stopped or the dose reduced by half.
Bone marrow transplantation failure or engraftment delay
Adults: 250 mcg/m^2 daily for 14 days as a 2-hour I.V. infusion. Same course may be repeated after 7 days off therapy if engraftment hasn't occurred. Third course of 500 mcg/m^2 daily for 14 days may be given after another 7 days off therapy if engraftment hasn't occurred.
Acute myelogenous leukemia
Adults: 250 mcg/m^2 daily by I.V. infusion over 4 hours. Start therapy about day 11 or 4 days after completion of induction therapy. Use only if bone marrow is hypoplastic (fewer than 5% blasts on day 10). Continue until absolute neutrophil count exceeds 1,500/mm^3 for 3 consecutive days or for a maximum of 42 days.
◇ *Myelodysplastic syndromes*
Adults: 15 to 500 mcg/m^2 daily by I.V. infusion over 1 to 12 hours.

◊ *Aplastic anemia*
Adults: 15 to 480 mcg/m^2 daily by I.V. infusion over 1 to 12 hours.

Pharmacodynamics
Immunostimulant action: A 127-amino acid glycoprotein manufactured by recombinant DNA technology in a yeast expression system. Differs from the natural human granulocyte macrophage-colony stimulating factor by the substitution of leucine for arginine at position 23. The carbohydrate moiety also may be different. Drug induces cellular responses by binding to specific receptors on cell surfaces of target cells. Blood counts return to normal or baseline levels within 2 to 10 days after stopping treatment.

Pharmacokinetics
• *Absorption:* Blood levels detectable within 5 minutes after S.C. administration; peak levels within 2 hours.
• *Distribution:* Bound to specific receptors on target cells.
• *Metabolism:* No information available.
• *Excretion:* No information available.

Contraindications and precautions
Contraindicated in patients with hypersensitivity to drug or its components or to yeast-derived products. Also contraindicated in those with excessive leukemic myeloid blasts in bone marrow or peripheral blood and in those receiving chemotherapy or radiotherapy.

Use cautiously in patients with impaired renal or hepatic function, preexisting cardiac disease or fluid retention, hypoxia, pulmonary infiltrates, or heart failure.

Interactions
Drug-drug. *Corticosteroids, lithium:* May potentiate myeloproliferative effects of sargramostim. Use cautiously together.

Adverse reactions
CNS: *malaise, CNS disorders, asthenia.*
CV: *blood dyscrasias, edema,* hemorrhage, supraventricular arrhythmia, pericardial effusion, *peripheral edema.*
GI: *nausea, vomiting, diarrhea, anorexia,* **hemorrhage,** *GI disorders, stomatitis.*
GU: *urinary tract disorder,* abnormal kidney function.
Hematologic: stimulation of hematopoiesis.
Hepatic: *liver damage.*
Musculoskeletal: *bone pain.*
Respiratory: *dyspnea, lung disorders,* pleural effusion.
Skin: *alopecia, rash.*
Other: *fever, mucous membrane disorder, sepsis.*

☑ Special considerations
• Stimulation of marrow precursors may result in rapid elevation of WBC count; biweekly monitoring of CBC count with differential, including examination for blast cells, is recommended.
• Transient rash and local injection site reactions may occur; no serious allergic or anaphylactic reactions have been reported.
• Drug can act as a growth factor for any tumor type, particularly myeloid malignancies.
• Unlabeled indications include to increase WBC counts in patients with myelodysplastic syndromes and in patients with AIDS on zidovudine; to decrease nadir of leukopenia secondary to myelosuppressive chemotherapy; to decrease myelosuppression in preleukemic patients; to correct neutropenia in patients with aplastic anemia; and to decrease transplant-associated organ system damage, particularly of the liver and kidneys.
• Drug is effective in accelerating myeloid recovery in patients receiving bone marrow purged from monoclonal antibodies.
• The effect of drug may be limited in patients who have received extensive radiotherapy to hematopoietic sites for treatment of primary disease in the abdomen or chest or who have been exposed to several drugs (alkylating drugs, anthracycline antibiotics, antimetabolites) before autologous bone marrow transplant.
• Refrigerate sterile powder, reconstituted solution, and diluted solution for injection. Don't freeze or shake. Don't use after expiration date.
• Doses up to 16 times the recommended dose have been administered with the following reversible adverse reactions: WBC counts up to 200,000/mm^3, dyspnea, malaise, nausea, fever, rash, sinus tachycardia, headache, and chills. The maximum dose that can be administered safely has yet to be determined.
• If overdose is suspected, monitor WBC count increase and respiratory symptoms.

Monitoring the patient
• Monitor CBC count with differential biweekly, including examination for blast cells.
• Monitor respiratory and hepatic status.

Information for the patient
• Warn patient about possible adverse reactions.
• Tell patient to immediately report any symptoms of respiratory problems.

Pediatric patients
• Safety and efficacy in children haven't been established; however, available data suggest that no differences in toxicity exist. The type and frequency of adverse reactions are comparable with those seen in adults.

Breast-feeding patients
• It's unknown if drug appears in breast milk; use with caution in breast-feeding women.

Reactions may be *common*, uncommon, *life-threatening*, or COMMON AND LIFE-THREATENING.

scopolamine hydrobromide
Isopto Hyoscine, Transderm-Scōp

Pharmacologic classification: anticholinergic
Therapeutic classification: antimuscarinic, cycloplegic mydriatic
Pregnancy risk category C

How supplied
Available by prescription only
Injection: 0.3 and 1 mg/ml in 1-ml vials and ampules; 0.4 mg/ml, 0.86 mg/ml in 0.5-ml ampules
Topical: Transdermal system 1.5 mg/72 hours
Ophthalmic solution: 0.25%

Indications, route, and dosage
Antimuscarinic, adjunct to anesthesia, prevention of nausea and vomiting
Adults: 0.3 to 0.6 mg I.M., S.C., or I.V. (after dilution with sterile water for injection) as a single dose.
Children: 0.006 mg/kg I.M., S.C., or I.V. (after dilution with sterile water for injection) as a single daily dose; maximum dose is 0.3 mg.
Prevention of nausea and vomiting associated with motion sickness
Adults: 1 transdermal patch applied behind the ear 4 hours before anticipated exposure to motion.
Cycloplegic refraction
Adults: 1 to 2 drops 0.25% solution in eye 1 hour before refraction.
Children: 1 drop 0.25% solution b.i.d. for 2 days before refraction.
Iritis, uveitis
Adults: 1 to 2 drops of 0.25% solution daily or up to t.i.d.
Children: 1 drop of 0.25% solution up to t.i.d.

Pharmacodynamics
Antimuscarinic action: Inhibits the muscarinic actions of acetylcholine on autonomic effectors, resulting in decreased secretions and GI motility; also blocks vagal inhibition of the SA node.
Mydriatic action: Competitively blocks acetylcholine at cholinergic neuroeffector sites, antagonizing the effects of acetylcholine on the sphincter muscle and ciliary body, thereby producing mydriasis and cycloplegia; these effects are used to produce cycloplegic refraction and pupil dilation to treat preoperative and postoperative iridocyclitis.

Pharmacokinetics
• *Absorption:* Rapidly absorbed when administered I.M. or S.C.; effects occur 15 to 30 minutes after I.M. or S.C. administration. Systemic drug absorption may occur from drug passage through nasolacrimal duct. Ophthalmic mydriatic effect peaks at 20 to 30 minutes after administration;

cycloplegic effects peak 30 to 60 minutes after administration.
• *Distribution:* Distributed widely throughout body tissues. Crosses placenta and probably blood-brain barrier.
• *Metabolism:* Probably metabolized completely in liver; exact metabolic fate unknown. Mydriatic and cycloplegic effects last 3 to 7 days.
• *Excretion:* Probably excreted in urine as metabolites.

Contraindications and precautions
Systemic form is contraindicated in patients with angle-closure glaucoma, obstructive uropathy, obstructive disease of the GI tract, asthma, chronic pulmonary disease, myasthenia gravis, paralytic ileus, intestinal atony, unstable CV status in acute hemorrhage, or toxic megacolon. Ophthalmic form is contraindicated in patients with hypersensitivity to drug and in those with shallow anterior chamber and angle-closure glaucoma.

Use systemic form cautiously in patients with autonomic neuropathy, hyperthyroidism, coronary artery disease, arrhythmias, heart failure, hypertension, hiatal hernia associated with reflux esophagitis, hepatic or renal disease, or ulcerative colitis; in children under age 6; or in patients in a hot or humid environment. Use ophthalmic form cautiously in elderly patients, in infants and children, and in those with cardiac disease.

Interactions
Drug-drug. *CNS depressants (sedative-hypnotics, tranquilizers):* Increased CNS depression. Avoid concomitant use.
Digoxin: Higher serum digoxin levels. Adjust dosage as needed.
Drugs with anticholinergic effects: Additive toxicity. Avoid concomitant use.
Oral potassium supplements (especially wax-matrix formulations): Increased potassium-induced GI ulcerations. Avoid concomitant use.
Drug-herb. *Jaborandi tree, pill-bearing spurge:* Decreased effect. Adjust dosage.
Squaw vine: Tannic acid content may decrease metabolic breakdown. Adjust dosage.
Drug-lifestyle. *Alcohol:* Increased CNS depression. Discourage use.

Adverse reactions
CNS: disorientation, restlessness, irritability, dizziness, drowsiness, headache, confusion, hallucinations, delirium.
CV: tachycardia; palpitations, ***paradoxical bradycardia (with systemic form).***
EENT: blurred vision, photophobia, increased intraocular pressure; dilated pupils, difficulty swallowing (with systemic form); ocular congestion (with prolonged use); conjunctivitis, eye dryness,

transient stinging and burning, edema (with ophthalmic form).
GI: dry mouth; *constipation, nausea, vomiting, epigastric distress* (with systemic form).
GU: urinary hesitancy, urine retention (with systemic form).
Respiratory: bronchial plugging, depressed respirations (with systemic form).
Skin: rash, flushing (with systemic form); dryness or contact dermatitis (with ophthalmic form).
Other: fever (with systemic form).

Adverse reactions may be caused by pending atropine-like toxicity and are dose-related. Individual tolerance varies greatly.

Many adverse reactions (such as dry mouth, constipation) are an expected extension of drug's pharmacologic activity.

☑ Special considerations

Besides the recommendations relevant to all anticholinergics, consider the following.

● Therapeutic doses may produce amnesia, drowsiness, and euphoria (desired effects for use as an adjunct to anesthesia). Reorient patient as necessary.
● Some patients (especially elderly patients) may experience transient excitement or disorientation.
● In ophthalmic use, apply pressure to the lacrimal sac for 1 minute after instillation to reduce risk of systemic drug absorption. Have patient lie down, tilt head back, or look at ceiling to aid instillation.
● Signs and symptoms of overdose include excitability, seizures, CNS stimulation; then depression and psychotic symptoms, such as disorientation, confusion, hallucinations, delusions, anxiety, agitation, and restlessness. Peripheral effects include dilated, nonreactive pupils; blurred vision; flushed, hot, dry skin; dryness of mucous membranes; dysphagia; decreased or absent bowel sounds; urine retention; hyperthermia; tachycardia; hypertension; and increased respiration.
● Treatment of overdose is primarily symptomatic and supportive, as needed. Maintain patent airway. If patient is awake and alert, induce emesis (or use gastric lavage); then use a sodium chloride cathartic and activated charcoal to prevent further drug absorption. In severe life-threatening cases, physostigmine may be given to block antimuscarinic effects. Give fluids, as needed, to treat shock; diazepam to control psychotic symptoms; and pilocarpine (instilled into eyes) to relieve mydriasis. If urine retention develops, catheterization may be necessary.

Monitoring the patient

● Monitor therapeutic response.
● Monitor respiratory status.

Information for the patient
Ophthalmic
● Advise patient to apply pressure to bridge of nose for about 1 minute after instillation.
● Advise patient not to close eyes tightly or blink for about 1 minute after instillation.
Topical
● Tell patient to wash hands after applying patch.
● Advise patient to use only one patch at a time.
● Patch delivers about 1 mg in 72 hours. Remove patch when antiemetic effect is no longer necessary.

Geriatric patients
● Use caution when administering drug to elderly patients. Lower doses are indicated.

Pediatric patients
● Use ophthalmic form cautiously, if at all, in infants and small children.

Breast-feeding patients
● Drug may appear in breast milk, possibly causing infant toxicity. Avoid drug in breast-feeding women; it may decrease milk production.

secobarbital sodium
Novosecobarb*, Seconal

Pharmacologic classification: barbiturate
Therapeutic classification: sedative-hypnotic, anticonvulsant
Controlled substance schedule II
Pregnancy risk category D

How supplied
Available by prescription only
Capsules: 100 mg

Indications, route, and dosage
Preoperative sedation
Adults: 200 to 300 mg P.O. 1 to 2 hours before surgery.
Children: 2 to 6 mg/kg P.O. (maximum dose is 100 mg).
Insomnia
Adults: 100 mg P.O., 100 to 200 mg I.M., or 50 to 250 mg I.V.

Pharmacodynamics
Sedative-hypnotic action: Acts throughout the CNS as a nonselective depressant with a rapid onset and short duration of action. Particularly sensitive to this drug is the reticular activating system, which controls CNS arousal. Drug decreases both presynaptic and postsynaptic membrane excitability by facilitating the action of gamma-aminobutyric acid. The exact cellular site and mechanisms of action are unknown.

Reactions may be *common*, uncommon, *life-threatening*, or COMMON AND LIFE-THREATENING.

Pharmacokinetics
• *Absorption:* After oral administration, 90% absorbed rapidly. Serum level after oral administration peaks between 2 and 4 hours. Rapid onset of action; within 15 minutes when administered orally. Peak effects seen 15 to 30 minutes after oral administration, 7 to 10 minutes after I.M. administration, and 1 to 3 minutes after I.V. administration. Levels of 1 to 5 mcg/ml needed for sedation; 5 to 15 mcg/ml needed for hypnosis. Hypnosis lasts for 1 to 4 hours after oral doses of 100 to 150 mg.
• *Distribution:* Distributed rapidly throughout body tissues and fluids; about 30% to 45% protein-bound.
• *Metabolism:* Oxidized in liver to inactive metabolites. Duration of action is 3 to 4 hours.
• *Excretion:* 95% of dose eliminated as glucuronide conjugates and other metabolites in urine. Drug has an elimination half-life of about 30 hours.

Contraindications and precautions
Contraindicated in patients with hypersensitivity to barbiturates and in those with porphyria or respiratory disease in which dyspnea or obstruction is evident. Use cautiously in patients with acute or chronic pain, depression, suicidal tendencies, history of drug abuse, or impaired hepatic or renal function.

Interactions
Drug-drug. *Antidepressants, antihistamines, narcotics, sedative-hypnotics, tranquilizers:* May potentiate CNS and respiratory depressant effects of these drugs. Use together cautiously.
Corticosteroids, digitoxin (not digoxin), doxycycline, griseofulvin, oral contraceptives, theophylline, other estrogens, other xanthines: Decreased therapeutic effects. Dosage adjustment of other drugs may be needed.
Disulfiram, MAO inhibitors, valproic acid: Decreased metabolism of secobarbital; increased toxicity. Monitor patient for toxicity. Adjust dosage.
Rifampin: Decreased secobarbital levels. Adjust dosage as needed.
Warfarin, other oral anticoagulants: Decreased therapeutic response. Increase in anticoagulant dosage may be needed.
Drug-lifestyle. *Alcohol:* May potentiate CNS and respiratory depressant effects. Discourage use.

Adverse reactions
CNS: *drowsiness, lethargy, hangover,* paradoxical excitement in elderly patients, somnolence, change in EEG patterns.
CV: hypotension (with I.V. use).
GI: nausea, vomiting.
Hematologic: exacerbation of porphyria.
Hepatic: decreased serum bilirubin levels.
Respiratory: *respiratory depression.*

Skin: rash, urticaria, ***Stevens-Johnson syndrome,*** tissue reactions, injection-site pain.
Other: *angioedema,* physical and psychological dependence.

☑ Special considerations
Besides the recommendations relevant to all barbiturates, consider the following.
• Use I.V. route of administration only in emergencies or when other routes are unavailable.
• Dilute secobarbital injection with sterile water for injection solution, normal saline injection, or Ringer's injection solution. Total I.V. dose shouldn't exceed 500 mg. Don't use if solution is discolored or if a precipitate forms.
• Avoid I.V. administration at a rate greater than 50 mg/15 seconds to prevent hypotension and respiratory depression. Have emergency resuscitative equipment on hand.
• Administer I.M. dose deep into large muscle mass to prevent tissue injury.
• Secobarbital sodium injection, diluted with lukewarm tap water to a concentration of 10 to 15 mg/ml, may be administered rectally in children. A cleaning enema should be administered before secobarbital enema.
• Drug may cause a false-positive phentolamine test. The physiologic effects of drug may impair absorption of cyanocobalamin C57.
• Signs and symptoms of overdose include unsteady gait, slurred speech, sustained nystagmus, somnolence, confusion, respiratory depression, pulmonary edema, areflexia, and coma. Typical shock syndrome with tachycardia and hypotension, jaundice, hypothermia, then fever, and oliguria may occur.
• In overdose, maintain and support ventilation and pulmonary function as necessary; support cardiac function and circulation with vasopressors and I.V. fluids as needed. If patient is conscious and gag reflex is intact, induce emesis (if ingestion was recent) with ipecac syrup. If not, perform gastric lavage while a cuffed endotracheal tube is in place to prevent aspiration. Then use activated charcoal or sodium chloride cathartic. Measure intake and output, vital signs, and laboratory parameters; maintain body temperature. Patient should be rolled from side to side every 30 minutes to avoid pulmonary congestion.
• Alkalinization of urine may be helpful in removing drug from body; hemodialysis may be useful in severe overdose.

Monitoring the patient
• Monitor hepatic and renal studies frequently to prevent possible toxicity.
• Monitor patient for adverse effects.

Information for the patient
• Emphasize danger of combining drug with alcohol. An excessive depressive effect is possi-

ble even if drug is taken the evening before ingestion of alcohol.

Geriatric patients
● Elderly patients are more susceptible to drug's effects and usually need lower doses. Confusion, disorientation, and excitability may occur in elderly patients.

Pediatric patients
● Drug may cause paradoxical excitement in children; use cautiously.

Breast-feeding patients
● Drug appears in breast milk. Don't use in breast-feeding women.

---

selegiline hydrochloride
(L-deprenyl hydrochloride)
Ataptryl, Carbex, Eldepryl, Selpak

Pharmacologic classification: MAO inhibitor
Therapeutic classification: antiparkinsonian
Pregnancy risk category C

How supplied
Available by prescription only
Capsules: 5 mg
Tablets: 5 mg

Indications, route, and dosage
Adjunctive treatment to levodopa-carbidopa in the management of symptoms associated with Parkinson's disease
Adults: 10 mg P.O. daily, taken as 5 mg at breakfast and 5 mg at lunch. After 2 or 3 days of therapy, begin gradual decrease of levodopa-carbidopa dose.

Pharmacodynamics
Antiparkinsonian action: Probably acts by selectively inhibiting MAO type B (found mostly in the brain). At higher-than-recommended doses, is a nonselective inhibitor of MAO, including MAO type A found in the GI tract. May also directly increase dopaminergic activity by decreasing the reuptake of dopamine into nerve cells. Has pharmacologically active metabolites (amphetamine and methamphetamine) that may contribute to this effect.

Pharmacokinetics
● *Absorption:* Rapidly absorbed; about 73% of dose absorbed.
● *Distribution:* After single dose, plasma levels below detectable levels (less than 10 ng/ml).
● *Metabolism:* Three metabolites detected in serum and urine; N-desmethylselegiline, L-amphetamine, and L-methamphetamine.

● *Excretion:* 45% of drug appears as a metabolite in urine after 48 hours.

Contraindications and precautions
Contraindicated in patients with hypersensitivity to drug and in those receiving meperidine and other opioids.

Interactions
Drug-drug. *Adrenergic drugs:* Increased pressor response. Use together cautiously.
Fluoxetine: Increased fluoxetine levels. Avoid concomitant use. Don't start selegiline for 5 weeks after stopping fluoxetine; don't start fluoxetine for 2 weeks after stopping selegiline.
Meperidine: Fatal interactions reported. Don't use together.
Drug-herb. *Cacao:* Potential vasopressor effects if used concurrently. Don't use together.
Ginseng: Possible adverse reactions, including headache, tremors, mania. Avoid concomitant use.
Drug-food. *Foods high in tyramine:* Possible hypertensive crisis. Avoid such foods.
Drug-lifestyle. *Alcohol:* Possible excessive depressant effect. Discourage use.

Adverse reactions
CNS: malaise, *dizziness,* increased tremor, chorea, loss of balance, restlessness, increased bradykinesia, facial grimacing, stiff neck, dyskinesia, involuntary movements, twitching, increased apraxia, behavioral changes, fatigue, headache, confusion, hallucinations, vivid dreams, anxiety, insomnia, lethargy.
CV: orthostatic hypotension, hypertension, hypotension, **arrhythmias**, palpitations, new or increased anginal pain, tachycardia, peripheral edema, syncope.
EENT: blepharospasm.
GI: dry mouth, *nausea,* vomiting, constipation, weight loss, abdominal pain, anorexia or poor appetite, dysphagia, diarrhea, heartburn.
GU: slow urination, transient nocturia, prostatic hyperplasia, urinary hesitancy, urinary frequency, urine retention, sexual dysfunction.
Skin: rash, hair loss, diaphoresis.

☑ Special considerations
● In some patients who experience an increase of adverse reactions associated with levodopa (including dyskinesias), reduction of levodopa-carbidopa is necessary. Most of these patients need a levodopa-carbidopa dose reduction of 10% to 30%.
● Limited experience with overdose suggests that symptoms may include hypotension and psychomotor agitation. Because selegiline becomes a nonselective MAO inhibitor in high doses, consider the possibility of symptoms of MAO inhibitor poisoning (drowsiness, dizziness, hyperactivity, agitation, seizures, coma, hypertension, hypo-

---

Reactions may be common, uncommon, *life-threatening,* or COMMON AND LIFE-THREATENING.

tension, cardiac conduction disturbances, and CV collapse). These symptoms may not develop immediately after ingestion (delays of 12 hours or more are possible).
• Provide supportive treatment; closely monitor patient for worsening of symptoms. Emesis or lavage may be helpful in the early stages of overdose treatment. Avoid phenothiazine derivatives and CNS stimulants; adrenergic drugs may provoke an exaggerated response. Diazepam may be useful in treating seizures.

Monitoring the patient
• Monitor patient for adverse effects.
• Watch for arrhythmias and hypertension.

Information for the patient
• Advise patient not to take more than 10 mg daily. There is no evidence that higher doses improve efficacy, and they may increase adverse reactions.
• Tell patient to move about cautiously at start of therapy because dizziness may occur, which can cause falls.
• Because drug is an MAO inhibitor, tell patient about possibility of an interaction with foods containing tyramine. Tell patient to immediately report signs or symptoms of hypertension, including severe headache. Reportedly, however, this interaction doesn't occur at recommended dose; at 10 mg daily, drug inhibits only MAO type B. Therefore, dietary restrictions appear unnecessary, provided that patient doesn't exceed recommended dose.
• Emphasize danger of combining drug with alcohol. An excessive depressant effect is possible even if drug is taken the evening before ingestion of alcohol.
• Advise patient to take second dose with lunch to avoid nighttime sedation.

Breast-feeding patients
• It's unknown if drug appears in breast milk. Use with caution in breast-feeding women.

---

senna
Black-Draught, Fletcher's Castoria, Nytilax, Senexon, Senokot, Senolax, X-Prep

Pharmacologic classification: anthraquinone derivative
Therapeutic classification: stimulant laxative
Pregnancy risk category C

How supplied
Available without a prescription
Tablets: 6 mg, 8.6 mg, 15 mg, 25 mg (as sennosides)
Granules: 15 mg, 20 mg/5 ml (as sennosides)
Liquid: 33.3 mg/ml
Suppositories: 30 mg (as sennosides)
Syrup: 8.8 mg/5 ml (as sennosides)

Indications, route, and dosage
Acute constipation, preparation for bowel examination
Black-Draught
Adults: 2 tablets or ¼ to ½ level tsp of granules mixed with water. Not recommended for children.
Other preparations
Adults and children ages 12 and over: Usual dose is 2 tablets, 1 tsp of granules dissolved in water, 1 suppository, or 10 to 15 ml syrup h.s. Maximum dose varies with preparation used.
Children ages 6 to 11: 1 tablet, ½ tsp of granules dissolved in water, ½ suppository h.s., or 5 to 10 ml syrup. Maximum dose is 2 tablets b.i.d. or 1 tsp of granules b.i.d.
Children ages 2 to 5: ½ tablet, ¼ tsp of granules dissolved in water. Maximum dose is 1 tablet b.i.d. or ½ tsp of granules b.i.d.
Children ages 1 to 5: 2.5 to 5 ml syrup h.s.
Children ages 1 to 12 months: 1.25 to 2.5 ml syrup h.s.

Pharmacodynamics
Laxative action: Has a local irritant effect on the colon, which promotes peristalsis and bowel evacuation. Also enhances intestinal fluid accumulation, thereby increasing the stool's moisture content.

Pharmacokinetics
• *Absorption:* Absorbed minimally. With oral administration, laxative effect in 6 to 10 hours; with suppository administration, laxative effect in 30 minutes to 2 hours.
• *Distribution:* May be distributed in bile, saliva, colonic mucosa, and breast milk.
• *Metabolism:* Absorbed portion of drug metabolized in liver.
• *Excretion:* Unabsorbed senna excreted mainly in feces; absorbed drug excreted in urine and feces.

Contraindications and precautions
Contraindicated in patients with ulcerative bowel lesions; nausea, vomiting, abdominal pain, or other symptoms of appendicitis or acute surgical abdomen; fecal impaction; or intestinal obstruction or perforation.

Interactions
None reported.

Adverse reactions
GI: *nausea,* vomiting, diarrhea, loss of normal bowel function with excessive use, *abdominal cramps* (especially in severe constipation), malabsorption of nutrients, "cathartic colon" (syndrome resembling ulcerative colitis radiological-

ly) with chronic misuse, possible constipation after catharsis, yellow or yellow-green cast to feces, diarrhea in breast-feeding infants of mothers receiving senna, darkened pigmentation of rectal mucosa with long-term use (usually reversible within 4 to 12 months after stopping drug), laxative dependence with excessive use.
GU: red-pink discoloration in alkaline urine; yellow-brown color to acidic urine.
Metabolic: protein-losing enteropathy, electrolyte imbalance (such as hypokalemia).

☑ Special considerations
● Protect drug from excessive heat or light.
● In the phenolsulfonphthalein excretion test, senna may turn urine pink to red, red to violet, or red to brown.

Monitoring the patient
● Monitor patient for therapeutic effect.
● Monitor patient for adverse effects.

Information for the patient
● Warn patient that drug may turn urine pink, red, violet, or brown, depending on urine pH.
● Advise patient that laxative use shouldn't exceed 1 week. Excessive use may result in dependence or electrolyte imbalance.
● Tell patient that bowel movement may have a yellow or yellow-green cast.

Geriatric patients
● Elderly persons often overuse laxatives and may be more prone to laxative dependency.

Pediatric patients
● Senna and other stimulant laxatives are used infrequently in children.

Breast-feeding patients
● Drug appears in breast milk. Diarrhea has been reported in breast-feeding infants.

---

sertraline hydrochloride
Zoloft

Pharmacologic classification: serotonin uptake inhibitor
Therapeutic classification: antidepressant
Pregnancy risk category B

How supplied
Available by prescription only
Tablets: 50 mg, 100 mg

Indications, route, and dosage
Depression, obsessive-compulsive disorder
Adults: 50 mg P.O. daily. Adjust dose as needed and tolerated (doses of 50 to 200 mg daily have

been used). Dosage adjustments should be made at intervals of no less than 1 week.
Children ages 13 to 17: 50 mg P.O. once daily.
Children ages 6 to 12: 25 mg P.O. once daily.
Panic disorder
Adults: 25 mg P.O. daily. Increase to 50 mg P.O. daily after 1 week.
✦ *Dosage adjustment.* A lower or less frequent dosage should be used in patients with hepatic impairment. Particular care should be used in patients with renal failure.

Pharmacodynamics
Antidepressant action: Probably acts by blocking the reuptake of serotonin (5-hydroxytryptamine; 5-HT) into presynaptic neurons in the CNS, prolonging the action of 5-HT.

Pharmacokinetics
● *Absorption:* Well absorbed after oral administration; absorption rate and extent enhanced when taken with food. Serum levels peak between 4½ and 8¼ hours after a dose.
● *Distribution:* In vitro studies indicate drug is more than 98% protein-bound.
● *Metabolism:* Probable hepatic metabolism; significant first-pass metabolism. N-desmethylsertraline is substantially less active than parent compound.
● *Excretion:* Excreted mostly as metabolites in urine and feces. Mean elimination half-life is 26 hours. Steady-state levels reached within 1 week of daily dosing in young, healthy patients.

Contraindications and precautions
Contraindicated in patients receiving MAO inhibitors. Use cautiously in patients at risk for suicide and in those with seizure disorders, major affective disorder, or diseases or conditions that affect metabolism or hemodynamic responses.

Interactions
Drug-drug. *Diazepam, tolbutamide:* Clearance decreased by sertraline. Significance unknown; monitor patient for increased drug effects.
MAO inhibitors: Possible serious mental status changes, hyperthermia, autonomic instability, rapid fluctuations of vital signs, delirium, coma, and death. Don't administer within 14 days after stopping MAO inhibitor. Allow 14 days after stopping sertraline before starting MAO inhibitor.
Warfarin, other highly protein-bound drugs: Possible interactions; increased plasma levels of sertraline or other highly bound drug. 8% increases in PT have occurred if drug is used with warfarin. Monitor patient closely.
Drug-lifestyle. *Alcohol:* Potential CNS depression. Discourage use.

Adverse reactions
CNS: *headache, tremor, dizziness, insomnia, somnolence,* paresthesia, hypoesthesia, *fatigue,*

Reactions may be *common,* uncommon, **life-threatening,** or COMMON AND LIFE-THREATENING.

nervousness, anxiety, agitation, hypertonia, twitching, confusion.
CV: palpitations, chest pain, hot flashes.
GI: *dry mouth, nausea, diarrhea, loose stools, dyspepsia,* vomiting, constipation, thirst, flatulence, anorexia, abdominal pain, increased appetite.
GU: *male sexual dysfunction,* polyuria, nocturia, dysuria.
Hepatic: elevated liver enzyme levels.
Metabolic: minor increases in serum cholesterol and triglycerides; decreased uric acid.
Musculoskeletal: myalgia.
Skin: rash, pruritus, *diaphoresis.*

☑ Special considerations
● Patients who respond during the first 8 weeks of therapy will probably continue to respond to drug, although some depressed patients have taken drug for longer than 16 weeks. If patients continue on drug for prolonged therapy, periodically monitor drug effectiveness. It's unknown if periodic dosage adjustments are necessary to maintain effectiveness.
● Drug may activate mania or hypomania in patients with cyclic disorders.
● Experience with sertraline overdose is limited. Treatment is supportive. Establish an airway and maintain adequate ventilation. Because the value of forced emesis or lavage is questionable, consider activated charcoal in sorbitol to bind drug in GI tract.
● There is no specific antidote for sertraline overdose. Monitor vital signs closely. Because drug has a large volume of distribution, hemodialysis, peritoneal dialysis, or forced diuresis probably isn't useful.

Monitoring the patient
● Monitor therapeutic response and adjust dose accordingly.
● Monitor patient for signs of mania or hypomania.

Information for the patient
● Tell patient to take drug once daily, in either the morning or evening, with or without food.
● Advise patient to avoid alcohol while taking drug and to call before taking OTC products.
● Although problems haven't been reported to date, advise patient to use caution when performing hazardous tasks that require alertness, such as driving and operating heavy machinery. Drugs that influence CNS may impair judgment.

Geriatric patients
● Plasma clearance of drug is slower in elderly patients. It may take 2 to 3 weeks of daily dosing before steady-state levels are reached. Monitor closely for dose-related side effects.

Pediatric patients
● Safety and efficacy in children with panic disorder haven't been established.

Breast-feeding patients
● It's unknown if drug appears in breast milk. Use with caution in breast-feeding women.

sibutramine hydrochloride monohydrate
Meridia

Pharmacologic classification: norepinephrine, serotonin, and dopamine reuptake inhibitor
Therapeutic classification: antiobesity drug
Controlled substance schedule IV
Pregnancy risk category C

How supplied
Available by prescription only
Capsules: 5 mg, 10 mg, 15 mg

Indications, route, and dosage
Management of obesity, including weight loss and maintenance of weight loss (should be used with reduced-calorie diet)
Adults: 10 mg P.O. once daily with or without food. May increase dose to 15 mg daily after 4 weeks if there is inadequate weight loss. Patients who don't tolerate the 10-mg dose may receive 5 mg daily. Doses above 15 mg daily aren't recommended.

Pharmacodynamics
Antiobesity action: Produces therapeutic effects by inhibiting the reuptake of norepinephrine, serotonin, and dopamine.

Pharmacokinetics
● *Absorption:* Rapidly absorbed from GI tract. Plasma levels of mono- and di-desmethyl metabolites M_1 and M_2 peak within 3 to 4 hours. On average, at least 77% of single oral dose is absorbed.
● *Distribution:* Distributed extensively into tissues, especially liver and kidneys, with relatively low transfer to fetus. In vitro, sibutramine, M_1, and M_2 are 97%, 94%, and 94%, respectively, bound to plasma proteins.
● *Metabolism:* Undergoes extensive first-pass metabolism by cytochrome P-450 3A4 isoenzyme to active desmethyl metabolites M_1 and M_2; elimination half-lives of M_1 and M_2 are 14 and 16 hours, respectively.
● *Excretion:* About 77% of oral dose excreted in urine.

Contraindications and precautions

Contraindicated in patients with hypersensitivity to drug or its inactive ingredients, in those with anorexia nervosa, and in those taking MAO inhibitors or other centrally acting appetite-suppressants.

Don't use drug in patients with history of coronary artery disease, heart failure, arrhythmias, stroke, severe renal failure, hepatic dysfunction, or history of seizures.

Use cautiously in patients with narrow-angle glaucoma.

Interactions

Drug-drug. *CNS depressants:* Enhanced CNS depression. Avoid concomitant use.

Dextromethorphan, dihydroergotamine, fentanyl, fluoxetine, fluvoxamine, lithium, MAO inhibitors, meperidine, paroxetine, pentazocine, sertraline, sumatriptan, tryptophan, venlafaxine: Possible hyperthermia, tachycardia, and loss of consciousness. Don't use together.

Drugs that inhibit cytochrome P-450 3A4 metabolism (erythromycin, ketoconazole): Increased effect of sibutramine. Adjust dosage.

Ephedrine, phenylpropanolamine, pseudoephedrine: Increased blood pressure or heart rate. Monitor patient carefully.

Drug-lifestyle. *Alcohol:* Enhanced CNS depression. Don't use together.

Adverse reactions

CNS: *headache, insomnia,* dizziness, nervousness, anxiety, depression, paresthesia, somnolence, CNS stimulation, emotional lability, migraine.

CV: tachycardia, vasodilation, hypertension, palpitation, chest pain, generalized edema.

EENT: thirst, *dry mouth, rhinitis, pharyngitis,* laryngitis, sinusitis, taste perversion, ear disorder, ear pain.

GI: *anorexia, constipation,* increased appetite, nausea, dyspepsia, gastritis, vomiting, abdominal pain, rectal disorder.

GU: dysmenorrhea, urinary tract infection, vaginal candidiasis, metrorrhagia.

Hepatic: elevated liver function tests.

Musculoskeletal: arthralgia, myalgia, asthenia, tenosynovitis, joint disorder, neck or back pain.

Respiratory: cough increase, laryngitis.

Skin: rash, sweating, herpes simplex, acne.

Other: flulike syndrome, *allergic reaction.*

☑ Special considerations

● Drug is recommended for obese patients with an initial body mass index of 30 kg/m^2 or more or 27 kg/m^2 or more in the presence of other risk factors (such as hypertension, diabetes, or dyslipidemia).

● Rule out organic causes of obesity before starting therapy.

● At least 2 weeks should elapse between stopping an MAO inhibitor and starting sibutramine, and vice versa.

● Weight loss can precipitate or exacerbate gallstone formation.

● Although not reported with sibutramine, some centrally acting weight-loss drugs have been associated with a rare but fatal condition known as primary pulmonary hypertension.

● If patient hasn't lost at least 4 lb in the first 4 weeks of treatment, reevaluate therapy to consider increasing dosage or stopping drug.

● There is no specific antidote for sibutramine overdose. Treatment should consist of general measures used in overdose management. Establish an airway, monitor cardiac and vital signs, and institute general symptomatic and supportive measures. Cautious use of beta blockers may be indicated to control elevated blood pressure or tachycardia. Benefits of forced diuresis and hemodialysis are unknown.

Monitoring the patient

● Measure blood pressure and heart rate before starting therapy, with dosage changes, and at regular intervals during therapy because drug is known to increase both blood pressure and heart rate.

● Monitor patient for adverse effects.

Information for the patient

● Advise patient to read package insert before starting therapy and to review it each time prescription is renewed.

● Advise patient to immediately report rash, hives, or other allergic reactions.

● Advise patient to disclose other prescription or OTC drugs being taken, especially other weight-reducing drugs, decongestants, antidepressants, cough suppressants, lithium, dihydroergotamine, sumatriptan, or tryptophan, because of the potential for drug interactions.

● Suggest that blood pressure and heart rate be monitored regularly. Emphasize importance of regular follow-up visits.

● Advise patient to use drug with a reduced calorie diet.

Geriatric patients

● Dosage selection for an elderly patient should be cautious, reflecting the greater frequency of decreased hepatic, renal, or cardiac function, and of concomitant disease or other drug therapy.

Pediatric patients

● Safety and efficacy in children under age 16 haven't been established.

Breast-feeding patients

● It's unknown if drug or metabolites appear in breast milk. Avoid use in breast-feeding women.

Reactions may be *common,* uncommon, **life-threatening**, or COMMON AND LIFE-THREATENING.

sildenafil citrate
Viagra

Pharmacologic classification: selective inhibitor of cyclic guanosine monophosphate-specific phosphodiesterase type 5
Therapeutic classification: therapy for erectile dysfunction
Pregnancy risk category B

How supplied
Available by prescription only
Tablets: 25 mg, 50 mg, 100 mg

Indications, route, and dosage
Erectile dysfunction
Adults: 50 mg P.O. as a single dose, p.r.n., 1 hour before sexual activity. However, may take drug 30 minutes to 4 hours before sexual activity. Based on effectiveness and tolerance by patient, may increase dose to maximum single dose of 100 mg or decrease dose to 25 mg. Maximum recommended dosing frequency is once daily.
✦ Dosage adjustment. In elderly patients, patients with hepatic impairment or severe renal impairment, and those concurrently taking potent cytochrome P-450 3A4 inhibitors, consider a starting dose of 25 mg.

Pharmacodynamics
Erectile action: Has no direct relaxant effect on isolated corpus cavernosum, but enhances the effect of nitric oxide (NO) by inhibiting phosphodiesterase type 5 (PDE5), which is responsible for degradation of cyclic guanosine monophosphate (cGMP) in the corpus cavernosum. When sexual stimulation causes local release of NO, inhibition of PDE5 by sildenafil causes increased levels of cGMP in the corpus cavernosum, resulting in smooth muscle relaxation and inflow of blood to the corpus cavernosum.

Pharmacokinetics
- *Absorption:* Rapidly absorbed after oral administration. Plasma levels peak in ½ to 2 hours (median, 1 hour); high-fat meal delays rate of absorption by about 1 hour and reduces peak levels by one third. Absolute bioavailability about 40%.
- *Distribution:* Widely distributed to body tissues; mean steady-state volume of distribution of 105 L. Both drug and major active metabolite are 96% bound to plasma proteins; protein-binding is independent of drug levels.
- *Metabolism:* Primary pathway for elimination is metabolism by the CYP 3A4 and CYP 2C9 hepatic microsomal isoenzymes. N-desmethylation converts drug into major circulating metabolite, which accounts for about 20% of sildenafil's pharmacologic effects.

- *Excretion:* About 80% of oral dose metabolized and excreted in feces; about 13% excreted in urine.

Contraindications and precautions
Contraindicated in patients with hypersensitivity to drug or its components and in those also using organic nitrates.
    Use with caution in patients who have had an MI, stroke, or life-threatening arrhythmias within the last 6 months or have a history of cardiac failure, coronary artery disease, or uncontrolled high or low blood pressure; in those with anatomic deformation of the penis; and in those predisposed to priapism (sickle cell anemia, multiple myeloma, leukemia), retinitis pigmentosa, bleeding disorders, or active peptic ulcers.

Interactions
Drug-drug. *Inhibitors of cytochrome P-450 isoforms 3A4 (cimetidine, erythromycin, itraconazole, ketoconazole):* Reduced clearance of sildenafil. Adjust dosage.
Nitrates: Enhanced hypotensive effects. Adjust nitrate dosage. Monitor blood pressure closely.
Rifampin: Reduced sildenafil plasma levels. Adjust dosage.
Drug-food. *High-fat meal:* Delayed absorption of drug and onset of action. Avoid ingesting with high-fat meal.

Adverse reactions
CNS: *headache,* dizziness.
CV: *flushing.*
EENT: nasal congestion, abnormal vision (photophobia, color blindness).
GI: dyspepsia, diarrhea.
GU: urinary tract infection.
Skin: rash.

☑ Special considerations
- Because cardiac risk is associated with sexual activity, evaluate patient's CV status before initiating therapy.
- In healthy volunteers, doses up to 800 mg produced adverse effects similar to those seen at lower doses, but at an increased rate. Use standard supportive measures to treat overdose. Renal dialysis probably won't increase clearance.

Monitoring the patient
- Monitor patient for adverse effects.
- Monitor cardiac status and vision changes.

Information for the patient
- Advise patient that high-fat meal will delay absorption and onset by 60 minutes.
- Tell patient that drug doesn't protect against sexually transmitted diseases and that he should use protective measures to prevent infection.
- Advise patient not to take drug with nitrates.
- Tell patient to report visual changes.

- Urge patient to call if erection lasts more than 4 hours.
- Advise patient that drug has no effect in the absence of sexual stimulation.

Geriatric patients
- Reduced drug clearance is seen in healthy elderly volunteers ages 65 and older. This reduction results in plasma levels about 40% greater than those in younger subjects.

Pediatric patients
- Drug shouldn't be used in children or neonates.

Breast-feeding patients
- Drug had only been used in men; it isn't indicated for use in women.

---

silver sulfadiazine
Silvadene, SSD AF, SSD Cream, Thermazene

Pharmacologic classification: synthetic anti-infective
Therapeutic classification: topical antibacterial
Pregnancy risk category B

How supplied
Available by prescription only
Cream: 1%

Indications, route, and dosage
Adjunct in the prevention and treatment of wound infection for second- and third-degree burns
Adults and children: Apply ⅟₁₆-inch (16 mm) thickness of ointment to cleansed and debrided burn wound once or twice daily. Reapply if accidentally removed.

Pharmacodynamics
Antibacterial action: Acts on bacterial cell membrane and bacterial cell wall. Has a broad spectrum of activity, including against gram-negative and gram-positive organisms.

Pharmacokinetics
- *Absorption:* Limited absorption with topical use.
- *Distribution:* None.
- *Metabolism:* None.
- *Excretion:* Excreted in urine.

Contraindications and precautions
Contraindicated in patients with hypersensitivity to drug and in premature and full-term neonates during first 2 months of life; drug may increase possibility of kernicterus. Also contraindicated in pregnant women at or near term. Use cautiously in patients with sulfonamide sensitivity.

Interactions
Drug-drug. *Collagenase, papain, sutilains:* Inactivated if used with drug. Avoid concomitant use.
Drug-lifestyle. *Sun exposure:* Enhanced photosensitivity reactions. Tell patient to take precautions.

Adverse reactions
Hematologic: *neutropenia.*
Skin: pain, burning, rash, pruritus, skin necrosis, *erythema multiforme,* skin discoloration.

☑ Special considerations
- Avoid drug contact with eyes and mucous membranes.
- Burned area should be covered with cream at all times.
- Continue treatment until site is healed or is ready for skin grafting.
- Delayed eschar separation may result when drug is used.
- To treat local overapplication, stop drug and clean area thoroughly.

Monitoring the patient
- Watch for signs of fungal superinfection.
- Monitor CBCs, serum sulfadiazine levels, and urine for crystalluria and calculi formation.

Information for the patient
- Advise patient about wound care and proper application.
- Tell patient that drug doesn't stain skin.
- Warn patient of potential photosensitivity.

Pediatric patients
- Drug is contraindicated in premature infants and infants under age 2 months.

Breast-feeding patients
- It's unknown if drug appears in breast milk. Avoid breast-feeding during and for several days after therapy.

---

simethicone
Gas-X, Mylicon, Phazyme

Pharmacologic classification: dispersant
Therapeutic classification: antiflatulent
Pregnancy risk category C

How supplied
Available without a prescription
Tablets (delayed-release; enteric-coated core): 60 mg, 95 mg
Tablets (chewable): 40 mg, 80 mg, 125 mg
Capsules: 125 mg
Drops: 40 mg/0.6 ml

Indications, route, and dosage
Flatulence, functional gastric bloating
Adults and children over age 12: 40 to 125 mg
P.O. after each meal and h.s.
Children ages 2 to 12: 40 mg (drops) P.O. q.i.d.
Children under age 2: 20 mg (drops) P.O. q.i.d.,
up to 240 mg/day.

Pharmacodynamics
Antiflatulent action: Acts as a defoamer by decreasing the surface tension of gas bubbles, thereby preventing the formation of mucus-coated gas
bubbles.

Pharmacokinetics
• *Absorption:* None.
• *Distribution:* None.
• *Metabolism:* None.
• *Excretion:* Excreted in feces.

Contraindications and precautions
Contraindicated in patients with hypersensitivity
to drug.

Interactions
Drug-drug. *Alginic acid:* Reduced therapeutic
effect of alginic acid. Adjust dosage.

Adverse reactions
GI: expulsion of excessive liberated gas as belching, rectal flatus.

☑ Special considerations
• Simethicone is found in many combination
antacid products.

Monitoring the patient
• Monitor therapeutic effect of drug.
• Monitor patient for adverse effects.

Information for the patient
• Tell patient to chew tablets thoroughly or to
shake suspension well before using.

Pediatric patients
• Drug isn't recommended as treatment for infant colic; has limited use in children.

simvastatin
Zocor

Pharmacologic classification: HMG-CoA
reductase inhibitor
Therapeutic classification: antilipemic,
cholesterol-lowering
Pregnancy risk category X

How supplied
Available by prescription only
Tablets: 5 mg, 10 mg, 20 mg, 40 mg, 80 mg

Indications, route, and dosage
Reduction of low-density lipoprotein (LDL)
and total cholesterol levels in patients with
primary hypercholesterolemia (types IIa and
IIb)
Adults: Initially, 5 to 10 mg daily in the evening.
Adjust dose q 4 weeks based on patient tolerance and response; maximum daily dose is 40
mg. Maximum daily dose for elderly patients is
20 mg.
✦ *Dosage adjustment.* For patients receiving
immunosuppressants, start with 5 mg/day; maximum daily dose is 10 mg. For patients with mild
to moderate renal insufficiency, give usual daily
dose; in those with severe renal impairment, start
therapy with 5 mg P.O. daily and closely monitor
patient.

Pharmacodynamics
Antilipemic action: Inhibits the enzyme 3-hydroxy-
3-methylglutaryl-coenzyme A (HMG-CoA) reductase. This hepatic enzyme is an early (and
rate-limiting) step in the synthetic pathway of cholesterol.

Pharmacokinetics
• *Absorption:* Readily absorbed; extensive hepatic extraction limits plasma availability of active inhibitors to 5% or less of dose. Individual
absorption varies considerably.
• *Distribution:* Parent drug and active metabolites more than 95% bound to plasma proteins.
• *Metabolism:* Hydrolysis occurs in plasma; at
least three major metabolites identified.
• *Excretion:* Excreted primarily in bile.

Contraindications and precautions
Contraindicated in patients with hypersensitivity
to drug and in those with active hepatic disease
or conditions that cause unexplained persistent
elevations of serum transaminase level; in pregnant and breast-feeding women; and in women
of childbearing age unless there is no risk of pregnancy.
   Use cautiously in patients with history of liver disease or who consume excessive amounts
of alcohol.

Interactions
Drug-drug. *Digoxin:* Elevated digoxin levels.
Closely monitor plasma digoxin levels at start of
simvastatin therapy.
*Drugs that decrease levels or activity of en-
dogenous steroids (such as cimetidine, ketoconazole, spironolactone):* Increased risk of endocrine dysfunction. Monitor patient closely.
*Erythromycin, fibric acid derivatives (such as
clofibrate, gemfibrozil), high doses of niacin (nicotinic acid; 1 g or more daily), immunosuppressants (such as cyclosporine):* Increased risk of
rhabdomyolysis. Monitor patient closely if use together can't be avoided. Limit daily dose of sim-

---

vastatin to 10 mg if patient must take cyclosporine.

Hepatotoxic drugs: Increased risk of hepatotoxicity. Monitor hepatic status closely.

Warfarin: Slightly enhanced anticoagulant effect. Monitor PT at start of therapy and during dosage adjustment.

Drug-lifestyle. *Alcohol:* Increased risk of hepatotoxicity. Discourage use.

Adverse reactions
CNS: headache, asthenia.
GI: abdominal pain, constipation, diarrhea, dyspepsia, flatulence, nausea, vomiting.
Hepatic: elevated liver enzyme levels.
Respiratory: upper respiratory tract infection.

☑ Special considerations
• Dosage adjustments should be made about every 4 weeks. If cholesterol levels decrease below target range, dosage may be reduced.
• Initiate drug only after diet and other nonpharmacologic therapies have proved ineffective. Patient should continue a cholesterol-lowering diet during therapy.
• There is no experience with simvastatin overdose and no known specific antidote. Treat symptomatically.

Monitoring the patient
• Perform liver function tests frequently at start of therapy and then periodically.
• Monitor therapeutic effect.

Information for the patient
• Tell patient that drug should be taken in the evening and may be taken without regard to meals.
• Because of possible impact of drug on liver function, advise patient to restrict alcohol intake.
• Tell patient to report adverse reactions, particularly muscle aches and pains.

Geriatric patients
• Most elderly patients respond to daily dose of 20 mg or less.

Pediatric patients
• Safety and efficacy in children haven't been established.

Breast-feeding patients
• It's unknown if drug appears in breast milk. Because of risk to infants, breast-feeding should be avoided during therapy.

sirolimus
Rapamune

Pharmacologic classification: macrocyclic lactone
Therapeutic classification: immunosuppressant
Pregnancy risk category C

How supplied
Available by prescription only
Oral solution: 1 mg/ml

Indications, route, and dosage
Prophylaxis, with cyclosporine and corticosteroids, of organ rejection in patients receiving renal transplants
Adults and adolescents ages 13 and older who weigh 40 kg (88 lb) or more: Initially, 6 mg P.O. as a one-time loading dose as soon as possible after transplantation; then maintenance dose of 2 mg P.O. once daily.
Adolescents ages 13 and older who weigh less than 40 kg: Initially, 3 mg/m2 P.O. as a one-time loading dose after transplantation; then maintenance dose of 1 mg/m2 P.O. once daily.
✦ *Dosage adjustment.* For patients with mild to moderate hepatic impairment, reduce maintenance dose by about one-third. It isn't necessary to reduce loading dose.

Pharmacodynamics
Immunosuppressant action: An immunosuppressant that inhibits T-lymphocyte activation and proliferation that occur in response to antigenic and cytokine stimulation. Also inhibits antibody formation.

Pharmacokinetics
• *Absorption:* Rapidly absorbed from GI tract. Mean peak levels in about 1 to 3 hours; oral bioavailability about 14%. Food decreases peak plasma levels and time to peak.
• *Distribution:* Extensively partitioned into formed blood elements. About 92% bound to plasma proteins.
• *Metabolism:* Extensively metabolized by mixed function oxidase system, primarily cytochrome P-450 3A4. Seven major metabolites identified in whole blood.
• *Excretion:* 91% excreted in feces and 2.2% in urine. Half-life about 62 hours.

Contraindications and precautions
Contraindicated in patients with hypersensitivity to active drug or its derivatives or components. Use with caution in patients with hyperlipidemia or impaired liver or renal function.

Reactions may be *common*, uncommon, **life-threatening**, or COMMON AND LIFE-THREATENING.

Interactions

Drug-drug. *Bromocriptine, cimetidine, clarithromycin, clotrimazole, danazol, erythromycin, fluconazole, indinavir, itraconazole, metoclopramide, nicardipine, ritonavir, verapamil, other drugs that inhibit CYP 3A4:* Decreased sirolimus metabolism; increased sirolimus levels. Monitor patient closely.

Carbamazepine, phenobarbital, phenytoin, rifabutin, rifapentine, other drugs that induce CYP 3A4: Increased sirolimus metabolism; decreased sirolimus blood levels. Monitor patient closely.

Cyclosporine (capsules, oral solution): Increased sirolimus levels. Administer sirolimus 4 hours after cyclosporine. After long-term administration, sirolimus may reduce cyclosporine clearance, leading to need for reduction in cyclosporine dose.

Diltiazem: Increased sirolimus levels. Monitor and reduce dosage of sirolimus, as necessary.

Ketoconazole: Increased rate and extent of sirolimus absorption. Avoid concomitant use.

Live virus vaccines (BCG, measles, mumps, oral polio, rubella, TY21a typhoid, varicella, yellow fever): Reduced effectiveness of vaccines. Avoid concomitant use.

Rifampin: Decreased sirolimus levels. Consider alternatives to rifampin.

Drug-food. *Grapefruit juice:* Decreased metabolism of sirolimus. Avoid concomitant use.

Adverse reactions

CNS: *headache, insomnia, tremor, anxiety, depression, asthenia,* malaise, syncope, confusion, dizziness, emotional lability, hypertonia, hypoesthesia, hypotonia, neuropathy, paresthesia, somnolence.

CV: *hypertension,* **heart failure, atrial fibrillation,** tachycardia, hypotension, *chest pain, edema,* **hemorrhage,** palpitations, peripheral vascular disorder, thrombophlebitis, thrombosis, vasodilation.

EENT: facial edema, *pharyngitis,* epistaxis, rhinitis, sinusitis, abnormal vision, cataract, conjunctivitis, deafness, ear pain, otitis media, tinnitus.

GI: *diarrhea, nausea, vomiting, constipation, abdominal pain, dyspepsia,* enlarged abdomen, ascites, peritonitis, anorexia, dysphagia, eructation, esophagitis, flatulence, gastritis, gastroenteritis, gingivitis, gum hyperplasia, ileus, mouth ulceration, oral candidiasis, stomatitis.

GU: dysuria, hematuria, albuminuria, **kidney tubular necrosis,** increased creatinine level, *urinary tract infection,* pelvic pain, glycosuria, increased BUN level, bladder pain, hydronephrosis, impotence, kidney pain, nocturia, oliguria, pyuria, scrotal edema, testis disorder, **toxic nephropathy,** urinary frequency, urinary incontinence, urine retention.

Hematologic: anemia, THROMBOCYTOPENIA, *leukopenia,* thrombotic thrombocytopenic purpura, ecchymosis, leukocytosis, polycythemia.

Hepatic: elevation in liver enzymes.

Metabolic: *hypercholesteremia, hyperlipidemia, hypokalemia, weight gain, hypophosphatemia, hyperkalemia,* hypervolemia, Cushing's syndrome, diabetes mellitus, acidosis, dehydration, hypercalcemia, hyperglycemia, hyperphosphatemia, hypocalcemia, hypoglycemia, hypomagnesemia, hyponatremia, weight loss.

Musculoskeletal: *back pain, arthralgia,* myalgia, arthrosis, bone necrosis, leg cramps, osteoporosis, tetany.

Respiratory: *dyspnea, cough, atelectasis, upper respiratory tract infection,* asthma, bronchitis, hypoxia, lung edema, pleural effusion, pneumonia.

Skin: *rash, acne,* hirsutism, fungal dermatitis, pruritus, skin hypertrophy, skin ulcer, sweating.

Other: *fever, pain, peripheral edema,* abscess, cellulitis, chills, flulike syndrome, hernia, infection, **sepsis,** lymphadenopathy, abnormal healing.

☑ Special considerations

● After transplantation, antimicrobials for prophylaxis of *Pneumocystis carinii* and *Cytomegalovirus* should be administered for 1 year and 3 months, respectively.

● Vaccinations may be less effective during sirolimus treatment. Avoid concomitant use of live vaccines.

● Drug may be used in a regimen with cyclosporine and corticosteroids.

● Only physicians experienced in immunosuppressive therapy and management of renal transplant patients should prescribe drug.

● Patients taking drug are more susceptible to infection and possible development of lymphoma, which may result from immunosuppression.

● Drug must be diluted before administration. After dilution, use product immediately.

● Store away from light, and refrigerate at 36° to 46° F (2° to 8° C). If necessary, bottles and pouches may be stored at room temperature (up to 77° F [25° C]) for several days. Drug can be kept in oral dosing syringe for 24 hours at room temperature or refrigerated at 36° to 46° F. A slight haze may develop during refrigeration, but this doesn't affect drug quality. If a haze develops, bring drug to room temperature and shake until haze disappears.

● There is limited experience with overdose. Provide general supportive care. Drug probably isn't dialyzable.

Monitoring the patient

● Monitor renal function because drug use with cyclosporine may cause an increase in serum creatinine levels. Dosage adjustment of immunosuppressive regimen may be needed.

● Monitor cholesterol and triglyceride levels during therapy. If hyperlipidemia is detected, initiate interventions, such as diet, exercise, and lipid-lowering drugs. If patient is on sirolimus and cy-

closporine is started as an HMG-CoA reductase inhibitor, watch for development of rhabdomyolysis.
• Monitor drug levels in children; in patients with hepatic impairment; during concurrent administration of drugs that induce or inhibit CYP 3A4; and if cyclosporine dosage is markedly reduced or stopped.

Information for the patient
• Advise woman to avoid pregnancy during therapy. Effective contraception is needed before, during, and for 12 weeks after therapy.
• Tell patient to take drug consistently with or without food to minimize drug absorption variability.
• Advise patient to take drug 4 hours after taking cyclosporine.
• Tell patient to wash area with soap and water if solution touches skin or mucous membranes and to rinse eyes with water if solution gets in eyes.

Geriatric patients
• Data suggest that dosage adjustments in elderly patients aren't necessary.

Pediatric patients
• Safety and efficacy of drug in children under age 13 haven't been established.

Breast-feeding patients
• It's unknown if drug appears in breast milk. Because of potential for adverse reactions in breast-feeding infants, stop either breast-feeding or drug.

sodium bicarbonate
Bell/ans, Neut, Soda Mint

Pharmacologic classification: alkalinizer
Therapeutic classification: systemic and urinary alkalinizer, systemic hydrogen ion buffer, oral antacid
Pregnancy risk category C

How supplied
Available by prescription only
Injection: 4% (2.4 mEq/5 ml), 4.2% (5 mEq/10 ml), 5% (297.5 mEq/500 ml), 7.5% (8.92 mEq/10 ml and 44.6 mEq/50 ml), 8.4% (10 mEq/10 ml and 50 mEq/50 ml)
Available without a prescription
Tablets: 325 mg, 520 mg, 650 mg

Indications, route, and dosage
Adjunct to advanced cardiac life support
Adults and children over age 2: Although no longer routinely recommended, inject either 300 to 500 ml of a 5% solution or 200 to 300 mEq of a 7.5% or 8.4% solution as rapidly as possible. Base further doses on subsequent blood gas values.

Children ages 2 and younger: 1 mEq/kg I.V. bolus of a 4.2% solution. Dose may be repeated q 10 minutes depending on blood gas values. Don't exceed daily dose of 8 mEq/kg.
Metabolic acidosis
Adults and children: Dose depends on blood carbon dioxide content, pH, and patient's clinical condition. Generally, administer 90 to 180 mEq/L I.V. during first hour; then adjust, p.r.n.
Urinary alkalization
Adults: 325 mg to 2 g P.O., up to q.i.d. Don't exceed 17 g in patients under age 60 or 8 g in patients over age 60.
Children: 1 to 10 mEq (84 to 840 mg)/kg daily.
Antacid
Adults: 300 mg to 2 g P.O. one to four times daily.

Pharmacodynamics
Alkalinizing buffering action: An alkalinizing drug that dissociates to provide bicarbonate ion. Bicarbonate in excess of that needed to buffer hydrogen ions causes systemic alkalinization and, when excreted, urinary alkalinization as well.
Oral antacid action: Taken orally, sodium bicarbonate neutralizes stomach acid by the above mechanism.

Pharmacokinetics
• *Absorption:* Well absorbed after oral administration as sodium ion and bicarbonate.
• *Distribution:* Bicarbonate occurs naturally; confined to systemic circulation.
• *Metabolism:* None.
• *Excretion:* Bicarbonate filtered and reabsorbed by kidney; less than 1% of filtered bicarbonate excreted.

Contraindications and precautions
Contraindicated in patients with metabolic or respiratory alkalosis; in those who are losing chlorides by vomiting or from continuous GI suction; in those receiving diuretics known to produce hypochloremic alkalosis; and in patients with hypocalcemia in which alkalosis may produce tetany, hypertension, seizures, or heart failure. Orally administered sodium bicarbonate is contraindicated in patients with acute ingestion of strong mineral acids.
    Use with extreme caution in patients with heart failure, renal insufficiency, or other edematous or sodium-retaining conditions.

Interactions
Drug-drug. *Amphetamines, ephedrine, pseudoephedrine, quinidine:* Increased half-life of these drugs (if urinary alkalinization occurs). Monitor patient closely and adjust dosages as needed.
Chlorpropamide, lithium, salicylates, tetracyclines: Increased urinary excretion of these drugs. Monitor patient closely and adjust dosages as needed.

Reactions may be *common*, uncommon, *life-threatening*, or COMMON AND LIFE-THREATENING.

Corticosteroids: Increased sodium retention. If concomitant use can't be avoided, use together cautiously.

Adverse reactions
GI: gastric distention, belching, flatulence.
Metabolic: *metabolic alkalosis,* hypernatremia, increased serum lactate levels, hyperosmolarity (with overdose).
Other: local pain and irritation at injection site.

☑ Special considerations
● Avoid extravasation of I.V. solutions. Addition of calcium salts may cause precipitate; bicarbonate may inactivate catecholamines in solution (epinephrine, phenylephrine, and dopamine).
● Discourage use as an oral antacid because of hazardous excessive systemic absorption.
● Drug may be used as an adjunct to treat hyperkalemia (with dextrose and insulin).
● Signs and symptoms of overdose include depressed consciousness and obtundation from hypernatremia, tetany from hypocalcemia, arrhythmias from hypokalemia, and seizures from alkalosis. Correct fluid, electrolyte, and pH abnormalities. Monitor vital signs and fluid and electrolytes closely.

Monitoring the patient
● Monitor vital signs regularly; when drug is used as urinary alkalinizer, monitor urine pH.
● Assess patient for milk-alkali syndrome if drug use is long-term.

Information for the patient
● Advise patient to avoid prolonged use as an oral antacid, and recommend nonabsorbable antacids.
● If patient takes oral dose form, tell patient to take drug 1 hour before or 2 hours after taking enteric-coated drugs because drug may cause enteric-coated products to dissolve in stomach.

Geriatric patients
● Elderly patients with heart failure or other fluid-retaining conditions are at greater risk for increased fluid retention; use drug with caution.

Pediatric patients
● Avoid rapid infusion (10 ml/minute) of hypertonic solutions in children under age 2.

Breast-feeding patients
● It's unknown if drug appears in breast milk. Use cautiously in breast-feeding women.

sodium chloride (NaCl)

Pharmacologic classification: electrolyte
Therapeutic classification: sodium and chloride replacement
Pregnancy risk category C

How supplied
Available by prescription only
Injection: 0.45% NaCl 25 ml, 50 ml, 150 ml, 250 ml, 500 ml, 1,000 ml; 0.9% NaCl 2 ml, 3 ml, 5 ml, 10 ml, 20 ml, 25 ml, 30 ml, 50 ml, 100 ml, 150 ml, 250 ml, 500 ml, 1,000 ml; 3% NaCl 500 ml; 5% NaCl 500 ml
Available without a prescription
Tablets: 650 mg, 1 g
Tablets (slow-release): 600 mg

Indications, route, and dosage
Water and electrolyte replacement in hyponatremia from electrolyte loss or severe NaCl depletion
Adults and children: Treatment is highly individualized based on frequent assessment of laboratory values and clinical picture. See manufacturer's recommendations for P.O. dosing.

Pharmacodynamics
Electrolyte replacement: Replaces deficiencies of the sodium and chloride ions in blood plasma.

Pharmacokinetics
● *Absorption:* Oral and parenteral NaCl absorbed readily.
● *Distribution:* Distributed widely.
● *Metabolism:* None significant.
● *Excretion:* Sodium and chloride eliminated primarily in urine, but also in sweat, tears, and saliva.

Contraindications and precautions
Contraindicated in patients with conditions in which sodium and chloride administration is detrimental. NaCl 3% and 5% injections are contraindicated in patients with increased, normal, or only slightly decreased serum electrolyte levels.
    Use cautiously in patients with heart failure, renal dysfunction, circulatory insufficiency, or hypoproteinemia and in elderly or postoperative patients.

Interactions
None reported.

Adverse reactions
CV: aggravation of heart failure; edema (if given too rapidly or in excess); thrombophlebitis.
Metabolic: hypernatremia and aggravation of existing metabolic acidosis (with excessive infu-

sion); serious electrolyte disturbances, loss of potassium.

Respiratory: *pulmonary edema* (if given too rapidly or in excess).

Other: local tenderness, abscess, tissue necrosis at injection site.

☑ Special considerations

• Use concentrated solutions (3% and 5%) only for correcting severe sodium deficits (sodium level below 120 mEq/ml). The solutions should be infused very slowly and with caution to avoid pulmonary edema. Observe patient constantly.

• Concentrated solutions (3.5 and 4 mEq/ml) are available for addition to parenteral nutrition solutions.

• Normal saline solution may be used in managing extreme dilution of hyponatremia and hypochloremia resulting from administration of sodium-free fluids during fluid and electrolyte therapy, and in managing extreme dilution of extracellular fluid after excessive water intake (for example, after several enemas).

• NaCl overdose causes serious electrolyte disturbances. Oral ingestion of large quantities irritates GI mucosa and may cause nausea and vomiting, diarrhea, and abdominal cramps.

• To treat oral overdose, empty stomach, give magnesium sulfate as a cathartic, and provide supportive therapy. Provide airway and ventilation, if necessary. Excessive I.V. administration requires stopping NaCl infusion.

Monitoring the patient

• Monitor changes in fluid balance, serum electrolyte disturbances, and acid-base imbalances.

• Watch for hypokalemia with administration of potassium-free solutions.

Information for the patient

• Inform patient of therapeutic goal.

• Advise patient to immediately report any change in respiratory status.

---

sodium ferric gluconate complex
Ferrlecit

Pharmacologic classification: macro-molecular iron complex
Therapeutic classification: hematinic
Pregnancy risk category B

How supplied

Available by prescription only
Injection: 62.5 mg elemental iron (12.5 mg/ml) in 5-ml ampules

Indications, route, and dosage

Iron deficiency anemia in patients undergoing long-term hemodialysis who are receiving supplemental erythropoietin therapy

Adults: Before initiating therapeutic doses, administer a test dose of 2 ml sodium ferric gluconate complex (25 mg elemental iron) diluted in 50 ml normal saline solution and given intravenously (I.V.) over 1 hour. If test dose is tolerated, give therapeutic dose of 10 ml (125 mg elemental iron) diluted in 100 ml normal saline solution and given I.V. over 1 hour. Most patients require a minimum cumulative dose of 1 g elemental iron administered at more than eight sequential dialysis treatments to achieve a favorable hemoglobin or hematocrit response.

Pharmacodynamics

Hematinic action: Restores total body iron content, which is critical for normal hemoglobin synthesis and oxygen transport. Iron deficiency in hemodialysis patients can be due to increased iron utilization (such as from erythropoietin therapy), blood loss (such as from fistula, retention in dialyzer, hematologic testing, menses), decreased dietary intake or absorption, surgery, iron sequestration caused by inflammatory process, and malignancy.

Pharmacokinetics

No information available.

Contraindications and precautions

Contraindicated in patients with hypersensitivity to drug or its components (such as benzyl alcohol). Also contraindicated in patients with anemias not associated with iron deficiency. Don't administer to patients with iron overload. Use cautiously in elderly patients.

Interactions

None reported.

Adverse reactions

CNS: asthenia, headache, fatigue, malaise, dizziness, paresthesia, agitation, insomnia, somnolence, syncope.

CV: hypotension, hypertension, tachycardia, *bradycardia,* angina, chest pain, *MI,* edema, flushing.

EENT: conjunctivitis, abnormal vision, rhinitis.

GI: nausea, vomiting, diarrhea, rectal disorder, dyspepsia, eructation, flatulence, melena, abdominal pain.

GU: urinary tract infection.

Hematologic: abnormal erythrocytes, anemia.

Metabolic: hyperkalemia, hypoglycemia, hypokalemia, hypervolemia.

Musculoskeletal: myalgia, arthralgia, back pain, arm pain, cramps.

Reactions may be *common,* uncommon, *life-threatening,* or COMMON AND LIFE-THREATENING.

Respiratory: dyspnea, coughing, upper respiratory tract infections, pneumonia, pulmonary edema.
Skin: pruritus, increased sweating, rash.
Other: injection site reaction, pain, fever, infection, rigors, chills, flulike syndrome, sepsis, *carcinoma, hypersensitivity reactions,* lymphadenopathy.

☑ Special considerations

• Potential life-threatening hypersensitivity reactions (characterized by cardiovascular collapse, cardiac arrest, bronchospasm, oral or pharyngeal edema, dyspnea, angioedema, urticaria, or pruritus sometimes associated with pain and muscle spasm of chest or back) may occur. Have adequate supportive measures readily available. Monitor patient closely during infusion.
• Profound hypotension associated with flushing, light-headedness, malaise, fatigue, weakness, or severe chest, back, flank, or groin pain has been reported after rapid I.V. administration of iron. These reactions aren't associated with hypersensitivity reactions and may be due to too rapid drug administration. Don't exceed recommended rate of administration (2.1 mg/minute). Monitor patient closely during infusion.
• Some adverse reactions in hemodialysis patients may be related to dialysis itself or to chronic renal failure.
• Check with patient about other potential sources of iron, such as nonprescription iron preparations and iron-containing multiple vitamins with minerals.
• Don't mix sodium ferric gluconate complex with other drugs or add to parenteral nutrition solutions. Use immediately after dilution in normal saline solution.
• Serum iron levels greater than 300 mcg/dl (with transferrin oversaturation) may indicate iron poisoning. Signs and symptoms include abdominal pain, diarrhea, or vomiting that progresses to pallor or cyanosis, lassitude, drowsiness, hyperventilation due to acidosis, and cardiovascular collapse. Treatment consists of supportive measures.
• Drug isn't dialyzable.

Monitoring the patient
• Monitor hemoglobin level and hematocrit during therapy.
• Monitor serum ferritin and iron saturation levels during therapy.

Information for the patient
• Abdominal pain, diarrhea, vomiting, drowsiness, or hyperventilation may indicate iron poisoning. Advise patient to immediately report any of these symptoms.

Geriatric patients
• It's unknown if patients ages 65 and older respond differently to drug than younger patients. In general, use cautiously in elderly patients because they may be taking other drugs or may have concomitant disease or decreased hepatic, renal, or cardiac function.

Pediatric patients
• Safety and effectiveness in children haven't been established.

Breast-feeding patients
• It's unknown if drug appears in breast milk. Because many drugs appear in breast milk, use with caution in breast-feeding women.

sodium fluoride
ACT, Fluorigard, Fluorinse, Fluoritab, Flura-Drops, Flura-Loz, Karidium, Karigel, Karigel-N, Luride, Luride Lozi-Tabs, Luride-SF Lozi-Tabs, Pediaflor, Phos-Flur, Point-Two, Prevident, Thera-Flur, Thera-Flur-N

Pharmacologic classification: trace mineral
Therapeutic classification: dental caries prophylactic
Pregnancy risk category C

How supplied
Available by prescription only
Tablets: 1 mg (sugar-free)
Tablets (chewable): 0.5 mg, 1 mg (sugar-free)
Drops: 0.125 mg/drop (30 ml), 0.125 mg/drop (60 ml, sugar-free), 0.25 mg/drop (19 ml), 0.25 mg/drop (24 ml, sugar-free), 0.5 mg/ml (50 ml)
Rinse: 0.09% (240 ml, 480 ml), 0.09% (480 ml, sugar-free)
Gel: 0.1% (65 g, 105 g, 122 g), 0.5% (24 g, 30 g, 60 g, 120 g, 130 g, 250 g), 1.23% (480 ml)
Gel drops: 0.5% (24 ml)
Available without a prescription
Rinse: 0.01% (180 ml, 300 ml, 360 ml, 480 ml, 540 ml, 720 ml, 960 ml, 1,740 ml); 0.02% (90 ml, 180 ml, 300 ml, 360 ml, 480 ml)
Gel: 0.1% (60 g, 120 g)

Indications, route, and dosage
Aid in prevention of dental caries
Oral
Children ages 6 months to 3 years: 0.25 mg daily.
Children ages 3 to 6: 0.5 mg daily.
Children ages 6 to 16: 1 mg daily.
✦ *Dosage adjustment.* If fluoride in the drinking water is below 0.3 ppm (mg/L), use dosage listed; if fluoride content is 0.3 to 0.6 ppm, use one-half of dosage; if fluoride content exceeds 0.6 ppm, don't use.

Topical

Adults and children over age 12: 10 ml of 0.09% (0.2% fluoride ion) rinse. Use once daily after thoroughly brushing teeth and rinsing mouth. Rinse around and between teeth for 1 minute, then spit out.

Children ages 6 to 12: 5 ml of 0.09% (0.2% fluoride ion) solution. Use once daily as a rinse.

Pharmacodynamics

Dental caries prophylactic action: Acts systemically before tooth eruption and topically afterward by increasing tooth resistance to acid dissolution, by promoting remineralization, and by inhibiting the cariogenic microbial process. Acidulation provides greater topical fluoride uptake by dental enamel than neutral solutions. When topical fluoride is applied to hypersensitive exposed dentin, the formation of insoluble materials within the dentinal tubules blocks transmission of painful stimuli.

Pharmacokinetics

- *Absorption:* Absorbed readily and almost completely from GI tract. Large amount of oral dose may be absorbed in stomach; rate of absorption may depend on gastric pH. Oral fluoride absorption may be decreased by simultaneous ingestion of aluminum or magnesium hydroxide. Simultaneous ingestion of calcium also may decrease absorption of large doses. Normal total plasma fluoride levels range from 0.14 to 0.19 mcg/ml.
- *Distribution:* Stored in bones and developing teeth after absorption. Skeletal tissue also has a high storage capacity for fluoride ions. Because of storage-mobilization mechanism in skeletal tissue, a constant fluoride supply may be provided. Although teeth have small mass, they also serve as storage sites. Fluoride deposited in teeth isn't released readily. Fluoride has been found in all organs and tissues with a low accumulation in noncalcified tissues. Fluoride distributed into sweat, tears, hair, and saliva; crosses placenta and is distributed into breast milk. Fluoride levels in milk range from about 0.05 to 0.13 ppm and remain fairly constant.
- *Metabolism:* Not metabolized.
- *Excretion:* Excreted rapidly, mainly in urine. About 90% of fluoride is filtered by glomerulus and reabsorbed by renal tubules.

Contraindications and precautions

Contraindicated in patients with hypersensitivity to fluoride or when intake from drinking water exceeds 0.6 ppm.

Interactions

Drug-drug. *Aluminum hydroxide, magnesium:* Impaired absorption of sodium fluoride. Avoid concomitant use.

Drug-food. *Dairy products:* Calcium fluoride formation with concomitant use of systemic fluorides. Use with caution.

Adverse reactions

CNS: headache, weakness.
GI: gastric distress.
Skin: hypersensitivity reactions (atopic dermatitis, eczema, urticaria).
Other: staining of teeth.

☑ Special considerations

- Fluoride supplementation must be continuous from infancy to age 14 to be effective.
- Tablets can be dissolved in mouth, chewed, swallowed whole, added to drinking water or fruit juice, or added to water in infant formula or other foods.
- Drops may be administered orally undiluted or added to fluids or food.
- Sodium fluoride may be preferred to stannous fluoride to avoid staining tooth surfaces. Neutral sodium fluoride also may be preferred to acidulated fluoride to avoid dulling of porcelain and ceramic restorations.
- Prolonged intake of drinking water containing a fluoride ion concentration of 0.4 to 0.8 ppm may result in increased density of bone mineral and fluoride osteosclerosis.
- An oral sodium fluoride dose of 40 to 65 mg/day has resulted in adverse rheumatic effects.
- Drug is used for investigational purposes to treat osteoporosis.
- In children, acute ingestion of 10 to 20 mg of sodium fluoride may cause excessive salivation and GI disturbances; 500 mg may be fatal. GI disturbances include salivation, nausea, abdominal pain, vomiting, and diarrhea. CNS disturbances include CNS irritability, paresthesia, tetany, hyperactive reflexes, seizures, and respiratory or cardiac failure (from calcium-binding effect of fluoride). Hypoglycemia and hypocalcemia are frequent laboratory findings.
- Using gastric lavage with 1% to 5% calcium chloride solution may cause the fluoride to precipitate. Administer glucose I.V. in saline solution; parenteral calcium administration may be indicated for tetany. Maintain adequate urine output.

Monitoring the patient

- Monitor patient for adverse effects.

Information for the patient

- Tell patient that tablets and drops should be taken with meals but not with dairy products.
- Advise patient that rinse and gel are most effective if used immediately after brushing or flossing and when taken at bedtime.
- Tell patient to expectorate (and not swallow) excess liquid or gel.

Reactions may be *common*, uncommon, *life-threatening*, or COMMON AND LIFE-THREATENING.

• Advise patient not to eat, drink, or rinse mouth for 15 to 30 minutes after application. Tell patient to use a plastic container—not glass—to dilute drops or rinse because the fluoride interacts with glass.
• Encourage patient to notify dentist if mottling of teeth occurs.
• Advise patient that, if there is a change in water supply or if patient moves to another area, a dentist should be contacted because excessive fluoride causes mottled tooth enamel. If patient uses a private well, the water should be tested for fluoride.
• Warn parents to treat fluoride tablets as a drug and to keep them away from children.

Pediatric patients
• Young children usually can't perform the rinse process necessary with oral solutions.
• Because prolonged ingestion or improper techniques may result in dental fluorosis and osseous changes, the dosage must be carefully adjusted according to amount of fluoride ion in drinking water.

Breast-feeding patients
• Very little sodium fluoride appears in breast milk. Levels in breast milk increase only when daily intake exceeds 1.5 mg.

sodium phosphates (sodium phosphate and sodium biphosphate)
Fleet Phospho-Soda

Pharmacologic classification: acid salt
Therapeutic classification: NaCl laxative
Pregnancy risk category C

How supplied
Available without a prescription
Solution: 18 g sodium phosphate and 48 g sodium biphosphate/100 ml

Indications, route, and dosage
Constipation
Adults: 20- to 30-ml solution mixed with 120 ml (4 oz) cold water.
Children ages 10 to 12: 10 ml solution mixed with 4 oz cold water.
Children ages 5 to 10: 5 ml solution mixed with 4 oz cold water.
Purgative action
Adults: 45-ml solution mixed with 4 oz cold water.

Pharmacodynamics
Laxative action: Exerts an osmotic effect in the small intestine by drawing water into the intesti-

nal lumen, producing distention that promotes peristalsis and bowel evacuation.

Pharmacokinetics
• *Absorption:* About 1% to 20% of oral dose of sodium and phosphate absorbed. With oral administration, action begins in 3 to 6 hours.
• *Distribution:* No information available.
• *Metabolism:* No information available.
• *Excretion:* No information available; probably excreted in feces and urine.

Contraindications and precautions
Contraindicated in patients with abdominal pain, nausea, vomiting, or other symptoms of appendicitis or acute surgical abdomen; intestinal obstruction or perforation; edema; heart failure; megacolon; or impaired renal function and in patients on sodium-restricted diets. Use cautiously in patients with large hemorrhoids or anal excoriations.

Interactions
Drug-drug. *Antacids:* Possible inactivation of both products. Avoid concomitant use.

Adverse reactions
GI: *abdominal cramping.*
Metabolic: fluid and electrolyte disturbances (hypernatremia, hyperphosphatemia) with daily use.
Other: laxative dependence with long-term or excessive use.

☑ Special considerations
• Dilute drug with water before taking orally (add 30 ml of drug to 120 ml [4 oz] of water); then follow with full glass of water.
• Drug isn't routinely used to treat constipation but is commonly used to evacuate bowel.
• Probable effects of overdose include abdominal pain and diarrhea.

Monitoring the patient
• Monitor serum electrolyte levels; when drug is given as NaCl laxative, up to 10% of sodium content may be absorbed.
• Monitor therapeutic effect.

Information for the patient
• Advise patient on how to mix drug and on dosing schedule.
• Warn patient that frequent or prolonged use of drug may lead to laxative dependence.

sodium polystyrene sulfonate
Kayexalate, SPS

Pharmacologic classification: cation-exchange resin
Therapeutic classification: potassium-removing resin
Pregnancy risk category C

How supplied
Available by prescription only
Oral powder: 1.25 g/5 ml suspension
Powder for oral or rectal administration: 453.6 g in 1-lb jar
Rectal administration: 1.25 g/5 ml, 15 g/60 ml suspension

Indications, route, and dosage
Hyperkalemia
Adults: 15 g P.O. daily to q.i.d. in water or sorbitol. Or give 30 to 50 g q.i.d. or q 6 hours as a retention enema.

Pharmacodynamics
Potassium-removing action: A cation-exchange resin that releases sodium in exchange for other cations in the GI tract. High levels of potassium ion are found in the large intestine and therefore are exchanged and eliminated.

Pharmacokinetics
- *Absorption:* Not absorbed. Onset of action varies from hours to days.
- *Distribution:* None.
- *Metabolism:* None.
- *Excretion:* Excreted unchanged in feces.

Contraindications and precautions
Contraindicated in patients with hypersensitivity to drug and in those with hypokalemia. Use cautiously in patients with marked edema or severe heart failure or hypertension.

Interactions
Drug-drug. *Antacids containing calcium and magnesium:* Possible metabolic alkalosis in patients with renal impairment. Monitor patient closely and avoid concomitant use.
Cardiac glycosides: Enhanced cardiac response. Monitor cardiac status closely.

Adverse reactions
GI: *constipation,* fecal impaction (in elderly patients), anorexia, gastric irritation, nausea, vomiting, *diarrhea* (with sorbitol emulsions).
Metabolic: *hypokalemia,* hypocalcemia, sodium retention, altered serum magnesium level.

☑ Special considerations
- Rectal route is recommended when vomiting, P.O. restrictions, or upper GI tract problems are present.
- Fecal impaction can be prevented in elderly patients by administering resin rectally. Cleaning enema should precede rectal administration.
- For rectal administration, mix polystyrene resin only with water and sorbitol. To prevent impactions, don't use other vehicles such as mineral oil for rectal administration. Ion exchange requires aqueous medium. Sorbitol content prevents impaction.
- Constipation is more likely to occur when drug is given with phosphate binders such as aluminum hydroxide.
- If hyperkalemia is severe, more drastic modalities should be added; for example, dextrose 50% with regular insulin I.V. push. Don't depend solely on polystyrene resin to lower serum potassium levels in severe hyperkalemia.
- Signs and symptoms of overdose include hypokalemia (irritability, confusion, arrhythmias, ECG changes, severe muscle weakness, and sometimes paralysis) and digitalis toxicity in digitalized patients. Drug may be discontinued or dose lowered when serum potassium level falls to the 4 to 5 mEq/L range.

Monitoring the patient
- Monitor serum potassium level at least once daily. Watch for other signs of hypokalemia.
- Monitor bowel status if rectal administration is being used.
- Watch for symptoms of other electrolyte deficiencies (magnesium, calcium) because drug is nonselective. Monitor serum calcium level in patients receiving sodium polystyrene therapy for more than 3 days. Supplementary calcium may be needed.

Information for the patient
- Advise patient of importance of following a prescribed low-potassium diet.
- Explain to patient the necessity of retaining enema. Retention for 6 to 10 hours is ideal, but 30 to 60 minutes is acceptable.

Geriatric patients
- Fecal impaction is more likely in elderly patients.

Pediatric patients
- Adjust dosage in children based upon a calculation of 1 mEq of potassium bound for each 1 g of resin.

Breast-feeding patients
- It's unknown if drug appears in breast milk. Use with caution in breast-feeding women.

---

somatropin
Genotropin, Humatrope, Norditropin,
Nutropin, Nutropin AQ, Serostim,
Saizen

Pharmacologic classification: anterior
pituitary hormone
Therapeutic classification: purified
growth hormone (GH)
Pregnancy risk category C

How supplied
Available by prescription only
Injection: 10 mg (30 IU)/2-ml vial
Powder for injection: 1.5 mg (4 IU), 4 mg (12 IU),
5 mg (13–15 IU), 5.8 mg (15 IU), 6 mg (18 IU),
8 mg (24 IU), 10 mg (26 IU)/vial with diluent or
as ready-mix

Indications, route, and dosage
**Long-term treatment of growth failure in chil-
dren with inadequate secretion of endogenous GH**
Children: Administer up to 0.06 mg/kg of body
weight of Humatrope S.C. or I.M. three times
weekly or 0.30 mg/kg of body weight of Nutropin
S.C. weekly in daily divided doses. Administer
0.06 mg/kg of Saizen S.C. or I.M. three times
weekly and stop when epiphyses are fused. Administer 0.024 to 0.034 mg/kg of Norditropin S.C.
six to seven times weekly.
**Growth failure associated with chronic renal
insufficiency up to time of renal transplantation in children**
Children: Administer 0.35 mg/kg of body weight
of Nutropin S.C. weekly in daily divided doses.
Turner's syndrome
Children: Administer up to 0.375 mg/kg of Nutropin or Nutropin AQ S.C. or I.M. in equally divided doses three to seven times weekly.
Cachexia
Children: Administer Serostim per kg of body
weight as follows: if greater than 55 kg (121 lb),
6 mg S.C. daily; if 45 to 55 kg (99 to 121 lb), 5
mg S.C. daily; if 35 to 45 kg (77 to 99 lb), 4 mg
S.C. daily.

Pharmacodynamics
Growth-stimulating action: Purified GH of recombinant DNA origin that stimulates skeletal,
linear bone, muscle, and organ growth.

Pharmacokinetics
• *Absorption:* Absorbed from injection site in a
similar fashion as somatrem (human GH).
• *Distribution:* Localizes to highly perfused or-
gans, notably liver and kidneys.
• *Metabolism:* Metabolized in liver.
• *Excretion:* Returned to systemic circulation as
amino acids.

Contraindications and precautions
Contraindicated in patients with closed epiphyses or an active underlying intracranial lesion.
Humatrope shouldn't be reconstituted with the
supplied diluent for patients with sensitivity to either m-cresol or glycerin.
 Use cautiously in children with hypothyroidism and in those whose GH deficiency results
from an intracranial lesion; these children should
be examined frequently for progression or recurrence of underlying disease.

Interactions
None reported.

Adverse reactions
CNS: headache, weakness.
CV: mild, transient edema.
Hematologic: *leukemia.*
Metabolic: mild hyperglycemia, hypothyroidism;
increased inorganic phosphorus, alkaline phos-
phatase, and parathyroid hormone levels.
Other: injection site pain, localized muscle pain,
antibody formation to GH.

☑ Special considerations
• Excessive glucocorticoid therapy inhibits growth-
promoting effect of somatropin. Adjust glucocorticoid replacement dose in patients with a coexisting corticotropin deficiency to avoid an inhibitory
effect on growth.
• Long-term overdose may result in signs and
symptoms of gigantism or acromegaly consistent with the effects of excess human GH.

Monitoring the patient
• Monitor child's height regularly. Regular monitoring of blood and radiologic studies is also necessary.
• Monitor patient's blood glucose levels regularly because GH may induce a state of insulin resistance.
• Periodically monitor thyroid function tests for
hypothyroidism, which may need treatment with
a thyroid hormone.

Information for the patient
• Inform parents that children with endocrine disorders, including GH deficiency, are more likely
to develop slipped capital epiphyses. Tell them to
call if they notice that their child is limping.

---

sotalol hydrochloride
Betapace

Pharmacologic classification: beta blocker
Therapeutic classification: anti-arrhythmic
Pregnancy risk category B

How supplied
Available by prescription only
Tablets: 80 mg, 120 mg, 160 mg, 240 mg

Indications, route, and dosage
Documented, life-threatening ventricular arrhythmias
Adults: Initially, 80 mg P.O. b.i.d. Increase dose q 2 to 3 days as needed and tolerated. Most patients respond to daily dose of 160 to 320 mg. A few patients with refractory arrhythmias have received as much as 640 mg daily.
✦ *Dosage adjustment.* For adults with renal failure and creatinine clearance above 60 ml/minute, no adjustment in dose interval is necessary. If creatinine clearance is 30 to 60 ml/minute, give q 24 hours; if 10 to 30 ml/minute, give q 36 to 48 hours; and if less than 10 ml/minute, individualize dosage.

Pharmacodynamics
Antiarrhythmic action: Nonselective beta blocker that depresses sinus heart rate, slows AV conduction, increases AV nodal refractoriness, prolongs the refractory period of atrial and ventricular muscle and AV accessory pathways in anterograde and retrograde directions, decreases cardiac output, and lowers systolic and diastolic blood pressure.

Pharmacokinetics
● *Absorption:* Well absorbed after oral administration, with bioavailability of 90% to 100%. After oral administration, plasma levels peak in 2½ to 4 hours; steady-state plasma levels in 2 to 3 days (after five to six doses when administered twice daily).
● *Distribution:* Not bound to plasma proteins; crosses blood-brain barrier poorly.
● *Metabolism:* Not metabolized.
● *Excretion:* Excreted primarily in urine unchanged.

Contraindications and precautions
Contraindicated in patients with hypersensitivity to drug and in those with severe sinus node dysfunction, sinus bradycardia, second- and third-degree AV block in the absence of an artificial pacemaker, congenital or acquired long QT interval syndrome, cardiogenic shock, uncontrolled heart failure, or bronchial asthma.

Use cautiously in patients with impaired renal function or diabetes mellitus.

Interactions
Drug-drug. *Antiarrhythmics:* Additive effects. Monitor patient closely; adjust dosage.
Calcium channel antagonists: Enhanced myocardial depression. Don't give with sotalol.
Catecholamine-depleting drugs (such as guanethidine, reserpine): Enhanced hypotensive effects. Monitor patient closely.
Clonidine: Enhanced rebound hypertensive effect seen after withdrawal. Stop sotalol several days before withdrawing clonidine.
Insulin, oral antidiabetics: Increased blood glucose levels; masked symptoms of hypoglycemia. Monitor patient closely; adjust dosage.
Drug-food. *Any food:* Increased absorption. Give drug on empty stomach.

Adverse reactions
CNS: asthenia, light-headedness, headache, dizziness, weakness, fatigue, sleep problems.
CV: *bradycardia, palpitations, chest pain, arrhythmias, heart failure, AV block, proarrhythmic events (ventricular tachycardia, PVCs, ventricular fibrillation),* edema, ECG abnormalities, hypotension.
GI: *nausea, vomiting,* diarrhea, dyspepsia.
Hepatic: elevated liver enzyme levels.
Metabolic: increased serum glucose level.
Respiratory: *dyspnea, bronchospasm.*

☑ Special considerations
● Make dosage adjustments slowly, allowing 2 to 3 days between dose increments for adequate monitoring of QT intervals and for drug plasma levels to reach steady-state.
● Because proarrhythmic events, such as sustained ventricular tachycardia or ventricular fibrillation, may occur at start of therapy and during dosage adjustments, patient should be hospitalized. Facilities and personnel should be available for cardiac rhythm monitoring and ECG interpretation.
● Electrolyte imbalances, such as hypokalemia or hypomagnesemia, may enhance QT interval prolongation and increase risk of serious arrhythmias such as torsades de pointes.
● Although patients receiving I.V. lidocaine have begun sotalol therapy without ill effect, other antiarrhythmics should be withdrawn before sotalol therapy begins. Sotalol therapy typically is delayed until two or three half-lives of the withdrawn drug have elapsed. After withdrawal of amiodarone, sotalol shouldn't be administered until QT interval normalizes.
● The most common signs and symptoms of overdose are bradycardia, heart failure, hypotension, bronchospasm, and hypoglycemia. If overdose occurs, stop sotalol and observe patient closely. Because of lack of protein-binding, hemodialy-

---

sis is useful in reducing sotalol plasma levels. Patients should be carefully observed until QT intervals are normalized.
• Atropine, another anticholinergic, a beta-adrenergic agonist, or transvenous cardiac pacing may also be used to treat bradycardia; transvenous cardiac pacing to treat second- or third-degree heart block; epinephrine to treat hypotension (depending on associated factors); aminophylline or an aerosol beta$_2$-receptor stimulant to treat bronchospasm; and direct current cardioversion, transvenous cardiac pacing, epinephrine, or magnesium sulfate to treat torsades de pointes.

Monitoring the patient
• Monitor cardiac status and serum electrolyte levels regularly, especially if patient is receiving diuretics.
• Monitor patient for adverse effects.

Information for the patient
• Explain to patient the importance of taking drug as prescribed, even when he is feeling well.
• Caution patient not to stop drug suddenly.

Pediatric patients
• Safety and effectiveness in children haven't been established.

Breast-feeding patients
• Drug may appear in breast milk. Stop either breast-feeding or drug, depending on importance of drug to mother.

sparfloxacin
Zagam

Pharmacologic classification: fluorinated quinolone
Therapeutic classification: broad-spectrum antibacterial
Pregnancy risk category C

How supplied
Available by prescription only
Tablets: 200 mg

Indications, route, and dosage
Acute bacterial exacerbation of chronic bronchitis caused by Staphylococcus aureus, Streptococcus pneumoniae, Chlamydia pneumoniae, Enterobacter cloacae, Klebsiella pneumoniae, Moraxella catarrhalis, Haemophilus influenzae, or H. parainfluenzae
Adults over age 18: 400 mg P.O. on first day as a loading dose; then 200 mg daily for total of 10 days of therapy (total, 11 tablets).
Community-acquired pneumonia caused by S. pneumoniae, M. catarrhalis, H. influenzae,

H. parainfluenzae, C. pneumoniae, *or* **Mycoplasma pneumoniae**
Adults over age 18: 400 mg P.O. on first day as a loading dose; then 200 mg daily for total of 10 days of therapy (total, 11 tablets).
♦ **Dosage adjustment.** For patients with renal impairment, if creatinine clearance is below 50 ml/minute, give a loading dose of 400 mg P.O.; then 200 mg P.O. q 48 hours for a total of 9 days of therapy (total, six tablets).

Pharmacodynamics
Antibactericidal action: Inhibits bacterial DNA gyrase and prevents DNA replication, transcription, repair, and deactivation in susceptible bacteria.

Pharmacokinetics
• *Absorption:* Well absorbed after oral administration; absolute bioavailability of 92%. Maximum plasma levels achieved 3 to 6 hours after dosing.
• *Distribution:* Volume of distribution is about 3.9 L/kg; distributed well into tissues. Level of drug in respiratory tissues at 2 to 6 hours after dosing is about three to six times greater than plasma.
• *Metabolism:* Metabolized by liver, primarily by phase II glucuronidation. Metabolism doesn't interfere with or use cytochrome P-450 system.
• *Excretion:* Excreted in both urine (50%) and feces (50%). Terminal elimination half-life varies between 16 and 30 hours; mean, 20 hours.

Contraindications and precautions
Contraindicated in patients with history of hypersensitivity or photosensitivity reactions to drug and in those who can't stay out of the sun. Don't use in patients with cardiac conditions that predispose them to arrhythmias.
    Use with caution in patients with known or suspected CNS disorders, such as seizures, toxic psychoses, or tremors.

Interactions
Drug-drug. *Antacids containing aluminum or magnesium, iron salts, sucralfate, zinc:* Interfere with GI absorption of sparfloxacin. Administer at least 4 hours apart.
Drug-lifestyle. *Sun exposure:* Photosensitivity reactions. Tell patient to take precautions.

Adverse reactions
CNS: asthenia, dizziness, headache, insomnia, *seizures,* somnolence.
CV: *QT interval prolongation,* vasodilatation.
EENT: dry mouth, taste perversion.
GI: abdominal pain, diarrhea, dyspepsia, flatulence, nausea, pseudomembranous colitis, vomiting.
GU: vaginal candidiasis.
Hematologic: elevated WBC.
Hepatic: elevated liver enzyme levels.
Musculoskeletal: tendon rupture.

Skin: photosensitivity, pruritus, rash.
Other: *hypersensitivity reactions.*

☑ **Special considerations**
• Because moderate to severe phototoxic reactions have occurred, patient should avoid exposure to sun, bright natural light, or ultraviolet light during therapy and for 5 days after therapy.
• Drug may produce false-negative culture results for *Mycobacterium tuberculosis.*
• If overdose is suspected, have patient avoid sunlight exposure for 5 days. Monitor ECG for prolonged QTc interval. It's unknown if drug is dialyzable.

Monitoring the patient
• Monitor cardiac status and watch for adverse CNS symptoms.
• Monitor renal function carefully in elderly patients and adjust dosages as needed.

Information for the patient
• Inform patient that drug may be taken with food, milk, or products that contain caffeine.
• Tell patient to take drug as prescribed, even if symptoms disappear.
• Advise patient to take drug with plenty of fluids and to avoid antacids, sucralfate, and products containing iron or zinc for at least 4 hours after each dose.
• Advise patient to avoid direct, indirect, and artificial ultraviolet light, even with sunscreen on, during treatment and for 5 days after treatment. Patient should stop drug and call if signs or symptoms of phototoxicity (skin burning, redness, swelling, blisters, rash, itching) occur.
• Advise patient to stop drug and report pain or inflammation; tendon rupture can occur with drug. Tell patient to rest and refrain from exercise until a diagnosis is made.

Geriatric patients
• Drug's pharmacokinetics aren't altered in elderly patients with normal renal function.

Pediatric patients
• Safety and effectiveness in children and adolescents under age 18 haven't been established. Quinolones, including sparfloxacin, may cause arthropathy and osteochondrosis.

Breast-feeding patients
• Drug appears in breast milk. Stop either breast-feeding or drug.

spectinomycin hydrochloride
Trobicin

Pharmacologic classification: aminocyclitol
Therapeutic classification: antibiotic
Pregnancy risk category NR

How supplied
Available by prescription only
Injection: 2-g vial with 3.2-ml diluent

Indications, route, and dosage
Uncomplicated gonorrhea in patients who are hypersensitive to penicillins or cephalosporins
Adults: 2 to 4 g I.M. single dose injected deeply into upper outer quadrant of the buttocks (4-g dose should be divided into two sites).
◇ *Disseminated gonorrhea*
Adults: 2 g I.M. b.i.d. for 3 to 7 days. Inject deeply into upper outer quadrant of buttocks.

Pharmacodynamics
Antibacterial action: Bacteriostatic effect results from binding of drug to 30S ribosomal subunits, thus inhibiting protein synthesis. Although drug is effective against many gram-positive and gram-negative organisms, it's used mostly against penicillin-resistant *Neisseria gonorrhoeae.*

Pharmacokinetics
• *Absorption:* Not absorbed orally. I.M. injection results in rapid absorption; levels peak in 1 and 2 hours for 2-g and 4-g doses, respectively.
• *Distribution:* No information available.
• *Metabolism:* No information available.
• *Excretion:* Most of dose excreted unchanged in urine. Elimination half-life ranges from 1 to 3 hours. Drug dose unchanged in renal failure.

Contraindications and precautions
Contraindicated in patients with hypersensitivity to drug.

Interactions
None reported.

Adverse reactions
CNS: insomnia, dizziness.
GI: nausea.
GU: decreased urine output and creatinine clearance, increased BUN level.
Hematologic: decreased hemoglobin and hematocrit levels.
Hepatic: transient increases in liver enzyme levels.
Skin: urticaria.
Other: fever, chills (may mask or delay symptoms of incubating syphilis), pain at injection site.

Reactions may be *common,* uncommon, **life-threatening**, or COMMON AND LIFE-THREATENING.

☑ Special considerations

- Obtain specimen for culture and sensitivity tests before starting therapy.
- Drug is usually reserved for patients with penicillin-resistant gonorrhea strains or for whom other drugs are contraindicated. Ceftriaxone is considered drug of choice for uncomplicated gonorrhea.
- To prepare drug, add supplied diluent to vial and shake until completely dissolved. Use reconstituted solution within 24 hours.
- Inject deep I.M. into upper outer quadrant of gluteal muscle. Give 2-g dose at single site; divide 4-g dose into two equal injections and give at two sites.
- Drug is ineffective against syphilis and may mask symptoms of incubating syphilis infection; also not effective in pharyngeal gonococcal infections.
- Lack of response to drug usually results from reinfection.

Monitoring the patient
- Monitor therapeutic response to drug.
- Monitor patient for adverse effects.

Information for the patient
- Advise patient that sexual partners must be treated.

Pediatric patients
- Because its safety in infants and children hasn't been established, drug isn't first choice in treatment of these patients. However, drug may be used in children for treatment of gonococcal infections in those hypersensitive to penicillins. A single dose of 40 mg/kg is recommended by the CDC. Drug shouldn't be used in neonates because of benzyl alcohol preservative.

Breast-feeding patients
- It's unknown if drug appears in breast milk; an alternative to breast-feeding is recommended during therapy.

spironolactone
Aldactone

Pharmacologic classification: potassium-sparing diuretic
Therapeutic classification: management of edema; antihypertensive; diagnosis of primary hyperaldosteronism; treatment of diuretic-induced hypokalemia
Pregnancy risk category NR

How supplied
Available by prescription only
Tablets: 25 mg, 50 mg, 100 mg

Indications, route, and dosage
Edema
Adults: 25 to 200 mg P.O. daily in divided doses.
Children: Initially, 3.3 mg/kg or 60 mg/m² P.O. daily in divided doses.
Hypertension
Adults: 50 to 100 mg P.O. daily in divided doses.
Diuretic-induced hypokalemia
Adults: 25 to 100 mg P.O. daily when oral potassium supplements are considered inappropriate.
Detection of primary hyperaldosteronism
Adults: 400 mg P.O. daily for 4 days (short test) or for 3 to 4 weeks (long test). If hypokalemia and hypertension are corrected, a presumptive diagnosis of primary hyperaldosteronism is made.
◇ Hirsutism
Adults: 50 to 200 mg P.O. daily.
◇ Premenstrual syndrome
Adults: 25 mg q.i.d. P.O. on day 14 of menstrual cycle.
◇ To decrease risk of metrorrhagia
Adults: 50 mg b.i.d. P.O. on days 4 through 21 of menstrual cycle.
◇ Acne vulgaris
Adults: 100 mg P.O. daily.

Pharmacodynamics
Diuretic and potassium-sparing action: Competitively inhibits aldosterone effects on distal renal tubules, increasing sodium and water excretion and decreasing potassium excretion. Used to treat edema associated with excessive aldosterone secretion, such as that with hepatic cirrhosis, nephrotic syndrome, and heart failure. Also used to treat diuretic-induced hypokalemia.
Antihypertensive action: Mechanism unknown. May block effect of aldosterone on arteriolar smooth muscle.
Diagnosis of primary hyperaldosteronism: Inhibits effects of aldosterone; therefore, correction of hypokalemia and hypertension is presumptive evidence of primary hyperaldosteronism.

Pharmacokinetics
- *Absorption:* About 90% of drug absorbed after oral administration. Gradual onset of action; maximum effect occurs on third day of therapy.
- *Distribution:* Drug and major metabolite, canrenone, are more than 90% plasma protein–bound.
- *Metabolism:* Rapidly and extensively metabolized to canrenone.
- *Excretion:* Canrenone and other metabolites excreted primarily in urine; small amount excreted in feces via biliary tract. Half-life of canrenone is 13 to 24 hours; half-life of parent compound is 1 to 2 hours.

Contraindications and precautions
Contraindicated in patients with anuria, acute or progressive renal insufficiency, or hyperkalemia. Use cautiously in patients with impaired renal

function, hepatic disease, or fluid and electrolyte imbalances.

Interactions
Drug-drug. *ACE inhibitors, drugs containing potassium (parenteral penicillin G), potassium supplements, other potassium-sparing diuretics:* Hyperkalemia. Monitor potassium levels closely.
Antihypertensives: Potentiated hypotensive effect; may be used to therapeutic advantage. Monitor blood pressure. Adjust dosage if needed.
Aspirin: Slightly decreased response to spironolactone. Monitor therapeutic effect; adjust dosage if needed.
NSAIDs (such as ibuprofen, indomethacin): Impaired renal function affecting potassium excretion. Monitor patient closely; adjust dosage as needed.
Drug-herb. *Licorice:* May block antiulcerative and aldosterone-like effects of licorice. Avoid ingesting together.
Drug-food. *Potassium-rich foods (such as citrus fruit, tomatoes), salt substitutes containing potassium:* Increased risk of hyperkalemia. Tell patient to use low-potassium salt substitutes and ingest high-potassium foods cautiously.

Adverse reactions
CNS: headache, drowsiness, lethargy, confusion, ataxia.
GI: diarrhea, gastric bleeding, ulceration, cramping, gastritis, vomiting.
GU: inability to maintain erection, gynecomastia, breast soreness and menstrual disturbances in women.
Hematologic: *agranulocytosis.*
Metabolic: *hyperkalemia,* dehydration, hyponatremia, transient elevation in BUN level, metabolic acidosis.
Skin: urticaria, maculopapular eruptions, hirsutism.
Other: drug fever.

☑ Special considerations
Besides the recommendations relevant to all potassium-sparing diuretics, consider the following.
• Drug should be taken with meals to enhance absorption.
• Diuretic effect may be delayed 2 to 3 days if drug is used alone; maximum antihypertensive effect may be delayed 2 to 3 weeks.
• Adverse reactions are related to dose levels and duration of therapy and usually disappear with withdrawal of drug; however, gynecomastia may persist.
• Drug is antiandrogenic and has been used to treat hirsutism in doses of 200 mg/day.
• Avoid unnecessary use of drug. Drug may induce tumors.
• Spironolactone therapy alters fluorometric determinations of plasma and urinary 17-hydroxy-

corticosteroid levels and may cause false elevations on radioimmunoassay of serum digoxin.
• Signs and symptoms of overdose are consistent with those of dehydration and electrolyte disturbance.
• Treatment of overdose is supportive and symptomatic. In acute ingestion, empty stomach by emesis or lavage. In severe hyperkalemia (over 6.5 mEq/L), reduce serum potassium levels with I.V. sodium bicarbonate or glucose with insulin. A cation exchange resin, sodium polystyrene sulfonate (Kayexalate), given orally or as a retention enema, may also reduce serum potassium levels.

Monitoring the patient
• Monitor potassium levels.
• Monitor therapeutic response and watch for symptoms of adverse effects.

Information for the patient
• Explain that maximal diuresis may not occur until day 3 of therapy and that diuresis may continue for 2 to 3 days after drug is withdrawn.
• Advise patient to immediately report mental confusion or lethargy.
• Explain that adverse reactions usually disappear after drug is stopped; gynecomastia, however, may persist.
• Caution patient to avoid such hazardous activities as driving until response to drug is known.

Geriatric patients
• Elderly patients are more susceptible to diuretic effects and may need lower doses to prevent excessive diuresis.

Pediatric patients
• When administering drug to children, crush tablets and administer in cherry syrup as an oral suspension.

Breast-feeding patients
• Canrenone, a metabolite, appears in breast milk. Drug's safety during breast-feeding hasn't been established. An alternative to breast-feeding is recommended during therapy.

stavudine (d4T)
Zerit

Pharmacologic classification: synthetic thymidine nucleoside analogue
Therapeutic classification: antiviral
Pregnancy risk category C

How supplied
Available by prescription only
Capsules: 15 mg, 20 mg, 30 mg, 40 mg

Indications, route, and dosage

Patients with HIV infection who have received prolonged prior zidovudine therapy
Adults: For patients weighing 60 kg (132 lb) or more, 40 mg P.O. q 12 hours; for patients weighing below 60 kg, 30 mg P.O. q 12 hours.
✦ *Dosage adjustment.* For patients with renal impairment, use the table below.

Creatinine clearance (ml/min)	Dosage for patients weighing ≥ 60 kg	Dosage for patients weighing < 60 kg
> 50	40 mg q 12 hours	30 mg q 12 hours
26 to 50	20 mg q 12 hours	15 mg q 12 hours
10 to 25	20 mg q 24 hours	15 mg q 24 hours

Pharmacodynamics

Antiviral action: Phosphorylated by cellular kinases to stavudine triphosphate, which exerts antiviral activity. Stavudine triphosphate inhibits HIV replication by two known mechanisms. First, it inhibits HIV reverse transcriptase by competing with the natural substrate deoxythymidine triphosphate. Second, it inhibits viral DNA synthesis by causing DNA chain termination because stavudine lacks the 3′-hydroxyl group necessary for DNA elongation. Stavudine triphosphate also inhibits cellular DNA polymerase beta and gamma and markedly reduces mitochondrial DNA synthesis.

Pharmacokinetics

● *Absorption:* Rapidly absorbed, with a mean absolute bioavailability of 86.4%. Plasma levels peak in 1 hour or less.
● *Distribution:* Mean volume of distribution is 58 L, suggesting distribution into extravascular space. Distributed equally between RBCs and plasma; binds poorly to plasma proteins.
● *Metabolism:* Not clearly defined.
● *Excretion:* Renal elimination accounts for about 40% of overall clearance, regardless of administration route; active tubular secretion in addition to glomerular filtration.

Contraindications and precautions

Contraindicated in patients with hypersensitivity to drug. Use cautiously in patients with impaired renal function or history of peripheral neuropathy and in pregnant women.

Interactions

Drug-drug. *Zidovudine:* Inhibited therapeutic effect of zidovudine. Avoid concomitant use.

Adverse reactions

CNS: *peripheral neuropathy, headache, malaise, insomnia, anxiety, depression, nervousness,* dizziness, *asthenia.*
CV: chest pain.
EENT: conjunctivitis.
GI: *abdominal pain, diarrhea, nausea, vomiting, anorexia,* dyspepsia, constipation, weight loss.
Hematologic: *neutropenia, thrombocytopenia,* anemia.
Hepatic: elevated liver enzyme levels, *hepatotoxicity.*
Musculoskeletal: *myalgia, back pain, arthralgia.*
Respiratory: *dyspnea.*
Skin: *rash, diaphoresis, pruritus,* maculopapular rash.
Other: *chills, fever.*

☑ Special considerations

● Patient may develop peripheral neuropathy, usually characterized by numbness, tingling, or pain in feet or hands. If symptoms develop, interrupt drug therapy. Symptoms may resolve if therapy is withdrawn promptly. Sometimes symptoms may worsen temporarily after drug is stopped. If symptoms resolve completely, resume treatment using the following dosage schedule: patients weighing 132 lb or more should receive 20 mg twice daily; patients weighing less than 132 lb should receive 15 mg twice daily. Manage significant elevations of hepatic transaminase levels in same way.
● Experience with adults who had received 12 to 24 times the recommended daily dose revealed no acute toxicity. Complications of long-term overdose include peripheral neuropathy and hepatic toxicity. It's unknown if drug is eliminated by peritoneal dialysis or hemodialysis.

Monitoring the patient

● Monitor patient for development of peripheral neuropathy, usually characterized by numbness, tingling, or pain in hands or feet.
● Monitor patient for adverse effects.

Information for the patient

● Inform patient that drug doesn't cure HIV infection and that he may continue to acquire illnesses associated with AIDS or AIDS-related complex, including opportunistic infections.
● Inform patient that drug doesn't reduce risk of transmitting HIV to others through sexual contact or blood contamination.
● Advise patient to report signs of peripheral neuropathy, such as tingling, burning, pain, or numbness in hands or feet, because dosage adjustments may be necessary. Counsel patient that this toxicity occurs with greater frequency in patients with history of peripheral neuropathy. Also advise patient not to use other drugs, including

OTC preparations, without calling first; some drugs can exacerbate peripheral neuropathy.
• Explain that long-term effects of drug are currently unknown.

Pediatric patients
• Safety and effectiveness for treatment of HIV in children haven't been established.

Breast-feeding patients
• It's unknown if drug appears in breast milk. Because of potential for adverse reactions from drug in breast-fed infants, women shouldn't breast-feed during therapy.

---

streptokinase
Kabikinase, Streptase

Pharmacologic classification: plasminogen activator
Therapeutic classification: thrombolytic enzyme
Pregnancy risk category C

How supplied
Available by prescription only
Injection: 250,000 IU, 600,000 IU, 750,000 IU, 1,500,000 IU in vials for reconstitution

Indications, route, and dosage
Lysis of coronary artery thrombi following acute MI
Adults: 1,500,000 IU by I.V. infusion over 60 minutes; intracoronary loading dose of 20,000 IU via coronary catheter, then a maintenance dose of 2,000 IU/minute for 60 minutes as an infusion.
Arteriovenous cannula occlusion
Adults: 250,000 IU in 2 ml I.V. solution by I.V. infusion pump into each occluded limb of the cannula over 25 to 35 minutes. Clamp off cannula for 2 hours; then aspirate contents of cannula, flush with saline solution, and reconnect.
Venous thrombosis, pulmonary embolism, arterial thrombosis and embolism
Adults: Loading dose of 250,000 IU I.V. infusion over 30 minutes. Sustaining dose: 100,000 IU/hour I.V. infusion for 72 hours for deep vein thrombosis and 100,000 IU/hour over 24 hours by I.V. infusion pump for pulmonary embolism.

Pharmacodynamics
Thrombolytic action: Promotes thrombolysis by activating plasminogen in two steps. First, plasminogen and streptokinase form a complex, exposing plasminogen-activating site, and, second, cleavage of peptide bond converts plasminogen to plasmin.
In treatment of acute MI, streptokinase prevents primary or secondary thrombus formation in microcirculation surrounding the necrotic area.

Pharmacokinetics
• *Absorption:* Plasminogen activation begins promptly after drug infusion or instillation; adequate activation of fibrinolytic system occurs in 3 to 4 hours.
• *Distribution:* Doesn't cross placenta, but antibodies do.
• *Metabolism:* Insignificant.
• *Excretion:* Removed from circulation by antibodies and reticuloendothelial system. Half-life is biphasic; initially, 18 minutes (from antibody action), and then extends up to 83 minutes. Anticoagulant effect may last for 12 to 24 hours after infusion ends.

Contraindications and precautions
Contraindicated in patients with ulcerative wounds, active internal bleeding, and recent CVA; recent trauma with possible internal injuries; visceral or intracranial malignant neoplasms; ulcerative colitis; diverticulitis; severe hypertension; acute or chronic hepatic or renal insufficiency; uncontrolled hypocoagulation; chronic pulmonary disease with cavitation; subacute bacterial endocarditis or rheumatic valvular disease; or recent cerebral embolism, thrombosis, or hemorrhage.
Also contraindicated within 10 days after intra-arterial diagnostic procedure or any surgery, including liver or kidney biopsy, lumbar puncture, thoracentesis, paracentesis, or extensive or several cutdowns. I.M. injections and other invasive procedures are contraindicated during streptokinase therapy.
Use cautiously in patients with arterial embolism that originates from the left side of heart.

Interactions
Drug-drug. *Aminocaproic acid:* Inhibited streptokinase-induced activation of plasminogen. Avoid concomitant use.
Anticoagulants: Possible hemorrhage. May be necessary to reverse effects of oral anticoagulants before beginning therapy.
Aspirin, indomethacin, phenylbutazone, other drugs affecting platelet activity: Increased risk of bleeding. Use together cautiously.

Adverse reactions
CNS: polyradiculoneuropathy, headache.
CV: reperfusion arrhythmias, *hypotension,* vasculitis.
EENT: periorbital edema.
GI: nausea.
Hematologic: *bleeding.*
Musculoskeletal: musculoskeletal pain.
Respiratory: minor breathing difficulty, *bronchospasm.*
Skin: urticaria, pruritus, flushing.
Other: phlebitis at injection site, hypersensitivity reactions (*anaphylaxis*), delayed hypersensitivity reactions (interstitial nephritis, serum sickness–like reactions), *angioedema, fever.*

Reactions may be *common*, uncommon, *life-threatening*, or COMMON AND LIFE-THREATENING.

☑ Special considerations
Besides the recommendations relevant to all thrombolytic enzymes, consider the following.
• Reconstitute vial with 5 ml normal saline injection, and further dilute to 45 ml; roll gently to mix. Don't shake. Use immediately; refrigerate remainder and discard after 8 hours. Store powder at room temperature.
• Rate of I.V. infusion depends on thrombin time and streptokinase resistance; higher loading dose may be needed in patients with recent streptococcal infection or recent treatment with streptokinase to compensate for antibody drug neutralization.
• Don't stop therapy for minor allergic reactions that can be treated with antihistamines or corticosteroids; about one-third of patients experience a slight temperature elevation, and some have chills. Symptomatic treatment with acetaminophen (but not aspirin or other salicylates) is indicated if temperature reaches 104° F (40° C). Patients may be pretreated with corticosteroids, repeating doses during therapy, to minimize pyrogenic or allergic reactions.
• If minor bleeding can be controlled by local pressure, don't decrease dose so that more plasminogen is available for conversion to plasmin.
• Antibodies to streptokinase can persist for 3 to 6 months or longer after initial dose; if further thrombolytic therapy is needed, consider urokinase.
• Indications of overdose include signs of potentially serious bleeding: bleeding gums, epistaxis, hematoma, spontaneous ecchymoses, oozing at catheter site, increased pulse, and pain from internal bleeding. Stop drug and restart when bleeding stops.

Monitoring the patient
• Watch for anaphylaxis, angioedema, bronchospasm, and bleeding.
• Monitor therapeutic effect.

Information for the patient
• Advise patient of potential adverse effects.
• Instruct patient to immediately report any breathing difficulty.

Geriatric patients
• Patients ages 75 and older have a greater risk of cerebral hemorrhage than younger patients because they are likely to have preexisting cerebrovascular disease.

Pediatric patients
• Safety and effectiveness in children haven't been established.

streptomycin sulfate

Pharmacologic classification: aminoglycoside
Therapeutic classification: antibiotic
Pregnancy risk category D

How supplied
Available by prescription only
Injection: 400 mg/ml

Indications, route, and dosage
Primary and adjunctive treatment in tuberculosis
Adults with normal renal function: 1 g or 15 mg/kg I.M. daily for 2 to 3 months; then 1 g two or three times weekly. Inject deeply into upper outer quadrant of buttocks or midlateral thigh. Maximum daily dose is 1 g.
Children with normal renal function: 20 to 40 mg/kg I.M. daily in divided doses injected deeply into large muscle mass, preferably in midlateral muscles of thigh. Give with other antituberculotics, but *not* with capreomycin, and continue until sputum specimen becomes negative. Maximum daily dose is 1 g. Or 25 to 35 mg/kg I.M. two to three times weekly (maximum dose is 1.5 g).
Enterococcal endocarditis
Adults: 1 g I.M. q 12 hours for 2 weeks; then 500 mg I.M. q 12 hours for 4 weeks with penicillin.
Tularemia
Adults: 1 to 2 g I.M. daily in divided doses injected deep into upper outer quadrant of buttocks. Continue until patient is afebrile for 7 to 14 days.
Plague
Adults: 2 g I.M. daily in divided doses injected deep into upper outer quadrant of buttocks for a minimum of 10 days.
◊ **Mycobacterium avium**
Adults: 11 to 13 mg/kg/day I.V. or 15 mg/kg/day I.M.
✦ **Dosage adjustment.** For adults and children with renal failure, initial dose is same as for those with normal renal function. Subsequent doses and frequency determined by renal function study results and blood serum levels; peak serum levels shouldn't exceed 20 to 25 mcg/ml, and trough levels should be 5 mcg/ml or less. Patients with a creatinine clearance over 50 ml/minute usually can tolerate drug daily; if creatinine clearance is 10 to 50 ml/minute, increase administration interval to q 24 to 72 hours. Patients with a creatinine clearance under 10 ml/minute may require 72 to 96 hours between doses.

Pharmacodynamics
Antibiotic action: Bactericidal. Binds directly to the 30S ribosomal subunit, thus inhibiting bacterial protein synthesis. Spectrum of activity includes many aerobic gram-negative organisms and some aerobic gram-positive organisms. Gen-

erally less active against many gram-negative organisms than is tobramycin, gentamicin, amikacin, or netilmicin. Also active against *Mycobacterium* and *Brucella.*

Pharmacokinetics

- *Absorption:* Absorbed poorly after oral administration; usually given parenterally. Serum levels peak 1 to 2 hours after I.M. administration.
- *Distribution:* Widely distributed after parenteral administration; poor intraocular penetration. Low CSF penetration, even in patients with inflamed meninges. Crosses placenta; 36% protein-bound.
- *Metabolism:* Not metabolized.
- *Excretion:* Excreted primarily in urine by glomerular filtration; small amounts may be excreted in bile and breast milk. Elimination half-life in adults is 2 to 3 hours. In severe renal damage, half-life may extend to 110 hours.

Contraindications and precautions

Contraindicated in patients with hypersensitivity to drug or other aminoglycosides and in those with labyrinthine disease. Never administer I.V. Use cautiously in patients with impaired renal function or neuromuscular disorders and in elderly patients.

Interactions

Drug-drug. *Amphotericin B, capreomycin, cephalosporins, cisplatin, methoxyflurane, polymyxin B, vancomycin, other aminoglycosides:* Increased hazard of nephrotoxicity, ototoxicity, and neurotoxicity. Avoid concomitant use.
Bumetanide, ethacrynic acid, furosemide, mannitol, urea: Increased risk of ototoxicity. Avoid concomitant use.
Dimenhydrinate, other antiemetics, other antivertigo drugs: May mask streptomycin-induced ototoxicity. Use cautiously together.
General anesthetics, neuromuscular blockers (such as succinylcholine, tubocurarine): Potentiated neuromuscular blockade. Avoid concomitant use.
Penicillin: Synergistic bactericidal effect against *Pseudomonas aeruginosa, Escherichia coli, Klebsiella, Citrobacter, Enterobacter, Serratia,* and *Proteus mirabilis;* however, drugs are physically and chemically incompatible and are inactivated when mixed or given together. Don't administer together.

Adverse reactions

CNS: *neuromuscular blockade.*
EENT: *ototoxicity.*
GI: vomiting, nausea.
GU: some *nephrotoxicity* (not as frequently as with other aminoglycosides).
Hematologic: eosinophilia, *leukopenia, thrombocytopenia.*
Respiratory: *apnea.*

Skin: *exfoliative dermatitis.*
Other: hypersensitivity reactions (rash, fever, urticaria, *angioedema*), *anaphylaxis.*

☑ Special considerations

Besides the recommendations relevant to all aminoglycosides, consider the following.
- Protect hands when preparing drug; drug irritates skin.
- In primary tuberculosis therapy, stop drug when sputum culture is negative.
- Because drug is dialyzable, patients undergoing hemodialysis may need dosage adjustments.
- Streptomycin may cause false-positive reaction in copper sulfate test for urine glucose (Benedict's reagent or Clinitest).
- Signs and symptoms of overdose include ototoxicity, nephrotoxicity, and neuromuscular toxicity. Remove drug by hemodialysis or peritoneal dialysis. Treatment with calcium salts or anticholinesterases reverses neuromuscular blockade.

Monitoring the patient

- Monitor patient for ototoxicity, nephrotoxicity, and neuromuscular toxicity.
- Monitor therapeutic effect.

Information for the patient

- Advise patient to report adverse reactions promptly.
- Encourage adequate fluid intake.
- Emphasize need for blood tests to monitor streptomycin levels and determine effectiveness of therapy.

Breast-feeding patients

- Because of the potential for serious adverse reactions in the infant, a decision should be made whether to discontinue breast-feeding or discontinue the drug.

---

succimer
Chemet

Pharmacologic classification: heavy metal
Therapeutic classification: chelating drug
Pregnancy risk category C

How supplied

Available by prescription only
Capsules: 100 mg

Indications, route, and dosage

Lead poisoning in children with blood lead levels above 45 mcg/dl
Children: Initially, 10 mg/kg or 350 mg/m² P.O. q 8 hours for 5 days. Higher starting doses aren't recommended. Frequency of administration may

be reduced to 10 mg/kg or 350 mg/m^2 q 12 hours for an additional 2 weeks of therapy. A course of treatment lasts 19 days, and repeated courses may be necessary if indicated by weekly monitoring of blood lead levels. A minimum of 2 weeks between courses is recommended unless blood lead levels mandate more prompt action.

✦ *Dosage adjustment.* Dose is administered q 8 hours for 5 days; then same dose q 12 hours for 14 days.

PEDIATRIC DOSAGES			
Weight		Dose (mg)	No. of Capsules
(lb)	(kg)		
18 to 35	8 to 15	100	1
36 to 55	16 to 23	200	2
56 to 75	24 to 34	300	3
76 to 100	35 to 44	400	4
> 100	> 45	500	5

Pharmacodynamics

Antidote action: Forms water-soluble chelates and increases urinary excretion of lead.

Pharmacokinetics

• *Absorption:* Rapidly but variably absorbed after oral administration; blood levels peak in 1 to 2 hours.
• *Distribution:* No information available.
• *Metabolism:* Rapidly and extensively metabolized.
• *Excretion:* Excreted 39% in feces as nonabsorbed drug; 9% in urine; 1% as carbon dioxide from lungs. About 90% of absorbed drug excreted in urine.

Contraindications and precautions

Contraindicated in patients with hypersensitivity to drug. Use cautiously in patients with impaired renal function.

Interactions

Drug-drug. *Other chelating drugs:* Unknown adverse effects. Don't administer together. Drug shouldn't be given until 4 weeks after chelating drug has been stopped.

Adverse reactions

CNS: *drowsiness, dizziness, sensory motor neuropathy, sleepiness, paresthesia, headache.*
CV: *arrhythmias.*
EENT: plugged ears, cloudy film in eyes, otitis media, watery eyes, sore throat, rhinorrhea, nasal congestion.
GI: *nausea, vomiting, diarrhea, loss of appetite, abdominal cramps, hemorrhoidal symptoms, metallic taste in mouth, loose stools.*

GU: decreased urination, difficult urination, proteinuria, candidiasis.
Hematologic: increased platelet count, intermittent eosinophilia.
Hepatic: *elevated serum AST, ALT, alkaline phosphatase levels.*
Metabolic: *elevated cholesterol levels.*
Musculoskeletal: *leg, kneecap, back, stomach, rib, or flank pain.*
Respiratory: cough, head cold.
Skin: papular rash, herpetic rash, mucocutaneous eruptions, pruritus.
Other: *flulike symptoms.*

☑ Special considerations

• Patients who have received ethylenediaminetetraacetic acid, with or without dimercaprol, may use succimer as subsequent therapy after an interval of 4 weeks. Use with other chelating drugs isn't recommended.
• Consider the possibility of allergic or other mucocutaneous reactions each time drug is used, including initial course.
• Elevated blood lead levels and associated symptoms may return rapidly after drug is stopped because of redistribution of lead from bone to soft tissues and blood.
• Don't use drug for prophylaxis of lead poisoning in a lead-containing environment.
• False-positive results for ketones in urine using nitroprusside reagents (Ketostix) and false decreased levels of serum uric acid and CK have been reported.
• In case of acute overdose, induce vomiting with ipecac syrup or perform gastric lavage; then use activated charcoal slurry and appropriate supportive therapy.

Monitoring the patient

• Monitor serum transaminase levels before and at least weekly during therapy. Patients with a history of hepatic disease should be monitored more closely.
• The severity of lead intoxication should be used as a guide for more frequent blood lead monitoring. This is measured by the initial blood lead level and the rate and degree of rebound of blood lead.
• Monitor patient at least once weekly for rebound blood lead levels.

Information for the patient

• Advise parents to maintain child's adequate fluid intake.
• Tell parents to report rash.
• Urge parents to identify and remove source of lead in environment.
• Tell parents to store capsules at room temperature, out of children's reach.

Pediatric patients
• For young children who can't swallow capsule, succimer capsule may be opened and sprinkled on a small amount of soft food, or medicated beads from capsules may be poured onto a spoon for administration and followed with a fruit drink.

Breast-feeding patients
• It's unknown if drug appears in breast milk. Breast-feeding should be discouraged because many drugs and heavy metals appear in breast milk.

succinylcholine chloride (suxamethonium chloride)
Anectine, Anectine Flo-Pack, Quelicin, Sucostrin

Pharmacologic classification: depolarizing neuromuscular blocker
Therapeutic classification: skeletal muscle relaxant
Pregnancy risk category C

How supplied
Available by prescription only
Injection: 20 mg/ml, 50 mg/ml, 100 mg/ml (powder for infusion); 500 mg, 1 g (sterile for I.V. infusion)

Indications, route, and dosage
To induce skeletal muscle relaxation; facilitate intubation, ventilation, or orthopedic manipulations; lessen muscle contractions in induced seizures
Dosage depends on the anesthetic used, patient's needs, and response. Doses are representative and must be adjusted. Paralysis is induced after inducing hypnosis with thiopental or other appropriate drug.
Adults: For short procedures, 0.6 mg/kg (range, 0.3 to 1.1 mg/kg) I.V. over 10 to 30 seconds; additional doses may be given if needed. For long procedures, 2.5 mg/minute (range, 0.5 to 10 mg/minute) continuous I.V. infusion; or 0.3 to 1.1 mg/kg by intermittent I.V. injection, then additional doses of 0.04 to 0.07 mg/kg, p.r.n.
Children: Administer 2 mg/kg I.V. for infants; for older children and adolescents, give 1 mg/kg I.V. or 3 to 4 mg/kg I.M. (don't exceed 150 mg).

Pharmacodynamics
Skeletal muscle relaxant action: Similar to acetylcholine (ACh), succinylcholine produces depolarization of the motor end-plate at the myoneural junction. Drug has a high affinity for ACh receptor sites and is resistant to acetylcholinesterase, thus producing a more prolonged depolarization at the motor end-plate. It also possesses histamine-releasing properties and reportedly stimulates the cardiac vagus and sympathetic ganglia.
A transient increase in intraocular pressure occurs immediately after injection and may persist after the onset of complete paralysis.

Pharmacokinetics
• *Absorption:* After I.V. administration, rapid onset of action (30 seconds); reaches peak within 1 minute; lasts for 2 to 3 minutes; gradually dissipates within 10 minutes. After I.M. administration, onset occurs within 2 to 3 minutes and lasts for 10 to 30 minutes.
• *Distribution:* After I.V. administration, distributed in extracellular fluid; rapidly reaches site of action. Crosses placenta.
• *Metabolism:* Rapidly metabolized by plasma pseudocholinesterase.
• *Excretion:* About 10% of drug excreted unchanged in urine.

Contraindications and precautions
Contraindicated in patients with hypersensitivity to drug and in those with abnormally low plasma pseudocholinesterase, angle-closure glaucoma, malignant hyperthermia, or penetrating eye injuries.
Use cautiously in elderly or debilitated patients; in those receiving quinidine or cardiac glycoside therapy; in those undergoing cesarean section; and in patients with respiratory depression, severe burns or trauma, electrolyte imbalances, hyperkalemia, paraplegia, spinal neuraxis injury, CVA, degenerative or dystrophic neuromuscular disease, myasthenia gravis, myasthenic syndrome of lung or bronchiogenic cancer, dehydration, thyroid disorders, collagen diseases, porphyria, fractures, muscle spasms, eye surgery, pheochromocytoma, or impaired renal, pulmonary, or hepatic function.

Interactions
Drug-drug. *Aminoglycoside antibiotics (such as amikacin, gentamicin, kanamycin, neomycin, streptomycin), antimalarials, cholinesterase inhibitors (demecarium, echothiophate, isoflurane), clindamycin, cyclophosphamide, general anesthetics, lincomycin, lithium, local anesthetics, nondepolarizing neuromuscular blockers, oral contraceptives, pancuronium, parenteral magnesium salts, phenelzine, phenothiazines, polymyxin antibiotics (colistin, polymyxin B sulfate), quinidine, quinine, thiotepa:* Enhanced or prolonged neuromuscular blocking effects. Use these drugs cautiously during surgical and postoperative periods. *Cardiac glycosides:* Possible arrhythmias. Use together cautiously.
Drug-herb. *Melatonin:* Potentiated blocking properties of succinylcholine. Don't use together.
Drug-lifestyle. *Neurotoxic insecticides:* Exposure can enhance or prolong neuromuscular

---

blocking effects. Patient shouldn't be exposed to these products.

Adverse reactions
CV: *bradycardia,* tachycardia, hypertension, hypotension, *arrhythmias,* flushing, *cardiac arrest.*
EENT: increased intraocular pressure.
Hematologic: myoglobinemia.
Metabolic: hyperkalemia.
Musculoskeletal: muscle fasciculation, *postoperative muscle pain.*
Respiratory: *prolonged respiratory depression, apnea,* bronchostriction.
Other: *malignant hyperthermia,* allergic or idiosyncratic hypersensitivity reactions (*anaphylaxis*).

☑ Special considerations
• Succinylcholine is drug of choice for short procedures (less than 3 minutes) and for orthopedic manipulations; use cautiously in fractures or dislocations.
• Duration of action is prolonged to 20 minutes with continuous I.V. infusion or when given with hexafluorenium bromide.
• Pretreatment of adult patients with tubocurarine (3 to 6 mg) might minimize muscle fasciculations.
• Repeated fractional doses of succinylcholine alone aren't advised; possible reduced response or prolonged apnea.
• Only trained anesthesia personnel should administer this drug.
• Emergency respiratory support (endotracheal equipment, ventilator, oxygen, atropine, neostigmine) should be available during administration.
• Drug shouldn't be mixed with alkaline solutions (thiopental, sodium bicarbonate, barbiturates).
• Usually administered I.V., drug may be administered I.M. if suitable vein is inaccessible. Give deep I.M., preferably high into deltoid muscle.
• Signs and symptoms of overdose include apnea or prolonged muscle paralysis, which may be treated with controlled respiration. Use a peripheral nerve stimulator to monitor effects and degree of blockade.

Monitoring the patient
• Monitor baseline electrolyte determinations and vital signs (check respirations every 5 to 10 minutes during infusion).
• Monitor patient for tachyphylaxis.
• Monitor patient for residual muscle weakness.

Information for the patient
• Reassure patient that postoperative stiffness is normal and will soon subside.

Geriatric patients
• Use with caution in elderly patients.

Breast-feeding patients
• It's unknown if drug appears in breast milk. Use with caution in breast-feeding women.

sucralfate
Carafate

Pharmacologic classification: pepsin inhibitor
Therapeutic classification: antiulcerative
Pregnancy risk category B

How supplied
Available by prescription only
Tablets: 1 g
Suspension: 1 g/10 ml

Indications, route, and dosage
Short-term (up to 8 weeks) treatment of duodenal ulcer, ◇ aspirin-induced gastric erosion
Adults: 1 g P.O. q.i.d. 1 hour before meals and h.s.
Maintenance therapy of duodenal ulcer
Adults: 1 g P.O. b.i.d.

Pharmacodynamics
Antiulcerative action: Has unique mechanism of action. Adheres to proteins at the ulcer site, forming a protective coating against gastric acid, pepsin, and bile salts. Also inhibits pepsin, exhibits a cytoprotective effect, and forms a viscous, adhesive barrier on the surface of the intact intestinal mucosa and stomach.

Pharmacokinetics
• *Absorption:* Only about 3% to 5% of dose absorbed. Drug activity isn't related to amount absorbed.
• *Distribution:* Acts locally, at ulcer site. Absorbed drug distributed to many body tissues, including liver and kidneys.
• *Metabolism:* None.
• *Excretion:* About 90% of dose excreted in feces; absorbed drug excreted unchanged in urine. Duration of effect is 6 hours.

Contraindications and precautions
No known contraindications. Use cautiously in patients with chronic renal failure.

Interactions
Drug-drug. *Antacids:* Decreased binding of drug to gastroduodenal mucosa, impairing effectiveness. Separate administration times of sucralfate and antacids by 30 minutes.
Cimetidine, digoxin, fat-soluble vitamins (A, D, E, K), phenytoin, quinidine, quinolones, ranitidine, tetracycline, theophylline: Decreased absorption of these drugs. Administer 2 hours apart; moni-

---

◇ Unlabeled clinical use

tor patient for therapeutic effect and adjust dosage as needed.

Adverse reactions
CNS: dizziness, sleepiness, headache, vertigo.
GI: *constipation,* nausea, gastric discomfort, diarrhea, bezoar formation, vomiting, flatulence, dry mouth, indigestion.
Musculoskeletal: back pain.
Skin: rash, pruritus.

☑ Special considerations
• Sucralfate may inhibit absorption of other drugs. Schedule administration of other drugs 2 hours before or after sucralfate.
• Drug is poorly water-soluble. For administration by nasogastric tube, have pharmacist prepare water-sorbitol suspension of sucralfate.
• Patients who have difficulty swallowing tablet may place it in 15 to 30 ml of water at room temperature, allow it to disintegrate, and then ingest resulting suspension. This method is particularly useful for patients with esophagitis and painful swallowing.
• Therapy lasting more than 8 weeks isn't recommended.
• Drug is as effective as H_2-receptor antagonists in treating ulcers.

Monitoring the patient
• Monitor patient for constipation.
• Monitor therapeutic effect.

Information for the patient
• Remind patient to take drug on empty stomach and at least 1 hour before meals.
• Advise patient to continue taking drug as directed, even after pain begins to subside, to ensure adequate healing.
• Tell patient that he may take an antacid 30 minutes before or 2 hours after sucralfate.
• Warn patient not to take drug for more than 8 weeks.

Breast-feeding patients
• Because it's unknown if drug appears in breast milk, risk to the breast-feeding infant must be weighed against benefits to mother.

---

sufentanil citrate
Sufenta

Pharmacologic classification: opioid
Therapeutic classification: analgesic, adjunct to anesthesia, anesthetic
Controlled substance schedule II
Pregnancy risk category C

How supplied
Available by prescription only
Injection: 50 mcg/ml

Indications, route, and dosage
Adjunct to general anesthetic
Adults: 1 to 8 mcg/kg I.V. administered with nitrous oxide and oxygen. Maintenance dose is 10 to 50 mcg.
Primary anesthetic
Adults: 8 to 30 mcg/kg I.V. administered with 100% oxygen and a muscle relaxant. Maintenance dose is 25 to 50 mcg.
Children: 10 to 25 mcg/kg I.V. administered with 100% oxygen and a muscle relaxant. Maintenance dose is up to 25 to 50 mcg.

Pharmacodynamics
Analgesic action: Has a high affinity for the opiate receptors with an agonistic effect to provide analgesia. Also used as an adjunct to anesthesia or as a primary anesthetic because of its potent CNS depressant effects.

Pharmacokinetics
• *Absorption:* After I.V. administration, more rapid onset of action (1½ to 3 minutes) than morphine or fentanyl.
• *Distribution:* Highly lipophilic; rapidly and extensively distributed in animals. More than 90% protein-bound; redistributed rapidly.
• *Metabolism:* Appears to be metabolized mainly in liver and small intestine. Relatively little accumulation. Elimination half-life of about 2½ hours.
• *Excretion:* Drug and metabolites excreted primarily in urine.

Contraindications and precautions
Contraindicated in patients with hypersensitivity to drug. Use cautiously in elderly or debilitated patients and in those with decreased respiratory reserve, head injuries, or renal, pulmonary, or hepatic disease.

Interactions
Drug-drug. *Anticholinergics:* Possible paralytic ileus. Monitor bowel status.
Cimetidine: Increased respiratory and CNS depression; confusion, disorientation, apnea, or seizures. Reduce sufentanil dosage.
General anesthetics: Severe CV depression. Use cautiously together.
Narcotic agonist-antagonist, single dose of an antagonist: Patients physically dependent on drug may experience acute withdrawal syndrome. Monitor patient closely.
Nitrous oxide: Possible CV depression when given with high doses of sufentanil. Use cautiously together.
Pancuronium: Possible dose-dependent elevation in heart rate during sufentanil and oxygen anesthesia. Use moderate doses of pancuronium or a less vagolytic neuromuscular blocker. The vagolytic effect of pancuronium may be reduced in patients given nitrous oxide with sufentanil. Sufentanil may produce muscle rigidity in-

---

Reactions may be *common,* uncommon, *life-threatening,* or COMMON AND LIFE-THREATENING.

volving all skeletal muscles (incidence and severity are dose-related). Choose a neuromuscular blocker appropriate for patient's CV status.
Other CNS depressants (antihistamines, barbiturates, benzodiazepines, general anesthetics, muscle relaxants, narcotic analgesics, phenothiazines, sedative-hypnotics, tricyclic antidepressants): Potentiated respiratory and CNS depression, sedation, and hypotensive effects of drug. Avoid concomitant use.
Other drugs extensively metabolized in liver (digitoxin, phenytoin, rifampin): Drug accumulation and enhanced effects. Use together with caution.
Drug-lifestyle. *Alcohol:* Possible additive effects. Discourage use.

Adverse reactions
CNS: chills, somnolence.
CV: *hypotension,* **bradycardia,** hypertension, **arrhythmias,** tachycardia.
GI: nausea, vomiting.
Metabolic: increased plasma amylase, lipase and serum prolactin levels.
Musculoskeletal: intraoperative muscle movement.
Respiratory: *chest wall rigidity, apnea, bronchospasm.*
Skin: *pruritus,* erythema.

☑ Special considerations
Besides the recommendations relevant to all opioids, consider the following recommendations.
• Sufentanil should be administered only by persons specifically trained in use of I.V. anesthetics.
• When used at doses exceeding 8 mcg/kg, postoperative mechanical ventilation and observation are essential because of extended postoperative respiratory depression.
• Compared with fentanyl, sufentanil has a more rapid onset and shorter duration of action.
• High doses can produce muscle rigidity. This effect can be reversed by administration of neuromuscular blockers.
• In patients weighing more than 20% above ideal body weight, determine dose based on ideal body weight.
• Signs and symptoms of acute overdose are probably similar to those occurring with other opioids, with less CV toxicity. The most common signs and symptoms of acute opiate overdose are CNS depression, respiratory depression, and miosis (pinpoint pupils). Other acute toxic effects include hypotension, bradycardia, hypothermia, shock, apnea, cardiopulmonary arrest, circulatory collapse, pulmonary edema, and seizures.
• To treat acute overdose, establish adequate respiratory exchange via a patent airway and ventilation, as needed; administer a narcotic antagonist (naloxone) to reverse respiratory depression. (Because the duration of action of sufentanil is longer than that of naloxone, repeated naloxone dosing is necessary.) Don't give naloxone unless patient has clinically significant respiratory or CV depression. Monitor vital signs closely.
• Provide symptomatic and supportive treatment (continued respiratory support, correction of fluid or electrolyte imbalance). Monitor laboratory parameters, vital signs, and neurologic status closely.

Monitoring the patient
• Monitor respiratory and cardiac status closely.

Information for the patient
• Advise patient of potential adverse effects.

Geriatric patients
• Lower dosages are usually indicated for elderly patients, who may be more sensitive to therapeutic and adverse effects of drug.

Pediatric patients
• Safety and efficacy in children under age 2 have been documented in only a limited number of patients (who were undergoing CV surgery).

Breast-feeding patients
• It's unknown if drug appears in breast milk.

---

sulfacetamide sodium
AK-Sulf Ointment, Bleph-10, Cetamide, Isopto Cetamide, Ocusulf-10, Sodium Sulamyd, Sulf-10, Sulfair 15, Sulfex*, Sulten-10

Pharmacologic classification: sulfonamide
Therapeutic classification: antibiotic
Pregnancy risk category C

How supplied
Available by prescription only
Ophthalmic solution: 1%, 10%, 15%, 30%
Ophthalmic ointment: 10%

Indications, route, and dosage
Inclusion conjunctivitis, corneal ulcers, trachoma, prophylaxis for ocular infection
Adults and children: Instill 1 or 2 drops of 10% solution into lower conjunctival sac q 2 to 3 hours during day, less often at night; or instill 1 or 2 drops of 15% solution into lower conjunctival sac q 1 to 2 hours initially, increasing interval as condition responds; or instill 1 drop of 30% solution into lower conjunctival sac q 2 hours. Instill ½ to 1 inch of 10% ointment into conjunctival sac q.i.d. and h.s. Ointment may be used at night along with drops during the day. Usual duration of treatment is 7 to 10 days.

Pharmacodynamics
Antibiotic action: Sulfonamides act by inhibiting the uptake of para-aminobenzoic acid, which is required in the synthesis of folic acid needed for bacterial growth.

Pharmacokinetics
• *Absorption:* Not readily absorbed from mucous membranes.
• *Distribution:* No information available.
• *Metabolism:* No information available.
• *Excretion:* No information available.

Contraindications and precautions
Contraindicated in patients with hypersensitivity to sulfonamides and in infants under age 2 months.

Interactions
Drug-drug. *Gentamicin sulfate ophthalmic solution, silver preparations:* Drug is incompatible with these drugs. Avoid concomitant use.
Tetracaine, other local anesthetics that are para-aminobenzoic acid derivatives: Decreased antibacterial activity of sulfacetamide. Avoid concomitant use.
Drug-lifestyle. *Sun exposure:* Enhanced photophobia. Tell patient to take precautions.

Adverse reactions
EENT: slowed corneal wound healing (ointment), pain (on instillation of eyedrops), headache or brow pain, photophobia, periorbital edema.
Hematologic: *agranulocytosis, aplastic anemia.*
Hepatic: *fulminant hepatic necrosis.*
Skin: *Stevens-Johnson syndrome.*
Other: hypersensitivity reactions (including itching or burning), overgrowth of nonsusceptible organisms.

☑ Special considerations
• Drug has largely been replaced by antibiotics for treating major infections, but it's still used in minor ocular infections.
• Purulent exudate interferes with sulfacetamide action; remove as much as possible from lids before instilling drug.
• Store in tightly closed, light-resistant container away from heat and light; don't use discolored (dark brown) solution.

Monitoring the patient
• Monitor therapeutic response.
• Monitor patient for adverse effects.

Information for the patient
• Warn patient that eyedrops may burn slightly.
• Caution patient against touching tip of tube or dropper to eye or surrounding tissue.
• Show patient how to instill drops correctly.

• Tell patient to watch for signs and symptoms of sensitivity, such as itching lids or constant burning, and to report them immediately.
• Tell patient to avoid sharing washcloths and towels with family members.
• Advise patient to wait 10 minutes before using another eye preparation.

Pediatric patients
• Use of drug in infants under age 2 months isn't recommended.

Breast-feeding patients
• Although orally ingested sulfonamides can appear in low levels in breast milk, no data are available concerning ophthalmic sulfacetamide. Because of the potential for serious adverse effects in breast-fed infants, women should not breast-feed while taking this drug.

---

sulfadiazine

Pharmacologic classification: sulfonamide
Therapeutic classification: antibiotic
Pregnancy risk category NR

How supplied
Available by prescription only
Tablets: 500 mg

Indications, route, and dosage
Urinary tract infection
Adults: Initially, 2 to 4 g P.O.; then 4 to 8 g/day in four to six divided doses.
Children ages 2 months and older: Initially, 75 mg/kg or 2 g/m² P.O.; then 120 mg/kg/day P.O. in four to six divided doses. Maximum daily dose is 6 g.
Rheumatic fever prophylaxis, as an alternative to penicillin
Children weighing over 30 kg (66 lb): 1 g P.O. daily.
Children weighing under 30 kg: 500 mg P.O. daily.
Adjunctive treatment in toxoplasmosis
Adults: 2 to 8 g daily P.O. in divided doses q 6 hours for 3 to 4 weeks and up to 6 months or longer in patients with AIDS; given with pyrimethamine 25 mg P.O. daily.
Children: 100 to 200 mg/kg P.O. daily in divided doses q 6 hours for 3 to 4 weeks; given with pyrimethamine 2 mg/kg daily for 3 days, then 1 mg/kg daily for 3 to 4 weeks.
Uncomplicated attacks of malaria
Adults: 500 mg P.O. q.i.d. for 5 days.
Children: 25 to 50 mg/kg P.O. q.i.d. for 5 days.
Nocardiasis
Adults: 4 to 8 g P.O. daily in divided doses q 6 hours for 6 weeks.

Reactions may be *common*, uncommon, **life-threatening**, or COMMON AND LIFE-THREATENING.

Asymptomatic meningococcal carrier
Adults: 1 g P.O. b.i.d. for 2 days.
Children ages 1 to 12: 500 mg P.O. b.i.d. for 2 days.
Children ages 2 to 12 months: 500 mg P.O. daily for 2 days.

Pharmacodynamics
Antibacterial action: Bacteriostatic. Inhibits formation of tetrahydrofolic acid from para-aminobenzoic acid (PABA), thus preventing bacterial cell synthesis of folic acid. Active against many gram-positive bacteria, *Chlamydia trachomatis,* many Enterobacteriaceae, and some strains of *Toxoplasma gondii* and *Plasmodium falciparum.*

Pharmacokinetics
• *Absorption:* Absorbed from GI tract after oral administration; serum levels peak at 2 hours.
• *Distribution:* Distributed widely into most body tissues and fluids, including synovial, pleural, amniotic, prostatic, peritoneal, and seminal fluids; poor CSF penetration. Crosses placenta; 32% to 56% protein-bound.
• *Metabolism:* Metabolized partially in liver.
• *Excretion:* Both unchanged drug and metabolites excreted primarily in urine by glomerular filtration; to a lesser extent by renal tubular secretion; some drug excreted in breast milk. Urine solubility of unchanged drug increases as urine pH increases.

Contraindications and precautions
Contraindicated in patients with hypersensitivity to sulfonamides, in those with porphyria, in infants under age 2 months (except in congenital toxoplasmosis), in pregnant women at term, and breast-feeding women.
    Use cautiously in patients with impaired renal or hepatic function, bronchial asthma, multiple allergies, G6PD deficiency, or blood dyscrasia.

Interactions
Drug-drug. *Oral anticoagulants:* Enhanced anticoagulant effects. Monitor patient closely; adjust dosage of anticoagulants.
Oral antidiabetics (sulfonylureas): Enhanced hypoglycemic effects. Monitor blood glucose level and adjust dosage as needed.
PABA: Antagonized effects of sulfonamides. Adjust dosage as needed.
Pyrimethamine, trimethoprim (folic acid antagonists with different mechanisms of action): Synergistic antibacterial effects; delays or prevents bacterial resistance. Adjust dosage as needed.
Drug-lifestyle. *Sun exposure:* Possible photosensitivity reactions. Tell patient to take precautions.

Adverse reactions
CNS: headache, mental depression, *seizures,* hallucinations.
GI: *nausea, vomiting, diarrhea,* abdominal pain, anorexia, stomatitis.
GU: elevated serum creatinine level, *toxic nephrosis* with oliguria and anuria, crystalluria, hematuria.
Hematologic: *agranulocytosis, aplastic anemia, hemolytic anemia, thrombocytopenia,* megaloblastic anemia, *leukopenia.*
Hepatic: elevated liver enzyme levels, jaundice.
Skin: generalized skin eruption, *erythema multiforme (Stevens-Johnson syndrome), epidermal necrolysis, exfoliative dermatitis,* photosensitivity, urticaria, pruritus.
Other: hypersensitivity reactions (*serum sickness, drug fever, anaphylaxis*), local irritation, extravasation.

☑ Special considerations
Besides the recommendations relevant to all sulfonamides, consider the following.
• Sulfadiazine is a less soluble sulfonamide; it's more likely to cause crystalluria. Avoid using drug with urine acidifiers and ensure adequate fluid intake. If adequate fluid intake can't be ensured, recommend sodium bicarbonate to reduce risk of crystalluria.
• Sulfadiazine alters urine glucose tests using cupric sulfate (Benedict's reagent or Clinitest).
• Signs and symptoms of overdose include dizziness, drowsiness, headache, unconsciousness, anorexia, abdominal pain, nausea, and vomiting. More severe complications, including hemolytic anemia, agranulocytosis, dermatitis, acidosis, sensitivity reactions, and jaundice, may be fatal.
• Treatment of overdose includes gastric lavage if ingestion has occurred within 4 hours; then correction of acidosis, forced fluids, and urinary alkalinization to enhance solubility and excretion. Treatment of renal failure as well as transfusion of appropriate blood products (in severe hematologic toxicity) may be needed.

Monitoring the patient
• Monitor therapeutic effect.
• Monitor patient for adverse effects.

Information for the patient
• Advise patient to take precautions against sun exposure.

Pediatric patients
• Contraindicated in children under age 2 months.

Breast-feeding patients
• Drug appears in breast milk. Don't give to breast-feeding women.

sulfamethoxazole
Gantanol

Pharmacologic classification: sulfonamide
Therapeutic classification: antibiotic
Pregnancy risk category C

How supplied
Available by prescription only
Tablets: 500 mg

Indications, route, and dosage
Urinary tract and systemic infections
Adults: Initially, 2 g P.O.; then 1 g P.O. b.i.d., up to t.i.d. for severe infections.
Children and infants over age 2 months: Initially, 50 to 60 mg/kg P.O.; then 25 to 30 mg/kg b.i.d. Maximum dose shouldn't exceed 75 mg/kg daily.
Lymphogranuloma venereum (genital, inguinal, or anorectal infection)
Adults: 1 g P.O. b.i.d. for 21 days.

Pharmacodynamics
Antibacterial action: Bacteriostatic. Acts by inhibiting formation of tetrahydrofolic acid from para-aminobenzoic acid (PABA), thus preventing bacterial cell synthesis of folic acid. Spectrum of action includes some gram-positive bacteria, *Chlamydia trachomatis*, many Enterobacteriaceae, and some strains of *Toxoplasma* and *Plasmodium*.

Pharmacokinetics
• *Absorption:* Absorbed from GI tract after oral administration; serum levels peak at 3 to 4 hours.
• *Distribution:* Distributed widely into most body tissues and fluids, including CSF, synovial, pleural, amniotic, prostatic, peritoneal, and seminal fluids. Crosses placenta; 50% to 70% protein-bound.
• *Metabolism:* Metabolized partially in liver.
• *Excretion:* Both unchanged drug and metabolites excreted primarily in urine by glomerular filtration; to a lesser extent by renal tubular secretion. Some drug excreted in breast milk. Urinary solubility of unchanged drug increases as urine pH increases. Elimination half-life in patients with normal renal function is 7 to 12 hours.

Contraindications and precautions
Contraindicated in patients with hypersensitivity to sulfonamides, in those with porphyria, in infants under age 2 months (except in congenital toxoplasmosis), in pregnant women at term, and in breast-feeding women. Use cautiously in patients with renal or hepatic impairment, bronchial asthma, severe allergies, G6PD deficiency, or blood dyscrasia.

Interactions
Drug-drug. *Oral anticoagulants:* Enhanced anticoagulant effects. Monitor patient closely.
Oral antidiabetic drugs (sulfonylureas): Enhanced hypoglycemic effects. Monitor serum glucose level.
PABA: Antagonizes sulfonamide effects. Adjust dosage as needed.
Pyrimethamine, trimethoprim: Synergistic antibacterial effects; delays or prevents bacterial resistance. Adjust dosage as needed.
Drug-lifestyle. *Sun exposure:* Possible photosensitivity reactions. Tell patient to take precautions.

Adverse reactions
CNS: headache, mental depression, *seizures,* hallucinations, aseptic meningitis, apathy.
EENT: tinnitus.
GI: *nausea, vomiting, diarrhea,* abdominal pain, anorexia, stomatitis, *pancreatitis,* pseudomembranous colitis.
GU: *toxic nephrosis with oliguria and anuria,* crystalluria, hematuria, interstitial nephritis.
Hematologic: *agranulocytosis, hemolytic anemia, aplastic anemia,* megaloblastic anemia, *thrombocytopenia, leukopenia.*
Hepatic: elevated liver enzyme levels, *jaundice.*
Skin: generalized skin eruption, *erythema multiforme (Stevens-Johnson syndrome), epidermal necrolysis, exfoliative dermatitis,* photosensitivity, urticaria, pruritus.
Other: hypersensitivity reactions (*serum sickness, drug fever, anaphylaxis*).

☑ Special considerations
• Recommendations for administration, preparation, and storage of drug and care and teaching of the patient during therapy with sulfamethoxazole are those common to all sulfonamides.
• Sulfamethoxazole alters results of urine glucose tests using cupric sulfate (Benedict's reagent or Clinitest).
• Signs and symptoms of overdose include dizziness, drowsiness, headache, unconsciousness, anorexia, abdominal pain, nausea, and vomiting. More severe complications, including hemolytic anemia, agranulocytosis, dermatitis, acidosis, sensitivity reactions, and jaundice, may be fatal.
• Treat overdose with gastric lavage if ingestion has occurred within 4 hours; then correction of acidosis, forced fluids, and I.V. fluids if urine output is low and renal function is normal. Treatment of renal failure and transfusion of appropriate blood products (in severe hematologic toxicity) may be needed.

Monitoring the patient
• Monitor therapeutic effect.
• Monitor patient for adverse effects.

Information for the patient
• Advise patient to avoid sun exposure.

Pediatric patients
• Drug is contraindicated in infants under age 2 months.

Breast-feeding patients
• Drug appears in breast milk. Don't give to breast-feeding women.

---

sulfasalazine
Azulfidine, Azulfidine EN-Tabs

Pharmacologic classification: sulfon-amide
Therapeutic classification: antibiotic
Pregnancy risk category B

How supplied
Available by prescription only
Tablets (with or without enteric coating): 500 mg

Indications, route, and dosage
Mild to moderate ulcerative colitis, adjunctive therapy in severe ulcerative colitis
Adults: Initially, 3 to 4 g P.O. daily in evenly divided doses. Maintenance dose is 2 g P.O. daily in divided doses q 6 hours. May need to start with 1 to 2 g initially, with a gradual increase in dose to minimize adverse reactions.
Children over age 2: Initially, 40 to 60 mg/kg P.O. daily, divided into three to six doses; then 30 mg/kg daily in four doses. Maximum daily dose is 2 g. May need to start at lower dose if GI intolerance occurs.

Pharmacodynamics
Antibacterial action: Exact mechanism unknown. Believed to be a prodrug metabolized by intestinal flora in the colon. One metabolite (5-aminosalicylic acid or mesalamine) is responsible for the anti-inflammatory effect; the other metabolite (sulfapyridine) may be responsible for antibacterial action and for some adverse effects.

Pharmacokinetics
• *Absorption:* Absorbed poorly from GI tract after oral administration; 70% to 90% transported to colon where intestinal flora metabolize drug to active ingredients (sulfapyridine [antibacterial] and 5-aminosalicylic acid [anti-inflammatory]); exert effects locally. Sulfapyridine absorbed from colon; only a small portion of 5-aminosalicylic acid absorbed.
• *Distribution:* Data lacking; drug and metabolites have been found in sera, liver, and intestinal walls. Parent drug and both metabolites cross placenta.
• *Metabolism:* Cleaved by intestinal flora in colon.

• *Excretion:* Systemically absorbed sulfasalazine excreted chiefly in urine; some parent drug and metabolites excreted in breast milk. Plasma half-life is about 6 to 8 hours.

Contraindications and precautions
Contraindicated in patients with hypersensitivity to salicylates or sulfonamides or to other drugs containing sulfur (such as thiazides, furosemide, or oral sulfonylureas); in those with porphyria or severe renal or hepatic dysfunction; during pregnancy and at term; in breast-feeding women; and in children under age 2. Sulfasalazine is also contraindicated in patients with intestinal or urinary tract obstructions because of risk of local GI irritation and crystalluria.
    Use cautiously in patients with mild to moderate renal or hepatic dysfunction, severe allergies, asthma, blood dyscrasia, or G6PD deficiency.

Interactions
Drug-drug. *Antacids:* Increased systemic absorption and possibility of toxicity. Avoid concomitant use.
Antibiotics that alter intestinal flora: Decreased sulfasalazine effectiveness. Avoid concomitant use.
Digoxin, folic acid: Reduced absorption of these drugs. Monitor therapeutic effect and adjust dosage as needed.
Oral anticoagulants: Enhanced anticoagulant effects. Dosage adjustment may be needed.
Oral antidiabetics (sulfonylureas): Enhanced hypoglycemic effect. Monitor blood glucose levels.
Urine acidifying drugs (ammonium chloride, ascorbic acid): Increased risk of crystalluria. Monitor urinary status closely.
Drug-lifestyle. *Sun exposure:* Increased photosensitivity reactions. Tell patient to take precautions.

Adverse reactions
CNS: headache, mental depression, ***seizures,*** hallucinations.
EENT: tinnitus.
GI: *nausea, vomiting, diarrhea, abdominal pain, anorexia,* stomatitis.
GU: toxic nephrosis with oliguria and anuria, crystalluria, hematuria, oligospermia, infertility.
Hematologic: ***agranulocytosis, aplastic anemia,*** megaloblastic anemia, ***thrombocytopenia,*** leukopenia, hemolytic anemia.
Hepatic: jaundice, elevated liver enzyme levels.
Skin: generalized skin eruption, ***erythema multiforme (Stevens-Johnson syndrome), epidermal necrolysis, exfoliative dermatitis,*** photosensitivity, urticaria, pruritus.
Other: ***hypersensitivity reactions,*** serum sickness, drug fever, ***anaphylaxis,*** bacterial and fungal superinfection.

☑ Special considerations
Besides the recommendations relevant to all sulfonamides, consider the following.
• Stop drug if signs of toxicity or hypersensitivity occur; if hematologic abnormalities are accompanied by sore throat, pallor, fever, jaundice, purpura, or weakness; if crystalluria is accompanied by renal colic, hematuria, oliguria, proteinuria, urinary obstruction, urolithiasis, increased BUN levels, or anuria; if severe diarrhea indicates pseudomembranous colitis; or if severe nausea, vomiting, or diarrhea persists.
• Most adverse effects involve GI tract; minimize reactions and facilitate absorption by spacing doses evenly and administering drug after food.
• Drug colors urine orange-yellow; may also color patient's skin orange-yellow.
• Don't give antacids together with enteric-coated sulfasalazine; they may alter absorption.
• Drug alters results of urine glucose tests using cupric sulfate (Benedict's reagent or Clinitest).
• Signs and symptoms of overdose include dizziness, drowsiness, headache, unconsciousness, anorexia, abdominal pain, nausea, and vomiting. More severe complications, including hemolytic anemia, agranulocytosis, dermatitis, acidosis, sensitivity reactions, and jaundice, may be fatal.
• Treat overdose with gastric lavage if ingestion has occurred within 4 hours; then correction of acidosis, forced fluids, and urinary alkalinization to enhance solubility and excretion. Treatment of renal failure and transfusion of appropriate blood products (in severe hematologic toxicity) may be needed.

Monitoring the patient
• Monitor patient for signs of toxicity and hypersensitivity.
• Monitor GI status.

Information for the patient
• Tell patient that drug normally turns urine orange-yellow. Warn him that skin may also turn orange-yellow and that drug may permanently stain soft contact lenses yellow.
• Advise patient not to take antacids simultaneously with sulfasalazine.
• Advise patient to take drug after meals to reduce GI distress and to facilitate passage into intestines.
• Tell patient to avoid prolonged exposure to sunlight because photosensitivity may occur; advise him to wear protective clothing and sunscreen.

Pediatric patients
• Drug is contraindicated in children under age 2.

Breast-feeding patients
• Drug appears in breast milk; use with caution in breast-feeding women.

sulfinpyrazone
Anturane

Pharmacologic classification: uricosuric
Therapeutic classification: renal tubular-blocking drug, platelet aggregation inhibitor
Pregnancy risk category NR

How supplied
Available by prescription only
Tablets: 100 mg
Capsules: 200 mg

Indications, route, and dosage
Chronic gouty arthritis and intermittent gouty arthritis; hyperuricemia associated with gout
Adults: Initially, 200 to 400 mg P.O. daily in two divided doses, gradually increasing to maintenance dose in 1 week. Maintenance dose is 400 mg P.O. daily in two divided doses; may increase to 800 mg daily or decrease to 200 mg daily.
◇ *Prophylaxis of thromboembolic disorders, including angina, MI, and transient (cerebral) ischemic attacks, and in patients with prosthetic heart valves*
Adults: 600 to 800 mg daily in divided doses to decrease platelet aggregation.

Pharmacodynamics
Uricosuric action: Sulfinpyrazone competitively inhibits renal tubule reabsorption of uric acid. Sulfinpyrazone inhibits adenosine diphosphate and 5-HT, resulting in decreased platelet adhesiveness and increased platelet survival time.

Pharmacokinetics
• *Absorption:* Absorbed completely after oral administration; plasma levels peak in 2 hours. Effects usually last 4 to 6 hours; may last up to 10 hours.
• *Distribution:* 98% to 99% protein-bound.
• *Metabolism:* Metabolized rapidly in liver.
• *Excretion:* Drug and metabolites eliminated in urine; about 50% excreted unchanged.

Contraindications and precautions
Contraindicated in patients with hypersensitivity to pyrazolone derivatives (including oxyphenbutazone and phenylbutazone) and in those with blood dyscrasia, active peptic ulcer, or symptoms of GI inflammation or ulceration. Use cautiously in patients with healed peptic ulcer and during pregnancy.

Interactions
Drug-drug. *Cholestyramine:* Decreased absorption of sulfinpyrazone. Sulfinpyrazone should be taken 1 hour before or 4 to 6 hours after cholestyramine.

Reactions may be *common*, uncommon, **life-threatening**, or COMMON AND LIFE-THREATENING.

Diazoxide, diuretics, pyrazinamide: Increased serum uric acid. Increase sulfinpyrazone dosage.
Nitrofurantoin, penicillin, sulfonylureas, other beta-lactam antibiotics: Decreased efficacy in treatment of urinary tract infections; increased systemic toxicity. Monitor patient closely.
Oral antidiabetics: Hypoglycemia. Monitor blood glucose levels.
Probenecid: Inhibited renal excretion of sulfinpyrazone. Adjust dosage.
Salicylates (in high doses): Blocked uricosuric effects of sulfinpyrazone. Avoid high doses of salicylates.
Warfarin: Increased bleeding. Monitor PT and INR.
Drug-lifestyle. *Alcohol:* Decreased effectiveness of drug. Discourage concomitant use.

Adverse reactions
GI: *nausea, dyspepsia,* epigastric pain, reactivation of peptic ulcerations.
GU: altered renal function test results, decreased urinary excretion of aminohippuric acid and phenolsulfonphthalein.
Hematologic: *blood dyscrasia* (such as anemia, leukopenia, *agranulocytosis, thrombocytopenia, aplastic anemia*).
Respiratory: bronchoconstriction in patients with aspirin-induced asthma.
Skin: rash.

☑ Special considerations
● Drug doesn't accumulate and tolerance doesn't develop; it's suitable for long-term use.
● Drug has no analgesic or anti-inflammatory actions.
● Drug may not be effective and should be avoided when creatinine clearance is less than 50 ml/minute.
● Drug should be administered with food, milk, or antacids to lessen GI upset.
● Sulfinpyrazone is used for investigational purposes to increase platelet survival time, to treat thromboembolic phenomena, and to prevent MI recurrence.
● Adequate hydration with high fluid intake will help to prevent formation of uric acid kidney stones.
● Signs and symptoms of overdose include nausea, vomiting, epigastric pain, ataxia, labored breathing, seizures, and coma. Treat supportively; induce emesis or use gastric lavage as appropriate. Treat seizures with diazepam, phenytoin, or both.

Monitoring the patient
● Monitor renal function and CBC routinely.
● Monitor serum uric acid levels and adjust dosage accordingly.

Information for the patient
● Explain that gouty attacks may increase during first 6 to 12 months of therapy; patient shouldn't stop drug without approval.
● Encourage patient to comply with dose regimen and to keep scheduled follow-up visits.
● Tell patient to drink 8 to 10 glasses of fluid each day and to take drug with food to minimize GI upset; warn patient to avoid alcoholic beverages, which decrease therapeutic effect.

Geriatric patients
● Elderly patients are more likely than younger patients to have glomerular filtration rates below 50 ml/minute; drug may be ineffective.

Breast-feeding patients
● Safety in breast-feeding women hasn't been established. It's unknown if drug appears in breast milk; an alternative to breast-feeding is recommended during therapy.

sulfisoxazole
Gantrisin

sulfisoxazole diolamine
Gantrisin (Ophthalmic Solution)

Pharmacologic classification: sulfonamide
Therapeutic classification: antibiotic
Pregnancy risk category C

How supplied
Available by prescription only
Tablets: 500 mg
Liquid: 500 mg/5 ml
Ophthalmic solution: 4%

Indications, route, and dosage
Urinary tract and systemic infections
Adults: Initially, 2 to 4 g P.O.; then 4 to 8 g P.O. daily in divided doses q 4 to 6 hours.
Children and infants over age 2 months: Initially, 75 mg/kg P.O.; then 150 mg/kg (or 4 g/m²) P.O. daily in divided doses q 4 to 6 hours. Maximum dose shouldn't exceed 6 g/24 hours.
Lymphogranuloma venereum (genital, inguinal, or anorectal infection)
Adults: 500 mg to 1 g q.i.d. for 3 weeks.
Conjunctivitis, corneal ulcer, superficial ocular infections; adjunct in systemic treatment of trachoma
Adults: Instill 1 to 2 drops in the lower conjunctival sac of affected eye daily q 1 to 4 hours, for 7 to 10 days.

Pharmacodynamics
Antibacterial action: Bacteriostatic. Acts by inhibiting formation of tetrahydrofolic acid from para-aminobenzoic acid (PABA), thus preventing bac-

terial cell synthesis of folic acid. Acts synergistically with folic acid antagonists such as trimethoprim, which block folic acid synthesis at a later stage, thus delaying or preventing bacterial resistance. Active against some gram-positive bacteria, *Chlamydia trachomatis,* many Enterobacteriaceae, and some strains of *Toxoplasma* and *Plasmodium.*

Pharmacokinetics
- *Absorption:* Absorbed readily from GI tract after oral administration; serum levels peak in 2 to 4 hours.
- *Distribution:* Distributed into extracellular compartments; CSF penetration is 8% to 57% of blood levels in uninflamed meninges. Drug crosses placenta; 85% protein-bound.
- *Metabolism:* Metabolized partially in liver.
- *Excretion:* Both unchanged drug and metabolites excreted primarily in urine by glomerular filtration; to a lesser extent by renal tubular secretion. Some drug excreted in breast milk. Urinary solubility of unchanged drug increases as urine pH increases. Plasma half-life in patients with normal renal function is about 4½ to 8 hours.

Contraindications and precautions
Contraindicated in patients with hypersensitivity to sulfonamides, in infants under age 2 months (except in congenital toxoplasmosis [with oral form only]), in pregnant women at term, and in breast-feeding women.

Use oral form cautiously in patients with impaired renal or hepatic function, severe allergies, bronchial asthma, or G6PD deficiency. Use ophthalmic form cautiously in patients with severely dry eyes.

Interactions
Drug-drug. *Oral anticoagulants:* Exaggerated anticoagulant effects. Monitor patient closely.
Oral antidiabetics (sulfonylureas): Enhanced hypoglycemic effects. Monitor serum glucose levels; adjust dosage as needed.
PABA: Antagonized effects of sulfonamides. Monitor patient closely.
Pyrimethamine, trimethoprim: Synergistic antibacterial effects; delays or prevents bacterial resistance. Monitor therapeutic effect.
Urine acidifying drugs (ammonium chloride, ascorbic acid): Increased risk of crystalluria. Monitor urinary status.
Drug-lifestyle. *Sun exposure:* Photosensitivity reactions. Tell patient to take precautions.

Adverse reactions
CNS: headache; mental depression, hallucinations, *seizures* (with oral administration).
CV: tachycardia, palpitations, syncope, cyanosis (with oral administration).
EENT: *ocular irritation, itching, chemosis, periorbital edema* (with ophthalmic form).

GI: *nausea, vomiting, diarrhea,* abdominal pain, anorexia, stomatitis, pseudomembranous colitis (with oral administration).
GU: *toxic nephrosis with oliguria and anuria, acute renal failure,* crystalluria, hematuria (with oral administration).
Hematologic: *agranulocytosis, aplastic anemia, thrombocytopenia, hemolytic anemia,* megaloblastic anemia, *leukopenia* (with oral administration).
Hepatic: elevated liver enzyme levels, jaundice (with oral administration), *hepatitis.*
Skin: *erythema multiforme, epidermal necrolysis, exfoliative dermatitis,* generalized skin eruption, photosensitivity, urticaria, pruritus (with oral administration); *Stevens-Johnson syndrome* (with ophthalmic form).
Other: hypersensitivity reactions (*serum sickness, drug fever, anaphylaxis*), overgrowth of nonsusceptible organisms (with ophthalmic form).

☑ Special considerations
Besides the recommendations relevant to all sulfonamides, consider the following.
- Sulfisoxazole-pyrimethamine is used to treat toxoplasmosis.
- Sulfisoxazole alters results of urine glucose tests using cupric sulfate (Benedict's reagent or Clinitest).
- Signs and symptoms of overdose include dizziness, drowsiness, headache, unconsciousness, anorexia, abdominal pain, nausea, and vomiting. More severe complications, including hemolytic anemia, agranulocytosis, dermatitis, acidosis, sensitivity reactions, and jaundice, may be fatal.
- Treat overdose with gastric lavage if ingestion has occurred within 4 hours; then correction of acidosis and forced fluids and urinary alkalinization to enhance solubility and excretion. Treatment of renal failure and transfusion of appropriate blood products (in severe hematologic toxicity) may be needed.

Monitoring the patient
- Monitor therapeutic effect.
- Monitor patient for adverse effects.

Information for the patient
- Tell patient to drink 8 oz (240 ml) of water with each oral dose and to take drug on empty stomach.
- Tell patient to take drug completely, as prescribed.
- Show patient how to use ophthalmic preparations. Warn patient not to touch tip of dropper or tube to any surface.
- Warn patient that ophthalmic solution may cause blurred vision immediately after application. Tell patient to gently close eyes and keep closed for 1 to 2 minutes.

Reactions may be *common,* uncommon, *life-threatening,* or COMMON AND LIFE-THREATENING.

• Tell patient to avoid prolonged exposure to sunlight because photosensitivity may occur; tell him to wear protective clothing and sunscreen.

Pediatric patients
• Drug is contraindicated in infants under age 2 months.

Breast-feeding patients
• Drug appears in breast milk. Don't give to breast-feeding women.

sulindac
Clinoril

Pharmacologic classification: NSAID
Therapeutic classification: nonnarcotic analgesic, antipyretic, anti-inflammatory
Pregnancy risk category NR

How supplied
Available by prescription only
Tablets: 150 mg, 200 mg

Indications, route, and dosage
Osteoarthritis, rheumatoid arthritis, ankylosing spondylitis
Adults: 150 mg P.O. b.i.d. initially; may increase to 200 mg P.O. b.i.d.
Acute subacromial bursitis or supraspinatus tendinitis, acute gouty arthritis
Adults: 200 mg P.O. b.i.d. for 7 to 14 days. Dose may be reduced as symptoms subside.

Pharmacodynamics
Analgesic, antipyretic, and anti-inflammatory actions: Mechanisms unknown. Thought to inhibit prostaglandin synthesis.

Pharmacokinetics
• *Absorption:* Rapidly and completely absorbed from GI tract.
• *Distribution:* Highly protein-bound.
• *Metabolism:* Drug is inactive; metabolized hepatically to active sulfide metabolite.
• *Excretion:* Excreted in urine. Half-life of parent drug about 8 hours; half-life of active metabolite is about 16 hours.

Contraindications and precautions
Contraindicated in patients with hypersensitivity to drug or in whom acute asthmatic attacks, urticaria, or rhinitis is precipitated by use of aspirin or NSAIDs. Avoid use during pregnancy.
Use cautiously in patients with history of ulcer or GI bleeding, renal dysfunction, compromised cardiac function, hypertension, or conditions predisposing to fluid retention.

Interactions
Drug-drug. *Antacids:* Delayed and decreased absorption of sulindac. Avoid concomitant use.
Anticoagulants, thrombolytics: Potentiated anticoagulation. Monitor patient closely.
Aspirin, diflunisal: Decreased plasma levels of active sulfide metabolite. Adjust dosage as necessary.
Dimethyl sulfoxide: Decreased plasma levels of active sulfide metabolite. Peripheral neuropathies also reported with this combination. Avoid concomitant use.
GI-irritating drugs (antibiotics, NSAIDs, corticosteroids): Potentiated adverse GI effects of sulindac. Use together with caution.
Highly protein-bound drugs (phenytoin, sulfonylureas, warfarin): Possible displacement of either drug; adverse effects. Monitor therapy closely for both drugs.
Lithium carbonate: Increased lithium serum levels and risks of adverse effects. Monitor serum lithium levels.
Probenecid: Increased plasma levels of sulindac and its inactive sulfane metabolite; sulindac may decrease uricosuric effect of probenecid. Avoid concomitant use.
Drug-food. *Any food:* Delayed and decreased absorption of sulindac. Monitor patient for drug effect.

Adverse reactions
CNS: dizziness, headache, nervousness, psychosis.
CV: hypertension, heart failure, palpitations, edema.
EENT: tinnitus, transient visual disturbances.
GI: *epigastric distress,* **peptic ulceration, GI bleeding, pancreatitis,** occult blood loss, nausea, constipation, dyspepsia, flatulence, anorexia, vomiting, diarrhea.
GU: increased BUN and serum creatinine levels, interstitial nephritis, **nephrotic syndrome, renal failure.**
Hematologic: prolonged bleeding time, **aplastic anemia, thrombocytopenia, agranulocytosis, neutropenia,** hemolytic anemia.
Hepatic: elevated liver enzymes.
Metabolic: hyperkalemia.
Skin: *rash,* pruritus.
Other: drug fever, **anaphylaxis, hypersensitivity syndrome,** angioedema.

☑ Special considerations
Besides the recommendations relevant to all NSAIDs, consider the following.
• Sulindac may be the safest NSAID for patients with mild renal impairment. It also may be less likely to cause further renal toxicity.
• Symptomatic improvement may take 7 days or longer.
• Signs and symptoms of overdose include dizziness, drowsiness, mental confusion, disorienta-

tion, lethargy, paresthesia, numbness, vomiting, gastric irritation, nausea, abdominal pain, headache, stupor, coma, and hypotension.
• To treat overdose, empty stomach immediately by inducing emesis with ipecac syrup or by gastric lavage. Administer activated charcoal via nasogastric tube. Provide symptomatic and supportive measures (respiratory support and correction of fluid and electrolyte imbalances). Dialysis is thought to be of minimal value because sulindac is highly protein-bound. Monitor laboratory parameters and vital signs closely.

Monitoring the patient
• Assess cardiopulmonary status frequently. Monitor vital signs, especially heart rate and blood pressure, to detect abnormalities.
• Assess fluid balance status. Monitor intake and output and daily weight. Observe for presence and amount of edema.
• Evaluate patient's response as evidenced by a reduction in symptoms.

Information for the patient
• Caution patient to avoid use of OTC preparations unless medically approved.
• Teach patient how to recognize signs and symptoms of possible adverse reactions; advise patient to report such adverse reactions.
• Advise patient to check weight two or three times weekly and to report weight gain of 3 lb (1.4 kg) or more within 1 week.
• Because drug causes sodium retention, advise patient to report edema and to have blood pressure checked routinely.
• Advise patient in safety measures; avoid hazardous activities that require alertness until CNS effects of drug are known.

Geriatric patients
• Patients over age 60 are more sensitive to drug's adverse effects. Use with caution.
• Because of its effect on renal prostaglandins, drug may cause significant fluid retention and edema in elderly patients and in those with heart failure.

Pediatric patients
• Safety of long-term use in children hasn't been established.

Breast-feeding patients
• Safe use during breast-feeding hasn't been established. Because it's unknown if drug appears in breast milk, avoid use in breast-feeding women.

sumatriptan succinate
Imitrex

Pharmacologic classification: selective 5-hydroxytryptamine ($5HT_1$)-receptor agonist
Therapeutic classification: antimigraine
Pregnancy risk category C

How supplied
Available by prescription only
Tablets: 25 mg, 50 mg
Injection: 12 mg/ml (0.5 ml in 1-ml prefilled syringe), 6-mg single-dose (0.5 ml in 2 ml) vial, and self-dose system kit
Nasal spray: 5 mg, 20 mg unit dose nasal spray device

Indications, route, and dosage
Acute migraine attacks (with or without aura)
Adults: 6 mg S.C. Maximum recommended dose is two 6-mg injections in 24 hours, separated by at least 1 hour, or 25 to 100 mg P.O. initially. If response isn't achieved in 2 hours, may give second dose of 25 to 100 mg. Additional doses may be used in at least 2-hour intervals. Maximum daily dose is 300 mg.

For nasal spray, administer single dose of 5 mg, 10 mg, or 20 mg once in one nostril; may repeat once after 2 hours for maximum daily dose of 40 mg. (A 10-mg dose may be achieved by the administration of a single 5-mg dose in each nostril.)

Pharmacodynamics
Antimigraine action: Selectively binds to a $5-HT_1$ receptor subtype found in the basilar artery and vasculature of dura mater, where drug presumably exerts its antimigraine effect. In these tissues, sumatriptan activates the receptor to cause vasoconstriction, an action correlating with the relief of migraine.

Pharmacokinetics
• *Absorption:* Bioavailability via S.C. injection is 97% of that obtained via I.V. injection. Peak level after S.C. injection in about 12 minutes.
• *Distribution:* Low protein-binding capacity (about 14% to 21%).
• *Metabolism:* About 80% of drug metabolized in liver, primarily to inactive indoleacetic acid metabolite.
• *Excretion:* Excreted primarily in urine, 20% as unchanged drug and partly as indoleacetic acid metabolite. Elimination half-life about 2 hours.

Contraindications and precautions
Contraindicated in patients with hypersensitivity to drug; in those with uncontrolled hypertension, ischemic heart disease (such as angina pectoris, Prinzmetal's angina, history of MI, or document-

ed silent ischemia), or hemiplegic or basilar migraine; within 14 days of MAO therapy; and in patients taking ergotamine.

Use cautiously in patients who may be at risk for coronary artery disease (CAD) (such as postmenopausal women or men over age 40) or in those with risk factors such as hypertension, hypercholesterolemia, obesity, diabetes, smoking, or family history. Use cautiously in women of childbearing age and in pregnant women.

Interactions
Drug-drug. *Ergot, ergot derivatives:* Prolonged vasospastic effects when given with sumatriptan. Don't use these drugs within 24 hours of sumatriptan therapy.
Drug-herb. *Horehound:* Enhanced serotonergic effects. Don't use together.

Adverse reactions
CNS: *dizziness, vertigo,* drowsiness, headache, anxiety, malaise, fatigue.
CV: *atrial fibrillation, ventricular fibrillation, ventricular tachycardia, MI,* pressure or tightness in chest.
EENT: discomfort of throat, nasal cavity or sinus, mouth, jaw, or tongue; altered vision.
GI: abdominal discomfort, dysphagia.
Musculoskeletal: myalgia, muscle cramps, neck pain.
Skin: flushing, diaphoresis.
Other: *tingling; warm or hot sensation; burning sensation; heaviness; pressure or tightness;* tight feeling in head; cold sensation; *injection site reaction.*

☑ Special considerations
• Don't use drug for management of hemiplegic or basilar migraine. Safety and effectiveness also haven't been established for cluster headache, which occurs in an older, predominantly male population.
• Don't give drug I.V. because coronary vasospasm may occur.
• Nasal spray is generally well tolerated; however, adverse reactions seen with other forms of drug can still occur.
• Drug has rarely caused serious or life-threatening arrhythmias, such as atrial and ventricular fibrillation, ventricular tachycardia, MI, and marked ischemic ST elevations. It also has rarely, but more frequently, caused chest and arm discomfort thought to represent angina pectoris. Because such coronary events can occur, consider administering first dose in an outpatient setting to patients in whom unrecognized CAD is comparatively likely (postmenopausal women; men over age 40; and patients with risk factors for CAD, such as hypertension, hypercholesterolemia, obesity, diabetes, smoking, and strong family history of CAD).

• Patient response to nasal spray may vary. The choice of dose should be made individually, weighing the possible benefit of the 20-mg dose with the potential for a greater risk of adverse effects.
• No specific overdose information is available. Drug would be expected to cause seizures, tremor, inactivity, erythema of extremities, reduced respiratory rate, cyanosis, ataxia, mydriasis, injection site reactions, and paralysis. Continue monitoring while signs and symptoms persist and for at least 10 hours thereafter. Effect of hemodialysis or peritoneal dialysis on serum levels of sumatriptan is unknown.

Monitoring the patient
• Monitor cardiac status closely.
• Monitor therapeutic effect.

Information for the patient
• Tell patient that drug may be given at any time during a migraine attack, but preferably as soon as symptoms begin. A second injection may be given if symptoms recur. Tell patient not to use more than two injections in 24 hours and to allow at least 1 hour between doses. Pain or redness at the injection site may occur but usually lasts less than 1 hour.
• Explain that drug is intended to relieve migraine, not to prevent or reduce number of attacks.
• Tell patient not to use a second nasal spray dose if there was no response to initial dose, unless directed otherwise.
• Explain that drug is available in a spring-loaded injector system that facilitates self-administration. Review detailed information with patient. Be sure he understands how to load injector, administer injection, and dispose of used syringes.
• Tell woman to call if she is pregnant or intends to become pregnant during therapy.
• Tell patient who feels persistent or severe chest pain to call immediately. Tell patient who experiences pain or tightness in the throat, wheezing, heart throbbing, rash, lumps, hives, or swollen eyelids, face, or lips to stop using drug and call immediately.

Pediatric patients
• Safety and effectiveness in children haven't been established.

Breast-feeding patients
• Drug appears in breast milk. Use with caution in breast-feeding women.

tacrine hydrochloride
Cognex

Pharmacologic classification: centrally acting reversible cholinesterase inhibitor
Therapeutic classification: psychotherapeutic drug (for Alzheimer's disease)
Pregnancy risk category C

How supplied
Available by prescription only
Capsules: 10 mg, 20 mg, 30 mg, 40 mg

Indications, route, and dosage
Mild to moderate dementia of the Alzheimer's type
Adults: Initially, 10 mg P.O. q.i.d. Maintain dose for at least 4 weeks, with every-other-week monitoring of transaminase levels beginning at week 4 of therapy. If patient tolerates treatment and transaminase levels remain normal, increase to 20 mg P.O. q.i.d. After 4 weeks, adjust dose to 30 mg P.O. q.i.d. If still tolerated, increase to 40 mg P.O. q.i.d. after another 4 weeks.
+ Dosage adjustment. In patients with ALT level two to three times the upper limit of normal, monitor ALT level weekly. If ALT level is three to five times the upper normal limit, reduce daily dose by 40 mg/day and monitor ALT level weekly. Resume dosage adjustment and every-other-week monitoring when ALT level returns to normal. If ALT level is above five times upper limit of normal, stop treatment and monitor ALT level. Watch for signs and symptoms associated with hepatitis. Rechallenge when ALT level is normal and monitor weekly.

Pharmacodynamics
Psychotherapeutic action: Presumably slows degradation of acetylcholine released by still-intact cholinergic neurons, thereby elevating acetylcholine levels in the cerebral cortex. If this theory is correct, the effects of tacrine may lessen as the disease process advances and fewer cholinergic neurons remain functionally intact. No evidence suggests that tacrine alters the course of the underlying dementia.

Pharmacokinetics
• *Absorption:* Rapidly absorbed after oral administration; maximum plasma levels within 1 to 2 hours. Absolute bioavailability about 17%. Food reduces bioavailability by about 30% to 40%; no food effect if given at least 1 hour before meals.
• *Distribution:* About 55% bound to plasma proteins.
• *Metabolism:* Undergoes first-pass metabolism; dose dependent. Extensively metabolized by cytochrome P-450 system to several metabolites; not all identified.
• *Excretion:* Elimination half-life about 2 to 4 hours.

Contraindications and precautions
Contraindicated in patients with hypersensitivity to drug or acridine derivatives. Also contraindicated in patients with tacrine-related jaundice that has been confirmed by an elevated total bilirubin level of more than 3 mg/dl and in patients with hypersensitivity reactions associated with ALT elevations.

Use cautiously in patients with sick sinus syndrome, bradycardia, history of hepatic disease, renal disease, Parkinson's disease, asthma, prostatic hyperplasia, or other urinary outflow impairment and in those at risk for peptic ulcer.

Interactions
Drug-drug. *Anticholinergics:* Reduced effect of anticholinergic. Adjust dosage as needed.
Cholinergic agonists (such as bethanechol), cholinesterase inhibitors, succinylcholine: Synergistic effect. Monitor therapeutic effect.
Cimetidine: Increased plasma level of tacrine. Adjust dosage.
Drugs that undergo extensive metabolism via cytochrome P-450: Drug interactions may occur. Avoid concomitant use.
NSAIDs: May contribute to GI irritation and gastric bleeding. Avoid concomitant use.
Theophylline: Increased average theophylline plasma levels. Monitor plasma theophylline levels.
Drug-food. *Any food:* Delayed drug absorption. Give drug 1 hour before meals.
Drug-lifestyle. *Smoking:* Decreased plasma levels of drug. Discourage smoking.

Adverse reactions
CNS: agitation, ataxia, insomnia, abnormal thinking, somnolence, depression, anxiety, *headache, dizziness,* fatigue, confusion, seizures.
CV: **bradycardia,** hypertension, palpitations, chest pain.
EENT: rhinitis.

Reactions may be *common,* uncommon, **_life-threatening_**, or COMMON AND LIFE-THREATENING.

GI: *nausea, vomiting, diarrhea,* dyspepsia, loose stools, changes in stool color, anorexia, abdominal pain, flatulence, constipation.
Hepatic: elevated liver enzyme levels, jaundice.
Metabolic: weight loss.
Musculoskeletal: myalgia.
Respiratory: upper respiratory tract infection, cough.
Skin: rash, facial flushing.
Other: increased sweating.

☑ **Special considerations**
• Tacrine as a cholinesterase inhibitor is likely to exaggerate succinylcholine-type muscle relaxation during anesthesia.
• Because of its cholinomimetic action, drug may have vagotonic effects on heart rate (such as bradycardia), which may be particularly important to patients with sick sinus syndrome.
• Rate of dosage escalation may be slowed if patient is intolerant to recommended adjustment schedule. However, don't accelerate dose incrementation plan.
• The incidence of transaminase elevations is higher among women. There are no other known predictors of risk of hepatocellular injury.
• If drug is stopped for 4 weeks or more, restart full dosage adjustment and monitoring schedule.
• Cognitive function can worsen after stopping drug abruptly or after a reduction in total daily dose of 80 mg/day or more.
• Overdose with cholinesterase inhibitors can cause a cholinergic crisis characterized by severe nausea, vomiting, salivation, sweating, bradycardia, hypotension, and seizures. Increasing muscle weakness may occur and can result in death if respiratory muscles are involved. Use general supportive measures. Tertiary anticholinergics such as atropine may be used as an antidote for tacrine overdose. I.V. atropine sulfate titrated to effect is recommended (initial dose of 1 to 2 mg I.V., with subsequent doses based on clinical response). It's unknown if tacrine or its metabolites can be eliminated by dialysis.

Monitoring the patient
• Monitor serum ALT levels every other week from at least week 4 to week 16 after initiation of therapy. Then monitoring may be decreased to every 3 months if ALT level is less than or equal to two times upper limit of normal. With each dosage adjustment, resume every-other-week monitoring.
• Monitor patient for adverse effects.

Information for the patient
• Tell patient and caregiver that drug should be taken between meals when possible. However, if GI upset occurs, drug may be taken with meals but this may reduce plasma levels.
• Inform patient and family that drug doesn't alter the underlying degenerative disease but can

alleviate symptoms. Effectiveness of therapy depends on drug administration at regular intervals.
• Remind caregiver that dosage adjustment is an integral part of safe use. An abrupt stop or a large reduction in daily dose (80 mg/day or more) may precipitate behavioral disturbances and a decline in cognitive function.
• Advise patient and caregiver to report significant adverse effects or changes in status immediately.

tacrolimus (FK506)
Prograf

Pharmacologic classification: bacteria-derived macrolide
Therapeutic classification: immunosuppressant
Pregnancy risk category C

How supplied
Available by prescription only
Capsules: 1 mg, 5 mg
Injection: 5 mg/ml

Indications, route, and dosage
Organ liver rejection prophylaxis
Adults: Initially, 0.05 to 0.1 mg/kg/day as a continuous I.V. infusion given no sooner than 6 hours after transplantation. I.V. route should be maintained only until patient can tolerate oral administration (usually within 2 to 3 days); then give 0.15 to 0.3 mg/kg/day P.O. in two divided doses q 12 hours, beginning 8 to 12 hours after stopping infusion. May use oral dosing originally, if tolerated. Administer doses at lower end of range, if possible.
Children: 0.1 mg/kg/day I.V. or 0.3 mg/kg/day P.O. given no sooner than 6 hours after transplantation. I.V. route should be maintained only until patient can tolerate oral administration (usually within 2 to 3 days); then give 0.3 mg/kg/day P.O. in two divided doses q 12 hours, beginning 8 to 12 hours after stopping infusion.

Pharmacodynamics
Immunosuppressant action: Exact mechanism unknown. Inhibits T-lymphocyte activation. Evidence suggests that drug binds to an intracellular protein, FKBP-12. A complex of tacrolimus-FKBP-12, calcium, calmodulin, and calcineurin then forms, inhibiting the phosphatase activity of calcineurin. This effect may prevent the generation of nuclear factor of activated T cells, a nuclear component thought to initiate gene transcription for the formation of lymphocyte activation and, therefore, to cause immunosuppression.

Pharmacokinetics
• *Absorption:* Absorption of oral drug from the GI tract varies. Absorption half-life in liver transplan

patients is about 5½ hours. Levels in blood and plasma peak in 1½ to 3½ hours. Absolute bioavailability is 14% to 17%. Food reduces absorption and bioavailability.

• *Distribution:* Bound to proteins, mainly albumin and alpha₁-acid glycoprotein, and is highly bound to erythrocytes. Protein-binding between 75% and 99%. Distribution of drug between whole blood and plasma depends on several factors, such as hematocrit, temperature of separation of plasma, drug level, and plasma protein level.
• *Metabolism:* Extensively metabolized by mixed-function oxidase system, primarily cytochrome P-450.
• *Excretion:* Less than 1% of dose excreted unchanged in urine. Ten possible metabolites identified in human plasma. Two metabolites, a demethylated and a double demethylated tacrolimus, shown to retain 10% and 7%, respectively, of inhibitory effect of tacrolimus on T-lymphocyte activation.

Contraindications and precautions
Contraindicated in patients with hypersensitivity to drug. I.V. form is contraindicated in those with hypersensitivity to castor oil derivatives. Use cautiously in patients with impaired renal or hepatic function.

Interactions
Drug-drug. *Antifungals, bromocriptine, calcium channel blockers, cimetidine, clarithromycin, danazol, diltiazem, erythromycin, methylprednisolone, metoclopramide:* Possible interference with tacrolimus metabolism. Reduced tacrolimus dosage may be needed.
Carbamazepine, phenobarbital, phenytoin, rifamycins: Decreased tacrolimus blood levels. Increase tacrolimus dosage.
Live vaccines: Active infection. Avoid concomitant use.
Nephrotoxic drugs (aminoglycosides, amphotericin B, cisplatin, cyclosporine): Increased risk of nephrotoxicity. Avoid use of tacrolimus and cyclosporine; stop one at least 24 hours before starting other. With elevated tacrolimus or cyclosporine levels, further dosing with other drug is usually delayed.
Other immunosuppressants (except adrenal corticosteroids): Increased susceptibility to infection. Avoid concomitant use.
Drug-food. *Any food:* Inhibited drug absorption. Take drug on empty stomach.
Grapefruit juice: Increased drug blood levels in liver transplant patients. Don't use together.

Adverse reactions
CNS: *headache, tremor, insomnia, paresthesia, asthenia.*
CV: *hypertension, peripheral edema.*
GI: *diarrhea, nausea, constipation, anorexia, vomiting, abdominal pain.*

GU: *abnormal renal function, increased creatinine or BUN levels, urinary tract infection, oliguria.*
Hematologic: *anemia, leukocytosis,* THROMBO-CYTOPENIA.
Hepatic: *abnormal liver function test results.*
Metabolic: *hyperkalemia, hypokalemia, hyperglycemia, hypomagnesemia.*
Musculoskeletal: *back pain.*
Respiratory: *pleural effusion, atelectasis, dyspnea.*
Skin: *pruritus, rash.*
Other: *pain, fever, ascites,* **anaphylaxis.**

☑ Special considerations
• Give adult patients doses at lower end of dosing range. Adjust dosage based on assessment of rejection and tolerance. Lower doses may be sufficient as maintenance therapy. Tacrolimus should be used with adrenal corticosteroids in early posttransplant period.
• Because of risk of anaphylaxis, reserve injection for patients unable to take capsules.
• Drug is being investigated for use in kidney, bone marrow, cardiac, pancreas, pancreatic island cell, and small bowel transplantation. It also may be used to treat autoimmune disease and severe recalcitrant psoriasis.
• Tacrolimus therapy is usually delayed 48 hours or longer in patients with postoperative oliguria.
• Because of risk of hyperkalemia (mild to severe hyperkalemia has been noted in 10% to 44% of liver transplant recipients given tacrolimus), monitor serum potassium levels and don't use potassium-sparing diuretics.
• Patients receiving drug are at increased risk for developing lymphomas and other malignancies, particularly of skin. Risk appears to be related to intensity and duration of immunosuppression rather than to use of any specific drug.
• A lymphoproliferative disorder (LPD) related to Epstein-Barr virus (EBV) has been reported in immunosuppressed organ transplant recipients. LPD risk appears greatest in young children who are at risk for primary EBV infection while immunosuppressed or who are switched to tacrolimus after long-term immunosuppressive therapy.
• Antihypertensive therapy may be needed to control blood pressure elevations associated with drug use. Likewise, therapy may be needed to control blood glucose elevations associated with drug use.
• Black renal transplant patients may need higher doses to maintain comparable whole blood trough drug levels.
• Dilute I.V. form with normal saline injection or 5% dextrose injection to a level between 0.004 and 0.02 mg/ml before use.
• Store diluted infusion solution in glass or polyethylene container and discard after 24 hours. Don't store in polyvinyl chloride container be-

cause of decreased stability and potential for extraction of phthalates.
• There is minimal experience with overdose. In patients who have received inadvertent overdose, no adverse reactions different from those reported in patients receiving therapeutic doses have been described. Follow general supportive measures and systemic treatment in all cases of overdose. Based on poor aqueous solubility and extensive erythrocyte and plasma protein-binding, tacrolimus probably isn't dialyzable to a significant extent.

Monitoring the patient
• Closely monitor patient with impaired renal function; dosage may need to be reduced. In patients with persistent elevations of serum creatinine level who are unresponsive to dosage adjustments, consider changing to another immunosuppressive therapy.
• Closely monitor patient experiencing post-transplant hepatic impairment because of increased risk of renal insufficiency related to high whole-blood levels of tacrolimus. Dosage adjustments may be needed.
• Continuously observe patient receiving drug I.V. for at least 30 minutes after start of infusion and frequently thereafter. Stop infusion if signs or symptoms of anaphylaxis occur. Have an aqueous solution of epinephrine 1:1,000 and a source of oxygen available at patient's bedside.

Information for the patient
• Tell patient to take capsules on empty stomach because food affects drug absorption.
• Inform patient of need for repeated laboratory tests during therapy to watch for adverse reactions and monitor drug effectiveness.
• Advise woman of childbearing age to call if she becomes pregnant or plans to become pregnant.

Pediatric patients
• Children without preexisting renal or hepatic dysfunction have needed and tolerated higher doses than adults to achieve similar blood levels. Children should receive high end of recommended adult I.V. and oral dosing ranges (0.1 mg/kg/day I.V. and 0.3 mg/kg/day P.O.). Dosage adjustments may be needed.

Breast-feeding patients
• Drug appears in breast milk. Avoid use in breast-feeding women.

tamoxifen citrate
Nolvadex, Nolvadex-D*, Tamofen*

Pharmacologic classification: nonsteroidal antiestrogen
Therapeutic classification: antineoplastic
Pregnancy risk category D

How supplied
Available by prescription only
Tablets: 10 mg, 20 mg
Tablets (enteric-coated): 20 mg*

Indications, route, and dosage
Dosage and indications may vary. Check current literature for recommended protocol.
Advanced breast cancer (men and postmenopausal women)
Adults: 20 to 40 mg P.O. b.i.d. Doses greater than 20 mg/day given as divided doses twice daily.
Adjunct treatment for breast cancer
Adults: 10 mg P.O. b.i.d. to t.i.d. for no more than 2 years.
Prevention of breast cancer in high risk women
Adults: 20 mg P.O. daily for 5 years.
◊ *Mastalgia*
Adults: 10 mg P.O. daily for 4 months.
◊ *Stimulation of ovulation*
Adults: 5 to 40 mg P.O. b.i.d. for 4 days.

Pharmacodynamics
Antineoplastic action: Exact mechanism unclear. May exert cytotoxic action by blocking estrogen receptors within tumor cells that need estrogen to thrive. The estrogen receptor-tamoxifen complex may be translocated into the nucleus of the tumor cell, where it inhibits DNA synthesis.

Pharmacokinetics
• *Absorption:* Well absorbed across GI tract after oral administration. Steady-state serum levels generally attained after 3 to 4 weeks.
• *Distribution:* Not fully established.
• *Metabolism:* Metabolized extensively in liver to several metabolites.
• *Excretion:* Excreted primarily in feces, mostly as metabolites. Distribution phase half-life is 7 to 14 hours. Secondary peak plasma levels occur 4 days after dose, probably because of enterohepatic circulation. Half-life of terminal elimination phase is more than 7 days.

Contraindications and precautions
Contraindicated in patients with hypersensitivity to drug and during pregnancy. Also contraindicated in women who are also taking coumarin-type anticoagulants and in women with a history of deep vein thrombosis or pulmonary edema. Use cautiously in patients with existing leukopenia or thrombocytopenia.

Interactions
Drug-drug. *Bromocriptine:* Elevated tamoxifen levels. Monitor tamoxifen levels. Adjust dosage.
Coumadin: Significant increase in anticoagulation effect. Adjust coumadin dosage.
Cytotoxic drugs: Increased thromboembolic events. Use together cautiously.
Estrogens: May interfere with therapeutic effect of drug. Monitor therapeutic effect.

Adverse reactions
GI: *nausea, vomiting, diarrhea.*
GU: *vaginal discharge* and bleeding, *irregular menses, increased BUN level, amenorrhea.*
Hematologic: leukopenia, *thrombocytopenia.*
Hepatic: elevated liver enzyme levels.
Metabolic: hypercalcemia; increased serum triglycerides and cholesterol levels, increased thyroxine level, *weight gain or loss.*
Musculoskeletal: temporary bone or tumor pain, brief exacerbation of pain from osseous metastases.
Skin: *skin changes.*
Other: *hot flashes, fluid retention.*

☑ Special considerations
• Initial adverse reactions (increased bone pain) may be associated with a good tumor response shortly after starting therapy.
• Analgesics are indicated to relieve pain.
• Adverse reactions are usually minor and well tolerated. They can usually be controlled by dosage reduction.
• Clotting factor abnormalities may occur with prolonged therapy at usual doses.
• Tamoxifen acts as an antiestrogen. Best results occur in patients with positive estrogen receptors.
• Drug is also used to treat breast cancer in men and advanced ovarian cancer in women.
• For sexually active women of childbearing potential, initiate tamoxifen during menses. In women with irregular menses, a negative pregnancy test immediately before therapy is sufficient.
• Variations on karyopyknotic index in vaginal smears and various degrees of estrogen effect on Papanicolaou smears have been seen in some postmenopausal women.
• Acute overdose hasn't been reported. No specific treatment is known. Treatment should include supportive measures.

Monitoring the patient
• Monitor WBC and platelet counts and periodic liver function tests.
• Monitor serum calcium levels; hypercalcemia may occur during initial therapy in patients with bone metastases.

Information for the patient
• Emphasize importance of continuing drug despite nausea and vomiting.

• Tell patient to promptly report vomiting if it occurs shortly after taking dose.
• Reassure patient that acute exacerbation of bone pain during therapy usually indicates drug will produce good response.
• Stress importance of swallowing enteric-coated tablets without crushing or breaking them.
• Advise women to avoid becoming pregnant during therapy. Also recommend barrier or nonhormonal contraceptive measures for sexually active patients during treatment period.

Breast-feeding patients
• It's unknown if drug appears in breast milk. However, because of potential for serious adverse reactions and carcinogenicity in infant, breast-feeding isn't recommended.

tamsulosin hydrochloride
Flomax

Pharmacologic classification: alpha$_{1A}$-antagonist
Therapeutic classification: benign prostatic hyperplasia (BPH) drug
Pregnancy risk category B

How supplied
Available by prescription only
Capsules: 0.4 mg

Indications, route, and dosage
BPH
Adult men: 0.4 mg P.O. once daily, administered 30 minutes after same meal each day. For those who fail to respond after 2 to 4 weeks, increase dose to 0.8 mg P.O. once daily. If either dosing regimen is interrupted for several days, restart therapy with the 0.4-mg once-daily dose.

Pharmacodynamics
Anti-BPH action: Selectively blocks alpha$_1$-receptors in the prostate, leading to relaxation of smooth muscles in the bladder neck and prostate, improving urine flow and reducing BPH symptoms.

Pharmacokinetics
• *Absorption:* Completely absorbed after oral administration under fasting conditions. Steady-state achieved by day 5 of once-daily dosing. Maximum levels achieved 4 to 5 hours under fasting conditions; 6 to 7 hours when given with food.
• *Distribution:* Most likely distributed into extracellular fluids and most tissues, including kidneys, prostate, gallbladder, heart, aorta, and brown fat; minimal distribution into brain, spinal cord, and testes. Extensively bound to plasma proteins but not thought to affect other highly bound drugs.
• *Metabolism:* Metabolized by cytochrome P-450 in liver; less than 10% excreted unchanged. Phar-

macokinetic profile of metabolites not established. Metabolites undergo extensive conjugation to glucuronide or sulfate before renal excretion.
• *Excretion:* 76% excreted in urine; about 21% excreted in feces. Elimination half-life 5 to 7 hours; apparent half-life from 9 to 15 hours secondary to rate-controlled absorption pharmacokinetics.

Contraindications and precautions
Contraindicated in patients with hypersensitivity to drug or its components.

Interactions
Drug-drug. *Alpha blockers:* Presumed to interact with drug. Don't use together.
Cimetidine: Decreased clearance of tamsulosin. Use together with caution, particularly if tamsulosin dose is over 0.4 mg.
Cytochrome P-450 metabolized drugs, warfarin: Inconclusive. Use together with caution.

Adverse reactions
CNS: *dizziness, headache,* insomnia, somnolence, asthenia.
CV: chest pain, syncope.
EENT: amblyopia, pharyngitis, *rhinitis,* sinusitis, tooth disorder.
GI: diarrhea, nausea.
GU: abnormal ejaculation, decrease in libido.
Musculoskeletal: back pain.
Respiratory: increased cough.
Other: *infection.*

☑ Special considerations
• Symptoms of BPH and carcinoma of the prostate are similar; rule out carcinoma before starting tamsulosin therapy.
• If treatment is interrupted for several days or more, restart therapy at 1 capsule daily.
• Overdose can lead to hypotension; support CV system. Keep patient in supine position; administer I.V. fluids if necessary. Initiate vasopressors, if needed, and monitor renal function, supporting as needed. Dialysis is unlikely to be beneficial.

Monitoring the patient
• Monitor patient for decreased blood pressure.
• Monitor patient for adverse effects.

Information for the patient
• Advise patient not to crush, chew, or open capsules.
• Tell patient to get up slowly from chair or bed during initiation of therapy.
• Advise patient not to drive or perform hazardous tasks during initiation of therapy and for 12 hours after initial dose or changes in dosage until response can be monitored.
• Tell patient to take drug about 30 minutes after same meal each day.

• Caution patient to avoid situations in which injury could occur due to syncope.

Pediatric patients
• Drug isn't indicated for use in children.

Breast-feeding patients
• Drug isn't indicated for use in women.

telmisartan
Micardis

Pharmacologic classification: angiotensin II antagonist
Therapeutic classification: antihypertensive
Pregnancy risk category C (D in second and third trimesters)

How supplied
Available by prescription only
Tablets: 40 mg, 80 mg

Indications, route, and dosage
Hypertension (used alone or with other antihypertensives)
Adults: 40 mg P.O. once daily. Blood pressure response is dose-related over a range of 20 mg to 80 mg daily.

Pharmacodynamics
Antihypertensive action: Inhibits vasoconstriction and aldosterone production by selectively blocking the binding of angiotensin II to its receptors.

Pharmacokinetics
• *Absorption:* Absolute bioavailability about 42% for 40-mg dose. Plasma levels peak in ½ to 1 hour after oral administration.
• *Distribution:* More than 99.5% bound to plasma proteins.
• *Metabolism:* Metabolized by glucuronide conjugation to inactive metabolite.
• *Excretion:* Half-life is about 24 hours. Majority excreted unchanged in feces via biliary excretion.

Contraindications and precautions
Contraindicated in patients hypersensitive to drug or its components. Use cautiously in patients with biliary obstruction disorders, renal stenosis, or renal or hepatic insufficiency and in those with an activated renin-angiotensin system, such as volume- or salt-depleted patients (for example, those being treated with high doses of diuretics).

Interactions
Drug-drug. *Digoxin:* Increased digoxin plasma levels. Monitor digoxin levels closely, especially when starting, adjusting, or stopping therapy.

Warfarin: Slightly decreased plasma warfarin levels. Adjust dosage as needed.
Drug-lifestyle. *Alcohol:* Diuresis; enhanced hypotensive effects of drug. Discourage use.

Adverse reactions
CNS: dizziness, pain, fatigue, headache.
CV: chest pain, hypertension, peripheral edema.
EENT: pharyngitis, sinusitis.
GI: abdominal pain, diarrhea, dyspepsia, nausea.
GU: urinary tract infection.
Hepatic: elevated liver enzyme levels.
Musculoskeletal: back pain, myalgia.
Respiratory: cough, upper respiratory tract infection.
Other: flulike symptoms.

☑ Special considerations
● Drugs that act on renin-angiotensin system can cause fetal and neonatal morbidity and death when administered to pregnant women. These problems haven't been detected when exposure has been limited to first trimester. If pregnancy is suspected, drug should be stopped.
● Most of the antihypertensive effect occurs within 2 weeks. Maximal blood pressure reduction is generally attained after 4 weeks. Diuretic may be added if blood pressure isn't controlled by drug alone.
● Renal function depends on activity of renin-angiotensin-aldosterone system (such as in patients with severe heart failure). Treatment with ACE inhibitors and angiotensin receptor antagonists has been associated with oliguria or progressive azotemia and (rarely) acute renal failure or death.
● Drug isn't removed by hemodialysis. Patients undergoing dialysis may develop orthostatic hypotension. Closely monitor blood pressure.
● Blood pressure response in blacks is noticeably less than in white patients.
● Data on overdose are limited. Most likely symptoms include hypotension, tachycardia, dizziness, and possibly bradycardia. Provide supportive treatment. Drug isn't removed by hemodialysis.

Monitoring the patient
● Monitor patient for hypotension after initiation of drug. Place patient in supine position if hypotension occurs and administer I.V. normal saline if necessary, as indicated.
● Monitor therapeutic effect.

Information for the patient
● Advise patient to report suspected pregnancy immediately.
● Inform woman of childbearing age of the consequences of second and third trimester exposure to drug.
● Tell patient that transient hypotension may occur. Advise patient to lie down if feeling dizzy and

to rise slowly from a lying or sitting position or when climbing stairs.
● Tell patient that drug may be taken without regard to meals.
● Tell patient that drug shouldn't be removed from blister-sealed packet until immediately before use.

Geriatric patients
● No significant difference has been reported in this age-group as compared to younger patients.

Pediatric patients
● Safety and effectiveness in children haven't been established.

Breast-feeding patients
● It's unknown if drug appears in breast milk. Assess risks and benefits before continuing drug in breast-feeding women.

---

temazepam
Restoril

Pharmacologic classification: benzodiazepine
Therapeutic classification: sedative-hypnotic
Controlled substance schedule IV
Pregnancy risk category X

How supplied
Available by prescription only
Capsules: 7.5 mg, 15 mg, 30 mg

Indications, route, and dosage
Insomnia
Adults: 7.5 to 30 mg P.O. 30 minutes before bedtime.
Elderly: Initiate at 7.5 mg P.O. h.s. until individual response is determined.
✦ Dosage adjustment. In debilitated patients, 7.5 mg P.O. h.s. until individual response is determined.

Pharmacodynamics
Sedative-hypnotic action: Depresses the CNS at the limbic and subcortical levels of the brain. Produces a sedative-hypnotic effect by potentiating the effect of the neurotransmitter gamma-aminobutyric acid on its receptor in the ascending reticular activating system, which increases inhibition and blocks both cortical and limbic arousal.

Pharmacokinetics
● *Absorption:* Well absorbed through GI tract when given orally. Levels peak in 1 hour 12 minutes to 1 hour 36 minutes (mean 1½ hours); onset of action in 30 to 60 minutes.

• *Distribution:* Widely distributed throughout body; 96% protein-bound.
• *Metabolism:* Metabolized in liver primarily to inactive metabolites.
• *Excretion:* Metabolites excreted in urine as glucuronide conjugates. Drug half-life is 4 to 20 hours.

Contraindications and precautions
Contraindicated in patients with hypersensitivity to drug or other benzodiazepines and during pregnancy. Use cautiously in patients with impaired renal or hepatic function, chronic pulmonary insufficiency, severe or latent mental depression, suicidal tendencies, or history of drug abuse.

Interactions
Drug-drug. *Antidepressants, antihistamines, barbiturates, general anesthetics, MAO inhibitors, narcotics, phenothiazines:* Potentiated CNS depressant effects. Avoid concomitant use.
Haloperidol: Decreased plasma level of haloperidol. Adjust dosage.
Levodopa: Decreased therapeutic effect of levodopa. Use together cautiously.
Oral contraceptives: Decreased half-life of temazepam. Adjust dosage.
Drug-lifestyle. *Alcohol:* Increased CNS depression. Discourage use.
Heavy smoking: Accelerated temazepam metabolism. Discourage use. Adjust dosage.

Adverse reactions
CNS: *drowsiness, dizziness, lethargy,* disturbed coordination, daytime sedation, confusion, nightmares, vertigo, euphoria, weakness, headache, fatigue, nervousness, anxiety, depression, minor changes in EEG patterns.
EENT: blurred vision.
GI: diarrhea, nausea, dry mouth.
Hepatic: elevated liver enzyme levels.
Other: physical and psychological dependence.

✓ Special considerations
Besides the recommendations relevant to all benzodiazepines, consider the following.
• Evaluate patient for cause of insomnia, commonly a symptom of an underlying disorder such as depression.
• Drug is useful for patients who have difficulty falling asleep or who awaken frequently in the night.
• Prolonged use isn't recommended; however, drug has proven effective for up to 4 weeks of continuous use.
• After long-term use, avoid stopping drug abruptly; gradually taper.
• Signs and symptoms of overdose include somnolence, confusion, hypoactive or absent reflexes, dyspnea, labored breathing, hypotension, bradycardia, slurred speech, unsteady gait or impaired coordination, and, ultimately, coma.

• To treat overdose, support blood pressure and respiration until drug effects subside; monitor vital signs. Mechanical ventilatory assistance via endotracheal tube may be needed to maintain a patent airway and support adequate oxygenation. Flumazenil, a specific benzodiazepine antagonist, may be useful. Use I.V. fluids and vasopressors, such as dopamine and phenylephrine, to treat hypotension as needed. If patient is conscious, induce emesis. Use gastric lavage if ingestion was recent, but only if an endotracheal tube is present to prevent aspiration. After emesis or lavage, use activated charcoal with a cathartic as a single dose. Don't use barbiturates if excitation occurs. Dialysis is of limited value.

Monitoring the patient
• Monitor hepatic function studies to prevent toxicity; lower doses are indicated in patients with hepatic dysfunction.
• Monitor patient for adverse effects.

Information for the patient
• Advise patient to seek approval before making changes in drug regimen.
• As necessary, teach patient safety measures to prevent injury, such as gradual position changes and supervised walking.
• Inform patient of risk of physical and psychological dependence with long-term use.
• Advise woman to call immediately if pregnancy is suspected.
• Emphasize potential for excessive CNS depression if drug is taken with alcohol.
• Tell patient that rebound insomnia may occur after stopping drug.

Geriatric patients
• Elderly patients are more susceptible to CNS depressant effects of drug. Use with caution.
• Lower doses are usually effective in elderly patients because of decreased elimination.
• Elderly patients who receive drug need supervision with walking and daily activities during initiation of therapy or after an increase in dosage.

Pediatric patients
• Safety in children under age 18 hasn't been established.

Breast-feeding patients
• Drug appears in breast milk. A breast-fed infant may become sedated, have feeding difficulties, or lose weight. Avoid use in breast-feeding women.

temozolomide
Temodar

Pharmacologic classification: alkylating drug
Therapeutic classification: antineoplastic
Pregnancy risk category D

How supplied
Available by prescription only
Capsules: 5 mg, 20 mg, 100 mg, 250 mg

Indications, route, and dosage
Refractory anaplastic astrocytoma that has relapsed after chemotherapy regimen containing a nitrosourea and procarbazine
Adults: Initial cycle: 150 mg/m² P.O. once daily for first 5 days of 28-day treatment cycle. Subsequent cycles: 100 to 200 mg/m² P.O. once daily for first 5 days of subsequent 28-day treatment cycles. Timing and dosage of subsequent cycles must be adjusted according to the absolute neutrophil count (ANC) and platelet count measured on cycle day 22 (expected nadir) and cycle day 29 (initiation of next cycle).
♦ Dosage adjustment. Based on the lowest of ANC and platelet results.
For ANC less than 1,000/mm³ or platelets less than 50,000/mm³: Hold therapy until ANC is greater than 1,500/mm³ and platelets are greater than 100,000/mm³. Reduce dosage by 50 mg/m² for subsequent cycle. Minimum dose is 100 mg/m².
For ANC 1,000 to 1,500/mm³ or platelets 50,000 to 100,000/mm³: Hold therapy until ANC is greater than 1,500/mm³ and platelets are greater than 100,000/mm³. Maintain prior dose for subsequent cycle.
For ANC greater than 1,500/mm³ and platelets greater than 100,000/mm³: Increase dosage to, or maintain at, 200 mg/m² for first 5 days of subsequent cycle.

Pharmacodynamics
Antineoplastic action: A prodrug rapidly hydrolyzed to the active form. Thought to interfere with DNA replication in rapidly dividing tissues, primarily through alkylation (methylation) of guanine nucleotides in the DNA structure.

Pharmacokinetics
• *Absorption:* Rapidly and completely absorbed from GI tract after oral administration; plasma levels peak in 1 hour.
• *Distribution:* 15% bound to plasma proteins.
• *Metabolism:* Undergoes spontaneous hydrolysis to active form and other metabolites. After 7 days, 38% of dose recovered in urine; 0.8% in feces.
• *Excretion:* Rapidly eliminated; elimination half-life of 1.8 hours.

Contraindications and precautions
Contraindicated in patients with hypersensitivity to drug or its components. Also contraindicated in patients allergic to dacarbazine, which is structurally similar to temozolomide. Use in pregnancy only if potential benefit to mother outweighs risk to fetus.

Interactions
Drug-drug. *Valproic acid:* Decreases oral clearance of temozolomide by about 5%. Use cautiously.
Drug-food. *Any food:* Reduces rate and extent of drug absorption, but no dietary restrictions with drug administration. Give drug on empty stomach to reduce nausea and vomiting.

Adverse reactions
CNS: amnesia, anxiety, asthenia, ataxia, confusion, *seizures,* coordination abnormality, depression, dizziness, fatigue, gait abnormality, headache, hemiparesis, insomnia, local seizures, paresis, paresthesia, somnolence.
CV: peripheral edema.
EENT: abnormal vision, diplopia, pharyngitis, sinusitis.
GI: abdominal pain, anorexia, constipation, diarrhea, dysphasia, nausea, vomiting.
GU: increased urinary frequency, urinary incontinence, urinary tract infection.
Hematologic: anemia, leukopenia, *neutropenia, thrombocytopenia.*
Metabolic: weight increase.
Musculoskeletal: back pain, myalgia.
Respiratory: coughing, upper respiratory tract infection.
Skin: pruritus, rash.
Other: hyperadrenocorticism, breast pain in women, fever, viral infection.

☑ Special considerations
• Women and elderly patients are at higher risk for developing myelosuppression.
• Nausea and vomiting, which may be self-limiting, are the most common side effects. Taking drug on empty stomach or at bedtime may lessen these effects. Usual antiemetics effectively control nausea and vomiting associated with temozolomide.
• Avoid skin contact with, or inhalation of, capsule contents if capsule is accidentally opened or damaged. Follow procedures for safe handling and disposal of antineoplastics.
• Neutropenia and thrombocytopenia have occurred after a single dose of 1,000 mg/m². Patient's hematologic status should be closely monitored and supportive therapies administered, as needed.

Monitoring the patient
• CBC should be obtained on days 22 and 29 of each treatment cycle. If ANC falls below 1,500/mm³ or platelet count falls below 100,000/mm³,

a weekly CBC should be obtained until counts have recovered.
• Monitor patient for adverse effects.

Information for the patient
• Emphasize importance of taking dose exactly as prescribed, usually on empty stomach or at bedtime.
• Stress importance of continuing drug despite nausea and vomiting.
• Tell patient to call immediately if vomiting occurs shortly after a dose is taken.
• Tell patient to promptly report sore throat, fever, unusual bruising or bleeding, rash, or seizures.
• Advise patient to avoid exposure to people with infections.
• Advise sexually active patient to use effective birth control measures during treatment because drug may cause birth defects.
• Tell patient to swallow capsules whole; don't break or crush.

Geriatric patients
• Severe neutropenia and thrombocytopenia are more common after first treatment cycle in patients ages 70 and older.

Pediatric patients
• Drug hasn't been evaluated for safety and efficacy in children.

Breast-feeding patients
• It's unknown if drug appears in breast milk. Women shouldn't breast-feed while receiving drug.

teniposide (VM-26)
Vumon

Pharmacologic classification: podophyllotoxin (cell cycle–phase specific, G_2 and late S phase)
Therapeutic classification: antineoplastic
Pregnancy risk category D

How supplied
Available by prescription only
Injection: 50 mg/5 ml ampules

Indications, route, and dosage
Dosage and indications may vary. Check current literature for recommended protocol.
Acute lymphoblastic leukemia induction therapy in childhood
Children: Optimum dosage hasn't been established. One protocol reported by manufacturer is 165 mg/m² I.V. teniposide with cytarabine 300 mg/m² I.V. twice weekly for eight or nine doses.

Pharmacodynamics
Antineoplastic action: Causes single- and double-stranded breaks in DNA and DNA protein cross-links, thus preventing cells from entering mitosis.

Pharmacokinetics
• *Absorption:* Not administered orally.
• *Distribution:* Over 99% bound to plasma proteins. Crosses blood-brain barrier to a limited extent.
• *Metabolism:* Metabolized extensively in liver.
• *Excretion:* About 4% to 12% of dose eliminated through kidneys as unchanged drug or metabolites. Terminal half-life of drug is 5 hours.

Contraindications and precautions
Contraindicated in patients with hypersensitivity to drug or to polyoxyethylated castor oil, an injection vehicle. Use only in pregnancy if benefit to mother outweighs risk to fetus.

Interactions
Drug-drug. *Methotrexate:* May increase effects of methotrexate. Monitor patient.
Sodium salicylate, sulfamethizole, tolbutamide: Potentiation of toxicity. Use together cautiously.

Adverse reactions
CV: hypotension from rapid infusion.
GI: *nausea, vomiting, mucositis, diarrhea.*
Hematologic: LEUKOPENIA, NEUTROPENIA, THROMBOCYTOPENIA, MYELOSUPPRESSION (dose-limiting), *anemia.*
Metabolic: elevated uric acid levels in blood and urine.
Skin: rash.
Other: *infection,* bleeding, *hypersensitivity reactions* (chills, fever, urticaria, tachycardia, **bronchospasm,** dyspnea, hypotension, flushing), *phlebitis, extravasation at injection site.*

☑ Special considerations
• Dilute with 5% dextrose injection USP or normal saline injection USP to give final teniposide levels of 0.1 mg/ml, 0.2 mg/ml, 0.4 mg/ml, or 1 mg/ml.
• Solutions containing levels of 0.1 mg/ml, 0.2 mg/ml, or 0.4 mg/ml are stable at room temperature for 24 hours. Solutions with a final level of 1 mg/ml should be administered within 4 hours of preparation.
• If teniposide solution contacts skin, immediately wash with soap and water. If drug contacts mucous membranes, immediately flush with water.
• Drug isn't to be administered through a membrane-type in-line filter; diluent may dissolve filter.

- Administer I.V. infusion over 30 to 60 minutes to prevent hypotension. Avoid I.V. push because of increased risk of hypotension.
- Use caution when handling and preparing solution; wear gloves.
- Use glass or polyolefin plastic bags or containers for infusion. Don't use polyvinyl chloride containers.
- Dose should be decreased in patients with renal or hepatic insufficiency and in patients with Down syndrome.
- Have diphenhydramine, hydrocortisone, epinephrine, and oral airway available in case of anaphylactic reaction.
- Signs and symptoms of overdose include myelosuppression, nausea, and vomiting. Treatment is usually supportive and includes transfusion of blood components, antiemetics, and antibiotics for infections that may develop.

Monitoring the patient
- Monitor blood pressure before infusion and at 30-minute intervals during infusion. If systolic blood pressure decreases below 90 mm Hg, stop infusion.
- Monitor CBC. Observe patient for signs of bone marrow depression.
- Monitor renal and hepatic function during therapy.
- Watch for chemical phlebitis at injection site.

Information for the patient
- Encourage adequate fluid intake to increase urine output and facilitate excretion of uric acid.
- Tell patient to avoid exposure to people with infections.
- Advise patient that hair should grow back after treatment ends.
- Tell patient to call promptly if a sore throat or fever develops or if unusual bruising or bleeding occurs.

Breast-feeding patients
- It's unknown if drug appears in breast milk. Because of risk of serious adverse reactions, mutagenicity, and carcinogenicity in infant, breast-feeding isn't recommended.

---

terazosin hydrochloride
Hytrin

Pharmacologic classification: selective alpha$_1$ blocker
Therapeutic classification: antihypertensive
Pregnancy risk category C

How supplied
Available by prescription only
Capsules: 1 mg, 2 mg, 5 mg, 10 mg

Indications, route, and dosage
Mild to moderate hypertension
Adults: Initially, 1 mg P.O. h.s. Adjust dosage and schedule according to patient response. Recommended range is 1 to 5 mg daily or divided b.i.d.

If therapy is stopped for several days or longer, reinstitute using the initial dosing regimen of 1 mg P.O. h.s. Slowly increase dosage until desired blood pressure is attained. Doses over 20 mg don't appear to further affect blood pressure.
Benign prostatic hyperplasia (BPH)
Adults: Initially, 1 mg P.O. h.s. Dosage may be adjusted upward based on patient response. Increase in a stepwise manner to 2 mg, 5 mg, and 10 mg. A daily dose of 10 mg may be required.

Pharmacodynamics
Antihypertensive action: Reduces blood pressure by selectively inhibiting alpha$_1$ receptors in vascular smooth muscle, thus reducing peripheral vascular resistance. Because of drug's selectivity for alpha$_1$ receptors, heart rate increases minimally. Significant decreases in serum cholesterol, low-density lipoprotein, and very-low-density lipoprotein cholesterol fractions occur during therapy; the significance of these changes is unknown, as is the mechanism by which they occur.

Terazosin doesn't significantly alter potassium or glucose levels; it's been used successfully with diuretics, beta blockers, and a combination of other antihypertensive regimens.
Hypertrophic action: Alpha blockade in nonvascular smooth muscle causes relaxation, notably in prostatic tissue, thereby reducing urinary symptoms in men with BPH.

Pharmacokinetics
- *Absorption:* Rapidly absorbed after oral administration; plasma levels peak in 1 to 2 hours. About 90% of oral dose is bioavailable; food doesn't appear to alter bioavailability.
- *Distribution:* About 90% to 94% plasma protein–bound.
- *Metabolism:* Drug metabolized in liver. Pharmacokinetics don't appear to be affected by hypertension, heart failure, or age.
- *Excretion:* About 40% of drug excreted in urine and 60% in feces; mostly as metabolites. Up to 30% excreted unchanged. Elimination half-life is about 12 hours.

Contraindications and precautions
Contraindicated in patients with hypersensitivity to drug.

Interactions
Drug-drug. *Diuretics, other antihypertensives:* Hypotension. Reduce dosage.
Drug-herb. *Butcher's broom:* Possible reduction in effects. Don't use together.

Reactions may be *common*, uncommon, *life-threatening*, or COMMON AND LIFE-THREATENING.

Adverse reactions

CNS: *asthenia, dizziness, headache,* nervousness, paresthesia, somnolence.
CV: *palpitations, peripheral edema,* orthostatic hypotension, tachycardia, syncope.
EENT: *nasal congestion,* sinusitis, blurred vision.
GI: *nausea.*
GU: impotence.
Musculoskeletal: back pain, muscle pain.
Respiratory: dyspnea.

☑ Special considerations

Besides the recommendations relevant to all alpha blockers, consider the following.
• Drug can cause marked hypotension, especially orthostatic hypotension, and syncope with first dose or during first few days of therapy. A similar response occurs if therapy is interrupted for more than a few doses.
• Terazosin causes small but significant decreases in hematocrit; WBC count; and hemoglobin, total protein, and albumin levels; the magnitude of these decreases hasn't been shown to worsen with time, suggesting the possibility of hemodilution.
• Signs and symptoms of overdose are exaggerated adverse reactions, particularly hypotension and shock. In case of overdose, treatment is symptomatic and supportive. Dialysis may not be helpful because drug is highly protein-bound.

Monitoring the patient
• Monitor blood pressure and cardiac status.
• Monitor patient for adverse effects.

Information for the patient
• Advise patient to take first dose at bedtime.
• Warn patient to avoid hazardous tasks that require alertness for 12 hours after first dose, when dosage is first increased, or when restarting dose after interruption of therapy.
• Caution patient to rise carefully and slowly from sitting and supine positions and to report dizziness, light-headedness, or palpitations. Dosage adjustment may be needed.

terbinafine hydrochloride
Lamisil

Pharmacologic classification: synthetic allylamine derivative
Therapeutic classification: antifungal
Pregnancy risk category B

How supplied
Available by prescription only
Cream: 1% in 15-g and 30-g containers
Tablets: 250 mg
Gel 1%: 5 g, 15 g, 30 g

Indications, route, and dosage
Interdigital tinea pedis (athlete's foot), tinea cruris (jock itch), or tinea corporis (ringworm) caused by Epidermophyton floccosum, Trichophyton mentagrophytes, *or* T. rubrum
Adults and children over age 12: For interdigital tinea pedis, apply to cover the affected and immediately surrounding areas b.i.d. until signs and symptoms are significantly improved (for most patients this occurs by day 7 of drug therapy); for tinea cruris or tinea corporis, apply to cover the affected and immediately surrounding areas once or twice daily until signs and symptoms are significantly improved (for most patients this occurs by day 7 of drug therapy). Treatment shouldn't exceed 4 weeks.
Onychomycosis of fingernails or toenails caused by dermatophytes (tinea unguium)
Adults and adolescents over age 12: For treatment of fingernails, give 250 mg/day P.O. for 6 weeks; for toenails, give 250 mg/day P.O. for 12 weeks.

Pharmacodynamics
Antifungal action: Exerts antifungal effect by inhibiting squalene epoxidase, a key enzyme in sterol biosynthesis in fungi. This action results in a deficiency in ergosterol and a corresponding accumulation of squalene within the fungal cell, causing fungal cell death.

Pharmacokinetics
Topical
• *Absorption:* Systemic absorption highly variable.
• *Distribution:* No information available.
• *Metabolism:* No information available.
• *Excretion:* About 75% of cutaneously absorbed drug eliminated in urine, predominantly as metabolites.
Oral
• *Absorption:* More than 70% of drug absorbed; food enhances absorption. Peak plasma level is 1 mcg/ml within 2 hours of drug intake.
• *Distribution:* Distributed to serum and skin. Plasma half-life about 36 hours; half-life in tissue 200 to 400 hours. More than 99% of drug bound to plasma proteins.
• *Metabolism:* First-pass metabolism is about 40%.
• *Excretion:* About 70% of dose eliminated in urine; clearance decreased by 50% in patients with hepatic cirrhosis and impaired renal function.

Contraindications and precautions
Contraindicated in patients with hypersensitivity to drug. Oral form is also contraindicated in patients with preexisting hepatic disease or impaired renal function (creatinine clearance of 50 ml/minute or less) and during pregnancy.

Interactions
None reported for topical form. For oral form:
Drug-drug. *Cimetidine:* Decreased terbinafine
clearance. Adjust dose.
Cyclosporine: Increased cyclosporine clearance.
Monitor cyclosporine level.
I.V. caffeine: Decreased clearance of caffeine.
Use together cautiously.
Rifampin: Increased clearance of terbinafine. Adjust dose of terbinafine.

Adverse reactions
CNS: *headache.*
EENT: taste disturbances, visual disturbances.
GI: diarrhea, dyspepsia, abdominal pain, nausea, flatulence.
Hematologic: decreased absolute lymphocyte count.
Hepatic: elevated liver enzyme levels.
Skin: *Stevens-Johnson syndrome,* irritation,
burning, pruritus, dryness.

☑ Special considerations
• Topical form of drug is for topical use only; not
for oral, ophthalmic, or intravaginal use.
• Diagnosis should be confirmed either by direct
microscopic examination of scrapings from infected tissue mounted in a solution of potassium
hydroxide or by culture.
Topical
• Duration of drug therapy should be for a minimum of 1 week and shouldn't exceed 4 weeks.
• Many patients treated with shorter durations
of therapy (1 to 2 weeks) continue to improve
during the 2 to 4 weeks after therapy has ended. As a consequence, patients shouldn't be considered therapeutic failures until they have been
observed for a period of 2 to 4 weeks off therapy. If successful outcome isn't achieved during
the posttreatment observation period, review diagnosis.
• Acute overdose with topical application is unlikely because of the limited absorption of topically applied drug and wouldn't be expected to
lead to a life-threatening situation.

Monitoring the patient
• Monitor patient for irritation or sensitivity to drug.
Stop therapy if irritation or sensitivity occurs and
institute appropriate treatment measures.
• For oral form, perform liver function tests for
patients receiving treatment for more than 6
weeks.

Information for the patient
• Advise patient to use drug as directed and to
avoid contact with eyes, nose, mouth, or other
mucous membranes.
• Stress importance of using drug for recommended treatment time.

• Tell patient to call if area of application shows
signs or symptoms of increased irritation or possible sensitization (redness, itching, burning, blistering, swelling, or oozing).
• Advise patient not to use occlusive dressings
unless directed.

Pediatric patients
• Safety and efficacy in children under age 12
haven't been established.

Breast-feeding patients
• Drug appears in breast milk. Stop either breast-feeding or drug, taking into account importance
of drug to mother. Breast-feeding women should
avoid application of cream to breast.

terbutaline sulfate
Brethaire, Brethine, Bricanyl

Pharmacologic classification: adrenergic
(beta$_2$ agonist)
Therapeutic classification: bronchodilator, premature labor inhibitor
(tocolytic)
Pregnancy risk category B

How supplied
Available by prescription only
Tablets: 2.5 mg, 5 mg
Aerosol inhaler: 200 mcg/metered spray
Injection: 1 mg/ml parenteral

Indications, route, and dosage
Relief of bronchospasm in patients with reversible obstructive airway disease
Adults and adolescents ages 15 and older: Administer 5 mg P.O. t.i.d. at 6-hour intervals. Reduce dose to 2.5 mg P.O. t.i.d. if side effects occur. Maximum daily dose is 15 mg. Or 0.25 mg
S.C. may be repeated in 15 to 30 minutes; maximum, 0.5 mg q 4 hours. Or two inhalations may
be given q 4 to 6 hours with 1 minute between
inhalations.
Adolescents ages 12 to 15: 2.5 mg P.O. t.i.d. Maximum daily dose is 7.5 mg. Or two inhalations
may be given q 4 to 6 hours with 1 minute between inhalations.
◇ *Premature labor*
Adults: Initially, 10 mcg/minute I.V. Titrate to maximum dose of 80 mcg/minute. Maintain at minimum effective dose for 4 hours. Maintenance
therapy until term is 2.5 mg P.O. q 4 to 6 hours.

Pharmacodynamics
Bronchodilator action: Acts directly on beta$_2$-adrenergic receptors to relax bronchial smooth
muscle, relieving bronchospasm and reducing
airway resistance. Cardiac and CNS stimulation
may occur with high doses.

Tocolytic action: When used in premature labor, terbutaline relaxes uterine smooth muscle, which inhibits uterine contractions.

Pharmacokinetics

• *Absorption:* 33% to 50% of oral dose absorbed through GI tract. Onset of action within 30 minutes, peaks within 2 to 3 hours, lasts for 4 to 8 hours. After S.C. injection, onset within 15 minutes, peaks within 30 to 60 minutes, lasts for 1½ to 4 hours. After oral inhalation, onset within 5 to 30 minutes, peaks within 1 to 2 hours, lasts for 3 to 4 hours.
• *Distribution:* Distributed widely throughout body.
• *Metabolism:* Partially metabolized in liver to inactive compounds.
• *Excretion:* After parenteral administration, 60% of drug excreted unchanged in urine, 3% in feces via bile, remainder in urine as metabolites. After oral administration, most of drug excreted as metabolites.

Contraindications and precautions

Contraindicated in patients with hypersensitivity to drug or sympathomimetic amines. Use cautiously in patients with CV disorders, hyperthyroidism, diabetes, or seizure disorders.

Interactions

Drug-drug. *Beta blockers:* Antagonized bronchodilating effects of terbutaline. Adjust dosage.
Bronchodilators (adrenergic stimulator type): May relieve acute bronchospasm in patients on long-term oral terbutaline therapy. May be used for this purpose.
MAO inhibitors (within 14 days of terbutaline), tricyclic antidepressants: Potentiated effects of terbutaline on vascular system. Use together with caution.
Sympathomimetics: Potentiated adverse CV effects. Avoid concomitant use.

Adverse reactions

CNS: *nervousness, tremor, drowsiness, dizziness, headache,* weakness.
CV: *palpitations,* tachycardia, **arrhythmias,** flushing.
EENT: dry and irritated nose and throat (with inhaled form).
GI: *vomiting, nausea,* heartburn.
Metabolic: hypokalemia (with high doses).
Respiratory: *paradoxical bronchospasm with prolonged usage,* dyspnea.
Skin: diaphoresis.

☑ Special considerations

Besides the recommendations relevant to all adrenergics, consider the following.
• Store injection solution away from light. Don't use if discolored.
• Give S.C. injection in lateral deltoid area.

• CV effects are more likely with S.C. route and when patient has arrhythmias.
• Most adverse reactions are transient; however, tachycardia may persist for a relatively long time.
• Patient may use tablets and aerosol together.
• Aerosol terbutaline produces minimal cardiac stimulation and tremors.
• Drug may reduce sensitivity of spirometry for diagnosis of bronchospasm.
• Signs and symptoms of overdose include exaggeration of common adverse reactions, particularly arrhythmias, seizures, nausea, and vomiting. Treatment requires supportive measures. If patient is conscious and ingestion was recent, induce emesis and follow with gastric lavage. If patient is comatose, after endotracheal tube is in place with cuff inflated, perform gastric lavage; then use activated charcoal to reduce drug absorption. Maintain adequate airway, provide cardiac and respiratory support, and monitor vital signs closely.

Monitoring the patient

• When drug is used for tocolytic therapy, monitor patient for CV effects, including tachycardia, for 12 hours after stopping drug. Monitor intake and output; fluid restriction may be necessary. Muscle tremor is common but may subside with continued use.
• Monitor neonate for hypoglycemia if mother used drug during pregnancy.
• Monitor patient for toxicity.

Information for the patient

• Show patient taking oral drug how to take pulse rate and tell him to report if pulse varies significantly from baseline.
• Advise patient to avoid simultaneous administration with adrenocorticoid aerosol. Separate administration times by 15 minutes.
• Instruct patient on proper use of inhaler.
• Advise patient to take a missed dose within 1 hour. After 1 hour, patient should skip dose and resume regular schedule. Patient shouldn't double dose.
• Advise patient to use drug only as directed. If drug produces no relief or if condition worsens, he should call promptly.
• Warn patient not to use OTC drugs without medical approval. Many cold and allergy remedies contain a sympathomimetic that may be harmful when combined with terbutaline.
• Advise patient to report decreased effectiveness. Excessive or prolonged use of aerosol form can lead to tolerance.

Geriatric patients

• Elderly patients are more sensitive to drug's effects; a lower dosage may be required.

Pediatric patients
● Drug isn't recommended for use in children under age 12.

Breast-feeding patients
● Drug appears in breast milk in minute amounts. Use with caution in breast-feeding women.

terconazole
Terazol 3, Terazol 7

Pharmacologic classification: triazole derivative
Therapeutic classification: antifungal
Pregnancy risk category C

How supplied
Available by prescription only
Vaginal cream: 0.4% in 45-g tube, 0.8% in 20-g tube with applicator
Vaginal suppositories: 80 mg

Indications, route, and dosage
Local treatment of vulvovaginal candidiasis (moniliasis)
Adults: 0.4%: 1 full applicator (5 g) intravaginally once daily h.s. for 7 consecutive days. 0.8%: 1 full applicator (5 g) intravaginally once daily h.s. for 3 consecutive days. Or insert 1 suppository vaginally h.s. for 3 consecutive days.

Pharmacodynamics
Antifungal action: Exact mechanism unknown. May disrupt fungal cell membrane permeability.

Pharmacokinetics
● *Absorption:* About 5% to 16% absorbed.
● *Distribution:* Mainly local effect.
● *Metabolism:* Metabolized mainly by oxidative N- and O-dealkylation, dioxolane ring cleavage, and conjugation pathways.
● *Excretion:* After oral administration, 32% to 56% of dose excreted in urine; 47% to 52% excreted in feces within 24 hours.

Contraindications and precautions
Contraindicated in patients with hypersensitivity to drug or its components.

Interactions
None reported.

Adverse reactions
CNS: headache.
GU: dysmenorrhea, pain of the female genitalia, vulvovaginal burning.
Skin: irritation, *pruritus,* photosensitivity.
Other: fever, chills, body aches.

☑ Special considerations
● Drug is only effective against vulvovaginitis caused by *Candida.* Diagnosis should be confirmed by cultures or potassium hydroxide smears.
● A persistent infection may be caused by reinfection. Evaluate patient for possible sources.
● Intractable candidiasis may be a sign of diabetes mellitus. Perform blood and urine glucose determinations to rule out undiagnosed diabetes mellitus.

Monitoring the patient
● Monitor therapeutic effect.

Information for the patient
● Tell patient to complete full course of therapy and to use drug continuously, even during menstrual period. Drug's therapeutic effect isn't affected by menstruation.
● Inform patient to report if drug causes burning or irritation.
● Advise patient to refrain from sexual intercourse or suggest partner use a condom to avoid reinfection.

Breast-feeding patients
● Safety hasn't been established. Because it's unknown if drug appears in breast milk, breast-feeding isn't recommended during therapy.

testosterone
Histerone 100, Malogen in Oil*, Tesamone, Testandro

testosterone cypionate
depAndro 100, depAndro 200, Depotest 100, Depotest 200, Depo-Testosterone, Duratest-100, Duratest-200

testosterone enanthate
Andro L.A. 200, Andropository 200, Delatestryl, Durathate-200, Everone 200

testosterone propionate
Malogen in Oil*

Pharmacologic classification: androgen
Therapeutic classification: androgen replacement, antineoplastic
Controlled substance schedule III
Pregnancy risk category X

How supplied
Available by prescription only
testosterone
Injection (aqueous suspension): 25 mg/ml, 50 mg/ml, 100 mg/ml

testosterone cypionate (in oil)
Injection: 100 mg/ml, 200 mg/ml
testosterone enanthate (in oil)
Injection: 100 mg/ml, 200 mg/ml
testosterone propionate (in oil)
Injection: 100 mg/ml

Indications, route, and dosage
Male hypogonadism
testosterone or testosterone propionate
Adults: 10 to 25 mg I.M. two or three times weekly.
testosterone cypionate or enanthate
Adults: 50 to 400 mg I.M. q 2 to 4 weeks.
Delayed puberty in males
testosterone or testosterone propionate
Children: 25 to 50 mg I.M. two or three times weekly for up to 6 months.
testosterone cypionate or enanthate
Children: 50 to 200 mg I.M. q 2 to 4 weeks for up to 6 months.
Postpartum breast pain and engorgement
testosterone or testosterone propionate
Adults: 25 to 50 mg I.M. daily for 3 to 4 days.
Inoperable breast cancer
testosterone propionate
Adults: 50 to 100 mg I.M. three times weekly.
testosterone cypionate or enanthate
Adults: 200 to 400 mg I.M. q 2 to 4 weeks.
testosterone
Adults: 100 mg I.M. three times weekly.
Postpubertal cryptorchidism
testosterone or testosterone propionate
Adults: 10 to 25 mg I.M. two or three times weekly.
Growth stimulation in Turner's syndrome
testosterone propionate
Adults: 40 to 50 mg/m² I.M. once monthly for 6 months.

Pharmacodynamics
Androgenic action: Endogenous androgen that stimulates receptors in androgen-responsive organs and tissues to promote growth and development of male sexual organs and secondary sexual characteristics.
Antineoplastic action: Exerts inhibitory, antiestrogenic effects on hormone-responsive breast tumors and metastases.

Pharmacokinetics
• *Absorption:* Testosterone and esters must be administered parenterally; inactivated rapidly by liver when given orally. Onset of action of cypionate and enanthate esters of testosterone somewhat slower than that of testosterone.
• *Distribution:* Drug is normally 98% to 99% plasma protein–bound, primarily to testosterone-estradiol binding globulin.
• *Metabolism:* Metabolized to several 17-ketosteroids by two main pathways in liver. Large portion of these metabolites form glucuronide and sulfate conjugates. Plasma half-life of testosterone ranges from 10 to 100 minutes. Cypionate and

enanthate esters have longer durations of action than testosterone.
• *Excretion:* Very little unchanged testosterone appears in urine or feces. About 90% of metabolized testosterone excreted in urine in the form of sulfate and glucuronide conjugates.

Contraindications and precautions
Contraindicated in men with breast or prostate cancer; in patients with hypercalcemia or cardiac, hepatic, or renal decompensation; during pregnancy; and in breast-feeding women. Use cautiously in elderly patients and in women of child-bearing age.

Interactions
Drug-drug. *Insulin, oral antidiabetics:* Hypoglycemia. Monitor blood glucose levels.
Oxyphenbutazone: Increased serum oxyphenbutazone levels. Monitor serum oxyphenbutazone levels.
Warfarin-type anticoagulants: Prolonged PT and INR. Monitor PT and INR.

Adverse reactions
CNS: headache, anxiety, depression, paresthesia, sleep apnea syndrome.
CV: edema.
GI: nausea.
GU: hypoestrogenic effects in women (flushing; diaphoresis; vaginitis, including itching, drying, and burning; vaginal bleeding; menstrual irregularities); androgenic effects in women (*acne, edema, oily skin, weight gain, hirsutism, hoarseness,* clitoral enlargement, deepening voice, decreased or increased libido); excessive hormonal effects in men (prepubertal—premature epiphyseal closure, *acne,* priapism, *growth of body and facial hair,* phallic enlargement; postpubertal—testicular atrophy, oligospermia, decreased ejaculatory volume, impotence, gynecomastia, epididymitis), increased serum creatinine.
Hematologic: elevated PT and INR; polycythemia; suppression of clotting factors.
Hepatic: reversible jaundice, cholestatic hepatitis, abnormal liver enzyme levels.
Metabolic: hypercalcemia; hypernatremia; hyperkalemia; hyperphosphatemia; hypercholesterolemia; abnormal results of glucose tolerance tests; decreased thyroid function tests and serum 17-ketosteroid levels.
Skin: pain and induration at injection site, local edema, hypersensitivity manifestations.

☑ Special considerations
Besides the recommendations relevant to all androgens, consider the following.
• When drug is used to treat male hypogonadism, initiate therapy with full therapeutic doses and taper according to patient tolerance and response. Administering long-acting esters (enanthate or cypionate) at intervals greater than every 2 to 3

weeks may cause hormone levels to fall below those found in normal adults.
- Inject deeply I.M., preferably into large muscle mass such as upper outer quadrant of gluteal muscle.
- Testosterone enanthate has been used for post-menopausal osteoporosis and to stimulate erythropoiesis.
- Solutions of long-acting esters (enanthate and cypionate) may become cloudy if a wet needle is used to draw up solution. This doesn't affect potency.

Monitoring the patient
- Carefully observe women for signs of excessive virilization. If possible, stop drug at first sign of virilization because some adverse effects (deepening of voice, clitoral enlargement) are irreversible.
- Patients with metastatic breast cancer should have regular determinations of serum calcium levels to avoid serious hypercalcemia.

Information for the patient
- Explain to woman that virilization may occur. Tell her to report androgenic effects immediately. Stopping drug prevents further androgenic changes but probably won't reverse those already present.
- Tell woman to report menstrual irregularities; drug may be stopped pending determination of the cause.
- Tell man to report too frequent or persistent penile erections.
- Advise patient to report persistent GI distress, diarrhea, or onset of jaundice.

Geriatric patients
- Observe elderly men for prostatic hyperplasia. Development of symptomatic prostatic hyperplasia or prostatic carcinoma mandates stopping drug.

Pediatric patients
- Use with extreme caution in children to avoid precocious puberty and premature closure of epiphyses. Obtain X-ray examinations every 6 months to assess skeletal maturation.

Breast-feeding patients
- It's unknown if drug appears in breast milk. An alternative to breast-feeding is recommended because of potential for severe adverse effects of androgens on infant.

testosterone transdermal system
Androderm, Testoderm, Testoderm TTS

Pharmacologic classification: androgen
Therapeutic classification: androgen replacement
Controlled substance schedule III
Pregnancy risk category X

How supplied
Available by prescription only
Transdermal system: 2.5 mg/day (Androderm), 4 mg/day (Testoderm), 5 mg/day (Androderm, Testoderm TTS), 6 mg/day (Testoderm)

Indications, route, and dosage
Primary or hypogonadotropic hypogonadism
Testoderm
Adult men ages 18 and older: Apply one 6-mg/day patch to scrotal area daily for 22 to 24 hours. If scrotal area is too small for 6-mg/day patch, start therapy with 4-mg/day patch.
Androderm
Adult men ages 18 and older: Two systems applied nightly for 24 hours, providing a total dose of 5 mg/day. Apply on dry area of skin on back, abdomen, upper arms, or thighs. Don't apply to scrotum.
    Note: Discontinue testosterone transdermal system if edema occurs.

Pharmacodynamics
Androgenic action: Releases testosterone, the endogenous androgen that stimulates receptors in androgen-responsive organs and tissues to promote growth and development of male sex organs and secondary sex characteristics.

Pharmacokinetics
- *Absorption:* After placement of transdermal system on scrotal skin, serum testosterone level increases to a maximum in 2 to 4 hours and returns toward baseline within about 2 hours after system removal. After application to nonscrotal skin, testosterone is absorbed during the 24-hour dosing period. Daily application of two Androderm systems at bedtime results in a serum testosterone level profile that mimics the normal circadian variation observed in healthy young men.
- *Distribution:* Circulating testosterone chiefly bound in serum to sex hormone–binding globulin and albumin.
- *Metabolism:* Metabolized to various 17-ketosteroids through two different pathways; major active metabolites are estradiol and dihydrotestosterone.
- *Excretion:* Little unchanged testosterone appears in urine or feces.

Contraindications and precautions
Contraindicated in patients with hypersensitivity to drug, in women, and in men with known or suspected breast or prostate cancer. Use cautiously in patients with preexisting renal, cardiac, or hepatic disease and in elderly men.

Interactions
Drug-drug. *Antidiabetics (such as insulin):* Enhanced hypoglycemic effect. Monitor blood glucose levels.
Oral anticoagulants: Increased anticoagulant effect. Monitor patient closely.
Oxyphenbutazone: Elevated serum levels of oxyphenbutazone. Monitor serum oxyphenbutazone levels.

Adverse reactions
CNS: *CVA.*
GU: *gynecomastia,* prostatitis, urinary tract infection, breast tenderness.
Metabolic: altered thyroid function tests.
Skin: acne, *pruritus.*
Other: discomfort, irritation.

☑ Special considerations
• Testoderm form of testosterone transdermal system doesn't produce adequate serum testosterone level if applied to nongenital skin.
• Edema with or without heart failure may be a serious complication in patients with preexisting cardiac, renal, or hepatic disease. In addition to discontinuing transdermal system, diuretic therapy may be needed.
• Gynecomastia commonly develops and occasionally persists in patients receiving treatment for hypogonadism.
• Topical adverse reactions decrease with duration of use.
• If patient hasn't achieved desired results within 8 weeks, another form of testosterone replacement therapy should be considered.
• Store transdermal system at room temperature.
• Testosterone levels of up to 11,400 ng/dl have been implicated in CVA. No other information is available.

Monitoring the patient
• Check hemoglobin levels and hematocrit periodically (to detect polycythemia) in patients on long-term androgen therapy.
• Check liver function, prostatic acid phosphatase, prostatic specific antigen, cholesterol, and high-density lipoproteins periodically.
• After 3 to 4 weeks of daily system use in patients receiving Testoderm, draw blood 2 to 4 hours after system application for determination of serum total testosterone. For patients receiving Androderm, monitor serum testosterone level the morning after regular evening application. Because of variability in analytical values among

diagnostic laboratories, this laboratory work and later analyses for assessing the effect of testosterone transdermal system should be performed at the same laboratory.

Information for the patient
• Show patient how to use system. For Testoderm, tell him to place system on clean, dry scrotal skin. Scrotal hair should be dry-shaved for optimal skin contact. Chemical depilatories shouldn't be used. For Androderm, tell patient to apply patches to clean, dry, designated areas. Avoid bony prominences such as shoulder and hip areas.
• Advise patient to report if nausea, vomiting, skin color changes, ankle edema, or too-frequent or persistent penile erections occur.
• Inform patient that topical testosterone preparations used by men have caused virilization in female partners. Changes in body hair distribution or significant increase in acne of female partner should be reported.

Geriatric patients
• Geriatric patients treated with androgens may be at increased risk for development of prostatic hyperplasia and prostatic carcinoma. Cautious use of system is required in this age-group.

Pediatric patients
• System hasn't been evaluated in boys under age 18.

Breast-feeding patients
• Drug is not appropriate for use in women.

tetanus immune globulin, human (TIG)
BayTet

Pharmacologic classification: immune serum
Therapeutic classification: tetanus prophylaxis
Pregnancy risk category C

How supplied
Available by prescription only
Injection: 250 units/ml in 1-ml vial or syringe

Indications, route, and dosage
Tetanus prophylactic dose
Adults and children over age 7: 250 units I.M.
Children under age 7: 4 units/kg I.M.
Tetanus treatment
Adults: Single doses of 3,000 to 6,000 units I.M. have been used. Optimal dose schedules aren't established. Don't give at same site as toxoid.

Pharmacodynamics
Antitetanus action: Provides passive immunity to tetanus. Antibodies remain at effective levels for 3 weeks or longer. Protects the patient for the incubation period of most tetanus cases.

Pharmacokinetics
- *Absorption:* Absorbed slowly.
- *Distribution:* No information available.
- *Metabolism:* No information available.
- *Excretion:* Serum half-life about 28 days.

Contraindications and precautions
Contraindicated in patients with hypersensitivity to thimerosal or TIG and in those with thrombocytopenia or any coagulation disorder that contraindicates I.M. injection unless potential benefits outweigh risks. Not recommended for use in immunoglobulin A deficiency. Don't give I.V.

Interactions
None reported.

Adverse reactions
GU: *nephrotic syndrome.*
Other: slight fever, *hypersensitivity reactions,* **anaphylaxis,** angioedema; pain, stiffness, erythema at injection site.

☑ Special considerations
- Obtain thorough history of injury, tetanus immunizations, last tetanus toxoid injection, allergies, and reactions to immunizations.
- Have epinephrine solution 1:1,000 available to treat allergic reactions.
- For wound management, use TIG for prophylaxis in patients with dirty wounds if patient has had fewer than three previous tetanus toxoid injections or if immunization history is unknown or uncertain.
- Give tetanus antitoxin when TIG isn't available.
- Don't confuse drug with tetanus toxoid, which should be given at the same time (but at different sites) to produce active immunization.
- Administer I.M. in deltoid muscle for adults and in anterolateral thigh for infants and small children. Don't inject I.V.
- Tetanus increases risks of severe morbidity and mortality in both mother and fetus if untreated. No fetal risk from use of immune globulin reported to date.
- TIG hasn't been associated with increased AIDS cases. The immune globulin is devoid of HIV. Immune globulin recipients don't develop antibodies to HIV.
- Store TIG between 36° and 46° F (2° and 8° C). Don't freeze.

Monitoring the patient
- Monitor patient for adverse effects.

Information for the patient
- Tell patient that available data indicate that TIG doesn't cause AIDS or hepatitis.
- Inform patient that he may experience some local pain, swelling, and tenderness at injection site. Recommend acetaminophen to alleviate these minor effects.
- Encourage patient to report headache, skin changes, or difficulty breathing.

Breast-feeding patients
- It's unknown if TIG appears in breast milk. Use with caution in breast-feeding women.

---

tetanus toxoid, adsorbed
tetanus toxoid

Pharmacologic classification: toxoid
Therapeutic classification: tetanus prophylaxis
Pregnancy risk category C

How supplied
Available by prescription only
tetanus toxoid, adsorbed
Injection: 5 to 10 Lf units of inactivated tetanus/ 0.5-ml dose, in 0.5-ml syringes and 5-ml vials
tetanus toxoid
Injection: 4 to 5 Lf units of inactivated tetanus/ 0.5-ml dose, in 0.5-ml syringes and 7.5-ml vials

Indications, route, and dosage
Primary immunization (tetanus toxoid, adsorbed)
Adults and children ages 1 and older: 0.5 ml I.M. 4 to 8 weeks apart for two doses, then a third dose 6 to 12 months after the second dose.
Children ages 2 to 12 months: 0.5 ml I.M. 4 to 8 weeks apart for three doses, then a fourth dose of 0.5 ml 6 to 12 months after the third dose. Booster dose is 0.5 ml I.M. q 10 years.
Primary immunization (tetanus toxoid)
Adults and children: 0.5 ml I.M. or S.C. 4 to 8 weeks apart for three doses, then a fourth dose 6 to 12 months after the third dose. Booster dose is 0.5 ml I.M. or S.C. q 10 years.

Pharmacodynamics
Tetanus prophylaxis action: Promotes active immunity by inducing production of tetanus antitoxin.

Pharmacokinetics
- *Absorption:* Absorbed slowly; fluid formulation provides quicker booster effect.
- *Distribution:* No information available.
- *Metabolism:* No information available.
- *Excretion:* No information available. Active immunity usually lasts 10 years. Adsorbed tetanus

---

toxoid usually produces more persistent antitoxin titers than fluid tetanus toxoid.

Contraindications and precautions
Contraindicated in immunosuppressed patients and in those with immunoglobulin abnormalities or severe hypersensitivity or neurologic reactions to the toxoid or its ingredients such as thimerosal. Also contraindicated in patients with thrombocytopenia or any coagulation disorder that would contraindicate I.M. injection unless potential benefits outweigh risks. Vaccination should be deferred in patients with acute illness and during polio outbreaks, except in emergencies.

Use adsorbed form cautiously in infants or children with cerebral damage, neurologic disorders, or history of febrile seizures.

Interactions
Drug-drug. *Chloramphenicol, corticosteroids, immunosuppressants:* May impair immune response to tetanus toxoid. Avoid concomitant administration of elective immunization.

Adverse reactions
CV: *tachycardia, hypotension.*
Skin: urticaria, pruritus, erythema, induration, nodule (at injection site).
Other: slight fever, chills, malaise, aches and pains, flushing, **anaphylaxis.**

☑ Special considerations
● Obtain thorough history of allergies and reactions to immunizations.
● Have epinephrine 1:1,000 solution available to treat allergic reactions.
● Determine tetanus immunization status and date of last tetanus immunization.
● Preferred I.M. injection site is deltoid or midlateral thigh in adults and children and midlateral thigh in infants.
● Preferably, tetanus immunization should be completed and maintained using several antigen preparations appropriate for patient's age, such as DTP, DT, or Td.
● Adsorbed toxoids induce higher antitoxin titers and, hence, more persistent antitoxin titers. Therefore, adsorbed tetanus toxoid is strongly recommended over tetanus toxoid for primary and booster immunizations.
● Don't confuse drug with tetanus immune globulin.
● These toxoids are used to prevent, not treat, tetanus infections.
● Store at 36° to 46° F (2° to 8° C). Don't freeze.

Monitoring the patient
● Monitor patient for adverse effects.

Information for the patient
● Tell patient to expect discomfort at injection site and a nodule that may develop at the site and persist for several weeks after immunization. Fever, general malaise, or body aches and pains are also possible.
● Advise patient not to use hot or cold compresses at injection site; they may increase severity of local reaction.
● Encourage patient to report distressing adverse reactions.
● Tell patient that immunization requires a series of injections. Stress importance of keeping scheduled appointments for subsequent doses.

Geriatric patients
● Elderly patients develop lower to normal antitoxin levels after tetanus immunization than younger patients. Skin test responsiveness may be delayed or reduced in elderly patients.

Breast-feeding patients
● It's unknown if tetanus toxoid appears in breast milk. Use with caution in breast-feeding women.

tetracycline hydrochloride
Novo-Tetra*, Panmycin, Sumycin, Tetracap, Tetracyn, Tetralan*

Pharmacologic classification: tetracycline
Therapeutic classification: antibiotic
Pregnancy risk category D (B for topical form)

How supplied
Available by prescription only
Capsules: 100 mg, 250 mg, 500 mg
Tablets: 250 mg, 500 mg
Suspension: 125 mg/5 ml
Topical solution: 2.2 mg/ml
Available without a prescription
Topical ointment: 3%*

Indications, route, and dosage
Infections caused by sensitive organisms
Adults: 1 to 2 g P.O. divided into two to four doses.
Children over age 8: 25 to 50 mg/kg P.O. daily, divided into two to four doses.
Uncomplicated urethral, endocervical, or rectal infection caused by Chlamydia trachomatis
Adults: 500 mg P.O. q.i.d. for at least 7 days.
Brucellosis
Adults: 500 mg P.O. q 6 hours for 3 weeks with streptomycin 1 g I.M. q 12 hours week 1 and daily week 2.
Gonorrhea in patients sensitive to penicillin
Adults: Initially, 1.5 g P.O.; then 500 mg q 6 hours for 4 days.
Syphilis in nonpregnant patients sensitive to penicillin
Adults: 500 mg P.O. q.i.d. for 14 days.

Acne
Adults and adolescents: Initially, 500 to 1,000 mg P.O. divided q.i.d.; then 125 to 500 mg P.O. daily or every other day; apply topical ointment generously to affected areas b.i.d. until skin is thoroughly wet.
◇ **Lyme disease**
Adults: 250 to 500 mg P.O. q.i.d. for 10 to 30 days.
◇ **Acute transmitted epididymitis (children over age 9);** ◇ **pelvic inflammatory disease;** ◇ Helicobacter pylori **(these indications use tetracycline as adjunctive therapy)**
Adults: 500 mg P.O. q.i.d. for 10 to 14 days.
Infection prophylaxis in minor skin abrasions and treatment of superficial infections caused by susceptible organisms
Adults and children: Apply topical ointment to infected area one to five times daily.

Pharmacodynamics
Antibacterial action: Bacteriostatic. Binds reversibly to ribosomal subunits, thus inhibiting bacterial protein synthesis. Spectrum of action includes many gram-negative and gram-positive organisms, *Mycoplasma, Rickettsia, Chlamydia,* and spirochetes.
   Useful against brucellosis, glanders, mycoplasma pneumonia infections (some clinicians prefer erythromycin), leptospirosis, early stages of Lyme disease, rickettsial infections (such as Rocky Mountain spotted fever, Q fever, and typhus fever), and chlamydial infections. Alternative to penicillin for *Neisseria gonorrhoeae,* but because of a high level of resistance in the United States, other alternative drugs should be considered.

Pharmacokinetics
• *Absorption:* 75% to 80% absorbed after oral administration; serum levels peak in 2 to 4 hours. Food or milk products significantly reduce oral absorption.
• *Distribution:* Widely distributed into body tissues and fluids, including synovial, pleural, prostatic, and seminal fluids, bronchial secretions, saliva, and aqueous humor; poor CSF penetration. Crosses placenta; 20% to 67% protein-bound.
• *Metabolism:* Not metabolized.
• *Excretion:* Excreted primarily unchanged in urine by glomerular filtration; plasma half-life is 6 to 12 hours in adults with normal renal function. Some drug excreted in breast milk. Only minimal amounts removed by hemodialysis or peritoneal dialysis.

Contraindications and precautions
Contraindicated in patients with hypersensitivity to tetracyclines. Use cautiously in patients with impaired renal or hepatic function. Use oral form cautiously in last half of pregnancy and in children under age 8.

Interactions
Drug-drug. *Antacids containing aluminum, bismuth, calcium, magnesium; laxatives containing magnesium, oral iron, sodium bicarbonate, zinc:* Decreased tetracycline absorption. Avoid concomitant use.
Cimetidine: Decreased absorption of tetracycline. Avoid concomitant use.
Digoxin: Increased bioavailability of digoxin. Lower dose of digoxin.
Methoxyflurane: Increased risk of nephrotoxicity. Avoid concomitant use.
Oral anticoagulants: Enhanced anticoagulant effect. Lower dosage of anticoagulant.
Oral contraceptives: Decreased contraceptive effectiveness. Advise secondary contraceptive during therapy.
Penicillin: Inhibited cell growth from bacteriostatic action. Give penicillin 2 to 3 hours before tetracycline.
Drug-food. *Dairy products, milk, other foods:* Decreased antibiotic absorption. Give antibiotic 1 hour before or 2 hours after such foods.
Drug-lifestyle. *Sun exposure:* Photosensitivity reactions. Tell patient to take precautions.

Adverse reactions
Unless noted, the following adverse reactions refer to oral form of drug.
CNS: dizziness, headache, *intracranial hypertension (pseudotumor cerebri).*
CV: pericarditis.
EENT: sore throat, glossitis, dysphagia.
GI: anorexia, *epigastric distress, nausea,* vomiting, *diarrhea,* esophagitis, oral candidiasis, stomatitis, enterocolitis, inflammatory lesions in anogenital region.
GU: elevated BUN levels.
Hematologic: neutropenia, eosinophilia.
Hepatic: elevated liver enzymes.
Skin: *candidal superinfection, maculopapular and erythematous rashes, urticaria, photosensitivity, increased pigmentation;* temporary stinging or burning on application; slight yellowing of treated skin, especially in patients with light complexions; severe dermatitis (with topical administration).
Other: *hypersensitivity reactions, permanent discoloration of teeth, enamel defects, and retardation of bone growth when used in children under age 8.*

☑ Special considerations
Besides the recommendations relevant to all tetracyclines, consider the following, which refer to topical use.
• Discontinue use if condition persists or worsens.
• To control the rate of flow, increase or decrease pressure of applicator against skin.
• Avoid contact with eyes, nose, and mouth.
• Solution should be used within 2 months.

Reactions may be *common*, uncommon, *life-threatening*, or COMMON AND LIFE-THREATENING.

• Tetracycline causes false-negative results in urine tests using glucose oxidase reagent (Diastix, Chemstrip uG, or glucose enzymatic test strip) and false elevations in fluorometric tests for urinary catecholamines.

• Signs and symptoms of overdose are usually limited to GI tract; give antacids or empty stomach by gastric lavage if ingestion occurs within 4 hours of treatment.

Monitoring the patient
• Monitor therapeutic effect.
• Monitor patient for adverse effects.

Information for the patient
• Advise patient to take drug 1 hour before or 2 hours after meals or drinking milk.
• Tell patient not to share drug with others.
• Tell patient that stinging may occur with topical use but resolves quickly; drug may stain clothing.
• Warn patient to avoid prolonged exposure to sunlight.
• Tell patient to report persistent nausea or vomiting or yellowing of skin or eyes.

Pediatric patients
• Don't use in children under age 8.

Breast-feeding patients
• Drug appears in breast milk; don't use in breast-feeding women.

tetrahydrozoline hydrochloride
Collyrium Fresh, Eyesine, Geneye, Mallazine Eye Drops, Murine Plus, Optigene 3, Tetrasine, Tyzine, Tyzine Pediatric, Visine

Pharmacologic classification: sympathomimetic
Therapeutic classification: vasoconstrictor, decongestant
Pregnancy risk category C

How supplied
Available by prescription only
Nasal solution: 0.05%, 0.1%
Available without a prescription
Ophthalmic solution: 0.05%

Indications, route, and dosage
Nasal congestion
Adults and children over age 6: Apply 2 to 4 drops of 0.1% solution in each nostril t.i.d. or q.i.d., p.r.n, or 3 to 4 sprays of 0.1% nasal solution in each nostril q.i.d., p.r.n.
Children ages 2 to 6: Apply 2 or 3 drops of 0.05% solution in each nostril q 4 to 6 hours, p.r.n.

Conjunctival congestion
Adults: 1 or 2 drops of ophthalmic solution in each eye b.i.d. to q.i.d.

Pharmacodynamics
Decongestant action: In ocular use, vasoconstriction is produced by local adrenergic action on the blood vessels of the conjunctiva. After nasal application, drug acts on alpha-adrenergic receptors in nasal mucosa to produce constriction, thereby decreasing blood flow and nasal congestion.

Pharmacokinetics
No information available.

Contraindications and precautions
Contraindicated in patients with hypersensitivity to drug or its components and in those with angle-closure glaucoma or other serious eye diseases and in patients on MAO inhibitor therapy. Nasal solution is contraindicated in those under age 2; 0.1% solution is contraindicated in those under age 6.

Use cautiously in patients with hyperthyroidism, hypertension, and diabetes mellitus. Also, use ophthalmic form cautiously in patients with cardiac disease.

Interactions
Drug-drug. *MAO inhibitors:* Increased adrenergic response and hypertensive crisis. Monitor blood pressure. Use cautiously together.

Adverse reactions
CNS: headache, drowsiness, insomnia, dizziness, tremor (with ophthalmic form).
CV: *arrhythmias* (with ophthalmic form), tachycardia, palpitations.
EENT: transient eye stinging, pupillary dilation, increased intraocular pressure, keratitis, lacrimation, eye irritation (with ophthalmic form); transient burning, stinging; sneezing, rebound nasal congestion with excessive or long-term use (with nasal form).

☑ Special considerations
• Excessive use of either preparation may cause rebound effect.
• Drug shouldn't be used for more than 4 days.
• Signs and symptoms of overdose include bradycardia, decreased body temperature, shocklike hypotension, apnea, drowsiness, CNS depression, and coma.
• Because of rapid onset of sedation, emesis isn't recommended unless induced early.
• Activated charcoal or gastric lavage may be used initially. Monitor vital signs and ECG. Treat seizures with I.V. diazepam

Monitoring the patient
- Monitor therapeutic effect.
- Monitor cardiac status.

Information for the patient
- Teach patient how to instill ophthalmic or nasal form and advise him not to share drug.
- Advise patient not to exceed recommended dose and to use drug only when needed.
- Tell patient to remove contact lenses before using drug.

Geriatric patients
- Don't use in elderly patients to treat redness and inflammation, which may represent more serious eye conditions.
- Use in glaucoma requires close medical attention.
- Elderly patients are more likely than younger patients to experience adverse reactions to sympathomimetics.

Pediatric patients
- The 0.1% nasal solution is contraindicated in children under age 6. All uses are contraindicated in children under age 2.

thalidomide
Thalomid

Pharmacologic classification: immuno-modulator
Therapeutic classification: antileprotic
Pregnancy risk category X

How supplied
Available by prescription only
Capsules: 50 mg

Indications, route, and dosage
Acute treatment of cutaneous manifestations of moderate to severe erythema nodosum leprosum (ENL)
Adults: 100 to 300 mg P.O. daily h.s. If patient weighs less than 50 kg (110 lb), start dosing at the lower end of range.
Maintenance therapy for prevention and suppression of the cutaneous manifestations of ENL recurrence
Adults: Up to 400 mg P.O. daily h.s. or in divided doses at least 1 hour after meals.

Pharmacodynamics
Antileprosy action: Exact mechanism unknown. Immunomodulatory product.

Pharmacokinetics
- *Absorption:* Slowly absorbed from GI tract; levels peak in 2.9 to 5.7 hours.
- *Distribution:* Not reported.

- *Metabolism:* Exact metabolic fate not known.
- *Excretion:* Mean half-life is 5 to 7 hours. Route of elimination not fully understood.

Contraindications and precautions
Contraindicated in patients with hypersensitivity to drug or its components; in pregnant women and those capable of becoming pregnant, except when alternative therapies are inappropriate and patient meets all conditions listed in the System for Thalidomide Education and Prescribing Safety (S.T.E.P.S.) program.

Interactions
Drug-drug. *Barbiturates, chlorpromazine, reserpine:* Enhanced sedative activity. Use cautiously together.
Drugs associated with peripheral neuropathy: Increased risk of peripheral neuropathy. Use cautiously together.
Drug-food. *Any food:* Decreased absorption of drug. Give at least 1 hour after meals at bedtime.
Drug-lifestyle. *Alcohol:* Increased sedation. Caution against using together.

Adverse reactions
CNS: *asthenia, drowsiness, somnolence, dizziness,* peripheral neuropathy, *headache,* agitation, insomnia, malaise, nervousness, *paresthesia,* tremor, vertigo.
CV: orthostatic hypotension, **bradycardia,** peripheral edema.
EENT: dry mouth, oral candidiasis, pharyngitis, sinusitis.
GI: abdominal pain, anorexia, constipation, *diarrhea,* flatulence, *nausea.*
GU: albuminuria, *hematuria,* impotence.
Hematologic: *neutropenia, increased HIV viral load,* anemia, *lymphadenopathy,* LEUKOPENIA.
Hepatic: abnormal liver function tests, increased AST.
Musculoskeletal: back pain, neck pain, neck rigidity.
Skin: acne, fungal dermatitis, nail disorder, pruritus, *rash, maculopapular rash, sweating.*
Other: *teratogenicity, hypersensitivity reactions,* facial edema, hyperlipidemia, lymphadenopathy, fever, chills, accidental injury, infection, pain.

☑ Special considerations
- Thalidomide must be administered in compliance with all of the terms outlined in the S.T.E.P.S. program, may be prescribed only by physicians registered with the S.T.E.P.S. program, and may be dispensed only by pharmacists registered with the S.T.E.P.S. program.
- All sexually mature patients (men or women) capable of reproduction must meet rigid S.T.E.P.S. program requirements, including ability to understand and carry out instructions, ability and willingness to comply with mandatory contraceptive measures (concurrent use of at least 2

*eactions may be *common*, uncommon, **life-threatening**, or COMMON AND LIFE-THREATENING.*

highly effective means of contraception), and a written acknowledgment of understanding of all warnings concerning the hazards of fetal exposure to thalidomide and the risk of contraception failure.

• Sexually mature women who haven't undergone a hysterectomy or who haven't been postmenopausal for at least 24 consecutive months (that is, who have had menses at some time in the preceding 24 consecutive months) are considered to be women of childbearing potential even with history of infertility.

• Immediately report suspected fetal exposure to FDA via MedWATCH at 1-800-FDA-1088, and to manufacturer.

• Corticosteroids may be administered with drug in patients with moderate to severe neuritis associated with severe ENL reaction. Corticosteroids can be tapered and stopped when neuritis improves.

• A patient with a history of requiring prolonged treatment to prevent recurrence of cutaneous ENL or who experiences flare during tapering should use minimum effective dose. Tapering should be attempted every 3 to 6 months at a dose reduction rate of 50 mg every 2 to 4 weeks.

Monitoring the patient

• Perform mandatory pregnancy test within 24 hours before therapy for women of childbearing potential, then weekly during first month of therapy, then monthly for women with regular menstrual cycles. If menstrual cycles are irregular, pregnancy testing continues every 2 weeks during therapy. Retesting is performed if menstrual changes occur, including missed menses.

• Perform CBC and differential before therapy and periodically thereafter. Patients with an absolute neutrophil count falling below 750/mm^2 while on treatment should be reevaluated.

• Monitor patient for signs and symptoms of neuropathy (such as numbness, tingling, or pain in hands or feet) at least once monthly during first 3 months of drug therapy, then periodically.

Information for the patient

• Warn patient of dangers of fetal exposure to any amount of thalidomide. Ascertain that S.T.E.P.S. program protocol has been fully followed and is understood by patient.

• Reinforce that blood and sperm donations are prohibited while taking thalidomide.

• Explain that at least two highly reliable means of contraception must be used simultaneously and continuously from at least 1 month before therapy until 1 month after completion of therapy.

• Advise woman to report signs or symptoms of pregnancy immediately without regard to probability or improbability of pregnancy.

• Inform woman of childbearing potential of mandatory pregnancy testing schedule.

• Inform woman that, if pregnancy occurs, drug must be stopped immediately.

• Caution patient that it isn't known if drug is present in ejaculate of men receiving drug; men receiving thalidomide must always use a latex condom when engaging in sexual activity with women of childbearing potential.

• Advise patient to read package insert carefully.

• Tell woman that, if she is taking drugs that reduce effectiveness of hormonal contraceptives (such as HIV-protease inhibitors, griseofulvin, rifampin, rifabutin, phenytoin, carbamazepine), she must use two other effective means of contraception.

• Stress importance of storing drug out of reach of children or others who may mistakenly take drug; drug should be stored at room temperature and protected from light.

• Advise patient to take drug only as prescribed.

• Caution patient against sharing drug with others, including those who also have a thalidomide prescription.

• Caution patient about potential for dizziness and orthostatic hypotension; advise patient to change position slowly when rising.

• Inform patient that drug frequently causes drowsiness and somnolence. Advise patient to avoid hazardous activities and alcohol or other drugs that might cause drowsiness.

• Tell patient to take drug at bedtime with a glass of water, at least 1 hour after the evening meal.

• Inform patient of signs and symptoms of peripheral neuropathy; tell him to report their occurrence immediately.

• Tell patient that drug has caused hypersensitivity reactions; advise him to call if erythematous macular rash, fever, tachycardia, hypotension, or other adverse reactions occur.

Geriatric patients

• There are no significant differences in safety and efficacy in elderly patients compared to younger patients.

Pediatric patients

• Safety and efficacy in children under age 12 haven't been established.

Breast-feeding patients

• It's unknown if drug appears in breast milk. Stop either drug or breast-feeding, depending on importance of drug to mother.

theophylline

Accurbron, Aquaphyllin, Asmalix,
Bronkodyl, Elixophyllin, Lanophyllin,
Quibron-T, Respbid, Slo-bid Gyrocaps,
Slo-Phyllin, Sustaire, Theobid
Duracaps, Theochron, Theoclear-80,
Theo-Dur, Theolair, Theo-Sav,
Theo-24, Theospan-SR, Theostat 80,
Theovent, Theo-X, T-Phyl, Uni-Dur,
Uniphyl

Pharmacologic classification: xanthine
derivative
Therapeutic classification: bronchodilator
Pregnancy risk category C

How supplied

Available by prescription only
Capsules: 100 mg, 200 mg
Capsules (extended-release): 50 mg, 60 mg, 65
mg, 75 mg, 100 mg, 125 mg, 130 mg, 200 mg,
250 mg, 260 mg, 300 mg
Tablets: 100 mg, 125 mg, 200 mg, 250 mg, 300
mg
Tablets (extended-release): 100 mg, 200 mg, 250
mg, 300 mg, 400 mg, 450 mg, 500 mg
Elixir: 50 mg/5 ml, 80 mg/15 ml
Syrup: 50 mg/5 ml, 80 mg/15 ml, 150 mg/15 ml
Dextrose 5% injection: 200 mg in 50 ml or 100
ml; 400 mg in 100 ml, 250 ml, 500 ml, or 1,000
ml; 800 mg in 250 ml, 500 ml or 1,000 ml

Indications, route, and dosage

**Symptomatic relief of bronchospasm in pa-
tients not currently receiving theophylline
who require rapid relief of acute symptoms**
Loading dose: 6 mg/kg anhydrous theophylline,
then:
Adults (nonsmokers): 3 mg/kg q 6 hours for two
doses; then 3 mg/kg q 8 hours.
Older adults with cor pulmonale: 2 mg/kg q 6
hours for two doses; then 2 mg/kg q 8 hours.
Adults with heart failure: 2 mg/kg q 8 hours for
two doses; then 1 to 2 mg/kg q 12 hours.
*Children and adolescents ages 9 to 16 and young
adult smokers:* 3 mg/kg q 4 hours for three doses; then 3 mg/kg q 6 hours.
Neonates and children ages 6 months to 9 years:
4 mg/kg q 4 hours for three doses; then 4 mg/kg
q 6 hours.
◊ *Neonates and infants under age 6 months:*
Dose is highly individualized. It's recommended
that serum theophylline levels be maintained below 10 mcg/ml in neonates and below 20 mcg/ml
in older infants.
Loading dose: 1 mg/kg for each 2 mcg/ml increase in theophylline level, then:
Infants ages 8 weeks to 6 months: 1 to 3 mg/kg
q 6 hours.
Infants ages 4 to 8 weeks: 1 to 2 mg/kg q 8 hours.

Neonates up to age 4 weeks: 1 to 2 mg/kg q 12
hours.
*Premature neonates (less than 40 weeks' ges-
tational age):* 1 mg/kg q 12 hours.
**Parenteral theophylline for patients not cur-
rently receiving theophylline**
Loading dose: 4.7 mg/kg (equivalent to 6 mg/kg
anhydrous aminophylline) I.V. slowly; then maintenance infusion:
Adults (nonsmokers): 0.55 mg/kg/hour (equivalent to 0.7 mg/kg/hour anhydrous aminophylline)
for 12 hours, then 0.39 mg/kg/hour (equivalent
to 0.5 mg/kg/hour anhydrous aminophylline).
Older adults with cor pulmonale: 0.47 mg/kg/hour
(equivalent to 0.6 mg/kg/hour anhydrous aminophylline) for 12 hours; then 0.24 mg/kg/hour (equivalent to 0.3 mg/kg/hour anhydrous aminophylline).
Adults with heart failure or liver disease: 0.39
mg/kg/hour (equivalent to 0.5 mg/kg/hour anhydrous aminophylline) for 12 hours; then 0.08 to
0.16 mg/kg/hour (equivalent to 0.1 to 0.2 mg/
kg/hour anhydrous aminophylline).
Children ages 9 to 16: 0.79 mg/kg/hour (equivalent to 1 mg/kg/hour anhydrous aminophylline)
for 12 hours; then 0.63 mg/kg/hour (equivalent
to 0.8 mg/kg/hour anhydrous aminophylline).
Infants and children ages 6 months to 9 years:
0.95 mg/kg/hour (equivalent to 1.2 mg/kg/hour
anhydrous aminophylline) for 12 hours; then 0.79
mg/kg/hour (equivalent to 1 mg/kg/hour anhydrous aminophylline).
   Switch to oral theophylline as soon as patient
shows adequate improvement.
**Symptomatic relief of bronchospasm in pa-
tients currently receiving theophylline**
Adults and children: Each 0.5 mg/kg I.V. or P.O.
(loading dose) increases plasma levels by 1
mcg/ml. Ideally, dose is based on current theophylline level and lean body weight. In emergency
situations, may use a 2.5 mg/kg P.O. dose of rapidly absorbed form if no obvious signs of theophylline toxicity are present.
**Prophylaxis of bronchial asthma, broncho-
spasm of chronic bronchitis, and emphysema**
Adults and children: Using rapidly absorbed dose
forms, initial dose is 16 mg/kg or 400 mg P.O. daily (whichever is less) divided q 6 to 8 hours; dose
may be increased in increments of about 25% at
2- to 3-day intervals. Using extended-release
dose forms, initial dose is 12 mg/kg or 400 mg
P.O. daily (whichever is less) divided q 8 to 12
hours; dose may be increased, if tolerated, by 2
to 3 mg/kg daily at 3-day intervals. Regardless
of dose form used, dose may be increased, if tolerated, up to the following maximum daily doses, without measurements of serum theophylline
level.
Adults and adolescents ages 16 and older: 13
mg/kg P.O. or 900 mg P.O. daily in divided
doses.
Adolescents ages 12 to 16: 18 mg/kg P.O. daily
in divided doses.

◊Reactions may be *common*, uncommon, **life-threatening**, or COMMON AND LIFE-THREATENING.

Children ages 9 to 12: 20 mg/kg P.O. daily in divided doses.

Children under age 9: 24 mg/kg P.O. daily in divided doses.

Note: Dosage individualization is needed. Use plasma peak and trough levels to estimate dose. Therapeutic range is 10 to 20 mcg/ml. All doses are based on theophylline anhydrous and lean body weight.

◊ *Cystic fibrosis*
Infants: 10 to 20 mg/kg I.V. daily.

◊ *Promotion of diuresis,* ◊ *treatment of Cheyne-Stokes respirations,* ◊ *paroxysmal nocturnal dyspnea*
Adults: 200 to 400 mg I.V. bolus (single dose).

Pharmacodynamics
Bronchodilator action: May act by inhibiting phosphodiesterase, elevating cellular cAMP levels, or antagonizing adenosine receptors in the bronchi, resulting in relaxation of the smooth muscle.

Increases sensitivity of the medullary respiratory center to carbon dioxide to reduce apneic episodes. Prevents muscle fatigue, especially that of the diaphragm. Also causes diuresis and cardiac and CNS stimulation.

Pharmacokinetics
• *Absorption:* Well absorbed. Rate and onset of action depend on dosage form; food may further alter rate of absorption, especially of some extended-release forms.
• *Distribution:* Distributed throughout extracellular fluids; equilibrium between fluid and tissues occurs within an hour of I.V. loading dose. Therapeutic plasma levels are 10 to 20 mcg/ml, but many patients respond to lower levels.
• *Metabolism:* Metabolized in liver to inactive compounds. Half-life is 7 to 9 hours in adults, 4 to 5 hours in smokers, 20 to 30 hours in premature infants, and 3 to 5 hours in children.
• *Excretion:* About 10% of dose excreted in urine unchanged. Other metabolites include 1,3-dimethyluric acid, 1-methyluric acid, and 3-methylxanthine.

Contraindications and precautions
Contraindicated in patients with hypersensitivity to xanthine compounds (caffeine, theobromine) and in those with active peptic ulcer and seizure disorders.

Use cautiously in elderly patients; in neonates, infants under age 1, and young children; and in patients with COPD, cardiac failure, cor pulmonale, renal or hepatic disease, peptic ulcer, hyperthyroidism, diabetes mellitus, glaucoma, severe hypoxemia, hypertension, compromised cardiac or circulatory function, angina, acute MI, or sulfite sensitivity.

Interactions
Drug-drug. *Allopurinol (high dose), calcium channel blockers, cimetidine, corticosteroids, erythromycin, interferon, mexiletine, oral contraceptives, propranolol, quinolones, troleandomycin:* Increased serum levels of theophylline. Monitor theophylline levels.
Barbiturates, charcoal, ketoconazole, phenytoin, rifampin: Decreased serum theophylline levels. Monitor patient and theophylline levels.
Beta blockers: Antagonistic pharmacologic effect. Monitor patient for effect.
Carbamazepine, isoniazid, loop diuretics: Increased or decreased theophylline levels. Monitor theophylline levels.
Lithium: Increased excretion of lithium. Monitor lithium levels.
Drug-herb. *Cacao tree:* Inhibited theophylline metabolism. Avoid ingesting large amounts of cocoa when using theophylline.
Caffeine, guarana: Additive CNS and CV effects. Avoid concomitant use.
Drug-food. *Any food:* Accelerated absorption. Administer Theo-24 on empty stomach.
Drug-lifestyle. *Smoking:* Increased elimination of theophylline; increased dosage requirements. Monitor theophylline response and serum levels.

Adverse reactions
CNS: *restlessness, dizziness, insomnia,* headache, irritability, ***seizures,*** muscle twitching.
CV: *palpitations, sinus tachycardia, extrasystoles,* flushing, marked hypotension, arrhythmias
GI: *nausea, vomiting,* diarrhea, epigastric pain.
Respiratory: tachypnea, ***respiratory arrest.***

☑ Special considerations
• Don't crush extended-release tablets. Some capsules are formulated to be opened and sprinkled on food.
• Obtain serum theophylline measurements in patients receiving long-term therapy. Ideal levels are between 10 and 20 mcg/ml, although some patients may respond adequately with lower serum levels. Check every 6 months. If levels are less than 10 mcg/ml, increase dosage by about 25% each day. If levels are 20 to 25 mcg/ml, decrease dosage by about 10% each day. If levels are 25 to 30 mcg/ml, skip next dose and decrease by 25% each day. If levels are more than 30 mcg/ml, skip next two doses and decrease by 50% each day. Repeat serum level determination.
• Theophylline increases plasma free fatty acids and urinary catecholamines. Depending on assay used, theophylline levels may be falsely elevated in the presence of furosemide, phenylbutazone, probenecid, theobromine, caffeine, tea, chocolate, cola beverages, and acetaminophen.
• Signs and symptoms of overdose include nausea, vomiting, insomnia, irritability, tachy

cardia, extrasystoles, tachypnea, or tonic-clonic seizures. Toxicity onset may be sudden and severe, with arrhythmias and seizures as the first signs. Induce emesis except in convulsing patients, then use activated charcoal and cathartics. Treat arrhythmias with lidocaine and seizures with I.V. diazepam; support respiratory and CV systems.

Monitoring the patient
- Monitor vital signs and observe for signs and symptoms of toxicity.
- Obtain serum theophylline measurements in patients receiving long-term therapy.

Information for the patient
- Advise patient regarding drugs and dosing schedule; if a dose is missed, it should be taken as soon as possible. Doses shouldn't be doubled.
- Advise patient to take drug at regular intervals around the clock.
- Tell patient to avoid excessive use of foods containing xanthine and beverages containing caffeine.
- Warn elderly patient of dizziness, a common reaction at start of therapy.
- Tell patient to take drug with food if GI upset occurs with liquid preparations or non-sustained-release forms.
- Advise patient to continue to use same brand of theophylline.

Pediatric patients
- Use with caution in neonates. Children usually need higher doses (on a mg/kg basis) than adults. Maximum recommended doses are 24 mg/kg/day in children under age 9; 20 mg/kg/day in children ages 9 to 12; 18 mg/kg/day in adolescents ages 12 to 16; 13 mg/kg/day or 900 mg (whichever is less) in adolescents and adults ages 16 and older.

Breast-feeding patients
- Drug appears in breast milk and may cause irritability, insomnia, or fretfulness in breast-fed infant. Stop either drug or breast-feeding.

---

thiabendazole
Mintezol

Pharmacologic classification: benzimidazole
Therapeutic classification: anthelmintic
Pregnancy risk category C

How supplied
Available by prescription only
Tablets (chewable): 500 mg
Oral suspension: 500 mg/5 ml

Indications, route, and dosage
Systemic infections with pinworm, roundworm, threadworm, whipworm, visceral larva migrans, trichinosis
Adults and children weighing 14 to 70 kg (30 to 154 lb): 22 mg/kg P.O. q 12 hours for 2 successive days.
Adults and children weighing over 70 kg: 1.5 g q 12 hours for 2 successive days. Maximum dose is 3 g daily.
Visceral larva migrans—Two doses daily for 7 successive days.
Trichinosis—Two doses daily for 2 to 4 successive days.
Cutaneous infestations with larva migrans (creeping eruption)
Adults and children: 25 mg/kg P.O. b.i.d. for 2 to 5 days. Maximum dose is 3 g daily. If lesions persist after 2 days, repeat course.
◊ *Dracunculiasis;* ◊ *infections caused by* **Angiostrongylus costaricensis**
Adults: 25 to 37.5 mg/kg P.O. b.i.d. (25 mg t.i.d. for *A. costaricensis*) for 3 successive days.
◊ *Capillariasis*
Adults: 25 mg/kg P.O. q 12 hours for 30 days.

Pharmacodynamics
Anthelmintic action: Kills susceptible helminths by inhibiting fumarate reductase. Drug of choice for *Strongyloides stercoralis* (threadworm) infections and may be useful in disseminated strongyloidiasis. Preferred for oral and topical therapy of *Ancylostoma braziliense, Toxocara canis,* and *T. cati.* Has shown activity in certain other nematode infections, but other drugs are preferred for the treatment of ascariasis, trichuriasis, uncinariasis, and enterobiasis.

Pharmacokinetics
- *Absorption:* Absorbed readily; serum levels peak in 1 to 2 hours.
- *Distribution:* Little information available.
- *Metabolism:* Metabolized almost completely by hydroxylation and conjugation.
- *Excretion:* About 90% of dose excreted in urine as metabolites within 48 hours; about 5% excreted in feces.

Contraindications and precautions
Contraindicated in patients with hypersensitivity to drug. Use cautiously in patients with renal or hepatic dysfunction, severe malnutrition, or anemia and in those who are vomiting.

Interactions
Drug-drug. *Aminophylline:* Elevated levels of both. Monitor patient closely.

Adverse reactions
CNS: impaired mental alertness, impaired coordination, numbness, *seizures,* drowsiness, *fatigue, headache,* giddiness, dizziness.

Reactions may be common, uncommon, **life-threatening**, or COMMON AND LIFE-THREATENING.

CV: *hypotension.*
EENT: tinnitus, blurry or yellow vision, dry mouth and eyes, xanthopsia.
GI: *anorexia, nausea, vomiting,* diarrhea, epigastric distress, cholestasis.
GU: hematuria, enuresis, crystalluria, malodorous urine.
Hematologic: LEUKOPENIA.
Hepatic: *jaundice, parenchymal liver damage,* elevated AST levels.
Metabolic: hyperglycemia.
Skin: *rash, pruritus,* **erythema multiforme, Stevens-Johnson syndrome.**
Other: lymphadenopathy, fever, flushing, chills, **angioedema, anaphylaxis.**

☑ Special considerations
● Drug may be given with milk, fruit juice, or food.
● Laxatives, enemas, and dietary restrictions are unnecessary.
● Signs and symptoms of overdose may include visual disturbances and altered mental status. Treat with induced emesis or gastric lavage if ingested within 4 hours; then provide supportive and symptomatic treatment.

Monitoring the patient
● Assess patient and review laboratory reports for signs of anemia, dehydration, or malnutrition before starting therapy.
● Monitor patient for adverse reactions, which usually occur 3 to 4 hours after drug is administered. Adverse effects are usually mild and related to dose and duration of therapy.

Information for the patient
● Warn patient that drug causes drowsiness or dizziness. Advise him to avoid driving or other hazardous activities during therapy.
● Teach patient signs and symptoms of hypersensitivity; tell him to call immediately if they occur.
● Tell patient to wash perianal area daily and to change undergarments and bedclothes daily.
● Explain routes of transmission, and encourage other household members and suspected contacts to be tested and, if necessary, treated.

Breast-feeding patients
● Safety hasn't been established. Because it's unknown if drug appears in breast milk, drug should not be used in breast-feeding women.

thiamine hydrochloride (vitamin B$_1$)
Biamine, Thiamilate

Pharmacologic classification: water-soluble vitamin
Therapeutic classification: nutritional supplement
Pregnancy risk category A (C if more than RDA)

How supplied
Available by prescription only
Injection: 1-ml prefilled (100 mg/ml), 1-ml vials (100 mg/ml), 2-ml vials (100 mg/ml)
Available without a prescription
Tablets: 50 mg, 100 mg, 250 mg
Tablets (enteric-coated): 20 mg

Indications, route, and dosage
Beriberi
Adults: 10 to 20 mg I.M., depending on severity (can receive up to 100 mg I.M. or I.V. for severe cases), t.i.d. for 2 weeks, then dietary correction and multivitamin supplement containing 5 to 30 mg thiamine daily in single or three divided doses for 1 month.
Children: 10 to 25 mg, depending on severity, I.M. daily for several weeks with adequate dietary intake.
Anemia secondary to thiamine deficiency; polyneuritis secondary to alcoholism, pregnancy, or pellagra
Adults and children: P.O. dosage is based on RDA for age-group.
Wernicke's encephalopathy
Adults: Initially, 100 mg I.V.; then 50 to 100 mg I.M. or I.V. daily.
"Wet beriberi" with myocardial failure
Adults and children: 10 to 30 mg I.V. for emergency treatment.

Pharmacodynamics
Metabolic action: Exogenous thiamine is needed for carbohydrate metabolism. Thiamine combines with ATP from thiamine pyrophosphate, a coenzyme in carbohydrate metabolism and transketolation reactions. This coenzyme is also necessary in the hexose monophosphate shunt during pentose utilization. One sign of thiamine deficiency is an increase in pyruvic acid. The body's need for thiamine is greater when the carbohydrate content of the diet is high. Within 3 weeks of total absence of dietary thiamine, significant vitamin depletion can occur. Thiamine deficiency can cause beriberi.

Pharmacokinetics
● *Absorption:* Absorbed readily after oral administration of small doses; after oral administration of a large dose, total amount absorbed is limited

to 4 to 8 mg. In alcoholics and in patients with cirrhosis or malabsorption, GI absorption of thiamine is decreased. When given with meals, drug's GI rate of absorption decreases, but total absorption remains the same. After I.M. administration, absorbed rapidly and completely.

• *Distribution:* Distributed widely into body tissues. When intake exceeds the minimal requirements, tissue stores become saturated. About 100 to 200 mcg/day of thiamine distributed into milk of breast-feeding women on normal diet.

• *Metabolism:* Metabolized in liver.

• *Excretion:* Excess thiamine excreted in urine. After administration of large doses (more than 10 mg), both unchanged thiamine and metabolites excreted in urine after tissue stores become saturated.

Contraindications and precautions
Contraindicated in patients with hypersensitivity to thiamine products.

Interactions
Drug-drug. *Alkaline solutions (bicarbonates, carbonates, citrates):* Thiamine is unstable in neutral or alkaline solutions. Don't use together.
Neuromuscular blockers: Enhanced effects of these drugs. Adjust dosage.
Sulfites: Incompatible with thiamine. Don't use together.

Adverse reactions
CNS: restlessness.
CV: *angioedema, CV collapse,* cyanosis.
EENT: tightness of throat (allergic reaction).
GI: nausea, hemorrhage.
Respiratory: pulmonary edema.
Skin: feeling of warmth, pruritus, urticaria, diaphoresis.
Other: weakness; tenderness and induration after I.M. administration.

☑ Special considerations
• The RDA of thiamine is as follows:
– *Neonates and infants up to age 6 months:* 0.3 mg daily.
– *Infants ages 6 months to 1 year:* 0.4 mg daily.
– *Children ages 1 to 3:* 0.7 mg daily.
– *Children ages 4 to 6:* 0.9 mg daily.
– *Children ages 7 to 10:* 1 mg daily.
– *Boys ages 11 to 14:* 1.3 mg daily.
– *Men ages 15 to 50:* 1.5 mg daily.
– *Men ages 51 and over:* 1.2 mg daily.
– *Women ages 11 to 50:* 1.1 mg daily.
– *Women ages 51 and over:* 1 mg daily.
– *Pregnant women:* 1.5 mg daily.
– *Breast-feeding women:* 1.6 mg daily.
• Give intradermal skin test before I.V. thiamine administration if sensitivity is suspected because anaphylaxis can occur. Keep epinephrine available when giving large parenteral doses.

• I.M. injection may be painful. Rotate injection sites and apply cold compresses to ease discomfort.
• Accurate dietary history is important during vitamin replacement therapy. Help patient develop a practical plan for adequate nutrition.
• Total absence of dietary thiamine can produce a deficiency state in about 3 weeks.
• Subclinical deficiency of thiamine or other B vitamins is common in patients who are poor, chronic alcoholics, or pregnant or who follow fad diets.
• Store thiamine in light-resistant, nonmetallic container.
• Drug therapy may produce false-positive results in the phosphotungstate method for determination of uric acid and in the urine spot tests with Ehrlich's reagent for urobilinogen.
• Large doses of thiamine interfere with the Schack and Waxler spectrophotometric determination of serum theophylline levels.
• Very large doses of thiamine administered parenterally may produce neuromuscular and ganglionic blockade and neurologic symptoms. Treatment is supportive.

Monitoring the patient
• Monitor patient for postadministration anaphylaxis.
• Monitor patient for adverse effects.

Information for the patient
• Inform patient about dietary sources of thiamine, such as yeast, pork, beef, liver, whole grains, peas, and beans.

Breast-feeding patients
• Thiamine (in amounts that don't exceed the RDA) is safe to use in breast-feeding women. It appears in breast milk and fulfills a nutritional requirement of infant.

thioguanine
(6-thioguanine, 6-TG)
Lanvis*

Pharmacologic classification: antimetabolite (cell cycle–phase specific, S phase)
Therapeutic classification: antineoplastic
Pregnancy risk category D

How supplied
Available by prescription only
Tablets (scored): 40 mg

Indications, route, and dosage
Dosage and indications may vary. Check current literature for recommended protocol.
Acute nonlymphocytic leukemias
Adults and children: Initially, 2 mg/kg/day P.O. (usually calculated to nearest 20 mg); then, if no

toxic effects occur, increase dosage gradually over 3 to 4 weeks to 3 mg/kg/day. Maintenance dose is 2 to 3 mg/kg/day P.O.

Pharmacodynamics
Antineoplastic action: Requires conversion intracellularly to active form to exert cytotoxic activity. Acting as a false metabolite, thioguanine inhibits purine synthesis. Cross-resistance exists between mercaptopurine and thioguanine.

Pharmacokinetics
- *Absorption:* After oral dose, absorption incomplete and variable. Average bioavailability is 30%.
- *Distribution:* Well distributed into bone marrow cells. Doesn't cross blood-brain barrier to any appreciable extent.
- *Metabolism:* Extensively metabolized to less active form in liver and other tissues.
- *Excretion:* Plasma levels decrease in biphasic manner; half-life of 15 minutes in initial phase and 11 hours in terminal phase. Excreted in urine, mainly as metabolites.

Contraindications and precautions
Contraindicated in patients with hypersensitivity to drug or mercaptopurine and in those whose disease has shown resistance to drug. Use cautiously in patients with renal or hepatic dysfunction.

Interactions
None reported.

Adverse reactions
GI: nausea, vomiting, stomatitis, diarrhea, anorexia.
Hematologic: *leukopenia, anemia, thrombocytopenia* (occurs slowly over 2 to 4 weeks).
Hepatic: *hepatotoxicity,* jaundice.
Metabolic: hyperuricemia.
Skin: rash.

☑ Special considerations
- Total daily dose can be given at one time.
- Give dose between meals to facilitate complete absorption.
- Dose modification may be needed in patients with renal or hepatic dysfunction.
- Avoid all I.M. injections when platelet count is less than 100,000/mm³.
- Signs and symptoms of overdose include myelosuppression, nausea, vomiting, malaise, hypertension, and diaphoresis. Treatment is usually supportive and includes transfusion of blood components and antiemetics. Induction of emesis may be helpful if performed soon after ingestion.

Monitoring the patient
- Monitor serum uric acid levels. Use oral hydration to prevent uric acid nephropathy. Alkalinize urine if serum uric acid levels are elevated.

- Monitor liver function tests. Stop drug if hepatotoxicity or hepatic tenderness occurs. Watch for jaundice, which may reverse if drug is stopped promptly.
- Conduct CBC daily during induction, then weekly during maintenance therapy.

Information for the patient
- Emphasize importance of continuing drug despite occurrence of nausea and vomiting.
- Tell patient to report promptly if vomiting occurs shortly after a dose is taken.
- Advise avoiding exposure to people with infections and tell patient to call immediately if signs of infection or unusual bleeding occur.
- Encourage adequate fluid intake to increase urine output and facilitate excretion of uric acid.
- Advise patient to use reliable contraceptive measures during therapy.

Breast-feeding patients
- It's unknown if drug appears in breast milk. Because of risk of serious adverse reactions, mutagenicity, and carcinogenicity in infant, breast-feeding isn't recommended.

thiopental sodium
Pentothal

Pharmacologic classification: barbiturate
Therapeutic classification: anesthetic
Controlled substance schedule III
Pregnancy risk category C

How supplied
Available by prescription only
Powder for injection: 2% (20 mg/ml): 1-g, 2.5-g, 5-g kits; 400-mg min-I-mix; 400-mg ready to mix syringe
2.5% (25 mg/ml): 500-mg, 1-g, 2.5-g, 5-g, 10-g kits; 250-mg, 500-mg min-I-mix; 250-mg, 500-mg ready to mix syringes

Indications, route, and dosage
General anesthetic for short-term procedures
Adults and children: 2 to 3 ml 2.5% solution (50 to 75 mg) administered I.V. for induction and repeated as a maintenance dose; however, dose is individualized.
Convulsive states after anesthesia
Adults: 75 to 125 mg (2 to 5 ml 2.5% solution) I.V.

Pharmacodynamics
Anesthetic action: Produces anesthesia by direct depression of the polysynaptic midbrain reticular activating system. Thiopental decreases presynaptic (via decreased neurotransmitter release) and postsynaptic excitation. These effects may be subsequent to increased gamma-aminobutyric acid (GABA) levels, enhanceme

of GABA effects, or a direct effect on GABA receptor sites.

Pharmacokinetics
- *Absorption:* I.V. produces peak brain levels in 10 to 20 seconds. Depth of anesthesia may increase for up to 40 seconds. Consciousness returns in 20 to 30 minutes.
- *Distribution:* Distributed throughout body; highest initial level occurs in vascular areas of brain, primarily gray matter; drug is 80% protein-bound. Redistribution primarily responsible for short duration of action.
- *Metabolism:* Metabolized extensively but slowly in liver.
- *Excretion:* Unchanged drug not excreted in significant amounts; duration of action depends on tissue redistribution.

Contraindications and precautions
Contraindicated in patients with hypersensitivity to drug, in those with acute intermittent or variegate porphyria but not other porphyrias, and whenever general anesthesia is contraindicated.

Use with extreme caution in status asthmaticus and use cautiously in patients with respiratory, cardiac, circulatory, renal, or hepatic dysfunction; severe anemia; shock; or myxedema because drug may worsen these conditions. Also use cautiously in patients with hypotension, Addison's disease, myasthenia gravis, or increased intracranial pressure and in breast-feeding women.

Interactions
Drug-drug. *Antihistamines, benzodiazepines, hypnotics, narcotics, phenothiazines, sedatives:* Increased CNS depressant effects. Avoid concomitant use.
Drug-lifestyle. *Alcohol:* Increased CNS depressant effects. Discourage use.

Adverse reactions
CNS: anxiety, restlessness, retrograde amnesia, prolonged somnolence, dose-dependent alteration in EEG patterns.
CV: thrombophlebitis, hypotension, tachycardia, peripheral vascular collapse, *myocardial depression, arrhythmias.*
GI: nausea and vomiting, abdominal pain; diarrhea, cramping.
Respiratory: coughing, sneezing, hiccups, *respiratory depression, apnea, laryngospasm, bronchospasm.*
Other: pain, swelling, ulceration, necrosis on extravasation (unlikely at levels less than 2.5%), gangrene after intra-arterial injection, *allergic reactions,* shivering, local irritation.
Note: Drug should be stopped if peripheral vascular collapse, respiratory arrest, or hypersensitivity occurs.

☑ Special considerations
- Solutions of succinylcholine, tubocurarine, or atropine shouldn't be mixed with thiopental but can be given to patient concomitantly.
- A small test dose (25 to 75 mg) may be administered to assess tolerance or unusual sensitivity.
- Signs and symptoms of overdose include respiratory depression, respiratory arrest, hypotension, and shock. Treat supportively, using mechanical ventilation, if needed; give I.V. fluids or vasopressors (dopamine, phenylephrine) for hypotension. Monitor vital signs closely.

Monitoring the patient
- Monitor patient for cardiac and respiratory reactions.

Information for the patient
- Inform patient of possible adverse reactions.

Geriatric patients
- Lower dosages may be indicated in elderly patients.

Pediatric patients
- Use cautiously in children.

---

thioridazine
Mellaril-S

thioridazine hydrochloride
Apo-Thioridazine*, Mellaril, Novo-Ridazine*, PMS Thioridazine*

Pharmacologic classification: phenothiazine (piperidine derivative)
Therapeutic classification: antipsychotic
Pregnancy risk category C

How supplied
Available by prescription only
Tablets: 10 mg, 15 mg, 25 mg, 50 mg, 100 mg, 150 mg, 200 mg
Oral concentrate: 30 mg/ml, 100 mg/ml (3% to 4.2% alcohol)
Suspension: 25 mg/5 ml, 100 mg/5 ml

Indications, route, and dosage
Psychosis
Adults: Initially, 50 to 100 mg P.O. t.i.d., with gradual increments up to 800 mg daily in divided doses, if needed. Dosage varies.
Dysthymic disorder (neurotic depression), dementia in elderly patients, behavioral problems in children
Adults: Initially, 25 mg P.O. t.i.d. Maintenance dose is 20 to 200 mg daily.
Children over age 2: Usually, 0.5 to 3 mg/kg/day P.O. in divided doses. Give 10 mg b.i.d. or t.i.d. to

---

children with moderate disorders and 25 mg b.i.d. or t.i.d. to hospitalized children.

Pharmacodynamics

Antipsychotic action: Thought to exert antipsychotic effects by postsynaptic blockade of CNS dopamine receptors, thereby inhibiting dopamine-mediated effects.

Has many other central and peripheral effects: Produces both alpha and ganglionic blockade and counteracts histamine- and serotonin-mediated activity. Most prevalent adverse reactions are antimuscarinic and sedative; drug causes fewer extrapyramidal effects than other antipsychotics.

Pharmacokinetics

• *Absorption:* Rate and extent of absorption vary with route. Oral tablet absorption erratic and variable; onset ranging from ½ to 1 hour. Oral concentrates and suspensions much more predictable.

• *Distribution:* Distributed widely into body, including breast milk. Effects peak in 2 to 4 hours; steady-state serum level within 4 to 7 days. 91% to 99% protein-bound.

• *Metabolism:* Metabolized extensively by liver; forms active metabolite mesoridazine; duration of action is 4 to 6 hours.

• *Excretion:* Mostly excreted as metabolites in urine; some excreted in feces via biliary tract.

Contraindications and precautions

Contraindicated in patients with hypersensitivity to drug and in those experiencing coma, CNS depression, or severe hypertensive or hypotensive cardiac disease.

Use cautiously in elderly or debilitated patients and in those with hepatic or CV disease, respiratory or seizure disorders, hypocalcemia, or severe reactions to insulin or electroconvulsive therapy, and in those who have been exposed to extreme cold or heat or organophosphate insecticides.

Interactions

Drug-drug. *Antacids containing aluminum and magnesium; antidiarrheals:* Decreased absorption; decreased therapeutic response to drug. Avoid concomitant use.

Antiarrhythmics (such as disopyramide, procainamide, quinidine): Increased risk of arrhythmias and conduction defects. Monitor patient closely; perform periodic ECG testing.

Appetite suppressants, sympathomimetics (such as ephedrine [commonly found in nasal sprays], epinephrine, phenylephrine, phenylpropanolamine): Decreased stimulatory and pressor effects. Monitor patient closely; check blood pressure regularly.

Atropine, other anticholinergics (such as antidepressants, antihistamines, antiparkinsonians, *MAO inhibitors, meperidine, phenothiazines):* Oversedation, paralytic ileus, visual changes, and severe constipation. Monitor patient closely.

Beta blockers: Increased thioridazine plasma levels and toxicity. Use together cautiously.

Bromocriptine: Antagonized effect on prolactin secretion. Use together cautiously.

Centrally acting antihypertensives (such as clonidine, guanabenz, guanadrel, guanethidine, methyldopa, reserpine): Inhibited therapeutic effect of these drugs. Monitor patient closely.

CNS depressants (such as analgesics, anesthetics [epidural, general, spinal], barbiturates, narcotics, parenteral magnesium sulfate, tranquilizers): Oversedation, respiratory depression, hypotension. Additive CNS effect. Avoid concomitant use.

Epinephrine: Epinephrine reversal. Avoid concomitant use.

High-dose dopamine: Decreased vasoconstriction. Monitor patient closely.

Levodopa: Decreased effectiveness; increased toxicity of levodopa. Avoid concomitant use.

Lithium: Severe neurologic toxicity with an encephalitis-like syndrome; decreased therapeutic response to thioridazine. Don't use together.

Metrizamide: Increased risk of seizures. Use together cautiously.

Nitrates: Possible hypotension. Monitor blood pressure.

Phenobarbital: Enhanced renal excretion; decreased therapeutic response to drug. Avoid concomitant use.

Phenytoin: Phenytoin toxicity. Don't use concomitantly.

Propylthiouracil: Increased risk of agranulocytosis. Avoid concomitant use.

Drug-food. *Caffeine:* Increased drug metabolism. Monitor patient for dosage adjustment.

Drug-lifestyle. *Alcohol:* Increased CNS depression. Avoid concomitant use.

Heavy smoking: Increased drug metabolism. Monitor patient for dosage adjustment.

Sun exposure: Photosensitivity reactions. Tell patient to take precautions.

Adverse reactions

CNS: extrapyramidal reactions (low incidence), *tardive dyskinesia, sedation* (high incidence), EEG changes, dizziness.

CV: *orthostatic hypotension,* tachycardia, ECG changes.

EENT: *ocular changes, blurred vision,* retinitis pigmentosa.

GI: *dry mouth, constipation,* increased appetite.

GU: *urine retention,* dark urine, menstrual irregularities, gynecomastia, inhibited ejaculation.

Hematologic: *transient leukopenia, **agranulocytosis,*** hyperprolactinemia.

Hepatic: cholestatic jaundice, elevated liver enzyme levels.

Metabolic: weight gain.
Skin: *mild photosensitivity,* allergic reactions.
    After abrupt withdrawal of long-term therapy: gastritis, nausea, vomiting, dizziness, tremor, feeling of warmth or cold, diaphoresis, tachycardia, headache, and insomnia.

☑ Special considerations
Besides the recommendations relevant to all phenothiazines, consider the following.
• Doses above 300 mg/day are usually reserved for adults with severe psychosis. Don't exceed 800 mg daily because of ophthalmic toxicity.
• Liquid formulations may cause a rash if skin contact occurs.
• Drug can cause pink to brown discoloration of patient's urine.
• Thioridazine is associated with a high risk of sedation, anticholinergic effects, orthostatic hypotension, photosensitivity reactions, and delayed or absent ejaculation. It has the lowest potential for extrapyramidal reactions of all phenothiazines.
• Oral formulations may cause stomach upset; give with food or fluid.
• Concentrate must be diluted in 2 to 4 oz (60 to 120 ml) of liquid, preferably water, carbonated drinks, fruit juice, tomato juice, milk, or pudding.
• All liquid formulations must be protected from light.
• Thioridazine causes false-positive test results for urinary porphyrins, urobilinogen, amylase, and 5-hydroxyindoleacetic acid because of darkening of urine by metabolites; also causes false-positive urine pregnancy results in tests using human chorionic gonadotropin as the indicator.
• CNS depression is characterized by deep, unarousable sleep and possible coma, hypotension or hypertension, extrapyramidal symptoms, abnormal involuntary muscle movements, agitation, seizures, arrhythmias, ECG changes, hypothermia or hyperthermia, and autonomic nervous system dysfunction.
• Treatment of CNS depression is symptomatic and supportive and includes maintaining vital signs, airway, stable body temperature, and fluid and electrolyte balance.
• Don't induce vomiting. Drug inhibits cough reflex, and aspiration may occur. Use gastric lavage, then activated charcoal and sodium chloride cathartics; dialysis doesn't help. Regulate body temperature as needed. Treat hypotension with I.V. fluids. Don't give epinephrine. Treat seizures with parenteral diazepam or barbiturates; arrhythmias with parenteral phenytoin (1 mg/kg with rate adjusted to blood pressure); and extrapyramidal reactions with benztropine at 1 to 2 mg or parenteral diphenhydramine at 10 to 50 mg. Contact local or regional poison information center for specific instructions.

Monitoring the patient
• Check patient regularly (at least once every 6 months) for abnormal body movements.
• Monitor therapeutic effect.

Information for the patient
• Explain risks of dystonic reactions and tardive dyskinesia, and tell patient to report abnormal body movements.
• Tell patient to avoid sun exposure and to wear sunscreen when going outdoors to prevent photosensitivity reactions. (Heat lamps and tanning beds also may cause skin burning or discoloration.)
• Warn patient not to spill liquid on skin; rash and irritation may result.
• Warn patient to avoid extremely hot or cold baths or exposure to temperature extremes, sunlamps, or tanning beds; drug may cause thermoregulatory changes.
• Advise patient to take drug exactly as prescribed and not to double missed doses.
• Explain that many drug interactions are possible.
• Tell patient not to stop taking drug suddenly; most adverse reactions may be relieved by dosage reduction. However, patient should call promptly if he experiences difficulty urinating, sore throat, dizziness, or fainting, or if visual changes develop.
• Warn patient to avoid hazardous activities that require alertness until effect of drug is established. Reassure patient that excessive sedation usually subsides after several weeks.
• Advise patient to maintain adequate hydration.
• Explain which fluids are appropriate for diluting concentrate and the dropper technique of measuring dose.

Geriatric patients
• Elderly patients tend to need lower doses, adjusted to individual response. Such patients also are more likely to experience adverse reactions, especially tardive dyskinesia and other extrapyramidal effects.

Pediatric patients
• Drug isn't recommended for children under age 2. For children over age 2, dose is 1 mg/kg/day in divided doses.

Breast-feeding patients
• Drug may appear in breast milk. Potential benefits to mother should outweigh potential harm to infant.

thiotepa
Thioplex

Pharmacologic classification: alkylating drug (cell cycle–phase nonspecific)
Therapeutic classification: antineoplastic
Pregnancy risk category D

How supplied
Available by prescription only
Injection: 15-mg vials

Indications, route, and dosage
Dosage and indications may vary. Check current literature for recommended protocol.
Breast and ovarian cancer, Hodgkin's disease, lymphomas
Adults and adolescents ages 12 and over: 0.2 mg/kg I.V. daily for 4 to 5 days, repeated q 2 to 4 weeks; or 0.3 to 0.4 mg/kg I.V. q 1 to 4 weeks.
Bladder tumor
Adults and adolescents ages 12 and over: 60 mg in 30 to 60 ml of normal saline solution (thiotepa in distilled water) instilled in bladder once weekly for 4 weeks.
Neoplastic effusions
Adults and adolescents ages 12 and over: 0.6 to 0.8 mg/kg intracavity or intratumor q 1 to 4 weeks.
◊ **Malignant meningeal neoplasm**
Adults: 1 to 10 mg/m² intrathecally, once to twice weekly.

Pharmacodynamics
Antineoplastic action: Exerts cytotoxic activity as an alkylating drug, cross-linking strands of DNA and RNA and inhibiting protein synthesis, resulting in cell death.

Pharmacokinetics
• *Absorption:* Incompletely absorbed across GI tract; absorption from bladder variable, ranging from 10% to 100% of instilled dose. Absorption increased by certain pathologic conditions. I.M. and pleural membrane absorption of thiotepa also variable.
• *Distribution:* Not known if drug or metabolites distributed into breast milk.
• *Metabolism:* Metabolized extensively in liver.
• *Excretion:* Drug and metabolites excreted in urine. Half-life is 2.4 hours.

Contraindications and precautions
Contraindicated in patients with hypersensitivity to drug and in those with severe bone marrow, hepatic, or renal dysfunction. Use cautiously in patients with impaired renal or hepatic function or bone marrow suppression.

Interactions
Drug-drug. *Pancuronium:* Prolonged effect. Monitor patient closely.

Pseudocholinesterase: Impaired activity of enzyme. Monitor patient closely.
Succinylcholine: Prolonged respirations and apnea. Don't use together.

Adverse reactions
CNS: headache, dizziness, blurred vision, fatigue, weakness.
EENT: *laryngeal edema,* conjunctivitis.
GI: *nausea, vomiting,* abdominal pain, anorexia.
GU: amenorrhea, decreased spermatogenesis, dysuria, urine retention, hemorrhagic cystitis.
Hematologic: *leukopenia* (begins within 5 to 30 days), *thrombocytopenia, neutropenia, anemia.*
Metabolic: hyperuricemia, decreased plasma pseudocholinesterase levels.
Respiratory: asthma.
Skin: hives, rash, dermatitis, alopecia.
Other: fever, hypersensitivity, *anaphylactic shock.*

☑ Special considerations
• Drug can be given by all parenteral routes, including direct injection into tumor.
• Stop drug or decrease dose if WBC count is below 4,000/mm³ or if platelet count is below 150,000/mm³.
• Drug may be mixed with procaine 2% or epinephrine 1:1,000, or both, for local use.
• Drug may be further diluted to larger volumes with normal saline solution, D_5W, or lactated Ringer's solution for administration by I.V. infusion, intracavitary injection, or perfusion therapy.
• Withhold fluids for 8 to 10 hours before bladder instillation. Instill 60 ml of drug into bladder by catheter; ask patient to retain solution for 2 hours. Volume may be reduced to 30 ml if discomfort is too great. Reposition patient every 15 minutes for maximum area contact.
• To prevent hyperuricemia with resulting uric acid nephropathy, allopurinol may be given; keep patient well hydrated.
• Avoid all I.M. injections when platelet count is less than 100,000/mm³.
• Use anticoagulants and aspirin products cautiously. Watch closely for signs of bleeding.
• Toxicity may be delayed and prolonged because drug binds to tissues and stays in body several hours.
• Signs and symptoms of overdose include nausea, vomiting, and precipitation of uric acid in renal tubules. Treatment is usually supportive and includes transfusion of blood components, antiemetics, hydration, and allopurinol.

Monitoring the patient
• Monitor uric acid.
• Monitor CBC weekly for at least 3 weeks after last dose.

Information for the patient
● Encourage patient to maintain an adequate fluid intake to facilitate uric acid excretion.
● Advise patient to avoid OTC products containing aspirin.
● Tell patient to avoid exposure to infections and to immediately report if infection occurs.
● Advise patient that hair should grow back after therapy has ended.
● Tell patient to report sore throat, fever, or unusual bruising or bleeding.
● Advise patient to use effective contraceptive measures; if pregnancy occurs, tell her to call immediately.

Breast-feeding patients
● It's unknown if drug appears in breast milk. Because of risk of serious adverse reactions, mutagenicity, and carcinogenicity in infant, breast-feeding isn't recommended.

---

thiothixene

thiothixene hydrochloride
Navane

Pharmacologic classification: thioxanthene
Therapeutic classification: antipsychotic
Pregnancy risk category C

How supplied
Available by prescription only
Capsules: 1 mg, 2 mg, 5 mg, 10 mg, 20 mg
Oral concentrate: 5 mg/ml (7% alcohol)

Indications, route, and dosage
Mild to moderate psychosis
Adults: Initially, 2 mg P.O. t.i.d.; may increase gradually to 15 mg daily.
Severe psychosis
Adults: Initially, 5 mg P.O. b.i.d.; may increase gradually to 20 to 30 mg daily. Maximum recommended daily dose is 60 mg.

Pharmacodynamics
Antipsychotic action: Thought to exert antipsychotic effects by postsynaptic blockade of CNS dopamine receptors, thereby inhibiting dopamine-mediated effects. Has many other central and peripheral effects; also acts as an alpha blocker. Most prominent adverse reactions are extrapyramidal.

Pharmacokinetics
● *Absorption:* Rapidly absorbed; I.M. onset of action 10 to 30 minutes.
● *Distribution:* Widely distributed into body. Effects peak 1 to 6 hours after I.M. administration; 91% to 99% protein-bound.
● *Metabolism:* Metabolized in liver.

● *Excretion:* Mostly excreted as parent drug in feces via biliary tract.

Contraindications and precautions
Contraindicated in patients with hypersensitivity to drug and in those experiencing circulatory collapse, coma, CNS depression, or blood dyscrasia. Use cautiously in elderly or debilitated patients; in those with history of seizure disorders, CV disease, heat exposure, glaucoma, or prostatic hyperplasia; and in those in a state of alcohol withdrawal.

Interactions
Drug-drug. *Antacids containing aluminum and magnesium, antidiarrheals:* Decreased absorption; decreased therapeutic response. Avoid concomitant use.
Antiarrhythmics (such as disopyramide, procainamide, quinidine): Increased cardiac arrhythmias and conduction defects. Monitor ECG periodically.
Appetite suppressants, sympathomimetics (such as ephedrine [commonly found in nasal sprays], epinephrine, phenylephrine, phenylpropanolamine): Decreased stimulatory and pressor effects. Adjust dosage.
Atropine, other anticholinergics (such as antidepressants, antihistamines, antiparkinsonians, MAO inhibitors, meperidine, phenothiazines): Oversedation, paralytic ileus, visual changes, and severe constipation. Monitor patient closely.
Beta blockers: Inhibited thiothixene metabolism, increasing plasma levels and toxicity. Use together with caution.
Bromocriptine: Antagonized effect on prolactin secretion. Monitor patient closely.
Centrally acting antihypertensives (such as clonidine, guanabenz, guanadrel, guanethidine, methyldopa, reserpine): Inhibited blood pressure response. Monitor patient closely.
CNS depressants (such as analgesics, anesthetics [epidural, general, spinal], barbiturates, narcotics, parenteral magnesium sulfate, tranquilizers): Oversedation, respiratory depression, and hypotension. Monitor patient closely.
Epinephrine: Epinephrine reversal. Avoid concomitant use. Monitor patient closely when concomitant use is necessary.
High-dose dopamine: Decreased effectiveness of dopamine. Monitor patient closely.
Levodopa: Decreased effectiveness and increased levodopa toxicity. Use together with caution.
Lithium: Severe neurologic toxicity with an encephalitis-like syndrome; decreased therapeutic response to thiothixene. Monitor patient closely.
Metrizamide: Increased risk of seizures. Use together cautiously.
Nitrates: Hypotension may occur. Monitor blood pressure regularly.

Phenobarbital: Enhanced renal excretion. Avoid concomitant use.

Phenytoin: Phenytoin toxicity. Avoid concomitant use.

Propylthiouracil: Increased risk of agranulocytosis. Avoid concomitant use.

Drug-herb. *Nutmeg:* Loss of symptom control. Avoid concomitant use.

Drug-food. *Caffeine:* Increased drug metabolism. Adjust dosage. Limit concomitant use.

Drug-lifestyle. *Alcohol:* Increased CNS depression. Discourage use.

Heavy smoking: Increased drug metabolism. Adjust dosage. Limit concomitant use.

Sun exposure: Photosensitivity reactions. Tell patient to take precautions.

Adverse reactions

CNS: *extrapyramidal reactions,* drowsiness, restlessness, agitation, insomnia, *tardive dyskinesia,* sedation, pseudoparkinsonism, EEG changes, dizziness.

CV: *hypotension,* tachycardia, ECG changes.

EENT: ocular changes, *blurred vision,* nasal congestion.

GI: *dry mouth, constipation.*

GU: *urine retention,* menstrual irregularities, gynecomastia, inhibited ejaculation.

Hematologic: *transient leukopenia,* leukocytosis, ***agranulocytosis.***

Hepatic: jaundice, elevated liver enzyme levels.

Metabolic: weight gain.

Skin: *mild photosensitivity,* allergic reactions, pain at I.M. injection site, sterile abscess.

Other: *neuroleptic malignant syndrome.*

After abrupt withdrawal of long-term therapy: gastritis, nausea, vomiting, dizziness, tremor, feeling of warmth or cold, diaphoresis, tachycardia, headache, insomnia.

☑ Special considerations

● Liquid and injectable formulations may cause a rash if skin contact occurs.

● Drug is associated with a high risk of extrapyramidal effects.

● Because stomach upset may occur, give drug with food or fluid.

● Dilute concentrate in 2 to 4 oz (60 to 120 ml) of liquid, preferably water, carbonated drinks, fruit juice, tomato juice, milk, or pudding.

● Photosensitivity reactions may occur; patient should avoid exposure to sunlight or heat lamps.

● Drug causes false-positive test results for urinary porphyrins, urobilinogen, amylase, and 5-hydroxyindoleacetic acid because of darkening of urine by metabolites; also causes false-positive urine pregnancy results in tests using human chorionic gonadotropin as the indicator.

● CNS depression is characterized by deep, unarousable sleep and possible coma, hypotension or hypertension, extrapyramidal symptoms, abnormal involuntary muscle movements, agitation, seizures, arrhythmias, ECG changes, hypothermia or hyperthermia, and autonomic nervous system dysfunction.

● Treatment of CNS depression is symptomatic and supportive and includes maintaining vital signs, airway, stable body temperature, and fluid and electrolyte balance.

● Don't induce vomiting. Drug inhibits cough reflex, and aspiration may occur. Use gastric lavage, then activated charcoal and sodium chloride cathartics; dialysis doesn't help. Regulate body temperature as needed. Treat hypotension with I.V. fluids. Don't give epinephrine. Seizures may be treated with parenteral diazepam or barbiturates, arrhythmias with parenteral phenytoin (1 mg/kg with rate titrated to blood pressure), and extrapyramidal reactions with benztropine at 1 to 2 mg or parenteral diphenhydramine at 10 to 50 mg.

Monitoring the patient

● Monitor blood pressure before and after parenteral administration.

● Check patient regularly (at least once every 6 months) for abnormal body movements.

Information for the patient

● Explain risks of dystonic reactions and tardive dyskinesia, and tell patient to report abnormal body movements.

● Tell patient to avoid sun exposure and to wear sunscreen when going outdoors to prevent photosensitivity reactions. (Heat lamps and tanning beds also may cause skin burning or discoloration.)

● Advise patient not to spill liquid on skin. Contact with skin may cause rash and irritation.

● Warn patient to avoid extremely hot or cold baths or exposure to temperature extremes, sunlamps, or tanning beds; drug may cause thermoregulatory changes.

● Tell patient to take drug exactly as prescribed, not to double missed doses, and not to share drug with others.

● Explain that many drug interactions are possible. Tell patient to call before taking any self-prescribed drug.

● Tell patient not to stop taking drug suddenly; most adverse reactions may be relieved by reducing dosage. However, patient should call if he experiences difficulty urinating, sore throat, dizziness, or fainting.

● Warn patient against hazardous activities that require alertness until effect of drug is established. Reassure patient that sedation usually subsides after several weeks.

● Tell patient not to drink alcohol or take other drugs that may cause excessive sedation.

● Explain which fluids are appropriate for diluting concentrate and the dropper technique of measuring dose.

• Recommend sugarless hard candy, chewing gum, or ice to alleviate dry mouth.
• Tell patient to shake concentrate before administration.

Geriatric patients
• Elderly patients tend to need lower doses, adjusted to individual response. Adverse reactions, especially tardive dyskinesia and other extrapyramidal effects, are more likely to develop in this age-group.

Pediatric patients
• Drug isn't recommended for children under age 12.

---

thrombin
Thrombinar, Thrombin-JMI, Thrombogen, Thrombostat

Pharmacologic classification: enzyme
Therapeutic classification: topical hemostatic
Pregnancy risk category C

How supplied
Available by prescription only
Powder: 1,000-, 5,000-, 10,000-, 20,000-, and 50,000-unit vials
Kit: 5,000, 10,000, 20,000 units with sprayer assembly

Indications, route, and dosage
Bleeding from parenchyma, cancellous bone, dental sockets, during nasal and laryngeal surgery, and in plastic surgery and skin-grafting procedures
Adults: Apply 100 units/ml of sterile isotonic saline solution or sterile distilled water to area where clotting is needed (or apply dry powder in bone surgery); in major bleeding, apply 1,000 to 2,000 units/ml sterile isotonic saline solution. Sponge blood from area before application, but avoid sponging area after application.

Pharmacodynamics
Hemostatic action: Catalyzes the conversion of fibrinogen to fibrin, one of the last stages of clot formation.

Pharmacokinetics
Not applicable.

Contraindications and precautions
Contraindicated in patients with hypersensitivity to thrombin or to bovine products. Don't inject thrombin or allow it to enter large blood vessels; death may result from severe intravascular clotting.

Interactions
None reported.

Adverse reactions
CV: *intravascular clotting* (could cause death if thrombin enters large vessels).
Other: hypersensitivity, fever.

☑ Special considerations
• Thrombostat can be stored at room temperature (59° to 86° F [15° to 30° C]). Thrombinar and Thrombin-JMI must be refrigerated at 36° to 46° F (2° to 8° C). Thrombogen must be used immediately upon reconstitution. If necessary, it can be refrigerated at 36° to 46° F for up to 3 hours. Thrombin may be used with absorbable gelatin sponge, but not oxidized cellulose; check label before using.
• Obtain patient history of reactions to thrombin or bovine products.
• Contents of a 5,000-unit vial dissolved in 5 ml saline solution are capable of clotting an equal volume of blood in less than 1 second, or 1,000 ml in less than 1 minute.

Monitoring the patient
• Observe patient for hypersensitivity reaction after administering.

Information for the patient
• Advise patient taking drug for GI hemorrhage to drink all prescribed milk and milk-thrombin solution.

Pediatric patients
• Safety in children hasn't been established.

---

thyroid, desiccated
Armour Thyroid, S-P-T

Pharmacologic classification: thyroid hormone
Therapeutic classification: thyroid drug
Pregnancy risk category A

How supplied
Available by prescription only
Tablets: 15 mg, 30 mg, 60 mg, 90 mg, 120 mg, 180 mg, 240 mg, 300 mg (Armour Thyroid)
Tablets (bovine): 30 mg, 60 mg, 120 mg (Thyrar)
Tablets (enteric-coated): 30mg, 60 mg, 120 mg, 180 mg
Capsules (pork): 60 mg, 120 mg, 180 mg, 300 mg (S-P-T, suspended in soybean oil)

Indications, route, and dosage
Adult hypothyroidism
Adults: Initially, 30 mg P.O. daily, increased by 15 mg q 14 to 30 days depending on disease severity until desired response is achieved. Usual main-

---

tenance dose is 60 to 180 mg P.O. daily as a single dose.

Congenital hypothyroidism
Children over age 12: Dose may approach adult dose (60 to 180 mg daily), depending on response.
Children ages 6 to 12: 60 to 90 mg P.O. daily.
Children ages 1 to 5: 45 to 60 mg P.O. daily.
Infants ages 6 to 12 months: 30 to 45 mg P.O. daily.
Neonates and infants ages 0 to 6 months: 15 to 30 mg P.O. daily.

Pharmacodynamics
Thyrotropic action: Affects protein and carbohydrate metabolism, promotes gluconeogenesis, increases the utilization and mobilization of glycogen stores, stimulates protein synthesis, and regulates cell growth and differentiation. The major effect of thyroid is to increase the metabolic rate of tissue.

Pharmacokinetics
● *Absorption:* Thyroid USP absorbed from GI tract.
● *Distribution:* Not fully understood. Highly protein-bound.
● *Metabolism:* Not fully understood.
● *Excretion:* Not fully understood.

Contraindications and precautions
Contraindicated in patients with hypersensitivity to drug and in those with acute MI uncomplicated by hypothyroidism, untreated thyrotoxicosis, or uncorrected adrenal insufficiency. Use cautiously in elderly patients and in patients with angina pectoris, hypertension, other CV disorders, renal insufficiency, or ischemia.

Interactions
Drug-drug. *Adrenocorticoids, corticotropin:* Changes in thyroid status. Dosage adjustments may be needed.
Anticoagulants: Altered anticoagulant effect. Reduced anticoagulant dosage may be needed.
Cholestyramine, colestipol: Decreased absorption. Monitor patient closely; adjust dosage.
Estrogens: Increased thyroid requirements. Adjust dosage.
Insulin, oral antidiabetics: May affect dosage requirements of these drugs. Monitor glucose levels; adjust dosage as needed.
I.V. phenytoin: May release free thyroid from thyroglobulin. Monitor patient closely; adjust dosage.
Somatrem: Accelerated epiphyseal maturation. Use together cautiously.
Sympathomimetics, tricyclic antidepressants: Increased effects of these drugs or of thyroid (desiccated); possible coronary insufficiency or cardiac arrhythmias. Monitor patient closely; adjust dosage.

Adverse reactions
CNS: *nervousness, insomnia,* tremor, headache.
CV: tachycardia, **arrhythmias, cardiac decompensation and collapse,** angina pectoris.
GI: diarrhea, vomiting.
GU: menstrual irregularities.
Metabolic: weight loss, heat intolerance.
Musculoskeletal: accelerated rate of bone maturation in infants and children.
Skin: allergic skin reactions, diaphoresis.

☑ Special considerations
Besides the recommendations relevant to all thyroid hormones, consider the following.
● Levothyroxine is considered drug of choice for thyroid hormone supplementation.
● Commercial preparations may have variable hormonal content and produce fluctuating liothyronine and levothyroxine levels. Because of this variability, the use of thyroid has decreased considerably.
● Enteric-coated tablets give unreliable absorption.
● Thyroid USP therapy alters ^{131}I thyroid uptake, protein-bound iodine levels, and liothyronine uptake.
● Evidence of overdose includes signs and symptoms of hyperthyroidism (weight loss, increased appetite, palpitations, nervousness, diarrhea, abdominal cramps, sweating, tachycardia, increased pulse and blood pressure, angina, cardiac arrhythmias, tremor, headache, insomnia, heat intolerance, fever, and menstrual irregularities).
● Treatment of acute overdose requires reduction of GI absorption and efforts to counteract central and peripheral effects, primarily sympathetic activity. Use gastric lavage or induce emesis (then activated charcoal, if less than 4 hours after ingestion). If patient is comatose or is having seizures, inflate cuff on endotracheal tube to prevent aspiration.
● Treatment of overdose may include oxygen and artificial ventilation to support respiration. It also should include appropriate measures to treat heart failure and control fever, hypoglycemia, and fluid loss.
● Propranolol may be used to combat many of the effects of increased sympathetic activity. Thyroid USP therapy should be withdrawn gradually over 2 to 6 days, then resumed at a lower dose.

Monitoring the patient
● Monitor patient's pulse rate and blood pressure. Thyroid may cause CV adverse effects.
● Digoxin levels should be monitored closely as patient becomes euthyroid.
● In children, sleeping pulse rate and basal morning temperature are guides to treatment.

Information for the patient
• Encourage patient to take daily dose at same time each day, preferably in morning to avoid insomnia.
• Advise patient to call if headache, diarrhea, nervousness, excessive sweating, heat intolerance, chest pain, increased pulse rate, or palpitations occur.
• Tell patient not to store drug in warm, humid areas such as bathroom to prevent deterioration.
• Warn patient not to switch brands or dose.

Geriatric patients
• Elderly patients are more sensitive to thyroid effects. In patients over age 60, initial dose should be 25% lower than usual recommended dose.

Pediatric patients
• Partial hair loss may occur during the first few months of therapy. Reassure child and parents that this is temporary.

Breast-feeding patients
• Minimal amounts of drug appear in breast milk. Use with caution in breast-feeding women.

---

thyrotropin (thyroid stimulating hormone, TSH)
Thytropar

Pharmacologic classification: anterior pituitary hormone
Therapeutic classification: thyrotropic hormone
Pregnancy risk category C

How supplied
Available by prescription only
Powder for injection: 10 IU/vial

Indications, route, and dosage
Diagnosis of thyroid cancer remnant with 131I *after surgery*
Adults and children: 10 IU I.M. or S.C. for 3 to 7 days.
Differential diagnosis of primary and secondary hypothyroidism
Adults and children: 10 IU I.M. or S.C. for 1 to 3 days.
In protein-bound iodine or 131I *uptake determinations for differential diagnosis of subclinical hypothyroidism or low thyroid reserve*
Adults and children: 10 IU I.M. or S.C.
Therapy for thyroid carcinoma (local or metastatic) with 131I
Adults and children: 10 IU I.M. or S.C. for 3 to 8 days.
To determine thyroid status of patient receiving thyroid
Adults and children: 10 IU I.M. or S.C. for 1 to 3 days.

Pharmacodynamics
Thyrotropic action: Produces increased uptake of iodine by the thyroid and increased formation and release of thyroid hormone.

Pharmacokinetics
• *Absorption:* Onset occurs within minutes after injection.
• *Distribution:* Concentrated primarily in thyroid gland.
• *Metabolism:* Not fully understood.
• *Excretion:* Excreted rapidly in urine.

Contraindications and precautions
Contraindicated in patients with hypersensitivity to drug and in those with coronary thrombosis or untreated Addison's disease. Use cautiously in patients with angina pectoris, heart failure, hypopituitarism, or adrenocortical suppression.

Interactions
None reported.

Adverse reactions
CNS: headache, fever.
CV: *tachycardia,* hypotension.
GI: nausea, vomiting.
Other: thyroid hyperplasia (with large doses), hypersensitivity reactions (postinjection flare, urticaria, ANAPHYLAXIS).

☑ Special considerations
Besides the recommendations relevant to all thyroid hormones, consider the following.
• Thyrotropin may cause thyroid hyperplasia.
• Three-day dose schedule may be used in longstanding pituitary myxedema or with prolonged use of thyroid medication.
• Thyrotropin therapy alters 131I thyroid uptake.
• Signs and symptoms of overdose include headache, irritability, nervousness, sweating, tachycardia, increased GI motility, and menstrual irregularities. Angina or heart failure may be aggravated. Shock may develop. Treatment includes administering propranolol (or another beta blocker) to treat adrenergic effects of hyperthyroidism. Adult dosage of propranolol is 1 mg over at least 1 minute, repeated every 2 to 5 minutes (maximum, 5 mg). Dosage in children is 0.01 to 0.1 mg/kg over 10 minutes (maximum, 1 mg). Monitor blood pressure and cardiac function.
• Exchange transfusions may be useful in acute overdose. Diuresis and dialysis are ineffective.

Monitoring the patient
• Monitor therapeutic effect.
• Monitor patient for symptoms of hypersensitivity.

Information for the patient
• Warn patient to report the following reactions: itching, redness, or swelling at injection site; rash;

---

tightness of throat or wheezing; chest pain; irritability; nervousness; rapid heartbeat; shortness of breath; or unusual sweating.

tiagabine hydrochloride
Gabitril

Pharmacologic classification: gamma aminobutyric acid (GABA) enhancer
Therapeutic classification: anticonvulsant
Pregnancy risk category C

How supplied
Available by prescription only
Tablets: 4 mg, 12 mg, 16 mg, 20 mg

Indications, route, and dosage
Adjunctive therapy in the treatment of partial seizures
Adults: Initially, 4 mg P.O. once daily. May increase total daily dose by 4 to 8 mg at weekly intervals until clinical response occurs or up to maximum of 56 mg/day. Give total daily dose in divided doses b.i.d. to q.i.d.
Adolescents ages 12 to 18: Initially, 4 mg P.O. once daily. May increase total daily dose by 4 mg beginning of week 2 and then by 4 to 8 mg/week at weekly intervals until clinical response is seen or up to maximum of 32 mg/day. Give total daily dose in divided doses b.i.d. to q.i.d.
✦ *Dosage adjustment.* In patients with impaired liver function, initial and maintenance doses or longer dosing intervals may be reduced.

Pharmacodynamics
Anticonvulsant action: Exact mechanism unknown. Thought to act by enhancing the activity of GABA, the major inhibitory neurotransmitter in the CNS. Binds to recognition sites associated with the GABA uptake carrier and may thus permit more GABA to be available for binding to receptors on postsynaptic cells.

Pharmacokinetics
• *Absorption:* Over 95% rapidly absorbed (plasma levels peak 45 minutes after oral dose in fasting state. Absolute bioavailability about 90%.
• *Distribution:* About 96% is bound to human plasma proteins, mainly to serum albumin and alpha-1 acid glycoprotein.
• *Metabolism:* Probably metabolized by cytochrome P-450 3A isoenzymes.
• *Excretion:* About 2% excreted unchanged; 25% and 63% of dose excreted into urine and feces, respectively. Half-life is about 7 to 9 hours.

Contraindications and precautions
Contraindicated in patients with hypersensitivity to drug or its components. Use cautiously in breast-feeding patients.

Interactions
Drug-drug. *Carbamazepine, phenobarbital, phenytoin:* Increased tiagabine clearance. Adjust dosage.
CNS depressants: Enhanced CNS effect. Avoid concomitant use.
Valproate: Decreased valproate level. Adjust valproate dosage.
Drug-lifestyle. *Alcohol:* Enhanced CNS effects. Discourage use.

Adverse reactions
CNS: *dizziness, asthenia, somnolence, nervousness,* tremor, difficulty with concentration and attention, insomnia, ataxia, confusion, speech disorder, difficulty with memory, paresthesia, depression, emotional lability, abnormal gait, hostility, language problems, agitation.
CV: vasodilation.
EENT: amblyopia, nystagmus, pharyngitis.
GI: abdominal pain, *nausea,* diarrhea, vomiting, increased appetite, mouth ulceration.
GU: urinary tract infection.
Musculoskeletal: myalgia, myasthenia.
Respiratory: increased cough.
Skin: rash, pruritus.
Other: flulike syndrome.

☑ Special considerations
• Never withdraw drug suddenly because seizure frequency may increase. Withdraw tiagabine gradually unless safety concerns require a more rapid withdrawal.
• A therapeutic range for plasma drug levels hasn't been established.
• Status epilepticus and sudden unexpected death in epilepsy have occurred in patients receiving tiagabine.
• Patients who aren't receiving at least one other enzyme-inducing antiepileptic at the time of tiagabine initiation may require lower doses or a slower dosage adjustment.
• The most common signs and symptoms of overdose include somnolence, impaired consciousness, impaired speech, agitation, confusion, speech difficulty, hostility, depression, weakness, and myoclonus.
• There is no specific antidote for overdose. If indicated, induce emesis or use gastric lavage. Observe usual precautions to maintain airway, and provide general supportive care.

Monitoring the patient
• Obtain plasma levels of drug before and after changes are made in therapeutic regimen.
• Monitor patient for adverse effects.

Information for the patient
• Advise patient to take drug only as prescribed.
• Tell patient to take drug with food.
• Warn patient that drug may cause dizziness, somnolence, and other signs and symptoms of

CNS depression. Advise patient to avoid driving and other potentially hazardous activities that require mental alertness until drug's CNS effects are known.
• Tell woman to call if pregnancy is being planned or suspected.
• Tell woman to disclose if she is planning to breast-feed because drug may appear in breast milk.

Geriatric patients
• Safety and effectiveness in this age-group haven't been established.

Pediatric patients
• Safety and effectiveness in children under age 12 haven't been established.

Breast-feeding patients
• Drug and metabolites may appear in breast milk. Use in breast-feeding women only if benefits clearly outweigh risks.

ticarcillin disodium
Ticar

Pharmacologic classification: extended-spectrum penicillin, alpha-carboxypenicillin
Therapeutic classification: antibiotic
Pregnancy risk category B

How supplied
Available by prescription only
Injection: 1 g, 3 g, 6 g
Pharmacy bulk package: 20 g, 30 g
I.V. infusion: 3 g

Indications, route, and dosage
Serious infections caused by susceptible organisms
Adults: 200 to 300 mg/kg I.V. daily, divided into doses given q 4 or 6 hours.
Children weighing less than 40 kg (88 lb): 200 to 300 mg/kg I.V. daily, divided into doses given q 4 to 6 hours.
Neonates weighing more than 2 kg (4.4 lb): 225 to 300 mg/kg/day, divided into doses given q 8 hours.
Neonates weighing less than 2 kg: 150 to 225 mg/kg/day, divided into doses given q 8 to 12 hours. Give prescribed dose I.M. or via I.V. infusion over 10 to 20 minutes.
Urinary tract infection
Adults: For patients with complicated infection, give 150 to 200 mg/kg I.V. daily, divided into doses q 4 to 6 hours; for treating uncomplicated infections, give 1 g I.V. or I.M. q 6 hours.
Children weighing less than 40 kg (88 lb): For patients with complicated infection, give 150 to 200

mg/kg/day by I.V. infusion divided into doses given every 4 to 6 hours.
For treating uncomplicated infections, give 50 to 100 mg/kg/day I.M. or direct I.V. divided into doses given every 6 to 8 hours.
✦ *Dosage adjustment.* For patient with renal failure, give initial loading dose of 3 g I.V. Then if patient receives hemodialysis, give 2 g I.V. q 12 hours and 3 g I.V. after each treatment. If he receives peritoneal dialysis, give 3 g I.V. q 12 hours. If he doesn't receive dialysis, give subsequent doses based on the table.

Creatinine clearance (ml/min)	Dosage in adults
> 60	3 g I.V. q 4 hours
30 to 60	2 g I.V. q 4 hours
10 to 30	2 g I.V. q 8 hours
< 10	2 g I.V. q 12 hours or 1 g I.M. q 6 hours
< 10 with hepatic failure	2 g I.V. q 24 hours or 1 g I.M. q 12 hours

Pharmacodynamics
Antibiotic action: Bactericidal. Adheres to bacterial penicillin-binding proteins, thus inhibiting bacterial cell-wall synthesis. Extended-spectrum penicillins are more resistant to inactivation by certain beta-lactamases, especially those produced by gram-negative organisms, but are still liable to inactivation by certain others.
Spectrum of activity includes many gram-negative aerobic and anaerobic bacilli, many gram-positive and gram-negative aerobic cocci, and some gram-positive aerobic and anaerobic bacilli. Drug may be effective against some strains of carbenicillin-resistant gram-negative bacilli.
In many cases, ticarcillin is more active (by weight) against *Pseudomonas aeruginosa* than is carbenicillin. Its primary use is in combination with an aminoglycoside to treat *P. aeruginosa* infections.
When ticarcillin is used alone, resistance develops rapidly. It's almost always used with other antibiotics (such as aminoglycosides).

Pharmacokinetics
• *Absorption:* Plasma levels peak 30 to 75 minutes after I.M. dose. About 86% of dose absorbed.
• *Distribution:* Distributed widely. Minimal CSF penetration with uninflamed meninges. Crosses placenta; 45% to 65% protein-bound.
• *Metabolism:* About 13% of dose metabolized by hydrolysis to inactive compounds.
• *Excretion:* 80% to 93% excreted in urine by renal tubular secretion and glomerular filtration; also excreted in bile and breast milk. Elimination half-life in adults is about 1 hour; in severe renal impairment, half-life extended to about 3 hours.

Removed by hemodialysis but not by peritoneal dialysis.

Contraindications and precautions
Contraindicated in patients with hypersensitivity to drug or other penicillins. Use cautiously in patients with other drug allergies, especially to cephalosporins, and in those with impaired renal function, hemorrhagic conditions, hypokalemia, and sodium restrictions.

Interactions
Drug-drug. *Aminoglycoside antibiotics:* Synergistic bactericidal effects against *P. aeruginosa, Escherichia coli, Klebsiella, Citrobacter, Enterobacter, Serratia,* and *Proteus mirabilis.* However, drugs are physically and chemically incompatible; inactivated when mixed or given together. Don't administer concomitantly. Adjust dosage for therapeutic response.
Clavulanic acid: Synergistic bactericidal effect against certain beta-lactamase-producing bacteria. Adjust dosage for therapeutic response.
Methotrexate: Elevated serum levels of methotrexate. Adjust dosage.
Probenecid: Increased serum levels of ticarcillin. Adjust dosage.

Adverse reactions
CNS: *seizures,* neuromuscular excitability.
GI: nausea, diarrhea, vomiting, pseudomembranous colitis.
Hematologic: leukopenia, eosinophilia, *neutropenia, thrombocytopenia,* hemolytic anemia, positive Coombs' test, prolonged PT and INR.
Hepatic: elevated liver enzyme levels.
Metabolic: hypokalemia, hypernatremia.
Other: hypersensitivity reactions (rash, pruritus, urticaria, chills, fever, edema, *anaphylaxis*), overgrowth of nonsusceptible organisms, pain at injection site, vein irritation, phlebitis.

☑ Special considerations
Besides the recommendations relevant to all penicillins, consider the following.
● Ticarcillin is almost always used with another antibiotic such as an aminoglycoside in life-threatening situations.
● Ticarcillin contains 5.2 mEq of sodium per gram of drug. Use with caution in patients with sodium restriction.
● Because drug is dialyzable, patients undergoing hemodialysis may need dosage adjustments.
● Ticarcillin alters tests for urinary or serum proteins; it interferes with turbidimetric methods that use sulfosalicylic acid, trichloroacetic acid, acetic acid, or nitric acid. Ticarcillin doesn't interfere with tests using bromophenol blue (Albustix, Albutest, Multistix).
● Drug may falsely decrease serum aminoglycoside levels.

● Signs and symptoms of overdose include neuromuscular hypersensitivity or seizures resulting from CNS irritation by high drug levels. Drug can be removed by hemodialysis.

Monitoring the patient
● Monitor serum electrolyte levels to prevent hypokalemia and hypernatremia.
● Monitor neurologic status. High levels of drug may cause seizures.
● Check CBC, differential, PT, and PTT. Drug may cause thrombocytopenia. Watch for signs of bleeding.

Information for the patient
● Warn patient about potential adverse reactions.
● Advise patient of need for monitoring.

Geriatric patients
● Half-life may be prolonged in elderly patients because of impaired renal function.

Pediatric patients
● Ticarcillin reconstituted for I.M. use with bacteriostatic water for injection containing benzyl alcohol shouldn't be used in neonates because of potential for toxicity. Children weighing more than 88 lb (40 kg) should receive adult dose.

Breast-feeding patients
● Drug appears in breast milk; use cautiously in breast-feeding women.

---

ticarcillin disodium/ clavulanate potassium
Timentin

Pharmacologic classification: extended-spectrum penicillin, beta-lactamase inhibitor
Therapeutic classification: antibiotic
Pregnancy risk category B

How supplied
Available by prescription only
Injection: 3 g ticarcillin and 100 mg clavulanic acid

Indications, route, and dosage
Infections of the lower respiratory tract, urinary tract, bones and joints, skin and skin structure, and septicemia when caused by susceptible organisms
Adults: 3.1 g (contains 3 g ticarcillin and 0.1 g clavulanate potassium) diluted in 50 to 100 ml D₅W, saline, or lactated Ringer's injection and administered by I.V. infusion over 30 minutes q 4 to 6 hours.
Children ages 3 months to 16 years weighing less than 60 kg (132 lb): For mild to moderate infections, 200 mg/kg/day (contains 3 g ti-

---

and 0.1 g clavulanate potassium) I.V. infusion given in divided doses q 6 hours. For severe infections, 300 mg/kg/day (contains 3 g ticarcillin and 0.1 g clavulanate potassium) I.V. given in divided doses q 4 hours.

✦ *Dosage adjustment.* For patient with renal failure, give a loading dose of 3.1 g (3 g ticarcillin with 100 mg clavulanate). Then if patient receives hemodialysis, give 2 g I.V. q 12 hours, and 3.1 g after treatment. If he receives peritoneal dialysis, give 3.1 g I.V. q 12 hours. If he doesn't receive dialysis, give subsequent doses based on the table.

Creatinine clearance (ml/min)	Dosage in adults
> 60	3.1 g I.V. q 4 hours
30 to 60	2 g I.V. q 4 hours
10 to 30	2 g I.V. q 8 hours
< 10	2 g I.V. q 12 hours
< 10 with hepatic failure	2 g I.V. q 24 hours

Pharmacodynamics

Antibiotic action: Ticarcillin is bactericidal; it adheres to bacterial penicillin-binding proteins, thus inhibiting bacterial cell wall synthesis. Extended-spectrum penicillins are more resistant to inactivation by certain beta-lactamases, especially those produced by gram-negative organisms, but are still liable to inactivation by certain others.

Clavulanic acid has only weak antibacterial activity and doesn't affect the action of ticarcillin. However, clavulanic acid has a beta-lactam ring and is structurally similar to penicillin and cephalosporins; it binds irreversibly with certain beta-lactamases, preventing inactivation of ticarcillin and broadening its bactericidal spectrum.

Spectrum of activity of ticarcillin includes many gram-negative aerobic and anaerobic bacilli, many gram-positive and gram-negative aerobic cocci, and some gram-positive aerobic and anaerobic bacilli. The combination of ticarcillin and clavulanate potassium is also effective against many beta-lactamase-producing strains, including *Staphylococcus aureus, Haemophilus influenzae, Neisseria gonorrhoeae, Escherichia coli, Klebsiella, Providencia,* and *Bacteroides fragilis,* but not *Pseudomonas aeruginosa.*

Pharmacokinetics

● *Absorption:* Only administered I.V.; plasma level peaks immediately after infusion is complete.
● *Distribution:* Distributed widely. Penetrates minimally into CSF with uninflamed meninges; clavulanic acid penetrates into pleural fluid, lungs, and peritoneal fluid. Ticarcillin sodium achieves high levels in urine. Protein-binding is 45% to 65% for ticarcillin, 22% to 30% for clavulanic acid; both cross placenta.
● *Metabolism:* About 13% of ticarcillin dose metabolized by hydrolysis to inactive compounds; clavulanic acid thought to undergo extensive metabolism, but fate unknown.
● *Excretion:* 83% to 90% of ticarcillin excreted in urine by renal tubular secretion and glomerular filtration; also excreted in bile and breast milk. Metabolites of clavulanate excreted in urine by glomerular filtration and in breast milk. Elimination half-life of ticarcillin in adults is about 1 hour and that of clavulanate is about 1 hour; in severe renal impairment, half-life of ticarcillin is extended to about 8 hours and that of clavulanate to about 3 hours. Both drugs are removed by hemodialysis but only slightly by peritoneal dialysis.

Contraindications and precautions

Contraindicated in patients with hypersensitivity to drug or other penicillins. Use cautiously in patients with other drug allergies, especially to cephalosporins, and in those with impaired renal function, hemorrhagic conditions, hypokalemia, or sodium restrictions.

Interactions

Drug-drug. *Aminoglycoside antibiotics:* Synergistic bactericidal effects against *Pseudomonas aeruginosa, Escherichia coli, Klebsiella, Citrobacter, Enterobacter, Serratia,* and *Proteus mirabilis.* However, drugs are physically and chemically incompatible; inactivated when mixed or given together. Don't give together.
Methotrexate: Elevated serum levels of methotrexate. Dosage adjustment may be needed.
Probenecid: Elevated ticarcillin serum level; no effect on clavulanate. Dosage adjustment may be needed.

Adverse reactions

CNS: *seizures,* neuromuscular excitability, headache, giddiness.
GI: nausea, diarrhea, stomatitis, vomiting, epigastric pain, flatulence, pseudomembranous colitis, taste and smell disturbances.
Hematologic: leukopenia, *neutropenia,* eosinophilia, *thrombocytopenia,* hemolytic anemia, anemia, positive Coombs' test, prolonged PT and INR.
Hepatic: elevated liver enzymes.
Metabolic: hypokalemia, hypernatremia.
Other: hypersensitivity reactions (rash, pruritus, urticaria, chills, fever, edema, *anaphylaxis*), overgrowth of nonsusceptible organisms, pain at injection site, vein irritation, phlebitis.

☑ Special considerations

Besides the recommendations relevant to all penicillins, consider the following.

• Ticarcillin disodium/clavulanate potassium is almost always used with another antibiotic such as an aminoglycoside in life-threatening situations.
• Administer aminoglycosides 1 hour before or after administration of ticarcillin disodium/clavulanate potassium.
• Ticarcillin contains 5.2 mEq of sodium per gram of drug. Use with caution in patients with sodium restriction.
• Because drug is dialyzable, patients undergoing hemodialysis may need dosage adjustments.
• Ticarcillin disodium/clavulanate potassium alters tests for urinary or serum proteins; it interferes with turbidimetric methods that use sulfosalicylic acid, trichloroacetic acid, acetic acid, or nitric acid. Ticarcillin disodium/clavulanate potassium doesn't interfere with tests using bromophenol blue (Albustix, Albutest, Multistix). It may falsely decrease serum aminoglycoside level.
• Signs and symptoms of overdose include neuromuscular hypersensitivity or seizures; ticarcillin and clavulanate potassium can be removed by hemodialysis.

Monitoring the patient
• Monitor serum electrolyte levels. Watch for signs of hypernatremia and hypokalemia.
• Monitor neurologic status. High blood levels of drug may cause seizures.

Information for the patient
• Warn patient about potential adverse reactions.
• Advise patient of need for monitoring.

Geriatric patients
• Half-life may be prolonged in elderly patients because of impaired renal function.

Breast-feeding patients
• Ticarcillin and clavulanate potassium appear in breast milk; use with caution in breast-feeding women.

---

ticlopidine hydrochloride
Ticlid

Pharmacologic classification: platelet aggregation inhibitor
Therapeutic classification: antithrombotic
Pregnancy risk category B

How supplied
Available by prescription only
Tablets (film-coated): 250 mg

Indications, route, and dosage
Reduction of risk of thrombotic stroke in patients with history of stroke, in those who
have experienced stroke precursors, or in those who are intolerant to aspirin therapy
Adults: 250 mg P.O. b.i.d. with meals.

Pharmacodynamics
Antithrombotic action: Blocks adenosine diphosphate-induced platelet-fibrinogen and platelet-platelet binding.

Pharmacokinetics
• *Absorption:* Over 80% rapidly absorbed after oral administration; plasma levels peak within 2 hours. Absorption enhanced by food.
• *Distribution:* 98% bound to serum proteins and lipoproteins.
• *Metabolism:* Extensively metabolized by liver. Over 20 metabolites identified; unknown if parent drug or active metabolites are responsible for pharmacologic activity.
• *Excretion:* 60% of drug excreted in urine and 23% in feces; only trace amounts of intact drug found in urine. After one dose, half-life is 12½ hours; with repeat dosing, half-life increases to 4 to 5 days.

Contraindications and precautions
Contraindicated in patients with hypersensitivity to drug and in those with hematopoietic disorders (such as neutropenia, thrombocytopenia, or disorders of hemostasis), active pathologic bleeding from peptic ulceration or active intracranial bleeding, or severely impaired hepatic function.

Interactions
Drug-drug. *Antacids:* Decreased plasma levels of ticlopidine. Separate administration times by at least 2 hours.
Aspirin: Potentiated effects of aspirin on platelets. Don't use together.
Cimetidine: Increased risk of ticlopidine toxicity. Avoid concomitant use.
Digoxin: Slightly decreased serum digoxin levels. Monitor serum digoxin levels.
Theophylline: Increased risk of theophylline toxicity. Monitor patient closely; adjust theophylline dosage as needed.
Drug-herb. *Red clover:* Increased risk of bleeding. Don't use together.

Adverse reactions
CNS: dizziness, *intracerebral bleeding,* peripheral neuropathy.
CV: vasculitis.
EENT: epistaxis, conjunctival hemorrhage.
GI: *diarrhea, nausea, dyspepsia, abdominal pain,* anorexia, vomiting, flatulence, bleeding, light-colored stools.
GU: hematuria, *nephrotic syndrome,* dark-colored urine.
Hematologic: prolonged bleeding time, *neutropenia, pancytopenia, agranulocytosis, immune thrombocytopenia.*

Hepatic: hepatitis, cholestatic jaundice, abnormal liver function test results.
Metabolic: *hyponatremia, increased serum cholesterol levels.*
Musculoskeletal: arthropathy, myositis.
Respiratory: *allergic pneumonitis.*
Skin: *rash,* pruritus, ecchymoses, maculopapular rash, urticaria, **thrombocytopenic purpura.**
Other: *hypersensitivity reactions,* postoperative bleeding, systemic lupus erythematosus, *serum sickness.*

☑ Special considerations
• If drug is being substituted for a fibrinolytic or anticoagulant, stop previous drug before starting ticlopidine.
• If necessary, methylprednisolone 20 mg I.V. has been shown to normalize the bleeding time within 2 hours. Platelet transfusions also may be necessary.
• Drug has been used for investigational purposes for many conditions, including intermittent claudication, chronic arterial occlusion, subarachnoid hemorrhage, primary glomerulonephritis, sickle cell disease, and uremic patients with AV shunts. When used preoperatively, drug may decrease graft occlusion in patients receiving coronary artery bypass grafts and reduce severity of decreased platelet count in patients receiving extracorporeal hemoperfusion during open heart surgery.
• Only one case of overdose has been reported. The patient, who had ingested over 6 g of drug, showed increased bleeding time and increased ALT levels. The patient recovered with supportive therapy alone.

Monitoring the patient
• Perform baseline liver function tests and repeat whenever liver dysfunction is suspected. Monitor patient closely, especially during first 4 months of treatment.
• Monitor CBC and WBC differential every 2 weeks for the first 3 months of therapy. Severe hematologic adverse events can occur with drug.
• After first 3 months of therapy, perform CBC and WBC differential determinations in patients showing signs of infection.

Information for the patient
• Tell patient to take drug with meals because food substantially increases bioavailability and improves GI tolerance.
• Advise patient to call if he is scheduled for elective surgery and to be prepared to discontinue drug 10 to 14 days before procedure.
• Inform patient of need to report for regular blood tests. Neutropenia can result in an increased risk of infection. Tell patient to report signs and symptoms of infection, such as fever, chills, and sore throat, immediately.

• Tell patient to immediately report yellow skin or sclera, severe or persistent diarrhea, rash, subcutaneous bleeding, light-colored stools, or dark urine.
• Emphasize that drug prolongs bleeding time. Tell patient to report unusual bleeding and to inform dentists and other health care providers that he is taking ticlopidine.
• Warn patient to avoid aspirin and products containing aspirin, which may also prolong bleeding. Advise him to call before taking OTC preparations because many contain aspirin.

Pediatric patients
• Safety and efficacy in children under age 18 haven't been established.

Breast-feeding patients
• It's unknown if drug appears in breast milk. Breast-feeding isn't recommended.

tiludronate disodium
Skelid

Pharmacologic classification: bisphosphonate analogue
Therapeutic classification: antihypercalcemic
Pregnancy risk category C

How supplied
Available by prescription only
Tablets: 200 mg

Indications, route, and dosage
Paget's disease
Adults: 400 mg P.O. once daily taken with 6 to 8 oz (180 to 240 ml) of water for 3 months, given 2 hours before or after meals.

Pharmacodynamics
Antihypercalcemic action: Thought to suppress bone resorption by reducing osteoclastic activity. Appears to inhibit osteoclasts through the following mechanisms: disruption of the cytoskeletal ring structure, possibly by inhibiting protein-tyrosine-phosphatase, thus leading to detachment of osteoclasts from the bone surface; and the inhibition of the osteoclastic proton pump.

Pharmacokinetics
• *Absorption:* Bioavailability of drug on empty stomach is 8%. Food and beverages other than water can reduce bioavailability by up to 90%.
• *Distribution:* Widely distributed in bone and soft tissue. Protein-binding is about 90% (mainly albumin).
• *Metabolism:* Doesn't appear to be metabolized.
• *Excretion:* Principally excreted in urine. Mean plasma half-life 150 hours.

Reactions may be *common,* uncommon, **life-threatening,** or COMMON AND LIFE-THREATENING.

Contraindications and precautions
Contraindicated in patients with hypersensitivity to drug or its components and in those with creatinine clearance below 30 ml/minute. Use cautiously in patients with upper GI disease, such as dysphagia, esophagitis, esophageal ulcer, or gastric ulcer.

Interactions
Drug-drug. *Aluminum antacids, calcium supplements, magnesium antacids:* Dramatically reduced bioavailability of tiludronate when administered 1 hour before tiludronate. Separate administration times by more than 1 hour.
Aspirin: Decreased bioavailability when taken 2 hours after tiludronate. Separate administration times by more than 2 hours.
Indomethacin: Increased bioavailability of tiludronate. Adjust dosage.
Drug-food. *Any food:* Delayed drug absorption. Don't give drug within 2 hours of meals.
Beverages (other than plain water): Reduced drug absorption. Don't give with drug.

Adverse reactions
CNS: anxiety, dizziness, headache, insomnia, involuntary muscle contractions, paresthesia, somnolence, vertigo.
CV: chest pain, hypertension.
EENT: cataracts, conjunctivitis, glaucoma, pharyngitis, sinusitis, rhinitis.
GI: anorexia, constipation, diarrhea, dry mouth, dyspepsia, flatulence, gastritis, nausea, tooth disorder, vomiting.
Metabolic: vitamin D deficiency.
Musculoskeletal: arthralgia, arthrosis, back pain.
Respiratory: bronchitis, coughing, crackles.
Skin: pruritus.
Other: edema, hyperparathyroidism, sweating, whole body pain.

☑ Special considerations
● Drug should be used in patients with Paget's disease who have serum alkaline phosphatase level at least twice the upper limit of normal or who are symptomatic or at risk for future complications of disease.
● Administer drug for 3 months to assess response.
● Hypocalcemia and other disturbances of mineral metabolism (such as vitamin D deficiency) should be corrected before initiating therapy.
● If hypocalcemia or renal insufficiency occurs, use standard treatment.
● Dialysis isn't beneficial for overdose.

Monitoring the patient
● Monitor therapeutic effect after 3 months.
● Monitor patient for adverse effects.

Information for the patient
● Tell patient to take drug with 6 to 8 oz (180 to 240 ml) of water.
● Advise patient that drug shouldn't be taken within 2 hours of eating.
● Advise patient to maintain adequate vitamin D and calcium intake.
● Inform patient that calcium supplements, aspirin, and indomethacin shouldn't be taken within 2 hours before or after drug.
● Tell patient that antacids containing aluminum and magnesium can be taken 2 hours after taking drug.

Geriatric patients
● Plasma levels may be higher in elderly patients. However, dosage adjustment isn't necessary.

Pediatric patients
● Safety and effectiveness in children haven't been established.

Breast-feeding patients
● It's unknown if drug appears in breast milk. Use cautiously in breast-feeding women.

---

timolol maleate
Blocadren, Timoptic, Timoptic-XE

Pharmacologic classification: beta blocker
Therapeutic classification: antihypertensive, adjunct in MI therapy, antiglaucoma drug
Pregnancy risk category C

How supplied
Available by prescription only
Tablets: 5 mg, 10 mg, 20 mg
Ophthalmic gel: 0.25%, 0.5%
Ophthalmic solution: 0.25%, 0.5%

Indications, route, and dosage
Hypertension
Adults: Initially, 10 mg P.O. b.i.d. Usual maintenance dose is 20 to 40 mg/day. Maximum dose is 60 mg/day. There should be an interval of at least 7 days between dosage increases.
Reduction of risk of CV mortality and reinfarction after MI
Adults: 10 mg P.O. b.i.d. initiated within 1 to 4 weeks after infarction.
Migraine headache
Adults: 10 mg P.O. daily b.i.d., then increase up to 20 mg; or 30-mg dose (10 mg P.O. in the morning and 20 mg P.O. in the evening).
Glaucoma
Adults: 1 drop of 0.25% or 0.5% solution to the conjunctiva once or twice daily; or 1 drop of 0.25% or 0.5% gel to the conjunctiva once daily.

◇ **Angina**
Adults: 15 to 45 mg P.O. daily given in three divided doses.

Pharmacodynamics
Antihypertensive action: Exact mechanism unknown. May reduce blood pressure by blocking adrenergic receptors (thus decreasing cardiac output), by decreasing sympathetic outflow from the CNS, and by suppressing renin release.
MI prophylactic action: Exact mechanism unknown. Produces a negative chronotropic and inotropic activity. This decrease in heart rate and myocardial contractility results in reduced myocardial oxygen consumption.
Antiglaucoma action: Beta-blocking action of timolol decreases production of aqueous humor, thereby decreasing intraocular pressure.

Pharmacokinetics
• *Absorption:* About 90% of oral dose absorbed from GI tract; plasma level peaks in 1 to 2 hours.
• *Distribution:* After oral administration, distributed throughout body; depending on assay method, drug is 10% to 60% protein-bound.
• *Metabolism:* About 80% of dose metabolized in liver to inactive metabolites.
• *Excretion:* Drug and metabolites excreted primarily in urine; half-life is about 4 hours. After topical application to eye, effects last up to 24 hours.

Contraindications and precautions
Contraindicated in patients with hypersensitivity to drug and in those with bronchial asthma, severe COPD, sinus bradycardia and heart block greater than first degree, cardiogenic shock, or heart failure.
    Use cautiously in patients with diabetes, hyperthyroidism, or respiratory disease (especially nonallergic bronchospasm or emphysema). Use oral form cautiously in patients with compensated heart failure and hepatic or renal disease. Use ophthalmic form cautiously in patients with cerebrovascular insufficiency.

Interactions
Drug-drug. *Beta-adrenergic stimulants, calcium channel blockers, cardiac glycosides:* Cardiac arrhythmias. Monitor cardiac status.
Fentanyl, general anesthetics: Excessive hypotension. Monitor blood pressure; adjust dosage.
Phenothiazines: Increased phenothiazine level. Monitor patient closely.
Xanthines: Antagonized xanthine effects. Monitor patient closely; adjust dosage as needed.
Other antihypertensives with NSAIDs: Antagonized antihypertensive effects. Dosage adjustment may be needed.

Adverse reactions
CNS: fatigue, lethargy, dizziness; depression, hallucinations, confusion (with ophthalmic form).

CV: *arrhythmias, bradycardia,* hypotension, *heart failure,* peripheral vascular disease, *pulmonary edema* (with oral administration); *CVA, cardiac arrest,* heart block, palpitations (with ophthalmic form).
EENT: minor eye irritation, decreased corneal sensitivity with long-term use, conjunctivitis, blepharitis, keratitis, visual disturbances, diplopia, ptosis (with ophthalmic form).
GI: nausea, vomiting, diarrhea (with oral administration).
GU: increased BUN level.
Hematologic: decreased hemoglobin level and hematocrit.
Metabolic: hyperkalemia, hyperuricemia, hyperglycemia.
Respiratory: dyspnea, *bronchospasm,* increased airway resistance (with oral administration); *asthma attacks in patients with history of asthma* (with ophthalmic form).
Skin: pruritus (with oral administration).

☑ Special considerations
Besides the recommendations relevant to all beta blockers, consider the following.
• Dosage adjustment may be needed for a patient with renal or hepatic impairment.
• Although controversial, drug may need to be stopped 48 hours before surgery in patients receiving ophthalmic timolol because systemic absorption occurs.
• Stop drug if response not attained after 6 to 8 weeks.
• Drug therapy may slightly increase BUN, serum potassium, uric acid, and blood glucose levels and may slightly decrease hemoglobin level and hematocrit.
• Signs and symptoms of overdose include severe hypotension, bradycardia, heart failure, and bronchospasm. After acute ingestion, empty stomach by induced emesis or gastric lavage and give activated charcoal to reduce absorption. Subsequent treatment is usually symptomatic and supportive.

Monitoring the patient
• Monitor renal and hepatic status.
• Monitor cardiac and respiratory status.

Information for the patient
• For ophthalmic form, teach patient proper method of eyedrop administration. Warn patient not to touch dropper to eye or surrounding tissue; tell him to lightly press lacrimal sac with finger after administration to decrease systemic absorption.
• Advise patient to invert ophthalmic gel container once before each use.
• Advise patient to administer other ophthalmic drugs at least 10 minutes before the ophthalmic gel.

Geriatric patients
● Elderly patients may need lower oral maintenance doses because of increased bioavailability or delayed metabolism; they also may experience enhanced adverse effects. Use cautiously because half-life may be prolonged in elderly patients.

Pediatric patients
● Safety and efficacy in children haven't been established; use only if potential benefit outweighs risk.

Breast-feeding patients
● Drug appears in breast milk. Because of potential for serious adverse reactions in breast-fed infants, an alternative to breast-feeding is recommended during therapy.

tioconazole
Vagistat-1

Pharmacologic classification: imidazole derivative
Therapeutic classification: antifungal
Pregnancy risk category C

How supplied
Available by prescription only
Vaginal ointment: 6.5%

Indications, route, and dosage
Vulvovaginal candidiasis
Adults: Insert 1 full applicator (about 4.6 g) intravaginally h.s. as a single dose.

Pharmacodynamics
Antifungal action: Tioconazole is a fungicidal imidazole that alters cell wall permeability.

Pharmacokinetics
● *Absorption:* Negligible.
● *Distribution:* No information available.
● *Metabolism:* No information available.
● *Excretion:* No information available.

Contraindications and precautions
Contraindicated in patients with hypersensitivity to drug or other imidazole antifungals (miconazole, ketoconazole) and in breast-feeding women.

Interactions
None reported.

Adverse reactions
GU: *burning, pruritus,* discharge, vaginal pain, dysuria, dyspareunia, vulvar edema, irritation.

☑ Special considerations
● Because drug is useful only for candidal vulvovaginitis, the diagnosis should be confirmed by potassium hydroxide smears or cultures before treatment with tioconazole.

Monitoring the patient
● Monitor therapeutic effect.
● Monitor patient for adverse effects.

Information for the patient
● Review correct use of drug with patient. She should insert drug high into vagina except during pregnancy. Detailed instructions for patient are available with product.
● Tell patient to avoid sexual intercourse during therapy or advise partner to use a condom to prevent reinfection.
● Warn patient to open applicator just before using product to avoid contamination.
● Tell patient to watch for and report irritation or sensitivity.
● Emphasize need for patient to continue therapy for full course, even if symptoms have improved, and during menstrual period.
● Advise patient to use a sanitary napkin to avoid staining of clothing.

Breast-feeding patients
● It's unknown if drug appears in breast milk. Advise patient to temporarily stop breast-feeding during therapy.

tirofiban hydrochloride
Aggrastat

Pharmacologic classification: GP IIb/IIIa receptor antagonist
Therapeutic classification: inhibitor of platelet aggregation
Pregnancy risk category B

How supplied
Injection: 50-ml vials (250 mcg/ml), 500-ml premixed single-dose (50 mcg/ml)

Indications, route, and dosage
Treatment, with heparin, of patients with acute coronary syndrome, including patients who are to be managed medically and those undergoing percutaneous transluminal coronary angioplasty (PTCA) or atherectomy
Adults: I.V. loading dose of 0.4 mcg/kg/minute for 30 minutes; then a continuous I.V. infusion of 0.1 mcg/kg/minute. Continue infusion through angiography and for 12 to 24 hours after angioplasty or atherectomy.
✦ *Dosage adjustment.* For patients with renal insufficiency (creatinine clearance under 30 ml/minute), use a loading dose of 0.2 mcg/kg/minute for 30 minutes; then a continuous infu-

sion of 0.05 mcg/kg/minute. Continue infusion through angiography and for 12 to 24 hours after angioplasty or atherectomy.

Pharmacodynamics
Platelet aggregation inhibitor action: Reversible antagonist of fibrinogen binding to the GP IIb/IIIa receptor on human platelets, producing a dose-dependent inhibition of platelet aggregation.

Pharmacokinetics
- *Absorption:* No information available.
- *Distribution:* 65% protein-bound. Volume of distribution ranges from 22 to 42 liters.
- *Metabolism:* Limited metabolism. Half-life is about 2 hours.
- *Excretion:* Renal clearance accounts for 39% to 69% of elimination; feces accounts for 25%.

Contraindications and precautions
Contraindicated in patients with hypersensitivity to drug or its components and in those with active internal bleeding or history of bleeding diathesis within the previous 30 days; past history of intracranial hemorrhage, intracranial neoplasm, arteriovenous malformation, or aneurysm; thrombocytopenia after prior exposure to drug; stroke within 30 days or history of hemorrhagic stroke; findings suggestive of aortic dissection; severe hypertension (systolic blood pressure over 180 mm Hg or diastolic blood pressure over 110 mm Hg); acute pericarditis; major surgical procedure or severe physical trauma within previous month. Also contraindicated when another parenteral GP IIb/IIIa inhibitor is also being used.

Use cautiously in patients with platelet count less than 150,000 mm^3 and in patients with hemorrhagic retinopathy.

Interactions
Drug-drug. *Clopidogrel, dipyridamole, NSAIDs, oral anticoagulants (warfarin), thrombolytics, ticlopidine:* Increased risk of bleeding. Monitor patient closely.
Levothyroxine, omeprazole: Increased renal clearance of tirofiban. Monitor patient.

Adverse reactions
CNS: dizziness, fever, headache.
CV: *bradycardia, coronary artery dissection,* edema, vasovagal reaction.
GI: nausea, *occult bleeding.*
GU: pelvic pain.
Hematologic: *bleeding, thrombocytopenia,* decreased hemoglobin level and hematocrit.
Musculoskeletal: leg pain.
Skin: sweating.
Other: bleeding at arterial access site.

☑ Special considerations
- Don't infuse at levels greater than 50 mcg/ml.

- Drug is associated with increases in bleeding rates, particularly at the site of arterial access for femoral sheath placement. Before pulling sheath, stop heparin for 3 to 4 hours and document activated clotting time under 180 seconds or APTT under 45 seconds. Sheath hemostasis should be achieved at least 4 hours before hospital discharge.
- Use of arterial and venous punctures, I.M. injections, urinary catheters, nasotracheal intubation and nasogastric tubes should be minimized. Avoid noncompressible I.V. access sites (for example, subclavian or jugular veins).
- In case of overdose, assess patient's condition and stop or adjust infusion. Drug is removed by dialysis.

Monitoring the patient
- Monitor hemoglobin level, hematocrit, and platelet counts before starting therapy, 6 hours after loading dose, and at least daily during therapy.

Information for the patient
- Advise patient to report chest discomfort or other adverse effects immediately.
- Inform patient that frequent blood sampling may be needed to evaluate therapy.

Pediatric patients
- Safety and effectiveness in children under age 18 haven't been established.

Breast-feeding patients
- It's unknown if drug appears in breast milk. Depending on importance of drug to mother, stop either breast-feeding or drug.

tobramycin

tobramycin ophthalmic
Tobrex

tobramycin sulfate
Nebcin

tobramycin solution for inhalation
TOBI

Pharmacologic classification: aminoglycoside
Therapeutic classification: antibiotic
Pregnancy risk category D

How supplied
Available by prescription only
Injection: 40 mg/ml, 10 mg/ml (pediatric)
Bulk powder for injection: 1.2 g
Ophthalmic solution: 0.3%
Ophthalmic ointment: 0.3%

Reactions may be *common*, uncommon, *life-threatening*, or COMMON AND LIFE-THREATENING.

Nebulizer solution for inhalation: single-use 5-ml (300-mg) ampule

Indications, route, and dosage

Serious infections caused by sensitive Escherichia coli, Proteus, Klebsiella, Enterobacter, Serratia, Staphylococcus aureus, Pseudomonas, Citrobacter, or Providencia
Adults and children with normal renal function: 3 mg/kg I.M. or I.V. daily, divided q 8 hours. Up to 5 mg/kg I.M. or I.V. daily, divided q 6 to 8 hours for life-threatening infections.
Neonates under age 1 week: Up to 4 mg/kg I.M. or I.V. daily, divided q 12 hours. For I.V. use, dilute in 50 to 100 ml normal saline solution or D₅W for adults and in less volume for children. Infuse over 20 to 60 minutes.

✦ *Dosage adjustment.* For patients with impaired renal function, initial dose is same as for those with normal renal function. Subsequent doses and frequency are determined by renal function study results and blood levels; keep peak serum levels between 4 and 10 mcg/ml and trough serum levels between 1 and 2 mcg/ml. Several methods have been used to calculate dosage in renal failure.

After a 1 mg/kg loading dose, adjust subsequent dosage by reducing doses administered at 8-hour intervals or by prolonging the interval between normal doses. Both of these methods are useful when serum levels of tobramycin can't be measured directly. They are based on either creatinine clearance (preferred) or serum creatinine level because these values correlate with drug's half-life.

To calculate reduced dosage for 8-hour intervals, use available nomograms; or, if patient's steady-state serum creatinine values are known, divide the normally recommended dose by patient's serum creatinine value. To determine frequency in hours for normal dosage (if creatinine clearance rate isn't available), divide the normal dose by patient's serum creatinine value. Dosage schedules derived from either method need careful clinical and laboratory observations of patient and should be adjusted as appropriate. These methods of calculation may be misleading in elderly patients and in those with severe wasting; neither should be used when dialysis is performed.

Hemodialysis removes 50% to 75% of a dose in 6 hours. In anephric patients maintained by dialysis, 1.5 to 2 mg/kg after each dialysis usually maintains therapeutic, nontoxic serum levels. Patients receiving peritoneal dialysis twice a week should receive a 1.5 to 2 mg/kg loading dose, then 1 mg/kg q 3 days. Those receiving dialysis q 2 days should receive a 1.5 mg/kg loading dose after first dialysis and 0.75 mg/kg after each subsequent dialysis.

◊ **Intrathecally or intraventricularly**
Adults: 3 to 8 mg q 18 to 48 hours.

Management of cystic fibrosis patients with Pseudomonas aeruginosa
Adults and children over age 6: 1 single-use ampule (300 mg) administered q 12 hours for 28 days, then off for 28 days, then on for 28 days as advisable. There is no dosage adjustment for age or renal failure.
External ocular infection caused by susceptible gram-negative bacteria
Adults and children: In mild to moderate infections, instill 1 or 2 drops into affected eye q 4 to 6 hours. In severe infections, instill 2 drops into affected eye hourly or apply a small amount of ointment into conjunctival sac t.i.d. or q.i.d.

Pharmacodynamics

Antibiotic action: Bactericidal. Binds directly to the 30S ribosomal subunit, thereby inhibiting bacterial protein synthesis. Spectrum of activity includes many aerobic gram-negative organisms, including most strains of *P. aeruginosa* and some aerobic gram-positive organisms. May act against some bacterial strains resistant to other aminoglycosides; many strains resistant to tobramycin are susceptible to amikacin, gentamicin, or netilmicin.

Pharmacokinetics

• *Absorption:* Absorbed poorly after oral administration; usually given parenterally. Serum levels peak 30 to 90 minutes after I.M. administration. Inhaled drug remains concentrated in airway, with serum level after 20 weeks of therapy 1.05 μg/ml 1 hour after dosing.
• *Distribution:* Distributed widely after parenteral administration; poor intraocular penetration. Low CSF penetration, even in patients with inflamed meninges. Minimal protein-binding; crosses placenta. Inhaled drug remains primarily concentrated in airway.
• *Metabolism:* Not metabolized.
• *Excretion:* Excreted primarily in urine by glomerular filtration; small amounts may be excreted in bile and breast milk. Elimination half-life in adults is 2 to 3 hours. In severe renal damage, half-life may extend to 24 to 60 hours. With inhalation use, unabsorbed drug probably eliminated in sputum.

Contraindications and precautions

Contraindicated in patients with hypersensitivity to drug or other aminoglycosides. Use injectable form cautiously in patients with impaired renal function or neuromuscular disorders and in elderly patients.

Interactions

Drug-drug. *Amphotericin B, capreomycin, cephalosporins, cisplatin, methoxyflurane, polymyxin B, vancomycin, other aminoglycosides:* Increased hazard of nephrotoxicity, ototoxicity, and neurotoxicity. Use cautiously together.

Bumetanide, ethacrynic acid, furosemide, mannitol, urea: Ototoxicity. Use cautiously together. Monitor patient closely.
Dimenhydrinate; other antiemetics, antivertigo drugs: May mask tobramycin-induced ototoxicity. Avoid concomitant use.
General anesthetics, neuromuscular blockers (such as succinylcholine, tubocurarine): Potentiated neuromuscular blockade. Use cautiously together. Monitor patient closely.
Penicillins: Synergistic bactericidal effect against *P. aeruginosa, E. coli, Klebsiella, Citrobacter, Enterobacter, Serratia,* and *Proteus mirabilis.* However, drugs are physically and chemically incompatible; inactivated when mixed or given together. Don't use together.

Adverse reactions
CNS: headache, lethargy, confusion, disorientation (with injectable form).
EENT: *ototoxicity* (with injectable form); blurred vision (with ophthalmic ointment); burning or stinging on instillation, lid itching or swelling, conjunctival erythema (with ophthalmic administration).
GI: vomiting, nausea, diarrhea (with injectable form).
GU: elevated BUN, nonprotein nitrogen, and serum creatinine levels; increased urinary excretion of casts; *nephrotoxicity* (with injectable form).
Hematologic: anemia, eosinophilia, **leukopenia, thrombocytopenia, granulocytopenia** (with injectable form).
Respiratory: *bronchospasm* (with inhalation form).
Skin: rash, urticaria, pruritus (with injectable form).
Other: fever, **hypersensitivity,** overgrowth of nonsusceptible organisms (with ophthalmic administration).

☑ Special considerations
Besides the recommendations relevant to all aminoglycosides, consider the following.
• For I.V. administration, the usual volume of diluent (normal saline injection or 5% dextrose injection) for adult doses is 50 to 100 ml. For children, the volume should be proportionately less. Infuse over 20 to 60 minutes.
• Don't premix tobramycin with other drugs; administer separately at least 1 hour apart.
• Stop ophthalmic preparation if keratitis, erythema, lacrimation, edema, or lid itching occurs.
• Because tobramycin is dialyzable, patients undergoing hemodialysis may need dosage adjustments.
• Inhalation form is an orphan drug used specifically for management of cystic fibrosis patients with *P. aeruginosa.*
• Signs and symptoms of overdose include ototoxicity, nephrotoxicity, and neuromuscular toxi-

city. Remove drug by hemodialysis or peritoneal dialysis. Treatment with calcium salts or anticholinesterases reverses neuromuscular blockade.

Monitoring the patient
• Monitor cardiac and respiratory status.
• Monitor therapeutic effect.

Information for the patient
• Advise patient that inhalation doses should be taken as close to 12 hours apart as possible and no less than 6 hours apart.
• Teach patient how to correctly use and maintain nebulizer.

tocainide hydrochloride
Tonocard

Pharmacologic classification: local anesthetic (amide type)
Therapeutic classification: ventricular antiarrhythmic
Pregnancy risk category C

How supplied
Available by prescription only
Tablets: 400 mg, 600 mg

Indications, route, and dosage
Suppression of symptomatic ventricular arrhythmias, including frequent premature ventricular tachycardia
Dosage must be individualized based on antiarrhythmic response and tolerance.
Adults: Initially, 400 mg P.O. q 8 hours. Usual dose is between 1,200 and 1,800 mg/day, divided into three doses. Drug may be administered on a twice daily regimen if patient is able to tolerate the t.i.d. regimen.
✦ **Dosage adjustment.** Patients with impaired renal or hepatic function may be adequately treated with less than 1,200 mg/day.
◇ **Myotonic dystrophy**
Adults: 800 to 1,200 mg P.O. daily.
◇ **Trigeminal neuralgia**
Adults: 20 mg/kg/day P.O. t.i.d.

Pharmacodynamics
Antiarrhythmic action: Structurally similar to lidocaine and possesses similar electrophysiologic and hemodynamic effects. A class IB antiarrhythmic that suppresses automaticity and shortens the effective refractory period and action potential duration of His-Purkinje fibers and suppresses spontaneous ventricular depolarization during diastole. Conductive atrial tissue and AV conduction aren't affected significantly at therapeutic levels.
Unlike quinidine and procainamide, doesn't significantly alter hemodynamics when adminis-

tered in usual doses. Exerts effects on the conduction system, causing inhibition of reentry mechanisms and cessation of ventricular arrhythmias; these effects may be more pronounced in ischemic tissue. Doesn't cause a significant negative inotropic effect. Direct cardiac effects are less potent than those of lidocaine.

Pharmacokinetics
• *Absorption:* Rapidly and completely absorbed from GI tract; unlike lidocaine, it undergoes negligible first-pass effect in liver. Serum levels peak in 30 minutes to 2 hours after oral administration. Bioavailability is nearly 100%.
• *Distribution:* Only partially known. Appears to be distributed widely and apparently crosses blood-brain barrier and placenta (however, is less lipophilic than lidocaine). Only about 10% to 20% of drug is bound to plasma protein.
• *Metabolism:* Apparently metabolized in liver to inactive metabolites.
• *Excretion:* Excreted in urine as unchanged drug and inactive metabolites. About 30% to 50% of orally administered dose excreted in urine as metabolites. Elimination half-life is about 11 to 23 hours, with initial biphasic plasma level decline similar to that of lidocaine. Half-life may be prolonged in patients with renal or hepatic insufficiency. Urine alkalinization may substantially decrease amount of unchanged drug excreted in urine.

Contraindications and precautions
Contraindicated in patients with hypersensitivity to drug or other amide-type local anesthetics and in those with second- or third-degree AV block in the absence of an artificial pacemaker. Use cautiously in patients with heart failure, diminished cardiac reserve, preexisting bone marrow failure, cytopenia, or impaired renal or hepatic function.

Interactions
Drug-drug. *Allopurinol:* Increased effects of tocainide. Adjust dosage.
Antiarrhythmics: Additive, synergistic, or antagonistic effects. Use together with caution.
Cimetidine, rifampin: Decreased elimination half-life and bioavailability of tocainide. Adjust dosage.
Lidocaine: Possible CNS toxicity. When concomitant use can't be avoided, use with caution.
Metoprolol: Additive effect on cardiac index, left ventricular function, and pulmonary wedge pressure. Monitor patient for decreased myocardial contractility and bradycardia.

Adverse reactions
CNS: *light-headedness, tremor,* paresthesia, *dizziness, vertigo,* drowsiness, fatigue, confusion, headache.
CV: hypotension, ***new or worsened arrhythmias, heart failure,*** palpitations.
EENT: blurred vision, tinnitus.

GI: *nausea, vomiting,* diarrhea, anorexia.
Hematologic: ***blood dyscrasias.***
Hepatic: abnormal liver function test results, hepatitis.
Respiratory: ***respiratory arrest, pulmonary fibrosis, pneumonitis, pulmonary edema.***
Skin: rash, diaphoresis.

☑ Special considerations
• Use cautiously and at lower doses in patients with hepatic or renal impairment.
• Adverse effects tend to be frequent and problematic.
• Drug is considered an oral lidocaine and may be used to ease transition from I.V. lidocaine to oral antiarrhythmic therapy.
• Effects of overdose include extensions of common adverse reactions, particularly those associated with CNS or GI tract. Treatment generally involves symptomatic and supportive care. In acute overdose, gastric emptying should be performed via emesis induction or gastric lavage.
• Respiratory depression necessitates immediate attention and maintenance of a patent airway with ventilatory assistance, if needed. Seizures may be treated with small incremental doses of a benzodiazepine, such as diazepam or a short- or ultrashort-acting barbiturate, such as pentobarbital or thiopental.

Monitoring the patient
• Perform a chest X-ray if pulmonary symptoms exist.
• Monitor blood levels; therapeutic levels range from 4 to 10 mcg/ml.
• Monitor periodic blood counts for the first 3 months of therapy and frequently thereafter. Perform CBC promptly if patient develops signs of infection.
• Observe patient for tremors—a possible sign that maximum safe dose has been reached.

Information for the patient
• Advise patient to report unusual bleeding or bruising, signs or symptoms of infection (such as fever, sore throat, stomatitis, or chills) or pulmonary symptoms (such as cough, wheezing, or exertional dyspnea).
• Tell patient he may take drug with food to lessen GI upset.
• Tell patient that drug may cause drowsiness or dizziness and that he should use caution while performing tasks that require alertness.

Geriatric patients
• Use with caution in elderly patients; increased serum drug levels and toxicity are more likely in this age-group. Monitor these patients carefully.
• Elderly patients are more likely to experience dizziness and should have assistance while walking.

Breast-feeding patients
• Safety in breast-feeding women hasn't been established. Because it's unknown if drug appears in breast milk, an alternative to breast-feeding is recommended during therapy.

tolazamide
Tolinase

Pharmacologic classification: sulfonylurea
Therapeutic classification: antidiabetic
Pregnancy risk category C

How supplied
Tablets: 100 mg, 250 mg, 500 mg

Indications, route, and dosage
Adjunct to diet to lower blood glucose levels in patients with type 2 diabetes mellitus
Adults: Initially, 100 mg P.O. daily with breakfast if fasting blood sugar (FBS) is less than 200 mg/dl; or 250 mg P.O. daily if FBS is more than 200 mg/dl. May adjust dosage at weekly intervals in increments of 100 to 250 mg based on blood glucose response. Maximum dose is 500 mg P.O. b.i.d. before meals.
Elderly: Initially, 100 mg P.O. daily.
✦ *Dosage adjustment.* For malnourished or underweight patients, initially 100 mg P.O. daily.

Pharmacodynamics
Antidiabetic action: Lowers blood glucose levels by stimulating insulin release from functioning beta cells of the pancreas. After prolonged administration, the drug's hypoglycemic effects appear to reflect extrapancreatic effects, possibly including reduction of basal hepatic glucose production and enhanced peripheral sensitivity to insulin.

Pharmacokinetics
• *Absorption:* Well absorbed from GI tract. Serum levels peak in 3 to 4 hours; onset of action within 4 to 6 hours.
• *Distribution:* Probably distributed into extracellular fluid.
• *Metabolism:* Probably metabolized by liver to several mildly active metabolites.
• *Excretion:* Excreted in urine primarily as metabolites, with small amounts excreted as unchanged drug; half-life is 7 hours.

Contraindications and precautions
Contraindicated in patients with hypersensitivity to drug or other sulfonylureas and in those with uremia; type 1 diabetes mellitus or diabetes that can be adequately controlled by diet; or type 2 diabetes mellitus complicated by ketosis, acidosis, coma, or other acute complications, such as major surgery, severe infection, or severe trauma. Also contraindicated in pregnant or breast-feeding women.
Use cautiously in elderly patients, in debilitated or malnourished patients, and in those with impaired renal or hepatic function or adrenal or pituitary insufficiency.

Interactions
Drug-drug. *Beta blockers (including ophthalmics):* Increased risk of hypoglycemia; may mask its symptoms (rising pulse rate and blood pressure), and prolong it by blocking gluconeogenesis. Use together cautiously.
Calcium channel blockers, corticosteroids, estrogens, isoniazid, oral contraceptives, phenothiazines, phenytoin, sympathomimetics, thiazide diuretics, thyroid hormones, triamterene: Decreased hypoglycemic effect. Monitor blood glucose level and adjust dosage accordingly.
Chloramphenicol, insulin, MAO inhibitors, NSAIDs, probenecid, salicylates, sulfonamides: Enhanced hypoglycemic effect. Monitor blood glucose level closely.
Oral anticoagulants: Increased hypoglycemic activity or enhanced anticoagulant effect. Monitor blood glucose level, PT, and INR.
Drug-lifestyle. *Alcohol:* Possible disulfiram-like reaction (nausea, vomiting, abdominal cramps, headaches). Discourage use.

Adverse reactions
CNS: weakness, fatigue, dizziness, vertigo, malaise, headache.
GI: nausea, vomiting, epigastric distress, heartburn.
Hematologic: *leukopenia, hemolytic anemia, thrombocytopenia, aplastic anemia, agranulocytosis, pancytopenia.*
Metabolic: *hyponatremia, hypoglycemia.*
Other: photosensitivity reactions.

☑ Special considerations
Besides the recommendations relevant to all sulfonylureas, consider the following.
• To avoid GI intolerance in those patients receiving doses of 500 mg/day or more and to improve control of hyperglycemia, divided doses are recommended; these are given before the morning and evening meals.
• Tablets may be crushed to ease administration.
• Use with caution in women of childbearing age. Drug isn't recommended for treatment of diabetes associated with pregnancy.
• Oral antidiabetics have been associated with an increased risk of CV mortality as compared to diet alone or diet and insulin therapy.
• *To change from insulin to oral therapy with tolazamide:* If insulin dose is under 20 units daily, insulin may be stopped and oral therapy started at 100 mg P.O. daily in the morning. If insulin dose is 20 to 40 units daily, insulin may be stopped and oral therapy started at 250 mg P.O. daily in the

morning. If insulin dose is over 40 units daily, decrease insulin dose by 50% and start oral therapy at 250 mg P.O. daily with breakfast. Increase doses as appropriate based on blood glucose response.

• Signs and symptoms of overdose include low blood glucose levels, tingling of lips and tongue, hunger, nausea, decreased cerebral function (lethargy, yawning, confusion, agitation, nervousness), increased sympathetic activity (tachycardia, sweating, tremor), and, ultimately, seizures, stupor, and coma.

• Mild hypoglycemia, without loss of consciousness or neurologic symptoms, responds to treatment with oral glucose and adjustments in drug doses and meal patterns. If the patient loses consciousness or develops neurologic symptoms, he should receive rapid injection of dextrose 50%, then a continuous infusion of dextrose 10% at a rate to maintain blood glucose levels greater than 100 mg/dl. Monitor patient for 24 to 48 hours.

Monitoring the patient
• Over time, patients may become unresponsive to therapy with this drug as well as other sulfonylureas; monitor patient appropriately.
• When substituting tolazamide for chlorpropamide therapy, monitor patient closely for 1 to 2 weeks because of chlorpropamide's prolonged retention in the body, which may result in hypoglycemia.

Information for the patient
• Advise patient to take drug at same time each day. Tell patient that if a dose is missed, it should be taken immediately, unless it's almost time to take next dose. Patient shouldn't double the dose.
• Warn patient to avoid alcohol when taking drug.
• Encourage patient to wear a medical identification bracelet or necklace.
• Recommend that patient take drug with food if drug causes GI upset.

Geriatric patients
• Elderly patients may be more sensitive to effects of drug because of reduced metabolism and elimination.
• Hypoglycemia causes more neurologic symptoms in elderly patients.
• Elderly patients usually need a lower initial dose.

Pediatric patients
• Drug is ineffective in type 1 diabetes mellitus. Safety and effectiveness in children haven't been established.

Breast-feeding patients
• It's unknown if drug appears in breast milk. Because of risk of hypoglycemia in breast-fed infant, a risk/benefit decision should be made to stop either drug or breast-feeding.

tolbutamide
Orinase

Pharmacologic classification: sulfonylurea
Therapeutic classification: antidiabetic
Pregnancy risk category C

How supplied
Available by prescription only
Tablets: 500 mg

Indications, route, and dosage
Adjunct to diet to lower blood glucose levels in patients with type 2 diabetes mellitus
Adults: Initially, 1 to 2 g P.O. daily as single dose or divided b.i.d. or t.i.d. May adjust dosage to maximum of 3 g P.O. daily.

Pharmacodynamics
Antidiabetic action: Lowers blood glucose levels by stimulating insulin release from functioning beta cells of the pancreas. After prolonged administration, drug's hypoglycemic effects appear to reflect extrapancreatic effects, possibly including reduction of basal hepatic glucose production and enhanced peripheral sensitivity to insulin.

Pharmacokinetics
• *Absorption:* Absorbed readily from GI tract; levels peak in 3 to 4 hours.
• *Distribution:* Probably distributed into extracellular fluid; 95% bound to plasma proteins.
• *Metabolism:* Metabolized in liver to inactive metabolites.
• *Excretion:* Drug and metabolites excreted in urine and feces. Half-life is 4½ to 6½ hours.

Contraindications and precautions
Contraindicated in patients with hypersensitivity to drug or other sulfonylureas; in patients with type 1 diabetes mellitus or diabetes that can be adequately controlled by diet; in patients with type 2 diabetes mellitus complicated by fever, ketosis, acidosis, coma, or other acute complications, such as major surgery, severe infection, or severe trauma; in patients with severe renal insufficiency; and in pregnant or breast-feeding women.

Use cautiously in elderly, debilitated, or malnourished patients and in those with impaired renal or hepatic function or porphyria.

Interactions
Drug-drug. *Anticoagulants:* Increased hypoglycemic activity or enhanced anticoagulant effect. Monitor blood glucose levels, PT, and INR.
Beta blockers (including ophthalmics): Increased risk of hypoglycemia; masks developing symptoms (such as rising pulse rate and blood pres-

sure), and may prolong hypoglycemia by blocking gluconeogenesis. Use together cautiously.

Calcium channel blockers, corticosteroids, estrogens, isoniazid, oral contraceptives, phenothiazines, phenytoin, sympathomimetics, thiazide diuretics, thyroid products, triamterene: Decreased hypoglycemic effect. Monitor blood glucose level and adjust dosage accordingly.

Chloramphenicol, insulin, monoamine oxidase inhibitors, NSAIDs, probenecid, salicylates, sulfonamides: Enhanced hypoglycemic effect by displacing tolbutamide from its protein-binding sites. Monitor blood glucose levels closely.

Drug-lifestyle. *Alcohol:* Possible disulfiram-like reaction (nausea, vomiting, abdominal cramps, headaches). Discourage use.

Adverse reactions

CNS: headache.
EENT: taste alterations.
GI: nausea, heartburn, epigastric distress.
Hematologic: *leukopenia,* hemolytic anemia, **thrombocytopenia, aplastic anemia, agranulocytosis, pancytopenia.**
Hepatic: hepatic porphyria.
Metabolic: hypoglycemia, dilutional hyponatremia, SIADH secretion.
Skin: rash, pruritus, erythema, urticaria.
Other: *hypersensitivity reactions,* disulfiram-like *reactions.*

☑ Special considerations

Besides the recommendations relevant to all sulfonylureas, consider the following.

● Elderly or debilitated patients and those with impaired renal or hepatic function usually need a lower initial dose.
● To avoid GI intolerance for those patients on larger doses and to improve control of hyperglycemia, divided doses given before the morning and evening meals are recommended.
● Patients should avoid taking drug at bedtime because of the potential for nocturnal hypoglycemia.
● Use with caution in women of childbearing age. Drug isn't recommended for treatment of diabetes associated with pregnancy.
● Oral antidiabetics have been associated with an increased risk of CV mortality as compared to diet alone or diet and insulin therapy.
● When substituting tolbutamide for chlorpropamide therapy, monitor patient closely for the first 2 weeks because of chlorpropamide's prolonged retention in the body, which may result in hypoglycemia.
● To change from insulin to oral therapy with tolbutamide: If insulin dose is under 20 units daily, insulin may be stopped and oral therapy started at 1 to 2 g daily. If insulin dose is 20 to 40 units daily, insulin dose is reduced 30% to 50% and oral therapy started as above. If insulin dose is over 40 units daily, insulin dose is decreased 20% and

oral therapy started as above. Further reductions in insulin dose are based on patient's response to oral therapy.

● Drug may give a false positive result for albumin in the urine if measured by the acidification-after-boiling test. There is no interference with the sulfosalicylic acid test.
● Signs and symptoms of overdose include low blood glucose levels, tingling of lips and tongue, hunger, nausea, decreased cerebral function (lethargy, yawning, confusion, agitation, nervousness), increased sympathetic activity (tachycardia, sweating, tremor), and, ultimately, seizures, stupor, and coma.
● Mild hypoglycemia, without loss of consciousness or neurologic symptoms, responds to treatment with oral glucose and dosage adjustments. If patient loses consciousness or develops neurologic symptoms, he should receive rapid injection of dextrose 50%, then a continuous infusion of dextrose 10% at a rate to maintain blood glucose levels greater than 100 mg/dl. Monitor patient for 24 to 48 hours.

Monitoring the patient

● Monitor therapeutic effect.
● Monitor patient for signs of adverse effects.

Information for the patient

● Advise patient to take drug at the same time each day.
● Inform patient that, if a dose is missed, it should be taken immediately unless it's almost time to take the next dose. Patient shouldn't double dose.
● Advise patient to avoid alcohol while taking drug because of prolonged hypoglycemic effect. Remind him that many foods and OTC drugs contain alcohol.
● Encourage patient to wear a medical identification bracelet or necklace.
● Suggest that patient take drug with food if it causes GI upset.

Geriatric patients

● Elderly patients may be more sensitive to effects of this drug because of reduced metabolism and elimination.
● Hypoglycemia causes more neurologic symptoms in elderly patients than in younger patients.
● Elderly patients usually need a lower initial dose.

Pediatric patients

● Drug is ineffective in type 1 diabetes mellitus. Safety and effectiveness in children haven't been established.

Breast-feeding patients

● Drug appears in breast milk. Because of risk of hypoglycemia in breast-fed infant, a decision should be made to stop either drug or breast-feeding.

Reactions may be *common,* uncommon, **life-threatening,** or COMMON AND LIFE-THREATENING.

tolcapone
Tasmar

Pharmacologic classification: catechol-O-methyltransferase (COMT) inhibitor
Therapeutic classification: antiparkinsonian
Pregnancy risk category C

How supplied
Available by prescription only
Tablets: 100 mg, 200 mg

Indications, route, and dosage
Adjunct to levodopa and carbidopa for treatment of signs and symptoms of idiopathic Parkinson's disease
Adults: Recommended initial dosage is 100 mg (preferred) or 200 mg P.O. t.i.d. If treatment is initiated with 200 mg t.i.d. and dyskinesias occur, a decrease in levodopa dose may be needed. Maximum daily dose is 600 mg. Always give with levodopa-carbidopa. The first tolcapone dose of the day should always be taken with the first levodopa-carbidopa dose of the day.

Pharmacodynamics
Antiparkinsonian action: Exact mechanism unknown. Thought to reversibly inhibit human erythrocyte COMT when given with levodopa-carbidopa, resulting in a decrease in the clearance of levodopa and a twofold increase in the bioavailability of levodopa. The decrease in clearance of levodopa prolongs the elimination half-life of levodopa from 2 to 3½ hours.

Pharmacokinetics
• *Absorption:* Rapidly absorbed; plasma levels peak within 2 hours. After oral administration, absolute bioavailability is 65%. Onset of effect occurs after first dose. Absorption decreases when given within 1 hour before or 2 hours after food, but can be given without regard to meals.
• *Distribution:* Over 99.9% bound to plasma proteins, primarily to albumin. Small steady-state volume of distribution.
• *Metabolism:* Completely metabolized before excretion. Main mechanism of metabolism is glucuronidation.
• *Excretion:* Only 0.5% of dose found unchanged in urine. Is a low-extraction-ratio drug with a systemic clearance of 7 L/hour. Elimination half-life is 2 to 3 hours. Dialysis isn't expected to affect clearance because of high protein-binding.

Contraindications and precautions
Contraindicated in patients with hypersensitivity to drug or its components; in those with liver disease or ALT or AST levels exceeding the upper limit of normal; patients withdrawn from therapy because of drug-induced hepatocellular injury; and patients with history of nontraumatic rhabdomyolysis or hyperpyrexia and confusion, possibly related to drug.
Use cautiously in patients with Parkinson's disease because syncope and orthostatic hypotension may worsen.

Interactions
Drug-drug. *Desipramine:* Increases adverse effects. Use cautiously together.
MAO inhibitors: Possible hypertensive crisis. Avoid concomitant use.

Adverse reactions
CNS: *dyskinesia, sleep disorder, dystonia, excessive dreaming, somnolence, dizziness, confusion,* headache, hallucinations, hyperkinesia, fatigue, falling, syncope, balance loss, depression, tremor, speech disorder, paresthesia.
CV: *orthostatic complaints,* chest pain, chest discomfort, palpitation, hypotension.
EENT: pharyngitis, tinnitus.
GI: *nausea, anorexia, diarrhea,* flatulence, *vomiting,* constipation, abdominal pain, dyspepsia, dry mouth.
GU: urinary tract infection, urine discoloration, hematuria, urinary incontinence, impotence.
Musculoskeletal: *muscle cramps,* myalgia, stiffness, arthritis, neck pain.
Respiratory: bronchitis, dyspnea, upper respiratory infections.
Skin: increased sweating, rash.

☑ Special considerations
• Because of risk of potentially fatal, acute fulminant liver failure, use drug only in patients on levodopa-carbidopa who don't respond to or who aren't suitable for other adjunctive therapy.
• Don't use drug until risks have been discussed and the patient has given a written informed consent.
• Safety of this drug hasn't been established for patients with creatinine clearance below 25 ml/minute.
• Diarrhea occurs commonly in patients treated with this drug. It may occur 2 weeks after therapy begins or after 6 to 12 weeks. Although diarrhea usually resolves when drug is stopped, hospitalization may be needed in rare cases.
• Dosage adjustments aren't needed in patients with mild to moderate renal dysfunction; use cautiously in patients with severe renal impairment.
• Stop drug in patients who fail to show clinical benefit within 3 weeks of treatment.
• Don't use drug with a nonselective MAO inhibitor.
• The highest dose administered is 800 mg t.i.d.; nausea, vomiting, and dizziness occurred. Provide supportive care and hospitalize patient, if indicated.

Monitoring the patient
- Monitor liver enzymes every 2 weeks for the first year of therapy, and then every 8 weeks. Stop drug if hepatic transaminase levels exceed the upper limit of normal or if patient appears jaundiced.
- Monitor therapeutic progress closely.

Information for the patient
- Advise patient to take drug exactly as prescribed.
- Warn patient about risk of orthostatic hypotension; tell him to use caution when rising from a seated or recumbent position.
- Caution patient to avoid hazardous activities until CNS effects of drug are known.
- Tell patient that nausea may occur and to report signs of liver injury immediately.
- Advise patient about risk of increased dyskinesia or dystonia.
- Inform patient that hallucinations may occur.
- Tell woman to report if pregnancy is being planned or is suspected during therapy.

Pediatric patients
- There is no identified potential use in children.

Breast-feeding patients
- Drug may appear in breast milk; use with caution in breast-feeding women.

---

tolmetin sodium
Tolectin, Tolectin DS

Pharmacologic classification: NSAID
Therapeutic classification: nonnarcotic analgesic, anti-inflammatory
Pregnancy risk category C

How supplied
Tablets: 200 mg, 600 mg
Capsules: 400 mg

Indications, route, and dosage
Rheumatoid arthritis and osteoarthritis, juvenile rheumatoid arthritis
Adults: Initially, 400 mg P.O. t.i.d. Maximum dose is 1,800 mg/day; usual dose ranges from 600 to 1,800 mg daily in three divided doses.
Children ages 2 and older: Initially, 20 mg/kg/day in three or four divided doses; usual dose ranges from 15 to 30 mg/kg/day in three or four divided doses.

Pharmacodynamics
Analgesic and anti-inflammatory actions: Exact mechanisms unknown. Thought that inhibition of prostaglandin synthesis may be responsible for anti-inflammatory effects of tolmetin. Drug also seems to possess analgesic and antipyretic activity.

Pharmacokinetics
- *Absorption:* Absorbed rapidly from GI tract; levels peak within 30 to 60 minutes.
- *Distribution:* Highly protein-bound.
- *Metabolism:* Metabolized in liver.
- *Excretion:* Essentially all drug excreted in urine within 24 hours as inactive metabolite or conjugates of tolmetin. Biphasic elimination; rapid phase with a half-life of 1 to 2 hours, then a slower phase with a half-life of about 5 hours.

Contraindications and precautions
Contraindicated in patients with hypersensitivity to drug or in whom acute asthmatic attacks, urticaria, or rhinitis is precipitated by aspirin or NSAIDs. Also contraindicated in breast-feeding women. Use cautiously in patients with renal or cardiac disease, GI bleeding, history of peptic ulcer, hypertension, and conditions predisposing to fluid retention.

Interactions
Drug-drug. *Anticoagulants, thrombolytics:* Increased risk of bleeding. Use caution when giving concomitantly.
Aspirin: Decreased plasma levels of tolmetin. Avoid concomitant use.
Highly protein-bound drugs (phenytoin, salicylates, sulfonamides, sulfonylureas, warfarin): Possible displacement of either drug and increased adverse effects. Monitor therapy closely for both drugs.
Methotrexate: Increased methotrexate toxicity. Avoid concurrent use. If given together, monitor patient closely.
Sodium bicarbonate: Reduced bioavailablity. Avoid concomitant use.
Other GI irritating drugs (such as antibiotics, corticosteroids, NSAIDs): Potentiated adverse GI effects of tolmetin. Use together cautiously.
Drug-food. *Any food:* Delayed and decreased absorption of tolmetin. Separate administration times.

Adverse reactions
CNS: headache, dizziness, drowsiness, asthenia, depression.
CV: chest pain, hypertension, edema.
EENT: tinnitus, visual disturbances.
GI: epigastric distress, peptic ulceration, occult blood loss, *nausea,* vomiting, abdominal pain, diarrhea, constipation, dyspepsia, flatulence, anorexia.
GU: urinary tract infection.
Hematologic: elevated BUN level, decreased hemoglobin level and hematocrit.
Metabolic: weight gain, weight loss.
Skin: irritation.
Other: *anaphylaxis.*

Reactions may be *common,* uncommon, *life-threatening,* or COMMON AND LIFE-THREATENING.

☑ Special considerations

Besides the recommendations relevant to all NSAIDs, consider the following.

• Therapeutic effect usually occurs within a few days to 1 week of therapy. Evaluate patient's response to drug as evidenced by relief of symptoms.

• Administer drug on empty stomach for maximum absorption. However, drug may be given with meals to lessen GI upset.

• Tolmetin falsely elevates results of urinary protein (pseudoproteinuria) in tests that rely on acid precipitation, such as those using sulfosalicylic acid. The drug doesn't interfere with tests for proteinuria using dye-impregnated reagent strips like Albustix or Unistix.

• Signs and symptoms of overdose include dizziness, drowsiness, mental confusion, and lethargy. For overdose, empty stomach immediately by inducing emesis or by gastric lavage; then use activated charcoal. Provide symptomatic and supportive measures (respiratory support and correction of fluid and electrolyte imbalances). Monitor laboratory parameters and vital signs closely. Alkalinization of urine via sodium bicarbonate ingestion may enhance renal excretion of tolmetin.

Monitoring the patient

• Assess cardiopulmonary status closely. Monitor vital signs closely, especially heart rate and blood pressure.

• Assess renal function periodically during therapy; monitor fluid intake and output and daily weight. Monitor patient for presence and amount of edema.

Information for the patient

• Explain that therapeutic effects may occur in 1 week but could take 2 to 4 weeks.

• Advise patient to avoid use of OTC products such as NSAIDs unless medically approved.

• Advise patient to report any signs of edema. Tell patient to routinely check weight and to report any significant weight gain or loss within 1 week.

• Tell patient to report adverse reactions.

Pediatric patients

• Safety and effectiveness in children under age 2 haven't been established.

Breast-feeding patients

• Drug appears in breast milk and may adversely affect neonates; avoid use in breast-feeding women.

tolterodine tartrate
Detrol

Pharmacologic classification: muscarinic receptor antagonist
Therapeutic classification: anticholinergic
Pregnancy risk category C

How supplied

Available by prescription only
Tablets: 1 mg, 2 mg

Indications, route, and dosage

Patients with overactive bladder with symptoms of urinary frequency, urgency, or urge incontinence

Adults: Initial dosage is 2 mg P.O. b.i.d. May lower to 1 mg b.i.d. based on response and tolerance.

✦ *Dosage adjustment.* In patients with significantly reduced hepatic function or who are currently taking a drug that inhibits the cytochrome P-450 3A4 isoenzyme system, recommended dose is 1 mg b.i.d.

Pharmacodynamics

Anticholinergic action: Competitive muscarinic receptor antagonist. Both urinary bladder contraction and salivation are mediated via cholinergic muscarinic receptors.

Pharmacokinetics

• *Absorption:* Well absorbed with about 77% bioavailability. Serum levels peak within 1 to 2 hours. Food increases bioavailability by 53%.

• *Distribution:* Volume of distribution is about 113 L. Drug is 96% protein-bound.

• *Metabolism:* Metabolized by liver primarily by oxidation by cytochrome P-450 2D6 pathway; pharmacologically active 5-hydroxymethyl metabolite formed.

• *Excretion:* Mostly recovered in urine; rest in feces. Less than 1% of dose recovered as unchanged drug; 5% to 14% recovered as active metabolite. Half-life is 1¾ to 3½ hours.

Contraindications and precautions

Contraindicated in patients with hypersensitivity to drug or its components and in those with urine or gastric retention or uncontrolled narrow-angle glaucoma. Use with caution in patients with significantly reduced hepatic or renal function.

Interactions

Drug-drug. *Cytochrome P-450 3A4 inhibitors such as antifungals (itraconazole, ketoconazole, miconazole), macrolide antibiotics (clarithromycin, erythromycin):* No data on interaction. However, don't give doses of tolterodine above 1 mg b.i

Fluoxetine: Inhibited metabolism of tolterodine. No dosage adjustment needed.
Drug-food. *Any food:* Increased absorption of tolterodine. No dosage adjustment needed.

Adverse reactions
CNS: paresthesia, vertigo, dizziness, *headache,* nervousness, somnolence, fatigue.
CV: hypertension, chest pain.
EENT: abnormal vision (including accommodation), xerophthalmia, pharyngitis, rhinitis, sinusitis.
GI: *dry mouth,* abdominal pain, constipation, diarrhea, dyspepsia, flatulence, nausea, vomiting.
GU: dysuria, micturition frequency, urine retention, urinary tract infection.
Metabolic: weight gain.
Musculoskeletal: arthralgia, back pain.
Respiratory: bronchitis, coughing, upper respiratory tract infection.
Skin: pruritus, rash, erythema, dry skin.
Other: flulike symptoms.

☑ Special considerations
• Food increases absorption of tolterodine, but no dosage adjustment is needed.
• Dry mouth is the most frequently reported adverse effect.
• Overdoses can result in severe central anticholinergic effects and should be treated accordingly. Perform ECG monitoring if an overdose occurs.

Monitoring the patient
• Monitor therapeutic effect.
• Monitor patient for signs of adverse effects.

Information for the patient
• Inform patient that antimuscarinics such as tolterodine may produce blurred vision.
• Caution patient to avoid hazardous activities until drug's effects are known.

Geriatric patients
• No overall differences in safety have been observed between older and younger patients.

Pediatric patients
• Safety and effectiveness in children haven't been established.

Breast-feeding patients
• It's unknown if drug appears in breast milk. Not recommended for use in breast-feeding women.

topiramate
Topamax

Pharmacologic classification: sulfamate-substituted monosaccharide
Therapeutic classification: antiepileptic
Pregnancy risk category C

How supplied
Available by prescription only
Tablets: 25 mg, 100 mg, 200 mg
Capsules: 15 mg, 25 mg, 50 mg

Indications, route, and dosage
Adjunctive therapy of partial onset seizures
Adults: Adjust to maximum daily dose of 400 mg in two divided doses. Adjustment schedule is as follows.

Week	A.M. dose	P.M. dose
1	None	50 mg
2	50 mg	50 mg
3	50 mg	100 mg
4	100 mg	100 mg
5	100 mg	150 mg
6	150 mg	150 mg
7	150 mg	200 mg
8	200 mg	200 mg

✦ *Dosage adjustment.* For patients with moderate to severe renal impairment, reduce dosage by 50%. A supplemental dose may be needed during hemodialysis.

Pharmacodynamics
Antiepileptic action: Mechanism unknown. Thought to block action potential, suggestive of a state-dependent sodium channel blocking action. May increase frequency at which gamma-aminobutyric acid (GABA) activates $GABA_A$ receptors as well as enhances the ability of GABA to induce a flux of chloride ions into neurons, suggesting that topiramate potentiates the activity of the inhibitory neurotransmitter. May also antagonize ability of kainate to activate the kainate/AMPA subtype of excitatory amino acid (glutamate) receptor. Also has weak carbonic anhydrase inhibitor activity, which is unrelated to drug's antiepileptic properties.

Pharmacokinetics
• *Absorption:* Rapidly absorbed; plasma levels peak about 2 hours after 400-mg oral dose. Relative bioavailability about 80% compared with a solution; not affected by food.
• *Distribution:* Plasma levels increase proportionately with dose; mean elimination half-life is

21 hours. Steady-state reached in 4 days in patients with normal renal function. 13% to 17% bound to plasma proteins.
• *Metabolism:* Not extensively metabolized.
• *Excretion:* About 70% of dose eliminated unchanged in urine. Mean plasma half-life is 21 hours.

Contraindications and precautions
Contraindicated in patients with history of hypersensitivity to drug or its components. Use cautiously in patients with hepatic or renal impairment because drug clearance may be decreased.

Interactions
Drug-drug. *Carbamazepine, phenytoin:* Decreased topiramate levels; increased phenytoin levels. Monitor patient closely; adjust dosage as needed.
Carbonic anhydrase inhibitors (acetazolamide, dichlorphenamide): Increased risk of renal stone formation. Avoid concomitant use.
Oral contraceptives: Compromised contraceptive effect. Advise second method of contraception during therapy.
Drug-lifestyle. *Alcohol:* Possible topiramate-induced CNS depression and other adverse cognitive and neuropsychiatric events. Discourage use.

Adverse reactions
CNS: abnormal coordination; agitation; apathy; asthenia; *ataxia; confusion;* depression; difficulty with concentration, attention, language, or memory; *dizziness;* emotional lability; euphoria; *fatigue; generalized tonic-clonic seizures;* hallucination; hyperkinesia; hypertonia; hypoesthesia; hypokinesia; insomnia; malaise, mood problems; *nervousness; nystagmus; paresthesia;* personality disorder; *psychomotor slowing;* psychosis; *somnolence; speech disorders;* stupor; *suicide attempts; tremor;* vertigo.
CV: chest pain, palpitations.
EENT: *abnormal vision,* conjunctivitis, *diplopia,* eye pain, epistaxis, hearing or vestibular problems, pharyngitis, sinusitis, taste perversion, tinnitus.
GI: abdominal pain, anorexia, constipation, diarrhea, dry mouth, dyspepsia, flatulence, gastroenteritis, gingivitis, *nausea,* vomiting.
GU: amenorrhea, dysuria, dysmenorrhea, leukorrhea, hematuria, impotence, intermenstrual bleeding, menstrual disorder, menorrhagia, micturition frequency, renal calculus, urinary incontinence, urinary tract infection, vaginitis.
Hematologic: anemia, leukopenia.
Metabolic: increased or decreased weight.
Musculoskeletal: back pain, leg pain, myalgia.
Respiratory: bronchitis, coughing, dyspnea, *upper respiratory tract infection.*
Skin: acne, alopecia, aggressive reaction, increased sweating, pruritus, rash.

Other: body odor, edema, fever, flulike symptoms, hot flashes, rigors.

☑ Special considerations
• Carefully review dosing schedule with patient to avoid under- or overmedication.
• If necessary, withdraw antiepileptic (including topiramate) gradually to minimize risk of increased seizure activity.
• Because of bitter taste, tablets shouldn't be broken.
• In acute overdose after recent ingestion, institute gastric lavage or emesis. Activated charcoal isn't recommended. Institute supportive treatment. Hemodialysis is an effective means of removing drug.

Monitoring the patient
• Monitor therapeutic effect.
• Monitor patient for adverse effects.

Information for the patient
• Tell patient to maintain adequate fluid intake during therapy because of potential for formation of renal stones.
• Advise patient to avoid hazardous activities until drug's effects are known.
• Tell patient drug may be taken without regard to meals.

Geriatric patients
• No age-related differences or adverse effects have been seen in elderly patients; however, age-related renal abnormalities should be considered.

Pediatric patients
• Safety and effectiveness in children haven't been established.

Breast-feeding patients
• It's unknown if drug appears in breast milk; use with caution in breast-feeding women.

topotecan hydrochloride
Hycamtin

Pharmacologic classification: semisynthetic camptothecin derivative
Therapeutic classification: antineoplastic
Pregnancy risk category D

How supplied
Available by prescription only
Injection: 4-mg single-dose vial

Indications, route, and dosage
Metastatic carcinoma of the ovary after failure of initial or subsequent chemotherapy
Adults: 1.5 mg/m²/day as an I.V. infusion given over 30 minutes for 5 consecutive days, starting

on day 1 of a 21-day cycle. Minimum of four cycles should be given.

✦ *Dosage adjustment.* In adults with renal impairment and creatinine clearance of 20 to 39 ml/minute, adjust dosage to 0.75 mg/m². In patients with mild renal impairment (creatinine clearance, 40 to 60 ml/minute), adjustment isn't needed. There are insufficient data available for a dosage recommendation for patients with creatinine clearance under 20 ml/minute. In the event of severe neutropenia occurring during any course, reduce dose by 0.25 mg/m² for subsequent courses. Or administer granulocyte colony–stimulating factor (G-CSF) starting from day 6 of subsequent courses (24 hours after completion of topotecan) before resorting to dosage reduction.

Small cell lung cancer sensitive disease after failure of first-line chemotherapy
Adults: 1.5 mg/m² I.V. infusion given over 30 minutes daily for 5 consecutive days, starting on day 1 of 21-day cycle. Minimum of four cycles should be given.

✦ *Dosage adjustment.* In patients with creatinine clearance of 20 to 39 ml/minute, dose is decreased to 0.75 mg/m². If severe neutropenia occurs, dose is decreased by 0.25 mg/m² for subsequent courses. Or if severe neutropenia occurs, G-CSF may be administered after the subsequent course (before resorting to dosage reduction) starting from day 6 of course (24 hours after completion of topotecan administration).

Pharmacodynamics
Antineoplastic action: Relieves torsional strain in DNA by inducing reversible single-strand breaks. Binds to the topoisomerase I–DNA complex and prevents religation of these single-strand breaks. The cytotoxicity of topotecan is thought to be due to double-strand DNA damage produced during DNA synthesis when replication enzymes interact with the ternary complex formed by topotecan, topoisomerase I, and DNA.

Pharmacokinetics
● *Absorption:* Given only I.V.
● *Distribution:* About 35% of drug is bound to plasma protein.
● *Metabolism:* Drug undergoes reversible pH-dependent hydrolysis of its lactone moiety; lactone form is pharmacologically active.
● *Excretion:* About 30% of drug excreted in urine. Terminal half-life is 2 to 3 hours.

Contraindications and precautions
Contraindicated in patients with hypersensitivity to drug or its components, in those with severe bone marrow depression, and in pregnant or breast-feeding women.

Interactions
Drug-drug. *Cisplatin:* Increased severity of myelosuppression. Use cautiously together.
G-CSF: Prolonged duration of neutropenia; if G-CSF is to be used, don't initiate until day 6 of course of therapy, 24 hours after completion of treatment with topotecan.

Adverse reactions
CNS: *fatigue, asthenia, headache,* paresthesia.
GI: *nausea, vomiting, diarrhea, constipation, abdominal pain, stomatitis, anorexia.*
Hematologic: NEUTROPENIA, LEUKOPENIA, THROMBOCYTOPENIA, *anemia.*
Hepatic: transient elevations of liver enzyme levels.
Respiratory: *dyspnea.*
Skin: *alopecia.*
Other: *sepsis,* fever.

☑ Special considerations
● Before administration of the first course, patient should have neutrophil count over 1,500 cells/mm³ and platelet count over 100,000 cells/mm³.
● Prepare drug under a vertical laminar flow hood and wear gloves and protective clothing. If drug solution contacts the skin, wash the skin immediately and thoroughly with soap and water. If mucous membranes are affected, flush areas thoroughly with water.
● Reconstitute each 4-mg vial with 4 ml sterile water for injection. Then dilute appropriate volume of reconstituted solution in either normal saline solution or D₅W before use.
● Protect unopened vials from light. Reconstituted vials are stable at about 68° to 77° F (20° to 25° C) and ambient lighting conditions for 24 hours.
● Bone marrow suppression (primarily neutropenia) is the dose-limiting toxicity of topotecan. The nadir occurs at about 11 days. If severe neutropenia occurs during therapy, reduce dosage by 0.25 mg/m² for subsequent courses. Or administer G-CSF after the subsequent course (before dose is reduced) starting from day 6 (24 hours after completion of topotecan administration). Neutropenia isn't cumulative over time.
● Thrombocytopenia occurred with a median duration of 5 days and platelet nadir at a median of 15 days; anemia occurred with a median nadir at day 15. Blood or platelet (or both) transfusions may be needed.
● Inadvertent extravasation with topotecan has been associated with only mild local reactions, such as erythema and bruising.
● The primary adverse effect associated with overdose is thought to be bone marrow suppression. Treatment should be supportive; there is no known antidote.

Monitoring the patient
• Frequent monitoring of peripheral blood cell counts is needed. Don't give patients subsequent courses of topotecan until neutrophil counts exceed 1,000 cells/mm³, platelet counts are over 100,000 cells/mm³, and hemoglobin levels are 9 mg/dl (with transfusion if needed).
• Monitor patient for adverse effects.

Information for the patient
• Advise patient to report any adverse effects immediately.

Pediatric patients
• Safety and effectiveness in children haven't been established.

Breast-feeding patients
• It's unknown if drug appears in breast milk, avoid use in breast-feeding women.

toremifene citrate
Fareston

Pharmacologic classification: nonsteroidal antiestrogen
Therapeutic classification: antineoplastic
Pregnancy risk category D

How supplied
Available by prescription only
Tablets: 60 mg

Indications, route, and dosage
Metastatic breast cancer in postmenopausal women with estrogen-receptor positive or unknown tumors
Adults: 60 mg P.O. once daily. Treatment is usually continued until disease progression is observed.

Pharmacodynamics
Antineoplastic action: Nonsteroidal triphenylethylene derivative that exerts antitumor effect by competing with estrogen for binding sites in the tumor. This blocks the growth-stimulating effects of endogenous estrogen in the tumor, causing an antiestrogenic effect.

Pharmacokinetics
• *Absorption:* Well absorbed after oral administration; not influenced by food. Plasma levels peak within 3 hours. Steady-state levels in about 4 to 6 weeks.
• *Distribution:* Apparent volume of distribution is 580 L; over 99.5% of drug binds to serum proteins, mainly albumin.
• *Metabolism:* Extensively metabolized, mainly by CYP 3A4, to N-demethyltoremifene, which is also antiestrogenic but with weak in vivo antitumor potency. Elimination half-life is about 5 days.

• *Excretion:* Eliminated in feces; about 10% excreted unchanged in urine. Slow elimination because of enterohepatic circulation.

Contraindications and precautions
Contraindicated in patients with hypersensitivity to drug. Avoid use in patients with history of thromboembolic diseases. Don't use drug long-term in patients with preexisting endometrial hyperplasia.

Interactions
Drug-drug. *Coumarin-like anticoagulants (such as warfarin):* Further prolongation of PT and INR. Monitor PT and INR closely.
Cytochrome P-450 3A4 enzyme inducers (such as carbamazepine, phenobarbital, phenytoin): Increased rate of toremifene metabolism. Adjust dosage as needed.
Cytochrome P-450 3A4-6 enzyme inhibitors (erythromycin, ketoconazole): Decreased toremifene metabolism. Adjust dosage as needed.
Drugs that decrease renal calcium excretion (such as thiazide diuretics): Increased risk of hypercalcemia. Monitor calcium levels closely.

Adverse reactions
CNS: dizziness, fatigue, depression.
CV: edema, **thromboembolism, heart failure, MI, pulmonary embolism.**
EENT: visual disturbances, glaucoma, ocular changes (such as dry eyes), *cataracts, abnormal visual fields.*
GI: *nausea,* vomiting.
GU: *vaginal discharge,* vaginal bleeding.
Hepatic: *elevated AST, alkaline phosphatase,* and bilirubin levels.
Metabolic: hypercalcemia.
Skin: *sweating.*
Other: *hot flashes.*

☑ Special considerations
• Drug causes fetal harm when given to pregnant women. If used during pregnancy, or if patient becomes pregnant while receiving toremifene, counsel her about potential hazard to fetus or risk of pregnancy loss.
• Overdose expected to produce increase of antiestrogenic effects (hot flashes), estrogenic effects (vaginal bleeding), or nervous system disorders (vertigo, dizziness, ataxia, and nausea). No specific antidote; treatment is symptomatic.

Monitoring the patient
• Obtain periodic CBC, calcium levels, and liver function tests.
• Monitor calcium levels closely for first weeks of treatment in patients with bone metastases because of increased risk of hypercalcemia and tumor flare.

Information for the patient
- Advise patient to take drug exactly as prescribed.
- Inform patient to report vaginal bleeding and other adverse effects.
- Warn patient that a disease flare-up may occur during first weeks of therapy. Reassure her that this doesn't indicate treatment failure.
- Advise patient to report leg or chest pain, severe headache, visual changes, or dyspnea.
- Inform patient with bone metastases of the signs and symptoms of hypercalcemia; tell her to call if they occur.

Geriatric patients
- No significant age-related differences in effectiveness or safety have been noted.

Breast-feeding patients
- It's unknown if drug appears in breast milk. Avoid use in breast-feeding women.

---

torsemide
Demadex

Pharmacologic classification: loop diuretic
Therapeutic classification: diuretic, antihypertensive
Pregnancy risk category B

How supplied
Available by prescription only
Tablets: 5 mg, 10 mg, 20 mg, 100 mg
Solution: 2-ml ampule (10 mg/ml), 5-ml ampule (10 mg/ml)

Indications, route, and dosage
Diuresis in patients with heart failure
Adults: Initially, 10 to 20 mg P.O. or I.V. once daily. If response is inadequate, double the dose until response is obtained. Maximum dose is 200 mg daily.
Diuresis in patients with chronic renal failure
Adults: Initially, 20 mg P.O. or I.V. once daily. If response is inadequate, double the dose until response is obtained. Maximum dose is 200 mg daily.
Diuresis in patients with hepatic cirrhosis
Adults: Initially, 5 to 10 mg P.O. or I.V. once daily with an aldosterone antagonist or a potassium-sparing diuretic. If response is inadequate, double the dose until response is obtained. Maximum dose is 40 mg daily.
Hypertension
Adults: Initially, 5 mg P.O. daily. Increase to 10 mg once daily in 4 to 6 weeks, if needed and tolerated. If response is still inadequate, add another antihypertensive.

Pharmacodynamics
Diuretic and antihypertensive actions: Loop diuretics enhance excretion of sodium, chloride, and water by acting on the ascending portion of the loop of Henle. Torsemide doesn't significantly alter glomerular filtration rate, renal plasma flow, or acid-base balance.

Pharmacokinetics
- *Absorption:* Absorbed with little first-pass metabolism; serum level peaks within 1 hour after oral administration.
- *Distribution:* Volume of distribution is 12 to 15 L in healthy patients and in those with mild to moderate renal failure or heart failure. In patients with hepatic cirrhosis, volume of distribution is about doubled. 97% to 99% bound to plasma protein.
- *Metabolism:* Metabolized in liver to inactive major metabolite and to two lesser metabolites that have some diuretic activity; for practical purposes, metabolism terminates drug action. Duration of action is 6 to 8 hours after oral or I.V. use.
- *Excretion:* From 22% to 34% of dose excreted unchanged in urine via active secretion of drug by proximal tubules.

Contraindications and precautions
Contraindicated in patients with hypersensitivity to drug or other sulfonylurea derivatives and in those with anuria. Use cautiously in patients with hepatic disease and associated cirrhosis and ascites.

Interactions
Drug-drug. *Cholestyramine:* Decreased torsemide absorption. Separate administration times by at least 3 hours.
Digoxin: Decreased torsemide clearance. Monitor patient closely.
Indomethacin, probenecid: Decreased diuretic effect. Monitor patient closely. If concomitant use can't be avoided, adjust dosage
Lithium: Lithium toxicity. Avoid concomitant use. If concomitant use can't be avoided, adjust dosage as needed.
NSAIDs: Renal dysfunction. Use together cautiously.
Ototoxic drugs (such as aminoglycosides): Increased potential for ototoxicity. Avoid concomitant use.
Salicylates: Reduced excretion of salicylates; possible salicylate toxicity. Avoid concomitant use.
Spironolactone: Decreased spironolactone clearance. Monitor patient closely.

Adverse reactions
CNS: asthenia, dizziness, headache, nervousness, insomnia, syncope.
CV: ECG abnormalities, chest pain, edema.
EENT: rhinitis, sore throat.
GI: diarrhea, constipation, nausea, dyspepsia.

---

actions may be *common,* uncommon, *life-threatening,* or COMMON AND LIFE-THREATENING.

GU: *excessive urination,* altered renal function tests.
Metabolic: altered electrolyte balance.
Musculoskeletal: arthralgia, myalgia.
Respiratory: cough.

☑ Special considerations
• Tinnitus and hearing loss (usually reversible) have been observed after rapid I.V. injection of other loop diuretics and also have been noted after oral torsemide administration. Inject drug slowly over 2 minutes; single doses shouldn't exceed 200 mg.
• In patients with CV disease, especially those receiving cardiac glycosides, diuretic-induced hypokalemia may be a risk factor for the development of arrhythmias. The risk of hypokalemia is greatest in patients with hepatic cirrhosis, brisk diuresis, inadequate oral intake of electrolytes, or concurrent therapy with corticosteroids or corticotropin. Perform periodic monitoring of serum potassium and other electrolytes.
• Excessive diuresis may cause dehydration, blood-volume reduction, and possibly thrombosis and embolism, especially in elderly patients.
• Although data specific to torsemide overdose are lacking, signs and symptoms would probably reflect excessive pharmacologic effect (dehydration, hypovolemia, hypotension, hyponatremia, hypokalemia, hypochloremic alkalosis, and hemoconcentration). Treatment should consist of fluid and electrolyte replacement.

Monitoring the patient
• Monitor fluid intake and output, serum electrolyte levels, blood pressure, weight, and pulse rate during rapid diuresis and routinely with long-term use. If fluid and electrolyte imbalances occur, stop drug until imbalances are corrected. Drug may then be restarted at a lower dose.
• Monitor patient for adverse effects.

Information for the patient
• Encourage patient to follow a high-potassium diet, including citrus fruits, tomatoes, bananas, dates, and apricots.
• Advise patient to take drug in the morning to prevent nocturia.
• Advise patient to change positions slowly to prevent dizziness.
• Inform patient to report ringing in ears immediately because this may indicate toxicity.
• Tell patient to call before taking OTC preparations.
• Advise patient to take protective measures against exposure to sunlight or ultraviolet light.

Geriatric patients
• Special dosage adjustment usually isn't needed. However, elderly patients are at greater risk for dehydration, blood-volume reduction, and pos-

sibly thrombosis and embolism with excessive diuresis.

Pediatric patients
• Safety and effectiveness in children under age 18 haven't been established.

Breast-feeding patients
• It's unknown if drug appears in breast milk. Use with caution in breast-feeding women.

tramadol hydrochloride
Ultram

Pharmacologic classification: synthetic derivative
Therapeutic classification: analgesic
Pregnancy risk category C

How supplied
Available by prescription only
Tablets: 50 mg

Indications, route, and dosage
Moderate to moderately severe pain
Adults: 50 to 100 mg P.O. q 4 to 6 hours, p.r.n. Maximum dose is 400 mg/day.
✦ *Dosage adjustment.* In patients with creatinine clearance below 30 ml/minute, increase dosing interval to q 12 hours; maximum daily dose is 200 mg.
  In patients with cirrhosis, recommended dose is 50 mg q 12 hours.

Pharmacodynamics
Analgesic action: Mechanism unknown. Centrally acting synthetic analgesic compound that isn't chemically related to opiates but is thought to bind to opioid receptors and inhibit reuptake of norepinephrine and serotonin.

Pharmacokinetics
• *Absorption:* Almost completely absorbed. Mean absolute bioavailability of a 100-mg dose is about 75%. Mean peak plasma levels at about 2 hours.
• *Distribution:* About 20% bound to plasma protein; may cross blood-brain barrier.
• *Metabolism:* Extensively metabolized.
• *Excretion:* About 30% of dose excreted unchanged in urine and 60% as metabolites. Half-life of drug is about 6 to 7 hours.

Contraindications and precautions
Contraindicated in patients with hypersensitivity to drug and in those with acute intoxication with alcohol, hypnotics, centrally acting analgesics, opioids, or psychotropic drugs. Use cautiously in patients at risk for seizures or respiratory depression; in those with increased intracranial pressure or head injury, acute abdominal conditions,

or impaired renal or hepatic function; and in patients physically dependent on opioids.

Interactions
Drug-drug. *Carbamazepine:* Increased tramadol metabolism. Patients receiving long-term carbamazepine therapy at doses up to 800 mg daily may need up to twice the recommended dose of tramadol.
CNS depressants: Additive effects. Use together with caution. Tramadol dosage may need to be reduced.
MAO inhibitors, neuroleptic drugs: Increased risk of seizures. Monitor patient closely.

Adverse reactions
CNS: *dizziness, vertigo, headache, somnolence, CNS stimulation, asthenia,* anxiety, confusion, coordination disturbance, euphoria, nervousness, sleep disorder, **seizures,** malaise.
CV: vasodilation.
EENT: visual disturbances.
GI: *nausea, constipation, vomiting,* dyspepsia, dry mouth, diarrhea, abdominal pain, anorexia, flatulence.
GU: urine retention, urinary frequency, increased creatinine clearance, proteinuria, menopausal symptoms.
Hematologic: decreased hemoglobin levels.
Hepatic: elevated liver enzyme levels.
Musculoskeletal: hypertonia.
Respiratory: *respiratory depression.*
Skin: *pruritus,* diaphoresis, rash.

☑ Special considerations
• Constipation is a common adverse reaction and may need laxative therapy.
• For better analgesic effect, give drug before patient has intense pain.
• Serious potential consequences of overdose are respiratory depression and seizures. Because naloxone will reverse some, but not all, of the symptoms caused by tramadol overdose, supportive therapy is recommended. Hemodialysis removes only a small percentage of drug.

Monitoring the patient
• Monitor patient at risk for seizures closely; drug has been reported to reduce seizure threshold.
• Monitor patient for drug dependence. Because drug dependence similar to codeine or dextropropoxyphene can occur, the potential for abuse exists.
• Monitor patient's CV and respiratory status and stop drug if respirations decrease or rate is below 12 breaths/minute or if patient exhibits signs of respiratory depression.

Information for the patient
• Advise patient to take drug only as prescribed and not to alter dose or dosing interval without approval.

• Caution ambulatory patient about getting out of bed or walking. Warn outpatient to avoid driving and other potentially hazardous activities that require mental alertness until adverse CNS effects of drug are known.
• Advise patient not to take OTC preparations unless instructed because drug interactions can occur.

Geriatric patients
• Use cautiously in elderly patients because serum levels are slightly elevated and the elimination half-life of drug is prolonged. Don't exceed daily dose of 300 mg in patients over age 75.

Pediatric patients
• Safety and effectiveness in children under age 16 haven't been established.

Breast-feeding patients
• Safety in breast-feeding women hasn't been established. Because it's unknown if drug appears in breast milk, it's not recommended for use in breast-feeding women.

trandolapril
Mavik

Pharmacologic classification: ACE inhibitor
Therapeutic classification: antihypertensive
Pregnancy risk category C (D in second and third trimesters)

How supplied
Available by prescription only
Tablets: 1 mg, 2 mg, 4 mg

Indications, route, and dosage
Hypertension
Adults: In patients not taking a diuretic, initially 1 mg for the nonblack patient and 2 mg for the black patient P.O. once daily. If control isn't adequate, dose can be increased at intervals of at least 1 week. Maintenance dose ranges from 2 to 4 mg daily for most patients; there is little experience with doses of more than 8 mg. Patients receiving once-daily dosing at 4 mg may use b.i.d. dosing.
   For patient receiving a diuretic, initially 0.5 mg P.O. once daily. Subsequent dosage adjustment made based on blood pressure response.
Heart failure post-MI or left ventricular dysfunction post-MI
Adults: Initially, 1 mg P.O. daily, adjusted to 4 mg P.O. daily. If patient can't tolerate 4 mg, continue at highest tolerated dose.
✦ Dosage adjustment. In adults with renal impairment (creatinine clearance under 30 ml/minute) or hepatic cirrhosis, initially 0.5 mg P.O. once daily; adjust to optimal response.

Pharmacodynamics

Antihypertensive action: Mechanism unknown. Thought to result primarily from inhibition of circulating and tissue ACE activity, thereby reducing angiotensin II formation, decreasing vasoconstriction and aldosterone secretion and increasing plasma renin. Decreased aldosterone secretion leads to diuresis, natriuresis, and a small increase in serum potassium.

Pharmacokinetics

• *Absorption:* Absolute bioavailability after oral administration is about 10% for trandolapril; 70% for its metabolite, trandolaprilat.
• *Distribution:* About 80% protein-bound.
• *Metabolism:* Metabolized by liver to active metabolite, trandolaprilat, and at least seven other metabolites.
• *Excretion:* About 66% excreted in feces; 33% in urine. Elimination half-lives of trandolapril and trandolaprilat are about 6 and 10 hours, respectively. Like all ACE inhibitors, trandolaprilat also has a prolonged terminal elimination phase.

Contraindications and precautions

Contraindicated in patients with hypersensitivity to drug and in those with history of angioedema related to previous treatment with an ACE inhibitor. Drug isn't recommended for use in pregnant women. Use cautiously in patients with impaired renal function, heart failure, or renal artery stenosis.

Interactions

Drug-drug. *Diuretics:* Increased risk of excessive hypotension. Stop diuretic or lower dose of trandolapril.
Lithium: Lithium toxicity. Avoid concomitant use. If concomitant use can't be avoided, adjust dosage.
Potassium-sparing diuretics, potassium supplements: Risk of hyperkalemia. Monitor serum potassium levels closely.
Drug-food. *Salt substitutes containing potassium:* Increased risk of hyperkalemia. Monitor serum potassium levels closely.

Adverse reactions

CNS: dizziness, headache, fatigue, drowsiness, insomnia, paresthesia, vertigo, anxiety.
CV: chest pain, *AV first-degree block, bradycardia,* edema, flushing, hypotension, palpitations.
EENT: epistaxis, throat inflammation.
GI: diarrhea, dyspepsia, abdominal distention, abdominal pain or cramps, constipation, vomiting, *pancreatitis.*
GU: urinary frequency, increased creatinine clearance and BUN level, impotence, decreased libido.
Hepatic: elevated liver enzyme levels.
Hematologic: *neutropenia,* leukopenia.

Metabolic: hyperkalemia, hyponatremia, hyperuricemia.
Respiratory: dry, persistent, tickling, nonproductive cough; dyspnea; upper respiratory tract infection.
Skin: rash, pruritus, pemphigus.
Other: *anaphylactoid reactions, angioedema.*

☑ Special considerations

• Angioedema associated with tongue, glottis, or larynx may be fatal because of airway obstruction. Appropriate therapy, such as S.C. epinephrine 1:1,000 (0.3 to 0.5 ml) and equipment to ensure a patent airway, should be readily available.
• If jaundice develops, stop drug because, although rare, ACE inhibitors have been associated with a syndrome of cholestatic jaundice, fulminant hepatic necrosis, and death.
• Although no information is available, it's thought that effects of overdose are similar to other ACE inhibitor overdose, with hypotension being the main adverse reaction. Because the hypotensive effect of trandolapril is achieved through vasodilation and effective hypovolemia, it's reasonable to treat trandolapril overdose by infusion of normal saline solution. In addition, renal function and serum potassium level should be monitored. Drug is removed by hemodialysis.

Monitoring the patient

• Assess patient's renal function before and periodically throughout therapy.
• Other ACE inhibitors have been associated with agranulocytosis and neutropenia. Monitor CBC with differential counts before therapy, especially in patients who have collagen vascular disease with impaired renal function.
• Monitor serum potassium levels and watch for jaundice.
• Monitor patient for hypotension. Excessive hypotension can occur when drug is given with diuretics. If possible, diuretic therapy should be stopped 2 to 3 days before starting trandolapril to decrease potential for excessive hypotensive response. If trandolapril doesn't adequately control blood pressure, diuretic therapy may be reinstituted with care.

Information for the patient

• Advise patient to report signs of infection (such as fever and sore throat) and the following signs or symptoms: easy bruising or bleeding; swelling of tongue, lips, face, eyes, mucous membranes, or extremities; difficulty swallowing or breathing; and hoarseness.
• Tell patient to avoid sodium substitutes; these products may contain potassium, which can cause hyperkalemia.
• Light-headedness can occur, especially during first few days of therapy. Tell patient to rise slowly to minimize this effect and to report symptoms.

If syncope occurs, tell patient to stop drug and call immediately.
- Advise patient to use caution in hot weather and during exercise. Inadequate fluid intake, vomiting, diarrhea, and excessive perspiration can lead to light-headedness and syncope.
- Tell woman to report suspected pregnancy immediately. Drug will need to be discontinued.

Pediatric patients
- Safety and effectiveness in children haven't been established.

Breast-feeding patients
- It's unknown if drug appears in breast milk; avoid use in breast-feeding women.

tranylcypromine sulfate
Parnate

Pharmacologic classification: MAO inhibitor
Therapeutic classification: antidepressant
Pregnancy risk category C

How supplied
Available by prescription only
Tablets: 10 mg

Indications, route, and dosage
Severe depression, ◊ panic disorder
Adults: 30 mg P.O. daily in divided doses. If there is no improvement after 2 weeks, increase dose in 10-mg/day increments q 1 to 3 weeks; maximum daily dose is 60 mg.

Pharmacodynamics
Antidepressant action: Endogenous depression is thought to result from low CNS levels of neurotransmitters, including norepinephrine and serotonin. Tranylcypromine inhibits effects of MAO, an enzyme that normally inactivates amine-containing substances, thus increasing their concentration and activity.

Pharmacokinetics
- *Absorption:* Rapidly and completely absorbed from GI tract. Serum levels peak at 1 to 3 hours; onset of therapeutic activity may not occur for 3 to 4 weeks.
- *Distribution:* Not fully understood. Dosage adjustments determined by therapeutic response and adverse reaction profile.
- *Metabolism:* Metabolized in liver.
- *Excretion:* Drug excreted primarily in urine within 24 hours; some drug excreted in feces via biliary tract. Half-life is 2½ hours (relatively short); enzyme inhibition prolonged and unrelated to half-life.

Contraindications and precautions
Contraindicated in patients receiving MAO inhibitors or dibenzazepine derivatives; sympathomimetics (such as amphetamines); some CNS depressants (such as narcotics and alcohol); selective serotonin reuptake inhibitors; antihypertensives, diuretics, antihistamines, sedatives, or anesthetics; bupropion hydrochloride, buspirone hydrochloride, dextromethorphan, or meperidine.

Also contraindicated in patients consuming cheese or other foods with a high tyramine or tryptophan content or excessive quantities of caffeine; in those with a confirmed or suspected cerebrovascular defect, pheochromocytoma, history of liver disease, severe impairment of renal function, CV disease, hypertension, or history of headache; and in those undergoing elective surgery.

Use cautiously in patients with renal disease, diabetes, seizure disorders, Parkinson's disease, or hyperthyroidism; in those at risk for suicide; and in patients receiving antiparkinsonians or spinal anesthetics.

Interactions
Drug-drug. *Amphetamines, ephedrine, phenylephrine, phenylpropanolamine, other related drugs:* May result in serious CV toxicity. Don't use together.
Barbiturates, dextromethorphan, narcotics, other sedatives: Increased CNS depressant effects. Reduce dosage if concomitant use can't be avoided.
Cocaine, local anesthetics containing vasoconstrictors: May precipitate hypertension. Should be avoided.
Disulfiram: Possible tachycardia, flushing, or palpitations. Don't use together. If concomitant use can't be avoided, use cautiously together.
General or spinal anesthetics normally metabolized by MAO inhibitors: Severe hypotension and excessive CNS depression. Tranylcypromine should be stopped for at least 1 week before using these drugs.
Local anesthetics (such as lidocaine, procaine): Decreased therapeutic effect; poor nerve block. Don't use together.
Meperidine: Circulatory collapse and death. Don't use together.
Tricyclic antidepressants: Enhanced adverse CNS effects. Wait at least 2 weeks before switching to these drugs.
Drug-herb. *Ginseng:* Possible adverse reactions, including headache, tremors, mania. Avoid concomitant use.
Drug-food. *Foods high in caffeine, tryptophan, tyramine:* Possible hypertensive crisis. Don't use together.
Drug-lifestyle. *Alcohol:* Potentiated CNS effects. Discourage use.

Reactions may be *common,* uncommon, **life-threatening**, or COMMON AND LIFE-THREATENING.

Adverse reactions

CNS: *dizziness,* headache, anxiety, agitation, paresthesia, drowsiness, weakness, numbness, tremor, jitters, confusion.
CV: *orthostatic hypotension, tachycardia,* paradoxical hypertension, palpitations, edema.
EENT: blurred vision, tinnitus.
GI: dry mouth, *anorexia,* nausea, diarrhea, constipation, abdominal pain.
GU: impotence, SIADH, urine retention, elevated urinary catecholamine levels, impaired ejaculation.
Hematologic: anemia, leukopenia, ***agranulocytosis, thrombocytopenia.***
Hepatic: elevated liver function test results, hepatitis.
Musculoskeletal: muscle spasm, myoclonic jerks.
Skin: rash.
Other: chills.

☑ Special considerations

• Consider the inherent risk of suicide until significant improvement of depressive state occurs. Closely supervise high-risk patients during initial drug therapy. To reduce risk of suicidal overdose, prescribe smallest quantity of tablets consistent with good management.
• Tranylcypromine may have a more rapid onset of antidepressant effect compared with other MAO inhibitors (7 to 10 days versus 21 to 30 days). MAO activity also returns rapidly to pretreatment values.
• Signs and symptoms of overdose include exacerbations of adverse reactions or an exaggerated response to normal pharmacologic activity; such signs and symptoms become apparent slowly (24 to 48 hours) and may persist for up to 2 weeks. Agitation, flushing, tachycardia, hypotension, hypertension, palpitations, increased motor activity, twitching, increased deep tendon reflexes, seizures, hyperpyrexia, cardiorespiratory arrest, or coma may occur. Death has occurred with doses of 350 mg.
• Treat symptomatically and supportively. Give 5 to 10 mg of phentolamine I.V. push for hypertensive crisis; treat seizures, agitation, or tremors with I.V. diazepam, tachycardia with beta blockers, and fever with cooling blankets. Monitor vital signs and fluid and electrolyte balance. Sympathomimetics (such as norepinephrine and phenylephrine) are contraindicated in hypotension because of MAO inhibitors.

Monitoring the patient

• Watch closely for suicidal risk.
• Monitor patient for adverse effects.

Information for the patient

• Warn patient to avoid taking alcohol and other CNS depressants or self-prescribed drugs, such as cold, hay fever, or diet preparations, without medical approval.
• To minimize daytime sedation, tell patient to take drug at bedtime.
• Explain that many foods and beverages containing tyramine or tryptophan (such as wines, beer, cheeses, preserved fruits, meats, and vegetables) may interact with drug. A list of foods to avoid can be obtained from the hospital dietary department or pharmacy.
• Tell patient to avoid hazardous activities that require alertness until full effect of drug on CNS is known.
• Inform patient to lie down after taking drug and to avoid abrupt postural changes, especially when arising, to prevent dizziness induced by orthostatic blood pressure changes.
• Tell patient to take drug exactly as prescribed, not to double a missed dose, and not to stop taking drug abruptly. Patient should promptly report any adverse reactions. Dosage reduction can relieve most adverse reactions.
• Tell patient to inform dentist or other health care providers about the use of an MAO inhibitor.
• Inform patient to call if severe headache, palpitations, tachycardia, sweating, tightness in throat and chest, dizziness, stiff neck, nausea, vomiting, or other unusual symptoms occur.
• Advise patient to store drug safely away from children.

Geriatric patients

• Drug isn't recommended for patients over age 60 because elderly patients have less compensatory reserve to cope with serious side effects of drug.

Pediatric patients

• Drug isn't recommended for children under age 16.

Breast-feeding patients

• Safety in breast-feeding women hasn't been established.

trastuzumab
Herceptin

Pharmacologic classification: monoclonal antibody to human epidermal growth factor receptor 2 protein (HER2)
Therapeutic classification: antineoplastic
Pregnancy risk category B

How supplied

Injection: lyophilized sterile powder containing 440 mg per vial

Indications, route, and dosage

Single-drug treatment of metastatic breast cancer in patients whose tumors overexpress

the HER2 protein and who have received one or more chemotherapy regimens for their metastatic disease, or with paclitaxel for metastatic breast cancer in patients whose tumors overexpress the HER2 protein and who haven't received chemotherapy for their metastatic disease
Adults: Initial loading dose 4 mg/kg I.V. over 90 minutes. Maintenance dose is 2 mg/kg I.V. weekly as a 30-minute I.V. infusion if initial loading dose is well tolerated.

Pharmacodynamics
Antineoplastic action: Recombinant DNA-derived monoclonal antibody that selectively binds to HER2, inhibiting the proliferation of human tumor cells that overexpress HER2. Protein overexpression is observed in 25% to 30% of primary breast cancers.

Pharmacokinetics
• *Absorption:* No information available.
• *Distribution:* Volume of distribution is about that of serum value (44 ml/kg). Between weeks 16 and 32, serum levels reached steady-state, with a mean trough of 79 mcg/ml and peak of 123 mcg/ml.
• *Metabolism:* No information available.
• *Excretion:* Half-life and clearance are dose-dependent. At recommended dosage, mean half-life is 5.8 days (range 1 to 32 days).

Contraindications and precautions
Use with caution in patients with hypersensitivity to drug or its components. Use cautiously in patients with preexisting cardiac dysfunction and in elderly patients.

Interactions
Drug-drug. *Paclitaxel:* Increases trastuzumab serum levels. Monitor patient closely; adjust dosage as needed.

Adverse reactions
CNS: depression, *headache, dizziness, insomnia, asthenia,* neuropathy, paresthesia, peripheral neuritis.
CV: heart failure, *peripheral edema,* tachycardia, edema.
EENT: *rhinitis, pharyngitis,* sinusitis.
GI: *anorexia, abdominal pain, diarrhea, nausea, vomiting.*
GU: urinary tract infection.
Hematologic: *leukopenia,* anemia.
Musculoskeletal: arthralgia, *back pain,* bone pain.
Respiratory: *dyspnea, increased cough.*
Skin: acne, herpes simplex, rash.
Other: *allergic reaction, chills, fever, flu syndrome, infection, pain.*

☑ Special considerations
• Trastuzumab administration can result in the development of ventricular dysfunction and heart failure. Before beginning therapy, patients should undergo a thorough baseline cardiac assessment, including history and physical examination and appropriate evaluation methods to identify those at risk for developing cardiotoxicity.
• Stopping treatment should be strongly considered in patients who develop a clinically significant decrease in left ventricular function.
• Drug should be used only in patients with metastatic breast cancer whose tumors have HER2 protein overexpression.
• Don't administer as an I.V. push or bolus. Reconstitute with diluent provided. Calculated dose should be added to an infusion bag containing 250 ml normal saline solution. Don't use D_5W solution. *Note:* If patient has known hypersensitivity to benzyl alcohol, drug may be reconstituted with sterile water for injection, used immediately, and unused portion discarded.
• A first-infusion symptom complex commonly consisting of chills or fever has been observed in about 40% of patients. Treat with acetaminophen, diphenhydramine, and meperidine (with or without reducing the rate of infusion). Other signs or symptoms may include nausea, vomiting, pain, rigors, headache, dizziness, dyspnea, hypotension, rash, and asthenia. These symptoms occur infrequently with subsequent infusions.

Monitoring the patient
• Watch for dyspnea, increased cough, paroxysmal nocturnal dyspnea, peripheral edema, or S_3 gallop, especially if patient is receiving drug with anthracyclines and cyclophosphamide.

Information for the patient
• Tell patient about risk of first dose infusion-associated adverse effects.
• Advise patient to immediately report symptoms of cardiac dysfunction, such as shortness of breath, increased cough, or peripheral edema.

Geriatric patients
• Risk of cardiac dysfunction may be increased in elderly patients.

Pediatric patients
• Safety and effectiveness in children haven't been established.

Breast-feeding patients
• Because human immunoglobulin G appears in breast milk and the potential for absorption harm to infant isn't known, women should be advised to stop breast-feeding during and for 6 months after therapy.

Reactions may be *common*, uncommon, **life-threatening**, or COMMON AND LIFE-THREATENING.

trazodone hydrochloride
Desyrel

Pharmacologic classification: triazolopyridine derivative
Therapeutic classification: antidepressant
Pregnancy risk category C

How supplied
Available by prescription only
Tablets: 50 mg, 100 mg
Tablets (film-coated): 50 mg, 100 mg
Dividose tablets: 150 mg, 300 mg

Indications, route, and dosage
Depression
Adults: Initial dose is 150 mg daily in divided doses, which can be increased by 50 mg/day q 3 to 4 days. Average dose ranges from 150 mg to 400 mg/day. Maximum dose is 400 mg/day in outpatients; 600 mg/day in hospitalized patients.
◇ *Alcoholism, adjunct treatment*
Adults: 50 mg to 100 mg P.O. daily.
◇ *Aggressive behavior*
Adults: 50 mg P.O. b.i.d.
◇ *Panic disorder*
Adults: 300 mg P.O. daily.

Pharmacodynamics
Antidepressant action: Thought to exert antidepressant effects by inhibiting reuptake of norepinephrine and serotonin in CNS nerve terminals (presynaptic neurons), which results in increased level and enhanced activity of these neurotransmitters in the synaptic cleft. Shares some properties with tricyclic antidepressants: Has antihistaminic, alpha-blocking, analgesic, and sedative effects as well as relaxant effects on skeletal muscle. Unlike tricyclic antidepressants, however, trazodone counteracts the pressor effects of norepinephrine, has limited effects on the CV system, and, in particular, has no direct quinidine-like effects on cardiac tissue; it also causes relatively fewer anticholinergic effects. Trazodone has been used in patients with alcohol dependence to decrease tremors and alleviate anxiety and depression. Adverse reactions are somewhat dose-related; incidence increases with higher dose levels.

Pharmacokinetics
• *Absorption:* Well absorbed from GI tract after oral administration. Peak effect occurs in 1 hour. Food delays absorption, extends peak effect of drug to 2 hours, and increases amount of drug absorbed by 20%.
• *Distribution:* Widely distributed in body; doesn't concentrate in any particular tissue, but small amounts may appear in breast milk. About 90% protein-bound. Proposed therapeutic drug levels haven't been established. Steady-state plasma levels reached in 3 to 7 days; onset of therapeutic activity occurs in 7 days.
• *Metabolism:* Metabolized by liver; more than 75% of metabolites excreted within 3 days.
• *Excretion:* Drug is mostly excreted in urine; the rest excreted in feces via biliary tract.

Contraindications and precautions
Contraindicated in patients with hypersensitivity to drug and during initial recovery phase of MI. Use cautiously in patients with cardiac disease and in those at risk for suicide.

Interactions
Drug-drug. *Antihypertensives (such as clonidine, guanabenz, guanadrel, guanethidine, methyldopa, reserpine):* Possible hypotension. If concomitant use can't be avoided, monitor patient closely and adjust dosage as needed.
CNS depressants (such as analgesics, anesthetics, barbiturates, narcotics, tranquilizers): Possible oversedation. Use together cautiously.
Digoxin, phenytoin: Increased serum levels of these drugs. Monitor digoxin and phenytoin levels.
Selective serotonin reuptake inhibitors: Serotonin syndrome. Use cautiously together.
Drug-herb. *St. John's wort:* Possible serotonin syndrome when used together. Avoid concomitant use.
Drug-lifestyle. *Alcohol:* Exacerbated CNS depression. Discourage concurrent use.

Adverse reactions
CNS: *drowsiness, dizziness,* nervousness, fatigue, confusion, tremor, weakness, hostility, anger, nightmares, vivid dreams, headache, insomnia, *generalized tonic-clonic seizures.*
CV: orthostatic hypotension, tachycardia, hypertension, prolonged conduction time on ECG, syncope, shortness of breath.
EENT: blurred vision, tinnitus, nasal congestion.
GI: dry mouth, dysgeusia, constipation, nausea, vomiting, anorexia.
GU: urine retention; priapism, possibly leading to impotence; decreased libido; hematuria.
Hematologic: anemia, decreased WBC counts.
Hepatic: elevated liver function test results.
Metabolic: altered serum glucose levels.
Skin: rash, urticaria, diaphoresis.

☑ Special considerations
• Consider the inherent risk of suicide until significant improvement of depressive state occurs. Closely monitor high-risk patients during initial drug therapy. To reduce risk of suicidal overdose, prescribe the smallest quantity of tablets consistent with good management.
• Administering drug with food helps to prevent GI upset and increases absorption.

- Adverse effects are more common when doses exceed 300 mg/day.
- 150-mg tablet may be broken on the scoring to obtain doses of 50 mg, 75 mg, or 100 mg.
- Tolerance to adverse effects (especially sedative effects) usually develops after 1 to 2 weeks of treatment.
- Drug has been used in alcohol dependence to decrease tremors and relieve anxiety and depression. Doses range from 50 to 75 mg daily.
- Drug has fewer adverse cardiac and anticholinergic effects than tricyclic antidepressants.
- Drug may cause prolonged, painful erections that may need surgical correction. Consider carefully before prescribing for men, especially those who are sexually active.
- Don't stop drug abruptly. However, discontinue drug at least 48 hours before surgical procedures.
- Sugarless chewing gum or hard candy or ice may relieve dry mouth.
- Drowsiness may require giving a major portion of the daily dose at bedtime or giving a reduced dose.
- The most common signs and symptoms of drug overdose are drowsiness and vomiting; other signs and symptoms include orthostatic hypotension, tachycardia, headache, shortness of breath, dry mouth, and incontinence. Coma may occur.
- Treatment of overdose is symptomatic and supportive and includes maintaining airway and stabilizing vital signs and fluid and electrolyte balance. Induce emesis if gag reflex is intact; then use gastric lavage (begin with lavage if emesis is unfeasible) and activated charcoal to prevent further absorption. Forced diuresis may aid elimination. Dialysis is usually ineffective.

Monitoring the patient
- Monitor blood pressure because hypotension may occur.
- Closely monitor high-risk patients during initial drug therapy.

Information for the patient
- Tell patient that full effects of drug may not become apparent for up to 2 weeks after therapy begins.
- Tell patient to take drug exactly as prescribed and not to double missed dose, not to share drug with others, and not to stop drug abruptly.
- Inform patient that drug may cause drowsiness or dizziness; advise patient not to participate in activities that require mental alertness until full effects of drug are known.
- Tell patient to avoid alcohol or medicinal elixirs while taking drug.
- Warn patient to store drug safely away from children.
- Suggest taking drug with food or milk if it causes stomach upset.

- To prevent dizziness, tell patient to lie down for about 30 minutes after taking the drug and avoid sudden postural changes, especially standing up.
- Tell patient that sugarless chewing gum or sugarless hard candy may relieve dry mouth.
- Advise patient to report unusual effects immediately and to report prolonged, painful erections, sexual dysfunction, dizziness, fainting, or rapid heartbeat.
- Tell patient that he should regard an involuntary erection lasting more than 1 hour as a medical emergency.

Geriatric patients
- Elderly patients usually need lower initial doses; they are more likely to develop adverse reactions. However, drug may be preferred in elderly patients because it has fewer adverse cardiac effects.

Pediatric patients
- Drug isn't recommended for children under age 18.

---

tretinoin (systemic)
Vesanoid

Pharmacologic classification: retinoid
Therapeutic classification: antineoplastic
Pregnancy risk category D

How supplied
Available by prescription only
Capsules: 10 mg

Indications, route, and dosage
Induction of remission in patients with acute promyelocytic leukemia (APL), French-American-British classification M3 (including the M3 variant), characterized by the presence of the t(15,17) translocation or the presence of PML/RAR alpha gene, who are refractory to or who have relapsed from anthracycline chemotherapy or for whom anthracycline-based chemotherapy is contraindicated
Adults and children ages 1 and older: 45 mg/m²/day P.O. administered as two evenly divided doses until complete remission is documented. Stop therapy 30 days after achievement of complete remission or after 90 days of treatment, whichever occurs first.

Pharmacodynamics
Antineoplastic action: Exact mechanism unknown. Produces an initial maturation of primitive promyelocytes derived from the leukemic clone, then a repopulation of bone marrow and peripheral blood by normal, polyclonal hematopoietic cells.

Pharmacokinetics
- *Absorption:* Well absorbed from GI tract.
- *Distribution:* About 95% bound to plasma protein.
- *Metabolism:* May induce its own metabolism.
- *Excretion:* Excreted in urine and feces.

Contraindications and precautions
Contraindicated in patients with hypersensitivity to retinoids or parabens used as preservatives in the gelatin capsule. Don't use in pregnant or breast-feeding women.

Interactions
Drug-drug. *Drugs that induce or inhibit hepatic cytochrome P-450 3A:* Altered pharmacokinetics. Avoid concomitant use.
Ketoconazole: Increased tretinoin plasma level when administered within 1 hour. Separate administration times by more than 1 hour.
Drug-food. *Any food:* Enhanced absorption of drug. Administer with food.

Adverse reactions
CNS: *malaise,* cerebral hemorrhage, dizziness, *paresthesia, headache, anxiety, insomnia, depression, confusion,* **cerebral hemorrhage,** intracranial hypertension, agitation, hallucination, abnormal gait, agnosia, aphasia, asterixis, cerebellar edema, cerebellar disorders, *seizures, coma,* CNS depression, dysarthria, encephalopathy, facial paralysis, hemiplegia, hyporeflexia, hypotaxia, no light reflex neurologic reaction, spinal cord disorder, tremor, leg weakness, unconsciousness, dementia, forgetfulness, somnolence, slow speech.
CV: *chest discomfort,* **arrhythmias,** *hypotension, hypertension, peripheral edema, phlebitis, edema,* **cardiac failure, cardiac arrest, MI,** enlarged heart, heart murmur, ischemia, **stroke,** myocarditis, pericarditis, secondary cardiomyopathy.
EENT: *ear fullness, visual disturbances, ocular disorders,* hearing loss, *mucositis.*
GI: **GI hemorrhage,** *nausea, vomiting, anorexia, abdominal pain, GI disorders, diarrhea, constipation, dyspepsia, abdominal distention,* hepatosplenomegaly, ulcer, unspecified liver disorder.
GU: *renal insufficiency,* **acute renal failure,** micturition frequency, dysuria, renal tubular necrosis, enlarged prostate.
Hematologic: leukocytosis, **hemorrhage, DIC.**
Hepatic: elevated liver function study results, **hepatitis.**
Metabolic: acidosis, hypothermia, fluid imbalance, hypercholesterolemia, hypertriglyceridemia, *weight increase, weight decrease.*
Musculoskeletal: flank pain, *myalgia, bone pain,* bone inflammation.
Respiratory: *pneumonia, upper respiratory tract disorders, dyspnea,* **respiratory insufficiency,** *pleural effusion, crackles, expiratory wheezing,* lower respiratory tract disorders, pulmonary infiltrate, bronchial asthma, pulmonary or larynx edema, unspecified pulmonary disease, pulmonary hypertension.
Skin: *flushing, skin mucous membrane dryness, pruritus, decreased sweating, alopecia, skin changes.*
Other: *fever, infections, shivering, pain, injection site reactions,* cellulitis, facial edema, pallor, lymph disorder, ascites.

☑ Special considerations
- Because patients with APL are generally at high risk and can have severe adverse reactions to tretinoin, administer drug in a facility with laboratory and supportive services sufficient to monitor drug tolerance and protect and maintain patients compromised by drug toxicity.
- About 25% of patients given drug have experienced retinoic acid-APL syndrome, characterized by fever, dyspnea, weight gain, radiographic pulmonary infiltrates, and pleural or pericardial effusions. This syndrome has occasionally been accompanied by impaired myocardial contractility and episodic hypotension with or without leukocytosis. Some patients have died because of progressive hypoxemia and multiorgan failure. The syndrome generally occurs during the first month of therapy. Treatment with high-dose corticosteroids at the first signs of the syndrome appear to reduce morbidity and mortality.
- Maintain supportive care, such as infection control and bleeding precautions, and provide prompt treatment.
- No overdose information available. Overdose with other retinoids has been associated with transient headache, facial flushing, cheilosis, abdominal pain, dizziness, and ataxia. These signs and symptoms have quickly resolved without apparent residual effects.

Monitoring the patient
- Monitor CBC and platelet counts regularly. Patients with high WBC counts at diagnosis are at greater risk for having further rapid increases in WBC counts. Rapidly evolving leukocytosis is associated with a higher risk of life-threatening complications.
- Monitor patients, especially children, for signs and symptoms of pseudotumor cerebri. Early signs and symptoms of pseudotumor cerebri include papilledema, headache, nausea, vomiting, and visual disturbances.
- Monitor cholesterol and triglyceride levels and liver function studies.
- Ensure that pregnancy testing and contraception counseling are repeated monthly throughout therapy.

Information for the patient
• Inform woman that a pregnancy test is needed within 1 week before therapy. When possible, therapy will be delayed until a negative result is obtained. Also tell her that effective contraception must be used during therapy and for 1 month after therapy ends. Contraception must be used even when there is history of infertility or menopause unless a hysterectomy has been performed. Tell patient that two forms of contraception should be used simultaneously unless abstinence is the chosen method. If pregnancy is suspected, tell patient to report this immediately.
• Advise patient on infection control and bleeding precautions. Tell patient to report signs or symptoms of infection (fever, sore throat, fatigue) or bleeding (easy bruising, nosebleeds, bleeding gums, melena). Also tell patient to record temperature daily.

Pediatric patients
• Safety and effectiveness in children under age 1 haven't been established.

Breast-feeding patients
• It's unknown if drug appears in breast milk. Because of potential for serious adverse reactions in breast-fed infants, drug shouldn't be given to breast-feeding women.

---

tretinoin (topical)
Avita, Renova, Retin-A, Retin-A Micro

Pharmacologic classification: vitamin A derivative
Therapeutic classification: antiacne
Pregnancy risk category C

How supplied
Available by prescription only
Cream: 0.025%, 0.05%, 0.1%
Gel: 0.025%, 0.01%
Solution: 0.05%
Microsphere gel: 0.1%

Indications, route, and dosage
Acne vulgaris (especially grades I, II, and III)
Adults and children: Clean affected area and lightly apply solution once daily h.s. or as directed.
◇ *Treatment of photodamaged skin (wrinkles)*
Adults: 0.05% solution or 0.025% to 0.1% cream applied daily for at least 4 months.

Pharmacodynamics
Antiacne action: Mechanism unknown. Appears to act as a follicular epithelium irritant, preventing horny cells from sticking together and therefore inhibiting the formation of additional comedones.

Pharmacokinetics
• *Absorption:* Limited with topical use.
• *Distribution:* None.
• *Metabolism:* None.
• *Excretion:* Minimal amount excreted in urine.

Contraindications and precautions
Contraindicated in patients with hypersensitivity to vitamin A or retinoic acid. Use cautiously in patients with eczema. Avoid contact of drug with eyes, mouth, angles of the nose, mucous membranes, or open wounds.

Interactions
Drug-drug. *Topical forms of benzoyl peroxide, resorcinol, salicylic acid, sulfur:* Increased risk of skin reactions. Use cautiously together.
Topical preparations containing high levels of alcohol, menthol, spices, or lime: May cause skin irritation. Avoid use together.
Drug-lifestyle. *Abrasive cleaners, medicated cosmetics, skin preparations containing alcohol:* Increased risk of skin irritation. Avoid concomitant use.
Sun exposure: Photosensitivity reactions. Tell patient to take precautions.

Adverse reactions
Skin: peeling, erythema, blisters, crusting, hyperpigmentation and hypopigmentation, contact dermatitis.
    Note: Stop drug if sensitization or extreme redness and blistering of skin occur.

☑ Special considerations
• Patient should know how to use drug and know of time needed for therapeutic effect, which normally occurs in 2 to 3 weeks but may take 6 weeks or more. Relapses generally occur within 3 to 6 weeks of stopping drug.
• Don't use drug in patients who can't or won't minimize sun exposure.
• Although tretinoin microsphere gel was developed to minimize dermal irritation, the skin of some patients may become excessively dry, red, swollen, blistered, or crusted.
• For possible overdose, stop use and rinse area thoroughly. Oral ingestion of drug may lead to the same adverse effects as those associated with excessive oral intake of vitamin A.

Monitoring the patient
• Monitor therapeutic effect.
• Monitor patient for possible relapse after drug is stopped.

Information for the patient
• Advise patient to apply sparingly to thoroughly clean, dry skin to minimize irritation, and to wash face with mild soap no more than once or twice daily. Stress importance of thorough removal of dirt and makeup before application and

---

of hand washing after each use, but warn against use of strong, medicated, or perfumed cosmetics, soaps, or skin cleansers.
• Explain that application may cause a temporary feeling of warmth. If discomfort occurs, tell patient to decrease amount, but not to stop drug.
• Stress that initial exacerbation of inflammatory lesions is common and that redness and scaling (usually occurring in 7 to 10 days) are normal skin responses; these disappear when drug is decreased or stopped.
• If severe local irritation develops, advise patient to stop drug temporarily and readjust dose when irritation or inflammation subsides.
• Caution patient to keep exposure to sunlight or ultraviolet rays to a minimum and, if sunburned, to delay therapy until sunburn fades. If patient can't avoid exposure to sunlight, recommend using a sunscreen with a sun protection factor of 15 or higher and wearing protective clothing.
• Advise patient to keep drug away from eyes, mouth, angles of nose, and mucous membranes or open wounds.

triamcinolone (systemic)
Aristocort, Kenacort

triamcinolone acetonide
Kenalog-10, Kenalog-40

triamcinolone diacetate
Aristocort

triamcinolone hexacetonide
Aristospan

Pharmacologic classification: glucocorticoid
Therapeutic classification: anti-inflammatory, immunosuppressant
Pregnancy risk category C

How supplied
Available by prescription only
triamcinolone
Tablets: 1 mg, 2 mg, 4 mg, 8 mg
triamcinolone acetonide
Injection: 3 mg/ml, 10 mg/ml, 40 mg/ml
triamcinolone diacetate
Injection: 25 mg/ml, 40 mg/ml
Syrup: 2 mg/5 ml
triamcinolone hexacetonide
Injection: 5 mg/ml, 20 mg/ml

Indications, route, and dosage
Adrenal insufficiency
triamcinolone
Adults: 4 to 12 mg P.O. daily, in single or divided doses.
Children: 117 mcg/kg or 3.3 mg/m² P.O. daily, in single or divided doses.

Severe inflammation or immunosuppression
triamcinolone
Adults: 8 to 16 mg P.O. daily, in single or divided doses.
Children: 416 mcg to 1.7 mg/kg or 12.5 to 50 mg/m² P.O. daily, in single or divided doses.
triamcinolone acetonide
Adults: Initially, 60 mg I.M. Additional doses of 20 to 100 mg may be given, p.r.n., at 6-week intervals. Or administer 2.5 to 15 mg intra-articularly, or up to 1 mg intralesionally, p.r.n.
Children ages 6 to 12: 0.03 to 0.2 mg/kg I.M. at 1- to 7-day intervals.
triamcinolone diacetate
Adults: 40 mg I.M. once weekly; or 2 to 40 mg intra-articularly, intrasynovially, or intralesionally q 1 to 8 weeks; or 4 to 48 mg P.O. divided q.i.d.
Children: 0.117 to 1.66 mg/kg/day P.O. divided q.i.d.
triamcinolone hexacetonide
Adults: 2 to 20 mg intra-articularly q 3 to 4 weeks, p.r.n.; or up to 0.5 mg intralesionally per square inch of skin.
Tuberculosis meningitis
triamcinolone
Adults: 32 to 48 mg P.O. daily.
Edematous states
triamcinolone
Adults: 16 to 48 mg P.O. daily.
Collagen diseases
triamcinolone
Adults: 30 to 48 mg P.O. daily.
Dermatologic disorders
triamcinolone
Adults: 8 to 16 mg P.O. daily.
Allergic states
triamcinolone
Adults: 8 to 12 mg P.O. daily.
Ophthalmic diseases
triamcinolone
Adults: 12 to 40 mg P.O. daily.
Respiratory diseases
triamcinolone
Adults: 16 to 48 mg P.O. daily.
Hematologic diseases
triamcinolone
Adults: 16 to 60 mg P.O. daily.
Neoplastic diseases
triamcinolone
Adults: 16 to 100 mg P.O. daily.

Pharmacodynamics
Anti-inflammatory action: Stimulates the synthesis of enzymes needed to decrease the inflammatory response. Suppresses the immune system by reducing activity and volume of the lymphatic system, thus producing lymphocytopenia (primarily of T lymphocytes), decreases immunoglobulin and complement levels, decreases passage of immune complexes through basement membranes, and possibly depresses reactivity of tissue to antigen-antibody interaction

An intermediate-acting glucocorticoid. The addition of a fluorine group in the molecule increases the anti-inflammatory activity, which is five times more potent than an equal weight of hydrocortisone. Has essentially no mineralocorticoid activity.

May be administered orally. The diacetate and acetonide salts may be administered by I.M., intra-articular, intrasynovial, intralesional or sublesional, and soft-tissue injection. Don't administer any of the parenteral suspensions I.V.

Pharmacokinetics

• *Absorption:* Absorbed readily after oral administration. After oral and I.V. administration, effects peak in about 1 to 2 hours. Suspensions for injection have variable onset and duration of action, depending on if injected into intra-articular space or muscle, and on blood supply to muscle. The diacetate suspension is slightly soluble, providing a prompt onset of action and a longer duration of effect (1 to 2 weeks). Triamcinolone acetonide is relatively insoluble and slowly absorbed. Its extended duration of action lasts for several weeks. Triamcinolone hexacetonide is relatively insoluble, is absorbed slowly, and has a prolonged action of 3 to 4 weeks.

• *Distribution:* Removed rapidly from blood and distributed to muscle, liver, skin, intestines, and kidneys. Extensively bound to plasma proteins (transcortin and albumin). Only unbound portion is active. Adrenocorticoids distributed into breast milk and through placenta.

• *Metabolism:* Metabolized in liver to inactive glucuronide and sulfate metabolites.

• *Excretion:* Inactive metabolites and small amounts of unmetabolized drug excreted by kidneys. Insignificant quantities of drug also excreted in feces. Biological half-life is 18 to 36 hours.

Contraindications and precautions

Contraindicated in patients with hypersensitivity to drug or its components and in those with systemic fungal infections.

Use cautiously in patients with GI ulcer, renal disease, hypertension, osteoporosis, diabetes mellitus, hypothyroidism, cirrhosis, diverticulitis, nonspecific ulcerative colitis, recent intestinal anastomosis, thromboembolic disorders, seizures, myasthenia gravis, heart failure, tuberculosis, ocular herpes simplex, emotional instability, or psychotic tendencies.

Interactions

Drug-drug. *Amphotericin B, cardiac glycosides, diuretics:* Enhanced hypokalemia; increased risk of toxicity. Avoid concomitant use.
Antacids, cholestyramine, colestipol: Decreased triamcinolone level. Avoid concomitant use. If concomitant use can't be avoided, adjust dosage.
Barbiturates, phenytoin, rifampin: Decreased corticosteroid effects. Monitor patient for drug effect.

Estrogens: Increased triamcinolone level. Monitor patient closely; adjust dosage.
Insulin, oral antidiabetics: Hyperglycemia. Monitor blood glucose levels.
Isoniazid, salicylates: Decreased effect of these drugs. Monitor patient for drug effect.
Oral anticoagulants: Decreased anticoagulant effect (rare). Monitor PT and INR.
Ulcerogenic drugs such as NSAIDs: Increased risk of GI ulceration. Avoid concomitant use. If concomitant use can't be avoided, monitor patient closely.

Adverse reactions

Most adverse reactions to corticosteroids are dose- or duration-dependent.
CNS: *euphoria, insomnia,* psychotic behavior, pseudotumor cerebri, vertigo, headache, paresthesia, *seizures.*
CV: *heart failure, thromboembolism,* hypertension, edema, *arrhythmias,* thrombophlebitis.
EENT: cataracts, glaucoma.
GI: peptic ulceration, GI irritation, increased appetite, pancreatitis, nausea, vomiting.
GU: increased urine glucose and calcium levels, menstrual irregularities.
Metabolic: hypokalemia, hyperglycemia, hypocalcemia, decreased T_3, and T_4 levels, hypercholesterolemia, carbohydrate intolerance.
Musculoskeletal: muscle weakness, osteoporosis.
Skin: delayed wound healing, acne, various skin eruptions, hirsutism.
Other: susceptibility to infections, growth suppression in children, cushingoid state (moonface, buffalo hump, central obesity), *acute adrenal insufficiency with increased stress (infection, surgery, or trauma) or abrupt withdrawal after long-term therapy.*

After abrupt withdrawal: rebound inflammation, fatigue, weakness, arthralgia, fever, dizziness, lethargy, depression, fainting, orthostatic hypotension, dyspnea, anorexia, hypoglycemia. *After prolonged use, sudden withdrawal may be fatal.*

☑ Special considerations

• Recommendations for use of triamcinolone and for care and teaching of patients during therapy are the same as those for all systemic adrenocorticoids.
• Triamcinolone suppresses reactions to skin tests; causes false-negative results in the nitroblue tetrazolium test for systemic bacterial infections; and decreases ^{131}I uptake and protein-bound iodine levels in thyroid function tests.
• Toxic signs and symptoms rarely occur if drug is used for less than 3 weeks, even at large doses. However, long-term use causes adverse physiologic effects, including suppression of the hypothalamic-pituitary-adrenal axis, cushingoid

---

eactions may be *common,* uncommon, *life-threatening,* or COMMON AND LIFE-THREATENING.

appearance, muscle weakness, and osteoporosis.

Monitoring the patient
• Monitor patient for bleeding and infection.
• Monitor cardiac status.

Information for the patient
• Tell patient to avoid aspirin during therapy; warn him of potential for GI bleeding.
• Advise patient of potential adverse effects.

Pediatric patients
• Long-term use of adrenocorticoids or corticotropin in children and adolescents may delay growth and maturation.

---

triamcinolone acetonide (oral and nasal inhalant)
Azmacort, Nasacort, Nasacort AQ, Tri-Nasal

Pharmacologic classification: glucocorticoid
Therapeutic classification: anti-inflammatory, antasthmatic
Pregnancy risk category C

How supplied
Available by prescription only
Oral inhalation aerosol: 100 mcg/metered spray, 240 doses/inhaler
Nasal aerosol: 50 mcg/metered spray, 55 mcg/metered spray

Indications, route, and dosage
Steroid-dependent asthma
Adults: 2 inhalations t.i.d. or q.i.d. Maximum dose is 16 inhalations daily.
Children ages 6 to 12: 1 or 2 inhalations t.i.d. or q.i.d. Maximum dose is 12 inhalations daily.
Rhinitis, allergic disorders, inflammatory conditions, nasal polyps
Adults: 2 sprays in each nostril daily; may increase dose to maximum of 4 sprays per nostril daily, if needed.

Pharmacodynamics
Anti-inflammatory action: Glucocorticoids stimulate the synthesis of enzymes needed to decrease the inflammatory response. Triamcinolone acetonide is used as an oral inhalant to treat bronchial asthma in patients who need corticosteroids to control symptoms.

Pharmacokinetics
• *Absorption:* Systemic absorption from the lungs is similar to oral administration. Levels peak in 1 to 2 hours.
• *Distribution:* After oral inhalation, 10% to 25% of drug distributed to lungs; rest is swallowed or

deposited in mouth. After nasal use, only a small amount reaches systemic circulation.
• *Metabolism:* Metabolized mainly by liver. Some that reaches lungs may be metabolized locally.
• *Excretion:* Major portion of dose eliminated in feces. Biological half-life is 18 to 36 hours.

Contraindications and precautions
Oral form is contraindicated in patients with hypersensitivity to drug or its components and in those with status asthmaticus. Nasal form is contraindicated in patients with hypersensitivity or untreated localized infections.
    Use oral form cautiously in patients with tuberculosis of the respiratory tract; untreated fungal, bacterial, or systemic viral infections; or ocular herpes simplex and in those receiving corticosteroids. Use oral and nasal forms with caution in breast-feeding women.

Interactions
None reported.

Adverse reactions
Most adverse reactions to corticosteroids are dose- or duration-dependent.
EENT: *oral candidiasis,* dry or irritated tongue or mouth, dry or irritated nose or throat, hoarseness.
Respiratory: cough, wheezing (with oral form).
Other: facial edema (with oral form).

☑ Special considerations
• Recommendations for use of triamcinolone and for care and teaching of patients during therapy are the same as those for all inhalant adrenocorticoids.

Monitoring the patient
• Monitor therapeutic effect.

Information for the patient
• Advise patient to rinse mouth or gargle after inhaler use.

Pediatric patients
• Safety and effectiveness haven't been established for children under age 12 for nasal aerosol and under age 6 for oral aerosol.

Breast-feeding patients
• Use drug with caution in breast-feeding women. It's unknown if drug appears in breast milk.

triamcinolone acetonide (topical)
Aristocort, Aristocort-A, Flutex, Kenalog, Kenalog in Orabase, Triacet, Triaderm*

Pharmacologic classification: topical adrenocorticoid
Therapeutic classification: anti-inflammatory
Pregnancy risk category C

How supplied
Available by prescription only
Cream, ointment: 0.025%, 0.1%, 0.5%
Lotion: 0.025%, 0.1%
Paste: 0.1%

Indications, route, and dosage
Inflammation of corticosteroid-responsive dermatoses
Adults and children: Apply cream, ointment, or lotion sparingly once to four times daily. Apply paste to oral lesions by pressing a small amount into lesion without rubbing until thin film develops. Apply b.i.d. or t.i.d. after meals and h.s.

Pharmacodynamics
Anti-inflammatory action: Glucocorticoids stimulate the synthesis of enzymes needed to decrease the inflammatory response. Triamcinolone acetonide is a synthetic fluorinated corticosteroid. The 0.5% cream and ointment are recommended only for dermatoses refractory to treatment with lower levels.

Pharmacokinetics
• *Absorption:* Absorption depends on potency of preparation, amount applied, and nature and condition of skin at application site. Ranges from about 1% in areas with thick stratum corneum (such as palms, soles, elbows, and knees) to as high as 36% in areas of thinnest stratum corneum (face, eyelids, and genitals). Absorption increases in areas of skin damage, inflammation, or occlusion. Some systemic absorption occurs, especially through oral mucosa.
• *Distribution:* After topical use, distributed throughout local skin layer. Drug absorbed into circulation; is rapidly distributed into muscle, liver, skin, intestines, and kidneys.
• *Metabolism:* After topical use, metabolized primarily in skin. Small amount that is absorbed into systemic circulation metabolized primarily in liver to inactive compounds.
• *Excretion:* Inactive metabolites excreted by kidneys, primarily as glucuronides and sulfates, but also as unconjugated products. Small amounts of metabolites also excreted in feces.

Contraindications and precautions
Contraindicated in patients with hypersensitivity to drug.

Interactions
None reported.

Adverse reactions
Metabolic: *hyperglycemia, glycosuria.*
Skin: *burning, pruritus, irritation, dryness, erythema, folliculitis, hypertrichosis, hypopigmentation, acneiform eruptions, perioral dermatitis, allergic contact dermatitis, maceration, secondary infection, atrophy, striae, miliaria (with occlusive dressings).*
Other: *hypothalamic-pituitary-adrenal axis suppression,* Cushing's syndrome.

☑ Special considerations
• Recommendations for use of triamcinolone, for care and teaching of patients during therapy, and for use in elderly patients, children, and breast-feeding women are the same as those for all topical adrenocorticoids.

Monitoring the patient
• Monitor therapeutic effect.
• Monitor patient for signs of adverse reactions.

Information for the patient
• Teach patient or family member how to apply drug.
• If an occlusive dressing is ordered, advise patient not to leave it in place longer than 12 hours each day and not to use occlusive dressings on infected or exudative lesions.
• Tell patient to stop drug and report signs of systemic absorption, skin irritation or ulceration, hypersensitivity, infection, or no improvement.

triamterene
Dyrenium

Pharmacologic classification: potassium-sparing diuretic
Therapeutic classification: diuretic
Pregnancy risk category B

How supplied
Available by prescription only
Capsules: 50 mg, 100 mg

Indications, route, and dosage
Edema
Adults: Initially, 100 mg P.O. b.i.d. after meals. Total daily dose shouldn't exceed 300 mg.

Pharmacodynamics
Diuretic action: Acts directly on the distal renal tubules to inhibit sodium reabsorption and potas-

sium excretion, reducing the potassium loss associated with other diuretic therapy.

Pharmacokinetics
• *Absorption:* Absorbed rapidly after oral administration, but extent varies. Diuresis usually begins in 2 to 4 hours. Diuretic effect may be delayed 2 to 3 days if used alone; maximum antihypertensive effect may be delayed 2 to 3 weeks.
• *Distribution:* About 67% protein-bound.
• *Metabolism:* Metabolized by hydroxylation and sulfation.
• *Excretion:* Drug and metabolites excreted in urine; half-life is 100 to 150 minutes.

Contraindications and precautions
Contraindicated in patients with hypersensitivity to drug; in those receiving other potassium-sparing drugs, such as spirolactone or amiloride hydrochloride; and in those with anuria, severe or progressive renal disease or dysfunction, severe hepatic disease, or hyperkalemia. Use cautiously in patients with impaired hepatic function or diabetes mellitus and in elderly or debilitated patients.

Interactions
Drug-drug. *ACE inhibitors (captopril, enalapril), potassium-containing drugs (parenteral penicillin G), potassium-sparing diuretics, potassium supplements:* Increased risk of hyperkalemia. Don't use together. If concomitant use can't be avoided, monitor potassium level and adjust dosage.
Antihypertensives: Potentiated hypotension. May be used to therapeutic advantage.
Cimetidine: Increased triamterene level. Adjust dosage.
Lithium: Decreased lithium clearance. Don't use together. If concomitant use can't be avoided, monitor patient closely and adjust lithium dosage as needed.
NSAIDs such as ibuprofen, indomethacin: Affect potassium excretion. Monitor patient closely.
Drug-food. *Salt substitutes containing potassium, potassium-rich foods:* Increased risk of hyperkalemia. Monitor serum potassium levels.
Drug-lifestyle. *Sun exposure:* Photosensitivity reactions. Tell patient to take precautions.

Adverse reactions
CNS: dizziness, weakness, fatigue, headache.
CV: hypotension.
GI: dry mouth, nausea, vomiting, diarrhea.
GU: transient elevation in BUN or creatinine levels, interstitial nephritis.
Hematologic: megaloblastic anemia related to low folic acid levels, ***thrombocytopenia.***
Hepatic: jaundice, increased liver enzyme abnormalities.
Metabolic: *hyperkalemia,* acidosis, hypokalemia, azotemia.
Musculoskeletal: muscle cramps.

Skin: photosensitivity, rash.
Other: *anaphylaxis.*

☑ Special considerations
• Recommendations for the use of triamterene and for care and teaching of the patient during therapy are the same as those for all potassium-sparing diuretics.
• Drug is commonly used with other, more effective diuretics to treat edema associated with excessive aldosterone secretion, hepatic cirrhosis, nephrotic syndrome, and heart failure.
• To minimize excessive rebound potassium excretion, withdraw drug gradually.
• Drug is less potent than thiazides and loop diuretics and is useful as an adjunct to other diuretic therapy. Usually used with potassium-wasting diuretics. Full effect is delayed 2 to 3 days when used alone.
• Drug therapy may interfere with enzyme assays that use fluorometry, such as serum quinidine determinations.
• Signs and symptoms of overdose include those indicative of dehydration and electrolyte disturbance. Treatment is supportive and symptomatic. For recent ingestion (less than 4 hours), empty stomach by induced emesis or gastric lavage. In severe hyperkalemia (more than 6.5 mEq/L), reduce serum potassium levels with I.V. sodium bicarbonate or glucose with insulin. A cation exchange resin, sodium polystyrene sulfonate (Kayexalate), given orally or as a retention enema, may also reduce serum potassium levels.

Monitoring the patient
• Monitor blood pressure, blood uric acid, CBC, and blood glucose, BUN, and serum electrolyte levels.
• Monitor patient for blood dyscrasia.

Information for the patient
• Tell patient to take drug after meals to minimize nausea.
• If a single daily dose is prescribed, advise patient to take it in the morning to prevent nocturia.
• Warn patient to avoid excessive ingestion of potassium-rich foods (such as citrus fruits, tomatoes, bananas, dates, and apricots), salt substitutes containing potassium, and potassium supplements to prevent serious hyperkalemia.
• Advise patient to avoid direct sunlight, wear protective clothing, and use a sunblock to prevent photosensitivity reactions.
• Tell patient that his urine may turn blue.
• Tell patient to immediately report if weakness, sore throat, headache, fever, bruising, bleeding, mouth sores, nausea, vomiting, or dry mouth occur or become severe.

Geriatric patients
• Elderly and debilitated patients need close observation because they are more suscepti-

drug-induced diuresis and hyperkalemia. Reduced dosages may be indicated.

Pediatric patients
● Use with caution; children are more susceptible to hyperkalemia.

Breast-feeding patients
● Drug may appear in breast milk. Safety during breast-feeding hasn't been established.

---

triazolam
Halcion

Pharmacologic classification: benzodiazepine
Therapeutic classification: sedative-hypnotic
Controlled substance schedule IV
Pregnancy risk category X

How supplied
Available by prescription only
Tablets: 0.125 mg, 0.25 mg

Indications, route, and dosage
Insomnia
Adults: 0.125 to 0.25 mg P.O. h.s. (0.5 mg P.O. h.s. only in exceptional patients; maximum dose is 0.5 mg).
Elderly: 0.125 mg P.O. h.s. May give up to 0.25 mg.

Pharmacodynamics
Sedative-hypnotic action: Depresses the CNS at the limbic and subcortical levels of the brain. Produces a sedative-hypnotic effect by potentiating the effect of the neurotransmitter gamma-aminobutyric acid on its receptor in the ascending reticular activating system, which increases inhibition and blocks both cortical and limbic arousal.

Pharmacokinetics
● *Absorption:* Well absorbed through GI tract after oral administration. Levels peak in 1 to 2 hours; onset of action at 15 to 30 minutes.
● *Distribution:* Distributed widely throughout body; 90% protein-bound.
● *Metabolism:* Metabolized in liver primarily to inactive metabolites.
● *Excretion:* Metabolites excreted in urine. Half-life of triazolam ranges from about 1½ to 5½ hours.

Contraindications and precautions
Contraindicated in patients with hypersensitivity to benzodiazepines and during pregnancy. Also contraindicated in patients taking ketoconazole, itraconazole, nefazodone, or any other drugs that impair the oxidative metabolism of triazolam by cytochrome P-450 3A.

Use cautiously in patients with impaired renal or hepatic function, chronic pulmonary insufficiency, sleep apnea, mental depression, suicidal tendencies, or history of drug abuse.

Interactions
Drug-drug. *Antidepressants, antihistamines, barbiturates, general anesthetics, MAO inhibitors, narcotics, phenothiazines:* Potentiated CNS depressant effect. Avoid concomitant use.
Cimetidine, isoniazid, oral contraceptives, possibly disulfiram: Increased triazolam plasma levels. Monitor triazolam levels.
Erythromycin: Decreased clearance of triazolam. Adjust dosage.
Haloperidol: Decreased haloperidol serum level. Don't use together. If concomitant use can't be avoided, adjust haloperidol dosage as necessary.
Levodopa: Decreased therapeutic effects of levodopa. Don't use together. If concomitant use can't be avoided, adjust levodopa dosage as needed.
Drug-food. *Grapefruit juice:* Increased triazolam levels. Don't give together.
Drug-lifestyle. *Alcohol:* Potentiated CNS depressant effects; risk of amnesia. Avoid concomitant use.
Heavy smoking: Decreased triazolam effectiveness. Discourage smoking.

Adverse reactions
CNS: *drowsiness, dizziness, headache,* rebound insomnia, amnesia, light-headedness, lack of coordination, mental confusion, depression, nervousness, ataxia, minor changes in EEG patterns.
GI: nausea, vomiting.
Hepatic: elevated liver enzymes.
Other: physical or psychological dependence.

☑ Special considerations
Besides the recommendations relevant to all benzodiazepines, consider the following.
● Onset of sedation or hypnosis is rapid; patient should be in bed when taking drug.
● Signs and symptoms of overdose include somnolence, confusion, hypoactive reflexes, dyspnea, labored breathing, hypotension, bradycardia, slurred speech, unsteady gait or impaired coordination, and, ultimately, coma.
● In case of overdose, support blood pressure and respiration until drug effects subside; monitor vital signs. Flumazenil, a specific benzodiazepine antagonist, may be useful. Mechanical ventilatory assistance via endotracheal tube may be needed to maintain a patent airway and support adequate oxygenation. Use I.V. fluids and vasopressors, such as dopamine and phenylephrine, to treat hypotension. If patient is conscious, induce emesis. Use gastric lavage if ingestion was recent, but only if an endotracheal

---

tube is present to prevent aspiration. After emesis or lavage, use activated charcoal with a cathartic as a single dose. Don't use barbiturates if excitation occurs. Dialysis is of limited value.

Monitoring the patient
• Monitor hepatic function studies to prevent toxicity.
• Monitor therapeutic effect.

Information for the patient
• Advise patient not to take OTC drugs or to change drug regimen without medical approval.
• Suggest other measures to promote sleep, such as drinking warm fluids, listening to quiet music, not drinking alcohol near bedtime, exercising regularly, and maintaining a regular sleep pattern.
• Advise patient that rebound insomnia may occur after stopping drug.
• To prevent falls, encourage safety precautions at start of therapy.
• Advise patient of potential for physical and psychological dependence.
• Advise woman to report suspected pregnancy immediately.
• Advise patient not to take drug when a full night's sleep and clearance of drug from body isn't possible before normal daily activities resume.

Geriatric patients
• Elderly patients are more susceptible to CNS depressant effects of drug. Use with caution.
• Elderly patients who receive drug need supervision with walking and daily activities during initiation of therapy or after an increase in dosage.

Pediatric patients
• Safety in children under age 18 hasn't been established.

Breast-feeding patients
• Drug appears in breast milk. A breast-fed infant may become sedated, have feeding difficulties, or lose weight. Avoid use in breast-feeding women.

triethanolamine polypeptide oleate-condensate
Cerumenex

Pharmacologic classification: oleic acid derivative
Therapeutic classification: ceruminolytic
Pregnancy risk category C

How supplied
Available by prescription only
Otic solution: 10% in 6-ml and 12-ml bottle with dropper

Indications, route, and dosage
Impacted cerumen
Adults and children: Fill ear canal with solution, and insert cotton plug. After 15 to 30 minutes, flush ear with warm water using a soft rubber bulb ear syringe. Don't expose ear canal to solution for more than 30 minutes.

Pharmacodynamics
Ceruminolytic action: Emulsifies and disperses accumulated cerumen.

Pharmacokinetics
No information available.

Contraindications and precautions
Contraindicated in patients with perforated eardrum, otitis media, or otitis externa.

Interactions
None reported.

Adverse reactions
EENT: ear erythema or itching.
Skin: severe eczema.

☑ Special considerations
• To determine allergic potential, do patch test: Place 1 drop of drug on inner forearm, then cover with small bandage; read in 24 hours. If reaction (redness, swelling) occurs, don't use drug.
• Moisten cotton plug with drug before insertion.
• Keep container tightly closed and away from moisture.
• Avoid touching ear with dropper.
• Signs and symptoms of overdose include vomiting and diarrhea, which, if protracted, may lead to fluid and electrolyte abnormalities. Evaluate patient for oral burns. In many cases, spontaneous emesis occurs; if it doesn't, it's unlikely that significant ingestion has occurred. Activated charcoal or a cathartic are unnecessary.
• Ocular exposure may result in transient eye irritation but usually no permanent damage. Treat eye exposure by irrigation with large amounts of tepid water for at least 15 minutes. Treat dermal exposure by washing exposed area.

Monitoring the patient
• Monitor therapeutic effect.
• Monitor patient for adverse effects.

Information for the patient
• Advise patient not to use drops more often than prescribed and to avoid touching ear with dropper.
• Teach patient correct application and storage.

---

trifluoperazine hydrochloride
Apo-Trifluoperazine,* Stelazine

Pharmacologic classification: phenothiazine (piperazine derivative)
Therapeutic classification: antipsychotic,
antiemetic
Pregnancy risk category C

How supplied
Available by prescription only
Tablets (regular and film-coated): 1 mg, 2 mg, 5
mg, 10 mg
Oral concentrate: 10 mg/ml
Injection: 2 mg/ml

Indications, route, and dosage
Anxiety states
Adults: 1 to 2 mg P.O. b.i.d. Increase dose, p.r.n.,
but don't exceed 6 mg/day.
Schizophrenia and other psychotic disorders
Adults: For outpatients, 1 to 2 mg P.O. b.i.d., increased, p.r.n. For hospitalized patients, 2 to 5
mg P.O. b.i.d.; may increase gradually to 40 mg
daily. For I.M. injection, 1 to 2 mg q 4 to 6 hours,
p.r.n.
*Children ages 6 to 12 (hospitalized or under close
supervision):* 1 mg P.O. daily or b.i.d.; may increase dose gradually to 15 mg daily. Or administer 1 mg I.M. once or twice daily.

Pharmacodynamics
Antipsychotic action: Thought to exert antipsychotic effects by postsynaptic blockade of CNS
dopamine receptors, thereby inhibiting dopamine-
mediated effects; antiemetic effects are attributed
to dopamine receptor blockade in the medullary
chemoreceptor trigger zone. Has many other central and peripheral effects; produces alpha and
ganglionic blockade and counteracts histamine-
and serotonin-mediated activity. Most prevalent
adverse reactions are extrapyramidal; has less
sedative and autonomic activity than aliphatic
and piperidine phenothiazines.

Pharmacokinetics
• *Absorption:* Rate and extent of absorption vary
with route. Oral tablet absorption erratic and variable, with onset of action ranging from ½ to 1 hour;
oral concentrate absorption much more predictable. I.M. drug absorbed rapidly. Peak effect
in 2 to 4 hours; steady-state serum levels within
4 to 7 days.
• *Distribution:* Distributed widely in body, including breast milk; 91% to 99% protein-bound.
• *Metabolism:* Metabolized extensively by liver,
but no active metabolites formed; duration of action is about 4 to 6 hours.
• *Excretion:* Mostly excreted in urine via kidneys;
some excreted in feces via biliary tract.

Contraindications and precautions
Contraindicated in patients with hypersensitivity
to phenothiazines and in patients experiencing
coma, CNS depression, bone marrow suppression, or liver damage. Use cautiously in elderly
or debilitated patients, in those exposed to extreme heat, and in patients with CV disease,
seizure disorders, glaucoma, or prostatic hyperplasia.

Interactions
Drug-drug. *Antacids containing aluminum and
magnesium; antidiarrheals:* Decreased absorption; decrease trifluoperazine effect. Avoid concomitant use.
*Antiarrhythmics, disopyramide, procainamide,
quinidine:* Increased risk of arrhythmias and conduction defects. Avoid concomitant use.
*Appetite suppressants, sympathomimetics (such
as ephedrine [commonly found in nasal sprays],
epinephrine, phenylephrine, phenylpropanolamine:* Decreased stimulatory and pressor effects.
Using epinephrine as a pressor drug in patients
taking trifluoperazine may result in epinephrine
reversal or further lowering of blood pressure.
Avoid concomitant use.
*Atropine, other anticholinergics (such as antide-
pressants, antihistamines, antiparkinsonians,
MAO inhibitors, meperidine, phenothiazines):*
Oversedation, paralytic ileus, visual changes, and
severe constipation. Avoid concomitant use.
Beta blockers: Increased trifluoperazine plasma
levels and toxicity. Avoid concomitant use.
Bromocriptine: Antagonized therapeutic effect on
prolactin secretion. Monitor patient closely.
*Centrally acting antihypertensives (such as cloni-
dine, guanabenz, guanadrel, guanethidine,
methyldopa, reserpine):* Inhibited blood pressure
response. Avoid concomitant use.
*CNS depressants (such as analgesics, anes-
thetics [epidural, general, spinal], barbiturates,
narcotics, parenteral magnesium sulfate, tranquilizers:* Possible oversedation, respiratory depression, and hypotension. Avoid concomitant
use.
High-dose dopamine: Decreased vasoconstriction. Monitor patient closely.
Levodopa: Decreased effectiveness and increased
toxicity of levodopa. Avoid concomitant use.
Lithium: Severe neurologic toxicity with encephalitis-like syndrome; decreases therapeutic response to trifluoperazine. Avoid concomitant use.
Metrizamide: Increased risk of seizures; additive
effects. Avoid concomitant use.
Nitrates: Possible hypotension. Avoid concomitant use.
Phenobarbital: Enhanced renal excretion; decreases trifluoperazine effect. Avoid concomitant
use.
Phenytoin: Increased risk of phenytoin toxicity.
Monitor phenytoin levels.

Reactions may be *common,* uncommon, *life-threatening,* or COMMON AND LIFE-THREATENING.

Propylthiouracil: Increased risk of agranulocytosis. Use together with caution.

Drug-food. *Caffeine:* Decreased therapeutic effect of drug. Avoid or limit concomitant use.

Drug-lifestyle. *Alcohol:* Additive effects. Discourage use.

Heavy smoking: Decreased therapeutic effects. Limit concomitant use when possible.

Sun exposure: Photosensitivity reactions. Tell patient to take precautions.

Adverse reactions

CNS: *extrapyramidal reactions, tardive dyskinesia,* pseudoparkinsonism, dizziness, drowsiness, insomnia, fatigue, headache.

CV: *orthostatic hypotension,* tachycardia, ECG changes.

EENT: ocular changes, *blurred vision.*

GI: *dry mouth, constipation,* nausea, weight gain.

GU: *urine retention,* menstrual irregularities, gynecomastia, inhibited lactation.

Hematologic: transient leukopenia, ***agranulocytosis.***

Hepatic: cholestatic jaundice, elevated liver function tests.

Skin: *photosensitivity,* allergic reactions, pain at I.M. injection site, sterile abscess, rash.

After abrupt withdrawal of long-term therapy: gastritis, nausea, vomiting, dizziness, tremor, feeling of warmth or cold, diaphoresis, tachycardia, headache, insomnia, anorexia, muscle rigidity, altered mental status, and evidence of autonomic instability.

☑ Special considerations

Besides the recommendations relevant to all phenothiazines, consider the following.

• Other drugs such as benzodiazepines are preferred for anxiety treatment. When drug is given for anxiety, don't exceed 6 mg daily for longer than 12 weeks. Some clinicians recommend using drug only for psychosis.

• Shake concentrate before administration.

• Worsening anginal pain has been reported in patients receiving trifluoperazine; however, ECG reactions are less common with drug than with other phenothiazines.

• Liquid and injectable formulations may cause a rash after contact with skin.

• Drug may cause pink to brown discoloration of urine or blue-grey skin.

• Drug is associated with a high risk of extrapyramidal symptoms and photosensitivity reactions.

• Oral formulations may cause stomach upset. Administer with food or fluid.

• Concentrate must be diluted in 2 to 4 oz (60 to 120 ml) of liquid, preferably water, carbonated drinks, fruit juice, tomato juice, milk, or pudding.

• Protect liquid formulation from light.

• Drug causes false-positive test results for urine porphyrins, urobilinogen, amylase, and 5-hydroxy-

indoleacetic acid levels from darkening of urine by metabolites; it also causes false-positive urine pregnancy results in tests using human chorionic gonadotropin as the indicator.

• CNS depression is characterized by deep, unarousable sleep and possible coma, hypotension or hypertension, extrapyramidal symptoms, dystonia, abnormal involuntary muscle movements, agitation, seizures, arrhythmias, ECG changes, hypothermia or hyperthermia, and autonomic nervous system dysfunction. Treatment is symptomatic and supportive and includes maintaining vital signs, airway, stable body temperature, and fluid and electrolyte balance.

• In overdose, don't induce vomiting. Drug inhibits cough reflex, and aspiration may occur. Use gastric lavage, then activated charcoal and sodium chloride cathartics; dialysis is usually ineffective. Regulate body temperature as needed. Treat hypotension with I.V. fluids. Don't give epinephrine.

• Treat seizures with parenteral diazepam or barbiturates, arrhythmias with parenteral phenytoin (1 mg/kg with rate titrated to blood pressure), extrapyramidal reactions with benztropine at 1 to 2 mg or parenteral diphenhydramine at 10 to 50 mg.

Monitoring the patient

• Monitor blood pressure before and after parenteral administration.

• Monitor patient regularly (at least once every 6 months) for abnormal body movements.

Information for the patient

• Explain risks of dystonic reactions, akathisia, and tardive dyskinesia, and tell patient to report abnormal body movements.

• Explain that many drug interactions are possible. Tell patient to call before taking any self-prescribed drugs.

• Tell patient that adverse reactions may be alleviated by a dosage reduction. Advise him to report difficulty urinating, sore throat, dizziness, or fainting.

• Warn man about inhibited ejaculation.

• Warn patient against hazardous activities that require alertness until effects of drug are known. Reassure patient that sedative effects usually subside in several weeks.

• Tell patient to avoid sun exposure and to wear sunscreen when going outdoors to prevent photosensitivity reactions. Explain that heat lamps and tanning beds also may cause skin burning or discoloration.

• Warn patient to avoid extremely hot or cold baths and exposure to temperature extremes, sunlamps, and tanning beds; drug may cause thermoregulatory changes.

• Tell patient to take drug exactly as prescribed and not to double missed doses, not to stop drug abruptly, and not to share drug with others.

- Advise patient to store drug in a safe place, away from children.
- Tell patient to avoid alcohol and other drugs that may cause excessive sedation.
- Inform patient that sugarless candy or gum, ice chips, or artificial saliva may relieve dry mouth.

Geriatric patients
- Elderly patients tend to need lower dosages, adjusted to effect. Adverse effects, especially tardive dyskinesia and other extrapyramidal effects and hypotension, are more likely to develop in such patients.

Pediatric patients
- Not recommended for children under age 6.

Breast-feeding patients
- Drug may appear in breast milk. Potential benefits to mother should outweigh potential harm to infant.

trihexyphenidyl hydrochloride
Apo-Trihex*, Artane, Artane Sequels, Trihexane, Trihexy-2, Trihexy-5

Pharmacologic classification: anticholinergic
Therapeutic classification: antiparkinsonian
Pregnancy risk category C

How supplied
Available by prescription only
Tablets: 2 mg, 5 mg
Capsules (sustained-release): 5 mg
Elixir: 2 mg/5 ml

Indications, route, and dosage
Idiopathic parkinsonism
Adults: 1 mg P.O. on first day, 2 mg on second day, then increase 2 mg q 3 to 5 days until total of 6 to 10 mg is given daily. Usually given t.i.d. with meals and, if needed, q.i.d. (last dose should be before bedtime). Postencephalitic parkinsonism may require 12 to 15 mg total daily dose. Patients receiving levodopa may need 3 to 6 mg daily. Sustained-release capsules shouldn't be used as initial therapy, but after the patient has been stabilized on the conventional dose forms. Sustained-release capsules can be dosed on a mg per mg of total daily dose and administered as a single dose after breakfast or in 2 divided doses 12 hours apart.
Drug-induced parkinsonism
Adults: 5 to 15 mg daily.

Pharmacodynamics
Antiparkinsonian action: Blocks central cholinergic receptors, helping to balance cholinergic activity in the basal ganglia. May also prolong the effects of dopamine by blocking dopamine reuptake and storage at central receptor sites.

Pharmacokinetics
- *Absorption:* Rapidly absorbed after oral administration; onset of action within 1 hour.
- *Distribution:* Crosses blood-brain barrier; little else known about distribution.
- *Metabolism:* Exact metabolic fate unknown; duration of effect is 6 to 12 hours.
- *Excretion:* Excreted in urine as unchanged drug and metabolites.

Contraindications and precautions
Contraindicated in patients with hypersensitivity to drug. Use cautiously in patients with impaired renal, cardiac, or hepatic function; glaucoma; obstructive disease of the GI or GU tract; or prostatic hyperplasia.

Interactions
Drug-drug. *Amantadine:* Amplified anticholinergic adverse effects of trihexyphenidyl, causing confusion and hallucinations. Monitor patient closely. When possible, avoid concomitant use.
Antacids, antidiarrheals: Decreased absorption of trihexyphenidyl. Avoid concomitant use.
CNS depressants (such as sedative-hypnotics, tranquilizers): Increased sedative effects of trihexyphenidyl. Avoid concomitant use.
Haloperidol, phenothiazines: Decreased antipsychotic effectiveness of these drugs; increased risk of anticholinergic adverse effects. Use together with caution. Monitor patient closely.
Levodopa: Synergistic anticholinergic effects. Adjust dosage of both drugs as needed.
Drug-lifestyle. *Alcohol:* May increase sedative effects. Discourage concomitant use.

Adverse reactions
CNS: nervousness, dizziness, headache, hallucinations, drowsiness, weakness.
CV: tachycardia.
EENT: blurred vision, mydriasis, increased intraocular pressure.
GI: *dry mouth,* nausea, constipation, vomiting.
GU: urinary hesitancy, urine retention.

☑ Special considerations
Besides the recommendations relevant to all anticholinergics, consider the following.
- Store drug in tight containers.
- Arrange for gonioscopic evaluation and close intraocular pressure monitoring, especially in patients over age 40.
- Tolerance to drug may develop, necessitating higher doses.
- Use drug with caution in hot weather because of increased risk of heat prostration.
- Signs and symptoms of overdose include central stimulation, then depression, with such psy-

chotic symptoms as disorientation, confusion, hallucinations, delusions, anxiety, agitation, and restlessness. Peripheral effects may include dilated, nonreactive pupils; blurred vision; flushed, dry, hot skin; dry mucous membranes; dysphagia; decreased or absent bowel sounds; urine retention; hyperthermia; headache; tachycardia; hypertension; and increased respiration.
• Treatment of overdose is primarily symptomatic and supportive, as needed. Maintain patent airway. If patient is alert, induce emesis (or use gastric lavage) and then use sodium chloride cathartic and activated charcoal to prevent further drug absorption. In severe cases, physostigmine may be administered to block antimuscarinic effects of trihexyphenidyl. Give fluids, as needed, to treat shock, diazepam to control psychotic symptoms, and pilocarpine (instilled into eyes) to relieve mydriasis. If urine retention occurs, catheterization may be necessary.

Monitoring the patient
• Monitor patient for urinary hesitancy.
• Monitor therapeutic effect.

Information for the patient
• Tell patient to avoid activities that require alertness until CNS effects of drug are known.
• Advise patient to report signs of urinary hesitation or urine retention.
• Tell patient to relieve dry mouth with cool drinks, ice chips, sugarless gum, or hard candy.
• Tell patient to take drug with food if GI upset occurs.

Geriatric patients
• Use caution when administering drug to elderly patients. Lower dosages are indicated.

Breast-feeding patients
• Drug may appear in breast milk, possibly resulting in infant toxicity. Drug also may decrease milk production. Avoid use in breast-feeding women.

trimethobenzamide hydrochloride
Tebamide, T-Gen, Ticon, Tigan, Trimazide

Pharmacologic classification: ethanolamine-related antihistamine
Therapeutic classification: antiemetic
Pregnancy risk category C

How supplied
Available by prescription only
Capsules: 100 mg, 250 mg
Suppositories: 100 mg, 200 mg
Injection: 100 mg/ml

Indications, route, and dosage
Treatment of nausea and vomiting
Adults: 250 mg P.O. t.i.d. or q.i.d.; or 200 mg I.M. or P.R. t.i.d. or q.i.d.
Children weighing 14 to 41 kg (30 to 90 lb): 100 to 200 mg P.O. or P.R. t.i.d. or q.i.d.
Children weighing under 14 kg: 100 mg P.R. t.i.d. or q.i.d.

Pharmacodynamics
Antiemetic action: Exact mechanism unknown. Weak antihistamine with limited antiemetic properties. Effects may occur in the chemoreceptor trigger zone of the brain; however, drug apparently doesn't inhibit direct impulses to the vomiting center.

Pharmacokinetics
• Absorption: About 60% of oral dose absorbed. After oral administration, action begins in 10 to 40 minutes; after I.M. administration, in 15 to 35 minutes.
• Distribution: No information available.
• Metabolism: About 50% to 70% of dose metabolized, probably in liver.
• Excretion: Drug excreted in urine and feces. After oral administration, duration of effect is 3 to 4 hours; after I.M. administration, 2 to 3 hours.

Contraindications and precautions
Contraindicated in patients with hypersensitivity to drug. Suppositories are contraindicated in patients with hypersensitivity to benzocaine hydrochloride or similar local anesthetic. Parenteral form is contraindicated in children, and suppositories are contraindicated in premature infants and neonates. Use cautiously in children.

Interactions
Drug-drug. Other CNS depressants (such as antihypertensives, belladonna alkaloids, phenothiazines, tricyclic antidepressants): Increased trimethobenzamide toxicity. Avoid concomitant use.
Drug-lifestyle. Alcohol: Increased sedative effects. Discourage use.

Adverse reactions
CNS: drowsiness, dizziness (in large doses), headache, disorientation, parkinsonian-like symptoms, depression, **coma, seizures.**
CV: hypotension.
EENT: blurred vision.
GI: diarrhea.
Hepatic: jaundice.
Musculoskeletal: muscle cramps.
Other: hypersensitivity reactions (pain, stinging, burning, redness, swelling at I.M. injection site).

☑ Special considerations
• Give I.M. dose by deep injection into upper outer gluteal quadrant to minimize pain and local irritation.
• Drug may be less effective against severe vomiting than other drugs.
• Drug has little or no value in treating motion sickness.
• Signs and symptoms of overdose may include severe neurologic reactions, such as opisthotonos, seizures, coma, and extrapyramidal reactions. Stop drug and provide supportive care.

Monitoring the patient
• Monitor frequency and volume of vomiting.
• Observe patient for signs and symptoms of dehydration.

Information for the patient
• Warn patient to avoid hazardous activities that require alertness because drug may cause drowsiness.
• Advise patient to avoid consuming alcohol to prevent additive sedation.
• Tell patient to report persistent vomiting.
• Advise patient using suppositories to remove foil and, if necessary, to moisten suppository with water for 10 to 30 seconds before inserting; tell patient to store suppositories in refrigerator.

Geriatric patients
• Use drug with caution in elderly patients because they may be more susceptible to adverse CNS effects.

Pediatric patients
• Use drug with caution in children. Don't administer to children with viral illness because drug may contribute to development of Reye's syndrome. Don't use in newborn or premature infants.

---

trimethoprim
Proloprim, Trimpex

Pharmacologic classification: synthetic folate antagonist
Therapeutic classification: antibiotic
Pregnancy risk category C

How supplied
Available by prescription only
Tablets: 100 mg, 200 mg

Indications, route, and dosage
Uncomplicated urinary tract infections
Adults: 100 mg P.O. q 12 hours or 200 mg q 24 hours for 10 days. Drug isn't recommended for children under age 12.

◊ *Pneumocystis carinii*
Adults: 5 mg/kg P.O. t.i.d. with dapsone 100 mg daily for 21 days.
✦ *Dosage adjustment.* If creatinine clearance is 15 to 30 ml/minute, give 50 mg every 12 hours. If creatinine clearance is below 15 ml/minute, manufacturer doesn't recommend use of this drug.

Pharmacodynamics
Antibacterial action: Usually bactericidal. By interfering with action of dihydrofolate reductase, drug inhibits bacterial synthesis of folic acid. Effective against many gram-positive and gram-negative organisms, including most Enterobacteriaceae organisms (except *Pseudomonas*), *Proteus mirabilis*, *Klebsiella*, and *Escherichia coli*.

Pharmacokinetics
• *Absorption:* Absorbed quickly and completely; serum levels peak in 1 to 4 hours.
• *Distribution:* Widely distributed. About 42% to 46% of dose is plasma protein-bound.
• *Metabolism:* Less than 20% of dose metabolized in liver.
• *Excretion:* Most of dose excreted in urine via filtration and secretion. In patients with normal renal function, elimination half-life is 8 to 11 hours; in patients with impaired renal function, half-life is prolonged.

Contraindications and precautions
Contraindicated in patients with hypersensitivity to drug and in those with documented megaloblastic anemia caused by folate deficiency. Use cautiously in patients with folate deficiency and impaired hepatic or renal function (especially those with creatinine clearance of 15 ml/minute or less).

Interactions
Drug-drug. *Phenytoin:* Increased serum phenytoin levels. Monitor phenytoin level; adjust dosage as needed.

Adverse reactions
GI: *epigastric distress, nausea, vomiting,* glossitis.
GU: increased BUN and serum creatinine levels.
Hematologic: **thrombocytopenia,** leukopenia, megaloblastic anemia, methemoglobinemia.
Hepatic: elevated liver enzyme levels.
Skin: *rash, pruritus,* exfoliative dermatitis.
Other: fever.

☑ Special considerations
• Drug is usually used with other antibiotics (especially sulfamethoxazole) because resistance develops rapidly when drug is used alone.
• Advanced age, malnourishment, pregnancy, debilitation, renal impairment, and prolonged high-

---

dose therapy increase risk of hematologic toxicity, as does use of drug with folate antagonistic drugs (such as phenytoin).

• Sore throat, fever, pallor, and purpura may be early signs and symptoms of serious blood disorders.

• Signs and symptoms of acute overdose include nausea, vomiting, dizziness, headache, confusion, and bone marrow depression. Treatment includes gastric lavage and supportive measures. Urine may be acidified to enhance drug elimination.

• Clinical effects of chronic toxicity caused by prolonged high-dose therapy include bone marrow depression, leukopenia, thrombocytopenia, and megaloblastic anemia. Treatment includes stopping drug and giving leucovorin—3 to 6 mg I.M. daily for 3 days or 5 to 15 mg P.O. daily until normal hematopoiesis returns.

Monitoring the patient
• Obtain urine specimen for culture and sensitivity tests before starting therapy.
• If patient is receiving drug with phenytoin, monitor serum phenytoin levels.
• Monitor blood counts regularly.

Information for the patient
• Advise patient to continue taking drug as directed, until it's completed, even if he is feeling better.
• Advise patient to report signs and symptoms of blood disorders (sore throat, fever, pallor, and purpura) immediately.

Geriatric patients
• Elderly patients may be more susceptible to hematologic toxicity.

Pediatric patients
• Safety in children under age 2 months hasn't been established. Effectiveness in children under age 12 hasn't been established; drug isn't recommended for children under age 12.

Breast-feeding patients
• Drug appears in breast milk. An alternative to breast-feeding is recommended during therapy.

trimipramine maleate
Surmontil

Pharmacologic classification: tricyclic antidepressant
Therapeutic classification: antidepressant, anxiolytic
Pregnancy risk category C

How supplied
Available by prescription only
Capsules: 25 mg, 50 mg, 100 mg

Indications, route, and dosage
Depression
Adults: For outpatients, give 75 mg/day P.O. in divided doses and increase to 200 mg/day; maintenance dose is 50 to 150 mg/day. Dose for inpatients is 100 mg/day in divided doses and increased, p.r.n. Maximum daily dose is 300 mg.
Elderly: 50 to 100 mg/day P.O.
Adolescents: 50 to 100 mg/day P.O.

Pharmacodynamics
Antidepressant action: Thought to exert its antidepressant effects by equally inhibiting reuptake of norepinephrine and serotonin in CNS nerve terminals (presynaptic neurons), which results in increased concentration and enhanced activity of these neurotransmitters in the synaptic cleft. Also has anxiolytic effects and inhibits gastric acid secretion.

Pharmacokinetics
• *Absorption:* Absorbed rapidly from GI tract after oral administration.
• *Distribution:* Distributed widely in body; 90% protein-bound. Effect peaks in 2 hours; steady-state within 7 days.
• *Metabolism:* Metabolized by liver; significant first-pass effect may explain variability of serum levels in different patients taking same dose.
• *Excretion:* Mostly excreted in urine; some excreted in feces via biliary tract.

Contraindications and precautions
Contraindicated in patients with hypersensitivity to drug, during acute recovery phase of MI, and in those receiving MAO inhibitor therapy within 14 days.
    Use cautiously in adolescents; in elderly or debilitated patients; in those receiving thyroid drugs; and in those with CV disease, increased intraocular pressure, hyperthyroidism, impaired hepatic function, or history of seizures, urine retention, or angle-closure glaucoma.

Interactions
Drug-drug. *Antiarrhythmics (disopyramide, procainamide, quinidine), pimozide, thyroid drugs:* Increased risk of arrhythmias and conduction defects. Monitor cardiac status. Use together cautiously.
Antihypertensives (such as clonidine, guanabenz, guanadrel, guanethidine, methyldopa, reserpine): Decreased hypotensive effect. Adjust dosage of antihypertensive drug.
Atropine, other anticholinergics (such as antihistamines, antiparkinsonians, meperidine, phenothiazines): Oversedation, paralytic ileus, visual changes, and severe constipation; additive effect. Avoid concomitant use.
Barbiturates: Decreased therapeutic efficacy of trimipramine. Monitor patient for drug effect.

Beta blockers, cimetidine, methylphenidate, oral contraceptives, propoxyphene: Increased trimipramine plasma levels and toxicity. Monitor trimipramine levels.

CNS depressants (such as analgesics, anesthetics, barbiturates, narcotics, tranquilizers): Oversedation; additive effect. Avoid concomitant use.

Disulfiram, ethchlorvynol: Risk of delirium and tachycardia. Use together cautiously.

Haloperidol, phenothiazines: Decreased therapeutic efficacy of trimipramine. Adjust dosage.

Metrizamide: Increased risk of seizures. Avoid concomitant use.

Selective serotonin reuptake inhibitors (fluoxetine, paroxetine, sertraline): Increased pharmacologic and toxic effects of trimipramine. Adjust dosage.

Sympathomimetics (such as ephedrine [commonly found in nasal sprays], epinephrine, phenylephrine, phenylpropanolamine): Increased blood pressure. Monitor blood pressure.

Warfarin: Increased risk of bleeding. Monitor PT and INR.

Drug-lifestyle. *Alcohol:* Additive CNS effects. Discourage use.

Heavy smoking: Decreased therapeutic efficacy. Limit or avoid concomitant use.

Sun exposure: Photosensitivity reactions. Tell patient to take precautions.

Adverse reactions

CNS: *drowsiness, dizziness,* paresthesia, ataxia, hallucinations, delusions, anxiety, agitation, insomnia, tremor, weakness, confusion, headache, EEG changes, **seizures,** extrapyramidal reactions.

CV: *orthostatic hypotension,* tachycardia, hypertension, **arrhythmias, heart block, MI, stroke,** prolonged conduction time on ECG.

EENT: *blurred vision,* tinnitus, mydriasis.

GI: *dry mouth, constipation,* nausea, vomiting, anorexia, paralytic ileus.

GU: *urine retention.*

Hematologic: decreased WBC counts, altered PT and INR.

Hepatic: elevated liver function test results.

Metabolic: altered serum glucose level.

Skin: rash, urticaria, photosensitivity, *diaphoresis.*

Other: *hypersensitivity reaction.*

After abrupt withdrawal of long-term therapy: possible nausea, headache, malaise (doesn't indicate addiction).

☑ Special considerations

Besides the recommendations relevant to all tricyclic antidepressants, consider the following.

● Consider the inherent risk of suicide until significant improvement of depressive state occurs. To reduce risk of suicidal overdose, prescribe smallest quantity of capsules consistent with good management.

● May give full dose at bedtime to offset daytime sedation.

● Drug also has been used to decrease gastric acid secretion in peptic ulcer disease. Safety and efficacy of drug in peptic ulcer disease hasn't been established.

● Watch for bleeding because drug may cause alterations in PT and INR.

● Don't stop drug abruptly. However, discontinue at least 48 hours before surgical procedures.

● Tolerance generally develops to drug's sedative effects.

● Manic or hypomanic episodes may occur in some patients, especially those with cyclic-type disorders, when taking drug.

● In overdose, the first 12 hours after acute ingestion are a stimulatory phase characterized by excessive anticholinergic activity (agitation, irritation, confusion, hallucinations, parkinsonian symptoms, seizure, urine retention, dry mucous membranes, pupillary dilation, constipation, and ileus). Then CNS depressant effects, including hypothermia, decreased or absent reflexes, sedation, hypotension, cyanosis, and cardiac irregularities (including tachycardia, conduction disturbances, and quinidine-like effects on the ECG.

● Severity of overdose is best indicated by prolongation of QRS complex beyond 100 milliseconds, which usually represents a serum level in excess of 1,000 ng/ml; serum levels generally aren't helpful. Metabolic acidosis may follow hypotension, hypoventilation, and seizures.

● Treatment of overdose is symptomatic and supportive and includes maintaining airway, stable body temperature, and fluid and electrolyte balance. Induce emesis with ipecac if patient is conscious; then use gastric lavage and activated charcoal to prevent further absorption. Dialysis is of little use. Physostigmine given I.V. slowly has been used to reverse most of the CV and CNS effects of overdose. Treat seizures with parenteral diazepam or phenytoin, arrhythmias with parenteral phenytoin or lidocaine, and acidosis with sodium bicarbonate. Don't give barbiturates because they may enhance CNS and respiratory depressant effects.

Monitoring the patient

● Closely monitor patients at high-risk for suicide during initial drug therapy.

● Monitor patient for adverse effects.

Information for the patient

● Advise patient to take full dose at bedtime to minimize daytime sedation.

● Explain that full effects of drug may not be seen for 4 to 6 weeks after therapy begins.

Reactions may be *common*, uncommon, **life-threatening**, or COMMON AND LIFE-THREATENING.

• Tell patient to take drug exactly as prescribed, not to double missed doses, not to stop drug suddenly, and not to share drug with others.
• Warn patient that drug may cause drowsiness or dizziness. Tell him to avoid activities that require mental alertness until the full effects of drug are known.
• Warn patient not to drink alcoholic beverages or medicinal elixirs while taking drug.
• Tell patient to store drug away from children.
• Suggest that patient take drug with food or milk if it causes stomach upset and ease dry mouth with sugarless chewing gum, hard candy, or ice.
• To prevent dizziness, advise patient to lie down for about 30 minutes after each dose and to avoid abrupt postural changes, especially when standing up.
• Tell patient to report adverse reactions promptly, especially confusion, movement disorders, rapid heartbeat, dizziness, fainting, or difficulty urinating.

Geriatric patients
• Elderly patients may be more vulnerable to adverse cardiac effects.

troleandomycin
Tao

Pharmacologic classification: macrolide antibiotic
Therapeutic classification: antibiotic
Pregnancy risk category C

How supplied
Available by prescription only
Capsules: 250 mg

Indications, route, and dosage
Pneumonia or respiratory tract infection caused by sensitive pneumococci or group A beta-hemolytic streptococci
Adults: 250 to 500 mg P.O. q 6 hours.
Children: 125 to 250 mg P.O. q 6 hours.

Pharmacodynamics
Antibacterial action: Inhibits bacterial protein synthesis by binding to 50S ribosomal subunit. Produces bacteriostatic effects on susceptible bacteria, including gram-positive cocci and bacilli and a few gram-negative organisms (Haemophilus influenzae, Neisseria gonorrhoeae, and N. meningitidis).

Pharmacokinetics
• Absorption: Absorbed rapidly but incompletely; serum levels peak in about 2 hours.
• Distribution: Distributed widely to body fluids, except to CSF.

• Metabolism: Metabolized in liver.
• Excretion: Excreted in bile, feces, and urine (10% to 25%).

Contraindications and precautions
Contraindicated in patients with hypersensitivity to drug. Use cautiously in patients with hepatic dysfunction.

Interactions
Drug-drug. Carbamazepine, methylprednisolone, theophylline: Decreased clearance of these drugs; possible risk of toxicity. Significance of decreased clearance of methylprednisolone is questionable; however, some clinicians recommend lower dosages of the corticosteroid.
Ergotamine: Risk of severe ischemic reactions and peripheral vasospasms. Avoid concomitant use.
Oral contraceptives: Risk of marked cholestatic jaundice. Use together cautiously.

Adverse reactions
GI: abdominal cramps, discomfort, vomiting, diarrhea.
Hematologic: eosinophilia, leukocytosis.
Hepatic: elevated liver enzymes, cholestatic jaundice.
Skin: urticaria, rash.
Other: anaphylaxis.

☑ Special considerations
• If patient is receiving drug with theophylline or carbamazepine, closely monitor serum theophylline or carbamazepine levels and assess patient often for signs and symptoms of theophylline or carbamazepine toxicity.
• Patient receiving drug together with methylprednisolone may need reduced dosages.
• Stop drug if liver function test values increase or if signs or symptoms of cholestatic hepatitis occur.
• Repeated courses of therapy or therapy exceeding 2 weeks may lead to allergic cholestatic hepatitis, as indicated by jaundice, right upper abdominal quadrant pain, fever, nausea, vomiting, eosinophilia, and leukocytosis.

Monitoring the patient
• Obtain culture and sensitivity tests before starting therapy.
• Monitor total serum bilirubin and AST, ALT, and serum alkaline phosphatase levels.

Information for the patient
• Advise patient to continue taking drug as directed, even if feeling better.
• For best absorption, advise patient to take drug on empty stomach 1 hour before or 2 hours after meals, with full glass of water.

• Advise patient to immediately report abdominal pain or nausea.

tromethamine
Tham

Pharmacologic classification: sodium-free organic amine
Therapeutic classification: systemic alkalinizer
Pregnancy risk category C

How supplied
Available by prescription only
Injection: 18 g/500 ml

Indications, route, and dosage
Correction of metabolic acidosis (associated with cardiac bypass surgery or with cardiac arrest)
Adults: Dosage depends on base deficit. Calculate as follows: ml of 0.3 molar tromethamine solution needed = body weight (in kg) × base deficit (in mEq/L) × 1.1. Total dose should be administered over at least 1 hour and shouldn't exceed 500 mg/kg for an adult.
   Usual dose of a 0.3 M solution (3.6 to 10.8 g tromethamine) may be administered into a large peripheral vein. If the chest is open, 55 to 165 ml of a 0.3 M solution (2 to 6 g tromethamine) has also been injected into ventricular cavity (not into cardiac muscle).
   For systemic acidosis during cardiac bypass surgery, usual single dose of a 0.3 M solution is 9 ml/kg (324 mg/kg tromethamine) or about 500 ml (18 g tromethamine) for most adults.
To titrate excess acidity of stored blood used to prime the pump-oxygenator during cardiac bypass surgery
Adults: Add 15 to 77 ml (500 mg to 2.5 g) of 0.3 M solution to each 500 ml of blood, depending on pH of blood.

Pharmacodynamics
Systemic alkalinizing action: As a weak base, acts as a proton acceptor to prevent or correct acidosis; reduces hydrogen ion concentration. Also acts as a weak osmotic diuretic, increasing the flow of alkaline urine.

Pharmacokinetics
• *Absorption:* Immediate absorption because drug is available for I.V. use only.
• *Distribution:* At pH of 7.4, about 25% of drug is un-ionized; this portion may enter cells to neutralize acidic ions of intracellular fluid.
• *Metabolism:* None.
• *Excretion:* Rapidly excreted renally as the bicarbonate salt.

Contraindications and precautions
Contraindicated in patients with anuria, uremia, or chronic respiratory acidosis and during pregnancy (except in acute, life-threatening situations). Use cautiously in patients with renal disease or poor urine output.

Interactions
Drug-drug. *Other CNS, respiratory depressants:* Risk of respiratory depression. Avoid concomitant use.

Adverse reactions
Hepatic: hemorrhagic hepatic necrosis.
Metabolic: hypoglycemia, *hyperkalemia* (with decreased urine output).
Respiratory: *respiratory depression.*
Other: venospasm; I.V. thrombosis; inflammation, necrosis, and sloughing (if extravasation occurs).

☑ Special considerations
• Administer drug by slow I.V. into the largest antecubital vein or via a large needle, indwelling catheter, or pump-oxygenator. If extravasation occurs, aspirate as much fluid as possible. Infiltrating area with 1% procaine hydrochloride to which hyaluronidase has been added may lessen extravasation and venospasm. Local injection of phentolamine can be used to reverse venospasm.
• Signs and symptoms of overdose include respiratory or systemic alkalosis, cardiac arrhythmias secondary to hypokalemia, respiratory depression, and hypoglycemia. Stop drug and correct pH; use decreased ventilation and systemic acidifiers, if necessary. Treat hypokalemia cautiously with potassium (serum potassium levels increase with correction of alkalosis), and hypoglycemia with I.V. glucose as needed.

Monitoring the patient
• Monitor vital signs, blood pH levels, carbon dioxide tension, and bicarbonate, glucose, and electrolyte levels before, during, and after infusion.
• Check infusion site frequently to avoid extravasation of solution and prevent tissue damage.

Information for the patient
• Explain drug to patient and family.
• Tell patient to report adverse reactions.

Geriatric patients
• Patients with severe renal dysfunction or chronic respiratory acidosis are at increased risk when receiving tromethamine; use drug with caution.

Pediatric patients
• Use drug cautiously; severe hepatic necrosis has occurred in infants and neonates after receiving a 1.2 M solution through umbilical vein.

Reactions may be *common*, uncommon, *life-threatening*, OR COMMON AND LIFE-THREATENING.

Hypoglycemia may occur when given to premature or full-term neonates.

tropicamide
I-Picamide, Mydriacyl, Ocu-Tropic, Opticyl, Tropicacyl

Pharmacologic classification: anticholinergic
Therapeutic classification: cycloplegic, mydriatic
Pregnancy risk category C

How supplied
Available by prescription only
Ophthalmic solution: 0.5%, 1%

Indications, route, and dosage
Cycloplegic refractions
Adults and children: Instill 1 or 2 drops of 1% solution in each eye; repeat in 5 minutes. If patient isn't examined within 30 minutes, an additional drop may be instilled into each eye.
Fundus examinations
Adults and children: Instill 1 or 2 drops of 0.5% solution in each eye 15 to 20 minutes before examination. May repeat q 30 minutes if necessary.
   Apply light finger pressure on lacrimal sac for 1 minute after instillation to minimize systemic absorption. Care should be taken to avoid contamination of the dropper tip.

Pharmacodynamics
Mydriatic action: Anticholinergic action prevents the sphincter muscle of the iris and the muscle of the ciliary body from responding to cholinergic stimulation, producing pupillary dilation (mydriasis) and paralysis of accommodation (cycloplegia).

Pharmacokinetics
• *Absorption:* Peak effect usually in 20 to 40 minutes.
• *Distribution:* No information available.
• *Metabolism:* No information available.
• *Excretion:* Recovery from cycloplegic and mydriatic effects usually in about 6 hours.

Contraindications and precautions
Contraindicated in patients with hypersensitivity to drug and in those with shallow anterior chamber or angle-closure glaucoma. Use cautiously in elderly patients.

Interactions
Drug-lifestyle. *Sun exposure:* May cause photophobia. Tell patient to take precautions.

Adverse reactions
CNS: confusion, somnolence, hallucinations, behavioral disturbances in children.

CV: edema.
EENT: *transient eye stinging on instillation,* increased intraocular pressure, hyperemia, irritation, conjunctivitis, *blurred vision, photophobia, dry throat.*
GI: dry mouth.
Skin: dryness.

☑ Special considerations
• Tropicamide is the shortest-acting cycloplegic, but its mydriatic effect is greater than its cycloplegic effect.
• Patients with highly pigmented irides may need higher strengths.
• Signs and symptoms of overdose include dry, flushed skin; dry mouth; dilated pupils; delirium; hallucination; tachycardia; and decreased bowel sounds. Treat accidental ingestion with emesis or activated charcoal. Use physostigmine to antagonize anticholinergic activity of tropicamide in severe toxicity and propranolol to treat symptomatic tachyarrhythmias unresponsive to physostigmine.

Monitoring the patient
• Monitor therapeutic effect.
• Monitor patient for symptoms of adverse reactions.

Information for the patient
• Advise patient to protect eyes from bright illumination for comfort.
• Advise patient not to touch dropper tip to any surface and to replace cap after use to avoid contamination.

Geriatric patients
• Use with caution in elderly patients to avoid triggering undiagnosed narrow-angle glaucoma.

Pediatric patients
• Infants and small children may be especially susceptible to CNS disturbances from systemic absorption. Psychotic reactions, behavioral disturbances, and cardiopulmonary collapse have been reported in children.

Breast-feeding patients
• It's unknown if drug appears in breast milk; use with extreme caution in breast-feeding women because of potential for CNS and cardiopulmonary effects in infants.

trovafloxacin mesylate
Trovan Tablets

alatrofloxacin mesylate
Trovan I.V.

Pharmacologic classification: fluoro-
quinolone derivative
Therapeutic classification: antibiotic
Pregnancy risk category C

How supplied
Available by prescription only
Tablets: 100 mg, 200 mg
Injection: 5 mg/ml, in 40 ml (200 mg) and 60 ml
(300 mg) vials

Indications, route, and dosage
For treatment of infections caused by suscepti-
ble microorganisms, the following doses are ad-
ministered once every 24 hours:
*Gynecologic and pelvic infections, compli-
cated intra-abdominal and postsurgical in-
fections*
Adults: 300 mg I.V. daily; then 200 mg P.O. daily
for 7 to 14 days.
Nosocomial pneumonia
Adults: 300 mg I.V. daily; then 200 mg P.O. daily
for 10 to 14 days.
Community-acquired pneumonia
Adults: 200 mg P.O. or I.V. daily; then 200 mg P.O.
daily for 7 to 14 days.
Complicated skin and diabetic foot infections
Adults: 200 mg P.O. or I.V. daily; then 200 mg P.O.
daily for 10 to 14 days.
✦ *Dosage adjustment.* Dosage adjustments are
unnecessary when switching from I.V. to oral
forms. An adjustment in dose isn't needed in patients with renal impairment; however, in patients
with mild to moderate hepatic disease (cirrhosis),
the following dose reductions are recommended: reduce 300 mg I.V. to 200 mg I.V.; reduce 200
mg I.V. or P.O. to 100 mg I.V. or P.O.; no reduction needed for 100 mg P.O.

Pharmacodynamics
Antibiotic action: Trovafloxacin is related to the
fluoroquinolones with in vitro activity against a
wide range of gram-positive and gram-negative
aerobic and anaerobic microorganisms. The bactericidal action of trovafloxacin results from inhibition of DNA gyrase and topoisomerase IV, two
enzymes involved in bacterial replication.

Pharmacokinetics
• *Absorption:* Well absorbed after oral administration; absolute bioavailability of about 88%.
Serum levels peak about 1 hour after oral administration; steady-state levels obtained by third
day of oral or I.V. administration.

• *Distribution:* Widely and rapidly distributed
throughout body, resulting in significantly higher
tissue levels than in plasma or serum. Mean plasma protein bound fraction about 76%; measurable levels in breast milk.
• *Metabolism:* Primarily metabolized by conjugation; minimal oxidative metabolism by cytochrome P-450. About 13% of dose appears in
urine as glucuronide ester, 9% as N-acetyl metabolite.
• *Excretion:* Primary route of elimination is fecal.
About 50% of oral dose excreted as unchanged
drug (43% in feces; 6% in urine).

Contraindications and precautions
Contraindicated in patients with hypersensitivity
to trovafloxacin, alatrofloxacin, or other quinolone
antimicrobials. Use cautiously in patients with history of seizures, psychosis, or increased intracranial pressure.

Interactions
Drug-drug. *Calcium carbonate, omeprazole:* Minor interactions that are probably not clinically
significant, including plasma level reductions by
these drugs. Monitor patient for possible adverse
effects.
I.V. morphine, sucralfate: Significantly reduced
trovafloxacin plasma levels. Avoid concomitant
use.
*Preparations containing aluminum, iron, mag-
nesium (such as antacids, minerals, vitamins):*
Significantly reduced drug bioavailability. Avoid
concomitant use.
Drug-lifestyle. *Caffeine:* Minor interactions that
are probably not clinically significant, including
plasma level reductions by caffeine. Monitor patient for possible adverse effects.

Adverse reactions
CNS: *dizziness,* light-headedness, headache,
seizures.
GI: diarrhea, nausea, vomiting, abdominal pain,
pseudomembranous colitis.
GU: vaginitis.
Hematologic: *bone marrow aplasia (anemia,
thrombocytopenia, leukopenia).*
Hepatic: *hepatic damage,* elevated hepatic
transaminases.
Musculoskeletal: arthralgia, arthropathy, myal-
gia.
Skin: pruritus, rash, injection site reaction (I.V.),
photosensitivity.

☑ Special considerations
• Drug has been associated with serious liver
damage leading to liver transplant or death. Reserve trovafloxacin for patients with serious infections and administer initial dose in an in-patient
facility. Don't use if a safer alternative is available.
Use shouldn't exceed 2 weeks' duration.

Reactions may be *common*, uncommon, **life-threatening**, or COMMON AND LIFE-THREATENING.

- I.V. drug should be administered as a 60-minute infusion.
- Changes in laboratory values during therapy don't produce clinical abnormalities, and levels generally return to normal 1 to 2 months after therapy ends.
- Oral form is more cost-effective and carries less risk; both forms have similar clinical efficacy and pharmacokinetics. Patients started with I.V. therapy may be switched to oral therapy when clinically indicated.
- Drug can be given as a single daily dose without regard for food.
- Administer I.V. morphine at least 2 hours after oral trovafloxacin in fasting state and at least 4 hours after oral trovafloxacin is taken with food.
- Alatrofloxacin is supplied in single-use vials which must be further diluted with a compatible solution, such as D₅W or 0.45% saline, before administration. Don't dilute drug with normal saline solution or lactated Ringer's solution. Follow package insert for specific instructions regarding preparation of desired dose.
- Trovafloxacin has a low order of acute toxicity. Signs and symptoms of toxicity include decreased activity and respiration, ataxia, ptosis, tremors, and seizures. Treat by emptying stomach and providing symptomatic and supportive treatment. Drug isn't efficiently removed by hemodialysis.

Monitoring the patient
- Perform periodic assessment of liver function because drug increases ALT, AST, and alkaline phosphatase levels.
- As with other quinolones, neurologic complications, such as seizures, psychosis, or increased intracranial pressure, may occur. Monitor patients with these preexisting conditions closely.

Information for the patient
- Inform patient that drug may be taken without regard to meals; however, tell him to take sucralfate, antacids containing citric acid buffered with sodium citrate, or products containing iron, aluminum, or magnesium (vitamin-minerals, antacids) at least 2 hours before or after a trovafloxacin dose.
- Advise patient who experiences dizziness or light-headedness to take drug with meals or at bedtime.
- Warn patient to avoid excessive sunlight or artificial ultraviolet light.
- Advise patient to stop treatment, refrain from exercise, and call if pain, inflammation, or rupture of a tendon occurs.
- Advise patient to stop treatment and call immediately at first sign of rash, hives, difficulty swallowing or breathing, or other symptoms suggesting an allergic reaction.
- Advise patient to report severe diarrhea because this could indicate pseudomembranous colitis.

Geriatric patients
- At recommended doses, drug is as well tolerated and efficacious in patients ages 65 and over as in younger patients.

Pediatric patients
- Safety and effectiveness in children under age 18 haven't been established.

Breast-feeding patients
- Drug appears in breast milk in measurable levels. Because of unknown effects in infants, evaluate risks of therapy and breast-feeding.

tuberculosis skin test antigens

tuberculin purified protein derivative (PPD)
Aplisol, Tubersol

tuberculin PPD multiple-puncture device
Aplitest (PPD), Mono-Vacc Test (Old Tuberculin), Tine Test (Old Tuberculin), Tine Test PPD

Pharmacologic classification: Mycobacterium tuberculosis and *Mycobacterium bovis* antigen
Therapeutic classification: diagnostic skin test antigen
Pregnancy risk category C

How supplied
Available by prescription only
tuberculin PPD
Injection (intradermal): 1 tuberculin unit/0.1 ml, 5 tuberculin units/0.1 ml, 250 tuberculin units/0.1 ml
tuberculin PPD multiple-puncture device
Test: 25 devices/pack

Indications, route, and dosage
Diagnosis of tuberculosis; evaluation of immunocompetence in patients with cancer or malnutrition
Adults and children: Intradermal injection of 5 tuberculin units/0.1 ml.

A single-use, multiple-puncture device is used for determining tuberculin sensitivity. All multiple-puncture tests are equivalent to or more potent than 5 tuberculin units of PPD.
Adults and children: Apply the unit firmly and without any twisting to the upper one-third of the forearm for about 3 seconds; this ensures stabilizing the dried tuberculin B in the tissue lymph. Exert enough pressure to ensure that all four tines have entered the skin of the test area and a circular depression is visible.

Pharmacodynamics

Diagnosis of tuberculosis: Administration to a patient with a natural infection with *M. tuberculosis* usually results in sensitivity to tuberculin and a delayed hypersensitivity reaction (after administration of old tuberculin or PPD). The cell-mediated immune reaction to tuberculin in tuberculin-sensitive individuals, which results mainly from cellular infiltrates of the dermis of the skin, usually causes local edema.

Evaluation of immunocompetence in patients with cancer or malnutrition: PPD is given intradermally with three or more antigens to detect anergy, the absence of an immune response to the test. The reaction may not be evident. Injection into a site subject to excessive exposure to sunlight may cause a false-negative reaction.

Pharmacokinetics

- *Absorption:* When PPD is injected intradermally or when a multiple-puncture device is used, a delayed hypersensitivity reaction is evident in 5 to 6 hours; peaks in 48 to 72 hours.
- *Distribution:* Injection must be given intradermally or by skin puncture; S.C. injection invalidates test.
- *Metabolism:* Not applicable.
- *Excretion:* Not applicable.

Contraindications and precautions

Severe reactions to tuberculin PPD are rare and usually result from extreme sensitivity to the tuberculin. Inadvertent S.C. administration of PPD may result in a febrile reaction in highly sensitive patients. Old tubercular lesions aren't activated by administration of PPD.

Interactions

Drug-drug. *Aminocaproic acid, systemic corticosteroids:* Possible false-negative reactions. Don't give test while other drugs are being used.

Live or inactivated viral vaccines (4 to 6 weeks preimmunization): Suppressed reaction to tuberculin. Wait more than 6 weeks before PPD test.

Topical alcohol: May inactivate PPD antigen and invalidate test. Don't use topical alcohol.

Adverse reactions

Other: local pain, pruritus, vesiculation, ulceration, or necrosis in some tuberculin-sensitive patients; hypersensitivity (immediate reaction may occur at the test site in the form of a wheal or flare that lasts less than a day, which shouldn't interfere with the PPD test reading at 48 to 72 hours); **anaphylaxis;** Arthus reaction.

☑ Special considerations

Tuberculin PPD

- Obtain history of allergies and previous skin test reactions before administration of the test.

- Epinephrine 1:1,000 should be available to treat rare anaphylactic reaction.
- Intradermal injection should produce a bleb 6 to 10 mm in diameter on skin. If bleb doesn't appear, retest at a site at least 5 cm from the initial site.
- Read test in 48 to 72 hours. An induration of 10 mm or greater is a significant reaction in patients who aren't suspected to have tuberculosis and who haven't been exposed to active tuberculosis, indicating present or past infection. An induration of 5 mm or more is significant in patients with AIDS or in those suspected to have tuberculosis or who have recently been exposed to active tuberculosis. An induration of 5 to 9 mm is inconclusive in patients not suspected of having been exposed to or having tuberculosis infection; therefore, test should be repeated if there is more than 10 mm of erythema without induration. The amount of induration at the site, not the erythema, determines the significance of the reaction.
- For either test, keep a record of the administration technique, manufacturer and tuberculin lot number, date and location of administration, date test is read, and the size of the induration in millimeters.

Multiple-puncture device

- Obtain history of allergies, especially to acacia (contained in the Tine Test as stabilizer), and reactions to skin tests.
- Report all known cases of tuberculosis to appropriate public health agency.
- Reaction may be depressed in patients with malnutrition, immunosuppression, or miliary tuberculosis.

Positive reaction: If vesiculation is present, the test may be interpreted as positive if induration is greater than 2 mm, but consider further diagnostic procedures.

Negative reaction: Induration is less than 2 mm. There is no reason to retest the patient unless the person is a contact of a patient with tuberculosis or there is clinical evidence of the disease.

Diagnosis of tuberculosis: PPD administration to a patient with a natural infection with *M. tuberculosis* usually results in sensitivity to tuberculin and a delayed hypersensitivity reaction after administration of old tuberculin or PPD. The cell-mediated immune reaction to tuberculin in tuberculin-sensitive individuals is seen as erythema and induration, which mainly results from cellular infiltrates of the dermis of the skin, usually causing local edema.

Diagnosis of immunocompetence in patients with such conditions as cancer or malnutrition: PPD is given intradermally with three or more antigens (such as Multitest CMI) to detect anergy.

- No evidence to date of adverse effects to fetus has been seen. The benefits of test are thought to outweigh potential risks to fetus.

Monitoring the patient
• Read test at 48 to 72 hours. Measure size of the largest induration in millimeters. A large reaction may cause the area around the puncture site to be indistinguishable.

Information for the patient
• Advise patient to report unusual adverse effects. Explain that induration will disappear in a few days.
• Reinforce the benefits of treatment if test is positive for tuberculosis.

Geriatric patients
• Elderly patients not having a cell-mediated immune reaction to the test may be anergic or they may test negative.

Breast-feeding patients
• Although it's unknown if drug appears in breast milk, there appears to be no risk to breast-feeding infants.

---

tubocurarine chloride

Pharmacologic classification: nondepolarizing neuromuscular blocker
Therapeutic classification: skeletal muscle relaxant
Pregnancy risk category C

How supplied
Available by prescription only
Injection: 3 mg/ml parenteral

Indications, route, and dosage
Adjunct to general anesthesia to induce skeletal muscle relaxation, facilitate intubation, and reduce fractures and dislocations
Dose depends on anesthetic used, individual needs, and response. Doses listed are representative and must be adjusted. Dose may be calculated on the basis of 0.165 mg/kg.
Adults: Initially, 6 to 9 mg I.V. or I.M., then 3 to 4.5 mg in 3 to 5 minutes if needed. Additional doses of 3 mg may be given, if needed, during prolonged anesthesia.
To assist with mechanical ventilation
Adults: Initially, 0.0165 mg/kg I.V. or I.M. (average 1 mg), then adjust subsequent doses to patient's response.
To weaken muscle contractions in pharmacologically or electrically induced seizures
Adults: Initially, 0.165 mg/kg I.V. or I.M. slowly. As a precaution, 3 mg less than the calculated dose should be administered initially.
Diagnosis of myasthenia gravis
Adults: Single I.V. or I.M. dose of 0.004 to 0.033 mg/kg.

Pharmacodynamics
Skeletal muscle relaxant action: Prevents acetylcholine from binding to receptors on motor endplate, thus blocking depolarization. Has histamine-releasing and ganglionic-blocking properties and is usually antagonized by anticholinesterase drugs.

Pharmacokinetics
• *Absorption:* After I.V. injection, rapid onset of muscle relaxation; peaks within 2 to 5 minutes. Duration is dose-related; effects usually begin to subside in 20 to 30 minutes. Paralysis may persist for 25 to 90 minutes. Subsequent doses have longer durations. After I.M. injection, onset of paralysis is unpredictable (10 to 25 minutes); duration is dose related.
• *Distribution:* After I.V. injection, distributed in extracellular fluid; rapidly reaches site of action. After tissue compartment is saturated, drug may persist in tissues for up to 24 hours; 40% to 45% is bound to plasma proteins, mainly globulins.
• *Metabolism:* Undergoes N-demethylation in liver.
• *Excretion:* About 33% to 75% of dose excreted unchanged in urine in 24 hours; up to 11% excreted in bile.

Contraindications and precautions
Contraindicated in patients with hypersensitivity to drug and in those for whom histamine release is a hazard (asthmatic patients). Use cautiously in elderly or debilitated patients; in those with impaired hepatic or pulmonary function, hypothermia, respiratory depression, myasthenia gravis, myasthenic syndrome of lung cancer or bronchiogenic carcinoma, dehydration, thyroid disorders, collagen diseases, porphyria, electrolyte disturbances, fractures, or muscle spasms; and in women undergoing cesarean section.

Interactions
Drug-drug. *Aminoglycoside antibiotics, beta blockers, calcium salts, clindamycin, depolarizing neuromuscular blocking drugs, furosemide, general anesthetics, lincomycin, local anesthetics, parenteral magnesium salts, polymyxin antibiotics, quinidine, quinine, thiazide diuretics, other nondepolarizing neuromuscular blocking drugs, other potassium-depleting drugs:* Enhanced or prolonged tubocurarine-induced neuromuscular blockade. Monitor patient closely; adjust dosage as needed.
Opioid analgesics, quinidine, quinine: Increased respiratory depressant effects. Use together cautiously.

Adverse reactions
CV: hypotension, *arrhythmias, cardiac arrest, bradycardia.*
GI: increased salivation.

Musculoskeletal: profound and prolonged muscle relaxation, idiosyncrasy, residual muscle weakness.
Respiratory: *respiratory depression or apnea, bronchospasm.*
Other: *hypersensitivity reactions.*

☑ Special considerations
● The margin of safety between therapeutic dose and dose causing respiratory paralysis is small.
● Allow effects of succinylcholine to subside before giving tubocurarine.
● Decrease dose if inhalation anesthetics are used.
● Use only fresh solution. Discard if discolored.
● Don't mix with barbiturates or other alkaline solutions in same syringe.
● I.V. administration requires direct medical supervision. Drug should be given I.V. slowly over 60 to 90 seconds or I.M. by deep injection in deltoid muscle. Tubocurarine is usually administered by I.V. injection, but if patient's veins are inaccessible, drug may be given I.M. in same dose as given I.V.
● Assess baseline tests of renal function and serum electrolyte levels before drug administration. Electrolyte imbalance (particularly potassium and magnesium) can potentiate effects of drug.
● Keep airway clear. Have emergency respiratory support equipment readily available.
● Be prepared for endotracheal intubation, suction, or assisted or controlled respiration with oxygen administration. Have available atropine and the antagonists neostigmine or edrophonium (cholinesterase inhibitors). A nerve stimulator may be used to evaluate recovery from neuromuscular blockade.
● Muscle paralysis follows drug administration in sequence: jaw muscles, levator eyelid muscles and other muscles of head and neck, limbs, intercostals and diaphragm, abdomen, trunk. Facial and diaphragm muscles recover first, then legs, arms, shoulder girdle, trunk, larynx, hands, feet, pharynx. Muscle function is usually restored within 90 minutes. Patient may find speech difficult until muscles of head and neck recover.
● Renal dysfunction prolongs drug action. Peristaltic action may be suppressed. Check for bowel sounds.
● Test for myasthenia gravis is considered positive if drug exaggerates muscle weakness.
● Drug doesn't affect consciousness or relieve pain; assess patient's need for analgesic or sedative.
● Signs and symptoms of overdose include apnea or prolonged muscle paralysis, which can be treated with controlled ventilation. Use a peripheral nerve stimulator to monitor effects and to determine nature and degree of blockade. Anticholinesterases may antagonize tubocurarine.

Atropine given before or with the antagonist counteracts its muscarinic effects.

Monitoring the patient
● Monitor respirations closely for early symptoms of paralysis.
● Monitor blood pressure, vital signs, and airway until patient recovers from drug effects. Ganglionic blockade (hypotension), histamine liberation (increased salivation, bronchospasm), and neuromuscular blockade (respiratory depression) are known effects of tubocurarine.
● After neuromuscular blockade dissipates, watch for residual muscle weakness.

Information for the patient
● Advise patient of potential adverse reactions.

Geriatric patients
● Administer cautiously to elderly patients.

Pediatric patients
● Administer cautiously to children.

Breast-feeding patients
● It's unknown if drug appears in breast milk. Use with caution in breast-feeding women.

typhoid vaccine
Vivotif Berna

Pharmacologic classification: vaccine
Therapeutic classification: bacterial vaccine
Pregnancy risk category C

How supplied
Available by prescription only
Oral vaccine: enteric-coated capsules of 2 to 6 $\times$ 10^9 colony-forming units of viable *Salmonella typhi* Ty-21a and 5 to 50 $\times$ 10^9 bacterial cells of nonviable *S. typhi* Ty-21a
Injection: suspension of killed Ty-2 strain of *S. typhi;* provides 8 units/ml in 5-ml and 10-ml vials
Powder for suspension: killed Ty-2 strain of *S. typhi;* provides 8 units/ml in 50-dose vial with 20 ml diluent/dose

Indications, route, and dosage
Primary immunization (exposure to typhoid carrier or foreign travel planned to area endemic for typhoid fever)
Parenteral
Adults and children over age 9: 0.5 ml S.C.; repeat in 4 or more weeks.
Infants and children ages 6 months to 9 years: 0.25 ml S.C.; repeat in 4 or more weeks.
Booster
Adults and children over age 10: 0.5 ml S.C. or 0.1 ml intradermally q 3 years.

Infants and children ages 6 months to 10 years: 0.25 ml S.C. or 0.1 ml intradermally q 3 years.
Oral
Adults and children over age 6: Primary immunization—1 capsule on alternate days (for example, days 1, 3, 5, 7) for four doses. Booster—repeat primary immunization regimen q 5 years.

Pharmacodynamics
Typhoid fever prophylaxis action: Promotes active immunity to typhoid fever in 70% to 90% of patients vaccinated.

Pharmacokinetics
No information available.

Contraindications and precautions
Contraindicated in patients with hypersensitivity to vaccine and in immunosuppressed patients. Vaccination should be deferred in patients with acute illness. Also, oral vaccine shouldn't be given to patients with acute GI distress (diarrhea or vomiting).

Interactions
Drug-drug. *Corticosteroids, immunosuppressants:* Impaired immune response to vaccine. Don't use together.
Phenytoin: Decreased antibody response to S.C. typhoid vaccine. Don't use together.
Sulfonamides, other anti-infectives active against S. typhi: Possible prevention of protective immune response. Don't use together.

Adverse reactions
CNS: malaise, headache.
GI: nausea, abdominal cramps, vomiting.
Musculoskeletal: myalgia.
Skin: rash, urticaria, swelling, pain, inflammation at injection site.
Other: *fever, anaphylaxis.*

☑ Special considerations
• Obtain thorough history of allergies and reactions to immunizations.
• Have epinephrine solution 1:1,000 available to treat allergic reactions.
• Shake vial thoroughly before withdrawing dose.
• Store injection at 36° to 50° F (2° to 10° C). Don't freeze.
• Store oral capsules at 36° to 46° F (2° to 8° C).
• Duration of vaccine-induced immunity is at least 2 years.

Monitoring the patient
• Monitor patient for adverse reaction, including anaphylaxis.

Information for the patient
• Tell patient to expect pain and inflammation at injection site, fever, malaise, headache, nausea, or difficulty breathing after vaccination. These re-

actions occur in most patients within 24 hours and may last for 1 to 2 days. Recommend acetaminophen for fever.
• Encourage patient to report adverse reactions.
• Tell patient traveling to area where typhoid fever is endemic to select food and water carefully. Vaccination isn't a substitute for careful selection of food.
• Inform patient that not all recipients of typhoid vaccine are fully protected. Travelers should take all necessary precautions to avoid infection.
• Advise patient that it's essential that all four doses of oral vaccine be taken at prescribed alternate-day interval to obtain a maximum protective immune response.
• Tell patient to take oral vaccine capsule about 1 hour before a meal with a cold or lukewarm (not exceeding body temperature) drink and to swallow capsule as soon as possible after placement in mouth. Remind patient not to chew capsule.

Pediatric patients
• Parenteral typhoid vaccine isn't indicated for those under age 6 months. Oral typhoid vaccine isn't indicated for children under age 6.

Breast-feeding patients
• It's unknown if vaccine appears in breast milk. Use with caution in breast-feeding women.

typhoid Vi polysaccharide vaccine
Typhim Vi

Pharmacologic classification: vaccine
Therapeutic classification: bacterial vaccine
Pregnancy risk category C

How supplied
Available by prescription only
Injection: 0.5-ml syringe, 20-dose vial, 50-dose vial

Indications, route, and dosage
Active immunization against typhoid fever
Adults and children ages 2 and older: 0.5 ml I.M. as a single dose. Reimmunization is recommended q 2 years with 0.5 ml I.M. as a single dose, if needed.

Pharmacodynamics
Antibacterial vaccine action: Promotes active immunity to typhoid fever.

Pharmacokinetics
• *Absorption:* Antibody levels usually remain elevated for 12 months after vaccination. Because of low occurrence of typhoid fever in United States, efficacy studies haven't been feasible.
• *Distribution:* No information available.

- *Metabolism:* No information available.
- *Excretion:* No information available.

Contraindications and precautions

Contraindicated in patients with hypersensitivity to any component of vaccine. Don't use to treat typhoid fever or give to those who are chronic typhoid carriers. Use cautiously in patients with thrombocytopenia or bleeding disorders and in those taking an anticoagulant because bleeding may occur after an I.M. injection in these individuals.

Interactions

None reported.

Adverse reactions

CNS: *headache, malaise.*
GI: nausea, diarrhea, vomiting.
Musculoskeletal: myalgia.
Other: *local injection site pain or tenderness, induration, erythema* at injection site; fever.

☑ Special considerations

- Delay administration of vaccine, if possible, in patients with febrile illnesses.
- Although anaphylaxis is rare, keep epinephrine readily available to treat anaphylactoid reactions.
- If vaccine is administered to immunosuppressed persons or persons receiving immunosuppressive therapy, the expected immune response may not be obtained.
- Persons who should receive vaccine include persons traveling to or living in areas of higher endemicity for typhoid fever.
- Administer as an I.M. injection into deltoid region in adults and in deltoid or vastus lateralis in children. Don't administer in gluteal region or areas where there may be a nerve trunk. Never inject I.V.

Monitoring the patient

- Monitor patient for adverse reactions.

Information for the patient

- Advise patient to take all necessary precautions to avoid contact with or ingestion of contaminated food and water.
- Inform patient that immunization should be given at least 2 weeks before expected exposure. Although an optimal reimmunization schedule hasn't been established, reimmunization with a single dose for U.S. travelers every 2 years, if exposure to typhoid fever is possible, is recommended at this time.

Pediatric patients

- Safety and effectiveness in children under age 2 haven't been established.

Breast-feeding patients

- It's unknown if drug appears in breast milk.

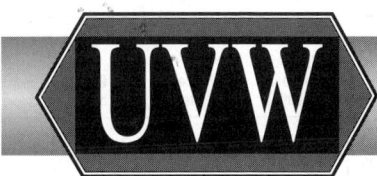

urea (carbamide)
Ureaphil

Pharmacologic classification: carbonic acid salt
Therapeutic classification: osmotic diuretic
Pregnancy risk category C

How supplied
Available by prescription only
Injectable: 40-g vial

Indications, route, and dosage
Reduction of intracranial or intraocular pressure
Adults: 1 to 1.5 g/kg as a 30% solution given by slow I.V. infusion over 1 to 2½ hours.
Children over age 2: 0.5 to 1.5 g/kg by slow I.V. infusion.
Children up to age 2: As little as 0.1 g/kg by slow I.V. infusion may be given. Maximum dose is 4 ml/minute.
   Maximum daily adult dose is 120 g. To prepare 135 ml of 30% solution, mix contents of a 40-g vial of urea with 105 ml of D_5W or $D_{10}W$ with 10% invert sugar in water. Each milliliter of 30% solution provides 300 mg of urea.
◊ *SIADH*
Adults: 80 g as a 30% solution I.V. over 6 hours.
◊ *Diuresis*
Adults and children over age 2: 500 mg to 1.5 g/kg as a 30% solution given by slow I.V. infusion over 30 minutes to 2 hours.
Children up to age 2: 100 mg to 1.5 g/kg as a 30% solution given by slow I.V. infusion over 30 minutes to 2 hours.

Pharmacodynamics
Diuretic action: Elevates plasma osmolality, enhancing the flow of water into extracellular fluid such as blood, and reducing intracranial and intraocular pressure.

Pharmacokinetics
• *Absorption:* I.V. urea produces diuresis and maximal reduction of intraocular and intracranial pressure within 1 to 2 hours; even though administered I.V., it's hydrolyzed and absorbed from GI tract.

• *Distribution:* Distributed into intracellular and extracellular fluid, including lymph, bile, and CSF.
• *Metabolism:* Hydrolyzed in GI tract by bacterial urease.
• *Excretion:* Excreted by kidneys.

Contraindications and precautions
Contraindicated in patients with severely impaired renal function, marked dehydration, frank hepatic failure, active intracranial bleeding, or sickle-cell disease with CNS involvement. Use cautiously in patients with cardiac disease or impaired renal or hepatic function and in pregnant or breast-feeding women.

Interactions
Drug-drug. *Lithium:* Enhanced renal excretion of lithium; lowered serum lithium levels. Monitor lithium levels closely.

Adverse reactions
CNS: *headache,* syncope, disorientation.
GI: *nausea, vomiting.*
Metabolic: altered electrolyte balance.
Other: irritation or necrotic sloughing with extravasation.

☑ Special considerations
Besides the recommendations relevant to all osmotic diuretics, consider the following.
• Avoid rapid I.V. infusion, which may cause hemolysis or increased capillary bleeding. Also avoid extravasation, which may cause reactions ranging from mild irritation to necrosis.
• Use only freshly reconstituted urea for I.V. infusion; solution turns to ammonia when left standing. Use within minutes of reconstitution.
• Don't administer through same infusion line as blood.
• Don't infuse into leg veins; this may cause phlebitis or thrombosis, especially in elderly patients.
• Maintain adequate hydration.
• If satisfactory diuresis doesn't occur in 6 to 12 hours, stop urea and reevaluate renal function.
• Urea has been used orally on an investigational basis for migraine prophylaxis, acute sickle-cell crisis prevention, and correction of SIADH.
• Signs and symptoms of overdose include unusually elevated BUN levels, polyuria, cellular dehydration, hypotension, and CV collapse. Stop infusion and institute supportive measures.

Monitoring the patient
- Monitor fluid and electrolyte balance.
- Monitor BUN levels frequently in patients with renal disease.
- Watch for signs and symptoms of hyponatremia or hypokalemia (muscle weakness, lethargy) as early indications of electrolyte depletion (before serum levels are reduced).
- Indwelling urinary catheter should be used in comatose patients to ensure bladder emptying. Use of an hourly urometer collection bag facilitates accurate measurement of urine output.

Information for the patient
- Advise patient of need to monitor fluid balance, electrolyte balance, and BUN level.
- Advise patient to report muscle weakness and lethargy.

Geriatric patients
- Elderly or debilitated patients will need close observation and may need lower doses. Excessive diuresis promotes rapid dehydration and hypovolemia, hypokalemia, and hyponatremia.

Breast-feeding patients
- It's unknown if drug appears in breast milk. Safety in breast-feeding women hasn't been established.

valacyclovir hydrochloride
Valtrex

Pharmacologic classification: synthetic purine nucleoside
Therapeutic classification: antiviral
Pregnancy risk category B

How supplied
Available by prescription only
Caplets: 500 mg

Indications, route, and dosage
Herpes zoster in immunocompetent patients
Adults: 1 g P.O. t.i.d. daily for 7 days.
Initial episode of genital herpes
Adults: 1 g P.O. b.i.d. for 10 days.
Recurrent genital herpes in immunocompetent patients
Adults: 500 mg P.O. b.i.d. for 5 days.
Chronic suppressive therapy of recurrent genital herpes
Adults: 1 g P.O. once daily.
✦ Dosage adjustment. For patients with renal impairment, see the table in the next column.

Creatinine clearance (ml/min)	Herpes zoster	Genital herpes
30 to 49	1 g q 12 hours	500 mg q 12 hours
10 to 29	1 g q 24 hours	500 mg q 24 hours
< 10	500 mg q 24 hours	500 mg q 24 hours

Pharmacodynamics
Antiviral action: Rapidly becomes converted to acyclovir. Acyclovir becomes incorporated into viral DNA and inhibits viral DNA polymerase, thus inhibiting viral multiplication.

Pharmacokinetics
- *Absorption:* Rapidly absorbed from GI tract; absolute bioavailability about 54.5%.
- *Distribution:* Protein-binding ranges from 13.5% to 17.9%.
- *Metabolism:* Rapidly and nearly completely converted to acyclovir and L-valine by first-pass intestinal or hepatic metabolism.
- *Excretion:* Excreted in urine and feces. Half-life is about 2½ to 3¼ hours.

Contraindications and precautions
Contraindicated in patients with hypersensitivity or intolerance to valacyclovir, acyclovir, or their components and in immunocompromised patients. Use cautiously in patients with impaired renal function and in those receiving other nephrotoxic drugs.

Interactions
Drug-drug. *Cimetidine, probenecid:* Reduced rate of renal clearance of acyclovir; increased acyclovir blood levels. Monitor patient for possible toxicity.

Adverse reactions
CNS: *headache,* dizziness, asthenia.
GI: *nausea,* vomiting, diarrhea, constipation, abdominal pain, anorexia.

☑ Special considerations
- Initiate therapy at first signs or symptoms of an episode, preferably within 24 hours after their onset; treatment is most effective when initiated within 48 hours of zoster rash onset.
- Glaxo-Wellcome (manufacturer) maintains an ongoing registry of women exposed to drug during pregnancy. Follow-up studies to date haven't shown an increased risk for birth defects in infants born to patients exposed to this drug during pregnancy. Physicians are encouraged to re-

port such exposures to the registrar at (800) 722-9292, extension 58465.
• Thrombotic thrombocytopenic purpura and hemolytic uremic syndrome have occurred, resulting in death in some patients with advanced HIV infection, and also in bone marrow transplant and renal transplant recipients participating in clinical trials of valacyclovir.
• No report of overdose. However, precipitation of acyclovir in renal tubules may occur when the solubility (2.5 mg/ml) is exceeded in the intratubular fluid. If acute renal failure and anuria occur, hemodialysis may be helpful until renal function is restored.

Monitoring the patient
• Monitor therapeutic effect.

Information for the patient
• Inform patient that drug may be taken without regard to meals.
• Advise patient to call immediately at the first sign of an episode.
• Tell patient to avoid contact with lesions and to avoid intercourse when lesions or symptoms are present.

Geriatric patients
• Dosage adjustment may be needed in elderly patients based on underlying renal status.

Pediatric patients
• Safety and effectiveness in children haven't been established.

Breast-feeding patients
• It's unknown if drug appears in breast milk. Use in breast-feeding women isn't recommended.

---

valproic acid
Depakene, Epival*

divalproex sodium
Depakote, Depakote Sprinkle

valproate sodium
Depacon

Pharmacologic classification: carboxylic acid derivative
Therapeutic classification: anticonvulsant
Pregnancy risk category D

How supplied
Available by prescription only
valproic acid
Capsules: 250 mg
Syrup: 250 mg/5 ml

divalproex sodium
Tablets (delayed-release): 125 mg, 250 mg, 500 mg
Capsules (sprinkle): 125 mg
valproate sodium
Injection: 5 ml single-dose vials

Indications, route, and dosage
Simple and complex absence seizures and mixed seizure types, ◊ tonic-clonic seizures
Adults and children: P.O.—initially, 15 mg/kg P.O. daily, divided b.i.d. or t.i.d.; may increase by 5 to 10 mg/kg daily at weekly intervals to maximum of 60 mg/kg daily divided b.i.d. or t.i.d.
   Note: Doses of divalproex sodium (Depakote) are expressed as valproic acid.
Adults and children: I.V.—initially, 10 to 15 mg/kg/day as a 60-minute I.V. infusion (rate 20 mg/minute or less). The dosage may increase by 5 to 10 mg/kg daily at weekly intervals to maximum of 60 mg/kg daily. Drug should be diluted in at least 50 ml of compatible diluent.
Mania
Adults: 750 mg P.O. in divided doses (divalproex sodium).
Migraine prophylaxis
Adults: 250 mg P.O. b.i.d. Some patients may benefit from doses up to 1 g daily.
◊ Status epilepticus refractory to I.V. diazepam
Adults: 400 to 600 mg P.R. q 6 hours.

Pharmacodynamics
Anticonvulsant action: Mechanism unknown; effects may be from increased brain levels of gamma-aminobutyric acid (GABA), an inhibitory transmitter. Also may decrease GABA's enzymatic catabolism. Onset of therapeutic effects may require a week or more. May be used with other anticonvulsants.

Pharmacokinetics
• *Absorption:* Valproate sodium and divalproex sodium quickly convert to valproic acid after administration of oral dose; plasma levels peak in 1 to 5 hours, 15 minutes to 2 hours with syrup, and immediately with I.V.; same bioavailability for all dose forms.
• *Distribution:* Distributed rapidly throughout body; 80% to 95% protein-bound.
• *Metabolism:* Metabolized by liver.
• *Excretion:* Excreted in urine; some drug excreted in feces and exhaled air. Breast milk levels are 1% to 10% of serum levels.

Contraindications and precautions
Contraindicated in patients with hypersensitivity to drug. Use cautiously in patients with history of hepatic dysfunction. Don't give valproate sodium injection to patients with hepatic disease or significant hepatic dysfunction.

Interactions
Drug-drug. *Clonazepam:* Absence seizures may occur. Avoid concomitant use.
Felbamate, salicylates: Increased valproate levels. Monitor valproate levels.
Lamotrigine: Increased valproate levels. Monitor valproate levels.
MAO inhibitors, oral anticoagulants, other CNS antidepressants: Potentiated effects of these drugs. Monitor patient closely.
Phenobarbital, phenytoin, primidone: Increased serum levels of these drugs; excessive somnolence. Monitor patient carefully.
Drug-lifestyle. *Alcohol:* Decreased valproic acid effectiveness; increases CNS adverse effects. Discourage use.

Adverse reactions
Because drug usually is used with other anticonvulsants, adverse reactions reported may not be caused by valproic acid alone.
CNS: *sedation,* emotional upset, depression, psychosis, aggressiveness, hyperactivity, behavioral deterioration, tremor, ataxia, headache, dizziness, incoordination.
EENT: nystagmus, diplopia.
GI: *nausea, vomiting, indigestion,* diarrhea, abdominal cramps, constipation, increased appetite and weight gain, anorexia, *pancreatitis.*
Hematologic: *thrombocytopenia,* increased bleeding time, petechiae, bruising, eosinophilia, *hemorrhage,* leukopenia, *bone marrow suppression.*
Hepatic: *elevated liver enzymes, toxic hepatitis.*
Musculoskeletal: muscle weakness.
Skin: rash, alopecia, pruritus, photosensitivity, *erythema multiforme.*

☑ Special considerations
• Administer drug with food to minimize GI irritation.
• Administer I.V. as 60-minute infusion with rate not exceeding 20 mg/minute.
• Use of valproate sodium injection for periods of more than 14 days hasn't been studied. Patients should be switched to oral products as soon as clinically feasible. When switching from I.V. to oral therapy or from oral to I.V. therapy, the total daily dose should be equivalent and given with the same frequency.
• Don't withdraw drug abruptly.
• Valproic acid may cause false-positive test results for urinary ketones.
• Signs and symptoms of overdose include somnolence and coma. Treat supportively. Maintain adequate urine output, and monitor vital signs and fluid and electrolyte balance carefully. Naloxone reverses CNS and respiratory depression but also may reverse anticonvulsant effects of valproic acid. Hemodialysis and hemoperfusion have been used.

Monitoring the patient
• Monitor plasma level and make dosage adjustments as needed; therapeutic range of drug is 50 to 100 mcg/ml.
• Watch for tremors; they may indicate need for dosage reduction.
• Evaluate liver function, platelet count, and PT at baseline and monthly intervals—especially during first 6 months.

Information for the patient
• Tell patient to swallow tablets or capsules whole to avoid local mucosal irritation. If necessary, take with food but not carbonated beverages because tablet may dissolve before swallowing, causing irritation and unpleasant taste.
• Warn patient to avoid alcohol while taking drug; may decrease drug's effectiveness and increase CNS adverse effects.
• Advise patient to avoid tasks that require mental alertness until CNS sedative effects are known. Drowsiness and dizziness may occur. Bedtime administration of drug may minimize CNS depression.
• Teach patient signs and symptoms of hypersensitivity and adverse effects and the need to report them.
• Advise patient not to stop drug suddenly, not to alter dose without approval, and to call before changing brand or using generic drug because therapeutic effect may change.
• Encourage patient taking anticonvulsants to wear a medical identification bracelet or necklace, listing drug and seizure disorders.

Geriatric patients
• Drug is eliminated more slowly in elderly patients; lower dosages are recommended.

Pediatric patients
• Not recommended for use in children under age 2; this age-group is at highest risk for adverse effects. Hyperexcitability and aggressiveness have occurred in a few children.

Breast-feeding patients
• Drug appears in breast milk in serum levels from 1% to 10%. An alternative to breast-feeding is recommended during therapy.

valrubicin
Valstar

Pharmacologic classification: anthracycline
Therapeutic classification: antineoplastic
Pregnancy risk category C

How supplied
Available by prescription only
Solution for intravesical instillation: 200 mg/5 ml

Indications, route, and dosage
**Intravesical therapy of BCG-refractory carci-
noma in situ (CIS) of the urinary bladder in
patients for whom immediate cystectomy
would be associated with unacceptable morbidity or mortality**
Adults: 800 mg intravesically once weekly for 6
weeks.

Pharmacodynamics
Antineoplastic action: Anthracycline exerts cytotoxic activity by penetrating cells and inhibiting
the incorporation of nucleosides into nucleic
acids, causes extensive chromosomal damage,
and arrests cell cycle in G_2. Also interferes with
the normal DNA breaking-resealing action of
DNA topoisomerase II, thereby inhibiting DNA
synthesis.

Pharmacokinetics
• *Absorption:* Only small quantities absorbed into
plasma after intravesical administration.
• *Distribution:* Penetrates into bladder wall after
intravesical administration. Systemic exposure
dependent on condition of bladder wall.
• *Metabolism:* Metabolites found in blood.
• *Excretion:* After retention, almost completely
excreted by voiding the instillate.

Contraindications and precautions
Contraindicated in patients with hypersensitivity
to drug or other anthracyclines or Cremophor EL
(polyoxyethyleneglycol triricinoleate). Also contraindicated in patients with urinary tract infections, small bladder capacity (unable to tolerate
a 75 mL instillation), or perforated bladder and in
those in whom the integrity of the bladder mucosa has been compromised.
Use cautiously in patients with severe irritable bladder symptoms.

Interactions
None reported.

Adverse reactions
CNS: asthenia, headache, malaise, dizziness.
CV: vasodilation, chest pain, peripheral edema.

GI: diarrhea, flatulence, nausea, vomiting, ab-
dominal pain.
GU: urinary retention, *urinary tract infection, uri-
nary frequency, dysuria, urinary urgency, blad-
der spasm,* hematuria, *bladder pain, urinary in-
continence,* pelvic pain, urethral pain, nocturia,
cystitis, local burning symptoms.
Hematologic: anemia.
Metabolic: hyperglycemia.
Musculoskeletal: myalgia, back pain.
Respiratory: pneumonia.
Skin: rash.
Other: fever.

☑ Special considerations
• In patients with severe irritable bladder symptoms, bladder spasm and spontaneous discharge
of the intravesical instillate may occur. Clamping
the urinary catheter isn't advised.
• For patients undergoing transurethral resection
of the bladder, evaluate bladder status before intravesical instillation of drug to avoid dangerous
systemic exposure.
• In case of bladder perforation, delay administration until bladder integrity has been restored.
• If there isn't a complete response of CIS to valrubicin treatment after 3 months or if CIS recurs,
cystectomy must be reconsidered because delaying cystectomy could lead to metastatic bladder cancer.
• Myelosuppression is possible if drug is inadvertently given systemically or if significant systemic exposure occurs after intravesical administration, such as in patients with bladder rupture
or perforation.
• Drug should be administered intravesically only
by those experienced in the use of intravesical
antineoplastics. Don't give I.V. or I.M.
• Use gloves during dose preparation and administration. Prepare and store solution in glass,
polypropylene, or polyolefin containers and tubing. It's recommended that polyethylene-lined administration sets be used. Don't use polyvinyl
chloride I.V. bags and tubing.
• Use proper procedures for handling and disposal of antineoplastics.
• Store unopened vials under refrigeration at 2°
to 8° C (36° to 46° F). Diluted drug is stable for
12 hours at temperatures up to 25° C (77° F).
• There is no known antidote for overdose. Anticipated complications associated with intravesical overdose would be consistent with irritable
bladder symptoms.

Monitoring the patient
• Monitor patient closely for disease recurrence
or progression by cystoscopy, biopsy, and urine
cytology every 3 months.
• If drug is administered when bladder rupture
or perforation is suspected, weekly monitoring of
CBC should be performed for 3 weeks. Myelo-

suppression begins during the first week, with the nadir by the second week, and recovery by the third week.

Information for the patient
• Advise patient that drug has been shown to induce complete response in only about 1 in 5 patients with refractory CIS. If there is no complete response of CIS to treatment after 3 months or if CIS recurs, discuss risks of cystectomy versus risks of metastatic bladder cancer with patient.
• Advise patient to retain drug for 2 hours before voiding, if possible. Instruct patient to void at the end of 2 hours.
• Instruct patient to maintain adequate hydration after treatment.
• Advise patient that major adverse reactions are related to irritable bladder symptoms that may occur during instillation and retention of drug and for a limited period after voiding. For the first 24 hours after administration, red-tinged urine is typical. Tell patient to report prolonged irritable bladder symptoms or prolonged passage of red-colored urine immediately.
• Advise a woman of childbearing age or a man and his partner to avoid pregnancy during treatment and to use effective contraception.

Pediatric patients
• Safety and effectiveness in children haven't been established.

Breast-feeding patients
• It's unknown if drug appears in breast milk. Because this drug is highly lipophilic and any exposure of infants to drug could cause serious health risks, women should stop breast-feeding before therapy begins.

valsartan
Diovan

Pharmacologic classification: angiotensin II antagonist
Therapeutic classification: antihypertensive
Pregnancy risk category X

How supplied
Available by prescription only
Capsules: 80 mg, 160 mg

Indications, route, and dosage
Hypertension, used alone or with other antihypertensives
Adults: Initially, 80 mg P.O. once daily as monotherapy in patients who aren't volume-depleted. Blood pressure reduction should occur in 2 to 4 weeks. If additional antihypertensive effect is needed, dose may be increased to 160 or 320 mg daily or add diuretic. (Addition of diuretic has greater

effect than dose increases beyond 80 mg.) Usual dose range is 80 to 320 mg daily.

Pharmacodynamics
Antihypertensive action: Blocks binding of angiotensin II to receptor sites in vascular smooth muscle and adrenal gland, which inhibits the pressor effects of the renin-angiotensin system.

Pharmacokinetics
• *Absorption:* Absolute bioavailability about 25%. Plasma level peaks 2 to 4 hours after dosing.
• *Distribution:* Isn't distributed extensively into tissues; 95% bound to serum proteins, mainly to serum albumin.
• *Metabolism:* Only about 20% is metabolized. Enzyme responsible for metabolism not yet identified; doesn't appear to be a cytochrome P-450 enzyme.
• *Excretion:* 83% of dose excreted through feces; about 13% in urine. Average elimination half-life is about 6 hours.

Contraindications and precautions
Contraindicated in patients with hypersensitivity to drug. Use cautiously in patients with renal or hepatic disease.

Interactions
Drug-drug. *Diuretics:* Increased risk of excessive hypotension. Use together with caution. Monitor patient closely.

Adverse reactions
CNS: fatigue, dizziness, headache.
CV: edema.
EENT: pharyngitis, rhinitis, sinusitis.
GI: abdominal pain, diarrhea, nausea.
Hematologic: neutropenia.
Metabolic: hyperkalemia.
Musculoskeletal: arthralgia.
Respiratory: cough, upper respiratory tract infection.
Other: viral infection.

☑ Special considerations
• Excessive hypotension can occur when drug is given with high doses of diuretics. Correct volume and salt depletions before therapy.
• Don't use in pregnant women because fetal and neonatal morbidity and death may occur.
• The most likely symptoms of overdose are hypotension and tachycardia; bradycardia could occur from parasympathetic (vagal) stimulation. If symptomatic hypotension should occur, provide supportive treatment.

Monitoring the patient
• Monitor fluid and electrolyte balance.
• Monitor cardiac status.

Information for the patient
- Advise woman to avoid pregnancy during therapy and to call immediately if pregnancy is suspected.
- Advise patient to report dizziness.

Geriatric patients
- Although no overall difference in efficacy or safety has been observed, greater sensitivity of some older patients to drug can't be ruled out.

Pediatric patients
- Safety and effectiveness in children haven't been established.

Breast-feeding patients
- It's unknown if drug appears in breast milk; use with caution in breast-feeding women.

vancomycin hydrochloride
Vancocin, Vancoled

Pharmacologic classification: glycopeptide
Therapeutic classification: antibiotic
Pregnancy risk category C

How supplied
Available by prescription only
Pulvules: 125 mg, 250 mg
Powder for oral solution: 1-g, 10-g bottles
Powder for injection: 500-mg, 1-g, 5-g vials; 10-g pharmacy bulk package

Indications, route, and dosage
Severe staphylococcal infections when other antibiotics are ineffective or contraindicated
Adults: 500 mg I.V. q 6 hours, or 1 g q 12 hours.
Children: 40 mg/kg I.V. daily divided q 6 hours.
Neonates: Initially, 15 mg/kg; then, 10 mg/kg I.V. q 12 hours for first week of life; then q 8 hours up to age 1 month.
Antibiotic-associated pseudomembranous and staphylococcal enterocolitis
Adults: 125 to 500 mg P.O. q 6 hours for 7 to 10 days.
Children: 40 mg/kg P.O. daily divided q 6 to 8 hours for 7 to 10 days. Don't exceed 2 g/day in children.
Endocarditis prophylaxis for dental, GI, biliary, and GU instrumentation procedures; surgical prophylaxis in patients allergic to penicillin
Adults: 1 g I.V., given slowly over 1 hour, starting 1 hour before procedure.
Children: 20 mg/kg, if child weighs less than 27 kg (60 lb); adult dose if child weighs more than 27 kg.

✦ *Dosage adjustment.* In renal failure, adjust dosage based on degree of renal impairment, severity of infection, and susceptibility of causative organism. Base dosage on serum levels of drug.
  Recommended initial dose is 15 mg/kg. Subsequent doses should be adjusted, p.r.n. Some clinicians use the following schedule.

Serum creatinine level (mg/dl)	Dosage in adults
< 1.5	1 g q 12 hours
1.5 to 5	1 g q 3 to 6 days
> 5	1 g q 10 to 14 days

Pharmacodynamics
Antibacterial action: Bactericidal. Hinders cell-wall synthesis and blocks glycopeptide polymerization. Spectrum of activity includes many gram-positive organisms, including those resistant to other antibiotics. Useful for *Staphylococcus epidermidis* and methicillin-resistant *S. aureus.* Also useful for penicillin-resistant *S. pneumococcus.*

Pharmacokinetics
- *Absorption:* Minimal systemic absorption with oral administration. However, drug may accumulate in patients with colitis or renal failure.
- *Distribution:* Distributed widely in body fluids, including pericardial, pleural, ascitic, synovial, and placental fluid. Will achieve therapeutic levels in CSF in patients with inflamed meninges. Therapeutic drug levels are 18 to 26 mcg/ml for 2-hour, postinfusion peaks; 5 to 10 mcg/ml for preinfusion troughs; values may vary depending on laboratory and sampling time.
- *Metabolism:* No information available.
- *Excretion:* When administered parenterally, excreted renally, mainly by filtration. When administered orally, excreted in feces. In patients with normal renal function, plasma half-life is 6 hours; in those with creatinine clearance of 10 to 30 ml/minute, plasma half-life is about 32 hours; if creatinine clearance is below 10 ml/minute, plasma half-life is 146 hours.

Contraindications and precautions
Contraindicated in patients with hypersensitivity to drug. Use cautiously in patients with impaired renal or hepatic function, preexisting hearing loss, or allergies to other antibiotics; in those receiving other neurotoxic, nephrotoxic, or ototoxic drugs; and in patients over age 60.

Interactions
Drug-drug. *Aminoglycosides, amphotericin B, capreomycin, cisplatin, colistin, methoxyflurane,*

polymyxin B: Additive effect on these drugs. Monitor closely; adjust dosages as needed.
Nondepolarizing muscle relaxants: Enhanced neuromuscular blockade. Use together with caution.

Adverse reactions
CV: hypotension.
EENT: tinnitus, ototoxicity.
GI: nausea.
GU: increased BUN and serum creatinine levels, *nephrotoxicity.*
Hematologic: *neutropenia,* eosinophilia.
Respiratory: wheezing, dyspnea.
Skin: "red-neck" syndrome with rapid I.V. infusion (maculopapular rash on face, neck, trunk, and extremities).
Other: chills, fever, *anaphylaxis,* superinfection, pain or thrombophlebitis at injection site.

☑ Special considerations
● Oral form isn't for systemic infections and can't be interchanged with I.V. form.
● If patient has preexisting auditory dysfunction or needs prolonged therapy, auditory function tests may be indicated before and during therapy.
● Obtain culture and sensitivity tests before starting therapy (unless drug is being used for prophylaxis).
● I.M. administration is contraindicated because drug is highly irritating.
● Hemodialysis and peritoneal dialysis remove only minimal drug amounts. Patients receiving these treatments need usual dose only once every 5 to 7 days; however, some dialysis centers are using high flux hemodialysis, which can remove up to 50% of vancomycin, creating a need for supplemental doses. Dose should be based on serum level of drug.
● Little information is available on acute toxicity of drug. Treatment includes providing supportive care and maintaining glomerular filtration rate. Hemodialysis and hemoperfusion have been used.

Monitoring the patient
● Monitor blood counts and BUN, serum creatinine, and drug levels.
● If patient develops maculopapular rash on face, neck, trunk, and upper extremities, slow infusion rate.

Information for the patient
● Advise patient receiving drug orally to continue taking as directed for full course of therapy, even when feeling better.
● Advise patient not to take antidiarrheals with drug unless prescribed.
● Instruct patient to promptly report onset of ringing in ears.

Geriatric patients
● Elderly patients may be more susceptible to drug's ototoxic effects. Monitor serum levels closely and adjust dosage as needed.

Breast-feeding patients
● Drug appears in breast milk. Use with caution in breast-feeding women.

varicella virus vaccine, live
Varivax

Pharmacologic classification: vaccine
Therapeutic classification: viral vaccine
Pregnancy risk category C

How supplied
Available by prescription only
Injection: Single-dose vial containing 1,350 plaque-forming units of Oka/Merck varicella virus

Indications, route, and dosage
Prevention of varicella-zoster (chickenpox) infections
Adults and children ages 13 and older: Administer 0.5 ml S.C.; then a second dose of 0.5 ml 4 to 8 weeks later.
Children ages 1 to 12: 0.5 ml S.C. as a single dose.

Pharmacodynamics
Antiviral vaccine action: Prevents chickenpox by inducing production of antibodies to varicella-zoster virus.

Pharmacokinetics
● *Absorption:* Antibodies usually noted 4 to 6 weeks after S.C. injection. Varicella antibodies have been detected 99.5% of the time 4 years postvaccination.
● *Distribution:* No information available.
● *Metabolism:* No information available.
● *Excretion:* No information available.

Contraindications and precautions
Contraindicated in patients with hypersensitivity to drug; in those with history of anaphylactoid reaction to neomycin, blood dyscrasia, leukemia, lymphomas, neoplasms affecting bone marrow or lymphatic system, primary and acquired immunosuppressive states, active untreated tuberculosis, or any febrile respiratory illness or other active febrile infection; and in pregnant women.

Interactions
Drug-drug. *Blood products, immune globulin:* May inactivate vaccine. Defer vaccination for at least 5 months after blood or plasma transfusions

---

or administration of immune globulin or varicella-zoster immune globulin.

Immunosuppressants: Increased risk of severe reactions to live virus vaccines. Postpone routine vaccination.

Salicylates: Potential for developing Reye's syndrome. Avoid use of salicylates for 6 weeks after vaccination.

Adverse reactions
Other: *fever, injection site reactions (swelling, redness, pain, rash),* varicella-like rash.

☑ Special considerations
- Have epinephrine readily available.
- Administer vaccine immediately after reconstitution. Discard if not used within 30 minutes.
- Vaccine contains a live attenuated virus. Children who develop a rash may be capable of transmitting virus.
- Vaccine has been safely and effectively used with measles, mumps, and rubella vaccine.
- Vaccine appears to be less effective in adults than in children.
- Studies are underway to determine how often herpes zoster occurs after a latent period.
- Pregnancy should be avoided for 3 months after receiving vaccine.

Monitoring the patient
- Monitor patient for rash; patient may be capable of transmitting virus.

Information for the patient
- Inform patient or parents about adverse reactions associated with vaccine.
- Caution woman of childbearing age to call if pregnancy is suspected before receiving vaccine.

Pediatric patients
- A safety study protocol program is available for children and adolescents (ages 12 to 17) with acute lymphocytic leukemia. Clinicians can enroll patients in this program by contacting Bio-Pharm Clinical Services at (215) 283-0897.
- Safety and efficacy in children under age 1 haven't been established.

Breast-feeding patients
- It's unknown if vaccine virus appears in breast milk; use cautiously in breast-feeding women.

varicella-zoster immune globulin (VZIG)
Pharmacologic classification: immune serum
Therapeutic classification: varicella-zoster prophylaxis
Pregnancy risk category C

How supplied
Available by prescription only
Injection: 10% to 18% solution of the globulin fraction of human plasma containing 125 units of varicella-zoster virus antibody in 2.5 ml or less

Indications, route, and dosage
Passive immunization of susceptible patients, primarily immunocompromised patients after exposure to varicella (chickenpox or herpes zoster)
Adults and children: 125 units per 10 kg of body weight I.M., to maximum of 625 units. Higher doses may be needed in immunocompromised adults.

Pharmacodynamics
Postexposure prophylaxis: Provides passive immunity to varicella-zoster virus.

Pharmacokinetics
- *Absorption:* After I.M. absorption, persistence of antibodies is unknown, but protection should last at least 3 weeks. Protection is sufficient to prevent or lessen severity of varicella infections.
- *Distribution:* No information available.
- *Metabolism:* No information available.
- *Excretion:* No information available.

Contraindications and precautions
Contraindicated in patients with thrombocytopenia, coagulation disorders, immunoglobulin A deficiency, or history of severe reaction to human immune serum globulin or thimerosal.

Interactions
Drug-drug. *Corticosteroids, immunosuppressants:* May interfere with immune response to this immune globulin. Whenever possible, avoid using these drugs during postexposure immunization period.
Live virus vaccines (such as those for measles, mumps, rubella): Drug may interfere with immune response. Don't administer live virus vaccines within 2 weeks before or 3 months after VZIG. If necessary to administer VZIG with a live virus vaccine, confirm seroconversion with follow-up serologic testing.

Adverse reactions
CNS: malaise, headache.
CV: chest tightness.
GI: GI distress.

GU: *nephrotic syndrome.*
Musculoskeletal: myalgia.
Respiratory: respiratory distress.
Skin: rash.
Other: *anaphylaxis,* discomfort at injection site, *angioedema, angioneurotic edema,* fever.

☑ Special considerations
● Have epinephrine solution 1:1,000 available to treat allergic reactions.
● For maximum benefit, administer VZIG within 96 hours of presumed exposure.
● Although usually used only in children under age 15, VZIG may be administered to adults, if needed.
● VZIG is recommended primarily for immuno-deficient patients under age 15 and certain infants exposed in utero, although use in other patients (especially immunocompromised patients of any age, normal adults, pregnant women, and premature and full-term infants) should be considered on a case-by-case basis. Not routinely recommended for use in immunocompetent pregnant women because chickenpox is much less severe than in immunosuppressed patients. Moreover, it won't protect fetus. VZIG isn't for use in immunodeficient patients with history of varicella, unless immunosuppression is due to bone marrow transplantation.
● Administer only by deep I.M. injection. Never administer I.V. Use gluteal muscle in infants and small children and deltoid or anterolateral thigh in adults and larger children. For patients over 22 lb (10 kg), give no more than 2.5 ml at a single injection site.

Monitoring the patient
● Monitor patient for immediate postadministration reactions, including anaphylaxis.

Information for the patient
● Advise patient that the chance of contracting AIDS or hepatitis from VZIG is very small.
● Inform patient that some local pain, swelling, and tenderness at injection site might be experienced. Acetaminophen may be taken to alleviate these minor effects.
● Encourage patient to immediately report severe reactions.

Breast-feeding patients
● It's unknown if VZIG appears in breast milk. Use cautiously in breast-feeding women.

vasopressin
Pitressin Synthetic

Pharmacologic classification: posterior pituitary hormone
Therapeutic classification: antidiuretic hormone, peristaltic stimulant, hemostatic
Pregnancy risk category C

How supplied
Available by prescription only
Injection: 0.5-ml and 1-ml ampules, 20 units/ml; 0.5-ml, 1-ml vials, 20 units/ml

Indications, route, and dosage
Nonnephrogenic, nonpsychogenic diabetes insipidus
Adults: 5 to 10 units I.M. or S.C. b.i.d. to q.i.d., p.r.n.
Children: 2.5 to 10 units I.M. or S.C. b.i.d. to q.i.d., p.r.n.
Postoperative abdominal distention
Adults: 5 units I.M. initially; then q 3 to 4 hours, increasing dose to 10 units, if needed. Reduce dosage for children proportionately.
To expel gas before abdominal X-ray
Adults: Inject 5 to 15 units S.C. at 2 hours; then again at 30 minutes before X-ray. Enema before first dose may also help to eliminate gas.
Upper GI tract hemorrhage
Adults: 0.2 to 0.4 units/minute I.V. or 0.1 to 0.5 units/minute intra-arterially.

Pharmacodynamics
Antidiuretic action: Used as an antidiuretic to control or prevent signs and complications of neurogenic diabetes insipidus. Acting primarily at the renal tubular level, drug increases cAMP, which increases water permeability at the renal tubule and collecting duct, resulting in increased urine osmolality and decreased urine flow rate.
Peristaltic stimulant action: Used to treat postoperative abdominal distention and to facilitate abdominal radiographic procedures, vasopressin induces peristalsis by directly stimulating contraction of smooth muscle in the GI tract.
Hemostatic action: In patients with GI hemorrhage, vasopressin, administered I.V. or intra-arterially into the superior mesenteric artery, controls bleeding of esophageal varices by directly stimulating vasoconstriction of capillaries and small arterioles.

Pharmacokinetics
● *Absorption:* Destroyed by trypsin in GI tract; must be given intranasally or parenterally.
● *Distribution:* Distributed throughout extracellular fluid, with no evidence of protein-binding.
● *Metabolism:* Most of dose destroyed rapidly in liver and kidneys.

• *Excretion:* About 5% of S.C. dose excreted unchanged in urine after 4 hours. Duration of action after I.M. or S.C. administration is 2 to 8 hours. Half-life, 10 to 20 minutes.

Contraindications and precautions
Contraindicated in patients with anaphylaxis or hypersensitivity to vasopressin or its components. Also contraindicated in patients with chronic nephritis accompanied by nitrogen retention. Use cautiously in patients with seizure disorders, migraine headache, asthma, CV or renal disease, heart failure, goiter with cardiac complications, arteriosclerosis, or fluid overload; in children and elderly or pregnant patients; and in preoperative or postoperative patients who are polyuric.

Interactions
Drug-drug. *Carbamazepine, chlorpropamide, clofibrate:* May potentiate vasopressin's antidiuretic effect. Monitor therapeutic effect.
Demeclocycline, epinephrine, heparin, lithium, norepinephrine: Decreased antidiuretic effect. Monitor therapeutic effect.
Drug-lifestyle. *Alcohol:* Reduced antidiuretic activity. Discourage use.

Adverse reactions
CNS: tremor, headache, vertigo.
CV: angina in patients with vascular disease; vasoconstriction, ***arrhythmias, cardiac arrest,*** myocardial ischemia, circumoral pallor, decreased cardiac output.
GI: abdominal cramps, nausea, vomiting, flatulence.
Skin: cutaneous gangrene, diaphoresis.
Other: *water intoxication* (drowsiness, listlessness, headache, confusion, weight gain, *seizures, coma),* hypersensitivity reactions (urticaria, angioedema, *bronchospasm, anaphylaxis*).

☑ Special considerations
Besides the recommendations relevant to all posterior pituitary hormones, consider the following.
• Never inject during first stage of labor; this may cause ruptured uterus.
• Use extreme caution to avoid extravasation because of risk of necrosis and gangrene.
• Signs and symptoms of overdose include drowsiness, listlessness, headache, confusion, anuria, and weight gain (water intoxication). Treatment requires water restriction and temporary withdrawal of vasopressin until polyuria occurs. Severe water intoxication may require osmotic diuresis with mannitol, hypertonic dextrose, or urea, either alone or with furosemide.

Monitoring the patient
• Establish baseline vital signs and intake and output ratio at initiation of therapy.
• Monitor patient's blood pressure twice daily. Watch for excessively elevated blood pressure

or lack of response to drug, which may be indicated by hypotension.
• Monitor fluid intake and output and daily weight.
• Observe for signs of early water intoxication—drowsiness, listlessness, headache, confusion, and weight gain—to prevent seizures, coma, and death.
• Monitor abdominal distention and GI function; a rectal tube will facilitate gas expulsion after vasopressin injection.

Information for the patient
• Advise patient to rotate injection sites.
• Tell patient to drink one or two glasses of water with each dose of vasopressin to reduce adverse reactions such as unusual paleness, nausea, abdominal cramps, and vomiting.
• Tell patient to call immediately if chest pain, confusion, fever, hives, rash, headache, problems with urination, seizures, weight gain, unusual drowsiness, wheezing, trouble with breathing, or swelling of face, hands, feet, or mouth occurs.

Geriatric patients
• Elderly patients show increased sensitivity to drug's effects. Use with caution.

Pediatric patients
• Children show increased sensitivity to drug's effects. Use with caution.

Breast-feeding patients
• It's unknown if drug appears in breast milk. Use with caution in breast-feeding women.

vecuronium bromide
Norcuron

Pharmacologic classification: nondepolarizing neuromuscular blocker
Therapeutic classification: skeletal muscle relaxant
Pregnancy risk category C

How supplied
Available by prescription only
Injection: 10 mg (with or without diluent), 20 mg (without diluent)

Indications, route, and dosage
Adjunct to anesthesia, to facilitate intubation, and to provide skeletal muscle relaxation during surgery or mechanical ventilation
Dose depends on anesthetic used, individual needs, and response. Doses are representative and must be adjusted.
Adults and children ages 10 and over: Initially, 0.08 to 0.1 mg/kg I.V. bolus. Higher initial doses (up to 0.3 mg/kg) may be used for rapid onset.

Maintenance doses of 0.01 to 0.015 mg/kg within 25 to 40 minutes of initial dose should be administered during prolonged surgical procedures. Maintenance doses may be given q 12 to 15 minutes in patients receiving balanced anesthetic.

Or, after the initial dosing of 0.08 to 0.1 mg/kg, a continuous infusion of 1 mcg/kg/minute may be initiated 20 to 40 minutes later.

Pharmacodynamics

Skeletal muscle relaxant action: Prevents acetylcholine from binding to receptors on motor endplate, thus blocking depolarization. Exhibits minimal CV effects and doesn't appear to alter heart rate or rhythm, systolic or diastolic blood pressure, cardiac output, systemic vascular resistance, or mean arterial pressure. Has little or no histamine-releasing properties.

Pharmacokinetics

● *Absorption:* After I.V. administration of 0.08 to 0.1 mg/kg, onset of action within 1 minute; action peaks at 3 to 5 minutes. Duration is about 25 to 40 minutes, depending on anesthetic used, dosage, and number of doses given.
● *Distribution:* After I.V. administration, distributed in extracellular fluid and rapidly reaches site of action. 60% to 90% plasma protein–bound. Volume of distribution decreased in children under age 1; may be decreased in elderly patients.
● *Metabolism:* Undergoes rapid and extensive hepatic metabolism.
● *Excretion:* Drug and metabolites appear to be primarily excreted in feces by biliary elimination; also excreted in urine.

Contraindications and precautions

Contraindicated in patients with hypersensitivity to vecuronium and bromides. Use cautiously in elderly patients and in patients with altered circulation caused by CV disease and edematous states, hepatic disease, severe obesity, bronchogenic carcinoma, electrolyte disturbances, or neuromuscular diseases.

Interactions

Drug-drug. *Aminoglycosides, clindamycin, depolarizing neuromuscular blockers, furosemide, general anesthetics, lincomycin, parenteral magnesium salts, polymyxin antibiotics, quinidine, quinine, thiazide diuretics, other nondepolarizing neuromuscular blockers, other potassium-depleting drugs:* Increased vecuronium-induced neuromuscular blockade. Don't use together. When concomitant use can't be avoided, use together with caution. Decrease dosage by 15%, especially with enflurane and isoflurane.
Anticholinesterases: Antagonized effects of vecuronium. Monitor patient closely. Adjust dosage as needed.

Narcotic (opioid) analgesics: Increased central respiratory depression. Monitor respiratory status closely.

Adverse reactions

Musculoskeletal: skeletal muscle weakness.
Respiratory: *prolonged, dose-related respiratory insufficiency or apnea.*

☑ Special considerations

● Have emergency respiratory support equipment immediately available.
● Administration of vecuronium must be accompanied by adequate anesthesia. Drug doesn't relieve pain or affect consciousness.
● Administer by rapid I.V. injection or I.V. infusion. Don't give I.M.
● Diluent supplied by manufacturer contains benzyl alcohol, which isn't intended for use in newborns.
● Don't mix in same syringe or give through same needle as barbiturates or other alkaline solutions.
● Protect solution from light.
● Signs and symptoms of overdose include prolonged duration of neuromuscular blockade, skeletal muscle weakness, decreased respiratory reserve, low tidal volume, and apnea. Treatment is supportive and symptomatic. Keep airway clear and maintain adequate ventilation.
● Use peripheral nerve stimulator to determine and monitor degree of blockade. Give anticholinesterase (edrophonium, neostigmine, or pyridostigmine) to reverse neuromuscular blockade and atropine or glycopyrrolate to overcome muscarinic effects.

Monitoring the patient

● Assess baseline serum electrolyte levels, acid-base balance, and renal and hepatic function before administration.
● Peripheral nerve stimulator may be used to identify residual paralysis during recovery and is especially useful during administration to high-risk patients.
● After procedure, monitor vital signs at least every 15 minutes until patient is stable, then every 30 minutes for next 2 hours. Monitor airway and pattern of respirations until patient has recovered from drug effects.
● Evaluate recovery from neuromuscular blockade by checking strength of patient's hand grip and his ability to breathe naturally, take deep breaths and cough, keep eyes open, and lift head keeping mouth closed.

Information for the patient

● Advise patient that drug won't relieve pain or affect consciousness.
● Inform patient that postprocedure monitoring will involve patient demonstrating hand grip, breathing, and coughing.

Reactions may be *common*, uncommon, *life-threatening*, or COMMON AND LIFE-THREATENING.

Geriatric patients
- Administer cautiously to elderly patients.

Pediatric patients
- Safety and efficacy haven't been established in infants under age 7 weeks. Infants ages 7 weeks to 1 year are more sensitive to neuromuscular blocking effects; less frequent administration may be needed. Higher doses may be needed in children ages 1 to 9.

Breast-feeding patients
- It's unknown if drug appears in breast milk. Use with caution in breast-feeding women.

---

venlafaxine hydrochloride
Effexor, Effexor XR

Pharmacologic classification: neuronal serotonin, norepinephrine, and dopamine reuptake inhibitor
Therapeutic classification: antidepressant
Pregnancy risk category C

How supplied
Available by prescription only
Capsules (extended-release): 37.5 mg, 75 mg, 150 mg
Tablets: 25 mg, 37.5 mg, 50 mg, 75 mg, 100 mg

Indications, route, and dosage
Depression
Adults: Initially, 75 mg P.O. daily, in two or three divided doses with food. Increase dosage as tolerated and needed in increments of 75 mg/day at intervals of no less than 4 days. For moderately depressed outpatients, usual maximum dose is 225 mg/day; in certain severely depressed patients, dose may be as high as 375 mg/day divided into three doses. For extended-release capsules, 75 mg P.O. daily, in a single dose. For some patients, it may be desirable to start at 37.5 mg P.O. daily for 4 to 7 days before increasing to 75 mg daily. Dosage may be increased at increments of 75 mg/day q 4 days to a maximum of 225 mg/day.
✦ *Dosage adjustment.* Reduce dosage by 50% in patients with impaired hepatic function. In patients with moderate renal impairment (glomerular filtration rate of 10 to 70 ml/minute), total daily dose should be reduced by 25%. In hemodialysis patients, reduce dosage by 50% and withhold drug until after dialysis treatment.

Pharmacodynamics
Antidepressant action: Thought to potentiate neurotransmitter activity in the CNS. Venlafaxine and its active metabolite, O-desmethylvenlafaxine (ODV) are potent inhibitors of neuronal serotonin

and norepinephrine reuptake and weak inhibitors of dopamine reuptake.

Pharmacokinetics
- *Absorption:* About 92% of drug absorbed after oral administration.
- *Distribution:* 25% to 29% protein-bound in plasma.
- *Metabolism:* Extensively metabolized in liver, with ODV the only major active metabolite.
- *Excretion:* About 87% of dose recovered in urine within 48 hours (5% as unchanged venlafaxine, 29% as unconjugated ODV, 26% as conjugated ODV, 27% as minor inactive metabolites).

Contraindications and precautions
Contraindicated in patients with hypersensitivity to drug and within 14 days of MAO inhibitor therapy. Use cautiously in patients with impaired renal or hepatic function, diseases or conditions that could affect hemodynamic responses or metabolism, or history of seizures or mania.

Interactions
Drug-drug. *Cimetidine, CNS-active drugs:* Pronounced increase in venlafaxine level in elderly patients and in those with hepatic dysfunction or preexisting hypertension. Use cautiously together.
MAO inhibitors: May precipitate a syndrome similar to neuroleptic malignant syndrome when used with venlafaxine. Don't start venlafaxine within 14 days of stopping an MAO inhibitor; don't start MAO inhibitor within 7 days of stopping venlafaxine.
Drug-herb. *Yohimbé:* Possible additive stimulation. Use together cautiously.

Adverse reactions
CNS: *headache, somnolence, dizziness, nervousness, insomnia,* anxiety, tremor, abnormal dreams, paresthesia, agitation, *asthenia.*
CV: hypertension, vasodilation.
EENT: blurred vision.
GI: *nausea, constipation,* vomiting, *dry mouth,* anorexia, diarrhea, dyspepsia, flatulence.
GU: *abnormal ejaculation,* impotence, urinary frequency, impaired urination.
Metabolic: weight loss.
Skin: *diaphoresis,* rash.
Other: yawning, chills, infection.

☑ Special considerations
- When ending therapy after more than 1 week, taper dose. If patient has received drug for at least 6 weeks, gradually taper dose over 2 weeks.
- Stop drug in patient who develops seizures.
- Symptoms of overdose may range from none (most commonly) to somnolence, generalized seizures, and prolongation of QT interval. Treatment should consist of general measures used in managing any antidepressant overdose (ensuring an adequate airway, providing oxygen

tion and ventilation, monitoring cardiac rhythm and vital signs). General supportive and symptomatic measures also are recommended. Use of activated charcoal, induction of emesis, or gastric lavage should be considered. No specific antidote is known for venlafaxine overdose.

Monitoring the patient
• Because drug is associated with sustained increases in blood pressure, regular monitoring of blood pressure is recommended. For patients who experience a sustained increase in blood pressure while receiving drug, either dose reduction or discontinuation should be considered.
• Monitor patients with major affective disorders; drug may activate mania or hypomania.

Information for the patient
• Caution patient not to operate hazardous machinery until drug's effects are known.
• Advise woman to call if pregnancy is planned or suspected during therapy.
• Instruct patient to call before taking other drugs, including OTC preparations, because of potential interactions.
• Tell patient to avoid alcohol while taking drug.
• Instruct patient to report rash, hives, or a related allergic reaction.

Pediatric patients
• Safety and effectiveness in children under age 18 haven't been established.

Breast-feeding patients
• Drug appears in breast milk. Because of the potential for serious adverse effects in the breast-fed infant, a decision should be made to discontinue the drug or discontinue breast-feeding.

---

verapamil hydrochloride
Calan, Calan SR, Isoptin, Isoptin SR, Verelan

Pharmacologic classification: calcium channel blocker
Therapeutic classification: antianginal, antihypertensive, antiarrhythmic
Pregnancy risk category C

How supplied
Available by prescription only
Tablets: 40 mg, 80 mg, 120 mg
Tablets (sustained-release): 120 mg, 180 mg, 240 mg
Capsules (sustained-release): 100 mg, 120 mg, 180 mg, 200 mg, 240 mg, 360 mg
Injection: 2.5 mg/ml

Indications, route, and dosage
Management of Prinzmetal's or variant angina or unstable or chronic stable angina pectoris
Adults: Initial dose, 80 to 120 mg P.O. t.i.d. Dosage may be increased at weekly intervals. Some patients may need up to 480 mg daily.
Supraventricular tachyarrhythmias
Adults: 0.075 to 0.15 mg/kg (5 to 10 mg) I.V. push over 2 minutes. If no response occurs, give a second dose of 10 mg (0.15 mg/kg) 15 to 30 minutes after the initial dose.
Children ages 1 to 15: 0.1 to 0.3 mg/kg (2 to 5 mg) as I.V. bolus over 2 minutes. Dose shouldn't exceed 5 mg. Dose may be repeated in 30 minutes if no response occurs (shouldn't exceed 10 mg).
Children under age 1: 0.1 to 0.2 mg/kg (0.75 to 2 mg) as I.V. bolus over 2 minutes. Dose may be repeated in 30 minutes if no response occurs.
Control of ventricular rate in digitalized patients with chronic atrial flutter or fibrillation
Adults: 240 to 320 mg P.O. daily in three to four divided doses.
Prophylaxis of repetitive paroxysmal supraventricular tachycardia (PSVT)
Adults: 240 to 480 mg/day given in three to four divided doses.
Hypertension
Adults: Usual starting dose is 80 mg P.O. t.i.d. Daily dose may be increased to 360 to 480 mg.
 Initiate therapy with sustained-release capsules at 180 mg (240 mg for Verelan) daily in the morning. A starting dose of 120 mg may be indicated in people who may have an increased response to verapamil. Adjust dosage based on clinical effectiveness 24 hours after dosing. Increase by 120 mg daily until a maximum dose of 480 mg daily is given. Sustained-release capsules should be given only once daily. Antihypertensive effects are usually seen within the first week of therapy. Most patients respond to 240 mg daily.

Pharmacodynamics
Antianginal action: Manages unstable and chronic stable angina by reducing afterload, both at rest and with exercise, thereby decreasing oxygen consumption. Also decreases myocardial oxygen demand and cardiac work by exerting a negative inotropic effect, reducing heart rate, relieving coronary artery spasm (via coronary artery vasodilation), and dilating peripheral vessels. The net result of these effects is relief of angina-related ischemia and pain. In patients with Prinzmetal's variant angina, verapamil inhibits coronary artery spasm, resulting in increased myocardial oxygen delivery.
Antihypertensive action: Reduces blood pressure mainly by dilating peripheral vessels. Drug's negative inotropic effect blocks reflex mechanisms that lead to increased blood pressure.

Reactions may be *common*, uncommon, *life-threatening*, or COMMON AND LIFE-THREATENING.

Antiarrhythmic action: Drug's combined effects on the SA and AV nodes help manage arrhythmias. Its primary effect is on the AV node; slowed conduction reduces the ventricular rate in atrial tachyarrhythmias and blocks reentry paths in paroxysmal supraventricular arrhythmias.

Pharmacokinetics

• *Absorption:* Absorbed rapidly and completely from GI tract after oral administration; however, only about 20% to 35% reaches systemic circulation because of first-pass effect. When administered orally, effects peak within 1 to 2 hours with conventional tablets; within 4 to 8 hours with sustained-release preparations. When administered I.V., effects occur within minutes after injection and usually last about 30 to 60 minutes (may last up to 6 hours). Therapeutic serum levels are 80 to 300 ng/ml.
• *Distribution:* Steady-state distribution volume in healthy adults ranges from about 4.5 to 7 L/kg; may increase to 12 L/kg in patients with hepatic cirrhosis. About 90% of circulating drug is bound to plasma proteins.
• *Metabolism:* Metabolized in liver.
• *Excretion:* Excreted in urine as unchanged drug and active metabolites. Elimination half-life normally 6 to 12 hours; increases to as much as 16 hours in patients with hepatic cirrhosis. In infants, elimination half-life may be 5 to 7 hours.

Contraindications and precautions

Contraindicated in patients with hypersensitivity to drug and in those with severe left ventricular dysfunction, cardiogenic shock, second- or third-degree AV block or sick sinus syndrome except in presence of functioning pacemaker, atrial flutter or fibrillation and accessory bypass tract syndrome, severe heart failure (unless secondary to verapamil therapy), and severe hypotension. In addition, I.V. verapamil is contraindicated in patients receiving I.V. beta blockers and in those with ventricular tachycardia.

Use cautiously in elderly patients and in patients with impaired renal or hepatic function or increased intracranial pressure.

Interactions

Drug-drug. *Beta blockers:* Additive effects leading to heart failure, conduction disturbances, arrhythmias, and hypotension, especially if high beta-blocker doses are used, if drugs are administered I.V., or if patient has moderately severe to severe heart failure, severe cardiomyopathy, or recent MI. Monitor cardiac status closely.
Carbamazepine: Increased serum carbamazepine levels and subsequent toxicity. Use together with caution; watch for signs of toxicity.
Cyclosporine: Increased serum levels of cyclosporine. Monitor therapeutic effect; adjust dosage of cyclosporine as needed.

Digoxin: May increase serum digoxin levels by 50% to 75% during first week of therapy. Adjust digoxin dosage; monitor cardiac status closely.
Disopyramide: Combined negative inotropic effects. Monitor patient closely.
Flecainide: May add to negative inotropic effect and prolong AV conduction. Monitor cardiac status.
Inhalation anesthetics: Excessive CV depression. Avoid concomitant use.
Lithium: May increase sensitivity of lithium effects. Adjust lithium dosage as needed.
Neuromuscular blockers: Drug may potentiate their action. Adjust dosage of neuromuscular blockers as needed; monitor patient closely.
Other antihypertensives, drugs that attenuate alpha-adrenergic response (such as methyldopa, prazosin), quinidine (to treat hypertrophic cardiomyopathy): Hypotension. Monitor blood pressure closely. Adjust dosage of either drug as needed.
Phenobarbital: May increase verapamil clearance. Monitor cardiac status.
Rifampin: May substantially reduce verapamil's oral bioavailability. Monitor therapeutic effect; adjust dosage of verapamil as needed.
Theophylline: Increased theophylline plasma levels. Monitor patient closely; adjust theophylline dosage as needed.
Drug-herb. *Black catechu:* May cause additive effects. Don't use together.
Yerba maté: May decrease clearance of yerba maté methylxanthines and cause toxicity. Use together cautiously.
Drug-food. *Any food:* Increased absorption. Patient should take drug with food.
Drug-lifestyle. *Alcohol:* Prolonged intoxication effect. Discourage use.

Adverse reactions

CNS: dizziness, headache, asthenia.
CV: *transient hypotension,* **heart failure, pulmonary edema, bradycardia, AV block, ventricular asystole, ventricular fibrillation,** peripheral edema.
GI: *constipation,* nausea.
Hepatic: elevated liver enzyme levels.
Skin: rash.

☑ Special considerations

• If verapamil is initiated in patient receiving carbamazepine, a 40% to 50% reduction in carbamazepine dosage may be necessary.
• Reduce dosage in patients with renal or hepatic impairment.
• If verapamil is added to therapy of patient receiving digoxin, reduce digoxin dosage by half and monitor subsequent serum drug levels.
• Use reduced dosages in patients with severely compromised cardiac function and in those receiving beta blockers.

- Stop disopyramide 48 hours before starting verapamil therapy and don't reinstitute until 24 hours after verapamil has been stopped.
- Generic sustained-release verapamil tablets may be substituted only for Isoptin SR and Calan SR, not Verelan capsules. The capsule formulation should be given only once daily. When using sustained-release tablets, doses over 240 mg should be given b.i.d.
- Effects of overdose are primarily extensions of adverse reactions. Heart block, asystole, and hypotension are the most serious reactions and require immediate attention.
- Treatment may include administering I.V. isoproterenol, norepinephrine, epinephrine, atropine, or calcium gluconate in usual doses. Adequate hydration should be ensured.
- In patients with hypertrophic cardiomyopathy, alpha-adrenergic drugs, such as methoxamine, phenylephrine, and metaraminol, should be used to maintain blood pressure. (Isoproterenol and norepinephrine should be avoided.) Inotropic drugs, such as dobutamine and dopamine, may be used if needed.
- If severe conduction disturbances, such as heart block and asystole, occur with hypotension that doesn't respond to drug therapy, cardiac pacing should be initiated immediately, with CPR measures as indicated.
- In patients with Wolff-Parkinson-White or Lown-Ganong-Levine syndrome and a rapid ventricular rate caused by hemodynamically significant antegrade conduction, synchronized cardioversion may be used. Lidocaine and procainamide may be used as adjuncts.

Monitoring the patient
- During long-term therapy with verapamil and digoxin, monitor ECG periodically to observe for AV block and bradycardia.
- Obtain periodic liver function tests.
- If patient is receiving I.V. verapamil, monitor ECG and blood pressure continuously.
- If verapamil is initiated in patient receiving carbamazepine, a 40% to 50% reduction in carbamazepine dosage may be necessary. Monitor patient closely for signs of toxicity.

Information for the patient
- Instruct patient to report signs of heart failure, such as swelling of hands and feet or shortness of breath.
- Urge patient who is receiving nitrate therapy while verapamil dosage is being adjusted to comply with prescribed therapy.

Geriatric patients
- Elderly patients may need lower doses. In elderly patients, administer I.V. doses over at least 3 minutes to minimize risk of adverse effects.

Pediatric patients
- Currently, only the I.V. form is indicated for use in children to treat supraventricular tachyarrhythmias.

Breast-feeding patients
- Drug appears in breast milk. To avoid possible adverse effects in infants, mother shouldn't breast-feed during therapy.

vidarabine
(adenine arabinoside)
Vira-A

Pharmacologic classification: purine nucleoside
Therapeutic classification: antiviral
Pregnancy risk category C

How supplied
Available by prescription only
Ophthalmic ointment: 3% in 3.5-g tube (equivalent to 2.8% vidarabine)

Indications, route, and dosage
Acute keratoconjunctivitis and recurrent epithelial keratitis caused by herpes simplex virus types 1 and 2
Adults and children: Administer ½-inch (1.3 cm) ointment into lower conjunctival sac five times daily at 3-hour intervals.

Pharmacodynamics
Antiviral action: Exact mechanism unknown Adenine analogue; presumably involves inhibition of DNA polymerase and viral replication by incorporation into viral DNA.

Pharmacokinetics
- *Absorption:* No systemic absorption occurs with ophthalmic use.
- *Distribution:* Only trace amounts of drug detected in aqueous humor if cornea is intact.
- *Metabolism:* Metabolized into active metabolite arabinosyl-hypoxanthine.
- *Excretion:* No information available.

Contraindications and precautions
Contraindicated in patients with hypersensitivity to drug and in those with sterile trophic ulcers. Use cautiously in patients receiving corticosteroids.

Interactions
None reported.

Adverse reactions
EENT: temporary burning, itching, mild irritation, pain, lacrimation, foreign body sensation, conjunctival injection, punctal occlusion, sensitivity, superficial punctate keratitis, photophobia.

Reactions may be *common*, uncommon, **life-threatening**, or COMMON AND LIFE-THREATENING.

Other: hypersensitivity reactions.

☑ Special considerations
● Drug proves effective only if patient has at least minimal immunocompetence.
● Definitive diagnosis of herpes simplex conjunctivitis should be made before administration of ophthalmic form.

Monitoring the patient
● Monitor therapeutic effect. If there are no signs of improvement after 7 days or if reepithelialization hasn't occurred in 21 days, consider other forms of therapy. Patients with severe cases may need longer treatment. Continue drug for 5 to 7 days, b.i.d., to prevent recurrence.
● Monitor patient for adverse effects.

Information for the patient
● Warn patient receiving ophthalmic ointment not to exceed recommended frequency or duration of therapy. Instruct him to wash hands before and after applying ointment, and warn him against allowing tip of tube to touch eye or surrounding area.
● Advise patient to wear sunglasses if photosensitivity occurs.
● Instruct patient to store ophthalmic ointment in tightly sealed, light-resistant container.

---

vinblastine sulfate (VLB)
Velban, Velbe*

Pharmacologic classification: vinca alkaloid (cell cycle–phase specific, M phase)
Therapeutic classification: antineoplastic
Pregnancy risk category D

How supplied
Available by prescription only
Injection: 10-mg vials (lyophilized powder), 1 mg/ml in 10-ml and 25-ml vials

Indications, route, and dosage
Dosage and indications may vary. Check current literature for recommended protocol.
Breast or testicular cancer, Hodgkin's and malignant lymphomas, choriocarcinoma, lymphosarcoma, neuroblastoma, lung cancer, mycosis fungoides, histiocytosis, Kaposi's sarcoma
Adults: 0.1 mg/kg or 3.7 mg/m^2 I.V. weekly or q 2 weeks. May be increased in weekly increments of 50 mcg/kg or 1.8 to 1.9 mg/m^2 to maximum dose of 0.5 mg/kg or 18.5 mg/m^2 I.V. weekly, based on response. Dose shouldn't be repeated if WBC count falls below 4,000/mm^3.

Children: 2.5 mg/m^2 I.V. as a single dose every week, increased weekly in increments of 1.25 mg/m^2 to maximum of 12.5 mg/m^2.

Pharmacodynamics
Antineoplastic action: Exerts cytotoxic activity by arresting the cell cycle in the metaphase portion of cell division, resulting in a blockade of mitosis. Drug also inhibits DNA-dependent RNA synthesis and interferes with amino acid metabolism, inhibiting purine synthesis.

Pharmacokinetics
● *Absorption:* Absorbed unpredictably across GI tract after oral administration; must be given I.V.
● *Distribution:* Distributed widely into body tissues. Drug crosses blood-brain barrier but doesn't achieve therapeutic levels in CSF.
● *Metabolism:* Metabolized partially in liver to an active metabolite.
● *Excretion:* Excreted primarily in bile as unchanged drug. Smaller portion excreted in urine. Triphasic plasma elimination; half-lives of 3.7 minutes, 1.6 hours, and 24.8 hours for alpha, beta, and terminal phases, respectively.

Contraindications and precautions
Contraindicated in patients with severe leukopenia, granulocytopenia (unless result of disease being treated), or bacterial infection. Use cautiously in patients with hepatic dysfunction.

Interactions
Drug-drug. *Erythromycin:* May cause toxicity of vinblastine. Watch closely for toxicity.
Mitomycin: Acute shortness of breath and severe bronchospasm. Use cautiously together.
Phenytoin: May result in lower plasma phenytoin levels. Increase dosage of phenytoin, as needed.

Adverse reactions
CNS: depression, *paresthesia, peripheral neuropathy and neuritis, numbness, loss of deep tendon reflexes, muscle pain and weakness, **seizures, CVA,** headache.*
CV: hypertension, ***MI.***
EENT: pharyngitis.
GI: *nausea, vomiting,* ulcer, bleeding, *constipation, ileus, anorexia,* diarrhea, abdominal pain, *stomatitis.*
Hematologic: *anemia,* **leukopenia** (nadir occurs days 4 to 10 and lasts another 7 to 14 days), **thrombocytopenia.**
Metabolic: hyperuricemia, *weight loss.*
Respiratory: ***acute bronchospasm,*** shortness of breath.
Skin: vesiculation, reversible alopecia.
Other: *irritation, phlebitis,* cellulitis, necrosis with extravasation.

☑ Special considerations
● Give an antiemetic before drug to reduce nausea.
● Drug may be administered by I.V. push injection over 1 minute into the tubing of a freely flowing I.V. infusion.
● Dilution into larger volume isn't recommended for infusion into peripheral veins. This method increases risk of extravasation. Drug may be administered as an I.V. infusion through a central venous catheter.
● Don't administer more frequently than every 7 days to allow review of effect on leukocytes before next dose. Leukopenia may develop.
● Reduced dosages may be needed in patients with liver disease.
● Prevent uric acid nephropathy with generous oral fluid intake and administration of allopurinol.
● Don't confuse vinblastine with vincristine or vindesine.
● Drug is less neurotoxic than vincristine.
● Signs and symptoms of overdose include stomatitis, ileus, mental depression, paresthesia, loss of deep reflexes, permanent CNS damage, and myelosuppression.
● Treatment is usually supportive and includes transfusion of blood components and appropriate symptomatic therapy.

Monitoring the patient
● Watch for life-threatening acute bronchospasm reaction. This reaction is most likely to occur in patients also receiving mitomycin.

Information for the patient
● Encourage adequate fluid intake to increase urine output and facilitate excretion of uric acid.
● Reassure patient that therapeutic response isn't immediate. Adequate trial is 12 weeks.
● Advise patient to avoid exposure to people with infections and to report signs of infection or unusual bleeding immediately.
● Reassure patient that hair should grow back after treatment has ended.

Geriatric patients
● Patients with cachexia or skin ulceration (which is more common in elderly patients) may be more susceptible to leukopenic effect of drug.

Breast-feeding patients
● It's unknown if drug appears in breast milk. However, because of risk of serious adverse reactions, mutagenicity, and carcinogenicity in infants, breast-feeding isn't recommended.

vincristine sulfate
Oncovin, Vincasar PFS

Pharmacologic classification: vinca alkaloid (cell cycle–phase specific, M phase)
Therapeutic classification: antineoplastic
Pregnancy risk category D

How supplied
Available by prescription only
Injection: 1 mg/1 ml, 2 mg/2 ml, 5 mg/5 ml multiple-dose vials; 1 mg/1 ml, 2 mg/2 ml preservative-free vials

Indications, route, and dosage
Dosage and indications may vary. Check current literature for recommended protocol.
Acute lymphoblastic and other leukemias; Hodgkin's disease; lymphosarcoma; reticulum cell, osteogenic, and other sarcomas; neuroblastoma; rhabdomyosarcoma; Wilms' tumor; lung and ◇ breast cancer
Adults: 1.4 mg/m² I.V. weekly.
Children: 2 mg/m² I.V. weekly. Maximum single dose (adults and children) is 2 mg.
Children weighing under 10 kg (22 lb) or with body surface area below 1 m²: 0.05 mg/kg once weekly.
✦ ***Dosage adjustment.*** Reduce dosage by 50% in patients with direct serum bilirubin level exceeding 3 ml/dl or other evidence of significant hepatic impairment.

Pharmacodynamics
Antineoplastic action: Exerts cytotoxic activity by arresting the cell cycle in the metaphase portion of cell division, resulting in a blockade of mitosis. Also inhibits DNA-dependent RNA synthesis and interferes with amino acid metabolites, inhibiting purine synthesis.

Pharmacokinetics
● *Absorption:* Absorbed unpredictably across GI tract after oral administration; must be given I.V.
● *Distribution:* Rapidly and widely distributed into body tissues; bound to erythrocytes and platelets. Drug crosses blood-brain barrier but doesn't achieve therapeutic levels in CSF.
● *Metabolism:* Extensively metabolized in liver.
● *Excretion:* Drug and metabolites primarily excreted into bile. Smaller portion eliminated through kidneys. Triphasic plasma elimination; half-lives of about 4 minutes, 2¼ hours, and 85 hours for distribution, second, and terminal phases, respectively.

Contraindications and precautions
Contraindicated in patients with hypersensitivity to drug and in those who have the demyeli-

nating form of Charcot-Marie-Tooth syndrome. Don't give to patients who are concurrently receiving radiation therapy through ports that include the liver. Use cautiously in patients with hepatic dysfunction, neuromuscular disease, or infection.

Interactions
Drug-drug. *Asparaginase:* Decreased hepatic clearance of vincristine. Adjust vincristine dosage.
Calcium channel blockers: Enhanced vincristine accumulation in cells. Monitor patient closely; adjust vincristine dosage.
Digoxin: Decreased digoxin levels. Monitor serum digoxin levels.
Methotrexate: Increased therapeutic effect of methotrexate. May require a lower dosage of methotrexate.
Mitomycin: Possible increased frequency of bronchospasm and acute pulmonary reactions. Avoid concomitant use.
Neurotoxic drugs: Increased neurotoxicity; additive effect. Monitor patient closely; adjust vincristine dosage as needed.
Phenytoin: May decrease plasma phenytoin levels. Monitor phenytoin levels.

Adverse reactions
CNS: *peripheral neuropathy,* sensory loss, *loss of deep tendon reflexes, paresthesia, wristdrop and footdrop,* **seizures, coma,** headache, ataxia, cranial nerve palsies, *jaw pain,* hoarseness, vocal cord paralysis, *muscle weakness and cramps.* Some neurotoxicities may be permanent.
CV: hypotension, hypertension.
EENT: diplopia, optic and extraocular neuropathy, ptosis, photophobia, transient cortical blindness, optical atrophy.
GI: diarrhea, *constipation, cramps,* ileus that mimics surgical abdomen, paralytic ileus, *nausea, vomiting,* anorexia, dysphagia, **intestinal necrosis,** stomatitis.
GU: urine retention, syndrome of inappropriate antidiuretic hormone, dysuria, acute uric acid neuropathy, polyuria.
Hematologic: anemia, *leukopenia, thrombocytopenia.*
Metabolic: *hyperuricemia,* hyponatremia, weight loss.
Respiratory: *acute bronchospasm,* dyspnea.
Skin: *reversible alopecia.*
Other: fever, severe local reaction with extravasation, *phlebitis,* cellulitis at injection site.

☑ Special considerations
● Drug may be administered by I.V. push injection over 1 minute into the tubing of a freely flowing I.V. infusion.
● Dilution into larger volumes isn't recommended for infusion into peripheral veins; this method increases risk of extravasation. Drug may be ad-

ministered as an I.V. infusion through a central venous catheter.
● Necrosis may result from extravasation. Manufacturer recommends treatment with moderate heat to the area and prompt administration of intradermal hyaluronidase. See package insert for additional recommendations.
● Because of potential for neurotoxicity, don't give drug more than once weekly. Children are more resistant to neurotoxicity than adults. Neurotoxicity is dose-related and usually reversible; reduce dosage if symptoms of neurotoxicity develop.
● Prevent uric acid nephropathy with generous oral fluid intake and administration of allopurinol. Alkalinization of urine may be required if serum uric acid level is increased.
● Reduced dosage may be needed in patients with obstructive jaundice or liver disease.
● Don't confuse vincristine with vinblastine or vindesine.
● Drug may cause SIADH secretion. Treatment requires fluid restriction and a loop diuretic.
● Management of patients mistakenly receiving intrathecal vincristine is a medical emergency. Prognosis is generally poor.
● Signs and symptoms of overdose include alopecia, myelosuppression, paresthesia, neuritic pain, motor difficulties, loss of deep tendon reflexes, nausea, vomiting, and ileus. Treatment is usually supportive and includes transfusion of blood components, antiemetics, enemas for ileus, phenobarbital for seizures, and other appropriate symptomatic therapy. Administration of calcium leucovorin at a dosage of 15 mg I.V. every 3 hours for 24 hours, then every 6 hours for 48 hours may help protect cells from the toxic effects of vincristine.

Monitoring the patient
● After administering drug, monitor patient for life-threatening bronchospasm reaction. It's most likely to occur in patients also receiving mitomycin.
● Watch for neurotoxicity by checking for depression of Achilles tendon reflex, numbness, tingling, footdrop or wristdrop, difficulty in walking, ataxia, and slapping gait. Also check ability to walk on heels.
● Monitor patient's bowel function. Patient should have stool softener, laxative, or water before dosing. Constipation may be an early indication of neurotoxicity.

Information for the patient
● Encourage adequate fluid intake to increase urine output and facilitate excretion of uric acid.
● Tell patient to call regarding use of laxatives if constipation or stomach pain occurs.
● Assure patient that hair should grow back after therapy ends.

Geriatric patients
● Elderly patients who are weak or bedridden may be more susceptible to neurotoxic effects. Use cautiously.

Breast-feeding patients
● It's unknown if drug appears in breast milk. However, because of risk of serious adverse reactions, mutagenicity, and carcinogenicity in infant, breast-feeding isn't recommended.

vinorelbine tartrate
Navelbine

Pharmacologic classification: semisynthetic vinca alkaloid
Therapeutic classification: antineoplastic
Pregnancy risk category D

How supplied
Available by prescription only
Injection: 10 mg/ml in 1-ml and 5-ml single-use vials

Indications, route, and dosage
Alone or as adjunct therapy with cisplatin for first-line treatment of ambulatory patients with nonresectable advanced non-small-cell lung cancer (NSCLC); alone or with cisplatin in stage IV of NSCLC; with cisplatin in stage III of NSCLC
Adults: 30 mg/m² I.V. weekly. In combination treatment, same dosage used with 120 mg/m² of cisplatin, given on days 1 and 29, then q 6 weeks.
✦ Dosage adjustment. Adjust dosage based on hematologic toxicity or hepatic insufficiency.

Pharmacodynamics
Antineoplastic action: Exerts antineoplastic effect by disrupting microtubule assembly, which disrupts spindle formation and prevents mitosis.

Pharmacokinetics
● *Absorption:* Only given I.V.
● *Distribution:* Drug binding to plasma constituents ranges from 79.6% to 91.2%. It demonstrates high binding to platelets and lymphocytes.
● *Metabolism:* Undergoes substantial hepatic metabolism.
● *Excretion:* About 18% of drug excreted in urine; 46% excreted in feces. Terminal phase half-life averages 27.7 to 43.6 hours.

Contraindications and precautions
Contraindicated in patients with pretreatment granulocyte counts below 1,000 cells/m³. Use with extreme caution in patients whose bone marrow may have been compromised by previous exposure to radiation or chemotherapy or whose bone marrow is still recovering from previous chemotherapy. Also use cautiously in patients with impaired hepatic function.

Interactions
Drug-drug. *Cisplatin:* Increased risk of bone marrow suppression. When concomitant use can't be avoided, use with caution. Monitor patient's hematologic status.
Mitomycin: Pulmonary reactions. Monitor patient's respiratory status.

Adverse reactions
CNS: *fatigue, peripheral neuropathy, asthenia.*
CV: chest pain.
GI: *nausea, vomiting, anorexia, diarrhea, constipation, stomatitis.*
Hematologic: **bone marrow suppression (agranulocytosis,** LEUKOPENIA, **thrombocytopenia,** anemia).
Hepatic: *abnormal liver function tests, bilirubinemia.*
Musculoskeletal: jaw pain, myalgia, arthralgia.
Respiratory: dyspnea.
Skin: *alopecia, rash, injection pain or reaction.*
Other: SIADH.

☑ Special considerations
● Dilute drug before administration. Administer I.V. over 6 to 10 minutes into side port of a free-flowing I.V. closest to I.V. bag, then flush with at least 75 to 125 ml of D_5W or normal saline solution.
● Drug can cause considerable irritation, localized tissue necrosis, and thrombophlebitis if extravasation occurs.
● Adjust dose based on hematologic toxicity or hepatic insufficiency, whichever results in a lower dose. Reduce dose by 50% if patient's granulocyte count falls below 1,500 cells/mm³ but exceeds 1,000 cells/mm³. If three consecutive doses are skipped because of granulocytopenia, stop further drug therapy.
● Drug may be a contact irritant and solution must be handled and administered with care. Use gloves. Avoid inhalation of vapors and contact with skin or mucous membranes, especially eyes. If contact occurs, wash with copious amounts of water for at least 15 minutes.
● The primary anticipated complications of overdose are bone marrow suppression and peripheral neurotoxicity. Treatment includes general supportive measures and appropriate blood transfusions and antibiotics as needed. There is no known antidote.

Monitoring the patient
● Check patient's granulocyte count before initiating therapy (should be 1,000 cells/mm³ or more for drug to be administered).
● Monitor patient closely for hypersensitivity reactions.

• Monitor patient's peripheral blood count and bone marrow to guide effects of therapy.

Information for the patient
• Tell patient not to take other drugs, including OTC preparations, unless instructed.
• Instruct patient to report signs and symptoms of infection (fever, chills, malaise) because drug has immunosuppressive activity.
• Tell woman to avoid becoming pregnant during therapy.

Pediatric patients
• Safety and effectiveness in children haven't been established.

Breast-feeding patients
• It's unknown if drug appears in breast milk. Because of risk of adverse effects in breast-fed infant, don't use drug in breast-feeding women.

vitamin A (retinol)
Aquasol A, Palmitate-A 5000

Pharmacologic classification: fat-soluble vitamin
Therapeutic classification: vitamin
Pregnancy risk category A (X if dose exceeds RDA)

How supplied
Available by prescription only
Capsules: 25,000 IU
Injection: 2-ml vials (50,000 IU/ml with 0.5% chlorobutanol, polysorbate 80, butylated hydroxyanisole, and butylated hydroxytoluene)
Available without a prescription, as appropriate
Capsules: 10,000 IU, 15,000 IU
Tablets: 5,000 IU

Indications, route, and dosage
Severe vitamin A deficiency with xerophthalmia
Adults and children over age 8: 500,000 IU P.O. daily for 3 days, then 50,000 IU P.O. daily for 14 days, then maintenance dose of 10,000 to 20,000 IU P.O. daily for 2 months, then adequate dietary nutrition and RDA vitamin A supplements.
Severe vitamin A deficiency
Adults and children over age 8: 100,000 IU P.O. or I.M. daily for 3 days, then 50,000 IU P.O. or I.M. daily for 14 days, then maintenance dose of 10,000 to 20,000 IU P.O. daily for 2 months, then adequate dietary nutrition and RDA vitamin A supplements.
Children ages 1 to 8: 17,500 to 35,000 IU I.M. daily for 10 days.
Infants under age 1: 7,500 to 15,000 IU I.M. daily for 10 days.
The RDA for vitamin A is as follows.

	Vitamin A RDA	Vitamin A and beta carotene RDA
Infants		
age 6 to 12 months	375 RE	1,875 IU
birth to 6 months	375 RE	1,875 IU
Children		
age 7 to 10	700 RE	3,500 IU
age 4 to 6	500 RE	2,500 IU
age 1 to 3	400 RE	2,000 IU
Males		
age 11 and over	1,000 RE	5,000 IU
Females		
age 11 and over	800 RE	4,000 IU
Pregnant	800 RE	4,000 IU
Breast-feeding	1,300 RE (1st 6 months)	6,500 IU
	1,200 RE (2nd 6 months)	6,000 IU

RE = retinol equivalents; IU = combination of retinol and beta-carotene.

Pharmacodynamics
Metabolic action: One IU of vitamin A is equivalent to 0.3 mcg of retinol or 0.6 mcg of betacarotene. Betacarotene, or provitamin A, yields retinol after absorption from the intestinal tract. Retinol's use with opsin, the red pigment in the retina, helps form rhodopsin, which is needed for visual adaptation to darkness. Vitamin A prevents growth retardation and preserves the integrity of the epithelial cells. Vitamin A deficiency is characterized by nyctalopia (night blindness), keratomalacia (necrosis of the cornea), keratinization and drying of the skin, low resistance to infection, growth retardation, bone thickening, diminished cortical steroid production, and fetal malformations.

Pharmacokinetics
• *Absorption:* In normal doses, absorbed readily and completely if fat absorption is normal. Larger doses, or regular doses in patients with fat malabsorption, low protein intake, or hepatic or pancreatic disease may be absorbed incompletely. Because vitamin A is fat-soluble, absorption needs bile salts, pancreatic lipase, and dietary fat.
• *Distribution:* Stored (primarily as palmitate) in Kupffer's cells of liver. Normal adult liver stores

are sufficient to provide vitamin A requirements for 2 years. Lesser amounts of retinyl palmitate are stored in kidneys, lungs, adrenal glands, retinas, and intraperitoneal fat. Vitamin A circulates bound to a specific alpha$_1$ protein, retinol-binding protein (RBP). Blood level assays may not reflect liver storage of vitamin A because serum levels depend partly on circulating RBP. Liver storage should be adequate before therapy ends. Distributed into breast milk; doesn't readily cross placenta.

• *Metabolism:* Metabolized in liver.
• *Excretion:* Retinol (fat-soluble) is conjugated with glucuronic acid and then further metabolized to retinal and retinoic acid. Retinoic acid is excreted in feces via biliary elimination. Retinal, retinoic acid, and other water-soluble metabolites excreted in urine and feces. Normally, no unchanged retinol excreted in urine, except in patients with pneumonia or chronic nephritis.

Contraindications and precautions

Oral form contraindicated in patients with malabsorption syndrome; if malabsorption is from inadequate bile secretion, oral route may be used with concurrent administration of bile salts (dehydrocholic acid).

Also contraindicated in those with hypervitaminosis A and hypersensitivity to any ingredient in product. I.V. route contraindicated except for special water-miscible forms intended for infusion with large parenteral volumes. I.V. push of vitamin A of any type also contraindicated (anaphylaxis or anaphylactoid reactions and death have resulted).

Use cautiously in pregnant women.

Interactions

Drug-drug. *Cholestyramine, mineral oil (prolonged use), neomycin:* Decreased absorption of vitamin A. Avoid concomitant use of mineral oil or neomycin. Daily vitamin A supplements have been recommended during long-term cholestyramine therapy.
Oral contraceptives: Significantly increased vitamin plasma levels. Adjust vitamin dosage.
Retinoids (such as etretinate, isotretinoin): Potential for additive adverse effects. Avoid concomitant use.
Warfarin: Large doses of vitamin A may interfere with hypoprothrombinemic effect of warfarin. Avoid concomitant use.

Adverse reactions

Adverse reactions usually occur only with toxicity.
CNS: irritability, headache, *increased intracranial pressure,* fatigue, lethargy, malaise.
EENT: papilledema, exophthalmos.
GI: anorexia, epigastric pain, vomiting, polydipsia.

GU: hypomenorrhea, polyuria.
Hepatic: jaundice, hepatomegaly, *cirrhosis,* elevated liver enzyme levels.
Musculoskeletal: slow growth, decalcification, hypercalcemia, periostitis, premature closure of epiphyses, migratory arthralgia, cortical thickening over the radius and tibia.
Skin: alopecia; dry, cracked, scaly skin; pruritus; lip fissures; erythema; inflamed tongue, lips, and gums; massive desquamation; increased pigmentation; night sweats.
Other: splenomegaly, *anaphylactic shock.*

☑ Special considerations

• Safety of amounts exceeding 5,000 IU/day (oral) or 6,000 IU/day (parenteral) during pregnancy is unknown.
• In any dietary deficiency, multiple vitamin deficiency should be suspected.
• Give vitamin A with bile salts to patients with malabsorption caused by inadequate bile secretion.
• Vitamin A given by I.V. push is contraindicated; can cause anaphylaxis and death.
• Use special water-miscible form of vitamin A when adding to large parenteral volumes.
• Vitamin A therapy may falsely increase serum cholesterol level readings by interfering with the Zlatkis-Zak reaction. Vitamin A has also been reported to falsely elevate bilirubin levels.
• In cases of acute toxicity, increased intracranial pressure develops within 8 to 12 hours; cutaneous desquamation follows in a few days. Toxicity can follow a single dose of 25,000 IU/kg, which in infants would represent about 75,000 IU and in adults over 2 million IU.
• Chronic toxicity results from administration of 4,000 IU/kg for 6 to 15 months. In infants (ages 3 to 6 months) this would represent about 18,500 IU/day for 1 to 3 months; in adults, 1 million IU/day for 3 days, 50,000 IU/day for more than 18 months, or 500,000 IU/day for 2 months.
• To treat toxicity, stop vitamin A if hypercalcemia persists; administer I.V. saline solution, prednisone, and calcitonin, if indicated. Perform liver function tests to detect possible liver damage.

Monitoring the patient
• Monitor therapeutic effect.
• Monitor patient for adverse effects.

Information for the patient
• Explain that patient must avoid prolonged use of mineral oil while taking drug because mineral oil reduces vitamin A absorption in the intestine.
• Tell patient not to exceed recommended dosage.
• Instruct patient to report promptly symptoms of overdose (nausea, vomiting, anorexia, malaise, drying or cracking of skin or lips, irritability, head-

---

Reactions may be *common*, uncommon, *life-threatening*, or COMMON AND LIFE-THREATENING.

ache, or loss of hair) and to stop drug immediately if they occur.
• Advise patient to consume adequate protein, vitamin E, and zinc, which, along with bile, are necessary for vitamin A absorption.
• Tell patient to store vitamin A in a tight, light-resistant container.

Geriatric patients
• Liquid preparations are available to administer by nasogastric tube.

Pediatric patients
• Liquid preparations may be mixed with fruit juice or cereal.

Breast-feeding patients
• Vitamin A appears in breast milk. The RDA of vitamin A for breast-feeding women in the United States is 1,300 and 1,200 retinol equivalents for the first 6 months and second 6 months, respectively. Unless the maternal diet is grossly inadequate, infants can usually obtain sufficient vitamin A from breast-feeding. The effect of large maternal doses of vitamin A on breast-fed infants is unknown.

vitamin E (alpha tocopherol)
Aquavit-E, d'Alpha E 1000

Pharmacologic classification: fat-soluble vitamin
Therapeutic classification: vitamin
Pregnancy risk category A (C if greater than RDA)

How supplied
Available without a prescription, as appropriate
Capsules: 100 IU, 200 IU, 400 IU, 1,000 IU
Tablets: 100 IU, 200 IU, 400 IU, 500 IU, 800 IU, 1,000 IU
Oral solution: 50 IU/ml
Drops: 15 IU/0.03 ml

Indications, route, and dosage
Vitamin E deficiency in premature infants and in patients with impaired fat absorption (including patients with cystic fibrosis); biliary atresia
Adults: 60 to 75 IU P.O. daily, depending on severity. Maximum dose is 300 IU/day.
Children: 1 unit/kg P.O. daily.
Premature neonates: 5 units P.O. daily.
Full-term neonates: 5 units P.O. per liter of formula.
    The RDA for vitamin E is as follows:
Infants up to age 6 months: 3 α-TE or 4 IU.
Children ages 6 months to 1 year: 4 α-TE or 6 IU.
Children ages 1 to 3: 6 α-TE or 9 IU.
Children ages 4 to 10: 7 α-TE or 10 IU.

Men over age 11: 10 α-TE or 15 IU.
Women over age 11: 8 α-TE or 12 IU.
Pregnant women: 10 α-TE or 15 IU.
Breast-feeding women: First 6 months, 12 α-TE or 18 IU; over 6 months, 11 α-TE or 16 IU.
    α-TE is alpha tocopherol equivalent (equal to 1 mg d-alpha-tocopherol or 1.49 IU).

Pharmacodynamics
Nutritional action: As a dietary supplement, exact biochemical mechanism unclear, although it's believed to act as an antioxidant. Vitamin E protects cell membranes, vitamin A, vitamin C (ascorbic acid), and polyunsaturated fatty acids from oxidation. It also may act as a cofactor in enzyme systems, and some evidence exists that it decreases platelet aggregation.

Pharmacokinetics
• *Absorption:* GI absorption depends on presence of bile. Only 20% to 60% of vitamin obtained from dietary sources is absorbed. As dose increases, the fraction of vitamin E absorbed decreases.
• *Distribution:* Distributed to all tissues; stored in adipose tissue.
• *Metabolism:* Metabolized in liver by glucuronidation.
• *Excretion:* Vitamin E excreted primarily in bile. Some enterohepatic circulation may occur. Small amounts of metabolites excreted in urine.

Contraindications and precautions
No known contraindications. Use cautiously in patients with liver or gallbladder disease.

Interactions
Drug-drug. *Cholestyramine, colestipol, mineral oil, sucralfate:* Increase vitamin E requirements. Give drugs at well-spaced intervals; monitor result.
Oral anticoagulants: Risk of hemorrhage after large doses of vitamin E. Avoid concomitant use.
Vitamin K: Vitamin E may have anti–vitamin K effects. Monitor therapeutic effect; adjust dosage as needed.

Adverse reactions
None reported with recommended doses. Hypervitaminosis E symptoms include fatigue, weakness, nausea, headache, blurred vision, flatulence, and diarrhea.

☑ Special considerations
• Give with bile salts if patient has malabsorption caused by lack of bile.
• Vitamin E has been used for investigational purposes to prevent retrolental fibroplasia and bronchopulmonary dysplasia in neonates and periventricular hemorrhage in premature infants, and to decrease the severity of hemolytic anemia in infants.

• Signs and symptoms of overdose include a possible increase in blood pressure. Treatment is generally supportive.

Monitoring the patient
• Monitor therapeutic effect.
• Monitor patient for hypervitaminosis E.

Information for the patient
• Tell patient about dietary sources of vitamin E.
• Instruct patient to swallow capsules whole and not to crush or chew them.
• Tell patient to store vitamin E in a tight, light-resistant container.

vitamin K derivatives

phytonadione
AquaMEPHYTON, Mephyton

Pharmacologic classification: vitamin K
Therapeutic classification: blood coagulation modifier
Pregnancy risk category C

How supplied
Available by prescription only
Tablets: 5 mg
Injection (aqueous colloidal solution): 2 mg/ml
Injection (aqueous dispersion): 10 mg/ml

Indications, route, and dosage
Hypoprothrombinemia secondary to vitamin K malabsorption or drug therapy, or when oral administration is desired and bile secretion is inadequate
Adults: 5 to 10 mg P.O. daily, or adjusted to patient's needs.
Hypoprothrombinemia secondary to vitamin K malabsorption, drug therapy, or excess vitamin A
Adults: 2 to 25 mg P.O. or parenterally, repeated and increased up to 50 mg, if needed.
Children: 5 to 10 mg P.O. or parenterally.
Infants: 2 mg P.O. or parenterally.
Hypoprothrombinemia secondary to effect of oral anticoagulants
Adults: 2.5 to 10 mg P.O., S.C., or I.M., based on PT and INR, repeated, if needed, 12 to 48 hours after oral dose or 6 to 8 hours after parenteral dose. In emergency, give 10 to 50 mg slow I.V., rate not to exceed 1 mg/minute, repeated q 6 to 8 hours, p.r.n.
Prevention of hemorrhagic disease in neonates
Neonates: 0.5 to 1 mg S.C. or I.M. immediately (within 1 hour) after birth, repeated in 2 to 3 weeks, if needed, especially if mother received oral anticoagulants or long-term anticonvulsant therapy during pregnancy.

Prevention of hypoprothrombinemia related to vitamin K deficiency in long-term parenteral nutrition
Adults: 5 to 10 mg I.M. weekly.
Children: 2 to 5 mg I.M. weekly.
The RDA for vitamin K is as follows:
Infants up to age 6 months: 5 mcg.
Children ages 6 months to 1 year: 10 mcg.
Children ages 1 to 3: 15 mcg.
Children ages 4 to 6: 20 mcg.
Children ages 7 to 10: 30 mcg.
Boys ages 11 to 14: 45 mcg.
Boys ages 15 to 18: 65 mcg.
Men ages 19 to 24: 70 mcg.
Men over age 24: 80 mcg.
Girls ages 11 to 14: 45 mcg.
Girls ages 15 to 18: 55 mcg.
Women ages 19 to 24: 60 mcg.
Women over age 24: 65 mcg.
Pregnant or breast-feeding women: 65 mcg.

Pharmacodynamics
Coagulation modifying action: Vitamin K is a lipid-soluble vitamin that promotes hepatic formation of active prothrombin and several other coagulation factors (specifically factors II, VII, IX, and X).
Phytonadione (vitamin K_1) is a synthetic form of vitamin K and is also lipid-soluble. Vitamin K doesn't counteract the action of heparin.

Pharmacokinetics
• *Absorption:* Phytonadione needs the presence of bile salts for GI tract absorption. Once absorbed, vitamin K enters blood directly. Onset of action after I.V. injection more rapid, but of shorter duration, than after S.C. or I.M. injection.
• *Distribution:* Concentrated in liver for a short time. Action of parenteral phytonadione begins in 1 to 2 hours; hemorrhage usually controlled within 3 to 6 hours, and normal prothrombin levels in 12 to 14 hours. Oral phytonadione begins to act within 6 to 10 hours.
• *Metabolism:* Metabolized rapidly by liver; little tissue accumulation occurs.
• *Excretion:* Limited data; high levels in feces; however, intestinal bacteria can synthesize vitamin K.

Contraindications and precautions
Contraindicated in patients with hypersensitivity to drug.

Interactions
Drug-drug. *Broad-spectrum antibiotics (especially cefoperazone, cefotetan):* May interfere with actions of vitamin K, producing hypoprothrombinemia. Avoid concomitant use; adjust dosage as needed.
Mineral oil: Inhibits absorption of oral vitamin K. Give drugs at well-spaced intervals; monitor result.

Oral anticoagulants: Antagonized effects of oral anticoagulants. Avoid concomitant use.

Adverse reactions
CNS: headache, dizziness, convulsive movements.
CV: transient hypotension after I.V. administration, rapid and weak pulse, ***arrhythmias.***
GI: nausea, vomiting.
Hematologic: *fatal kernicterus, severe hemolytic anemia in neonates.*
Hepatic: hyperbilirubinemia.
Respiratory: *bronchospasm,* dyspnea.
Skin: diaphoresis, flushing, erythema, urticaria, pruritus, allergic rash.
Other: cramplike pain, *anaphylaxis and anaphylactoid reactions* (usually after too-rapid I.V. administration), pain, swelling, hematoma at injection site.

☑ Special considerations
● When I.V. administration is unavoidable, inject drug very slowly, not exceeding 1 mg/minute.
● If severity of condition warrants I.V. infusion, mix with preservative-free normal saline solution, D_5W, or dextrose 5% in normal saline solution.
● Stop drug if allergic or severe CNS reactions appear.
● Excessive use of vitamin K may temporarily defeat oral anticoagulant therapy; higher doses of oral anticoagulant or interim use of heparin may be needed.
● Phytonadione for hemorrhagic disease in infants causes fewer adverse reactions than do other vitamin K analogues; phytonadione is the vitamin K analogue of choice to treat oral anticoagulant overdose.
● Patients receiving phytonadione who have bile deficiency need concurrent use of bile salts to ensure adequate absorption.
● Phytonadione can falsely elevate urine steroid levels.
● Excessive doses of vitamin K may cause hepatic dysfunction in adults; in neonates and premature infants, large doses may cause hemolytic anemia, kernicterus, and death. Treatment of overdose is supportive.

Monitoring the patient
● During I.V. administration, watch for flushing, weakness, tachycardia, and hypotension; shock may follow. Deaths have occurred.
● Monitor PT and INR to determine effectiveness.
● Monitor patient response, and watch for adverse effects; failure to respond to vitamin K may indicate coagulation defects or irreversible hepatic damage.

Information for the patient
● For patient receiving oral form, explain rationale for drug therapy and stress importance of complying with medical regimen and keeping follow-up appointments.
● Tell patient to take a missed dose as soon as possible (but not if it's almost time for next dose) and to report missed doses.

Pediatric patients
● Don't exceed recommended dosage. Hemolysis, jaundice, and hyperbilirubinemia in newborns, particularly premature infants, may be related to vitamin K administration.

Breast-feeding patients
● It's unknown if vitamin K appears in breast milk. Use with caution in breast-feeding women.

warfarin sodium
Coumadin

Pharmacologic classification: coumarin derivative
Therapeutic classification: anticoagulant
Pregnancy risk category X

How supplied
Available by prescription only
Tablets: 1 mg, 2 mg, 2.5 mg, 3 mg, 4 mg, 5 mg, 6 mg, 7.5 mg, 10 mg
Injection: 5 mg/vial

Indications, route, and dosage
Pulmonary emboli, deep vein thrombosis, MI, rheumatic heart disease with heart valve damage, atrial arrhythmias
Adults: Initially, 2 to 5 mg P.O. or I.V.; then daily PT and INR are used to establish optimal dose. Usual maintenance dose is 2 to 10 mg P.O. daily.

Pharmacodynamics
Anticoagulant action: Inhibits vitamin K–dependent activation of clotting factors II, VII, IX, and X, which are formed in the liver; has no direct effect on established thrombi and can't reverse ischemic tissue damage. However, may prevent additional clot formation, extension of formed clots, and secondary complications of thrombosis.

Pharmacokinetics
● *Absorption:* Rapidly and completely absorbed from GI tract.
● *Distribution:* Highly bound to plasma protein, especially albumin; crosses placenta but doesn't appear to accumulate in breast milk.
● *Metabolism:* Hydroxylated by liver into inactive metabolites.
● *Excretion:* Metabolites reabsorbed from bile and excreted in urine. Half-life of parent drug is 1 to 3 days, but is highly variable. Because therapeutic effect is relatively more dependent on clotting factor depletion (factor X has half-lif

40 hours), PT won't peak for 1½ to 3 days despite use of a loading dose. Duration of action is 2 to 5 days—more closely reflecting drug's half-life.

Contraindications and precautions

Contraindicated in pregnant patients; in patients with bleeding or hemorrhagic tendencies, GI ulcerations, severe hepatic or renal disease, severe uncontrolled hypertension, subacute bacterial endocarditis, aneurysm, ascorbic acid deficiency, history of warfarin-induced necrosis, threatened abortion, eclampsia, preeclampsia, regional or lumbar block anesthesia, polycythemia vera, and vitamin K deficiency; in those in whom diagnostic tests or therapeutic procedures have potential for uncontrolled bleeding; in unsupervised patients with senility, alcoholism, psychosis, or lack of cooperation; and after recent eye, brain, or spinal cord surgery.

Use cautiously in patients with diverticulitis, colitis, hypertension, hepatic or renal disease, drainage tubes in any orifice, infectious disease or disturbance of intestinal flora, trauma, indwelling catheters, known or suspected deficiency in protein C or S, heart failure, severe diabetes, vasculitis, polycythemia vera, or risk of hemorrhage. Also use cautiously in patients who have had surgery resulting in large exposed surface, in those concurrently using NSAIDs, and in breast-feeding women.

Interactions

Oral anticoagulants interact with many drugs; thus, changes in drug regimen, including use of OTC compounds, need careful monitoring. The most significant interactions follow.
Drug-drug. *Allopurinol, cefotetan, danazol, diflunisal, erythromycin, glucagon, heparin, miconazole, quinidine, sulindac, vitamin E:* Increased anticoagulant effects. Monitor patient closely.
Amiodarone, anabolic steroids, chloramphenicol, cimetidine, clofibrate, dextrothyroxine, disulfiram, metronidazole, salicylates, streptokinase, sulfonamides, urokinase, other thyroid preparations: Markedly increased anticoagulant effect. Don't use together.
Barbiturates: May inhibit anticoagulant effect for several weeks after barbiturate withdrawal; fatal hemorrhage can occur after cessation of barbiturate effect. If barbiturates are withdrawn, reduce anticoagulant dosage.
Carbamazepine, corticosteroids, ethchlorvynol, griseofulvin, oral contraceptives, vitamin K: Possible decreased anticoagulant effect. Monitor patient closely.
Chloral hydrate: Increased or decreased warfarin anticoagulant effect. Monitor therapy closely; avoid concomitant use when possible.
Cholestyramine: Decreased anticoagulant effect when used together. Separate administration times by 6 hours.

Ethacrynic acid, indomethacin, mefenamic acid, phenylbutazone, sulfinpyrazone: Increased anticoagulant effect; severe GI irritation (may be ulcerogenic). If possible, avoid using together.
Glutethimide, rifampin: Significantly decreased anticoagulant effect. Avoid concomitant use.
Drug-herb. *Angelica sinensis:* Significantly prolonged PT. Don't use together.
Mother wort, red clover: Increased risk of bleeding. Don't use together.
Drug-food. *Enteral products, foods containing vitamin K:* May impair anticoagulation. Patients should maintain consistent daily intake of leafy green vegetables.
Drug-lifestyle. *Acute alcohol intoxication:* Increased anticoagulant effect. However, one or two drinks daily are unlikely to affect warfarin response. Discourage use together.
Chronic alcohol abuse: Decreased anticoagulant effect. Discourage use.

Adverse reactions

GI: anorexia, nausea, vomiting, cramps, *diarrhea,* mouth ulcerations, sore mouth.
GU: hematuria.
Hematologic: prolonged PT, INR, and partial thromboplastin time; HEMORRHAGE (with excessive dosage).
Hepatic: hepatitis, elevated liver function tests, jaundice.
Skin: dermatitis, urticaria, necrosis, gangrene, alopecia, *rash.*
Other: *fever,* enhanced uric acid excretion.

☑ Special considerations

● Store drug in light-resistant container at controlled room temperature (59° to 86° F [15° to 30° C]). After reconstitution, injection is stable for 4 hours at controlled room temperature.
● I.V. drug provides an alternative for patients who can't tolerate or receive oral form. I.V. dosage is the same as P.O. dosage. Administer over 1 to 2 minutes into peripheral vein.
● Discard solution that contains a precipitate.
● Warfarin causes false-negative serum theophylline levels.
● Signs and symptoms of overdose vary with severity and may include internal or external bleeding or skin necrosis of fat-rich areas, but most common sign is hematuria. Excessive prolongation of PT and INR or minor bleeding mandates withdrawal of drug; withholding one or two doses may be adequate in some cases.
● Treatment to control bleeding may include oral or I.V. phytonadione (vitamin K_1) and, in severe hemorrhage, fresh frozen plasma or whole blood. Use of phytonadione may interfere with subsequent oral anticoagulant therapy.

Monitoring the patient

● Monitor therapeutic effect.
● Watch for abnormal bleeding.

Information for the patient
• Warn patient to avoid taking OTC products containing aspirin, other salicylates, or drugs that may interact with the anticoagulant, causing an increase or decrease in drug action, and to call before stopping or starting any of these OTC preparations.
• Advise patient not to substantially alter daily intake of leafy green vegetables (asparagus, broccoli, cabbage, lettuce, turnip greens, spinach, or watercress) or of fish, pork or beef liver, green tea, or tomatoes. These foods contain vitamin K, and widely varying daily intake may alter drug's anticoagulant effect.
• Instruct patient to inform all other health care providers (including dentists) about use of warfarin.
• Instruct woman to call if planning pregnancy or if pregnancy occurs.
• Tell patient to report any unusual bruising or bleeding.

Geriatric patients
• Elderly patients are more susceptible than younger patients to effects of anticoagulants and are at increased risk for hemorrhage; this may be due to altered hemostatic mechanisms or age-related deterioration of hepatic and renal functions.

Pediatric patients
• Infants, especially neonates, may be more susceptible to anticoagulants because of vitamin K deficiency. Safety and efficacy haven't been established in children under age 18.

Breast-feeding patients
• Although drug doesn't appear in breast milk, use with caution in breast-feeding women.

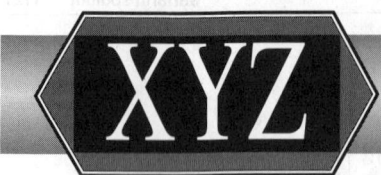

xylometazoline hydrochloride
Otrivin, Otrivin Pediatric Nasal Drops

Pharmacologic classification: sympathomimetic
Therapeutic classifications: decongestant, vasoconstrictor
Pregnancy risk category C

How supplied
Available without a prescription
Nasal drops: 0.05%, 0.1% (pediatric use)
Nasal spray: 0.1%

Indications, route, and dosage
Nasal congestion
Adults and children over age 12: Apply 2 or 3 drops or sprays of 0.1% solution to nasal mucosa q 8 to 10 hours, not to exceed three times in 24 hours.
Infants and children ages 6 months to 12 years: Apply 2 or 3 drops of 0.05% solution to nasal mucosa q 8 to 10 hours, not to exceed three times in 24 hours.
Infants under age 6 months: 1 drop of 0.05% solution in each nostril q 6 hours, p.r.n., under medical direction.

Pharmacodynamics
Decongestant action: Acts on alpha-adrenergic receptors in nasal mucosa to produce constriction, thereby decreasing blood flow and nasal congestion.

Pharmacokinetics
No information available.

Contraindications and precautions
Contraindicated in patients with hypersensitivity to drug and in those with angle-closure glaucoma. Use cautiously in patients with hyperthyroidism, cardiac disease, hypertension, diabetes mellitus, and advanced arteriosclerosis.

Interactions
Drug-drug. *Tricyclic antidepressants:* May potentiate pressor effects of tricyclic antidepressants if significant systemic absorption occurs. Use together with caution.

Adverse reactions
EENT: transient burning, stinging; dryness or ulceration of nasal mucosa; sneezing; rebound nasal congestion, irritation (with excessive or long-term use).

☑ Special considerations
• Nasal spray is less likely to cause systemic absorption and is more effective if 3 to 5 minutes elapse between sprays and nose is cleared before next spray.
• Signs and symptoms of overdose include somnolence, sedation, sweating, CNS depression with hypertension, bradycardia, decreased cardiac output, rebound hypotension, CV collapse, depressed respirations, coma. Because of rapid onset of sedation, emesis isn't recommended in therapy unless given early. Activated charcoal or gastric lavage may be used initially. Monitor vital signs and ECG. Treat seizures with I.V. diazepam.

Monitoring the patient
• Watch carefully for adverse effects in patients with CV disease, diabetes mellitus, or hyperthyroidism.
• Monitor therapeutic effect.

Information for the patient
• Advise patient that drug should only be used for short-term relief of symptoms and for no longer than 3 to 5 days.
• Inform patient of proper administration technique. For spray, hold head upright and sniff spray briskly; for drops, apply to the dependent or lower nostril, while in a lateral, head-low position. The patient should remain in that position for about 5 minutes and then repeat procedure on other side.
• Advise patient that only one person should use dropper bottle or nasal spray.
• Caution patient not to exceed recommended dosage to avoid rebound congestion.
• Advise patient to report insomnia, dizziness, weakness, tremor, or irregular heartbeat.

Geriatric patients
• Use with caution in elderly patients with cardiac disease, diabetes mellitus, or poorly controlled hypertension.

Pediatric patients
● Children may be prone to greater systemic absorption, with resultant increase in adverse effects. Use cautiously.

Breast-feeding patients
● It's unknown if drug appears in breast milk.

yellow fever vaccine
YF-Vax

Pharmacologic classification: vaccine
Therapeutic classification: viral vaccine
Pregnancy risk category C

How supplied
Available by prescription only
Injection: Live, attenuated 17D yellow fever virus in 1-dose, 5-dose, 20-dose, and 100-dose vials, with diluent; supplied only to designated yellow fever vaccination centers authorized to issue yellow fever vaccination certificates

Indications, route, and dosage
Primary vaccination
Adults and children over age 6 months: 0.5 ml deep S.C. Booster dose is 0.5 ml S.C. q 10 years.

Pharmacodynamics
Yellow fever prophylaxis: Promotes active immunity to yellow fever.

Pharmacokinetics
● *Absorption:* Immunity usually develops within 7 to 10 days; lasts for 10 years or longer.
● *Distribution:* No information available.
● *Metabolism:* No information available.
● *Excretion:* No information available.

Contraindications and precautions
Contraindicated in patients with hypersensitivity to chicken or eggs, in those with cancer or gamma globulin deficiency, in immunosuppressed patients, and in those receiving corticosteroid or radiation therapy. Also contraindicated in pregnant women and in infants under age 4 months, except in high-risk areas. Information regarding these areas can be obtained from the Centers for Disease Control and Prevention, Division of Vector-Borne Infectious Diseases, at (970) 221-6400.

Interactions
Drug-drug. *Blood, plasma transfusion:* May impair effectiveness. Defer vaccination for 2 months.
Cholera vaccines: Administration simultaneously or 1 to 3 weeks apart may result in lower than normal antibody responses to both vaccines. Give more than 3 weeks apart.

Corticosteroids, immunosuppressants: May impair immune response to vaccine. Avoid concomitant use.

Adverse reactions
Musculoskeletal: myalgia.
Other: *anaphylaxis, fever, malaise,* headache, mild swelling, pain (at injection site).

☑ Special considerations
● Have epinephrine solution 1:1,000 available to treat allergic reactions.
● Don't administer yellow fever vaccine less than 1 month before or after immunization with other live virus vaccines except for live, attenuated measles virus vaccine; BCG vaccine and hepatitis B vaccine may also be given concurrently.
● Whenever possible, administer cholera and yellow fever vaccines at least 3 weeks apart; however, if time constraints require it, they may be given simultaneously.
● Because of theoretical risk of maternal-fetal transmission of infection through vaccination, don't give yellow fever vaccine to pregnant women unless they are at high risk for exposure in an epidemic focus. There are no data that exhibit teratogenicity or ill effects in fetus after maternal immunization.
● Reconstitute vaccine only with diluent provided. Follow package insert carefully for reconstitution directions. Swirl and agitate reconstituted vial but don't shake vigorously to avoid foaming of suspension. Use vaccine within 60 minutes of preparation.
● Unreconstituted vials must be stored between –22° and 41° F (–30° and 5° C). Don't use unless shipping case contains some dry ice upon arrival.
● Discard unused reconstituted vaccine.

Monitoring the patient
● Watch for postadministration anaphylaxis.

Information for the patient
● Advise patient to expect some pain or swelling at injection site and fever or general malaise after injection. Recommend acetaminophen to alleviate fever.
● Advise patient to report adverse reactions.
● Inform patient about need for revaccination in 10 years to maintain his traveler's vaccination certificate.

Pediatric patients
● Never give vaccine to children under age 4 months. Vaccination of children ages 4 to 9 months may be needed in high-risk areas or when travel to high-risk areas can't be postponed and a high level of protection against mosquito exposure isn't feasible.

Breast-feeding patients
• It's unknown if vaccine appears in breast milk. Use with caution in breast-feeding women.

zafirlukast
Accolate

Pharmacologic classification: leukotriene receptor antagonist
Therapeutic classification: antasthmatic
Pregnancy risk category B

How supplied
Available by prescription only
Tablets: 20 mg

Indications, route, and dosage
Prophylaxis and long-term treatment of asthma
Adults and children ages 12 and older: 20 mg P.O. b.i.d. taken 1 hour before or 2 hours after meals.

Pharmacodynamics
Antasthmatic action: Selectively competes for leukotriene receptor (LTD_4 and LTE_4) sites, blocking inflammatory action.

Pharmacokinetics
• *Absorption:* Rapidly absorbed after oral administration. Plasma levels peak 3 hours after dosing.
• *Distribution:* Over 99% of drug is protein-bound to plasma proteins, predominantly albumin.
• *Metabolism:* Extensively metabolized through cytochrome P-450 2C9 (CYP 2C9) system. Drug also inhibits the CYP 3A4 and CYP 2C9 isoenzymes.
• *Excretion:* Primarily excreted in feces. Mean terminal half-life is about 10 hours.

Contraindications and precautions
Contraindicated in patients with hypersensitivity to drug or its components. Use cautiously in elderly patients and in patients with hepatic impairment.

Interactions
Drug-drug. *Aspirin, erythromycin, theophylline:* Increased plasma levels of zafirlukast. If concomitant use can't be avoided, monitor plasma levels and adjust dosage.
Warfarin: Increased PT and INR. Monitor PT and INR; adjust dosage of anticoagulant.

Adverse reactions
CNS: asthenia, dizziness, *headache.*
GI: abdominal pain, diarrhea, dyspepsia, nausea, vomiting.
Hepatic: elevated liver enzyme levels.
Musculoskeletal: back pain, myalgia.

Other: accidental injury, fever, infection, pain.

☑ Special considerations
• Drug isn't indicated for reversal of bronchospasm in acute asthma attacks.
• Drug is known to inhibit CYP 3A4 and CYP 2C9 in vitro; it's reasonable to use appropriate clinical monitoring when drugs metabolized by this isoenzyme system are administered together.
• There is no experience with zafirlukast overdose. For overdose, treat patient symptomatically and provide supportive measures, as needed. If indicated, remove unabsorbed drug from GI tract.

Monitoring the patient
• Monitor therapeutic effect.
• Monitor patient for adverse effects.

Information for the patient
• Tell patient that drug is used for long-term treatment of asthma and to keep taking drug even if his symptoms disappear.
• Advise patient to continue taking other antasthmatics as prescribed.
• Instruct patient not to take drug with food. Drug should be taken 1 hour before or 2 hours after meals.

Geriatric patients
• Drug clearance is reduced in elderly patients; use with caution.

Pediatric patients
• Safety and efficacy in children under age 12 haven't been established.

Breast-feeding patients
• Drug appears in breast milk. Don't use in breast-feeding women.

zalcitabine (dideoxycytidine, ddC)
Hivid

Pharmacologic classification: nucleoside analogue
Therapeutic classification: antiviral
Pregnancy risk category C

How supplied
Available by prescription only
Tablets (film-coated): 0.375 mg, 0.75 mg

Indications, route, and dosage
Patients with advanced HIV infection (CD4 count below 300 cells/mm³) who have demonstrated significant clinical or immunologic deterioration
Adults weighing 30 kg (66 lb) or more: 0.75 mg P.O. q 8 hours. Can be taken with zidovudine (200 mg P.O. q 8 hours).

✦ Dosage adjustment. Adjustment may be necessary in patients with impaired renal function (creatinine clearance below 55 ml/minute). For adults with renal failure, use this table.

Creatinine clearance (ml/min)	Dosage
> 40	0.75 mg P.O. q 8 hours
10 to 40	0.75 mg P.O. q 12 hours
< 10	0.75 mg P.O. q 24 hours

Pharmacodynamics

Antiviral action: Active against HIV. Within cells, drug is converted by cellular enzymes into its active metabolite, dideoxycytidine 5'-triphosphate. Inhibits replication of HIV by blocking viral DNA synthesis. Also inhibits reverse transcriptase by acting as an alternative for the enzyme's substrate, deoxycytidine triphosphate.

Pharmacokinetics

• *Absorption:* Mean absolute bioavailability above 80%; food decreases rate and extent of absorption.
• *Distribution:* Steady-state volume of distribution is 0.534 to 0.127 L/kg. Drug enters CNS.
• *Metabolism:* Doesn't appear to undergo significant hepatic metabolism; phosphorylation to the active form occurs within cells.
• *Excretion:* Primarily excreted by kidneys; about 70% of dose appears in urine within 24 hours. Mean elimination half-life is 2 hours.

Contraindications and precautions

Contraindicated in patients with hypersensitivity to drug or its components. Use cautiously in patients with preexisting peripheral neuropathy, impaired renal function, hepatic failure, or history of pancreatitis, heart failure, or cardiomyopathy.

Interactions

Drug-drug. *Cimetidine, probenecid:* Decreased elimination of zalcitabine. Monitor patient closely; adjust dosage as needed.
Drugs that cause peripheral neuropathy (such as chloramphenicol, cisplatin, dapsone, didanosine, disulfiram, ethionamide, glutethimide, gold salts, hydralazine, iodoquinol, isoniazid, metronidazole, nitrofurantoin, phenytoin, ribavirin, vincristine): Increased risk of peripheral neuropathy. Monitor patient closely; adjust dosage as needed.
Drugs that may impair renal function (aminoglycosides, amphotericin, foscarnet): Increased risk of zalcitabine-induced adverse effects. Limit concomitant use; monitor patient closely.
Pentamidine: Risk of pancreatitis. Avoid concomitant use.

Adverse reactions

CNS: *peripheral neuropathy, headache, fatigue,* dizziness, confusion, ***seizures,*** impaired concentration, amnesia, insomnia, mental depression, tremor, hypertonia, anxiety.
EENT: pharyngitis, cough, ocular pain, abnormal vision, ototoxicity, nasal discharge.
GI: nausea, vomiting, diarrhea, abdominal pain, anorexia, constipation, stomatitis, esophageal ulcer, glossitis, ***pancreatitis.***

☑ Special considerations

• If drug is stopped because of toxicity, resume recommended dosage for zidovudine alone, which is 100 mg every 4 hours.
• If symptoms indicating peripheral neuropathy occur, stop drug if symptoms are bilateral and persist beyond 72 hours. If these symptoms persist or worsen beyond 1 week, permanently stop drug. However, if all findings relevant to peripheral neuropathy have resolved to minor symptoms, drug may be reintroduced at 0.375 mg P.O. every 8 hours.
• When drug alone is only treatment, peripheral neuropathy has occurred in 17% to 31% of patients. The peripheral neuropathy seen with zalcitabine therapy is a sensorimotor neuropathy, initially characterized by numbness and burning in the extremities. If drug isn't withdrawn, symptoms can progress to sharp, shooting pain or severe, continuous burning pain requiring narcotic analgesics; pain may or may not be reversible.
• Women of childbearing age should use an effective contraceptive while taking drug.
• There is little experience with acute overdose and it's unknown if drug is dialyzable. Treat overdose symptomatically.
• Patients who had long-term exposure to doses about six times higher than the current recommended dosage experienced peripheral neuropathy within 10 weeks; patients exposed to twice the recommended dosage experienced peripheral neuropathy within 12 weeks.

Monitoring the patient

• Watch for toxic effects. Toxic effects of drug may cause abnormalities in several laboratory tests, including CBC, leukocyte count, reticulocyte count, granulocyte count, hemoglobin level, platelet count, and AST, ALT, and alkaline phosphatase levels.
• Monitor patient for peripheral neuropathy.

Information for the patient

• Explain that drug doesn't cure HIV infection and that HIV can still be transmitted. Opportunistic infections may continue to occur despite use of drug.
• Tell patient that drug may cause peripheral neuropathy and life-threatening pancreatitis. Review signs and symptoms of these reactions, and instruct patient to report them immediately.

Pediatric patients
● Safety and efficacy in children under age 13 haven't been established.

Breast-feeding patients
● It's unknown if drug appears in breast milk. Because of risk of transmitting virus, HIV-positive women shouldn't breast-feed.

---

zaleplon
Sonata

Pharmacologic classification: pyrazolopyrimidine
Therapeutic classification: hypnotic
Controlled substance schedule IV
Pregnancy risk category C

How supplied
Available by prescription only
Capsules: 5 mg, 10 mg

Indications, route, and dosage
Short-term treatment for insomnia
Adults: 5 to 20 mg P.O. daily, immediately before bedtime.
Elderly: 5 to 10 mg P.O. daily, immediately before bedtime; doses exceeding 10 mg aren't recommended.
✦ *Dosage adjustment.* For debilitated patients, initially 5 mg P.O. daily, immediately before bedtime; doses over 10 mg aren't recommended. For patients with mild to moderate hepatic failure or those receiving cimetidine concomitantly, 5 mg by P.O. daily immediately before bedtime.

Pharmacodynamics
Hypnotic action: Hypnotic with a chemical structure unrelated to benzodiazepines; interacts with the gamma-aminobutyric acid BZ receptor complex in the CNS. Modulation of this complex is hypothesized to be responsible for sedative, anxiolytic, muscle relaxant, and anticonvulsant effects of benzodiazepines.

Pharmacokinetics
● *Absorption:* Rapidly and almost completely absorbed; levels peak within 1 hour. Dosing after a high-fat or heavy meal delays peak levels by about 2 hours.
● *Distribution:* Distributed substantially into extravascular tissues. Plasma protein-binding about 60%.
● *Metabolism:* Extensively metabolized, primarily by aldehyde oxidase and, to a lesser extent, CYP 3A4 to inactive metabolites. Less than 1% of dose excreted unchanged in urine.
● *Excretion:* Rapidly excreted, with a mean half-life of about 1 hour.

Contraindications and precautions
Contraindicated in patients with severe hepatic impairment. Use cautiously in elderly and debilitated patients, in those with compromised respiratory function, and in those with signs and symptoms of depression.

Interactions
Drug-drug. *Carbamazepine, phenobarbital, phenytoin, rifampin, and other drugs that affect CYP 3A4 enzyme:* Reduce bioavailability and peak levels of zaleplon by about 80%. Consider alternative hypnotic.
Cimetidine: Increases zaleplon bioavailability and peak levels by 85%. For patient taking cimetidine, use initial zaleplon dose of 5 mg.
CNS depressants (imipramine, thioridazine): Possible additive CNS effects. Use cautiously together.
Drug-food. *Heavy meals, high-fat foods:* Prolong absorption, delaying peak zaleplon levels by about 2 hours; sleep onset may be delayed. Separate administration from meals.
Drug-lifestyle. *Alcohol:* Concurrent use may increase CNS effects. Discourage use.

Adverse reactions
CNS: *headache,* amnesia, dizziness, somnolence, depression, hypertonia, nervousness, depersonalization, hallucinations, vertigo, difficulty concentrating, anxiety, paresthesia, hypoesthesia, tremor, asthenia, migraine, malaise.
CV: chest pain, peripheral edema.
EENT: abnormal vision, conjunctivitis, eye pain, ear pain, hyperacusis, epistaxis, parosmia.
GI: constipation, dry mouth, anorexia, dyspepsia, nausea, abdominal pain, colitis.
GU: dysmenorrhea.
Musculoskeletal: arthritis, myalgia, back pain.
Respiratory: bronchitis.
Skin: pruritus, rash, photosensitivity reaction.
Other: fever.

☑ Special considerations
● Because drug works rapidly, it should only be ingested immediately before bedtime or after patient has gone to bed and has experienced difficulty falling asleep.
● Don't administer drug with or after a high-fat or heavy meal.
● Limit hypnotics use to 7 to 10 days. Reevaluate patient if hypnotics are to be taken for more than 2 to 3 weeks.
● Initiate treatment only after careful evaluation of patient because sleep disturbances may be a symptom of an underlying physical or psychiatric disorder.
● Adverse reactions are usually dose-related. Use the lowest effective dose.
● Potential for drug abuse and dependence exists. Don't give drug in quantities exceeding 1-month supply.

Reactions may be *common*, uncommon, *life-threatening*, or COMMON AND LIFE-THREATENING.

- Overdose signs and symptoms usually include exaggerated CNS depressant effects of drug, ranging from drowsiness to coma. Use immediate gastric lavage when appropriate and general supportive measures for symptomatic management.

Monitoring the patient
- Closely monitor therapeutic effect.
- Monitor patients for signs of adverse effects, especially patients with compromised respiratory function due to preexisting illness, and elderly or debilitated patients.

Information for the patient
- Advise patient that drug works rapidly and should only be taken immediately before bedtime or after patient has gone to bed and has experienced difficulty falling asleep.
- Advise patient to take drug only if he will be able to sleep for at least 4 undisturbed hours.
- Caution patient that drowsiness, dizziness, lightheadedness, and difficulty with coordination most frequently occur within 1 hour after taking drug.
- Advise patient to avoid performing activities that require mental alertness until CNS effects of drug are known.
- Advise patient to avoid alcohol while taking drug and to call before taking any prescription or OTC drugs.
- Tell patient not to take drug after a high-fat or heavy meal.
- Advise patient to report any continued sleep problems despite use of drug.
- Notify patient that dependence can occur and that drug is recommended for short-term use only.
- Warn patient not to abruptly stop drug because withdrawal symptoms (including unpleasant feelings, stomach and muscle cramps, vomiting, sweating, shakiness, and seizures) may occur.
- Notify patient that insomnia may recur for a few nights after stopping drug, but should resolve on its own.
- Advise patient that drug may cause changes in behavior and thinking, including outgoing or aggressive behavior, loss of personal identity, confusion, strange behavior, agitation, hallucinations, worsening of depression, or suicidal thoughts. Tell patient to call immediately if any of these symptoms occur.

Geriatric patients
- Elderly patients appear to be more sensitive to the effects of hypnotics. Monitor these patients closely for impaired motor or cognitive performance.

Pediatric patients
- Safety and effectiveness in children haven't been established.

Breast-feeding patients
- A small amount of drug appears in breast milk. Avoid use in breast-feeding women.

zanamivir
Relenza

Pharmacologic classification: neuraminidase inhibitor
Therapeutic classification: antiviral
Pregnancy risk category B

How supplied
Available by prescription only
Powder for inhalation: 5 mg per blister

Indications, route, and dosage
Uncomplicated acute illness due to influenza virus in patients who have been symptomatic for no more than 2 days
Adults and adolescents ages 12 and older: Two oral inhalations (one 5-mg blister per inhalation for a total dose of 10 mg) twice daily using the Diskhaler inhalation device for 5 days. Two doses should be taken on the first day of treatment provided there are at least 2 hours between doses. Subsequent doses should be about 12 hours apart (in the morning and evening) at about the same time each day.

Pharmacodynamics
Antiviral action: Most likely inhibits neuraminidase on the surface of the influenza virus, potentially altering virus particle aggregation and release. With the inhibition of neuraminidase, the virus can't escape from its host cell to attack others, thereby inhibiting the process of viral proliferation.

Pharmacokinetics
- *Absorption:* About 4% to 17% of orally inhaled drug systemically absorbed; serum levels peak 1 to 2 hours after a 10-mg dose.
- *Distribution:* Less than 10% plasma protein–binding.
- *Metabolism:* Not metabolized; excreted by kidneys as unchanged drug.
- *Excretion:* Excreted unchanged in urine within 24 hours. Unabsorbed drug excreted in feces; serum half-life ranges from 2.5 to 5.1 hours.

Contraindications and precautions
Contraindicated in patients with hypersensitivity to drug or its components. Use cautiously in patients with severe or decompensated COPD, asthma, or other underlying respiratory disease.

Interactions
None reported.

Adverse reactions
CNS: headache, dizziness.
EENT: nasal signs and symptoms; sinusitis; ear, nose, and throat infections.
GI: diarrhea, nausea, vomiting.
Respiratory: bronchitis, cough.

☑ Special considerations
• Patient with underlying respiratory disease should have a fast-acting bronchodilator available in case of wheezing while taking zanamivir. Patients scheduled to use an inhaled bronchodilator for asthma should use their bronchodilator before taking zanamivir.
• Safety and efficacy of drug haven't been established in patients who begin treatment after 48 hours of symptoms.
• Safety and efficacy of drug haven't been established for influenza prophylaxis. Use of zanamivir shouldn't affect the evaluation of patients for their annual influenza vaccination.
• Lymphopenia, neutropenia, and a rise in liver enzyme and CK levels have been reported during therapy.
• Signs and symptoms of overdose include exaggeration of drug's adverse reactions.

Monitoring the patient
• Monitor patient for bronchospasm and decline in lung function. Stop drug, as needed, in such situations.
• Monitor therapeutic effect.

Information for the patient
• Advise patient to carefully read instructions regarding proper use. Tell him to keep Diskhaler level when loading and inhaling, always check inside mouthpiece to make sure it's free of foreign objects, exhale fully before putting mouthpiece in mouth, close lips around mouthpiece, breathe in steadily and deeply, and hold breath for a few seconds after inhaling to prolong drug's presence in lungs.
• Advise patient with underlying respiratory disease who is scheduled to use an inhaled bronchodilator to do so before taking zanamivir. Tell patient to have a fast-acting bronchodilator available in case of wheezing while taking zanamivir.
• Advise patient that it's important to finish entire 5-day course of treatment even if feeling better.
• Advise patient that drug hasn't been shown to reduce risk of transmitting influenza virus to others.

Pediatric patients
• Safety and effectiveness in children under age 12 haven't been established.

Breast-feeding patients
• It's unknown if drug appears in breast milk. Because many drugs appear in breast milk, use with caution in breast-feeding women.

zidovudine (AZT)
Retrovir

Pharmacologic classification: thymidine analogue
Therapeutic classification: antiviral
Pregnancy risk category C

How supplied
Available by prescription only
Capsules: 100 mg
Tablets: 300 mg
Syrup: 50 mg/5 ml
Injection: 10 mg/ml

Indications, route, and dosage
Symptomatic HIV, AIDS, or advanced AIDS-related complex
Adults and children over age 12: 100 mg P.O. q 4 hours (600 mg daily dose). Or administer by I.V. infusion 1 to 2 mg/kg (at constant rate over 1 hour) q 4 hours for total of 6 mg/kg/day.
Children ages 3 months to 12 years: 180 mg/m^2 q 6 hours (720 mg/m^2/day). Don't exceed 200 mg q 6 hours.
Asymptomatic HIV infection (CD4 count below 500 cells/mm^3)
Adults and children over age 12: 100 mg P.O. q 4 hours while awake (for total of five doses or 500 mg daily). Or administer 1 mg/kg I.V. over 1 hour q 4 hours while awake (5 mg/kg daily).
Children ages 3 months to 12 years: 180 mg/m^2 q 6 hours (720 mg/m^2 P.O. daily) in divided doses q 6 hours. Don't exceed 200 mg q 6 hours.
Maternal-fetal transmission of HIV
Adults: Maternal dosing: Give 100 mg P.O. q 4 hours while awake (for total of five doses daily) until onset of labor. During labor and delivery, administer 2 mg/kg I.V. over 1 hour, then a continuous infusion of 1 mg/kg/hour until clamping of umbilical cord. Infant dosing: 2 mg/kg P.O. q 6 hours starting 12 hours after birth and continuing until 6 weeks of age; or administer 1.5 mg/kg via I.V. infusion over 30 minutes q 6 hours.
✦ Dosage adjustment. Because drug is partially removed by dialysis, dosage adjustment may be needed in affected patients. Dosage adjustment also may be warranted in patients with decreased liver function.

Pharmacodynamics
Antiviral action: Converted intracellularly to an active triphosphate compound that inhibits reverse transcriptase (an enzyme essential for retroviral DNA synthesis), thereby inhibiting viral replication. When used in vitro, drug inhibits certain other viruses and bacteria; however, this has undetermined clinical significance.

Pharmacokinetics

• *Absorption:* Absorbed rapidly from GI tract. Average systemic bioavailability 65% of dose (drug undergoes first-pass metabolism).

• *Distribution:* Preliminary data reveal good CSF penetration. About 36% of dose plasma protein-bound.

• *Metabolism:* Metabolized rapidly to inactive compound.

• *Excretion:* Parent drug and metabolite excreted by glomerular filtration and tubular secretion in kidneys. Urine recovery of parent drug and metabolite is 14% and 74%, respectively. Elimination half-lives of these compounds, 1 hour.

Contraindications and precautions

Contraindicated in patients with hypersensitivity to drug. Use cautiously in patients in advanced stages of HIV and in those with severe bone marrow suppression, renal insufficiency, or hepatomegaly, hepatitis, or other risk factors for hepatic disease.

Interactions

Drug-drug. *Acyclovir:* Severe drowsiness and lethargy. Use cautiously together.

Drugs that are nephrotoxic or affect bone marrow function or formation of bone marrow elements (such as amphotericin B, dapsone, doxorubicin, flucytosine, ganciclovir, interferon, pentamidine, vinblastine, vincristine): May increase risk of toxicity of these drugs. Use cautiously together.

Probenecid: Impaired elimination of zidovudine. Monitor patient closely; adjust dosage as necessary.

Adverse reactions

CNS: headache, *seizures,* paresthesia, malaise, asthenia, insomnia, dizziness, somnolence.
EENT: taste perversion.
GI: nausea, anorexia, abdominal pain, vomiting, constipation, diarrhea, dyspepsia.
Hematologic: *severe bone marrow suppression (resulting in anemia), agranulocytosis, thrombocytopenia.*
Musculoskeletal: myalgia.
Skin: *rash,* diaphoresis.
Other: *fever.*

☑ Special considerations

• Neither optimum duration of treatment nor dosage for optimum effectiveness and minimum toxicity is known.

• I.V. dosage equivalent to 100 mg P.O. every 4 hours is about 1 mg/kg I.V. every 4 hours.

• Store undiluted injection, capsules, and syrup at room temperature (77° F [25° C]); protect from light. Dilute I.V. form to less than 4 mg/ml with D₅W before administering. Don't mix with solutions containing protein. To minimize potential for microbial contamination, administer within 8 hours of mixing if left at room temperature or within 24 hours if refrigerated (36° to 46° F [2° to 8° C]).

• Drug doesn't cure HIV infection or AIDS but may reduce morbidity resulting from opportunistic infections and thus prolong patient's life.

Monitoring the patient

• Monitor CBC and platelet count at least every 2 weeks. Significant anemia (hemoglobin level less than 7.5 g/dl or reduction of over 25% of baseline) or significant neutropenia (granulocyte count below 750 cells/mm³ or reduction of more than 50% from baseline) may need interruption of drug until evidence of bone marrow recovery occurs. In patients with less severe anemia or neutropenia, a dosage reduction may be adequate.

• Watch for signs and symptoms of opportunistic infection (including pneumonia, meningitis, and sepsis).

Information for the patient

• Because drug frequently causes a low RBC count, advise patient that he may need blood transfusions or epoetin alfa therapy during treatment.

• Instruct patient on proper drug administration; explain importance of maintaining an adequate blood level.

• Warn patient not to take other drugs for AIDS (especially from the "street") without medical approval.

• Advise patient that drug doesn't reduce the ability to transmit HIV.

Breast-feeding patients

• Drug appears in breast milk. To avoid transmitting HIV to infant, HIV-positive women shouldn't breast-feed.

zileuton
Zyflo Filmtab

Pharmacologic classification: 5-lipoxygenase inhibitor
Therapeutic classification: antasthmatic
Pregnancy risk category C

How supplied

Available by prescription only
Tablets: 600 mg

Indications, route, and dosage
Prophylaxis and long-term treatment of asthma

Adults and children ages 12 and older: 600 mg P.O. q.i.d.

Pharmacodynamics
Antasthmatic action: Inhibits enzyme responsible for formation of leukotrienes, thus reducing inflammatory response.

Pharmacokinetics
- *Absorption:* Rapidly absorbed with oral administration; mean time to peak levels is 1.7 hours.
- *Distribution:* Apparent volume of distribution is 1.2 L/kg. 93% bound to plasma proteins, primarily albumin.
- *Metabolism:* Oxidatively metabolized by cytochrome P-450 system. Several active and inactive metabolites identified.
- *Excretion:* Elimination predominantly via metabolism with a mean terminal half-life of 2½ hours.

Contraindications and precautions
Contraindicated in patients with hypersensitivity to drug or its components and in those with active hepatic disease or transaminase elevations at least three times upper limit of normal. Use with caution in patients with hepatic impairment or history of heavy alcohol use.

Interactions
Drug-drug. *Drugs metabolized by the CYP 3A4 isoenzyme (cyclosporine, dihydropyridine calcium channel blockers, estradiol, ethinyl, prednisone):* No formal interaction studies have been conducted. Administer with caution.
Propranolol, other beta blockers: Increased beta-blocker effect. Monitor patient; reduce dosage of beta blocker.
Theophylline: Decreased theophylline clearance (on average, serum theophylline levels double). Reduce theophylline dosage; monitor serum levels.
Warfarin: Increased PT and INR. Monitor PT and INR; adjust dosage of anticoagulant.

Adverse reactions
CNS: malaise, asthenia, dizziness, headache, insomnia, nervousness, somnolence.
CV: chest pain.
EENT: conjunctivitis.
GI: abdominal pain, constipation, dyspepsia, flatulence, nausea.
GU: urinary tract infection, vaginitis.
Hematologic: *leukopenia.*
Hepatic: elevated liver enzyme levels.
Musculoskeletal: arthralgia, hypertonia, myalgia, neck pain and rigidity.
Skin: pruritus.
Other: accidental injury, fever, lymphadenopathy, pain.

☑ Special considerations
- Drug may be taken with meals and at bedtime.
- Drug isn't indicated for use in the reversal of bronchospasm in acute asthma attacks.

- There are limited data on acute overdose. Drug isn't removed by dialysis. If overdose occurs, treat patient symptomatically and provide supportive measures. If indicated, eliminate unabsorbed drug by emesis or gastric lavage.

Monitoring the patient
- Obtain liver enzyme levels at baseline, once a month for the first 3 months, then every 2 to 3 months for the remainder of the first year, and periodically thereafter.
- Monitor patient for adverse effects.

Information for the patient
- Advise patient that drug is used for long-term treatment of asthma and to continue taking drug even if his symptoms disappear.
- Caution patient that drug isn't a bronchodilator and shouldn't be used to treat an acute asthma attack.
- Advise patient to continue taking other antasthmatics.
- Instruct patient to call if short-acting bronchodilator isn't effective in relieving symptoms.
- Advise patient to call immediately if signs and symptoms of hepatic dysfunction develop (right upper quadrant pain, nausea, fatigue, pruritus, jaundice, malaise).
- Advise patient to avoid alcohol and to call before taking OTC or new prescription drugs.

Pediatric patients
- Safety and effectiveness in children under age 12 haven't been studied.

Breast-feeding patients
- It's unknown if drug appears in breast milk. Use with caution in breast-feeding women.

zinc
Orazinc, Verazinc, Zinc 15, Zinc-220, Zincate, Zinca-Pak

zinc sulfate (ophthalmic)
Eye-Sed

Pharmacologic classification: trace element, miscellaneous anti-infective
Therapeutic classification: nutritional supplement, topical anti-infective
Pregnancy risk category C

How supplied
Available by prescription only
Injection: 10 ml (1 mg/ml), 30 ml (1 mg/ml with 0.9% benzyl alcohol), 5 ml (5 mg/ml); 10 ml (5 mg/ml)
Capsules: 220 mg (50 mg zinc)
Available without a prescription, as appropriate
Tablets: 66 mg (15 mg zinc), 110 mg (25 mg zinc), 200 mg (47 mg zinc)

Reactions may be *common,* uncommon, ***life-threatening,*** or COMMON AND LIFE-THREATENING.

Capsules: 220 mg (50 mg zinc)
Solution: 15 ml (0.25%)

Indications, route, and dosage
RDA of zinc is 15 mg/day P.O. for adults and 0.3 mg/kg/day P.O. for children.
Metabolically stable zinc deficiency
Adults: 2.5 to 4 mg/day I.V.; add 2 mg/day for acute catabolic states.
Stable zinc deficiency with fluid loss from the small bowel
Adults: Add 12.2 mg/L of total parenteral nutrition solution or 17.1 mg/kg of stool or ileostomy output.
Zinc deficiency
Children under age 5: 100 mcg/kg/day I.V.
Premature infants: 300 mcg/kg/day I.V.
Dietary supplementation
Adults: 25 to 50 mg P.O. daily.
For relief of minor eye irritation
Adults: 1 to 2 drops ophthalmic solution into eye b.i.d. to q.i.d. Patients should report irritation that persists for more than 3 days.

Pharmacodynamics
Metabolic action: Zinc serves as a cofactor for more than 70 different enzymes. It facilitates wound healing, normal growth rates, and normal skin hydration and helps maintain the senses of taste and smell.
　Adequate zinc provides normal growth and tissue repair. In patients receiving total parenteral nutrition with low plasma levels of zinc, dermatitis has been followed by alopecia. Zinc is an integral part of many enzymes important to carbohydrate and protein mobilization of retinal-binding protein.
　Zinc sulfate ophthalmic solution exhibits astringent and weak antiseptic activity, which may result from precipitation of protein by the zinc ion and by clearing mucus from the outer surface of the eye. Drug has no decongestant action and produces mild vasodilation.

Pharmacokinetics
● *Absorption:* Zinc sulfate is absorbed poorly from the GI tract; only 20% to 30% of dietary zinc is absorbed. After administration, zinc resides in muscle, bone, skin, kidneys, liver, pancreas, retina, prostate, and particularly RBCs and WBCs. Binds to plasma albumin, alpha-2 macroglobulin, and some plasma amino acids, including histidine, cysteine, threonine, glycine, and asparagine.
● *Distribution:* Major zinc stores in skeletal muscle, skin, bone, and pancreas.
● *Metabolism:* Zinc is a cofactor in many enzymatic reactions; is needed for synthesis and mobilization of retinal binding protein.
● *Excretion:* After parenteral administration, 90% excreted in stool, urine, and sweat. After oral use, major route of excretion is secretion into duode-
num and jejunum. Small amounts excreted in urine (0.3 to 0.5 mg/day) and sweat (1.5 mg/day).

Contraindications and precautions
Parenteral use of zinc sulfate is contraindicated in patients with renal failure or biliary obstruction (and requires caution in all patients); monitor zinc plasma levels frequently. Don't exceed prescribed dosages. In patients with renal dysfunction or GI malfunction, trace metal supplements may need to be reduced, adjusted, or omitted. Hypersensitivity may result. Routine use of zinc supplementation during pregnancy isn't recommended.
　Administering copper in the absence of zinc or administering zinc in the absence of copper may result in decreased serum levels of either element. When only one trace element is needed, it should be added separately and serum levels monitored closely. To avoid overdose, administer multiple trace elements only when clearly needed. In patients with extreme vomiting or diarrhea, large amounts of trace element replacement may be needed. Excessive intake in healthy persons may be deleterious.

Interactions
Drug-drug. *Certain proteins, methylcellulose suspensions:* Precipitation of these drugs. Avoid concomitant use.
Fluoroquinolones, tetracyclines: Impaired antibiotic absorption. Avoid concomitant use.
Sodium borate: Precipitation of zinc borate when using ocular preparation. Glycerin may prevent interaction.
Drug-herb. *Acacia:* Zinc ophthalmic solution may precipitate acacia. Avoid concomitant use.
Drug-food. *Dairy products:* Possible reduction in zinc absorption. Don't use together.

Adverse reactions
CNS: restlessness.
GI: distress and irritation, nausea, vomiting with high doses, gastric ulceration, diarrhea.
Skin: rash.
Other: dehydration.

☑ Special considerations
● Results may not appear for 6 to 8 weeks in zinc-depleted patients.
● Zinc decreases absorption of tetracyclines and fluoroquinolones.
● Calcium supplements may confer a protective effect against zinc toxicity.
● Because of potential for infusion phlebitis and tissue irritation, an undiluted direct injection must not be administered into a peripheral vein.
● Don't exceed prescribed dosage of oral zinc; if oral zinc is administered in single 2-g doses, emesis will occur.
● If ophthalmic use causes increasing irritation, stop drug.

- Signs and symptoms of severe toxicity include hypotension, pulmonary edema, diarrhea, vomiting, jaundice, and oliguria. If toxicity occurs, stop drug and provide support measures.

Monitoring the patient
- Monitor patient for severe vomiting and dehydration, which may indicate overdose.

Information for the patient
- Advise patient not to take zinc with dairy products, which can reduce zinc absorption.
- Teach patient how to instill ophthalmic solution and to prevent contamination. Tell him to avoid contacting lip of container with other surface and to tightly close container after use.
- Warn patient about self-medication with zinc sulfate ophthalmic solution, which shouldn't continue longer than 3 days. Patient should report increased irritation or redness.
- Advise patient that GI upset may occur after oral administration but may decrease if zinc is taken with food. Tell him to avoid foods high in calcium, phosphorus, or phytate during therapy.

---

zolmitriptan
Zomig

Pharmacologic classification: selective 5-hydroxytryptamine receptor agonist
Therapeutic classification: antimigraine drug
Pregnancy risk category C

How supplied
Available by prescription only
Tablets: 2.5 mg, 5 mg

Indications, route, and dosage
Acute migraine headaches with or without aura
Adults: Initially, 2.5 mg or less P.O. A dose lower than 2.5 mg can be achieved by manually breaking a 2.5 mg tablet in half. If headache returns after initial dose, a second dose may be given after 2 hours. Maximum dose is 10 mg in 24-hour period.
✦ **Dosage adjustment.** In patients with liver disease, use doses under 2.5 mg.

Pharmacodynamics
Antimigraine action: Binds with high affinity to recombinant 5-HT$_{1D}$ and 5-HT$_{1B}$ receptors, aborting migraine headaches by causing constriction of cranial blood vessels and inhibition of pro-inflammatory neuropeptide release.

Pharmacokinetics
- *Absorption:* Well absorbed after oral administration; plasma level peaks in 2 hours. Mean absolute bioavailability about 40%.

- *Distribution:* Apparent volume of distribution is 7 L/kg. Plasma protein–binding is 25%.
- *Metabolism:* Drug is converted to an active N-desmethyl metabolite. Time to maximum concentration for the metabolite is 2 to 3 hours. Mean elimination half-life of zolmitriptan and active N-desmethyl metabolite is 3 hours.
- *Excretion:* Mean total clearance is 31.5 ml/minute/kg; one-sixth is renal clearance. The renal clearance is greater than the glomerular filtration rate, suggesting renal tubular secretion. About 65% of dose excreted in urine, 30% in feces.

Contraindications and precautions
Contraindicated in patients with hypersensitivity to drug or its components; in those with uncontrolled hypertension, ischemic heart disease (angina pectoris, history of MI or documented silent ischemia), or other significant heart disease (including Wolff-Parkinson-White syndrome).

Avoid use within 24 hours of other 5-HT$_1$ agonists or drugs containing ergot, or within 2 weeks of stopping MAO inhibitor therapy. Also avoid use in patients with hemiplegic or basilar migraine.

Use cautiously in patients with liver disease and in pregnant or breast-feeding women.

Interactions
Drug-drug. *Cimetidine:* Doubled half-life of zolmitriptan. Monitor patient closely.
Drugs containing ergot: Additive vasospastic reactions. Avoid concomitant use.
Fluoxetine, fluvoxamine, paroxetine, sertraline: Possible weakness, hyperreflexia, and incoordination. Use cautiously together.
MAO inhibitors: Increased plasma levels of zolmitriptan. Monitor zolmitriptan levels; adjust dosage as needed. Avoid use of drug within 2 weeks of stopping MAO inhibitor therapy.
Oral contraceptives: Increased mean plasma levels of zolmitriptan. Adjust dosage as needed.

Adverse reactions
CNS: somnolence, vertigo, *dizziness,* hyperesthesias, paresthesia, asthenia.
CV: palpitations, pain or heaviness in chest, *pain, tightness, or pressure in the neck, throat, or jaw.*
GI: dry mouth, dyspepsia, dysphagia, nausea.
Musculoskeletal: myalgia.
Skin: sweating.
Other: warm or cold sensations.

☑ Special considerations
- Drug isn't intended for prophylactic therapy of migraine headaches or for use in hemiplegic or basilar migraines.
- Safety of drug hasn't been established for cluster headaches.
- Serious cardiac events, including some that have been fatal, have occurred rarely after use of 5-HT$_1$ agonists. Events reported have includ-

ed coronary artery vasospasm, transient myocardial ischemia, MI, ventricular tachycardia, and ventricular fibrillation.

● There is no specific antidote for overdose. If severe intoxication occurs, intensive care procedures are recommended, including establishing and maintaining a patent airway, ensuring adequate oxygenation and ventilation, and monitoring and supporting CV system. The effect of hemodialysis or peritoneal dialysis on drug plasma levels is unknown.

Monitoring the patient
● Monitor blood pressure in patients with liver disease.
● Monitor therapeutic effect.

Information for the patient
● Advise patient that drug is intended to relieve migraine symptoms, not prevent them.
● Advise patient to take drug only as prescribed and not to take a second dose unless instructed. If a second dose is indicated, he should take it 2 hours after initial dose.
● Advise patient to immediately report pain or tightness in chest or throat, heart throbbing, rash, skin lumps, or swelling of face, lips, or eyelids.
● Caution woman to avoid pregnancy during therapy.
● Advise patient that drug shouldn't be taken with other migraine drugs.

Geriatric patients
● No information available for this age-group. Pharmacokinetic disposition is similar to that seen in younger adults.

Pediatric patients
● Safety and effectiveness in children haven't been established.

Breast-feeding patients
● It's unknown if drug appears in breast milk. Use with caution in breast-feeding women.

zolpidem tartrate
Ambien

Pharmacologic classification: imidazopyridine
Therapeutic classification: hypnotic
Controlled substance schedule IV
Pregnancy risk category B

How supplied
Available by prescription only
Tablets: 5 mg, 10 mg

Indications, route, and dosage
Short-term management of insomnia
Adults: 10 mg P.O. immediately before bedtime.

✦ *Dosage adjustment.* In elderly or debilitated patients or patients with hepatic insufficiency, 5 mg P.O. immediately before bedtime. Maximum daily dose is 10 mg.

Pharmacodynamics
Hypnotic action: Hypnotic with a chemical structure unrelated to benzodiazepines, barbiturates, or other drugs with known hypnotic properties; however, it interacts with a gamma-aminobutyric acid (GABA)-benzodiazepine or omega-receptor complex and shares some of the pharmacologic properties of the benzodiazepines. It exhibits no muscle relaxant or anticonvulsant properties.

Pharmacokinetics
● *Absorption:* Absorbed rapidly from GI tract; mean peak concentration time of 1½ hours. Food delays absorption.
● *Distribution:* Protein-binding is about 92.5%.
● *Metabolism:* Converted to inactive metabolites in liver.
● *Excretion:* Primarily eliminated in urine; elimination half-life about 2½ hours.

Contraindications and precautions
No known contraindications. Use cautiously in patients with conditions that could affect metabolism or hemodynamic response and in those with decreased respiratory drive, depression, or history of alcohol or drug abuse.

Interactions
Drug-drug. *Other CNS depressants:* Enhanced CNS depression of zolpidem. Avoid concomitant use.
Drug-lifestyle. *Alcohol:* Excessive CNS depression. Use together cautiously.

Adverse reactions
CNS: daytime drowsiness, light-headedness, abnormal dreams, amnesia, dizziness, *headache,* hangover, sleep disorder, lethargy, depression.
CV: palpitations, chest pain.
EENT: sinusitis, pharyngitis, dry mouth.
GI: nausea, vomiting, diarrhea, dyspepsia, constipation, abdominal pain.
Musculoskeletal: back pain, myalgia, arthralgia.
Skin: rash.
Other: flulike symptoms, *hypersensitivity reactions.*

☑ Special considerations
● Limit drug therapy to 7 to 10 days; reevaluate patient if drug is to be taken for over 2 weeks.
● Because sleep disturbance may be a sign or symptom of a physical or psychiatric disorder, initiate symptomatic treatment of insomnia only after careful evaluation of patient.
● Zolpidem has CNS-depressant effects similar to other sedative-hypnotic drugs. Because of its

rapid onset of action, drug should be given immediately before going to bed.
● Dosage adjustments may be needed when drug is given with other CNS depressants because of the potentially additive effects.
● Prevent hoarding or self-overdosing by hospitalized patients who are depressed, suicidal, or known to abuse drug.
● Symptoms may range from somnolence to light coma. CV and respiratory compromise also may occur. Use general symptomatic and supportive measures, along with immediate gastric lavage when appropriate. Give I.V. fluids as needed. Flumazenil may be useful. Monitor and treat hypotension and CNS depression. Withhold sedatives after zolpidem overdose even if excitation occurs.

Monitoring the patient
● Closely monitor patient with history of addiction to or abuse of drugs or alcohol because of risk of habituation and dependence.
● Monitor patient for hypersensitivity reactions.

Information for the patient
● Tell patient not to take drug with or immediately after a meal.
● Stress importance of taking drug only as prescribed; inform patient of potential drug dependency associated with hypnotics taken for long periods.
● Inform patient that tolerance may occur if drug is taken for more than a few weeks.
● Warn patient against use of alcohol or other sleep preparations during therapy to avoid serious adverse effects.
● Caution patient to avoid activities that require alertness, such as driving, until adverse CNS effects of drug are known.
● Tell patient not to increase dose and to call if he feels drug is no longer effective.

Geriatric patients
● Impaired motor or cognitive performance after repeated exposure or unusual sensitivity to sedative-hypnotics may occur in elderly patients. Recommended dose is 5 mg rather than 10 mg.

Pediatric patients
● Safety and effectiveness in children under age 18 haven't been established.

Breast-feeding patients
● Because drug appears in breast milk, its use in breast-feeding women isn't recommended.

Reactions may be *common*, uncommon, *life-threatening*, or COMMON AND LIFE-THREATENING.

Pharmacologic classes

adrenergics, direct and indirect acting

albuterol sulfate, arbutamine hydrochloride, bitolterol mesylate, brimonidine tartrate, dobutamine hydrochloride, dopamine hydrochloride, ephedrine, ephedrine hydrochloride, ephedrine sulfate, epinephrine, epinephrine bitartrate, epinephrine hydrochloride, epinephryl borate, isoetharine hydrochloride, isoetharine mesylate, isoproterenol, isoproterenol hydrochloride, isoproterenol sulfate, metaproterenol sulfate, metaraminol bitartrate, naphazoline hydrochloride, norepinephrine bitartrate, phenylephrine hydrochloride, pirbuterol acetate, pseudoephedrine hydrochloride, pseudoephedrine sulfate, ritodrine hydrochloride, salmeterol xinafoate, terbutaline sulfate, tetrahydrozoline hydrochloride, xylometazoline hydrochloride

Beta-receptor activation is associated with the activation of adenylate cyclase and the accumulation of cAMP; the cellular consequences of alpha-receptor activation are less well understood.

Alpha$_1$ receptors are located on smooth muscle and glands and are excitatory; alpha$_2$ receptors are prejunctional regulatory receptors in the CNS and postjunctional receptors in many peripheral tissues. Beta$_1$ receptors are located in cardiac tissues and are excitatory; beta$_2$ receptors are located primarily on smooth muscle and glands and are inhibitory.

Adrenergic drugs may mimic the naturally occurring catecholamines norepinephrine, epinephrine, and dopamine or may function by stimulating the release of norepinephrine.

Pharmacology

Most actions of clinically useful adrenergic drugs involve peripheral excitatory actions on glands and vascular smooth muscle; cardiac and CNS excitatory actions; peripheral inhibitory actions on smooth muscle of the bronchial tree and blood vessels supplying skeletal muscles and gut; and metabolic and endocrine effects. Because different tissues respond in varying degrees to adrenergic agonists, differences in the actions of catecholamines are attributed to the presence of different receptor types within the tissues (alpha and beta).

Clinical indications and actions

Most drugs act on two or more receptor sites; the net effect is the sum of alpha and beta activity. Dopaminergic and serotonergic activity may occur, possibly stimulating receptors in the CNS to release histamine.

Temporary appetite suppression is another effect, often resulting in a rebound weight gain after patient develops tolerance to the anorexic effect, or after withdrawal of the drug. Other uses include support of blood pressure, suppression of urinary incontinence and enuresis, and relief from pain of dysmenorrhea.

Hypotension

Alpha agonists (norepinephrine, metaraminol, phenylephrine, and pseudoephedrine) cause arteriolar and venous constriction, resulting in increased blood pressure. This action helps support blood pressure in hypotension and in management of serious allergic conditions. Topical formulations are used to induce local vasoconstriction (decongestion), arrest superficial hemorrhage (styptic), stimulate radial smooth muscle of the iris (mydriasis), and (with local anesthetics) localize anesthesia and prolong duration of action. Ophthalmic preparations reduce aqueous humor production and increase uveoscleral outflow.

Cardiac stimulation

Beta$_1$ agonists (dobutamine) act primarily in the heart, producing a positive inotropic effect. Because they increase heart rate, enhance AV conduction, and increase the strength of the heartbeat, beta$_1$ agonists may be used to restore heartbeat in cardiac arrest and for heart block in syncopal seizures (not treatment of choice), or to treat acute heart failure and cardiogenic or other types of shock. Their use in shock is somewhat controversial because beta$_1$ agonists induce lipolysis (increase of free fatty acids in plasma), which promotes a metabolic acidosis, and because they favor arrhythmias, which pose a special threat in cardiogenic shock.

Bronchodilation

Beta$_2$ agonists (albuterol, bitolterol, isoetharine, metaproterenol, salmeterol, pirbuterol, and te' taline) act primarily on smooth muscle of the bronchial tree, vasculature, intestines, and uterus. They also induce hepatic and muscle glycogenolysis, which results in hyperglycemia (sometimes useful in insulin overdose) and hyperlactic acidemia.

Some are used as bronchodilators, some as vasodilators. They are also used to relax the uterus, to delay delivery in premature labor, and for dysmenorrhea. Some degree of cardiostimulation may occur because all $beta_2$ agonists have some degree of $beta_1$ activity.

Renal vasodilation
Dopamine is currently the only commercially available sympathomimetic with significant dopaminergic activity, although some other sympathomimetics appear to act on dopamine receptors in the CNS. Dopamine receptors are prominent in the periphery (splanchnic and renal vasculature), where they mediate vasodilation, which is useful in inducing diuresis in patients with acute renal failure, heart failure, and shock.

Overview of adverse reactions
Patients who are more sensitive to the effects of these drugs include elderly persons, infants, and patients with thyrotoxicosis or CV disease.

The alpha agonists commonly produce CV reactions. An excessive increase in blood pressure is a major adverse reaction of systemically administered alpha agonists. Exaggerated pressor response may occur in hypertensive or elderly patients, which may evoke vagal reflex responses resulting in bradycardia and AV block. Alpha agonists also interfere with lactation and may cause nausea, vomiting, sweating, piloerection, rebound congestion or miosis, difficult urination, and headache. Ophthalmic use may cause mydriasis, photophobia, burning, stinging, and blurring.

The beta agonists most frequently cause tachycardia, palpitations, and other arrhythmias. Their other effects include premature atrial and ventricular contractions; tachyarrhythmias, and myocardial necrosis. Reflex tachycardia and palpitations occur with $beta_2$ agonists because of decreased blood pressure.

Metabolic reactions to beta agonists include hyperglycemia, increased metabolic rate, hyperlactic acidosis, and local and systemic acidosis (decreased bronchodilator response).

Respiratory reactions include increased perfusion of nonfunctioning portions of lungs (COPD); mucus plugs may develop as a result of increased mucus secretion. Other reactions include tremors, vertigo, insomnia, sweating, headache, nausea, vomiting, and anxiety.

The centrally acting adrenergics have similar effects, which may also be associated with dry mouth, flushing, diarrhea, impotence, hyperthermia (excessive doses), agitation, anorexia, dizziness, dyskinesia, and changes in libido.

Chronic use of adrenergics in children may cause endocrine disturbances that arrest growth; however, growth usually rebounds after withdrawal of drug.

☑ Special considerations
Parenteral preparations
● If used as a pressor drug, recommend correction of fluid volume depletion before administration. Adrenergics aren't a substitute for blood, plasma, fluid, or electrolytes.
● Blood pressure, pulse, and respiratory and urine output should be monitored carefully during therapy.
● Tachyphylaxis or tolerance may develop after prolonged or excessive use.

Inhalation therapy
● The preservative sodium bisulfite is present in many adrenergic formulations. Patients with a history of allergy to sulfites should avoid drugs that contain this preservative.
● Patient should take drug when arising in morning and before meals to reduce fatigue by improving ventilation.
● For unknown reasons, paradoxical airway resistance (manifested by sudden increase in dyspnea) may result from repeated excessive use of isoetharine. If this occurs, stop drug and use alternative therapy (such as epinephrine).
● Adrenergic inhalation may be alternated with other drugs (corticosteroids, other adrenergics), if necessary, but shouldn't be given simultaneously because of danger of excessive tachycardia.
● Don't use discolored or precipitated solutions.
● Protect solutions from light, freezing, and heat. Store at controlled room temperature.
● Systemic absorption, though infrequent, can follow applications to nasal and conjunctival membranes. If symptoms of systemic absorption occur, stop drug.
● Prolonged or too-frequent use may cause tolerance to bronchodilating and cardiac stimulant effect. Rebound bronchospasm may follow end of drug effect.

Information for the patient
Inhalation therapy
● Instruct patient in correct use of nebulizer and warn him to use lowest effective dose.
● Inform patient that most inhalers need to be shaken before use; instruct patient in proper use.
● Explain that overuse of adrenergic bronchodilators may cause tachycardia, headache, nausea and dizziness, loss of effectiveness, possible paradoxical reaction, and cardiac arrest.
● Tell patient to call if bronchodilator causes dizziness, chest pain, or lack of therapeutic response to usual dose.
● Tell patient to avoid other adrenergic drugs unless prescribed.

• Inform patient that saliva and sputum may appear pink after inhalation treatment.
• Instruct patient to begin treatment with first symptoms of bronchospasm.
• Caution patient to keep spray away from eyes.
• Tell patient not to discard drug applicator. Refill units are available.

Nasal therapy
• Instruct patient to blow nose gently (with both nostrils open) to clear nasal passages well, before administration of drug.
• Show patient proper method of instillation.
– Drops: Tell patient to tilt head back while sitting or standing up, or to lie on bed with head over side. He should stay in position a few minutes to permit drug to spread through nose.
– Spray: Tell patient, with head upright, to squeeze bottle quickly and firmly to produce one or two sprays into each nostril; wait 3 to 5 minutes, blow nose, and repeat dose.
– Jelly: Tell patient to place in each nostril and sniff it well back into nose.
• Advise patient not to use nasal decongestant for longer than 5 days.

Ophthalmic therapy
• To avoid excessive systemic absorption, tell patient to apply pressure to lacrimal sac during and for 1 to 2 minutes after instillation of drops.
• Inform patient that after instillation of ophthalmic preparation, pupils of eyes will be very large and eyes may be more sensitive to light than usual. Advise patient to use dark glasses until pupils return to normal.
• Warn patient to use drug only as directed.
• Instruct patient to call if no relief occurs or condition worsens.
• Tell patient to store drug away from heat and light and out of reach of children.
• Tell patient not to use for longer than 72 hours without first calling.

Geriatric patients
• Elderly patients may be more sensitive to therapeutic and adverse effects of some adrenergics and may require lower doses.

Pediatric patients
• Lower doses of adrenergics are recommended in children.

Pregnant patients
• Pregnancy risk categories range from B to D in this group. Refer to specific package insert for manufacturer recommendations.

Breast-feeding patients
• The use of adrenergics during breast-feeding usually isn't recommended.

Representative combinations

Ephedrine sulfate with belladonna extract, boric acid, zinc oxide, beeswax, and cocoa butter: Wyanoids Relief Factor.

Epinephrine with benzalkonium chloride: Glaucon; with pilocarpine: E-Pilo.

Naphazoline with antazoline phosphate, boric acid, phenylmercuric acetate, and carbonate anhydrous: Vasocon-A Solution; with pheniramine maleate: Naphcon-A; with phenylephrine hydrochloride, pyrilamine maleate, and phenylpropanolamine hydrochloride: 4-Way Long Lasting Spray; with polyvinyl alcohol: Albalon.

Pseudoephedrine with chlorpheniramine maleate: Chlor-Trimeton; with codeine phosphate and guaifenesin: Deproist Expectorant with Codeine, Guiatussin DAC, Isoclor Expectorant, Novahistine Expectorant, Robitussin-DAC; with dextromethorphan and acetaminophen: Contac Severe Cold and Flu Nighttime; with dextromethorphan, acetaminophen, and guaifenesin: Vicks 44M Cough, Cold, and Flu Relief; with dexbrompheniramine: Disophrol, Drixoral; with dexchlorpheniramine: Polaramine; with guaifenesin: Robitussin-PE, Zephrex; with hydrocodone bitartrate: De-Tuss, Detussin Liquid, Entuss-D, Tussend; with triprolidine: Actagen, Actamin, Actifed, Allerfrim Tablets, Aprodine, Cenafed Plus, Triposed.

See also *antihistamines* and *barbiturates*.

---

adrenocorticoids (nasal and oral inhalation)

Nasal: **beclomethasone dipropionate, budesonide, dexamethasone sodium phosphate, flunisolide, fluticasone propionate, triamcinolone acetonide**

Oral: **beclomethasone dipropionate, budesonide, dexamethasone sodium phosphate, flunisolide, triamcinolone acetonide**

Topical administration through oral aerosol and nasal spray delivers adrenocorticoids to sites of inflammation in the nasal passages or the tracheobronchial tree. Because smaller doses are administered, less drug is absorbed systemically, with fewer systemic adverse effects.

Pharmacology

Inhaled glucocorticoid is absorbed through the nasal mucosa or through the trachea, bronchi, and alveoli. The anti-inflammatory effects of the glucocorticoids depend on the direct local action of the corticosteroid. Glucocorticoids stimulate transcription of messenger RNA in individual cell nuclei to synthesize enzymes that decrease

COMPARING NASAL ADRENOCORTICOIDS

Drug	Half-life (hr)	Indications	Pediatric daily dose	Adult daily dose
beclomethasone	15	Rhinitis Allergic disorders Nasal polyposis	**Nasal aerosol** < age 6: Not recommended Ages 6 to 12: 42 to 50 mcg t.i.d. to q.i.d. Maximum dose: 500 mcg/day **Nasal solution** < age 6: Not recommended Ages 6 to 12: 42 to 100 mcg b.i.d. Maximum dose: 500 mcg/day	**Nasal aerosol** 42 to 50 mcg b.i.d. to q.i.d. Maximum dose: 1,000 mcg/day **Nasal solution** 42 to 100 mcg b.i.d. Maximum dose: 600 mcg/day
budesonide	2	Rhinitis Allergic disorders	**Nasal powder** < age 6: Not recommended Ages 6 to 12: 200 to 400 mcg/day Maximum dose: 400 mcg/day **Nasal solution** < age 6: Not recommended Ages 6 to 12: 100 to 400 mcg/day Maximum dose: 400 mcg/day	**Nasal powder** 200 to 400 mcg/day Maximum dose: 800 mcg/day **Nasal solution** 100 to 400 mcg/day Maximum dose: 800 mcg/day
dexamethasone	3.2	Rhinitis Allergic disorders	**Nasal aerosol** < age 6: Not recommended Ages 6 to 12: 100 to 200 mcg b.i.d. Maximum dose: 800 mcg/day	**Nasal aerosol** 100 to 200 mcg b.i.d. to t.i.d. Maximum dose: 1,200 mcg/day
flunisolide	1 to 2	Rhinitis Allergic disorders	**Nasal solution** < age 6: Not recommended Ages 6 to 14: 25 to 50 mcg b.i.d. Maximum dose: 200 mcg/day	**Nasal solution** 25 to 50 mcg b.i.d. to t.i.d. Maximum dose: 400 mcg/day
triamcinolone	1 to 7	Rhinitis Allergic disorders	**Nasal aerosol** < age 12: Not recommended > age 12: 110 mcg once daily Maximum dose: 440 mcg/day	**Nasal aerosol** 110 mcg once daily Maximum dose: 440 mcg/day

flammation. These enzymes stimulate biochemical pathways that decrease the inflammatory response by stabilizing leukocyte lysosomal membranes, which prevent the release of destructive acid hydrolases from leukocytes; inhibiting macrophage accumulation in inflamed areas; reducing leukocyte adhesion to the capillary endothelium; reducing capillary wall permeability and edema formation; decreasing complement components; antagonizing histamine activity and release of kinin from substrates; reducing fibroblast proliferation, collagen deposition, and scar tissue formation; and by other unknown mechanisms. (See *Comparing nasal adrenocorticoids* and *Comparing oral inhalation adrenocorticoids*.)

Clinical indications and actions
Nasal inflammation
Nasal solutions are used to relieve symptoms of seasonal or perennial rhinitis when antihistamines and decongestants are ineffective; to treat in-flammatory conditions of the nasal passages; and to prevent recurrence after surgical removal of nasal polyps.
Chronic bronchial asthma
Aerosols treat chronic bronchial asthma not controlled by bronchodilators and other nonsteroidal drugs.

Overview of adverse reactions
Local sensations of nasal burning and irritation (in about 10% of patients), sneezing attacks immediately after the nasal application (in about 10% of patients), and transient mild nosebleeds (in 10% to 15% of patients) have occurred. It's unknown if these reactions are an effect of the nasal solution or of the dryness it induces in the nasal passages. Localized candidal infections of the nose or pharynx have occurred rarely.

Localized infections with *Candida albicans* or *Aspergillus niger* have occurred commonly in the

COMPARING ORAL INHALATION ADRENOCORTICOIDS

Drug	Half-life (hr)	Indications	Pediatric daily dose	Adult daily dose
beclomethasone	15	Chronic bronchial asthma	**Inhalation aerosol** < age 6: Not recommended Ages 6 to 12: 84 to 100 mcg t.i.d. to q.i.d. or 168 mcg b.i.d. Maximum dose: 840 to 1,000 mcg/day **Inhalation capsules** < age 6: Not recommended Ages 6 to 14: 100 mcg b.i.d. or q.i.d. Maximum dose: 500 mcg/day **Inhalation powder** < age 6: Not recommended Ages 6 to 14: 100 mcg b.i.d. or q.i.d. Maximum dose: 500 mcg/day	**Inhalation aerosol** 84 to 100 mcg t.i.d. to q.i.d. or 168 to 200 mcg b.i.d. Maximum dose: 1,000 mcg/day **Inhalation capsules** 200 mcg t.i.d. or q.i.d. **Inhalation powder** Not recommended
budesonide	2	Chronic bronchial asthma	**Inhalation powder** < age 6: Not recommended Ages 6 to 12: 200 to 400 mcg b.i.d. Maximum dose: 800 mcg/day **Inhalation suspension** < age 3 months: Not recommended Ages 3 months to 12 years: 25 mcg to 1 mg b.i.d. Maximum dose: Not specified	**Inhalation powder** 200 to 400 mcg b.i.d. Maximum dose: 1,600 mcg/day **Inhalation suspension** 1 to 2 mg b.i.d. Maximum dose: Not specified
dexamethasone	3.2	Not recommended because of frequent adverse effects		
flunisolide	1 to 2	Chronic bronchial asthma	**Inhalation aerosol** < age 4: Not recommended > age 4: 500 mcg b.i.d. Maximum dose: 2 mg/day	**Inhalation aerosol** 500 mcg b.i.d. Maximum dose: 2 mg/day
triamcinolone	1 to 7	Chronic bronchial asthma	**Inhalation aerosol** < age 6: Not recommended Ages 6 to 12: 100 to 200 mcg t.i.d. or q.i.d. Maximum dose: 1.2 mg/day	**Inhalation aerosol** 200 mcg t.i.d. or q.i.d. Maximum dose: Not specified

mouth and pharynx and occasionally in the larynx.

Systemic absorption may occur, potentially leading to hypothalamic-pituitary-adrenal (HPA) axis suppression. This is more likely with large doses or with combined nasal and oral corticosteroid therapy.

Hypersensitivity reactions are possible. Also, some patients may be intolerant of the fluorocarbon propellants in the preparations.

☑ Special considerations
• Full therapeutic benefit requires regular use and is usually evident within a few days, although a few patients may need up to 3 weeks of therapy for maximum benefit. Therapy should be stopped in the absence of significant symptomatic improvement within recommended time frame (varies per drug used).
• Use of nasal or oral inhalation therapy may allow a patient to stop systemic corticosteroid therapy.
• After the desired clinical effect is obtained, maintenance dose should be reduced to the smallest amount necessary to control symptoms.
• Drug should be stopped if patient develops signs of systemic absorption (including Cushing's syndrome, hyperglycemia, or glycosuria), muco-

sal irritation or ulceration, hypersensitivity, or infection. (If antifungals or antibiotics are being used with corticosteroids and the infection doesn't respond immediately, stop corticosteroids until the infection is controlled.)

Information for the patient
Nasal therapy
- Instruct patient to use only as directed. Inform him that full therapeutic effect isn't immediate but requires regular use of inhaler.
- Encourage patient with blocked nasal passages to use an oral decongestant 30 minutes before intranasal corticosteroid to ensure adequate penetration. Advise patient to clear nasal passages of secretions before using inhaler.
- Instruct patient to shake inhaler before use as directed.
- Instruct patient to clean inhaler according to manufacturer's instructions.

Oral therapy
- Instruct patient to use only as directed.
- Advise patient receiving bronchodilators by inhalation to use the bronchodilator before the corticosteroid to enhance penetration of the corticosteroid into the bronchial tree. He should wait several minutes to allow time for the bronchodilator to relax the smooth muscle.
- Instruct patient to shake inhaler before use as directed.
- Instruct patient to hold breath for a few seconds to enhance placement and action of drug and to wait 1 minute before taking subsequent puffs.
- Tell patient to rinse mouth with water after using the inhaler to decrease the chance of oral fungal infections. Tell him to check nasal and oral mucous membranes frequently for signs of fungal infection.
- Instruct patient to clean inhaler properly.
- Warn asthmatic patient not to increase use of corticosteroid inhaler during a severe asthma attack, but to call for adjustment of therapy, possibly by adding a systemic corticosteroid.
- Inform patient that drug is for preventative therapy, not to abort an acute attack.

Either nasal or oral therapy
- Tell patient to report decreased response; adjusting dosage or stopping drug may be needed.
- Instruct patient to observe for adverse effects, and if fever or local irritation develops, to stop drug and report the effect promptly.

Geriatric patients
- Many elderly patients have conditions that could be aggravated by excessive use of corticosteroid inhalant therapy. Elderly patients have a reduced ability to metabolize and eliminate drugs; monitor these patients closely for adverse effects.

Pediatric patients
- In children, nasal or oral inhalant corticosteroid therapy may be successfully substituted for systemic corticosteroid therapy. However, the risk of HPA axis suppression and Cushing's syndrome still exists.

Pregnant patients
- Corticosteroids shouldn't be used in pregnant women, especially in large doses or for long periods of time. They should be used only when potential benefits outweigh potential risks.

Breast-feeding patients
- It's unknown if corticosteroids appear in breast milk. They may cause growth suppression in infants. Use with caution in breast-feeding women.

Representative combinations
None.

adrenocorticoids (systemic)

Glucocorticoids: **betamethasone, betamethasone sodium phosphate, betamethasone sodium phosphate and betamethasone acetate, cortisone acetate, dexamethasone, dexamethasone acetate, dexamethasone sodium phosphate, hydrocortisone, hydrocortisone acetate, hydrocortisone cypionate, hydrocortisone sodium phosphate, hydrocortisone sodium succinate, methylprednisolone, methylprednisolone acetate, methylprednisolone sodium succinate, prednisolone, prednisolone acetate, prednisolone sodium phosphate, prednisolone tebutate, prednisone, triamcinolone, triamcinolone acetonide, triamcinolone diacetate, triamcinolone hexacetonide**

Mineralocorticoid: **fludrocortisone acetate**

Active adrenocortical extracts were first prepared in 1930; by 1942, chemists had isolated 28 steroids from the adrenal cortex.

The adrenocortical hormones are classified according to their activity into two groups: the glucocorticoids and the mineralocorticoids. The glucocorticoids regulate carbohydrate, lipid, and protein metabolism; inflammation; and the body's immune responses to diverse stimuli. The mineralocorticoids regulate electrolyte homeostasis. Many corticosteroids exert both kinds of activity.

(See *Comparing systemic adrenocorticoids,* pages 1142 and 1143.)

Pharmacology

Corticosteroids dramatically affect almost all body systems. They are thought to act by controlling the rate of protein synthesis; they react with receptor proteins in the cytoplasm of sensitive cells to form a steroid-receptor complex. Steroid receptors have been identified in many tissues. The steroid-receptor complex migrates into the nucleus of the cell, where it binds to chromatin. Information carried by the steroid of the receptor protein directs the genetic apparatus to transcribe RNA, resulting in the synthesis of specific proteins that serve as enzymes in various biochemical pathways. Because the maximum pharmacologic activity lags behind peak blood levels, the effects of corticosteroids may result from modification of enzyme activity rather than from direct action by the drugs.

Glucocorticoids stimulate transcription of messenger RNA in individual cell nuclei to synthesize enzymes that decrease inflammation. These enzymes stimulate biochemical pathways that decrease the inflammatory response by stabilizing leukocyte lysosomal membranes, which prevent the release of destructive acid hydrolases from leukocytes; inhibiting macrophage accumulation in inflamed areas; reducing leukocyte adhesion to the capillary endothelium; reducing capillary wall permeability and edema formation; decreasing complement components; antagonizing histamine activity and release of kinin from substrates; reducing fibroblast proliferation, collagen deposition, and scar tissue formation; and by other unknown mechanisms.

Mineralocorticoids act renally at the distal tubules to enhance the reabsorption of sodium ions (and thus water) from the tubular fluid into the plasma, and the urinary excretion of both potassium and hydrogen ions. The primary features of excess mineralocorticoid activity are positive sodium balance and expansion of the extracellular fluid volume; normal or slight increase in the level of sodium in the plasma; hypokalemia; and alkalosis. In contrast, deficiency of mineralocorticoids produces sodium loss, hyponatremia, hyperkalemia, contraction of the extracellular fluid volume, and cellular dehydration.

Clinical indications and actions
Inflammation

A major pharmacologic use of glucocorticoids is treatment of inflammation. The anti-inflammatory effects depend on the direct local action of the corticosteroids. Glucocorticoids decrease the inflammatory response by stabilizing leukocyte lysosomal membranes, which prevent the release of destructive acid hydrolases from leukocytes;

inhibiting macrophage accumulation in inflamed areas; reducing leukocyte adhesion to the capillary endothelium; reducing capillary wall permeability and edema formation; decreasing complement components; antagonizing histamine activity and release of kinin from substrates; reducing fibroblast proliferation, collagen deposition, and subsequent scar tissue formation; and by other unknown mechanisms.

Immunosuppression

Exact mechanisms of action are unknown. Glucocorticoids reduce activity and volume of the lymphatic system, producing lymphocytopenia, decreasing immunoglobulin and complement levels, decreasing passage of immune complexes through basement membranes, and possibly depressing reactivity of tissue to antigen-antibody interaction.

Adrenal insufficiency

Combined mineralocorticoid and glucocorticoid therapy is used in treating adrenal insufficiency and in salt-losing forms of congenital adrenogenital syndrome.

Rheumatic and collagen diseases; other severe diseases

Glucocorticoids are used to treat rheumatic and collagen diseases (arthritis, polyarteritis nodosa, systemic lupus erythematosus); thyroiditis; severe dermatologic diseases, such as pemphigus, exfoliative dermatitis, lichen planus, and psoriasis; allergic reactions; ocular disorders (such as inflammations); respiratory diseases (asthma, sarcoidosis, lipid pneumonitis); hematologic diseases (autoimmune hemolytic anemia, idiopathic thrombocytopenia); neoplastic diseases (leukemias, lymphomas); and GI diseases (ulcerative colitis, regional enteritis, celiac disease). They also can be used in the treatment of myasthenia gravis, organ transplants, nephrotic syndrome, and septic shock.

Antenatal use in preterm labor

Dexamethasone and betamethasone have been used as short-course I.M. therapy in women with preterm labor to hasten fetal maturation of lungs and cerebral blood vessels.

Hypercalcemia

Glucocorticoids are used to treat hypercalcemia secondary to sarcoidosis, vitamin D intoxication, multiple myeloma, and breast cancer in postmenopausal women.

Cerebral edema

High-dose parenteral glucocorticoid administration may decrease cerebral edema in brain tumors and neurosurgery.

◊ Acute spinal cord injury

Large I.V. doses of glucocorticoids, when given shortly after injury, may improve motor and sensory function in patients with acute spinal cord injury.

COMPARING SYSTEMIC ADRENOCORTICOIDS

Drug	Glucocorticoid dose (mg)	Glucocorticoid activity	Mineralocorticoid activity	Plasma half-life (hr)	Biological half-life (hr)
betamethasone, oral	0.6	20 to 30	0	3 to 5	36 to 54
betamethasone acetate	0.6	20 to 30	0	3 to 5	36 to 54
betamethasone sodium phosphate	0.6	20 to 30	0	3 to 5	36 to 54
cortisone acetate	25	0.8	2	0.5	8 to 12
dexamethasone, oral	0.5 to 0.75	20 to 30	0	3 to 4.5	36 to 54
dexamethasone acetate	0.5 to 0.75	20 to 30	0	3 to 4.5	36 to 54
dexamethasone sodium phosphate	0.5 to 0.75	20 to 30	0	3 to 4.5	36 to 54
hydrocortisone, oral	20	1	2	1.5 to 2	8 to 12
hydrocortisone acetate	20	1	2	1.5 to 2	8 to 12
hydrocortisone cypionate	20	1	2	1.5 to 2	8 to 12
hydrocortisone sodium phosphate	20	1	2	1.5 to 2	8 to 12
hydrocortisone sodium succinate	20	1	2	1.5 to 2	8 to 12
methyl prednisolone, oral	4	5	0	> 3.5	18 to 36
methyl prednisolone acetate	4	5	0	> 3.5	18 to 36
methylprednisolone sodium succinate	4	5	0	> 3.5	18 to 36
prednisolone, oral	5	4	0	2.1 to 3.5	18 to 36
prednisolone acetate	5	4	0	2.1 to 3.5	18 to 36
prednisolone sodium phosphate	5	4	0	2.1 to 3.5	18 to 36
prednisolone tebutate	5	4	1	2.1 to 3.5	18 to 36
prednisone	5	4	1	3.4 to 3.8	18 to 36
triamcinolone, oral	4	5	1	2 to > 5	18 to 36
triamcinolone acetonide	4	5	1	2 to > 5	18 to 36
triamcinolone diacetate	4	5	1	2 to > 5	18 to 36
triamcinolone hexacetonide	4	5	0	2 to > 5	18 to 36

Onset of action	Peak	Duration
Unknown	1 to 2 hr	3.25 days
1 to 3 hours	Unknown	Unknown
Rapid	Unknown	1 to 2 wk
Rapid (P.O.); slow (I.M.)	2 hr (P.O.) 20 to 48 hr (I.M.)	1.25 to 1.5 days
Unknown	1 to 2 hr	2.75 days
Unknown	8 hr	1 to 3 wk
Rapid	Unknown	3 days to 3 wk
Unknown	1 hr	1.25 to 1.5 days
Unknown	24 to 48 hr	3 days to 4 wk
Unknown	1 to 2 hr	Unknown
Rapid	1 hr	Unknown
Rapid	1 hr	Variable
Unknown	1 to 2 hr	1.25 to 1.5 days
Slow	4 to 8 days	1 to 5 wk
Rapid	Unknown	Unknown
Unknown	1 to 2 hr	1.25 to 1.5 days
Slow	Unknown	3 days to 4 wk
Rapid	1 hr	3 days to 3 wk
Slow	Unknown	1 to 3 wk
Unknown	1 to 2 hr	Unknown
Unknown	1 to 2 hr	2.25 days
Slow	Unknown	1 to 6 wk
Slow	1 to 2 hr	1 to 8 wk
Unknown	Unknown	3 to 4 wk

Overview of adverse reactions

Suppression of the hypothalamic-pituitary-adrenal (HPA) axis is the major effect of systemic therapy with corticosteroids. When administered in high doses or for prolonged therapy, the glucocorticoids suppress release of corticotropin from the pituitary gland; subsequently, the adrenal cortex stops secreting endogenous corticosteroids. The degree and duration of HPA axis suppression produced by the drugs are highly variable among patients and depend on the dose, frequency and time of administration, and duration of therapy.

Patients with a suppressed HPA axis resulting from exogenous glucocorticoid administration who abruptly stop therapy may experience severe withdrawal symptoms, such as fever, myalgia, arthralgia, malaise, anorexia, nausea, desquamation of skin, orthostatic hypotension, dizziness, fainting, dyspnea, and hypoglycemia. Therefore, corticosteroid therapy should always be withdrawn gradually.

Adrenal suppression may last for as long as 12 months in patients who have received large doses for prolonged periods. Until complete recovery occurs, patients subjected to stress may show signs and symptoms of adrenal insufficiency and may need glucocorticoid and mineralocorticoid replacement therapy.

Cushingoid symptoms, the effects of excessive glucocorticoid therapy, may develop in patients receiving large doses of glucocorticoids over several weeks or longer. These include moon face, central obesity, striae, hirsutism, acne, ecchymoses, hypertension, osteoporosis, muscle atrophy, sexual dysfunction, diabetes, cataracts, hyperlipidemia, peptic ulcer, increased susceptibility to infection, and fluid and electrolyte imbalances.

Other adverse reactions to normal or high doses of corticosteroids may include CNS effects (euphoria, insomnia, psychotic behavior, pseudotumor cerebri, mental changes, nervousness, restlessness), CV effects (heart failure, hypertension, edema), GI effects (peptic ulcer, irritation, increased appetite), metabolic effects (hypokalemia, sodium retention, fluid retention, weight gain, hyperglycemia, osteoporosis), dermatologic effects (delayed wound healing, acne, skin eruptions, striae), and immunosuppression (increased susceptibility to infection).

☑ Special considerations

• Patient may experience sudden weight gain, edema, change in blood pressure, or change in electrolyte status.
• During times of physiologic stress (trauma, surgery, infection), patient may need additional corticosteroids and may experience signs of corticosteroid withdrawal; patients who were previously corticosteroid-dependent may need s▿

---

temic corticosteroids to prevent adrenal insufficiency.
• Reduce drug gradually in long-term therapy. Rapid reduction may cause withdrawal symptoms.
• Know patient's psychological history and watch for behavioral changes.
• Patient should be observed for infection or delayed wound healing.

Information for the patient
• Tell patient to take the adrenocorticoid as prescribed. Give him instructions on what to do if a dose is missed.
• Warn patient not to stop drug abruptly.
• Inform patient of drug's therapeutic and adverse effects; tell him to report complications immediately.
• Tell patient to carry medical identification noting need for more adrenocorticoids during stress.

Geriatric patients
• Many elderly patients have conditions that could easily be aggravated by corticosteroid therapy. Elderly patients have a reduced ability to metabolize and eliminate drugs; monitor these patients closely.

Pediatric patients
• Long-term administration of glucocorticoids in children may retard bone growth. Signs and symptoms of adrenal suppression in children include retardation of linear growth, delayed weight gain, low plasma cortisol levels, and lack of response to corticotropin stimulation. Alternate-day therapy is recommended to minimize growth suppression.

Pregnant patients
• Glucocorticoids may cause fetal abnormalities if given to pregnant women. Avoid use if possible.

Breast-feeding patients
• Women who are taking corticosteroids shouldn't breast-feed.

Representative combinations
Betamethasone sodium phosphate with betamethasone acetate: Celestone Soluspan.
   Dexamethasone sodium phosphate with lidocaine hydrochloride: Decadron with Xylocaine.

adrenocorticoids (topical)

alclometasone dipropionate, amcinonide, betamethasone benzoate, betamethasone dipropionate, betamethasone valerate, clobetasol propionate, clocortolone pivalate, desonide, desoximetasone, dexamethasone, dexamethasone sodium phosphate, diflorasone diacetate, fluocinolone acetonide, fluocinonide, flurandrenolide, fluticasone propionate, halcinonide, halobetasol propionate, hydrocortisone, hydrocortisone acetate, hydrocortisone butyrate, hydrocortisone valerate, methylprednisolone acetate, triamcinolone acetonide

Since topical hydrocortisone was introduced in the 1950s, numerous analogues have been developed to provide a wide range of potencies in creams, ointments, lotions, and gels.

Pharmacology
The anti-inflammatory effects of topical glucocorticoids depend on the direct local action of the corticosteroid. Although the exact mechanism of action is unknown, many researchers believe that glucocorticoids stimulate transcription of messenger RNA in individual cell nuclei to synthesize enzymes that decrease inflammation. These enzymes stimulate biochemical pathways that decrease the inflammatory response by stabilizing leukocyte lysosomal membranes, which prevents the release of destructive acid hydrolases from leukocytes; inhibiting macrophage accumulation in inflamed areas; reducing leukocyte adhesion to the capillary endothelium; reducing capillary wall permeability and edema formation; decreasing complement components; antagonizing histamine activity and release of kinin from substrates; reducing fibroblast proliferation, collagen deposition, and subsequent scar tissue formation; and by other unknown mechanisms.

Topical corticosteroids are minimally absorbed systemically and cause fewer adverse effects than systemically administered corticosteroids. Fluorinated derivatives are absorbed to a greater extent than other topical corticosteroids. The degree of absorption depends on the site of application, the amount applied, the relative potency, the presence of an occlusive dressing (may increase penetration by 10%), the condition of the skin, and the vehicle carrying the drug. Topical corticosteroids are used to relieve pruritus, inflammation, and other signs of corticosteroid-responsive dermatoses.

COMPARATIVE POTENCY OF TOPICAL CORTICOSTEROIDS

Topical corticosteroid preparations can be grouped according to relative anti-inflammatory activity. The following list arranges groups of topical corticosteroids in decreasing order of potency (based mainly on vaso-constrictor assay or clinical effectiveness in psoriasis). Preparations within each group are approximately equivalent.

Group	Drug	Concentration (%)
I	betamethasone dipropionate (Diprolene)	0.05
	betamethasone dipropionate (Diprolene AF)	0.05
	clobetasol propionate (Temovate)	0.05
	diflorasone diacetate (Psorcon)	0.05
II	amcinonide (Cyclocort)	0.1
	betamethasone dipropionate ointment (Diprosone)	0.05
	desoximetasone (Topicort)	0.05, 0.25
	diflorasone diacetate (Florone, Maxiflor)	0.05
	fluocinonide (Lidex)	0.05
	fluocinonide gel	0.05
	halcinonide (Halog)	0.1
III	betamethasone benzoate gel	0.025
	betamethasone dipropionate cream (Diprosone)	0.05
	betamethasone valerate ointment (Valisone)	0.1
	diflorasone diacetate cream (Florone, Maxiflor)	0.05
	triamcinolone acetonide cream (Aristocort)	0.5
IV	desoximetasone (Topicort LP)	0.05
	fluocinolone acetonide (Synalar-HP)	0.2
	fluocinolone acetonide ointment (Synalar)	0.025
	flurandrenolide (Cordran)	0.05
	fluticasone propionate (Cutivate)	0.005, 0.05
	triamcinolone acetonide ointment (Aristocort, Kenalog)	0.1
V	betamethasone benzoate cream	0.025
	betamethasone dipropionate lotion (Diprosone)	0.05
	betamethasone valerate cream or lotion (Valisone)	0.1
	fluocinolone acetonide cream (Synalar)	0.025
	flurandrenolide (Cordran)	0.05
	hydrocortisone butyrate (Locoid)	0.1
	hydrocortisone valerate (Westcort)	0.2
	triamcinolone acetonide cream or lotion (Kenalog)	0.1
VI	alclometasone dipropionate (Aclovate)	0.05
	desonide (Tridesilon)	0.05
	fluocinolone acetonide solution (Synalar)	0.01

Ointments are preferred for dry, scaly areas; solutions, gels, aerosols, and lotions for hairy areas. Creams can be used for most areas except those in which dampness may cause maceration. Gels and lotions can be used for moist lesions; however, gels may contain alcohol, which can dry and irritate the skin. The topical preparations are classified by potency into six groups: group I is the most potent, group VI the least potent. (See *Comparative potency of topical corticosteroids*.)

Clinical indications and actions

The topical adrenocorticoids relieve inflammatory and pruritic skin disorders, including localized neurodermatitis, psoriasis, atopic or seborrheic dermatitis, the inflammatory phase of xerosis, anogenital pruritus, discoid lupus erythemato-sus, lichen planus, granuloma annulare, and lupus erythematosus.

These drugs may also relieve irritant or allergic contact dermatitis; however, relief of acute dermatosis may require systemic adrenocorticoids.

Rectal disorders responsive to this class of drugs include ulcerative colitis, cryptitis, inflamed hemorrhoids, postirradiation or factitial proctitis, and pruritus ani.

Oral lesions, such as nonherpetic oral inflammatory and ulcerative lesions and routine gingivitis, may respond to treatment with topical adrenocorticoids.

OTC formulations of the topical corticosteroids are indicated for minor skin irritation such as itching; rash due to eczema, dermatitis, insect bites, poison ivy, poison oak, or poison sumac; or dermatitis due to exposure to soaps, detergents, cosmetics, and jewelry.

Overview of adverse reactions

Local effects include burning, itching, irritation, dryness, folliculitis, striae, miliaria, acne, perioral dermatitis, hypopigmentation, hypertrichosis, allergic contact dermatitis, secondary infection, and atrophy.

Systemic absorption may occur, leading to hypothalamic-pituitary-adrenal (HPA) axis suppression.

The risk of adverse reactions increases with the use of occlusive dressings or more potent corticosteroids, in patients with liver disease, and in children (because of their greater ratio of skin surface to body weight).

Prolonged application around the eyes may lead to cataracts or glaucoma.

☑ Special considerations

● Wash hands before and after applying drug.
● Gently clean area of application. Washing or soaking area before application may increase drug penetration.
● Apply sparingly in a light film; rub in lightly. Avoid contact with eyes, unless using an ophthalmic product.
● Avoid prolonged application in areas near eyes, genitals, rectum, on the face, and in skin folds. High-potency topical corticosteroids are more likely to cause striae and atrophy in these areas because of their higher rates of absorption.
● Monitor response; observe area of inflammation.
● Don't apply occlusive dressings over topical corticosteroids.
● Stop drug if patient develops signs of systemic absorption.

Information for the patient

● Instruct patient on use of drug.
● Instruct patient to stop drug and report local or systemic adverse reactions, worsening condition, or persistent symptoms.
● Warn patient not to use OTC topical products other than those specifically recommended.
● Tell patient to apply a missed dose as soon as it's remembered, and continue on with regular schedule of application. However, if it's almost time for the next application, tell him to wait and continue with regular schedule. He shouldn't apply a double dose.

Geriatric patients

● In elderly patients, loss of collagen may lead to friable and transparent skin with increased epidermal permeability to water and certain chemicals. In these patients, topically applied drugs such as corticosteroid creams may have a greater effect locally. Elderly patients also have a reduced ability to metabolize and eliminate

drugs and may have higher plasma drug levels and more adverse reactions. Monitor these patients closely.

Pediatric patients

● To minimize risk, limit topical corticosteroid therapy in children to the minimum amount necessary for therapeutic efficacy. Advise parents not to use tight-fitting diapers or plastic pants on a child being treated in the diaper area because such garments may serve as occlusive dressings. Children may be more susceptible to topical corticosteroid-induced HPA-axis suppression and Cushing's syndrome than adults because of a greater skin surface–to–body weight ratio.

Pregnant patients

● It's unknown if topical corticosteroids affect fertility. Safe use during pregnancy hasn't been established.

Breast-feeding patients

● Use with caution in breast-feeding women.

Representative combinations

Betamethasone with clotrimazole: Lotrisone.
Betamethasone dipropionate with clotrimazole: Lotrisone.
Dexamethasone with neomycin sulfate: NeoDecadron Cream; with neomycin sulfate and polymyxin B sulfate: Dexacidin Ointment.
Flurandrenolide with neomycin: Cordran.
Hydrocortisone with iodoquinol: Vytone Cream; with iodochlorhydroxyquin: Vioform-Hydrocortisone Cream, AP, Corque Cream, Hysone; with neomycin: Hydrocortisone-Neomycin; with pramoxine: Pramosone, Zone-A Forte; with neomycin and polymyxin B: Cortisporin Cream; with neomycin, bacitracin, and polymyxin B sulfate: Cortisporin Ointment; with neomycin sulfate and polymyxin B sulfate: Cortisporin; with dibucaine: Corticaine; with pyrilamine maleate, pheniramine maleate, and chlorpheniramine maleate: HC Derma-Pax; with benzoyl peroxide and mineral oil: Vanoxide-HC; with lidocaine and glycerin: Lida-Mantle-HC; with sulfur and salicylic acid: Therac Lotion.
Triamcinolone acetonide with nystatin: Myco II, Myco-Biotic II, Mycogen II, Mycolog-II, Myco-Triacet II, Mykacet, Mytrex, Nystatin-Triamcinolone Acetonide, N.G.T.; with neomycin, gramicidin, and nystatin: Myco-Triacet II, Tri-Statin II.

alpha blockers

carvedilol, dihydroergotamine mesylate, doxazosin mesylate, ergotamine tartrate, phentolamine mesylate, prazosin hydrochloride, tamsulosin hydrochloride, terazosin hydrochloride, tolazoline hydrochloride

Drugs that block the effects of peripheral neurohormonal transmitters (norepinephrine, epinephrine, and related sympathomimetic amines) on adrenergic receptors in various effector systems are designated as adrenergic blockers. Just as adrenoreceptors are classified into two subtypes—alpha and beta—so too are the blocking drugs. Essentially, those drugs that antagonize mydriasis, vasoconstriction, nonvascular smooth-muscle excitation, and other adrenergic responses caused by alpha receptor stimulation are termed alpha blockers.

Pharmacology
Nonselective alpha antagonists
Ergotamine, phentolamine, and tolazoline antagonize both alpha$_1$ and alpha$_2$ receptors. Generally, alpha blockade results in tachycardia, palpitations, and increased secretion of renin due to the abnormally large amounts of norepinephrine (transmitter "overflow") released from adrenergic nerve endings as a result of the concurrent blockade of alpha$_1$ and alpha$_2$ receptors. The effects of norepinephrine are clinically counterproductive to the major uses of nonselective alpha blockers, which include treating peripheral vascular disorders such as Raynaud's disease, acrocyanosis, frostbite, acute atrial occlusion, phlebitis, phlebothrombosis, diabetic gangrene, shock, and pheochromocytoma.
Selective alpha antagonists
Alpha$_1$ blockers have readily observable effects and are currently the only alpha-adrenergic drugs with known clinical uses. They decrease vascular resistance and increase venous capacitance, thereby lowering blood pressure and causing pink warm skin, nasal and scleroconjunctival congestion, ptosis, orthostatic and exercise hypotension, mild to moderate miosis, and interference with ejaculation. They also relax nonvascular smooth muscle, notably in the prostate capsule, thereby reducing urinary symptoms in men with benign prostatic hyperplasia (BPH). Because alpha$_1$ blockers don't block alpha$_2$ receptors, they don't cause transmitter overflow. In theory, alpha$_1$ blockers should be useful in the same conditions as nonselective alpha blockers; however, doxazosin, prazosin, and terazosin are approved for treating hypertension. Terazosin and doxazosin are approved in treatment of prostatic outflow obstruction secondary to BPH.

Alpha$_2$ blockers produce more subtle physiologic effects and currently have no therapeutic applications. Yohimbine is one such drug.

Clinical indications and actions
Peripheral vascular disorders
Alpha blockers are indicated for treating peripheral vascular disorders, including Raynaud's disease, acrocyanosis, frostbite, acute atrial occlusion, phlebitis, and diabetic gangrene. Dihydroergotamine and ergotamine have been used to treat vascular headaches. Prazosin has been used to treat Raynaud's disease. Phentolamine is indicated to treat dermal necrosis caused by extravasation of norepinephrine, dopamine, or phenylephrine (alpha agonists).
Hypertension
Tolazoline is used to treat persistent pulmonary hypertension in neonates. Prazosin, carvedilol, doxazosin, and terazosin are used in managing essential hypertension. Phentolamine is used to control hypertension and is a useful adjunct in surgical treatment of pheochromocytoma.
BPH
Terazosin, tamsulosin, and doxazosin are used to control mild to moderate urinary obstructive symptoms in men with BPH.

Overview of adverse reactions
Nonselective alpha antagonists typically cause orthostatic hypotension, tachycardia, palpitations, fluid retention (from excess renin secretion), nasal and ocular congestion, and aggravation of the signs and symptoms of respiratory infection. These drugs are contraindicated in patients with severe cerebral and coronary atherosclerosis and in those with renal insufficiency.

Selective alpha antagonists may cause severe orthostatic hypotension and syncope, especially with the first dose; most common adverse effects of alpha$_1$ blockade are dizziness, headache, and malaise.

☑ Special considerations
- Monitor vital signs, especially blood pressure.
- Administer dose at bedtime to reduce potential for dizziness or light-headedness.
- To avoid first-dose syncope, begin with small dose.

Information for the patient
- Warn patient about orthostatic hypotension. Tell him to avoid sudden changes to upright position.
- Advise patient to sit in bed, and then dangle legs at bedside for a full minute, before attempting to stand upright.
- Tell patient to promptly report dizziness or irregular heartbeat.
- Advise patient to take dose at bedtime to reduce potential for dizziness or light-headedness

• Warn patient to avoid driving and other hazardous tasks that require mental alertness until effects of drug are known.
• Reassure patient that adverse effects, including dizziness, should lessen after several doses.
• Tell patient that alcohol use, excessive exercise, prolonged standing, and exposure to heat will intensify adverse effects.
• Advise patient of the reason for taking drug (hypertension versus BPH).

Geriatric patients
• Hypotensive effects may be more pronounced in elderly patients.

Pediatric patients
• Safety and efficacy of many of these drugs haven't been established in children. Refer to specific drug monographs for more information.

Pregnant patients
• Avoid use in pregnancy.

Breast-feeding patients
• Women who are taking these drugs shouldn't breast-feed.

Representative combinations
None.

aminoglycosides

amikacin sulfate, gentamicin sulfate, kanamycin sulfate, neomycin sulfate, netilmicin sulfate, streptomycin sulfate, tobramycin sulfate

Aminoglycoside antibiotics were discovered during the search for drugs to treat serious penicillin-resistant, gram-negative infections. Streptomycin, derived from soil actinomycetes, was the first therapeutically useful aminoglycoside. Bacterial resistance to this prototype and adverse reactions soon led to the development of kanamycin, gentamicin, neomycin, netilmicin, tobramycin, and amikacin.

The basic structure of aminoglycosides is an aminocyclitol nucleus joined with one to two amino sugars by glycosidic linkage, hence the name aminoglycosides.

Aminoglycosides share certain pharmacokinetic properties, such as poor oral absorption, poor CNS penetration, and renal excretion as well as serious adverse reactions and toxicity. Clinical use may require close monitoring of serum levels.

Pharmacology
Aminoglycosides are bactericidal. Although the exact mechanism of action is unknown, the drugs appear to bind directly and irreversibly to 30S ribosomal subunits, inhibiting bacterial protein synthesis. Bacterial resistance to aminoglycosides may be from decreased bacterial cell-wall permeability, low affinity of the drug for ribosomal binding sites, or enzymatic degradation by microbial enzymes.

Aminoglycosides are active against many aerobic gram-negative organisms and some aerobic gram-positive organisms; they don't kill fungi, viruses, or anaerobic bacteria.

Gram-negative organisms susceptible to aminoglycosides include *Acinetobacter, Citrobacter, Enterobacter, Escherichia coli, Klebsiella,* indole-positive and indole-negative *Proteus, Providencia, Pseudomonas aeruginosa, Salmonella, Serratia,* and *Shigella.* Streptomycin is active against *Brucella, Calymmatobacterium granulomatis, Francisella tularensis, Haemophilus influenzae, H. ducreyi, Pasteurella multocida,* and *Yersinia pestis.*

Susceptible aerobic gram-positive organisms include *Staphylococcus aureus* and *S. epidermidis.* Streptomycin is active against *Nocardia, Erysipelothrix, Enterococcus faecalis,* and some mycobacteria, including *Mycobacterium tuberculosis, M. marinum,* and certain strains of *M. kansasii* and *M. leprae.*

Paromomycin is active against protozoa, especially *Entamoeba histolytica* and is somewhat effective against *Taenia saginata, Hymenolepsis nana, Diphyllobothrium latum,* and *Taenia solium.* Neomycin and paromomycin have some activity against *Acanthamoeba.*

Aminoglycosides aren't systemically absorbed after oral administration to patients with intact GI mucosa and, with few exceptions, are used parenterally for systemic infections; intraventricular or intrathecal administration is necessary for CNS infections. Kanamycin and neomycin are given orally for bowel sterilization.

Aminoglycosides are distributed widely throughout the body after parenteral administration; CSF levels are minimal even in patients with inflamed meninges. Over time, aminoglycosides accumulate in body tissue, especially the kidney and inner ear, causing drug saturation. The drug is released slowly from these tissues. Most aminoglycosides are minimally protein-bound and aren't metabolized. They don't penetrate abscesses well.

Aminoglycosides are excreted primarily in urine, chiefly by glomerular filtration; neomycin is chiefly excreted unchanged in feces when taken orally. Elimination half-life ranges between 2 and 4 hours and is prolonged in patients with decreased renal function. (See *Aminoglycosides: Renal function and half-life.*)

Clinical indications and actions
Aminoglycosides are used for infections caused by susceptible aerobic gram-negative bacilli, in-

AMINOGLYCOSIDES: RENAL FUNCTION AND HALF-LIFE

The aminoglycosides, which are excreted by the kidneys, have significantly prolonged half-lives in patients with end-stage renal disease. Knowing this can help you assess the patient's potential for drug accumulation and toxicity. Nephrotoxicity, a major hazard of therapy with aminoglycosides, is clearly linked to serum concentrations that exceed the therapeutic concentrations listed in the table below. Therefore, monitoring peak and trough levels is essential for safe use of these drugs.

Drug and administration	Half-life Normal renal function	Half-life End-stage renal disease	Therapeutic concentrations (mcg/ml) Peak	Therapeutic concentrations (mcg/ml) Trough
amikacin I.M., I.V.	2 to 3 hr	24 to 60 hr	16 to 32	< 10
gentamicin I.M., I.V., topical	2 hr	24 to 60 hr	4 to 8	< 2
kanamycin I.M., I.V., topical	2 to 3 hr	24 to 60 hr	15 to 40	< 10
neomycin oral, topical	2 to 3 hr	12 to 24 hr	Not applicable	Not applicable
netilmicin I.M., I.V.	2 to 2.7 hr	< 10 hr	6 to 10	< 2
streptomycin I.M., I.V.	2.5 hr	100 hr	20 to 30	Not applicable
tobramycin I.M., I.V., topical	2 to 2.5 hr	24 to 60 hr	4 to 8	< 2

cluding septicemia; postoperative, pulmonary, intra-abdominal, and serious, recurrent urinary tract infections; and infections of skin, soft tissue, bones, and joints. They also can be used (unlabeled) for infections from aerobic gram-negative bacillary meningitis (not susceptible to other antibiotics); because of poor CNS penetration, drugs are given intrathecally or intraventricularly (in ventriculitis).

Oral kanamycin is used orally and neomycin is used orally or as a retention enema as an adjunct therapy to inhibit ammonia-forming bacteria in the GI tract of patients with hepatic encephalopathy.

Gentamicin encapsulated in liposomes is being evaluated for treatment of disseminated *Mycobacterium avium* complex infections.

Tobramycin, in an inhalant form in nebulizer treatments, has been used to treat chronic lung infections.

Aminoglycosides are combined with other antibacterials in many other types of infection, including serious staphylococcal infections (with an antistaphylococcal penicillin); serious *P. aeruginosa* infections (with such drugs as an antipseudomonal penicillin or cephalosporin); enterococcal infections, including endocarditis (with such drugs as penicillin G, ampicillin, or vancomycin); serious *Klebsiella* infections (with a

cephalosporin); nosocomial pneumonia (with a cephalosporin); anaerobic infections involving *Bacteroides fragilis* (with such drugs as clindamycin, metronidazole, cefoxitin, doxycycline, chloramphenicol, or ticarcillin); tuberculosis (parenteral amikacin, kanamycin, or streptomycin with other antituberculotics); and pelvic inflammatory disease (PID) (gentamicin with clindamycin)

Aminoglycosides are also used as initial empiric therapy in febrile, leukopenic compromised host (with an antipseudomonal penicillin or cephalosporin).

Overview of adverse reactions

Systemic reactions: Ototoxicity and nephrotoxicity are the most serious complications of aminoglycoside therapy. Ototoxicity involves both vestibular and auditory functions and usually is related to persistently high serum drug levels. Damage is reversible only if detected early and if drug is stopped promptly.

Any aminoglycoside may cause usually reversible nephrotoxicity. The damage results in tubular necrosis. Mild proteinuria and casts are early signs of declining renal function; elevated serum creatinine levels follow several days after the decline has begun. Nephrotoxicity usually begins on day 4 to 7 of therapy and appears to be dose-related.

Neuromuscular blockade results in skeletal weakness and respiratory distress similar to that seen with the use of neuromuscular blockers like tubocurarine and succinylcholine.

Oral aminoglycoside therapy most often causes nausea, vomiting, and diarrhea. Less common adverse reactions include hypersensitivity reactions (ranging from mild rashes, fever, and eosinophilia to fatal anaphylaxis); hematologic reactions include hemolytic anemia, transient neutropenia, leukopenia, and thrombocytopenia. Transient elevations of liver function values also occur.

Local reactions: Parenterally administered forms of aminoglycosides may cause vein irritation, phlebitis, and sterile abscess.

☑ Special considerations
● Don't give an aminoglycoside to patient with history of hypersensitivity reactions to any aminoglycoside.
● Obtain results of culture and sensitivity tests before giving first dose.
● Monitor vital signs, electrolyte levels, and renal function studies before and during therapy; be sure patient is well hydrated to minimize chemical irritation of renal tubules; watch for signs of declining renal function.
● Peak and trough serum levels should be kept at recommended concentrations, especially in patients with decreased renal function. Draw blood for peak level 1 hour after I.M. injection (30 minutes to 1 hour after I.V. infusion); for trough level, draw sample just before the next dose. Time and date all blood samples. Don't use heparinized tube to collect blood samples; it interferes with results.
● The patient's hearing should be evaluated before and during therapy; monitor patient for tinnitus, vertigo, or hearing loss.
● Avoid using aminoglycosides with other ototoxic or nephrotoxic drugs.
● Usual duration of therapy is 7 to 10 days; if no response occurs in 3 to 5 days, drug should be stopped and cultures repeated for reevaluation of therapy.
● Patients on long-term therapy—especially elderly and debilitated patients and others receiving immunosuppressive or radiation therapy—should be closely monitored for possible bacterial or fungal superinfection; watch especially for fever.
● Oral aminoglycosides may be absorbed systemically in patients with ulcerative GI lesions; significant absorption may endanger patients with decreased renal function.
● Don't add or mix other drugs with I.V. infusions (particularly penicillins, which will inactivate aminoglycosides); the two groups are chemically and physically incompatible. If other drugs must be given I.V., temporarily stop infusion of primary drug.

● Solutions should always be clear, colorless to pale yellow (in most cases, darkening indicates deterioration), and free of particles; don't give solutions containing precipitates or other foreign matter.
● Too-rapid I.V. administration may cause neuromuscular blockade. I.V. drug should be infused continuously or intermittently over 30 to 60 minutes for adults, 1 to 2 hours for infants; dilution volume for children is determined individually.
● Amikacin, gentamicin (without preservatives), kanamycin, and tobramycin have been given intrathecally or intraventricularly. Some clinicians prefer intraventricular administration to ensure adequate CSF levels in treatment of ventriculitis.

Information for the patient
● Tell patient signs and symptoms of hypersensitivity and other adverse reactions to aminoglycosides.
● Teach signs and symptoms of bacterial or fungal superinfection to elderly and debilitated patients and others with low resistance from immunosuppressants or irradiation; emphasize need to report these signs promptly.

Geriatric patients
● Elderly patients usually have decreased renal function and are at greater risk for nephrotoxicity; many need lower drug dosage and longer dosing intervals. These patients are also susceptible to ototoxicity and superinfection.

Pediatric patients
● Half-life of aminoglycosides is prolonged in neonates and premature infants because of immaturity of their renal systems; dosage alterations may be needed in infants and children.

Pregnant patients
● Pregnancy risk category D. Drugs cross the placenta, creating the potential for fetal toxicity; may cause congenital deafness.

Breast-feeding patients
● Recommend an alternative to breast-feeding during therapy. Small amounts of drug appear in breast milk.

Representative combinations
Neomycin with polymyxin B sulfates and bacitracin: Foille Plus, Mycitracin, Neosporin; with polymyxin B sulfates and gramicidin: Neosporin; with polymyxin B sulfates and hydrocortisone: Cortisporin, Drotic, Octicair, Otocort; with dexamethasone sodium phosphate: Neo-Decadron; with flurandrenolide: Cordran SP.
See also *adrenocorticoids (topical)*.

androgens

danazol, fluoxymesterone, methyl-testosterone, testosterone, testosterone cypionate, testosterone enanthate, testosterone propionate, testosterone transdermal system

Testosterone is the endogenous androgen (male sex hormone). The testosterone esters (cypionate, enanthate, propionate), methyltestosterone, and fluoxymesterone are synthetic derivatives with greater potency or longer duration of action than testosterone.

Pharmacology

Testosterone promotes maturation of the male sexual organs and the development of secondary sexual characteristics (facial and body hair, vocal cord thickening). Testosterone also causes the growth spurt of adolescence and terminates growth of the long bones by closing the epiphyses (growth plates at the ends of bones). Testosterone promotes retention of calcium, nitrogen, phosphorus, sodium, and potassium and enhances anabolism (tissue building). Through negative feedback on the pituitary, exogenously administered testosterone (and other androgenic drugs) decreases endogenous testosterone production and to some degree inhibits spermatogenesis in men. Androgens repeatedly stimulate production of erythrocytes, apparently by enhancing the production of erythropoietic stimulating factor.

Clinical indications and actions

Androgen deficiency

Androgens (testosterone, all testosterone esters, methyltestosterone, fluoxymesterone) are used to treat androgen deficiency resulting from testicular failure or castration, or gonadotropin or luteinizing hormone–releasing hormone deficiency of pituitary origin. Methyltestosterone and testosterone cypionate are also used to treat male climacteric symptoms and impotence when these are caused by androgen deficiency.

Delayed male puberty

All androgens may be used to stimulate the onset of puberty when it's significantly delayed and psychological support proves insufficient.

Breast cancer

Testosterone, all testosterone esters, and fluoxymesterone are indicated for palliative treatment of metastatic breast cancer in women during the first 5 postmenopausal years. Androgens also may be used in premenopausal women with metastatic disease if the tumor is hormone responsive.

Postpartum breast engorgement

Fluoxymesterone, testosterone, methyltestosterone, and testosterone propionate are used to treat painful postpartum breast engorgement in non-breast-feeding women.

Hereditary angioedema

Danazol is indicated in the prophylaxis of angioedema attacks.

Endometriosis

Danazol is indicated for palliative treatment of endometriosis. Danazol relieves pain and helps resolve endometrial lesions in 30% to 80% of patients who receive it. Endometriosis usually recurs 8 to 12 months after danazol is stopped.

Fibrocystic breast disease

Danazol is indicated for palliative treatment of fibrocystic breast disease unresponsive to simple therapy. It usually relieves pain before it reduces nodularity. Fibrocystic breast disease recurs in about half of patients treated successfully with danazol, usually 1 year after stopping drug.

◊ Danazol has been used for the palliative treatment of virginal breast hypertrophy, gynecomastia, and excessive menstrual blood loss; contraception in men (with testosterone) and women; treatment of alpha$_1$-antitrypsin deficiency, systemic lupus erythematosus, gynecomastia in men, and Melkersson-Rosenthal syndrome; management of patients with hemophilia A (factor VIII deficiency, classic hemophilia), hemophilia B (factor IX deficiency, Christmas disease), and idiopathic thrombocytopenia purpura (ITP).

Overview of adverse reactions

The most common adverse reactions associated with androgen therapy are extensions of the hormonal action. In men, frequent and prolonged erections, bladder irritability (causing frequent urination), and gynecomastia (swelling or tenderness of breast tissue) may occur. In women, clitoral enlargement, deepening of the voice, growth of facial or body hair, unusual hair loss, and irregular or absent menses may occur. Note that virilization, including hirsutism, deepening of the voice, and clitoral enlargement, may be irreversible even when the drug is promptly stopped. Oily skin or acne occurs commonly in both sexes.

Metabolic adverse reactions include retention of fluid and electrolytes (occasionally resulting in edema), increased serum calcium levels (hypercalcemia may occur, especially in women receiving the drug for breast cancer metastatic to bone), decreased blood glucose levels, and increased serum cholesterol levels.

Long-term administration of androgens may cause loss of libido and suppression of spermatogenesis in men. Serious, although rare, hepatic dysfunction, including hepatic necrosis and hepatocellular carcinoma, has been reported in prolonged androgen administration.

☑ Special considerations
• Don't administer androgens to men with breast or prostatic cancer or symptomatic prostatic hypertrophy; to patients with severe cardiac, renal, or hepatic disease; or to patients with undiagnosed abnormal genital bleeding.
• Hypercalcemia symptoms may be difficult to distinguish from symptoms of the condition being treated unless anticipated and thought of as a cluster. Hypercalcemia is most likely to occur in women with breast cancer, particularly when metastatic to bone.
• Priapism in men indicates that dosage is excessive.
• Yellowing of the skin or sclera of the eyes may indicate hepatic dysfunction resulting from administration of androgens.

Information for the patient
• Warn patient against using androgens to improve athletic performance. Androgens are now classified as Schedule III controlled substances and their distribution is regulated by the Drug Enforcement Agency.
• Tell patient to report GI upset.
• Tell woman that virilization, including hirsutism, deepening of voice, and clitoral enlargement, may not be reversible.
• Explain to woman that drug may cause menstrual cycle irregularities (if she is premenopausal) or withdrawal bleeding (if she is postmenopausal).

Geriatric patients
• Elderly men receiving androgens may be at increased risk for prostatic hypertrophy and prostatic carcinoma. Androgens are contraindicated in the presence of prostatic hypertrophy with obstruction because they can aggravate this condition.

Pediatric patients
• Observe children receiving androgens carefully for excessive virilization and precocious puberty. Androgen therapy may cause premature epiphyseal closure and short stature. Regular X-ray examinations of hand bones may be used to monitor skeletal maturation during therapy.

Pregnant patients
• Don't administer androgens during pregnancy because they may cause masculinization of female fetus or other fetal harm.

Breast-feeding patients
• The amount of androgen that appears in breast milk is unknown. Because androgens may induce premature sexual development (in men) or virilization (in women), women who are receiving androgens shouldn't breast-feed.

Representative combinations
Fluoxymesterone with ethinyl estradiol: Halodrin.
    Testosterone cypionate with estradiol cypionate: De-Comberol, depAndrogyn, Depo-Testadiol, Depotestogen, Duo-Cyp, Duratestin, Menoject-L.A., Test-Estro Cypionate.
    Testosterone enanthate with estradiol valerate: Andrest 90-4, Andro-Estro 90-4, Androgyn L.A., Duo-Gen L.A., Duogex L.A.*, Neo-Pause*, Teev, Valertest No. 1.

---

angiotensin-converting enzyme (ACE) inhibitors

benazepril hydrochloride, captopril, enalapril maleate, fosinopril sodium, lisinopril, moexipril hydrochloride, quinapril hydrochloride, ramipril, trandolapril

---

ACE inhibitors are used to manage hypertension, and most are used to treat heart failure. Captopril is indicated for the prevention of diabetic nephropathy, and captopril and lisinopril are useful in improving survival in patients after an MI.

Pharmacology
ACE inhibitors prevent the conversion of angiotensin I to angiotensin II, a potent vasoconstrictor. Besides decreasing vasoconstriction, and thus reducing peripheral arterial resistance, inhibition of angiotensin II decreases adrenocortical secretion of aldosterone. This results in decreased sodium and water retention and extracellular fluid volume.

Clinical indications and actions
ACE inhibitors are used to treat hypertension; their antihypertensive effects are secondary to decreased peripheral resistance and decreased sodium and water retention.
    ACE inhibitors are used to manage heart failure; they decrease systemic vascular resistance (afterload) and pulmonary capillary wedge pressure (preload). They are also used post-MI to decrease mortality and prevent diabetic nephropathy. (See *ACE inhibitors: Dosage forms and dosages.*)

Overview of adverse reactions
The most common adverse effects of therapeutic doses of ACE inhibitors are headache, fatigue, hypotension, tachycardia, dysgeusia, proteinuria, hyperkalemia, rash, cough, and angioedema of the face and extremities. Severe hypotension may occur at toxic drug levels. ACE inhibitors should be used cautiously in patients with impaired renal function or serious autoimmune disease, and

ACE INHIBITORS: DOSAGE FORMS AND DOSAGES

Drug	Dosage forms	Initial adult dose	Target adult dose	Special dosages
benazepril	Tablets: 5, 10, 20, 40 mg	HTN: 10 mg q.d.	20 to 40 mg in single or divided dose	5 mg q.d.[a]
captopril	Tablets: 12.5, 25, 50, 100 mg (scored)	HTN: 25 mg b.i.d. or t.i.d. HF: 25 mg t.i.d. LVD post-MI: 12.5 mg t.i.d. Diabetic nephropathy: 25 mg t.i.d.	25 to 150 mg in single or divided dose 50 to 100 mg t.i.d. 50 mg t.i.d. 25 mg t.i.d.	6.25 to 12.5 mg b.i.d. or t.i.d.[b]
enalapril, enalaprilat	Tablets: 2.5 (scored), 5 (scored), 10, 20 mg Injection: 1.25 mg/ml	HTN: 5 mg P.O. q.d. or enalaprilat I.V. 0.625 mg over 5 or more min HF: 2.5 mg q.d. or b.i.d. Asymptomatic LVD: 2.5 mg b.i.d.	P.O.: 10 to 40 mg in single or divided dose or I.V. (enalaprilat) 1.25 mg (over more than 5 minutes) q 6 hr 2.5 to 10 mg b.i.d. 10 mg b.i.d.	P.O.: 2.5 mg q.d.[c]
fosinopril	Tablets: 10, 20 mg	HTN: 10 mg q.d. HF: 10 mg q.d.	20 to 40 mg in single or divided dose 20 to 40 mg q.d.	10 mg q.d.[d]
lisinopril	Tablets: 5 (Zestril scored), 10, 20, 40 mg	HTN: 10 mg q.d. HF: 5 mg q.d. Post-MI: Within 24 hr of MI symptom, give 5 mg, then 5 mg at 24 hr, then 10 mg at 48 hr, then 10 mg q.d.	20 to 40 mg q.d. 5 to 20 mg q.d. 10 mg q.d. for 6 weeks	2.5 to 5 mg q.d.[e]
moexipril	Tablets: 7.5, 15 mg	HTN: 7.5 mg q.d.	7.5 to 30 mg in single or divided dose	3.75 mg q.d.[f]
quinapril	Tablets: 5, 10, 20, 40 mg (scored)	HTN: 10 mg q.d. HF: 5 mg b.i.d.	20 to 80 mg in single or divided dose 10 to 20 mg b.i.d.	2.5 or 5 mg q.d.[g]
ramipril	Capsules: 1.25, 2.5, 5, 10 mg	HTN: 2.5 mg q.d. HF post-MI: 2.5 mg b.i.d.	2.5 to 20 mg in single or divided dose 5 mg b.i.d.	1.25 mg q.d.[h]
trandolapril	Tablets: 1, 2, 4 mg	HTN: Caucasian—1 mg q.d.; African American—2 mg q.d. Heart failure post-MI: 1 mg q.d. LVD post-MI: 1 mg q.d.	2 to 4 mg q.d. 1 to 4 mg q.d. 1 to 4 mg q.d.	0.5 mg q.d.[i]

HTN = hypertension; HF = heart failure; LVD = left ventricular dysfunction; MI = myocardial infarction.
[a] Consider if creatinine clearance < 30 ml/min.
[b] Consider if renal impairment, hyponatremia, or hypovolemia.
[c] Consider if HTN and creatinine clearance ≤ 30 ml/min or concurrent diuretic; also consider if CHF and creatinine clearance ≤ 30 ml/min, serum creatinine > 3 mg/dl, or serum sodium < 130 mEq/L.
[d] Use cautiously if concurrent diuretic.
[e] In HTN: consider 5-mg dose if creatinine clearance ≤ 10 to 30 ml/min or concurrent diuretic; 2.5-mg dose if creatinine clearance < 10 ml/min. In CHF: consider 2.5-mg dose if creatinine clearance ≤ 30 ml/min, serum creatinine > 3 mg/dl, or serum sodium < 130 mEq/L.
[f] Consider if creatinine clearance < 40 ml/min.
[g] Consider 2.5-mg dose if creatinine clearance 10 to 30 ml/min and 5-mg dose if creatinine clearance 30 to 60 ml/min or concurrent diuretic.
[h] Consider if creatinine clearance < 40 ml/min or serum creatinine > 2.5 mg/dl.
[i] Consider if concurrent diuretic, hepatic cirrhosis, or creatinine clearance < 30 ml/min.

in patients taking other drugs known to depress WBC count or immune response.

☑ Special considerations
- Stop diuretic therapy 2 to 3 days before beginning ACE inhibitor therapy to reduce risk of hypotension; if drug doesn't adequately control blood pressure, reinstate diuretics. If diuretics can't be stopped, initiate ACE inhibitor at the lowest possible dose.
- Periodic monitoring of WBC count is necessary.
- Lower doses are needed in patients with impaired renal function.
- Use potassium supplements with caution because ACE inhibitors may cause potassium retention.
- Watch for feelings of light-headedness, especially in first few days, because dosage may need adjustment; signs of infection, such as sore throat and fever, because drugs may decrease WBC count; facial swelling or difficulty breathing because drugs may cause angioedema; and loss of taste, which may necessitate discontinuing drug.

Information for the patient
- Tell patient that drug may cause a dry, persistent, tickling cough; it's reversible when therapy ends.
- Advise patient to avoid sudden position changes to minimize orthostatic hypotension.
- Instruct patient to sit up in bed slowly, and then dangle legs at bedside for a full minute before attempting to stand upright.
- Tell patient to report feelings of light-headedness, especially in first few days; signs of infection, such as sore throat and fever; facial swelling or difficulty breathing; and loss of taste.
- Warn patient to call before taking OTC cold preparations.
- Tell patient to call if troublesome cough develops.
- Instruct woman to promptly report pregnancy.
- Tell patient not to take salt substitutes containing potassium without medical approval.

Geriatric patients
- Elderly patients may need lower doses because of impaired drug clearance. These patients may be more sensitive to hypotensive effects.

Pediatric patients
- Safety and efficacy of ACE inhibitors in children haven't been established; use only if potential benefit outweighs risk.

Pregnant patients
- Stop ACE inhibitors if pregnancy is detected. Drug may harm or cause fetal death during the second or third trimesters.

Breast-feeding patients
- Captopril and enalapril appear in breast milk. An alternative to breast-feeding is recommended during therapy.

Representative combinations
Captopril with hydrochlorothiazide: Capozide.
   Benazepril hydrochloride with amlodipine: Lotrel; with hydrochlorothiazide: Lotensin HCT.
   Enalapril with hydrochlorothiazide: Vaseretic.
   Lisinopril with hydrochlorothiazide: Prinzide, Zestoretic.

angiotensin II receptor antagonists

candesartan, irbesartan, losartan, telmisartan, valsartan

The angiotensin II receptor antagonists (AIIRAs) are a class of antihypertensive drugs that are used as monotherapy and with other antihypertensives. In comparison to ACE inhibitors, AIIRAs are associated with fewer adverse effects, such as cough and angioedema.

Pharmacology
Angiotensin II is a potent vasoconstrictor formed from angiotensin I by the angiotensin-converting enzyme (ACE). Angiotensin II plays an important role in the pathophysiology of hypertension. It causes vasoconstriction, increased aldosterone secretion, cardiac stimulation, and reabsorption of sodium by the kidneys. AIIRAs exert their therapeutic effects by blocking binding of angiotensin II to the AT_1 receptor.

AT_1 receptors are found in many tissues throughout the body, including vascular smooth muscle and the adrenal gland. Blockade of AT_1 receptors by AIIRAs results in vasodilation, decreased aldosterone secretion, a two- to threefold rise in plasma renin activity, and an increase in angiotensin II. The increase in renin and angiotensin II is due to removal of the negative feedback of angiotensin II and isn't enough to overcome the antihypertensive effects of AIIRAs. Another type of receptor exists called the AT_2 receptor. It's unknown what the AT_2 receptor's role is, but it doesn't appear to be involved in cardiovascular homeostasis. AIIRAs are 1,000- to 20,000-fold more selective for AT_1 than AT_2 receptors.

Unlike ACE inhibitors, AIIRAs don't have any effect on ACE or bradykinin. ACE catalyzes the formation of angiotensin II and is responsible for the degradation of bradykinin. Bradykinin is thought to be responsible for the cough and angioedema associated with ACE inhibitor therapy; AIIRAs are less likely than ACE inhibitors to cause cough and angioedema.

Clinical indications and actions

Hypertension

All AIIRAs are indicated for the treatment of hypertension. They can be used as monotherapy or with other drugs. AIIRAs exert their antihypertensive effects by blocking binding of angiotensin II to the AT_1 receptor.

◊ Heart failure

AIIRAs may be beneficial in the treatment of heart failure. Heart failure is associated with elevated levels of angiotensin II and aldosterone. ACE inhibitors have been shown to decrease mortality in patients with heart failure. The beneficial effects of ACE inhibitors are thought to be related to inhibition of the renin-angiotensin-aldosterone system (RAAS). AIIRAs may prove to have effects on mortality similar to those of ACE inhibitors in patients with heart failure. Until more information is available, AIIRAs should be reserved for patients unable to tolerate ACE inhibitors. (See *Comparing angiotensin II receptor antagonists,* pages 1156 and 1157.)

Overview of adverse reactions

AIIRAs are well tolerated, with adverse effects similar to those of placebo. 2.3% to 3.3% of patients receiving AIIRAs stopped therapy because of adverse reactions compared to 2% to 6.1% of patients receiving placebo. Reported adverse effects include dizziness, insomnia, headache, fatigue, anxiety or nervousness, diarrhea, dyspepsia or heartburn, nausea or vomiting, arthralgia, back or leg pain, muscle cramps, myalgia, upper respiratory tract infection, cough, nasal congestion, sinusitis, pharyngitis, rhinitis, influenza, bronchitis, viral infection, edema, chest pain, rash, tachycardia, urinary tract infection, peripheral edema, and albuminuria.

Symptomatic hypotension may occur in patients who are volume- or salt-depleted (such as those treated with diuretics). These conditions should be corrected before drug administration, and a lower starting dose should be used.

As with ACE inhibitors, AIIRAs can cause deterioration in renal function, including oliguria, acute renal failure, and progressive azotemia. Patients whose renal function may depend on the RAAS (such as those with heart failure, volume depletion, or unilateral or bilateral renal artery stenosis) are at increased risk for this effect.

A more than 2 g/dl decrease in hemoglobin was observed in 0.8% of patients taking telmisartan compared to 0.3% of patients receiving placebo. Decreases of more than 20% in hemoglobin level and hematocrit were observed in 0.4% to 0.8% of valsartan patients compared to 0.1% of patients receiving placebo.

Serum potassium level increases of more than 20% were observed in valsartan patients compared to 2.9% of patients receiving placebo.

Occasional increases in liver function test results have occurred in patients treated with valsartan.

☑ Special considerations

● Use extreme caution when using angiotensin II receptor antagonists with potassium supplements or potassium-sparing diuretics
● Use caution in volume-depleted patients (patients taking diuretics). Correct condition before giving drug, and use a lower starting dose.
● Use with caution in patients with hepatic dysfunction; losartan needs dosage adjustment.
● Use with caution in patients whose renal function may be dependent on the RAAS (such as patients with heart failure or renal artery stenosis); a worsening of renal function may occur.
● Telmisartan increases peak digoxin levels about 49% and troughs about 20%. Monitor digoxin levels more frequently when initiating, adjusting, or stopping telmisartan.

Information for the patient

● Tell woman of childbearing age about risk of exposure to AIIRAs during the second and third trimesters. Inform patient that adverse effects on fetus aren't likely when intrauterine exposure is limited to the first trimester.
● Tell woman to report pregnancy immediately.
● Tell patient not to stop taking drug unless directed.
● Instruct patient to take missed doses as soon as he remembers unless it's almost time for the next dose.
● Tell patient to report if signs of allergy or dizziness occur while taking drug.

Geriatric patients

● No dosage adjustments are needed in elderly patients. No differences in efficacy or safety have been observed with losartan, candesartan, or telmisartan when older and younger patients were compared.

Pediatric patients

● Safety and efficacy in children below age 18 haven't been established.

Pregnant patients

● Pregnancy risk category C in the first trimester and D in the second and third trimesters. Drugs that act on the RAAS have been associated with fetal and neonatal injury, and death when intrauterine exposure occurred during the second or third trimester of pregnancy. Stop AIIRAs in patients that become pregnant.

Breast-feeding patients

● It's unknown if AIIRAs appear in breast milk. Because of potential risk to infant, a decision should be made to stop either drug or breast-feeding.

COMPARING ANGIOTENSIN II RECEPTOR ANTAGONISTS

Drug	Oral bioavailability	Effect of food	Prodrug	Metabolized by CYP-450 isoenzymes	Protein binding
candesartan	15%	No effect	Yes	Unknown	> 99%
irbesartan	60% to 80%	No effect	No	Yes, CYP 2C9	90%
losartan	33%	↓AUC ~ 10%	Yes	Yes, CYP 2C9 and CYP 3A4	~ 99%
telmisartan	42% to 58%	↓AUC 6% to 20%	No	No	> 99.5%
valsartan	25%	↓AUC ~ 40%	No	Unknown	95%

Representative combinations

Hydrochlorothiazide and losartan: Hyzaar; hydrochlorothiazide and valsartan: Diovan HCT.

anticholinergics

Belladonna alkaloids: atropine sulfate, hyoscyamine sulfate, scopolamine hydrobromide

Semi-synthetic and synthetic quaternary anticholinergics: anisotropine, clidinium, glycopyrrolate, ipratropium bromide, mepenzolate bromide, methscopolamine, propantheline bromide

Tertiary synthetic and semisynthetic (antispasmodic) derivatives: dicyclomine hydrochloride, homatropine, oxybutynin, pirenzepine, tolterodine tartrate

Antiparkinsonians: benztropine mesylate, biperiden hydrochloride, biperiden lactate, trihexyphenidyl hydrochloride

Anticholinergics are used to treat various spastic conditions, including acute dystonic reactions, muscle rigidity, parkinsonism, and extrapyramidal disorders. They also are used to reverse neuromuscular blockade, to prevent nausea and vomiting resulting from motion sickness, as adjunctive treatment for peptic ulcer disease and other GI disorders, and preoperatively to decrease secretions and block cardiac reflexes. Belladonna alkaloids are naturally occurring anticholinergics that have been used for centuries. Many semisynthetic alkaloids and synthetic anticholinergic compounds are available; however, most offer few advantages over naturally occurring alkaloids.

Pharmacology

Anticholinergics competitively antagonize the actions of acetylcholine and other cholinergic agonists at muscarinic and nicotinic receptors within the parasympathetic nervous system and smooth muscles that lack cholinergic innervation. Lack of specificity for site of action increases the hazard of adverse effects in association with therapeutic effects.

Antispasmodics are structurally similar to anticholinergics; however, their anticholinergic activity usually occurs only at high doses. Their mechanism of action is unknown, but they are believed to directly relax smooth muscle.

Clinical indications and actions

Hypersecretory conditions

Many anticholinergics (atropine, belladonna leaf, glycopyrrolate, hyoscyamine, levorotatory alkaloids of belladonna, and mepenzolate) are used therapeutically for their antisecretory properties; these properties derive from competitive blockade of cholinergic receptor sites, causing decreased gastric acid secretion, salivation, bronchial secretions, and sweating.

GI tract disorders

Some anticholinergics (atropine, belladonna leaf, glycopyrrolate, hyoscyamine, levorotatory alkaloids of belladonna, mepenzolate, and propantheline) as well as the antispasmodic dicyclomine treat spasms and other GI tract disorders. These drugs competitively block acetylcholine's actions at cholinergic receptor sites. Antispasmodics presumably act by a nonspecific, direct spasmolytic action on smooth muscle. These drugs are useful in treating pylorospasm, ileitis, and irritable bowel syndrome.

Sinus bradycardia

Atropine is used to treat sinus bradycardia caused by drugs, poisons, or sinus node dysfunction. It blocks normal vagal inhibition of the SA node and causes an increase in heart rate.

T½ (hr)	Dosing interval	Uricosuric effect
9	q.d. to b.i.d.	No
11 to 15	q.d.	No
2 (6 to 9 for active metabolite)	q.d. to b.i.d.	Yes
24	q.d.	No
6	q.d.	No

Dystonia and parkinsonism
Biperiden, benztropine, and trihyphenidyl hydrochloride are used to treat acute dystonic reactions and drug-induced extrapyramidal adverse effects. They act centrally by blocking cholinergic receptor sites, balancing cholinergic activity with dopamine activity.

Perioperative use
Atropine, glycopyrrolate, and hyoscyamine are used postoperatively with anticholinesterase drugs to reverse nondepolarizing neuromuscular blockade. These drugs block muscarinic effects of anticholinesterases by competitively blocking muscarinic receptor sites.

Atropine, glycopyrrolate, and scopolamine are used preoperatively to decrease secretions and block cardiac vagal reflexes. They diminish secretions by competitively inhibiting muscarinic receptor sites; they block cardiac vagal reflexes by preventing normal vagal inhibition of the SA node.

Bronchospasm
Atropine and ipratropium are potent bronchodilators and are used to treat antigen-, methacholine-, histamine-, or exercise-induced bronchospasm (oral inhalation and I.M. atropine). Oral inhalation of atropine or ipratropium is effective in the treatment of chronic bronchitis and asthma; oral inhalation of atropine sulfate has been used for the short-term treatment and prevention of bronchospasm associated with chronic bronchial asthma, bronchitis, and COPD.

Genitourinary tract disorders
Atropine, oxybutynin, and propantheline have been used to treat reflex neurogenic bladder.

Poisoning
Atropine is used to reverse the cholinergic effects of toxic exposure to organophosphate, carbamate anticholinesterase pesticides, and cholinomimetic plants and fungi.

Motion sickness
Scopolamine is effective in preventing nausea and vomiting associated with motion sickness. Its exact mechanism of action is unknown, but it's thought to affect neural pathways originating in the labyrinth of the ear.

Overview of adverse reactions
Dry mouth, decreased sweating or anhidrosis, headache, mydriasis, blurred vision, cycloplegia, urinary hesitancy and urine retention, constipation, palpitations, and tachycardia most commonly occur with therapeutic doses and usually disappear once drug is stopped.

Signs and symptoms of drug toxicity include CNS signs resembling psychosis (disorientation, confusion, hallucinations, delusions, anxiety, agitation, and restlessness) and such peripheral effects as dilated, nonreactive pupils; blurred vision; hot, dry, flushed skin; dry mucous membranes; dysphagia; decreased or absent bowel sounds; urine retention; hyperthermia; tachycardia; hypertension; and increased respiration.

☑ Special considerations
• Monitor vital signs, urine output, and visual changes; watch for signs of impending toxicity.
• Constipation may be relieved by stool softeners or bulk laxatives.

Information for the patient
• Teach patient how and when to take drug.
• Warn patient to avoid driving and other hazardous activities if he experiences dizziness, drowsiness, or blurred vision.
• Advise patient to avoid alcoholic beverages because they may cause additive CNS effects.
• Advise patient to consume plenty of fluids and dietary fiber to help avoid constipation.
• Tell patient to promptly report dry mouth, blurred vision, rash, eye pain, significant changes in urine volume, or pain or difficulty on urination.
• Warn patient that drug may cause increased sensitivity or intolerance to high temperatures, resulting in dizziness.
• Instruct patient to report confusion and rapid or pounding heartbeat.
• Advise woman to report pregnancy or intent to conceive.
• Warn patient to avoid OTC drugs such as Benadryl or Nytol (they also have anticholinergic activity).

Geriatric patients
• Lower doses are usually indicated in elderly patients. Patients over age 40 may be more sensitive to the effects of these drugs. Administer cautiously to elderly patients.

Pediatric patients
• Safety and effectiveness in children haven't been established.

Pregnant patients
• Safety of anticholinergic therapy during pregnancy hasn't been determined. Use in pre-

women only when drug's benefits to woman outweigh potential risks to fetus.

Breast-feeding patients
• Some anticholinergics may appear in breast milk, possibly resulting in infant toxicity. Breast-feeding women should avoid these drugs. Anticholinergics may decrease milk production.

Representative combinations
Atropine with meperidine: Atropine and Demerol; with scopolamine hydrobromide (hyoscine hydrobromide), hyoscyamine sulfate, and phenobarbital: Antispasmodic Elixir, Bellalphen, Donnatal, Donnatal No. 2, Haponal, Kinesed, Phenobarbital with Belladonna Alkaloids Elixir, Spasmolin; with scopolamine hydrobromide (hyoscine hydrobromide), hyoscyamine sulfate, kaolin, pectin, sodium benzoate, alcohol, and powdered opium: Donnagel-PG; with phenazopyridine, hyoscyamine, and scopolamine: Urogesic; with hyoscyamine, methenamine, phenyl salicylate, methylene blue, and benzoic acid: Urised; with scopalamine hydrobromide, hyoscyamine hydrobromide, and phenobarbital: Barbidonna No. 2 Tablets, Barbidonna Tablets, Barophen, Belladonna Alkaloids with Phenobarbital Tablets, Donnamor, Donnapine, Donnatal Extentabs, Hyosophen Tablets, Malatal Tablets, Spasmophen, Spasquid, Susano.

Belladonna alkaloids with ergotamine tartrate, caffeine, and phenacetin: Wigraine; with phenobarbital: Chardonna-2, Butibel Elixir; with powdered opium: B&O Supprettes No. 15A, B&O Supprettes No. 16A.

Belladonna extract with butabarbital: Butibel.

Hyoscyamine sulfate with phenobarbital: Levsin with Phenobarbital, Levsin-PB, Bellacane Tablets.

antihistamines

astemizole, azelastine hydrochloride, brompheniramine maleate, cetirizine hydrochloride, chlorpheniramine maleate, clemastine fumarate, cyclizine hydrochloride, cyclizine lactate, cyproheptadine hydrochloride, dimenhydrinate, diphenhydramine hydrochloride, fexofenadine hydrochloride, hydroxyzine, loratadine, meclizine hydrochloride, promethazine hydrochloride, trimeprazine tartrate, tripelennamine hydrochloride, triprolidine hydrochloride

Antihistamines, synthetically produced H_1-receptor antagonists, were discovered in the late 1930s and proliferated rapidly during the next decade. They have many applications related specifically to chemical structure, their widespread use testifying to their versatility and relative safety. Some antihistamines are used primarily to treat rhinitis or pruritus, whereas others are used more often for their antiemetic and antivertigo effects; still others are used as sedative-hypnotics, local anesthetics, and antitussives.

Pharmacology
Antihistamines are structurally related chemicals that compete with histamine for H_1-receptor sites on the smooth muscle of the bronchi, GI tract, uterus, and large blood vessels, binding to the cellular receptors and preventing access and subsequent activity of histamine. They don't directly alter histamine or prevent its release. Also, antihistamines antagonize the action of histamine that causes increased capillary permeability and resultant edema and suppress flare and pruritus associated with the endogenous release of histamine.

Clinical indications and actions
Allergy
Most antihistamines (azelastine, brompheniramine, chlorpheniramine, clemastine, cyproheptadine, diphenhydramine, promethazine, and triprolidine) are used to treat allergic symptoms, such as rhinitis and urticaria. By preventing access of histamine to H_1-receptor sites, they suppress histamine-induced allergic symptoms.
Pruritus
Cyproheptadine, hydroxyzine, and trimeprazine are used systemically. It's believed that these drugs counteract histamine-induced pruritus by a combination of peripheral effects on nerve endings and local anesthetic and sedative activity.

Tripelennamine and diphenhydramine are used topically to relieve itching associated with minor skin irritation. Structurally related to local anesthetics, these compounds prevent initiation and transmission of nerve impulses.
Vertigo, nausea, and vomiting
Cyclizine, dimenhydrinate, and meclizine are used only as antiemetics and antivertigo drugs; their antihistaminic activity hasn't been evaluated. Diphenhydramine and promethazine are used as antiallergenic and antivertigo drugs and as antiemetics and antinauseants. Although the mechanisms aren't fully understood, antiemetic and antivertigo effects probably result from central antimuscarinic activity.
Sedation
Diphenhydramine and promethazine are used for their sedative action; the mechanism of antihistamine-induced CNS depression is unknown.
Suppression of cough
Diphenhydramine syrup is used as an antitussive. The cough reflex is suppressed by a direct effect on the medullary cough center.

Dyskinesia
The central antimuscarinic action of diphenhy-dramine reduces drug-induced dyskinesias and parkinsonism through inhibition of acetylcholine (anticholinergic effect).

Overview of adverse reactions
At therapeutic dosage levels, all antihistamines except astemizole and loratadine are likely to cause drowsiness and impaired motor function during initial therapy. Also, their anticholinergic action usually causes dry mouth and throat, blurred vision, and constipation. Antihistamines that are also phenothiazines, such as prometh-azine, may cause other adverse effects, includ-ing cholestatic jaundice (thought to be a hyper-sensitivity reaction) and may predispose patients to photosensitivity; patients taking such drugs should avoid prolonged exposure to sunlight.
 Toxic doses elicit a combination of CNS de-pression and excitation as well as atropine-like symptoms, including sedation, reduced mental alertness, apnea, CV collapse, hallucinations, tremors, seizures, dry mouth, flushed skin, and fixed, dilated pupils. Toxic effects reverse when drug is stopped. Used appropriately, in correct doses, antihistamines are safe for prolonged use.

☑ Special considerations
● Don't use antihistamines during an acute asth-ma attack because they may not alleviate the symptoms, and antimuscarinic effects can cause thickening of secretions.
● Use antihistamines with caution in elderly pa-tients and in those with increased intraocular pres-sure, hyperthyroidism, CV or renal disease, dia-betes, hypertension, bronchial asthma, urine re-tention, prostatic hypertrophy, bladder neck obstruction, or stenosing peptic ulcers.
● Monitor blood counts during long-term thera-py; watch for signs of blood dyscrasias.
● Antihistamines should be taken with food to re-duce GI distress; sugarless gum, hard candy, or ice chips may be used to relieve dry mouth; in-crease fluid intake or humidify air to decrease ad-verse effect of thickened secretions.
● If tolerance develops to one antihistamine, an-other may be substituted.
● Some antihistamines may mask ototoxicity from high doses of aspirin and other salicylates.

Information for the patient
● Advise patient to take drug with meals or snack to prevent gastric upset and to use any of the fol-lowing measures to relieve dry mouth: warm wa-ter rinses, artificial saliva, ice chips, or sugarless gum or candy. Tell him to avoid overusing mouth-wash, which may add to dryness (because of al-cohol content) and destroy normal flora.
● Warn patient to avoid hazardous activities, such as driving or operating machinery, until extent of CNS effects are known and to call before using

alcohol, tranquilizers, sedatives, pain relievers, or sleep aids.
● Warn patient to stop taking antihistamines 4 days before diagnostic skin tests to preserve ac-curacy of tests.

Geriatric patients
● Elderly patients are usually more sensitive to adverse effects of antihistamines and are espe-cially likely to experience a greater degree of dizziness, sedation, hypotension, and urine re-tention.

Pediatric patients
● Children, especially those under age 6, may experience paradoxical hyperexcitability with rest-lessness, insomnia, nervousness, euphoria, tremors, and seizures.

Pregnant patients
● Safe use of antihistamines during pregnancy hasn't been established. Some manufacturers recommend that drugs not be used during the third trimester of pregnancy due to the risk of se-vere reactions (i.e., seizures) in neonates and premature infants.

Breast-feeding patients
● Antihistamines shouldn't be used in breast-feeding women.

Representative combinations
Carbinoxamine maleate with pseudoephedrine and dextromethorphan: Carbodec DM, Pseudo-Car DM, Rondec-DM, Tussafed; with pseu-doephedrine hydrochloride: Rondec, Rondec-TR; with pseudoephedrine and guaifenesin: Brex-in L.A.
 Chlorpheniramine with phenylephrine and phenylpropanolamine: Naldecon; with dex-tromethorphan: Vicks Formula 44 Cough Mixture; with codeine and guaifenesin: Tussar SF; with ac-etaminophen: Coricidin; with pseudoephedrine and dextromethorphan: Rhinosyn-DM; with pseu-doephedrine, dextromethorphan, and aceta-minophen: Co-Apap; with phenylpropanolamine: Contac 12-Hour, Ornade, Resaid S.R., Triaminic-12, Dura-Vent; with pseudoephedrine hydro-chloride: Cophene No. 2, Rescon, Chlordrine S.R., Chlorphendrine SR, Colfed-A, Duralex, Klerist-D, Kronofed-A, ND Clear, Pseudo-Clor, Rescon-ED, Time-Hist, Chlorpheniramine Maleate/Pseudoephedrine HCl.
 Diphenhydramine with pseudoephedrine: Ben-adryl Allergy Decongestant, Benylin DM; with ac-etaminophen: Tylenol Severe Allergy.
 Promethazine with codeine: Phenergan with Codeine; with dextromethorphan: Phenergan with Dextromethorphan; with phenylephrine: Phener-gan VC; with phenylephrine and codeine: Phen-ergan VC with Codeine.

Pyrilamine maleate with codeine: Tricodene Cough and Cold; with phenylephrine and codeine: Codimal; with phenylephrine and dextromethorphan: Codimal DM; with phenylephrine, dextromethorphan, and acetaminophen: Robitussin Night Relief; with phenylephrine and hydrocodone: Codimal; with phenylpropanolamine, chlorpheniramine maleate, and dextromethorphan: Tricodene Forte, Tricodene NN, Triminol Cough.

Triprolidine with pseudoephedrine and codeine: Actifed with Codeine, CoActifed*; with pseudoephedrine: Actagen, Actifed, Allerfrin, Novafed, Triacin-C, Triafed with Codeine, Trifed-C, Trifed-C Cough, Triofed, Triposed.

---

barbiturates

amobarbital, amobarbital sodium, aprobarbital, butabarbital sodium, mephobarbital, metharbital, phenobarbital, pentobarbital sodium, phenobarbital sodium, primidone, secobarbital sodium

---

Barbituric acid was compounded more than 100 years ago in 1864. The first hypnotic barbiturate, barbital, was introduced into medicine in 1903. Although barbiturates have been used extensively as sedative-hypnotics and anxiolytics, benzodiazepines are the current drugs of choice for sedative-hypnotic effects. Phenobarbital remains effective for anticonvulsant therapy as well as mephobarbital and metharbital. A few short-acting barbiturates are used as general anesthetics.

Pharmacology

Barbiturates are structurally related compounds that act throughout the CNS, particularly in the mesencephalic reticular activating system, which controls the CNS arousal mechanism. Barbiturates induce an imbalance in central inhibitory and facilitatory mechanisms, which, in turn, influence the cerebral cortex and the reticular formation. Barbiturates decrease both presynaptic and postsynaptic membrane excitability.

The exact mechanism of action of barbiturates at these sites isn't known, nor is it clear which cellular and synaptic actions result in sedative-hypnotic effects. Barbiturates can produce all levels of CNS depression, from mild sedation, to coma, to death. Barbiturates exert their effects by facilitating the actions of gamma-aminobutyric acid (GABA). Barbiturates also exert a central effect, which depresses respiration and GI motility. Barbiturates have no analgesic action and may increase the reaction to painful stimuli at subanesthetic doses. The principal anticonvulsant mechanism of action is reduction of nerve transmission and decreased excitability of

the nerve cell. Barbiturates also raise the seizure threshold.

Clinical indications and actions
Seizure disorders

Phenobarbital is used in the prophylactic treatment and acute management of seizure disorders. It's used mainly in tonic-clonic and partial seizures. At anesthetic doses, all barbiturates have anticonvulsant activity. Phenobarbital is an effective parenteral drug for status epilepticus (with airway support). Mephobarbital and metharbital may also be used.

Barbiturates suppress the spread of seizure activity produced by epileptogenic foci in the cortex, thalamus, and limbic systems by enhancing the effects of GABA.

Sedation, hypnosis

Most currently available barbiturates are used as sedative-hypnotics for short-term (up to 2 weeks) treatment of insomnia because of their nonspecific CNS effects.

Barbiturates aren't used routinely as sedatives. Barbiturate-induced sleep differs from physiologic sleep by decreasing the rapid-eye-movement sleep cycles.

Preanesthesia sedation

Barbiturates are also used as preanesthetic sedatives and for relief of anxiety.

Psychiatric use

Barbiturates (especially amobarbital) have been used parenterally in narcoanalysis and narcotherapy and in identifying schizophrenia.

Overview of adverse reactions

Drowsiness, lethargy, vertigo, headache, and CNS depression are common with barbiturates. After hypnotic doses, a hangover effect, subtle distortion of mood, and impairment of judgment or motor skills may continue for many hours. After a decrease in dose or discontinuation of barbiturates used for hypnosis, rebound insomnia or increased dreaming or nightmares may occur. Barbiturates cause hyperalgesia in subhypnotic doses. Hypersensitivity reactions (rash, fever, serum sickness) aren't common, and are more likely to occur in patients with a history of asthma or allergies to other drugs; reactions include urticaria, rash, angioedema, and Stevens-Johnson syndrome. Barbiturates can cause paradoxical excitement at low doses, confusion in elderly patients, and hyperactivity in children. High fever, severe headache, stomatitis, conjunctivitis, or rhinitis may precede skin eruptions. Because of the potential for fatal consequences, stop barbiturates if dermatologic reactions occur.

Withdrawal symptoms may occur after as little as 2 weeks of uninterrupted therapy. Symptoms of abstinence usually occur within 8 to 12 hours after the last dose, but may be delayed up to 5 days. They include weakness, anxiety, nausea, vomiting, insomnia, hallucinations, and possibly seizures.

☑ Special considerations
- Doses of barbiturates must be individualized.
- Don't use barbiturates in nephritic patients or in those with porphyria, liver impairment, severe respiratory disease, or previous addiction to barbiturates.
- Barbiturates should be used cautiously, if at all, in patients who are mentally depressed or have suicidal tendencies or history of drug abuse.
- Avoid administering barbiturates to patients with status asthmaticus.
- Parenteral solutions are highly alkaline and contain organic solvents (propylene glycol); infuse at 100 mg/minute or less; avoid extravasation, which may cause local tissue damage and tissue necrosis; inject I.V. or deep I.M. only. Don't exceed 5 ml per I.M. injection site to avoid tissue damage.
- Too-rapid I.V. administration of barbiturates may cause respiratory depression, apnea, laryngospasm, or hypotension. Have resuscitative measures available. Assess I.V. site for signs of infiltration or phlebitis.
- Drug may be given P.R. if oral or parenteral route is inappropriate; don't give intra-arterially or S.C.
- Assess level of consciousness before and frequently during therapy to evaluate effectiveness of drug. Monitor neurologic status for possible alterations or deteriorations and note seizure character, frequency, and duration for changes.
- Vital signs should be checked frequently, especially during I.V. administration.
- Patient's sleeping patterns should be assessed before and during therapy to ensure effectiveness of drug.
- Safety measures (side rails, assistance when out of bed, call light within reach) should be used to prevent falls and injury.
- Consider airway support during I.V. administration.
- Anticipate possible rebound confusion and excitatory reactions in patient.
- Patients should be monitored for complaints of constipation. Advise diet high in fiber, if indicated.
- PT and INR should be carefully monitored in patients taking anticoagulants; dosage of anticoagulant may need adjustment to counteract possible interaction.
- Abrupt discontinuation may cause withdrawal symptoms; discontinue slowly.
- Death is common with an overdose of 2 to 10 g; it may occur at much smaller doses if alcohol is also ingested.

Information for the patient
- Warn patient to avoid concurrent use of other drugs with CNS depressant effects, such as antihistamines, analgesics, and alcohol, because they will have additive effects and result in increased drowsiness. Instruct patient to call before taking OTC cold or allergy preparations.
- Caution patient not to change dose or frequency without approval; stopping drug abruptly may trigger rebound insomnia, with increased dreaming, nightmares, or seizures.
- Warn patient against driving and other hazardous activities that require alertness while taking barbiturates. Instruct him in safety measures to prevent injury.
- Tell a woman that barbiturates can cause physical or psychological dependence (addiction), and that these effects may be transmitted to the fetus; withdrawal symptoms can occur in a neonate whose mother took barbiturates in the third trimester.
- Instruct patient to report skin eruption or other marked adverse reaction.
- Explain that a morning hangover is common after therapeutic use of barbiturates.

Geriatric patients
- Elderly patients and patients receiving subhypnotic doses may experience hyperactivity, excitement, confusion, depression, or hyperalgesia. Use with caution in this age-group.

Pediatric patients
- Premature infants are more susceptible to the depressant effects of barbiturates because of immature hepatic metabolism. Children receiving barbiturates may experience hyperactivity, excitement, or hyperalgia.

Pregnant patients
- Barbiturates may cause fetal harm. Postpartum hemorrhage and hemorrhagic disease of the newborn have occurred. The latter can be reversed with vitamin K therapy. If barbiturates are taken in the last trimester of pregnancy, neonates may exhibit withdrawal symptoms.

Breast-feeding patients
- Barbiturates appear in breast milk and may result in infant CNS depression. Use with caution in breast-feeding women.

Representative combinations
Amobarbital with secobarbital: Tuinal 100 mg Pulvules, Tuinal 200 mg Pulvules.

Butabarbital with acetaminophen: Sedapap; with belladonna: Butibel.

Phenobarbital with CNS stimulants: Quadrinal; with ergotamine tartrate: Bellergal-S; with phenytoin: Dilantin Kapseals; with aminophylline and ephedrine hydrochloride: Mudrane; with belladonna: Butibel, Butibel Elixir, Chardonna-2; with atropine: Antrocol; with hyoscyamine: Bellacane, Levsin-PB, Levsin with Phenobarbital; with ASA and codeine phosphate: Phenaphen with Codeine No. 3, Phenaphen with Codeine No. 4; with

ropine, hyoscyamine, and scopolamine hydrobromide: Antispasmodic Elixir, Barbidonna, Barbidonna No. 2, Barophen, Belladonna Alkaloids with Phenobarbital Tablets, Donnamor, Donnapine, Donnatal, Donnatal No. 2, Donnatal Extentabs, Hyosophen, Kinesed, Malatal, Phenobarbital with Belladonna Alkaloids Elixir, Spasmophen, Spasquid, Susano.
See also *anticholinergics (belladonna alkaloids)*.

benzodiazepines

alprazolam, chlordiazepoxide hydrochloride, clonazepam, clorazepate dipotassium, diazepam, estazolam, flurazepam hydrochloride, lorazepam, midazolam hydrochloride, oxazepam, quazepam, temazepam, triazolam

Benzodiazepines, synthetically produced sedative-hypnotics, gained popularity in the early 1960s, replacing barbiturates as the treatment of choice for anxiety, convulsive disorders, and sedation. These drugs are preferred over barbiturates because therapeutic doses produce less drowsiness, respiratory depression, and impairment of motor function, and toxic doses are less likely to be fatal.

Pharmacology
Benzodiazepines are a group of structurally related chemicals that selectively act on polysynaptic neuronal pathways throughout the CNS. Their precise sites and mechanisms of action aren't completely known. However, the benzodiazepines enhance or facilitate the action of gamma-aminobutyric acid (GABA), an inhibitory neurotransmitter in the CNS. The drugs appear to act at the limbic, thalamic, and hypothalamic levels of the CNS. These drugs produce anxiolytic, sedative, hypnotic, skeletal muscle relaxant, and anticonvulsant effects. All of the benzodiazepines have CNS-depressant activities; however, individual derivatives act more selectively at specific sites, allowing them to be subclassified into five categories based on their predominant clinical use.

Clinical indications and actions
Seizure disorders
Four of the benzodiazepines (diazepam, clonazepam, clorazepate, and parenteral lorazepam) are used as anticonvulsants. Their anticonvulsant properties are derived from an ability to suppress the spread of seizure activity produced by epileptogenic foci in the cortex, thalamus, and limbic systems by enhancing presynaptic inhibition. Clonazepam is useful in the adjunctive treatment of petit mal variant (Lennox-Gastaut syn-

drome), myoclonic, or akinetic seizures. Benzodiazepines are also useful adjuncts for the prophylactic management of partial seizures with elementary symptomatology (Jacksonian seizures), psychomotor seizures, and absence seizures. Parenteral diazepam is indicated to treat status epilepticus.
Anxiety, tension, and insomnia
Most benzodiazepines (alprazolam, chlordiazepoxide, clorazepate, diazepam, estazolam, flurazepam, lorazepam, oxazepam, quazepam, temazepam, and triazolam) are useful as anxiolytics or sedative-hypnotics. They have a similar mechanism of action: they are believed to facilitate the effects of GABA in the ascending reticular activating system, increasing inhibition and blocking both cortical and limbic arousal.

They are used to treat anxiety and tension that occur alone or as an adverse effect of a primary disorder. They aren't recommended for tension associated with everyday stress. The choice of a specific benzodiazepine depends on individual metabolic characteristics of the drug. For instance, in patients with depressed renal or hepatic function, alprazolam, lorazepam, or oxazepam may be selected because they have a relatively short duration of action and have no active metabolites.

The sedative-hypnotic properties of chlordiazepoxide, clorazepate, diazepam, lorazepam, and oxazepam make these the drugs of choice as preoperative drugs and as adjuncts in the rehabilitation of alcoholics.
Surgical adjuncts for conscious sedation or amnesia
Diazepam, midazolam, and lorazepam have amnestic effects. The mechanism of action is unknown. Parenteral administration before such procedures as endoscopy or elective cardioversion causes impairment of recent memory and interferes with the establishment of memory trace, producing anterograde amnesia.
Skeletal muscle spasm, tremor
Because oral forms of diazepam and chlordiazepoxide have skeletal muscle relaxant properties, they are commonly used to treat neurologic conditions involving muscle spasms and tetanus. The mechanism of action is unknown, but they are believed to inhibit spinal polysynaptic and monosynaptic afferent pathways.
◊ Schizophrenia
Benzodiazepines have been used as an adjunct to antipsychotic drugs in the management of schizophrenia.
◊ Cancer chemotherapy–induced nausea and vomiting
Benzodiazepines have been used as an adjunct to control nausea and vomiting associated with emetogenic cancer chemotherapy.

◊ **Neonatal opiate withdrawal**
Parenteral diazepam has been used to relieve agitation associated with neonatal opiate withdrawal.

Overview of adverse reactions
Therapeutic dosage of the benzodiazepines usually causes drowsiness and impaired motor function, which should be monitored early in treatment and which may or may not be persistent. GI discomfort, such as constipation, diarrhea, vomiting, and changes in appetite, with urinary alterations also have been reported. Visual disturbances and CV irregularities also are common. Continuing problems with short-term memory, confusion, severe depression, shakiness, vertigo, slurred speech, staggering, bradycardia, shortness of breath or difficulty breathing, and severe weakness usually indicate a toxic dose level. Prolonged or frequent use of benzodiazepines can cause physical dependency and withdrawal syndrome when drug is stopped.

☑ Special considerations
• Benzodiazepines shouldn't be used in patients with chronic pulmonary insufficiency, sleep apnea, or depressive neuroses or psychotic reactions without predominant anxiety, or in acute alcohol intoxication.
• Level of consciousness and neurologic status should be assessed before and frequently during therapy. Watch for paradoxical reactions, especially early in therapy.
• Sleep patterns and quality should be observed. Watch for changes in seizure character, frequency, or duration.
• Vital signs should be assessed frequently during therapy. Significant changes in blood pressure and heart rate may indicate impending toxicity.
• Drugs should be given with milk or immediately after meals to prevent GI upset. Give antacid, if needed, at least 1 hour before or after dose to prevent interaction and ensure maximum drug absorption and effectiveness.
• Renal and hepatic function should be periodically monitored to ensure adequate drug removal and prevent cumulative effects.
• Safety measures must be instituted (raised side rails and ambulatory assistance) to prevent injury. Anticipate possible rebound excitement reactions.
• After prolonged use, abrupt discontinuation may cause withdrawal symptoms; discontinue gradually.

Information for the patient
• Warn patient to avoid use of alcohol or other CNS depressants, such as antihistamines, analgesics, MAO inhibitors, antidepressants, and barbiturates, to prevent additive depressant effects.

• Caution patient to take drug as prescribed and not to give drug to others. Tell him not to change the dose or frequency and to call before taking OTC cold or allergy preparations that may potentiate CNS depressant effects.
• Warn patient to avoid activities requiring alertness and good psychomotor coordination until CNS response to drug is known. Instruct him in safety measures to prevent injury.
• Tell patient to avoid using antacids, which may delay drug absorption, unless prescribed.
• Be sure patient understands that benzodiazepines are capable of causing physical and psychological dependence with prolonged use.
• Warn patient not to stop taking drug abruptly to prevent withdrawal symptoms after prolonged therapy.
• Tell patient that smoking decreases drug's effectiveness. Encourage him to stop smoking during therapy.
• Tell patient to report adverse effects. These are often dose-related and can be relieved by dosage adjustments.
• Inform woman of childbearing age who is taking drug to report if she suspects pregnancy or intends to become pregnant during therapy.

Geriatric patients
• Because they are sensitive to CNS effects, elderly patients receiving benzodiazepines need lower doses. Use with caution in this age-group.
• Parenteral administration of these drugs is more likely to cause apnea, hypotension, bradycardia, and cardiac arrest in elderly patients.
• Elderly patients may show prolonged elimination of benzodiazepines, except possibly of oxazepam, lorazepam, temazepam, and triazolam.

Pediatric patients
• Because children, particularly very young ones, are sensitive to CNS depressant effects of benzodiazepines, use with caution. A neonate whose mother took a benzodiazepine during pregnancy may exhibit withdrawal symptoms.

Pregnant patients
• Benzodiazepines can cause fetal harm if used during pregnancy. Risk of congenital malformation increases if drug is given during first trimester. Use of benzodiazepines during labor may cause neonatal flaccidity.

Breast-feeding patients
• Safe use in breast-feeding women hasn't been established. Breast-fed infants of mothers who use a benzodiazepine may show sedative effects, have feeding difficulties, and lose weight.

Representative combinations
Chlordiazepoxide with amitriptyline hydrochloride: Limbitrol DS; with clidinium bromide: Libre

beta blockers

Beta₁ blockers: **acebutolol, atenolol, betaxolol hydrochloride, bisoprolol, esmolol, metoprolol tartrate**

Beta₁ and beta₂ blockers: **carteolol hydrochloride, carvedilol, labetalol, levobunolol hydrochloride, metipranolol hydrochloride, nadolol, penbutolol sulfate, pindolol, propranolol, sotalol, timolol maleate**

Beta blockers were first used in the early 1960s; they are now widely used to treat hypertension, angina pectoris, and arrhythmias. These drugs are well tolerated by most patients.

Pharmacology

Beta blockers are chemicals that compete with beta agonists for available beta-receptor sites; individual drugs differ in their ability to affect beta receptors. Some available drugs are considered nonselective; that is, they block both beta₁ receptors in cardiac muscle and beta₂ receptors in bronchial and vascular smooth muscle. Several drugs are cardioselective and in lower doses primarily inhibit beta₁ receptors. Some beta blockers have intrinsic sympathomimetic activity and simultaneously stimulate and block beta receptors, decreasing cardiac output; still others also have membrane-stabilizing activity, which affects cardiac action potential. (See *Comparing beta blockers.*)

Clinical indications and actions

Hypertension
Most beta blockers are used to treat hypertension. Although the exact mechanism is unknown, the action is thought to result from decreased cardiac output, decreased sympathetic outflow from the CNS, and suppression of renin release.

Angina
Propranolol, atenolol, nadolol, and metoprolol are used to treat angina pectoris; they decrease myocardial oxygen needs through the blockade of catecholamine-induced increases in heart rate, blood pressure, and the extent of myocardial contraction.

Arrhythmias
Propranolol, acebutolol, sotalol, and esmolol are used to treat arrhythmias; they prolong the refractory period of the AV node and slow AV conduction.

Glaucoma
The mechanism by which betaxolol, levobunolol, metipranolol, and timolol reduce intraocular pressure is unknown, but the drug effect is at least partially caused by decreased production of aqueous humor.

MI
Timolol, propranolol, atenolol, and metoprolol are used to prevent MI in susceptible patients.

Migraine prophylaxis
Propranolol and timolol are used to prevent recurrent attacks of migraine and other vascular headaches. The exact mechanism is unknown, but it's thought to result from inhibition of vasodilation of cerebral vessels.

Other uses
Some beta blockers have been used as anxiolytics, for managing subaortic stenosis, as adjunctive therapy of bleeding esophageal varices or pheochromocytomas, and to treat portal hypertension or essential tremors. Carvedilol is used to treat heart failure with cardiac glycosides, diuretics, or ACE inhibitors.

Overview of adverse reactions

Therapeutic doses may cause bradycardia, fatigue, and dizziness; some cause other CNS disturbances, such as nightmares, depression, memory loss, or hallucinations. Impotence, cold extremities, and elevated cholesterol levels also may occur. Severe hypotension, bradycardia, heart failure, or bronchospasm usually indicates toxic dose levels.

☑ Special considerations

● Apical pulse rate should be checked daily. Monitor blood pressure, ECG, heart rate and rhythm frequently; be alert for progression of AV block or severe bradycardia.
● Patients with heart failure must be weighed regularly; watch for gains of more than 5 lb (2.27 kg) per week.
● Signs of hypoglycemic shock are masked; watch diabetic patients for sweating, fatigue, and hunger. Tachycardia in hyperthyroidism is also masked.
● Don't stop these drugs before surgery for pheochromocytoma; before any surgical procedure, notify anesthesiologist that patient is taking a beta blocker.
● Glucagon may be prescribed to reverse signs and symptoms of beta blocker overdose.
● Don't dispense to patients with asthma, sinus bradycardia, first-degree heart block, cardiogenic shock, or overt cardiac failure.

Information for the patient

● Explain rationale for therapy, and emphasize importance of taking drug as prescribed, even when patient is feeling well.
● Warn patient that stopping drug abruptly can exacerbate angina or precipitate MI.
● Teach patient to minimize dizziness from orthostatic hypotension by taking dose at bedtime, and by rising slowly and avoiding sudden position changes.
● Advise patient to call before taking OTC cold preparations.

COMPARING BETA BLOCKERS

Drug	Half-life (hr)	Lipid solubility	Membrane-stabilizing activity	Intrinsic sympathomimetic activity
Nonselective				
carteolol	6	Low	0	++
carvedilol	7 to 10	High	Unknown	0
labetalol	6 to 8	Moderate	0	0
metipranolol	4	Low to moderate	0	0
nadolol	20	Low	0	0
penbutolol	5	High	0	+
pindolol	3 to 4	Moderate	+	+++
propranolol	4	High	++	0
timolol	4	Low to moderate	0	0
Beta₁-selective				
acebutolol	3 to 4	Low	+	+
atenolol	6 to 7	Low	0	0
betaxolol	14 to 22	Low	+	0
bisoprolol	9 to 12	Low	0	0
esmolol	0.15	Low	0	0
metoprolol	3 to 7	Moderate	♦	0

♦ Only in higher-than-usual doses.
+ Activity that drug possesses in comparison to other beta blockers.

Geriatric patients
• Elderly patients may need lower maintenance doses of beta blockers; they also may experience enhanced adverse effects.

Pediatric patients
• Safety and efficacy of beta blockers in children haven't been established; use only if potential benefit outweighs risk.

Pregnant patients
• Pregnancy risk category C or D. Beta blocker therapy should be avoided in pregnant women. Atenolol has been associated with intrauterine growth retardation.

Breast-feeding patients
• Beta blockers appear in breast milk. Recommendations for breast-feeding vary with individual drugs.

Representative combinations
Atenolol with chlorthalidone: Tenoretic.
  Bisoprolol with hydrochlorothiazide: Ziac Tablets.
  Metoprolol with hydrochlorothiazide: Lopressor HCT.
  Pindolol with hydrochlorothiazide: Viskazide.
  Propranolol hydrochloride with hydrochlorothiazide: Inderide, Inderide LA.
  Timolol with hydrochlorothiazide: Timolide.

calcium channel blockers

amlodipine besylate, bepridil hydrochloride, diltiazem hydrochloride, felodipine, isradipine, nicardipine hydrochloride, nifedipine, nimodipine, nisoldipine, verapamil hydrochloride

Calcium channel blockers (also called slow channel calcium antagonists or slow channel blockers) were introduced in the United States in the early 1980s. They have become increasingly popular as a treatment for classic and variant angina and are now the preferred drugs for Prinzmetal's variant angina (vasospastic angina). They are used as antihypertensives. Verapamil has proved effective in the acute treatment of supraventricular tachycardias (SVTs). (See *Comparing oral calcium channel blockers*, page 1166.)

Pharmacology
The main physiologic action of calcium channel blockers is to inhibit calcium influx across the slow channels of myocardial and vascular smooth muscle cells. By inhibiting calcium influx into these cells, calcium channel blockers reduce intracellular calcium levels. This, in turn, dilates coronary arteries, peripheral arteries, and arterioles, and slows cardiac conduction.
  When used to treat Prinzmetal's variant angina, calcium channel blockers inhibit coronary

COMPARING ORAL CALCIUM CHANNEL BLOCKERS

Drug	Onset of action	Peak serum level	Half-life	Therapeutic serum level
bepridil	1 hr	2 to 3 hr	24 hr	1 to 2 ng/ml
diltiazem	15 min	30 min	3 to 4 hr	50 to 200 ng/ml
felodipine	2 to 5 hr	2.5 to 5 hr	11 to 16 hr	Unknown
nicardipine	20 min	1 hr	8.6 hr	28 to 50 ng/ml
nifedipine	5 to 30 min	30 min to 2 hr	2 to 5 hr	25 to 100 ng/ml
nimodipine	Unknown	< 1 hr	1 to 2 hr	Unknown
nisoldipine	Unknown	6 to 12 hr	7 to 12 hr	Unknown
verapamil	30 min	1 to 2.2 hr	6 to 12 hr	80 to 300 ng/ml

spasm, increasing oxygen delivery to the heart. Peripheral artery dilation leads to a decrease in total peripheral resistance; this reduces afterload, which, in turn, decreases myocardial oxygen consumption. Inhibition of calcium influx into the specialized cardiac conduction cells (specifically, those in the SA and AV nodes) slows conduction through the heart. This effect is most pronounced with verapamil and diltiazem.

Clinical indications and actions
Angina
Calcium channel blockers are useful in managing Prinzmetal's variant angina, chronic stable angina, and unstable angina. In Prinzmetal's variant angina, they inhibit spontaneous and ergonovine-induced coronary spasm, thereby increasing coronary blood flow and maintaining myocardial oxygen delivery. In unstable and chronic stable angina, their effectiveness presumably stems from their ability to reduce afterload.
Arrhythmias
Of the calcium channel blockers, verapamil and diltiazem have the greatest effect on the AV node, slowing the ventricular rate in atrial fibrillation or flutter and converting SVT to normal sinus rhythm.
Hypertension
Because they dilate systemic arteries, most of these drugs are useful in mild to moderate hypertension.
Other uses
Calcium channel blockers (especially verapamil) may also prove to be effective as a hypertrophic cardiomyopathy therapy adjunct by improving left ventricular outflow as a result of negative inotropic effects and possibly improved diastolic function. They have been used to treat peripheral vascular disorders, subarachnoid hemorrhage (nimodipine), and as adjunctive therapy in the treatment of esophageal spasm. They also have been used prophylactically in the treatment of migraine headaches.

Overview of adverse reactions
Verapamil may adversely affect the conduction system, causing bradycardia and various degrees of heart block and exacerbating heart failure; hypotension also may occur after rapid I.V. administration. Prolonged oral verapamil therapy may cause constipation.

Adverse effects of nifedipine include hypotension, reflex tachycardia, peripheral edema, flushing, light-headedness, and headache.

Diltiazem most commonly causes anorexia, nausea, various degrees of heart block, bradycardia, heart failure, and peripheral edema.

☑ Special considerations
● Monitor cardiac rate and rhythm and blood pressure carefully when initiating therapy or increasing dose.
● Use of calcium supplements may decrease the effectiveness of calcium channel blockers.
● Use cautiously in patients with impaired left ventricular function.

Information for the patient
● Tell patient not to stop drug abruptly; gradual dose reduction may be needed.
● Instruct patient to report irregular heartbeat, shortness of breath, swelling of hands and feet, pronounced dizziness, constipation, nausea, or hypotension.
● Warn patient not to double the dose.

Geriatric patients
● Use with caution in this age-group because the half-life of calcium channel blockers may be increased as a result of decreased clearance.

Pediatric patients
● Adverse hemodynamic effects of parenteral verapamil have been observed in neonates and infants. Safety and effectiveness of diltiazem and nifedipine haven't been established.

Pregnant patients
● Pregnancy risk category C. Avoid use in pregnant women.

Breast-feeding patients
● Calcium channel blockers (verapamil and diltiazem) may appear in breast milk. To avoid possible adverse effects in infants, women shouldn't breast-feed during therapy.

Representative combinations
Amlodipine and benazepril hydrochloride: Lotrel.

cephalosporins

First-generation cephalosporins: cefadroxil, cefazolin sodium, cephalexin monohydrate, cephalothin sodium, cephradine

Second-generation cephalosporins: cefaclor, cefamandole nafate, cefmetazole sodium, cefonicid sodium, cefotetan disodium, cefoxitin sodium, cefprozil, cefuroxime axetil, cefuroxime sodium

Third-generation cephalosporins: cefdinir, cefixime, cefoperazone sodium, cefotaxime sodium, cefpodoxime proxetil, ceftazidime, ceftibuten, ceftizoxime sodium, ceftriaxone sodium

Fourth-generation cephalosporin: cefepime hydrochloride

Cephalosporins are beta-lactam antibiotics first isolated in 1948 from the fungus *Cephalosporium acremonium.* Their mechanism of action is similar to that of penicillins, but their antibacterial spectra differ.

Pharmacology
Cephalosporins are chemically and pharmacologically similar to penicillin; their structure contains a beta-lactam ring, a dihydrothiazine ring, and side chains, and they act by inhibiting bacterial cell-wall synthesis, causing rapid cell lysis. (See *Comparing cephalosporins,* page 1168.)

The sites of action for cephalosporins are enzymes known as penicillin-binding proteins (PBP). The affinity of certain cephalosporins for PBP in various microorganisms helps explain the differing spectra of activity in this class of antibiotics.

Bacterial resistance to beta-lactam antibiotics is conferred most significantly by production of beta-lactamase enzymes (by both gram-negative and gram-positive bacteria) that destroy the beta-lactam ring and thus inactivate cephalosporins;

decreased cell-wall permeability and alteration in binding affinity to PBP also contribute to bacterial resistance.

Cephalosporins are bactericidal; they act against many gram-positive and gram-negative bacteria, and some anaerobic bacteria; they don't kill fungi or viruses.

First-generation cephalosporins act against many gram-positive cocci, including penicillinase-producing *Staphylococcus aureus* and *S. epidermidis; Streptococcus pneumoniae, S. agalactiae* (group B streptococci), and *S. pyogenes* (group A beta-hemolytic streptococci); susceptible gram-negative organisms include *Klebsiella pneumoniae, Escherichia coli, Proteus mirabilis,* and *Shigella.*

Second-generation cephalosporins are effective against all organisms attacked by first-generation drugs and have additional activity against *Branhamella catarrhalis, Haemophilus influenzae, Enterobacter, Citrobacter, Providencia, Acinetobacter, Serratia,* and *Neisseria; Bacteroides fragilis* is susceptible to cefotetan and cefoxitin.

Third-generation cephalosporins are less active than first- and second-generation drugs against gram-positive bacteria, but more active against gram-negative organisms, including those resistant to first- and second-generation drugs; they have the greatest stability against beta-lactamases produced by gram-negative bacteria. Susceptible gram-negative organisms include *E. coli, Klebsiella, Enterobacter, Providencia, Acinetobacter, Serratia, Proteus, Morganella,* and *Neisseria;* some third-generation drugs are active against *B. fragilis* and *Pseudomonas.*

The fourth-generation cephalosporin, cefepime, is active against a wide range of gram-positive and gram-negative bacteria. Susceptible gram-negative organisms include *Enterobacter sp., E. coli, K. pneumoniae, P. mirabilis,* and *Pseudomonas aeruginosa;* susceptible gram-positive organisms include *S. aureus* (methicillin-susceptible strains only), *S. pneumoniae,* and *Streptococcus pyogenes* (Lancefield's group A streptococci).

Oral absorption of cephalosporins varies widely; many must be given parenterally. Most are distributed widely into the body, the actual amount varying with individual drugs. CSF penetration by first- and second-generation drugs is minimal; third-generation drugs achieve much greater penetration; and although the fourth-generation drug, cefepime, is known to cross the blood-brain barrier, it isn't known to what degree. Cephalosporins cross the placenta. Degree of metabolism varies with individual drugs; some aren't metabolized at all, and others are extensively metabolized.

Cephalosporins are excreted primarily in urine, chiefly by renal tubular effects; elimination half-life ranges from ½ to 10 hours in patients with normal renal function. Some drug is excreted in b

COMPARING CEPHALOSPORINS

Drug and route	Elimination half-life (hr)		Sodium (mEq/g)	CSF penetration
	Normal renal function	End-stage renal disease		
cefaclor oral	0.5 to 1	3 to 5.5	No data available	No
cefadroxil oral	1 to 2	20 to 25	No data available	No
cefamandole I.M., I.V.	0.5 to 2	12 to 18	3.3	No
cefazolin I.M., I.V.	1.2 to 2.2	3 to 7	2.0 to 2.1	No
cefdinir P.O.	1.5	16	No data available	No data available
cefepime I.M., I.V.	2	17 to 21	No data available	Yes
cefixime oral	3 to 4	11.5	No data available	Unknown
cefmetazole I.V.	1.2	Unknown	2	Unknown
cefonicid I.M., I.V.	3.5 to 5.8	11	3.7	No
cefoperazone I.M., I.V.	1.5 to 2.5	1.3 to 2.9	1.5	Sometimes
cefotaxime I.M., I.V.	1 to 1.5	3 to 11	2.2	Yes
cefotetan I.M., I.V.	2.8 to 4.6	13 to 35	3.5	No
cefoxitin I.M., I.V.	0.5 to 1	6.5 to 21.5	2.3	No
cefpodoxime oral	2 to 3	9.8	No data available	Unknown
cefprozil oral	1 to 1.5	5.2 to 5.9	No data available	Unknown
ceftazidime I.M., I.V.	1.5 to 2	35	2.3	Yes
ceftibuten oral	2.4	13.4 to 22.3	No data available	Unknown
ceftizoxime I.M., I.V.	1.5 to 2	30	2.6	Yes
ceftriaxone I.M., I.V.	5.5 to 11	15.7	3.6	Yes
cefuroxime I.M., I.V.	1 to 2	15 to 22	2.4	Yes
cephalexin oral	0.5 to 1	19 to 22	No data available	No
cephalothin I.M., I.V.	0.5 to 1	19	2.8	No
cephapirin I.M., I.V.	0.5 to 1	1.0 to 1.5	2.4	No
cephradine oral, I.M., I.V.	0.5 to 2	8 to 15	6	No

milk. Most cephalosporins can be removed by hemodialysis or peritoneal dialysis. Patients on dialysis may need dosage adjustment.

Clinical indications and actions

Parenteral cephalosporins: Cephalosporins are used to treat serious infections of the lungs, skin, soft tissue, bones, joints, urinary tract, blood (septicemia), abdomen, and ◊ heart (endocarditis).

Third-generation cephalosporins (except moxalactam and cefoperazone) and the second-generation drug cefuroxime are used to treat CNS infections caused by susceptible strains *of N. meningitidis, H. influenzae,* and *S. pneumoniae;* meningitis caused by *E. coli* or *Klebsiella* can be treated by ceftriaxone, cefotaxime, or ceftizoxime.

First-generation and some second-generation cephalosporins also can be given prophylactically to reduce postoperative infection after surgical procedures classified as contaminated or potentially contaminated; third-generation drugs aren't usually indicated.

Penicillinase-producing *N. gonorrhoeae* can be treated with cefoxitin, cefotaxime, ceftriaxone, ceftizoxime, or cefuroxime.

Oral cephalosporins: Cephalosporins can be used to treat otitis media and infections of the respiratory tract, urinary tract, skin, and soft tissue.

Ceftriaxone, cefotaxime, or cefuroxime axetil has been used in the treatment of ◊ Lyme disease. Cefepime, ◊ ceftazidime, and ◊ ceftriaxone have been used parenterally for empiric anti-infective therapy of probable bacterial infections in febrile neutropenic patients.

Overview of adverse reactions

Hypersensitivity reactions range from mild rash, fever, and eosinophilia to fatal anaphylaxis, and are more common in patients with penicillin allergy. Hematologic reactions include positive direct and indirect antiglobulin (Coombs' test), thrombocytopenia or thrombocythemia, transient neutropenia, reversible leukopenia, adverse renal effects, nausea, vomiting, diarrhea, abdominal pain, glossitis, dyspepsia, tenesmus, and minimal elevation of liver function test results.

Local venous pain and irritation are common after I.M. injection; such reactions occur more often with higher doses and long-term therapy.

Disulfiram-type reactions occur when cefamandole, cefoperazone, moxalactam, cefonicid, or cefotetan are administered within 48 to 72 hours of alcohol ingestion.

Bacterial and fungal superinfection results from suppression of normal flora.

☑ Special considerations

● Review patient's history of allergies.
● Watch for possible hypersensitivity reactions or other adverse effects.

● Perform renal function studies; doses of certain cephalosporins must be lowered in patients with severe renal impairment. In decreased renal function, monitor BUN levels, serum creatinine levels, and urine output for significant changes.
● Monitor PT and platelet counts and assess patient for signs of hypoprothrombinemia, which may occur, with or without bleeding, during therapy with cefamandole, cefepime, cefoperazone, cefonicid, or cefotetan (usually in elderly, debilitated, or malnourished patients).
● Monitor patients on long-term therapy for possible bacterial and fungal superinfection, especially elderly and debilitated patients, and others receiving immunosuppressants or radiation therapy.
● Monitor susceptible patients receiving sodium salts of cephalosporins for possible fluid retention; consult individual drug entry for sodium content.
● Cephalosporins cause false-positive results in urine glucose tests using cupric sulfate solutions (Benedict's reagent or Clinitest); glucose oxidase tests aren't affected. Consult individual drug entries for other possible test interactions.
● Give cephalosporins at least 1 hour before giving bacteriostatic antibiotics (tetracyclines, erythromycins, and chloramphenicol); these drugs inhibit bacterial cell growth, decreasing cephalosporin uptake by bacterial cell walls.
● Give oral cephalosporin at least 1 hour before or 2 hours after meals for maximum absorption.
● Refrigerate oral suspensions; shake well before administering to assure correct dose.
● I.M. dose should be given deep into large muscle mass (gluteal or midlateral thigh); rotate injection sites.
● Don't add or mix other drugs with I.V. infusions—particularly aminoglycosides, which will be inactivated if mixed with cephalosporins; if other drugs must be given I.V., temporarily stop infusion of primary drug.
● Adequate dilution of I.V. infusion and rotation of the site every 48 hours help minimize local vein irritation; use of small-gauge needle in largest available vein may be helpful.

Information for the patient
● Explain disease process and rationale for therapy.
● Teach signs and symptoms of hypersensitivity and other adverse reactions, and emphasize need to report any unusual effects.
● Teach signs and symptoms of bacterial and fungal superinfection to elderly and debilitated patients and others with low resistance from immunosuppressants or irradiation; emphasize need to report these signs and symptoms promptly.
● Advise patient using oral contraceptives to use additional form of contraception during therapy.

• Warn patient not to ingest alcohol in any form within 72 hours of treatment with cefamandole, cefoperazone, moxalactam, cefonicid, or cefotetan.

• Advise patient to add yogurt or buttermilk to diet to prevent intestinal superinfection resulting from suppression of normal intestinal flora.

• Advise diabetic patient to monitor urine glucose level with Diastix, Chemstrip uG, or glucose enzymatic test strip and not to use Clinitest.

• Tell patient to take oral drug with food if GI irritation occurs.

• Teach patient how and when to take drug; urge patient to complete entire prescribed regimen, to comply with instructions for around-the-clock dosing, and to keep follow-up appointments.

• Tell patient to check expiration date of drug, to discard unused drug, and to store correctly.

Geriatric patients
• Elderly patients are susceptible to superinfection and to coagulopathies. These patients commonly have renal impairment and may require lower doses of cephalosporins. Use with caution in this age-group.

Pediatric patients
• Serum half-life is prolonged in neonates and in infants up to age 1.

Pregnant patients
• Safety during pregnancy hasn't been established. Use only when clearly needed.

Breast-feeding patients
• Cephalosporins appear in breast milk; use with caution in breast-feeding women.

Representative combinations
None.

---

diuretics, loop

bumetanide, ethacrynate sodium, ethacrynic acid, furosemide, torsemide

---

Loop diuretics are sometimes referred to as high-ceiling diuretics because they produce a peak diuresis greater than that produced by other drugs. Loop diuretics are particularly useful in edema associated with heart failure, hepatic cirrhosis, and renal disease. Ethacrynic acid was synthesized during the search for compounds that might interact with renal sulfhydryl groups like mercurial diuretics. Unfortunately, ethacrynic acid is associated with ototoxicity and GI reactions and is used less frequently. Structurally similar to furosemide, bumetanide is about 40 times more

potent. Torsemide is the newest loop diuretic. (See *Comparing loop diuretics.*)

Pharmacology
Loop diuretics inhibit sodium and chloride reabsorption in the ascending loop of Henle, thus increasing renal excretion of sodium, chloride, and water; like thiazide diuretics, loop diuretics increase excretion of potassium. Loop diuretics produce greater maximum diuresis and electrolyte loss than thiazide diuretics.

Clinical indications and actions
Edema
Loop diuretics effectively relieve edema associated with heart failure. They may be useful in patients refractory to other diuretics; because furosemide and bumetanide may increase glomerular filtration rate, they are useful in patients with renal impairment. I.V. loop diuretics are used adjunctively in acute pulmonary edema to decrease peripheral vascular resistance. Loop diuretics also are used to treat edema associated with hepatic cirrhosis and nephrotic syndrome.

Hypertension
Loop diuretics are used in patients with mild to moderate hypertension, although thiazides are the initial diuretics of choice in most patients. Loop diuretics are preferred in patients with heart failure or renal impairment; used I.V., they are a helpful adjunct in managing hypertensive crises.

◊ Loop diuretics have been used to increase excretion of calcium in patients with hypercalcemia.

◊ Loop diuretics have been used to enhance the elimination of drugs or toxic substances after intoxication.

Overview of adverse reactions
The most common adverse effects associated with therapeutic doses of loop diuretics are metabolic and electrolyte disturbances (particularly potassium depletion), hypochloremic alkalosis, hyperglycemia, hyperuricemia, and hypomagnesemia. Rapid parenteral administration of loop diuretics may cause hearing loss (including deafness) and tinnitus. High doses may produce profound diuresis, leading to hypovolemia and CV collapse.

☑ Special considerations
• Advise safety measures for all ambulatory patients until response to diuretic is known.

• Patients taking cardiac glycosides are at increased risk for digitalis toxicity from potassium depletion.

• Patients with hepatic disease are especially susceptible to diuretic-induced electrolyte imbalance; in extreme cases, stupor, coma, and death can result.

COMPARING LOOP DIURETICS

Drug and route	Onset	Peak	Duration	Usual dosage
bumetanide				
I.V.	≤ 5 min	15 to 45 min	4 to 6 hr	0.5 to 1 mg ≤ t.i.d
P.O.	30 to 60 min	1 to 2 hr	½ to 1 hr	0.5 to 2 mg/day
ethacrynic acid				
I.V.	≤ 5 min	¼ to ½ hr	2 hr	50 mg/day
P.O.	≤ 30 min	2 hr	6 to 8 hr	50 to 100 mg/day
furosemide				
I.V.	≤ 5 min	½ to 1 hr	2 hr	20 to 40 mg q 2 hr, p.r.n.
P.O.	30 to 60 min	1 to 2 hr	6 to 8 hr	20 to 80 mg ≤ b.i.d.
torsemide				
I.V.	≤ 10 min	≤ 60 min	6 to 8 hr	5 to 20 mg/day
P.O.	≤ 60 min	60 to 120 min	6 to 8 hr	5 to 20 mg/day

• Consider possible dosage adjustment in the following circumstances: reduced dosage for patients with hepatic dysfunction; increased dosage in patients with renal impairment, oliguria, or decreased diuresis (inadequate urine output may result in circulatory overload, causing water intoxication, pulmonary edema, and heart failure); increased dosage of insulin or oral hypoglycemics in diabetic patients; and reduced dosage of other antihypertensives.

• Monitor blood pressure and pulse rate (especially during rapid diuresis), establish baseline values before therapy, and watch for significant changes.

• Establish baseline and periodically review CBC, including WBC count; serum electrolyte, carbon dioxide; magnesium; BUN and creatinine levels; and liver function test results.

• Diuretics should be taken in the morning so major diuresis occurs before bedtime. To prevent nocturia, don't prescribe diuretics for use after 6 p.m.

• Watch for signs of excessive diuresis (hypotension, tachycardia, poor skin turgor, and excessive thirst).

• Monitor patient for edema and ascites.

Information for the patient

• Explain the rationale for therapy and diuretic effect of these drugs (increased volume and frequency of urination).

• Teach patient signs of adverse effects, especially hypokalemia (weakness, fatigue, muscle cramps, paresthesia, confusion, nausea, vomiting, diarrhea, headache, dizziness, or palpitations), and importance of reporting such symptoms promptly.

• Advise patient to eat potassium-rich foods.

• Tell patient to report increased edema or weight or excess diuresis (more than 2-lb. [0.9-kg] weight loss per day).

• With initial doses, caution patient to change position slowly, especially when rising to upright position, to prevent dizziness from orthostatic hypotension.

• Instruct patient to call at once if he experiences chest, back, or leg pain; shortness of breath; or dyspnea.

• Inform patient that photosensitivity may occur. Caution patient to take protective measures, such as sunscreens and protective clothing, against exposure to ultraviolet light or sunlight.

Geriatric patients

• Elderly and debilitated patients need close observation because they are more susceptible to drug-induced diuresis. In elderly patients, excessive diuresis can quickly lead to dehydration, hypovolemia, hypokalemia, and hyponatremia and may cause circulatory collapse. Reduced dosages may be indicated.

Pediatric patients

• Use loop diuretics with caution in neonates; ethacrynic acid and ethacrynate sodium shouldn't be used in infants. The usual pediatric dose can be used, but dosing intervals should be extended.

Pregnant patients

• Safety during pregnancy is unknown. Avoid use if possible.

Breast-feeding patients

• Don't use loop diuretics in breast-feeding women.

Representative combinations
None.

---

diuretics, potassium-sparing

amiloride hydrochloride, spironolactone, triamterene

Potassium-sparing diuretics are less potent than many others; in particular, amiloride and triamterene have little clinical effect when used alone. However, they protect against potassium loss and are used with more potent diuretics. Spironolactone, an aldosterone antagonist, is particularly useful in patients with edema and hypertension associated with hyperaldosteronism.

Pharmacology
Amiloride and triamterene act directly on the distal renal tubules, inhibiting sodium reabsorption and potassium excretion, thereby reducing potassium loss. Spironolactone competitively inhibits aldosterone at the distal renal tubules, also promoting sodium excretion and potassium retention.

Clinical indications and actions
Edema
All potassium-sparing diuretics are used to manage edema associated with hepatic cirrhosis, nephrotic syndrome, and heart failure.
Hypertension
Amiloride and spironolactone are used to treat mild and moderate hypertension; the exact mechanism is unknown. Spironolactone may block the effect of aldosterone on arteriolar smooth muscle.
Diagnosis of primary hyperaldosteronism
Because spironolactone inhibits aldosterone, correction of hypokalemia and hypertension is presumptive evidence of primary hyperaldosteronism.
Other uses
Amiloride has been used to correct metabolic alkalosis produced by thiazide and other kaliuretic diuretics.
◊ Amiloride has been used with hydrochlorothiazide in patients with recurrent calcium nephrolithiasis.
◊ Amiloride has been used to manage lithium-induced polyuria secondary to lithium-induced nephrogenic diabetes insipidus.
Spironolactone has been used to aid in the treatment of hypokalemia and for prophylaxis of hypokalemia in patients taking cardiac glycosides.
◊ Spironolactone has been used in the treatment of precocious puberty, female hirsutism, and as an adjunct to treatment in myasthenia gravis and familial periodic paralysis.

Overview of adverse reactions
Hyperkalemia is the most important adverse reaction; it may occur with all drugs in this class and could lead to arrhythmias. Other adverse reactions include nausea, vomiting, headache, weakness, fatigue, bowel disturbances, cough, and dyspnea.

Potassium-sparing diuretics are contraindicated in patients with serum potassium levels above 5.5 mEq/L, in those receiving other potassium-sparing diuretics or potassium supplements, and in patients with anuria, acute or chronic renal insufficiency, diabetic nephropathy, or known hypersensitivity to the drug. They should be used cautiously in patients with severe hepatic insufficiency because electrolyte imbalance may precipitate hepatic encephalopathy, and in patients with diabetes, who are at increased risk of hyperkalemia.

☑ Special considerations
● Administer diuretics in morning to ensure that major diuresis occurs before bedtime. To prevent nocturia, don't prescribe diuretics for use after 6 p.m.
● Establish safety measures for ambulatory patients until response is known; diuretics may cause orthostatic hypotension, weakness, ataxia, and confusion.
● Consider possible dosage adjustments in the following circumstances: reduced dosages for patients with hepatic dysfunction and for those taking other antihypertensives; increased dosages for patients with renal impairment; and changes in insulin requirements for diabetic patients.
● Watch for hyperkalemia and arrhythmias; measure serum potassium and other electrolyte levels frequently, and check for significant changes. Monitor the following at baseline and at periodic intervals: CBC including WBC count; carbon dioxide, BUN, and creatinine levels; and especially liver function test results.
● Monitor vital signs, intake and output, weight, and blood pressure daily; check patient for edema, oliguria, or lack of diuresis, which may indicate drug tolerance.
● Monitor patient with hepatic disease in whom mild drug-induced acidosis may be hazardous; watch for mental confusion, lethargy, or stupor. Patients with hepatic disease are especially susceptible to diuretic-induced electrolyte imbalance; in extreme cases, coma and death can result.
● Watch for other signs of toxicity.

Information for the patient
● Explain signs and symptoms of possible adverse effects and importance of reporting unusual effect.
● Tell patient to report increased edema or weight or excess diuresis (more than 2-lb. [0.9-kg] weight loss per day) and to record weight each morning

after voiding and before dressing and breakfast, using same scale.
• Teach how to minimize dizziness from orthostatic hypotension by avoiding sudden postural changes.
• Advise patient to avoid potassium-rich food and potassium-containing salt substitutes or supplements, which increase the hazard of hyperkalemia.
• Advise patient to take drug at same time each morning to avoid interrupted sleep from nighttime diuresis.
• Advise patient to take drug with or after meals to minimize GI distress.
• Caution patient to avoid hazardous activities, such as driving or operating machinery, until response to drug is known.
• Tell patient to call before taking OTC drugs; many contain sodium and potassium and can cause electrolyte imbalance.

Geriatric patients
• Elderly and debilitated patients need close observation because they are more susceptible to drug-induced diuresis and hyperkalemia. Reduced dosages may be indicated.

Pediatric patients
• Children are more susceptible to hyperkalemia. If indicated, use drugs with caution.

Pregnant patients
• Safety during pregnancy is unknown.

Breast-feeding patients
• Drug may appear in breast milk. Safety hasn't been established.

Representative combinations
Amiloride with hydrochlorothiazide: Moduretic.
   Spironolactone with hydrochlorothiazide: Aldactazide.
   Triamterene with hydrochlorothiazide: Dyazide, Maxzide.

diuretics, thiazide

bendroflumethiazide, chlorothiazide, hydrochlorothiazide, hydroflumethiazide, methyclothiazide

diuretics, thiazide-like

chlorthalidone, indapamide, metolazone

Thiazide diuretics were discovered and synthesized as an outgrowth of studies on carbonic anhydrase inhibitors. Until the 1950s, organic mercurials were the only effective diuretics available;

though potent, they were also toxic. Introduction of the thiazides in 1957 proved a major advance because these were the first potent, and safe, diuretics.

Pharmacology
Thiazide diuretics interfere with sodium transport across tubules of the cortical diluting segment of the nephron, thereby increasing renal excretion of sodium, chloride, water, potassium, and calcium. Bicarbonate, magnesium, phosphate, bromide, and iodide excretion also increase. These drugs may also decrease excretion of ammonia, causing increased serum ammonia levels. Long-term thiazide therapy can cause mild metabolic alkalosis associated with hypokalemia and hypochloremia.

The exact mechanism of the antihypertensive effect of thiazides is unknown; however, it's thought to be partially caused by direct arteriolar dilatation. Thiazides initially decrease extracellular fluid volume, plasma volume, and cardiac output; extracellular fluid volume and plasma volume revert to near baseline levels in several weeks but remain slightly below normal. Cardiac output returns to normal or slightly above. Total body sodium remains slightly below pretreatment levels. Peripheral vascular resistance is initially elevated but falls below pretreatment levels with long-term diuretic therapy. (See *Comparing thiazide diuretics*, page 1174.)

In patients with diabetes insipidus, thiazides cause a paradoxical decrease in urine volume and increase in renal concentration of urine, possibly because of sodium depletion and decreased plasma volume, which leads to an increase in renal water and sodium reabsorption. In addition, thiazides can cause hyperglycemia, exacerbation of diabetes mellitus, or precipitation of diabetes mellitus.

Clinical indications and actions
Edema
Thiazide diuretics are used to treat edema associated with right-sided heart failure, mild to moderate left-sided heart failure, nephrotic syndrome and, with spironolactone, to treat edema and ascites secondary to hepatic cirrhosis. Thiazides may also be used to control edema during pregnancy except if caused by renal disease. This treatment isn't indicated for mild edema.

Efficacy and toxicity profiles of thiazide and thiazide-like diuretics are equivalent at comparable doses; the single exception is metolazone, which may be more effective in patients with impaired renal function. Usually, thiazide diuretics are less effective than loop diuretics in patients with renal insufficiency.
Hypertension
Thiazide diuretics are commonly used for initial management of all degrees of hypertension. Used alone, they reduce mean blood pressure by

COMPARING THIAZIDE DIURETICS

Drug	Equivalent dose	Onset	Peak	Duration
bendroflumethiazide	5 mg	Within 2 hr	4 hr	6 to 12 hr
chlorothiazide	500 mg	Within 2 hr	4 hr	6 to 12 hr
hydrochlorothiazide	50 mg	Within 2 hr	4 to 6 hr	6 to 12 hr
methyclothiazide	5 mg	Within 2 hr	4 to 6 hr	24 hr

10 to 15 mm Hg; in mild hypertension, thiazide diuresis alone will usually reduce blood pressure to desired levels. However, in moderate to severe hypertension that doesn't respond to thiazides alone, therapy with another antihypertensive is necessary.

◇ **Diabetes insipidus**
In diabetes insipidus, thiazides cause a paradoxical decrease in urine volume; urine becomes more concentrated, possibly because of sodium depletion and decreased plasma volume. Thiazides are particularly effective in nephrogenic diabetes insipidus.

◇ **Other uses**
Thiazides are used for prophylaxis of renal calculi formation associated with hypercalciuria and in the treatment of electrolyte disturbances associated with renal tubular necrosis.

Overview of adverse reactions
Therapeutic doses of thiazide diuretics cause electrolyte and metabolic disturbances, the most common being potassium depletion; patients may need dietary supplementation.

Other abnormalities include hypochloremic alkalosis, hypomagnesemia, hyponatremia, hypercalcemia, hyperuricemia, elevated cholesterol levels, and hyperglycemia. Overdose of thiazides may produce lethargy that can progress to coma within a few hours.

☑ Special considerations
• Thiazides and thiazide-like diuretics (except metolazone) are ineffective in patients with a glomerular filtration rate below 25 ml/minute.
• Because thiazides may cause adverse lipid effects, consider an alternative drug in patients with significant hyperlipidemia.
• Monitor intake and output, weight, and serum electrolyte levels regularly.
• Monitor serum potassium levels; consult a dietitian to provide high-potassium diet. Foods rich in potassium include citrus fruits, tomatoes, bananas, dates, and apricots. Watch for signs of hypokalemia (for example, muscle weakness or cramps). Patients also taking a cardiac glycoside have an increased risk of digitalis toxicity from the potassium-depleting effect of these diuretics.

• Thiazides may be used with potassium-sparing diuretics or potassium supplements to prevent potassium loss.
• Monitor blood glucose values in diabetic patients. Thiazides may cause hyperglycemia and a need to adjust insulin or oral hypoglycemic dosages.
• Monitor serum creatinine and BUN levels regularly. Drug isn't as effective if these levels are more than twice the normal limit.
• Monitor blood uric acid levels, especially in patients with history of gout; thiazides may cause an increase in uric acid levels.
• Advise patient to take drug in the morning to prevent nocturia.
• Antihypertensive effects last for about 1 week after stopping drug.

Information for the patient
• Explain rationale of therapy and diuretic effects of these drugs (increased volume and frequency of urination).
• Instruct patient to report joint swelling, pain, or redness; these signs may indicate hyperuricemia.
• Warn patient to call immediately if signs of electrolyte imbalance occur; these include weakness, fatigue, muscle cramps, paresthesia, confusion, nausea, vomiting, diarrhea, headache, dizziness, and palpitations.
• Tell patient to report increased edema, excess diuresis, or weight loss (more than a 2-lb. [0.9-kg] weight loss per day); advise him to record weight each morning after voiding and before dressing and breakfast, using the same scale.
• Advise patient to take drug with food to minimize gastric irritation, to eat potassium-rich foods, and not to add salt to other foods. Recommend use of salt substitutes.
• Tell patient to take drug only as prescribed and at the same time each day to prevent nighttime diuresis and interrupted sleep.
• Counsel patient to avoid smoking because nicotine increases blood pressure.
• Tell patient to call before taking OTC drugs.
• Warn patient about photosensitivity reactions.

With initial doses
- Caution patient to change position slowly, especially when rising to upright position, to prevent dizziness from orthostatic hypotension.
- Instruct patient to call immediately if he experiences chest, back, or leg pain; shortness of breath; or dyspnea.

Geriatric patients
- Elderly and debilitated patients need close observation and may require reduced dosages. They are more sensitive to excess diuresis because of age-related changes in CV and renal function. In elderly patients, excess diuresis can quickly lead to dehydration, hypovolemia, hyponatremia, hypomagnesemia, and hypokalemia.

Pediatric patients
- Safety and effectiveness in children haven't been established for all thiazide diuretics. Indapamide and metolazone aren't recommended for use in children.

Pregnant patients
- Thiazides cross the placenta and appear in cord blood. Benefits must be weighed against risks. Teratogenic effects may occur. Some clinicians recommend avoiding drug in the first trimester. Routine use isn't recommended if patient has mild edema.

Breast-feeding patients
- Thiazides appear in breast milk. Safety and effectiveness in breast-feeding women haven't been established.

Representative combinations
Chlorthalidone with atenolol: Atenolol/Chlorthalidone Tablets, Tenoretic; with reserpine: Regroton.
Hydrochlorothiazide with bisoprolol: Ziac Tablets; with deserpidine: Oreticyl; with guanethidine monosulfate: Esimil; with hydralazine: Apresazide, Hydrochlorothiazide/Hydralazine Caps; with hydralazine hydrochloride and reserpine: Hydrap-ES Tablets, Marpres Tablets, Tri-Hydroserpine Tablets; with methyldopa: Aldoril, Methyldopa/Hydrochlorothiazide Tablets; with propranolol: Inderide, Propranolol/Hydrochlorothiazide Tablets; with reserpine: Hydrochlorothiazide/Reserpine Tablets, Hydropres, Hydro-Serp, Hydroserpine; with hydralazine and reserpine: Ser-Ap-Es, Unipres; with spironolactone: Aldactazide; with timolol maleate: Timolide; with triamterene: Dyazide, Maxzide; with amiloride hydrochloride: Moduretic.
Hydroflumethiazide with reserpine: Salutensin Tablets.

estrogens

dienestrol, diethylstilbestrol, diethylstilbestrol diphosphate, esterified estrogens, estradiol, estradiol cypionate, estradiol valerate, estrogen and progestin, estrogenic substances (conjugated), estropipate, ethinyl estradiol

Estrogens were first discovered in the urine of humans and animals in 1930. Since then, numerous synthetic modifications of the naturally occurring estrogen molecules and completely synthetic estrogenic compounds have been developed.

Estrogens have several uses: treatment of symptoms of menopause, atrophic vaginitis, breast cancer, and other diseases; prophylaxis of osteoporosis; and contraception when used with progestins.

Pharmacology
Estrogens are hormones secreted by ovarian follicles and also by the adrenals, corpus luteum, placenta, and testes. Conjugated estrogens and estrogenic substances are normally obtained from the urine of pregnant mares. Other estrogens are manufactured synthetically. Of the six naturally occurring estrogens, three (estradiol, estrone, and estriol) are present in significant quantities.

Estrogens promote the development and maintenance of the female reproductive system and secondary sexual characteristics. Estrogens inhibit release of pituitary gonadotropins and also have various metabolic effects, including retention of fluid and electrolytes, retention and deposition in bone of calcium and phosphorus, and mild anabolic activity. They also increase high-density lipoproteins and decrease low-density lipoproteins.

Estrogens and estrogenic substances administered as drugs have effects related to endogenous estrogen's mechanism of action. They can mimic the action of endogenous estrogen when used as replacement therapy or produce such useful effects as inhibiting ovulation or inhibiting growth of certain hormone-sensitive cancers.

Use of estrogens isn't without risk. Long-term use is associated with an increased risk of endometrial cancer, gallbladder disease, and thromboembolic disease. Elevations in blood pressure often occur as well.

Clinical indications and actions

Moderate to severe vasomotor symptoms of menopause

Levels of endogenous estrogens are markedly reduced after menopause. This commonly results in vasomotor symptoms, such as hot flashes and dizziness. Diethylstilbestrol, estradiol cypionate, and ethinyl estradiol serve to mimic the action of endogenous estrogens in preventing these symptoms.

Atrophic vaginitis, kraurosis vulvae

Diethylstilbestrol stimulates development, cornification, and secretory activity in vaginal tissues.

Carcinoma of the breast

Conjugated estrogens, diethylstilbestrol, esterified estrogens, estradiol, and ethinyl estradiol inhibit the growth of hormone-sensitive cancers in certain carefully selected men and postmenopausal women.

Carcinoma of the prostate

Conjugated estrogens, diethylstilbestrol, esterified estrogens, estradiol, estradiol valerate, and ethinyl estradiol inhibit growth of hormone-sensitive cancer tissue in men with advanced disease.

Prophylaxis of postmenopausal osteoporosis

Conjugated estrogens replace or augment activity of endogenous estrogen in causing calcium and phosphate retention and preventing bone decalcification.

Contraception

Estrogens are used with progestins for ovulation control to prevent conception.

Overview of adverse reactions

Acute reactions: Changes in menstrual bleeding patterns (spotting, prolongation or absence of bleeding), abdominal cramps, swollen feet or ankles, bloated sensation (fluid and electrolyte retention), breast swelling and tenderness, weight gain, nausea, loss of appetite, headache, photosensitivity, loss of libido.

With long-term administration: Increased blood pressure (sometimes into the hypertensive range), thromboembolic disease, cholestatic jaundice, benign hepatomas. Risk of thromboembolic disease increases markedly with cigarette smoking, especially in women over age 35.

☑ Special considerations

● Don't use estrogens in patients with thrombophlebitis or thromboembolic disorders; cancer of the breast, reproductive organs, or genitals; or undiagnosed abnormal genital bleeding.

● Use with caution in patients with hypertension, asthma, mental depression, bone disease, blood dyscrasias, gallbladder disease, migraine, seizures, diabetes mellitus, amenorrhea, heart failure, hepatic or renal dysfunction, or a family history of breast or genital tract cancer. Develop ment or worsening of these conditions may require stopping drug.

● Give patient package insert describing estrogen adverse reactions; also provide verbal explanation.

● Monitor patients with diabetes mellitus for loss of diabetes control.

● If patient is receiving a warfarin-type anticoagulant, PT and INR must be monitored for anticoagulant dosage adjustment.

● Estrogen therapy is usually administered cyclically. The drugs are usually given once daily for 3 weeks, then 1 week without the drugs; this regimen is repeated as needed.

Information for the patient

● Warn patient to report adverse reactions immediately.

● Tell man on long-term therapy about possible gynecomastia and impotence.

● Explain to patient on cyclic therapy for postmenopausal symptoms that, although withdrawal bleeding may occur in week off drug, fertility hasn't been restored; ovulation doesn't occur.

● Diabetic patients should report symptoms of hyperglycemia or glycosuria.

● Tell woman who is planning to breast-feed not to take estrogens.

Geriatric patients

● Postmenopausal women with long-term estrogen use have an increased risk of endometrial cancer if they have a uterus. This risk can be reduced by adding a progestin to the regimen.

Pediatric patients

● Because of the effects of estrogen on epiphyseal closure, estrogens should be used with caution in adolescents whose bone growth isn't complete. Estrogens aren't used in children.

Pregnant patients

● Estrogens are contraindicated for use in pregnancy.

Breast-feeding patients

● Estrogens are contraindicated in breast-feeding women.

Representative combinations

Estradiol cypionate with testosterone cypionate and chlorobutanol: Depo-Testadiol, Duo-Cyp, Menoject, testosterone cypionate and estradiol cypionate, depAndrogyn, Depotestogen, Duratestin, Test-Estro Cypionate.

Estradiol valerate with testosterone enanthate: Deladumone, Delatestadiol, Teev, Testosterone Enanthate and Estradiol Valerate Injection, Valertest.

Estrogen with methyltestosterone: Estratest, Estratest H.S.

Estrogenic substances (conjugated) with meprobamate: Milprem, PMB; with methyltestosterone: Premarin with Methyltestosterone; with medroxyprogesterone: Premphase, Prempro.

Ethinyl estradiol with norethindrone: Brevicon, Genora 1/35, Jenest, Loestrin Fe 1.5/30, ModiCon, Nelova 1/35E, Ortho-Novum 1/35, Ortho-Novum 7/7/7, Ortho-Novum 10/11; with norgestimate: Cyclen; with ethynodiol diacetate: Demulen 1/35, Demulen 1/50; with desogestrel: Desogen, Marvelon; with norgestrel: Lo/Ovral, Ovral; with levonorgestrel: Levlen, Min-Ovral, Nordette, Tri-Levlen, Triphasil, Triquilar.

Ethynodiol diacetate with ethinyl estradiol: Demulen 1/35, Demulen 1/50.

fluoroquinolones

ciprofloxacin, enoxacin, lomefloxacin, norfloxacin, ofloxacin, levofloxacin, sparfloxacin, trovafloxacin mesylate

Fluoroquinolones are broad-spectrum, systemic antibacterial drugs active against a wide range of aerobic gram-positive and gram-negative organisms. Gram-positive aerobic bacteria include *Staphylococcus aureus, S. epidermis, S. saprophyticus, S. hemolyticus,* penicillinase- and non-penicillinase-producing staphylococci as well as some methicillin-resistant strains; *Streptococcus pneumoniae;* group A (beta) hemolytic streptococci *(S. pyogenes);* group B streptococci *(S. agalactiae);* alpha hemolytic streptococci; groups C, F, and G streptococci and nonenterococcal group D streptococci; and *Enterococcus faecalis.*

Fluoroquinolones are active against gram-positive aerobic bacilli, including *Corynebacterium, Listeria monocytogenes,* and *Nocardia asteroides.* They are effective against gram-negative aerobic bacteria including, but not limited to, *Neisseria meningitidis* and most strains of penicillinase- and non-penicillinase-producing *N. gonorrhoeae, Haemophilus influenzae, H. parainfluenzae, H. ducreyi, Moraxella catarrhalis* and, most clinically important, *Enterobacteriaceae, Pseudomonas aeruginosa, Vibrio cholerae,* and *V. parahaemolyticus.*

Certain fluoroquinolones are active against *Chlamydia trachomatis, Mycoplasma hominis, Mycoplasma pneumoniae, Legionella pneumophila,* and *Mycobacterium avium-intracellulare.*

Pharmacology

Fluoroquinolones produce a bactericidal effect by inhibiting intracellular DNA topoisomerase II (DNA gyrase) or topoisomerase IV. These enzymes are essential catalysts in the duplication, transcription, and repair of bacterial DNA.

Clinical indications and actions

Fluoroquinolones are indicated for the treatment of the following infections when caused by susceptible organisms: bone and joint infections, bacterial bronchitis, endocervical and urethral chlamydial infections, bacterial gastroenteritis, endocervical and urethral gonorrhea, intra-abdominal infections, pelvic inflammatory disease, bacterial pneumonia, bacterial prostatitis, acute sinusitis, skin and soft-tissue infections, typhoid fever, bacterial urinary tract infections, chancroid, meningococcal carriers, and bacterial septicemia. Fluoroquinolones may be used for the prevention of bacterial urinary tract infections and as empiric therapy for febrile neutropenia.

Overview of adverse reactions

CNS stimulation (acute psychosis, agitation, hallucinations, tremors), hepatotoxicity, hypersensitivity reactions, interstitial nephritis, phlebitis, pseudomembranous colitis, and tendinitis or tendon rupture are observed rarely but require medical attention.

CNS adverse effects (dizziness, headache, nervousness, drowsiness, insomnia), gastrointestinal reactions, and photosensitivity may occur but don't require medical attention unless they persist or become intolerable.

☑ Special considerations

• The risk-benefit ratio of therapy with fluoroquinolones should be considered on an individual basis when any of the following conditions are present: seizure disorders, cerebral ischemia, severe hepatic dysfunction, or renal insufficiency.
• Monitor renal and liver function test results in patients with impaired renal or hepatic function.
• Achilles and other tendon ruptures have been reported. Stop drug if patient experiences pain, inflammation, or rupture of a tendon.

Information for the patient

• Instruct patient to take drug as prescribed and to complete full course of therapy.
• Tell patient to take drug with an 8-oz (240-ml) glass of water.
• Advise patient that enoxacin and norfloxacin should be taken on an empty stomach.
• Instruct patient that if a dose is missed, the next dose should be taken as soon as possible; tell him not to double the dose.
• Advise patient to avoid antacids or sucralfate while taking oral fluoroquinolones.
• Tell patient taking fluoroquinolones to call before using other drugs.

Geriatric patients

• Adverse reactions haven't occurred in this age-group. However, because renal function deteriorates over time, elderly patients may need a reduction in daily dose.

Pediatric patients
- Fluoroquinolones aren't recommended for use in children because they can cause joint problems.

Pregnant patients
- Pregnancy risk category C. Effects during pregnancy aren't fully known. These drugs cross the placenta and may cause arthropathies.

Breast-feeding patients
- Fluoroquinolones may appear in breast milk. Use in breast-feeding women isn't recommended.

Representative combinations
None.

histamine (H)₂-receptor antagonists

cimetidine, famotidine, nizatidine, ranitidine, ranitidine bismuth citrate

The introduction of H₂-receptor antagonists has revolutionized the treatment of peptic ulcer disease. These drugs structurally resemble histamine and competitively inhibit histamine's action on gastric H₂ receptors. Cimetidine, approved for clinical use in 1977, is the prototype of this class.

Pharmacology
All H₂-receptor antagonists inhibit histamine's action at H₂ receptors in gastric parietal cells, reducing gastric acid output and concentration regardless of the stimulant (histamine, food, insulin, caffeine, betazole, pentagastrin) or basal conditions.

Clinical indications and actions
Duodenal ulcer
Cimetidine, famotidine, nizatidine, and ranitidine are used to treat acute duodenal ulcer and to prevent ulcer recurrence. Ranitidine bismuth citrate is used with clarithromycin to treat active duodenal ulcer associated with *Helicobacter pylori* infection.
Gastric ulcer
Cimetidine, famotidine, nizatidine, and ranitidine are indicated for acute gastric ulcer. However, the benefits of long-term therapy (over 8 weeks) with these drugs remain unproven.
Hypersecretory states
Cimetidine, famotidine, nizatidine, and ranitidine are used to treat hypersecretory states such as Zollinger-Ellison syndrome. Because patients with these conditions need much higher doses than patients with peptic ulcer disease, they may experience more pronounced adverse effects.

Reflux esophagitis
Cimetidine, famotidine, nizatidine, and ranitidine are used to provide short-term relief from gastroesophageal reflux in patients who don't respond to conventional therapy (lifestyle changes, antacids, diet modification). They act by raising the stomach pH. Some clinicians prefer to combine the H₂-receptor antagonist with metoclopramide, but further study is needed to confirm effectiveness of the combination.
◊ **Stress ulcer prophylaxis**
Cimetidine, famotidine, nizatidine, and ranitidine are used to prevent stress ulcers in critically ill patients, particularly those in intensive care units. However, some health care providers prefer intensive antacid therapy for such patients.
◊ **Other uses**
H₂-receptor antagonists have been used for short-bowel syndrome, for prophylaxis for allergic reactions to I.V. contrast medium, and to eradicate *Helicobacter pylori* in treatment of peptic ulcers. Ranitidine bismuth citrate with clarithromycin is used to treat *H. pylori*.

H₂-receptor antagonists also may be used for relief of occasional heartburn, acid indigestion, or sour stomach.

Overview of adverse reactions
H₂-receptor antagonists rarely cause adverse reactions. However, mild transient diarrhea, neutropenia, dizziness, fatigue, arrhythmias, and gynecomastia have been reported.

Cimetidine may inhibit hepatic enzymes, thereby impairing the metabolism of certain drugs. Ranitidine may also produce this effect, but to a lesser extent. Famotidine and nizatidine haven't been shown to inhibit hepatic enzymes or drug clearance.

☑ Special considerations
- Give single daily dose at bedtime, twice-daily doses morning and evening, and multiple doses with meals and at bedtime. Most clinicians prefer the once-daily dose at bedtime regimen for improved compliance.
- When administering drugs I.V., don't exceed recommended infusion rates because this may increase the risk of adverse CV effects. Continuous I.V. infusion may yield better suppression of acid secretion.
- Because antacids may decrease drug absorption, give them at least 1 hour apart from H₂-receptor antagonists.
- Patients with renal disease may need a modified schedule.
- Avoid stopping these drugs abruptly.
- Many investigational uses for these drugs (particularly cimetidine) are being evaluated. Ranitidine bismuth citrate shouldn't be prescribed alone for the treatment of active duodenal ulcers.
- Symptomatic response to therapy doesn't rule out gastric malignancy.

• Tagamet may result in reversible decreased sperm levels in men.

Information for the patient
• Instruct patient to avoid smoking during therapy because smoking stimulates gastric acid secretion and worsens the disease.

Geriatric patients
• Use caution when administering these drugs to elderly patients because of the increased risk of adverse reactions, particularly those affecting the CNS. Dosage adjustment is needed in patients with impaired renal function.

Pediatric patients
• Safety and efficacy in children haven't been established.

Pregnant patients
• Effects of these drugs in pregnant women aren't fully known.

Breast-feeding patients
• H_2-receptor antagonists may appear in breast milk. Benefit-to-risk ratio must be considered.

Representative combinations
None.

HMG-CoA reductase inhibitors

atorvastatin, cerivastatin, fluvastatin, lovastatin, pravastatin, simvastatin

The 3-hydroxy-3-methyl-glutaryl-coenzyme A (HMG-CoA) reductase inhibitors, also known as the statins, are a highly effective drug class that has become first-line pharmacologic therapy for the management of hypercholesterolemia.

Pharmacology
The statins lower cholesterol by competitively inhibiting the enzyme HMG-CoA reductase. This is an enzyme that catalyzes the conversion of HMG-CoA to mevalonate, which is an early rate-limiting step in cholesterol biosynthesis. The statins decrease low-density lipoprotein cholesterol (LDL-C), total cholesterol (total-C), apoprotein B (apo-B), very low-density lipoprotein (VLDL) cholesterol, and plasma triglycerides, and increase high-density lipoprotein cholesterol (HDL-C).

Coronary artery disease may be caused by increased levels of total cholesterol, apoprotein B, and LDL cholesterol as well as by decreased levels of HDL cholesterol. In addition, cardiovascular morbidity and mortality have been shown to vary directly with the level of total-C and

LDL-C, and inversely with the level of HDL-C. The mechanism by which the statins lower LDL-C may be related to both a reduction of VLDL cholesterol and an induction of the LDL receptor, which result in reduced synthesis or increased breakdown of LDL-C.

The statins are highly effective at lowering total-C and LDL-C in patients with heterozygous familial and nonfamilial forms of hypercholesterolemia. Initial cholesterol-lowering effects are seen within 1 to 2 weeks, with maximum lowering effects observed within 4 to 6 weeks. Because cholesterol synthesis occurs mainly at night, single daily doses of statins (except atorvastatin) should be given in the evening or at bedtime. Lovastatin should be taken with the evening meal because food increases its absorption.

Clinical indications and actions
All of the statins are indicated for the treatment of primary hypercholesterolemia. All except fluvastatin are indicated for mixed dyslipidemia. Atorvastatin is indicated for hypertriglyceridemia and primary dysbetalipoproteinemia. Atorvastatin and simvastatin are indicated for homozygous familial hyperlipidemia. Pravastatin is indicated for the primary prevention of coronary events. All the statins except atorvastatin and cerivastatin are indicated for the secondary prevention of cardiovascular events.

The efficacy of the statins in these disorders is related to their effects on total-C, LDL-C, apo-B, VLDL cholesterol, triglycerides, and HDL-C. The statins work by competitively inhibiting HMG-CoA reductase.

◊ **Other uses**
Lovastatin is used to treat diabetic dyslipidemia, nephrotic hyperlipidemia, neck artery disease, familial beta dysbetalipoproteinemia, and familial combined hyperlipidemia.

Pravastatin is used to treat heterozygous familial hypercholesterolemia, diabetic dyslipidemia in type 2 diabetes mellitus, hypercholesterolemia secondary to the nephrotic syndrome, homozygous familial hypercholesterolemia in patients with reduced LDL receptor activity.

Simvastatin is used to treat heterozygous familial hypercholesterolemia, familial combined hyperlipidemia, diabetic dyslipidemia in type 2 diabetes mellitus, hyperlipidemia secondary to the nephrotic syndrome, and homozygous familial hypercholesterolemia in patients with defective LDL receptors.

Overview of adverse reactions
The statins are well tolerated and have very few adverse effects. About 1% to 3% of patients discontinue therapy because of adverse effects. The most common reasons for stopping therapy are asymptomatic increases in serum transaminase levels and mild, nonspecific GI adverse effects.

Photosensitivity and hepatotoxicity may occasionally occur. Transient and mild increase in CK levels may also occur.

About 0.1% to 0.5% of patients taking lovastatin develop a myopathy, characterized by myalgia, or muscle weakness associated with CK levels more than 10 times the upper limit of normal.

Lovastatin and simvastatin may cause insomnia.

Although rare, a hypersensitivity syndrome may occur characterized by one or more of the following: anaphylaxis, angioedema, lupus-like syndrome, polymyalgia rheumatica, vasculitis, purpura, thrombocytopenia, leukopenia, hemolytic anemia, positive antinuclear antibodies, an increased erythrocyte sedimentation rate, eosinophilia, arthritis, asthenia, photosensitivity, fever, chills, flushing, malaise, dyspnea, toxic epidermal necrolysis, erythema multiforme, and dermatomyositis.

☑ Special considerations:

• Statins are contraindicated in patients with active liver disease or unexplained persistent elevations of liver function test results.

• Statins should be used with caution in patients who consume large quantities of alcohol and in patients with a history of liver disease.

• Liver function test results should be monitored before the initiation of statins, at 6 and 12 weeks after initiation of treatment, after a dosage adjustment, and periodically (semiannually) thereafter. Stop drug if AST level increases more than three times the upper limit of normal.

• Patients with renal insufficiency taking pravastatin should be monitored closely.

• The absorption of lovastatin increases with food; patient should take with evening meal. All other statins, except atorvastatin, may be taken without regard to meals, but should be taken in the evening or at bedtime because most cholesterol synthesis occurs during the night.

• The risk of myopathy increases when statins are taken with cyclosporine, erythromycin, gemfibrozil, fibric acid derivatives, azole antifungals, or lipid-lowering doses of niacin. Because of increased risk of myopathy, avoid concurrent use of statins and fibrates.

• Consider myopathy in any patient with diffuse myalgias, muscle tenderness, weakness, or CK levels more than 10 times the upper limit of normal. Drug should be stopped if markedly elevated CK levels occur or if myopathy is suspected. Don't exceed 20 mg/day of lovastatin or 10 mg/day of simvastatin in patients taking cyclosporine or itraconazole.

• Consider withholding or stopping statins in patients with risk factors for renal failure secondary to rhabdomyolysis, including severe acute infection, sepsis, hypotension, major surgery, trauma, uncontrolled seizures, and severe metabolic, endocrine, or electrolyte disorders.

Information for the patient

• Warn patient that statin drugs may cause photosensitivity; tell him to avoid prolonged exposure to sun and other sources of ultraviolet light, to wear protective clothing, and to use sunscreens until tolerance is determined.

• Instruct woman of childbearing age on the potential hazards of statin drugs in pregnancy. Tell patient to stop drug immediately and to call if she becomes pregnant.

• Tell patient to promptly call if he experiences any unexplained muscle pain, tenderness, or weakness, especially if accompanied by malaise or fever.

• Instruct patient on the importance of adhering to dietary recommendations.

• Tell patient that lovastatin should be taken with the evening meal and that fluvastatin, pravastatin, and simvastatin may be taken without regard to meals but should be taken in the evening or at bedtime for best results. Tell patient that atorvastatin may be taken without regard to meals and at anytime of the day.

Geriatric patients

• Plasma levels don't vary with age for cerivastatin, fluvastatin, and atorvastatin. In patients over age 70, the adequate area under the curve increases with lovastatin and simvastatin. For pravastatin, patients over age 65 show a greater effect on LDL-C, total-C, and LDL-HDL ratio compared to patients below age 65.

Pediatric patients

• Safety and efficacy in children below age 18 haven't been established; use isn't recommended. Atorvastatin in doses up to 80 mg/day for 1 year has been used in 8 children, none below age 9, with homozygous familial hypercholesterolemia. No problems were noted.

Pregnant patients

• Pregnancy risk category X. Contraindicated during pregnancy. Cholesterol is essential for fetal development; drugs that inhibit cholesterol synthesis may have adverse effects on the developing fetus. If a woman becomes pregnant while taking a statin, stop drug immediately.

Breast-feeding patients

• The statins appear in breast milk. Because of the potential adverse effects on infant, don't use in breast-feeding women.

Representative combinations
None.

nitrates

amyl nitrite, isosorbide dinitrate, isosorbide mononitrate, nitroglycerin

Nitrates have been recognized as effective vasodilators for more than 100 years. The best known drug of this group, nitroglycerin, remains the therapeutic mainstay for classic and variant angina. With the availability of an I.V. nitroglycerin form, the drug's use in reducing afterload and preload in various cardiac disorders has been generated renewed enthusiasm. Various other dosage forms of nitroglycerin and other nitrates also are available, thereby improving and extending their clinical usefulness.

Pharmacology

The major pharmacologic property of nitrates is vascular smooth muscle relaxation, resulting in generalized vasodilation. Venous effects predominate; however, nitroglycerin produces dose-dependent dilation of both arterial and venous beds. Nitrates are metabolized to a free radical nitric oxide, thought to be an endothelium-derived relaxing factor (EDRF), which is usually impaired in patients with coronary artery disease. Decreased peripheral venous resistance results in venous pooling of blood and decreased venous return to the heart (preload); decreased arteriolar resistance reduces systemic vascular resistance and arterial pressure (afterload). These vascular effects lead to reduction of myocardial oxygen consumption, promoting a more favorable oxygen supply-to-demand ratio. (Although nitrates reflexively increase heart rate and myocardial contractility, reduced ventricular wall tension results in a net decrease in myocardial oxygen consumption.) In the coronary circulation, nitrates redistribute circulating blood flow along collateral channels and preferentially increase subendocardial blood flow, improving perfusion to the ischemic myocardium.

Nitrates relax all smooth muscle—not just vascular smooth muscle—regardless of autonomic innervation, including bronchial, biliary, GI, ureteral, and uterine smooth muscle.

Clinical indications and actions
Angina pectoris

By relaxing vascular smooth muscle in both the venous and arterial beds, nitrates cause a net decrease in myocardial oxygen consumption; by dilating coronary vessels, they lead to redistribution of blood flow to ischemic tissue. Although systemic and coronary vascular effects may vary slightly, depending on which nitrate is used, both smooth muscle relaxation and vasodilation probably account for nitrates' value in treating angi-

na. Because individual nitrates have similar pharmacologic and therapeutic properties, the best nitrate to use in a specific situation depends mainly on the onset of action and duration of effect needed.

Sublingual nitroglycerin is considered the drug of choice to treat acute angina pectoris because of its rapid onset of action, relatively low cost, and well-established effectiveness. Lingual or buccal nitroglycerin and other rapidly acting nitrates (amyl nitrite and sublingual or chewable isosorbide dinitrate) also may prove useful for this indication. Amyl nitrite is rarely used because it's expensive, inconvenient, and carries a high risk of adverse effects. Sublingual, lingual, or buccal nitroglycerin or sublingual or chewable isosorbide dinitrate typically prove effective in circumstances likely to provoke an angina attack.

Long-acting nitrates and beta blockers usually are considered the drugs of choice for prophylaxis of angina pectoris. Nitrates with a relatively long duration of effect include oral preparations of isosorbide mononitrate, pentaerythritol tetranitrate, and oral or topical nitroglycerin.

The effectiveness of oral nitrates is debatable, although isosorbide dinitrate and nitroglycerin generally are now considered effective. However, the effectiveness of pentaerythritol tetranitrate and topical nitroglycerin preparations hasn't been fully determined. Some experts believe oral nitrates are ineffective or less effective than rapidly acting I.V. nitrates in reducing frequency of angina and increasing exercise tolerance. Also, prolonged use of oral nitrates may cause cross-tolerance to sublingual nitrates.

I.V. nitroglycerin may be used to treat unstable angina pectoris, Prinzmetal's angina, and angina pectoris in patients who haven't responded to recommended doses of nitrates or a beta blocker.

Sedatives may be useful in the adjunctive management of angina pectoris associated with psychogenic factors. However, if combination therapy is needed, each drug should be adjusted individually; fixed combinations of oral nitrates and sedatives should be avoided.

Acute MI

The hemodynamic effects of I.V., sublingual, or topical nitroglycerin may prove beneficial in treating left-sided heart failure and pulmonary congestion associated with acute MI. However, the drugs' effects on morbidity and mortality in patients with these conditions are controversial.

I.V., sublingual, and topical nitroglycerin and isosorbide dinitrate are effective adjunctive drugs in managing acute and chronic heart failure. Sublingual administration can quickly reverse the signs and symptoms of pulmonary congestion in acute pulmonary edema; however, the I.V. form may control hemodynamic status more accurately.

Other uses

I.V. nitroglycerin is used to control perioperative hypertension, hypertensive emergencies, heart failure, and pulmonary edema associated with MI.

◊ I.V. nitroglycerin has been used to treat severe hypertension, hypertensive crises; other forms have been used to treat refractory heart failure. Nitroglycerin also has been used for relief of pain, dysphagia, and spasm in patients with diffuse esophageal spasm without gastroesophageal reflux.

Overview of adverse reactions

Headache is most common early in therapy; it may be severe, but usually diminishes rapidly. Orthostatic hypotension, dizziness, weakness, and transient flushing may occur. In patients sensitive to hypotensive effects, nausea, vomiting, weakness, restlessness, pallor, cold sweats, tachycardia, syncope, or CV collapse may occur. Dosage reduction may control GI upset; therapy should be discontinued if blurred vision, dry mouth, or rash develops. Tolerance and dependence can occur with repeated, prolonged use.

Tolerance to both the vascular and antianginal effects of the drugs can develop, and cross-tolerance between the nitrates and nitrites has been demonstrated. Tolerance is associated with a high or sustained plasma drug level and occurs with oral, I.V., and topical therapy. It rarely occurs with intermittent sublingual use. However, patients taking oral isosorbide dinitrate or topical nitroglycerin haven't exhibited cross-tolerance to sublingual nitroglycerin.

To prevent tolerance, the lowest effective dose and an intermittent dosing schedule should be used. A nitrate-free interval of 10 to 12 hours daily may also be helpful.

☑ Special considerations

Oral form

● Provide a dosage regimen that incorporates a 10- to 12-hour nitrate-free interval.

● Best absorption will occur if taken on an empty stomach (1 hour before or 2 hours after meals) and with a full glass of water.

● Dosage should be adjusted to patient response. Patients should avoid switching brands after they are stabilized on a particular formulation.

Buccal form

● The tablet should be placed between the upper lip or cheek and gum.

● Dissolution rate varies, but will usually range from 3 to 5 hours. Hot liquids will increase dissolution rate and should be avoided.

● Patient shouldn't use buccal form at bedtime because of risk of aspiration.

Sublingual form

● Only the sublingual and translingual forms should be used to relieve acute angina attack. Although a burning sensation was formerly an indication of drug's potency, many current preparations don't produce this sensation.

Translingual spray

● Only the sublingual and translingual forms should be used to relieve acute angina attack. The translingual form should be sprayed onto or under the tongue. Patient shouldn't inhale the spray.

Topical form

● To apply ointment, spread in uniform thin layer to any hairless part of the skin except distal parts of arms and legs (absorption won't be maximal at these sites). Don't rub in. Cover with plastic film to aid absorption and to protect clothing. If using Tape-Surrounded Appli-Ruler (TSAR) system, keep TSAR on skin to protect patient's clothing and ensure that ointment remains in place. If serious adverse reactions develop in patients using ointment or transdermal system, remove product at once or wipe ointment from skin. Avoid contact with ointment.

● Remove transdermal patch before defibrillation. Because of the patch's aluminum backing, electric current may cause patch to explode.

● Don't administer with sildenafil (Viagra).

Information for the patient

● Instruct patient to avoid alcohol while taking nitrates because severe hypotension and CV collapse may occur.

● Instruct patient to sit when taking nitrates to prevent injury from transient episodes of dizziness, syncope, or other signs of cerebral ischemia that the drug may cause.

● Advise patient to treat headache with aspirin or acetaminophen.

● Tell patient to report blurred vision, dry mouth, or persistent headache.

● Warn patient not to stop taking drug abruptly because this may cause withdrawal symptoms.

Pediatric patients

● Safety and effectiveness in children haven't been established.

Pregnant patients

● Pregnancy risk category C. Safety during pregnancy isn't adequately known. Use only if clearly indicated.

Breast-feeding patients

● It's unknown if drug appears in breast milk; use with caution in breast-feeding women.

Representative combinations

None.

nonsteroidal anti-inflammatory drugs (NSAIDs)

celecoxib, choline magnesium salicylate, diclofenac potassium, diclofenac sodium, diflunisal, etodolac, fenoprofen calcium, flurbiprofen sodium, ibuprofen, indomethacin, indomethacin sodium trihydrate, ketoprofen, ketorolac meclofenamate, mefenamic acid, tromethamine, nabumetone, naproxen, naproxen sodium, oxaprozin, piroxicam, rofecoxib, salsalate, sulindac, tolmetin sodium

NSAIDs are a growing class of drugs that are prescribed widely for their analgesic and anti-inflammatory effects; some members of this class have an antipyretic effect.

Pharmacology

The analgesic effect of NSAIDs may result from interference with the prostaglandins involved in pain. Prostaglandins appear to sensitize pain receptors to mechanical stimulation or to other chemical mediators (e.g., bradykinin and histamine). NSAIDs inhibit synthesis of prostaglandins peripherally and possibly centrally. Their anti-inflammatory action also may contribute indirectly to their analgesic effect.

Like the salicylates, the anti-inflammatory effects of NSAIDs may result in part from inhibition of prostaglandin synthesis and release during inflammation. The exact mechanism has not been established, but the anti-inflammatory effect of NSAIDs correlates with their ability to inhibit prostaglandin synthesis.

The antipyretic effect may be due to suppression of prostaglandin synthesis in the CNS (probably the hypothalamus).

Clinical indications and actions

NSAIDs are used principally for symptomatic relief of pain and inflammation. These drugs usually provide temporary relief of mild to moderate pain, especially that associated with inflammation. NSAIDs are used to treat low-intensity pain of headache, arthralgia, myalgia, neuralgia, and mild to moderate pain from dental or surgical procedures or dysmenorrhea.

Oral NSAIDs also are used for long-term treatment of rheumatoid arthritis, juvenile arthritis, and osteoarthritis. In osteoarthritis, NSAIDs are used primarily for analgesia. NSAIDs offer only symptomatic treatment for rheumatoid conditions, and don't reverse or arrest the disease process. NSAIDs reduce pain, stiffness, swelling, and tenderness.

Overview of adverse reactions

Adverse reactions to oral NSAIDs chiefly involve the GI tract, particularly erosion of the gastric mucosa. Most common symptoms are dyspepsia,. heartburn, epigastric distress, nausea, and abdominal pain. GI symptoms usually occur in the first few days of therapy, and often subside with continuous treatment. They can be minimized by giving NSAIDs with meals or food, antacids, or large quantities of water or milk.

CNS adverse effects (headache, dizziness, drowsiness) also may occur. Flank pain with other signs and symptoms of nephrotoxicity occasionally has been reported. Fluid retention may aggravate preexisting hypertension or heart failure. NSAIDs shouldn't be used in patients with renal insufficiency.

☑ Special considerations

● Use NSAIDs cautiously in patients with history of GI disease, increased risk of GI bleeding, or decreased renal function.
● Patients with known "triad" symptoms (aspirin hypersensitivity, rhinitis or nasal polyps, and asthma) are at high risk of bronchospasm.
● NSAIDs may mask the signs and symptoms of acute infection.
● Administer oral NSAIDs with a full 8-oz (240-ml) glass of water to assure adequate passage into stomach.
● Tablets may be crushed and mixed with food or fluids to aid swallowing, and with antacids to minimize gastric upset.
● Watch for signs and symptoms of bleeding. Assess bleeding time if surgery is needed.
● Monitor ophthalmic and auditory function before and periodically during therapy to prevent toxicity.
● Monitor CBC, platelets, PT, and hepatic and renal function studies periodically to detect abnormalities.
● Use of an NSAID with an opioid analgesic has an additive effect. Lower doses of the opioid analgesic may be possible.

Information for the patient

● Tell patient to take drug with 8 oz (240 ml) of water 30 minutes before or 2 hours after meals, or with food or milk if gastric irritation occurs.
● Explain that taking drug as directed is necessary to achieve the desired effect; 2 to 4 weeks of treatment may be needed before benefit is seen.
● Advise patient on long-term NSAID therapy to arrange for monitoring of laboratory parameters, especially BUN and serum creatinine levels, liver function test results, and CBC.
● Warn patient with current rectal bleeding or history of rectal bleeding to avoid using rectal NSAID suppositories. Because they must be retained in the rectum for at least 1 hour, they may cause irritation and bleeding.

• Warn patient that use of alcoholic beverages while on NSAID therapy may cause increased GI irritation and, possibly, GI bleeding.

Geriatric patients
• Patients over age 60 may be more susceptible to the toxic effects of NSAIDs because of decreased renal function, resulting in NSAID accumulation.
• The effects of NSAIDs on renal prostaglandins may cause fluid retention and edema, a significant drawback for elderly patients, especially those with heart failure.

Pediatric patients
• Don't use long-term NSAID therapy in children under age 14; safety in this age-group hasn't been established.

Pregnant patients
• Pregnant patients should avoid all NSAIDs, especially during the third trimester when prostaglandin inhibition may cause prolonged gestation, dystocia, and delayed parturition.

Breast-feeding patients
• Most NSAIDs appear in breast milk; NSAID therapy isn't recommended during breast-feeding.

Representative combinations
Diclofenac sodium and misoprostol: Arthrotec.

---

nucleoside reverse transcriptase inhibitors

didanosine, lamivudine, stavudine, zalcitabine

Nucleoside reverse transcriptase inhibitors are antivirals that act specifically against HIV.

Pharmacology
These drugs suppress HIV replication by inhibition of HIV DNA polymerase. Competitive inhibition of nucleoside reverse transcriptase inhibits DNA viral replication by chain termination, competitive inhibition of reverse transcriptase, or both.

Clinical indications and actions
Nucleoside reverse transcriptase inhibitors are indicated for the treatment of HIV infection or AIDS. These drugs may also be used for the prevention of maternal-fetal HIV transmission and of HIV infection after occupational exposure (such as needlesticks or other parenteral exposures).

Overview of adverse reactions
Because of the complexity of HIV infection, it's often difficult to distinguish between disease-related symptoms and adverse drug reactions.

The most frequently reported adverse effects of nucleoside reverse transcriptase inhibitors are anemia, leukopenia, and neutropenia. Thrombocytopenia occurs less frequently.

Rare adverse effects include hepatotoxicity, myopathy, and neurotoxicity. The occurrence of any of these adverse effects requires prompt medical attention. The following adverse effects don't need medical attention unless they persist or are bothersome: headache, severe insomnia, myalgias, nausea, or hyperpigmentation of nails.

☑ Special considerations
• The risk-benefit ratio of therapy with nucleoside reverse transcriptase inhibitors should be considered on an individual basis when any of the following conditions are present: alcoholism, cardiac disease, hypertriglyceridemia, pancreatitis, bone marrow suppression, fluid overload, folic acid or vitamin B_{12} deficiency, liver dysfunction, peripheral neuropathy, or renal or hepatic dysfunction. These conditions may predispose the patient to adverse drug reactions during treatment.
• The bone marrow suppressant action of these drugs may cause increased susceptibility to certain microbial infections; this effect may be accentuated by other drugs that also cause bone marrow suppression.

Information for the patient
• Tell patient to take drug as prescribed; not to take more or less than instructed; and to finish the full course.
• Instruct patient not to miss a dose. If a dose is missed, he should take the next dose as soon as possible, but he shouldn't double the dose.
• Advise patient to adhere to follow-up appointments because blood tests are needed to evaluate the response to drug.
• Tell patient to call before taking other drugs.
• Instruct patient to floss and brush teeth carefully to prevent bleeding from gums.
• Tell patient to avoid sexual intercourse or to use a condom to decrease the risk of HIV transmission.

Geriatric patients
• Safety and effectiveness of these drugs in elderly patients are unknown. Anecdotal evidence suggests that elderly patients respond well to this therapy, but that they may experience a more prolonged half-life of elimination.

Pediatric patients
• Nucleoside reverse transcriptase inhibitors may be used in children ages 3 months and older. The half-life of these drugs may be prolonged in newborns; otherwise the drugs' pharmacokinetic and safety profiles children and adults are similar.

Pregnant patients
● Pregnancy risk category C (didanosine, B). The risk of HIV transmission to fetus is decreased when these drugs are used during pregnancy. There is no evidence of teratogenicity or ill effects in newborns. Drug crosses placenta and decreases perinatal transmission of HIV.

Breast-feeding patients
● It's unknown if these drugs appear in breast milk. Use in breast-feeding mothers isn't recommended. Risks and benefits to mother and infant must be considered in each case.

Representative combinations
Lamivudine and zidovudine: Combivir.

opioids

alfentanil hydrochloride, codeine phosphate, codeine sulfate, difenoxin hydrochloride, diphenoxylate hydrochloride, fentanyl citrate, hydrocodone hydromorphone hydrochloride, levomethadyl acetate hydrochloride, meperidine hydrochloride, methadone hydrochloride, morphine sulfate, oxycodone hydrochloride, oxymorphone hydrochloride, propoxyphene hydrochloride, propoxyphene napsylate, remifentanil hydrochloride, sufentanil citrate

Opioids, previously called narcotic agonists, are usually understood to include natural and semisynthetic alkaloid derivatives from opium and their synthetic surrogates, whose actions mimic those of morphine. Most of these drugs are classified as Schedule II by the Federal Drug Enforcement Agency because they have a high potential for addiction and abuse. (See *Comparing opioids,* page 1186.)

Pharmacology
Opioids act as agonists at specific opiate receptor binding sites in the CNS and other tissues; these are the same receptors occupied by endogenous opioid peptides (enkephalins and endorphins) to alter CNS response to painful stimuli. Opiate agonists don't alter the cause of pain, but only the patient's perception of pain; they relieve pain without affecting other sensory functions. Opiate receptors are present in highest levels in the limbic system, thalamus, striatum, hypothalamus, midbrain, and spinal cord.

Opioids produce respiratory depression by a direct effect on the respiratory centers in the brain stem, resulting in decreased sensitivity and responsiveness to increases in carbon dioxide ten-

sion. These drugs' antitussive effects are mediated by a direct suppression of the cough reflex center. They cause nausea, probably by stimulation of the chemoreceptor trigger zone in the medulla oblongata; through orthostatic hypotension, which causes dizziness; and possibly by increasing vestibular sensitivity.

Opioids also cause drowsiness, sedation, euphoria, dysphoria, mental clouding, and EEG changes; higher than usual analgesic doses cause anesthesia. Most opioids cause miosis, although meperidine and its derivatives may also cause mydriasis or no pupillary change.

Because opioids decrease gastric, biliary, and pancreatic secretions and delay digestion, constipation is a common adverse reaction. At the same time, these drugs increase tone in the biliary tract and may cause biliary spasms. Some patients may have no biliary effects, whereas others may have biliary spasms that increase plasma amylase and lipase levels up to 15 times upper limit of normal.

Opioids increase smooth muscle tone in the urinary tract and induce spasms, causing urinary urgency. These drugs have little CV effect in a supine patient, but may cause orthostatic hypotension when the patient assumes upright posture. These drugs also are associated with histamine release or peripheral vasodilation, including pruritus, flushing, red eyes, and sweating. These effects are often mistakenly attributed to allergy and should be evaluated carefully.

The opiates can be divided chemically into three groups: phenanthrenes (codeine, hydrocodone, hydromorphone, morphine, oxycodone, and oxymorphone); diphenylheptanes (levomethadyl, methadone, and propoxyphene); and phenylpiperidines (alfentanil, diphenoxylate, fentanyl, meperidine, remifentanil, and sufentanil). If a patient is hypersensitive to an opioid, agonist-antagonist, or antagonist of a given chemical group, use extreme caution when considering using another drug from the same chemical group; however, a drug from the other groups might be well tolerated.

Some of the opioids are well absorbed after oral or rectal administration; others must be administered parenterally. I.V. dosing is the most rapidly effective and reliable; absorption after I.M. or S.C. dosing may be erratic. Opioids vary in onset and duration of action; they are removed rapidly from the bloodstream and distributed, in decreasing order of concentration, into skeletal muscle, kidneys, liver, intestinal tract, lungs, spleen, and brain; they readily cross the placenta.

Opioids are metabolized mainly in the microsomes in the endoplasmic reticulum of the liver (first-pass effect) and also in the CNS, kidneys, lungs, and placenta. They undergo conjugation with glucuronic acid, hydrolysis, oxidation, or N-dealkylation. They are excreted primarily in the urine; small amounts are excreted in the feces.

COMPARING OPIOIDS

Drug	Route	Onset	Peak	Duration
alfentanil	I.V.	Immediate	Not available	Not available
codeine	I.M., P.O., S.C.	15 to 30 min	30 to 60 min	4 to 6 hr
fentanyl	I.M., I.V.	7 to 8 min	Not available	1 to 2 hr
hydrocodone	P.O.	30 min	60 min	4 to 6 hr
hydromorphone	I.M., I.V., S.C.	15 min	30 min	4 to 5 hr
	P.O., rectal	30 min	60 min	4 to 5 hr
meperidine	I.M.	10 to 15 min	30 to 50 min	2 to 4 hr
	P.O.	15 to 30 min	60 min	2 to 4 hr
	S.C.	10 to 15 min	40 to 60 min	2 to 4 hr
methadone	I.M., P.O., S.C.	30 to 60 min	30 to 60 min	4 to 6 hr†
morphine	I.M.	≤ 20 min	30 to 60 min	3 to 7 hr
	P.O., rectal	≤ 20 min	≤ 60 min	3 to 7 hr
	S.C.	≤ 20 min	50 to 90 min	3 to 7 hr
oxycodone	P.O.	15 to 30 min	30 to 60 min	4 to 6 hr
oxymorphone	I.M., S.C.	10 to 15 min	30 to 60 min	3 to 6 hr
	I.V.	5 to 10 min	30 to 60 min	3 to 6 hr
	rectal	15 to 30 min	30 to 60 min	3 to 6 hr
propoxyphene	P.O.	20 to 60 min	2 to 2½ hr	4 to 6 hr
remifentanil	I.V.	Immediate	Not available	Not available
sufentanil	I.V.	1.3 to 3 min	Not available	Not available

† Due to cumulative effects, duration of action increases with repeated doses.

Clinical indications and actions

The opioids produce varying degrees of analgesia and have antitussive, antidiarrheal, and sedative effects. Response is dose-related and varies with each patient.

Analgesia

Opioids may be used in the symptomatic management of moderate to severe pain associated with acute and some chronic disorders, including renal or biliary colic, MI, acute trauma, postoperative pain, and terminal cancer. They also may be used to provide analgesia during diagnostic and orthopedic procedures and during labor. Drug selection, route of administration, and dosage depend on a variety of factors. For example, in mild pain, oral therapy with codeine or oxycodone usually suffices. In acute pain of known short duration, such as that associated with diagnostic procedures or orthopedic manipulation, a short-acting drug such as meperidine or fentanyl is effective. These drugs are often given to alleviate postoperative pain, but because they influence CNS function, special care should be taken to monitor the course of recovery and to detect early signs of complications. Opioids are commonly used to manage severe, chronic pain associated with terminal cancer; management of this type requires careful evaluation of drug used, dosage needed, and route of administration.

Pulmonary edema

Morphine, meperidine, oxymorphone, hydromorphone, and other similar drugs have been used to relieve anxiety in patients with dyspnea associated with acute pulmonary edema and acute left-sided heart failure. These drugs shouldn't be used to treat pulmonary edema resulting from a chemical respiratory stimulant. Opioids decrease peripheral resistance, causing pooling of blood in the extremities and decreased venous return, cardiac workload, and pulmonary venous pressure; blood is thus shifted from the central to the peripheral circulation.

Preoperative sedation

Routine use of opioids for preoperative sedation in patients without pain isn't recommended because it may cause complications during and after surgery. To allay preoperative anxiety, a barbiturate or benzodiazepine is equally effective, with a lower risk of postoperative vomiting.

Anesthesia

Certain opioids, including alfentanil, fentanyl, remifentanil, and sufentanil, may be used for induction of anesthesia, as an adjunct in the maintenance of general and regional anesthesia, or as a primary anesthetic in surgery.

Cough suppression

Some opioids, most commonly codeine and its derivative, hydrocodone, are used as antitussives to relieve dry, nonproductive cough.

Diarrhea

Diphenoxylate and other opioids are used as antidiarrheals. All opioids cause constipation to some degree; however, only a few are indicated for this use. Usually, opiate antidiarrheals are empirically combined with antacids, absorbing products, and belladonna alkaloids in commercial preparations.

Overview of adverse reactions

Respiratory depression and, to a lesser extent, circulatory depression (including orthostatic hypotension) are the major hazards of treatment with opioids. Rapid I.V. administration increases the risk and severity of these adverse effects. Respiratory arrest, shock, and cardiac arrest have occurred. It's likely that equianalgesic doses of individual opiates produce a comparable degree of respiratory depression, but its duration may vary. Other adverse CNS effects include dizziness, visual disturbances, mental clouding or depression, sedation, coma, euphoria, dysphoria, weakness, faintness, agitation, restlessness, nervousness, seizures and, rarely, delirium and insomnia. Adverse effects seem to be more prevalent in ambulatory patients and those not experiencing severe pain. Adverse GI effects include nausea, vomiting, and constipation as well as increased biliary tract pressure that may result in biliary spasm or colic. Tolerance, psychological dependence, and physical dependence (addiction) may follow prolonged, high-dose therapy (more than 100 mg morphine daily for more than 1 month).

Use opiate agonists with extreme caution during pregnancy and labor because they readily cross the placenta. Premature infants appear especially sensitive to the respiratory and CNS depressant effects of these drugs when used during delivery.

Opiate agonists have a high potential for addiction and should always be administered with caution in patients prone to physical or psychic dependence. The agonist-antagonists have a lower potential for addiction and abuse, but the possibility still exists.

☑ Special considerations

• Administer with extreme caution to patients with head injury, increased intracranial pressure, seizures, asthma, COPD, alcoholism, prostatic hypertrophy, severe hepatic or renal disease, acute abdominal conditions, arrhythmias, hypovolemia, or psychiatric disorders, and to elderly or debilitated patients. Reduced dosages may be needed.

• Resuscitative equipment and a narcotic antagonist (naloxone) should be available. Be prepared to provide ventilation and gastric lavage.

• Parenteral administration of opiates provides better analgesia than oral administration. I.V. administration should be given by slow injection, preferably in diluted solution. Rapid I.V. injection increases the risk of adverse effects.

• Parenteral injections by I.M. or S.C. route should be given cautiously to patients who are chilled, hypovolemic, or in shock because decreased perfusion may lead to accumulation of the drug and toxic effects. Rotate I.M. or S.C. injection sites to avoid induration.

• A regular dosing schedule (rather than "as needed for pain") is preferred to alleviate the symptoms and anxiety that accompany pain.

• Duration of respiratory depression may be longer than the analgesic effect. Monitor patient closely with repeated dosing.

• With long-term administration, the patient's respiratory status should be evaluated before each dose. Because severe respiratory depression may occur (especially with accumulation from prolonged dosing), watch for respiratory rate below the patient's baseline level. The patient should be evaluated for restlessness, which may be a sign of compensatory response for hypoxia.

• Opiates or agonist-antagonists may cause orthostatic hypotension in ambulatory patients. The patient should sit or lie down to relieve dizziness or fainting.

• Because opiates depress respiration when used postoperatively, encourage patient to turn, cough, and deep-breathe to avoid atelectases.

• If gastric irritation occurs, give oral products with food; food delays absorption and onset of analgesia.

• Opiates may mask signs and symptoms of an acute abdominal condition or worsen gallbladder pain.

• Because of their antitussive activity, opiates are used to control persistent, exhausting cough or dry, nonproductive cough.

• The first sign of tolerance to the therapeutic effect of opioid agonists or agonist-antagonists is usually a shortened duration of effect.

• Preservative-free morphine (Astramorph, Duramorph) is available for epidural or intrathecal use.

Information for the patient

• Instruct patient to use drug with caution and to avoid hazardous activities that require full alertness and coordination.

• Tell patient to avoid alcohol when taking opioid agonists because it will cause additive CNS depression.

• Explain that the opiate may cause constipation. Suggest measures to increase dietary fiber and recommend a stool softener.

- If patient's condition allows, instruct him to breathe deeply, cough, and change position every 2 hours to avoid respiratory complications.
- Encourage patient to void at least every 4 hours to avoid urine retention.
- Tell the patient to take drug as prescribed and to call if significant adverse effects occur.
- Tell patient not to increase dose if he isn't experiencing the desired effect, but to call for prescribed dosage adjustment.
- Tell patient that, if he misses a dose, to take the missed dose as soon as he remembers unless it's almost time for the next dose. If this is the case, he should skip the missed dose and return to the regular dosing schedule. He shouldn't double a dose.
- Tell patient to call immediately for emergency help if he thinks he or someone else has taken an overdose.
- Explain signs and symptoms of overdose to patient and family.

Geriatric patients
- Lower doses are usually indicated for elderly patients, who may be more sensitive to the therapeutic and adverse effects of drug.

Pediatric patients
- Safety and effectiveness in children haven't been established. Use care when administering to children.

Pregnant patients
- Meperidine and oxymorphone hydrochloride are classified as pregnancy risk category B, but D if used for a prolonged time or if high doses are given at term. Most opioids are listed as pregnancy risk category C. Giving an opiate shortly before delivery may cause respiratory depression in the neonate. Monitor this stage of delivery closely and be prepared to resuscitate neonate.

Breast-feeding patients
- Codeine, meperidine, methadone, morphine, and propoxyphene appear in breast milk; use with caution in breast-feeding women. Methadone has caused physical dependence in breast-feeding infants of women maintained on methadone.

Representative combinations
Codeine with acetaminophen: Aceta with Codeine, Acetaminophen with Codeine Oral Solution, Acetaminophen with Codeine Tablets, Capital with Codeine, Margesic No. 3, Phenaphen with Codeine, Phenaphen with Codeine No. 4, Tylenol with Codeine, Tylenol with Codeine No. 4; with caffeine: Fioricet with Codeine; with calcium iodide and alcohol: Calcidrine.

Codeine phosphate with guaifenesin: Cheracol, Guiatuss AC, Guiatussin with Codeine Liquid, Mytussin AC, Robitussin A-C, Tolu-Sed Cough; with iodinated glycerol: Tussi-Organidin NR; with triprolidine hydrochloride and pseudoephedrine hydrochloride: Actifed with Codeine.

Codeine with aspirin: Aspirin with Codeine No. 3, Aspirin with Codeine No. 4, Empirin with Codeine.

Codeine and aspirin with caffeine and butalbital: Fiorinal with Codeine; with carisoprodol: Soma Compound with Codeine.

Dihydrocodeine with acetaminophen and caffeine: Synalgos-DC.

Fentanyl with droperidol: Fentanyl Citrate and Droperidol, Innovar.

Hydrocodone bitartrate with acetaminophen: Anexsia 5/500 Tablets, Anexsia 7.5/650 Tablets, Anexsia 10/660 Tablets, Bancap HC, Co-Gesic, Damason-P, Dolacet, Duocet, Hydrocet, Hydrocodone Bitartrate and Acetaminophen Tablets, Hydrogesic, Hy-Phen, Lorcet-HD, Lorcet Plus, Lortab, Lortab Elixir, Vicodin, Vicodin ES, Zydone; with aspirin: Lortab ASA, Panasal 5/500; with aspirin and caffeine: Damason-P; with aspirin, acetaminophen, and caffeine: Hyco-Pap; with guaifenesin: Hycotuss Expectorant Syrup (with alcohol); with guaifenesin and pseudoephedrine hydrochloride: Detussin Expectorant, Entuss-D; with guaifenesin and phenindamine tartrate: P-V-Tussin tablets; with guaifenesin and phenylephrine: Donatussin DC; with potassium guaiacolsulfonate: Codiclear DH, Entuss-D Liquid; with pseudoephedrine hydrochloride: Detussin Liquid; with homatropine methylbromide: Hycodan; with phenylephrine hydrochloride and pyrilamine maleate: Codimal DH; with phenylpropanolamine hydrochloride: Hycomine; with phenylephrine hydrochloride, pyrilamine maleate, chlorpheniramine maleate salicylamide, citric acid, and caffeine: Citra Forte; with pheniramine maleate, pyrilamine maleate, potassium citrate, and ascorbic acid: Citra Forte; with phenylephrine hydrochloride, phenylpropanolamine hydrochloride, pheniramine maleate, pyrilamine maleate, and alcohol: Ru-Tuss with hydrocodone; with guaifenesin and alcohol: S-T Forte; with phenyltoloxamine: Tussionex.

Hydromorphone with guaifenesin: Dilaudid Cough.

Meperidine with promethazine: Mepergan, Mepergan Fortis; with atropine sulfate: Atropine and Demerol Injection.

Oxycodone hydrochloride with acetaminophen: Oxycocet*, Oxycodone with Acetaminophen Capsules, Percocet, Percocet-Demi, Roxicet, Roxicet 5/500 Caplets, Roxicet Oral Solution, Roxilox Capsules, Tylox; with aspirin: Oxycodone with Aspirin Tablets, Roxiprin Tablets; with oxycodone terephthalate and aspirin: Percodan, Percodan-Demi.

Propoxyphene with acetaminophen: Darvocet-N, E-Lor Tablets, Lorcet, Propacet 100, Propoxyphene Napsylate and Acetaminophen, Wygesic.

Propoxyphene napsylate with acetaminophen: Darvocet-N 50, Darvocet-N 100, Propacet 100; with aspirin: Propoxyphene HCl Compound Capsules; with aspirin and caffeine: Darvon Compound, Propoxyphene Compound, PC-Cap.

opioid (narcotic) agonist-antagonists

buprenorphine hydrochloride, butorphanol tartrate, nalbuphine hydrochloride, pentazocine hydrochloride

The term "narcotic (or opiate) agonist-antagonist" is somewhat imprecise. This class of drugs has varying degrees of agonist and antagonist activity. These drugs are potent analgesics, with somewhat less addiction potential than the pure narcotic agonists.

Pharmacology
The detailed pharmacology of these drugs is poorly understood. Each drug is believed to act on different opiate receptors in the CNS to a greater or lesser degree, thus yielding slightly different effects. Like the opioid agonists, these drugs can be divided into related chemical groups. Buprenorphine, butorphanol, and nalbuphine are phenanthrenes, like morphine, whereas pentazocine falls into a unique class, the benzmorphans.

Clinical indications and actions
Pain
Opioid agonist-antagonists primarily are used as analgesics, particularly in patients at high risk for drug dependence or abuse. Some are used as preoperative or preanesthetic drugs, to supplement balanced anesthesia, or to relieve prepartum pain.
◊ **Other uses**
Buprenorphine has been used to reverse fentanyl-induced anesthesia. Buprenorphine and naloxone have been used to reduce opiate consumption in patients who are physically dependent on opiates.

Overview of adverse reactions
Major hazards of opioid agonist-antagonists are respiratory depression, apnea, shock, and cardiopulmonary arrest, possibly causing death. All opioid agonist-antagonists can cause respiratory depression, but the severity of such depression each drug can cause has a "ceiling"; for example, each drug depresses respiration to a certain point, but increased doses don't depress it further. All of the opioid agonist-antagonists have been reported to cause withdrawal symptoms after abrupt discontinuation of long-term use; they

appear to have some addiction potential, but less than that of the pure opioid agonists.

CNS effects are the most common adverse reactions and may include drowsiness, sedation, light-headedness, dizziness, hallucinations, disorientation, agitation, euphoria, dysphoria, insomnia, confusion, headache, tremor, miosis, seizures, and psychic dependence. CV reactions may include tachycardia, bradycardia, palpitations, chest wall rigidity, hypertension, hypotension, syncope, and edema. GI reactions may include nausea, vomiting, and constipation (most common), dry mouth, anorexia, and biliary spasms (colic). Other effects include urine retention or hesitancy, decreased libido, flushing, rash, pruritus, and pain at the injection site.

Opioid agonist-antagonists can produce morphine-like dependence and thus have abuse potential. Psychic and physiologic dependence with drug tolerance can develop upon long-term, repeated administration. Patients with dependence or tolerance to narcotic agonist-antagonists usually experience an acute abstinence syndrome or withdrawal signs and symptoms, the severity of which is related to the degree of dependence, abruptness of withdrawal, and the drug used.

Commonly, signs and symptoms of withdrawal include yawning, lacrimation, and sweating (early); mydriasis, piloerection, facial flushing, tachycardia, tremor, irritability, and anorexia (intermediate); and muscle spasms, fever, nausea, vomiting, and diarrhea (late).

☑ Special considerations
● Opioid agonist-antagonists are contraindicated in patients with hypersensitivity to any drug of the same chemical group. Use with extreme caution in patients with supraventricular arrhythmias. Avoid use or administer drug with extreme caution in patients with head injury or increased intracranial pressure because neurologic parameters are obscured and during pregnancy and labor because drug readily crosses placenta (premature infants are especially sensitive to respiratory and CNS depressant effects of opioid agonist-antagonists).
● Use opioid agonist-antagonists cautiously in patients with renal or hepatic dysfunction because drug accumulation or prolonged duration of action may occur; in patients with pulmonary disease (asthma, COPD) because drug depresses respiration and suppresses cough reflex; in patients undergoing biliary tract surgery because drug may cause biliary spasm; in patients with convulsive disorders because drug may precipitate seizures; in elderly and debilitated patients, who are more sensitive to both therapeutic and adverse drug effects; and in patients prone to physical or psychic addiction because of the high risk of addiction.

- Opioid agonist-antagonists have a lower potential for abuse than opioid agonists, but the risk still exists.
- Before administration, visually inspect all parenteral products for particles and discoloration and note strength of solution.
- Parenteral administration of opioid agonist-antagonists provides better analgesia than does oral dosing. I.V. dosing should be given by very slow injections, preferably in diluted solution. Rapid I.V. injection increases risk of adverse effects.
- Give I.M. or S.C. injections cautiously to patients who are chilled, hypovolemic, or in shock; decreased perfusion may lead to accumulation.
- The opioid agonist-antagonists as well as the opioids, antagonists can reverse the desired effects of opioids; thus, members of different pharmacologic groups (for example, meperidine and buprenorphine) shouldn't be prescribed at the same time.
- Have resuscitative equipment and an opioid antagonist (naloxone) available; ventilation and gastric lavage may be needed.
- Patient tolerance may develop to the opiate agonist activity but doesn't develop to opiate antagonist activity.
- A regular dosing schedule (rather than "as needed for pain") is preferable to alleviate the symptoms and anxiety that accompany pain.
- The duration of respiratory depression may be longer than the analgesic effect. Monitor patient closely with repeated dosing.
- During long-term administration, regularly evaluate the patient's respiratory status. Because severe respiratory depression may occur (especially with accumulation with long-term dosing), watch for respiratory rate that is less than the patient's baseline respiratory rate. Also evaluate patient for restlessness, which may be a compensatory response to hypoxia.
- Opioid agonist-antagonists may cause orthostatic hypotension in ambulatory patients. Advise patient to sit or lie down to relieve dizziness or fainting.
- Because opioid agonist-antagonists can depress respiration when used postoperatively, strongly encourage patient to turn, cough, and deep breathe to avoid atelectases. Monitor respiratory status.
- Oral opioid agonist-antagonists may be taken with food to prevent gastric irritation. Food will delay absorption and the onset of analgesia.
- Opioid agonist-antagonists may mask signs and symptoms of an acute abdominal condition or worsen gallbladder pain.
- The first sign of tolerance to the therapeutic effect of opioid agonist-antagonists is usually a reduced duration of effect.

Information for the patient
- Warn ambulatory patient to be cautious when performing tasks that require alertness, such as driving, if he is taking an opioid agonist-antagonist.
- Warn patient not to stop taking drug abruptly if he has been taking it for a prolonged period or at a high dose.
- Tell patient not to increase dose if it isn't producing desired effect but to call for prescribed dosage adjustment.
- Tell patient to avoid alcohol when taking drug because additive CNS depression will occur.
- Tell patient that constipation may result. Suggest measures to increase dietary fiber or recommend a stool softener.
- Instruct patient not to take a double dose. Tell him to take a missed dose as soon as he remembers unless it's almost time for next dose. If this is the case, tell him to skip the missed dose and return to regular dosing schedule.
- Tell patient to call for emergency help if he thinks he or someone else has taken an overdose.
- Explain signs of overdose to patient and his family.
- Instruct patient to breathe deeply, cough, and change position every 2 hours to avoid respiratory complications.
- Encourage patient to void at least every 4 hours to avoid urine retention.
- Tell patient to take drug as prescribed and to promptly report significant adverse effects.
- Inform woman taking drug to call promptly if she is planning or suspects pregnancy; warn her that fetus may become addicted to drug.

Geriatric patients
- Lower doses are usually indicated for elderly patients, who may be more sensitive to the therapeutic and adverse effects of these drugs.

Pediatric patients
- Neonates may be more susceptible to the respiratory depressant effects of opiate agonist-antagonists.

Pregnant patients
- Most drugs in this class are pregnancy risk category C. Administering these drugs to the mother shortly before delivery may cause respiratory depression in neonate. Monitor neonate closely and be prepared to resuscitate.

Breast-feeding patients
- These drugs usually aren't recommended for use in breast-feeding women.

Representative combinations
Pentazocine with acetaminophen: Talacen; with aspirin: Talwin Compound; with naloxone: Talwin Nx.

penicillins

Natural penicillins: penicillin G benzathine, penicillin G potassium, penicillin G procaine, penicillin G sodium, penicillin V potassium

Aminopenicillins: amoxicillin trihydrate with clavulanate potassium, ampicillin, ampicillin sodium with sulbactam sodium, ampicillin trihydrate

Penicillinase-resistant penicillins: cloxacillin sodium, dicloxacillin sodium, methicillin sodium, nafcillin sodium, oxacillin sodium

Extended-spectrum penicillins: carbenicillin indanyl sodium, mezlocillin sodium, piperacillin sodium, piperacillin sodium with tazobactam sodium, ticarcillin disodium, ticarcillin with clavulanate potassium

---

Penicillins are very effective antibiotics with low toxicity. Their activity was first discovered by Sir Alexander Fleming in 1928, but they weren't developed for use against systemic infections until 1940. Penicillin is naturally derived from *Penicillium chrysogenum.* New synthetic derivatives are created by chemical reactions that modify their structure, resulting in increased GI absorption, resistance to destruction by beta-lactamase (penicillinase), and a broader spectrum of susceptible organisms.

Pharmacology

The basic structure of penicillin is a thiazolidine ring connected to a beta-lactam ring that contains a side chain. This nucleus is the main structural requirement for antibacterial activity; modifications of the side chain alter penicillin's antibacterial and pharmacologic effects.

Penicillins are generally bactericidal. They inhibit synthesis of the bacterial cell wall, causing rapid cell lysis, and are most effective against fast-growing susceptible bacteria.

The sites of action for penicillins are enzymes known as penicillin-binding proteins (PBPs). The affinity of certain penicillins for PBPs in various microorganisms helps explain differing spectra of activity in this class of antibiotics.

Bacterial resistance to beta-lactam antibiotics is conferred most significantly by bacterial production of beta-lactamase enzymes, which destroy the beta-lactam ring and thus inactivate penicillin; decreased cell-wall permeability and alteration in binding affinity to PBPs also contribute to such resistance.

Oral absorption of penicillin varies widely; the most acid labile is penicillin G. Side-chain modifications in penicillin V, ampicillin, amoxicillin, and other orally administered penicillins are more stable in gastric acid and permit better absorption from the GI tract. (See *Comparing penicillins,* page 1192.)

Penicillins are distributed widely throughout the body; CSF penetration is minimal but is enhanced in patients with inflamed meninges. Most penicillins are only partially metabolized. With the exception of nafcillin, penicillins are excreted primarily in urine, chiefly through renal tubular effects; nafcillin undergoes enterohepatic circulation and is excreted chiefly through the biliary tract.

Clinical indications and actions
Natural penicillins

Penicillin G is the prototype of this group; derivatives such as penicillin V are more acid stable and thus better absorbed by the oral route. All natural penicillins are vulnerable to inactivation by beta-lactamase–producing bacteria. Natural penicillins act primarily against gram-positive organisms.

Clinical indications for natural penicillins include streptococcal pneumonia, enterococcal and nonenterococcal group D endocarditis, diphtheria, anthrax, meningitis, tetanus, botulism, actinomycosis, syphilis, relapsing fever, Lyme disease, rat-bite fever, and Whipple's disease. Natural penicillins are used prophylactically against pneumococcal infections, rheumatic fever, bacterial endocarditis, and neonatal group B streptococcal disease.

Susceptible aerobic gram-positive cocci include non-penicillinase-producing *Staphylococcus aureus, S. epidermis;* nonenterococcal group D streptococci; groups A, B, C, D, G, H, K, L, and M streptococci; *Streptococcus viridans;* and enterococcus (usually with an aminoglycoside). Susceptible aerobic gram-negative cocci include *Neisseria meningitidis* and non-penicillinase-producing *N. gonorrhoeae.*

Susceptible aerobic gram-positive bacilli include *Corynebacterium* (both diphtheria and opportunistic species), *Listeria,* and *Bacillus anthracis.* Susceptible anaerobes include *Peptococcus, Peptostreptococcus, Actinomyces, Clostridium, Fusobacterium, Veillonella,* and non-beta-lactamase–producing strains of *S. pneumoniae.* The drugs are also active against some gram-negative aerobic bacilli, including strains of *Haemophilus influenzae, Pasteurella multocida, Streptobacillus moniliformis,* and *Spirillum minus.*

Susceptible spirochetes include *Treponema pallidum, T. pertenue, Leptospira, Borrelia recurrentis,* and possibly *B. burgdorferi.*

COMPARING PENICILLINS

Drug	Route	Adult dosage	Frequency	Penicillinase-resistant
amoxicillin	P.O.	250 to 500 mg 3 g with 1 g probenecid for gonorrhea	q 8 hr Single dose	No
amoxicillin/ clavulanate potassium	P.O.	250 mg 500 mg	q 8 hr q 12 hr	Yes
ampicillin	I.M., I.V. P.O.	2 to 14 g daily 250 to 500 mg 2.5 g with 1 g probenecid (for gonorrhea)	Divided doses given q 4 to 6 hr q 6 hr Single dose	No
ampicillin sodium/ sulbactam sodium	I.M., I.V.	1.5 to 3 g	q 6 to 8 hr	Yes
carbenicillin	P.O.	382 to 764 mg	q 6 hr	No
cloxacillin	P.O.	250 mg to 1 g	q 6 hr	Yes
dicloxacillin	P.O.	125 to 500 mg	q 6 hr	Yes
mezlocillin	I.M., I.V.	3 to 4 g	q 4 to 6 hr	No
nafcillin	I.M., I.V. P.O.	250 mg to 2 g 500 mg to 1 g	q 4 to 6 hr q 6 hr	Yes
oxacillin	I.M., I.V. P.O.	250 mg to 2 g 500 mg to 1 g	q 4 to 6 hr q 6 hr	Yes
penicillin G benzathine	I.M.	1.2 to 2.4 million units	Single dose	No
penicillin G potassium	I.M., I.V.	200,000 to 4 million units	q 4 hr	No
penicillin G procaine	I.M.	600,000 to 1.2 million units 4.8 million units with 1 g probenecid (for syphilis)	q 1 to 3 days Single dose for primary, secondary, and early latent syphilis; weekly for 3 weeks for late latent syphilis	No
penicillin G sodium	I.M., I.V.	200,000 to 4 million units	q 4 hr	No
penicillin V potassium	P.O.	250 to 500 mg	q 6 to 8 hr	No
piperacillin	I.M., I.V.	100 to 300 mg/kg daily	Divided dose given q 4 to 6 hr	No
piperacillin sodium/ tazobactam sodium	I.V.	3.375 g	q 6 hr	Yes
ticarcillin	I.M., I.V.	150 to 300 mg/kg daily	Divided doses given q 3 to 6 hr	No
ticarcillin/ clavulanate potassium	I.V.	3.1 g	q 4 to 6 hr	Yes

Aminopenicillins

Aminopenicillins (amoxicillin and ampicillin) offer a broader spectrum of activity, including many gram-negative organisms. Like natural penicillins, aminopenicillins are vulnerable to inactivation by penicillinase. They are primarily used to treat septicemia, gynecologic infections, infections of the urinary, respiratory, and GI tracts; and infections of skin, soft tissue, bones, and joints. Their activity spectrum includes *Escherichia coli, Proteus mirabilis, Shigella, Salmonella, S. pneumoniae, N. gonorrhoeae, H. influenzae, S. aureus, S. epidermidis* (non-penicillinase-producing staphylococci), and *Listeria monocytogenes.*

Penicillinase-resistant penicillins

Penicillinase-resistant penicillins (cloxacillin, dicloxacillin, oxacillin, and nafcillin) are semisynthetic penicillins designed to remain stable against hydrolysis by most staphylococcal penicillinases and thus are the drugs of choice against susceptible penicillinase-producing staphylococci. They also retain activity against most organisms susceptible to natural penicillins. Clinical indications are much the same as for aminopenicillins.

Extended-spectrum penicillins

Extended-spectrum penicillins (carbenicillin, mezlocillin, piperacillin, and ticarcillin), as their name implies, offer a wider range of bactericidal action than the other three classes, are used in hard-to-treat gram-negative infections, and are usually given with aminoglycosides. They are used most often against susceptible strains of *Enterobacter, Klebsiella, Citrobacter, Serratia, Bacteroides fragilis,* and *Pseudomonas aeruginosa;* their gram-negative spectrum also includes *Proteus vulgaris, P. mirabilis, Providencia rettgeri, Salmonella, Shigella,* and *Morganella morganii.* These penicillins are also vulnerable to destruction by beta-lactamase or penicillinases.

Overview of adverse reactions

Systemic reactions: Hypersensitivity reactions range from mild rash, fever, and eosinophilia to fatal anaphylaxis. Hematologic reactions include hemolytic anemia, transient neutropenia, leukopenia, and thrombocytopenia.

Certain adverse reactions are more common with specific classes of penicillin: bleeding episodes are usually seen at high-dose levels of extended-spectrum penicillins; acute interstitial nephritis is reported most often with methicillin; GI adverse effects are most common with but not limited to ampicillin. High doses, especially of penicillin G, irritate the CNS in patients with renal disease, causing confusion, twitching, lethargy, dysphagia, seizures, and coma. Hepatotoxicity is most common with penicillinase-resistant penicillins; hyperkalemia and hypernatremia with extended-spectrum penicillins.

Jarisch-Herxheimer reaction (chills, fever, headache, myalgia, tachycardia, malaise, sweating, hypotension, and sore throat) can occur when penicillin G is used in secondary syphilis and is attributed to release of endotoxin following spirochete death.

Local reactions: Local irritation from parenteral therapy may be severe enough to require stopping drug or giving drug by subclavian catheter if therapy is to continue.

☑ Special considerations

● Assess patient's history of allergies.
● A negative history for penicillin hypersensitivity doesn't preclude future allergic reactions; patient should be monitored continuously for possible allergic reactions or other adverse effects.
● Reduce dosage in patients with renal impairment based on creatinine clearance and manufacturer's guidelines.
● Assess level of consciousness, neurologic status, and renal function when high doses are used; excessive blood levels can cause CNS toxicity.
● Monitor vital signs, electrolytes, and renal function studies; monitor body weight for fluid retention with extended-spectrum penicillins for possible hypokalemia or hypernatremia.
● Coagulation abnormalities, even frank bleeding, can follow high doses, especially of extended-spectrum penicillins. PT and platelet counts should be monitored, and patient should be assessed for signs of occult or frank bleeding.
● Patients on long-term therapy should be monitored for possible superinfection, especially elderly and debilitated patients and others receiving immunosuppressants or radiation therapy; monitor these patients closely, and watch for fever.

Oral and parenteral administration
● Give penicillins at least 1 hour before giving bacteriostatic antibiotics (tetracyclines, erythromycins, and chloramphenicol); these drugs inhibit bacterial cell growth, decreasing rate of penicillin uptake by bacterial cell walls.
● Refrigerate oral suspensions; shake well before administering to assure correct dose.
● Give oral penicillin at least 1 hour before or 2 hours after meals to enhance gastric absorption; food may or may not decrease absorption.
● Administer I.M. dose deep into large muscle mass (gluteal or midlateral thigh); rotate injection sites to minimize tissue injury; don't inject more than 2 g of drug per injection site. Apply ice to injection site for pain.
● Don't add or mix other drugs with I.V. infusions—particularly aminoglycosides, which will be inactivated if mixed with penicillins; they are chemically and physically incompatible. If other drugs must be given I.V., temporarily stop infusion of primary drug.
● Infuse I.V. drug continuously or intermittently (over 30 minutes) and assess I.V. site frequently to prevent infiltration or phlebitis; rotate infusion site q 48 hours; intermittent I.V. infusion may be diluted in 50 to 100 ml sterile water, normal

saline solution, D_5W, D_5W and 0.45% saline, or lactated Ringer's solution.

Information for the patient
• Explain disease process and rationale for therapy.
• Teach signs and symptoms of hypersensitivity and other adverse reactions, and emphasize need to report unusual reactions.
• Teach signs and symptoms of bacterial and fungal superinfection, especially to elderly and debilitated patients and others with low resistance due to immunosuppressants or irradiation; emphasize need to report signs of infection.
• Teach patient how and when to take drugs; urge him to complete entire prescribed regimen, to comply with instructions for around-the-clock dosing, and to keep follow-up appointments.
• Tell patient to check expiration date of drug, discard unused drug, and not give it to family members or friends.
• Advise patient using oral contraceptives to use a back-up form of contraception during therapy.

Geriatric patients
• Use with caution; elderly patients are susceptible to superinfection.
• Many elderly patients have renal impairment, which decreases excretion of penicillins; use a lower dose in elderly patients who have diminished creatinine clearance.

Pediatric patients
• Specific dosage recommendations have been established for most penicillins.

Pregnant patients
• Safety of penicillins during pregnancy hasn't been definitely established. However, penicillin G has been used for syphilis without adverse effects, and amoxicillin and ampicillin have been used for urinary tract infections without adverse effects.

Breast-feeding patients
• Consult individual drug recommendations.

Representative combinations
Amoxicillin with clavulanate potassium: Augmentin.
Ampicillin sodium with sulbactam sodium: Unasyn.
Penicillin G benzathine with penicillin G procaine: Bicillin C-R, Bicillin C-R 900/300.
Piperacillin sodium with tazobactam sodium: Zosyn.
Ticarcillin disodium with clavulanate potassium: Timentin.

phenothiazines

Aliphatic derivatives: chlorpromazine hydrochloride, promethazine hydrochloride, trimeprazine, triflupromazine

Piperazine derivatives: fluphenazine hydrochloride, perphenazine, prochlorperazine, trifluoperazine hydrochloride

Piperidine derivatives: mesoridazine besylate, thioridazine

The phenothiazines were originally synthesized by European scientists seeking aniline-like dyes in the late 1800s. Several decades later, in the 1930s, promethazine was identified and found to have sedative, antihistaminic, and narcotic-potentiating effects. Chlorpromazine was synthesized in the 1950s; this drug proved to have many effects, among them strong antipsychotic activity.

Pharmacology
Phenothiazines are classified in terms of chemical structure: the aliphatic drug (chlorpromazine) has a greater sedative, hypotensive, allergic, and convulsant activity; the piperazines (perphenazine, prochlorperazine, fluphenazine, and trifluoperazine) are more likely to produce extrapyramidal symptoms; the piperidines (thioridazine and mesoridazine) have intermediate effects. Thioxanthenes are chemically similar to phenothiazines and pharmacologically similar to piperazine phenothiazines. Promethazine is a derivative that has antihistamine qualities.

All antipsychotics have fundamentally similar mechanisms of action; they are believed to function as dopamine antagonists, blocking postsynaptic dopamine receptors in various parts of the CNS; their antiemetic effects result from blockage of the chemoreceptor trigger zone. They also produce varying degrees of anticholinergic and alpha-adrenergic receptor blocking actions. The drugs are structurally similar to tricyclic antidepressants (TCAs) and share many adverse reactions.

All antipsychotics have equal clinical efficacy when given in equivalent doses; choice of specific therapy is determined primarily by the individual patient's response and adverse reaction profile. A patient who doesn't respond to one drug may respond to another.

Onset of full therapeutic effects requires 6 weeks to 6 months of therapy; therefore, dosage adjustment is recommended at not less than weekly intervals.

Clinical indications and actions

Psychoses
The phenothiazines (except promethazine) and thiothixene are indicated to treat agitated psychotic states. They are especially effective in controlling hallucinations in schizophrenic patients, the manic phase of manic-depressive illness, and excessive motor and autonomic activity.

Nausea and vomiting
Chlorpromazine, perphenazine, promethazine, and prochlorperazine are effective in controlling severe nausea and vomiting induced by CNS disturbances. They don't prevent motion sickness or vertigo.

◇ Anxiety
Chlorpromazine, mesoridazine, promethazine, prochlorperazine, and trifluoperazine also may be used for short-term treatment of moderate anxiety in selected nonpsychotic patients, for example, to control anxiety before surgery.

Severe behavior problems
Chlorpromazine and thioridazine are indicated to control combativeness and hyperexcitability in children with severe behavior problems. They also are used in hyperactive children for short-term treatment of excessive motor activity with labile moods, impulsive behavior, aggressiveness, attention deficit, and poor tolerance of frustration. Mesoridazine is used to manage hypersensitivity and to promote cooperative behavior in patients with mental deficiency and chronic brain syndrome.

Tetanus
Chlorpromazine is an effective adjunct in treating tetanus.

Porphyria
Because of its effects on the autonomic nervous system, chlorpromazine is effective in controlling abdominal pain in patients with acute intermittent porphyria.

Intractable hiccups
Chlorpromazine has been used to treat patients with intractable hiccups. The mechanism is unknown.

Neurogenic pain
Fluphenazine is a useful adjunct, managing selected chronic pain states.

Allergies and pruritus
Because of their potent antihistaminic effects, many of these drugs (including promethazine and trimeprazine) are used to relieve itching or symptomatic rhinitis.

Overview of adverse reactions
Phenothiazines may produce extrapyramidal symptoms (dystonic movements, torticollis, oculogyric crises, parkinsonian symptoms) from akathisia during early treatment to tardive dyskinesia after long-term use.

In rare cases, a neuroleptic malignant syndrome resembling severe parkinsonism may occur, consisting of rapid onset of hyperthermia, muscular hyperreflexia, marked extrapyramidal and autonomic dysfunction, arrhythmias, and sweating.

Other adverse reactions are similar to those seen with TCAs, including sedative and anticholinergic effects, orthostatic hypotension, reflex tachycardia, fainting, dizziness, arrhythmias, anorexia, nausea, vomiting, abdominal pain, local gastric irritation, seizures, endocrine effects, hematologic disorders, ocular changes, skin eruptions, and photosensitivity. Allergic manifestations are usually marked by elevation of liver enzyme levels progressing to obstructive jaundice.

The piperidine derivatives have the most pronounced CV effects; the piperazine derivatives have the least. Parenteral administration is often associated with CV effects because of more rapid absorption. Seizures are common with aliphatic derivatives.

☑ Special considerations
● Phenothiazines are contraindicated in patients with hypersensitivity to phenothiazines and related compounds.
● Use with caution in patients with cardiac disease (arrhythmias, heart failure, angina pectoris, valvular disease, or heart block).
● Also use cautiously in patients with encephalitis, Reye's syndrome, head injury, epilepsy, or other seizure disorders.
● Use phenothiazines cautiously in patients with glaucoma, prostatic hypertrophy, paralytic ileus, urine retention, hepatic or renal dysfunction, Parkinson's disease, pheochromocytoma, or hypocalcemia.
● Vital signs should be checked regularly for decreased blood pressure (especially before and after parenteral therapy) or tachycardia; observe patient carefully for other adverse reactions.
● Monitor intake and output for urine retention or constipation, which may require dosage reduction.
● Monitor bilirubin levels weekly for first 4 weeks; monitor CBC, ECG (for quinidine-like effects), liver and renal function studies, and electrolyte levels (especially potassium).
● Baseline eye examinations are needed, and periodically thereafter, especially in patients on long-term therapy.
● Monitor patient for mood changes to monitor progress; benefits may not be apparent for several weeks.
● Monitor patient for involuntary movements. Check patient receiving prolonged treatment at least once every 6 months.
● Don't withdraw drug abruptly; although physical dependence doesn't occur with antipsychotics, rebound exacerbation of psychotic symptoms may occur, and many drug effects persist.
● Manufacturer's instructions for reconstitution, dilution, administration, and storage of drugs must

be carefully followed; slightly discolored liquids may or may not be acceptable to use.

Information for the patient
• Explain rationale and anticipated risks and benefits of therapy, and that full therapeutic effect may not occur for several weeks.
• Teach signs and symptoms of adverse reactions and importance of reporting unusual effects, especially involuntary movements.
• Tell patient to avoid beverages and drugs containing alcohol, and not to take other drugs, especially CNS depressants and OTC products, without approval.
• Instruct diabetic patients to monitor blood glucose level because drug may alter insulin needs.
• Tell patient how and when to take drug, not to increase dose without approval, and never to stop drug abruptly; suggest taking full dose at bedtime if daytime sedation is troublesome.
• Advise patient to lie down for 30 minutes after first dose (1 hour if I.M.) and to rise slowly from sitting or supine position to prevent orthostatic hypotension.
• Warn patient to avoid tasks such as driving that require mental alertness and psychomotor coordination until full effects of drug are known; emphasize that sedative effects will lessen after several weeks.
• Advise patient to take drug with milk or food to minimize GI distress. Warn him that oral concentrates and solutions will irritate skin, and tell him not to crush or open sustained-release products, but to swallow them whole.
• Warn patient that photosensitivity reactions (burns and abnormal hyperpigmentation) may occur.
• Tell patient to avoid exposure to extremes of heat or cold because of risk of hypothermia or hyperthermia induced by alteration in thermoregulatory function.
• Explain that phenothiazines may cause pink to brown discoloration of urine.

Geriatric patients
• Lower doses are indicated in elderly patients, who are more sensitive to therapeutic and adverse effects, especially cardiac toxicity, tardive dyskinesia, and other extrapyramidal effects. Adjust dosage to patient response.

Pediatric patients
• Unless otherwise specified, antipsychotics aren't recommended for children under age 12; use with caution for nausea and vomiting because acutely ill children (suffering from chickenpox, measles, CNS infections, or dehydration) are at greatly increased risk for dystonic reactions.

Pregnant patients
• Safety of phenothiazines during pregnancy hasn't been established.

Breast-feeding patients
• Most phenothiazines appear in breast milk and have a direct effect on prolactin levels. If possible, women shouldn't breast-feed while taking antipsychotics. Benefit to mother must outweigh risk to infant.

Representative combinations
None.

progestins

hydroxyprogesterone caproate, medroxyprogesterone acetate, megestrol acetate, norethindrone, norethindrone acetate, norgestrel, progesterone

Progesterone is the endogenous progestin, secreted by the corpus luteum within the female ovary. Several synthetic progesterone derivatives with greater potency or duration of action have been synthesized. Some of these derivatives also possess weak androgenic or estrogenic activity. The progestins are used to treat dysfunctional uterine bleeding and certain cancers. They also are used as contraceptives, either alone or with estrogens.

Pharmacology
Progesterone is formed from steroid precursors in the ovary, testis, adrenal cortex, and placenta. Luteinizing hormone stimulates the synthesis and secretion of progesterone from the corpus luteum. Progesterone causes secretory changes in the endometrium, changes in the vaginal epithelium, increases in body temperature, relaxation of uterine smooth muscle, stimulation of growth of breast alveolar tissue, inhibition of gonadotropin release from the pituitary, and withdrawal bleeding (in the presence of estrogens). The synthetic progesterone derivatives have these properties as well.

Clinical indications and actions
Hormonal imbalance, female
Hydroxyprogesterone, medroxyprogesterone, norethindrone, and progesterone are indicated to treat amenorrhea and dysfunctional uterine bleeding resulting from hormonal imbalance. Hydroxyprogesterone also is indicated to produce desquamation and a secretory endometrium.
Endometriosis
Norethindrone and norethindrone acetate are indicated to treat endometriosis.
Carcinoma
Hydroxyprogesterone, medroxyprogesterone, and megestrol are indicated in the adjunctive and palliative treatment of certain types of metastat-

ic tumors. They aren't considered primary therapy. See individual drugs for specific indications.

Contraception
Norethindrone, medroxyprogesterone acetate, and norgestrel are approved for use with estrogens or alone as oral contraceptives.

Progestins are no longer indicated to detect pregnancy (because of teratogenicity) or to treat threatened or habitual abortion, for which they aren't effective.

Overview of adverse reactions
The most common adverse effect is a change in menstrual bleeding pattern, ranging from spotting or breakthrough bleeding to complete amenorrhea. Other reactions include breast tenderness and secretion, weight changes, increases in body temperature, edema, nausea, acne, somnolence, insomnia, hirsutism, hair loss, depression, cholestatic jaundice, and allergic reactions (rare). Some patients taking parenteral progestins also have suffered localized reactions at the injection site.

☑ Special considerations
• Progestins are contraindicated during pregnancy and in patients with thromboembolic disorders, breast cancer, undiagnosed abnormal vaginal bleeding, or severe hepatic disease.
• Use cautiously in patients with diabetes mellitus, cardiac or renal disease, seizure disorder, migraine, or mental depression.
• Give oil injections deep I.M. in gluteal muscles. I.M. injections may be painful; observe injection site for sterile abscess formation.
• Glucose tolerance may be altered in diabetic patients. Monitor patient closely because antidiabetic may need to be adjusted.
• When used as an oral contraceptive, progestins are administered daily without interruption, regardless of menstrual cycle.
• Use of progestins may lead to gingival bleeding and hyperplasia.
• A woman who is exposed to progestins during the first 4 months of pregnancy or who becomes pregnant while receiving progestins should be informed of potential risks to fetus.
• Because oral contraceptive combinations contain progestins, the precautions associated with oral contraceptives should be considered in patients receiving progestins.

Information for the patient
• Tell patient that GI distress may subside with use (after a few cycles).
• Instruct patient receiving progestins to have a full physical examination, including a gynecologic examination and a Papanicolaou test, every 6 to 12 months.
• Advise patient to stop drug and call immediately if migraine or visual disturbances occur, or if sudden severe headache or vomiting develops.

• Teach patient how to perform breast self-examination.
• Tell patient to call promptly if period is missed or unusual bleeding occurs and to call and stop drug immediately if pregnancy is suspected.
• Advise patient who misses a dose to take the missed dose as soon as possible or omit it.
• Advise patient who misses consecutive doses when progestins are used as a contraceptive to stop drug and use an alternative contraceptive method until period begins or pregnancy is ruled out.
• Inform patient that drug may cause possible dental problems (tenderness, swelling, or bleeding of gums). Advise patient to brush and floss teeth, massage gums, and have dentist clean teeth regularly. Tell her to check with dentist if there are questions about care of teeth or gums or if tenderness, swelling, or bleeding of gums is noticed.
• Advise patient to use extra care to avoid pregnancy when starting drug as an oral contraceptive and for at least 3 months after stopping drug.
• Advise patient to keep an extra 1-month supply available.
• Tell patient to keep tablets in original container.
• Emphasize importance of not giving drug to anyone else.

Pregnant patients
• Pregnancy risk category X. Potential adverse effects include masculinization of female fetus, hypospadias in male fetus, and potential cardiovascular and limb defects.

Breast-feeding patients
• Detectable amounts of progestins have been found in breast milk. Effects on breast-feeding infants are unknown.

Representative combinations
Hydroxyprogesterone caproate with estradiol valerate: Hylutin.

Norethindrone acetate with ethinyl estradiol: Brevicon, Loestrin 1.5/30, Loestrin Fe 1.5/30, Loestrin 21 1/20, Loestrin Fe 1/20, Modicon, Norinyl 1 + 35, Ortho 1/35*, Ortho 7/7/7*, Ortho 10/11*, Ortho-Novum 7/7/7, Ovcon-35, Ovcon-50, Tri-Norinyl; with mestranol: Norinyl 1 + 50, Ortho-Novum 1/50, Ortho-Novum 1/35.

Norgestrel with ethinyl estradiol: Lo/Ovral, Ovral.

protease inhibitors

indinavir, nelfinavir, saquinavir, ritonavir

Protease inhibitors are antivirals that act specifically against HIV through inhibition of HIV protease.

Pharmacology
Protease inhibitors bind to the protease active site and inhibit the activity of HIV protease. This enzyme is needed for the proteolysis of viral polyprotein precursors into individual functional proteins found in infectious HIV. The net effect is formation of noninfectious, immature viral particles.

Clinical indications and actions
HIV infection or AIDS
Protease inhibitors are indicated, as monotherapy or with nucleoside analogues, for the treatment of HIV infection or AIDS.
◇ Postexposure prophylaxis after occupational exposure to HIV
Protease inhibitors may be used with zidovudine and lamivudine for postexposure prophylaxis of HIV infection.

Overview of adverse reactions
The most frequently reported adverse effects of protease inhibitors, for which immediate medical attention should be sought, are kidney stones, diabetes or hyperglycemia, ketoacidosis, and paresthesia. Frequently reported adverse effects that don't need medical attention unless they persist or are bothersome include generalized weakness, GI disturbances, headache, insomnia, and taste perversion. Less frequent adverse effects include dizziness and somnolence.

☑ Special considerations
● The risk-benefit ratio of therapy with protease inhibitors should be considered when hemophilia or liver dysfunction is present.
● Indinavir may cause nephrolithiasis. Patient should drink at least 48 oz (1.5 L) of fluids per day.

Information for the patient
● Instruct patient to take drug as prescribed and to finish full course.
● Tell patient that, if he misses a dose, he should take the next dose as soon as possible and shouldn't double the dose.
● Tell patient that drug should be taken with plenty of water 1 or 2 hours before meals
● Advise patient to drink about 48 oz (1.5 L) of water daily while on drug.

● Instruct patient to call before taking other drugs or OTC products.

Geriatric patients
● Safety and efficacy haven't been evaluated.

Pediatric patients
● Refer to specific drug monographs for dosing information.

Pregnant patients
● Pregnancy risk category B or C. Drug can produce hyperbilirubinemia; use with caution in pregnant patients to prevent adverse effects in newborns.

Breast-feeding patients
● It's unknown how much of these drugs appears in breast milk. Use in breast-feeding women isn't recommended. However, risks and benefits to mother and infant must be considered in each case.

Representative combinations
None.

selective serotonin reuptake inhibitors (SSRIs)

fluoxetine, sertraline, paroxetine

Fluoxetine, sertraline, and paroxetine are antidepressant, antiobsessional, antipanic drugs that selectively inhibit the reuptake of serotonin with little or no effect on other neurotransmitters such as norepinephrine or dopamine.

Pharmacology
The antidepressant, antiobsessional, antipanic actions of these drugs are thought to be related to the potent and selective inhibition of serotonin uptake, but not of norepinephrine or dopamine uptake, in the CNS. These drugs lack affinity for alpha-adrenergic receptors and muscarinic receptors.

Clinical indications and actions
SSRIs are used in the treatment of major depression, obsessive compulsive disorder (OCD), bulimia nervosa, premenstrual dysphoric disorders, and panic disorders.
◇ Fluoxetine has been used for the treatment of bipolar disorder, symptomatic management of cataplexy, and management of alcohol dependence.
◇ Paroxetine and sertraline have been used for the treatment of premature ejaculation, chronic headache, and noncombat-related, chronic posttraumatic stress disorder (PTSD). Paroxe-

tine has been used to treat symptoms of diabetic neuropathy.

Overview of adverse reactions

Frequent adverse effects include headache, tremor, dizziness, sleep disturbances, GI disturbances, and sexual dysfunction. Less frequent adverse effects include bleeding (red spots on skin, nose bleeds), akathisia (restlessness), breast tenderness or enlargement, extrapyramidal effects, dystonia, fever, hyponatremia, mania or hypomania, palpitations, serotonin syndrome, skin rash, hives, and itching.

☑ Special considerations

• Hyponatremia is usually due to inappropriate secretion of antidiuretic hormone. This problem is most often seen in elderly patients and in those taking diuretics.

• Serotonin syndrome, characterized by diarrhea, fever, palpitations, mood swings or behavioral changes, restlessness, shaking, and shivering, may be accompanied by hypertension and seizures. This syndrome is most commonly seen within days after dosage increases or concurrent administration of a serotonergic drug.

Information for the patient

• Tell patient that this drug may take 4 to 5 weeks to produce full benefit.

• Advise patient to take drug as prescribed and, if he misses a dose, not to double the next dose.

• Instruct patient to stop drug and call immediately if a rash or hives develop while taking drug.

• Warn patient to avoid alcohol and not to use drugs or substances that have serotonergic activity.

• Tell patient to use caution during activities requiring alertness, such as driving, because drug may cause drowsiness and impairment of judgment, thinking, or motor skills.

Geriatric patients

• SSRIs are safe and effective in elderly patients. However, elderly patients are more sensitive to insomniac effects of SSRIs.

Pediatric patients

• Safety and efficacy of SSRIs in children are unknown. However, there is evidence of beneficial response after SSRI therapy for depression or obsessive compulsive disorders in this age-group. Children appear to be more susceptible than adults to the behavioral adverse reactions of SSRIs (for example, mania, social inhibition, irritability, restlessness, and insomnia).

Pregnant patients

• Pregnancy risk category C. There is no evidence of teratogenicity or ill effects in newborns of mothers treated with SSRIs during the first trimester or throughout gestation. Effects of SSRIs on labor and delivery are unknown.

Breast-feeding patients

• SSRIs appear in breast milk and may cause diarrhea and sleep disturbance in newborns. Use of SSRIs in breast-feeding women isn't recommended; however, risks and benefits to mother and infant must be considered in each case.

Representative combinations

None.

sulfonamides

co-trimoxazole (trimethoprim-sulfamethoxazole), sulfadiazine, sulfamethoxazole, sulfasalazine, sulfisoxazole

Sulfonamides were the first effective drugs used to treat systemic bacterial infections. The prototype, sulfanilamide, was discovered in 1908 and first used clinically in 1933. Since then, many derivatives have been synthesized, and many therapeutic milestones have been reached, including improved solubility of sulfonamides in urine (which reduces renal toxicity) and discovery of the advantages of combinations such as triple sulfa and, especially, of combined trimethoprim and sulfamethoxazole (co-trimoxazole). Development of other major antibiotics has reduced the clinical impact of sulfonamides; however, introduction of the combination drug co-trimoxazole has increased their usefulness in certain infections.

Pharmacology

Sulfonamides are bacteriostatic. Their mechanism of action correlates directly with the structural similarities they share with para-aminobenzoic acid. They inhibit biosynthesis of folic acid, which is needed for cell growth; susceptible bacteria are those that synthesize folic acid.

Sulfonamides are well absorbed from the GI tract after oral administration, except for sulfasalazine, which is absorbed minimally by the oral route. Sulfonamides are distributed widely into tissues and fluids, including pleural, peritoneal, synovial, and ocular fluids; some, including sulfisoxazole, penetrate CSF. Sulfonamides readily cross the placenta and are found in low levels in breast milk. Sulfonamides are metabolized by the liver and the parent drug, and metabolites are excreted in urine by glomerular filtration. Hemodialysis removes both sulfamethoxazole and sulfisoxazole, but peritoneal dialysis removes only sulfisoxazole.

Clinical indications and actions

Bacterial infections

When first introduced, sulfonamides were active against many gram-positive and gram-negative organisms; over time, many bacteria have become resistant. Currently, sulfonamides are active against some strains of staphylococci, streptococci, *Nocardia asteroides* and *N. brasiliensis*, *Clostridium tetani* and *C. perfringens*, *Bacillus anthracis*, *Escherichia coli*, and *Neisseria gonorrhoeae* and *N. meningitidis*. Resistance to sulfonamides is common if therapy continues beyond 2 weeks; resistance to one sulfonamide usually means cross-resistance to others.

Sulfonamides are used to treat urinary tract infections caused by *E. coli*, *Proteus mirabilis* and *P. vulgaris*, *Klebsiella*, *Enterobacter*, and *Staphylococcus aureus*, and genital lesions caused by *Haemophilus ducreyi* (chancroid). They are the drugs of choice in nocardiosis, usually with surgical drainage or with other antibiotics, including ampicillin, erythromycin, cycloserine, or minocycline. Sulfonamides are also used to treat otitis media and may be used as alternative therapy to tetracyclines against *Chlamydia trachomatis* (lymphogranuloma venereum). Sulfadiazine is used to eradicate meningococci from the nasopharynx of asymptomatic carriers of *N. meningitidis*.

Co-trimoxazole is used to treat infections of the urinary tract, respiratory tract, and ear; to treat chronic bacterial prostatitis; and to prevent traveler's diarrhea and recurrent urinary tract infection in women.

Parasitic infections

Sulfonamides with pyrimethamine are used to treat toxoplasmosis; certain sulfonamides are used with quinine and pyrimethamine to treat chloroquine-resistant *Plasmodium falciparum* malaria.

Co-trimoxazole is also used to treat *Pneumocystis carinii* pneumonia.

Inflammations

Sulfasalazine, used to treat inflammatory bowel disease, is cleaved in the intestine to sulfapyridine and 5-aminosalicylic acid.

Plague

Co-trimoxazole is recommended by the CDC for anti-infective prophylaxis in adults ages 18 and older and children ages 2 months and older who are at high risk for exposure to pneumonic plague.

Overview of adverse reactions

Sulfonamides cause adverse reactions affecting many organs and systems. Many are considered to be caused by hypersensitivity, including the following: rash, fever, pruritus, erythema multiforme, erythema nodosum, Stevens-Johnson syndrome, Lyell's syndrome, exfoliative dermatitis, photosensitivity, joint pain, conjunctivitis, leukopenia, and bronchospasm. Hematologic reactions include granulocytopenia, thrombocytopenia, agranulocytosis, hypoprothrombinemia, and, in G6PD deficiency, hemolytic anemia. Renal effects usually result from crystalluria (precipitation of the sulfonamide in the renal system). GI reactions include anorexia, stomatitis, pancreatitis, diarrhea, and folic acid malabsorption. Oral therapy commonly causes nausea and vomiting. Hepatotoxicity and CNS reactions (dizziness, confusion, headache, ataxia, drowsiness, and insomnia) are rare.

☑ Special considerations

● Assess patient's history of allergies; don't give a sulfonamide to patient with history of hypersensitivity reactions to sulfonamides or to other drugs containing sulfur.

● Sulfonamides are contraindicated in patients with severe renal or hepatic dysfunction, in those with porphyria, and during pregnancy, at term, and during breast-feeding. Sulfonamides may cause kernicterus in infants because these drugs displace bilirubin at the binding site, cross the placenta, and are excreted in breast milk. Don't use in infants under age 2 months (except in treatment of congenital toxoplasmosis as adjunctive therapy with pyrimethamine).

● Administer sulfonamides with caution to patients with the following conditions: mild to moderate renal or hepatic impairment; urinary obstruction because of the risk of drug accumulation; severe allergies; asthma; blood dyscrasia; or G6PD deficiency.

● Continuously monitor patient for possible hypersensitivity reactions or other adverse effects; patients with AIDS have a much higher risk of adverse reactions.

● Cultures and sensitivity tests should be obtained before giving first dose, but therapy may begin before laboratory tests are complete; check test results periodically to assess drug efficacy. Monitor urine cultures, CBCs, and urinalysis before and during therapy.

● Monitor patients on prolonged therapy for superinfection, especially elderly and debilitated patients and others receiving immunosuppressants or radiation therapy.

● Sulfonamides may interact with other drugs (oral anticoagulants, cyclosporine, digoxin, folic acid, hydantoins, methotrexate, and sulfonylureas) and may alter test results; consult specific drug monographs for possible test interactions.

● Give oral dose with full glass (8 oz [240 ml]) of water, and force fluids (12 to 16 glasses/day) depending on drug; patient's urine output should be at least 1,500 ml/day.

● Follow manufacturer's directions for reconstitution, dilution, and storage of drugs; check expiration dates.

● Give oral sulfonamide at least 1 hour before or 2 hours after meals for maximum absorption.

● Shake oral suspensions well before administering to ensure correct dose.

Information for the patient

• Teach signs and symptoms of hypersensitivity and other adverse reactions, and emphasize need to report these; specifically urge patient to report bloody urine, difficulty breathing, rash, fever, chills, or severe fatigue.

• Teach signs and symptoms of bacterial and fungal superinfection to elderly and debilitated patients and others with low resistance from immunosuppressants or irradiation; emphasize need to report any of these signs and symptoms.

• Advise diabetic patient that sulfonamides may increase effects of oral hypoglycemic. Tell him not to monitor urine glucose levels with Clinitest; sulfonamides alter results of tests using cupric sulfate.

• Advise patient to avoid exposure to direct sunlight because of risk of photosensitivity reaction.

• Tell patient to take oral drug with a full glass (8 oz [240 ml]) of water and to drink at least 12 to 16 glasses of water daily depending on drug; explain that tablet may be crushed and swallowed with water to ensure maximum absorption.

• Teach patient how and when to take drugs; urge him to complete entire regimen, to comply with instructions for around-the-clock dosing, and to keep follow-up appointments.

• Teach patient to check expiration date of drug and how to store drug; tell him to discard unused drug.

• For sulfasalazine, inform patient to take with food if GI irritation occurs; tell him that it may cause an orange-yellow discoloration of urine or skin and may permanently stain soft contact lenses yellow.

• Caution patient to take protective measures (for example, sunscreen, protective clothing) against exposure to ultraviolet light or sunlight until tolerance is determined because photosensitization may occur.

Geriatric patients

• Use with caution; elderly patients are susceptible to bacterial and fungal superinfection, are at greater risk for folate deficiency anemia after sulfonamide therapy, and commonly are at greater risk for renal and hematologic effects because of diminished renal function.

Pediatric patients

• Sulfonamides are contraindicated in infants under age 2 months unless there is no therapeutic alternative.

• Give sulfonamides with caution to children with fragile X chromosome associated with mental retardation; they are vulnerable to psychomotor depression from folate depletion.

Pregnant patients

• Safety during pregnancy hasn't been established. Cleft palate, other bony abnormalities, and kernicterus in infant may occur.

Breast-feeding patients

• Because sulfonamides appear in breast milk, a decision should be made to either stop drug or breast-feeding, taking into account importance of drug to mother. Premature infants, infants with hyperbilirubinemia, and those with G6PD deficiency are at risk for kernicterus.

Representative combinations

Sulfadiazine with sulfamerazine and sulfamethazine: Triple Sulfa.

Sulfamethizole with sulfathiazole, sulfacetamide, sulfabenzamide, and urea: Triple Sulfa, V.V.S., Trysul, Gyne-Sulf, Sultrin.

Sulfamethoxazole with phenazopyridine hydrochloride: Azo Gantanol, Azo-Sulfamethoxazole; with trimethoprim: Bactrim, Cotrim, cotrimoxazole, Septra, SMZ-TMP.

Sulfisoxazole with erythromycin ethylsuccinate: Pediazole; with phenazopyridine hydrochloride: Azo Gantrisin.

Sulfadoxine with pyrimethamine: Fansidar.

---

sulfonylureas

acetohexamide, chlorpropamide, glimepiride, glipizide, glyburide, tolazamide, tolbutamide

---

In 1942, a sulfonamide, an antibacterial, was discovered to have hypoglycemic effects. Subsequent experiments showed that this drug didn't exert similar effects in pancreatectomized animals. Later, tolbutamide was introduced and soon became popular for managing certain diabetic patients. Sulfonylureas are useful only in patients with mild to moderately severe type 2 diabetes mellitus. These drugs can be used only in patients with functioning beta cells of the pancreas.

Pharmacology

The sulfonylurea antidiabetics are sulfonamide derivatives that exert no antibacterial activity.

Sulfonylureas lower blood glucose levels by stimulating insulin release from the pancreas. These drugs work only in the presence of functioning beta cells in the islet tissue of the pancreas. After prolonged administration, they produce hypoglycemia through significant extrapancreatic effects, including reduction of hepatic glucose production and enhanced peripheral sensitivity to insulin. The latter may result from an increase in the number of insulin receptors or from changes in events after insulin binding. (See *Comparing oral antidiabetics*, page 1202.)

The sulfonylureas are divided into first-generation drugs (chlorpropamide) and second-generation drugs (glyburide, glipizide, and glimepiride). Although their mechanisms of action are similar, the second-generation drugs car-

COMPARING ORAL ANTIDIABETICS

Typically, sulfonylureas have similar actions and produce similar effects. They differ mainly in duration of action and dosage.

Drug	Usual daily dosage	Onset	Peak	Duration
First generation				
acetohexamide (Dymelor)	500 mg once daily or b.i.d.	1 hr	2 hr	12 to 24 hr
chlorpropamide (Diabenese)	250 mg once daily	1 hr	3 to 6 hr	24 to 60 hr
tolazamide (Tolinase)	250 mg once daily or b.i.d.	4 to 6 hr	6 to 10 hr	12 to 24 hr
tolbutamide (Orinase)	1,000 mg b.i.d. or t.i.d.	½ to 1 hr	4 to 8 hr	6 to 12 hr
Second generation				
glimepiride (Amaryl)	1 to 4 mg once daily	1 hr	2 to 3 hr	24 hr
glipizide (Glucotrol)	5 mg once daily	1 to 3 hr	2 to 3 hr	10 to 24 hr
glyburide (DiaBeta, Micronase)	5 mg once daily	2 hr	3 to 4 hr	12 to 24 hr

ry a more lipophilic side chain, are more potent, and cause fewer adverse reactions. Their most important differences are their durations of action.

Clinical indications and actions

Type 2 diabetes mellitus

Sulfonylureas are used to manage mild to moderately severe, stable, nonketotic type 2 diabetes mellitus that can't be controlled by diet alone. Sulfonylureas stimulate insulin release from the pancreas. After long-term therapy, extrapancreatic hypoglycemic effects include reduced hepatic glucose production, an increased number of insulin receptors, and changes in insulin binding.

◇ **Neurogenic diabetes insipidus**

Chlorpropamide has been used in selected patients to treat neurogenic diabetes insipidus. The drug appears to potentiate the effect of minimal levels of antidiuretic hormone.

Overview of adverse reactions

Dose-related adverse effects, which usually aren't serious and respond to decreased dosages, include headache, nausea, vomiting, anorexia, heartburn, weakness, and paresthesia. Hypoglycemia may follow excessive doses, increased exercise, decreased food intake, or consumption of alcohol. Signs and symptoms of overdose include anxiety; chills; cold sweats; confusion; cool, pale skin; difficulty concentrating; drowsiness; excessive hunger; headache; nausea; nervousness;

rapid heartbeat; shakiness; unsteady gait; weakness; and unusual fatigue.

☑ Special considerations

● Sulfonylureas should be given 30 minutes before the morning meal for once-daily dosing, or 30 minutes before the morning and evening meals for twice-daily dosing.

● Contraindicated in patients with type 1 diabetes mellitus; brittle or severe diabetes; diabetes mellitus adequately controlled by diet; and type 2 diabetes mellitus complicated by ketosis, acidosis, diabetic coma, Raynaud's gangrene, renal or hepatic impairment, or thyroid or other endocrine dysfunction.

● Use cautiously in patients with sulfonamide hypersensitivity.

● Chlorpropamide shouldn't be used in elderly patients.

● Monitor patients transferring from insulin therapy to a sulfonylurea for urine glucose and ketones at least three times daily, before meals; emphasize the need for testing a double-voided specimen. Patients may need hospitalization during such changes in therapy.

● Patients transferring from another sulfonylurea (except chlorpropamide) usually need no transition period.

● Patients with type 2 diabetes mellitus may need insulin therapy during periods of increased stress, such as infection, fever, surgery, or trauma. Monitor patients closely for hyperglycemia in these situations.

Information for the patient
- Teach patient about the nature of the disease.
- Emphasize importance of following therapeutic regimen and adhering to specific diet, weight reduction, exercise, and personal hygiene recommendations. Patient also should know how to avoid infections and test for glycosuria and ketonuria; he should know signs and symptoms of hypoglycemia (fatigue, excessive hunger, profuse sweating, and numbness of extremities) and hyperglycemia (excessive thirst or urination and excessive urine glucose or ketones).
- Inform patient that drug relieves symptoms but doesn't cure the disease.
- Discourage patient from consuming moderate to large amounts of alcohol while taking sulfonylureas; disulfiram-type reactions are possible.

Geriatric patients
- Elderly patients and those with renal insufficiency may be more sensitive to these drugs because of decreased metabolism and excretion. They usually need lower doses and should be closely monitored.
- Hypoglycemia may be more difficult to recognize in elderly patients, although it usually causes neurologic symptoms in such patients. Drugs with prolonged duration of action should be avoided in elderly patients.

Pediatric patients
- Oral antidiabetics aren't effective in type 1 diabetes mellitus.

Pregnant patients
- Don't use sulfonylurea antidiabetics during pregnancy because of prolonged, severe hypoglycemia lasting from 4 to 10 days in neonates born to mothers taking these drugs. Also, use of insulin permits more rigid control of blood glucose levels, which should reduce the risk of congenital abnormalities, mortality, and morbidity caused by abnormal glucose levels.

Breast-feeding patients
- Oral antidiabetics appear in breast milk in minimal amounts and may cause hypoglycemia in breast-fed infants.

Representative combinations
None.

tetracyclines

demeclocycline hydrochloride, doxycycline hyclate, minocycline hydrochloride, oxytetracycline hydrochloride, tetracycline hydrochloride

Tetracycline antibiotics were discovered during the random screening of soil samples for antibiotic-producing microorganisms. The prototype, chlortetracycline, was discovered in 1948; tetracycline was developed in 1952. Structural modifications that enhanced both antibacterial activity and pharmacokinetic parameters led to development of doxycycline in 1966 and minocycline in 1972.

Usually well tolerated with few serious adverse effects, tetracyclines have an unusually broad spectrum of antibacterial activity, including gram-negative and gram-positive anaerobic and aerobic bacteria, *Chlamydia,* and protozoa; longer-acting tetracyclines have enhanced activity against *Chlamydia* and *Legionella.*

Demeclocycline has a higher risk of severe photosensitivity reactions. Because of its renal effects, it is rarely prescribed, ◊ although it as been used in the treatment of SIADH secretion.

Pharmacology
Tetracyclines are bacteriostatic but may be bactericidal against certain organisms. They bind reversibly to 30S and 50S ribosomal subunits, inhibiting bacterial protein synthesis. Bacterial resistance to tetracyclines is usually mediated by plasmids (R-factor resistance), which decrease bacterial cell-wall permeability; this is the most important cause of resistance by staphylococci, streptococci, most aerobic gram-negative organisms, and *Pseudomonas aeruginosa.* With two exceptions, cross-resistance occurs with all tetracyclines; doxycycline is active against *Bacteroides fragilis,* and minocycline is active against *Staphylococcus aureus, Acinetobacter,* and Enterobacteriaceae.

Tetracyclines attack many pathogens; they aren't antifungal or antiviral.

Susceptible gram-positive organisms include *Bacillus anthracis, Actinomyces israelii, Clostridium perfringens, C. tetani, Listeria monocytogenes,* and *Nocardia.* Initial but transient activity exists against staphylococci and streptococci; infections caused by these organisms are usually treated with other drugs.

Susceptible gram-negative organisms include *Bartonella bacilliformis, Calymmatobacterium granulomatis, Francisella tularensis, Leptotrichia buccalis, Neisseria meningitidis, Pasteurella multocida, Legionella pneumophila, Brucella, Vibrio cholerae, Yersinia enterocolitica, V. parahaemolyticus, Y. pestis, Bordetella pertussis, Haemoph-*

ilus influenzae, H. ducreyi, Campylobacter fetus, Spirillum minus, Streptobacillus moniliformis, Shigella, and many other common pathogens.

Other susceptible organisms include *Rickettsia akari, R. typhi, R. prowazekii, R. tsutsugamushi, Coxiella burnetii, Chlamydia trachomatis, C. psittaci, Mycoplasma pneumoniae, M. hominis, Leptospira, Treponema pallidum, T. pertenue,* and *Borrelia recurrentis.*

Tetracyclines are absorbed systemically after oral administration, chiefly from the duodenum; with the exception of doxycycline and minocycline, absorption is decreased by food, milk, and divalent and trivalent cations. Oral absorption of tetracyclines is affected by chelation with certain minerals such as calcium (doxycycline is least involved); chelation causes tetracyclines to localize in bones and teeth. Because of hepatotoxicity and thrombophlebitis, only doxycycline and, to a lesser extent, minocycline, are used I.V.

Tetracyclines are distributed widely into body tissues and fluid, but CSF penetration is minimal; lipid-soluble minocycline and doxycycline penetrate fluids and tissues better; all tetracyclines cross the placenta.

Tetracyclines are excreted primarily in urine, chiefly by glomerular filtration; some drug is excreted in breast milk, and some inactivated drug is excreted in feces. Unlike other tetracyclines, minocycline undergoes enterohepatic circulation and is excreted in feces.

Oxytetracycline is moderately hemodialyzable; other tetracyclines are removed only minimally by hemodialysis or peritoneal dialysis.

Clinical indications and actions
Bacterial, antiprotozoal, rickettsial, and fungal infections
Tetracyclines are used as first-line therapy for chlamydial infections and are the drugs of choice for lymphogranuloma venereum, nonlymphogranuloma venereum strains of *C. trachomatis* in sexually transmitted diseases, psittacosis, and nongonococcal urethritis if the primary pathogen is probably *M. hominis* or *C. trachomatis.* They are also the drugs of choice for rickettsial infections (Rocky Mountain spotted fever, scrub and endemic typhus, rickettsial pox, and Q fever) and brucellosis. Tetracyclines also are used to treat infections caused by *Campylobacter*, mycoplasma pneumonia (after Legionnaire's disease is ruled out), pertussis, and cholera (in United States only).

Tetracyclines are second-line drugs in therapy of syphilis, actinomycosis, listeriosis, chancroid, and infections caused by *Pasteurella multocida* and *Yersinia pestis.* They also provide economical prophylaxis in chronic pulmonary disease.

Tetracyclines are used orally to treat inflammatory acne vulgaris, topically for mild to moderate inflammatory acne, and as eyedrops for superficial eye infections, inclusion conjunctivitis, and prophylaxis of ophthalmia neonatorum.

Individual tetracyclines are more effective against certain species or strains of a particular organism.

◇ Diuretic drug in SIADH
Demeclocycline causes diuresis by blocking antidiuretic hormone–induced reabsorption of water in the distal convoluted tubules and collecting ducts of the kidneys.

Sclerosing drug
Parenteral tetracycline hydrochloride has been administered by intracavitary injection as a sclerosing drug in pleural or pericardial effusion. Parenteral doxycycline hyclate has been used as a sclerosing drug to control pleural effusions associated with metastatic tumors.

Other uses
◇ Oral doxycycline and oral tetracycline have been used to treat Lyme disease.

Tetracycline is used as an adjunct to therapy for *Helicobacter pylori* infection.

◇ Tetracycline is used to treat various GI infections, including balantidiasis caused by *Balantidium coli,* Whipple's disease, blind-loop syndrome, and tropical sprue.

Doxycycline is used for the suppression or prophylactic treatment of malaria caused by *Plasmodium falciparum* (chloroquine-resistant or sulfadoxine and pyrimethamine–resistant) in individuals traveling for less than 4 months.

Overview of adverse reactions
The most common adverse effects of tetracyclines involve the GI tract, are dose-related, and include anorexia; flatulence; nausea; vomiting; bulky, loose stools; epigastric burning; and abdominal discomfort.

Hypersensitivity reactions are infrequent; they manifest as urticaria, rash, pruritus, eosinophilia, and exfoliative dermatitis.

Photosensitivity reactions may be severe; they commonly occur with demeclocycline, rarely with minocycline.

Renal effects are minor and include occasional elevations in BUN levels (without rise in serum creatinine level) and a reversible diabetes insipidus syndrome (reported only with demeclocycline); renal failure has been attributed to Fanconi's syndrome after use of outdated tetracycline.

Rare adverse effects include hepatotoxicity (often in pregnant women receiving more than 2 g/day I.V.), leukocytosis, thrombocytopenia, hemolytic anemia, leukopenia, neutropenia, and atypical lymphocytes. There also have been reports of vaginal candidiasis, microscopic thyroid discoloration (after long-term use), lightheadedness, dizziness, drowsiness, vein irritation (after I.V. use), and permanent discoloration of teeth in children under age 8.

Drug use with oral contraceptives can decrease contraceptive's effectiveness and increase the risk of pregnancy.

☑ Special considerations
• Assess patient's allergic history; don't give tetracycline antibiotics to patient with history of hypersensitivity reactions to other tetracyclines; monitor patient continuously for this and other adverse reactions.
• Obtain cultures and sensitivity tests before giving first dose, but don't delay therapy; check cultures periodically to assess drug efficacy.
• Monitor vital signs, electrolytes, and renal function studies before and during therapy.
• Check expiration dates. Outdated tetracyclines may cause nephrotoxicity.
• Watch for bacterial and fungal superinfection, especially in elderly or debilitated patients and in those receiving immunosuppressants or radiation therapy; watch especially for oral candidiasis. If symptoms occur, stop drug.
• Tetracyclines may interfere with certain laboratory tests; consult specific drug monograph.
• Give oral drugs 1 hour before or 2 hours after meals for maximum absorption; don't give with food, milk or other dairy products, sodium bicarbonate, iron compounds, or antacids, which may impair absorption.
• Give water with and after oral drug to facilitate passage to stomach because incomplete swallowing can cause severe esophageal irritation; don't administer within 1 hour of bedtime to prevent esophageal reflux.
• Follow manufacturer's directions for reconstitution and storage; keep product refrigerated and out of light.
• Avoid I.V. administration of drug in patients with decreased renal function.
• I.V. administration during pregnancy or in patients with renal impairment, especially when dose exceeds 2 g/day, can cause hepatic failure.
• Monitor I.V. injection sites and rotate routinely to reduce local irritation. I.V. administration may cause severe phlebitis.

Information for the patient
• Explain disease process and rationale for therapy.
• Teach signs and symptoms of adverse reactions, and emphasize need to report these promptly; urge patient to report unusual effects.
• Teach signs and symptoms of bacterial and fungal superinfection to elderly and debilitated patients and to others with low resistance from immunosuppressants or irradiation.
• Advise patient using oral contraceptives to use a back-up method of contraception during therapy.
• Advise patient to avoid direct sunlight and to use a sunscreen to prevent photosensitivity reactions.

• Tell patient to take oral tetracyclines with a full glass (8 oz [240 ml]) of water (to facilitate passage to the stomach) 1 hour before or 2 hours after meals for maximum absorption, and not less than 1 hour before bedtime (to prevent irritation from esophageal reflux).
• Emphasize that taking drug with food, milk or other dairy products, sodium bicarbonate, or iron compounds may interfere with absorption. Tell patient to take antacids 3 hours after tetracycline.
• Stress importance of completing prescribed regimen exactly as prescribed and keeping follow-up appointments.
• Tell patient that doxycycline and minocycline may be taken with food.
• Instruct patient to check expiration date before use.

Geriatric patients
• Some elderly patients have decreased esophageal motility; use tetracyclines cautiously and watch for local irritation from slowly passing oral dosage forms. Elderly patients are more susceptible to superinfection.

Pediatric patients
• Don't use in children under age 8 unless there's no alternative. Tetracyclines can cause permanent discoloration of teeth, enamel hypoplasia, and a reversible decrease in bone calcification.
• Reversible decreases in bone calcification have been reported in infants.

Pregnant patients
• Tetracyclines may cause fetal toxicity in pregnant women.

Breast-feeding patients
• Avoid use of tetracyclines in breast-feeding women.

Representative combinations
Oxytetracycline with polymyxin B sulfate: Terramycin with Polymyxin B.
Tetracycline hydrochloride with citric acid: Achromycin V.

thrombolytic enzymes

alteplase, anistreplase, reteplase (recombinant), streptokinase, urokinase

When a thrombus obstructs a blood vessel, permanent damage to the ischemic area may occur before the body can dissolve the clot. Thrombolytics were developed in the hope that speeding lysis of the clot would prevent permanent ischemic damage. Thrombolytic activity attributable to streptokinase was described in 1933; this

COMPARING THROMBOLYTIC ENZYMES

Thrombolytic enzymes dissolve clots by accelerating the formation of plasmin by activated plasminogen. Plasminogen activators, found in most tissues and body fluids, help plasminogen (an inactive enzyme) convert to plasmin (an active enzyme), which dissolves the clot. Doses of these enzymes may vary according to the patient's condition.

Drug	Action	Initial dose	Maintenance therapy
alteplase	Directly converts plasminogen to plasmin	*I.V. bolus:* 6 to 10 mg over 1 to 2 min	*I.V. infusion:* 60 mg/hr in the 1st hr; then 20 mg/hr for the next 2 hr for a total of 100 mg
anistreplase	Directly converts plasminogen to plasmin	*I.V. push:* 30 units over 2 to 5 min	Not necessary
reteplase	Enhances the cleavage of plasminogen to generate plasmin	Double I.V. bolus injection of 10 + 10 units	Not necessary
streptokinase	Indirectly activates plasminogen, which converts to plasmin	*Intracoronary bolus:* 15,000 to 20,000 IU *I.V. bolus:* none needed	*Intracoronary infusion:* 2,000 to 4,000 IU/min over 1 hr; total dose 140,000 IU *I.V. infusion:* 1,500,000 units over 1 hr
urokinase	Directly converts plasminogen to plasmin	*Intracoronary bolus:* none needed	*Intracoronary infusion:* 2,000 units/lb/hr (4,400 units/kg/hr); rate of 15 ml of solution/hr for total of 12 hr (total volume shouldn't exceed 200 ml)

compound's effects have since been studied on various kinds of clots. It's unclear whether such drugs significantly reduce thrombosis-induced ischemic damage in all situations for which the drugs are currently used. (See *Comparing thrombolytic enzymes*.)

Pharmacology
Streptokinase is a proteinlike substance produced by group C beta-hemolytic streptococci; urokinase is an enzyme isolated from human kidney tissue cultures. Alteplase is a tissue-type plasminogen activator synthesized by recombinant DNA technology. Anistreplase is an anisoylated streptokinase-plasminogen activated complex; it's a fibrinolytic enzyme (plasminogen) plus activator complex (streptokinase) with the activator temporarily blocked by an anisoyl group. Reteplase is a recombinant-plasminogen activator. Thrombolytic enzymes act to lyse clots chiefly by converting plasminogen to plasmin; in contrast, anticoagulants act by preventing thrombi from developing. Thrombolytics are more likely to produce clinical bleeding than are oral anticoagulants.

Clinical indications and actions
Alteplase, streptokinase, and urokinase are used to treat acute pulmonary thromboembolism; strep-

tokinase and urokinase are used to treat deep vein thrombosis, acute arterial thromboembolism, and acute coronary arterial thrombosis and to clear arteriovenous cannula occlusion and venous catheter obstruction. Anistreplase, alteplase, reteplase, streptokinase, and urokinase are indicated in acute MI. These drugs are administered in an attempt to lyse coronary artery thrombi, which may result in improved ventricular function and decreased risk of heart failure. Alteplase is used in the management of acute ischemic stroke.

Overview of adverse reactions
Adverse reactions to these drugs are essentially an extension of their actions; hemorrhage is the most common adverse effect. These drugs cause bleeding twice as often as does heparin. Streptokinase is more likely than urokinase to cause an allergic reaction. Information regarding hypersensitivity to alteplase is limited.

☑ Special considerations
• Thrombolytic therapy requires medical supervision with continuous clinical and laboratory monitoring.
• Thrombolytics act only on fibrin clots, not those formed by a precipitated drug.

• Instructions for reconstitution must be followed precisely and solution passed through a filter 0.45 microns or smaller to remove solution filaments; don't use with dextran because it can interfere with coagulation as well as blood typing and cross-matching.

• Obtain pretherapy baseline determinations of thrombin time, APTT, PT, INR, hematocrit, and platelet count for subsequent blood monitoring. During systemic thrombolytic therapy, as in pulmonary embolism or venous thrombosis, PT, INR, or thrombin time after 4 hours of therapy should be about twice the pretreatment value.

• Administer drugs by infusion pump to ensure accuracy; I.M. injections are contraindicated because of increased risk of bleeding at injection site.

• Monitor vital signs frequently. Monitor patient for blood pressure alterations in excess of 25 mm Hg and any change in cardiac rhythm. Check pulses, color, and sensitivity of extremities every hour. Monitor patient for excessive bleeding every 15 minutes for first hour, every 30 minutes for second through eighth hours; then at least once every 8 hours. Stop therapy if bleeding is evident; pretreatment with heparin or drugs affecting platelets increases risk.

• Watch for hypersensitivity as well as hemorrhage; keep available typed and crossmatched packed RBCs and whole blood, aminocaproic acid to treat bleeding, and corticosteroids to treat allergic reactions.

• Keep involved extremity in straight alignment to prevent bleeding from infusion site. Establish precautions to prevent injury and avoid unnecessary handling of patient because bruising is likely.

• At end of infusion, remaining dose should be flushed from pump tubing with I.V. 5% dextrose or normal saline solution.

• Continuous heparin infusion usually is started with the prescribed thrombolytic.

• Before using thrombolytic to clear an occluded catheter, try to gently aspirate or flush with heparinized saline solution. Avoid forcible flushing or vigorous suction, which could rupture catheter or expel clot into the circulation.

• When treating MI or CVA, the sooner treatment is started, the greater the benefit.

Information for the patient
• Explain rationale for treatment and procedure, and necessity for bed rest.
• Advise patient to be alert for signs of bleeding.
• When using these drugs to clear catheter, tell patient to exhale and hold breath any time catheter isn't connected to prevent air entering open catheter.

Geriatric patients
• Patients ages 75 and older are at greater risk for cerebral hemorrhage because they are more likely to have preexisting cerebrovascular disease.

Pediatric patients
• Safety in children hasn't been established.

Pregnant patients
• Thrombolytics should be used during pregnancy only if clearly indicated.

Breast-feeding patients
• Safety hasn't been established.

Representative combinations
None.

tricyclic antidepressants (TCAs)

amitriptyline hydrochloride, clomipramine hydrochloride, desipramine hydrochloride, doxepin hydrochloride, imipramine hydrochloride, imipramine pamoate, nortriptyline hydrochloride, protriptyline, trimipramine maleate

The inherent mood-elevating activity of TCAs was discovered during research with iminodibenzyl, a compound originally investigated for sedative, analgesic, antihistaminic, and antiparkinsonian effects. Clinical trials in 1958 with the class prototype, imipramine, found no antipsychotic activity, but showed marked mood-elevating effects.

Pharmacology
Although the precise mechanism of their CNS effects isn't established, TCAs may exert their effects by inhibiting reuptake of the neurotransmitters norepinephrine and serotonin in CNS nerve terminals (presynaptic neurons), resulting in increased levels and enhanced activity of neurotransmitters in the synaptic cleft. TCAs also have antihistaminic, sedative, anticholinergic, vasodilatory, and quinidine-like effects; the drugs are structurally similar to phenothiazines and share similar adverse effects.

Individual TCAs differ somewhat in their degree of CNS inhibitory effect. The tertiary amines (amitriptyline, doxepin, imipramine, and trimipramine) exert greater sedative effects; tertiary amines and protriptyline have more profound effects on cardiac conduction, whereas desipramine has the least anticholinergic activity. All of the currently available TCAs have equal clinical efficacy when given in equivalent therapeutic doses; choice of specific therapy is determined primarily by pharmacokinetic properties and the patient's adverse reaction profile. Patients may respond to some TCAs and not others; if a patient doesn't respond to one drug, another should be tried.

Clinical indications and actions
Depression
TCAs are used to treat major depression and dysthymic disorder. Depressed patients who are also anxious are helped most by the more sedating drugs: doxepin, imipramine, and trimipramine. Protriptyline has a stimulant effect that evokes a favorable response in withdrawn, depressed patients.

Obsessive-compulsive disorder (OCD)
Clomipramine is used in the treatment of OCD.

Enuresis
Imipramine is used for enuresis in children over age 6.

Severe, chronic pain
TCAs, especially amitriptyline, desipramine, doxepin, imipramine, and nortriptyline, are useful in the management of severe, chronic pain.

◇ Other psychiatric disorders
TCAs have been used to treat phobic disorders with panic attacks and eating disorders (bulimia nervosa), and in the short-term treatment of duodenal or gastric ulcer.

Overview of adverse reactions
Adverse reactions to TCAs are similar to those seen with phenothiazine antipsychotics, including varying degrees of sedation, anticholinergic effects, and orthostatic hypotension. The tertiary amines have the strongest sedative effects; tolerance to these effects usually develops in a few weeks. Protriptyline has the least sedative effect (and may be stimulatory), but shares with the tertiary amines the most pronounced effects on blood pressure and cardiac tissue. Desipramine has a greater margin of safety in patients with prostatic hypertrophy, paralytic ileus, glaucoma, and urine retention because of its relatively low level of anticholinergic activity.

☑ Special considerations
• TCAs impair ability to perform tasks such as driving that require mental alertness.
• Monitor vital signs regularly for decreased blood pressure or tachycardia; observe patient carefully for adverse reactions and report changes. ECG should be obtained in patients over age 40 before initiating therapy. Advise having the patient take the first dose in the office to allow close observation for adverse reactions.
• Watch for anticholinergic adverse reactions, which may need dosage reduction.
• Caregiver should be sure patient swallows each dose of drug when given; as depressed patients begin to improve, they may hoard pills for suicide attempt.
• Observe patients for mood changes to monitor progress; benefits may not occur for 3 to 6 weeks.

• Don't withdraw full dose of drug abruptly; gradually reduce dosage over a period of weeks to avoid rebound effect or other adverse reactions.
• Carefully follow manufacturer's instructions for reconstitution, dilution, and storage of drugs.
• Investigational uses include peptic ulcer treatment, migraine prophylaxis, and allergy. Potential toxicity has, to date, outweighed most advantages.
• Because suicidal overdose with TCAs is commonly fatal, prescribe only small amounts. If possible, entrust a reliable family member with drug and warn him to store drug safely away from children.

Information for the patient
• Explain rationale for therapy and anticipated risks and benefits; also explain that full therapeutic effect may not occur for several weeks.
• Teach signs and symptoms of adverse reactions and importance of reporting them.
• Tell patient to avoid beverages and drugs containing alcohol and not to take other drugs or OTC products without calling first.
• Teach patient how and when to take drug; tell him not to increase dose without calling, and never to stop drug abruptly.
• Tell patient to lie down for 30 minutes after first dose and to rise slowly to avoid orthostatic hypotension.
• Advise taking drug with milk or food to minimize GI distress; suggest taking full dose at bedtime if daytime sedation is troublesome.
• Urge diabetic patients to monitor blood glucose level because drug may alter insulin needs.
• Advise patient to avoid tasks that require mental alertness until full effect of drug is known.
• Warn patient that excessive exposure to sunlight, heat lamps, or tanning beds may cause burns and abnormal hyperpigmentation.
• Recommend sugarless gum or hard candy, artificial saliva, or ice chips to relieve dry mouth.
• Advise patient that unpleasant adverse effects (except dry mouth) generally diminish over time.

Geriatric patients
• Use lower doses because these patients are more sensitive to therapeutic and adverse effects of TCAs.

Pediatric patients
• TCAs aren't recommended for children under age 12.

Pregnant patients
• Safety during pregnancy hasn't been established. Fetal malformations, urine retention, CNS effects (lethargy), developmental delay, and withdrawal symptoms have occurred in neonates born to mothers who took TCAs during pregnancy.

Breast-feeding patients
• Safety in breast-feeding women hasn't been established.

Representative combinations
Amitriptyline hydrochloride with perphenazine: Etrafon, Triavil; with chlordiazepoxide: Limbitrol.

vitamins

Fat-soluble: **vitamin A (retinol), vitamin A acid (retinoic acid), vitamin D, vitamin D_2 (ergocalciferol), vitamin D_3 (calcipotriene), vitamin E, vitamin K (phytonadione)**

Water-soluble: **vitamin B_1 (thiamine), vitamin B_2 (riboflavin), vitamin B_3 (niacin), vitamin B_6 (pyridoxine), vitamin B_9 (folic acid, folacin), vitamin B_{12} (cyanocobalamin), vitamin C (ascorbic acid)**

Vitamins are chemically unrelated organic compounds that are needed for normal growth and maintenance of metabolic functions. Because the body is unable to synthesize many vitamins, it must obtain them from exogenous sources. Vitamins don't furnish energy and aren't essential building blocks for the body; however, they are essential for the transformation of energy and for the regulation of metabolic processes.

Vitamins are classified as fat-soluble or water-soluble, and the Food and Nutrition Board of the National Research Council determines the recommended daily allowances (RDAs) for each. These allowances represent amounts that will provide adequate nutrition in most healthy persons; they aren't minimum requirements. Note that a diet that includes ample intake of the four basic food groups will provide sufficient quantities of vitamins. If needed, vitamins should be used as an adjunct to a regular diet and not as a food substitute.

Controversy has existed for years over the vitamin issue. Some argue that vitamin supplementation is unnecessary; some advise moderate supplementation; still others advocate the use of megavitamins. The public should be warned against self-medication with vitamins because the safety and efficacy of their long-term use haven't been established.

Pharmacology
Vitamins are available as single drugs or with several other vitamins with or without minerals, trace elements, iron, fluoride, or other nutritional supplements. Usually, diets deficient in one vitamin are also deficient in other vitamins of similar dietary source. Malabsorption syndromes also affect the usage of several vitamins as do certain disease states that increase metabolic rates. Therefore, multiple vitamin therapy may prove rational and useful in these situations.

Fat-soluble vitamins are absorbed with dietary fats and stored in the body in moderate amounts; they aren't normally excreted in urine. Long-term ingestion leads to excessive build-up of these drugs and toxicity.

Water-soluble vitamins aren't stored in the body in any appreciable amounts and are excreted in urine. These drugs seldom cause toxicity in patients with normal renal function.

Both types of vitamins are needed for the maintenance of normal structure and metabolic functions of the body. (See *Recommended daily allowances for adults ages 23 to 50*, page 1210.)

Clinical indications and actions
Vitamin deficiency or malabsorption; conditions of metabolic stress
Vitamin supplementation is needed when deficiencies exist, in malabsorption syndrome, in hypermetabolic disease states, during pregnancy and lactation, and in elderly patients, alcoholics, and dieters. Multiple vitamins may be indicated for patients taking oral contraceptives, estrogens, prolonged antibiotic therapy, or isoniazid and for those receiving prolonged total parenteral nutrition.

Patients with increased metabolic requirements, such as infants and those suffering severe injury, trauma, major surgery, or severe infection, also need supplementation. Prolonged diarrhea, severe GI disorders, malignancy, surgical removal of sections of GI tract, obstructive jaundice, cystic fibrosis, and other conditions leading to reduced or poor absorption are indications for multiple vitamin therapy. Refer to specific monographs for specific indications.

Overview of adverse reactions
Common adverse reactions seen with both water-soluble and fat-soluble vitamins include nausea, vomiting, diarrhea, tiredness, weakness, headache, loss of appetite, rash, and itching.

☑ Special considerations
• Monitoring may be needed. See specific monographs for details.
• Vitamins containing iron may cause constipation and black, tarry stools.

Information for the patient
• Stress importance of adequate dietary intake of food pyramid. Vitamins aren't food substitutes.
• Tell patient to take vitamins only as directed, not to exceed RDA, and to take with food, milk, or after meals to reduce chance of stomach upset.
• Store vitamins away from heat and light and out of reach of children.

◇ Unlabeled clinical use

RECOMMENDED DAILY ALLOWANCES FOR ADULTS AGES 23 TO 50

Vitamin	Men	Women	Pregnant women†	Lactating women†
A	1,000 mcg	800 mcg	800 mcg	1,300 mcg
B_1	1.5 mg	1.1 mg	1.5 mg	1.6 mg
B_2	1.7 mg	1.3 mg	1.6 mg	1.8 mg
B_6	2 mg	1.6 mg	2.2 mg	2.1 mg
B_{12}	2 mcg	2 mcg	2.2 mcg	2.6 mcg
C	60 mg	60 mg	70 mg	95 mg
D	200 IU	200 IU	400 IU	400 IU
E	15 IU	12 IU	15 IU	18 IU
K	80 mcg	65 mcg	65 mcg	65 mcg
folic acid	200 mcg	180 mcg	400 mcg	280 mcg
niacin	19 mg	15 mg	17 mg	20 mg

† First 6 months.

• Advise patient to take with food or after meals to reduce GI distress associated with vitamin therapy.
• Warn patient that vitamins with iron may cause constipation and black, tarry stools.
• Tell patient to read all label directions. Warn him not to take large doses unless prescribed.
• Inform patient that liquid vitamins may be mixed with food or juice.
• Advise patient not to refer to vitamins or other drugs as candy and to avoid taking them indiscriminately.

Pediatric patients
• RDAs vary with age. Excessive amounts of vitamins, particularly in neonates, may be toxic.

Pregnant patients
• Vitamin supplementation during pregnancy should be done under medical supervision.

Breast-feeding patients
• RDAs may be increased in breast-feeding women.

Representative combinations
The following list includes selected combinations that are available only by prescription.

B vitamins (oral) niacin (B_3), pantothenic acid (B_5), pyridoxine (B_6), and cyanocobalamin (B_{12}), with folic acid (B_9), iron, manganese, zinc, and 13% alcohol: Megaton Elixir; with thiamine (B_1), riboflavin (B_2), ferric pyrophosphate, and 15% alcohol: Senilezol Liquid; with thiamine (B_1), riboflavin (B_2), ascorbic acid, and folic acid: B-C with Folic Acid, Berocca, B-Plex, Strovite; with thiamine (B_1), riboflavin (B_2), ascorbic acid, folic acid, and biotin: Nephrocaps.

Multivitamins (oral) vitamins E, thiamine (B_1), riboflavin (B_2), niacin (B_3), pantothenic acid (B_5), pyridoxine (B_6), cyanocobalamin (B_{12}), ascorbic acid, and folic acid: Cefol Filmtabs; with vitamins A, D, E, thiamine (B_1), riboflavin (B_2), niacin (B_3), pantothenic acid (B_5), pyridoxine (B_6), cyanocobalamin (B_{12}), ascorbic acid, iron, and folic acid: Centrum Jr. with Iron, Cerovite Jr., Hi-Po-Vites, Monocaps, Quintabs-M, Unicap Sr., Unicomplex-T&M Tablets.

Multivitamins (parenteral) vitamins A, D, E, thiamine (B_1), riboflavin (B_2), niacin (B_3), pantothenic acid (B_5), pyridoxine (B_6), anocobalamin (B_{12}), ascorbic acid, biotin, and folic acid: Berocca Parenteral Nutrition, M.V.I.-12.

Multivitamins with fluoride (oral) vitamins A, D, thiamine (B_1), riboflavin (B_2), niacin (B_3), pantothenic acid (B_5), pyridoxine (B_6), cyanocobalamin (B_{12}), ascorbic acid, folic acid, and fluoride: Mulvidren-F Softab Tablets, Polytabs-F, Polyvitamin Fluoride; vitamins A, D, E, thiamine (B_1), riboflavin (B_2), niacin (B_3), pyridoxine (B_6), cyanocobalamin (B_{12}), ascorbic acid, folic acid, and fluoride: Florvite, Poly-Vi-Flor, Vi-Daylin/F.

Physician assistants' prescribing authority by state

The prescribing authority of physician assistants (PAs) is constantly changing as regulations are either continually implemented or in the process of being passed. Consult the respective state board for the most current laws and regulations on the prescribing authority for PAs. As of July 2000, PAs held the prescribing authorities indicated by the map below.

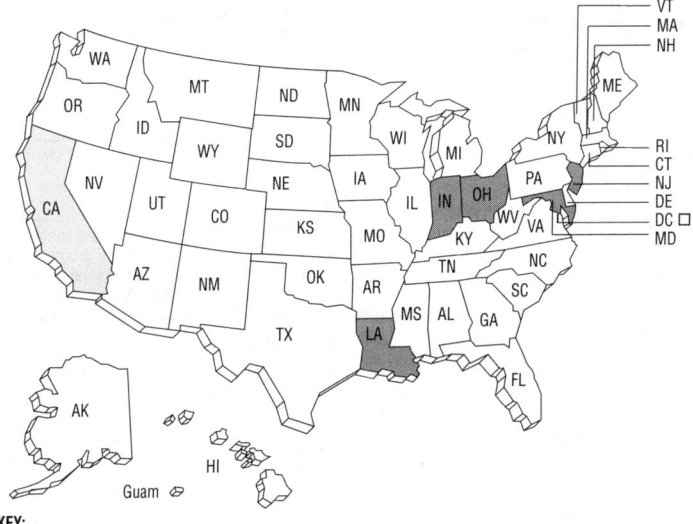

KEY:

☐ No physician signature required.

☐ Written prescription transmittal orders.

■ Physician signature required.

ALABAMA

PAs may prescribe noncontrolled drugs from board-approved formulary.

ALASKA

PAs may prescribe Schedule III to V controlled substances. The prescription must be written and signed by PA and include the collaborating physician's name and Drug Enforcement Administration (DEA) number.

ARIZONA

PAs may prescribe noncontrolled and controlled drugs. However, Schedule II and III drugs are limited to a 72-hour supply and Schedule IV and V drugs to a 34-day supply. Refills cannot be prescribed and DEA registration is required. Except for samples, dispensed drugs must be prepackaged by physician or pharmacist.

ARKANSAS

PAs may prescribe noncontrolled and controlled Schedule III-V medications as delegated by a physician.

CALIFORNIA

PAs may administer or provide medications to a patient, or transmit orally or in writing on a patient's record or in a transmittal order, a prescription from a supervising physician based on protocol or on patient-specific order. PAs may prescribe noncontrolled and controlled (Schedule II-V) drugs. PAs may hand the patient a properly labeled drug prepackaged by pharmacist, physician, or manufacturer. Medical records containing a prescription must be countersigned by supervising physician within 7 days.

COLORADO

PAs may prescribe controlled and noncontrolled substances using the supervising physician's forms. All drugs dispensed by PAs must be unit doses prepackaged by pharmacist or physician.

CONNECTICUT

PAs may prescribe noncontrolled and controlled (Schedule IV-V) drugs and dispense drugs in outpatient or nonprofit clinics. They may also order Schedule II and III drugs for inpatients.

DELAWARE

PAs may prescribe therapeutic drugs (Schedule II-V and legend drugs) as delegated by the physician, consistent with board rules.

DISTRICT OF COLUMBIA

PAs may prescribe noncontrolled drugs.

FLORIDA

PAs may prescribe drugs from formulary adopted by medical and osteopathic boards.

GEORGIA

PAs may prescribe noncontrolled and Schedule III-V drugs as delegated by physicians. DEA registration is required. PAs may also dispense drugs in public or nonprofit health facilities.

HAWAII

PAs may prescribe noncontrolled and controlled (Schedule III-V) drugs as delegated by a physician.

IDAHO

PAs may prescribe noncontrolled and controlled substances Schedule III-V.

ILLINOIS

PAs may prescribe noncontrolled and controlled substances Schedule III-V.

INDIANA

PAs have no prescribing authority. PAs may only use or dispense drugs prescribed or approved by the supervising physician. They may not dispense controlled substances.

IOWA

PAs may prescribe controlled substances (except Schedule II stimulants and depressants) and dispense drugs under certain conditions.

KANSAS

PAs may verbally (by telephone) transmit a prescription for Schedule III to V controlled substance (Schedule II drug only in emergency). Prescription for noncontrolled substances may be transmitted verbally (by phone) or in writing. Prescription-only drugs may be supplied to patients if directly ordered by the physician, authorized in written protocol, or in an emergency.

KENTUCKY

PAs can prescribe for legend drugs.

LOUISIANA

PAs have no prescribing or dispensing authority.

MAINE

PAs may prescribe and dispense drugs and medical devices, including Schedules III-V controlled substances. DEA registration is required.

MARYLAND

PAs may write medication orders in either a hospital, correctional facility, or a public health clinic and only pursuant to that institution's policy. All medication orders are reviewed and countersigned by the supervising physician within 48 hours if the care is rendered without direct supervision of the physician. At this time, there is no statutory authority for a PA to request or receive drug samples.

MASSACHUSETTS

PAs may prescribe controlled substances (Schedules II to V).

MICHIGAN

PAs may prescribe noncontrolled and controlled (Schedule III-V) drugs. Schedule II drugs (7-day supply) may be prescribed as discharge medication. The names of the PA and supervising physician must be included on the prescription.

MINNESOTA

NCCPA-certified PAs may prescribe controlled and noncontrolled drugs.

MISSISSIPPI

PAs have prescribing authority without controlled substances.

MISSOURI

PAs may not prescribe or dispense any drug, medicine, device, or therapy without the consultation of the supervising physician. Regulations to clarify prescriptive authority are pending.

MONTANA

PAs may prescribe and dispense drugs, including Schedule II-V controlled substances, as delegated by a physician. Schedule II controlled substances are limited to a 34-day supply.

NEBRASKA

PAs prescribe medications under the supervision of a physician. PAs may prescribe medications, including 72-hour supply of Schedule II controlled substances, in the supervising physician's name if authority is assigned by that physician.

NEVADA

With board approval, PAs may prescribe and dispense noncontrolled and controlled (Schedule II-V) drugs and devices as required by the supervising physician. Registration with pharmacy board required.

NEW HAMPSHIRE

PAs may prescribe noncontrolled and controlled (Schedule II-V) drugs. They must pass pharmacy law examination.

NEW JERSEY

PAs may prescribe medications, other than controlled substances, only in an inpatient setting and must provide specific information on the prescription blanks with required physician signature.

NEW MEXICO

PAs may prescribe, administer, and distribute Schedules II-V under direction of the supervising physician and within parameters of board-approved formulary and guidelines.

NEW YORK

PAs may write and sign prescriptions for noncontrolled and controlled substances Schedule III-V on the prescription blanks of the supervising physician.

NORTH CAROLINA

PAs may prescribe controlled drugs in Schedules II-V (Schedule II and III limited to 7-day supply). Pharmacy Board approval required for compounding and dispensing drugs.

NORTH DAKOTA

PAs may prescribe Schedule III to V controlled substances. They may also dispense prepackaged medications (Schedules IV and V and noncontrolled substances) prepared by pharmacist acting on the physician's written order and labeled to show names of PA and physician. Dispensing must be authorized by and within preestablished guidelines of the supervising physician.

OHIO

PAs do not have prescribing or dispensing authority.

OKLAHOMA

PAs may transmit oral or written prescriptions for noncontrolled drugs on board-approved formulary.

OREGON

PAs may prescribe drugs, including Schedule III to V controlled substances, as determined by the physician and approved by board. DEA registration is required. PAs may apply for emergency dispensing authority for medications prepackaged by pharmacist.

PENNSYLVANIA

PAs may prescribe and dispense drugs from a formulary which excludes parenterals except insulin and allergy kits. PAs may prescribe Schedule III-V drugs, which are limited to a 30-day supply unless they are for chronic conditions.

RHODE ISLAND

PAs may prescribe drugs, including Schedule II-V. They must register with the state drug control office and DEA.

SOUTH CAROLINA

PAs may prescribe drugs, including Schedule V controlled substances.

SOUTH DAKOTA

PAs may prescribe drugs, including Schedules II-V substances. Schedule II drugs are limited to a 48-hour supply.

TENNESSEE

PAs may prescribe noncontrolled and Schedule II-V drugs.

TEXAS

PAs may sign or complete presigned prescription blanks if delegated this task under standing orders. Limited to medically underserved areas, practices with preponderance of medically indigent patients, a physician's primary practice site, hospital, or other location or when physician is present.

UTAH

PAs may prescribe noncontrolled and controlled Schedule II-V drugs. Any limitations on prescribing may be made in the delegation agreement. Prescriptions for Schedule II and III medications require chart cosignature.

VERMONT

PAs may prescribe drugs, including Schedule II-V, authorized by physician in job description and the formulary.

VIRGINIA

PAs may prescribe noncontrolled drugs and devices on board-approved formulary.

WASHINGTON

Certified PAs may write and sign prescriptions, including controlled substances in Schedules II to V; using the supervisor's DEA number with suffix or own number. PAs may dispense medications from office supplies (for osteopathic PAs), limited to 48-hour supply.

WEST VIRGINIA

PAs with 2 years of experience who have completed board-approved pharmacology course and maintain NCCPA certification may prescribe controlled (Schedule III to V) and noncontrolled drugs from formulary. Schedule III drugs are limited to 72-hour supply. DEA registration is required. PAs may dispense samples and, under certain conditions, legend drugs.

WISCONSIN

PAs may prepare prescription order for controlled substances Schedule II-V in situations specified in written protocols and, when practical, after consultation with the physician. The physician must review and sign records within certain time limits.

WYOMING

Physicians may delegate prescribing (including Schedules II-V) to PAs; dispensing of prepackaged drugs in rural areas is allowed when pharmacy services are unavailable. The supervising physician's DEA number must be used when prescribing controlled substances.

Guidelines for use of selected antimicrobials

This table provides guidelines for the first-line (denoted by the numeral 1) and second-line (numeral 2) management of selected organisms and should be used as a general reference only. Use patient condition, sensitivities, institutional policies, and recent research when initiating new therapy.

Organism	Aminoglycosides				Cephalosporins									
	Amikacin	Gentamicin	Netilmicin	Tobramycin	Cefazolin	Cefepime	Cefixime	Cefoperazone	Cefotaxime	Cefoxitin	Ceftazidime	Ceftizoxime	Ceftriaxone	Cefuroxime
Acinetobacter	1	1	1	1							2			
Bacillus anthracis														
Bacteroides fragilis								2		2				
Borrelia burgdorferi (skin)													1	2
Campylobacter jejuni														
Chlamydia pneumoniae														
Chlamydia psittaci														
Chlamydia trachomatis														
Citrobacter freundii		1		1										
Clostridium difficile														
Clostridium perfringens					2					2	2	2	2	
Enterobacter sp.	1	1	1	1			2		2	2		2	2	
Enterococcus faecalis														
Enterococcus faecium														
Escherichia coli	2	2	2	2	1	1	1	1	1	1	1	1	1	1
Haemophilus influenzae*	1	1	1	1						1		1	1	
Haemophilus influenzae†						2								2
Klebsiella pneumoniae (UTI)					1		1		1	1		1	1	1
Klebsiella pneumoniae (pneumonia)	2	2	2	2			1	1	1	1	1	1	1	1
Legionella pneumophila														
Listeria monocytogenes		1		1										
Moraxella catarrhalis					2	2	2	2	2	2	2	2	2	2
Mycoplasma pneumoniae														
Neisseria gonorrhoeae							1						1	
Nocardia asteroides														
Pneumocystis carinii														
Proteus mirabilis					2	2	2	2	2	2	2	2	2	2
Proteus vulgaris							1	1	1			1	1	1
Pseudomonas aeruginosa	2	2	2	1		2		1			1			
Serratia marcescens	2	2	2	2				2	1			2	2	1
Shigella sp.														
Staphylococcus aureus					1									
Staphylococcus saprophyticus														
Streptococcus pneumoniae									2			2		
Streptococcus pyogenes (group A)					1	1	1		1	1		1	1	1
Streptococcus (anaerobic sp.)														
Streptococcus (viridans group)		1											2	
Vibrio cholerae														

* Life-threatening   † Non-life-threatening

Miscellaneous											Penicillins								
Azithromycin	Aztreonam	Clarithromycin	Clindamycin	Erythromycin	Imipenem/Cilastatin	Meropenem	Metronidazole	Quinupristin/Dalfopristin	Trimethoprim/Sulfamethoxazole	Vancomycin	Amoxicillin	Ampicillin	Mezlocillin	Nafcillin	Oxacillin	Penicillin G	Piperacillin	Piperacillin/Tazobactam	Ticarcillin
					1	1			2										
		2	2													1			
			2				1											2	
2		2		2							1								
				1															
2		2		2															
1				2															
	2				1	1			1									2	2
							1			2									
			2													1			
	2				1	1			1								2	2	2
										2	1	1				1			
							2			1	1	1							
	2				2	2			2				2				2		2
	2				2	2			2										
2		2							1										
	2								1									2	
	2				2	2			2										2
2		2	1																
									2			1				1			
2		2							1										
2		2	1																
									1										
									1										
									1			1							
					2	2			1										
	2				2	2								1			1	1	1
	2				2	2			1										
									1				2						
			2						2	1				1	1			2	
			2																
										1	1	1				1			
2		2	2	2							1	1				1			
			2													1			
2		2	2	2												1			
									2										

(continued)

	Combination with β-lactamase inhibitors			Tetracyclines		Fluoroquinolones						
	Amoxicillin/Clavulanic acid	Ampicillin/Sulbactam	Ticarcillin/Clavulanic acid	Doxycyline	Minocycline	Ciprofloxacin	Levofloxacin	Norfloxacin	Ofloxacin	Sparfloxacin	Trovafloxacin
Acinetobacter						2	2		2	2	2
Bacillus anthracis				1		1					
Bacteroides fragilis	2	2	2								2
Borrelia burgdorferi (skin)				1							
Campylobacter jejuni						2	2		2	2	2
Chlamydia pneumoniae				1		2	2		2	2	2
Chlamydia psittaci				1							
Chlamydia trachomatis				1			2		2		2
Citrobacter freundii						1	2		2	2	2
Clostridium difficile											
Clostridium perfringens				2							
Enterobacter sp.			2			1					
Enterococcus faecalis											
Enterococcus faecium				2							
Escherichia coli	1	1				2	2		2	2	2
Haemophilus influenzae*	1	1	1			1	1	1	1	1	1
Haemophilus influenzae†	1	1		1				2			
Klebsiella pneumoniae (UTI)	2	2	2			1	1	1	1	1	1
Klebsiella pneumoniae (pneumonia)	2	2	2			2	2	2	2	2	2
Legionella pneumophila						2	1	2	2	1	1
Listeria monocytogenes											
Moraxella catarrhalis	1			2							2
Mycoplasma pneumoniae				1							2
Neisseria gonorrhoeae						2	2		2		2
Nocardia asteroides					2						
Pneumocystis carinii											
Proteus mirabilis											2
Proteus vulgaris	2					1	1	1	1	1	1
Pseudomonas aeruginosa			1			2					2
Serratia marcescens						2	2	2	2	2	2
Shigella sp.				2		1	1	1	1	1	1
Staphylococcus aureus	2	2	2			2	2		2	2	2
Staphylococcus saprophyticus						2	2	1	2	2	2
Streptococcus pneumoniae				1			1			1	1
Streptococcus pyogenes (group A)											
Streptococcus (anaerobic sp.)											
Streptococcus (viridans group)											
Vibrio cholerae				1		1	1		1	1	1

* Life-threatening   † Non-life-threatening

Selected analgesic combination products

Many common analgesics are combinations of two or more generic drugs. This table gives you the components of common nonnarcotic analgesics and narcotic and opioid analgesic products.

Nonnarcotic analgesics	
Trade name	*Generic drugs*
Allerest No-Drowsiness Tablets, Coldrine, Ornex No Drowsiness Caplets, Sinus-Relief Tablets, Sinutab Without Drowsiness	• acetaminophen 325 mg • pseudoephedrine hydrochloride 30 mg
Amaphen, Anoquan, Butace, Endolor, Esgic, Femcet, Fioricet, Fiorpap, Isocet, Medigesic, Repan	• acetaminophen 325 mg • caffeine 40 mg • butalbital 50 mg
Anacin, Gensan	• aspirin 400 mg • caffeine 32 mg
Arthritis Foundation Nighttime, Extra Strength Tylenol PM, Midol PM	• acetaminophen 500 mg • diphenhydramine 25 mg
Ascriptin	• aspirin 325 mg • magnesium hydroxide 50 mg • aluminum hydroxide 50 mg • calcium carbonate 50 mg
Ascriptin A/D	• aspirin 325 mg • magnesium hydroxide 75 mg • aluminum hydroxide 75 mg • calcium carbonate 75 mg
Cama, Arthritis Pain Reliever	• aspirin 500 mg • magnesium oxide 150 mg • aluminum hydroxide 125 mg
COPE	• aspirin 421 mg • caffeine 32 mg • magnesium hydroxide 50 mg • aluminum hydroxide 25 mg
Doan's P.M. Extra Strength	• magnesium salicylate 500 mg • diphenhydramine 25 mg
Esgic-Plus	• acetaminophen 500 mg • caffeine 40 mg • butalbital 50 mg
Excedrin Extra Strength	• aspirin 250 mg • acetaminophen 250 mg • caffeine 65 mg
Excedrin P.M. Caplets	• acetaminophen 500 mg • diphenhydramine citrate 38 mg
Fiorinal†, Fiortal†, Lanorinal†	• aspirin 325 mg • caffeine 40 mg • butalbital 50 mg
Midrin	• isometheptene mucate 65 mg • dichloralphenazone 100 mg • acetaminophen 325 mg
Phrenilin	• acetaminophen 325 mg • butalbital 50 mg

(continued)

---

* Available in Canada only. † Controlled substance schedule III.

Nonnarcotic analgesics *(continued)*

Trade name	Generic drugs
Phrenilin Forte, Sedapap	• acetaminophen 650 mg • butalbital 50 mg
Sinus Excedrin Extra Strength	• acetaminophen 500 mg • pseudoephedrine hydrochloride 30 mg
Sinutab Regular*	• acetaminophen 325 mg • chlorpheniramine 2 mg • pseudoephedrine hydrochloride 30 mg
Sinutab Maximum Strength	• acetaminophen 500 mg • pseudoephedrine hydrochloride 30 mg • chlorpheniramine maleate 2 mg
Tecnal*	• aspirin 330 mg • caffeine 40 mg • butalbital 50 mg
Vanquish	• aspirin 227 mg • acetaminophen 194 mg • caffeine 33 mg • aluminum hydroxide 25 mg • magnesium hydroxide 50 mg

Narcotic and opioid analgesics

Trade name	Controlled substance schedule	Generic drugs
Aceta with Codeine	III	• acetaminophen 300 mg • codeine phosphate 30 mg
Anexsia 7.5/650, Lorcet Plus	III	• acetaminophen 650 mg • hydrocodone bitartrate 7.5 mg
Azdone, Damason-P	III	• acetaminophen 500 mg • hydrocodone bitartrate 5 mg
Capital with Codeine, Tylenol with Codeine Elixir	V	• acetaminophen 120 mg • codeine phosphate 12 mg/5 ml
Darvocet-N 50	IV	• acetaminophen 325 mg • propoxyphene napsylate 50 mg
Darvocet-N 100, Propacet 100	IV	• acetaminophen 650 mg • propoxyphene napsylate 100 mg
E-Lor, Genagesic, Wygesic	IV	• acetaminophen 650 mg • propoxyphene hydrochloride 65 mg
Empirin With Codeine No. 3	III	• aspirin 325 mg • codeine phosphate 30 mg
Empirin With Codeine No. 4	III	• aspirin 325 mg • codeine phosphate 60 mg
Flioricet With Codeine	III	• acetaminophen 325 mg • butalbital 50 mg • caffeine 40 mg • codeine phosphate 30 mg
Fiorinal With Codeine	III	• aspirin 325 mg • butalbital 50 mg • caffeine 40 mg • codeine phosphate 30 mg

* Available in Canada only.

Narcotic and opioid analgesics *(continued)*

Trade name	Controlled substance schedule	Generic drugs
Innovar Injection	II	• droperidol 2.5 mg • fentanyl citrate 0.05 mg/ml
Lorcet 10/650	III	• acetaminophen 650 mg • hydrocodone bitartrate 10 mg
Lortab 2.5/500	III	• acetaminophen 500 mg • hydrocodone bitartrate 2.5 mg
Lortab 5/500	III	• acetaminophen 500 mg • hydrocodone bitartrate 5 mg
Lortab 7.5/500	III	• acetaminophen 500 mg • hydrocodone bitartrate 7.5 mg
Percocet 5/325	II	• acetaminophen 325 mg • oxycodone hydrochloride 5 mg
Percodan-Demi	II	• aspirin 325 mg • oxycodone hydrochloride 2.25 mg • oxycodone terephthalate 0.19 mg
Percodan, Roxiprin	II	• aspirin 325 mg • oxycodone hydrochloride 4.5 mg • oxycodone terephthalate 0.38 mg
Phenaphen/Codeine No. 3	III	• acetaminophen 325 mg • codeine phosphate 30 mg
Phenaphen/Codeine No. 4	III	• acetaminophen 325 mg • codeine phosphate 60 mg
Propoxyphene Napsylate/ Acetaminophen	IV	• propoxyphene napsylate 100 mg • acetaminophen 650 mg
Roxicet	II	• acetaminophen 325 mg • oxycodone hydrochloride 5 mg
Roxicet 5/500	II	• acetaminophen 500 mg • oxycodone hydrochloride 5 mg
Roxicet Oral Solution	II	• acetaminophen 325 mg • oxycodone hydrochloride 5 mg/5 ml
Talacen	IV	• acetaminophen 650 mg • pentazocine hydrochloride 25 mg
Talwin Compound	IV	• aspirin 325 mg • pentazocine hydrochloride 12.5 mg
Tylenol With Codeine No. 2	III	• acetaminophen 300 mg • codeine phosphate 15 mg
Tylenol With Codeine No. 3	III	• acetaminophen 300 mg • codeine phosphate 30 mg
Tylenol With Codeine No. 4	III	• acetaminophen 300 mg • codeine phosphate 60 mg
Tylox	II	• acetaminophen 500 mg • oxycodone hydrochloride 5 mg
Vicodin, Zydone	III	• acetaminophen 500 mg • hydrocodone bitartrate 5 mg
Vicodin ES	III	• acetaminophen 750 mg • hydrocodone bitartrate 7.5 mg

* Available in Canada only.

Topical drugs

This table shows commonly used topical drugs and their indications, dosages, and actions. It also provides special considerations for topical administration.

	Drug	Indications and dosage
Antibacterials and antifungals	**alcohol, ethyl and isopropyl**	*To disinfect skin, instruments, and ampules:* Disinfect, p.r.n. Isopropyl alcohol is superior to ethyl alcohol as an anti-infective (70%). *Antipyresis:* Apply 25% solution. *Anhidrosis:* Apply 50% solution p.r.n.
	hydrogen peroxide (PerOxyl)	*Cleaning wounds:* Use 1.5% to 3% solution, p.r.n. *Mouthwash for necrotizing ulcerative gingivitis:* Gargle with 3% solution, p.r.n. *Cleaning minor wounds or irritations of the mouth or gums:* Use 1.5% gel, p.r.n. *Cleaning douche:* Use 2% solution q.i.d., p.r.n.
Antiseptics and germicidals	**benzalkonium chloride** (Benza, Zephiran Chloride)	*Preoperative disinfection of unbroken skin:* Apply 1:750 tincture or spray. *Disinfection of mucous membranes and denuded skin:* Apply 1:10,000 to 1:5,000 aqueous solution. *Irrigation of vagina:* Instill 1:5,000 to 1:2,000 aqueous solution. *Irrigation of deep infected wounds:* Instill 1:20,000 to 1:3,000 aqueous solution. *Irrigation of urinary bladder and urethra:* 1:5,000 to 1:20,000 aqueous solution.
	chlorhexidine gluconate (Hibiclens, Hibistat, Peridex)	*Surgical hand scrub, hand wash, hand rinse, skin wound cleanser:* Use 0.5% to 4% strength, p.r.n. *Gingivitis:* Use 0.12% strength (Peridex oral rinse), p.r.n.
	hexachlorophene (pHisoHex, Septisol)	*Surgical scrub, bacteriostatic skin cleanser:* Use 0.23% to 3% concentrations, p.r.n.
	iodine	*Preoperative disinfection of skin (small wounds and abraded areas):* Apply p.r.n.
	povidone-iodine (ACU-dyne, Aerodine, Betadine, Betagen, Biodine, Efodine, Iodex, Operand, Polydine)	*Preoperative skin preparation and scrub; germicide for surface wounds; postoperative application to incisions; prophylactic application to urinary meatus of catheterized patients; miscellaneous disinfection:* Apply p.r.n., or use as scrub, p.r.n.
Keratolytics	**podophyllum resin** (Pod-Ben 25, Podocon)	*Venereal warts:* Apply podophyllum resin preparation to the lesion, cover with waxed paper, and bandage. The first application should remain on skin for 30 to 40 minutes; subsequent applications may last 1 to 4 hours, depending on lesion and patient's condition. Wash lesion to remove medication. Repeat at weekly intervals, if indicated. *Multiple superficial epitheliomatosis and keratosis:* Apply daily with applicator and allow to dry. Remove necrotic tissue before each application.
	salicylic acid (Calicylic, Compound W, DuoFilm, Freezone, Gordofilm, Hydrisalic, Keralyt, Occlusal, Off-Ezy, Sal-Acid, Wart-Off)	*Scaling dermatoses, hyperkeratosis, calluses, warts:* Apply to affected area and cover with occlusive dressing at night.
Protectants	**benzoin tincture compound**	*Demulcent and protectant (cutaneous ulcers, bedsores, cracked nipples, fissures of lips and anus):* Apply locally once daily or b.i.d.
	zinc oxide with calamine and gelatin (Dome-Paste)	*Protectant (lesions or injuries of lower legs or arms):* Wrap the wet bandage in place and retain for about 1 week. Dome-Paste, in 3″ to 4″ bandages, can be applied directly to arm or leg.
Wet dressings, soaks	**aluminum acetate, aluminum sulfate** (Boropak Powder, Burow's Solution, Domeboro Powder)	*Mild skin irritation from exposure to soaps, chemicals, diaper rash, acne, eczema:* Apply p.r.n. *Skin inflammation, contact dermatoses:* Mix powder or tablet with 1 pint of lukewarm water. Apply to loose dressing q 15 to 30 minutes for 4 to 8 hours.

Action	Special considerations
Antibacterial effect through reduction of surface tension of bacterial cell walls, inhibiting bacterial growth. Also antipyretic and astringent effects.	• Avoid contact with eyes and mucous membranes. • Contraindicated in patients taking disulfiram if used over large surface area. • Don't apply to open wounds.
Antibacterial effect through oxidation.	• Don't instill into closed body cavities or abscesses because released gas cannot escape. • Store in a tightly capped, dark container in a cool, dry place. • Don't confuse with peroxide (6% to 20%) used for bleaching hair.
Cationic surface action producing bacteriostatic or bactericidal effect, depending on the concentration used.	• Don't use with occlusive dressings or packs. • Inactivated by anionic compounds such as soap. • Rinse area thoroughly after each application. • Skin inflammation and irritation may require lower concentration or discontinuation.
Persistent antimicrobial effect against gram-negative and gram-positive bacteria.	• Avoid contact with eyes, ears, and mucous membranes. Rinse well if drug enters eyes or ears. • May cause deafness if drug enters middle ear.
Bacteriostatic effect against staphylococci and other gram-positive bacteria, probably due to inhibition of bacterial membrane-bound enzymes.	• Don't use on broken skin, skin lesions, burns, wounds, or under occlusive dressings. Do not use around eyes or mucous membranes. • Discontinue promptly if CNS irritability occurs. • Rinse thoroughly after use. • Don't use in infants; use cautiously in children.
Germicidal effect against bacteria, fungi, and viruses, probably due to disruption of microorganism proteins.	• Don't cover after application to avoid irritation. • Iodine stains skin and clothing. • Toxic if ingested; sodium thiosulfate is an antidote.
Germicidal effect against bacteria, fungi, and viruses; has same action as iodine without its irritating effects.	• Contraindicated in patients with known sensitivity to iodine. • Don't use around eyes; do not use full-strength solution on mucous membranes. May stain skin and mucous membranes. • Avoid using solution that contains a detergent when treating open wounds.
Caustic and erosive action from disruption of epithelial cell division.	• Shouldn't be used in pregnant patients. • May be toxic if applied to large surface area or applied too frequently. • Wash hands thoroughly after applying. • Protect surrounding area with petrolatum. • Wash off thoroughly with soap and water after prescribed time. • May cause abnormal pigmentation. • To be applied by a health care provider only.
Causes desquamation of cornified epithelium by increasing hydration.	• Don't use on birthmarks, moles, or areas with hair follicle involvement. • Don't use in aspirin-sensitive patients. • Hydrate skin for at least 5 minutes before application. • Apply emollient to surrounding skin for protection. • Wash off thoroughly after overnight use.
Protects skin from external environment by coating action.	• Clean and dry area before applying. • Useful in protection of skin from adhesive.
Protects skin by forming occlusive barrier.	• Watch for signs of infection. • Warn patient not to shower or bathe with gel on. • Remove by soaking in warm water. Remove all of previous application before reapplying. • Apply with nap of hair to avoid folliculitis. • Don't use with constrictive bandage.
Reduces friction and provides soothing relief through astringent action.	• Avoid use around eyes and mucous membranes. • Don't use with occlusive dressings. • Discontinue if irritation occurs.

Immunization schedule

The current childhood immunization schedule as approved by the American Academy of Family Physicians, the American Academy of Pediatrics, and the Advisory Committee on Immunization Practices encompasses recent changes in recommendations. These guidelines were developed so the recommended immunization schedule would minimize adverse reactions while preserving effectiveness and maximizing patient compliance. The schedule may be appropriately altered wtih the use of currently licensed combination vaccines.

The following includes important information to consider when immunizing children.

Vaccine	Age											
	Birth	1 mo.	2 mos.	4 mos.	6 mos.	12 mos.	15 mos.	18 mos.	24 mos	4-6 yrs.	11-12 yrs.	14-16 yrs.
Hepatitis B[1]	Hep B-1											
			Hep B-2			Hep B-3					Hep B	
Diphtheria and tetanus toxoids and acellular pertussis[2] (DTaP, DTP)			DTaP	DTaP	DTaP		DTaP			DTaP	Td	
Haemophilus influenzae type b[3]			Hib	Hib	Hib	Hib						
Poliovirus[4]			IPV	IPV		IPV				IPV		
Measles, mumps, rubella[5]							MMR			MMR	MMR	
Varicella virus[6]							Var				Var	
Hepatitis A[7]										Hep A		

☐ Range of acceptable ages for vaccination.

☐ "Catch-up" vaccination.

[1]**Hepatitis B:** Children and adolescents who were not immunized against hepatits B in infancy may begin the series at any time. The series should be initiated or completed at age 11 or 12 in any child who has not previously received three doses of hepatitis B. The second dose should be administered at least 1 month after the first dose, and the third dose should be given at least 4 months after the first dose and at least 2 months after the second dose.

Infants born to hepatitis B surface antigen (HBsAg)-negative mothers should receive hepatitis B vaccine by age 2 months. The second dose is given at least 1 month after the first. The third dose is given at least 4 months after the first dose and at least 2 months after the second dose, but not before 6 months of age for infants.

Infants born to HBsAg-positive mothers should receive 0.5 ml of hepatitis B immune globulin (HBIG) within 12 hours of birth, and either 5 mcg of Recombivax HB (Merck) or 10 mcg of Engerix-B (SmithKline Beecham) at a separate site. The second dose is given at age 1 to 2 months and the third dose at age 6 months.

Infants born to mothers with unknown HBsAg status should receive 5 mcg of Recombivax HB (Merck) or 10 mcg of Engerix-B (SmithKline Beecham) within 12 hours of birth. Blood should be drawn at the time of delivery to determine the mother's HBsAg status. If positive, the baby should receive 0.5 ml of HBIG as soon as possible and no later than age 1 week. The dosage and timing of subsequent vaccine doses should be based upon the mother's HBsAg status.

[2]**DTP:** DTaP is the recommended vaccine for all doses in the series. Children who have received one or more doses of the whole-cell DTP may complete the series with DTaP. To combat compliance issues in patients who are unlikely to return at age 15 to 18 months, the fourth dose of the vaccine may be given as early as age 12 months, as long as 6 months have elapsed since the third dose. Td is recommended at age 11 to 12, provided that at least 5 years have elapsed since the last dose of DTP, DTaP, or DT. Routine Td boosters are recommended every 10 years for adults.

[3]**H. influenzae type B:** Three *H. influenzae* type b (Hib) vaccines are licensed for use in infants. They are given at age 2, 4, 6, and 12 to 15 months unless the PRP-OMP (PedvaxHIB [Merck]) is used, in which case a dose at age 6 months is not necessary. Any Hib conjugate vaccine may be used as a booster dose at age 12 to 15 months. Because some combination products may induce a lower immune response to the Hib vaccine, DTaP/Hib combination products shouldn't be used for primary immunization in infants at 2, 4, or 6 months of age unless FDA-approved for these ages.

[4]**Poliovirus:** Inactivated poliovirus vaccine (IVP) is given at age 2, 4, 6 to 18 months, and 4 to 6.

Oral polio vaccine (OPV) is no longer recommended for routine immunizations. However, OPV may still be appropriate in special circumstances, such as when parents don't accept the number of injections the child receives or late immunization would call for too many injections, for imminent travel to polio-endemic areas, and when mass vaccination campaigns are needed to control outbreaks. OPV shouldn't be used in immunocompromised children or those in close contact with immunocompromised persons.

[5]**Measles, Mumps, Rubella:** The second dose is recommended at age 4 to 6 before school entry, but may be administered at any visit, as long as both doses are given at or after age 12 months, and at least 1 month has elapsed between the first and second doses. Those who haven't received the second dose should complete the schedule by age 11 or 12.

[6]**Varicella virus:** Varicella vaccine may be administered on or after age 12 months to any child who lacks a reliable history of varicella and who hasn't been previously vaccinated. Children ages 13 and older must be given two doses of the vaccine at least 1 month apart.

[7]**Hepatitis A:** Specific changes in the schedule over the course of the past year include: suspending use of the rotavirus vaccine; using inactivated polio vaccine (IPV) for all four doses of the vaccine instead of the oral polio vaccine (OPV); and recommending Hepatitis A virus vaccine in certain states where the disease is most prevalent. (Hepatitis A can be transmitted from person to person or through contaminated food or water and can cause fever, jaundice, anorexia, and nausea.)

Therapeutic drug monitoring guidelines

Drug	Laboratory test monitored	Therapeutic ranges of test
aminoglycoside antibiotics (amikacin, gentamicin, tobramycin)	Serum amikacin peak trough Serum gentamicin/tobramycin peak trough Serum creatinine	20 to 25 mcg/ml 5 to 10 mcg/ml 4 to 8 mcg/ml 1 to 2 mcg/ml 0.6 to 1.3 mg/dl
amphotericin B	Serum creatinine BUN Serum electrolytes (especially potassium and magnesium) Liver function tests CBC with differential and platelets	0.6 to 1.3 mg/dl 5 to 20 mg/dl Potassium: 3.5 to 5 mEq/L Magnesium: 1.5 to 2.5 mEq/L Sodium: 135 to 145 mEq/L Chloride: 98 to 106 mEq/L * *****
antibiotics	WBC with differential Cultures and sensitivities	*****
biguanides (metformin)	Serum creatinine Fasting serum glucose Glycosolated hemoglobin CBC	0.6 to 1.3 mg/dl 70 to 110 mg/dl 5.5% to 8.5% of total hemoglobin *****
clozapine	WBC with differential	*****
digoxin	Serum digoxin Serum electrolytes (especially potassium, magnesium, and calcium) Serum creatinine	0.8 to 2 ng/ml Potassium: 3.5 to 5 mEq/L Magnesium: 1.7 to 2.1 mEq/L Sodium: 135 to 145 mEq/L Chloride: 98 to 106 mEq/L Calcium: 8.6 to 10 mg/dl 0.6 to 1.3 mg/dl
diuretics	Serum electrolytes Serum creatinine BUN Uric acid Fasting serum glucose	Potassium: 3.5 to 5 mEq/L Magnesium: 1.7 to 2.1 mEq/L Sodium: 135 to 145 mEq/L Chloride: 98 to 106 mEq/L Calcium: 8.6 to 10 mg/dl 0.6 to 1.3 mg/dl 5 to 20 mg/dl 2 to 7 mg/dl 70 to 110 mg/dl
erythropoietin	Hematocrit	Female: 36% to 48% Male: 42% to 52%
ethosuximide	Serum ethosuximide	40 to 100 mcg/ml
gemfibrozil	Serum lipids	Total cholesterol: < 200 mg/dl LDL: < 130 mg/dl HDL: Female: 40 to 75 mg/dl Male: 37 to 70 mg/dl Triglycerides: 10 to 160 mg/dl

Note: ***** For those areas marked with asterisks, the following values can be used:

Hemoglobin: Female: 12 to 16 g/dl
         Male: 14 to 18 g/dl
Hematocrit: Female: 37% to 48%
         Male: 42% to 52%
RBCs: 4 to 5.5 × 10^6/mm³
WBCs: 5 to 10 × 10^3/mm³

Differential: Neutrophils: 45% to 74%
         Bands: 0% to 8%
         Lymphocytes: 16% to 45%
         Monocytes: 4% to 10%
         Eosinophils: 0% to 7%
         Basophils: 0% to 2%

Monitoring guidelines

Wait until the administration of the third dose to check drug levels. Obtain blood for peak level 30 minutes after I.V. infusion or 60 minutes after I.M. administration. For trough levels, draw blood just before next dose. Dosage may need to be adjusted accordingly. Recheck after three doses. Monitor serum creatinine and BUN levels and urine output for signs of decreasing renal function.

Monitor serum creatinine, BUN, and serum electrolyte levels at least weekly during therapy. Also, regularly monitor blood counts and liver function tests during therapy.

Specimen cultures and sensitivities will determine the cause of the infection and the best treatment. Monitor WBC with differential weekly during therapy.

Check renal function and hematologic parameters before initiating therapy and at least annually thereafter. If the patient has impaired renal function, don't use metformin because it may cause lactic acidosis. Monitor response to therapy by periodically evaluating fasting glucose and glycosolated hemoglobin levels. A patient's home monitoring of blood glucose levels helps monitor compliance and response.

Obtain WBC with differential before initiating therapy, weekly during therapy, and 4 weeks after discontinuing the drug.

Check serum digoxin levels at least 12 hours, but preferably 24 hours, after the last dose is administered. To monitor maintenance therapy, check drug levels at least 1 to 2 weeks after therapy is initiated or changed. Make any adjustments in therapy based on entire clinical picture, not solely on drug levels. Also, check electrolyte levels and renal function periodically during therapy.

To monitor fluid and electrolyte balance, perform baseline and periodic determinations of serum electrolyte, serum calcium, BUN, uric acid, and serum glucose levels.

After therapy is initiated or changed, monitor the hematocrit twice weekly for 2 to 6 weeks until stabilized in the target range and a maintenance dose determined. Monitor hematocrit regularly thereafter.

Check drug level 8 to 10 days after therapy is initiated or changed.

Therapy is usually withdrawn after 3 months if response is inadequate. Patient must be fasting to measure triglyceride levels.

(continued)

* For those areas marked with one asterisk, the following values can be used:

ALT: 7 to 56 U/L
AST: 5 to 40 U/L
Alkaline phosphatase: 17 to 142 U/L
LD: 60 to 220 U/L
GGTP: < 40 U/L
Total bilirubin: 0.2 to 1 mg/dl

Drug	Laboratory test monitored	Therapeutic ranges of test
heparin	Activated partial thromboplastin time (APTT)	1.5 to 2 times control
HMG-CoA reductase inhibitors (fluvastatin, lovastatin, pravastatin, simvastatin)	Serum lipids	Total cholesterol: < 200 mg/dl LDL: < 130 mg/dl HDL: Female: 40 to 75 mg/dl Male: 37 to 70 mg/dl Triglycerides: 10 to 160 mg/dl
	Liver function tests	*
insulin	Fasting serum glucose Glycosylated hemoglobin	70 to 110 mg/dl 5.5% to 8.5% of total hemoglobin
lithium	Serum lithium Serum creatinine CBC Serum electrolytes (especially potassium and sodium) Fasting serum glucose Thyroid function tests	0.5 to 1.4 mEq/L 0.6 to 1.3 mg/dl ***** Potassium: 3.5 to 5 mEq/L Magnesium: 1.7 to 2.1 mEq/L Sodium: 135 to 145 mEq/L Chloride: 98 to 106 mEq/L 70 to 110 mg/dl TSH: 0.2 to 5.4 microU/ml T_3: 80 to 200 ng/dl T_4: 5.4 to 11.5 mcg/dl
methotrexate	Serum methotrexate CBC with differential Platelet count Liver function tests Serum creatinine	Normal elimination: < 10 micromol 24 hours postdose < 1 micromol 48 hours postdose < 0.2 micromol 72 hours postdose ***** 150 to 450 × 10^3/mm^3 * 0.6 to 1.3 mg/dl
phenytoin	Serum phenytoin CBC	10 to 20 mcg/ml *****
potassium chloride	Serum potassium	3.5 to 5 mEq/L
procainamide	Serum procainamide Serum N-acetylprocainamide CBC	4 to 8 mcg/ml (procainamide) 5 to 30 mcg/ml (combined procainamide and NAPA) *****
quinidine	Serum quinidine CBC Liver function tests Serum creatinine Serum electrolytes (especially potassium)	2 to 6 mcg/ml ***** * 0.6 to 1.3 mg/dl Potassium: 3.5 to 5 mEq/L Magnesium: 1.7 to 2.1 mEq/L Sodium: 135 to 145 mEq/L Chloride: 98 to 106 mEq/L
sulfonylureas	Fasting serum glucose Glycosylated hemoglobin	70 to 110 mg/dl 5.5% to 8.5% of total hemoglobin
theophylline	Serum theophylline	10 to 20 mcg/ml

Note: ***** For those areas marked with asterisks, the following values can be used:

Hemoglobin: Female: 12 to 16 g/dl
            Male: 14 to 18 g/dl
Hematocrit: Female: 37% to 48%
          Male: 42% to 52%
RBCs: 4 to 5.5 × 10^6/mm^3
WBCs: 5 to 10 × 10^3/mm^3

Differential: Neutrophils: 45% to 74%
           Bands: 0% to 8%
           Lymphocytes: 16% to 45%
           Monocytes: 4% to 10%
           Eosinophils: 0% to 7%
           Basophils: 0% to 2%

Monitoring guidelines

When drug is given by continuous I.V. infusion, check APTT every 4 hours in the early stages of therapy. When drug is given by deep S.C. injection, check APTT 4 to 6 hours after injection.

Perform liver function tests at baseline, 6 to 12 weeks after therapy is initiated or changed, and periodically thereafter. If adequate response isn't achieved within 6 weeks, consider changing the therapy.

Monitor response to therapy by evaluating serum glucose and glycosolated hemoglobin levels. Glycosolated hemoglobin level is a good measure of long-term control. A patient's home monitoring of blood glucose levels helps measure compliance and response.

Checking blood lithium levels is crucial to the safe use of the drug. Obtain serum lithium levels immediately before next dose. Monitor levels twice weekly until stable. Once at steady state, levels should be checked weekly; when the patient is on the appropriate maintenance dose, levels should be checked every 2 to 3 months. Monitor serum creatinine, serum electrolyte, and fasting serum glucose levels; CBC; and thyroid function tests before therapy is initiated and periodically during therapy.

Monitor methotrexate levels according to dosing protocol. Monitor CBC with differential, platelet count, and liver and renal function tests more frequently when therapy is initiated or changed and when methotrexate levels may be elevated, such as when the patient is dehydrated.

Monitor serum phenytoin levels immediately before next dose and 2 to 4 weeks after therapy is initiated or changed. Obtain a CBC at baseline and monthly early in therapy. Watch for toxic effects at therapeutic levels. Adjust the measured level for hypoalbuminemia or renal impairment, which can increase free drug levels.

Check level weekly after oral replacement therapy is initiated until stable and every 3 to 6 months thereafter.

Measure procainamide levels 6 to 12 hours after a continuous infusion is started or immediately before the next oral dose. Combined (procainamide and NAPA) levels can be used as an index of toxicity when renal impairment exists. Obtain CBC periodically during longer-term therapy.

Obtain levels immediately before next oral dose and 30 to 35 hours after therapy is initiated or changed. Periodically obtain blood counts, liver and kidney function tests, and serum electrolyte levels.

Monitor response to therapy by periodically evaluating fasting glucose and glycosolated hemoglobin levels. A patient's home monitoring of blood glucose levels helps measure compliance and response.

Obtain serum theophylline levels immediately before next dose of sustained-release oral product and at least 2 days after therapy is initiated or changed.

(continued)

* For those areas marked with one asterisk, the following values can be used:

ALT: 7 to 56 U/L
AST: 5 to 40 U/L
Alkaline phosphatase: 17 to 142 U/L
LD: 60 to 220 U/L
GGTP: < 40 U/L
Total bilirubin: 0.2 to 1 mg/dl

Drug	Laboratory test monitored	Therapeutic ranges of test
thyroid hormone	Thyroid function tests	TSH: 0.2 to 5.4 microU/ml T_3: 80 to 200 ng/dl T_4: 5.4 to 11.5 mcg/dl
vancomycin	Serum vancomycin	20 to 35 mcg/ml (peak) 5 to 10 mcg/ml (trough)
	Serum creatinine	0.6 to 1.3 mg/dl
warfarin	INR	For an acute MI, atrial fibrillation, treatment of pulmonary embolism, prevention of systemic embolism, tissue heart valves, valvular heart disease, or prophylaxis or treatment of venous thrombosis: 2 to 3 For mechanical prosthetic valves or recurrent systemic embolism: 2.5 to 3.5

Note: ***** For those areas marked with asterisks, the following values can be used:

Hemoglobin: Female: 12 to 16 g/dl
　　　　　　 Male: 14 to 18 g/dl
Hematocrit: Female: 37% to 48%
　　　　　　 Male: 42% to 52%
RBCs: 4 to 5.5 × 10^6/mm^3
WBCs: 5 to 10 × 10^3/mm^3

Differential: Neutrophils: 45% to 74%
　　　　　　　 Bands: 0% to 8%
　　　　　　　 Lymphocytes: 16% to 45%
　　　　　　　 Monocytes: 4% to 10%
　　　　　　　 Eosinophils: 0% to 7%
　　　　　　　 Basophils: 0% to 2%

Monitoring guidelines

Monitor thyroid function tests every 2 to 3 weeks until appropriate maintenance dose is determined.

Serum vancomycin levels may be checked with the third dose administered, at the earliest. Draw peak levels ½ hour after the I.V. infusion is completed. Draw trough levels immediately before the next dose is administered. Renal function can be used to adjust dosing and intervals.

Check INR daily, beginning 3 days after therapy is initiated. Continue checking it until therapeutic goal is achieved, and monitor it periodically thereafter. Also, check levels 7 days after any change in warfarin dose or concomitant, potentially interacting therapy.

* For those areas marked with one asterisk, the following values can be used:

ALT: 7 to 56 U/L
AST: 5 to 40 U/L
Alkaline phosphatase: 17 to 142 U/L
LD: 60 to 220 U/L
GGTP: < 40 U/L
Total bilirubin: 0.2 to 1 mg/dl

Antidotes to poisoning or overdose

The table below summarizes the major uses and dosage recommendations for selected antidotes. For more information about specific antidotes, contact your local poison information center.

Antidote and dosages	Type of poisoning or overdose	General considerations
acetylcysteine (Mucomyst, Mucosil) *Adults and children:* 140 mg/kg P.O. diluted to a 5% concentration in soft drinks or juice, given within 16 to 24 hr after ingestion. Follow loading dose with 17 additional doses of 70 mg/kg q 4 hr unless acetaminophen assay reveals a nontoxic level (repeat if dose is vomited within 1 hr).	acetaminophen	• Activated charcoal will adsorb the antidote if both are present in the gut. If charcoal is used, it must be aspirated before the antidote is given. • If patient is unable to retain the oral dose, administer by duodenal intubation. • If patient is seen within 1 hour of ingestion, perform gastric lavage.
activated charcoal (Actidose-Aqua, Liqui-Char) *Adults and children:* 5 to 10 times the weight of the ingested poison. Minimum dose is 20 to 30 g (½ cup of lightly packed powder) in 250 ml of water (to make a slurry); repeat as soon as possible. Most adults can tolerate doses of 120 g. For best results, use within 30 min of ingestion.	All oral poisonings except those caused by iron, cyanide, organic solvents, mineral acids, or corrosive agents	• Induce emesis before giving activated charcoal. After ipecac-induced vomiting, patient may be intolerant of activated charcoal for 1 to 2 hr. • Repeated doses may not provide additional benefit unless the poison undergoes enterohepatic recycling. • Activated charcoal may adsorb other orally administered antidotes. • Contraindicated in patients at risk for aspiration and patient with ileus or intestinal obstruction.
amyl nitrite inhalants (Step I) *Adults:* Inhale for 30 sec q min until an I.V. sodium nitrite infusion is available. **sodium nitrite** (Step II) *Adults:* 300 mg in 10-ml solution given I.V. at a rate of 2.5 to 5 ml/min (if symptoms reappear, administer half the original dose in 2 hr). *Children:* Depends on hemoglobin level. **sodium thiosulfate** (Step III) *Adults:* 12.5 g in 50-ml solution given I.V. over 10 min (if symptoms reappear, give half the original dose of sodium nitrite again in 2 hr). *Children:* Depends on hemoglobin level.	Cyanide	• Nitrites cause vasodilation. Hypotension is a common adverse reaction.
atropine sulfate *Adults:* 1 to 6 mg I.V. for pesticides (may repeat q 5 to 60 min until signs of atropinization appear, such as dilated pupils, flushed face, or tachycardia). *Children:* 0.05 mg/kg for pesticides (may repeat q 10 to 30 min until signs of atropinization appear).	Anticholinesterase substances, organophosphate pesticides, carbamate pesticides	• Large doses (up to 2,000 mg over several days) may be required. • Sudden cessation of atropine may cause pulmonary edema. • Maintain adequate ventilation to prevent cardiac arrhythmias. • A cholinesterase reactivator, such as pralidoxime, is also given in organophosphate poisoning; a cholinesterase reactivator is also given in carbamate poisoning when severe respiratory depression and severe muscle weakness exist.

Antidote	Type of poisoning or overdose	General considerations
calcium disodium edetate (Calcium Disodium Versenate, EDTA) *Adults and children:* 1,000 mg/m²/ day I.V. or I.V. for 5 days. Infuse I.V. dose over 8 to 12 hr. I.M. dose should be divided into equal doses spaced 8 to 12 hr apart. Give second course after 2 to 4 days' rest.	Chromium, lead, manganese, nickel, zinc, cadmium, cobalt	• Most experts recommend that calcium disodium edetate be used in conjunction with dimercaprol for the treatment of severe lead poisoning. • Rapid injection may precipitate renal failure. • I.M. route is preferred by some clinicians because I.V. route has been associated with fatality.
deferoxamine mesylate (Desferal) *Adults and children:* 1,000 mg I.M. or I.V. (< 15 mg/kg/hr initially), then 500 mg q 4 hr for two doses. Subsequent doses of 500 mg q 4 to 12 hr may be given, depending on patient response; maximum dosage 6,000 mg daily.	Iron	• Renal excretion of compound will cause the urine to turn reddish pink.
digoxin immune Fab (Digibind) *Adults:* Depends on amount of digoxin or digitoxin to be neutralized. If unable to determine dosage using manufacturer-supplied dosage formulas, 760 mg I.V. may be infused over 30 min.	digoxin, digitoxin	• Use is reserved for severe overdose only. • If possible, first obtain serum digoxin and digitoxin concentrations. • If cardiac arrest seems imminent, give dose as a bolus injection. • Monitor serum potassium levels carefully. • Monitor cardiac rate and rhythm.
dimercaprol (BAL in oil) *Adults:* For arsenic or gold poisoning, 3 mg/kg I.M. q 4 hr for first 2 days, then q 6 hr on day 3, followed by 3 mg/kg q 12 hr for 10 days or until recovery; for mercury poisoning, 5 mg/kg I.M. initially, followed by 2.5 mg/kg once or twice daily for 10 days.	Mercury, arsenic, gold, lead (in conjunction with calcium disodium edetate)	• Dimercaprol must be given promptly to be effective. • Contraindicated in iron, cadmium, selenium, and uranium toxicity. • Use requires that patient has adequate renal and hepatic function to excrete toxins.
flumazenil (Romazicon) *Adults:* Initially, give 0.2 mg I.V. over 30 sec. If patient doesn't reach the desired level of consciousness after 30 sec, give 0.3 mg over 30 sec. If response is inadequate, give 0.5 mg over 30 sec; repeat doses of 0.5 mg at 1-min intervals until 3 mg has been given.	Benzodiazepines	• Most patients respond to cumulative doses between 1 and 3 mg; rarely, patients who partially respond after 3 mg may require more. Don't give more than 5 mg in a 5-min period initially, and don't give more than 3 mg/hr. • Contraindicated in patients who also have severe cyclic antidepressant overdose. • Use with caution in cases of mixed overdose.
naloxone hydrochloride (Narcan) *Adults:* 0.4 to 2 mg I.V. bolus to reverse the narcotic effect (may need to repeat dose q 2 to 3 min). *Children:* 0.01 mg/kg I.V. bolus. Give subsequent dose of 0.1 mg/kg if needed.	Opiates: morphine, heroin, methadone, meperidine, oxycodone, codeine, diphenoxylate, fentanyl, propoxyphene	• Time of action is shorter than that of narcotic; observe patient for recurring narcosis. Repeat doses or a continuous infusion may be necessary. • If no response occurs after 10 mg has been administered, depression may be caused by a drug or disease that doesn't respond to naloxone.
penicillamine (Cuprimine) *Adults:* 500 mg to 1,500 mg/day for 1 to 2 months. *Children:* 30 to 40 mg/kg/day P.O. for 1 to 6 months. Doses above 500 mg should be divided b.i.d.	Heavy metals	• Penicillamine should be used in patients with minimal signs and symptoms and positive serum lead levels. • Use only if patient can't take succimer or calcium disodium edetate.

(continued)

Antidote	Type of poisoning or overdose	General considerations
physostigmine salicylate (Antilirium) *Adults:* 0.5 to 2 mg I.V. slowly over 2 to 3 min (repeat with a 1-mg to 2-mg dose in 20 min if symptoms are still present; repeat with a 1-mg to 4-mg dose if life-threatening symptoms reappear). *Children:* 0.02 mg/kg slow I.V. over 2 to 3 min (repeat within 5 min if symptoms recur); maximum dosage is 2 mg.	Anticholinergics; tricyclics (amitriptyline, doxepin, imipramine, nortriptyline); antihist-amines; some antiemetics, antiparkinsonian agents, and phenothiazines	• Use is reserved for severe poisoning (coma, hallucinations, delirium, tachycardia, arrhythmias, and hypertension). • Rapid I.V. injection may cause bradycardia and hypersalivation with respiratory difficulties and convulsions. • Physostigmine can produce a cholinergic crisis. If so, atropine should be used as an antidote.
pralidoxime chloride (Pralidoxime Chloride, Protopam Chloride) *Adults:* 1 to 2 g I.V. as 15- to 30-min infusion in 100 ml of 0.9% sodium chloride; repeat dose in 1 hr if muscle weakness persists. Additional doses may be needed q 3 to 8 hr in severe cases. *Children:* 20 to 40 mg/kg/dose, administer as above.	Organophosphate pesticides	• Best if given within 24 hr after exposure; is still effective within 36 to 48 hr. • Pesticide absorption through the skin is possible—wash patient and remove contaminated clothing, or symptoms may reappear within 48 to 72 hr. • Drug has no anticholinergic effects. • Use with atropine.
protamine sulfate *Adults:* 5 ml of a 1% solution slow I.V. over 10 min (give 1 to 1.5 mg protamine for each 100 units of heparin consumed).	heparin	• Maximum dosage is 50 mg (as a single dose).
succimer (Chemet) *Adults and children:* 10 mg/kg q 8 hr for 5 days; then 10 mg/kg q 12 hr for 14 days. A course of treatment lasts 19 days; repeated courses should be separated by 2 weeks unless blood levels indicate the need for prompt treatment.	Heavy metals	• Don't give until patient is no longer exposed to heavy metals hazard.
vitamin K analogue (AquaMEPHYTON) *Adults:* Usual initial dose is 2.5 to 10 mg I.M., S.C., or P.O. (if patient is not vomiting); it may be as high as 25 mg, or, rarely, 50 mg. Monitor patient response or PT to determine need for subsequent doses. If results unsatisfactory 6 to 8 hr after parenteral dose or 12 to 48 hr after P.O. dose, repeat.	warfarin	• Fresh whole blood may be necessary to stop bleeding.

Creatinine clearance calculations

In adults with stable renal function, the following formulas will provide a reliable estimate of creatinine clearance (Cl_{Cr}) except:

Patients with falsely low serum creatinine (such as paraplegic patients with muscle wasting) will give an artificially high predicted creatinine clearance.

Patients with rapidly increasing serum creatinine (over 0.5 to 0.7 mg/dl/day) will give an unreliable estimate of creatinine clearance.

Adults (age 18 and older)

Method 1*:

Estimated creatinine clearance, Cl_{Cr} (ml/minute):

$$\text{Male } Cl_{Cr} = \frac{(140 - \text{age})\,(\text{IBW})}{(72)\,(\text{SrCr})}$$

Female Cl_{Cr} = (Estimated male Cl_{Cr}) (0.85)

where age = in years
IBW = ideal body weight in kilograms:
IBW (Male) = 50 + [(2.3) (height in inches over 5 feet)]
IBW (Female) = 45.5 + [(2.3) (height in inches over 5 feet)]
   Note: The use of the patient's IBW is recommended except when the patient's actual body weight is less than IBW.
SrCr = Serum creatinine in mg/dl

Method 2†:

Estimated creatinine clearance, Cl_{Cr} (ml/minute/1.73 m^2):

$$\text{Male } Cl_{Cr} = \frac{98 - [(0.8)\,(\text{age} - 20)]}{\text{SrCr}}$$

Female Cl_{Cr} = (Estimated male Cl_{Cr}) (0.90)

where age is in years, SrCr is serum creatinine in mg/dl.

---

*Cockroft, D.W., and Gault, M.H. "Prediction of Creatinine Clearance From Serum Creatinine," *Nephron* 16:31, 1976.
†Jelliffe, R.W. "Creatinine Clearance: Bedside Estimate," *Ann Intern Med* 79:604, 1973.

Herbal medicines

Plants have been used to cure disease for thousands of years, but the recent popularity of herbal medicines means that many of your patients need reliable information on using these substances appropriately. Most botanical products, vitamins, minerals, amino acids, and mammalian tissue abstracts are currently regulated only under the Dietary Supplement Health and Education Act of 1994. This act limits the FDA's authority to require proof of efficacy, safety, or quality before these products are sold commercially. And that means that herbal medicines have many unknown and undocumented risks. Remind your patient to disclose all medications he takes at each visit.

Names	Reported uses	Forms and dosages
Aloe (aloe vera, burn plant, plant of immortality)	*External:* burns/sunburn, cuts, skin irritations, wounds, abrasions *Internal:* constipation	*External:* gels, creams, lotions *Internal:* not recommended
Angelica (dong-quai, tang-kuei)	Gynecologic disorders, post-menopausal symptoms, menstrual discomfort	Fluid extract, tablets, capsules, injection; no consistently reported dosage
Cayenne pepper (Capsicum, capsaicin, chili pepper, pepper sauce, hot pepper)	*External:* pain, including shingles, stump pain, diabetic neuropathy, cluster headache, arthritis *Internal:* stimulation of stomach secretions	*External:* creams, gels, ointment, lotion, 0.025%-0.075% *Internal:* diet as tolerated; supplements not recommended
Chamomile	Treatment of stomach maladies including gastrointestinal (GI) spasms and inflammatory conditions of the GI tract, sedation	Teas most common; also capsules and liquid. For tea, dose is 2-3 grams (1 tablespoon) of dried flowers t.i.d. or q.i.d.
Cranberry (marsh apple, mountain cranberry)	Prevention of urinary tract infections (UTIs), possible antitumor effects	Capsules: 475-500 mg, 1-2 capsules per day P.O. Juices: 10-16 oz per day Powdered concentrates
Echinacea (American cone flower, coneflower, hedgehog, snakeroot)	Wound-healing agent and nonspecific immunostimulant for upper respiratory infections and UTIs	Capsules: 125, 355, and 500 mg P.O. t.i.d. Tablets: 335 mg P.O. t.i.d. Tincture: 0.75-1.5 ml P.O. 2-5 times per day
Feverfew (bachelors' button, febrifuge plant)	Prophylaxis of migraine headache, antipyretic for treating fever, toothache, psoriasis, insect bites, asthma, rheumatism and menstrual problems	Capsules: 380 mg (pure leaf); 250 mg (leaf extract) P.O. Liquid Tablets No consensus for dosage exists.
Flax (flaxseed, linseed, lint bells, linium)	*External:* inflammation *Internal:* constipation, irritable bowel, diverticulitis, functional disorders of the colon, hypercholesterolemia	*External:* 30-50 grams of flax meal applied as a poultice *Internal:* 1-2 tablespoons of oil or seeds daily in 2 or 3 divided doses P.O.
Garlic (allium, stinking rose, nectar of the gods, camphor of the poor)	Antimicrobial, lowers cholesterol and blood pressure, antiplatelet agent	600-900 mg daily P.O.
Ginger (Zingiber)	Antiemetic for morning sickness, motion sickness, postoperative nausea; anti-inflammatory, antitumor, antioxidant, antimicrobial agent	Varies with disease Antiemetic: 500-1,000 mg in 4 divided doses P.O.

Inform him that herbal medicines may interact adversely with his existing medications, and make him aware of the variable quality of products produced in the "alternative" industry. He should agree to monitor the goals of therapy with you; if he hasn't achieved those goals after a sufficient time, suggest he consider conventional pharmacotherapy. Be sure to tell him to watch for any unusual reactions to any medication, particularly alternative ones, and to report them promptly.

Considerations	Information for the patient
Internal use produces a cathartic action and has resulted in painful intestinal contractions, electrolyte imbalance, hemorrhagic diarrhea, and kidney damage.	Tell patient with a history of allergy to aloe, garlic, onion, or tulips not to use aloe. Warn against internal use. Can cause severe burning in patients undergoing dermabrasion or chemical peel.
Avoid in pregnancy and during breast-feeding because of possible uterine stimulation. Prolongs PT. Avoid use with anticoagulants. Human study data are lacking.	Tell diabetic patient she may exhibit poor glycemic control; instruct patient to monitor for signs of bleeding and warn of potential carcinogenic risk.
Topical application as a counterirritant produces a "heat" sensation. Repeated applications produce analgesia due to neuronal depletion of substance P, a mediator of pain transmission between periphery and spinal cord. Burning and itching diminish with continued use. Commercially available capsaicin preparations proved effective topical analgesics for some pain syndromes.	Pain relief may take up to 28 days. Avoid contact with eyes, mucous membranes, or nonintact skin. If contact occurs, flush area with cool running water as long as needed until burning sensation subsides. Used orally, capsicum has the potential to reduce the effectiveness of antihypertensives and may promote hypertensive crisis when used with MAO inhibitors.
Theoretical potential exists for decreased absorption of certain medications from antispasmodic activity. Excessive anticoagulation may occur when used with other anticoagulants.	Avoid use in pregnancy because of potential abortifacient and teratogenic effects. Instruct atopic patients to avoid use because of potential allergic reactions.
Has the potential to enhance the elimination of some drugs normally excreted in urine. Consumption of large quantities may cause diarrhea. Cranberry, which prevents bacteria from embedding in bladder walls, may be an important agent for prophylaxis in patients prone to UTIs.	Counsel diabetic patient to use sugar-free juices. Encourage patient to drink sufficient fluids and to call if urinary symptoms worsen or don't resolve.
Activity shown against influenza, herpes, and *Candida*. Adverse effects, except possible allergy, are uncommon. No documented drug interactions. Prolonged use may lead to overstimulation of the immune system and possible immune suppression.	Instruct patient not to use echinacea for more than 8 weeks; therapy for 10-14 days probably is sufficient. Advise patient with HIV/AIDS, collagen disease, multiple sclerosis, tuberculosis, and other autoimmune diseases not to use echinacea.
Adverse effects include allergic reactions, mouth ulcers, and postfeverfew syndrome (withdrawal symptoms of aches, pains, and joint and muscle stiffness). Avoid use during pregnancy and lactation.	Instruct patient to taper off the agent and to use proven therapies for migraine before using feverfew.
Adverse effects include diarrhea, nausea, and flatulence. May diminish absorption of other medications. Contraindicated in pregnancy, breast-feeding, ileus, and prostate cancer.	Instruct patient to refrigerate the oil and to never ingest immature seed because of potential toxicity. Overdose signs and symptoms include tachypnea, paralysis, and convulsions.
Adverse effects include contact dermatitis, dizziness, garlic odor, hypothyroidism, GI irritation, nausea, and vomiting. Potential drug interactions exist with antiplatelet therapy or anticoagulants. Avoid use in pregnant women and patients with GI disorders.	Advise patient that chronic or excessive use might cause decreased hemoglobin production or lysis of blood cells. Also advise patient using garlic to lower cholesterol that proven regimens should be part of his plan.
Overdose may produce CNS depression and arrhythmias. Ginger may enhance the effect of anticoagulants.	Advise patient considering ginger for morning sickness that the teratogenic potential is largely unstudied and to avoid ginger in large doses in pregnancy. Also advise her to watch for signs of bleeding and tell her that no consensus exists for dosing or monitoring.

(continued)

Names	Reported uses	Forms and dosages
Ginkgo biloba (EGB 761, GBE, GBX, Rokan, Tebonin, Ginkogink)	Cerebrovascular disease and peripheral vascular insufficiency resulting in short-term memory loss, vertigo, tinnitus, intermittent claudication; dementia	Vascular: 120-160 mg daily in 2 or 3 divided doses P.O. Dementia: 120-240 mg daily in 2 or 3 divided doses P.O.
Ginseng (five fingers, tartar root, Western ginseng, seng and sang, Asian Ginseng)	Improvement of stamina, concentration, healing, work efficiency, and well-being; aphrodisiac; sleep aid; antidepressant; antistress agent	200-600 mg ginseng extract daily P.O.
Green tea (tea, matsu-cha)	Prevention of cancer, dental caries, hypercholesterolemia, atherosclerosis; diuretic; stimulant; astringent; antibacterial	6-10 cups of tea per day
Kava (sakau, kawa, awa, kava-kava, tonga)	Treatment of anxiety, stress, and restlessness	90-110 mg dried kava extract P.O. t.i.d.
Ma huang (ephedra, Chinese ephedra, Teamster's tea, desert tea, popotillo, natural ecstacy)	CNS stimulant, appetite suppressant, treatment of asthma, colds, flu, nasal congestion	Tablets: 7 mg P.O. Teas: Unknown
Milk thistle (Mary thistle, Marian thistle, Lady's thistle, Holy thistle, silymarin)	Liver disease, including cirrhosis and chronic hepatitis; gallstones; liver protectant from toxins (death cap mushroom, halothane, psychotropic drugs)	420-800 mg P.O. daily as a single dose or in 2 or 3 divided doses
Nettle (stinging nettle, common nettle, greater nettle)	Diuretic, BPH, allergic rhinitis, bladder irrigation, gout	Tincture: ¼-1 teaspoon b.i.d. P.O. Capsules: 150-300 mg b.i.d. P.O.
Passion flower (passion fruit, granadilla, water lemon, maypop)	Sedative	4-8 grams (3-6 teaspoons) as a tea daily in divided doses
Peppermint (brandy mint, balm mint, menthol)	*External:* Common cold, arthritis, other musculoskeletal problems *Internal:* Irritable bowel syndrome, dyspepsia	*External:* 3 or 4 times per day as menthol in creams, rubs, and so forth *Internal:* Teas—1 tablespoon in 160 ml 3 or 4 times per day P.O.
Saw palmetto (sabal, American dwarf palm tree, Serenoa repens, LSESR)	BPH	320 mg daily in divided doses (160 mg b.i.d.) P.O.
St. John's wort (Hypericum, amber, chassediable, devil's scourge, goat weed)	Mild to moderate depression; anxiety; viral infection	300 mg (standardized to 0.3% Hypericum) t.i.d. for 4-6 weeks P.O.
Tea tree oil (Australian tea tree oil, melaleuca alternifolia, melaleuca oil, tea tree)	Local antiseptic; treatment of burns, cuts, athlete's foot, and various other cutaneous conditions	Topical application in various concentrations (0.4%-100%)

By Christine K. O'Neil, PharmD, Assistant Professor, Duquesne University Mylan School of Pharmacy, Pittsburgh, Pa. Juan R. Avila, PharmD, Medical Therapeutics Liaison, Sanofi-Synthelabo Pharmaceuticals, New York. C.W. Fetrow, PharmD, Coordinator, Pharmacokinetics, Outpatient Anticoagulation, and Drug Evaluation Services, St. Francis Medical Center, Pittsburgh, Pa.

Considerations	Information for the patient
Studies have shown that ginkgo extract produces arterial and venous vasoactive changes that increase tissue perfusion and cerebral blood flow. Adverse reactions are uncommon, but there have been reports of seizures in children and bleeding complications. Potential drug interactions may exist with antiplatelet therapy or anticoagulants.	Avoid use in children and pregnancy. Warn patient to monitor for unusual bleeding or bruising. If applied externally, gingko may cause irritation or blistering of the skin or mucous membranes. Results may not be evident for 6-8 weeks.
Avoid in pregnancy or during breast-feeding. Patients with cardiovascular disease, hypertension, hypotension, diabetes, or concurrent steroid therapy should avoid use. Drug interactions may exist with agents that inhibit MAO (phenelzine, St. John's wort, selegeline).	Counsel patient that large doses may be fatal and not to use for long periods. Use of coffee or tea may enhance CNS effects. Patient should watch for signs of ginseng toxicity, which include diarrhea, hypertension, restlessness, insomnia, and skin eruptions.
Concomitant administration with milk may inhibit the antioxidant effect. A patient taking doxorubicin may experience enhanced antitumor activity.	Patient with "green-tea asthma" should avoid use because of immunoglobulin E–mediated allergic reactions.
Kava doesn't appear to cause physiologic dependence. Expect enhanced sedative effects if combined with other CNS depressants (alcohol, benzodiazepines, and opioid analgesics). Heavy use may cause nutritional deficiencies, skin dermopathy, blood dyscrasias, pulmonary hypertension, and dopamine antagonism.	Counsel patient to avoid with pregnancy and during breast-feeding and not to use in children under age 12. Advise patient to avoid alcohol while using. Kava is generally well tolerated except in high doses or for long-term use.
Adverse reactions appear to be dose-related and include anxiety, cardiac arrhythmia and infarction, insomnia, psychosis, stroke, urine retention, and uterine contractions. Avoid use in individuals with hypertension, diabetes, cardiac disease, prostatic enlargement, cerebrovascular disease, or pregnancy.	Caution patient to watch for such signs and symptoms as chest pain or shortness of breath. Advise patient not to exceed 24 mg/day or more than 8 mg in 6 hours or to use ephedra for more than 7 days. Avoid use with other CNS stimulants such as caffeine.
Historic use and clinical trials indicate a promising role for milk thistle in acute and chronic liver disease. Because there are no allopathic alternatives, a trial of milk thistle may be warranted in life-threatening situations.	Advise patient that concentrations of 70%-80% are necessary because of poor bioavailability. Patient with liver disease should seek advice of a specialist before pursuing this therapy.
Adverse reactions are rare but include edema, oliguria, and stomach irritation. Avoid in pregnancy and during breast-feeding. Treat for heart failure and BPH only under a physician's supervision. Only proven action is diuresis.	Tell patient that the plant causes intense burning if it rubs against the skin. Advise him to eat food high in potassium to replenish electrolytes lost through diuresis.
Adverse effects and drug interactions are unknown. Avoid in pregnancy and lactation.	Warn patient of the potential for oversedation.
Patients with gastroesophageal reflux disease should avoid because peppermint may exacerbate it. Peppermint teas and mentholated ointment shouldn't be used in infants and small children. Menthol can cause sensitization and allergic reactions.	Advise patient not to apply topical mentholated products to broken skin. Menthol is generally recognized as safe when used externally. Internal use of peppermint for purposes other than flavoring isn't recommended.
Adverse events include minor GI reactions, decreased libido, hypertension, back pain, dysuria, and headache. Appears to be well tolerated and has demonstrated greater efficacy than placebo and equal efficacy to finasteride in improving symptoms of BPH.	Advise patient to take with morning and evening meals to minimize GI disturbances. Those seeking to use saw palmetto for BPH should do so only after diagnosis.
There are numerous case reports and clinical trials evaluating the efficacy and safety of St. John's wort. Most trials contain design flaws, but overall suggest that St. John's wort may be beneficial for depression. Adverse reactions are uncommon but include photosensitivity, constipation, dizziness, dry mouth, restlessness, and sleep disturbances.	Advise patient to take precautions against sun exposure. Caution that the possibility of serotonin syndrome exists when this herb is used with other serotoninergic drugs such as the serotonin reuptake inhibitors, trazodone, tricyclic antidepressants, and amphetamines. Avoid concurrent use with MAO inhibitors, alcoholic beverages, opioids, sympathomimetics, OTC cold and flu medications, and tyramine-containing foods such as chocolate, aged cheeses, and beer. Avoid in pregnancy and during breast-feeding; don't use in children.
Topical application hasn't been shown to be toxic, but ingesting the oil can produce CNS depression and GI irritation. The oil's antimicrobial activity has been well documented, but only anecdotal evidence exists for its efficacy in treating skin maladies.	Advise patient of the various product concentrations. Those with a propensity for contact dermatitis should probably avoid the use of tea tree oil.

Contact numbers and Web sites for pharmaceutical companies, agencies, and organizations

Pharmaceutical Companies	Main Number	Medical Product Information Number	Web site Address
Abbott Laboratories	(847) 937-6100	(800) 633-9110	www.abbott.com
Alcon Laboratories, Inc.	(817) 293-0450	(800) 757-9195	www.alconlabs.com
Allergan, Inc.	(714) 246-4500	(800) 433-8871	www.allergan.com
ALRA Laboratories, Inc.	(800) 248-ALRA		
ALZA Corp.	(800) 227-9953	(800) 634-8977	www.alza.com
Amgen, Inc.	(805) 447-1000	(800) 772-6436	www.amgen.com
AstraZeneca, Inc.	(800) 942-0424	(800) 355-6044	www.astrazeneca.com
Aventis Pharma			www2.aventis.com
Aventis Pharmaceuticals	(816) 966-5000		www.aventispharma-us.com
Baker Norton Pharmaceuticals, Inc.	(800) 347-4774	(305) 575-6244	www.ivax.com
Baxter Healthcare Co.	(818) 956-3200	(818) 507-5496	www.baxter.com
Bayer Co. Pharmaceutical	(800) 468-0894	(800) 288-8371	www.bayerus.com
Allergy	(509) 489-5656		www.bayer-ag.de
Biological	(510) 705-5000		
Bedford Laboratories	(440) 232-3320	(800) 521-5169	
Beiersdorf, Inc.	(203) 563-5800	(800) 227-4703	www.beiersdorf.com
Berlex Laboratories	(973) 694-4100		
Beutlich LP Pharmaceuticals	(800) 238-8542		www.beutlich.com
Blansett Pharmacal	(800) 379-9299		
Boehringer Ingelheim	(203) 798-9988	(800) 243-0127	www.boehringer-ingelheim.com
Braintree Laboratories	(800) 874-6756		www.braintreelabs.com
Bristol-Myers Squibb Co.	(609) 897-2000	(800) 332-2056	www.bms.com
Westwood-Squibb	(800) 333-0950		
Carnrick Laboratories	(888) CARNICK		www.elanpharma.com
Cephalon, Inc.	(610) 344-0200		www.cephalon.com
Cetylite Industries, Inc.	(800) 257-7740	(856) 665-6111	www.cetylite.com
Chiron Therapeutics	(510) 655-8730	(800) 244-7668	www.chiron.com
Dupont Pharmaceuticals Co.	(302) 992-5000	(800) 474-2762	www.dupontmerck.com
Dura Pharmaceuticals, Inc.	(619) 457-2553		www.durapharm.com
Duramed Pharmaceuticals, Inc.	(800) 543-8338		www.duramed.com
Eli Lilly and Co.	(317) 276-2000	(800) 545-5979	www.lilly.com
Ferring Pharmaceuticals	(888) 793-6367	(888) 337-7464	www.ferringusa.com
The Fielding Pharmaceutical Co., Inc.	(314) 567-5462		www.fieldingcompany.com
Flemming and Co.	(314) 343-8200		www.flemingcompany.com
Forest Pharmaceuticals, Inc.	(314) 493-7000	(800) 947-5227	www.frx.com
Fujisawa USA, Inc.	(847) 317-8800	(800) 888-7704	www.fujisawausa.com
Galderma Laboratories, Inc.	(817) 263-2600		www.galderma.com
Gate Pharmaceuticals	(215) 256-8400		www.gatepharma.com
Glaxo Wellcome, Inc.	(888) 825-5249	(800) 334-0089	www.glaxowellcome.com
Glenwood Western Medical	(800) 237-9083		www.glenwood-llc.com
ICN Pharmaceuticals, Inc.	(800) 556-1937		www.icnpharm.com
Immunex Corp.	(800) 466-8639		www.immunex.com
Ion Laboratories, Inc.	(817) 589-7257		

Pharmaceutical Companies	Main Number	Medical Product Information Number	Web site Address
Janssen Pharmaceutica, Inc.	(800) JANSSEN		www.janssen.com
Key Pharmaceuticals	(908) 298-4000	(800) 526-4099	www.schering-plough.com
Knoll Pharmaceutical Co.	(800) 526-1072	(800) 526-0221	www.basf.com
3M Pharmaceuticals	(800) 328-0255	(800) 364-3577	www.3m.com
Marlyn Neutraceuticals	(800) 899-4499		www.naturallyvitamins.com
McNeil Consumer Products Co.	(215) 273-7000		www.tylenol.com
Medeva Pharmaceuticals	(716) 274-5300	(800) 234-5535	www.medeva.com
Merck & Co., Inc.	(800) 672-6372	(800) 672-6372	www.merck.com
Merz Pharmaceuticals	(910) 856-2003		www.merzusa.com
Mission Pharmacal Co.	(210) 696-8400		www.missionpharmacal.com
Monarch Pharmaceuticals	(800) 546-4906	(284) 656-5299	www.monarchpharm.com
Monsanto	(847) 982-7000	(800) 323-4204	www.monsanto.com
Muro Pharmaceutical, Inc.	(800) 225-0974		
Mylan Pharmaceuticals	(800) 82-MYLAN		www.mylan.com
Novartis	(973) 781-8300	(800) 742-2422	www.novartis.com
Novartis Pharmaceuticals	(888) 631-8184	(888) 669-6682	www.novartis.com
Novartis Consumer Health	(800) 452-0051		www.novartis.com
Novo Nordisk Pharmaceuticals	(609) 987-5800	(800) 727-6500	www.novo.dk
Organon, Inc.	(800) 631-1253		www.organon.com
Ortho Biotech, Inc.	(800) 325-7504		
Ortho-McNeil Pharmaceutical Co.	(800) 682-6532		www.ortho-mcneil.com
Ortho Dermatological Division	(800) 426-7762	(800) 426-7762	
Paddock Laboratories	(800) 328-5113		www.paddocklabs.com
Par Pharmaceutical, Inc.	(800) 828-9393	(914) 425-7100	www.parpharm.com
Parke-Davis	(800) 223-0432	(973) 540-4381	www.parke-davis.com
Pasteur Merlieux Connaught Rhone Poulenc Group	(800) 822-2463		www.us.pmc-vacc.com
Pedinol Pharmacal, Inc.	(516) 293-9500		www.pedinol.com
Person & Covey, Inc.	(800) 423-2341		
Pfizer Consumer Health Care	(973) 887-2100	(800) 438-1985	www.pfizer.com
Pfizer, Inc./Labs Division	(800) 438-1985	(800) 438-1985	www.pfizer.com
Pharmaceutical Associates, 2055, Inc.	(800) 845-8210		
Pharmacia & Upjohn Co.	(888) 768-5501	(616) 833-8244	www.pnu.com
Procter & Gamble Pharmaceutical, Inc.	(800) 836-0658	(800) 836-0658	www.pg.com
Purdue Pharma L.P.	(203) 853-0123	(800) 733-1333	www.pharma.com
Respa Pharmaceuticals	(630) 462-9986		
Roche Pharmaceuticals	(973) 235-5000	(800) 526-6367	www.roche.com
Ross Products Division	(800) 624-7677		www.ross.com
Roxane Laboratories, Inc.	(800) 848-0120	(800) 962-8364	www.roxane.com
Rystan Co., Inc.	(973) 256-3737		
SCS	(847) 982-7000	(800) 323-4204	www.monsanto.com
Sandoz Pharmaceuticals	(973) 503-7500		www.novartis.com
Sanofi Winthrop Pharmaceuticals, Inc.	(212) 551-4000	(800) 446-6267	
Savage Laboratories	(516) 454-7677		www.savagelabs.com
Scandipharm, Inc.	(205) 991-8085	(800) 950-8080	www.scandipharm.com
Schering-Plough	(908) 298-4000	(800) 526-4099	www.schering-plough.com

Pharmaceutical Companies	Main Number	Medical Product Information Number	Web site Address
Schwarz Pharma, Inc.	(800) 558-5114		www.schwarzpharma.com
G.D. Searle & Co.	(800) 323-4204		www.searlehealthnet.com
Serono Laboratories	(800) 283-8088		www.seronousa.com
Shire Richwood Inc.	(606) 282-2100		www.shiregroup.com
Smith Kline Beecham Consumer Health Care	(800) Beecham	(800) 456-6670	www.sb.com
Smith Kline Beecham Pharmaceuticals	(800) 366-8900	(800) 751-5231	www.sb.com
Solvay Pharmaceuticals, Inc.	(770) 578-9000		www.solvay.com
Star Pharmaceuticals, Inc.	(954) 971-9704		www.starpharm.com
Stiefel Laboratories, Inc.	(305) 443-3800	(800) 327-3858	www.stiefel.com
TAP Pharmaceuticals, Inc.	(800) 622-2011	(800) 622-2011	
Teva Pharmaceuticals USA	(888) TEVA-USA		www.tevapharmusa.com
Tyson and Associates, Inc.	(800) 318-9766		
US Bioscience, Inc.	(800) 872-4672		www.usbio.com
Upsher-Smith Laboratories, Inc.	(800) 654-2299		www.upsher-smith.com
Warner Chilcott, Inc.	(800) 521-8813	(800) 521-8813	www.wclabs.com
Warner Lambert Co.	(800) 223-0182		www.warner-lambert.com
WE Pharmaceuticals, Inc.	(800) 262-9555		
Wyeth-Ayerst Laboratories	(800) 934-5556		

Agencies and organizations	Main Number	Web site Address
Agency for Health Care Policy Research and Quality	(301) 594-1364	www.ahcpr.gov
Centers for Disease Control and Prevention	(800) 311-3435	www.cdc.gov
F-D-C Reports	(800) 332-2181	www.fdcreports.com
Institute for Safe Medication Practices	(215) 947-7797	www.ismp.org
National Cancer Institute	(800) 4-CANCER	www.nci.nih.gov
National Institutes of Health	(301) 496-2351	www.nih.gov
National Library of Medicine	(888) 346-3656	www.nlm.nih.gov
U.S. Food and Drug Administration	(888) INFO-FDA	www.fda.gov
World Health Organization	(202) 974-3000	www.who.org

Physician Assistant's Drug Handbook
Photoguide to tablets and capsules

This photoguide provides full-color photographs of some of the most commonly prescribed tablets and capsules in the United States. Shown in actual size, the drugs are organized alphabetically by trade or generic name for quick reference. Page numbers direct you to drug information.

Accupril (page 903)	10 mg	20 mg
Adalat CC (extended-release) (page 759)	30 mg	
Allegra (page 449)	60 mg	
Altace (page 915)	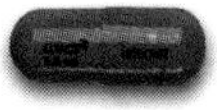 2.5 mg	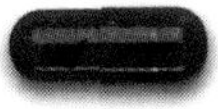 5 mg
Ambien (page 1133)	5 mg	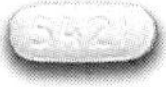 10 mg
amitriptyline hydrochloride (page 58)	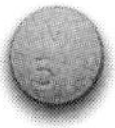 25 mg	50 mg
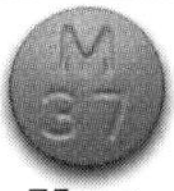	75 mg	
	100 mg	
amoxicillin trihydrate (page 66)	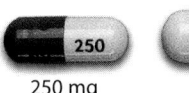 250 mg	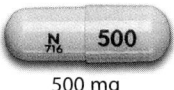 500 mg

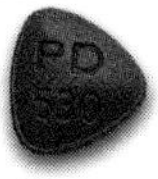

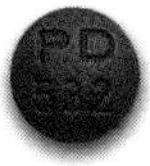

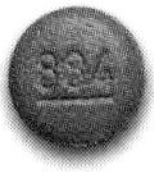

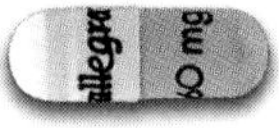

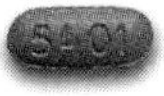

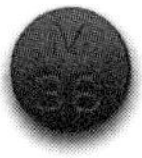

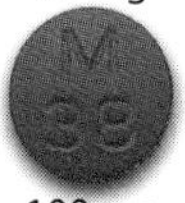

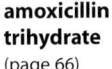

Amoxil
(page 66)

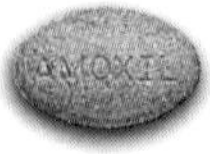

125 mg
(chewable)

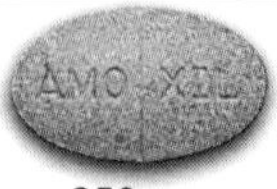

250 mg
(chewable)

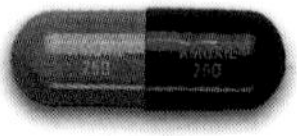

250 mg

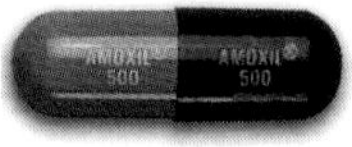

500 mg

atenolol
(page 88)

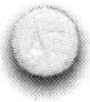

25 mg

Ativan
(page 633)

0.5 mg

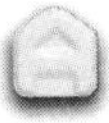

1 mg

Augmentin
(page 65)

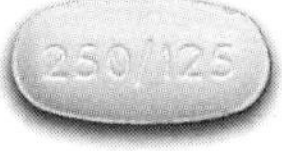

250 mg/125 mg

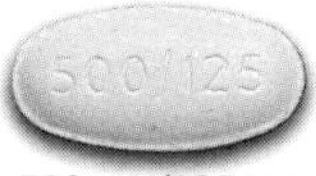

500 mg/125 mg

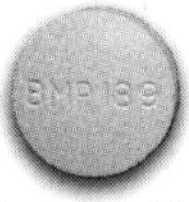

125 mg/31.25 mg
(chewable)

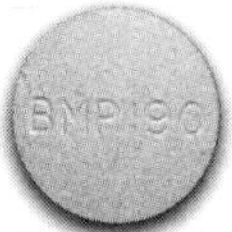

250 mg/62.5 mg
(chewable)

Axid
(page 767)

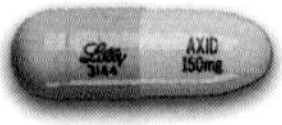

150 mg

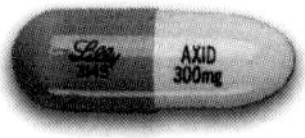

300 mg

Biaxin
(page 235)

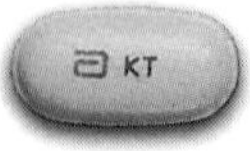

250 mg

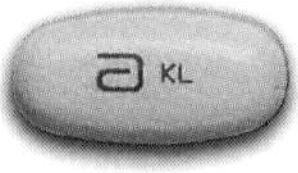

500 mg

Bumex
(page 134)

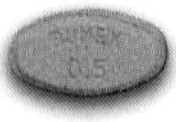

0.5 mg

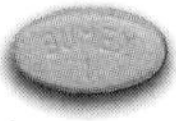

1 mg

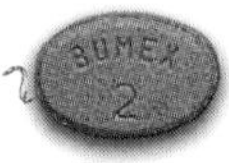

2 mg

BuSpar
(page 139)

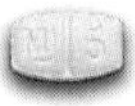

5 mg

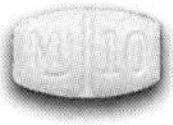

10 mg

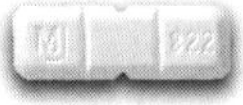

15 mg

Calan (page 1108)	40 mg	80 mg	 120 mg

Capoten (page 155)	12.5 mg	25 mg	

Carafate (page 985)	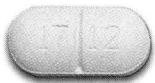 1 g		

Cardizem (page 332)	 30 mg	60 mg	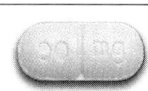 90 mg

Cardizem CD (extended-release) (page 332)	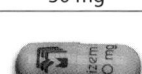 120 mg	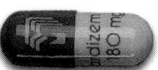 180 mg	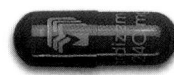 240 mg

Cardura (page 362)	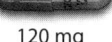 1 mg	 2 mg	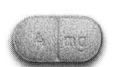 4 mg

Ceclor (page 169)	250 mg	500 mg	

Ceftin (page 194)	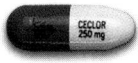 250 mg	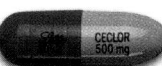 500 mg	

Cefzil (page 187)	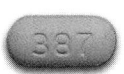 250 mg		

Celebrex (page 196)	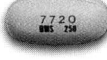 100 mg	 200 mg	

cephalexin monohydrate (page 197)	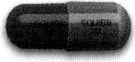 250 mg	 500 mg	

cimetidine
(page 226)

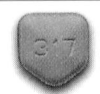 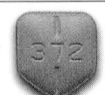

300 mg 400 mg

Cipro
(page 227)

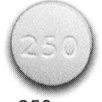 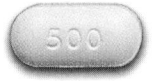 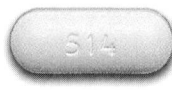

250 mg 500 mg 750 mg

Claritin
(page 632)

10 mg

Compazine
(page 880)

5 mg 10 mg

Cordarone
(page 56)

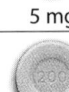

200 mg

Coreg
(page 165)

3.125 mg 6.25 mg 12.5 mg

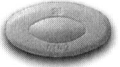

25 mg

Coumadin
(page 1119)

1 mg 2 mg 2.5 mg

  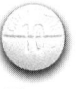

5 mg 7.5 mg 10 mg

Cozaar
(page 635)

25 mg 50 mg

**cyclobenzaprine
hydrochloride**
(page 267)

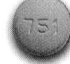

10 mg

Darvocet-N 100
(page 888)

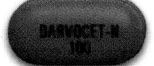

100 mg/650 mg

Daypro
(page 789)

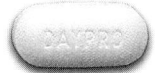

600 mg

Deltasone
(page 871)

2.5 mg   5 mg   10 mg

20 mg

Depakote
(page 1097)

 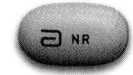 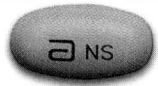

125 mg   250 mg   500 mg

Depakote Sprinkle
(delayed-release)
(page 1097)

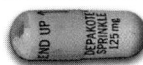

125 mg

DiaBeta
(page 502)

1.25 mg   2.5 mg   5 mg

Diflucan
(page 454)

 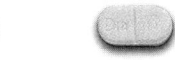

100 mg   150 mg   200 mg

Dilacor XR
(page 332)

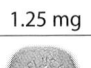 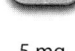 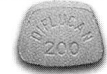

180 mg   240 mg

Dilantin Infatabs
(page 837)

 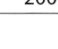

50 mg

Dilantin Kapseals
(page 837)

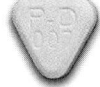 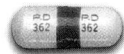

100 mg

doxepin hydrochloride (page 363)

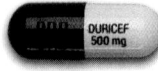

75 mg

Duricef (page 170)

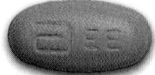

500 mg

E.E.S. (page 403)

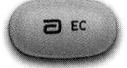

400 mg

Effexor (page 1107)

 25 mg   37.5 mg   50 mg

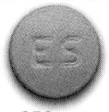 75 mg 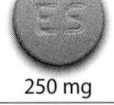 100 mg

Ery-Tab (delayed-release) (page 403)

 250 mg   333 mg

Erythrocin Stearate Filmtab (page 403)

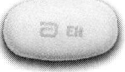

250 mg

Erythromycin Base Filmtab (page 403)

 250 mg   500 mg

Estrace (page 410)

1 mg 2 mg

Fiorinal with Codeine (page 1218)

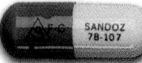

325 mg aspirin, 50 mg butalbital, 40 mg caffeine, 30 mg codeine phosphate

Floxin
(page 777)

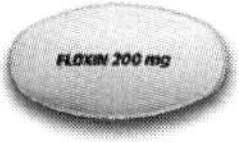

200 mg 300 mg 400 mg

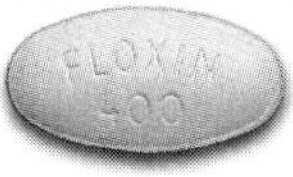

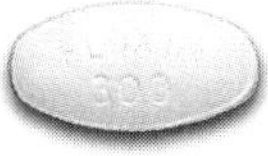

Fosamax
(page 35)

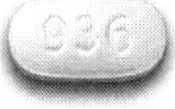

10 mg 40 mg

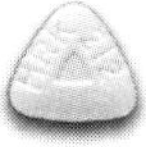

furosemide
(page 486)

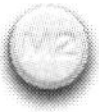

20 mg

glipizide
(page 499)

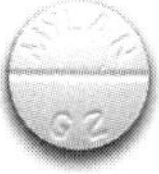

10 mg

Glucophage
(page 672)

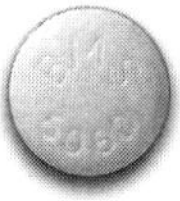

500 mg 850 mg

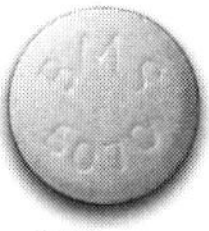

Glucotrol
(page 499)

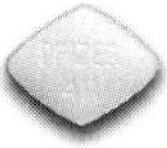

5 mg 10 mg

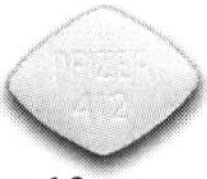

Glucotrol XL
(page 499)

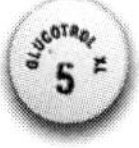

5 mg 10 mg

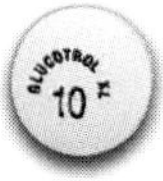

Glynase PresTab
(page 502)

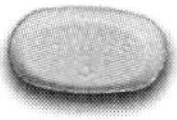

3 mg 6 mg

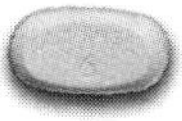

hydrocodone bitartrate and acetaminophen
(page 1188)

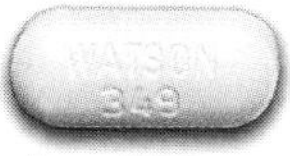

5 mg/500 mg 7.5 mg/500 mg 7.5 mg/750 mg

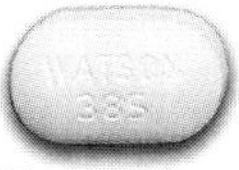

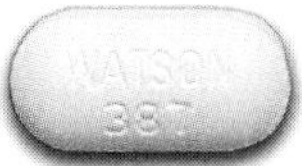

Hytrin
(page 1008)

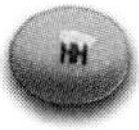

1 mg 2 mg 5 mg

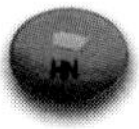

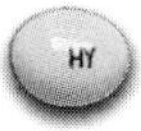

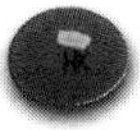

10 mg

Inderal
(page 889)

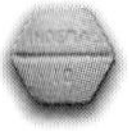

10 mg

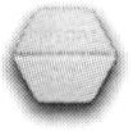

20 mg

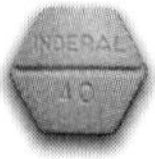

40 mg

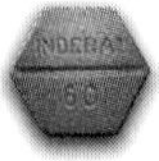

60 mg

K-Dur
(page 861)

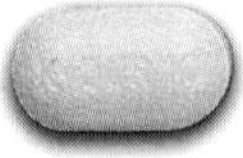

10 mEq

20 mEq

Klonopin
(page 244)

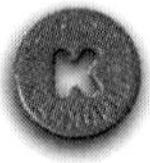

0.5 mg

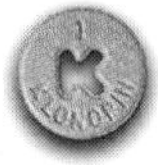

1 mg

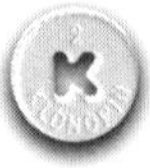

2 mg

Lanoxin
(page 325)

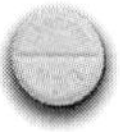

0.125 mg

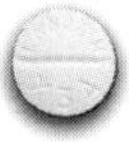

0.25 mg

Lasix
(page 486)

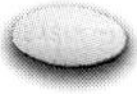

20 mg

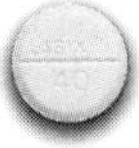

40 mg

Levaquin
(page 613)

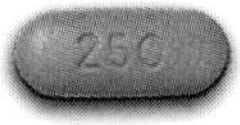

250 mg

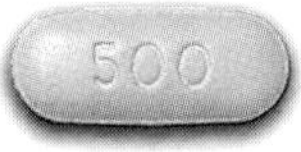

500 mg

Levoxyl
(page 616)

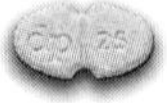

0.025 mg

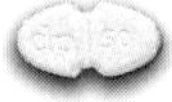

0.050 mg

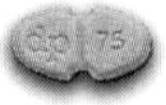

0.075 mg

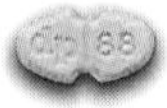

0.088 mg

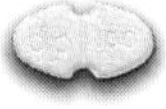

0.1 mg

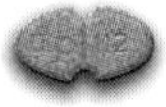

0.112 mg

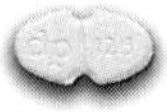

0.125 mg

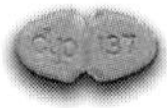

0.137 mg

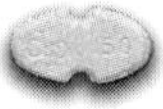

0.15 mg

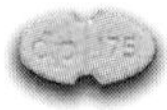

0.175 mg

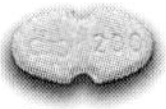

0.2 mg

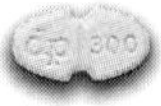

0.3 mg

Lipitor
(page 89)

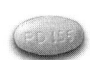 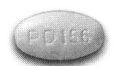 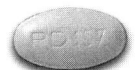

10 mg   20 mg   40 mg

Lodine
(page 428)

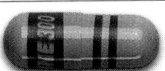 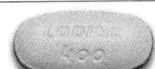

200 mg   300 mg   400 mg

Lopid
(page 494)

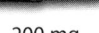

600 mg

Lorabid
(page 631)

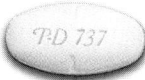

400 mg

Lorcet 10/650
(page 1219)

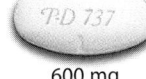

10 mg/650 mg

Lotensin
(page 109)

5 mg   10 mg   20 mg

40 mg

Macrobid
(page 762)

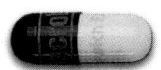

75/25 mg

methylphenidate hydrochloride
(page 686)

5 mg   10 mg   20 mg

20 mg
(sustained-release)

Mevacor
(page 636)

10 mg   20 mg   40 mg

Micro-K Extencaps
(controlled-release)
(page 861)

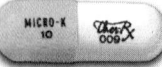

10 mEq (750 mg)

Micronase
(page 502)

  2.5 mg

  5 mg

Monopril
(page 483)

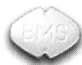 10 mg

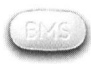 20 mg

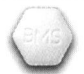 40 mg

Motrin
(page 544)

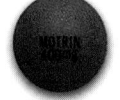 400 mg

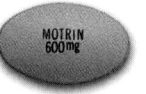 600 mg

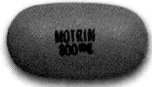 800 mg

Naprosyn
(page 743)

  250 mg

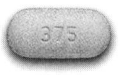 375 mg

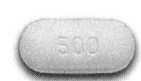 500 mg

naproxen
(page 743)

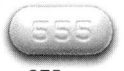 375 mg

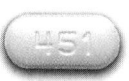 500 mg

Nitrostat
(page 764)

  0.3 mg

  0.4 mg

  0.6 mg

Nolvadex
(page 1001)

  10 mg

nortriptyline hydrochloride
(page 773)

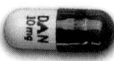 10 mg

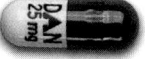 25 mg

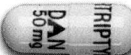 50 mg

Norvasc
(page 60)

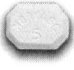 5 mg

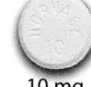 10 mg

Oruvail
(page 588)

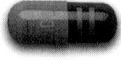 100 mg

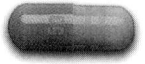 150 mg

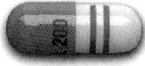 200 mg

Pamelor
(page 773)

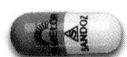

10 mg

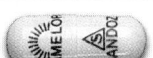

25 mg

50 mg

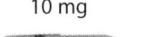
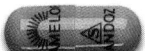

75 mg

Paxil
(page 807)

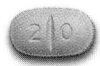

20 mg

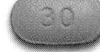

30 mg

PCE
(page 403)

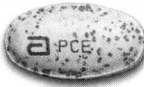

333 mg

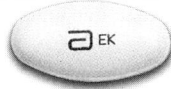

500 mg

Pepcid
(page 435)

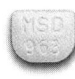

20 mg

40 mg

Percocet 5/325
(page 1219)

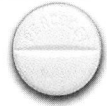

5 mg/325 mg

potassium chloride
(controlled-release)
(page 861)

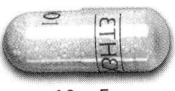

10 mEq

Pravachol
(page 866)

10 mg

20 mg

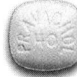

40 mg

Premarin
(page 417)

0.3 mg

0.625 mg

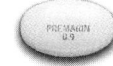

0.9 mg

1.25 mg

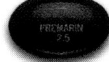

2.5 mg

Prevacid
(page 598)

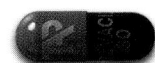

15 mg

30 mg

Prilosec
(page 780)

10 mg   20 mg

Prinivil
(page 624)

5 mg   10 mg   20 mg

Procardia XL
(extended-release)
(page 759)

30 mg   60 mg   90 mg

**propoxyphene
napsylate with
acetaminophen**
(page 1218)

100 mg/650 mg

Provera
(page 655)

2.5 mg   5 mg   10 mg

Prozac
(page 464)

10 mg   20 mg

Relafen
(page 732)

500 mg   750 mg

Risperdal
(page 932)

1 mg   2 mg   3 mg

4 mg

Roxicet
(page 1218)

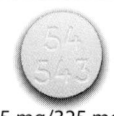

5 mg/325 mg

Serzone
(page 747)

50 mg

100 mg

150 mg

200 mg

Sinemet
(page 612)

10 mg/100 mg

25 mg/250 mg

Sinemet CR
(extended-release)
(page 612)

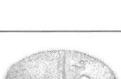

25 mg/100 mg

Slo-bid Gyrocaps
(extended-release)
(page 1022)

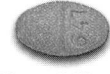

50 mg

75 mg

100 mg

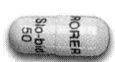

200 mg

300 mg

Sumycin
(page 1017)

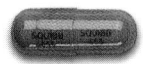

250 mg

Tagamet
(page 226)

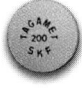

200 mg

300 mg

Tenormin
(page 88)

25 mg

50 mg

100 mg

Theo-Dur
(extended-release)
(page 1022)

100 mg

200 mg

300 mg

450 mg

Ticlid
(page 1041)

250 mg

Toprol XL
(page 695)

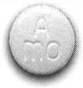 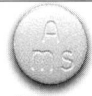 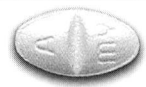

50 mg   100 mg   200 mg

Toradol
(page 590)

10 mg

Trental
(page 821)

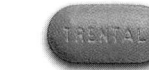

400 mg

Trimox
(page 66)

 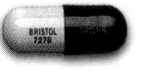

250 mg   500 mg

Tylenol with Codeine No. 3
(page 1219)

300 mg/30 mg

Ultram
(page 1061)

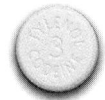

50 mg

Valium
(page 312)

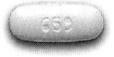

2 mg   5 mg   10 mg

Vasotec
(page 381)

2.5 mg   5 mg   10 mg

20 mg

Veetids
(page 816)

 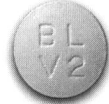

250 mg   500 mg

verapamil hydrochloride
(extended-release)
(page 1108)

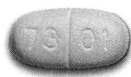

180 mg

Verelan
(sustained-release)
(page 1108)

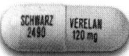   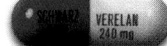

120 mg   240 mg

Viagra
(page 961)

      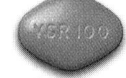

25 mg   50 mg   100 mg

Vioxx
(page 940)

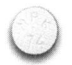   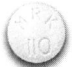

12.5 mg   25 mg

Xanax
(page 39)

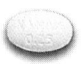

0.25 mg   0.5 mg   1 mg

Zantac
(page 916)

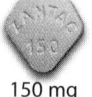   

150 mg   300 mg

Zantac EFFERdose
(page 916)

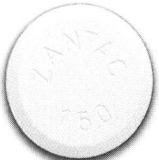

150 mg

Zestril
(page 624)

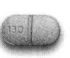

5 mg   10 mg   20 mg

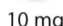

40 mg

Zocor
(page 963)

  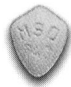

5 mg   10 mg   20 mg

Zoloft
(page 958)

 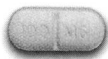

50 mg   100 mg

Zovirax
(page 27)

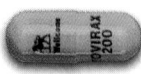 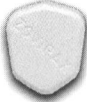 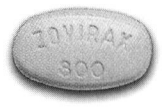

200 mg   400 mg   800 mg

Zyrtec
(page 202)

5 mg   10 mg

Acknowledgments

We would like to thank the following companies for granting us permission to include their drugs in the full-color photoguide.

Abbott Laboratories
Biaxin®
Depakote®
Depakote® Sprinkle
E.E.S.®
Ery-Tab®
Erythrocin Stearate Filmtab®
Erythromycin Base Filmtab®
Hytrin®
PCE®

AstraZeneca LP
Nolvadex®
Prilosec®
Tenormin®
Toprol XL®
Zestril®

Aventis Pharmaceuticals
Allegra®
Carafate®
Cardizem®
Cardizem® CD
DiaBeta®
Lasix®
Slo-Bid™ Gyrocaps®
Trental®

Bayer Corporation
Adalat CC®
Cipro®

Bristol-Myers Squibb Company
BuSpar®
Capoten®
Cefzil®
Duricef®
Estrace®
Glucophage®
Monopril®
Pravachol®
Serzone®
Sumycin®
Trimox®
Veetids®

DuPont Pharmaceuticals Company
Coumadin®

Eli Lilly and Company
Axid®
Ceclor®
Darvocet-N® 100
Prozac®

Endo Pharmaceuticals, Inc.
Percocet® 5/325

ESI Lederle Division of American Home Products
atenolol

Ethex Corporation
potassium chloride

Forest Pharmaceuticals, Inc.
Lorcet® 10/650

Glaxo Wellcome, Inc.
Ceftin®
Lanoxin®
Zantac®
Zantac® EFFERdose®
Zovirax®

Janssen Pharmaceutica, Inc.
Risperdal®

Jones Pharma
Levoxyl®

King Pharmaceuticals, Inc.
Altace®
Lorabid®

KV Pharmaceutical Company
Micro-K Extencaps®

McNeil-PPC, Inc.
Motrin®

Medeva Pharmaceuticals
methylphenidate hydrochloride

Merck & Co., Inc.
Cozaar®
Fosamax®
Mevacor®
Pepcid®
Prinivil®
Sinemet®
Sinemet® CR
Vasotec®
Vioxx®
Zocor®

Mylan Pharmaceuticals, Inc.
amitriptyline hydrochloride
cimetidine
cyclobenzaprine hydrochloride
doxepin hydrochloride
furosemide
glipizide
naproxen
propoxyphene napsylate with acetaminophen

Novartis Pharmaceuticals Corporation
Fiorinal® with Codeine
Lotensin®
Pamelor®

Novopharm USA, Inc., Division of Novopharm Limited
amoxicillin trihydrate

Ortho-McNeil Pharmaceutical
Floxin®
Levaquin®
Tylenol® with Codeine No. 3
Ultram®

Pfizer, Inc.
Cardura®
Diflucan®
Glucotrol®
Glucotrol XL®
Norvasc®
Procardia XL®
Viagra®
Zithromax®
Zoloft®
Zyrtec®

Pharmacia & Upjohn
Deltasone®
Glynase®
Micronase®
Provera®
Xanax®

Procter and Gamble Pharmaceuticals, Inc.
Macrobid®

Roche Laboratories, Inc.
Bumex®
Klonopin®
Naprosyn®
Ticlid®
Toradol®
Valium®

Roxane Laboratories, Inc.
Roxicet™

Schein Pharmaceutical, Inc.
nortriptyline hydrochloride

**Schering-Plough
Corporation/Key
Pharmaceuticals, Inc.**
Claritin®
K-Dur®
Theo-Dur®

Schwarz Pharma
Verelan®

G.D. Searle & Company
Ambien®
Calan®
Celebrex®
Daypro®

**SmithKline Beecham
Pharmaceuticals**
Amoxil®
Augmentin®
Compazine®
Coreg®
Dyazide®
Paxil®
Relafen®
Tagamet®

Tap Pharmaceuticals, Inc.
Prevacid®

Teva Pharmaceuticals USA
cephalexin

**Warner-Lambert
Company**
Accupril®
Dilantin® Infatabs
Dilantin® Kapseals®
Lipitor®
Lopid®
Nitrostat®

Watson Pharma Inc.
Dilacor XR®
hydrocodone bitartrate and
acetaminophen

**Wyeth-Ayerst
Laboratories**
Ativan®
Cordarone®
Effexor®
Inderal®
Lodine®
Oruvail®
Premarin®

**Zenith Goldline
Pharmaceuticals**
verapamil hydrochloride

Index

Brucellosis, tetracycline for, 1017
budesonide, 133-134
Bufferin, 86
Bulimia, amitriptyline for, 58
bumetanide, 134-135
Bumex, 134, **C2**
Buminate 5%, 30
Buminate 25%, 30
Buprenex, 135
buprenorphine hydrochloride, 135-137
bupropion hydrochloride, 137-139
Burkitt's lymphoma, methotrexate for, 681
Burns
  albumin, human, for, 30
  dibucaine for, 316
  ethyl chloride for, 427
  gentamicin for, 495
  lidocaine for, 618
  neomycin for, 750
  nitrofurazone for, 763
Burow's Solution, 1220t
Bursitis, sulindac for, 995
BuSpar, 139, **C2**
buspirone hydrochloride, 139-140
busulfan, 140-141
Butace, 1217t
butoconazole nitrate, 141-142
butorphanol tartrate, 142-143
Byclomine, 320

C

Cachexia, somatropin for, 973
Cafergot, 401
Caffedrine, 144
caffeine, 144-145
Calan, 1108, **C3**
Calan SR, 1108
Calciday-667, 149
Calciferol, 399
Calcijex, 147
Calcimar (salmon), 146
calcipotriene, 145-146
calcitonin, 146-147
calcitriol, 147-148
calcium acetate, 149-152
calcium carbonate, 149-152
Calcium channel blockers, 1165-1167
calcium chloride, 149-152
calcium citrate, 149-152
Calcium Disodium Versenate, 375
calcium EDTA, 375-376
calcium glubionate, 149-152
calcium gluceptate, 149-152
calcium gluconate, 149-152
calcium lactate, 149-152

calcium phosphate, tribasic, 149-152
calcium polycarbophil, 148-149
calcium salts, 149-152
Calculus formation
  allopurinol for, 37
  aluminum carbonate for, 44
CaldeCORT, 535
Calicylic, 1220t
Calm-X, 334
Caloric supplementation
  dextrose for, 310
  fat emulsions for, 436
Cal-Plus, 149
Caltrate 600, 149
Cama, 1217t
Camptosar, 572
Cancer, bumetanide for, 134. *See also specific type.*
candesartan cilexetil, 152-153
Candidal infections
  amphotericin B for, 69, 70
  amphotericin B cholesteryl sulfate complex for, 71
  fluconazole for, 455
  nystatin for, 775
Candidiasis
  amphotericin B for, 69
  butoconazole for, 141
  clotrimazole for, 249
  econazole for, 375
  fluconazole for, 454-455
  itraconazole for, 584
  terconazole for, 1012
  tioconazole for, 1045
capecitabine, 153-154
Capillariasis
  mebendazole for, 652
  thiabendazole for, 1024
Capital with Codeine, 1218t
Capoten, 155, **C3**
capsaicin, 154-155
captopril, 155-156
Carafate, 985, **C3**
carbachol, 156-157
carbamazepine, 157-159
carbamide, 754
carbamide, 1095-1096
carbamide peroxide, 159-160
Carbatrol, 157
Carbex, 956
Carbolith, 625
carboplatin, 160-161
Carboptic, 156
Carcinoma in situ, valrubicin for, 1099
Cardene, 754
Cardene SR, 754
Cardiac arrest, epinephrine for, 389
Cardiac bypass surgery, tromethamine for, 1086

Cardiac glycoside toxicity, cholestyramine for, 219
Cardiac output, increasing
  dobutamine for, 348
  dopamine for, 356
Cardiac vagal reflexes, blocking
  atropine for, 93
  glycopyrrolate for, 505
Cardiomyopathy, doxorubicin-induced, dexrazoxane for, 304
Cardioquin, 905
Cardiotonic use, calcium salts for, 150
Cardioversion, diazepam for, 312
Cardizem, 332, **C3**
Cardizem CD, 332, **C3**
Cardizem SR, 332
Cardura, 362, **C3**
carisoprodol, 161-163
carmustine, 163-164
carteolol hydrochloride, 164-165
Cartrol, 164
carvedilol, 165-167
cascara sagrada, 167-168
cascara sagrada aromatic fluidextract, 167-168
Casodex, 121
castor oil, 168-169
Castration
  esterified estrogens for, 409
  estradiol for, 410
  estradiol/norethindrone transdermal system for, 412
  estropipate for, 419
Cataflam, 317
Cataplexy, fluoxetine for, 464
Catapres, 245
Catapres-TTS, 245
Cataract removal
  diclofenac for, 317
  ketorolac for, 591
Catheter patency, heparin for, 523
Caverject, 41
CCNU, 629-630
Cebid Timecelles, 82
Ceclor, 169, **C3**
Ceclor CD, 169
Cecon, 82
Cedax, 190
CeeNU, 629
cefaclor, 16°
cefadroxi'
cefar

Dosage form, 4
Dovonex, 145
doxacurium chloride, 359-361
doxapram hydrochloride, 361-362
doxazosin mesylate, 362-363
doxepin hydrochloride, 363-365, **C6**
doxercalciferol, 365-366
Doxil, 366, 368
doxorubicin hydrochloride, 366-368
doxorubicin hydrochloride liposomal, 368-370
Doxy 100, 370
Doxy 200, 370
Doxy Caps, 370
doxycycline, 370-372
doxycycline calcium, 370-372
doxycycline hyclate, 370-372
doxycycline monohydrate, 370-372
Dracunculiasis
mebendazole for, 652
thiabendazole for, 1024
Dramamine, 334
Drenison, 469
Drisdol, 399
Dristan 12 Hr Spray, 794
dronabinol, 372-373
droperidol, 373-374
Droxia, 540
Drug administration, 4
Drug allergy, 5
Drug interactions, 4-5
Drug intoxication, mannitol for, 647
Drug monitoring guidelines, 1224-1229t
Drug properties, 3-4
Drug therapy
in children, 8-11
in elderly patients, 11-13
D-S-S, 351
DT, 340-341
d4T, 978-980
DTaP, 341-342
DTIC, 277-278
DTIC-Dome, 277
DTP, 341-342
DTwP, 341
Dulcolax, 123
Dull-C, 82
Dumping syndrome, octreotide for, 776
Duodenal ulcer
cimetidine for, 226
famotidine for, 435
lansoprazole for, 598
misoprostol for, 712
nizatidine for, 767
omeprazole for, 780-781

Duodenal ulcer *(continued)*
rabeprazole for, 910
ranitidine bismuth citrate for, 917
ranitidine for, 916
sucralfate for, 985
DuoFilm, 1220t
Duphalac, 594
Durabolin, 740
Duragesic-25, 442
Duragesic-50, 442
Duragesic-75, 442
Duragesic-100, 442
Duralith, 625
Duralone-40, 687
Duralone-80, 687
Duramist Plus, 794
Duramorph, 723
Duratest-100, 1012
Duratest-200, 1012
Durathate-200, 1012
Duration, 794
Duricef, 170, **C6**
Duvoid, 118
$D_{2.5}W$, 310
D_5W, 310
$D_{10}W$, 310
$D_{20}W$, 310
$D_{25}W$, 310
$D_{30}W$, 310
$D_{38}W$, 310
$D_{40}W$, 310
$D_{50}W$, 310
$D_{60}W$, 310
$D_{70}W$, 310
Dycill, 318
Dymenate, 334
Dynabac, 344
Dynacin, 707
DynaCirc, 583
Dynapen, 318
Dyrenium, 1074
Dysautonomia, bethanechol for, 118
Dyslipidemia
atorvastatin for, 89
cerivastatin for, 200
Dysmenorrhea
diclofenac for, 317
ibuprofen for, 544
indomethacin for, 557
ketoprofen for, 588
naproxen for, 743
rofecoxib for, 940
Dyspepsia, activated charcoal for, 26
Dysthymic disorder, thioridazine for, 1028-1029
Dystonic reaction, benztropine for, 112

E

Ear infection
chloramphenicol for, 205
neomycin for, 750
Eating disorders, fluoxetine for, 464
E-Base, 403
Eclampsia, magnesium sulfate for, 645
EC-Naprosyn, 743
econazole nitrate, 375
Econochlor, 205
Econopred, 870
Ecotrin, 86
Ectosone, 116
Edecrin, 421
Edema
acetazolamide for, 24
amiloride for, 50
bumetanide for, 134
captopril for, 155
chlorthalidone for, 216
ethacrynic acid for, 421
furosemide for, 486
hydrochlorothiazide for, 532
indapamide for, 555
mannitol for, 646
metolazone for, 693
neomycin for, 750
spironolactone for, 977
triamcinolone for, 1071
triamterene for, 1074
edetate calcium disodium, 375-376
edetate disodium, 376-377
edrophonium chloride, 378-379
EDTA, 376-377
EEG preparation, chloral hydrate for, 203
E.E.S., 403, **C6**
efavirenz, 379-381
Effexor, 1107, **C6**
Effexor XR, 1107
Efidac/24, 893
Efodine, 1220t
Efudex, 462
Elavil, 58
Eldepryl, 956
Elderly patients, drug therapy in, 11-13
Elimite, 825
Elixophyllin, 1022
Ellence, 392
E-Lor, 1218t
Elspar, 84
Eltroxin, 616
Emcyt, 412
Emo-Cort, 535
Emphysema
ipratropium for, 570
salmeterol for, 949

---

t refers to a table; **boldface** refers to full-color photographs.

---

t refers to a table; **boldface** refers to full-color photographs.

Iron overload from transfusions, deferoxamine for, 291
Irritable bowel syndrome
calcium polycarbophil for, 148
dicyclomine for, 320
octreotide for, 776
propantheline for, 886
psyllium for, 895
Ischemic complications, enoxaparin for, 384
Ischemic heart disease
isosorbide for, 579
papaverine for, 805
Ischemic stroke, alteplase for, 43
ISG, 552-553
Ismelin, 516
ISMO, 581
Isocet, 1217t
isoniazid, 575-577
isophane insulin suspension, 561-565
isophane insulin suspension and insulin injection (50% isophane insulin and 50% insulin injection), 561-565
isophane insulin suspension and insulin injection (70% isophane insulin and 30% insulin injection), 561-565
isoproterenol, 577-579
isoproterenol hydrochloride, 577-579
isoproterenol sulfate, 577-579
Isoptin, 1108
Isoptin SR, 1108
Isopto Carbachol, 156
Isopto Carpine, 840
Isopto Cetamide, 987
Isopto Frin, 834
Isopto Homatropine, 529
Isopto Hyoscine, 953
Isordil, 579
Isordil Tembids, 579
Isordil Titradose, 579
isosorbide dinitrate, 579-581
isosorbide mononitrate, 581-582
Isosporiasis
co-trimoxazole for, 261
pyrimethamine for, 900
Isotamine, 575
isotretinoin, 582-583
isradipine, 583-584
Isuprel, 577
Isuprel Mistometer, 577
itraconazole, 584-585

Iveegam, 552

J

Jenamicin, 495
Juvenile arthritis
ibuprofen for, 544
naproxen for, 743
piroxicam for, 852
tolmetin for, 1054

K

K-8, 861
K-10, 861
Kabikinase, 980
Kalium Durules, 861
Kaochlor S-F, 861
Kaon, 861
Kaon-Cl, 861
Kaon-Cl-10, 861
Kaopectate, 95
Kaopectate Advanced Formula, 95
Kaopectate Maximum Strength, 95
Kaopectate II, 630
Kaposi's sarcoma
alitretinoin for, 36
dactinomycin for, 279
daunorubicin citrate liposomal for, 288
doxorubicin hydrochloride liposomal for, 368
interferon for, 565
paclitaxel for, 798
vinblastine for, 1111
Karidium, 969
Karigel, 969
Karigel-N, 969
Kasof, 351
Kato, 861
Kawasaki syndrome, aspirin for, 86
Kay Ciel, 861
Kayexalate SPS, 972
K+ Care ET, 861
K+ Care KCL, 861
K-Dur, 861, **C8**
Keflex, 197
Keftab, 197
Kefurox, 194
Kefzol, 173
K-Electrolyte, 861
Kenacort, 1071
Kenalog, 1074
Kenalog-10, 1071
Kenalog-40, 1071
Kenalog in Orabase, 1074
Keppra, 608
Keralyt, 1220t
Keratinization disorders, isotretinoin for, 582

Keratitis
clotrimazole for, 249
cromolyn sodium for, 263
itraconazole for, 584
vidarabine for, 1110
Keratoconjunctivitis
cromolyn sodium for, 263
vidarabine for, 1110
Keratoplasty rejection, dexamethasone for, 299
Kerlone, 117
Ketalar, 586
ketamine hydrochloride, 586-587
ketoconazole, 587-588
ketoprofen, 588-589
ketorolac tromethamine, 590-591
ketorolac tromethamine (ophthalmic), 591
ketotifen fumarate, 592
Key-Pred-25, 869
Key-Pred SP, 869
KI, 860-861
K-Ide, 861
Kidney cancer, medroxyprogesterone for, 655
Kidney transplantation
azathioprine for, 97
basiliximab for, 105
cyclosporine for, 273
daclizumab for, 278
dactinomycin for, 279
lymphocyte immune globulin for, 639-640
misoprostol for, 712
muromonab-CD3 for, 729
mycophenolate for, 730
sirolimus for, 964
K-Lease, 861
K-Long, 861
Klonopin, 244, **C8**
K-Lor, 861
Klor-Con, 861
Klor-Con/EF, 861
Klorvess, 861
Klotrix, 861
K-Lyte, 861
K-Lyte/Cl Powder, 861
K-Med 900, 861
Knee replacement surgery
ardeparin for, 81
enoxaparin for, 384
K-Norm, 861
Koffex DM, 309
Kondon's Nasal, 386
Kondremul, 707
Kondremul Plain, 707
Konsyl, 895
Konsyl-D, 895
K-Pek, 95

---

t refers to a table; **boldface** refers to full-color photographs.

---

t refers to a table; **boldface** refers to full-color photographs.

---

t refers to a table; **boldface** refers to full-color photographs.

---

t refers to a table; **boldface** refers to full-color photographs.

---

t refers to a table; **boldface** refers to full-color photographs.